CLINICAL SPORTS MEDICINE

We dedicate this fifth edition to the Clinical Sports Medicine community—we are proud to be in a family of clinicians who are absolutely unwavering in prioritising patient care.

BRUKNER & KHAN'S
CLINICAL SPORTS MEDICINE

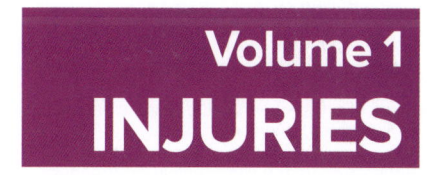

Volume 1
INJURIES

5TH EDITION

Peter Brukner
Ben Clarsen
Jill Cook
Ann Cools
Kay Crossley
Mark Hutchinson
Paul McCrory
Roald Bahr
Karim Khan

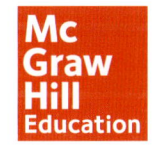

McGraw Hill Education

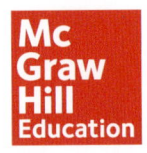

Notice
Medicine is an ever-changing science. As new research and clinical experience broaden our knowledge, changes in treatment and drug therapy are required. The editors and the publisher of this work have checked with sources believed to be reliable in their efforts to provide information that is complete and generally in accord with the standards accepted at the time of publication. However, in view of the possibility of human error or changes in medical sciences, neither the editors, nor the publisher, nor any other party who has been involved in the preparation or publication of this work warrants that the information contained herein is in every respect accurate or complete. Readers are encouraged to confirm the information contained herein with other sources. For example, and in particular, readers are advised to check the product information sheet included in the package of each drug they plan to administer to be certain that the information contained in this book is accurate and that changes have not been made in the recommended dose or in the contraindications for administration. This recommendation is of particular importance in connection with new or infrequently used drugs.

First published 1993
Second edition 2001
Revised second edition 2002
Third edition 2006
Revised third edition 2009
Fourth edition 2012

Text © 2017 McGraw-Hill Education (Australia) Pty Ltd
Additional owners of copyright are acknowledged in on-page credits.

Every effort has been made to trace and acknowledge copyrighted material. The authors and publisher tender their apologies should any infringement have occurred.

Reproduction and communication for educational purposes
The Australian Copyright Act 1968 (the Act) allows a maximum of one chapter or 10% of the pages of this work, whichever is the greater, to be reproduced and/or communicated by any educational institution for its educational purposes provided that the institution (or the body that administers it) has sent a Statutory Educational notice to Copyright Agency and been granted a licence. For details of statutory educational and other copyright licences contact: Copyright Agency, 66 Goulburn Street, Sydney NSW 2000. Telephone: (02) 9394 7600. Website: www.copyright.com.au

Reproduction and communication for other purposes
Apart from any fair dealing for the purposes of study, research, criticism or review, as permitted under the Act, no part of this publication may be reproduced, distributed or transmitted in any form or by any means, or stored in a database or retrieval system, without the written permission of McGraw-Hill Education (Australia) Pty Ltd, including, but not limited to, any network or other electronic storage.

Enquiries should be made to the publisher via www.mcgraw-hill.com.au or marked for the attention of the permissions editor at the address below.

National Library of Australia Cataloguing-in-Publication entry : (hardback)
Creator: Brukner, Peter, author
Title: Brukner & Khan's clinical sports medicine: injuries / Peter Brukner [and eight others]
Edition: 5th edition
ISBN: 9781743761380 (hardback)
Notes: Includes index
Subjects: Sports medicine,
             Sports injuries
Other Creators/Contributors: Khan, Karim, author
Dewey Number: 617.1027

Published in Australia by
McGraw-Hill Education (Australia) Pty Ltd
Level 2, 82 Waterloo Road, North Ryde NSW 2113
Product manager: Yani Silvana
Content developer: Isabella Mead
Senior content producers: Claire Linsdell, Daisy Patiag
Copy editors: Lindsey Langston, Gillian Armitage, Jess Ní Chuinn, Martina Edwards, Leanne Poll
Proofreader: Paul Leslie
Indexer: Russell Brooks
Medical illustrator: Vicky Earle
Cover design: Simon Rattray
Printed in China on 80 gsm matt art by CTPS

Foreword to the first edition (1993)

Sport in Australia is ingrained in the national consciousness more widely, deeply and indelibly than almost anywhere else in the world. When a prominent sportsperson sustains a sporting injury, either traumatically or from overuse, becomes excessively fatigued, or fails to live up to expectations, this assumes national importance. It is even more relevant nowadays with greater individual participation in sporting activities. The same type of problems occur for recreational athletes, middle-aged people wanting to become fit, or older people wishing to sustain a higher level of activity in their later years.

In *Clinical Sports Medicine* the authors take sport and exercise medicine out of the realm of the elite athlete and place it fairly and squarely where it belongs–as a subspecialty to serve everyone in the community who wishes to be active.

The book is organised in a manner that is sensible and usable. The chapters are arranged according to the anatomical region of the symptom rather than diagnostic categories. This results in a very usable text for the sports physician, general/family practitioner, physiotherapist, masseur, or athletic trainer whose practice contains many active individuals.

Practical aspects of sports medicine are well covered–care of the sporting team and concerns that a clinician might have when travelling with a team. In all, this is an eminently usable text which is timely in its production and will find an important place among clinicians involved in the care of active individuals.

JOHN R SUTTON MD, FRACP
Professor of Medicine, Exercise Physiology and Sports Medicine
Faculty of Health Sciences
University of Sydney
Past President, American College of Sports Medicine

This foreword was written by the late Professor John Sutton before his untimely death in 1996; we honour the memory of this champion of the integration of science, physical activity promotion and multidisciplinary patient care.

Foreword to the fifth edition

Twenty-four years after the publication of the first edition, the salient point made by Professor John Sutton in his foreword remains true–in *Clinical Sports Medicine* the authors take sports and exercise medicine out of the realm of the elite athlete and present it in the service of everyone in the community who wishes to remain active.

A search for the fourth edition in our university library revealed very well used and even threadbare copies and illustrated how indispensable this resource is to students and practitioners alike. This fifth edition continues the clear focus of previous editions: 'helping clinicians help patients', transcending professional boundaries to enable best practice.

The authors of *Clinical Sports Medicine: Injuries* include the very top names in sports and musculoskeletal physiotherapy, sports medicine and sport science from around the world–in short, the community that takes care of active people everywhere, including the recreational or competitive sportsperson. The truly interdisciplinary nature of professional practice in sports medicine is revealed in this book. Indeed, this fifth edition includes specific chapters on key but often overlooked aspects of professional development; namely working in collaborative teams and how to develop your career. To achieve this, it draws on real-life lessons from around the world.

Clinical Sports Medicine: Injuries builds on the high-quality, evidence-based content of previous editions, with 15 new or substantially revised chapters. It is beautifully illustrated, combining aesthetics and evidence in a partnership that provides accessible learning to all readers. Practice pearls and step-by-step illustrations of physical activity for every joint are supported by more than 550 new and innovative illustrations, and line drawings superimposed on selected photographs to aid understanding.

A striking feature of *Clinical Sports Medicine* has always been the authors' relentless commitment to 'clinical'. This is a useful book; one to be consulted between patients or even while the patient is with you. The colour-coded sections develop, one on another. Part A–Fundamental principles–has been completely rewritten and the cadre of expert authors added new chapters on Pain, Core stability, Patient-reported outcomes (for use in the clinic), Training and Return to sport. Each of the 24 chapters in Part B–Regional problems–stands alone, flowing logically from functional anatomy to the broader, expert clinical perspective on the specific management of more than 100 major conditions. These chapters include the key aspects of injury epidemiology, clinical risk factors and interventions across sports; they cover the common presentations but also provide commentary on the atypical. One aim and notable focus throughout the book is to make evidence accessible to busy practitioners to aid their decision making. Best available evidence, consensus statements and cautionary notes are provided throughout in an eye-catching and succinct way. Part C–Practical sports medicine–closes out Volume 1 with five chapters for those working in various sport settings.

This is a unique book. The variety of illustrations and their contribution to the understanding of form, function, concepts, intervention and management, in combination with decades of the cumulative wisdom of practitioners, teachers and researchers, ensures that this is an indispensable work.

Dr Emma K. Stokes FTCD
Associate Professor | Deputy Head
Department of Physiotherapy, School of Medicine, Trinity College, Dublin
President, World Confederation for Physical Therapy

Brief contents

PART A FUNDAMENTAL PRINCIPLES

1 Sport and exercise medicine: the team approach 2
2 Integrating evidence into shared decision making with patients 9
3 Sports injuries: acute 13
4 Sports injuries: overuse 29
5 Pain: why and how does it hurt? 55
6 Pain: the clinical aspects 65
7 Beware: conditions that masquerade as sports injuries 77
8 Introduction to clinical biomechanics 85
9 Biomechanical aspects of injury in specific sports 121
10 Training programming and prescription 139
11 Core stability 153
12 Preventing injury 165
13 Recovery 189
14 Clinical assessment: moving from rote to rigorous 201
15 How to make the diagnosis 209
16 Patient-reported outcome measures in sports medicine 231
17 Treatment of sports injuries 239
18 Principles of sports injury rehabilitation 277
19 Return to play 285

PART B REGIONAL PROBLEMS

20 Sports concussion 296
21 Headache 317
22 Face, eyes and teeth 331
23 Neck pain 347
24 Shoulder pain 377
25 Elbow and arm pain 439
26 Wrist pain 463
27 Hand and finger injuries 489
28 Thoracic and chest pain 507
29 Low back pain 521
30 Buttock pain 567
31 Hip pain 593
32 Groin pain 629
33 Anterior thigh pain 659
34 Posterior thigh pain 679
35 Acute knee injuries 713
36 Anterior knee pain 769
37 Lateral, medial and posterior knee pain 805
38 Leg pain 825
39 Calf pain 847
40 Pain in the Achilles region 865
41 Acute ankle injuries 893
42 Ankle pain 917
43 Foot pain 937

PART C PRACTICAL SPORTS MEDICINE

44 The younger athlete 974
45 Military personnel 991
46 Periodic medical assessment of athletes 1003
47 Working and travelling with teams 1017
48 Career development 1027

Contents

Foreword to the first edition	v	Co-authors	xxx
Foreword to the fifth edition	vi	Other contributors	xxxvi
Preface	xxv	Acknowledgments	xxxvii
About the authors	xxvii	Guided tour of your book	xxxviii
Editors	xxix		

PART A   FUNDAMENTAL PRINCIPLES

1 Sport and exercise medicine: the team approach
with Paul Dijkstra and Stefano Della Villa — 2

The SEM team	2
Multiskilling, roles, responsibilities and communication	3
The sport and exercise medicine model	3
The challenges of management	4
Diagnosis	4
Treatment	5
Meeting individual needs	5
The coach, the athlete and the clinician	5
'Love thy sport' (and physical activity!)	6

2 Integrating evidence into shared decision making with patients
with Steven J Kamper and Catherine Sherrington — 9

What is evidence-based practice?	9
Why is the evidence-based practice concept controversial?	10
Challenges to EBP	10
Implementing EBP	10
Accessing research	10
Retrieving articles	11
Published appraisals	11
Interpreting research about treatment effects	11
Risk of bias	11
Research about other types of clinical questions	12

3 Sports injuries: acute
with Stuart Warden — 13

Pathophysiology and initial management	13
Bone	15
Fracture	15
Periosteal contusion	16
Hyaline cartilage	17
Chondral and osteochondral injuries	17
Fibrocartilage	18
Acute tear	18
Herniation of nucleus pulposus from intervertebral disc	18
Joint	18
Dislocation/subluxation	18
Ligament	19
Sprain/tear	19
Muscle	21
Strain/tear	21
Contusion	23
Myositis ossificans	24
Acute compartment syndrome	24
Cramp	25
Tendon	25
Tear/rupture	25
Fascia	26
Tear/rupture	26
Bursa	26
Traumatic bursitis	26
Nerve	26
Neuropraxia	26

Fat pad	26
Bruise/contusion	26
Skin	27

4   Sports injuries: overuse
with Stuart Warden   29

Bone stress injury	29
Pathophysiology	30
Epidemiology	31
Risk factors	31
Diagnosis	34
Classification of bone stress injuries	37
Management	38
Osteitis and periostitis	42
Apophysitis	43
Articular cartilage	43
Joint	43
Ligament	43
Muscle	43
Myofascial pain: trigger points or just sore spots of unknown origin?	43
Chronic compartment syndrome	45
Exercise-induced muscle soreness	45
Tendon	46
Tendon overuse injury (tendinopathy) —with Jill Cook, Craig Purdam	46
Principles of rehabilitating lower limb tendinopathy	50
Enthesopathy	51
Bursa	51
Nerve	52
Skin	52
Blisters	52
Skin infections	52
But it's not that simple	53
Pain: where is it coming from?	53
Masquerades	53
The kinetic chain	53

5   Pain: why and how does it hurt?
by Lorimer Moseley   55

What is pain?	55
What is nociception? Clue—nociception is not pain!	56
Sensitisation of primary nociceptors ('peripheral sensitisation')	57
Sensitisation of spinal nociceptors ('central sensitisation')	58
The brain decides	59
The brain corrects the spinal cord	60
The brain is different in those with persistent pain	60
Treating someone in pain—a complex system requires a comprehensive approach	61

6   Pain: the clinical aspects
with Ebonie Rio   65

Input-dominated pain	65
Pain and musculoskeletal tissues	66
Less well characterised input-dominated pain—referred pain	66
Neuropathic pain	68
Centrally dominated pain	69
Central sensitisation	69
Motor adaptation to pain	72
Treatment options for patients with pain	72
Language	75
Summary	75

7   Beware: conditions that masquerade as sports injuries
with Nick Carter and Mark Hutchinson   77

How to recognise a condition masquerading as a sports injury	77
Conditions masquerading as sports injuries	78
Summary	84

8   Introduction to clinical biomechanics
with Christian Barton, Natalie Collins and Kay Crossley   85

'Ideal' lower limb biomechanics—the basics	85
Lower limb joint motion	85
Ideal neutral stance position	88
'Ideal' biomechanics with movement—running	90
Loading (heel strike to foot flat)	90
Midstance (foot flat to heel off)	91
Propulsion (heel off to toe off)	92
Initial swing	92
Terminal swing	93
Angle and base of gait	93
Landing point relative to centre of mass	94
Influence of gait velocity	94
Comparing heel and forefoot strike patterns	94
Influence of fatigue on running biomechanics	95

Contents

Lower limb biomechanical assessment in the clinical setting	95
Structural ('static') biomechanical assessment	96
Functional lower limb tests	100
Dynamic movement assessment (e.g. running biomechanics)	104
Sport-specific assessment	105
Summary of the lower limb biomechanical assessment	105
Clinical assessment of footwear—the Footwear Assessment Tool	105
Conditions related to suboptimal lower limb biomechanics	106
Management of lower limb biomechanical abnormalities	108
Biofeedback and movement pattern retraining	108
Foot orthoses	109
Taping	112
Upper limb biomechanics—with W Ben Kibler	114
The biomechanics of throwing	114
The kinetic chain	116
Normal biomechanics of the scapula in throwing	117
Abnormal scapular biomechanics and physiology	118
Clinical significance of scapular biomechanics in shoulder injuries	118
Changes in throwing arm with repeated throwing	119
Common biomechanical abnormalities specific to throwing	120

9 Biomechanical aspects of injury in specific sports
with Ben Clarsen   121

Cycling—with Phil Burt	121
Relationship between risk factors and loading	121
Knee pain	121
Low back pain	123
Cricket fast bowling—with Alex Kountouris	125
Golf—with Roger Hawkes	128
Wrist pain	128
Shoulder pain	129
Hip pain	130
Low back pain	130
Rowing—with Fiona Wilson	130
Low back pain	130
Chest wall pain	132
Wrist and forearm pain	132
Knee pain	133
Swimming—with Elsbeth van Dorssen	133
Swimming biomechanics	133
Shoulder pain	133
Medial knee pain	136
Tennis—with Babette Pluim	136
Lateral elbow pain	136
Shoulder injuries	137

10 Training programming and prescription
with Darren Burgess   139

Principles of training	139
Periodisation	139
Overload	140
Specificity	140
Individualisation	140
Conditioning training	142
Endurance training	142
Speed training	143
Agility training	144
Resistance training	144
Flexibility training	149
Training load management for performance enhancement	150

11 Core stability
by Paul Hodges   153

Introduction	153
Rationale for motor control training for lumbopelvic dysfunction	154
Motor control training to optimise core stability—key principles and common misconceptions	155
Optimal motor control requires a balance between movement and stiffness	155
Optimal lumbopelvic control involves three main neural strategies	155
Optimal motor control requires a whole system, not a single muscle	156
Motor control training involves rehabilitation of whole system	156
Motor control training involves a motor learning approach	157
Interplay between motor control and biology of pain	158

Implications of the role of trunk muscles in respiration and bladder and bowel function	159
Is motor control training effective for everyone or is it more effective when targeted to specific individuals?	159
Principles of the clinical application of motor control training	160
Assessment of motor control for core stability	160
Training of motor control for core stability	161
Training of motor control for core stability for prevention of pain and injury	164
Considerations for training of motor control for core stability in athletes	164
Conclusion	164

12 Preventing injury
with Roald Bahr, Ben Clarsen and Grethe Myklebust — **165**

A conceptual approach to injury prevention	165
The inciting event	166
Risk management: applying prevention models to your team	166
Reviewing the literature—risk identification and assessment	167
Developing an injury surveillance program within the team	168
Season analysis—risk profiling the training and competition program	170
The periodic medical assessment—mapping current problems and intrinsic risk factors	171
Developing and initiating a targeted prevention program	172
Preventing hamstring strains	173
Injury mechanisms	173
Risk factors	173
Prevention programs	173
Preventing ankle sprains—with Evert Verhagen	174
Injury mechanisms	175
Risk factors	175
Prevention programs	175
Preventing acute knee injuries	177
Injury mechanisms	177
Risk factors	177
Prevention programs	177
Preventing overuse injuries	181
Stretching	181

Structured training programs	182
Technique modification	182
Nutritional strategies to prevent stress fractures	182
Modification of extrinsic risk factors	182
Managing load to prevent injury—with Tim Gabbett	183
The relationship between load and injury	183
Monitoring the rate of load increase	184
Monitoring the acute:chronic load ratio	184
Monitoring athletes' response to load—the traffic-light approach	185
Protective equipment	187
Appropriate surfaces—with John Orchard	187
Natural grass versus artificial turf	187

13 Recovery
with Shona Halson and Phil Glasgow — **189**

Assessing recovery	189
Active recovery	189
After high-intensity short-duration exercise	190
After longer-duration exercise—active recovery and metabolite clearance	190
Psychological effects of active recovery	191
Massage	191
Massage and blood flow	191
Massage, muscle tone and viscoelasticity	191
Massage and delayed onset muscle soreness (DOMS)	191
Cellular and structural effects of massage	192
Psychological effects of massage	192
Neuromuscular electrical stimulation	193
NMES and blood flow	193
NMES and performance	193
NMES and muscle soreness	193
Stretching	193
Sleep	194
Water immersion	195
Compression	196
Nutrition—with Graeme Close	196
Replacing fluids	197
Replacing fuel	197
Repair	198
Pulling the different threads together—practical considerations for the clinician	199
Summary	200

14 Clinical assessment: moving from rote to rigorous
by Chad Cook — 201

- Why is differential diagnosis important? — 201
- Differential diagnosis: a three-step process — 201
- How to calculate an accurate diagnosis — 202
  - Reliability — 202
  - Sensitivity and specificity — 202
  - Positive and negative predictive values — 202
  - Likelihood ratio — 203
  - Clinical utility — 203
- The formal diagnostic assessment — 206
  - The role of bias in influencing diagnostic metrics — 206
  - Challenges to making a diagnosis — 206
- Final thoughts and guidance — 207

15 How to make the diagnosis
with Ali Guermazi, Jon Patricios and Bruce Forster — 209

- Does 'diagnosis' mean 'tissue diagnosis'? — 209
- Keys to accurate diagnosis — 210
- History — 211
  - Allow enough time — 211
  - Be a good listener — 211
  - Know the sport — 211
  - Discover the exact circumstances of the injury — 211
  - Obtain an accurate description of symptoms, both at the time of injury and at the initial consultation — 211
  - History of a previous similar injury — 212
  - Other injuries — 212
  - General health — 212
  - Work and leisure activities — 212
  - Consider why the problem has occurred — 212
  - Training/activity history — 213
  - Equipment — 213
  - Technique — 213
  - Overtraining — 213
  - Psychological factors — 213
  - Nutritional factors — 213
  - Drugs: prescription and others — 213
  - History of exercise-induced anaphylaxis — 213
  - Determine the importance of the sport to the athlete — 213
  - Differential diagnosis — 213
- Physical examination — 213
  - Develop a routine — 214
  - Where relevant, examine the other side — 214
  - Consider possible causes of the injury — 214
  - Attempt to reproduce the patient's symptoms — 214
  - Assess local tissues — 214
  - Assess for referred pain — 214
  - Assess neural mechanosensitivity — 214
  - Examine the spine — 214
  - Biomechanical examination — 214
  - Functional testing — 214
  - The examination routine — 214
  - Differential diagnosis — 221
- Diagnostic imaging — 221
  - The five imaging-related habits of highly effective sports medicine clinicians — 221
- Specific imaging modalities — 223
  - Conventional radiography — 224
  - MRI: massive blessing for active patients — 224
  - Ultrasound scan (for diagnosis) — 227
  - CT scanning — 229
  - Radioisotopic bone scan — 229

16 Patient-reported outcome measures in sports medicine
with Natalie Collins, Kay Crossley and Ewa M Roos — 231

- What are PROMs? — 231
- Why is it important to use appropriate PROMs in sports medicine? — 231
- Considerations for what constitutes a 'good' PROM for use in sports medicine — 232
  - Is the PROM easy to use in a sports medicine setting? — 232
  - Does the PROM evaluate dimensions that are relevant for the patient? — 233
  - Do all items within a PROM measure the same construct? — 233
  - Can the PROM be trusted to detect true change in the patient and be free from error? — 233
  - Is the PROM sensitive enough to detect real change in the patient's condition? — 234
- Summary — 235

17 Treatment of sports injuries
with Ben Clarson — 239

- Therapeutic exercise — 241
  - Stimulation of repair and remodelling: mechanotherapy — 241

Altering biomechanics: motor-control training	245
Exercise-induced hypoalgesia	246
Acute injury management	247
Protection	247
Optimal loading	247
Ice	248
Compression	248
Elevation	250
Do no HARM!	250
Manual treatments	250
Joint techniques: mobilisation and manipulation	251
Soft tissue therapy—**with Robert Granter**	252
Dry needling	256
Neurodynamic techniques	258
Taping—with Sam Blanchard	259
Proposed mechanisms of taping	259
Evidence of efficacy	259
Practical considerations	260
Electrophysical agents—with Nick Gardiner, Adam Gledhill, Lawrence Mayhew and Vasileios Korakakis	261
Therapeutic ultrasound	261
Transcutaneous electrical nerve stimulation	262
Neuromuscular stimulators	262
Interferential stimulation	262
Laser	262
Electromagnetic therapy	263
Extracorporeal shockwave therapy	263
Therapeutic medication in musculoskeletal injury—with Noel Pollock	264
Analgesics	264
Nonsteroidal anti-inflammatory drugs (NSAIDs)	264
Medications for neuropathic pain and central sensitisation	267
Local anaesthetic injections	268
Traumeel	269
Actovegin	269
Sclerosant	269
Prolotherapy	269
Mechanical and high-volume injections	269
Hyaluronic acid	269
Corticosteroids	270
Other medications	271
Nutraceuticals in injury management —with Noel Pollock	272
Glucosamine, chondroitin and omega-3 fatty acids	272
Vitamin D	273
Green tea/polyphenols	273
Autologous blood, blood products and cell therapy—with Robert-Jan de Vos	273
Autologous blood injections	273
Platelet-rich plasma	273
Cell therapy	274
Surgery	274
Arthroscopic surgery	274
Open surgery	275

18 Principles of sports injury rehabilitation
with Håvard Moksnes and Phil Glasgow 277

General principles	277
An essential element—effective planning	278
Goal setting and targeted interventions	279
Phases of rehabilitation	280
Phase 1: Acute	280
Phase 2: Restore activities of daily living	281
Phase 3: Returning to sports activities	282
Phase 4: Prevention of re-injury	282
When rehabilitation doesn't go according to plan	283

19 Return to play
with Ian Shrier 285

Strategic Assessment of Risk and Risk Tolerance framework for RTP decision making	286
Step 1: Tissue health	286
Step 2: Tissue stresses	287
Step 3: Risk tolerance modifiers	287
Return-to-play decision making—beyond risk for injury	287
Applying the StARRT framework	287
Assessing across outcomes and probabilities	288
Additional perspectives	289
Who should be the decision maker?	290
Clinicians	290
Athletes	292
The coach	292
Family, friends, agents	292
Management	292
A multidisciplinary approach	292
Summary	293

Contents

PART B REGIONAL PROBLEMS

20 Sports concussion
with Paul McCrory, Michael Makdissi,
Gavin Davis and Michael Turner ... 296

Definition ... 296
Prevention of concussion ... 297
The initial impact: applied pathophysiology ... 298
Management of the concussed athlete ... 298
    On-field management ... 298
    Confirming the diagnosis ... 300
    Determining when the player can return
        safely to competition ... 306
    The risk of premature return to play and
        concussion sequelae ... 309
The 'difficult' concussion ... 310
    Clinical assessment ... 311
    Treatment ... 311
Children and concussion in sport ... 311

21 Headache
with Toby Hall ... 317

Headache in sport ... 317
Clinical approach to the patient with
    headache ... 318
    History ... 318
    Clinical measurement of headache ... 319
    Examination ... 320
Primary headache ... 320
    Migraine ... 320
    Primary exercise headache ... 322
Secondary headache ... 322
    Cervicogenic headache ... 322
    Post-traumatic headache ... 328
    Post-traumatic migraine ... 328
    External compression headache ... 328
    High-altitude headache ... 328
    Hypercapnia headache ... 329

22 Face, eyes and teeth
with Rodney French, Geoffrey St George,
Ian Needleman and Steffan Griffin ... 331

Functional anatomy ... 331
Clinical assessment ... 331
Lacerations and contusions ... 332
    Immediate management of lacerations ... 332
    Management of larger lacerations ... 332
    Additional considerations ... 333
Nose ... 333
    Epistaxis (nosebleed) ... 333
    Nasal fractures ... 334
    Septal haematoma ... 334
Ear ... 335
    Auricular haematoma ... 335
    Perforated eardrum ... 335
    Otitis externa ... 336
Eyes ... 336
    Assessment of the injured eye ... 336
    Corneal injuries: abrasions and foreign body ... 338
    Subconjunctival haemorrhage ... 338
    Eyelid injuries ... 339
    Hyphaema ... 339
    Lens dislocation ... 339
    Vitreous haemorrhage ... 339
    Retinal haemorrhage ... 339
    Retinal detachment ... 340
    Prevention of eye injuries ... 340
Teeth ... 340
    Nature of injuries ... 340
    Emergency management ... 340
    Dental management and follow-up ... 341
    Prevention ... 341
Fractures of facial bones ... 343
    Orbital fracture +/- globe trauma ... 343
    Fractures of the zygomaticomaxillary
        complex ... 343
    Maxillary fractures ... 344
    Mandibular fractures ... 344
    Temporomandibular injuries ... 345
Prevention of facial injuries ... 346

23 Neck pain
by Gwendolen Jull and Deborah Falla ... 347

Anatomical considerations ... 347
Clinical perspective ... 349
    History ... 350
    Patient-reported outcome measures ... 352

Imaging	353
Physical examination	353
Performance-based outcome measures	364
Management of mechanical neck pain	**365**
Sport and functional modifications	365
Education	366
Pain management	367
Manual therapy	367
Neural tissue mobilisation	369
Training motor function	370
Training sensorimotor control	373
Maintenance program	374
Neck pain conditions	**374**
Cervicogenic headache	374
Acute wry neck	374
Cervical nerve injury	374
Conclusion	**375**

24 Shoulder pain
by Ann MJ Cools — 377

Functional anatomy and biomechanics	**377**
Static stabilisers	377
Dynamic stabilisers	379
The role of the scapula in normal shoulder function	379
Causes of shoulder pain—overview	**380**
Acute versus overuse shoulder pain	380
Impingement	380
Clinical approach	**382**
History	383
Physical examination	383
Special tests—diagnostic testing and symptom modification tests	388
Screening of the kinetic chain	396
Key outcome measures	397
Investigations	**397**
Radiography	401
Arthrography	401
Ultrasound	401
Magnetic resonance imaging	401
Diagnostic arthroscopy	402
General treatment and rehabilitation guidelines for the most common shoulder injuries in athletes	**402**
Rotator cuff injuries	**402**
Rotator cuff tendinopathy	402
Rotator cuff tears	406
Shoulder instability	**407**
Traumatic shoulder instability—TUBS	407
Acquired sport-specific instability—AIOS	408
Atraumatic multidirectional instability—AMBRI	411
Rehabilitation guidelines for shoulder instability—overview	412
Biceps-related pathology and SLAP lesions	**414**
Pathomechanics of biceps-related shoulder pain	414
Clinical features	415
Pathological glenohumeral internal rotation deficit	**417**
Pathomechanics of GIRD	417
Treatment of GIRD	417
Scapular dyskinesis	**419**
Rehabilitation of scapular dyskinesis—a scapular rehabilitation algorithm	420
Fractures of the clavicle	**424**
Special note—immature skeleton	426
Acromioclavicular joint injuries	**426**
Acute acromioclavicular joint injuries	426
Chronic acromioclavicular joint pain	426
Less common causes of shoulder pain	**429**
Other muscle tears around the shoulder	429
Adhesive capsulitis—'frozen shoulder'	429
Neurovascular injuries	429
Less common fractures around the shoulder	432
Snapping scapula	432
Special considerations for the overhead athlete	**433**
Kinetic chain integration	433
The thrower's program	435
Return to play following shoulder injury	437

25 Elbow and arm pain
with Bill Vicenzino, Alex Scott, Simon Bell and Nebojsa Popovic — 439

Anatomy	**439**
Ligaments	439
Muscles	440
Lateral elbow pain	**440**
History	440
Examination	441
Investigations	442
Lateral elbow tendinopathy	443
Other causes of lateral elbow pain	451
Medial elbow pain	**451**
Flexor/pronator tendinopathy	452

Contents

Medial collateral ligament sprain	452
Posterior elbow pain	**454**
Olecranon bursitis	454
Triceps tendinopathy	455
Posterior impingement	455
Acute elbow injuries	**456**
Fractures	456
Posterior dislocation	457
Acute rupture of the medial collateral ligament	459
Tendon ruptures	459
Hyperextension injuries	460
Forearm pain	**460**
Fracture of the radius and ulna	460
Stress fractures	460
Entrapment of the posterior interosseous nerve (radial tunnel syndrome)	460
Pronator teres syndrome (median nerve entrapment)	461
Forearm compartment pressure syndrome	461
Upper arm pain	**461**
Myofascial pain	461
Stress reaction of the humerus	462

26 Wrist pain
with Gregory Hoy and Hamish Anderson — **463**

Clinical approach	**463**
History	463
Physical examination	466
Key outcome measures	466
Investigations	466
Radial column problems	**470**
Fracture of the distal radius	470
Fracture of the scaphoid	472
Fracture of the trapezium	475
Radial epiphyseal injury (gymnast's wrist)	476
De Quervain's tenosynovitis	476
Intersection syndrome	477
Radial sensory nerve compression	478
Central column problems	**478**
Ganglions	478
Dislocation of the carpal bones	479
Scapholunate dissociation	479
Kienböck's disease	479
Impingement syndromes	481
Ulnar column problems	**481**
Ulnar styloid fracture	481
Fracture of the hook of hamate	481
Triquetral fracture	482
Lunotriquetral dissociation	482
Triangular fibrocartilage complex tear	483
Distal radio-ulnar joint instability	484
Extensor carpi ulnaris tendon injuries	484
General tendinopathies around the wrist	485
Causes of wrist numbness and hand pain	**485**
Carpal tunnel syndrome	485
Ulnar nerve compression	486
Surgery for wrist conditions	**486**
Wrist rehabilitation	**487**
Wrist splinting	487
Post-immobilisation wrist rehabilitation	487

27 Hand and finger injuries
with Hamish Anderson and Gregory Hoy — **489**

Clinical approach	**489**
History	489
Physical examination	489
Key outcome measures	492
Investigations	492
Principles of treatment	**492**
Oedema control	493
Exercises	494
Taping and splinting	494
Metacarpal fractures	**494**
Fracture of the base of the first metacarpal	494
Fractures of the other metacarpals	496
Fractures of phalanges	**497**
Proximal phalanx fractures	497
Middle phalanx fractures	497
Distal phalanx fractures	498
Dislocations of the carpo-metacarpal joints	**498**
Dislocations of the finger joints	**499**
Dislocations of the PIP joint	499
Dislocations of the DIP joint	499
Ligament and tendon injuries	**499**
Sprain of the ulnar collateral ligament of the first MCP joint	499
Sprain of the radial collateral ligament of the first MCP joint	500
Capsular sprain of the first MCP joint	500
PIP joint sprains	501
Mallet finger	501

Chronic swan neck deformity	503
Boutonnière deformity	503
Avulsion of the flexor digitorum profundus tendon ('jersey finger')	504
Lacerations and infections of the hand	504
Overuse conditions of the hand and fingers	**505**
Surgical referrals following hand injury	**505**
Exercises for the hand	505

28 Thoracic and chest pain
with Kevin Singer and Jeff Boyle — 507

Thoracic pain	**507**
Assessment	508
Thoracic intervertebral joint disorders	511
Costovertebral and costotransverse joint disorders	511
Scheuermann's disease	512
Thoracic intervertebral disc prolapse	512
T4 syndrome	514
Postural imbalance of the neck, shoulder and upper thoracic spine	514
Chest pain	**514**
Clinical assessment	516
Rib trauma	516
Referred pain from the thoracic spine	517
Sternoclavicular joint problems	517
Costochondritis	518
Stress fracture of the ribs	518
Side strain—with Andrew Nealon	519
Conclusion	520

29 Low back pain
by Peter O'Sullivan and Alex Kountouris with Joel Press and Maria Reese — 521

Epidemiology	**521**
The multidimensional nature of low back pain	523
Triage	**523**
Serious pathology	523
Specific pathoanatomical diagnoses	523
Low back pain without a pathoanatomical diagnosis	526
Factors contributing to low back pain	**526**
Physical factors	526
Lifestyle factors	526
Psychosocial factors	526
Neurophysiological factors	527
Individual considerations	528
Clinical approach	**528**
History	528
Physical examination	530
Investigations	534
Management of specific LBP disorders	**535**
Stress fracture of the pars interarticularis/lumbar spondylolysis	535
Spondylolisthesis	543
Acute radiculopathy +/– nerve root compression	545
Vertebral endplate oedema (Modic type 1 changes)	547
Management of non-specific LBP disorders	**548**
Clinical approach	548
Acute severe low back pain	549
Subacute low back pain	551
Recurrent/persistent low back pain: a clinical sub-grouping approach	555
Rehabilitation following low back pain	**563**
Sporting technique	563
Optimal motor control	563
Flexibility	563
Conclusion	**563**

30 Buttock pain
with Adam Meakins — 567

Clinical approach	**567**
History	568
Physical examination	569
Key outcome measures	573
Investigations	573
Myofascial buttock pain	**574**
Examination	575
Treatment of myofascial buttock pain	575
Referred pain from lumbar spine	**576**
Examination	576
Treatment	576
Proximal hamstring tendinopathy	**577**
Functional anatomy	577
Examination	578
Treatment	578
Sacroiliac joint dysfunction	**581**
Functional anatomy	582
Clinical features	583
Treatment	585

Contents

Less common causes of buttock pain	585
Piriformis syndrome	585
Ischiofemoral impingement	587
Posterior thigh compartment syndrome	587
Proximal hamstring tendon rupture	588
Avulsion fracture of ischial tuberosity	589
Conditions not to be missed	589
Spondyloarthropathies	589
Stress fracture of the sacrum	590

31 Hip pain
with Joanne Kemp, Kay Crossley, Rintje Agricola, Anthony Schache and Michael Pritchard — 593

Epidemiology	593
Functional anatomy and biomechanics	593
Morphology	594
Acetabular labrum	594
Ligaments of the hip	596
Chondral surfaces	596
Muscle function	596
Clinical approach	598
History	598
Physical examination	601
Key outcome measures	603
Investigations	603
Predisposing factors for pain	604
Local factors	606
Remote factors	606
Systemic factors	607
Femoroacetabular impingement	607
Types of FAI—cam and pincer impingement	607
Prevalence of FAI	607
Aetiology	608
Association with pain and pathology	608
Labral tears	610
Pathology	610
Ligamentum teres tears	612
Synovitis	612
Chondropathy	613
Hip instability	614
Treatment of hip impairments	614
Principles of rehabilitation of the injured hip	614
Nine principles of rehabilitation for hip pain patients	615
Surgical management of the injured hip	621

Lateral hip pain—with Alison Grimaldi	622
Greater trochanteric pain	622
Iliac crest pain	623
Examination of the patinet with lateral hip pain	623
Treatment of the patinet with lateral hip pain	625

32 Groin pain
with Adam Weir, Per Hömlich and Kristian Thorborg — 629

Anatomy	629
Pubic symphysis	629
Hip adductors	630
Hip flexors	630
Inguinal region	631
Summary of anatomy	631
Epidemiology	631
Incidence—soccer	631
Incidence—elite sports other than soccer	631
Prevalence	631
Distribution of acute injuries	631
Risk factors	632
Terminology and definitions	632
Classification	633
Clinical overview	634
History	634
Clinical examination	635
Imaging	639
Acute groin injuries	642
Diagnosis	642
Longstanding groin pain	643
Adductor-related groin pain	643
Iliopsoas-related groin pain	650
Inguinal-related groin pain	652
Pubic-related groin pain	654
Complete adductor avulsions	654
Less common injuries	654
Obturator neuropathy	654
Other nerve entrapments	655
Stress fractures of the neck of the femur	655
Stress fracture of the inferior pubic ramus	656
Referred pain to the groin	656
Prevention of groin injuries	657
Possible prevention strategies	657

33 Anterior thigh pain
with Zuzana Machotka — 659

- Epidemiology — 660
- Functional anatomy and biomechanics — 660
- Clinical approach — 661
  - History — 661
  - Physical examination — 661
  - Key outcome measures — 664
  - Investigations — 664
- Quadriceps contusion — 664
  - Treatment of quadriceps contusion — 666
  - Complications related to contusion — 670
- Quadriceps strain — 671
  - Distal quadriceps muscle strain — 671
  - Proximal rectus femoris strain — 672
  - Complete rectus femoris tear — 673
  - Avulsion injury — 673
  - Prevention — 674
- Less common causes — 674
  - Stress fracture of the femur — 674
  - Lateral femoral cutaneous nerve injury ('meralgia paraesthetica') — 676
  - Femoral nerve injury — 676
  - Referred pain — 677

34 Posterior thigh pain
with Carl Askling and Anthony Schache — 679

- Functional anatomy — 679
- Clinical approach — 681
  - History — 681
  - Physical examination — 682
  - Investigations — 684
  - Integrating the clinical assessment and investigation to make a diagnosis — 685
- Acute hamstring muscle strains — 685
  - Epidemiology — 686
  - Type I and type II acute hamstring strains—not all acute hamstring injuries are the same! — 686
  - Type I acute hamstring strain: sprinting-related — 688
  - Type II acute hamstring strain: stretch-related (dancers) — 689
  - Prognosis of hamstring injuries — 689
  - Management of hamstring injuries — 690
- Risk factors for acute hamstring strain — 703
  - Intrinsic risk factors — 703
  - Extrinsic risk factors — 705
- Prevention of hamstring strains — 705
  - Eccentric hamstring strength training — 705
  - Balance exercises/proprioception training — 705
  - Sport-specific training — 706
  - A promising clinical approach for the high-risk athlete — 706
- Referred pain to posterior thigh — 707
  - Trigger points — 707
  - Lumbar spine — 708
  - Sacroiliac complex — 709
- Other hamstring injuries — 709
  - Avulsion of the hamstring from the ischial tuberosity—with Raj Subbu and Fares Haddad — 709
  - Upper hamstring tendinopathy — 710
- Less common causes — 711
  - Nerve entrapments — 711
  - Ischial bursitis — 711
  - Adductor magnus strains — 711
  - Compartment syndrome of the posterior thigh — 711
  - Vascular — 712

35 Acute knee injuries
with Richard Frobell, Randall Cooper, Hayden Morris and Mark Hutchinson — 713

- Functional anatomy — 713
- Clinical approach — 714
  - 'Does this patient have a significant knee injury?' — 714
  - History — 714
  - Physical examination — 716
  - Key outcome measures — 717
  - Investigations — 722
- Meniscal injuries — 723
  - Clinical features — 724
  - Treatment — 726
  - Rehabilitation after meniscal surgery — 727
- Medial (tibial) collateral ligament injury — 729
  - Treatment — 729
- Anterior cruciate ligament injuries — 737
  - Anatomy of the ACL — 737

xix

Contents

Mechanism of ACL injury	737
Clinical features	738
Surgical or conservative treatment of the torn ACL?	740
Surgical treatment	742
Combined injuries	744
Rehabilitation after ACL injury	745
Problems encountered during ACL rehabilitation	748
Outcomes after ACL treatment	750
Partial ACL tear	755
Prevention of ACL injuries	755
ACL rupture in children with open physes	755
Posterior cruciate ligament injuries	755
Clinical features	756
Treatment	757
Lateral collateral ligament tears	759
Posterolateral corner injuries	759
Articular cartilage damage	760
Epidemiology	760
Quantifying chondral injury	761
Management	761
Acute patellar trauma	762
Fracture of the patella	762
Patella dislocation	762
Less common causes	765
Patellar tendon rupture	765
Bursal haematoma	767
Fat pad impingement	767
Fracture of the tibial plateau	767
Superior tibiofibular joint injury	767
Ruptured hamstring tendon	767

36 Anterior knee pain
by Kay Crossley, Jill Cook with Sallie Cowan, Adam Culvenor, Sean Docking, Michael Rathleff and Ebonie Rio — 769

Clinical approach	770
History	770
Physical examination	771
Patient-reported outcome measures	774
Investigations	775
Patellofemoral pain	775
What is patellofemoral pain?	776
What is patellofemoral osteoarthritis?	777
Functional anatomy	778
Factors that may contribute to patellofemoral pain	778
Treatment of PFP	782
Patellofemoral instability	792
Primary patellofemoral instability	792
Secondary patellofemoral instability	793
Patellar tendinopathy	793
Nomenclature	793
Clinical features	793
Investigations	794
Management: is the athlete still competing?	794
Sudden, acute patellar tendon pain	801
Less common causes of anterior knee pain	801
Fat pad irritation/impingement	801
Osgood–Schlatter lesion	802
Sinding-Larsen–Johansson lesion	802
Quadriceps tendinopathy	802
Bursitis	802
Synovial plica	803

37 Lateral, medial and posterior knee pain
with Mark Hutchinson — 805

Lateral knee pain	805
Clinical approach	806
Iliotibial band friction syndrome	809
Lateral meniscus abnormality	813
Less common causes of lateral knee pain	814
Medial knee pain	816
Patellofemoral syndrome	817
Medial meniscus abnormality	817
Osteoarthritis and chondral injuries of the medial compartment of the knee	818
Less common causes of medial knee pain	819
Posterior knee pain	820
Clinical evaluation	820
Baker's cyst	822
Biceps femoris tendinopathy	823
Popliteus tendinopathy	823
Other causes of posterior knee pain	824

38 Leg pain
with Mark Hutchinson, Walter Kim and Matt Hislop — 825

Clinical approach	825
Role of biomechanics	826
History	826
Physical examination	828
Key outcome measures	832
Investigations	832

Medial tibial stress fracture of the tibia	836
Assessment	836
Treatment	837
Prevention of recurrence	837
Stress fracture of the anterior cortex of the tibia	838
Treatment	838
Medial tibial stress syndrome	839
Risk factors	839
Treatment	839
Chronic exertional compartment syndrome	841
Pathogenesis	841
Clinical features	841
Deep posterior compartment syndrome	842
Anterior and lateral exertional compartment syndromes	843
Outcomes of exertional compartment syndrome surgery	844
Rehabilitation following compartment syndrome surgery	845
Less common causes	845
Stress fracture of the fibula	845
Referred pain	845
Nerve entrapments	845
Vascular entrapments	846
Developmental issues	846
Periosteal contusion	846
Fractured tibia and fibula	846

39 Calf pain
with Tamim Khanbhai, Matt Hislop and Jeff Boyle **847**

Anatomy	847
Clinical approach	849
History	849
Physical examination	850
Key outcome measures	853
Investigations	853
Gastrocnemius muscle strains	853
Acute strain	853
Soleus muscle strains	856
Accessory soleus	858
Claudicant-type calf pain	859
Vascular causes	859
Less common causes	862
Neuromyofascial causes	862
Nerve entrapments	862
Superficial compartment syndrome	863
Conditions not to be missed	863

40 Pain in the Achilles region
with Jill Cook, Karin Silbernagel, Steffan Griffin, Håkan Alfredson and Jon Karlsson **865**

Clinical perspective	865
History	866
Physical examination	868
Key outcome measures (PROMs)	872
Investigations	872
Midportion Achilles tendinopathy	872
Pathology	872
Predisposing factors for Achilles tendinopathy	876
Treatment of midportion Achilles tendinopathy	877
Medications	884
Electrophysical agents	884
Surgical treatment	884
Insertional Achilles tendinopathy including retrocalcaneal bursitis—the 'enthesis organ'	884
Anatomy and the key role of compression	884
Clinical assessment	886
Treatment	886
Retrocalcaneal bursitis	886
Achilles (superficial calcaneal) bursitis	887
Posterior impingement syndrome —with Susan Mayes	887
Sever's disease	888
Other causes of pain in the Achilles region (gradual onset)	888
Accessory soleus	888
Referred pain	888
Acute Achilles tendon rupture (complete)	889
Clinical approach	889
History	889
Physical examination	890
Key outcome measures	890
Investigations	890
Rehabilitation of Achilles tendon ruptures	890

41 Acute ankle injuries
with Pieter D'Hooghe, Evert Verhagen and Jon Karlsson **893**

Functional anatomy	893
Clinical perspective	894
History	895
Examination	895

xxi

Investigations	897
Lateral ligament injuries	899
Treatment and rehabilitation of lateral ligament injuries	900
Initial management	900
Treatment of grade III injuries	903
Less common causes	904
Medial (deltoid) ligament injuries	904
Significant ankle fractures	905
Lateral malleolar fracture with syndesmotic injury (Maisonneuve fracture)	905
Persistent pain after ankle sprain—'the difficult ankle'	905
Clinical approach to the difficult ankle	906
Osteochondral lesions of the talar dome	906
Avulsion fracture of the base of the fifth metatarsal	908
Other fractures	910
Impingement syndromes	911
Tendon dislocation or rupture	911
Other causes of the difficult ankle	912
Sinus tarsi syndrome	914
Complex regional pain syndrome type 1	914

42 Ankle pain
with Karen Holzer and Jon Karlsson — 917

Medial ankle pain	917
History	917
Examination	918
Key outcome measures	918
Investigations	918
Tibialis posterior tendinopathy	923
Flexor hallucis longus tendinopathy	924
Tarsal tunnel syndrome	926
Medial malleolar stress fracture	928
Medial calcaneal nerve entrapment	928
Other causes of medial ankle pain	929
Lateral ankle pain	929
Examination	929
Peroneal tendinopathy	929
Sinus tarsi syndrome	931
Anterolateral impingement	932
Posterior impingement syndrome	933
Stress fracture of the talus	933
Referred pain	933
Anterior ankle pain	934
Anterior impingement of the ankle	934
Tibialis anterior tendinopathy	935
Anterior inferior tibiofibular ligament (AITFL) injury	936

43 Foot pain
with Karl Landorf, Stephen Simons, Christopher Jordan and Michael Rathleff — 937

Rearfoot pain	937
History	937
Examination	939
Investigations	939
Patient-reported outcome measures	940
Plantar fasciopathy (formerly called 'plantar fasciitis')	941
Fat pad contusion	946
Calcaneal stress fracture	947
First branch of lateral plantar nerve (Baxter's nerve) entrapment	947
Midfoot pain	948
Clinical approach to midfoot pain	949
Investigations	949
Navicular stress fracture	949
Midtarsal joint sprains	952
Lisfranc joint injuries	952
Tibialis posterior tendinopathy (distal pain presentation)	955
Less common causes of midfoot pain	955
Forefoot pain	958
Clinical perspective	958
Stress fractures of the neck of metatarsals I–IV	959
Special metatarsal stress fracture: base of the second MT	961
Fractures of the fifth metatarsal	961
MTP joint synovitis	965
First MTP joint sprain ('turf toe')	966
Hallux limitus	967
Hallux valgus	967
Sesamoid injuries	968
Plantar plate tear—**with Kent Sweeting**	969
Corns and calluses	970
Morton's interdigital neuroma	970
Plantar warts	971
Onychocryptosis	972
Less common causes of forefoot pain	972

PART C PRACTICAL SPORTS MEDICINE

44 The younger athlete
with Nebojsa Popovic, Bojan Bukva, Nicola Maffulli and Dennis Caine — **974**

The young athlete is unique — 974
- Nonlinearity of growth — 974
- Maturity-associated variation — 975
- Unique response to skeletal injury — 975

Management of musculoskeletal conditions — 976
- Acute fractures — 976
- Overuse injuries of the physis — 979
- Shoulder pain — 979
- Elbow pain — 980
- Wrist pain — 980
- Back pain and postural abnormalities — 981
- Hip pain — 982
- Knee pain — 984
- Painless abnormalities of gait — 986
- Foot pain — 988

45 Military personnel
with Stephan Rudzki, Tony Delaney and Erin Macri — **991**

Special military culture — 991
Epidemiology of military injuries — 992
Common military injuries — 993
- Overuse injuries of the lower limb — 994
- Blister injuries — 994
- Parachuting injuries — 995
- The ageing defence forces — 995

Injury prevention in the military — 996
- Injury surveillance — 996
- Sex as a risk factor for injury — 997
- Body composition — 998
- Previous injury — 998
- Weekly running distance — 999
- Running experience — 1000
- Competitive behaviours — 1000
- Warm-up/stretching — 1000
- Conclusion — 1001

46 Periodic medical assessment of athletes
with Stephen Targett and Ben Clarsen — **1003**

Why perform the medical assessment? — 1003
- Identification of medical conditions that contraindicate participation in sport — 1003
- Assessment of known injuries and illnesses — 1006
- Review of current medications and supplements — 1007
- Education — 1007
- Baseline testing — 1007
- Development of athlete rapport — 1008
- Screening — 1008

Who is being assessed? — 1011
- Sport and position — 1011
- Geographical location — 1011
- Age — 1012
- Sex — 1012
- Available resources — 1012

When to perform a PMA — 1012
What to include in the template — 1013
Other issues to consider — 1013
- Consent — 1013
- Clearance or restriction from play — 1013
- Who should perform the PMA? — 1014
- Pre-employment medical assessment — 1014
- Insurance medical assessment — 1014
- Action points from the PMA — 1014

Summary — 1015

47 Working and travelling with teams
with Liam West — **1017**

The medical support team — 1017
Key attributes of a successful medical team — 1017
Medical indemnity and trauma training — 1018
Where does the medical team work? — 1018
Medical equipment — 1018
Team care throughout the season — 1018
- Core principles providing care for a team — 1018

Contents

Emergency action plans	1020
Preparing to travel	1021
1. Before travel	1021
2. During travel	1022
3. On arrival	1022
4. Journey home	1022
Jet lag	1023
Air travel and jet lag	1023
Pathophysiology	1023
Prevention of jet lag	1023
Symptomatic treatment for jet lag	1025

48 Career development
with Michael Davison — **1027**

Development of sport and exercise medicine	1027
The adoption of exercise medicine in the sports medicine movement	1028
Increased resources in sport	1028
Proficiency in a second or third language	1028
Widening the scope of practice—dual qualifications and subspecialist courses	1028
Sports therapy, sports and exercise science and sports rehabilitation	1029
Men and women have a place in sport and exercise medicine	1029
Key behaviours for a successful and interesting career	1029
Lessons from around the world	1031
Ummukulthoum Bakare—football medicine enthusiast and sports injury prevention strategist, West Africa	1031
Dr Liam West—the rookie doctor, Northern Europe and Australia	1031
Hans-Wilhelm Müller-Wohlfahrt—the team and celebrity doctor, Bavaria, Central Europe	1033
Rod Whiteley—sports physiotherapist who has moved across continents for his career, Middle East via Australasia and Major League Baseball	1033
Roald Bahr—Professor of Sports Medicine, the Nordic countries	1034

Quotation sources	1035
Index	1039

Preface

'Helping clinicians help patients' has been the clear focus of *Clinical Sports Medicine* from its inception. This edition brings you more authors, more artwork and more evidence. We are fortunate that many reading this will already have *Clinical Sports Medicine* in their library, so you are asking, 'What's new?'

- *The complete focus on sports injuries for 1034 pages.* So many advances, we had to make a volume just for injuries. We decided to call it *Injuries*.
- *The giants of sports medicine and sports physiotherapy joining us on the front cover–our seven editors.* You know their work and now they have distilled their best for your benefit (see below and on the Editors page).
- *The artwork.* Vicky Earle's artwork is recognised the world over, the way Dr Frank Netter's was in the 1900s. You may not know the name, but you have seen the tendons, the groin entities and the *BJSM* covers. Five hundred new illustrations to clarify our field.
- *Fifteen new chapters.* (See new content, below.)
- *More than 4000 references*–the solid foundation. As Chapter 2 tells us, we do not yet have all the evidence we would like to have, and clinical advances can outpace the science, but ultimately the scientific method underpins quality care.
- *The unprecedented complementary social media*–Facebook, Twitter, Instagram and the www.clinicalsportsmedicine.com website. This content will have shelf life until 2020 and we will continually update it with the existing digital methods and those that have not yet been invented.

Editors and authors

Volume 1–Injuries reflects the generosity of seven sports physiotherapy and sports medicine editors. Ben Clarsen (senior editor), Jill Cook, Ann Cools, Kay Crossley, Mark Hutchinson, Paul McCrory and Roald Bahr share their passion for helping patients and educating clearly. Our 121 chapter authors and contributors represent 19 countries. Recruited for their first edition, alongside editors Cools and Clarsen, are Rintje Agricola, Hamish Anderson, Sam Blanchard, Jeffrey Boyle, Darren Burgess, Phil Burt, Bojan Buvka, Graeme Close, Natalie Collins, Chad Cook, Adam Culvenor, Michael Davison, Stefano Della Villa, Pieter D'Hooghe, Paul Dijkstra, Sean Docking, Deborah Falla, Rodney French, Tim Gabbett, Phil Glasgow, Adam Gledhill, Alison Grimaldi, Fares Haddad, Toby Hall, Shona Halson, Roger Hawkes, Greg Hoy, Steven Kamper, Vasileios Korakakis, Alex Kountouris, Karl Landorf, Adam Meakins, Håvard Moksnes, Grethe Myklebust, Andrew Nealon, Ian Needlman, Kieran O'Sullivan, Peter O'Sullivan, Jon Patricios, Noel Pollock, Nebojsa Popovic, Michael Rathleff, Ebonie Rio, Ewa Roos, Stephen Simons, Geoffrey St George, Raj Subbu, Stephen Targett, Kristian Thorborg, Elsbeth van Dorssen, Stuart Warden, Adam Weir, Liam West and Fiona Wilson.

New content

Five years is a long time in our field. Major advances, such as high quality evidence for physiotherapy rehabilitation in the management of acute knee injuries, new algorithms for the treatment of shoulder pain and fresh space for the biopsychosocial model are included. The shoulder and knee will remain the shoulder and knee for the next 100 years but chapters can be completely renovated between editions, by new authors. The following chapters have new authors with new diagnostic approaches and new treatments to benefit the clinician.

Preface

- Chapter 1: Paul Dijkstra and Stefano Della Villa outline the **team approach** to sports medicine.
- Chapters 3 and 4: Stuart Warden shares the latest mechanistic understanding of **acute** and **overuse injury**.
- Chapter 6: Ebonie Rio builds on Lorimer Moseley's chapter on **pain** (Chapter 5) for the clinician.
- Chapter 9: Experts in their fields share decades each of experience in assessing patients for **sport-specific biomechanical errors**.
- Chapter 10: Darren Burgess gives clinicians insight into the principles that underpin **training** at the very top level of sport and how these apply at the community level.
- Chapter 11: Paul Hodges summarises 20 years of thinking about **core stability**.
- Chapter 14: Chad Cook clarifies the numerical basis that should underpin clinical reasoning and **assessment**.
- Chapter 15: Ali Guermazi partners with fellow radiologist Bruce Forster, and clinician Jon Patricios, to simplify accurate **diagnosis** including MRI interpretation for every clinician.
- Chapter 16: Natalie Collins launches *Clinical Sports Medicine* squarely into the world of PROMs–**patient-reported outcome measures.**
- Chapter 17: Ben Clarsen threw away the fourth edition chapter and built a new **treatment** chapter with international leaders in the different disciplines.
- Chapter 19: Ian Shrier outlines the StARRT model for **return to play.**
- Chapter 21: Toby Hall brings a very practical physiotherapy focus to **headache**.
- Chapter 23: Together with Deborah Falla, Gwen Jull unravels **neck pain** and provides detailed treatment principles and tips.
- Chapter 24: Ann Cools shares her 20 years' experience in assessing and managing **shoulder pain**.
- Chapters 26 and 27: Greg Hoy led the extensive revision of the **wrist pain** and **hand and finger injuries** chapters, highlighting new treatments and new conditions.
- Chapter 29: Peter O'Sullivan incorporates the biopsychosocial approach to **back pain** assessment and management. See the very clinical patient triage outline in Figure 29.2.
- Chapter 30: Adam Meakins describes and illustrates (51 images) how to treat **buttock pain** using exercises as the foundation.
- Chapter 32: Adam Weir skilfully extracted the most useful clinical discoveries from the first world conference on **groin pain**.
- Chapter 35: Sports **knee** surgeons and physiotherapists combine to highlight what is working and what is not working for patients in this rapidly changing field.
- Chapter 43: Karl Landorf and Michael Rathleff are the world leaders on plantar fasciopathy. They provide a major new section inside the important **foot pain** chapter.
- Chapter 46: Stephen Targett applies his vast experience of **periodic medical assessment** to issues such as cardiac clearance, and giving advice that influences contracts worth millions of dollars when doing professional athlete transfer medicals.
- Chapter 47: Liam West hit the refresh button on **working and travelling with teams** and included essentials such as indemnity and emergency preparation.
- Chapter 48: Michael Davison introduces the junior clinician to the global world of sports medicine and sports physiotherapy–A 'how to' on **career development**. (Spoiler alert: hard work is involved!)

No single profession has all the answers required to treat every ill or injured athlete or enthusiast. *Volume 1–Injuries* was created by a champion team. We are confident that, whatever your training, *Clinical Sports Medicine* fifth edition will reinforce and refine existing knowledge and techniques, and introduce useful new approaches for your clinical practice as well as for your teaching of our wonderful vocation.

About the authors

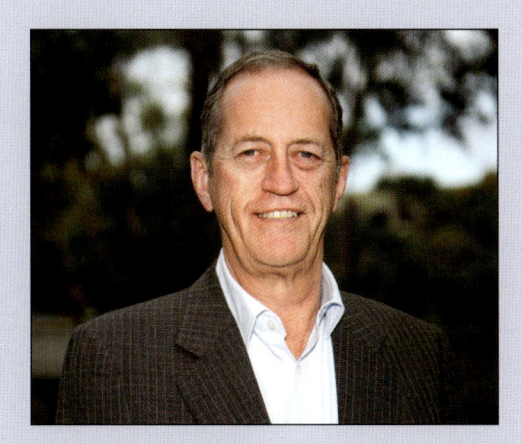

Peter Brukner

OAM, MBBS, DRCOG, FACSEP, FASMF, FACSM, FFSEM (Ireland, Hon), FFSEM (UK, Hon)

Sport and Exercise Medicine physician

Team Doctor, Australian cricket team

Head, Sports Medicine and Sports Science, Liverpool Football Club, UK 2010–12

Founding Partner, Olympic Park Sports Medicine Centre, Melbourne, Australia

Professor of Sports Medicine, La Trobe University, Melbourne, Australia

Associate Professor, Centre for Health, Exercise and Sports Medicine, The University of Melbourne, Australia

Honorary Fellow, Faculty of Law, The University of Melbourne, Australia

Adjunct Professor, School of Human Movement Studies, The University of Queensland Australia

Adjunct Professor, Liverpool John Moores University, UK

Visiting Professor, Lee Kong Chian School of Medicine, Singapore

Visiting Associate Professor, Stanford University, USA 1997

Executive Member, Australian College of Sports Physicians 1985–2000

President, Australian College of Sports Physicians 1991–92, 1999–2000

Board of Trustees, American College of Sports Medicine 2000–02

State and Federal Council Member, Sports Medicine Australia 1984–90

Team physician

Socceroos 2007–10, Asian Cup Finals 2007, World Cup Finals 2010

Australian Olympic Team, Atlanta 1996, Sydney 2000

Australian Commonwealth Games team, Edinburgh 1986, Kuala Lumpur 1998

Australian team, World Student Games, Edmonton 1983, Kobe 1985, Zagreb 1987

Australian Athletics team 1990–2000, World Championships Tokyo 1991, Gothenburg 1995, Seville 1999

Australian team, World Cup Athletics, Havana 1992

Australian Men's Hockey team 1995–96

Australian team, World Swimming Championships, Madrid 1986

Melbourne Football Club (AFL) 1987–90

Collingwood Football Club (AFL) 1996

Books (co-author)

Food for Sport 1987

Stress Fractures 1999

Drugs in Sport—What the GP Needs to Know 1996, 2000

The Encyclopedia of Exercise, Sport and Health 2004

Essential Sports Medicine 2005

Clinical Sports Anatomy 2010

Editorial boards

British Journal of Sports Medicine

Clinical Journal of Sport Medicine

Current Sports Medicine Reports

The Physician and Sportsmedicine

Editor

Sport Health 1990–95

Awards

Medal of the Order of Australia 2006

Inaugural Honour Award, *Australian College of Sports Physicians* 1996

Citation Award, *American College of Sports Medicine* 2000

Honorary Fellowship, *Faculty of Sports and Exercise Medicine (Ireland)* 2012

About the authors

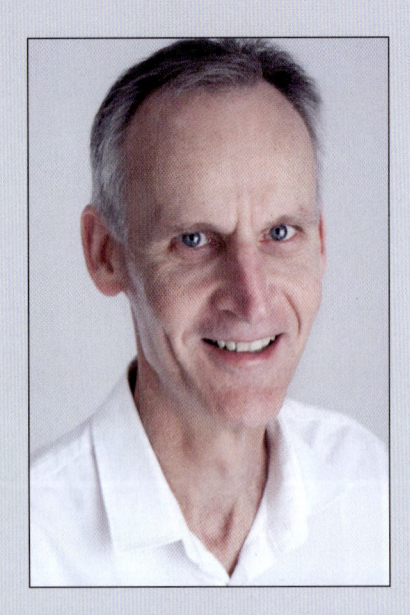

Karim Khan

MD, PhD, MBA, FACSEP, FSMA, DipSportMed (CASEM), FACSM, FFSEM (Ireland, Hon), FFSEM (UK, Hon)

Sport and Exercise Medicine physician

Professor, University of British Columbia, (Department of Family Practice and School of Kinesiology) Vancouver, Canada

Co-Director, Centre for Hip Health and Mobility, University of British Columbia, Vancouver, Canada

Adjunct Professor: Professor, School of Allied Health, College of Science Health and Engineering, La Trobe University, Melbourne, Australia

Visiting Professor, School of Human Movement Studies, The University of Queensland, Brisbane, Australia

Clinical Professor, Centre for Musculoskeletal Studies, School of Surgery, University of Western Australia, Perth, Australia

Exercise is Medicine Committee, American College of Sports Medicine 2009–11

Medical Education Committee, American College of Sports Medicine 2002–04

Research Evaluation Committee, American College of Sports Medicine 2005–07

Director of Research and Education, Aspetar Orthopaedic and Sports Medicine Hospital, Qatar 2013–15

Sports Medicine Advisory Board to the International Olympic Committee 2015–

Team physician

Olympic Games Sydney 2000, Basketball Competition Venue

Australian Women's Basketball (The Opals) 1991–96

The Australian Ballet Company 1991–96

The Australian Ballet School 1991–96

Australian team, World Student Games 1993

Australian team, Junior World Cup Hockey 1993

Editor-in-chief

British Journal of Sports Medicine 2008–

BMJ Open Sport and Exercise Medicine 2015–

Sport Health 1995–97

Books (co-author)

Physical Activity and Bone Health 2001

The Encyclopedia of Exercise, Sport and Health 2004

Editorial boards

The BMJ (International Advisory Board) 2008–14

Scandinavian Journal of Medicine and Science in Sport 2007–10

British Journal of Sports Medicine (North American Editor) 2005–07

Journal of Science and Medicine in Sport 1997–2001

Year Book of Sports Medicine 2008–10

Clinical Journal of Sport Medicine 2003–06

Selected awards

Prime Minister's Medal for Service to Australian Sport 2000

Sports Medicine Australia Fellows' Citation for Service 2005

Honorary Fellowship, Faculty of Sports and Exercise Medicine (Ireland) 2011

Honorary Fellowship, Faculty of Sport and Exercise Medicine (UK) 2014

Editors

Ben Clarsen PT, MSc, PhD
Specialist sports physiotherapist, Norwegian Olympic Training Centre (Olympiatoppen); Postdoctoral Research Fellow, Oslo Sports Trauma Research Center, Norwegian School of Sport Sciences; Team Physiotherapist, London Olympic Games 2012, UCI Road Cycling Professional Tour 2005–07, UCI World Road Cycling Championships 2004–12; Senior Editor for *Volume 1—Injuries*

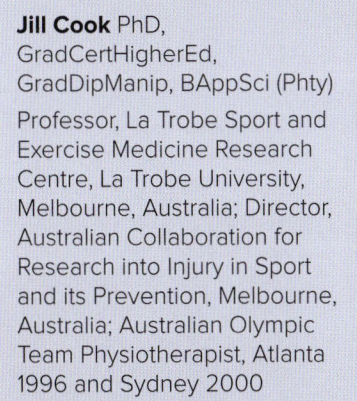

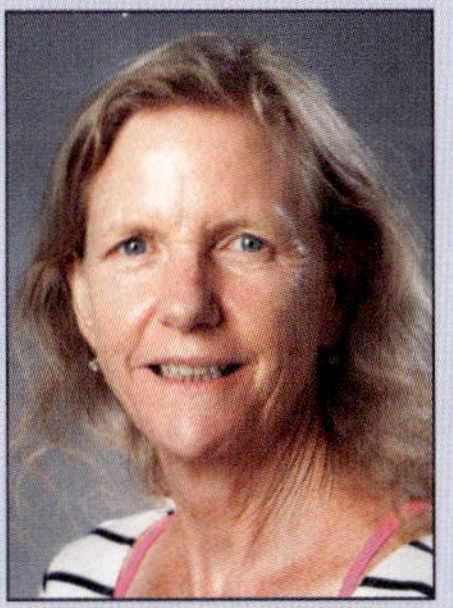

Jill Cook PhD, GradCertHigherEd, GradDipManip, BAppSci (Phty)
Professor, La Trobe Sport and Exercise Medicine Research Centre, La Trobe University, Melbourne, Australia; Director, Australian Collaboration for Research into Injury in Sport and its Prevention, Melbourne, Australia; Australian Olympic Team Physiotherapist, Atlanta 1996 and Sydney 2000

Ann MJ Cools PT, PhD
Associate Professor, Department of Rehabilitation Sciences and Physiotherapy, Faculty of Medicine and Health Sciences, Ghent University, Belgium; Research Consultant, Department of Occupational and Physical Therapy and Institute of Sports Medicine, Bispebjerg Hospital, University of Copenhagen, Denmark

Kay Crossley BAppSci(Physio), PhD
Professor and Director, La Trobe Sport and Exercise Medicine Research Centre, School of Allied Health, College of Science, Health and Engineering, La Trobe University, Melbourne, Australia; Australian Olympic Team Physiotherapist, Sydney 2000

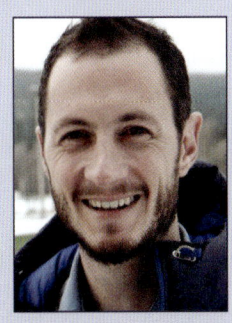

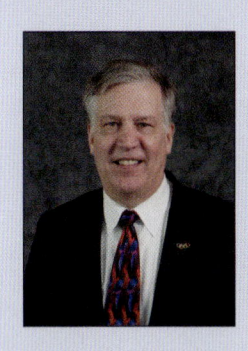

Mark R Hutchinson MD, FACSM
Professor of Orthopaedics and Sports Medicine and Head Team Physician, University of Illinois at Chicago, Chicago, Illinois; Volunteer Team Physician, United States, Olympic Games, Rio de Janeiro, 2016

Paul McCrory MBBS, PhD, FRACP, FACSEP, FFSEM, FACSM, FRSM, GradDipEpidStats
Consultant Neurologist, Internist and Sport and Exercise Physician; NHMRC Practitioner Fellow, The Florey Institute of Neuroscience and Mental Health, Melbourne Brain Centre—Austin Campus, Melbourne, Australia

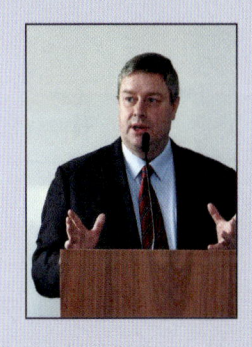

Roald Bahr MD, PhD
Professor and Chair, Oslo Sports Trauma Research Center; Chair, Department of Sports Medicine, Norwegian School of Sport Science; Chief Medical Officer, Olympiatoppen and Norwegian Olympic Training Center; Head, Aspetar Injury and Illness Prevention Program, Aspetar, Orthopaedic and Sports Medicine Hospital, Doha, Qatar

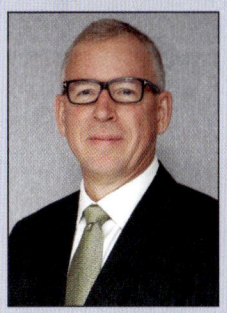

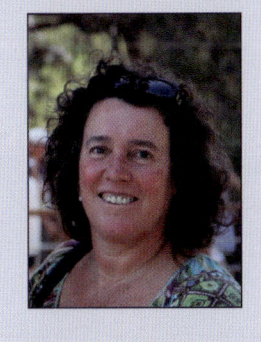

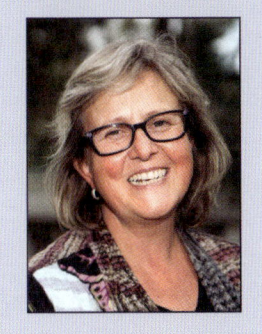

Co-authors

Rintje Agricola MD, PhD
Department of Orthopaedic Surgery, Erasmus University Medical Centre, Rotterdam, The Netherlands

Håkan Alfredson MD, PhD
Professor in Sports Medicine, Sports Medicine Unit, University of Umeå, Sweden; Orthopaedic Surgeon, Alfredson Tendon Clinic Inc. Umeå, Sweden; Orthopaedic Surgeon, Pure Sports Medicine Clinic, London, England & University College London Hospital, Institute of Sport, Exercise and Health (ISEH), London, UK

Hamish Anderson BA, BSc(Occ Thy), CHT(USA), AHTA full member
Certified Hand Therapist, Melbourne, Australia

Carl Askling PhD, PT
Vice-President, Swedish Sports Trauma Research Group, Swedish School of Sport and Health Sciences and Department of Molecular Medicine and Surgery, Karolinska Institutet, Stockholm, Sweden

Christian J Barton PhD, BPhysio (Hons)
Post-Doctoral Research Fellow, La Trobe Sport and Exercise Medicine Research Centre Melbourne, Australia; Clinical Director, Complete Sports Care, Melbourne, Australia

Simon Bell FRCS, FRACS, FAOrthA, PhD
Associate Professor of Orthopaedic Surgery, Monash University and Melbourne Shoulder and Elbow Centre, Melbourne, Australia

Mario Bizzini PhD, MSc, PT
Research Associate, FIFA—Medical Assessment & Research Centre (F-MARC), Human Performance Lab, Swiss Concussion Center, Schulthess Clinic, Zürich, Switzerland; Sports Physiotherapist to Swiss Football World Cup and Olympic Teams

Sam Blanchard BSc (Physiotherapy), MSc, ACPSEM Gold, IFSPT
Academy Clinical Lead Physiotherapist & Women's Lead Physiotherapist, BT Sport Scottish Rugby, UK

Jeffrey Boyle BSc (Physiotherapy), Grad Dip Manipulative Therapy, PhD
Fellow, Australian College of Physiotherapists (Sports Physiotherapy); Associate Professor, Curtin University; Principal Physiotherapist, Fremantle Football Club, Australia

Darren Burgess PhD
Head of High Performance, Port Adelaide Football Club, Australia

Bojan Bukva MD, PhD
Pediatric Surgeon and Pediatric Orthopaedic Surgeon; Sports Physician in National Sports Medicine Program, Aspetar Orthopaedic and Sports Medicine Hospital, Doha, Qatar

Phil Burt BSc (Hons)
Lead Physiotherapist, British Cycling; Consultant Physiotherapist, Team Sky Pro Cycling Team, UK

Nick Carter MB ChB, MRCP
Consultant in Rheumatology and Rehabilitation, Medical Defence Services, Medical Rehabilitation Centre, Headley Court, UK

Dennis Caine PhD
Emeritus Professor, University of North Dakota, Department of Kinesiology and Public Health Education, University of North Dakota, Grand Forks, USA

Graeme Close PhD
Sports Nutrition Consultant, Professor of Human Physiology, Liverpool John Moores University, UK; England Rugby and Everton FC

Natalie Collins BPhty (Hons), M. Sports Physio, PhD
School of Health and Rehabilitation Sciences, The University of Queensland, Brisbane, Australia

Chad E Cook PT, PhD, MBA
Professor and Program Director, Division of Physical Therapy, Department of Orthopaedics, Duke Clinical Research Institute, Duke University, USA

Randall Cooper B. Physio, M. Physio, FACP
Adjunct Lecturer, La Trobe University Sport and Exercise Medicine Research Centre, Melbourne, Australia

Sallie Cowan BAppSci(Physio), GradDipManipTher, PhD
Senior Research Fellow, Musculoskeletal Physiotherapist, School of Physiotherapy, The University of Melbourne, Australia

Adam Culvenor BPhysio (Hons), PhD
Post-doctoral Research Fellow, La Trobe Sport and Exercise Medicine Research Centre, La Trobe University, Melbourne, Australia; and Institute of Anatomy, Paracelsus Medical University, Salzburg, Austria

Co-authors

Gavin Davis MBBS, FRACS (Neurosurgery)
Associate Professor Neurosurgery, Cabrini Hospital, Melbourne, Australia; Chairman, Department of Surgical Specialties, Cabrini Hospital; Consultant Neurosurgeon, Austin and Box Hill Hospitals; University of Notre Dame, Australia

Michael Davison MA (Oxon), MBA
Managing Director, Isokinetic Medical Group, London, UK; FIFA Medical Centre of Excellence; Consultant, San Antonio Spurs, Brooklyn Nets, *The Daily Telegraph*, and Football Research Group

Robert-Jan de Vos MD, PhD
Sports Physician, Erasmus MC University Medical Centre, Department of Orthopaedics and Sports Medicine, Rotterdam, The Netherlands; Club Doctor at Excelsior Football Club, Rotterdam, The Netherlands

Tony J Delaney RFD, MBBS, FACSP
Sports Physician, Narrabeen Sports and Exercise Medicine Clinic, Academy of Sport, Sydney, Australia; Visiting Senior Specialist, Sports Medicine Clinic, 1st Health Support Battalion, Holsworthy Military Area and Fleet Base East Health Centre, New South Wales, Australia; Chair, Australian Defence Force Sports, Rehabilitation and Musculoskeletal Consultative Group

Stefano Della Villa MD
Isokinetic Medical Group, FIFA Medical Centre of Excellence, Italy

Pieter PRN D'Hooghe MD, MSc, MBA
Orthopaedic Surgeon, Aspetar Orthopaedic and Sports Medicine Hospital, Doha, Qatar

H Paul Dijkstra MBChB, BSc (Hons) (Pharmacology), MPhil (Sports Medicine), FFSEM (UK)
Specialist Sport and Exercise Medicine Physician; Director of Medical Education at Aspetar, Qatar Orthopaedic and Sports Medicine Hospital, Doha, Qatar

Sean Docking BAppSci, B. Physiot (Hons), M. Sports Physio, PhD
Post-doctoral Research Fellow, La Trobe University Sport and Exercise Medicine Centre, La Trobe University; The Australian Collaboration for Research into Injury in Sport and its Prevention, Melbourne, Australia

Jiri Dvorak MD
Senior Consultant, Spine Unit, Schulthess Clinic Zürich; Professor of Neurology, University of Zürich, Switzerland

Deborah Falla BPhty (Hons), PhD
Professor and Chair in Rehabilitation Science and Physiotherapy, School of Sport, Exercise and Rehabilitation Sciences, College of Life and Environmental Sciences, University of Birmingham, UK

Bruce Forster MSc, MD, FRCPC
SPECIAL IMAGING CO-AUTHOR/EDITOR
Professor and Head, Department of Radiology, Faculty of Medicine, University of British Columbia; Regional Medical Director, Medical Imaging; Regional Department Head, Dept. of Radiology / Diagnostic Imaging; Vancouver Coastal Health / Providence Health Care, Canada

Rodney French MD, MEd, FRCSC
Clinical Associate Professor, Division of Plastic Surgery, UBC Faculty of Medicine, Vancouver, Canada

Richard Frobell PhD
Associate Professor, Orthopedics, Clinical Sciences, Lund University, Lund, Sweden

Tim Gabbett PhD, PhD
Principal of Gabbett Performance Solutions and consultant to international athletes Commonwealth Games (2002 and 2006) and Olympic Games (2000, 2004 and 2008)

Nick Gardiner BSc (Hons) Sports Therapy, PGCHE, MSST
BSc Sports Therapy Course Leader, London Metropolitan University; Founder of Fit for Sport, Sports Therapy and Injury Clinic, London, UK

Phil Glasgow PhD, MTh, MRes, MCSP
Head of Sports Medicine, Sport Northern Ireland Sports Institute, UK

Adam Gledhill MSc, PhD
Senior Lecturer, Sport and Exercise Therapy, Musculoskeletal Health Research Group and Centre for Sport Performance, Leeds Beckett University, Leeds, UK

Co-authors

Robert Granter BSocSci, AdDipRemMass (Myotherapy)
Myotherapist, Head of Soft Tissue Therapy Services Australian Olympic Team 1996 and 2000; Head of Massage Therapy Services, Melbourne 2006 Commonwealth Games

Steffan Griffin BSc (Hons)
College of Medical and Dental Sciences, University of Birmingham, Birmingham, UK; *BJSM* Associate Editor; USEMS President and BASEM executive member,

Alison Grimaldi BPhty, MPhty(Sports), PhD
Principal Physiotherapist, Physiotec Physiotherapy, Brisbane, Australia; Adjunct Research Fellow, School of Health & Rehabilitation Sciences, University of Queensland, Brisbane, Australia

Ali Guermazi MD, PhD
SPECIAL IMAGING CO-AUTHOR/EDITOR
Professor of Radiology; Vice Chair, Academic Affairs; Assistant Dean, Office of Diversity; Director, Quantitative Imaging Center (QIC); Boston University School of Medicine, Boston, Massachusetts, USA

Fares S Haddad BSc (Hons), MBBS, MD(Res), MCh(Orth), FRCS(Orth), FFSEM
Professor of Orthopaedic and Sports Surgery, Divisional Clinical Director, University College London Hospitals; Director, ISEH, UK

Toby Hall PhD, MSc, FACP
Adjunct Associate Professor, Director of Manual Concepts, Curtin University, Perth, Australia; Senior Teaching Fellow, University of Western Australia, Western Australia, Australia

Shona Halson PhD
Senior Physiologist, Department of Physiology, Australian Institute of Sport, Australia; Sports Science Team Summer Olympic Games in Beijing 2008, London 2012 and Rio de Janeiro 2016

Roger A Hawkes MB ChB, Dip Sports Med, FFSEM (UK)
Chief Medical Officer, European Tour (Golf)

Matthew Hislop MBBS, MSc, FACSP
Sport and Exercise Medicine Physician, Brisbane; Sports and Exercise Medicine Specialists, Brisbane, Australia; Queensland Rugby League State of Origin Team Physician; Australian Olympic Doctor London 2012; Medical Director Brisbane International Tennis Tournament

Paul Hodges PhD, MedDr, DSc, BPhty (Hons), FACP
Professor & NHMRC Senior Principal Research Fellow, Director, NHMRC Centre of Clinical Research Excellence in Spinal Pain, Injury & Health, School of Health & Rehabilitation Sciences, University of Queensland, Brisbane, Australia

Per Hölmich MD, DMSc
Professor of Orthopedic Surgery, Sports Ortopedic Research Center—Copenhagen (SORC-C), Department of Orthopedic Surgery, Copenhagen University Hospital, Amager-Hvidovre, Denmark; The Aspetar Sports Groin Pain Center, Doha, Qatar

Karen Holzer MBBS, FACSP, PhD
Sport and Exercise Medicine Physician, South Yarra Sports Medicine, Melbourne, Australia; Australian Team Doctor, World Track and Field Championships, Helsinki 2005, and Olympic Games, Beijing 2008

Greg Hoy FRACS, FAOrthA, FACSP
Hand and Upper Limb Surgeon, Melbourne Orthopaedic Group, Melbourne, Australia

Christopher Jordan MD,
Assistant Director, South Bend-Notre Dame Sports Medicine Fellowship, University of Notre Dame, South Bend, USA

Gwendolen Jull AO MPhty, PhD, FACP
Emeritus Professor; Physiotherapy, School of Health and Rehabilitation Sciences, The University of Queensland, Australia

Astrid Junge PhD
Professor for Prevention and Sport, MSH University, Hamburg, Germany; Head of Research, FIFA-Medical Assessment and Research Centre (F-MARC) and Schulthess Clinic, Zürich, Switzerland

Steven J Kamper BSc (Hons), BAppSc, PhD
Senior Research Fellow, The George Institute for Global Health, Australia

Jon Karlsson MD, PhD
SPECIAL SURGERY CO-AUTHOR/EDITOR
Professor of Sports Traumatology, Sahlgrenska Academy, Gothenburg; IFK Gothenburg football; Ortopedic Surgeon, Sahlgrenska University Hospital, Sweden

Joanne Kemp PhD, MSportsPhysio, BAppSci(Physio)
APA Sports Physiotherapist, Research Fellow, La Trobe Sports Exercise Medicine Research Centre;

School of Allied Health; College of Science, Health and Engineering, La Trobe University, Melbourne, Australia

Tamim Khanbhai MBBS, FFSEM (UK)
Sport and Exercise Medicine Physician, Defence Medical Rehabilitation Centre, Headley Court, Epsom, Surrey, UK; Club Doctor, West Ham United, UK

W Ben Kibler MD
Orthopedic Surgeon; Medical Director, Shoulder Center of Kentucky, Lexington Clinic, Lexington, Kentucky, USA; Team Physician, Lexington Legends/Kansas City Royals baseball teams Transylvania University, Lexington, Kentucky, USA; Medical Consultant, Women's Tennis Association

Walter Kim MD
Orthopaedic Surgeon, University of Illinois at Chicago, USA

Vasileios Korakakis PT, PhD, MSc, OMT, DipMDT
Senior Sports Physiotherapist, Aspetar Orthopaedic and Sports Medicine Hospital, Doha, Qatar

Alex Kountouris BAppSci(Physio), PostGradDip Sports Physio, PhD
Sports Science & Sports Medicine Manager, Cricket Australia; Physiotherapist, Australian Men's Cricket Team

Karl B Landorf Dip App Sc (Pod), Grad Cert Clin Instr, Grad Dip Ed, PhD
Associate Professor in Podiatry, School of Allied Health, La Trobe University, Australia

Zuzana Machotka MPhysio (Musc and Sports), BPhysio
Clinical Researcher/Physiotherapist, International Centre for Allied Health Evidence, University of South Australia, Adelaide, Australia; Australian Paralympic Winter Team

Erin M Macri MSc(Kin), MPT, MSc
Registered Physical Therapist, PhD candidate, Experimental Medicine Program, University of British Columbia, Centre for Hip Health and Mobility, Vancouver, Canada; OARSI Scholar, Boston University, USA

Nicola Maffulli MD, MS, PhD, FRCP, FRCS(Orth)
Department of Musculoskeletal Surgery, University of Salerno School of Medicine, Salerno, Italy; Centre for Sports and Exercise Medicine, Queen Mary University of London, London, UK

Michael Makdissi BSc (Hons), MBBS, PhD, FACSP
Sport and Exercise Medicine Physician, Olympic Park Sports Medicine Centre, Melbourne, Australia; Team Doctor, Hawthorn Football Club (Australian Football League)

Lawrence Mayhew MSc, MCSP, FHEA
Senior Lecturer, Sports and Exercise Medicine and Physiotherapy, Musculoskeletal Health Research Group, Leeds Beckett University, Leeds, UK; Physiotherapist (Women's), England Football Association

Adam Meakins BSc (Hons) Physiotherapy
Lead Physiotherapist, Perform for Sport, Bushey, Herts. UK; Extended Scope Practitioner, West Herts. NHS Trust; Author of The Sports Physio Blog, http://thesportsphysio.wordpress.com

Håvard Moksnes Bachelor of Physiotherapy, PhD
Clinical Sports Physiotherapist, Norwegian Olympic Training Center (Olympiatoppen) & the Norwegian Sports Medicine Center (Idrettens Helsesenter); Co-director of the IOC Diploma in Sports Physical Therapie; The Norwegian Alpine Skiing Team 'Attacking Vikings' and Norwegian Athletics

Hayden Morris MBBS, DipAnat, FRACS
Orthopaedic Surgeon, Park Clinic Orthopaedics and Olympic Park Sports Medicine Centre, Melbourne, Australia

G Lorimer Moseley BAppSc(Phty) (Hons) PhD
Professor of Clinical Neuroscience & Foundation Chair in Physiotherapy, University of South Australia, Adelaide, Australia

Grethe Myklebust PT, PhD
Professor, Oslo Sport Trauma Research Center, Norwegian School of Sport Sciences, Oslo, Norway; Specialist in Sports Physiotherapy; Physiotherapist at the Seoul Olympics in 1988 and Sydney Olympics in 2000

Andrew Nealon BAppSc(Phty)
Principal, Aspire Physiotherapy Centre, Holgate, NSW, Australia; Head of Medical, Central Coast Mariners Football Club

Co-authors

Ian Needleman BDS, MSc, PhD, MRDRCS, FDSRCS, FFPH, FHEA
Centre for Oral Health and Performance, UCL Eastman Dental Institute, London, UK

John W Orchard MD, PhD, FACSEP, FFSEM, FACSM
Sport and Exercise Medicine Physician; Adjunct Professor, School of Public Health, University of Sydney; Chief Medical Officer, Cricket Australia

Kieran O'Sullivan BSc, M Manip Ther, PhD, Postgrad Dip Teaching & Learning
Lecturer, University of Limerick, Ireland; Lead Physiotherapist, Sports Spine Centre, Aspetar Orthopaedic and Sports Medicine Centre, Doha, Qatar

Peter O'Sullivan Dip Physio, Grad Dip Manip Ther, PhD, FACP
Professor, School of Physiotherapy and Exercise Science, Curtin University, Perth; Specialist Musculoskeletal Physiotherapist, Bodylogic Physiotherapy, Perth, Australia

Jon Patricios MBBCh, MMedSci, FACSM, FFSEM (UK), FFIMS
Sports Physician, Morningside Sports Medicine and Waterfall Sports Orthopaedic Surgery; Director of Sports Concussion, South Africa; Consultant to World Rugby, South African Rugby, Kaizer Chiefs Football Club and Team Didata cycling

Babette M Pluim MD, PhD
Chief Medical Officer, Royal Netherlands Lawn Tennis Association; Team Physician, Dutch Davis Cup and Fed Cup teams; Sports Physician, Amsterdam Collaboration on Health and Safety in Sports, IOC Research Centre for Prevention of Injury and Protection of Athlete Health, VUmc/AMC, Amsterdam, The Netherlands

Noel Pollock MBBCh, MSc, FFSEM
Sport and Exercise Medicine Physician; Team Doctor with British Athletics; Great Britain team doctor at six World Championships, the Beijing Paralympic Games and 2016 Summer Olympic Games, Rio de Janeiro

Nebojsa Popovic MD, PhD
Orthopaedic Sugeon and former Acting Chief Medical Officer, Aspetar Orthopaedic and Sports Medicine Hospital, Doha, Qatar; Chief Medical Officer for Yugoslavia, Summer Olympic Games, Seoul 1988 and Barcelona 1992

Joel M Press MD
Professor, Physical Medicine and Rehabilitation, Feinberg/Northwestern School of Medicine; Medical Director, Spine and Sports Rehabilitation Centers, Rehabilitation Institute of Chicago, USA; Reva and David Logan Distinguished Chair of Musculoskeletal Rehabilitation

Michael Pritchard BMedSci, MBBS (Hons), FRACS (Orth)
Orthopaedic Surgeon, St John's Hospital, Hobart, Australia

Craig Purdam Dip Physio, Postgrad Dip Sports Physio, MSc (Sports Physio)
Specialist Sports Physiotherapist; Adjunct Professor, University of Canberra; Head of Physical Therapies, Australian Institute of Sport; Australian Olympic Team Physiotherapist (x5)

Michael Skovdal Rathleff Bachelor of Physiotherapy, PhD
Senior Researcher, Research Unit for General Practice in Aalborg and Department of Clinical Medicine, Aalborg University, Denmark; Department of Occupational Therapy and Physiotherapy, Department of Clinical Medicine, Aalborg University Hospital, Denmark

Maria Reese MD
Specialist in Physical Medicine (Physiatry), Rehabilitation Institute of Chicago, Illinois, USA

Ebonie Rio B App Sci, B Physiot (Hons), M Sports Physio, PhD
Post-doctoral Research Fellow, La Trobe University Sport and Exercise Medicine Centre; The Australian Collaboration for Research into Injury in Sport and its Prevention; Victorian Institute of Sport, Australia

Ewa M Roos PT, PhD
Professor and Head of Research, Research Unit for Musculoskeletal Function and Physiotherapy, Institute of Sports Science and Clinical Biomechanics, University of Southern Denmark, Denmark

Stephan Rudzki MBBS, GradDipSportSc, MPH, PhD, FACSP
Brigadier, Australian Defence Force, Joint Health Command; Director, General Army Health Services, Canberra, Australia

Co-authors

Anthony Schache BPhysio (Hons), PhD
Physiotherapist, Olympic Park Sports Medicine Centre and Richmond Football Club (AFL); Research Fellow, Hugh Williamson Gait Laboratory, Royal Children's Hospital, Melbourne, and Faculty of Engineering, The University of Melbourne, Australia

Alex Scott BSc(PT), MSc, PhD
Associate Professor, Department of Physical Therapy, University of British Columbia, Canada

Catherine Sherrington PhD, MPH, BAppSc(Physio)
Professorial Research Fellow, George Institute for Global Health, Sydney Medical School, University of Sydney, Australia

Ian Shrier MD, PhD
Associate Professor, McGill University; Centre for Clinical Epidemiology, Lady Davis Institute, Jewish General Hospital, Montreal, Canada

Karin Grävare Silbernagel PT, ATC, PhD
Assistant Professor, Department of Physical Therapy, University of Delaware, USA

Stephen M Simons MD, FACSM
Director of Sports Medicine, Saint Joseph Regional Medical Center. Mishawaka, Indiana; Co-Director, South Bend-Notre Dame Sports Medicine Fellowship, USA

Kevin Singer PhD, PT
Emeritus Professor, School of Surgery, The University of Western Australia, Australia

Geoffrey St George BDS, DGDP (UK), MSc, FDS (RCSEd), FDS (Rest Dent)
Centre for Oral Health and Performance, UCL Eastman Dental Institute, London, UK

Raj Subbu MBBch MRCS, BSci (Hons) PGMedEDCert
Sports Research Fellow, Institute of Sport Exercise and Health, London; Watford FC & Fulham FC, UK

Kent Sweeting BHlthSc (Pod) (Hons)
Podiatrist and Director, Performance Podiatry & Physiotherapy; Director, Queensland Orthotic Laboratory, Brisbane, Australia

Stephen Targett MB ChB, FACSEP
Sport and Exercise Medicine Physician; Clinical Lead Athlete Screening, Aspetar Hospital, Doha, Qatar

Kristian Thorborg PT, PhD
IOC Sports Medicine Copenhagen; Sports Orthopedic Research Center—Copenhagen (SORC-C), Amager-Hvidovre Hospital, Copenhagen University, Denmark

Michael Turner MB BS, MD, FFSEM (UK and Ireland)
Chief Medical Advisor, Lawn Tennis Association; Chief Medical Advisor, British Horseracing Authority, UK

Elsbeth van Dorssen MD, MSc
Sports Medicine Physician and Team Doctor KNZB (Royal Dutch Swimming Federation), The Netherlands; Paralympic Games, Rio de Janeiro 2016

Evert Verhagen PhD
Department of Public and Occupational Health, VU University Medical Center, Amsterdam, The Netherlands

Bill Vicenzino PhD, MSc, Grad Dip Sports Phty, BPhty
Professor, Chair in Sports Physiotherapy; Director of MPhty (Musculoskeletal, Sports Phty), School of Health and Rehabilitation Sciences, The University of Queensland, Australia

Stuart Warden BPhysio (Hons), PhD, FACSM
Professor and Associate Dean for Research, School of Health and Rehabilitation Sciences, Indiana University, Indianapolis, USA

Adam Weir MBBS, PhD
Aspetar Orthopaedic and Sports Medicine Hospital, Doha, Qatar; Amsterdam Center of Evidence Based Sports Medicine, Academic Medical Center, Amsterdam, The Netherlands

Liam West BSc (Hons), MBBCh, ECOSEP(ac), DipSEM
Junior Doctor, Royal Melbourne Hospital, Melbourne, Australia; Head Doctor, Williamstown Football Club

Fiona Wilson BSc, MSc, MA, PhD
Assistant Professor & Chartered Physiotherapist, Discipline of Physiotherapy, School of Medicine, Trinity College Dublin, The University of Dublin, Dublin, Ireland

Other contributors

Richard Allison BSc, MSc, PhD
Senior Sports Dietitian, Aspetar Orthopaedic and Sports Medicine Hospital, Doha, Qatar

Ummukulthoum Bakare PT
Sports Physiotherapist; Secretary, Nigeria Sports Physiotherapy Association; Chief Physiotherapist, Lagos University Teaching Hospital; Member, Medical and Scientific Commission, Nigeria Olympic Committee; Team Physiotherapist, All Africa Games 2015, Paralympic Team, Rio de Janeiro 2016

Tone Bere PT, PhD
Research Co-ordinator, Department of Orthopaedics, Oslo University Hospital, Norway

Inge De Wandele PT, PhD
Center for Medical Genetics, Department of Rehabilitation Sciences and Physiotherapy, Ghent University, Ghent, Belgium

John DiFiori MD
NBA Director of Sports Medicine; Professor and Chief, Division of Sports Medicine and Non-Operative Orthopaedics, David Geffen School of Medicine, UCLA; Head Team Physician, UCLA Department of Intercollegiate Athletics, Los Angeles, USA

Allison Ezzat PT, MCISc, MSc, PhD candidate
British Columbia Children's Hospital Research Institute, School of Population and Public Health, University of British Columbia, Canada

Anna Frohm PT, PhD
Swedish Sports Confederation, Elite Performance, Head of Sports Medicine and Karolinska Institut, Department of Neurobiology, Care Sciences and Society, Section of Physiotherapy

Sue Mayes BAppSc (Phty), Grad Dip Sports Physiotherapy, PhD(c)
Principal Physiotherapist, The Australian Ballet

Francis O'Connor MD, MPH, FACSM
Professor and Chair, Military and Emergency Medicine Uniformed Services University of the Health Sciences Bethesda, USA

Seth O'Neill MSc, BSc, MACP, MCSP
Lecturer, University of Leicester, UK

Matthew Stride MRCP (UK), DipSEM MSc, FFSEM, CES
Consultant Sport and Exercise Medicine, Isokinetic London, UK; Team Doctor Brentford Football Club

Markus Walden MD, PhD
Orthopaedic Surgeon, Department of Orthopaedics, Hässleholm, Sweden; Member of Football Research Group (FRG), Linköping University, Sweden; Team Physician, IFK Kristianstad (handball), Sweden

Medical illustrator

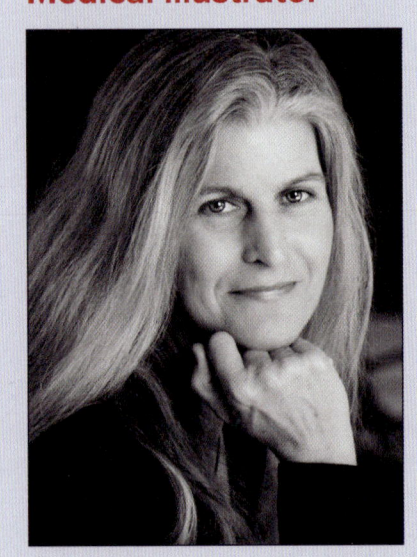

Vicky Earle BSc (AAM), MET, Cert TBDL

Vicky, an international award winning medical illustrator, has worked with renowned researchers, sports medicine physicians and surgeons around the globe. She has created thousands of illustrations for medical and scientific textbooks and journals, as well as artwork for legal litigation, video, animation and websites on a variety of topics. Vicky's keen interest in *Clinical Sports Medicine* stems not only from a great appreciation of the human body and its capabilities, but also from years of racing experience as a championship rower, a world-class paddler, and a rock climbing enthusiast—and knowing first-hand the many injuries that accompany these activities.

Acknowledgments

Allow me to thank you for being part of this wonderful sports medical book family. I cherish the privilege to have partnered with you to blend science with practice.

This page allows us to say 'thank you'. We open with a quote from one of our chapter authors because it captures the spirit of the large and diverse team that has created Volume 1 of this fifth edition of *Clinical Sports Medicine*. Every single colleague went beyond the call of duty during their busy lives at the peak of great careers.

This highlights that the global sports medicine and sports physiotherapy community is generous and patient focused. Our community shares the wonderful compelling goal of making life better for athletes and for recreational individuals. We share a passion: the joy of physical activity, the love of sport, the conviction that these are elements of medicine at its very best. Here we say 'thank you' to every contributor for allowing us to guide your passion into these pages and the digital elements that complement them.

On the topic of professions in our field, please indulge us a personal note from two medical doctors. To leaders in physiotherapy/physical therapy, we thank you for having embraced the value of physical activity and sport from your profession's beginnings. Physiotherapy/physical therapy has established a very substantial evidence base, along with other disciplines, so that our field—sport and exercise medicine—is recognised as a critical pillar in health. The PEDro database is just one example we can point to if people ask 'What is the scientific basis of the field?' Your profession has been generous to us personally by educating us, and by welcoming us to share our humble opinions with you. We are honoured and grateful to the President of the World Confederation for Physical Therapy for reading this edition and vouching for its value in the foreword and on the back cover. Dr Emma Stokes, we salute you and wish you every success as you execute a shared vision for a very proud, difference-making profession.

Specific thanks for this edition of *Volume 1–Injuries* go to chapter co-authors listed, with their affiliations, on pages xxx–xxxv. We are both humbled and privileged to be sharing cover authorship with seven amazing colleagues and friends: Ben Clarsen, Jill Cook, Ann Cools, Kay Crossley, Mark Hutchinson, Paul McCrory and Roald Bahr. Vicky Earle, our medical illustrator, is part of this book's DNA (three editions now).

The University of British Columbia (Department of Family Practice–Faculty of Medicine, as well as the Faculty of Education–School of Kinesiology) provided essential support (KK), as did La Trobe University in establishing the Sport and Exercise Medicine Research Centre.

We have passed the silver anniversary of McGraw-Hill writing a snail-mail letter to Peter Brukner in 1990 wondering if he thought a sports medicine book might be in order; we are very fortunate for more than 25 years of remarkable support. Nicole Meehan and Robert Ashworth are passionate about this book. Isabella Mead and Yani Silvana always reached out with offers of help. The copy-editing team have added great value for the reader.

We dedicate this fifth edition to the *Clinical Sports Medicine* community. We are proud to be in a family of clinicians who are absolutely unwavering in prioritising patient care. Lastly, to our very, very patient friends and families, 'Yes, it is finished (for now)'. Diana and Heather, thank you for the many editions you have shared us with. Let's leave the conversation about the fifth edition of *Volume 2–Exercise Medicine* (for 2018 release) for another day.

Guided tour of your book

The principal text in its field, this first volume of the fifth edition of *Clinical Sports Medicine* continues to provide readers with quality up-to-date content. The engaging material has been contributed by leading experts from around the world. Look out for these key features, which are designed to enhance your learning.

Premium, up-to-date content

Treatment and rehabilitation is emphasised. Part A—Fundamental Principles includes 12 chapters that are either brand new or written by new authors. The chapters in Part B, which address regional problems, provide clinical solutions via clear text, abundant clinical photos (e.g. physical examination), relevant imaging and customised medical illustrations.

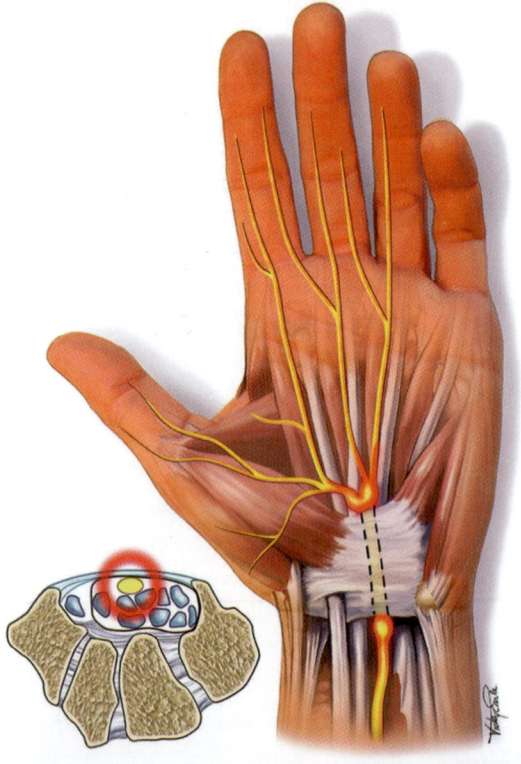

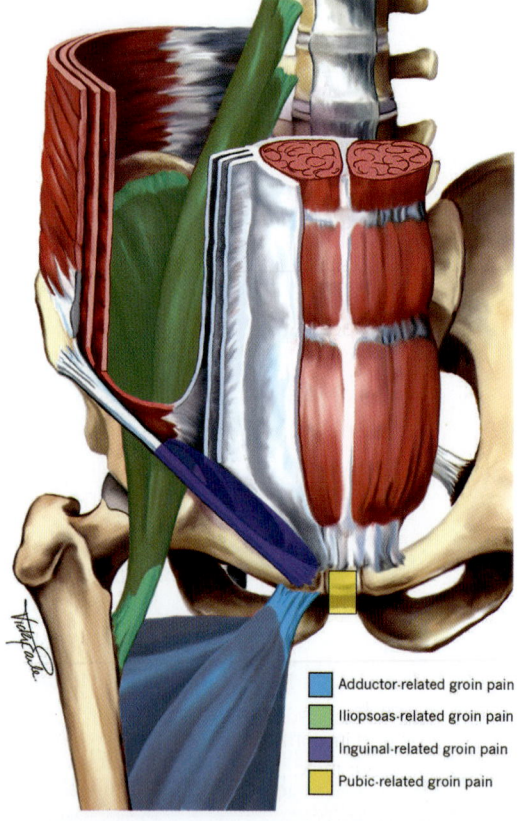

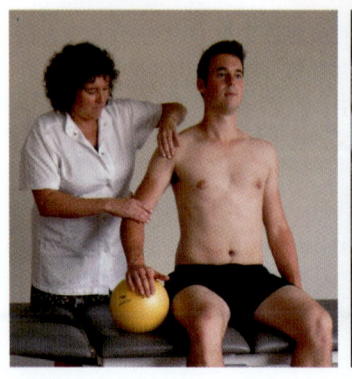

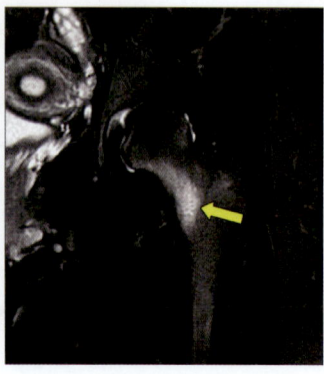

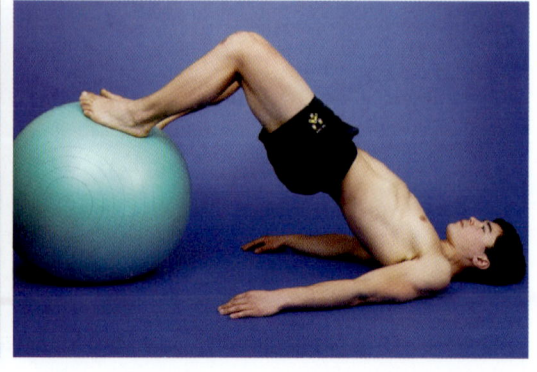

- Adductor-related groin pain
- Iliopsoas-related groin pain
- Inguinal-related groin pain
- Pubic-related groin pain

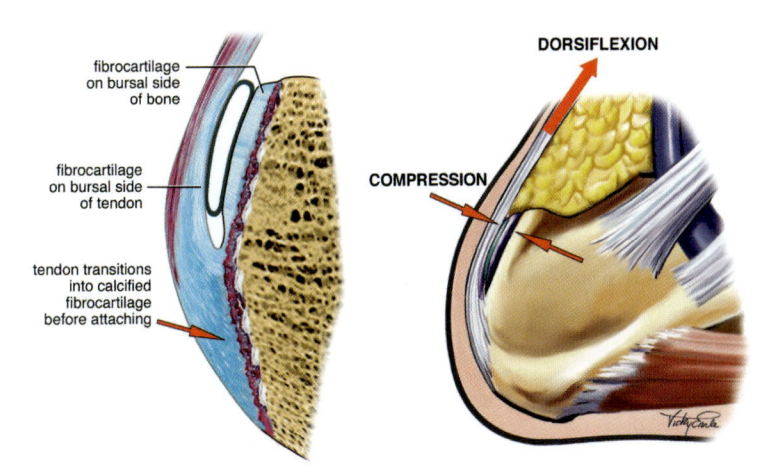

Tables

New tables summarise vast amounts of evidence to provide take-home messages. Primary sources are readily available.

Table 36.6c Remote factors that can contribute to patellofemoral pain syndrome and their possible mechanisms—increased knee valgus/tibial external rotation

Increased apparent knee valgus/tibial external rotation	Possible contributing factors	Confirmatory assessments
	Structural: • genu varum • tibial varum • coxa varum	Radiographic: • long leg X-ray Clinical assessment: • goniometer/inclinometer
	Inadequate strength/control: • hip external rotators • hip extensors • hip abductors • quadriceps • hamstrings • lumbopelvic muscles	Clinical assessment: • manual muscle test • hand-held dynamometer • biofeedback
	Altered movement patterns	Biomechanical/gait assessment (Chapter 8): • can the patient correct the movement pattern when asked to focus on it?

Practice Pearl

Practice pearls are a valuable feature that provide clinical tips and important information to keep in the forefront of your mind.

PRACTICE PEARL

In the large majority of these hamstring strains, the injured muscle is the biceps femoris (reported as 76–87%). Semimembranosus injury is uncommon; semitendinosus injury is rare.

Contributors

The 121 **world-renowned contributors** bring a truly global perspective to the book.

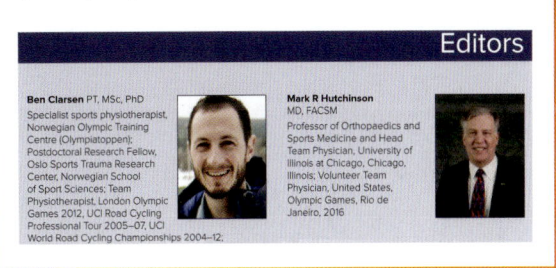

Editors

Ben Clarsen PT, MSc, PhD
Specialist sports physiotherapist, Norwegian Olympic Training Centre (Olympiatoppen); Postdoctoral Research Fellow, Oslo Sports Trauma Research Center, Norwegian School of Sport Sciences; Team Physiotherapist, London Olympic Games 2012, UCI Road Cycling Professional Tour 2005–07, UCI World Road Cycling Championships 2004–12;

Mark R Hutchinson MD, FACSM
Professor of Orthopaedics and Sports Medicine and Head Team Physician, University of Illinois at Chicago, Chicago, Illinois; Volunteer Team Physician, United States, Olympic Games, Rio de Janeiro, 2016

References

Over 4000 carefully chosen references. A comprehensive list of references for each chapter can be found here: **www.mhhe.com/au/CSM5e.**

PART A

Fundamental principles

Chapter 1

Sport and exercise medicine: the team approach

with PAUL DIJKSTRA and STEFANO DELLA VILLA

You may have the greatest bunch of individual stars in the world, but if they don't play together, the club won't be worth a dime.
Babe Ruth (1895–1948)

Sport and exercise medicine (SEM) is evolving as a specialist medical discipline that includes a variety of tasks and responsibilities.[1-7] These include:

- injury and illness prevention
- injury diagnosis, treatment and rehabilitation
- management of medical problems
- performance enhancement through training
- nutrition and psychology
- exercise prescription in health and in chronic disease states
- exercise prescription in special subpopulations
- medical care of sporting teams and events
- medical care in situations of altered physiology, such as at altitude, environmental extremes, or at depth
- dealing with ethical issues, such as the problem of drug abuse in sport.

SEM has been defined as the scope of medical practice that focuses on:

1. prevention, diagnosis treatment and rehabilitation of injuries that occur during physical activity
2. prevention, diagnosis, and management of medical conditions that occur during or after physical activity
3. promotion and implementation of regular physical activity in the prevention, treatment and rehabilitation of chronic diseases of lifestyle.[8]

Because of the growing breadth of content, SEM traditionally lends itself to being practised by a multidisciplinary team of professionals with specialised skills who provide optimal care for the athlete and improve each other's knowledge and skills. The sporting adage that a 'champion team' would always beat a 'team of champions' applies to sport and exercise medicine. This team approach can be implemented in a multidisciplinary SEM clinic or by individual practitioners of different disciplines collaborating by cross-referral. However, the real-world application of this multiskilled team approach poses significant challenges– some of which are eloquently dealt with by the specialist SEM physician. SEM is now an official medical specialty in many countries and this has significantly changed the level of care to athletes and also patients suffering from chronic disease.

THE SEM TEAM

The most appropriate sports medicine team depends on the setting. Clubs and sporting bodies increasingly employ specialist SEM physicians, with the primary role being the comprehensive health management of the athlete to facilitate optimal performance. This includes the diagnosis and treatment of injuries and illnesses associated with exercise to ultimately improve performance. In an isolated rural community the sports medicine team may consist of a family physician or a physiotherapist/physical therapist alone. In a populous city, the team may consist of a number of clinicians and sports scientists working together and may include:

- specialist SEM physician
- family physician
- physiotherapist/physical therapist
- soft tissue therapist
- exercise specialist for exercise prescription
- other medical specialists with an interest in SEM
- orthopaedic surgeon, rheumatologist, radiologist, cardiologist, etc.
- podiatrist
- dietitian/nutritionist

- psychologist
- sports trainer/athletic trainer
- other professionals such as osteopaths, chiropractors, exercise physiologists, biomechanists, nurses, occupational therapists, orthotists, optometrists
- coach
- fitness adviser.

In the Olympic polyclinic, an institution that aims to serve all 10 000 athletes at the games, the sports medicine team includes 160 practitioners (Table 1.1).

Multiskilling, roles, responsibilities and communication

There are, of course, distinct differences in roles and responsibilities when clinicians are employed by sporting organisations or clubs as opposed to providing care in the form of a once-off expert opinion for a specific athlete's injury or illness. Equally, medical teams contracted by the local organising committees (LOCs) of smaller or major events have very specific roles and skills depending on the size of the event. Multiskilling, where practitioners in the team each develop skills in a particular area of sports medicine, is important but may also pose challenges in areas of considerable amount of overlap between the different practitioners. The key is always effective teamwork with clear roles and responsibilities, leadership and communication. This 'multiskilling' might be of use if the practitioner is geographically isolated or is travelling alone with sporting teams.

The concept of effective teamwork is best illustrated by example. When an athlete presents with an overuse injury of the lower limb, the specialist SEM (or other physician) will have the diagnostic responsibility but the sport-specific therapist, podiatrist or biomechanist might have a better knowledge of clinical biomechanical assessment, the functional relationship between abnormal biomechanics and the development of the injury and how to correct any biomechanical cause. However, it is essential that all the practitioners have a basic understanding of lower limb biomechanics and are able to perform a clinical assessment.

Similarly, for the athlete who presents complaining of excessive fatigue and poor performance, the dietitian is best able to assess the nutritional state of the athlete and determine if a nutritional deficiency is responsible for the patient's symptoms. However, other practitioners such as the SEM physician, physiotherapist/physical therapist or trainer must also be aware of the possibility of nutritional deficiency as a cause of tiredness and be able to perform a brief nutritional assessment.

Table 1.1 The clinical team structure at the London 2012 Olympic Games polyclinic

Administration/organisation
• Chief Medical Officer
• Deputy Chief Medical Officer and Chief Athlete Services (sports physician)
• Director of Clinical Services—polyclinic (sports physician)
• Director of Nursing
• Director of Physiotherapy/Physical therapy
• Director of Remedial Massage
• Director of Podiatric Services
• Director of Dental Services
• Director of Emergency Services

Consulting
• Medical practitioners: sports physicians; orthopaedic surgeons; general practitioners; rehabilitation specialists; emergency medicine specialists; ear, nose and throat specialists; gynaecologists; dermatologists; ophthalmologists; ophthalmic surgeons; radiologists; amputee clinic physicians; spinal clinic physicians
• Physiotherapists/Physical therapists
• Soft tissue therapists
• Podiatrists
• Optometrists
• Pharmacists
• Dentists
• Interpreters

The sport and exercise medicine model

The model for the delivery of effective healthcare is changing with an increased focus on individualised medical care and case managing. The traditional medical model (Fig. 1.1) has the physician as the primary contact practitioner with subsequent referral to other medical and paramedical practitioners. The early SEM model (Fig. 1.2) is different. The athlete's primary professional contact is often with a physiotherapist/physical therapist; however, it is just as likely to be a trainer, SEM physician or soft tissue therapist. It is essential that all practitioners in the healthcare team understand their own strengths and limitations and are aware of who else can improve management of the patient.

This improved SEM model recognises the multidisciplinary nature of the athlete's 'primary professional contact' but still emphasises the reductionist approach, with each discipline potentially operating

PART A Fundamental principles

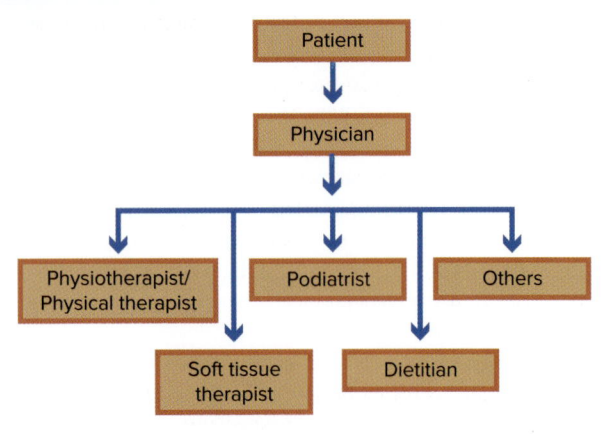

Figure 1.1 The traditional medical model

in its own specialist silo with little focus on holistic athlete health management, effective communication integration and understanding to facilitate decision making. The athlete and coach are often ill equipped to integrate the different contributions in these settings of increasing complexity and multispecialists. They often rely on expert case managers with a very good sport-specific understanding (in big teams the specialist SEM physician) to provide 'health leadership', effectively and efficiently communicating and integrating the contributions of all the key role players in the so-called *integrated performance health management and coaching model*.[9] This new model emphasises the importance of an integrated approach in communication and management to athlete health problems. The focus is on operational integration of the health management and coaching to improve performance with one accountable 'case manager'.

THE CHALLENGES OF MANAGEMENT

The secret of success in SEM is to take a broad view of the patient and his or her problem. The narrow view may provide short-term amelioration of symptoms but will ultimately lead to failure. Examples of a narrow view may include a runner who presents with shin pain, is diagnosed as having a stress fracture of the tibia and is treated with rest until pain-free.

Although it is likely that in the short term the athlete will improve and return to activity there remains a high likelihood of recurrence of the problem on resumption of activity. The clinician must always ask 'Why has this injury/illness occurred?' The cause may be obvious, for example, a recent sudden doubling of training load, or it may be subtle and, in many cases, multifactorial.

The greatest challenge of SEM is to identify and correct the cause of the injury/illness. The runner with shin pain arising from a stress fracture may have abnormal biomechanics, inappropriate footwear, had a change in the training surface, or a change in the quantity or quality of training. In medicine, there are two main challenges: diagnosis and treatment. In SEM it is necessary to diagnose both the problem and the cause. Treatment then needs to be focused on both these areas.

Diagnosis

Every attempt should be made to diagnose the precise anatomical, pathological and functional cause of the presenting problem. Knowledge of anatomy (especially surface anatomy) and an understanding of the pathological and functional processes likely to occur in athletes often permits a precise diagnosis. Thus, instead of using a purely descriptive term such as 'shin splints', the practitioner

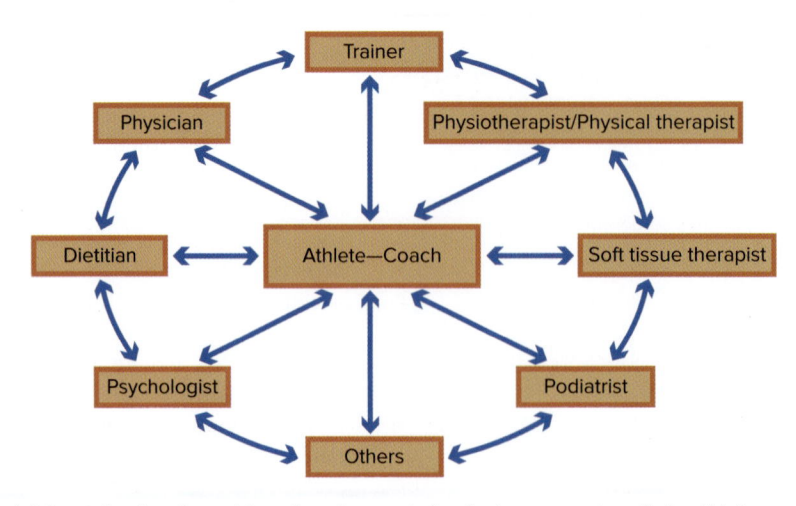

Figure 1.2 The SEM model. In professional sport the player's agent also features prominently in athlete–coach interaction

should attempt to diagnose which of the three underlying causes it could be–stress fracture, chronic compartment syndrome or periostitis–and use the specific term. Accurate diagnosis guides precise treatment.

Some clinical situations do not allow a precise anatomical and pathological diagnosis. For example, in many cases of low back pain, it is clinically impossible to differentiate between potential sites of pathology. In situations such as these it is necessary to establish a functional diagnosis, monitor symptoms and signs through careful clinical assessment and correct any abnormalities present (e.g. hypomobility) using appropriate treatment techniques.

As mentioned, diagnosis of the presenting problem should be followed by diagnosis of the cause of the problem. American orthopaedic surgeon Ben Kibler coined the term 'victim' for the presenting problem and 'culprit' for the cause.[10] Diagnosis of the cause often requires a good understanding of biomechanics, technique, training, nutrition and psychology. Just as there may be more than one pathological process contributing to the patient's symptoms, a combination of factors may cause the problem.

As with any branch of medicine, diagnosis depends on careful clinical assessment, which consists of obtaining a history, physical examination and investigations. The most important of these is undoubtedly the history but, unfortunately, this is often neglected. It is essential that the sports clinician be a good listener and develop skills that enable him or her to elicit the appropriate information from the athlete. Once the history has been taken, an examination can be performed. It is essential to develop examination routines for each joint or region and to include in the examination an assessment of any potential causes.

Investigations should be regarded as an adjunct to, rather than a substitute for, adequate history and examination.[11] The investigation must be appropriate to the athlete's problem, provide additional information and should only be performed if it will affect the diagnosis and/or treatment.

Treatment
Ideally, treatment has at least three components: discussing the planned treatment with the athlete, coach and key role players (also in the context of the immediate and future performance goals); treatment of the presenting injury/illness; and treatment to correct the cause. Generally, no single form of treatment will correct the majority of SEM problems. A combination of different forms of treatment will usually give the best results.

Therefore, it is important for the clinician to be aware of the variety of treatments and to appreciate when their use may be appropriate. It is also important to develop as many treatment skills as possible or, alternatively, ensure access to others with particular skills. It is essential to evaluate the effectiveness of treatment constantly. If a particular treatment is not proving to be effective, it is important firstly to reconsider the diagnosis. If the diagnosis appears to be correct, other treatments should be considered.

Meeting individual needs
Every patient is a unique individual with specific needs. Without an understanding of this, it is not possible to manage the athlete appropriately. The patient may be an Olympic athlete whose selection depends on a peak performance at forthcoming trials. The patient may be a non-competitive business executive whose jogging is an important means of coping with the stress of everyday life. The patient may be a club tennis player whose weekly competitive game is as important as a Wimbledon final is to a professional. Alternatively, the patient may be someone to whom sport is not at all important but whose low back pain causes discomfort at work.

The cost of treatment should also be considered. Does the athlete merely require a diagnosis and reassurance that he or she has no major injury? Or does the athlete want twice-daily treatment in order to be able to play in an important game? Treatment depends on the patient's situation, not purely on the diagnosis.

THE COACH, THE ATHLETE AND THE CLINICIAN
The relationship between the coach, the athlete and the clinician is shown in Figure 1.3. The clinician obviously needs to develop a good relationship with the athlete. A feeling of mutual trust and confidence would lead to the athlete feeling that he or she can confide in the clinician and the clinician feeling that the athlete will comply with advice.

As the coach is directly responsible for the athlete's training and performance, it is essential to involve the

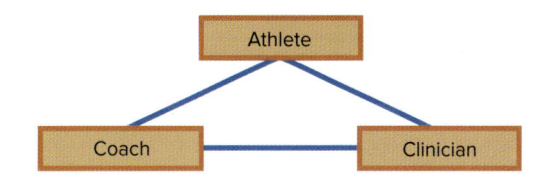

Figure 1.3 The relationship between the coach, the athlete and the clinician

coach in clinical decision making. Involving the coach in the decision-making process is essential for athlete compliance. The coach will also be a valuable aid in supervising the recommended treatment or rehabilitation program. Discussion with the coach may help to establish a possible technique-related cause for the injury. Unfortunately, some coaches have a distrust of clinicians; however, it is essential for the coach to understand that the clinician is also aiming to maximise the performance and health of the athlete. When major injuries occur, professional athletes' agents will also be involved in discussions. It is therefore crucial that clinicians understand the performance environment and develop skills in communication and management to complement optimal decision making in challenging situations.

'LOVE THY SPORT' (AND PHYSICAL ACTIVITY!)

To be a successful SEM clinician it is essential to be an advocate for physical activity. A good understanding of a sport confers two advantages. First, if the clinician understands the physical demands and technical aspects of a particular sport, this will improve his or her understanding of possible causes of injury and facilitate development of sport-specific rehabilitation programs. Second, it will result in the athlete having increased confidence in the clinician. The best way to understand the sport is to attend training and competition and ideally to participate in the sport. Thus, it is essential to be on site, not only to be available when injuries occur, but also to develop a thorough understanding of the sport and its culture.

The case manager approach

The Isokinetic group of sports medicine clinics in Italy and the United Kingdom adopt the case manager approach to rehabilitation of the injured athlete. Here the group's founder, sports physician Dr Stefano della Villa, explains the Isokinetic philosophy.

The final result of our job, as a sport physician, is when the athlete is able to play again; as fast, as strong and as powerful as before. Everything in the middle is just a ring in the chain. Despite everyone being aware of this, in real life the situation is completely different.

Most of the time, sports physicians are unable to follow the patient during the long process from injury to return to play. A long list of practical issues may become obstacles along the way, including:

- the length of the process, especially if it is post-surgery
- the number of professionals involved, from the surgeon to the team coach and all those in the middle
- logistical issues during the recovery process—the needs of the patient during recovery to use different facilities and environments such as consultation rooms, gyms, pools and pitches, all of which may well be located in different areas
- pressure from the outside—family, friends, agent, manager, other players, coaches, fitness team, traditional media and social media.

In my opinion, this long list is not the biggest obstacle to overcome. That obstacle is our way of thinking as doctors. The key is to change this paradigm: we need to forget the injury and to re-focus on the recovery from the first moment after the injury. We must do it, from the very beginning, when we explain the recovery process to the patient.

Medical training and its influence

Studying at university does not help the sports physician to follow the approach described above. During our time at university we learn a lot about anatomy and symptoms of diseases. The real challenge for a student is to be prepared and ready to make the right diagnosis. However, the right diagnosis does not have value without a strategy to ensure the patient returns to sport. The right diagnosis is crucial, but it is only the first step. Then the process begins and the patient goes through different steps, such as in the following example of an injury that requires surgical treatment:

- imaging
- surgical procedure
- pain management and prevention of deep venous thrombosis
- post-surgical protocols
- recovery of activities of daily living (ADL)
- recovery of range of motion
- recovery of strength
- recovery of coordination and proprioception
- recovery of match fitness
- restoration of specific sports skills
- prevention of re-injury.

We believe the sports physician should always be in charge and control all of these steps (Fig. 1.4). This, however, is not what happens in the sports medicine community. Apart from a few examples in professional sports, most of the time responsibility is shared during the recovery process, without central coordination. In the end this means that no one person is responsible. Many professionals are involved in this process, as it must be, but each of them is focused only on

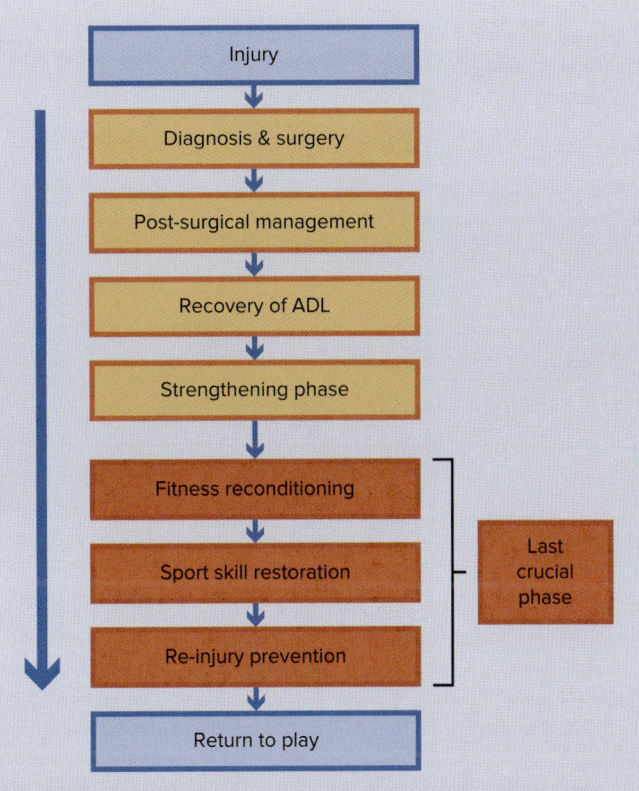

Sport and exercise medicine: the team approach CHAPTER 1

```
Injury
  ↓
Diagnosis & surgery
  ↓
Post-surgical management
  ↓
Recovery of ADL
  ↓
Strengthening phase
  ↓
Fitness reconditioning  ⎤
  ↓                     ⎥
Sport skill restoration ⎬ Last crucial phase
  ↓                     ⎥
Re-injury prevention    ⎦
  ↓
Return to play
```

Figure 1.4 From injury to return to play

their single job and there is a need for a leader to coordinate all of them.

The case manager concept
We believe that the management of sports injuries can be visualised like a symphony. Many musicians are involved, but they need a conductor—a director of the orchestra. This person is able to deal with the first violin and all the other elements. Based on our experience, our medical group has defined this role as that of the 'case manager'—the manager of each specific patient and their recovery from injury.

We strongly believe in the concept 'patient first' and we put the patient at the centre of our attention. We also understand that after a bad injury the patient needs a project, a plan and a conductor who is able to drive them through the potentially long recovery process.

The facilities for the sports recovery process
Utilising this new approach, sports physicians should always be a step ahead in the process. During the diagnosis process they must look ahead to the next possible steps. They need to have a vision of the future for the patient and understand where there could be obstacles on the road to recovery. They need to anticipate problems but, more importantly, consider when there will be key decision points. This will include the times when the path and speed of the recovery can change, such as the options for surgery and the surgeon. Both before, and at the time of, the surgery they must plan the post-surgical management, right up to completion of the final phase. This can include seeking activities that may ordinarily appear in a future phase of rehabilitation and bringing them forward to operate in parallel with earlier phase activities. An example might be using a pool early to maintain cardiorespiratory fitness, while working to regain strength in the injured limb. Therefore, having the appropriate facilities is a first and major step in planning effective rehabilitation.

We believe for an athlete to fully complete their rehabilitation, they need access to a proper facility consisting of medical offices, rehabilitation gyms, rehabilitation pools and sports fields. The use of these specific areas at well-defined moments in the pathway is critical for the best functional outcome. For example, using a pool-based environment allows the early introduction of sport-specific movement patterns, such as kicking or heading in football (Fig. 1.5).

These exercises will be introduced again in the later phases, both in the gym and on the field, creating a type of continuum in the recovery process. It is a form of stimulation

7

PART A Fundamental principles

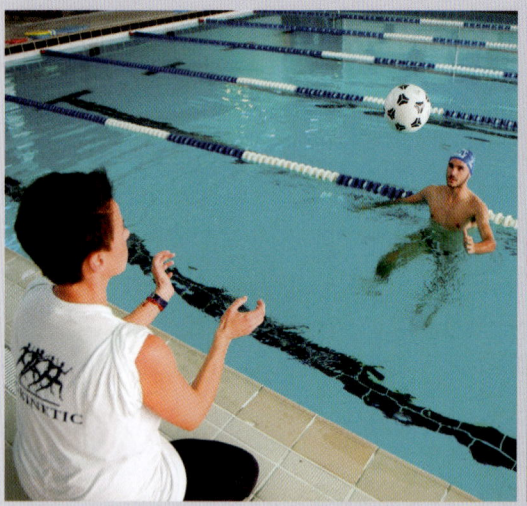

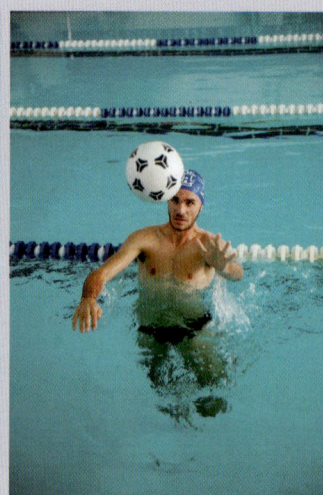

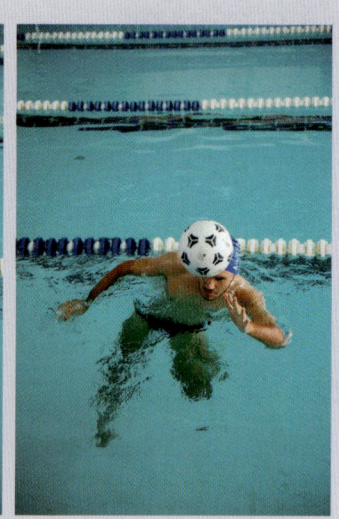

Figure 1.5 Neuroplasticity exercises in the pool. Heading a football with partial-body submersion allows safe football-specific movement patterns while in the early phases of rehabilitation

and is thought to favour the re-education of motor skills. In fact, after the injury there may be a process of joint de-efferentation and central disorganisation. The early introduction of some complex stimuli is recommended to solve neuromuscular impairments.

The rehabilitation gym is still considered the main rehabilitation area. Aside from the classical range of motion and strength exercises, it is useful and important to introduce more neuromuscular exercises. These exercises should not only consider the affected joint, but also the whole kinetic chain and the biomechanical connection among different joints.

According to our philosophy, we progressively introduce sport-specific movements on a real sports field, to better restore players' self-confidence in a supervised environment. The on-field rehabilitation (OFR) offers three main advantages: the complete recovery of specific movement patterns, metabolic reconditioning and a real education of the athlete in prevention strategies.

Teamwork and communication

With regard to the sports medicine team, we think it should at least consist of a sports medicine physician, a physical therapist and a conditioning specialist. Together they follow the player from injury to return to play.

The final key point of a good strategy is to have a shared working method within the clinical team. Within our philosophy the physician should act as the case manager. He or she is in charge of controlling the process, from the beginning to the end, communicating regularly and coordinating the team around the patient, and planning a customised protocol. Having a strong and consistent communication model within the team is critical for success. Frequent clinical updates are important to constantly monitor patient's improvements and solve eventual complications. In fact, the strength of a sports medicine group has to be measured in the management of difficult cases, when both logistical considerations and clinical skills are required.

REFERENCES

References for this chapter can be found at www.mhhe.com/au/CSM5e

Chapter 2

Integrating evidence into shared decision making with patients

with STEVEN J KAMPER and CATHERINE SHERRINGTON

Incredibly, some scientifically educated medical school graduates still see evidence as inferior to intuition and experience: those are the ones who give me chills.

Dr Harriet Hall

Case: introduction

Your patient is Mrs J, a 55-year-old woman with knee pain. She complains of pain, stiffness and mechanical symptoms consistent with a meniscal tear. She has had an X-ray in which the radiologist notes degenerative changes consistent with osteoarthritis.

Question
Should you recommend surgical or non-surgical management?

WHAT IS EVIDENCE-BASED PRACTICE?

Evidence-based practice (EBP), also known as evidence-based medicine (EBM), is the dominant paradigm under which healthcare professionals across the world are now expected to practice. We use the term 'practice' to avoid the ambiguity in the word 'medicine' (which is sometimes used to refer only to the work of medical doctors). Clinicians and researchers from McMaster University in Canada in the 1980s and 90s are credited with developing the ideas behind EBP and championing the movement. The most commonly used definition comes from David Sackett[1] and it highlights the integration of three elements: best available evidence from well-conducted and relevant scientific research, clinical expertise, and patient values and preferences[2] (Fig. 2.1).

Evidence-based practice should provide better patient outcomes than so-called 'eminence-based practice' whereby the opinion of the clinician alone defines an optimal management decision. In the caricature of eminence-based practice, inappropriate and outdated methods and practices were perpetuated from senior to junior clinicians and personal clinical experience weighed more heavily than quality research evidence. We acknowledge that many clinicians provided wonderful evidence-based practice before the term 'evidence-based practice' was coined.

Today, healthcare systems and consumers expect practice to be grounded in science. This mirrors the progression to today's technology-supported world from a society based on semi-mystical beliefs and paternalism. EBP, however, asks more than just acceptance of a scientific world view; it requires explicit understanding and integration of the three elements.

'Evidence-based practice' is the integration of best research evidence with clinical expertise and patient values—David Sackett

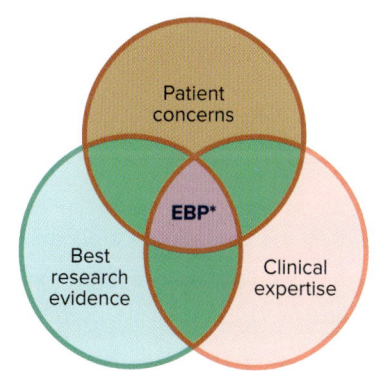

Figure 2.1 Schematic illustration of how clinical skills, evidence from research and patient desire should overlap to provide the 'quality decision' for the patient
*evidence-based practice

PART A Fundamental principles

WHY IS THE EVIDENCE-BASED PRACTICE CONCEPT CONTROVERSIAL?

Superficially, the principles of EBP are straightforward and few argue that it represents a superior model to a paternalistic opinion-based medical model. In general, clinicians have positive attitudes towards EBP. Yet debate over the merit of EBP occupies space in numerous high-profile medical journals. In particular, there is contention when research evidence conflicts with clinical opinion that is based on observation and recall of patient outcomes.

> **PRACTICE PEARL**
>
> To accept the primacy of relevant high-quality research evidence requires acceptance of the flawed nature of one's own observations and recollections.

Also, engagement with EBP requires the clinician to be continually up-to-date as new scientific evidence emerges. This represents a substantial, perpetual commitment when compared to the alternative of basing decisions only on one's clinical expertise and prior academic training.

Many critics of EBP accuse its practitioners of focusing only on research results. This is an inappropriate criticism of EBP because EBP by definition integrates the best available research evidence *with* clinical expertise to guide treatment of individual patients.

> **PRACTICE PEARL**
>
> All three elements of EBP (not one alone), guide the final informed and shared decision about the treatment course.

CHALLENGES TO EBP

Four barriers facing clinicians who embrace EBP are:
- lack of access to digestible evidence
- inadequate skills to appraise and interpret published research[3, 4]
- limited patient understanding of clinical issues–health literacy
- lack of time to address the above.

A lack of access to research, inadequate computer and internet services, and the inability to locate and retrieve

> **Case: eminence-based practice**
>
> You ask a senior colleague for advice regarding Mrs J. He has seen lots of these cases and says that Mrs J. needs to get her meniscus sorted out with an arthroscopy, the sooner the better.

articles may become less problematic with time. Clinicians' self-perceived inability to locate, appraise, synthesise and integrate research into practice reflects limitations in their training. As a newcomer to the curriculum, EBP is squeezed in behind the established curriculum. Of course, it should be naturally integrated into all clinical teaching and supplemented with formal training in technical issues such as performing or interpreting meta-analysis. As with all elements of clinical practice, 'time' limits clinicians in accessing evidence, synthesising evidence to plan best practice, and in sharing all the evidence with the patient in a 10, 20 or even 30-minute consultation. We stress that 'shared decision making' means that patient scheduling must include time for the patient to truly engage, consider and discuss the options.

IMPLEMENTING EBP

Here we outline some first steps and resources[2, 5, 6] for clinicians aiming to follow EBP guidelines.

Accessing research

Continuously updated and freely available databases including the Physiotherapy Evidence Database (PEDro), PubMed and the Cochrane Library index health and medical literature. Their search interfaces are intuitive. These resources can be accessed via personal computers as well as tablet and mobile devices. Designing and carrying out searches of these databases is a particular skill in itself, but one that is easily learned using these free websites and their 'help' resources.

The PubMed database cites more than 24 million references in all areas of biomedicine and it provides free access to abstracts. Its 'clinical queries' feature can greatly assist in locating relevant articles (www.ncbi.nlm.nih.gov/pubmed/clinical).

The Physiotherapy Evidence Database (PEDro) indexes more than 30 000 clinical practice guidelines, systematic reviews and randomised controlled trials (RCTs) relevant to physiotherapy.[6] Two important features of PEDro are its specificity to physiotherapy research and study design, which means that searches are more likely to find relevant studies and the methodological quality rating of all RCTs via the PEDro scale.

The Cochrane Library houses carefully conducted systematic reviews that provide the most robust evidence related to the effectiveness of interventions and diagnostic tests. Cochrane reviews are all conducted according to rigorous standards and processes to ensure maximum reliability of results. Cochrane reviews are freely accessible from all IP addresses within the countries that pay a subscription fee, as well as in developing countries.

Retrieving articles

While databases such as PEDro and PubMed provide the article abstract, this is rarely enough to appraise the reliability and applicability of a study so it is necessary to access the full text. A recent change in scientific publishing toward the 'open-access model', comes with a trend toward increasing availability of free, full-text versions of articles. This is likely to increase in the future. Currently, research articles are freely available from large general medical journals such as the *British Medical Journal* and specialty journals published by the BioMed Central (BMC) and Public Library of Science (PLoS) groups, among others. Some other individual journals make selected content or material greater than one year old freely available. An index of freely available journals can be found at www.freemedicaljournals.com. Clinicians working in universities or large hospitals will have access to the full text articles of journals for which their institution pays a subscription fee and some professional associations pay subscription fees to relevant journals so that content is available to members.

Published appraisals

In addition to complete reports of original research studies, some journals publish short summaries, including critical appraisal of studies published elsewhere. These include the *British Journal of Sports Medicine*, *Evidence-based Medicine* and the *Journal of Physiotherapy*. The Cochrane Library also includes lay-language summaries of their systematic reviews. The advantage of these short summaries is that the quality of the study and reliability of the evidence is appraised and reported along with the findings themselves.

Interpreting research about treatment effects

The top level of evidence for questions regarding the effectiveness of an intervention comes from a systematic review of RCTs; evidence from an individual RCT occupies the level underneath (Fig. 2.2). Systematic reviews of RCTs provide the highest level of evidence[1, 2, 5] because a well-designed and conducted RCT design overcomes many of the sources of bias associated with other study types; appropriate synthesis of the findings of all available RCTs relevant to a particular question gives the most accurate estimate of the size of the treatment effect. However, the strength of the evidence depends on the number and quality of the RCTs in the systematic review.

Why prioritise RCTs over case series or observational studies when it comes to determining the effect of treatment? The key issue with observational studies is that

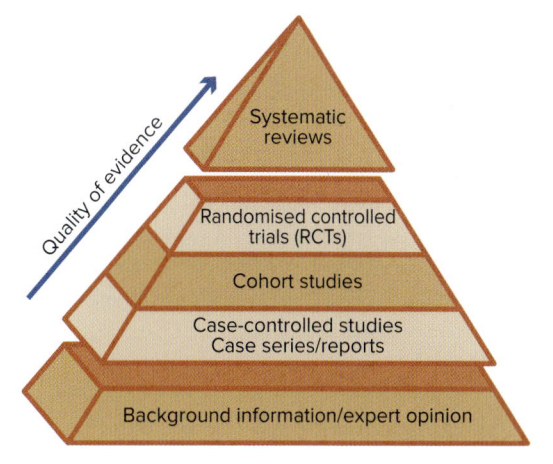

Figure 2.2 Hierarchy of evidence about the effects of treatment

we do not know what would have happened to patients if they received a different treatment or no treatment at all. It is also not enough to compare the response to treatment in one study with the response to another treatment (or no treatment) in another study, as there may be important unmeasured differences between the two samples.

Risk of bias

All research studies are not created equal; some are more likely to give a reliable answer to the question than others.[5, 6] All RCTs indexed on the PEDro database are rated for

Case: initial search

A search of the Cochrane Library using the words 'knee and arthritis' returns 33 records. One is a Cochrane systematic review titled 'Arthroscopic debridement for knee osteoarthritis' published in 2008. The authors conclude that debridement is no different to sham surgery (based on one RCT) and no different to arthroscopic lavage (two RCTs).

Case: second search

You recognise that the systematic review is a bit old and not completely specific to patients with meniscal pathology, so you look further. A search of PEDro using the keywords 'arthritis and surgery' specifying the method 'clinical trial' and the body part 'lower leg or knee' returns 10 studies. One is an RCT titled 'Surgery versus physical therapy for a meniscal tear and osteoarthritis', from 2013. The authors found that there was no difference between the meniscectomy group and the physiotherapy group in terms of pain and disability at 6 months.

methodological quality. In practice, this means that trained raters have gone through every trial and scored whether it satisfies each of a list of criteria (the PEDro scale) that are reported on the PEDro website. (www.pedro.org.au).

The Cochrane risk of bias tool has many commonalities with the PEDro scale and is used to assess the quality of trials in many Cochrane reviews. Each item of the quality scale relates to an issue that could result in biased study results; for each criterion that is not met, the risk that the study results are biased is greater. Examples of items that might bias a study result include:

1. whether the researcher deciding whether patients were included in the study knew to which group they would be assigned (concealed allocation)
2. whether the intervention and control groups were comparable at baseline
3. whether a large proportion of the patients who began in the study remained until follow-up was complete.

Research about other types of clinical questions

Not all clinical questions relate to the effectiveness of treatments. For example, there are also relevant clinical questions about predicting the likelihood of good or poor outcomes in a patient or about the accuracy of a diagnostic test. These types of questions are fundamentally different to those about the effect of treatment, so it makes sense that the study design is different.

Questions about prediction or risk require that investigators recruit a large group of people who are at the same stage of the disease process. These participants are then followed over time to see who does well and who does not (i.e. a prospective cohort study). The investigators need to measure all the factors that might be relevant in determining the patients' future outcome (e.g. body weight in people with osteoarthritis) and make sure not too many of the participants drop out over the course of the study. A prospective cohort study can be useful to help a clinician provide evidence-based advice to patients about what to expect regarding their recovery.

Questions about diagnosis should be addressed using a study that compares the results of a diagnostic test (the index test) with the results of an accepted standard for the diagnosis (the reference standard or gold standard), at the same time. For example, a study might compare Lachman's test for anterior cruciate rupture (detailed in Chapter 35) with MRI assessment (reference standard) in the same patients. The accuracy of the reference standard is key to the quality of a diagnostic study.

A second critical design feature of diagnostic studies is that the person performing the index test does not know the results of the reference standard. If the tester knows whether or not the patient has the condition it may bias their interpretation of the index test. So in the example, the person performing the Lachman's test should not know the results of the MRI assessment.

A final important feature concerns how the patients in the study sample are assembled. Ideally, all the patients in the sample should represent those that present for care, which means that diagnosis is unknown before the test is performed. The Cochrane Library now includes systematic reviews of diagnostic test studies.

Case: appraisal

Looking at the PEDro scale score for the RCT you find that six of the 10 criteria were met. This indicates moderate quality, but there is the potential for bias due to certain factors, including the lack of blinding of outcome assessors and the fact that randomisation was not concealed. Further, a significant proportion of the patients randomised to the physical therapy intervention later crossed over and received surgery.

Case: decision

Based on the evidence from the review and the RCT, you are doubtful of the benefits of surgery for Mrs J. You note, however, the moderate quality of the RCT and the issue of crossover and following discussion with Mrs J decide to trial a 2–3 month program of physical therapy prior to reviewing her condition.

REFERENCES

References for this chapter can be found at www.mhhe.com/au/CSM5e

Chapter 3

Sports injuries: acute

with STUART WARDEN

> *After feeling discomfort in my hamstring after the first round last night and then again in the semi-final tonight, I was examined by the Chief Doctor of the National Championships and diagnosed with a grade I tear.*
> Usain Bolt, posted on Twitter 6 weeks before the Rio 2016 Olympic Games

Participation in sports and athletic endeavours has well-known health and wellness benefits. Unfortunately, participation is also associated with a risk of injury. Sporting injuries can occur during either competition or training and can affect any type of musculoskeletal connective tissue (Table 3.1). Injury to these tissues may be categorised as being either acute or overuse, based on the mechanism of injury and rapidity of symptom onset. The current chapter discusses acute injuries, whereas overuse injuries are described in the subsequent chapter (Chapter 4).

An acute injury refers to an injury that occurs during a single, identifiable traumatic event. They arise when the force applied to a tissue generates stresses and/or strains that are greater than the tissue can withstand. The net result is tissue failure which generates macroscopic damage and the rapid onset of symptoms, such as pain and loss of function. The severity of the symptoms depends on the tissue injured and the extent of the damage.

Forces applied to a tissue can be derived from either extrinsic (i.e. from outside the body, such as from a direct blow or collision with an external object) or intrinsic (i.e. from inside the body, such as from muscle contractile forces, or joint and tissue biomechanics) sources. Thus, acute injuries are frequently categorised as having extrinsic or intrinsic causes. Knowing the cause of acute injury has implications with regard to injury prevention as extrinsically generated forces may be modified by altering equipment, playing surface or sport rules, while intrinsically generated forces require an individual athlete's characteristics and capabilities to be considered (such as muscle strength, endurance and flexibility, motor control, joint range, biomechanics and proprioception). However, as an acute injury always results in intrinsic changes, an individual athlete's characteristics and capabilities need to be considered in all instances of acute injury in order to facilitate return to participation and prevent re-injury.

When a force is applied to a tissue, the nature of the force being applied (such as the direction, magnitude and rate of loading) and the mechanical properties of the tissue in the direction of loading determine whether the tissue fails. The latter is determined by a combination of innate (non-modifiable) and environmental (modifiable) factors. Modifiable factors alter the safety factor between usual and injurious loads by either increasing or decreasing genetically endowed tissue strength. Modifiable factors include:

1. previous loading history and subsequent tissue adaptation
2. the presence and degree of any underlying microscopic tissue damage (overuse injury)
3. history of previous acute injury to the tissue and extent of mechanical strength recovery.

PATHOPHYSIOLOGY AND INITIAL MANAGEMENT

An acute injury initiates a common sequence of preliminary processes, irrespective of the specific tissue injured. Haematoma formation from damaged blood vessels gives way to an acute inflammatory response involving fluid exudation and phagocytosis. Fluid exudation contributes to oedema formation (i.e. swelling) and the delivery of white blood cells to the injured site, while phagocytosis aids the removal of damaged tissue and cellular debris. Swelling occurring within a joint is referred to as an 'effusion' and usually takes place slowly over the course of 12–24 hours. More rapidly occurring joint swelling (e.g. within the first 2–3 hours after injury)

PART A Fundamental principles

Table 3.1 Classification of sporting injuries

Site	Acute injuries	Overuse injuries
Bone	Fracture (including growth plate) Periosteal contusion	Stress injury (including stress reaction and stress fracture) Osteitis, periostitis Apophysitis, enthesopathy Osteophyte/bone spur
Hyaline cartilage	Chondral/osteochondral injury	Chondropathy (e.g. softening, fibrillation, fissuring, chondromalacia)
Fibrocartilage	Acute tear (including meniscal, labral, and intra-articular and intervertebral discs) Herniation of nucleus pulposus from intervertebral disc	Degenerative tear Herniation of nucleus pulposus from intervertebral disc Chondropathy (e.g. softening, fibrillation, fissuring, chondromalacia)
Joint	Dislocation Subluxation	Synovitis Osteoarthritis/osteoarthrosis Instability
Ligament	Sprain/tear (grades I–III)	Inflammation
Muscle	Strain/tear Contusion Cramp Acute compartment syndrome	Chronic compartment syndrome Delayed onset muscle soreness Focal tissue thickening/fibrosis
Tendon	Tear (partial or complete)	Tendinopathy (includes paratenonitis, tenosynovitis, tendinosis and tendinitis)
Fascia	Tear (partial or complete)	Fasciopathy (includes fasciitis and fasciosis)
Bursa	Traumatic bursitis	Bursitis/bursosis
Nerve	Neuropraxia	Entrapment Minor nerve injury/irritation Adverse neural tension
Fat pad	Bruise/contusion	Impingement/irritation
Skin	Laceration Abrasion Puncture wound	Blister Callus

indicates the effusion contains blood (i.e. haemarthrosis) and that an intra-articular structure has been damaged.

The acute inflammatory response to injury stimulates nociceptors to activate pain pathways. Pain is the body's way of protecting the injured site from further damage and leads to muscle inhibition and functional limitation. Muscle inhibition is also influenced by swelling. Reactive muscle spasm serves as an additional protective mechanism to further reduce potentially injurious loading, but also contributes to pain.

The acute inflammatory phase has the goals of protecting the damaged tissue from further injury, preparing the injured site for repair and stimulating the recruitment and activation of reparative cells. The inflammatory phase is generally thought to persist for 48–72 hours; however, the duration within a particular individual can vary, and can be influenced by the tissue damaged, the severity of the damage and early management. Signs that acute inflammation is persistent include ongoing pain at rest and/or night, prolonged (>30 minutes) morning pain and stiffness and ongoing swelling that changes in volume according to recent activity.

Early management of acute injuries has historically centred on the PRICE acronym, which stands for protection, rest, ice, compression and elevation. Ice, compression and elevation are universally accepted, despite a lack of strong evidence for their efficacy,[1] and are introduced to reduce pain, decrease blood flow and swelling and slow cellular metabolism to reduce risk of secondary injury (e.g. cell death due to hypoxia).

Similarly, there is general consensus for some degree of protection and rest immediately after injury; however, there is increasing acknowledgement that their duration should be limited due to the known detrimental effects of prolonged immobilisation and unloading of connective tissues. Instead, early loading is being increasingly advocated and shown as an important component of the early management of acute injuries. As a result, there are calls for the PRICE acronym to be changed to POLICE whereby 'rest' is replaced by 'optimal loading' (see Chapter 17).[2]

Optimal loading aims to take advantage of the responsiveness of musculoskeletal tissues to mechanical stimuli. It involves introducing progressive functional loading to stimulate connective tissue synthesis and promote healing, but without causing further damage. Optimal loading is principally guided by pain, with the induction of pain during loading indicating that tissue-level forces are too great for the current level of healing and that the load should be reduced to a pain-free level.

BONE
Fracture

There is a large safety factor between the forces bone is exposed to during athletic activities and the forces required to generate a fracture. In the absence of a bone pathology that is causing generalised or localised bone fragility, large forces are required to fracture a bone. Such forces can result from direct trauma such as a blow or indirect trauma such as an awkward fall or twisting motion.

Traumatic fractures can be dichotomised as either closed (simple) or open (compound). The skin is intact over the fracture site in closed fractures, whereas in open fractures skin integrity is lost, often due to penetration from within by the fractured bone. The presence of a skin wound in open fractures that is continuous with the fracture site enables pathogens to enter and contribute to bone infection. Thus, individuals with an open fracture should be treated with prophylactic antibiotic therapy.

Within the dichotomy of open and closed fractures, fractures can be further classified according to their fracture pattern (Fig. 3.1), location in terms of both the affected bone and the location within that bone, amount and type of displacement of the fractured ends of the bone, and/or the specific name of the fracture. For instance, a Colles' fracture refers to a fracture of the distal radius with dorsal (posterior) and radial displacement of the distal fracture segment, whereas a Smith's fracture also refers to a fracture of the distal radius, but with ventral (anterior) displacement of the distal segment.

The immature skeleton presents some unique fractures because of its lower mineralisation and presence of unfused

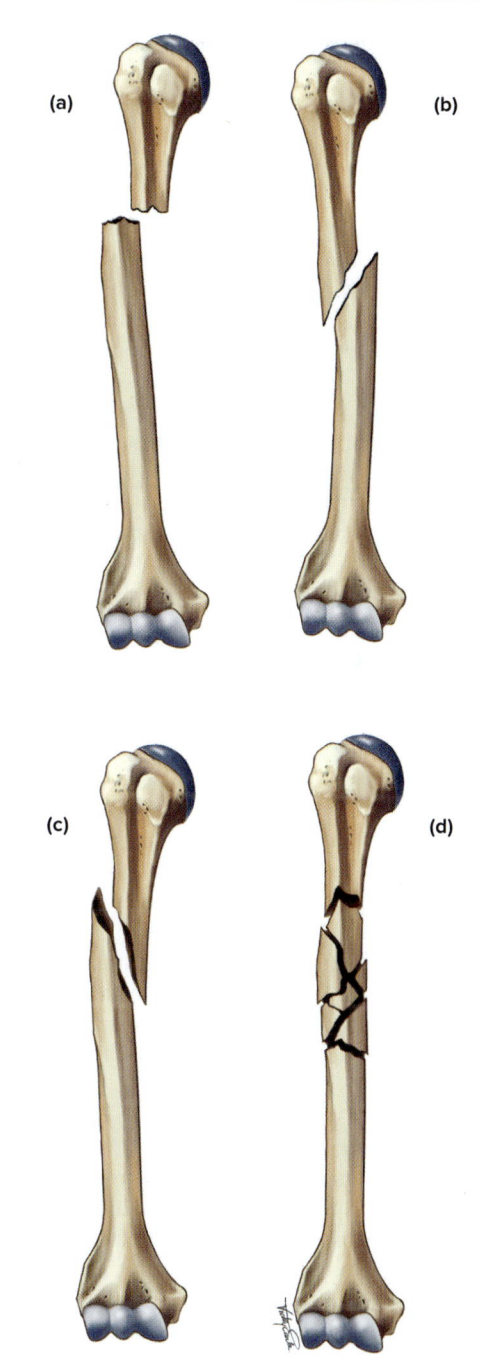

Figure 3.1 Types of fracture (a) Transverse (b) Oblique (c) Spiral (d) Comminuted

secondary ossification centres with interposed growth plates. The lower mineralisation of the immature skeleton makes it more flexible than the adult skeleton and, consequently, susceptible to buckling. When a sufficient bending force is applied to an immature bone the cortex on the side that the bone is bending toward is exposed to compressive forces and buckles, while the cortex on the opposite side cracks open due to tensile forces. The resultant greenstick fracture is named according to how a green (i.e. fresh) stick buckles and cracks when bent. When the injurious force causes axial compressive loading of an immature bone as opposed to bending, the result can be the development of a torus or buckle fracture characterised by buckling and bulging of the cortex on all sides.

Growth plate fractures in children and adolescents present a particular problem and are discussed in detail in Chapter 43. The most common growth plate fracture is an avulsion fracture. Unfused secondary ossification centres represent an area of relative weakness in the young skeleton. They serve to develop bony prominences, such as tubercles and epicondyles, upon which tendons and ligaments attach. With an appropriate tensile pull from a tendon or ligament, a secondary ossification centre can be pulled away from the rest of the bone at its growth plate resulting in the development of an avulsion fracture. Avulsion fractures can also occur in the adult skeleton when extreme tensile forces at the insertion site of a tendon or ligament pull off a portion of bone.

The primary aim of fracture management is to allow the fracture to heal in the most anatomical position possible so that the mechanical function of the bone can be restored. If the fracture is displaced, it should be reduced to realign the bone fragments back to their anatomical position. A fracture that heals in an abnormal position (i.e. mal-united fracture) can lead to the long-term development of secondary complications, such as osteoarthritis.

Reduction is typically extremely painful and resisted by muscle spasm. Thus, it is usually performed under a short-acting anaesthetic, sedative or nerve block and with muscle relaxants. Once the fragments are reduced, the fracture needs to be held in place to permit fracture gap bridging. The method of stabilisation depends on the stability of the fracture. Stable fractures may be managed with a simple sling, cast or fracture brace, whereas more rigid stabilisation is required for unstable fractures that do not readily maintain their reduced position. Rigid stabilisation may consist of open reduction and internal fixation (ORIF) wherein the fracture site is opened surgically, reduced and fixed using metal plates, rods, screws, pins, and/or wires. ORIF has the advantage of allowing earlier introduction of forces across the fracture site. However, the trade-offs include:

- potential hardware loosening, failure and irritation
- opening the fracture site to the possibility for infection
- excessive stabilisation of the fracture leading to insufficient fragment micromotion and atrophic non-union
- peri-implant fracture resulting from regional osteoporosis due to stress shielding.

In addition to reducing a fracture and providing an environment that is permissive of bone regeneration, it is necessary to assess and monitor for other possible complications of fracture. Infection and mal-union have already been mentioned. Other acute complications that need consideration include acute compartment syndrome (discussed later), associated injuries (e.g. nerve, vessel), deep venous thrombosis/pulmonary embolism, and delayed or non-union.

Soft tissue injury, such as ligament or muscle damage, is often associated with a fracture and may cause more long-term problems than the fracture itself. Thus, it is important to address any concomitant soft tissue injury. Occasionally, deep venous thrombosis and pulmonary embolism may occur after a fracture, especially a lower limb fracture. This should be prevented by early movement and active muscle contraction.

Delayed or non-union of a fracture causes persistent pain and disability, and can be caused by excessive or insufficient fracture site stabilisation, presence of a complicated fracture type (e.g. open or highly comminuted fractures), insufficient or disrupted blood supply (e.g. due to abnormal regional anatomy or the presence of comorbid conditions such as diabetes) and lifestyle factors (e.g. smoking, excessive alcohol intake and poor nutrition), to name a few. Management options for delayed or non-united fractures include non-surgical treatments, such as low-intensity pulsed ultrasound and electromagnetic therapies (Chapter 16), as well as surgical treatments, such as bone graft or bone graft substitute, internal fixation and/or external fixation. In the future, biological compounds and small molecule pharmaceuticals may become available. Specific fractures that are common in athletes are discussed in Part B chapters.

Periosteal contusion

The periosteum is a dense, fibrous tissue that is firmly attached to the outer surface of bones and is both highly vascular and innervated. At subcutaneous skeletal sites (such as the medial surface of the tibia and iliac crest), the periosteum is susceptible to acute trauma from a direct blow with an external object, such as a ball, stick, opponent or playing surface. The blow damages periosteal blood vessels resulting in the development of a subperiosteal haematoma, otherwise known as a periosteal contusion. The confined space beneath the periosteum limits the spread of the haematoma, occasionally leading to the development of a palpable lump. The raised periosteum is tensed and inflamed/irritated, stimulating its plentiful nociceptive nerve endings to cause considerable pain, especially upon palpation and on contraction of muscles attaching to the injured region.

A periosteal contusion at the iliac crest, often referred to as a 'hip pointer' injury, can be extremely painful because of involvement of the cluneal nerve which runs along the iliac crest. Management of periosteal contusions focuses initially on minimising the extent of the haematoma using conventional first aid approaches followed by a gradual return to activity. Protective equipment (such as shin guards and padding) should be considered for future prevention.

HYALINE CARTILAGE
Chondral and osteochondral injuries

Hyaline, or articular, cartilage lines the articular surface of bone regions forming synovial joints. It provides a smooth, lubricated surface allowing for low-friction gliding and possesses unique viscoelastic properties which facilitate the absorption and distribution of loads to the underlying subchondral bone. In fulfilling these roles, hyaline cartilage is principally exposed to compressive loads. Acute joint subluxation or dislocation (discussed below) and acute ligament sprain or rupture (discussed later) can lead to locally high compressive forces and the superimposition of shearing forces due to excessive joint translation. The net result can be development of an acute chondral (cartilage), as shown in Figure 3.2a and b, or osteochondral injury, with the latter involving both the articular cartilage and underlying (subchondral) bone (Fig. 3.2c).

Articular cartilage is radiolucent and therefore most chondral injuries are not visible on conventional radiology. As a result, these injuries have historically been underdiagnosed. With the advent of magnetic resonance imaging and direct visualisation via arthroscopy, it has become clear that chondral injuries are far more common than previously realised. Clinicians must maintain a high index of suspicion for chondral involvement if an apparently 'simple joint sprain' remains painful and swollen for longer than expected, despite the presence of normal X-rays. Common sites for chondral and osteochondral injuries are the femoral condyles, superior articular surface of the talus, capitellum of the humerus and patella.

Chondral injuries are a concern due to their poor healing and their contribution to the development of premature osteoarthritis. Articular cartilage has limited regenerative and repair capacity due to its avascular nature. As larger lesions or defects have lower probability of healing, classification systems have been developed to quantify the severity of chondral damage and guide prognosis. Chondral lesion severity is determined by the depth the injury extends towards the underlying bone and the size of cartilage affected, whereas osteochondral lesion severity is determined by the continuity of the overlying cartilage

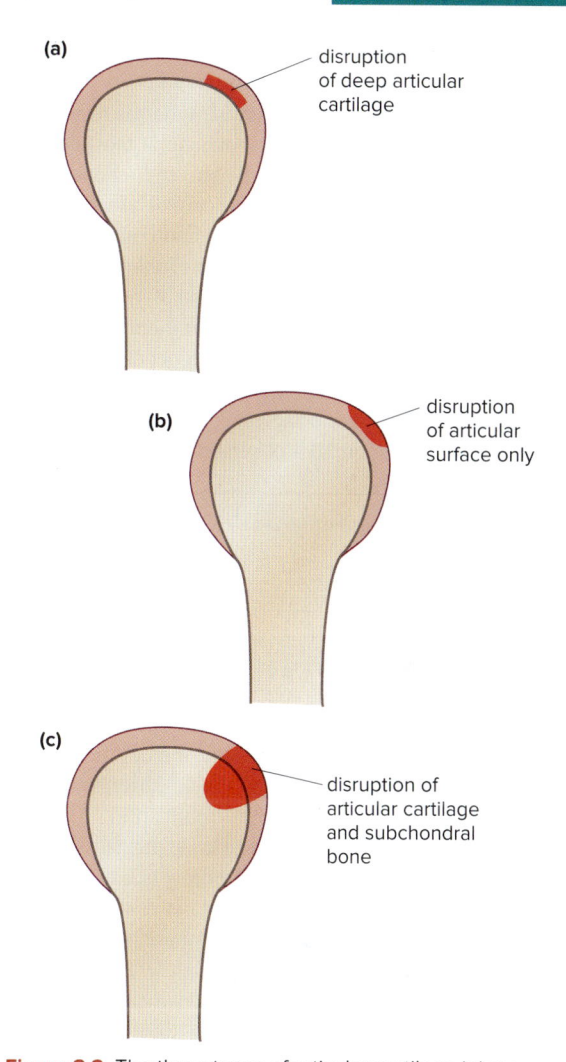

Figure 3.2 The three types of articular cartilage injury

and stability of the lesion. Scales generally extend from 0 (normal) to a high score of 4 (exposed bone for chondral injuries; fragment displacement for osteochondral lesions), with higher scores indicating greater damage and a worse prognosis.

Chondral and osteochondral injuries in young active individuals represent a therapeutic challenge. The goal of treatment is to restore the structural integrity and function of the affected surface so that it can withstand the significant stresses associated with athletic endeavours. The hope is to permit a return to participation while minimising cartilage degeneration and the need for early arthroplasty (joint replacement). Treatment options for chondral injuries range from palliative techniques (such as chondroplasty to smooth loose edges of damaged cartilage and arthroscopic washout to remove debris) to techniques aimed at stimulating cartilage repair or restoration. Reparative techniques include bone marrow stimulation techniques such as abrasion arthroplasty, drilling and microfracture, whereas restorative approaches include autologous osteochondral mosaicplasty, osteochondral allograft transplantation, and chondrocyte and mesenchymal stem cell-based therapies wherein cells are implanted into the cartilage lesion and covered with a periosteal or collagen-membrane cover. Treatment choice depends upon the size of the chondral or osteochondral lesion, with great debate continuing as to the most effective approach. Ultimately, return to sport depends on a range of factors, including athlete age, duration of symptoms, level of play, repair tissue morphology, lesion size, type and location, and the number of surgeries and concomitant procedures.[3]

FIBROCARTILAGE
Acute tear

Fibrocartilage consists of a mixture of fibrous and cartilaginous tissue in varying proportions, which provide it with both toughness and elasticity. Fibrocartilage forms a range of structures in different joints with varying functions, but roles generally include enhancing joint stability, contributing to shock absorption and distribution and promoting joint lubrication. Example fibrocartilage structures include the knee menisci, glenoid and acetabular labrums, triangular fibrocartilage complex (TFCC) at the radio-carpal joint, volar plates of the digits, and articular discs within the acromioclavicular and sternoclavicular joints.

Given the predominantly mechanical roles of fibrocartilage structures in enhancing joint congruency and distributing stresses, it is not surprising that they are at risk of acute injury when excessive forces are introduced. For instance, the knee menisci are at risk when rotation is superimposed onto a flexed and loaded knee, whereas a fall onto an outstretched hand can acutely injure the TFCC at the radio-carpal joint. Joint fibrocartilage structures can be injured in isolation; however, simultaneous injury with associated joint structures (e.g. ligaments and joint capsule) is common due to their close anatomical and mechanical relationships. For instance, it is common for a knee meniscus and the anterior cruciate ligament to be simultaneously injured as they share a common mechanism of injury (i.e. rotating on a flexed and loaded knee). Similarly, during shoulder dislocation it is common for the anterior glenoid labrum to be simultaneously injured with the glenohumeral ligaments and joint capsule due to their anatomical connections and forces being introduced.

Signs and symptoms of acute fibrocartilage injury are region- and injury-specific, but generally include pain and swelling in the affected joint combined with joint clicking, catching or locking. The latter joint events are often delayed in their presentation, occurring once the initial acute symptoms have subsided and normal use of the joint has recommenced. Joint clicking, catching or locking can contribute to reflex muscle inhibition and the sensation of the joint 'giving way' during load bearing.

Management of acute fibrocartilage injuries depends on the type, size and location of damage. Management options are dichotomised into conservative and surgical, with surgical options including repair, removal and replacement of the damaged fibrocartilaginous structure. Surgery is an option for individuals who have failed to respond to conservative management, but is also frequently used as a first-line management approach, particularly for injuries in regions that have limited healing potential. The latter regions include the relatively avascular zones within the inner two-thirds of the menisci and the central region of the TFCC.

Herniation of nucleus pulposus from intervertebral disc

Herniation of the nucleus pulposus in athletes most commonly occurs secondary to damage accumulation within the disc in response to repetitive flexion and/or rotational loading. Thus, the vast majority of disc herniations are overuse injuries, despite the onset of symptoms often occurring relatively spontaneously and in response to an apparently trivial loading event. However, it is possible to acutely prolapse or herniate an otherwise healthy intervertebral disc with sufficient compressive and flexion force. This can occur during contact sports when the spine is axially loaded while in a flexed position, such as when driven into the ground when being tackled. The disc may protrude or herniate radially beyond the usual margins of the annulus fibrosis or herniate through the vertebral body endplate into the vertebral body to form a Schmorl's node.

JOINT
Dislocation/subluxation

Joint stability depends on the interaction between the passive, active and neural subsystems. Muscles and tendons combine to form the active subsystem, which is controlled by the neural subsystem, to provide dynamic joint stability. When the force applied to a joint exceeds the capabilities of the active subsystem or when the active and/or neural subsystems are compromised, loads are transferred to the passive subsystem. The passive subsystem consists of non-contractile connective tissues, which includes the bony anatomy, joint capsule, ligaments and fibrocartilage joint structures (e.g. labrum, volar plates, menisci).

Excessive load placed on the passive subsystem can cause the bones forming a joint to abnormally translate or luxate relative to one another. When the bones are forced to completely separate so that the articulating surfaces are no longer in contact it is referred to as dislocation (Fig. 3.3a). Subluxation (partial dislocation) refers to when the bones shift relative to one another, but the articulating surfaces remain partially in contact (Fig. 3.3b).

Luxation of a joint invariably results in damage to passive subsystem structures. The structures damaged and extent of damage depends on the direction and magnitude of the luxation force and the inherent stability of the joint created by the passive subsystem. The hip joint is inherently stable because the large ball shape of the femoral head is well encased in a reciprocating socket-shaped acetabulum and the bones are supported by a strong joint capsule that is reinforced by robust ligaments. Thus, considerably more force is required to luxate the hip joint compared to a less stable joint, such as the shoulder.

The shoulder lacks inherent stability because the large humeral head outsizes the small, shallow glenoid fossa and the joint possesses a thin, loose capsule that is minimally supported by ligaments. The heightened force required to luxate inherently stable joints (such as the hip, elbow, ankle and subtalar joints) means that subluxation or dislocation of these joints is more likely to be associated with damage beyond that to the joint capsule and ligaments, including fractures and damage to cartilage, vessels and nerves.

A dislocated joint is readily identifiable by gross deformity with complete loss of joint function. The individual presents with significant, acute pain and often has the afflicted limb cradled or held. Following a neurovascular screen to assess for nerve and blood vessel damage, the dislocated joint should be reduced as quickly as possible. In most cases, this can be performed by applying gradual and controlled distraction of the joint while simultaneously moving the joint through a passive range of motion. When distraction is unable to overcome the opposing muscle spasm and the joint does not readily reduce, use of an injected muscle relaxant or general anaesthetic may be required.

After reduction, all dislocated joints should be X-rayed for the presence of an accompanying fracture and the joint should be protected to allow the joint capsule and ligaments time to heal. However, early protected mobilisation is encouraged to promote functional healing, and training of the active and neural subsystems should commence as early as possible and progress to functional activities so that these subsystems may compensate for the reduced stability afforded by the damage to the passive subsystem. Unfortunately, in some joints (such as the shoulder), active and neural subsystem training is often insufficient to prevent re-dislocation or chronic subluxation, necessitating eventual surgical reconstruction of the damaged capsule and ligaments.

LIGAMENT
Sprain/tear

Ligaments typically span joints to connect articulating bones, and present as either discrete extra-articular structures or thickenings of the joint capsule. Their structure consisting of tightly packed bundles of collagen arranged nearly in parallel along the longitudinal axis of the ligament is designed to resist tensile loads. Ligaments function to provide passive stability and guide what directions of motion are available at a joint. When force is applied to a joint that attempts to move the bones in a direction they are not designed to move, passive tension rises in ligaments on the side of the joint being gapped open. When the load is sufficient, and dynamic joint stabilisation afforded by the active and neural subsystems is insufficient, collagen fibres within ligaments begin to yield resulting in an acute ligament injury (commonly referred to as a 'sprain').

Ligament sprains range in severity from mild injuries involving tearing of only a few fibres to complete tears of the ligament where ligament continuity and its stabilising role is completely lost. Based on the number of fibres torn and the subsequent degree of joint instability, ligament sprains are classified into three grades (Fig. 3.4), each representing an increase in injury severity (Table 3.2).

Management of acute ligament sprains is summarised in Figure 3.5. Initial management consists of first aid techniques to minimise bleeding and swelling (Chapter 17). For grade I and II sprains, subsequent treatment aims to promote tissue healing, prevent joint stiffness, protect against further damage and strengthen muscle to provide dynamic joint stability. Return to sport usually takes place before tissue level healing is complete, with healing of collagen in a partial

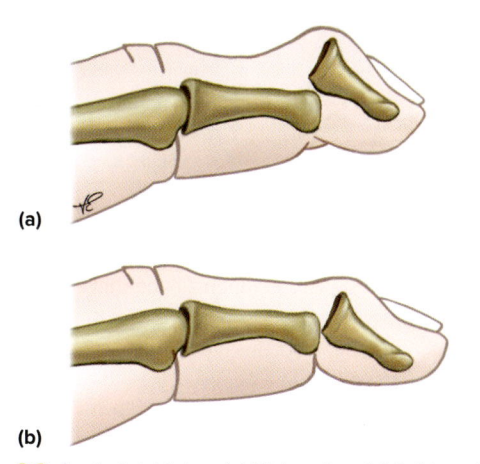

Figure 3.3 Acute joint injury (a) Dislocation (b) Subluxation

PART A   Fundamental principles

Table 3.2 Classification of ligament injuries

Grade	Pathology	Clinical findings
I	Disruption of some collagen fibres	• Localised tenderness on palpation • Minimal inflammation (swelling) • Normal range and end feel on ligament stress test, but test may be painful • Little functional deficit
II	Disruption of considerable proportion of collagen fibres	• Significant tenderness on palpation • Can be considerable inflammation (swelling) involving the whole joint (effusion) • Increased joint play on ligament stress test (increased ligament laxity), but a definite end point is present • Moderate functional deficit
III	Complete disruption of all collagen fibres	• Audible 'pop' may have been heard at the time of injury • Often immediately painful, but may become pain-free a short time after the injurious event due to simultaneous disruption of nociceptors (pain returns thereafter due to effusion and inflammatory mediators activating alternative nociceptors) • Can be considerable swelling which may occur rapidly due to bleeding into the joint (haemarthrosis) • Significantly increased joint play on ligament stress test with no discernible end point • Significant functional deficit

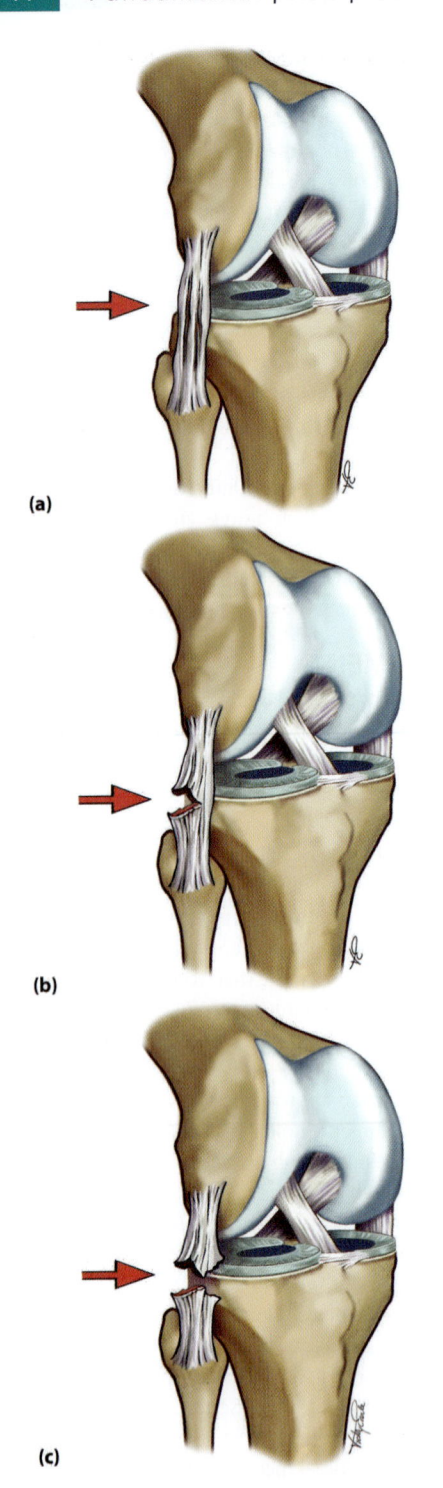

Figure 3.4 Ligament sprains (a) Grade I (b) Grade II (c) Grade III

ligament tear taking several months.[4, 5] Earlier return to sport is facilitated by the use of bracing or taping to help protect against re-injury. Rehabilitation (especially neuromuscular training) should continue in some form following return to sport as injury risk is heightened, and individuals often have ongoing objective mechanical laxity and subjective instability. For instance, as much as one-third of individuals report ongoing pain and subjective instability one year following acute ankle sprain, while up to a third report at least one re-sprain within a period of 3 years.[6]

The treatment of a grade III sprain may be either conservative or surgical. For example, the torn medial collateral ligament of the knee and the torn lateral

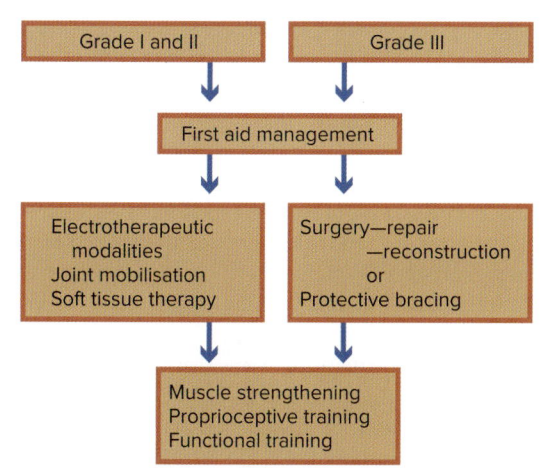

```
         Grade I and II              Grade III
               │                        │
               ▼                        ▼
              ┌─────────────────────────┐
              │   First aid management  │
              └─────────────────────────┘
               │                        │
               ▼                        ▼
    ┌──────────────────┐    ┌──────────────────────┐
    │ Electrotherapeutic│    │ Surgery—repair       │
    │    modalities    │    │   —reconstruction    │
    │ Joint mobilisation│    │         or           │
    │ Soft tissue therapy│   │  Protective bracing  │
    └──────────────────┘    └──────────────────────┘
               │                        │
               ▼                        ▼
              ┌─────────────────────────┐
              │ Muscle strengthening    │
              │ Proprioceptive training │
              │ Functional training     │
              └─────────────────────────┘
```

Figure 3.5 Management of acute ligament sprains

ligament of the ankle may be treated conservatively with full or partial immobilisation. Alternatively, the two ends of a torn ligament can be reattached surgically and the joint then fully or partially immobilised for approximately 6 weeks. In certain instances (e.g. anterior cruciate ligament rupture), torn ligament tissue is not amenable to primary repair and surgical ligament reconstruction may be required (Chapter 35).

During the past few decades, there have been mounting efforts to develop tissue engineering strategies that encourage ligament regeneration (as opposed to repair) so that the final product matches that of native ligament. Strategies have included the use of growth factors, cell-based therapies, gene transfer and therapy, and the use of scaffolding materials of varying origin.[7] While these approaches have shown promise in preclinical studies, translation to clinical populations remains lacking and is required before clinical utility.

MUSCLE

Muscle injuries are among the most common injuries in sports, accounting for up to half of all sport-related injuries at the elite level. They result from either intrinsic or extrinsic causes, with the former contributing to muscle strains/tears and the later resulting in contusions.

Strain/tear

A muscle is strained or torn when excessive tensile and/or shear forces within the muscle cause muscle fibres and their surrounding connective tissue to fail. Muscles consist of a hierarchy of active contractile elements and passive non-contractile connective tissue. The actin and myosin machinery responsible for producing active contractile forces form myofibrils which are housed in elongated, rod-shaped cells called muscle fibres. The cell membrane of the muscle fibre (i.e. sarcolemma) attaches to a basal membrane surrounded by a connective tissue sheath called the endomysium. Groups of muscle fibres bundle together to form fascicles encased in a connective tissue sheath called the perimysium. The fascicles in turn combine to form the muscle which is surrounded by a final dense sheath of connective tissue called the epimysium.

During muscle contraction, actin and myosin form cross-bridges to generate force, which is transmitted either via the surrounding connective tissue or directly to an attached tendon and subsequently the skeleton, to produce motion. In muscle strains, excessive tensile force results in muscle fibre failure, which ruptures its cell membrane and the basal membrane to which the membrane attaches, damages the surrounding connective tissue sheaths and tears blood vessels contained within the connective tissue sheaths. Depending on the severity of the injury, the net result can be pain on active contraction and passive stretch of the muscle, a reduction in strength due to pain-inhibition, decreased range of motion due to muscle spasm and loss of function.

Muscle strains most commonly occur within the hamstring, quadriceps and gastrocnemius muscles, as these muscles are exposed to the highest amounts of total tension. Total tension is the sum of active tension generated by muscle fibre contractile forces and passive tension due to stretch on the connective tissue components. Active tension can be high in the hamstring, quadriceps and gastrocnemius muscles as these muscles often contract eccentrically and they contain a high proportion of type-II (fast-twitch) muscle fibres–both factors associated with the generation of greater active tension. Passive tension is also often high in these muscles as they are biarthrodial (cross two joints) and are often required to contract while on passive stretch over more than one joint.

To guide prognosis, muscle strains have historically been graded using a three-tiered system, with increasing grade suggesting a greater severity of injury requiring longer recovery.[8] A minor strain causing localised pain but no or minimal loss of strength is referred to as a grade I injury and suggests the involvement of a small number of muscle fibres. A grade II strain involves a greater number of muscle fibres and is clinically evident by greater pain, swelling and loss of strength, while a complete tear of the muscle is classified as a grade III injury. In addition to these three grades, a grade 0 injury has been described wherein an athlete presents with a clinical syndrome of muscle abnormality, but without imaging evidence of pathology.

Grading systems provide an indication of the severity or extent of muscle damage; however, the variable recovery time for individuals with similarly graded injuries suggest that other factors influence prognosis. With advances in magnetic resonance imaging and ultrasonography, it is now possible to also classify or categorise injuries in terms of their anatomical location and the type/s of tissue involved. The role of imaging in predicting recovery time from muscle strains remains unclear.[9] However, there is increasing recognition of the benefits of combining clinical and radiological findings, which has resulted in the generation of a number of 'new' muscle injury grading and classification systems (Table 3.3 and Fig. 3.6).[8, 10-12] These systems have yet to be convincingly validated,[13] but may represent a new era in understanding and establishing prognosis for muscle strains.

Common to the new muscle strain grading systems is the recognition that strains involving tendinous components of the muscle have a worse prognosis. Muscle strains most commonly occur at or near the musculotendinous junction, which appears as an area of relative weakness in skeletally mature individuals. The traditional view of the muscle-tendon unit involved a relatively distinct separation between the muscle belly and the free tendon at the end via which active contractile forces are transmitted to the bone. However, advanced imaging and anatomical dissection studies have clearly shown that tendinous structures extend deeply into the muscle belly and that some muscles also have isolated central tendinous structures within the muscle belly itself.

It is well established that muscle strains involving concomitant damage to the free tendon (e.g. proximal hamstring tendon) require a longer recovery time than strains isolated to the musculoskeletal junction. However, the presence of and damage to intramuscular and central tendons may explain why some individuals with historically labelled 'muscle belly strains' have a slower than expected recovery. The presence of intramuscular and central tendinous structures means that musculotendinous junctions occur throughout a greater length of a muscle and that 'muscle belly strains' still represent an injury occurring at one or more of these junctions. As tendinous structures have a slower healing rate than muscle tissue, a muscle strain that also involves damage to intramuscular or central tendinous structures has the potential to delay healing and return to play.[13] Indeed, a recent cohort study reported that strains of the biceps femoris muscle with and without central tendon disruption required contrasting median recovery times of 72 and 21 days, respectively.[14]

Table 3.3 Comparison of classification systems for acute muscle injuries

O'Donoghue, 1962[8]	Chan et al., 2012[10]	Müller-Wohlfahrt et al., 2013[11]	Pollock et al., 2014[12]

1. Mild
No appreciable tissue tearing, no loss of function or strength, only a low-grade inflammatory response
2. Moderate
Tissue damage, strength of the musculotendinous unit reduced, some residual function
3. Severe
Complete tear of musculotendinous unit, complete loss of function
	1. Proximal musculotendinous junction
	2. Muscle
	  A. Proximal
	  B. Middle
	  C. Distal
	    a. Intramuscular
	    b. Myofascial
	    c. Myofascial/perifascial
	    d. Myotendinous
	    e. Combined
	3. Distal musculotendinous junction
		A. Indirect muscle disorder/injury
		Functional muscle disorder
		Type 1: Overexertion-related muscle disorder
		  1A: Fatigue-induced muscle disorder
		  1B: Delayed onset muscle soreness (DOMS)
		Type 2: Neuromuscular muscle disorder
		  2A: Spine-related neuromuscular
		  2B: Muscle-related neuromuscular
		Structural muscle injury
		Type 3: Partial muscle tear
		  3A: Minor partial muscle tear
		  3B: Moderate partial muscle tear
		Type 4: (Sub)total tear
		  Subtotal or complete muscle tear
		  Tendinous avulsion
		B. Direct muscle injury
		  Contusion
		  Laceration
			0a. Focal neuromuscular injury with normal MRI
			0b. Generalised muscle soreness (DOMS) with normal MRI
			1. Small injuries (tears)
			2. Moderate injuries (tears)
			3. Extensive tears
			4. Complete tears
			  a. Myofascial injury
			  b. Within muscle usually at musculotendinous junction
			  c. Extends into tendon

Sports injuries: acute   CHAPTER 3

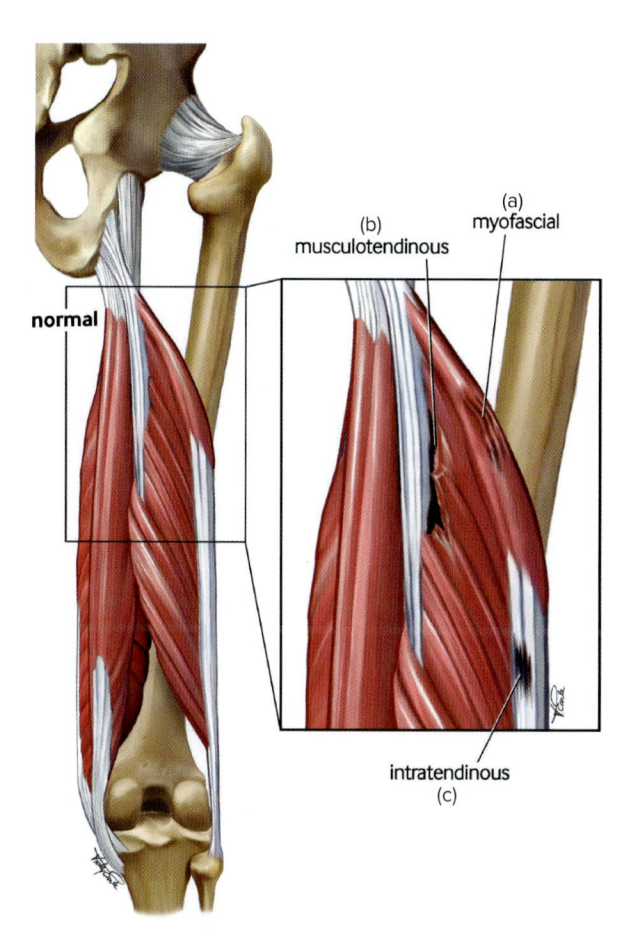

Figure 3.6 Letter classification based on the anatomical site of muscle injury within the British Athletics Classification system described by Pollock et al.[12] (a) Myofascial (b) Musculotendinous (c) Intratendinous

Subsequent management allows for increased exercise intensity, neuromuscular training at faster speeds and larger amplitudes and the initiation of eccentric resistance training. The final stage of recovery progresses to high-speed neuromuscular training and eccentric resistance training in a lengthened position in preparation for return to sport.[16]

Contusion

Muscle contusion is the medical term for a muscle bruise, and refers to bleeding and subsequent haematoma formation within a muscle and its surrounding connective tissue sheaths. Contusions occur when a muscle is compressed against the underlying bone by a blunt, external force. The force can result from a direct blow or collision with an external object, such as an opposing player, teammate or piece of equipment. Thus, they are common in contact sports and sports involving the use of rapidly moving hard objects (e.g. sticks and balls).

The most common site for muscle contusion is the quadriceps, with contusions at this site being referred to as a 'corked thigh', 'charley horse' or 'dead leg'. Other common sites for contusion include the gastrocnemius and gluteal muscles; however, a contusion can occur in any muscle exposed to a blunt compressive force.

Muscle compression causes muscle fibre damage and rupture of microvessels. The released blood clots to form a haematoma that initiates an acute inflammatory reaction aimed at removing the haematoma and damaged tissue and initiating a repair response. The haematoma may form either within (i.e. intramuscular) or between (i.e. intermuscular) the fascial coverings of the muscle. Intramuscular contusions are more self-limiting as the rise in pressure within the confines of the fascial compartment reduces blood flow, but they are also generally more painful and more restrictive because muscle contraction results in further rises in compartment pressure and stimulation of nociceptors.

In contrast, intermuscular contusions are generally less painful as the fascial sheath is damaged which allows the haematoma to spread to relieve compartment pressure. Intermuscular haematomas are generally more evident externally as the blood is able to travel distally due to gravity and into the subcutaneous tissues resulting in a visible bruise.

Initial management of a muscle contusion involves assessing for presence of an acute compartment syndrome (discussed below), controlling bleeding to reduce secondary injury (i.e. muscle fibre hypoxia) and protecting the injured site from further injury. Techniques include compression and ice with the muscle placed in a pain-free stretched position to help stop the bleeding and reduce muscle spasm. Techniques such as heat, alcohol and

The goal of management of an acute muscle strain is to return the athlete to activity at the prior level of performance and with minimal risk for re-injury. This requires the underlying pathology and the changes it introduces (i.e. pain, swelling, weakness, reduced range of motion), be addressed. It also requires causative risk factors be addressed, with a previous muscle injury being the single largest risk factor for a future strain.

Acute management of muscle strains focuses on minimisation of pain and oedema, restoration of neuromuscular control at slow speeds and prevention of excessive scar formation while protecting the healing fibres from excessive lengthening. Recommended early techniques include: 1) ice and compression; 2) mobilisation and motion, within pain limits and while avoiding aggressive stretching techniques; and 3) gentle massage of the affected muscle peripheral to the lesion.[15]

vigorous massage, which have the potential to increase blood flow and/or cause a rebleed, should be avoided in the acute and subacute stages. Subsequent management focuses on restoring muscle function via progressive stretching and strengthening. The use of protective equipment in the form of force dissipating and dispersing padding should be considered to prevent re-injury upon return to activity. However, the reduction in injury risk gained by using protective equipment will need to be weighed against any associated reduction in athlete mobility and performance.

Myositis ossificans

Myositis ossificans is a form of heterotrophic ossification and refers to the formation of bone within a muscle. It is an infrequent complication of a contusion injury wherein bone-forming osteoblasts invade the haematoma and begin to lay down bone. The cause remains unknown; however, risk factors include severe contusions that limit joint range of motion (e.g. thigh contusions that limit knee flexion to <45°), repeat contusion injury and inappropriate initial management that causes a rebleed.

Myositis ossificans should be suspected in muscle contusions that do not resolve in the expected time. Particular signs and symptoms include initial improvements in range and pain followed by subsequent deterioration and ongoing or reappearance of inflammatory symptoms (i.e. resting, morning and night pain). The bone grows from 2–4 weeks after injury at which time an area of calcification may be visible on X-ray (Fig. 3.7a) or ultrasound (Fig. 3.7b) and a firm lump may be felt. Once active bone formation ceases the area of calcification gets slowly reabsorbed. As myositis ossificans is self-limiting, management is typically conservative and consists of anti-inflammatory approaches and non-painful stretching and strengthening.

Acute compartment syndrome

Muscles in the extremities are surrounded by a strong, thick connective tissue called fascia. The fascia serves as an attachment site for muscle, aids in force transmission and forms non-distensible compartments that facilitate muscle-pump mediated venous return. Injury leading to swelling or bleeding into one of the fascial compartments (usually the flexor compartment of the forearm or anterior compartment of the lower leg) can result in the development of acute compartment syndrome.

Acute compartment syndrome occurs when interstitial pressure within a compartment exceeds perfusion pressure leading to the onset of ischaemia and, ultimately, cellular anoxia and death. It is characterised by pain that is out of proportion to the inciting injury, pain on passive stretch and at rest, paraesthesia and pulselessness (although the

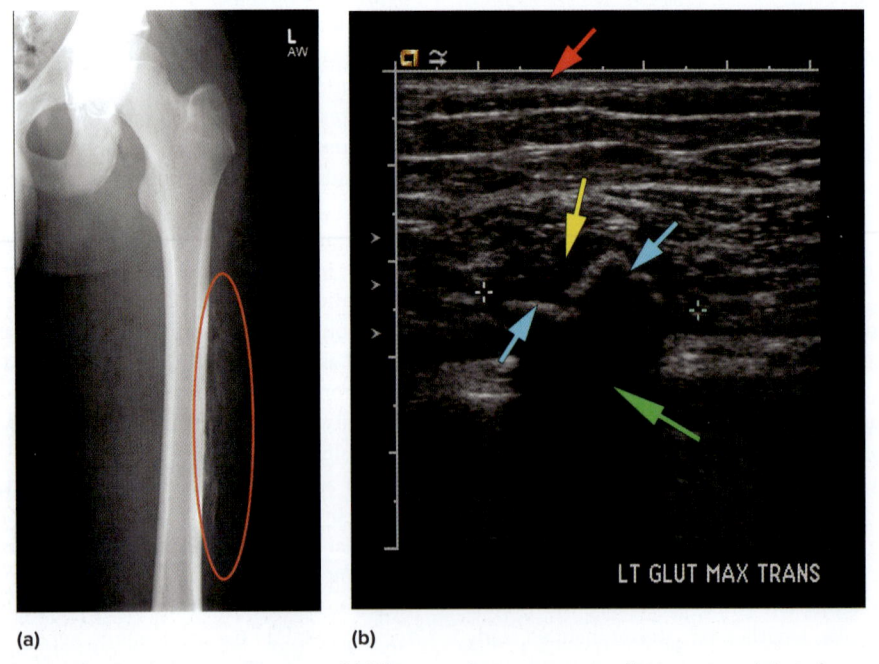

Figure 3.7 Myositis ossificans (a) X-ray appearance (b) Ultrasound appearance: yellow arrow points to haematoma within gluteal muscle; blue arrows to calcification within gluteal muscle; green arrow to acoustic shadowing, characteristic of calcification. Red arrow is skin and then subcutaneous fat, and below it are layers of gluteal muscles

latter is a late finding as the interstitial pressure needs to be high enough to occlude arterial flow). Acute compartment syndrome represents a medical emergency that may require urgent fasciotomy (i.e. release of the fascia surrounding the muscle compartment) in order to prevent permanent, irreversible damage.[17] Hence, referral to an orthopaedic emergency specialist is recommended.

Cramp

Muscle cramps are sudden, painful, involuntary contractions characterised by repetitive firing of motor unit action potentials. When they occur during or immediately after exercise in healthy individuals with no underlying metabolic, neurological or endocrine pathology, they are referred to as 'exercise associated muscle cramps' (EAMC).[18] EAMC are usually temporary (lasting <60 seconds), but are often incapacitating and tend to recur if activity at the same exercise intensity level is continued without an adequate recovery period. Thus, EAMC can significantly impair athletic performance. The most common sites for EAMC are in the calf and foot muscles, followed by the hamstring and quadriceps muscles.

EAMC were historically thought to be due to dehydration and/or electrolyte depletion, but this hypothesis has not been supported by scientific evidence. As EAMC most commonly occur towards the end of or after fatiguing exercise, or following a rapid increase in exercise intensity, fatigue appears to be a significant contributing factor. The current leading theory is that EAMC result from abnormal neuromuscular control at the spinal level in response to fatiguing exercise.[18] This theory ascribes EAMC to increased excitatory and decreased inhibitory afferent inputs to motor neurons during fatigue. The net result is sustained motor neuron activity and the production of a cramp-inducing discharge.

Immediate treatment of EAMC aims to reduce motor neuron activity, with the most popular and effective technique being passive stretching. Passive stretching increases the Golgi tendon organ's inhibitory activity to reduce muscle electromyographic activity within 10–20 seconds and provide symptomatic relief. Ideally, passive tension should be maintained to the affected muscle for up to 20 minutes or until fasciculation ceases.[19] If the EAMC were particularly intense or prolonged, icing while the muscle is on stretch may be considered to offset any potential delayed onset muscle soreness resulting from microscopic muscle fibre damage. Other potential methods of reducing motor neuron activity during EAMC include electrical stimulation of tendon afferents and antagonist contraction to induce reciprocal inhibition.

The incomplete knowledge of the aetiology of EAMC has limited the development of preventative strategies. Fluid and electrolyte replacement has not been shown to be beneficial, consistent with the now debunked dehydration-electrolyte imbalance theory. In contrast, strategies aimed at modulating fatigability and altering neuromuscular control may be beneficial. Fatigability may be modified by improving generalised conditioning and endurance, and ensuring and maintaining adequate carbohydrate reserves. Neuromuscular control may be targeted by performing plyometric and eccentric exercises, which may elicit changes in muscle spindle and Golgi tendon organ firing to enhance efficiency and sensitivity of reflexive and descending pathways used for neuromuscular control. Regular stretching is also recommended as EAMC frequently occur when the muscle is in its shortened position, while massage and treatment of myofascial trigger points may improve muscle efficiency and reduce fatigability.

TENDON
Tear/rupture

Tendons connect muscle to bone and function to transmit muscle contractile forces necessary for motion. They consist of parallel collagen fibres that are more tightly packed than in ligaments, which endow tendons with the consummate ability to resist tensile loading. The tensile strength of tendon is so great that acute tear or rupture of a normal, healthy tendon is relatively rare, with forces more likely to cause an avulsion fracture or failure at the musculotendinous junction (i.e. muscle strain).

Tendons that do acutely fail usually have some form of underlying pathology (i.e. tendinosis). The pathology is usually asymptomatic, such that the tendon failure appears to occur without warning. As the presence of pathology increases with age, tendon ruptures most frequently occur in middle-aged and older athletes. The two most commonly ruptured tendons are the Achilles and supraspinatus tendons, with ruptures involving either a portion (partial rupture) or the full thickness (complete rupture) of the respective tendon (Fig. 3.8). Partial ruptures are characterised by the sudden onset of pain, localised tenderness and a loss of tendon function that is inversely related to the size of the tear. In contrast, complete ruptures are associated with total loss of tendon function and acute pain, but the pain often settles quickly due to concomitant damage of nociceptor afferents.

Diagnosis of tendon ruptures can be confirmed using imaging, with both ultrasonography and magnetic resonance imaging being useful at distinguishing between partial and complete rupture. Partial tendon ruptures may be managed conservatively using progressive rehabilitation; however, complete ruptures may be treated by surgical repair to restore tendon continuity and function, followed by rehabilitation or by rehabilitation alone.

PART A Fundamental principles

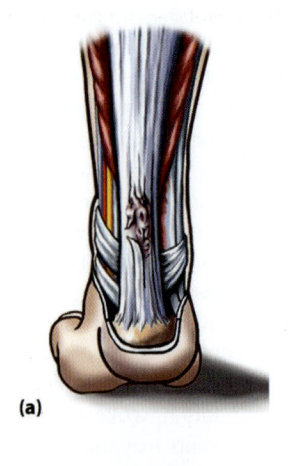

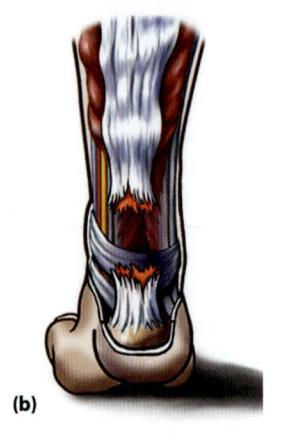

Figure 3.8 Tendon rupture (a) Partial (b) Complete

FASCIA
Tear/rupture
Fascia is a dense, regular connective tissue consisting of closely packed bundles of collagen fibres. It divides muscles into compartments and forms specific force-transmitting structures, such as the iliotibial band (ITB) and plantar fascia. Most injuries to fascia are associated with overuse, with prominent conditions being ITB syndrome (Chapter 37) and plantar fasciopathy (Chapter 43). Acute sprain or rupture of fascia is rare, but has been reported.

BURSA
Traumatic bursitis
Bursae are small, synovial membrane-lined sacs that are filled with an inner layer of viscous fluid. They are frequently found between bone and overlying connective tissues (such as tendon, muscle and skin) where they function to provide cushioning and facilitate movement by reducing friction. Most injuries to bursae are associated with overuse (Chapter 4), but occasionally a direct fall onto a bursa may result in acute traumatic bursitis due to bleeding into the bursa. The management of acute haemorrhagic bursitis involves the application of ice and compression. Aspiration may be considered if the condition does not resolve, but corticosteroid injection is rarely indicated.

NERVE
Neuropraxia
Major acute nerve injuries are unusual in athletes. Specific nerves are susceptible to compression injury because of their subcutaneous location, including the ulnar nerve at the elbow and common peroneal nerve at the neck of the fibula. Similarly, some nerves are vulnerable to being co-injured with other tissues, such as axillary nerve injury during shoulder dislocation and radial nerve injury with humeral shaft fracture.

The most common acute nerve injury in athletes is a 'stinger' or 'burner'. A stinger or burner results from an overstretching injury to the brachial plexus that conveys the nerve supply to the arm. Overstretching can occur when the head is forcibly bent away from the shoulder while the shoulder is simultaneously depressed. This can occur when an athlete is driven into the playing surface during a high-contact sport, such as ice hockey, rugby, wrestling and various football codes.

Symptoms are a stinging or burning sensation that spreads from the shoulder to the hand, which may be associated with numbness in the sensory distribution of the involved nerves. The paraesthesia is often temporary, disappearing in minutes and usually within hours; however, injuries that are more serious can result in longer lasting symptoms involving the loss of both sensory and motor function due to blockage of nerve conduction. The later type of injury, known as 'neuropraxia', usually resolves spontaneously but slowly.

FAT PAD
Bruise/contusion
Fat pads consist of closely packed adipose cells surrounded by fibrous septa, which commonly divide the fat pad into separate compartments. The function of fat pads is not well established and may vary according to anatomical location. However, they appear to have roles in cushioning and facilitating joint lubrication. It is in their cushioning role that fat pads are susceptible to acute compression injury. In particular, the calcaneal fat pad under the heel and the infrapatellar fat pad located behind the patellar tendon can be acutely injured. The plantar fat pad can be injured during landing onto the heel from a height, while the infrapatellar fat pad can be injured by landing on the knees or pinching the fat pad between the femoral

condyles, proximal tibia and inferior pole of the patella during knee hyperextension. The infrapatellar fat pad is also often acutely injured when creating portals during knee arthroscopic surgery.

Fat pads are well vascularised and innervated. The blood supply contributes to haematoma formation (contusion) in response to acute injury, but also enables fat pad injuries to readily heal. The rich innervation of fat pads means that they can be a significant source of pain, with the infrapatellar fat pad being reported to be the most pain evoking structure in the knee.[20] The integrity and function of the calcaneal fat pad may be compromised if its organised compartments are disrupted; however, this is rare, with compression injuries sufficient to fracture the calcaneus not damaging the fibrous septa.[21] Management of fat pad injuries, beyond acute care techniques, includes externally padding using heel cups or knee pads and using tape to limit radial expansion of the calcaneal fat pad or unload the infrapatellar fat pad. These injuries can take considerable time to heal.

SKIN

Acute skin injuries are common in athletes, particularly those competing in contact sports and cycling. Open wounds may be caused by a scraping (abrasion), cutting (laceration) or piercing (puncture) force. Possible damage to underlying structures, such as tendons, muscles, blood vessels and nerves, should always be considered. The principles of treatment of all open wounds are shown in Table 3.4.

Table 3.4 Principles of treatment of all open wounds

Principle	Details
1. Stop any associated bleeding	Apply a pressure bandage directly to the injured part and elevate it. If the wound is open and clean, bring the wound edges together using adhesive strips or sutures. A contaminated wound should not be closed.
2. Prevent infection	Remove all dirt and contamination by simple irrigation. Extensively wash and scrub with antiseptic solution as required as soon as possible. If the wound is severely contaminated, prophylactic antibiotic therapy should be commenced (e.g. flucloxacillin, 500 mg orally four times a day). If anaerobic organisms are suspected (e.g. wound inflicted by a bite), add an antibiotic such as metronidazole (400 mg orally three times a day).
3. Immobilisation (where needed)	This applies when the wound is over a constantly moving part, for example, the anterior aspect of the knee. Certain lacerations, such as pretibial lacerations, require particular care and strict immobilisation to encourage healing.
4. Check tetanus status	All contaminated wounds, especially penetrating wounds, have the potential to become infected with *Clostridium tetani*. Tetanus immunisation consists of a course of three injections over 6 months given during childhood. Further tetanus toxoid boosters should be given at 5 to 10 year intervals. In the case of a possible contaminated wound, a booster should be given if none has been administered within the previous 5 years.

REFERENCES

References for this chapter can be found at www.mhhe.com/au/CSM5e

Chapter 4

Sports injuries: overuse

with STUART WARDEN

During training, I suffered a stress fracture. It was madness that I carried on and ran the 800 metres and 1500 metres, but because it's the Olympics, you run through the pain. You never know if you'll have another chance at the Olympics, so unless you can't actually walk you carry on, because you don't want to be asking yourself, 'What if?'
Dame Kelly Holmes, MBE, DBE, 800 and 1500 m gold medallist, Athens 2004 Olympic Games

Overuse injuries present three distinct challenges to the clinician—diagnosis, understanding of why the injury occurred and treatment. Diagnosis requires taking a comprehensive history of the onset, nature and site of the pain along with a thorough assessment of potential risk factors, for example training and technique. Careful examination may reveal which anatomical structure is affected. It is often helpful to ask patients to perform the manoeuvre that produces their pain.

The skilled clinician must seek a cause for every overuse injury. The cause may be quite evident, such as a sudden doubling of training quantity, poor footwear or an obvious biomechanical abnormality, or it may be more subtle, such as running on a cambered surface, muscle imbalance or leg length discrepancy. The causes of overuse injuries are usually divided into extrinsic factors, such as training, surfaces, shoes, equipment and environmental conditions, and intrinsic factors, such as age, gender, malalignment, leg length discrepancy, muscle imbalance, muscle weakness, lack of flexibility and body composition. Possible factors in the development of overuse injuries are shown in Table 4.1.

Treatment of overuse injuries will usually require addressing of the cause as well as specific additional elements such as activity modification, specific exercises to promote tissue repair, soft tissue therapy and pharmacologic agents where appropriate (Chapter 17).

Table 4.1 Overuse injuries: predisposing factors

Extrinsic factors	Intrinsic factors
Training errors	Malalignment
• excessive volume	• pes planus
• excessive intensity	• pes cavus
• rapid increase	• rearfoot varus
• sudden change in type	• tibia vara
• excessive fatigue	• genu valgum
• inadequate recovery	• genu varum
• faulty technique	• patella alta
Surfaces	• femoral neck anteversion
• hard	• tibial torsion
• soft	Leg length discrepancy
• cambered	Muscle imbalance
Shoes	Muscle weakness
• inappropriate	Lack of flexibility
• worn out	• generalised muscle tightness
Equipment	• focal areas of muscle thickening
• inappropriate	• restricted joint range of motion
Environmental conditions	
• hot	
• cold	Sex, size, body composition
• humid	Other
Psychological factors	• genetic factors
Inadequate nutrition	• endocrine factors
	• metabolic conditions

BONE STRESS INJURY

A bone stress injury (BSI) represents the inability of bone to withstand repetitive mechanical loading, which results in structural fatigue and localised bone pain and tenderness. It occurs along a pathology continuum beginning with a stress reaction, which can progress to a stress fracture and ultimately a complete bone fracture.

PART A Fundamental principles

Pathophysiology

BSIs result from an imbalance between the formation and removal of load-induced damage. A theoretical model is presented in Figure 4.1. Bones deform in response to loading, with the amount of deformation (expressed in terms of strain) depending on the magnitude of load applied and the ability of bone to resist deformation. While the safety factor between exercise-induced strains and those required for complete bone fracture is large, exercise-induced strains can generate microscopic damage (termed 'microdamage').[1] The threshold for microdamage formation depends on the interaction between the number of bone-loading/-strain cycles, the load/strain magnitude and the speed at which load/strain is introduced (strain rate).

Microdamage serves as a stimulus for targeted remodelling.[2] Targeted remodelling involves activation of remodelling units consisting of advancing front-of-bone-resorbing osteoclasts which remove the damage, followed by rows of bone-forming osteoblasts which deposit layers of new bone. Targeted remodelling maintains homeostasis between damage formation and its removal to preserve bone mechanical properties and enable a bone to adapt over time to meet changing demands. The adaptation decreases bone strain for a given load,[3, 4] which means greater loads can be tolerated before the threshold for microdamage formation is surpassed.

Remodelling normally removes damage approximately as fast as it occurs and a reserve exists whereby additional remodelling units can be activated in response to increased microdamage formation. Thus, changes in loading are generally well tolerated. However, remodelling is time dependent and, if insufficient time is given to adapt to a new mechanical stimulus, progressively more damage may form as a result of feedforward between remodelling and damage formation. Feedforward results from resorption preceding formation in remodelling so that an increase in the number of active remodelling units locally reduces bone mass and the energy absorbing capacity of the bone, which potentiates further damage formation.

Accumulating microdamage may combine to initiate the BSI pathology continuum, which includes stress reactions, stress fractures and ultimately complete fracture (Fig. 4.1). Stress reactions are characterised by increased bone turnover associated with periosteal and/or marrow

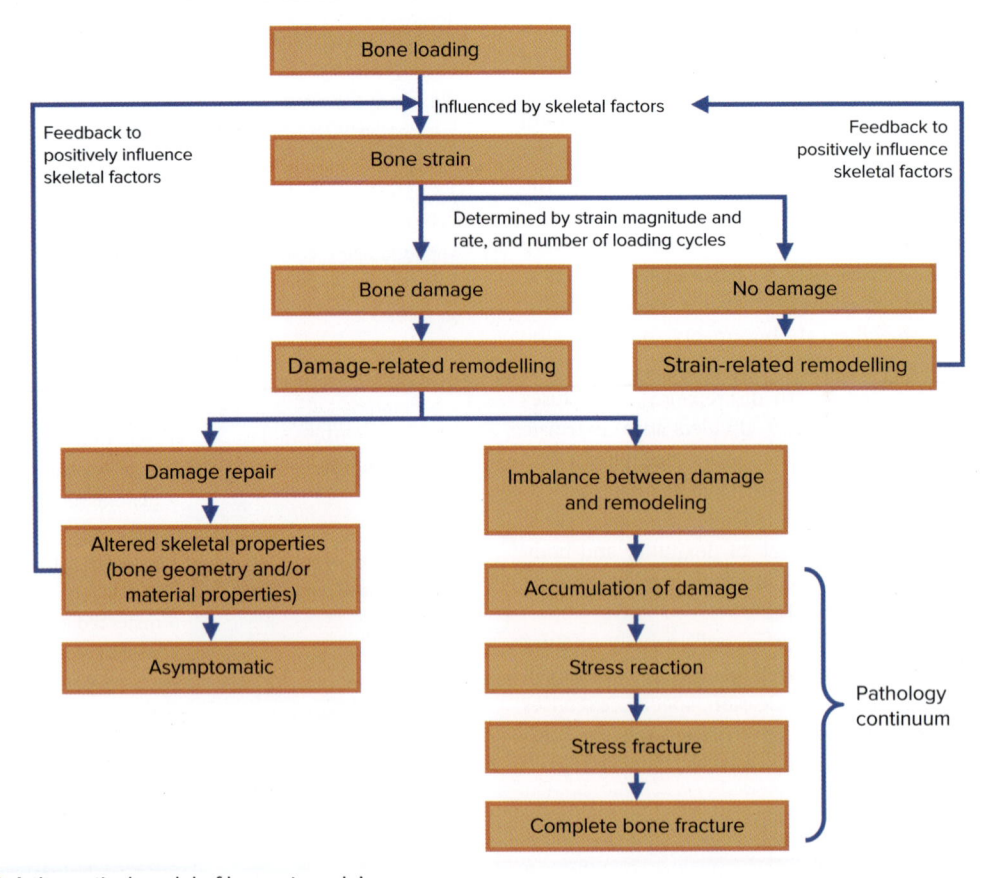

Figure 4.1 A theoretical model of bone stress injury
REPRINTED WITH KIND PERMISSION FROM SPRINGER SCIENCE+BUSINESS MEDIA, *CURRENT OSTEOPOROSIS REPORTS* 2006;4(3):103–9

Sports injuries: overuse — CHAPTER 4

oedema, whereas stress fractures have the addition of a discernible fracture line.

Epidemiology

As BSIs develop in response to repetitive mechanical loading, it is not surprising they frequently occur in athletes. In athletes, BSIs cause a considerable loss of participation time and are a significant source of frustration, particularly when they occur in the lead up to a major event or competition. Between one- and two-thirds of runners have a history of a BSI,[5, 6] while the one-year cumulative incidence of BSIs in cross-country and track and field athletes ranges between 5% and 21%.[7, 8] Also of note is the high recurrence rate of BSIs, with half of track and field athletes reporting a history of BSIs on more than one occasion and 10-13% of cross-country and track and field athletes with a history of a BSI sustaining a subsequent BSI when followed for 1-2 years.[6, 7]

BSIs are site specific, occurring at sites exposed to repetitive mechanical loading. Given their association with mechanical loading, BSIs predominantly occur at weight-bearing sites, with the most common sites being the tibia, the metatarsals and the fibula. The exact location depends on how the skeleton is loaded, with different activities resulting in different loading patterns within different bones. For example, long distance runners typically use a rearfoot strike pattern to preferentially load long bones (tibia, fibula, femur), whereas sprinters use a forefoot strike pattern to introduce relatively greater loads to the bones of the feet. As a result of the differential bone loading, distance runners are at a greater risk of developing long BSIs, whereas sprinters are more prone to BSIs of the tarsals and metatarsals.[7]

Although BSIs predominantly occur at weight-bearing sites, they also occur in response to repetitive loading at non weight-bearing sites.[9] For instance, rowers repetitively load their rib cage during the drive phase of the rowing stroke and, consequently, are at heightened risk of generating BSIs in their ribs (see Chapter 9).[10] Similarly, throwing athletes are at risk of developing humeral diaphysis BSIs as they repetitively expose their humerus to significant loads during the throwing motion.[4, 11] As BSIs can occur at both weight-bearing and non weight-bearing sites, they can occur in virtually any bone (Fig. 4.2). Thus, they need to be considered in the differential diagnosis of all presenting injuries.

Risk factors

BSIs can be viewed as occurring when the mechanical stimulus at a specific bone site repetitively exceeds the threshold for microdamage formation. As the bone

Site of stress fracture	Associated sport/activity
Coracoid process of scapula	Trapshooting
Scapula	Running with hand weights
Humerus	Throwing; racquet sports
Olecranon	Throwing; pitching
Ulna	Racquet sports (esp. tennis); gymnastics; volleyball; swimming; softball; wheelchair sports
Ribs—1st	Throwing; pitching
Ribs—2nd–10th	Rowing; kayaking
Pars interarticularis	Gymnastics; ballet; cricket fast bowling; volleyball; springboard diving
Pubic ramus*	Distance running; ballet
Femur—neck	Distance running; jumping; ballet
Femur—shaft	Distance running
Patella	Running; hurdling
Tibia—plateau	Running
Tibia—shaft	Running; ballet
Fibula	Running; aerobics; race-walking; ballet
Medial malleolus*	Running; basketball
Calcaneus	Long-distance military marching
Talus	Pole vaulting
Navicular	Sprinting; middle-distance running; hurdling; long jump; triple jump; football
Metatarsal—general	Running; ballet; marching
Metatarsal—2nd base	Ballet
Metatarsal—5th	Tennis; ballet
Sesamoid bone—foot	Running; ballet; basketball; skating

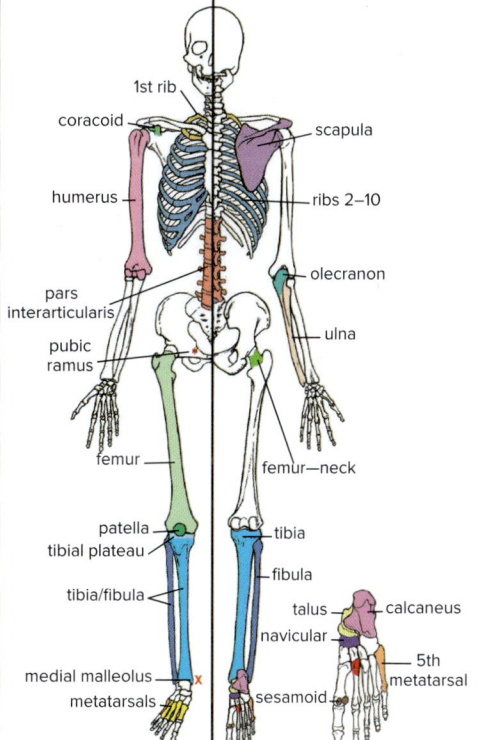

Figure 4.2 Stress fracture site and common associated activity

31

mechanical stimulus is dependent on the interaction between the applied load and the ability of the bone to resist deformation, risk factors for BSIs can be grouped into two categories:
1. factors modifying the load being applied to a bone
2. factors modifying the ability of a bone to resist load without damage accumulation (Fig. 4.3).

Factors modifying the load applied to a bone

The load applied to a bone during athletic activities represents the summation of external and internal forces, and has magnitude, rate, frequency, duration and direction components. These components influence bone strain magnitude, rate, frequency, duration and location, respectively. Factors modifying the load applied to a bone include biomechanical, training and muscle factors, playing surface and shoes and inserts (orthoses and insoles).

Biomechanical factors

Faulty biomechanics can contribute to BSI risk, and can be dichotomised into those related to abnormal forces and abnormal motions. Increased forces on a normally aligned skeleton can result in abnormal bone loading, with athletes exhibiting high ground reaction force (GRF) magnitudes and rates, and high accelerations during the early stance phase of running gait being proposed to be at heightened BSI risk. Alternatively, normal forces applied to a malaligned skeleton can also abnormally load bone. Altered movement patterns have the potential to alter the magnitude and/or rate of bone loading, and also alter the direction a bone is loaded and the subsequent distribution of strain within the bone.

The net result may be increased loading of a less accustomed bone site. Statically assessed biomechanical variables that have been implicated in BSI development include external rotation range of motion of the hip,[13] leg length discrepancy,[14] and both pes planus[15] and cavus.[16] Dynamically assessed variables implicated in BSI development include greater peak hip adduction, knee internal rotation and peak rearfoot eversion in the frontal plane during running[17-19] and less knee flexion in the sagittal plane.[20] Having the combination of abnormal forces coupled with a malaligned lower limb is thought to further amplify BSI risk.

Training factors

Chronic introduction of high absolute load magnitudes, rates and accelerations may reduce bone fatigue life, particularly

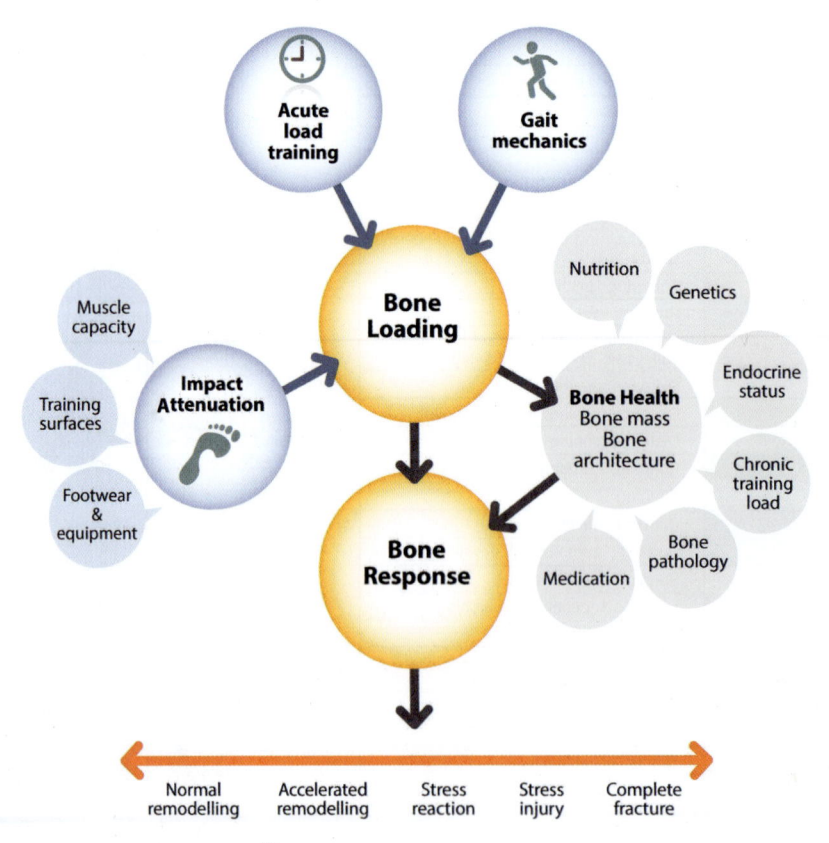

Figure 4.3 Risk factors for bone stress injuries[12]

when the number of loading cycles is high (i.e. running long distances). However, the influence of these variables may be most prominent when an athlete attempts to progress their training. Increases in running speed increase GRFs and their rates of introduction,[21] while increases in the duration and/or frequency of training sessions increase the total number of bone-loading cycles. In the absence of a change in the load-bearing capacity of a bone, altered loading associated with large changes in training may contribute to microdamage accumulation and the generation of a BSI.

Evidence from military studies confirms that individuals exposed to large changes in physical activity have a heightened BSI risk. For instance, recruits with a lesser history of regular physical activity prior to the commencement of standardised basic training (i.e. those with larger changes in physical activity levels) are at a greater risk of developing a BSI.[22-24] While most athletes do not introduce changes in their bone-loading environment to the same extremes as many military recruits, change is a frequent and required means of inducing adaptation. Incrementing training too rapidly or frequently relative to an athlete's usual activities is thought to be central to disrupting the balance between bone microdamage formation and removal.

Muscle factors

Training changes may independently contribute to BSI development, but the relative risk associated with the change may be compounded by muscle factors. An intimate mechanical relationship exists between muscle and bone and the general hypothesis is that muscle is generally protective of BSIs, particularly those occurring in the lower extremity. During impact loading, muscle acts as an active shock attenuator helping to reduce loads as they are transmitted proximally.

When muscles are dysfunctional (weakened, fatigued or altered in their activation patterns) their ability to attenuate loads becomes compromised leading to increased loading of the skeleton. For instance, fatigue results in a decrease in shock attenuation,[25, 26] increase in GRF loading rates and peak accelerations,[27, 28] and increase in bone strain magnitude and rate.[29, 30] In addition, fatigue can lead to altered kinematics, which may alter the direction a bone is loaded resulting in increased bone strain at less accustomed bone sites.[31] Further support for a protective role of muscle in stress fracture development comes from prospective clinical studies which demonstrated that BSI susceptibility was directly related to muscle size[14, 32, 33] and strength.[34]

Playing surface

Playing surface has historically been considered a contributor to BSI risk, with participation on harder surfaces such as asphalt hypothesised to increase loading compared to participating on softer surfaces such as grass, rubber and sand. However, the interaction between playing surface and injury risk is complex. Athletes alter their leg stiffness when running on surfaces of differing compliance apparently to maintain a constant vertical excursion of their centre of mass.[35] Leg stiffness decreases when running on stiffer surfaces to normalise to some extent GRF magnitude; however, GRF loading rates do appear to be systematically increased when running on surfaces that are less compliant.[36]

Ultimately, what may be important with regards to BSI risk is whether there has been a recent change in running surface that an athlete has yet to become accustomed to. Changes may include increased participation on:

1. less compliant surfaces, which may increase bone strain magnitudes and rate[37]
2. very compliant surfaces (such as sand), which may increase energy expenditure and influence muscle-related risk factors and kinematics[38, 39]
3. downhill slopes, which may decrease shock attenuation[40] and increase loading magnitudes and rates[41]
4. altered terrain, which may alter kinematics to load less accustomed skeletal sites.[42]

Shoes and inserts

The role of shoes and inserts (orthoses and insoles) on bone loading and BSI risk is a topic of ongoing debate. Located at the foot–ground interface, shoes and inserts act as filters that theoretically attenuate ground impact forces. In addition, they have the potential to influence motion of the foot and ankle and the subsequent mechanics proximally in the kinetic chain. Via these two mechanisms, shoes and inserts may influence bone loading and have an effect on BSI risk.

Factors influencing the ability of the bone to resist load without damage accumulation

The amount and rate of strain engendered when a load is applied to a bone is dependent upon the ability of the bone to resist deformation in the direction of loading. For a given applied load, less rigid bones experience greater strain and at a faster rate than more rigid bones and, thus, are more susceptible to microdamage and BSI formation. Skeletal features that influence bone rigidity include the amount of bone material present (mass) and its distribution (structure). There is strong evidence that both contribute to BSI risk[14, 23, 33, 43, 44] and therefore it is important to consider modifiable factors that may contribute to these skeletal characteristics. Three modifiable factors in athletes that may impact the ability of bone to resist loading and contribute to BSI risk are physical activity history, energy availability, and calcium and vitamin D status.

PART A Fundamental principles

Physical activity history

A longer history of physical activity appears to be protective against the development of a BSI.[22-24, 45, 46] An improved ability of the skeleton to resist loading likely contributes to the reduced BSI risk in individuals with a prior history of physical activity. The skeleton responds and adapts to mechanical loading in a site-specific manner to increase its rigidity in the direction of loading. It principally does this during the growing years by preferentially depositing small amounts of new bone on the outer periosteal surface at a distance from the bending axes. As the rigidity of a unit area of bone is proportional to the fourth power of its distance from a bending axis, the addition of a small amount of mass to the outer surface of a bone results in a disproportionate increase in bone strength. The net result is a decrease in the bone strain engendered in response to a given load and increase in bone fatigue life.[3]

Energy availability

Gender factors contribute to BSI susceptibility, with females being at greater risk.[47] The cause for the higher incidence of BSIs in females appears to relate to the interrelationships between energy availability, menstrual function and bone mass–otherwise known as the female athlete triad. While athletes can have one or more components of the triad, low energy availability appears to be the central factor.[48] Low energy availability results from insufficient dietary intake to meet exercise energy expenditure. It can result from low dietary energy intake (whether inadvertent, intentional or psychopathological) and/or excessive exercise energy expenditure. The menstrual and skeletal changes associated with low energy availability reduce the ability of bone to resist load and/or impair its ability to repair microdamage. The net result is heightened BSI risk, particularly in elite female long distance runners where the difference between dietary energy intake and exercise energy expenditure is often small and the incidence of menstrual dysfunction is elevated.

Calcium and vitamin D status

Calcium combines with phosphate to form hydroxyapatite crystals to endow bone with rigidity, while vitamin D contributes by promoting calcium absorption in the gut and reabsorption in the kidneys. Prospective studies provide evidence for roles of both low calcium and vitamin D in BSIs,[49, 50] and a large randomised controlled trial demonstrated a 20% reduction in BSI incidence in female Navy recruits with suboptimal baseline daily calcium intake when they were supplemented with daily calcium and vitamin D.[51] Overall, the data suggest that athletes should ensure sufficient calcium and vitamin D intakes to meet or exceed the current recommended dietary allowances of 1000–1300 mg and 600 IU (for individuals aged 14–50 years), respectively.[52]

Diagnosis

BSIs often present with a history consistent with an overuse injury–the gradual onset of activity-related pain. As BSIs occur along a pathology continuum, signs and symptoms may vary depending upon what point along the continuum the athlete presents. An astute clinician may be able to diagnose the pathology at the stress reaction stage. However, some patients may not present until the pathology has progressed to a stress fracture where there is actual cortical disruption. The earlier within the continuum an athlete presents and a diagnosis is made, the more likely the pathology may respond quickly and favourably to management. Thus, bone as the tissue of origin of an athlete's symptoms needs to be considered at all times during differential diagnosis to ensure prompt diagnosis and management.

The diagnostic features of a stress fracture are shown in Table 4.2.

History

A thorough history is the first step to the diagnosis of a BSI. In most instances, individuals with a BSI have a consistent and predictable history that centres on pain. At the start of the pathology continuum, pain is usually described as a mild diffuse ache that occurs after a specific amount of activity and at specific times (depending on which bone is afflicted and when loaded during activity). The pain does not tend to resolve or 'warm-up' as activity is continued and only abates once activity (i.e. bone loading) is ceased.

As the initial pain often subsides soon after activity completion and is not present during rest it is often ignored at first. However, with continued training and progression of the pathology the pain may become more severe and localised and occur at an earlier stage. It may also persist for longer periods following the completion of activity and begin to be present during activities that involve lower levels of bone loading, such as walking. Eventually, the pain can result in activity restriction or the

Table 4.2 Diagnostic features of a stress fracture

- Localised pain and tenderness over the fracture site.
- A history of a recent change in training or taking up a new activity.
- X-ray appearance often normal or there may be a periosteal reaction (Fig. 4.4).
- Abnormal appearance on MRI (Fig. 4.5), radioisotopic bone scan (scintigraphy) (Fig. 4.7) or CT scan (Fig. 4.8).

need to cease training altogether. At this more advanced stage, any associated inflammatory response to the injury may also occasionally contribute to resting and night pain.

Examination

On physical examination, the most obvious feature of a BSI is localised bony tenderness. Certain bones (such as the tibia, fibula and metatarsals) lend themselves well to palpation because of their well-defined anatomical boundaries and the absence of overlying muscle. In these relatively subcutaneous bones, precise and thorough palpation is required as tenderness may be localised with adjacent areas being completely pain-free. Occasionally redness, swelling and warmth from an associated inflammatory reaction may also be felt, along with periosteal thickening and callus formation in longer-standing BSIs.

Direct palpation is obviously not possible at deeper sites (such as the femur and pars interarticularis of the spine), with symptoms at these sites possibly being provoked by specific bone-loading tests, such as hopping,[53] the fulcrum test for the femoral shaft,[54] or the one-legged hyperextension test for the pars interarticularis.[55] However, the sensitivity and specificity of these bone-loading tests have either not been investigated or disputed.[56] Likewise, the application of a vibrating tuning fork or therapeutic ultrasound for the clinical diagnosis of BSIs is not supported.[57]

Imaging

Imaging plays a significant role in the diagnosis. Imaging options include plain radiography, bone scan, computed tomography (CT), magnetic resonance imaging (MRI) and, more recently, ultrasound.

Plain radiographs have poor sensitivity and may not detect stress injury until the injury has developed along the bone stress continuum.[58, 59] Although some old textbooks suggested that stress fractures become visible on plain radiographs after 2–6 weeks, prospective studies prove that some stress fractures remain invisible on plain radiography. Radiographic changes, when present, include subtle focal periosteal bone formation (Fig. 4.4), or, later, frank cortical defects.

In countries where physicians have ready access to MRI, this is generally the first line investigation of bone stress injuries. MRI is sensitive in detecting pathophysiological changes in soft tissue, bone and marrow associated with bone related stress injuries. It can reveal abnormalities in these structures before plain radiographic changes and has comparable sensitivity to a bone scan.[58] Other advantages of MRI for bone imaging are its multiplanar capability (which helps the clinician precisely define the location and extent of injury), lack of exposure to ionising radiation and significantly less imaging time than a three-phase bone scan.

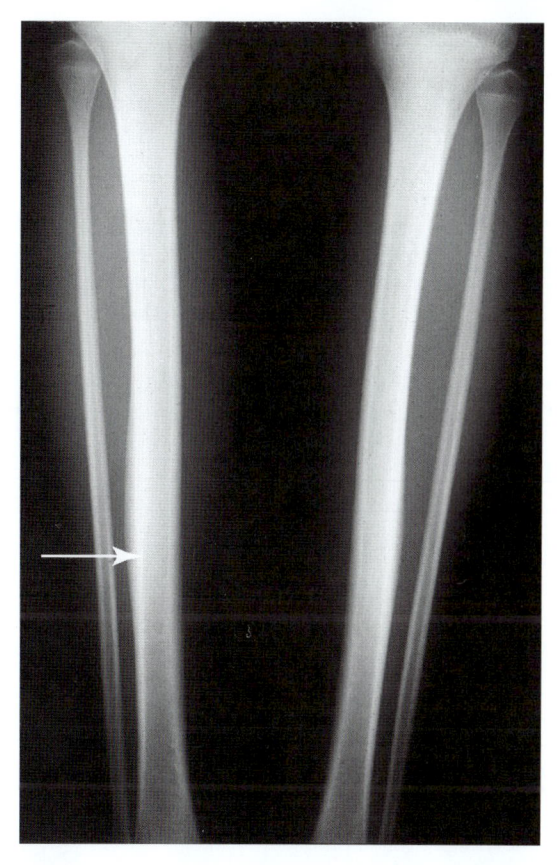

Figure 4.4 X-ray showing periosteal new bone formation indicative of a stress fracture

The typical MRI appearance of a stress fracture shows periosteal and marrow oedema plus or minus the actual fracture line (Fig. 4.5). Several fat-suppression techniques such as short tau inversion recovery are used to maximise the sensitivity of MRI in bone stress injuries.[60]

Various grading systems for stress fractures based on MRI appearances have been suggested.[61] The most commonly used systems [62-64] are shown in Table 4.3.

Attempts have been made to use the MRI appearance to predict return to play (RTP). In a prospective study involving 34 fractures among 211 college athletes, MRI grading severity, lower bone mineral density (BMD) and the fracture site (trabecular > cortical bone) were important variables associated with time to return to sport.[64] The mean time to full return to sport for grade 4 BSIs (31.7 +/− 3.7 weeks) was significantly higher compared with grade 3 (18.8 +/− 2.9 weeks), grade 2 (13.5 +/− 2.1 weeks) and grade 1 injuries (11.4 +/− 4.5 weeks). Among grade 3 and 4 injuries, the mean time to return to sport was significantly longer for those at sites high in trabecular versus cortical bone (38.1 +/− 6.4 vs 18.8 +/− 2.1 weeks, respectively).[64]

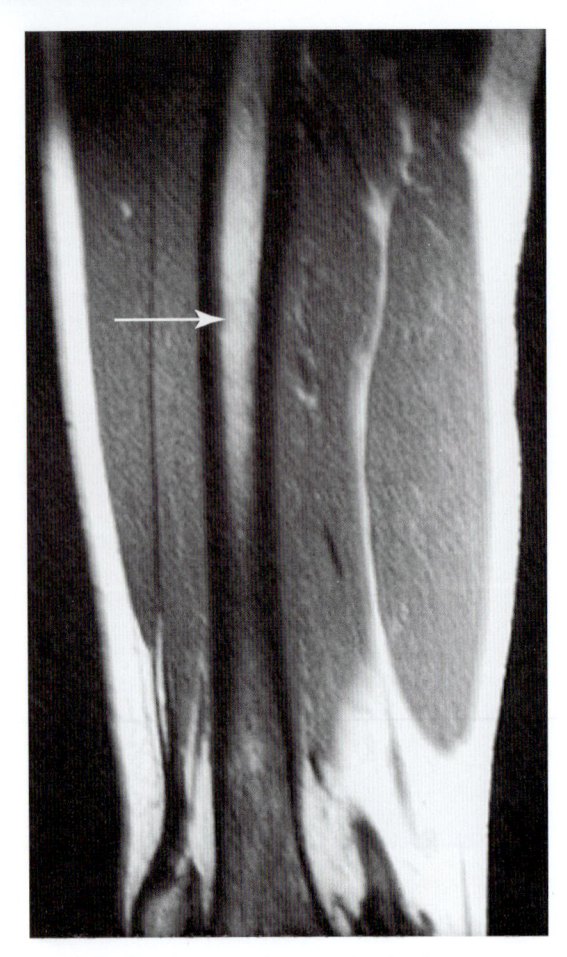

PART A   Fundamental principles

It should be recognised that the above values are based on the average time taken to return to sport. However, as illustrated in Figure 4.6, this fails to reflect the wide variation among individuals–particularly those with higher MRI-grade injuries or injuries located in high-risk sites (covered in the section 'Classification of bone stress injuries').[65] Care should therefore be taken in making definitive return-to-sport predictions based on imaging alone, except perhaps in the case of mild stress reactions in low-risk sites.

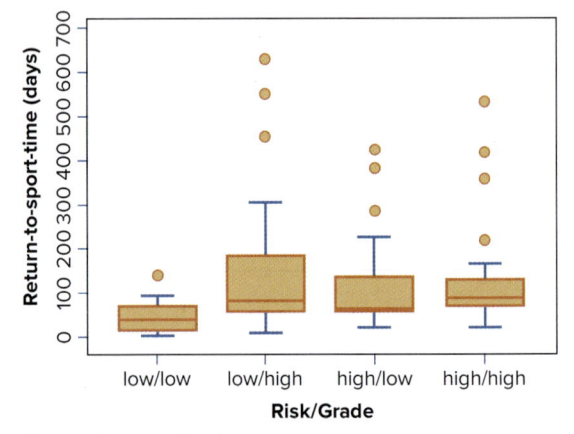

Figure 4.5 MRI of a stress fracture showing bony oedema (white)

(Dots indicate outliers).

Figure 4.6 Return-to-sport times for BSIs grouped according to a combination of their location (low risk/high risk) and MRI grade (low: grades 1 and 2; high: grades 3 and 4)[66]

Table 4.3 MRI grading scales for BSIs

Grade	Fredericson et al.[62]	Arendt et al.[63]	Nattiv et al.[64]
1	Mild to moderate periosteal oedema on T2 Normal marrow on T2 and T1	Positive signal change on STIR	Mild marrow or periosteal oedema on T2 T1 normal*
2	Moderate to severe periosteal oedema on T2 Marrow oedema on T2 but not T1	Positive STIR plus positive T2	Moderate marrow or periosteal oedema plus positive T2 T1 normal
3	Moderate to severe periosteal oedema on T2 Marrow oedema on T2 and T1	Positive STIR plus positive T2 and T1	Severe marrow or periosteal oedema on T2 and T1
4	Moderate to severe periosteal oedema on T2 Marrow oedema on T2 and T1 Fracture line present	Fracture line present on T2 or T1	Severe marrow or periosteal oedema on T2 and T1 Fracture line present on T2 or T1

STIR: short T1 inversion recovery
*Radiograph results are often negative at all grades; they may be normal, or a periosteal reaction may be evident

Sports injuries: overuse — CHAPTER 4

Beck and colleagues in their study included grading systems for radiography, isotope bone scan, CT scan, as well as MRI and found that only the MRI grading system had any relationship to clinical severity.[67]

A radioisotopic bone scan was the most important diagnostic test for athletic stress fractures in the 1990s.[60] The technical aspects of this modality are outlined in Chapter 15. The appearance of a BSI on a bone scan is a focal area of increased uptake (Fig. 4.7).

Note that bone scans lack specificity for stress fractures– bony abnormalities such as tumours, especially osteoid osteoma and osteomyelitis, have similar appearances. It may also be difficult to precisely localise the site of the area of increased uptake. Increased uptake can occur in non-painful sites, indicating subclinical accelerated remodelling. As with plain film, CT and MR imaging, imaging appearance returns to normal after clinical resolution because of ongoing bony remodelling.[60]

CT is less sensitive than a bone scan or MRI in the early detection of a BSI.[58, 59] However, it is more sensitive than both radiographs and MRI for the detection of cortical fracture lines. CT is thus well suited to demonstrate stress fractures of the sacrum, pars interarticularis, tarsal navicular and longitudinal stress fractures of the tibia.[58]

A CT scan will clearly image the fracture (Fig. 4.8) and differentiate between a stress fracture (positive bone scan, clear fracture line) and a stress reaction (positive bone scan and negative CT scan). CT can also distinguish a BSI and other causes of hot bone scans such as osteoid osteoma and osteomyelitis.

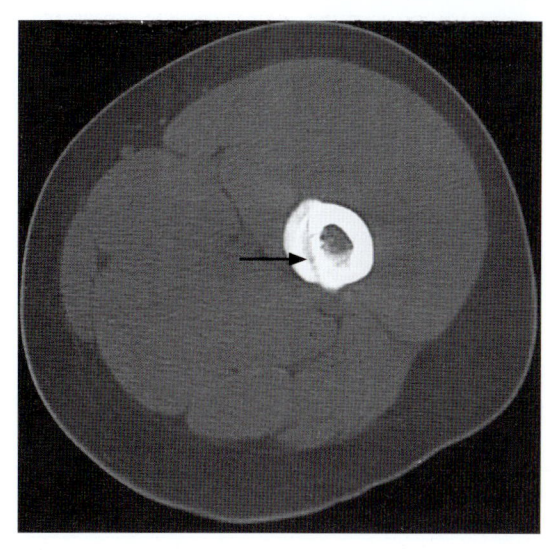

Figure 4.8 CT scan of a stress fracture showing a cortical defect (arrowed)

Ultrasound has some potential in the diagnosis of stress fractures but it is not ready for routine clinical use.[59]

Ultimately, athletes who display clinical signs and symptoms of a possible BSI require imaging to confirm suspicions and make a definitive diagnosis. Briefly, in most clinical settings, plain radiographs remain the first line of imaging for BSIs because of their low cost and wide availability; however, radiographs are limited by their planar nature and low spatial resolution, which contribute to extremely low sensitivity. CT also lacks sensitivity, but may be utilised in specific cases where demonstration of a fracture line may affect treatment. In contrast, bone scintigraphy has high sensitivity, but is limited by low specificity and the use of extremely high ionising radiation doses. Of the imaging modalities currently available, MRI is the modality of choice because of its superior contrast resolution, lack of exposure to ionising radiation, and its combined high sensitivity and specificity.

The different imaging appearances of the various stages of the BSI continuum are shown in Table 4.4.

Classification of bone stress injuries

BSIs can be dichotomised into either low or high-risk groups according to their location (Table 4.5).[68] Low-risk BSIs predominantly occur on the compression side of a bone's bending axis, and have a favourable natural history in that recovery occurs with a low incidence of complications and without the need for aggressive intervention (such as surgery and/or prolonged modified weight-bearing). In contrast, high-risk BSIs often occur on the tension side of a bone's bending axis, and present treatment challenges demanding specific attention

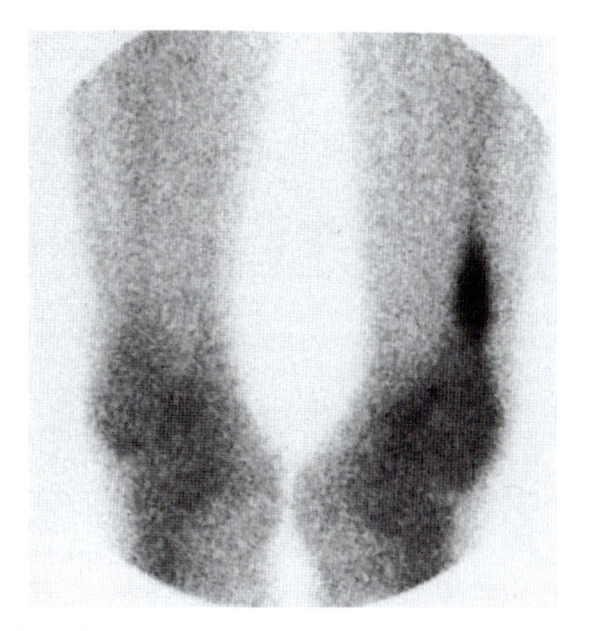

Figure 4.7 Radioisotopic bone scan of a stress fracture
COURTESY OF ZS KISS

PART A Fundamental principles

Table 4.4 Imaging findings with different phases of the BSI continuum

Clinical features	Early bone stress	Stress reaction	Stress fracture
Local pain	Nil	Usually	Always
Local tenderness	Nil	Usually, if superficial	Usually, if superficial
X-ray appearance	Normal	Normal	May be abnormal (periosteal reaction or cortical defect in cortical bone, sclerosis in trabecular bone)
Radioisotopic bone scan appearance	Increased uptake	Increased uptake	Increased uptake
CT scan appearance	Normal	Normal	Features of stress fracture (as for X-ray)
MRI appearance	May show increased high signal	Increased high signal	Increased high signal ± cortical defect

Table 4.5 Low-risk and high-risk BSIs

Low risk	High risk
Posteromedial tibia	Femoral neck
Fibula/lateral malleolus	Anterior cortex of the tibia
Femoral shaft	Medial malleolus
Pelvis	Talus (lateral process)
Calcaneus	Navicular
Diaphysis of second to fourth metatarsals	Proximal diaphysis of the fifth metatarsal
	Base of second metatarsal
	Great-toe sesamoids

because they are prone to delayed or non-union and/or are at high risk for progression to complete fracture.

Management

This section focuses on general management principles for a low-risk BSI, such as one occurring at the posteromedial border of the tibia. The management of specific high-risk BSIs is summarised in Table 4.6 and detailed management is included in chapters covering different regions of the body.

Low-risk BSIs represent relatively straightforward management problems in the sense that they readily heal without complication. A two-phase approach consisting of modified activity followed by a gradual resumption of activity forms the cornerstone of management. While the overarching goal is to return the athlete to his or her

Table 4.6 Stress fractures that require specific treatment other than rest

Stress fracture	Treatment
Femoral neck	Non-displaced: initial bed rest for 1 week, then gradual weight-bearing Displaced: surgical fixation
Anterior tibial cortex	Non weight-bearing on crutches for 6–8 weeks or intramedullary screw fixation
Medial malleolus	Non weight-bearing cast immobilisation for 6 weeks or surgical fixation
Talus (lateral process)	Non weight-bearing cast immobilisation for 6 weeks or surgical excision of fragment
Navicular	Non weight-bearing cast immobilisation for 6–8 weeks or surgery
Metatarsal—2nd base	Non weight-bearing for 2 weeks; partial weight-bearing for 2 weeks
Metatarsal—5th base	Cast immobilisation or percutaneous screw fixation
Sesamoid bone of the foot	Non weight-bearing for 4 weeks

pre-injury level of function in the shortest time possible without compromising tissue level healing, it is generally acknowledged that there is more to the successful management of athletes with a BSI. The high recurrence rate of BSIs indicates that a central goal for clinicians when managing low-risk BSIs should be to identify and modify potential risk factors for future BSIs. Using the concept that BSIs occur when the load being applied exceeds a bone's ability to resist the load without microdamage accumulation, runners with a BSI require strategies to either reduce the load being introduced or increase the load-bearing capacity of their skeleton.

Phase 1. Initial management
Activity modification
There is no question that temporary discontinuation of usual activity and the introduction of a variable period of modified activity is required in the initial management of low-risk BSIs in order to permit tissue-level healing and prevent pathology progression. However, the duration and extent of activity modification is highly variable and is decided upon on an individual basis using pain as the principal guiding variable. The presence of pain either during or after an activity indicates that the pathological site is being excessively loaded for the current stage of healing and that loading needs to be titrated.

In the initial stages of BSI management, the goal is for the athlete to be pain-free during and after usual activities of daily living (ADLs). Cushioned shoes and/or insoles may provide assistance with dissipating impact forces during ADLs in athletes with a rearfoot or leg BSI,[67, 68] whereas athletes with a BSI within the mid or forefoot may consider wearing a stiff soled shoe to reduce bending forces and symptoms.[69]

Walking should be minimised to that essential to perform ADLs and must use a normal gait pattern. If a normal gait pattern cannot be used or symptoms are produced either during or after walking, partial weight-bearing via the use of assistive gait devices should be considered. Alternatively, a pneumatic leg brace may be introduced to promote pain-free gait in the case of BSIs of the fibula or posteromedial border of the tibia.[70] If a pain-free normal gait pattern cannot be achieved, a short period in a walking boot or of non weight-bearing may be considered. However, in each scenario progression to unassisted pain-free gait should be sought as soon as possible.

Athletes need to be pain-free not only during, but also after activities. The presence of resting and/or night pain is a sign that the underlying pathology may have an inflammatory component. While resting pain does not typically require specific intervention as it is usually short term and abates with activity modification, some athletes may consider non-steroidal anti-inflammatory drugs (NSAIDs) or other analgesics. The use of these agents should be discouraged beyond a few days because of their ability to mask pain and subsequently influence activity progression and their potential to impede tissue-level healing when taken for prolonged periods.[71]

Identification and initial management of potential risk factors
The initial period following BSI diagnosis is a useful time to evaluate and begin addressing potential contributing factors as it is often the time when an athlete gives most attention. A detailed activity history is important. Consider not only usual and recent changes in activity frequency, duration and intensity, but also unusual or new participation in physical activities beyond running. BSI risk reflects the sum of all bone loading and loading from non-running activities may be enough to push an athlete beyond their injury threshold. Note should also be taken of any recent changes in running surfaces, shoes/inserts or technique. By combining knowledge of recent running progressions with knowledge of lifelong physical activity history, it may be possible to provide a runner returning from a BSI with advice with regards to future running program design. For instance, novice runners with a minimal physical activity history may need to progress their training program at a slower rate so as to not overload the skeleton and disrupt the homeostasis between microdamage formation and removal.

History taking in an injured athlete should also assess factors influencing the ability of their skeleton to resist loading. It is essential to obtain a history of the patient's general health, medications and personal habits to ensure that there are no factors that may influence bone health. A past history of BSIs (and other bone injuries) and current body mass index of less than 19 are strong risk factors for BSIs that require assessment and thorough exploration.[6, 8]

A full dietary history should be taken with particular attention paid towards the possible presence of deficits in energy intake and/or eating disorders, and calcium and vitamin D intake. A maternal family history of osteoporosis or low bone mineral density should be explored and a detailed menstrual history should be taken in female runners including their age of menarche and subsequent menstrual status. Identification of any issues of concern warrants appropriate referral when indicated, remembering that consultation for a BSI may be the first time that an athlete's issues associated with their relative energy deficiency are identified.

In addition to history taking, initial assessment and management of potential factors influencing bone loading can be explored. To guide the interventions and formulate an initial biomechanical impression of the athlete, it is important to gather as much circumstantial evidence as possible. Such evidence may come from recent videos of the athlete running, assessment of their shoe wear pattern, their history of overuse injuries and whether there is a unilateral predominance, static posture and alignment, and hip, knee and foot mechanics during non-painful activities such as walking or single-leg squats.

Depending on the individual athlete and the preliminary examination findings, initial biomechanical interventions can be introduced to maintain what the athlete already has or address suspected deficits. Activities can include muscle strength, endurance and control training and interventions for muscle length and joint mobility. Key areas to consider include control, endurance and strength at the hip, knee and ankle, core stability, and strength of the intrinsic and extrinsic muscles of the foot. The activities may need to be modified in order to be pain-free, and are often performed in non or partial weight-bearing.

Maintenance of physical conditioning

Maintaining conditioning during recovery is important for as seamless a return to activity as the athlete's pathology permits. Conditioning activities should be introduced early and can include cycling, swimming, deep-water running and anti-gravity treadmill training. The latter two methods may be most specific in running athletes as they more closely reproduce the neuromuscular recruitment patterns involved in running. Anti-gravity treadmill training is not introduced until a runner is pain-free during both walking and ADLs. In the interim, deep-water running can be introduced as long as the athlete is pain-free both during and after sessions.

Accelerating tissue healing

It would be beneficial to provide an athlete with a means of accelerating healing of their BSI. While there are no proven methods of accelerating BSI healing, a number of candidate methods have been proposed. Low intensity (<1.0 W/cm^2) pulsed ultrasound (LIPUS) therapy currently has the greatest support given its observed beneficial effects on complete bone fractures.[72] LIPUS has been effective in stimulating union in 98% and 94% of BSIs displaying delayed and non-union, respectively.[73] However, the benefits of LIPUS on uncomplicated BSIs currently remain unclear. Extracorporeal shock wave therapy and electromagnetic and capacitive coupled electric fields have also been considered as modalities for promoting BSI repair, but studies of their effects have principally been limited to recalcitrant BSIs. At this stage, the use of electrotherapeutic agents to accelerate BSI healing cannot be recommended.

A number of pharmaceutical agents may facilitate BSI healing but currently none are accepted as standard treatment. They include bisphosphonates[74] and the anabolic therapies parathyroid hormone and anti-sclerostin antibody therapy. Parathyroid hormone, when administered intermittently, promotes osteoblastogenesis and osteoblast survival. Anti-sclerostin antibody therapy inhibits osteocyte-secretion of sclerostin to facilitate Wnt signalling and subsequently promote osteoblast proliferation and function. Both agents stimulate bone formation and accelerate fracture healing in preclinical models. Whether the same fracture healing benefits carry over to humans and to BSIs currently remains unknown.[75]

Phase 2. Return to running

Beginning and progressing initial running

A graduated running program can be used in low-risk BSIs to introduce controlled loading and facilitate a return to activity in a timely, yet safe manner. While loading is central to the development of low-risk BSIs, recovery is best met by a balance between rest from aggravating activities and performance of appropriate loading. Appropriate loading can be defined as loading that does not provoke BSI symptoms either during or after completion of an activity. Once an athlete with a low-risk BSI becomes pain-free during unassisted walking, they can start reintroducing running-related loads. While there is no established protocol for returning to running during recovery from a low-risk BSI, a prescriptive program to facilitate the return of a recreational athlete to 30 minutes of running is provided in Table 4.7. The program consists of a pre-entry stage and three running stages.

Once the athlete is completely pain-free for five consecutive days during usual activities, they leave the pre-entry stage (stage 0) and commence deliberate progressive loading. Stage 1 introduces loading in 30-minute sessions separated by rest days. Sessions in this stage consist of increasing durations of jogging (defined as running at 50% of normal pace) and decreasing durations of walking. The pace of running is progressed in stage 2 until the athlete can run for 30 minutes at their usual pace, with stage 3 consisting of running on two consecutive days followed by a rest day. The last stage incorporates individualised running until there is complete return to desired running activities.

Progress through each stage of the graduated running program is determined by BSI provocation. If an athlete is able to complete a session with no BSI symptoms and they do not experience latent symptoms, they can progress to the next level during the ensuing session. However, if BSI symptoms are experienced during or after a session, the athlete must stop the session and at the next session return to the last level they were able to successfully complete.

Sports injuries: overuse — CHAPTER 4

Table 4.7 Graduated running program to return a runner to 30 minutes of pain-free running[12]

Stage 0	Pre-entry to graduated running program	
	Pain during walking in normal ADLs	
Stage 1	**Initial loading and jogging (50% normal pace) with increasing duration**	
Level	A	Walk 30 minutes
	B	Rest
	C	Walk 9 minutes and jog 1 minute (x3)
	D	Rest
	E	Walk 8 minutes and jog 2 minutes (x3)
	F	Rest
	G	Walk 7 minutes and jog 3 minutes (x3)
	H	Rest
	I	Walk 6 minutes and jog 4 minutes (x3)
	J	Rest
	K	Walk 4 minutes and jog 6 minutes (x3)
	L	Rest
	M	Walk 2 minutes and jog 8 minutes (x3)
	N	Rest
Stage 2	**Running with increasing intensity**	
Level	A	Jog 30 minutes
	B	Rest
	C	Run 30 minutes at 60% normal pace
	D	Rest
	E	Run 30 minutes at 60% normal pace
	F	Rest
	G	Run 30 minutes at 70% normal pace
	H	Rest
	I	Run 30 minutes at 80% normal pace
	J	Rest
	K	Run 30 minutes at 90% normal pace
	L	Rest
	M	Run 30 minutes at full pace
	N	Rest
Stage 3	**Running on consecutive days**	
Level	A	Run 30 minutes at full pace
	B	Run 30 minutes at full pace
	C	Rest
	D	Run 30 minutes at full pace
	E	Run 30 minutes at full pace
	F	Rest
	G	Run 30 minutes at full pace
Stage 4	**Return to running**	

Using a graduated loading program that is strictly guided by pain, the athlete and clinician can facilitate recovery while being relatively confident that there is no pathology progression. This requires the full understanding of the athlete regarding the appropriate progression through the program and adherence to the set pain levels. Patients with lower grade BSIs may be able to progress more quickly through a graduated loading program and the total duration of their program may be reduced from that outlined. Program duration should be based on the expected time course for recovery and, thus, all patients should perform individualised programs.

Anti-gravity treadmill training

When available, an anti-gravity treadmill may initially be used in the place of overground running as anti-gravity treadmill training may allow an athlete to run at higher intensities earlier during recovery, but with lower bone loading. Thereby, anti-gravity treadmill training can be used to maintain fitness while protecting the BSI site. Anti-gravity treadmills consist of a treadmill with an air-filled pressure-controlled chamber that surrounds the lower half of the body from the waist down. Pressure in the chamber is modulated to unweight the runner in 1% increments so that they are running with between 100% and 20% body weight.

Runners with a low-risk BSI can start anti-gravity treadmill training once they are pain-free during walking and ADLs for at least a week. A typical starting point is to jog every other day three times for five minutes with between 50% and 70% body weight and one-minute recovery between repetitions. This is performed for an initial week to acclimatise to anti-gravity treadmill training while symptoms are monitored for provocation. How to progress from this initial stage is currently somewhat of an art rather than a science; however, a proposed progression is, over the next 2 weeks, to increase the duration of each run to a total of 20–30 minutes, the body weight percentage by 5–10% and the running speed.[76] The progression continues thereafter as long as there are no BSI symptoms until the athlete is running at their usual speed and duration with 90% body weight. Once this is achieved, ground running is introduced and relatively quickly progressed over a couple of weeks to normal durations and intensities.

Running gait retraining

Despite a slow, progressive return to a running program, the persistence of faulty mechanics may hinder the healing process or contribute to elevated risk for a repeat injury. Therefore, it is important to identify and address any underlying mechanics when treating a runner with a BSI. Using the hypothesis that bone loading is directly related to GRF and acceleration parameters, interventions that reduce GRFs and shock during running gait may represent a means of decreasing BSI risk. By reducing the magnitude and rate of bone loading, the number of loading cycles until microdamage accumulation and fatigue failure may be increased. A number of gait retraining techniques are currently being investigated to reduce bone loading during running, including:

- the use of accelerometer-based biofeedback to encourage reductions in loading magnitude and rate[77, 78]
- increasing stride rate to reduce stride length and, subsequently, vertical excursion and velocity of the centre of mass, and GRFs and tibial accelerations[79-81]
- modifying initial contact to encourage a more forefoot, rather than heel or rearfoot, strike pattern.[82, 83]

These gait retraining techniques should not be taken lightly. Athletes have typically been running with their particular gait pattern for many years and the ability of an athlete's musculoskeletal system to adapt to the nuances of their particular gait should not be underestimated. However, a history of repeat BSIs and the accumulating loss of running time is a sign that gait retraining should be considered. In doing so, it must be remembered that, when inducing a change in gait, there is always the potential of altering injury risk at an alternative site. Thus, transitioning to a new running gait should be performed slowly and may be benefited by a preconditioning program.

Running program design

Incrementing a training program too rapidly or frequently relative to an athlete's usual activities can contribute to the generation of a BSI by upsetting the balance between bone microdamage formation and its removal. Unfortunately, there is no accepted algorithm for how much an individual can modify their training program before excessively heightening their BSI risk. The historical rule of thumb has been to change a training program by no more than 10% per week to reduce injury risk. However, this 'rule' is not generalisable on an individual basis, with different runners being able to tolerate more or less change before development of an injury.[84]

In order to provide an athlete returning from a BSI with appropriate advice regarding the design and advancement of their running program, it is important that they recall as much as they can of their pre-injury training regime. This should include information on changes in any feature that may have altered the load being introduced to the skeleton, including training intensity, duration, frequency, type, surface, technique, shoes and so on. In addition, recovering athletes should be encouraged to maintain a training diary containing these data, to not only track their training progress, but also to provide reliable data regarding their training program for future reference.

In addition to the obvious limiting of the magnitude and number of training variables changed at any one given time, the use of cyclic training methods should be encouraged. Cyclic training may involve the introduction of rest periods into a training program, or the replacement of overground training sessions with lower bone-loading activities such as deep-water running or anti-gravity treadmill training. This may involve a monthly regime of 3 weeks of training and 1 week of rest or low-load activities.

Healing of bone stress injuries

Healing is assessed clinically by the absence of local tenderness and functionally by the ability to perform the precipitating activity without pain. It is not useful to attempt to monitor healing with X-ray or radioisotopic bone scan.[85] CT scan appearances of healing stress fractures can be deceptive as in some cases the fracture is still visible well after clinical healing has occurred.[86] Figure 4.9 shows the relationship between imaging appearance and the various stages of bone stress.

Osteitis and periostitis

Osteitis (impaction trauma or primary inflammation of bone) and periostitis (abnormal histological appearance of periosteal collagen) are also considered overuse injuries. The condition known as osteitis pubis occurs in the pubic bones of the pelvis and is characterised by deep-seated pain and tenderness of the symphysis pubis with generalised increased uptake on the radioisotopic bone

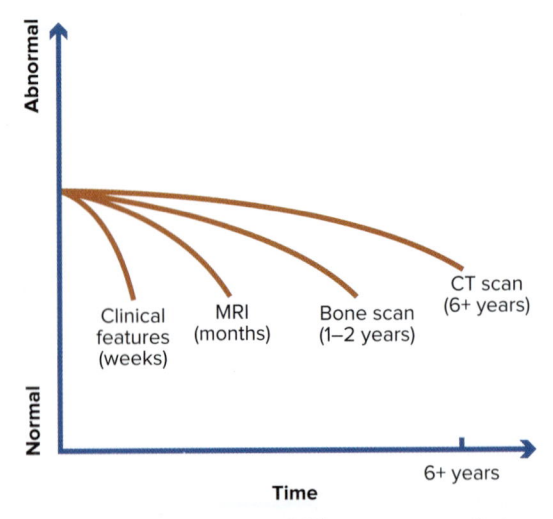

Figure 4.9 MRI, bone scan and CT scan return to their normal appearance well after clinical union occurs

scan. The exact pathogenesis of this injury remains in debate (Chapter 32).

Periostitis occurs commonly, mainly at the medial border of the tibia, a condition often known as 'shin splints'. In this condition, tenderness along the medial border of the tibia at the interface between the muscles and their bony attachments corresponds with an area of increased uptake on the bone scan.

The treatment of periostitis consists of local symptomatic therapy as well as unloading the muscle contraction on the periosteum. In the shin, strain may be reduced by altering the biomechanics through controlling excessive pronation. Soft tissue therapy and stretching may also be effective.

Apophysitis

Bony injury may occur at the attachment of the strong, large tendons to the growth areas. This condition is called 'apophysitis' and the most common examples are Osgood-Schlatter disease at the attachment of the patellar tendon to the tibial tuberosity and Sever's disease at the attachment of the Achilles tendon to the calcaneus. A full description of apophysitis is given in Chapter 44.

ARTICULAR CARTILAGE

Overuse injury can affect the articular cartilage lining of joints, particularly in osteoarthritis. Changes range from microscopic inflammatory changes to softening, fibrillation, fissuring and, ultimately, to gross visible changes. In younger people, this pathology can arise at the patella (patellofemoral syndrome), but it is important to note that the pain of patellofemoral syndrome can occur in the presence of normal joint surfaces. This very common condition is discussed in Chapter 36.

JOINT

Inflammatory changes in joints associated with overuse are classified as synovitis or capsulitis. Examples of these problems are the sinus tarsi syndrome of the subtalar joint and synovitis of the hip joint.

Impingement syndromes occur when a bony abnormality, either congenital or acquired, causes two bony surfaces to impinge on each other (e.g. femoro-acetabular impingement at hip, posterior impingement at ankle) or impinge on a structure passing between them (e.g. supraspinatus tendon in shoulder) causing damage to that structure. Treatment requires either removal of the structural abnormality or modification of biomechanics to relieve the impingement.

LIGAMENT

Overuse injuries of ligaments are uncommon, but may occur as a result of excessive load.

Injury to the medial ulnar collateral ligament of the elbow in baseball pitchers is the most common ligamentous overuse injury.[87]

MUSCLE

Muscle may respond to overuse in a number of ways, including myofascial pain, chronic compartment syndromes and exercise-induced muscle soreness.

Myofascial pain: trigger points or just sore spots of unknown origin?

The clinical phenomenon of localised palpatory muscle pain is one that is well known to sports medicine practitioners. The concept of myofascial pain caused by trigger points is a popular explanatory model with several putative pathophysiological mechanisms having been proposed to explain these findings.

The trigger point model

The myofascial trigger point theory was pioneered by Travell and Simons over 30 years ago.[88] The theory postulated by Travell and Simons has, until recent times, had widespread acceptance. Trigger points are classified as either active or latent, with only active trigger points being symptomatic. Active trigger points are thought to be tender to palpation, generate a local twitch response on stimulation and create a predictable pattern of referred pain on compression.

The term myofascial pain syndrome is commonly used to describe the clinical signs thought to represent active trigger points. As per Travell's original description, this is characterised by:

1. localised areas of deep muscle tenderness or hyperirritability, referred to as 'trigger points'–palpable taut bands within the muscle associated with muscle inhibition, intolerance to stretch, as well as autonomic symptoms such as vasoconstriction or dilation
2. a predictable, discrete reference zone of deep aching pain which is worsened by palpation of the trigger point. This may be located in the immediate region of or remote from, the trigger point.

Dommerholt expanded on Travell's theory, postulating a role for excessive release of acetylcholine from dysfunctional neuromuscular endplates, causing taut bands and subsequent muscle ischaemia. This muscle ischaemia was thought to precipitate an energy crisis in the muscle, causing the release of pro-inflammatory molecules, thereby activating nociceptive neurons.[89] Newer theories currently subject to research include the principle of neurogenic inflammation leading to sensitisation of innervated muscle,[90] secondary allodynia secondary to irritation of deeper structures such as ligament or bone (central sensitisation),[91] descending inhibitory pain modulation,[92] and diffuse noxious inhibitory control.[93]

Despite the abundance of hypothesised theories regarding the pathophysiology of myofascial trigger points, their existence is not widely accepted in the medical literature. Furthermore, much of the research to date is limited by significant methodological flaws.[90] Consequently, despite many years of research endeavour, the diagnosis, treatment and pathophysiological mechanisms underlying localised palpatory muscle pain remains an area of vigorous debate.[90, 94] Despite this, the lack of definitive anatomical or biochemical evidence has not prevented the concept of trigger points from achieving popularity among sports and musculoskeletal medicine clinicians.

While many alternative hypotheses of myofascial trigger points have been proposed since Travell's original description, none have been widely accepted. Consequently, there are no generally accepted diagnostic criteria for myofascial trigger points.[95] Meakins articulated a key component of this controversy by coining the term 'sore spots of unknown origin'.[92] This reflects the unreliability of identifying taut bands in skeletal muscle[96-99] while acknowledging the acceptable reliability of localising muscle tenderness based on patient feedback, presumably through the removal of the subjective phenomenon of palpatory pareidolia.[100]

A diagnosis of trigger points causing pain must only be made following the appropriate exclusion of alternative diagnoses. Failure to respond to appropriate treatment should necessitate a review of the diagnosis.

Pain from trigger points

The onset of pain from trigger points may follow either an acute or subacute pattern. Some patients may be able to recall the onset of pain, often noting a precipitating event, while others will report a gradual onset of pain over time. Where a precipitating event is recalled, the initial amplitude of pain is often only minor, with a subsequent progressive increase over time.

In contrast, the onset of pain due to acute mechanical tissue trauma, as with a ruptured ankle ligament, displays a very rapid onset to near maximal severity (though exceptions such as meniscal tears do exist). Subacute onset trigger point pain may be more difficult to identify on history, as patients often present following many months of pain. In this situation, identification of aetiological or exacerbating factors, such as inappropriate loads or sustained postures, is useful.

Fluctuations in pain, over the course of a day or longer periods, are typical of trigger points and suggestive that acute tissue trauma is not involved. Fluctuations usually follow particular events, such as lying on a particular side in bed or computer-based work. This is quite distinct from the diurnal variation as seen in inflammatory conditions. While the pain of trigger points has a different temporal pattern to that of tissue trauma, it is important to note that trigger points are often secondary to and therefore frequently coexist with acute tissue trauma.

The spatial distribution of pain also differs between that of trigger points and localised tissue trauma. Travell describes predictable referred pain patterns attributed to myofascial trigger points,[97] derived from the injection of hypertonic saline into muscle. As referred pain tends to be poorly localised, patients often indicate the location of referred pain with a wave of the hand. Direct stimulation of tissue nociceptors in contrast, as may occur with a ligament rupture, typically results in more precisely located pain, able to be indicated with a pointed finger.

Clinical features

Recent years have seen attempts to utilise medical imaging techniques in the detection of myofascial trigger points. Unique features of localised elliptical hypoechogenicity corresponding to palpable findings have been demonstrated with sonoelastography,[98-100] while magnetic resonance elastography has demonstrated the ability to identify increased tissue stiffness in muscle.[101, 102] A lack of control groups in this research, however, limits the ability to draw firm conclusions regarding the role of myofascial trigger points in these findings.

While Travell describes palpable taut bands in muscle as a diagnostic feature of trigger points,[97] several controlled studies have found this finding to be unreliable and therefore not recommended.[103-106]

In contrast, the identification of localised muscle tenderness based on patient feedback has shown acceptable inter-examiner reliability,[96] presumably by removing the subjective phenomenon of palpatory pareidolia. Thus, on the basis of existing research, the clinical identification of trigger points should be based primarily on localisation of maximally tender points within muscle. Consideration also may be given to the reproduction of any referred pain patterns.

Treatment

Evidence for the effectiveness of trigger point treatments is inconclusive.[107] Despite widespread anecdotal reports of effectiveness, systematic reviews and blinded randomised placebo-controlled studies show no clinical worthwhile effect of these treatments over sham, standard care or exercise therapy.[108-110] The apparent contradiction between the anecdotal experience of many clinicians and research findings may be explained by the phenomenon of the localised twitch response, an involuntary localised transient contraction within the muscle being treated. Many experienced practitioners elicit multiple twitch responses when treating a muscle. In contrast, much of the research conducted on trigger point therapy has not placed any emphasis on the localised twitch response, failing to account for its presence or absence in findings of efficacy.

A variety of methods of treating trigger points have been described in the literature, with the most effective method unclear. These include spray and stretch, digital ischaemic pressuring, dry needling, wet needling, proprioceptive neuromuscular facilitation and muscular 'stripping'. Published research on these methods is frequently sparse, confounded by methodological limitations or both.

The most rigorously researched of the above methods are dry needling, wet needling and digital ischaemic pressure. Wet needling is generally considered to be at least equal to alternative methods. In many jurisdictions, however, injection therapy is limited to appropriately qualified medical practitioners. The application of dry needling has been shown to be a reasonable alternative. Subsequent digital ischaemic pressure applied immediately following needling therapy may further improve efficacy.

Dry needling and other techniques used in the treatment of trigger points are discussed in Chapter 17.

Chronic compartment syndrome

Chronic compartment syndrome (CCS) refers to the intermittent and reversible pathologic elevation of compartment pressures following exertion.[111] The condition usually affects the lower leg but may also occur in the forearm in the sports of tennis, rock climbing and weightlifting.[112]

The muscles of the lower leg are divided into a number of compartments by fascial sheaths, which are relatively inelastic thickenings of collagenous tissue. Exercise raises the intracompartmental pressure and may cause local muscle swelling and accumulation of fluid in the interstitial spaces. The tight fascia prevents expansion. This impairs the blood supply and causes pain with exertion. Compression of neurological structures may also contribute to the clinical presentation. Muscle hypertrophy may also precipitate CCS.

The main symptom of CCS is pain that commences during activity and ceases with rest. This differs from other overuse injuries such as tendinopathies, where pain may be present with initial exercise, then diminish as the affected area warms up, only to return following cessation of activity. The role of imaging in the diagnosis of CCS is unclear.[113]

The gold standard for diagnosis of CCS has always been measurement of compartment pressures at rest and during pain-provoking exercise. Compartment pressure testing is described in Chapter 15. In recent years, various authors have expressed reservations regarding the reliability and validity of these tests.[114-116]

Surgical treatment–fasciotomy (release of the fascia) or fasciectomy (removal of the fascia)–has always been the mainstay of treatment of compartment syndromes. Results of surgery are often disappointing with a high incidence of recurrence of exercise-related leg pain. The role of surgery is now being questioned.[117]

A biomechanical basis of the exercise-related leg pain has been suggested by Franklyn-Miller,[118] and changes in running gait has shown promising initial results in the management of these patients.[119]

Exercise-induced muscle soreness

Exercise-induced muscle soreness is a common complaint during or immediately following vigorous unaccustomed exercise. Muscle soreness that develops 24–48 hours after unaccustomed high-intensity activity is known as delayed onset muscle soreness (DOMS). DOMS appears to be more severe after activities that involve eccentric muscle contractions; that is, when muscle contracts whilst simultaneously lengthening. Activities that involve both high muscle forces and eccentric muscle contractions, such as skiing and downhill running, are a common cause of DOMS in untrained individuals.

The exact cause of acute exercise-induced muscle soreness and DOMS is unclear. Although debate in the literature about the mechanism of muscle soreness is ongoing, the general consensus is that the soreness is caused by microtrauma of muscle cells and connective tissue. Microtrauma is followed by a local inflammatory process within the extracellular space which sensitises nerve endings via mechanical, chemical or thermal stimulation.[120-122]

Signs and symptoms

Exercise-induced muscle soreness is often accompanied by muscle stiffness, ache and mild cramping. Symptoms can persist for several hours post exercise before resolving.[121] DOMS is characterised by tenderness on palpation and a sense of stiffness with physical activity. Soreness can peak around 48 hours after exercise. Resolution of symptoms can take up to 10 days.[120] Soreness can vary from mild discomfort to incapacitating pain; this is largely dependent on the intensity and volume of training, as well as the actual inducing event.

Importantly, DOMS can be associated with muscle strength deficits, which may affect physical performance. Strength deficits associated with DOMS are typically greatest between 24 and 48 hours after activity.[123, 124] A reduction in muscle power and reduced joint range of motion may also affect an athlete's performance. Local muscle swelling and intracellular proteins in the blood are also common signs.[120, 123-125] Exercise-induced muscle soreness and DOMS are often associated with elevated levels of creatine kinase in the blood. However, given the self-limiting nature of acute muscle soreness and DOMS, blood tests are rarely warranted and the clinical interpretation of such tests is unclear.[125]

Management

Management strategies in the treatment of DOMS focus on encouraging healing and recovery of the inflamed and damaged muscle tissue. Intense exercise during the symptomatic period can potentially cause more micro-trauma and muscle injury, particularly as strength, power and coordination of movement are compromised. Therefore, during the symptomatic period, training and competition performance should be modified accordingly.

Common modalities used to treat exercise-induced muscle soreness and DOMS include massage, cryotherapy, stretching and active recovery. The management of DOMS is described in Chapter 13.

Prevention of exercise-induced muscle soreness and delayed onset muscle soreness

Prevention of exercise-induced muscle soreness should be centred on a properly planned training program, which adequately addresses strength, power, endurance and quality of movement. Adequate periods of training and conditioning are needed before individuals participate in strenuous activity to ensure the exercise-induced muscle soreness is minimised and more serious injuries are prevented. DOMS occurs less in those who train regularly, although even trained individuals may become sore after an unaccustomed exercise bout. There is little evidence to support the use of static stretching to prevent acute muscle soreness and DOMS.[121] Variable results have been shown with preventative approaches such as the use of vitamins C and E and protein supplements.[126] Understanding an athlete's current training volume including exercise intensity, duration, rate of progression and recovery will provide a context for understanding and preventing future episodes of muscle soreness.

TENDON
Tendon overuse injury (tendinopathy)

with JILL COOK, CRAIG PURDAM

Tendon overuse injuries provide a major proportion of the sports clinician's workload. The clinical presentation is straightforward in many cases–the patient presents with tendon pain during or after activity (Table 4.8) and loading tests demonstrate increased pain with increased load.

In the 1980s, the underlying pathology was often referred to as 'tendinitis'–this was associated with a belief that cellular inflammation contributed to the pathological process. Histopathological studies in the 1990s indicated that inflammatory cells were absent in patients who underwent surgery for tendon pain. Recently, low levels of inflammatory cells and markers have been demonstrated, but it is unlikely that inflammation is a key driver of tendon pathology and a resident cell-driven process remains the best-supported pathoaetiology.

The pathological findings at surgery are consistent with 'tendinosis'. The boxed item illustrates tendon pathology–'tendinosis'–at the anatomical level (Fig. 4.10) and at two microscopic levels (Figs. 4.11 and 4.12). The pathology is also summarised in Table 4.9.

A contemporary model of a continuum of tendon pathology

Tendon authorities Jill Cook and Craig Purdam have proposed that tendon pathology should be considered as a continuum.[127] They contend that the dichotomy of 'normal' and 'degenerative tendinosis' is too simplistic. Importantly, their three-part classification has implications for treatment, and so it is summarised here and illustrated (Fig. 4.13).

Stage 1. Reactive tendinopathy

This refers to the non-inflammatory response of tendon cells and matrix proteins to an acute tensile or compressive overload. Tendon cells become activated and may proliferate in this stage–they become more prominent–consistent with the appearance of cells that

Table 4.8 Clinical presentation of patients with overuse tendon pain (tendinosis)

- Pain after exercise or, more frequently, the following morning upon rising.
- It can be pain-free at rest and initially becomes more painful with use.
- Athletes can 'run through' the pain or the pain disappears when they warm up, only to return after exercise when they cool down.
- Athletes are able to continue to train fully in the early stages of the condition; this may interfere with the healing process.
- Examination reveals local tenderness and/or thickening.
- Frank swelling and crepitus may be present, although crepitus is more usually a sign of associated tenosynovitis (it is not 'inflammatory fluid').

Sports injuries: overuse   CHAPTER 4

Tendinosis: what is it?

This box illustrates the pathology found at end-stage tendinopathy—when symptoms have been present for at least 3 months. The illustration (Fig. 4.10) is based on pathological specimens (Figs 4.11 and 4.12) obtained at surgery for chronic sports-related tendon pain.

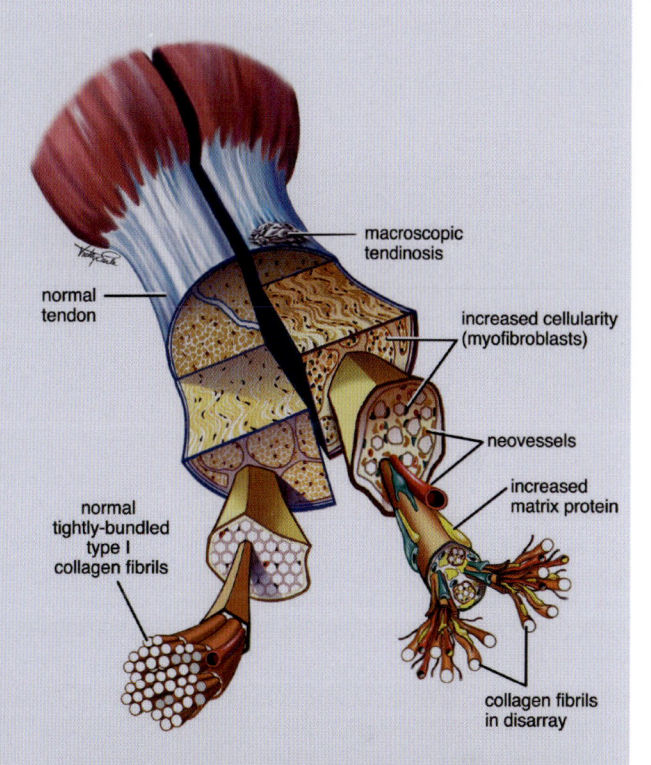

Figure 4.10 The contrasting features of normal tendon (left side) and tendinosis (right side). Characteristic features at this macroscopic level are the collagen fibres of different sizes in disarray, abnormal cell numbers (decreased and increased), abnormally prominent blood vessels and an increase in matrix proteins

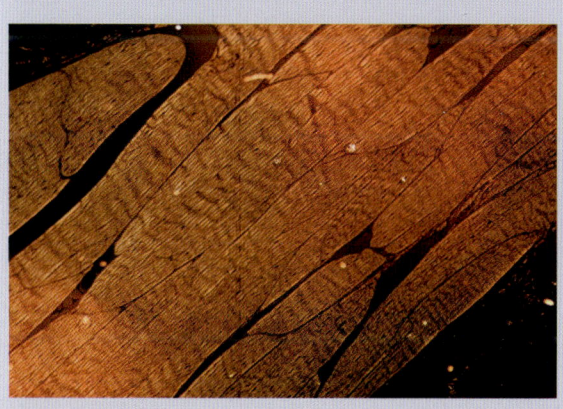

(a) (b)

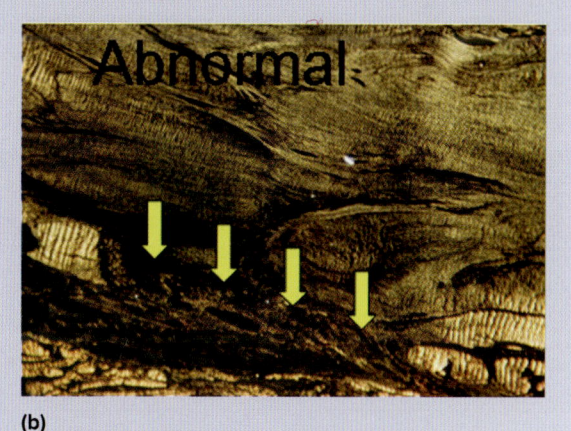

Figure 4.11 Under polarised light microscopy: (a) normal tendon has tightly bundled parallel collagen fibrils with a characteristic golden reflectivity; (b) a specimen from a patient with chronic patellar tendinopathy showing collagen fibril separation and frank discontinuity within some fibrils

continued

PART A Fundamental principles

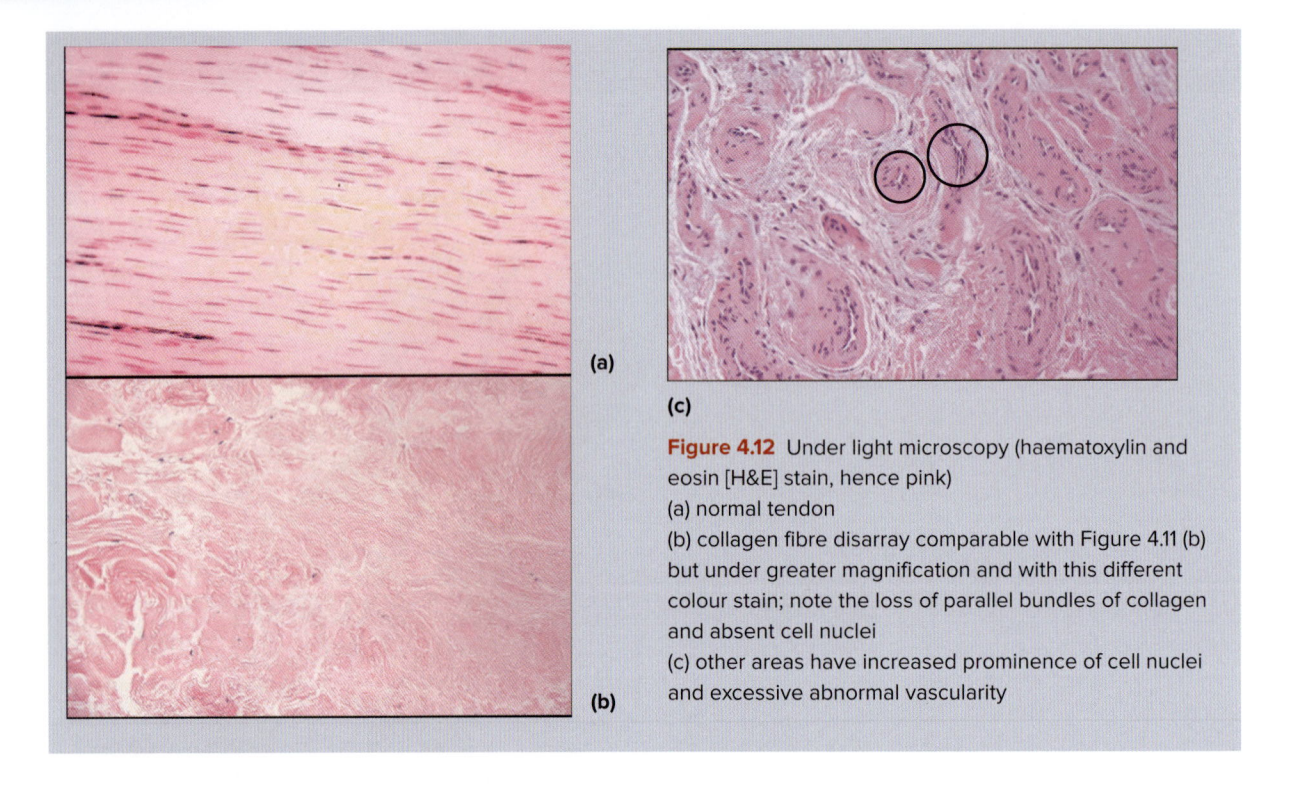

Figure 4.12 Under light microscopy (haematoxylin and eosin [H&E] stain, hence pink)
(a) normal tendon
(b) collagen fibre disarray comparable with Figure 4.11 (b) but under greater magnification and with this different colour stain; note the loss of parallel bundles of collagen and absent cell nuclei
(c) other areas have increased prominence of cell nuclei and excessive abnormal vascularity

Table 4.9 Five elements of normal tendon compared with the characteristic elements of end-stage tendon overuse injury

Tendon element	Normal tendon	Changes that occur in response to excessive tendon loading
Cells—tenocytes	Tendon cells are spindle-shaped and nuclei cluster in longitudinal chains on microscopy	Tissue has proliferation of cells with abnormally rounded nuclei (Fig. 4.12c) and areas with fewer than normal cell numbers (Fig. 4.12b)
Ground substance or 'matrix' proteins	The ground substance in the matrix is minimal and is not visible when stained for light microscopic viewing	Increased amount of ground substance/matrix proteins which stain and are visible under light microscopy
Collagen	Linear and tightly bundled and has a characteristic crimp under polarised light	Disrupted—both longitudinally and in its bundles (Fig. 4.12b)
Nerves	Minimal intratendinous nerves, some innervation of connective tissue in and around the tendon	Abnormal ingrowth of nerves (mostly sympathetic) and a preponderance of neuropeptides
Vessels	Minimal vascularity when examined histologically or by using ultrasound	Prominent vessels histologically or using ultrasound (Fig. 4.12c)

are producing repair proteins, especially proteoglycans. This results in a short-term thickening of a portion of the tendon that reduces stress. This differs from the normal tendon adaptation to tensile load that generally occurs through tendon stiffening with little change in thickness. This is seen clinically in the acutely overloaded tendon and is more common in the younger person. It also arises when there is trauma to a tendon, such as a direct blow.

At this stage, both ultrasound and MRI show mild fusiform swelling–greater tendon diameter with little disruption of the collagen fascicles. The change in imaging appearance is mainly derived from the increase in bound water within the matrix proteins (proteoglycans).

Sports injuries: overuse — CHAPTER 4

will reveal more focal changes of hypoechogenicity on ultrasound. There may be a mild increase in vascularity on colour or Doppler ultrasound. MRI reveals a swollen tendon with increased signal.

Stage 3. Degenerative tendinopathy
This is the stage that is present in patients who undergo surgery for chronic tendon pain–it is the 'end stage' of tendon overuse injury. The matrix and cell changes described in stages 1 and 2 may progress so that areas of apoptosis (absent cell nuclei due to cell death) are evident. Large areas of matrix are disordered and filled with cells, vessels, matrix breakdown products and disordered type I, II and III collagen. The structure of the tendon is heterogeneous–degenerative pathology is interspersed between other stages of pathology and normal tendon.

This pathology exists in the older person, or the younger person or elite athlete with long-term tendon overload. Typically, it is seen in a middle-aged, recreational athlete with focal tendon swelling and pain (e.g. mid-Achilles region). The tendon may have focal nodular areas with or without general thickening. This is the type of tendon that may rupture if the degenerative pathology is extensive.

In this stage, compromised matrix and vascular changes are obvious on ultrasound scans as hypoechogenic regions with few reflections from collagen fascicles. Larger vessels are usually prominent on Doppler ultrasound. MRI shows increased tendon size and intratendinous signal. The changes are more focal than spread throughout the tendon.

Reactive on degenerative tendon
Degenerative tendinopathy exists in a tendon that has normal tissue. When these tendons are overloaded, the degenerative part of the tendon is unlikely to take load because of a lack of matrix structure, so the load is borne by the normal part of the tendon. Overload can induce a reactive change in this normal tendon, resulting in a reactive on degenerative tendon.

Other terms associated with overuse tendon injuries
Although the most-used clinical label for tendon overuse injuries is 'tendinopathy' as above and is used in specific chapters of this book (i.e. Achilles tendinopathy), the terms 'paratenonitis', 'partial tear' and 'tendinitis' need definition.

Paratenonitis
This term includes peritendinitis, tenosynovitis (single layer of areolar tissue covering the tendon) and tenovaginitis (double-layered tendon sheath). This

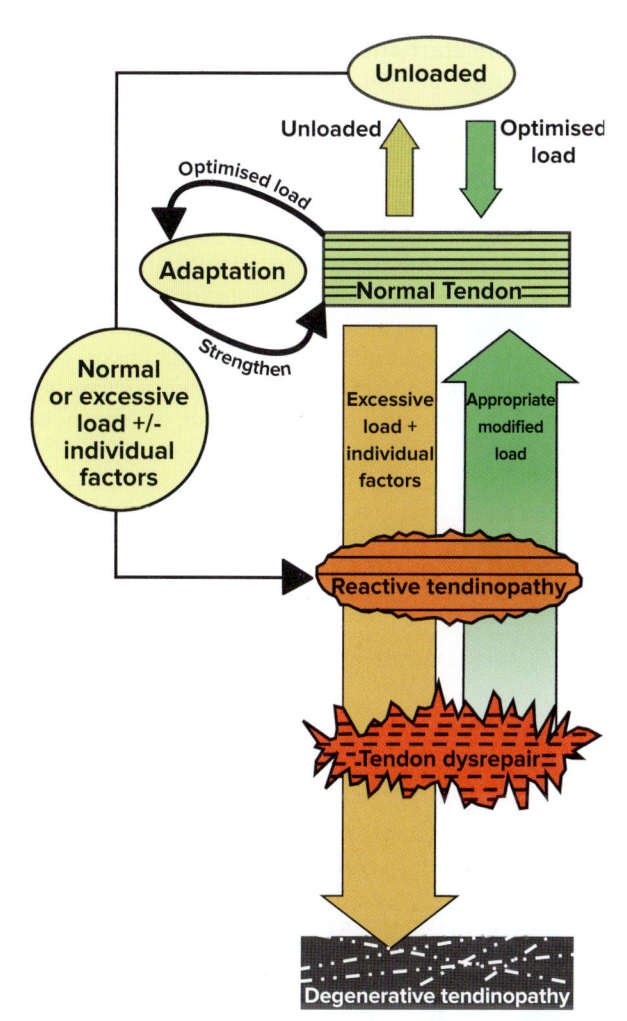

Figure 4.13 The Cook–Purdam model to help clinicians understand the relationship between loading/unloading and the several stages of tendon pathology
REDRAWN FOR *CLINICAL SPORTS MEDICINE*. REPRODUCED WITH PERMISSION FROM *BRITISH JOURNAL OF SPORTS MEDICINE*[127]

Stage 2. Tendon dysrepair
This describes a worsening tendon pathology with greater matrix breakdown. Tendon cells are more prominent and take on a rounded appearance (chondrocytic). Protein production increases–both matrix proteoglycans and collagen. As a result of these changes, collagen separates and the matrix becomes somewhat disorganised. The disruption of the matrix may allow for some ingrowth of vessels and nerves.

This is seen clinically in overloaded tendons in the young, but it may appear across a spectrum of ages and loading environments. The transition from the previous stage may be difficult to detect clinically, but imaging

PART A Fundamental principles

occurs in situations where the tendon rubs over a bony prominence and/or where repeated movement directly irritates the paratenon. Uncommonly, it can coexist with partial tears and tendinosis.

Partial tears
The term 'partial tear of a tendon' should be reserved for a macroscopically evident subcutaneous partial tear of a tendon, an uncommon acute, not overuse, injury, at least in the Achilles and patellar tendon (see Chapter 3). The distinction on imaging between tendon degeneration and partial tear is difficult because there are no definite signs that allow a clear distinction and diagnosis is reliant on radiologist expertise.

Principles of rehabilitating lower limb tendinopathy
Before starting
Ensure that the diagnosis is correct and the pain is from the tendon. Tendon pain will respond best to the loading program described.

Decide the start and end of the program
Start at the functional level and capacity of the person. This can be determined from a comprehensive examination of function and its relationship to pain. The program should end at the functional level required for the person to return to their desired activity level. This can be determined from their history; both the sport that the person has been involved in as well as the sport or activity and level they want to return to. The sport and the level will determine how much endurance is required for the tendon, associated muscle and kinetic chain.

A schematic of tendon rehabilitation, improving tendon capacity with progressive loads, is shown in Figure 4.14.[128]

Stages of rehabilitation
Stage 1. Isometric exercise
Isometrics are a great way to relieve tendon pain, hence a good spot to start as most clinical presentations are for tendon pain. Isometric exercises result in pain relief in

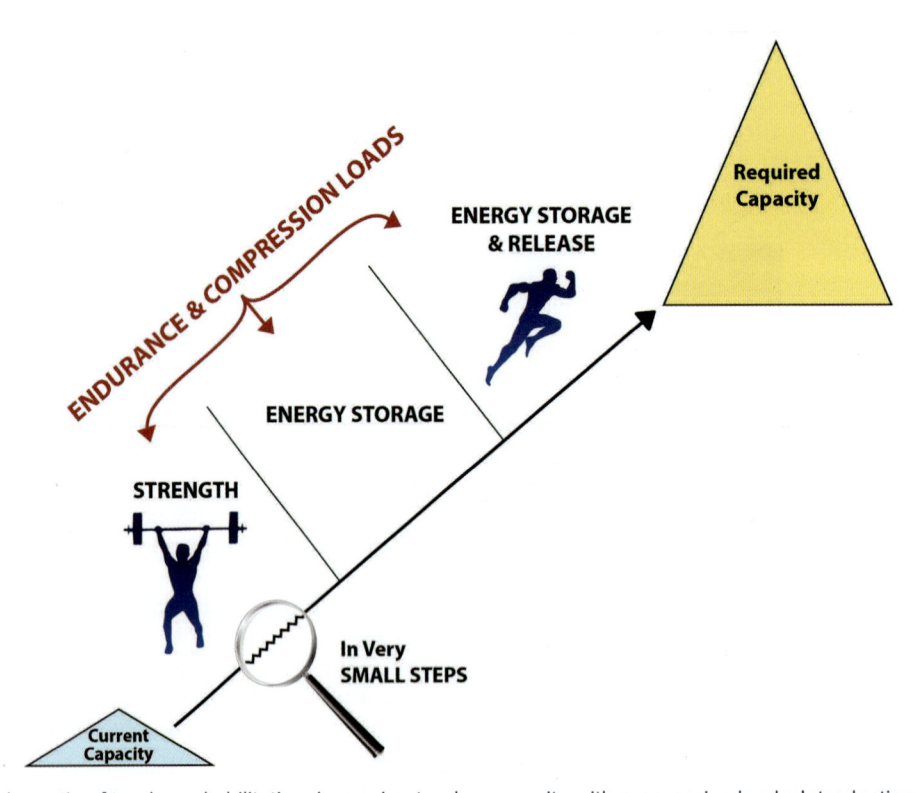

Figure 4.14 Schematic of tendon rehabilitation, improving tendon capacity with progressive loads. Introduction and progression of endurance and compressive loads are critical within each stage. The start and end points of rehabilitation will vary between individuals
WITH PERMISSION FROM *BRITISH JOURNAL OF SPORTS MEDICINE*[128]

7-10 days in a reactive on degenerative tendon, but can take up to 6-8 weeks in a purely reactive tendon.

Isometrics have been shown to immediately relieve patellar tendon pain more than isotonic exercise and the pain relief was sustained for 45 minutes.[129] Rio et al. also showed in this study that isometric exercise normalised cortical inhibition that was excessive in patellar tendinopathy, whereas isotonic exercise had no effect on cortical inhibition.[129]

Clinically, isometrics are therefore used to manage pain in the reactive or reactive on degenerative phase of tendon pathology. The research protocol in young, jumping men was four repetitions of 45 second holds at 70% of maximal voluntary contraction and this level of loading is appropriate for the painful athletic tendon.[129] This level of loading may be too much for the older person with clinical tendinopathy, and varying both the load and time held is necessary. Using body weight loads for longer holds is a simple place to start and adding weights often requires equipment. As isometrics may need to be done more than once a day, doing them at home is the best option. Hiring gym equipment such as a seated calf raise for a few months can help adherence to regular isometric exercise.

Stage 2. Isotonic exercise

Once the pain has settled and/or is stable at a low level, isotonic exercises can be started. These are slow and heavy concentric/eccentric exercises directed at improving strength in the muscle tendon unit. These are best performed with a slightly longer eccentric component (e.g. three-second concentric, four-second eccentric) for brain plasticity. These should be performed for every muscle in the kinetic chain that has a functional deficit–most likely the anti-gravity muscles such as the calf (gastrocnemius and soleus), quadriceps and gluteal muscles. Hamstrings are clearly addressed as a priority in hamstring tendinopathy.

Isotonic exercises should be continued until there is good strength in the affected musculotendinous unit and the agonists in kinetic chain function. This can take up to 12 weeks in a profoundly unloaded limb. An endurance set is added if the person requires higher levels of endurance for their activity. Endurance can also be added with weight-bearing exercise, such as stair climbing for either Achilles or patellar tendinopathy.

> **PRACTICE PEARL**
>
> Performing a bout of isometrics before isotonic exercises increases maximum voluntary contraction, most likely due to cortical pain inhibition.[129]

Stage 3. Energy storage exercise

Once the muscles are stronger, the tendon can be loaded with energy storage exercises. To store energy in a tendon you need to do faster eccentric exercises, initially with a slower release (concentric phase), but building to stage 4 with quick energy storage and faster release. As these exercises place high loads on the tendon they are best completed only 2-3 times a week. These faster exercises need to be controlled in terms of numbers and/or time, started at a low level and gradually increased.

> **PRACTICE PEARL**
>
> It is essential to continue isotonic exercises at least two days a week throughout the entire rehabilitation program, as well as after the athlete has returned to full training and competition. Continued isometric loading before isotonic exercises may also be helpful throughout the whole program.

Stage 4. Sport-specific energy storage and release exercise

Once the tendon can tolerate high-energy storage loads, then functional activity-specific exercises can be introduced in a clinical setting. These will replace stage 3 exercises and can only be completed 2-3 times a week. Once the tendon is tolerant to training numbers of high-level functional activities then the person can return to a controlled training environment and from there to a graduated return to competition.

Enthesopathy

Enthesopathies occur at the bone-tendon junction, such as the Achilles tendon insertion onto the calcaneus. Enthesopathies are similar to tendinopathies in that they are primarily degenerative in nature. Treatment principles are the same.

BURSA

The body contains many bursae situated usually between bony surfaces and overlying tendons. Their role is to facilitate movement of the tendon over the bony surface. All bursae are susceptible to injury. Typically, injuries to bursae are overuse injuries resulting from excessive shearing and/or compressive forces.[130, 131]

Overuse injuries in bursae are quite common, particularly at the subacromial bursa,[132] the greater trochanteric bursa,[133] the bursa deep to the iliotibial band at the knee,[131, 133] and the retrocalcaneal bursa separating the Achilles tendon from the calcaneus.[134] Overuse pathologies affecting bursae commonly couple with other local pathologies such as tendinopathies and impingement syndromes.[135, 136] Symptoms include localised pain and swelling and typically increase with activity. Conservative approaches to treatment are often trialled first.

Treatment involves removal of irritating loads, reduction of inflammation and a progressive return to pain-free activity. Specific treatments including ice, electrical stimulation, iontophoresis and gentle stretching. Once initial inflammation subsides, a stretching and strengthening program for the surrounding tissues and muscles can commence. NSAIDs are widely prescribed for these conditions and corticosteroid injections, often guided by ultrasound, are considered where conservative approaches have failed.

NERVE

Nerve entrapment syndromes occur in athletes as a result of swelling in the surrounding soft tissues or anatomical abnormalities. These may affect the suprascapular nerve, the posterior interosseous, ulnar and median nerves in the forearm, the obturator nerve in the groin, the posterior tibial nerve at the tarsal tunnel on the medial aspect of the ankle and, most commonly, the interdigital nerves, especially between the third and fourth toes, a condition known as Morton's neuroma. This condition is not a true neuroma but rather a nerve compression. These nerve entrapments occasionally require surgical decompression.

Chronic mild irritation of a nerve may result in damage manifested by an increase in neural mechanosensitivity. These may be the primary cause of the patient's symptoms or may contribute to symptoms. This concept is discussed more fully in Chapters 5 and 6.

SKIN

The skin's integrity is constantly challenged by athletic activity, weather conditions and pathogenic organisms.

Blisters

The skin of many athletes is subjected to friction-related forces and compounded by perspiration.[137, 138] Exposure to shearing and compressive forces can lead to mechanical separation of the epidermal cell layers. Hydrostatic pressure causes further separation and allows plasma-like fluid or sweat into the space to form a blister.[137] The repair process starts 24 hours post incident and blisters generally heal in approximately five days.[137] Blisters may occur at any site of friction with an external source, such as shoes or sporting equipment.

Blisters are common in marathon runners, rowers, race walkers, triathletes, hikers and in military populations. Foot blisters are painful and can have an impact on sporting performance. Sock type, race, previous hiking or military experience and certain orthopaedic foot conditions predict the development of foot blisters in the military population.[138]

Foot blisters can be prevented by wearing-in new shoes, wearing socks and smearing petroleum jelly over the sock at sites of friction. Strategies to prevent blisters also serve to prevent callus. Symptomatic callus can be pared down with a scalpel blade, taking care not to lacerate the normal skin.

At the first sign of a blister, the aggravating source should be removed and either adhesive tape applied over the blistered area or blister pads should be applied. Blister pads prevent blisters by acting as a barrier between skin and shoe.

Treatment of blisters involves prevention of infection by the use of antiseptics and protection with sticking plaster. Fluid-filled blisters may be punctured and drained.

Skin infections

Almost any cutaneous infection can afflict athletes. However, their activities place these individuals at higher risk to develop and subsequently transmit their skin ailment to competitors. Athletes acquire infections as a result of their interaction with other athletes and with the environment in which they compete. An athlete's skin is often macerated from sweating which promotes common infections in sports including bacterial, fungal and viral infections, but parasites can also afflict the athlete.[139]

Dermatitis

An athlete's skin suffers repeated exposure to trauma, heat, moisture and numerous allergens and chemicals. These factors combine with other unique and less well-defined genetically predisposing factors in the athlete's skin to cause both allergic contact dermatitis (ACD) and irritant contact dermatitis (ICD). As with other cases of contact dermatitis, these eruptions in athletes present as a spectrum of acute to subacute to chronic dermatitis. Recognising the unique environmental irritants and allergens encountered by athletes is paramount to facilitate appropriate therapy and prevention.[140]

Skin cancers

Skin cancers are not true overuse injuries, but perhaps can be described as 'overexposure.' Nevertheless, athletes are particularly vulnerable as many sports involve prolonged exposure to sun during training and games.

The incidence of melanoma and non-melanoma skin cancers is increasing worldwide. Ultraviolet light exposure is the most important risk factor for cutaneous melanoma and non-melanoma skin cancers. Non-melanoma skin cancer includes basal cell carcinoma and squamous cell carcinoma. Constitutive skin colour and genetic factors, as well as immunological factors, play a role in the development of skin cancer. Ultraviolet light also causes sunburn and photoaging damage to the skin. Studies conducted within athletic populations have found that certain sports are associated with increased risk for skin cancers.[141]

Athletes should take care to avoid excessive exposure to ultraviolet light and in particular should avoid sunburn.

BUT IT'S NOT THAT SIMPLE

Although it is important to have a good understanding of the conditions outlined in this chapter and Chapter 3, three important additional components are necessary for successful management of patients with sporting injuries.

Pain: where is it coming from?

The pain your patient feels at a particular site may not necessarily be emanating from that site. It is essential to understand pain, which is the topic of Chapters 5 and 6.

Masquerades

There are many medical conditions whose presentation may mimic a sporting injury. While many of these conditions are relatively rare, it is nevertheless important to keep them at the back of your mind. If the clinical pattern does not seem to fit the obvious diagnosis, then think of the conditions that may masquerade as sporting injuries. These are described in Chapter 7.

The kinetic chain

Every athletic activity involves movements of joints and limbs in coordinated ways to perform a task. These activities include running, jumping, throwing, stopping or kicking. The tasks may include throwing a ball, hitting a ball, kicking a ball, jumping over an object, or propelling the body through air or water. Individual body segments and joints, collectively called links, must be moved in certain specific sequences to allow efficient accomplishment of the tasks.

The sequencing of the links is called the kinetic chain of an athletic activity.[142] Each kinetic chain has its own sequence but the basic organisation includes proximal to distal sequencing, a proximal base of support or stability, and successive activation of each segment of the link and each successive link. The net result is generation of force and energy in each link, summation of the developed force and energy through each of the links, and efficient transfer of the force and energy to the terminal link.

Injuries or adaptations in some areas of the kinetic chain can cause problems not only locally but distantly, as distal links must compensate for the lack of force and energy delivered through the more proximal links. This phenomenon, called catch-up, is both inefficient in the kinetic chain and dangerous to the distal link because it may cause more load or stress than the link can safely handle. These changes may result in anatomical or biomechanical situations that increase injury risk, perpetuate injury patterns or decrease performance. For example, a tennis player with stiffness of the lumbar spine may overload the rotator cuff muscles while serving to generate sufficient power and, thus, develop a tear of the rotator cuff muscles.

These deficits in the kinetic chain must be identified and corrected as part of the treatment and rehabilitation process. We will be constantly returning to the theme of the kinetic chain throughout the following chapters.

REFERENCES

References for this chapter can be found at www.mhhe.com/au/CSM5e

Chapter 5

Pain: why and how does it hurt?

by LORIMER MOSELEY

> *...then, [Mr Hammerhead Shark] his shirt covered in blood, spun around and hit his knee on the table, at which point he swore and yelled 'My knee! My knee!', the whole time unfussed about the hammer stuck in his neck.*
>
> G Lorimer Moseley, *Painful Yarns. Metaphors and stories to help understand the biology of pain*

Even the simplest biological organisms can protect themselves from threatening stimuli–by altering their path of movement away from the source of the threat.[1] As evolution has honed us into more and more sophisticated creatures, we have also honed this fundamental capacity to protect ourselves from threat. Indeed, perhaps our most sophisticated protective strategy is pain. In this chapter, some of the 'fearful and wonderful complexity' of pain is conveyed, by:

- outlining a contemporary definition of pain that is contrary to conventional definitions but which integrates the huge amount of research that has been undertaken since our conventional definitions were established
- introducing the idea of nociception and describing some of what is known about the biological mechanisms that underpin nociception
- providing a conceptual framework with which to make sense of pain within the context of clinical practice.

WHAT IS PAIN?

Almost everyone experiences pain. Those who do not experience pain, as the rest of us know it, are at a distinct disadvantage in life and are likely to die young without living fast. Pain is an unpleasant sensory and emotional experience that is felt in the body and motivates us to do something to escape it. These two characteristics of pain–its unpleasantness and its anatomical focus–are what makes it such an effective protector.

Pain alerts us to tissue damage or the threat thereof. Pain makes us seek care. Pain stops us competing, keeps us seeking a cure, compels us to prioritise pain relief above almost everything else. That's the rub–pain changes our behaviour. In fact, if the brain concludes that there is

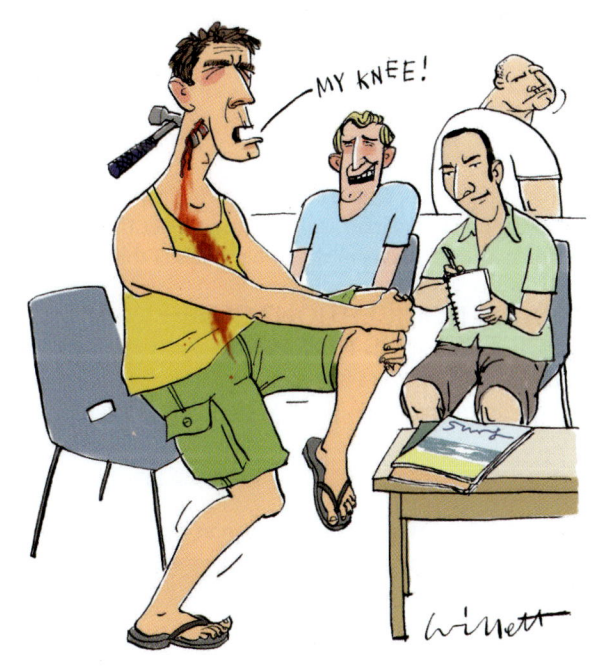

COURTESY OF MALCOLM WILLETT

something more important than protecting a body part then it makes the executive decision to *not* produce pain. Therein lies the key to really understanding pain; it is as simple and as difficult as this–if *the brain* concludes that a body part is in danger and needs protecting and you, the organism, ought to know about it, then *the brain* will make that body part hurt.[2]

There is a critical caveat here, one that was overlooked in the fourth edition of this book. This convention to ascribe pain to the brain is flawed, because a brain, on its own, almost certainly would not and probably could not, produce pain. This position has been criticised, with merit and additional pieces have been authored that critique it.[3] The caveat, then, is this: to attribute it all to the brain is simplistic and denies the role of physiological mechanisms that extend beyond the brain. However, as much as we know now, networks of brain cells (neuronal and non-neuronal) are the most obvious 'last step' and the emergence of consciousness (and therefore pain) is likely to be most closely related to their activation.

With that rather perplexing caveat out of the way, let's consider what is *good* about this concept of pain. This concept of pain integrates a vast body of basic, applied and clinical research. It differs greatly from conventional theories, which have changed little since the 17th century when René Descartes was ridiculed for suggesting that we were not made from four bodily humours.[4]

> **PRACTICE PEARL**
>
> The critical concept is that pain is not a measure of tissue damage, but an indicator of the brain's conviction about the need to protect certain tissue.

To better understand pain as the protective output of the brain, not as a marker of tissue damage, let us consider several contrasts between the two models (Table 5.1).

WHAT IS NOCICEPTION? CLUE—NOCICEPTION IS NOT PAIN!

At the risk of sounding a bit repetitive, let us start by saying that nociception is not pain. Nociception refers to the detection, transmission and processing of noxious stimuli. A noxious stimulus is one that is actually or potentially damaging. The neurons that detect noxious stimuli and transmit a nociceptive message to the spinal cord are called nociceptors ('danger receptors').

Nociceptors are high threshold neurons, which means that they respond to stimuli that are approaching or surpassing that which is damaging to the tissue in which the neuron resides. Nociceptors are mostly thin neurons and many are not myelinated. They fall into three nerve fibre types: Abeta (β)(fast, myelinated neurons), Adelta (slow, myelinated neurons), C (very slow, unmyelinated neurons; see [5] for full review).

Nociceptors are located in almost all the tissues of the body, with the notable exception of the brain. This network of neurons, can be considered a very thorough surveillance system. Of course, the surveillance function of the peripheral nervous system is much more comprehensive than nociceptors alone—it is just that nociceptors are always surveying the anatomical landscape for dangerous events. All such events fall into one or more of three categories: thermal, chemical or mechanical. Thus, nociceptors have specialised receptors in their cell walls that are cold-sensitive, hot-sensitive, chemosensitive or mechanosensitive.

Humans have low-threshold neurons that are solely interested in one modality or another, such as thermo-sensitive Aβ fibres, which inform brainstem areas of even tiny fluctuations in tissue temperature—fluctuations that are well within a safe operating range. In contrast, nociceptors are most often bimodal or multimodal. That is, they are responsive to thermal and mechanical input, or to thermal, mechanical and chemical input. These nociceptors, which are situated in the tissues of

Table 5.1 Contrasts between (a) pain as a protective output of the brain and (b) pain as a marker of tissue damage

A Pain as a protective output of the brain	B Pain as a marker of tissue damage
Pain is in consciousness.	Damage is in the body.
One cannot be in pain and not know about it.	One can be severely damaged and not know about it.
No brain, no pain.	No body, no damage.
Pain is affected by what else is at stake.	Damage is not affected by what else is at stake.
Pain is affected by who is in the area.	Damage is not affected by who is in the area.
Pain is affected by beliefs.	Damage is not (well, not directly).
Pain can occur in a body part that does not exist.	Damage cannot occur in a body part that does not exist.
Pain can occur in a body part that is not damaged.	Damage can occur in a body part that is not painful.
Pain can occur without activation of nociceptors (see next section).	Damage cannot (excepting local anaesthetic or pre-injury nociceptor death).

the body, are called primary nociceptors (see [6, 7] for review).

Primary nociceptors are also different to other peripheral neurons in that they project to neurons in the dorsal horn of the spinal cord, not directly to thalamic or cortical structures. The neurons with which primary nociceptors synapse in the spinal cord are called secondary or spinal nociceptors and the synapse is open to modulatory input from other peripheral inputs and from descending neurons (see below). That the nociceptive system is polymodal and has a 'relay station' in the spinal cord raises two very important issues.

That primary nociceptors are multimodal and only project as far as the spinal cord clearly shows that the nociceptive system, per se, is not able to transmit information specific to each modality. That is, the nociceptive system does not tell the brain that something is 'dangerously hot', or 'dangerously cold' or 'dangerously squashed'. Rather, the nociceptive system has the apparently simple task of telling the brain that something is 'dangerous'. It is the non-nociceptive inputs (including non-somatosensory cues[8]) that provide critical information about the nature of the danger.

The polymodal characteristic also means that if a stimulus is both dangerously hot and dangerously squashing, it evokes quicker firing of primary nociceptors, which effectively tells the spinal nociceptor that something is 'doubly dangerous'. To consider a clinical example, if a primary nociceptor is activated by chemicals released by an inflammatory event and the tissues are then poked and prodded, the addition of a mechanical input to the chemical input will increase firing of nociceptors to a greater extent than either would alone.

That primary nociceptive input is open to modulation at the spinal 'relay station' (better conceptualised as a spinal 'processing station') means that other peripheral input can decrease noxious input. Peripheral input at the spinal relay station is from interneurons that are activated by wide diameter peripheral neurons (Aβ fibres) from the same or adjacent area. This is why one can, for example, 'rub it better', or, in a more sophisticated way, put TENS on it. In fact, TENS was born from Melzack and Wall's famous gate control theory of 1965.[9] Moreover, the spinal relay station can be modulated by descending input from supraspinal structures and it is this descending input that arguably represents a more important and potent modulatory influence.[10]

Sensitisation of primary nociceptors ('peripheral sensitisation')

Primary nociceptors become sensitised in the presence of chemical irritants, that is, they are subsequently activated at a lower threshold than is ordinarily required. The most common chemical irritants are generated by the tissues themselves when they are injured. These injured tissues are often referred to as 'inflammatory soup' because there are many chemicals involved and the exact ingredients of any particular soup will vary, depending upon the particular situation/injury/context/chemical stimuli and, critically, person.

Figure 5.1 depicts typical inflammation-mediated sensitisation of primary nociceptors. This 'peripheral sensitisation' is exactly that—nociceptors become responsive

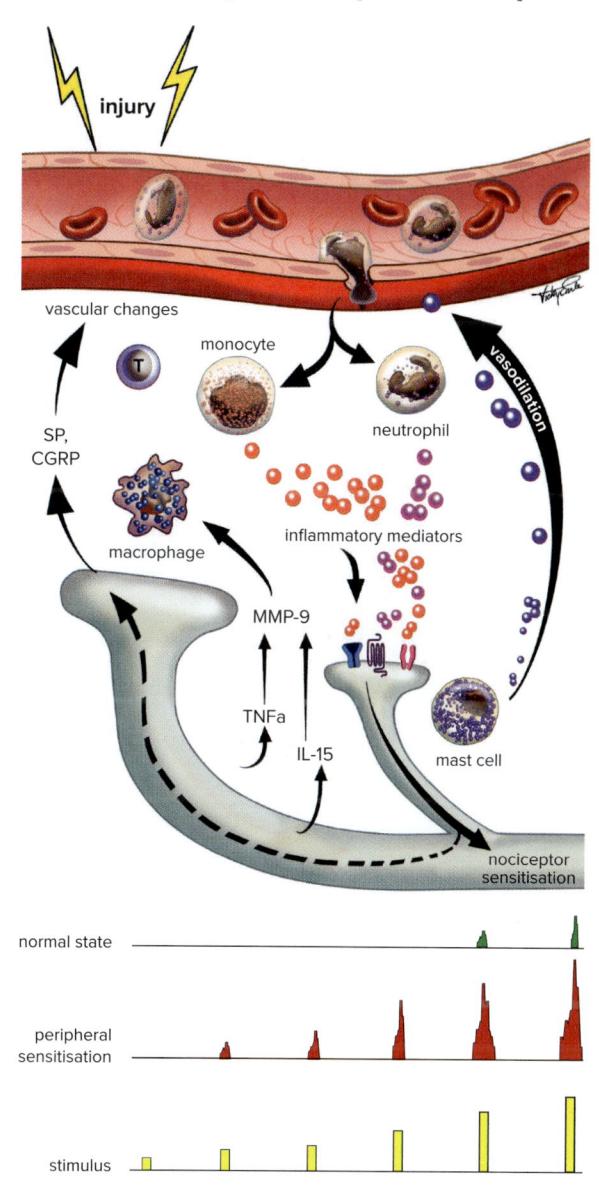

Figure 5.1 A simplified illustration of the connection between nerve terminals and vasculature. The green (normal) and red (sensitised) bars depict nociceptor responses to test stimuli (yellow bars). When there is peripheral sensitisation (red bars), even tiny stimuli evoke responses

PART A   Fundamental principles

to stimuli that are not normally evocative. One obvious example is that of sunburn: sunburnt skin hurts when you get into a shower of 40°C because nociceptors are sensitised sufficiently to be activated by a thermal stimulus 4–5°C cooler than that which would normally be required. That peripherally sensitised tissues are heat-sensitive is a very important phenomenon for the reasoning clinician because sensitisation of the spinal nociceptor does not result in heat sensitivity (Fig. 5.2). Therefore, if one has concluded that there is a peripheral problem and one can heat the culprit tissues to 42°C, one can confirm the conclusion or question it, by determining whether the tissues are more sensitive in the presence of thermal stimuli that *normally* do not activate nociceptors (Fig. 5.2).

Another aspect of sunburn, the reddening of the skin, is an important aspect of peripheral sensitisation. Reddening of the skin is a sign of neurogenic inflammation (Figs 5.1, 5.2). When nociceptors are activated, an impulse is transmitted along every branch of the nociceptor. If an impulse transmits 'in the wrong direction' and arrives at another terminal branch, then it causes the release of chemicals that in themselves are inflammatory and cause vasodilation.[5] This mechanism is responsible for the flare one gets around a skin wound or scratch. It is an important mechanism if the nociceptor is being activated proximally, for example, in the dorsal root ganglion or in the spinal cord, because it means that the tissues become inflamed as a consequence of action potentials being propagated elsewhere–in this situation, the tissues are not generating the inflammation.

Sensitisation of spinal nociceptors ('central sensitisation')

When spinal nociceptors are active for some time, they too become sensitised. Many biological processes that can contribute to 'central sensitisation' have been uncovered, and while in-depth discussion is beyond the scope of this chapter, there are several resources that discuss central

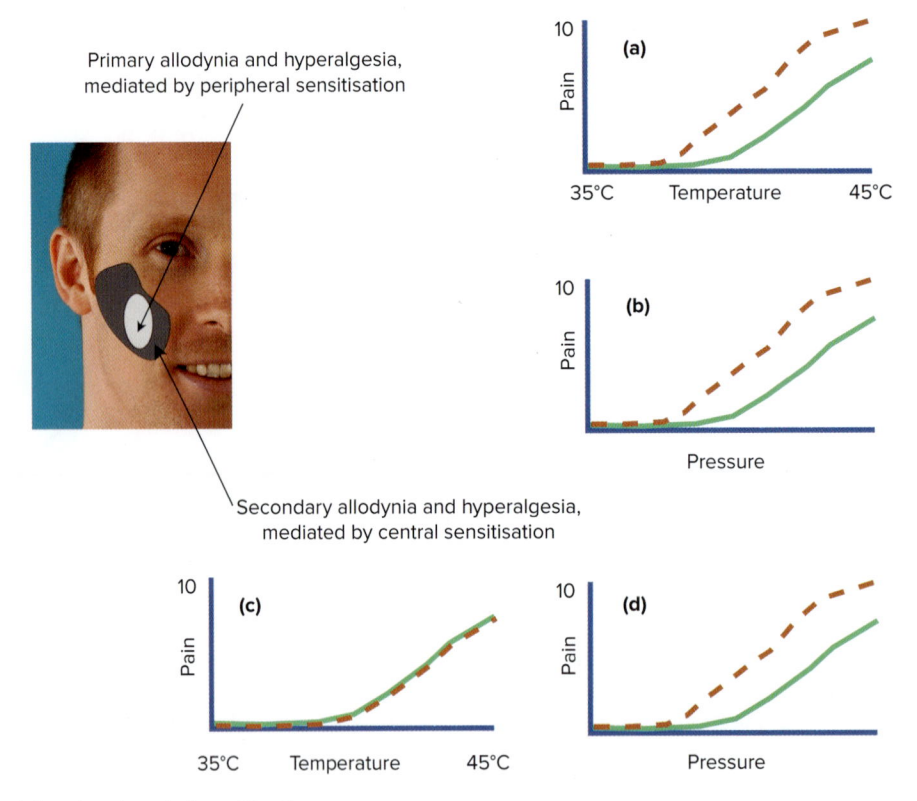

Figure 5.2 Peripheral and central sensitisation.
Presuming an injury within the lightly shaded zone, the presence of inflammation in the area and activation of primary nociceptors will lead to peripheral sensitisation. This will manifest as primary allodynia and hyperalgesia, as represented by a shift in the thermal pain threshold so that pain is evoked at lower temperatures than normal (a) and a similar shift in the mechanical pain threshold so that pain is evoked at lower pressures than normal (b). If central sensitisation ensues, the surrounding area, here represented by the dark shaded zone, will not be heat sensitive (c) but will be mechanically sensitive (d).

Pain: why and how does it hurt? CHAPTER 5

> ### A note on the evolution of meaning of central sensitisation
>
> There has been a shift in the common understanding of central sensitisation, from that presented above, to that presented below. That is, many people with persistent pain have reduced pain thresholds across half or all of their body. The most obvious biological substrate for this sensitivity is the central nervous system. As a result, the term central sensitisation has been commandeered to explain this phenomenon.[13] This is understandable but may also be problematic because it takes us away from likely candidate adaptations or problems, to a very generic and exclusion-based approach. One can describe 'new central sensitisation' as 'reduced pain thresholds not explainable by peripheral sensitisation'. In this chapter, the former definition of the term is used because it describes a series of biological adaptations that are well understood at a molecular level.

sensitisation in more detail and are listed at the end of the chapter. Central sensitisation manifests as mechanical sensitivity beyond the area of injury and peripheral sensitisation (Fig. 5.2). In short, central sensitisation means that the spinal cord 'upregulates' nociceptive input at the spinal cord (see[10-12] for reviews). This has implications for the biopsychosocial model of pain that is illustrated in Chapter 29.

THE BRAIN DECIDES

As illustrated earlier, pain emerges from the brain and reflects the brain's evaluation of threat to body tissue and the subsequent need for action. As mentioned in the earlier caveat, it is true to say that this perspective is 'neurocentric'[3] insofar as pain does not emerge from a nervous system, sitting in isolation from the rest of our biology. The truth is, of course, that pain emerges into consciousness from the entire person. This acknowledgement, however, is perhaps more philosophical than a sport and exercise medicine textbook permits. To iterate, we can avoid this difficulty by conceding that although it is not just a brain that evaluates this input and creates an experience, to conceptualise it this way is faithful to much of our understanding and is far more applicable than a more precise but philosophically challenging conceptualisation.

Spinal nociceptors are important informants about danger to body tissue, but, ultimately, nociception is neither sufficient nor necessary for pain (see Table 5.1). Modern conceptual models of pain highlight this critical role of the brain. One framework that makes this clear is that of cortical representations (see[7] for a clinician-friendly review). According to this framework, an individual will experience, for example, ankle pain when a network of brain cells, distributed across the brain, is activated. That network of brain cells, then, is considered the neural representation of that individual's ankle pain. As it is a unique and distributed network, one might call it a neuro*tag*.[7] Each of the brain cells that constitute this ankle pain neurotag also contribute to other neurotags and activation or otherwise, of this ankle pain neurotag is open to modulation at every synapse of every constituent brain cell. This brings an enormous complexity to the neurobiology of pain, although pain is simply one expression of the neurobiology of consciousness, which no one fully understands (see above). For a more in-depth review of this neurotag-based concept as it applies to performance, sports medicine and rehabilitation (see Wallwork et al).[14, 15]

This conceptual framework means that anything that is represented by that individual's brain *and* which provides credible evidence about the danger to which the ankle is currently exposed, should modulate activity of the 'ankle pain neurotag'. In more clinical terms, anything that provides credible information about the likely danger level should modulate ankle pain. Credible information may relate to likely consequences of damage–ankle damage is more dangerous to a top-level dancer than it is to an archer, a fact that will upregulate the ankle pain neurotag in the dancer. However, a top-level dancer might have the long-held belief that his/her body is indestructible, which would downregulate the ankle pain neurotag; a top-level archer may not have this belief. As you can see, it is a very complex system.

Credible information might relate to other sensory cues–damaging one's ankle on the bend in the final of the 200 m in front of a screaming crowd may very well lead to those same cues upregulating the ankle pain neurotag when those sensory cues occur again. Clearly, this neural complexity has important implications for rehabilitation; the neuroscience of pain and protection suggests that rehabilitation of this individual with ankle pain is not complete until the athlete has been exposed to every credible 'byte' of information that implies danger to the ankle.[14, 15]

Hopefully the reader can now appreciate why Descartes' idea, that we have pain receptors in the tissues and pain signals are transmitted to the brain,[4] is as inadequate as it is popular. While its simplicity may be seductive, the ever-increasing body of evidence suggests it simply does not hold up. If, as a clinician or patient, one is to accept the true complexity of pain as evidenced by a huge amount of experimental and clinical literature (see[16] for review) and to conceptualise pain by the representation framework, then one must also accept that activity in spinal nociceptors is one of many contributors to pain. The truly modern day clinician should be open to non-tissue contributions (i.e. differential modulation exerted by other systems, for example, immune upregulation, central sensitisation and central downregulation) and be alert to evidence of their influence.

Charles Darwin suggested that young scientists should write down the results that do not support their current beliefs because they are the results that are most forgettable.[17] As clinicians we should do the same (see also [18]). With regard to pain, this might mean taking note of:

- when the same mechanical input flares a condition one day and not the next
- when pain is worse in competition than it is in training
- when strength, endurance, control and flexibility are exemplary but the athlete still 'tweaks' a hamstring running at 90% effort
- when a 20-second manual therapy technique increases hip range of motion by 25°.

Sure, one might squeeze some such findings into a Descartian framework, but they arguably fit more easily in a modern knowledge-based framework and Ockham's razor* compels us to look there first.

THE BRAIN CORRECTS THE SPINAL CORD

There are several hundred projections from the brain to the spinal nociceptor. Projections originate throughout the brain and have both facilitatory and inhibitory effects. Structures within the brainstem, for example, the periaqueductal grey (PAG) are important relay stations between the brain and the spinal nociceptor.[19] Such a powerful modulatory capacity evokes, not surprisingly, powerful modulation.

Many experiments have investigated the circumstances under which the brain modulates the spinal nociceptors. We can easily summarise them here using the same language as above: if the *entire package* of credible evidence of danger is different from that suggested by spinal nociceptor input, the brain will 'correct' the spinal cord by either inhibiting spinal nociceptors or facilitating them.

Those familiar with principles of motor control will recognise the same principles also in the pain system. In motor control, this idea of re-afference and sensory-motor feedback loops is well established–a motor command generates an efferent copy that is then compared to sensory feedback of the movement (from vision and proprioceptors) and any discrepancy between the predicted and actual outcome is used to correct the motor command.[20]

Going back to our example of ankle pain, we can describe it thus: activation of the brain's ankle pain neurotag also triggers its efferent copy, the latter of which is compared to spinal nociceptive input, triggering correcting descending modulation to adjust ascending 'danger' input (Fig. 5.3). This kind of feedback loop is common in human physiology.

> **PRACTICE PEARL**
>
> In short, if the brain concludes that the need to protect tissues is greater than spinal nociceptor activity would suggest, it will facilitate the spinal nociceptor. If the brain concludes the need to protect is less than spinal nociceptor activity would suggest, it will inhibit it.

The effects of such correction will be different if the spinal cord itself is sensitised. That is, if non-tissue factors are increasing the brain's evaluation of danger to a particular tissue, such that the brain upregulates the spinal cord, it has the capacity to maintain or indeed instigate, central sensitisation. There is potential here for a vicious cycle of increasing nociception → increased perceived danger → increased descending facilitation → increased nociception. Thus, it is all the more important for the clinician to evaluate *every* factor that is contributing to the perception of threat to tissues because *any* credible evidence of danger has the potential to upregulate the spinal nociceptor (see [18, 21] for reviews).

THE BRAIN IS DIFFERENT IN THOSE WITH PERSISTENT PAIN

In much the same way that spinal nociceptors adapt to become more sensitive, so too do the brain cells that underpin pain[22-25] (Wand et al.[26] have reviewed the cortical changes in people with back pain). That is, the more the pain neurotag is active, the better it gets at being active. This manifests in more and more advanced hyperalgesia and allodynia, extended across modalities and exhibiting 'over-generalisation'.

Over-generalisation refers to that phenomenon in which pain begins to be evoked by more innocuous stimuli, in different contexts and under different circumstances.[27-29] Spreading pain, unpredictable pain, and pain that is less

---

*Ockham's razor is attributed to William of Ockham (14th century), although it was thought to be 'invented' well before his time. Its earliest and most enduring iteration is 'Entities must not be multiplied beyond necessity' or far more commonly now 'The simplest answer is probably the correct one'.

Pain: why and how does it hurt? CHAPTER 5

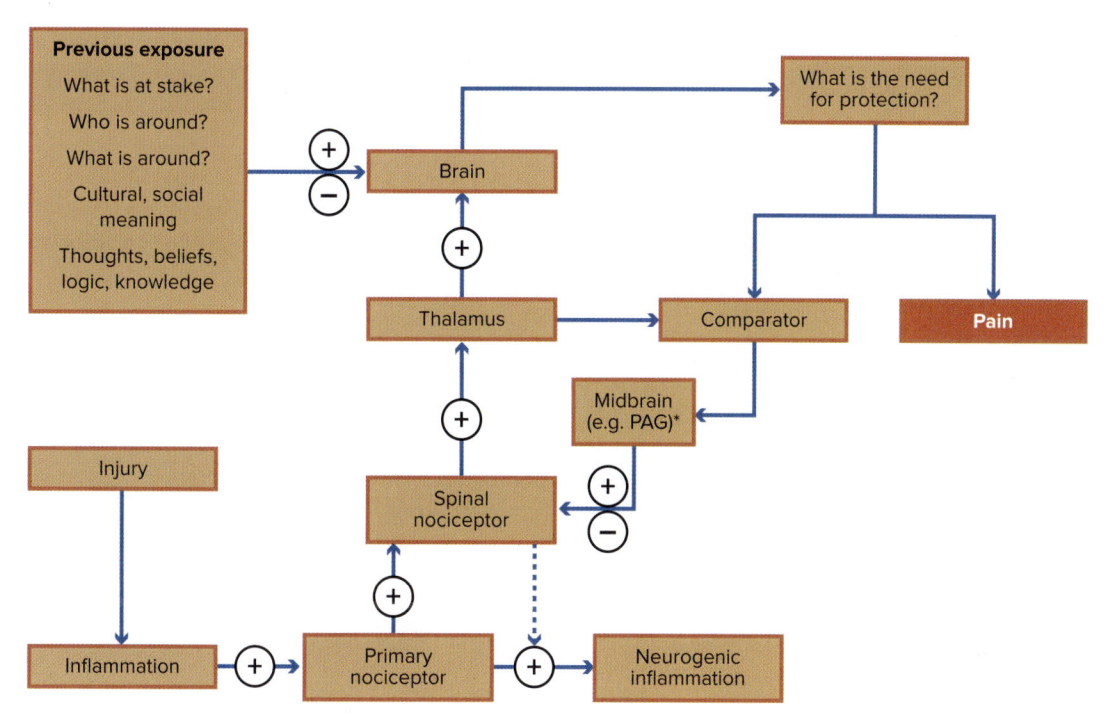

Figure 5.3 Feedback loops within the nociceptive system and the endpoint of pain: injury excites primary nociceptors. Injury-induced inflammation activates and sensitises primary nociceptors (peripheral sensitisation).
Activation of nociceptors causes neurogenic inflammation in nearby areas and excites spinal nociceptors. Spinal nociceptors project to thalamic nuclei, which then project to the brain. A complex evaluative process occurs within the brain, whereby every byte of information that provides credible evidence about the actual danger faced by the tissues in question is able to upregulate or downregulate the pain neurotag. This process permits the brain to determine 'What is the need for protection?' The final 'decision' leads to activation of the pain neurotag and pain emerges into consciousness. Simultaneously, as though a bifurcation of a single neural output, the determined need for protection is sent to a 'comparator', where it is used as a reference for the spinal nociceptor input. This comparator then modulates midbrain structures and thence in turn the spinal nociceptor to 'correct' its activation level. Thus, descending modulation can be facilitatory or inhibitory. The broken line from spinal nociceptor towards neurogenic inflammation refers to the possibility of tissue inflammation evoked by descending facilitation. That is, excessive facilitation of the spinal nociceptor in the absence of primary nociceptor activity is thought to activate the primary nociceptor antidromically, which induces neurogenic inflammation in the periphery.

and less related to tissue state and activity are cardinal signs of cortical dysfunction.

The full mechanisms and manifestations of cortical sensitivity are not as well understood as the changes in the spinal nociceptor are understood, but they are, at least theoretically, likely to be of far more widespread impact for the clinician and patient. Suffice it to state here that the complexity of pain and the adaptability of the nervous system mean that the modern clinician needs to think well beyond the tissues when dealing with anyone in pain. Indeed, common changes in the sensitivity of the nociception/pain system can be mediated at various levels of the neuraxis (Table 5.2).

TREATING SOMEONE IN PAIN—A COMPLEX SYSTEM REQUIRES A COMPREHENSIVE APPROACH

This chapter is not designed to provide a comprehensive guide to treating the patient in pain. Instead, it provides an account of pain that can underpin the assessment and management of people in pain, whatever the 'clinical toolbox' of the clinician. One implication of what we now know about pain is that there are certainly 'many ways to skin a cat' insofar as there are many ways to decrease credible evidence of danger and increase credible evidence of safety (see Moseley and Butler[21] for a step-by-step approach to doing this).

61

PART A Fundamental principles

Table 5.2 Clinical patterns of increased sensitivity to peripheral stimuli and possible underlying mechanisms

Clinical manifestation	Possible underlying cause
Mechanical allodynia: mechanical stimuli that do not normally evoke pain now do	Peripheral sensitisation, central sensitisation, cortical modulation
Thermal allodynia: heat pain threshold is decreased	Peripheral sensitisation, cortical modulation
Hyperalgesia: normally painful stimuli are now more painful	Peripheral sensitisation, central sensitisation, cortical modulation
Primary hyperalgesia	Hyperalgesia attributed to peripheral sensitisation
Secondary hyperalgesia	Hyperalgesia attributed to central sensitisation (or simply not attributable to peripheral sensitisation)

The best practice approach to rehabilitation integrates the complexity of the individual, and targets aspects of normal and altered physiology associated with pain (Fig. 5.4). The model is most established for the management of people in chronic pain[2] but can also be applied to the sporting and performance context.[14, 15] This is extremely relevant to sport and exercise medicine because (i) active people often present with these

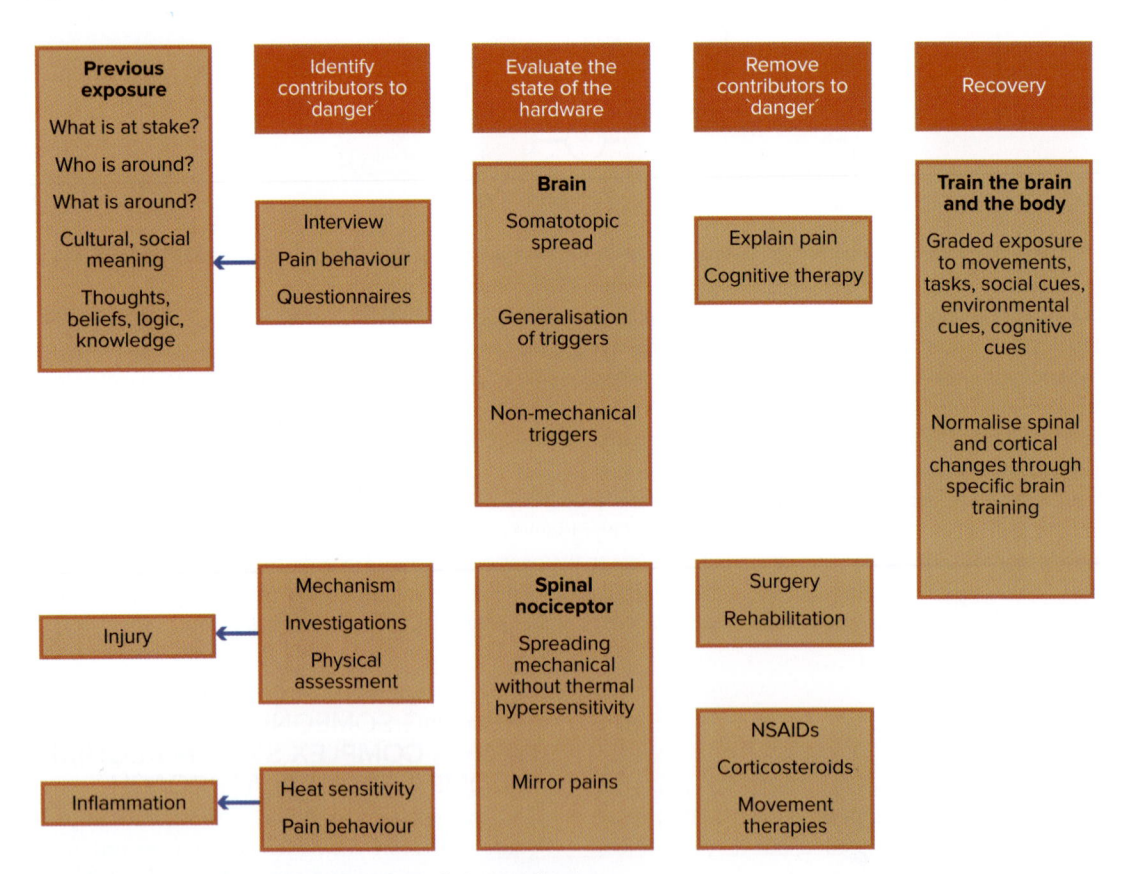

Figure 5.4 Major contributions to pain and their clinical implications.
The left column lists the major contributions to the brain's evaluation of danger to tissues, which determines pain and descending modulation. The second column suggests mechanisms with which to assess the major contributions, thereby identifying key triggers. The middle column suggests signs of spinal and cortical sensitisation, so as to determine the state of the nociceptive system. The fourth column suggests approaches to minimise the impact of the triggers that have been identified. (Note that this extends beyond physical approaches to include cognitive and educational approaches.) The final column recommends avenues to recovery. (Note the emphasis on training both the body and the brain, via specific techniques and graded exposure to physical and non-physical triggers.)

symptoms and (ii) the skillset and credibility of those working in this field is well suited to motivating people in pain to embrace a multifactorial approach to management. Because the biological mechanisms that underpin pain are the same for acute and chronic pain, albeit with increasing sensitivity as pain persists, the model outlined is applicable across patient groups. In Chapter 6, Dr Ebonie Rio outlines approaches to several clinical scenarios to show how the principles outlined here can underpin work in the clinic.

REFERENCES

References for this chapter can be found at www.mhhe.com/au/CSM5e

Chapter 6

Pain: the clinical aspects

with EBONIE RIO

Understanding pain biology changes the way people think about pain, reduces its threat value and improves their management of it.
David Butler & Lorimer Moseley, *Explain Pain*

Chapter 5 provided the complex foundational elements of pain science. In this chapter, we share how clinicians can apply this knowledge to better manage patients.[1] Being a clinician would be straightforward if the location of pain always revealed the precise area of pathology and pain had a tissue basis. But this is commonly not the case!

It is useful to consider the contributions to a patient's pain. For example, is there peripheral sensitisation? Is there central sensitisation? Is there referral? Are there cortical contributions? Are there changes in cortical representations? No matter what the answer to these questions, pain is a sign that the brain is urging protection. Identifying the relative importance of different contributions allows you to target your treatment accordingly.

Let's consider a patient with longstanding back pain. Historically, clinicians developed a list of differential diagnoses to classify injury or disease. In this case the options include muscle strain, disc injury or facet joint injury. Working from such a list of differential diagnoses relies on several assumptions. First, that knowledge of the affected structure is important to the assessment and diagnosis. Second, that it is possible to accurately confirm the diagnosis (i.e. that a gold standard exists). Third, that making a tissue diagnosis will inform treatment. Contrary to these 1980s opinions, none of those assumptions appear correct today.

A complementary approach is to consider an overarching classification (e.g. 'the patient had an episode of back pain') that focuses on *the pain experience and contributing factors* as a distinct clinical entity. With this foundation, the clinician can add information about the state of specific anatomical structures and determine the best treatment approach (which may change over time).

This broader perspective of painful events, which encourages assessment by body region and type of threat, is based on the neuroscience that body movements are represented on motor homunculi and body surfaces are represented on sensory homunculi (Fig. 6.1). While the chapters of this book are arranged to permit region-specific assessment and treatment of what we consider predominantly nociceptive-driven (or input-dominated) presentations, this chapter aims to help clinicians to know when to consider centrally dominated pain in their assessment and management. So, what is meant by 'input-dominated pain' and 'centrally dominated pain'?

INPUT-DOMINATED PAIN

Let's begin with the most common type of pain that brings the patient to a clinician in this field–pain from a musculoskeletal injury. This is 'input-dominated pain' and it is distinguished from 'centrally dominated pain' (discussed in the next section). When learning about concepts like this, it is helpful to artificially distinguish ends of a spectrum. Of course input-dominated and centrally dominated pains occur together, but let's put them in very distinct boxes to start with. In this context, 'input dominated' is a term used to get the clinician to appreciate the nociceptive contribution. The input is the sensory information from the periphery that has stimulated a nociceptor (a receptor capable of transducing and encoding noxious stimuli).

PART A   Fundamental principles

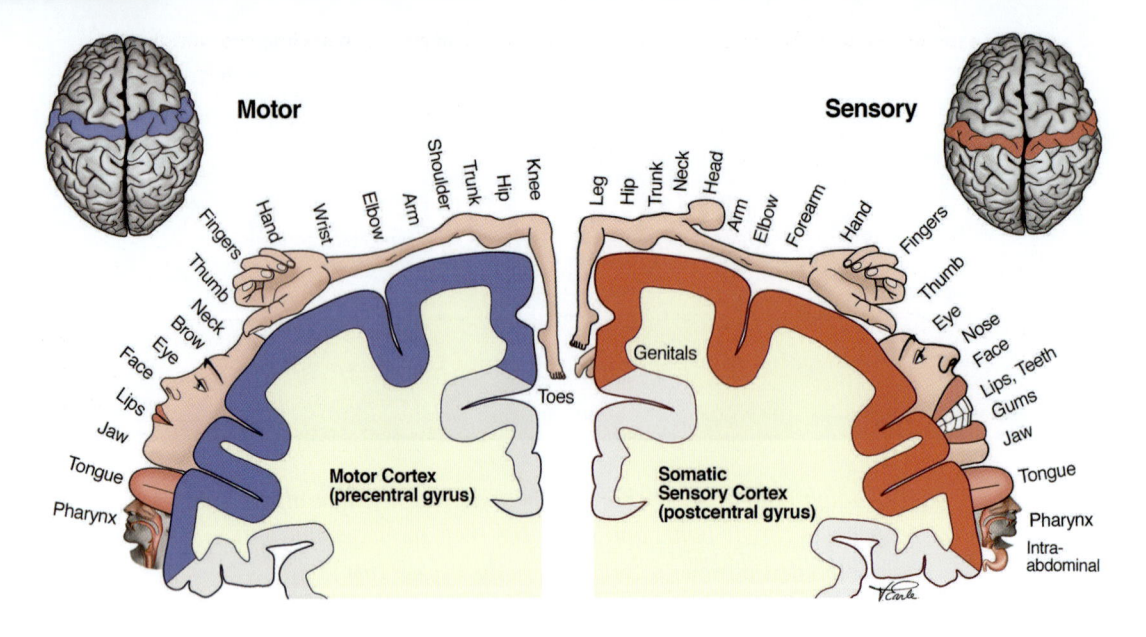

Figure 6.1 Motor and sensory homunculi

Pain and musculoskeletal tissues

Pain is what makes a person go to see a clinician. Acute incidents or injuries are generally associated with nociceptive sensory inputs from tissues. Many patients will report that their pain has affected their function in sporting, occupational or everyday activities. The clinician should evaluate the status of musculoskeletal structures as per a normal clinical encounter (see Chapter 14) and consider the following:

1. joints, including ligaments
2. bones
3. muscles and fascia
4. tendons
5. neural structures (see below).

In acute states, pain associated with nociceptive contributions is thought by clinicians to be fairly closely linked with injury and the repair process. As explained in Chapter 5, the relationship between tissue status (damage), afferent impulses (i.e. impulses perceived as noxious), and pain is not predictable or linear. Afferent impulses may overemphasise the danger associated with an injury at first (e.g. severe pain of an ankle sprain), but this can quickly diminish. The patient can be pain-free at 2 weeks post-injury, but not fully healed for 6 weeks. It is important to avoid thinking of pain presentations purely in terms of the length of time of symptoms. An example of this is pain associated with the patellar tendon (see Chapter 36), where pain is intimately linked with patellar tendon load, implying a nociceptive contribution even though pain can persist for years. In this example, the pain experience is of course modulated (as all pain is an output), yet there appears evidence of a nociceptive contribution.

Table 6.1 demonstrates examples of nociceptive pain descriptors and clinical examples.

> **PRACTICE PEARL**
>
> It is essential that the clinician eliminates sinister causes such as cancer (see Chapter 7).

Less well characterised input-dominated pain—referred pain

Referred pain is an example of nociceptive input-dominated pain. It can be thought of as an error in the brain's processes that determine where, exactly, it should hurt. That is, the location of the dangerous event is 'misread' by the brain. An example of referred pain is pain in the neck or left arm when it is the heart that is the structure under threat. Another common example is leg pain when nociceptive input arises from a structure in the back or the ascending projections normally associated with that structure. An extreme case of referred pain is 'phantom pain' where pain appears to be localised in a limb that is no longer part of the body (e.g. after amputation). This is also a good example of the discrepancy between apparent input and the experience of pain.

Pain: the clinical aspects — CHAPTER 6

Table 6.1 Clinical examples of terminology and tissue-based examples of pain with nociceptive contributions[2]

Nociceptive pain descriptors	Tissue-based examples
Patients describe an incident that fits with anatomical location	Ankle sprain may injure ligaments, fascia, muscles, tendon, bone and neural structures via mechanical, ischaemic and/or inflammatory processes
Patient reports clear aggravating and easing factors as well as consistent and clear pain reproduction on movement (or testing) of target tissues	Testing of the involved ligaments reproduces pain
Pain usually eases as the injury settles	Initially someone may present with a limp and this reduces over time, perhaps with appropriate treatment that may include activity modification, ice, compression and optimal loading (graduated exercise progression)

Four case scenarios where referred pain is a common culprit!

- A patient presents with a long history of intermittent, dull, occipital headaches. The patient is thoroughly investigated for eye problems and the presence of intracranial pathology. All tests are normal.
- A patient presents with a history of an ache in the right shoulder that is difficult to localise and is associated with pain on the medial aspect of the upper arm. There is some neck stiffness and tightness in the trapezius muscle.
- A 35-year-old executive complains of episodes of sharp, left-sided chest pain related to activity. The patient has already undergone extensive cardiac investigations that were all normal.
- A young athlete presents with a history of recurrent episodes of buttock and hamstring pain. There is no history of an acute tear and the patient describes the pain as deep-seated and dull with occasional sharp cramping in the hamstring. Examination of the hamstring shows some mild tenderness but full stretch and strength.

These clinical presentations are common in sport and exercise medicine practice. All of the patients are likely to be experiencing referred pain and treatment needs to take this into account.

It is important to keep in mind that there is always a reason for pain (response to perceived threat). Because pain is the end point of a complex danger-relevant processing system, it means that when the tissue that hurts seems normal, we may need to look elsewhere rather than presume the patient is not in pain.

Consider that the brain is wrongly locating a dangerous event–that there is a noxious contributor in an area that does not hurt (and the pain is felt at a remote distance to the noxious contributor). There are common patterns and mechanisms of referred pain. Two of these are 'radicular referred pain' and 'somatic referred pain'. Being familiar with these will stand the young clinician in very good stead. You will make many diagnoses and help many patients who your colleagues will consider 'difficult' or even 'crazy'. (We don't condone terms like 'crazy' about patients, but patients have reported to us that they were told this or they felt crazy, so the term is used here to emphasise the burden that undiagnosed referred pain can have.)

Radicular pain

The concept of radicular pain is increasingly taught to undergraduate health professionals, and it is pain associated with nerve root compression or irritation. It has the characteristic quality of sharp, shooting pain in a relatively narrow band, known as a dermatome. Dermatomes are mapped out and can be used to determine the segmental level of the nerve root compromise. Dermatomes themselves are variable both between and within individuals–they move in line with shifting receptor fields of spinal neurons.[3,4] (Fig. 6.2). Nonetheless, current convention tells us that if the radicular pain is associated with compression of the nerve root, it will usually be accompanied by neurological abnormalities, e.g. paraesthesia corresponding to a reasonably typical dermatomal distribution or muscle weakness corresponding to a reasonably typical myotome.

Irritation of the dorsal root ganglion can evoke a similar distribution of pain, although the shooting pain may be delayed for several seconds and will sometimes

PART A Fundamental principles

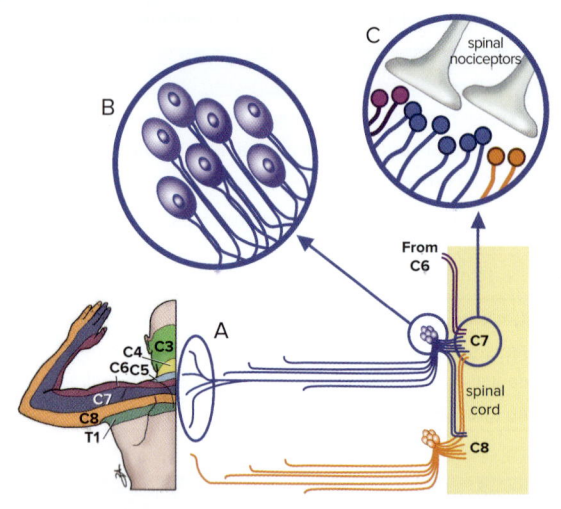

Figure 6.2 Radicular pain runs in well-characterised narrow bands according to which nerve root is affected. The left panel shows the dermatomal distribution of the neck region. The image also explains mechanisms that can underpin radicular pain—convergence of multiple incoming nociceptors. Note that radicular pain within the peripheral supply of a single spinal segment can occur via convergence of multiple branches of single nociceptors (A). Radicular pain can also occur via nociceptors within the dorsal root ganglion of that peripheral nerve (B). Pain can occur within the adjacent spinal nerve root territory via convergence within the dorsal horn, where projections from levels above (C6) or below (C8) can terminate alongside those from the spinal segment concerned (C)

reverberate (see Butler and Moseley 2013[5] for more on this). That nerve root irritation and dorsal root ganglion irritation evoke pain in the area normally supplied by the affected nerve is intuitively sensible. The spinal neurons that convey the danger message have no method by which to differentiate where along the primary nociceptor the activity was generated, which leaves the brain allocating the danger to the target tissues.

Somatic pain

The other type of referred pain–the one that is largely ignored in traditional medical (i.e. MBBS, MD) teaching–is often called somatic referred pain. The mechanisms that underpin somatic referred pain are not as structurally simple as radicular referred pain. This is because the 'disrupted transmission' occurs within the central nervous system. This might happen at the dorsal horn in the spinal cord, in the thalamus or in the brain itself (Fig. 6.3). For example, visceral and musculoskeletal afferents converge in the case of left arm pain evoked by cardiac problems. Similarly, immune mechanisms form functional connections with contralateral spinal nociceptors and as such might evoke 'mirror pains' at the identical site on the opposite limb.

It can be helpful for the young clinician to conceptualise somatic referred pain as the brain attempting to localise the pain in response to ambiguous input (Fig. 6.3). As a result, the patient explains that the boundaries of pain seem indistinct, and that the pain can move. There is a large amount of variability between how individuals tell their story of this type of pain.

Two structures that are widely held by clinicians to be common contributors to somatic referred pain are (i) joints and (ii) myofascial trigger points (although the evidence concerning popular treatments for the latter is somewhat fragile). The growing ambiguity or *imprecision*, that seems to accompany somatic referred pain increases as the usual intracortical inhibitory mechanisms break down in persistent pain. The longer pain persists, the more 'bodily real estate' it tends to consume. Indeed, the attribution of danger to a particular area of *space*, in addition to body,[6-8] is consistent with this loss of inhibition in brain areas dedicated to spatial localisation of body parts.[10]

Neuropathic pain

Neuropathic pain can be difficult to categorise and is defined as pain arising as a direct consequence of a lesion or disease affecting the somatosensory system.[10] In contrast to pain that arises from activating nociceptive afferents (discussed above as pain with nociceptive contribution), pain can arise by activity generated without adequate stimulation of sensory nerve endings and is probably best described as a characteristic rather than a diagnosis. However, neuropathic pain can occur concurrently with nociceptive contributions to pain, that is, initial trauma can damage peripheral musculoskeletal tissue as well as neural tissue. This provides a mixed clinical picture that makes it more challenging for the clinician to unravel the contributor(s) to pain.

There is no gold standard or even clinical test for neuropathic pain. It represents clusters of features that may or may not have a history of injury or illness preceding the symptoms. Clinically, many find it useful to grade according to the level of certainty with which it can be determined in a patient[10] (definite, probably, possible). This is based on the premise of pain distribution being consistent with dermatomes (that is, corresponding to peripheral innervation patterns or representations). Causes of neuropathic pain include diabetes, malignant disease, trauma and ischaemia. People presenting with pain (often to a musculoskeletal clinician) may have diabetes or an undiagnosed malignancy, so the clinician must remain alert to this possibility when a patient presenting with what would be expected to be

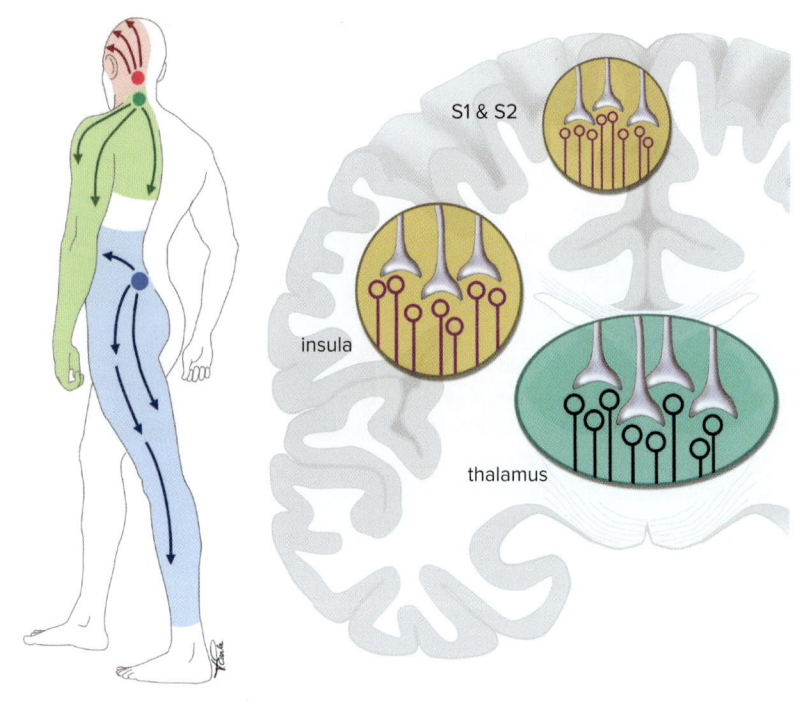

Figure 6.3 Somatic pain is an important type of input-dominated pain. As in the illustration of the person on the left side of the figure, pain can be referred in non-radicular patterns such as within a limb or 'quadrant'. Nociceptive signals converge in higher centres, e.g. thalamus, insula, and primary (S1) and secondary (S2) somatosensory areas.

input-dominated pain (e.g. local tissue trauma) reports ongoing pain with neuropathic features.

The clinical features of neuropathic pain may include burning or shooting pain, hypersensitivity, expansion of receptive fields, deep aching, motor deficits, abnormal neurological examination and spontaneous pain.[2, 11, 12] A patient with neuropathic pain may experience both sensory loss (cold, warmth and pinprick) and the presence of certain hyperphenomena such as tingling or prickling sensations. However, clinical neurological testing may not be sensitive enough to detect the afferent (sensory) changes. There is no gold standard to identify neuropathic pain, nor consensus over whether neuropathic pain questionnaires should be used in clinical practice. Of the available questionnaires, PainDETECT and LANSS[13] have the best clinical applicability as well as acceptable sensitivity and specificity.

CENTRALLY DOMINATED PAIN

These classifications merely aim to assist clinicians to form a treatment path. This is because people who have reduced thresholds to the way they perceive stimuli that is contributing to their pain (perhaps even a main driver) require individual approaches. The term 'centrally dominated pain' refers to clusters of clinical features and includes sensory findings (both positive and negative findings). It is often thought of as pain that persists beyond usual time frames (however, this is difficult to quantify and could mean treatment was inappropriately directed) or as pain that is experienced without stimuli.

This is where it gets tricky as reduced sensory thresholds are also observed even in acute situations such as an ankle sprain. Thus, centrally dominated pain refers to the pain of a subgroup of people who have not responded to many traditional treatments. Unfortunately many people experience persistent pain and there are no tests that can identify people early that are at risk of persistent pain. The language strategies provided at the end of this chapter aim to help clinicians reduce their negative impact (and perhaps even have a positive impact) on their patient interactions. (Note that neuropathic pain has elements of both input-dominated and centrally dominated pain but it is included below.) Many conditions may have elements of neuropathic pain.

Central sensitisation

The expert sport and exercise clinician recognises that the relationship between pain and tissue damage becomes more tenuous as pain persists.[14] As pain persists, the central nervous system (CNS) switches to a state of spinal hypersensitivity, which generates allodynia (e.g. the experience of pain from non-noxious stimuli such as light touch) and the descending control pathways shift to excitation rather than inhibition.

Central sensitisation results from a complex cascade of physiological events involving all levels of the CNS and many areas of the brain[15] (see Chapter 5 for more detail). Often the patient has a reduced pain threshold that is not explained by peripheral sensitisation. (Note that the clinical finding of lowered pain threshold can be explained by one of two mechanisms—central or peripheral sensitisation. This amplified neural signalling and potential for evoked pain via non-nociceptive channels elicits pain hypersensitivity and may represent a shift in the main contributor to pain. Neural impulses may be spontaneous.

These features can be difficult to clinically assess and have been mainly reported using equipment such as qualitative sensory testing, which is expensive and time consuming. Light touch testing (e.g. with von Frey filaments) and two-point discrimination testing require practice to obtain reasonable reliability and repeatability and also rely on the assumption that there are established normative data–which there are not! This may sound very negative, but it is important for clinicians to put everything together in the clinical picture. The clinician should be alert to the possibility of central sensitisation when pain persists beyond the 'normal healing' time frames for an injury. At the same time, please listen to the voice saying that you also need to watch for 'red flags' (masquerades– see Chapter 7) at that point too. Unfortunately, no simple clinical tests provide confirmation that the pain presentation is centrally dominated. The clinician needs to take a reading from a cluster of signs and symptoms.

Another clue that pain may be centrally dominated is that it may respond poorly to treatments such as manual therapy, because CNS changes may have altered neural function (e.g. a light touch may evoke pain).

After an injury (e.g. ankle sprain), a period of increased sensitivity is an adaptation that reduces the risk of secondary injury and provides an opportunity for tissue to heal;[14] however, persistent hypervigilance can substantially impair quality of life. The concept of threat and pain is summarised in the previous chapter and also detailed in the book *Explain Pain*[1, 5] (Fig. 6.4). Remember that the relationship between perceived threat and pain is true of all pain presentations, not just chronic pain states.

Table 6.2 assists clinicians to interpret information obtained in their subjective assessment and to guide pain classification. It includes common assessment techniques

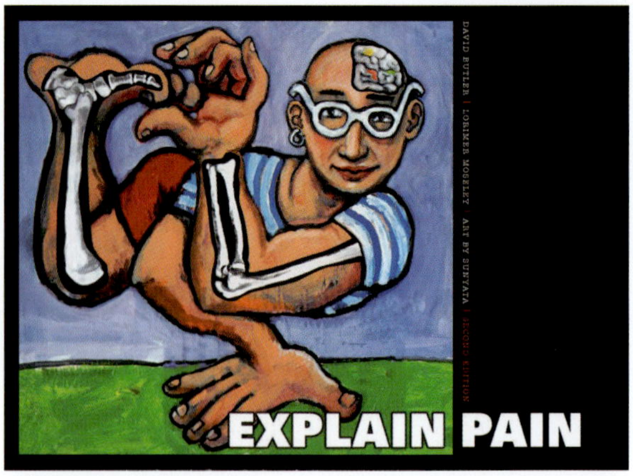

Figure 6.4 *Explain Pain* is a book by Dr David Butler and Professor Lorimer Moseley, but the term 'explain pain' has increasingly been used to refer to an approach to treating centrally dominated pain. We recommend it as part of the essential library for the *Clinical Sports Medicine* community

and tools that may be used to assess sensory processing and pain.

It can be difficult to classify patients but some consideration of the primary contributors to their clinical presentation may assist with efficacious treatment selection. Figure 6.5 aims to assist clinicians with their clinical reasoning process. Of note, clinicians may be persistent in trying to identify a tissue-based diagnosis with ongoing pain. Conversely and of no benefit to patients, many are told the pain is all in their head! There are a number of patterns that can assist with using Figure 6.5. Here is a list of clinical symptoms and signs to assist with identifying centrally dominated pain presentations (refer to *Explain Pain* for greater detail):[1, 5]

- loss of two-point discrimination[17]
- language of pain–'everything hurts'
- cold sensitivity
- tenderness to palpation away from injury site (secondary hyperalgesia)
- multiple diagnoses including myofascial syndrome, fibromyalgia
- red flags (see Chapter 7), including history of traumatic events, anxiety/depressive states
- cyclical or seasonal presentation (without links to changes in load or mechanical stimulus).

Table 6.3 includes common assessment techniques and tools that may be used to assess sensory processing and pain.

Pain: the clinical aspects CHAPTER 6

Table 6.2 Questions that clinicians can use to guide their approach to patients with pain. Note there generally exists a crossover among contributors to pain[2, 11, 14, 16]

Question	Examples of responses	Clinical reasoning
Onset: was there an initial incident/injury and when was it?	Some people report a clear onset of pain, others do not. Some individuals do not report pain even from a clear episode of severe trauma	Is the tissue a predominant driver of the pain? (No recollection of pain makes this less likely but not impossible) Overuse presentations (of input-dominated pain) may not have a sudden onset In the case of persistent pain, the incident may be a long time ago (may or may not be due to centrally dominated pain)
Where is the pain? Does it move around or spread?	Localised pain Within dermatomal distribution Pain that does not fit a dermatomal or myotomal distribution	May reflect nociceptive including compression of neural tissue May be referred (e.g. from the spine or viscera) Potential centrally dominated or neuropathic pain
Can you describe the symptoms?	Burning, electric shock-like, shooting, crushing, paraesthesia, and pins and needles Specific clusters of symptoms such as sweating, swelling, glossy skin, together with burning pain may reflect increased sympathetic activity	May reflect neuropathic pain (input dominated) These features are characteristic of complex regional pain syndrome. This is an example of centrally dominated pain
Does anything provoke the pain? (Examples given include visual and mechanical stimuli.)	No	If the patient has pain without a physical stimulus, consider centrally dominated pain such as neuropathic pain, rheumatological causes, sensitisation, inflammation or a sinister cause (see Chapter 7) Even being at rest may irritate some nociceptive pain (including neural irritation, for example, if your ulnar nerve has pressure when your elbow rests on something) People may report that pain swaps sides, or limbs or 'pain has a mind of its own' Pain may be unpredictable, non-mechanical and non-anatomical in response to movement Possible to have movement-related memory pain that is reinforced by cognitive emotional factors Some patients with centrally dominated pain experience pain with visual stimuli
Does the patient report hyperexcitability of response to stimuli?	Yes Pain with light touch (mechanical) Cold allodynia (thermal) Chemical stimuli Wind-up-like pain (abnormal temporal summation, that is, the perceived increase in pain intensity over time when the stimulus is repeated above a critical rate) or aftersensations (persistence of pain after termination of a painful stimulus)	Possibly centrally dominated or neuropathic pain. Chemical and cold allodynia can be difficult to assess in the clinic. Patients can report hypersensitivity to cold Described following repetitive noxious or non-noxious stimuli (like light touch can evoke pain)

71

PART A   Fundamental principles

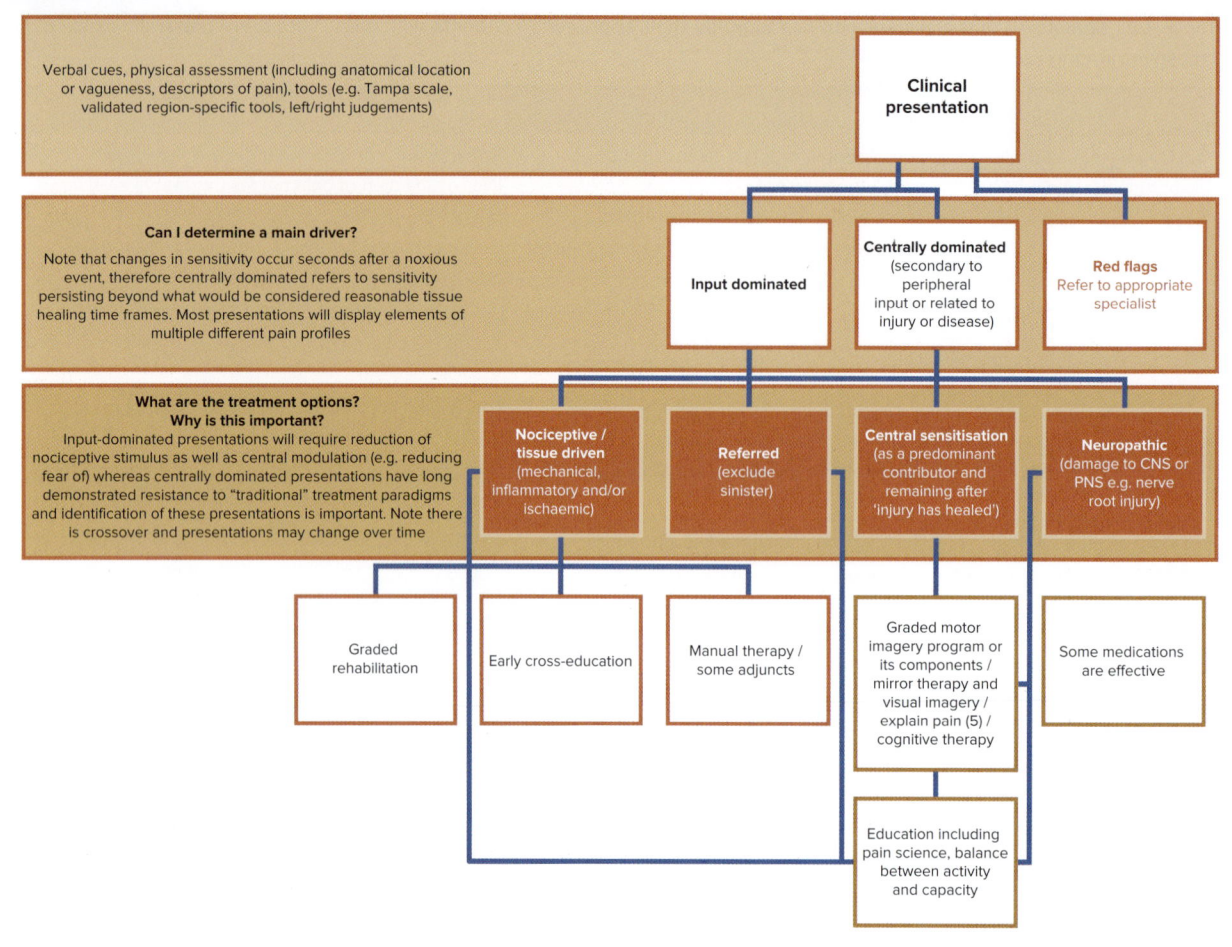

Figure 6.5 Flowchart to assist with clinical presentation and treatment path

MOTOR ADAPTATION TO PAIN

It is important for the clinician to appreciate that there are movement changes with pain–technically, 'motor adaptations.' Understanding what may underpin abnormal movement can allow appropriate rehabilitation (see Chapter 18).

Clinicians will recall examples of what pain scientists call the *pain–spasm–pain model*–pain increases muscle activity which in turn causes pain.[21] Consider secondary muscle spasm associated with some forms of back pain. In contrast, the *pain-adaptation model* postulates that pain actually reduces activation of agonist muscles and increases activation of antagonist muscles[22] to limit movement and avoid provoking pain and further damaging tissues. An example of this would be inhibition of the quadriceps to limit patellar movement in cases of patellofemoral pain.

Both of these types of motor change may reduce movement variability and that abnormal pattern may in turn increase the likelihood of recurrence of pain.[14, 20, 23, 24] Importantly, a so-called 'protective movement-related pain memory' may even hamper some attempts at rehabilitation for some patients.[1, 25]

Limiting movement can be effective in reducing pain in the short term and as long as there is a perceived threat, motor outputs may serve to protect the part. These changes in motor learning occur at multiple levels of the motor neuroaxis (e.g. motor unit, spinal cord, brain), so the patient may need to relearn appropriate motor patterns (i.e. reprogram motor outputs) after a period of sustained protection. The expert clinician builds this in to the progressive rehabilitation and exercise prescription (see Chapter 18).

Treatment options for patients with pain

CNS modulation occurs with all sensory input–memories, thoughts, fears and expectations will influence and shape the output. There are many ways to treat people with centrally dominated pain and many aspects of the

Pain: the clinical aspects — CHAPTER 6

Table 6.3 Tools for sensory processing and pain reporting

Clinical manifestation	Definition	Clinical examples	Tools
Allodynia	Stimuli that do not normally evoke pain (non-noxious stimuli) are now capable of evoking pain	Jumping can be painful for someone with patellar tendinopathy. Walking may be painful for someone who has sprained their lateral ankle	Observation. Physical assessment, including palpation. Note that allodynia is a normal and protective response to injury, but can also be part of persistent pain states
Hyperalgesia (primary and secondary)	Stimuli that are normally painful now evoke more pain. Lowering of pain threshold response to noxious stimuli	Primary hyperalgesia—peripheral sensitisation. Secondary hyperalgesia—attributed to central sensitisation	Pressure pain algometer to detect mechanical hyperalgesia. Qualitative sensory testing can examine the presence of thermal and mechanical hyperalgesia by checking thresholds and detection
Pain during function	Patient reports pain during activity. Using a functional test enables re-testing of the task		Visual analogue scale. Numerical rating scale (e.g. 0–10). Multidimensional descriptors such as McGill Pain questionnaire[18]. Specific questionnaires for diagnosis, e.g. VISA-P for patellar tendinopathy[19]
Disrupted motor imagery performance	Accuracy and time to recognise left and right body images	This test has three steps: 1. Initial spontaneous judgment 2. Mentally match image to mimic posture shown (requires intact working body schema/cortical representation) 3. Confirm or deny initial judgment. This is impaired in some conditions such as Complex Regional Pain Syndrome and phantom limb pain[20]	Android and iPhone apps can test this—for example Recognise

PART A   Fundamental principles

Be alert to the onset of centrally dominated pain

As an injury progresses from acute to chronic, the nature of the pain may change in some patients with centrally dominated pain becoming more likely as pain persists.

Let's take the example of an ankle sprain. In the acute setting with pain, swelling and disability, the major contributions to the pain are nociceptive input dominated.

In this example, the clinician has the benefit of the patient reporting that he or she had rolled the ankle, the presence of swelling in the area and perhaps their limping gait, to guide clinical assessment. The combination of subjective information and physical signs points to a tissue-based diagnosis, which helps the clinician formulate a management plan based on the philosophy that this is input dominated/nociceptive. Appropriate language that avoids fear mongering, and education to guide exercise and analgesic behaviours will be beneficial (or at least do no harm as the body heals).

If the person continues to limp after several months, is afraid to use the ankle, describes pain without activity or pain with clothes against his or her ankle and perhaps there are skin changes, the clinician may start to think that the presentation has changed from input dominated to centrally dominated. In the former, the ligaments would be expected to be 'healed' after this period of time. However, there is no cut off for a transition to a centrally dominant picture (e.g. not greater than 3 months, as many texts will indicate).

The important point to make here is that manual techniques aimed at the ankle joint could easily make pain worse. The treatment path may need to be very creative and use techniques such as graded motor imagery to begin moving the virtual ankle before the physical ankle is re-introduced to rehabilitation. This is never easy, and the clinician must always remember the possibility of a missed diagnosis (such as a fracture) or a sinister cause, yet not continue to hunt for a tissue-based diagnosis when some contributors to pain cannot be scanned (such as beliefs and feelings).

treatment are different to that used for nociceptive pain (Fig. 6.5).

Education

Most patients with pain will benefit from accurate education about perceived threat and pain. The clinician must avoid potentially harmful language such as 'bone on bone' changes in osteoarthritis or 'massive disc rupture/herniation' in back pain.

Identification of centrally dominated pain is important because evidence suggests the best way to help patients lies in skilled practitioners and appropriate resources. In the future, strategies need to be improved that target all aspects of CNS changes, including cortical reorganisation.[14, 20] It is possible to achieve a positive outcome; ion channels can change in minutes (see[26] for review) and movement-specific motor maps can shift over days and even minutes.[27, 28] This suggests that patients may benefit from rapid neurological changes which equate to symptom relief (usually less pain) as the nervous system is restored to a less sensitive state.

Manual therapy

Touch can have anti-nociceptive effects[29] and can also benefit patients in conjunction with exercise in some conditions such as shoulder disorders.[30] In mechanical neck pain, with or without headache, the Cochrane review concluded that manual therapy should only be done in conjunction with exercise and that mobilisation or manipulation alone was less effective.[31] Inaccurate statements from clinicians such as 'putting your spine back in place' should be avoided. Acupuncture has been shown to have short-term effects on pain.[32]

The remaining chapters of the book will direct the reader to appropriate and evidence-based techniques. Given the potential for anti-nociceptive effects, it stands to reason this may be an appropriate part of management for someone that has nociceptive contributions to pain, but less so for someone demonstrating sensitivity (e.g. when light touch is painful).

Medications

Medications may modify pain. Examples include medications that block inflammatory drivers, blunt neural sensitisation or promote neural plasticity. This topic is covered in Chapter 17.

Exercise/progressive loading

Following the initial period of unloading after an acute injury (or after prolonged changes to movement as a protective strategy), it is critical for patients to move and reload tissue in a gradual manner that promotes progressive tissue adaptation. Rest reduces capacity[33] in musculoskeletal tissues. (See Mechanotherapy in Chapter 17).

In nociceptive presentations, the clinician may focus more on local tissue reloading whereas, when pain is more centrally dominant, the exercise program may need to drop to below that which provokes them and take a backseat to techniques such as graded motor imagery (GMI) and 'explain pain'. This is described in

Table 6.4 Language that may be unhelpful and and how to rephrase it (adapted from *Explain Pain*—see text for more detail)[5]

Unhelpful language that may amplify pain experience or interfere with progress	Potential rephrasing that may be clinically appropriate	Considerations/rationale
'It's bone on bone in there.'	'Your MRI shows age- and load-appropriate changes.'	Asymptomatic pathology is common[36, 37] and focus on pathology (that may or may not be relevant for the patient's presentation) can be negative
'Your scan shows degeneration.'	'Your scan shows adaptations to age and load.'	Conversely, targeted education that demonstrates adaptation can improve outcomes[38]
'You have no core strength.'	'Your trunk muscles could be stronger.'	The body has remarkable ability to heal/adapt and, in many cases, to function better than prior to a medical incident. Treatment should facilitate this
'Your pelvis is out.'	'I am a complete idiot.'	OK—you can see Lorimer Moseley's influence here. But we are making a serious point and humour is a powerful communication tool, whether in textbooks or with patients

the GMI handbook where the GMI program is part of rehabilitation. When symptoms worsen, the techniques used are more focused on motor/functional empathy and implicit motor imagery such as left/right judgments, and as symptoms improve, the techniques are directed more towards mirror therapy and actual exposure to load. The start point can be established between the clinician and the patient by listening to their current activity and how well they tolerate it. Ultimately, clinicians should be assisting patients and athletes to restore function.

Graded motor imagery/explain pain/cognitive therapy/sensory discrimination training

Some people will not benefit from manual therapy or exercise as touch or movement may trigger their pain. In this instance, pain science education is essential. The goal of this approach is to help patients understand the concepts of threat and related body responses. Fundamental concepts include extinction of pain/signal and desensitisation with the aim of reducing the patient's feelings of helplessness.[14]

Some patients may benefit from the use of mirror therapy, visual distortion (e.g. minimising lens), graded motor imagery (GMI), and strategies that stimulate sensory and motor representations with context.[14]. These methods are very well described in the book *Explain Pain* (see Fig. 6.6).[5]

Language

Language is a powerful tool and has potential for both negative and positive impacts.[5, 34, 35] Skilful communication can better engage a patient in his or her own care decisions and this can improve outcomes. Table 6.4 provides some examples of language that may be considered unhelpful and how they can be rephrased.

SUMMARY

In many cases in sport and exercise medicine, physical assessment is aimed at establishing a structural diagnosis to guide an effective treatment plan in the hope that someone will fully recover. The expert clinician appreciates pain as a protective output, maintains a level of vigilance for when it is necessary to take a broader approach, assesses the various contributors to the patient's pain and considers secondary factors that may act to modulate it at the peripheral and/or central levels (see Fig. 6.3). This approach, which incorporates advances in pain science, will mean fewer patients are given inappropriate treatment that is missing an important element of their condition.

PART A   Fundamental principles

INTEGRATION OF EXPLAIN PAIN EDUCATION WITH THREE STAGES OF GRADED MOTOR IMAGERY

Recognise App
LEFT/RIGHT DISCRIMINATION
Quick judgements of left or right images

Recognise Flash Cards
EXPLICIT MOTOR IMAGERY
Rehearsing imagined movements

Mirror Box
MIRROR THERAPY
Using a Mirror Box to create the illusion of therapeutic movement

GRADED PHYSICAL REHABILITATION

ONGOING EXPLAIN PAIN EDUCATION

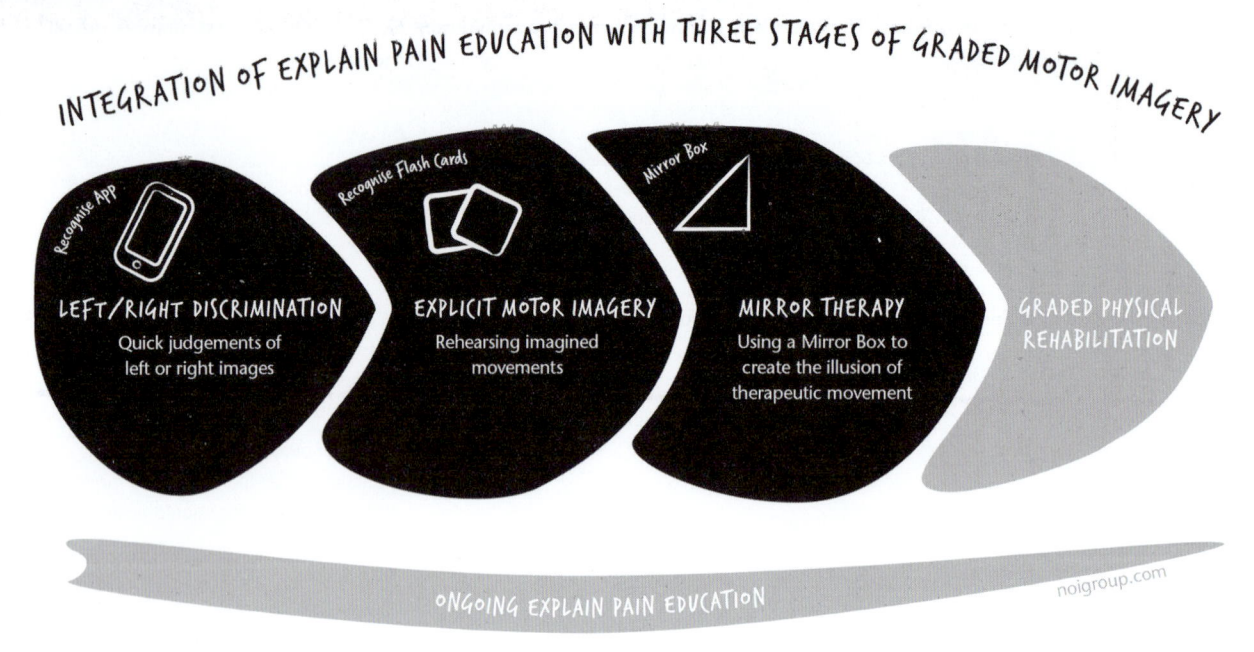

noigroup.com

Figure 6.6 'Explain pain' education, and the specific details of teaching graded motor imagery, is outside the scope of this book. We recommend that clinicians carefully consider this element when addressing painful conditions.
WITH PERMISSION FROM DAVID BUTLER AND LORIMER MOSELEY, *EXPLAIN PAIN*

REFERENCES

References for this chapter can be found at www.mhhe.com/au/CSM5e

Chapter 7

Beware: conditions that masquerade as sports injuries

with NICK CARTER and MARK HUTCHINSON

Belgian decathlete Thomas Van der Plaetsen had testicular cancer diagnosed because abnormal levels of the HCG hormone were detected on a routine doping test in 2014. After treatment, 2016 saw him win the European Championships and compete at the Rio 2016 Olympic Games.

Not every patient who presents to the sport and exercise medicine clinician has a sports-related condition. Sport and exercise medicine has its share of conditions that must not be missed—'red flag' conditions that may appear at first to be rather benign. For example, a patient diagnosed with a minor 'calf strain' may have a deep venous thrombosis or a young basketball player with proximal anterior tibial pain who has been labelled as having Osgood-Schlatter disease may have an osteosarcoma or giant cell tumur of the proximal tibia. In this chapter we:

- outline a clinical approach that should maximise your chances of recognising a condition that is 'masquerading' as a sports-related condition
- describe some of these conditions to illustrate how they can present.

HOW TO RECOGNISE A CONDITION MASQUERADING AS A SPORTS INJURY

Three key factors will assist the clinician to avoid missing an atypical or masquerading condition. The first is keeping an open mind to the possibility. Too often, we become more rigid regarding our initial diagnosis rather than being open to consider other possibilities. Sometimes a fresh perspective from a colleague can be helpful in this regard.

The second and perhaps most important key is obtaining a detailed and complete history and physical examination. If you do not ask the question or consider a broader differential diagnosis, it is impossible to pick up the subtle clues pointing to a less likely but masquerading condition. Indeed, if the concept of a masquerading condition is not triggered from the history and examination, it is unlikely that appropriate investigations to make the diagnosis will be ordered. For example, if a patient presents with tibial pain and it is, in fact, due to hypercalcaemia secondary to lung cancer, a bone scan of the tibia looking for stress fracture will usually not help with the diagnosis, but a history of weight loss, occasional haemoptysis and associated abdominal pain may. In a basketball player with shoulder pain, the history of associated arm tightness and the physical finding of prominent superficial veins are important clues to axillary vein thrombosis; a grey-scale ultrasound scan looking for rotator cuff tendinopathy will not provide the diagnosis.

> **PRACTICE PEARL**
>
> In sports medicine, it may seem simple to jump to the obvious conclusion regarding a specific diagnosis but if more in-depth questions or a thorough physical exam are not completed, it is difficult to be alert to a less common or 'non-obvious' diagnosis.

A third important key that points to masquerading conditions is when the clinical progression does not fit the pattern expected of the more common diagnosis or condition. When this occurs, consider alternative less common conditions. For example, the lingering contusion that should have resolved long ago could represent an underlying blood dyscrasia or tumour of the soft tissue or bone.

> **PRACTICE PEARL**
>
> You must ask yourself, 'Could this be a rare condition or unusual manifestation?' When the question is asked, then other options are entertained and the appropriate diagnosis can be conceived.

Ultimately, successful diagnosis of masquerading conditions requires keeping an open mind, performing a complete history and exam, and recognition of discrepancies between the patient's clinical features and clinical progress compared to what should be expected by the more typical diagnosis.

Conditions masquerading as sports injuries

Table 7.1 lists some of the conditions that may masquerade as sport and exercise medicine conditions. These are outlined below.

Bone and soft tissue tumours

Primary malignant tumours of bone and soft tissues are rare but when they occur it is most likely to be in the younger age group (second to third decade). Osteosarcoma can present at the distal or proximal end of long bones, more commonly in the lower limb, producing joint pain. Patients often recognise that pain is aggravated by activity and hence present to the sports medicine clinic. The pathological diagnosis of osteosarcoma is dependent on the detection of tumour-producing bone and so an X-ray may reveal a moth-eaten appearance with new bone formation in the soft tissues and lifting of the periosteum (Fig. 7.1). In young patients, the differential diagnosis includes osteomyelitis. It is recommended that any child or adolescent with bone pain be X-rayed.

Another presentation of tumour is when a patient presents with a mild injury that won't get better or with an atypical finding on radiographs taken when a fracture occurs. If fractures occur with relatively low energy or when they do not have an appropriate mechanism of injury masqueraders should be considered. They may also present as progressive pain rather than pain that improves with rest and treatment.

Malignant tumours (e.g. of the breast, lung and prostate) may metastasise to bone. Patients may not recognise that a previously treated malignancy could be related to limb pain. Breast carcinoma may also present as a frozen shoulder. An accurate history is, therefore, central to making an accurate diagnosis. Red flag signs for malignancy or infection include prominent night pain, often being woken at night with pain, fever, loss of appetite, weight loss and malaise. Patients exhibiting these symptoms should be examined and investigated thoroughly to determine the cause. In the sports population, patients with metastatic disease are more likely older and have more complex medical histories.

Giant cell tumours, aneurismal bone cysts and unicameral bone cysts are benign or less aggressive bone tumours that can present in a similar fashion with pain and failure to resolve in a time frame expected of a simple contusion or traumatic injury. Osteoid osteoma is a benign bone tumour that often presents as exercise-related bone pain and tenderness and is frequently misdiagnosed as a stress fracture. It can occasionally be seen on plain radiographs (Fig. 7.2a). The bone scan appearance is similar to that of a stress fracture, although the isotope uptake is more intense and widespread. This condition is characterised clinically by the presence of night pain and by the abolition of symptoms with the use of aspirin. The tumour has a characteristic appearance on CT scan (Fig. 7.2b) with a central nidus.

Ultimately, like malignant tumours of bone, the examiner should be vigilant regarding atypical complaints and failure to progress along normal healing timelines expected of simple contusions, stress fractures or frank fractures. Care should be taken to thoroughly interpret all radiographs for other potential causes of bone weakening that led to a fracture in the first place.

As for atypical bone pathologies, when soft tissue lesions present with an unusual history or do not progress as expected, the clinician should readily consider a broader differential diagnosis.

Synovial cell sarcoma frequently involves the larger lower joints such as the knee and ankle. Patients present with pain, often at night or with activity, maybe with instability and swelling. As a masquerader, these present as chronic swelling and pain that does not resolve with standard treatment. Like synovial sarcoma, synovial chondromatosis and pigmented villonodular synovitis are benign tumours of the synovium[1] found mainly in

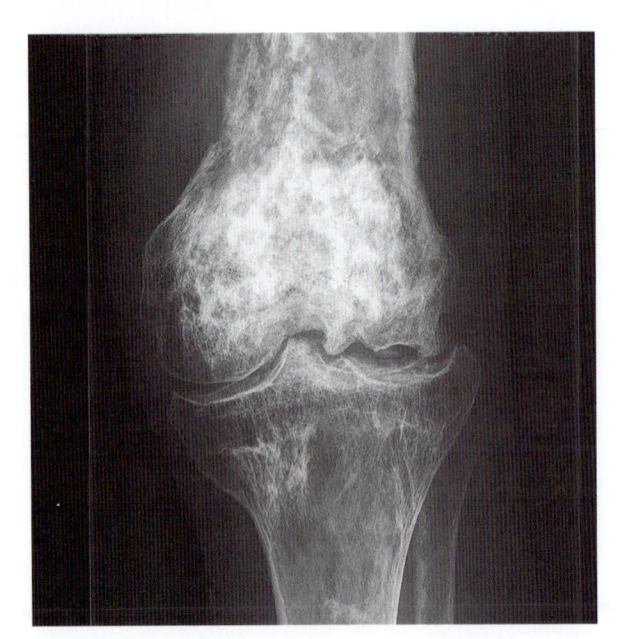

Figure 7.1 X-ray of an osteosarcoma in the distal femur

Beware: conditions that masquerade as sports injuries — CHAPTER 7

Table 7.1 Conditions that may masquerade as sport and exercise medicine conditions

CONDITION	
Bone and soft tissue tumours	• Osteosarcoma • Synovial sarcoma • Synovial chondromatosis • Pigmented villonodular synovitis • Rhabdomyosarcoma • Osteoid osteoma • Ganglion cyst
Rheumatological	• Inflammatory monoarthritis • Inflammatory polyarthritis • Inflammatory low back pain (e.g. sacroiliitis) • Enthesopathies (e.g. psoriatic, reactive arthritis)
Disorders of muscle	• Dermatomyositis • Polymyositis • Muscular dystrophy
Endocrine	• Dysthyroidism • Hypercalcaemia • Hypocalcaemia • Hyperparathyroidism • Diabetes • Cushing's syndrome • Acromegaly
Vascular	• Venous thrombosis (e.g. deep venous thrombosis, axillary vein thrombosis) • Artery entrapment (e.g. popliteal artery entrapment) • Peripheral vascular disease
Genetic	• Marfan syndrome • Haemochromatosis
Granulomatous diseases	• Tuberculosis • Sarcoidosis
Infection	• Osteomyelitis • Septic arthritis • Shingles • Lyme disease
Regional pain syndromes	• Complex regional pain syndrome • Fibromyalgia/myofascial pain syndrome

PART A   Fundamental principles

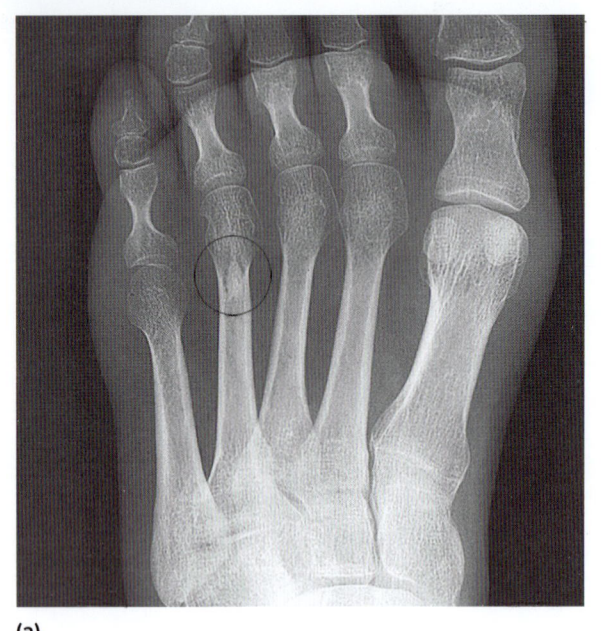

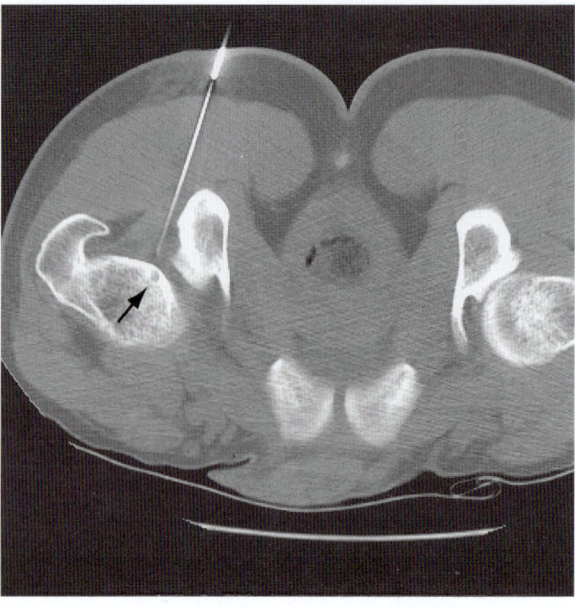

Figure 7.2 Osteoid osteoma (a) Radiograph showing sclerotic focus in distal fourth metacarpal (b) Transverse image from a CT scan demonstrating an osteoid osteoma. Note the lytic lesion in the anterior cortex of the femoral neck (arrow), with radiofrequency probe in position for ablation

the knee, which present with mechanical symptoms, persistent swelling, and failure to respond to basic rest, ice and anti-inflammatory regimens.

Direct trauma to muscle tissue can lead to a contusion, haematoma or myositis ossificans. Myositis generally presents with the classic history of direct trauma and swelling. Heat or ultrasound can exacerbate the process. Imaging studies show calcification within the muscle that should not be in continuity with the bone itself. Biopsies should be performed with caution, as there are case reports in the literature of the active edge of myositis ossificans being misread as osteosarcoma. Even less typically, trauma may result in haemorrhage into an indolent, underlying rhabdomyosarcoma. The clinician should consider alternative diagnoses in patients with hematomata that is slow to resolve or when the history of trauma does not fit with the clinical signs.

The most common of benign soft tissue tumours are ganglion cysts. These cysts are lined by connective tissue, contain mucinous fluid and are found mainly around the wrist, hand, knee and foot. They may be attached to a joint capsule or tendon sheath and may have a connection to the synovial cavity. They are usually asymptomatic but can occasionally cause pain and cosmetic deformity (Chapter 26).[2] However, ganglion cysts may also represent an important clue regarding other underlying, masquerading disease processes such as osteoarthritis or chronic tendinopathy.

Rheumatological conditions

Inflammatory musculoskeletal disorders in patients presenting to the sports medicine clinic frequently masquerade as a traumatic or mechanical condition. Low back pain of ankylosing spondylitis, psoriatic enthesopathy[3] presenting as patellar tendinopathy or flitting arthritis in early rheumatoid arthritis are common examples.

Effective management of athletes presenting with musculoskeletal complaints requires a structured history, physical examination and definitive diagnosis to distinguish soft tissue problems from joint problems and an inflammatory syndrome from a non-inflammatory syndrome. Clues to a systemic inflammatory aetiology may include constitutional symptoms, morning stiffness, elevated acute-phase reactants and progressive symptoms despite modification of physical activity. The mechanism of injury or lack thereof, is also a clue to any underlying disease. In these circumstances, more complete work-up is reasonable, including radiographs, MR imaging and laboratory testing for autoantibodies.[4]

When patients present with an acutely swollen knee without a history of precipitant trauma or patellar tendinopathy without overload, the clinician may be alerted to the possibility that these could be inflammatory in origin. Prominent morning joint or back stiffness, night pain or extra-articular manifestations of rheumatological conditions (e.g. skin rashes, nail abnormalities–Fig. 7.3), bowel disturbance, eye involvement (conjunctivitis, iritis) or urethral discharge may all provide clues.

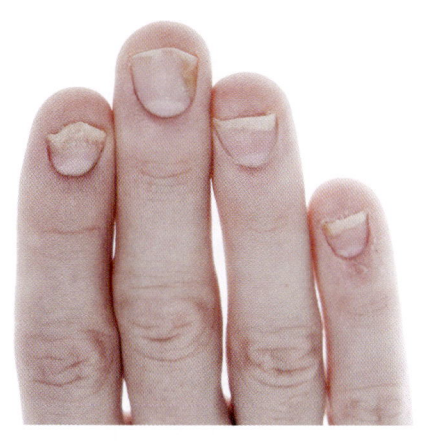

Figure 7.3 Typical appearance of nails in a patient with psoriatic arthropathy

Inflammation of entheses (e.g. in lateral elbow pain, patellar tendinopathy–Fig. 7.4), insertional Achilles tendinopathy and plantar fasciopathy) is almost universal among those with HLA (human leukocyte antigens) B27-related, seronegative (for rheumatoid factor) arthropathies. Enthesopathy is usually associated with other joint or extra-articular involvement, although a subgroup exists with enthesitis as the sole presentation.[2]

Muscle disorders

Dermatomyositis and polymyositis are inflammatory connective tissue disorders characterised by proximal limb girdle weakness, often without pain. Dermatomyositis, unlike polymyositis, is also associated with a photosensitive skin rash in light-exposed areas (hands and face). In the older adult, dermatomyositis may be associated with malignancy in approximately 50% of cases. The primary malignancy may be easily detectable or occult. In the younger adult, weakness may be profound (e.g. unable to rise from the floor) but in the early stages may manifest only as underperformance in training or competition.

Dermatomyositis and polymyositis may also be associated with other connective tissue disorders such as systemic lupus erythematosus or systemic sclerosis, and muscle abnormality is characterised by elevated creatine kinase levels and electromyographic (EMG) and muscle biopsy changes.

Endurance athletes may complain of myalgia and fatigue that is out of proportion with their training schedule. The differential diagnosis to explain these symptoms is broad. Mitochondrial myopathies, though uncommon, may present with cramping and muscle pain.[5] Consider myoglobinuria in these patients. Referral to a specialist neurologist for investigations and diagnosis will be necessary.[6]

Regional limb girdle dystrophies such as limb girdle dystrophy and facio-scapulo-humeral dystrophy may also present with proximal limb girdle weakness in young adults. They are also associated with characteristic EMG changes. Ultimately, when an athlete complains of muscle fatigue, aches and pains that fail to respond in a normal time frame expected with the patterns of training, a broader differential diagnosis needs to be considered

Endocrine disorders

Occasionally, the source of the masquerading symptoms in athletes is underlying endocrine disorders and pathologies. Disorders of thyroid function may present with a variety of rheumatological conditions.[7] Proximal muscle weakness with elevated creatine kinase and fibromyalgia may develop with hypothyroidism. Hyperthyroidism is associated with thyroid acropachy (soft tissue swelling and periosteal bone changes), adhesive capsulitis and painless proximal muscle weakness.[4] Hyperparathyroidism may be associated with the deposition of calcium pyrophosphate in joints. Patients may develop acute pseudogout or a polyarticular inflammatory arthritis resembling rheumatoid arthritis. X-rays of the wrists or knees may demonstrate chondrocalcinosis of the menisci or triangular fibrocartilage complex (Fig. 7.5).

Adhesive capsulitis or septic arthritis may be the presenting complaint in patients with diabetes mellitus and those with other endocrine disorders such as acromegaly may develop premature osteoarthritis or carpal tunnel syndrome. Patients with hypercalcaemia secondary to malignancy (e.g. of the lung) or other conditions such as hyperparathyroidism can present with bone pain as well as constipation, confusion and renal calculi. A proximal

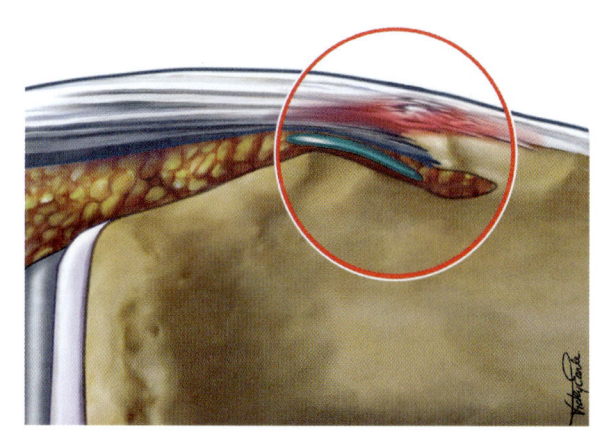

Figure 7.4 Enthesopathy (such as at the distal patellar tendon shown here) should alert the clinician to consider the possibility of an underlying spondyloarthropathy

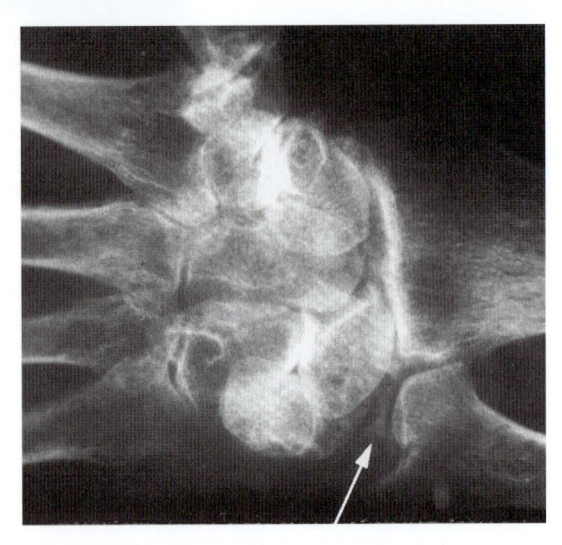

Figure 7.5 Chondrocalcinosis of the triangular fibrocartilage (arrow) in calcium pyrophosphate dehydrate deposition disease

myopathy may develop in patients with primary Cushing's syndrome or after corticosteroid use. When symptoms of myalgia, joint stiffness and swelling do not resolve, a more in-depth laboratory work-up hunting for masqueraders is appropriate and indicated.

Vascular disorders
Patients with venous thrombosis or arterial abnormalities (Fig. 7.6) may present with limb pain and swelling aggravated by exercise. Calf, femoral or axillary veins are common sites for thrombosis. While a precipitant cause may be apparent (e.g. recent surgery or air travel), consider also the thrombophilias such as the antiphospholipid syndrome or deficiencies of protein C, protein S, antithrombin III or factor V Leiden. When athletes with no other risk factors for thrombosis develop a blood clot, more extensive work-up is necessary to look for the masquerading underlying cause, which in turn will guide treatment.

The claudicant pain of peripheral vascular disease is most likely to be first noticed with exercise and so patients may present to the sports medicine practitioner. Remember also that arteriopathy can occur in patients with diabetes. Various specific vascular entrapments are also found, such as popliteal artery entrapment, which presents as exercise-related calf pain and thoracic outlet syndrome.

Genetic disorders
Various genetic disorders have been associated with an increased risk of injury and in some cases catastrophic injuries in athletes. Ehlers Danlos with its increased ligamentous laxity has been associated with increased risk of ligament injuries. Osteogenesis imperfect has been associated with an increased fracture risk. Down's syndrome is associated with odontoid hypoplasia with inherent increased risk of cervical spine injuries. Marfan syndrome has been associated with sudden cardiac death. Marfan syndrome is an autosomal dominant disorder of fibrillin characterised by musculoskeletal, cardiac and ocular abnormalities.[8] Musculoskeletal problems are common due to joint hypermobility, ligament laxity, scoliosis or spondylolysis. In patients with the Marfanoid habitus, referral for echocardiography and ophthalmological opinion should be considered as sudden cardiac death or lens dislocation may result.

Haemochromatosis is an autosomal recessive disorder of iron handling, which results in iron overload. Patients may present with a calcium pyrophosphate arthropathy with characteristic involvement of the second and third metacarpophalangeal joints and hook-shaped osteophytes seen on X-ray of these joints. While ferritin levels are raised in patients with haemochromatosis, it is important to remember that ferritin may also be elevated in athletes taking iron supplements or in response to any acute inflammatory illness.[9] Fasting transferrin levels and detection of the HFE gene are central to the diagnosis of inherited haemochromatosis. Once again, considering a broad differential diagnosis based on clinical presentation and history may help make these genetic diagnoses, which in turn will allow the clinician to better counsel the athlete regarding risks of participation in certain sports.

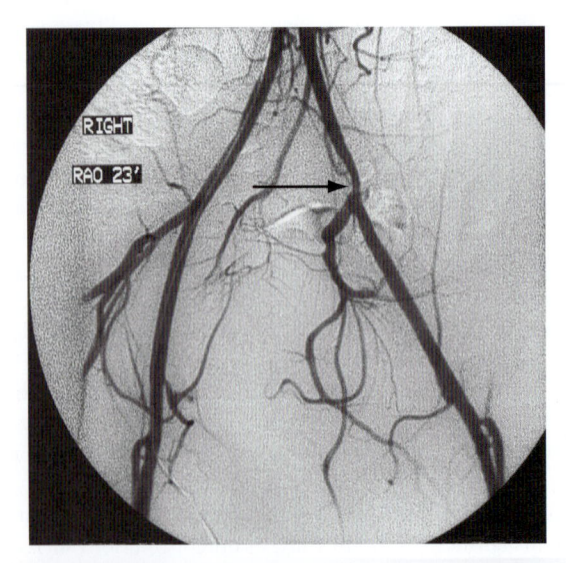

Figure 7.6 Angiogram showing common iliac artery stenosis (arrow)

Granulomatous diseases

Granulomatous diseases such as tuberculosis and sarcoidosis have been called 'the great mimickers' or great 'masqueraders' secondary to their ability to present in many varied and atypical fashions. They can look like tumours, inflammation, infection or traumatic injuries. Tuberculosis is a granulomatous mycobacterial infection. Musculoskeletal involvement includes chronic septic arthritis and Pott's spine fracture.

Patients with acute sarcoidosis can present with fevers, lower limb (commonly) rash and ankle swelling. The rash of erythema nodosum (Fig. 7.7) may be mistaken for cellulitis and antibiotics have frequently been prescribed in error. The diagnosis is easily made by chest X-ray, which shows changes of bilateral hilar lymphadenopathy. The clinician should remember that the differential diagnosis of bilateral hilar lymphadenopathy includes tuberculosis and lymphoma. Chronic sarcoidosis is a systemic disorder involving the lungs, central nervous system, skin, eyes and musculoskeletal system. Patients can present with chronic arthropathy together with bone cysts or with bone pain due to hypercalcaemia.

Infection

Bone and joint infections, while uncommon, may have disastrous consequences if the diagnosis is missed. Bone pain in children, worse at night or with activity, should alert the clinician to the possibility of osteomyelitis. Bone infection near a joint may result in a reactive joint effusion.

Septic arthritis is rare in the normal joint. In arthritic or diabetic joints or joints that recently underwent arthroscopy, sepsis is much more common. Rapid joint destruction may follow if left untreated.

Even though *Staphylococcus aureus* is the causative organism in more than 50% of cases of acute septic joints, it is imperative that joint aspiration for Gram stain, and culture and blood cultures are taken before commencement of antibiotic treatment. Once-only or repeated joint lavage may be considered in patients receiving intravenous antibiotic treatment. The immunocompromised patient may present with a chronic septic arthritis. In this situation, tuberculosis or fungal infections should be considered. In suspected cases of septic arthritis, the patient should be admitted to hospital.[10]

Another cause of arthritis is Lyme disease, a common arthropod-borne infection in some countries including the US. Hallmarks of Lyme disease are erythema migrans (EM), disruption of electrical conduction of cardiac muscle, the development of neurological abnormalities and episodes of arthritis. Intermittent episodes of arthritis develop several weeks or months after infection and, despite adequate antibiotic therapy, symptoms persist in 10% of patients with arthritis. The severity of arthritis can range from mild to moderate inflammation of the joints and tendons months after infection, to a chronic, debilitating osteoarthropathy complete with destruction of cartilage and erosion of bone in a subset of these individuals within a few years. In severe cases, the highly inflammatory aspects of Lyme arthritis can lead to cartilage and bone erosion with permanent joint dysfunction. The diagnosis of Lyme disease is clinical and serological tests should be used to confirm the clinical diagnosis.[11]

Pain syndromes

Complex regional pain syndrome type I is a post-traumatic phenomenon characterised by localised pain out of proportion to the injury, vasomotor disturbances, oedema and delayed recovery from injury. The vasomotor disturbances of an extremity manifest as vasodilatation (warmth, redness) or vasoconstriction (coolness, cyanosis, mottling).[12] Early mobilisation, use of motor imagery and avoidance of surgery are important keys to successful management (see also Chapter 6).

Myofascial pain syndromes develop secondary to either acute or overuse trauma. They present as regional pain associated with the presence of one or more active trigger points (Chapter 4).

Fibromyalgia is a chronic pain syndrome characterised by widespread pain, chronic fatigue, decreased pain threshold, sleep disturbance, psychological distress and characteristic tender points. It is often associated with other symptoms including irritable bowel syndrome, dyspareunia, headache, irritable bladder, and subjective joint swelling and pain. Fibromyalgia is diagnosed on the examination finding of 11 of 18 specific tender point sites in a patient with widespread pain. Chronic fatigue syndrome has many similarities to fibromyalgia[10] and may be the same disease process. It may present as excessive post-exercise muscle soreness but is always

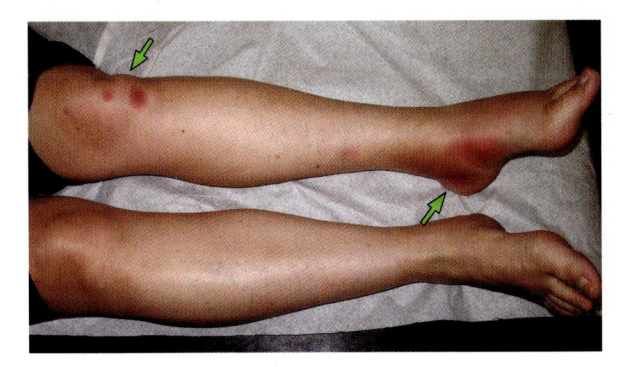

Figure 7.7 Erythema nodosum in acute sarcoidosis.
PHOTO COURTESY OF DR RAHEEM B KHERANI

associated with excessive fatigue. There is evidence that exercise improves global wellbeing in women with this condition.[13]

SUMMARY

In summary, it is important for the clinician to be on constant alert for potential masqueraders when dealing with athletic injuries. Clearly, common things are common; most of the time the clinician will be correct with the first and most likely diagnosis. However, when the history or physical examination is not classic and an athlete fails to improve and heal in the expected time frame of the more common diagnosis, a broader differential diagnosis including masquerading causes should be considered. Stay open minded to the potential if not likelihood of important masquerading pathologies.

REFERENCES

References for this chapter can be found at www.mhhe.com/au/CSM5e

Chapter 8

Introduction to clinical biomechanics

with CHRISTIAN BARTON, NATALIE COLLINS and KAY CROSSLEY

> *Mo Farah has nine key elements to his running technique that have allowed him to become Britain's greatest ever runner.*
> www.telegraph.co.uk, 16 September 2013

The term 'biomechanics' can be used in a variety of ways. In this book, biomechanics refers to the description, analysis and assessment of human movement during sporting activities.[1] Broadly, biomechanics can be broken into three categories, including 'kinematics' (movement we can see), 'kinetics' (forces driving the movement) and 'neuromotor' (muscle function controlling forces and movement). This chapter will focus primarily on the actual movement occurring in the body segments (kinematics). Our approach can be referred to as 'subjective biomechanical analysis'. We aim to describe movement such as running or squatting as it appears to visual observation. This reflects how clinicians assess and treat, and it can be done with the assistance of video analysis and without expensive laboratory equipment.

The aims of this chapter are to:

- outline the basics of 'ideal' lower limb biomechanics
- explain the ideal biomechanics with running
- describe lower limb biomechanical assessment in the clinical setting
- outline how to clinically assess footwear
- review the best available evidence associating biomechanical factors with injuries, as well as sharing clinical opinions as to which technical factors in sports contribute to specific injuries
- discuss how to manage biomechanical abnormalities detected in the assessment
- explain normal and abnormal upper limb biomechanics.

We address lower limb and upper limb biomechanics separately for the learner's convenience, but the experienced clinician will consider the close relationship between the upper and lower limbs during a variety of functional tasks.

Ultimately, biomechanical evaluation should be completed based on task specificity to ensure the clinician is confident in the accuracy of information obtained.

'IDEAL' LOWER LIMB BIOMECHANICS—THE BASICS

Here we discuss ideal structural characteristics, including available joint range of motion and stance position. Note that each individual has his or her own mechanical make-up due to structural characteristics (anatomy), and may never achieve the 'ideal' position or biomechanical function. Table 8.1 and Figure 8.1 provide reference for ideal joint range of motion and planes of movement respectively.

Lower limb joint motion

The *hip joint* is formed between the femoral head and acetabulum. The ball-and-socket structure of this joint permits motion in all three planes.

The *knee joint* is formed between the tibial plateau and femoral condyles. Primarily a hinge joint, the knee allows flexion and extension in the sagittal plane. The knee also permits some rotation in the transverse plane. This secondary motion is particularly important to allow the knee to lock into an extended position for stance stability, and to unlock when moving into flexion for shock absorption.

The *ankle joint* (between the shank and rearfoot) consists primarily of two articulations, the *talocrual joint* and the *subtalar joint* (STJ). The talocrual joint is formed between the talus and the mortise of the tibia and fibula malleoli. Its axis of motion is predominantly in the frontal plane which allows dorsiflexion and plantarflexion motion in the sagittal plane (Fig. 8.2a and b).[2]

PART A Fundamental principles

Table 8.1 A guide to lower limb joint ranges of motion when in neutral positions

Joint	Plane	Assessment position	Available range
Hip	Sagittal	Supine	Flexion = 120°
		Prone	Extension = 20°
	Frontal	Supine	Abduction = 40°; adduction = 25°
	Transverse	Supine/prone±hip flexion/extension	Internal rotation = 45°; external rotation = 45°
Knee	Sagittal	Supine	Flexion = 135°; extension = 0°
	Frontal		None
	Transverse	Full extension	None
		70° flexion	45° rotation
Foot and ankle (triplanar)*	Sagittal	Supine	Plantarflexion = 45°; dorsiflexion = 20°
	Frontal		Supination = 45–60°; pronation = 15–30°
First metatarsophalangeal (MTP)	Sagittal	Supine	Plantarflexion = 45°; dorsiflexion = 70°

*Refers to combined motion of the talocrual, subtalar, midtarsal and metatarsal break joints

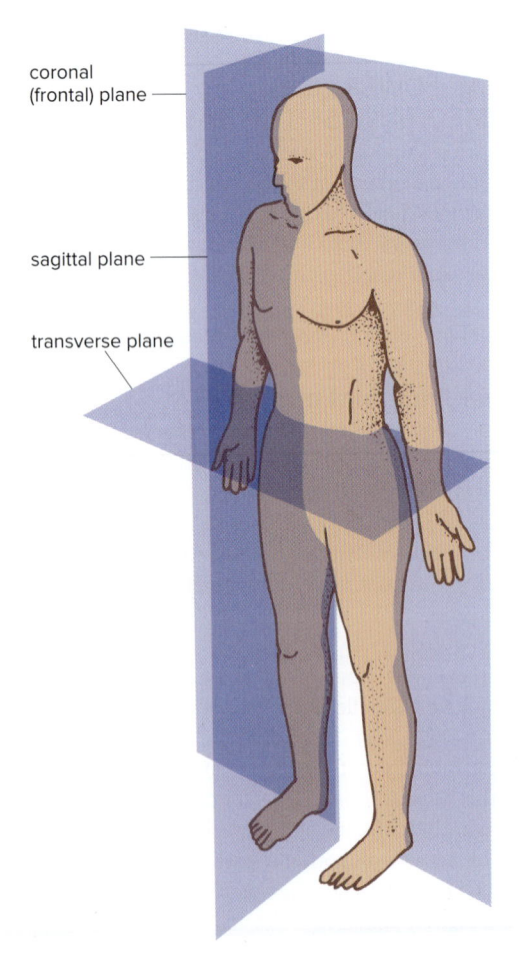

Figure 8.1 Anatomical planes of the body

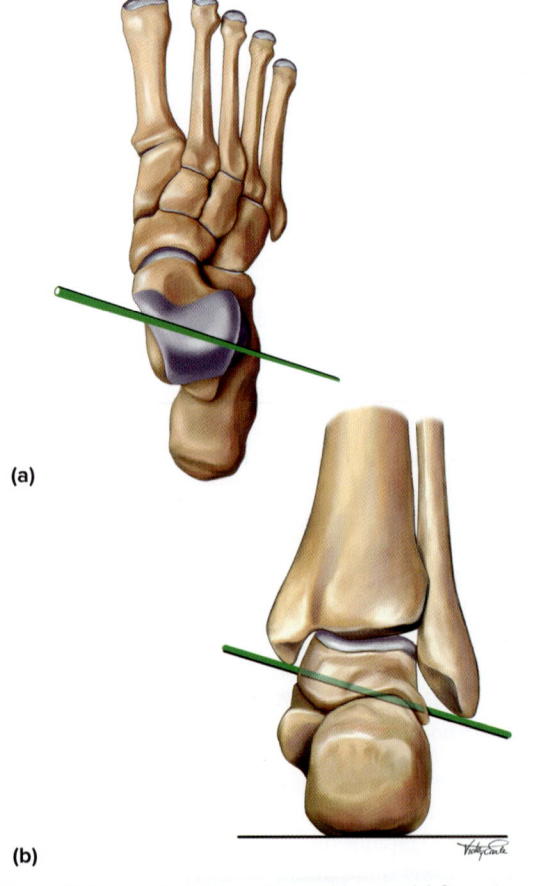

Figure 8.2 Axis of motion of the ankle joint (a) Superior view (b) Posterior view

86

Introduction to clinical biomechanics CHAPTER 8

The STJ is formed between the calcaneus and talus. The three articular facets of the STJ allow for complex triplanar motions of pronation and supination. The axis of motion runs posteriorly and inferiorly in the sagittal plane (40–50°), and laterally in the transverse plane (20–25°)[2] (Fig. 8.3a–d). During pronation, the STJ axis provides primarily eversion, which is combined with dorsiflexion and abduction (Fig. 8.3d). During supination, the STJ axis provides primarily inversion, which is combined with plantarflexion and adduction (Fig. 8.3c).

The *midtarsal joint* is formed between the midfoot and rearfoot, and consists of two articulations, the *calcaneocuboid joint* and the *talonavicular joint*. These articulations provide two joint axes. The oblique axis allows large amounts of sagittal plane (dorsiflexion/plantarflexion) and transverse plane (abduction/adduction) motion, while the longitudinal axis allows small amounts of frontal plane (eversion and inversion) motion (Fig. 8.4a and b).

Importantly, the orientation between these two axes allows the role of the foot to change during weight-bearing. As the rear foot everts, the two axes align so they are more parallel, unlocking the foot and allowing it to conform to the surface and/or absorb the ground reaction force (GRF). Conversely, as the rearfoot inverts, the two axes converge, locking the foot into a supinated position and allowing it to function as a rigid lever for propulsion.[2]

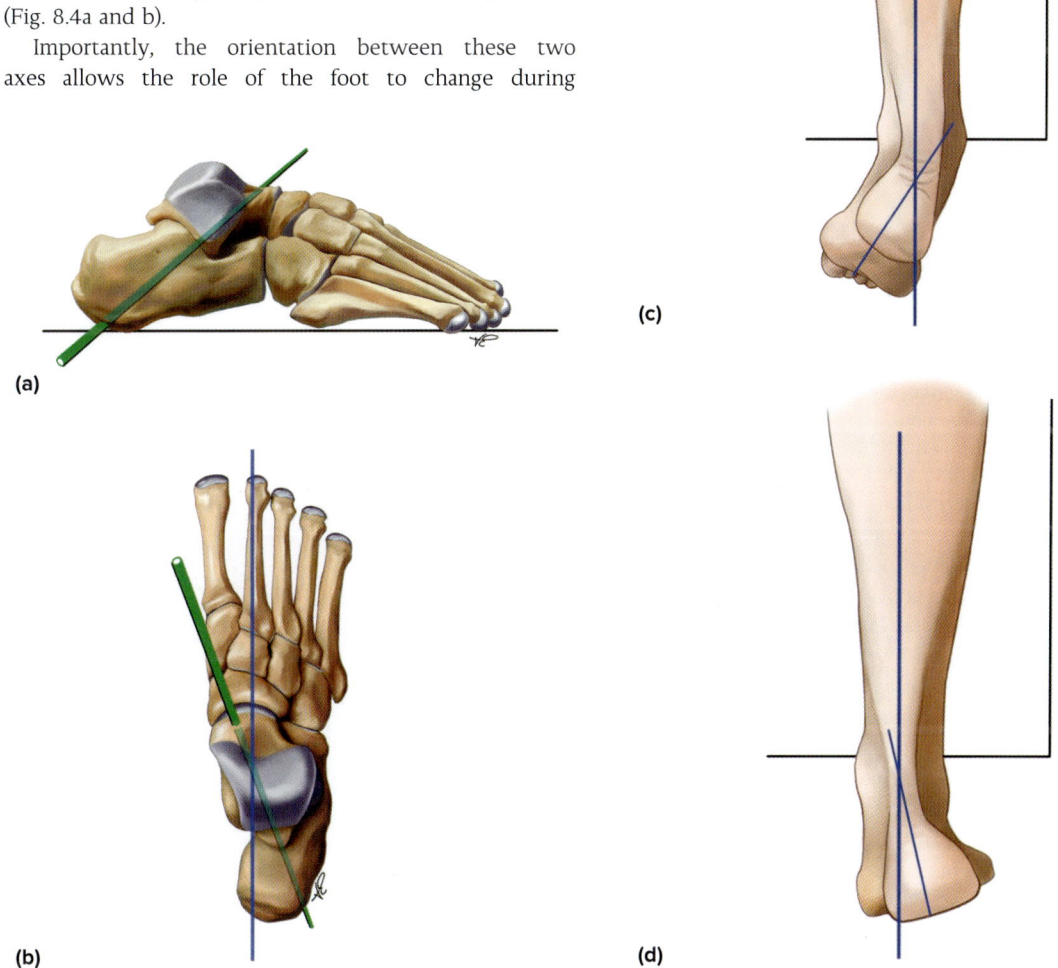

Figure 8.3 Axis of motion of the subtalar joint (a) Lateral view. Angle of inclination approximately 50° to transverse plane (b) Superior view. Angle between axis of motion of subtalar joint and longitudinal axis of the rearfoot is approximately 15° (c) Supination at subtalar joint with 20° calcaneal inversion (d) Pronation at subtalar joint with 10° calcaneal inversion

87

PART A   Fundamental principles

(a)

(b)

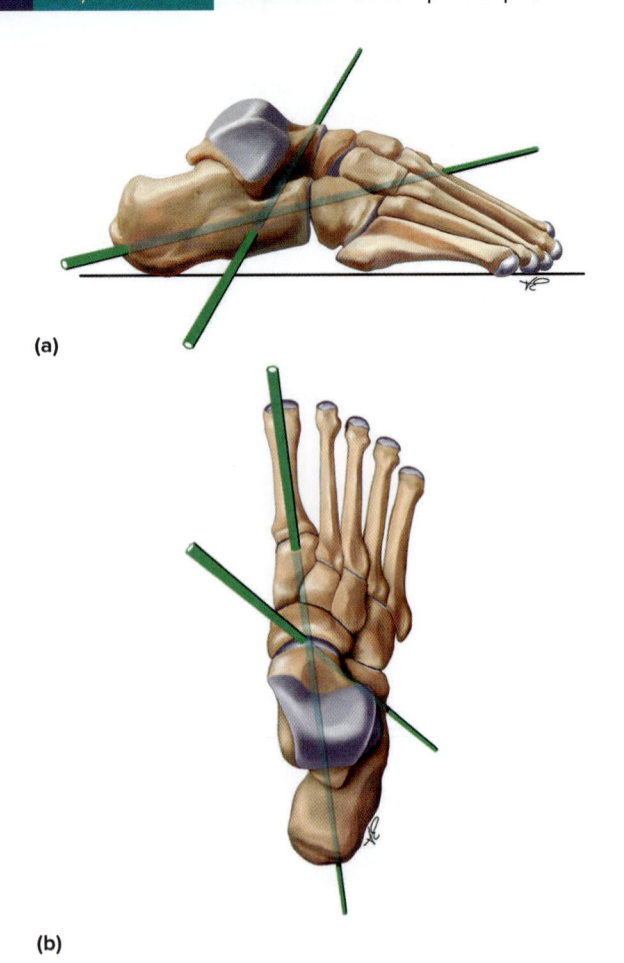

Figure 8.4 Oblique and longitudinal axis of midtarsal joint (a) Lateral view (b) Superior view

The *midtarsal (or Lisfranc) joints* are formed between the distal tarsal bones of the midfoot (cuneiforms and cuboid) and the five metatarsal bones (forefoot). The axis of motion for these joints runs primarily in the transverse plane in an oblique direction (Fig. 8.5a and b). This leads primarily to sagittal plane motion (flexion/extension), although some frontal plane motion (eversion/inversion) does occur medially (adduction, Fig. 8.5c) and laterally (abduction, Fig. 8.5d).

The *first metatarsophalangeal joint* (MTPJ) is formed between the head of the first metatarsal and the base of the proximal phalanx. The primary motion that occurs at this joint is in the sagittal plane (flexion/extension) (Fig. 8.6). In particular, extension of this joint is essential to optimise function of the windlass mechanism (see below) during gait.

Ideal neutral stance position

To examine stance position, have the patient adopt a normal, comfortable, standing posture. Ideal neutral stance occurs when the joints of the lower limbs and feet are symmetrically aligned, with the weight-bearing

(a)

(b)

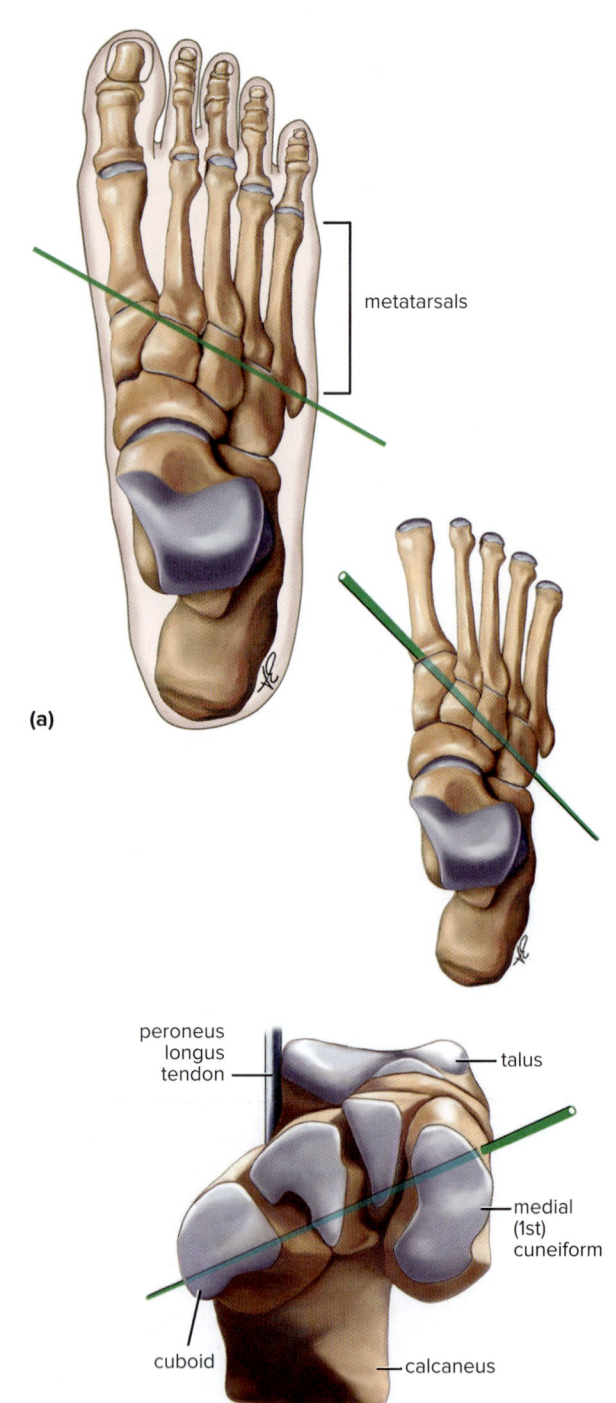

Figure 8.5 (a) midtarsal joints—the joints between the distal tarsal bones of the midfoot (cuneiforms and cuboid) and the five metatarsal bones (forefoot) (b) The metatarsal break (frontal plane). The axis of motion runs as shown (green rod)

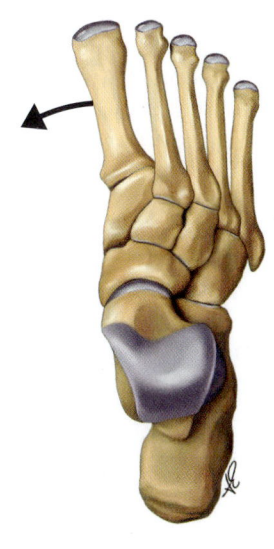

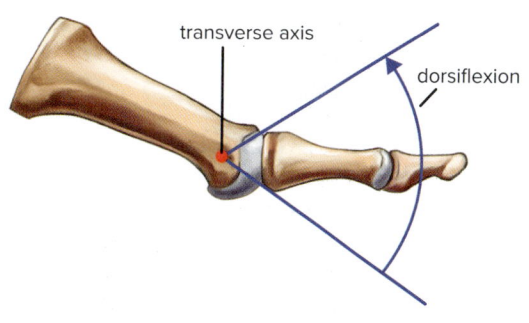

Introduction to clinical biomechanics CHAPTER 8

Figure 8.6 Motion of the hallux around the transverse axis of the first metatarsophalangeal joint

(c)

(d)

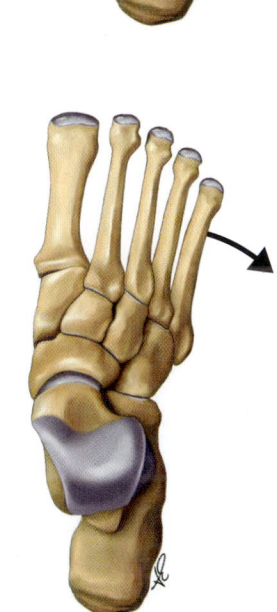

Figure 8.5 (cont.) Frontal plane motion of the metatarsal break showing that the forefoot can (c) adduct and (d) abduct

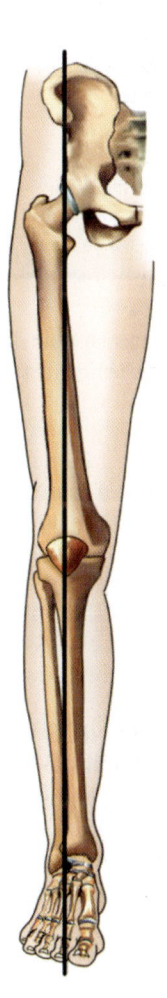

Figure 8.7 The alignment of the lower limb in neutral position. The weight-bearing line runs through the anterior superior iliac spine, patella and second metatarsal. The calcaneus is in line with the tibia, and the forefoot is perpendicular to the calcaneus

line passing through the anterior superior iliac spine, the patella and the second metatarsal (Fig. 8.7).

When the feet are in a symmetrical position, the subtalar (talocalcaneal) joint is neither pronated nor supinated, and the midtarsal joint (talonavicular and calcaneocuboid joints) is maximally pronated so that the first and second metatarsal heads are in contact with the ground. The long axis of the forefoot through the second metatarsal is perpendicular to the bisection of the heel (Fig. 8.8) and in line with the tibial tuberosity. The ankle joint is neither plantarflexed nor dorsiflexed, and the tibia is perpendicular

89

PART A Fundamental principles

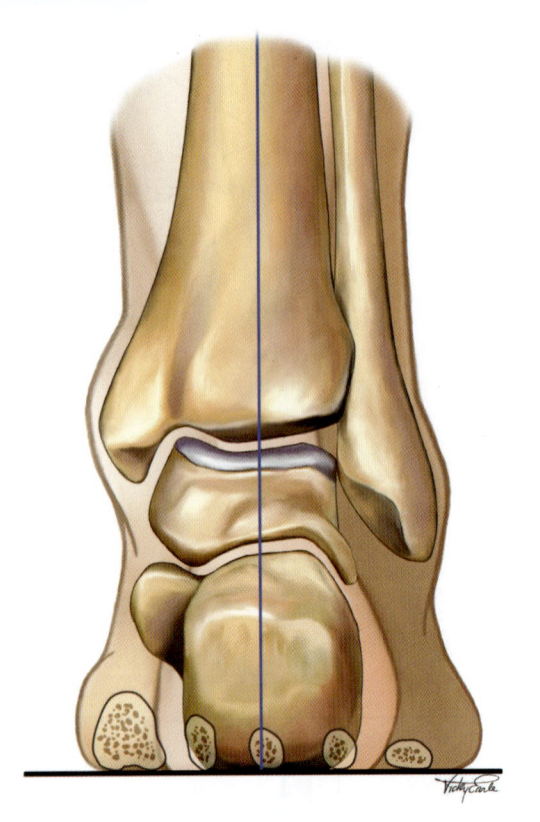

Figure 8.8 Normal relationship between the forefoot and rearfoot when the foot is in neutral stance

to the supporting surface in the sagittal and frontal plane. The knee is fully extended (but not hyper extended) and in slight valgus alignment. The hips are in a neutral position (neither internally nor externally rotated, neither flexed nor extended). The left and right anterior superior iliac spines of the pelvis are level. A slight anterior tilt of the pelvis is normal. More specific objective descriptions of ideal alignment are outlined in the assessment section.

'IDEAL' BIOMECHANICS WITH MOVEMENT—RUNNING

As injury mechanisms for many overuse injuries can be associated with theoretically suboptimal lower limb biomechanics, the clinician must know how to assess lower limb biomechanics during running. We focus first on the heel strike pattern of running as this is the predominant pattern for the majority of runners.[3] We will then consider how biomechanics is altered when running with a forefoot strike pattern.

Although we focus on ideal running biomechanics, ideal walking biomechanics are similar to heel strike running patterns outlined below. The most important biomechanical feature that distinguishes running from walking is the airborne or 'float' phase of running, where neither foot is in contact with the ground.[2] Additionally, vertical GRFs during running are double that of walking,[2,4] the pelvis is in greater anterior tilt,[5] and sagittal plane excursions of the knee and hip are increased. Ultimately, this leads to greater stress on structures of the lower limb.

The heel strike pattern of running can be split into a number of phases (Fig. 8.9), each of which will be discussed below.

Loading (heel strike to foot flat)

With the leg swinging toward the line of progression, and the foot supinated, the rearfoot (heel) contacts the ground in slight inversion (0-5°).[2,6-8] At heel strike, the pelvis is level, in slight anterior tilt (10°), and internally rotated; the hip is externally rotated (5-10°) and flexed (20-30°); and the knee is flexed (10°). Due to the laterally directed line of the GRF produced by heel strike, a cascade of events occurs to assist shock absorption. First, the rearfoot begins to evert, accompanied by tibial and femoral (hip) internal rotation, and hip adduction. This is combined with knee flexion, which peaks at around 45° as a result of the GRF line passing posterior to the knee joint.[9,10] Each of these motions is controlled by eccentric muscle activity which helps to dissipate the GRF. In addition, there may be contralateral pelvic drop, although this should be minimal (approximately 5°).[10] The gluteal musculature should actively control this motion and further dissipate the GRF.

Initial rearfoot eversion also results in more parallel alignment of the midtarsal joints (i.e. calcaneocuboid and talonavicular), causing them to unlock.[2] Importantly, this allows the forefoot to make solid contact with the ground at foot flat[11] and allows the foot to adapt during loading to potentially uneven or unstable terrain.[2]

Although motions that comprise foot pronation are normal, they should not be excessive or rapid (i.e. hyperpronation). Excessive motion will place strain on structures designed to control foot pronation, such as the plantar fascia, tibialis posterior muscle and intrinsic foot musculature.[2] Excessive pronation also increases medial GRF, accentuating more proximal motion at the knee, hip and pelvis, and increasing load on ligamentous and muscular structures responsible for proximal control.[2]

The clinician should carefully note proximal motion during this early phase of stance. Excessive contralateral pelvic drop and/or hip adduction/internal rotation may increase strain on structures required to control it, such as the iliotibial band (ITB), gluteal musculature and tensor fascia latae (TFL) muscle. Additionally, this may also place increased or altered loading on the lumbar spine, tibiofemoral joint and patellofemoral joint (PFJ). Any

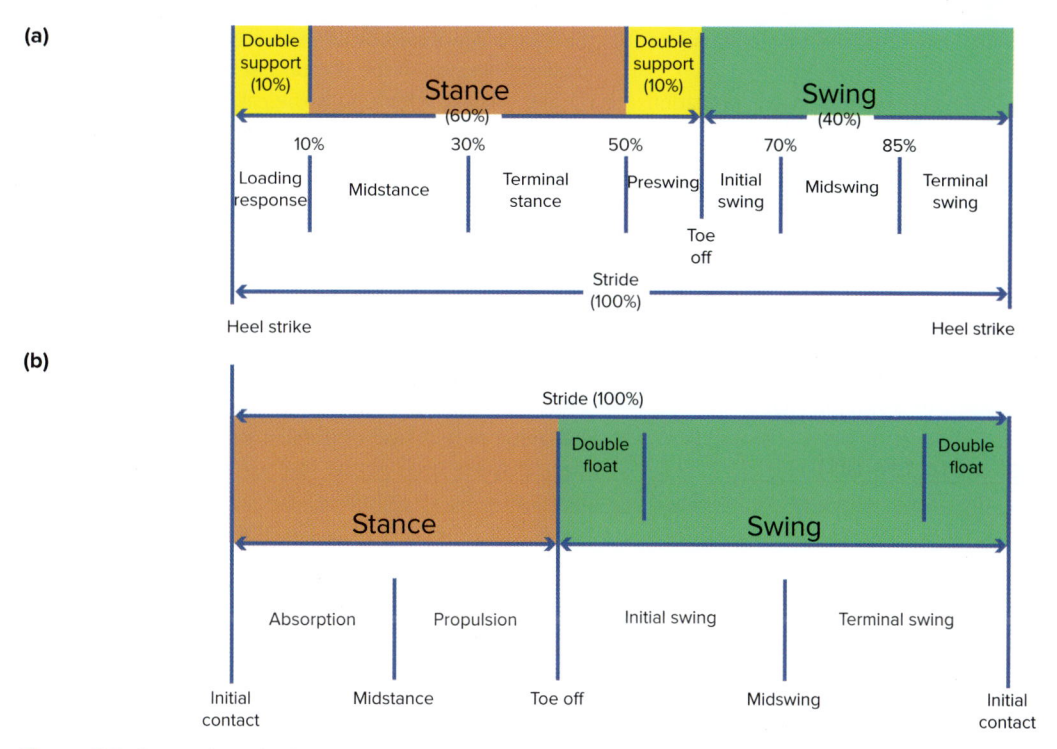

Introduction to clinical biomechanics CHAPTER 8

Figure 8.9 Gait cycle with phases and individual components (a) Walking (b) Running
ADAPTED FROM DUGAN AND BHAT[2]

excessive anterior tilting of the pelvis may place excessive strain on the lumbar spine and/or hamstring musculature, and may impair gluteal function.

Conversely, inadequate pronation or excessive supination may lead to an excessive or prolonged laterally directed GRF,[2] resulting in a less mobile foot and poorer shock absorption capacity. This may be associated with lower limb stress fractures,[12] or increase the incidence of lateral ankle sprain and chronic ankle instability.[13, 14]

Midstance (foot flat to heel off)

The beginning of midstance is indicated by the forefoot making contact with the ground, normally in a neutral transverse plane position (i.e. not abducted or adducted).[6] Lower limb biomechanical function during midstance involves a transition from biomechanics required for shock absorption following loading, to biomechanics required for propulsion. During this time, the ankle moves towards maximal dorsiflexion (approximately 20°) to allow forward motion of the tibia and the centre of mass (COM) to pass over the stance leg.[15] Excessive ankle dorsiflexion can lead to increased strain on the plantar fascia, Achilles tendon, and associated gastrocnemius and soleus musculature. At the same time, the hip and knee are moving from flexion towards extended positions, assisting forward motion of the body's COM.

Maximal foot pronation followed by maximal ankle dorsiflexion should be reached immediately after the body's COM has passed anterior to the stance limb.[11] Peak rearfoot eversion should reach approximately 10°,[6, 16] and peak forefoot abduction approximately 5°.[6] The rearfoot then begins to invert and the forefoot adducts, causing the foot to supinate, and the tibia and femur to externally rotate.[11] This external rotation action is assisted by force transmission from the externally rotating pelvis, which results from momentum of the swinging contralateral limb.

There are a number of things for the clinician to consider during this phase. Excessive pronation, or delayed/failed transition from shock absorption to propulsion actions by the lower limb, may be detrimental to a number of structures. Firstly, this will place excessive strain on structures responsible for controlling pronation and may increase the risk of conditions such as plantar fasciopathy, Achilles and tibialis posterior tendinopathies, proximal tibial periostitis, or tibial stress fractures due to excessive pull of the tibialis posterior and long flexors. Also, continued instability of the foot may lead to development of first MTPJ abnormalities, including hallux valgus, sesamoid pain and/or excessive interdigital compression (Morton's neuroma). If left untreated, over time this instability may also lead to metatarsal or sesamoid stress fractures.

More proximally, excessive or prolonged pronation may also result in abnormal transverse and frontal plane motion at the hip and knee due to a delay in external rotation. Ultimately, this can place excessive strain on many structures such as the PFJ, patellar tendon (both conditions discussed in Chapter 36), ITB (Chapter 37), and musculature that control this motion. Conversely, the same proximal anomalies may result due to inadequate pelvic and hip control. The source of the biomechanical dysfunction may need to be determined through further structural and functional tests (see assessment section below).

Propulsion (heel off to toe off)

Following heel off, the foot continues to supinate. Importantly, as this occurs, inversion of the rearfoot causes the transverse tarsal joint axes to converge.[2] This convergence of joint axes causes the midfoot to lock into position, creating a rigid lever.[2] Concurrently, the stance limb continues to externally rotate, the hip reaches maximal extension of between 0 and 10°,[5, 15, 17] and the knee flexes once more due to hamstring muscle contraction.[15, 17] Additionally, acceleration of the stance limb is provided through plantar flexion at the ankle, produced by the gastrocnemius and soleus complex.[18] This same gastrocnemius and soleus activity, along with the tibialis posterior and intrinsic foot musculature activity, continues to actively assist supination of the foot, and maintain its function as a rigid lever.[2] Passively, rigidity of the foot is supported by the windlass mechanism, that is, increased tension of the plantar fascia due to extension of the metatarsals, which pulls the calcaneus and metatarsal heads together (Fig. 8.10).[2] By toe off, the rearfoot should be inverted to approximately 10°, and the forefoot adducted approximately 5°.[6]

Failure of normal propulsion will cause an inefficient gait pattern. This can limit performance and predispose to injury for several reasons. First, the peroneal musculature may be forced to work harder to stabilise the medial and lateral columns of the foot which can lead to peroneal tendinopathy and/or stress fracture of the fibula.

Second, impaired supination may lead to toe off via the lateral rays instead of the first ray. This may compress the transverse arch of the foot excessively, and lead to interdigital nerve compression (Morton's neuroma) and risk of lateral forefoot stress fracture.

Third, reduced propulsion from the stance limb may increase reliance on the swing phase to produce forward momentum. To achieve this, the hip flexors, rectus femoris and iliopsoas will generate more rapid hip flexion, increasing the potential for tendinopathies. Additionally, to compensate for impaired propulsion, pelvic and trunk rotation may increase, leading to increased strain on spinal structures.

Initial swing

Following ipsilateral toe off, the body is thrust into the first 'float' phase where neither limb is in contact with the ground. Rectus femoris and iliopsoas muscle activity continue the forward momentum of the now swinging

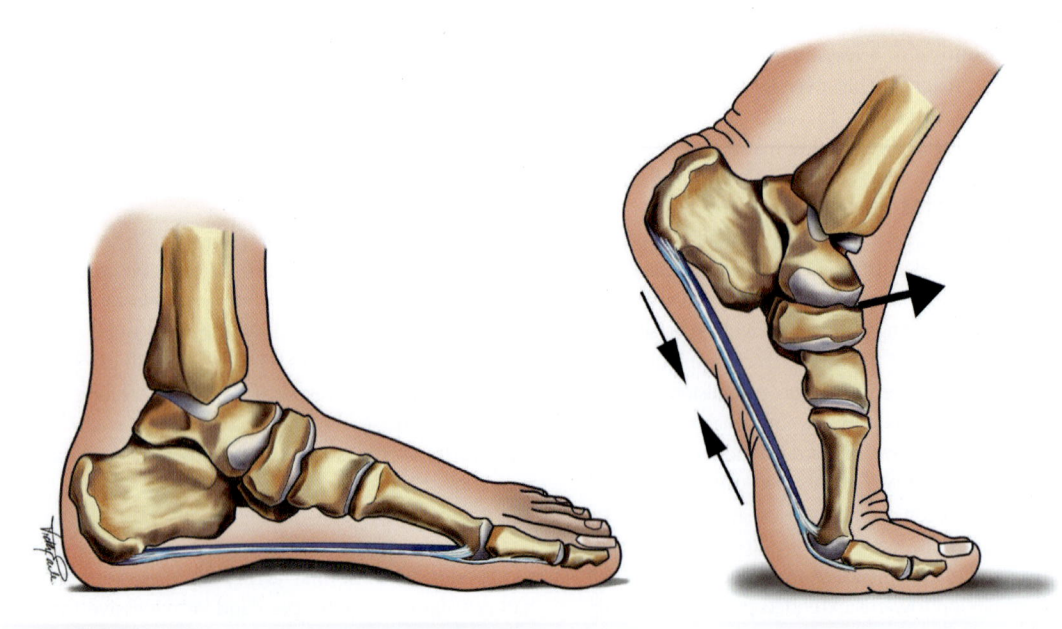

Figure 8.10 The windlass mechanism comes into play after heel off. Metatarsal extension increases tension on the plantar fascia, and forces the transverse tarsal joint into flexion which increases stability at push off

Introduction to clinical biomechanics   CHAPTER 8

limb.[19] As the limb advances, the pelvis moves with it, thrusting the hip into abduction and external rotation, which is in turn controlled by the hip adductors.[19] The tibialis anterior contracts to begin dorsiflexing the foot in preparation for terminal swing.[19] While these motions continue, they are aided by the addition of a new stable support when the contralateral limb strikes the ground and commences its own *loading* phase. Continuation of normal swing at this time relies on the ability of the contralateral gluteal musculature to dissipate the GRF produced by this event and prevent the pelvis dropping on the swing side. Failure to do so will increase the work required by the hip and knee flexors to clear the swinging limb, possibly leading to overuse injury.

Terminal swing

Following contralateral toe off, the body is thrust into the second 'float' phase. During this time the ipsilateral swinging hip reaches maximal flexion (approximately 30°),[5, 9] before being brought under control by the hamstring and gluteal musculature.[19] The same hamstring activity slows the rapidly extending knee in preparation for heel strike. At the same time, the hip adductors, which have been working eccentrically to control abduction of the swinging limb, begin to work concentrically to adduct the hip and bring it toward the midline.[19]

Angle and base of gait

The angle of gait is the angle between the longitudinal bisection of the foot and the line of progression (Fig. 8.11). The normal angle of gait is approximately 10° abducted from the line of progression in walking. Abducted gait describes an angle of gait greater than 10°. The angle of gait reflects the hip and tibial transverse plane positions. The base of gait is the distance between the medial aspect of the heels (Fig. 8.11). A normal base of gait is approximately 2.5-3 cm.

Changes from the normal angle and base of gait may be secondary to structural abnormalities or, more commonly, as compensation for another abnormality. For example, a wide base of gait may be necessary to increase stability. As running velocity increases, the angle and base of gait decrease. With faster running, the angle of gait approaches zero and foot strike is on the line of progression. This limits deviation of the COM as the lower limbs move beneath the body, thus allowing more efficient locomotion (Fig. 8.12).

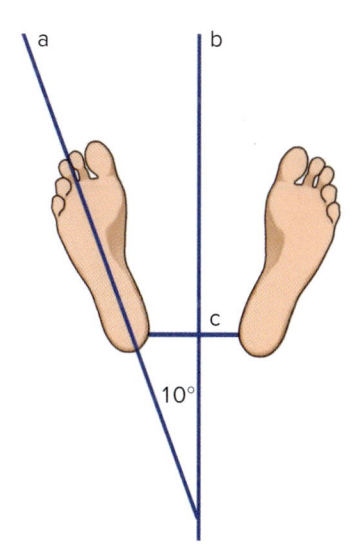

Figure 8.11 The angle of gait is the angle between (a) the long axis at the foot and (b) the line of progression. (c) Base of gait is the distance between the medial aspects of the heels

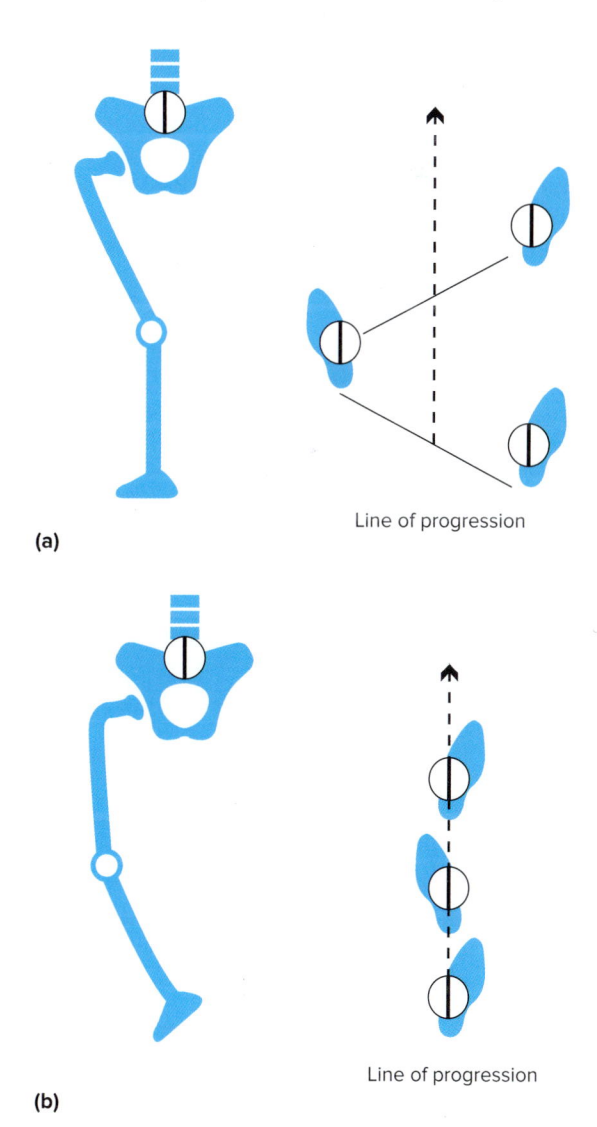

Figure 8.12 Angle and base of gait (a) Walking (b) Running

93

PART A Fundamental principles

Landing point relative to centre of mass

Greater distance between foot strike point and COM (i.e. overstride) has been reported to increase lower limb joint loads,[20] and as a result is thought to increase the risk of running injury development. When measuring this clinically, we suggest this distance should not exceed more than one third of a foot length (Fig. 8.13), with greater than a foot length considered a marked overstride. During sprinting, the foot should land almost directly under the COM.

Influence of gait velocity

Increased gait velocity influences a number of biomechanical factors. As gait velocity is increased, greater emphasis is placed on the swinging actions of the upper limbs, trunk and lower limbs to produce forward momentum.[2] This difference has significant implications for the flexibility and eccentric muscle control requirements of these structures (e.g. ipsilateral hamstrings strain during late swing). Greater excursion of the proximal joints (knee, hip and pelvis) also occurs with increased velocity, placing increased reliance on eccentric muscle control.[19, 21] At the foot and ankle, the bones making up the rearfoot, midfoot and forefoot all reduce their excursions in all three planes with increased velocity.[22] This indicates the need for stiffer joint structures with increased speed and a greater demand on intrinsic foot musculature control.[22]

In slower running, the stance phase takes longer than the swing phase. As running speed increases, stance phase and flight phase times approach each other until the stance phase becomes shorter than the swing phase in sprinting (Fig. 8.14).[2]

Additionally, as running velocity increases, foot strike patterns may be altered. As mentioned previously, foot strike patterns are similar between slow running and walking for most individuals (Fig. 8.15). During faster running (striding), the foot may strike with the heel and forefoot simultaneously prior to heel off (midfoot strike), or may strike with the forefoot initially followed by heel lowering to the surface prior to heel off (forefoot strike). In sprinting, weight-bearing is maintained on the forefoot from contact to toe off, although the heel may lower to the supporting surface at midstance. In some individuals, this pattern can commence even at slower running speeds, or immediately upon initiation of a run. In particular, some habitual barefoot runners often have a natural forefoot strike pattern regardless of velocity.[3]

Comparing heel and forefoot strike patterns

Changing from a heel strike to a forefoot strike pattern has significant implications for lower limb biomechanics and assessment. This has become particularly important

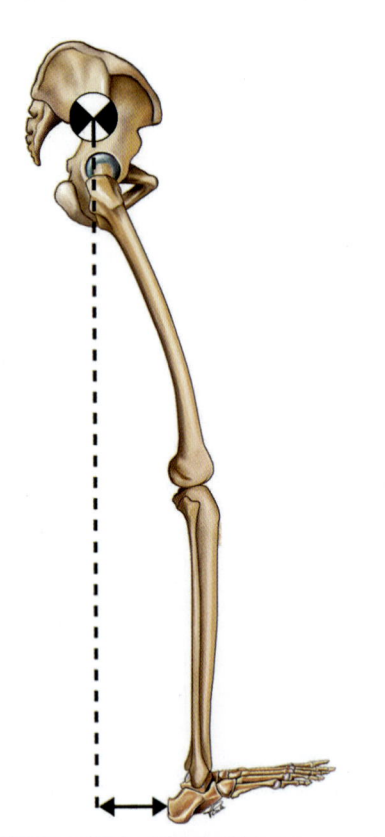

Figure 8.13 Heel to COM distance at initial contact during running[20]

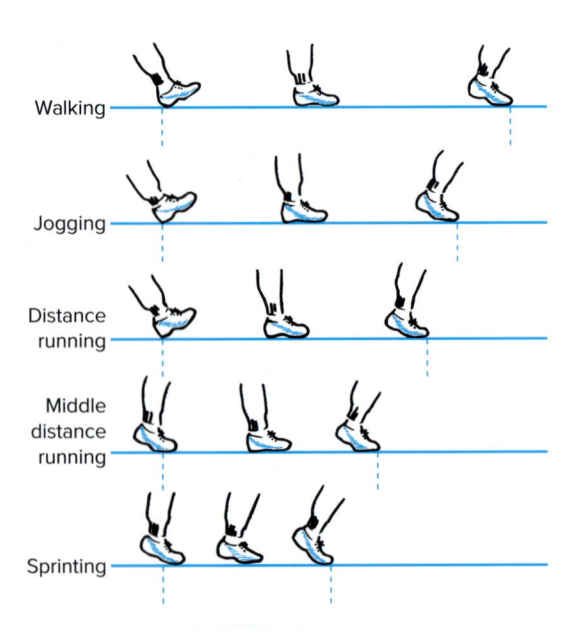

Figure 8.14 Pattern of the stance phase during different speeds of walking and running

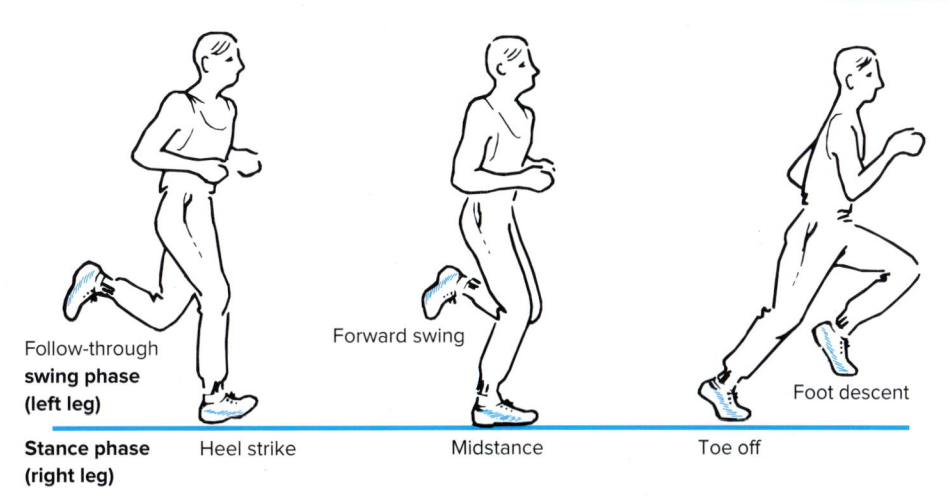

Introduction to clinical biomechanics CHAPTER 8

Follow-through
**swing phase
(left leg)**   Forward swing

Stance phase   Heel strike   Midstance   Toe off   Foot descent
(right leg)

Figure 8.15 The swing and stance phases of running

to clinical practice with the recent popularity of *Born to Run*[23] and many runners choosing to transition from a habitual heel to a forefoot strike. Firstly, forefoot strike patterns result in slight plantar flexion of the foot at impact, followed by dorsiflexion as the heel lowers to the ground.[2] This means that the ankle joint is more compliant and able to absorb GRF in the sagittal plane, and can lead to a reduction in vertical GRF and loading rates following foot strike.[3, 6] Additionally, forefoot striking has also been reported to reduce knee and hip joint loads, and these changes are often used to justify transition toward a forefoot strike for hip and knee injuries.[24] However, concurrent increases to joint loads at the ankle indicate potential detrimental increases to tissue stresses distally,[24] which fits with many anecdotal reports of Achilles tendinopathy, plantar fasciopathy and metatarsal stress fractures as a result of transitioning from heel to forefoot strike.

Influence of fatigue on running biomechanics

Some runners will report pain that only occurs following prolonged activity. For example, an individual with patellofemoral pain (Chapter 36) may report no pain during the early stages of a run, but cease running due to severe pain after five kilometres. This can make clinical assessment difficult, since the condition may result from suboptimal biomechanics that only occur with fatigue. For example, excessive hip adduction during running in the individual with patellofemoral pain may occur due to poor gluteal muscle endurance. Therefore, the clinician should evaluate functional biomechanics both at baseline and following fatigue and/or onset of pain. In the clinical setting, this means scheduling the appointment so that the patient can be seen before and immediately after a run, or having them run to a fatigued state before attending the clinic.

LOWER LIMB BIOMECHANICAL ASSESSMENT IN THE CLINICAL SETTING

This section aims to help the junior clinician develop a routine for efficient lower limb biomechanical assessment. There is no single best way to assess biomechanics and the experienced clinician will vary his or her assessment depending on the clinical presentation.

For this example, consider the patient to have patellofemoral pain–a condition that warrants assessment of the entire kinetic chain.

> **PRACTICE PEARL**
>
> Two guiding principles will help with the efficiency of the office assessment and ensure it is appropriately comprehensive.
>
> 1. Examine from distal to proximal (start at the foot and then examine proximally to the pelvis and trunk).
> 2. Examine the patient in 'static stance' first before increasingly challenging him or her with 'functional' tests before moving to fully 'dynamic' or 'sport-specific' tests as appropriate (see Fig. 8.16 for the concept of the hierarchy). These terms are explained below.

Thorough biomechanical assessment may require the patient to stand, walk, run, land on two feet and land on one leg only. Assessment during 'function' (playing sports, executing certain sporting activities such as a kick or a pirouette) may also be relevant.

We explain each of these steps in the order that many experienced clinicians perform the assessment. The major elements in the assessment are:

- structural (static) biomechanical assessment (Fig. 8.17a–g)
- functional lower limb tests–single-leg stance, heel raise, squat and landing (Fig. 8.18a–g)

95

PART A Fundamental principles

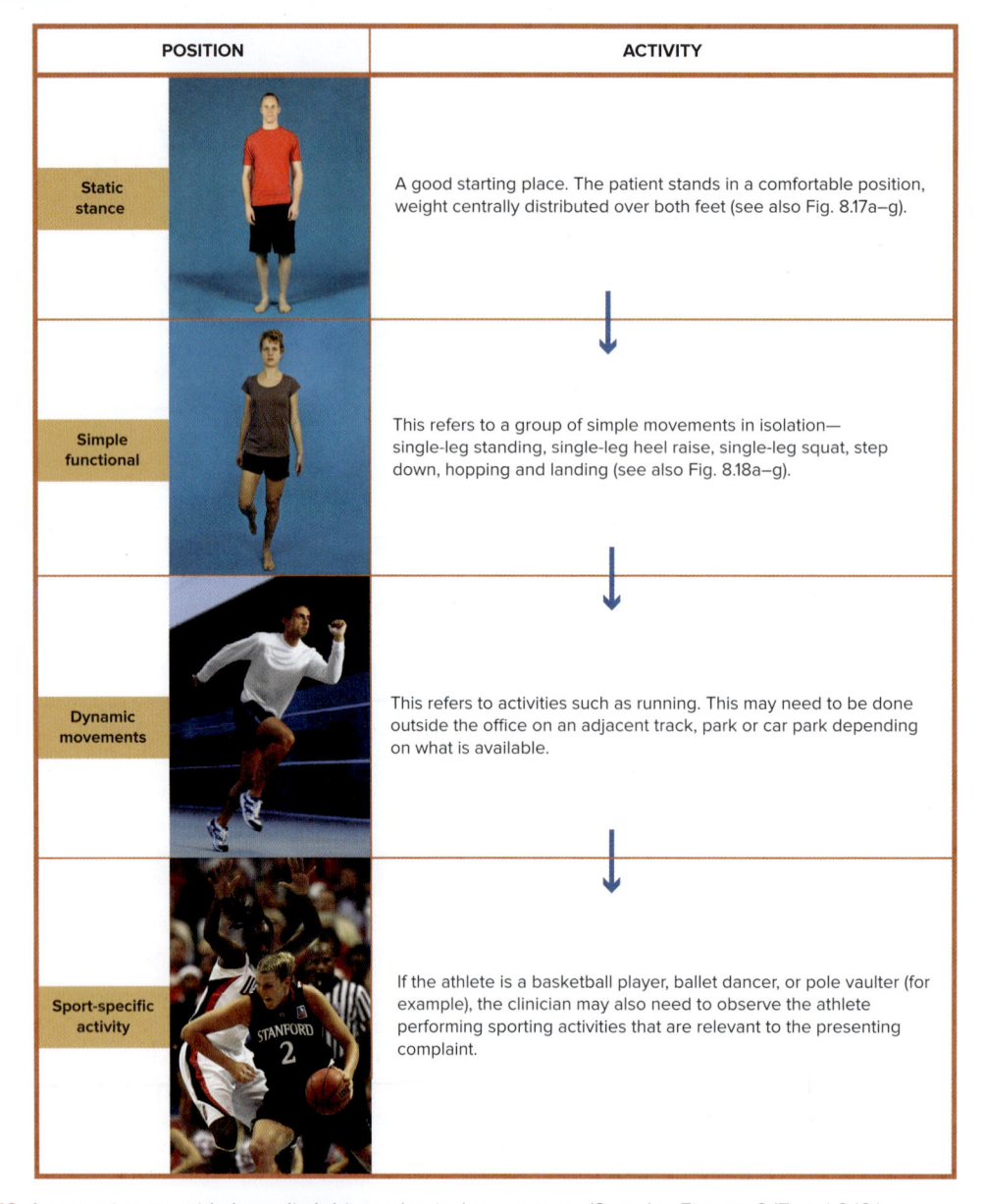

POSITION		ACTIVITY
Static stance		A good starting place. The patient stands in a comfortable position, weight centrally distributed over both feet (see also Fig. 8.17a–g).
Simple functional		This refers to a group of simple movements in isolation—single-leg standing, single-leg heel raise, single-leg squat, step down, hopping and landing (see also Fig. 8.18a–g).
Dynamic movements		This refers to activities such as running. This may need to be done outside the office on an adjacent track, park or car park depending on what is available.
Sport-specific activity		If the athlete is a basketball player, ballet dancer, or pole vaulter (for example), the clinician may also need to observe the athlete performing sporting activities that are relevant to the presenting complaint.

Figure 8.16 An overview to guide lower limb biomechanical assessment (See also Figures 8.17 and 8.18.)

- assessment of a patient's running biomechanics ('dynamic assessment')
- detailed sport-specific tests as indicated by the above tests and the clinical presentation.

Structural ('static') biomechanical assessment

The clinician performs the assessment of static stance by critically viewing the foot, ankle, knee and pelvis (Fig. 8.17a).

Foot

Inspect the foot subjectively (does it look abnormal?), quantify posture using the six item Foot Posture Index (FPI) below and also pay attention to first MTP range of motion (Fig. 8.17b).

Foot Posture Index

Quantify standing foot posture objectively with the FPI, a test that reflects foot posture at the rearfoot, midfoot and forefoot, as well as an overall impression of foot

96

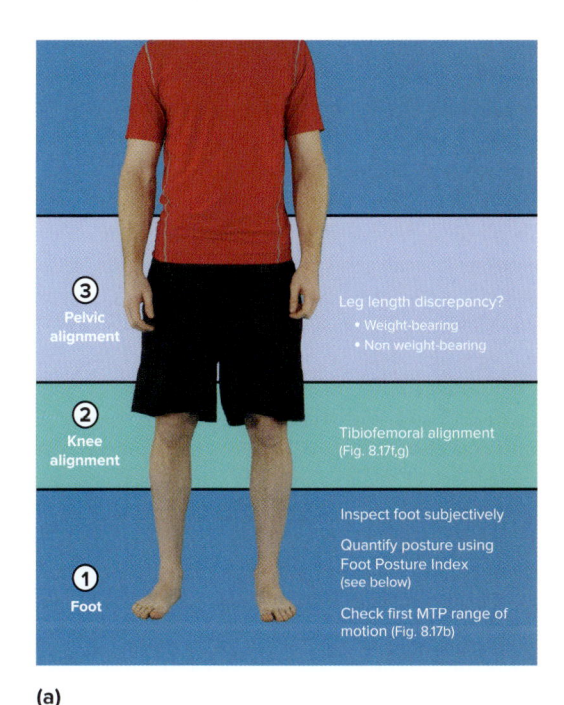

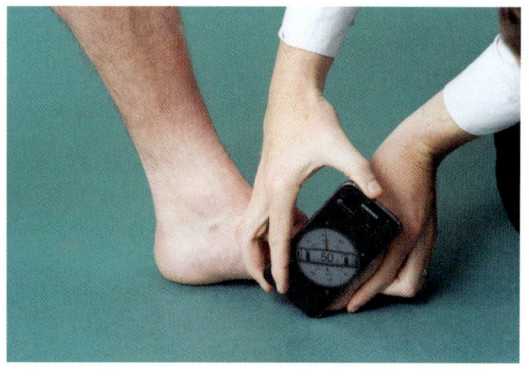

Introduction to clinical biomechanics CHAPTER 8

Figure 8.17 Static assessment of the lower limb (a) With the patient in this comfortable position, static stance examination begins at the foot. The examiner then assesses the ankle, knee and hip/pelvis (b) Jack's test for first MTPJ dorsiflexion range of motion. Normal range of motion is approximately 50° relative to the floor

The Foot Posture Index [26]—a rapid, quantitative measure of static foot biomechanics

Each of the six items in the FPI is scored as −2 (highly supinated), −1 (supinated), 0 (neutral), +1 (pronated) or +2 (highly pronated); this leads to sums between −12 (highly supinated) and +12 (highly pronated).[26]

Talar head palpation
The talar head is palpated on the anterior aspect of the ankle. If the head can be felt equally on the medial and lateral side, a neutral score (0) is given. If greater prominence is felt medially, a pronated score is given (+2 defined by only medial prominence felt) and if greater prominence is felt laterally, a supinated score is given (−2 defined by only lateral prominence felt).

Supra and infra lateral malleolar curvature
A neutral score for this item is given if the curves above and below the lateral malleolus are equal when viewed posteriorly. If the curve above the malleolus is flatter, a pronated score is given (+2 defined by completely flat) and if the curve below the malleolus is flatter, a supinated score is given (−2 defined by completely flat).

Calcaneal frontal plane position
A neutral score is given if the rearfoot is perpendicular to the floor. A more valgus rearfoot relative to the floor is given a pronated score (+2 defined by >5°) and a more varus rearfoot relative to the floor is given a supinated score (−2 defined by >5°).

Bulging in the region of the talonavicular joint (TNJ)
A neutral score is given if the skin immediately superficial to the TNJ is flat. If the TNJ is bulging, a pronated score is given (+2 defined by marked bulging) and if the TNJ area is concave (indented) a supinated score is given (−2 defined by marked concavity).

Height and congruence of the medial longitudinal arch
A neutral score is given if the arch shape is uniform and similarly shaped to the circumference of a circle. If the arch is flattened and lowered, a pronated score is given (+2 defined by the mid-portion of the arch making contact with the floor). If the arch is high, a supinated score is given (−2 defined by an acutely angled posterior end of the arch).

Abduction/adduction of the forefoot on the rearfoot
A neutral score is given when the forefoot can be seen equally on the medial and lateral side when viewed from behind the axis of the rearfoot. If more of the forefoot is visible laterally than medially, a pronated score is given (+2 defined by only lateral forefoot visible) and if more of the forefoot is visible medially than laterally, a supinated score is given (−2 defined by only medial forefoot visible).

The total FPI score for the normal healthy population is 2.4 (i.e. slightly pronated).[28] *Thus, scores of 0 to +5 are considered neutral. A score of +6 to +9 is considered pronated, ≥+10 highly pronated, −1 to −4 supinated and −5 to −12 highly supinated.*

type. It requires no equipment and takes approximately 2 minutes to complete.[25, 26, 27]

Additional background information about the FPI, including definitions and pictures of various foot types for each item, are shown in the user guide and manual.[25] Note that, as with any clinical skill, training and experience are important. The clinician should rate at least 30 individuals with a broad range of foot types before applying the FPI clinically.[29, 30, 31]

Jack's test for first metatarsophalangeal joint (MTPJ) range (plantar fascia integrity)

The clinician can rapidly assess the first MTPJ and also the integrity of the plantar fascia using 'Jack's test' (Fig. 8.17b).[32] The normal range of first MTPJ dorsiflexion motion should be around 50° relative to the floor. As the first ray dorsiflexes, tightening of an intact plantar fascia should cause the rearfoot to invert. If the rearfoot does not move, it suggests poor plantar fascia integrity which can result in inadequate supination during the propulsive phase of gait. Additionally, increased resistance to or a reduction in motion may result from the presence of a valgus aligned forefoot.[33] Both these structural issues can be corrected using orthoses, taping and/or corrective exercise.

Ankle dorsiflexion

Accurate ankle dorsiflexion in weight-bearing using an inclinometer provides a more useful measure of range of motion at this important joint than does a rough assessment when the patient is lying on a treatment couch. This ankle biomechanical assessment is best done with the knee both extended and flexed (Fig. 8.17c and d). Normal ankle dorsiflexion range with the knee flexed is 45° and with the knee extended is 40°.[30] We recommend that clinicians have an inclinometer readily available (Fig. 8.17c and d)–it adds a great deal of accuracy to measurements and reduces assessment time.

An alternative way of quickly assessing weight-bearing ankle dorsiflexion is to have the patient perform the 'knee-to-wall' test (Fig. 8.17e). This provides an efficient outcome measure for ankle dorsiflexion range when gastrocnemius tightness is not a concern and this can be

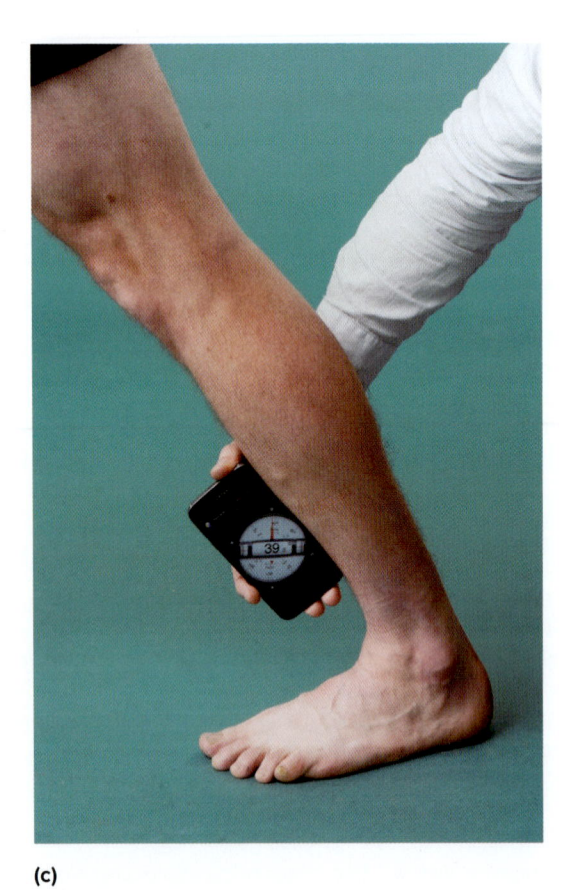

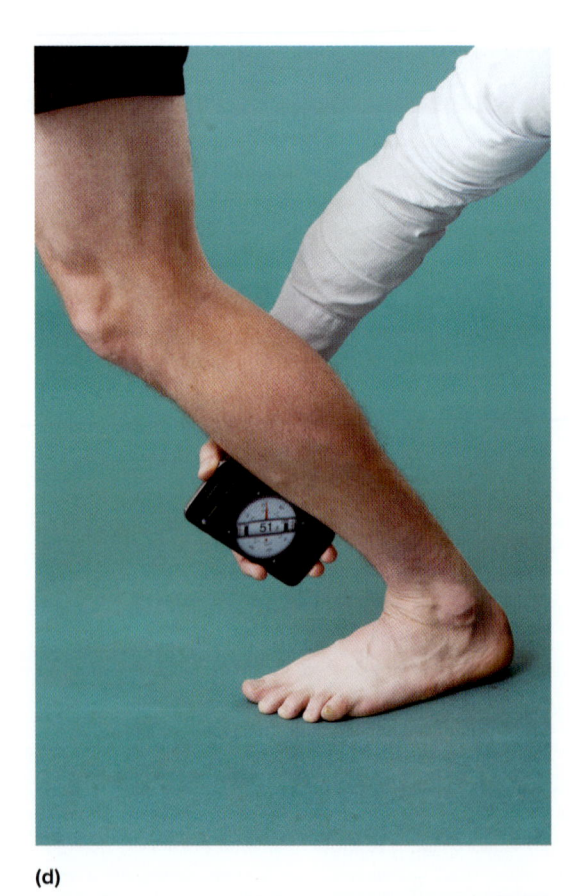

Figure 8.17 (cont.) (c) Assessing ankle dorsiflexion in weight-bearing with the knee extended (d) Assessing ankle dorsiflexion in weight-bearing with the knee flexed

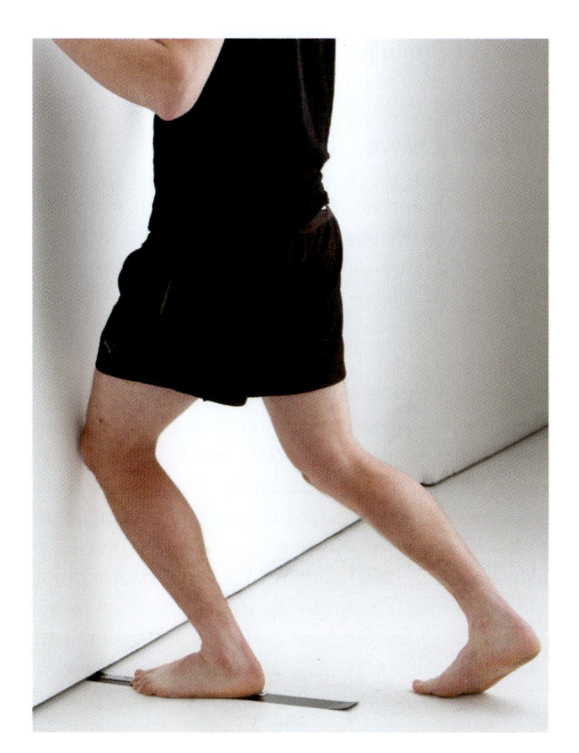

Introduction to clinical biomechanics   CHAPTER 8

Assessment of tibiofemoral alignment at the knee

Tibiofemoral joint alignment may reflect genu varum or valgum (Fig. 8.17f and g). This can also be measured using an inclinometer, which compares favourably to the gold standard radiographic measure.[34]

Leg length assessment

Discrepancies in leg length are extremely common, existing in up to 70% of the normal population.[35] Nevertheless, leg length discrepancy has long been thought to be a risk factor for a range of musculoskeletal conditions, including low back pain, hip and knee osteoarthritis, and lower limb stress fractures.[35, 36]

Laboratory studies have shown that leg length differences alter the distribution of mechanical stress within the body, particularly by increasing the magnitude of forces through the shorter limb.[37] However, prospective risk-factor studies in athletes are lacking and what constitutes a clinically significant leg length difference remains unknown. Subsequently, the extent to which leg length differences should be

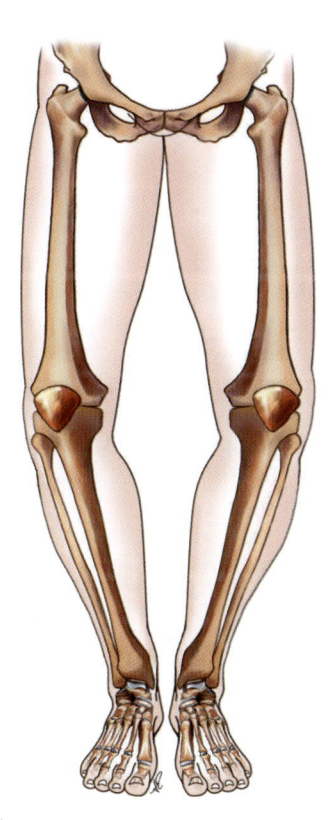

(e)

Figure 8.17 (cont.) (e) The knee-to-wall test. It is useful to have a line on the floor that continues up the wall. The patient lines up their second toe and mid-calcaneus on the horizontal line and lunges their patella toward the vertical line. This minimises the likelihood of going into pronation to achieve greater range of motion (ROM). The distance from the wall to the second toe is recorded

PRACTICE PEARL

If ankle dorsiflexion range differs in knee extension and flexion by more than 5°, it suggests there is limitation of dorsiflexion with the knee extended; this points to gastrocnemius tightness. If foot pronation is excessive to achieve normal ankle dorsiflexion range (i.e. 45°) with the knee bent, excessive pronation may be occurring during functional activities to achieve full functional movement (e.g. when running).

particularly useful following lateral ankle sprain. With the knee-to-wall test, clinicians can determine whether there are side-to-side differences or if ankle dorsiflexion is restricted. 'Normal' values will vary depending on the size of the patient and their sport-specific demands, but, as a general rule of thumb, the distance from the wall to the second toe should be greater than 8–10 cm.

(f)

Figure 8.17 (cont.) Static assessment of the lower limb—alignment at the knee (f) Genu varum

PART A   Fundamental principles

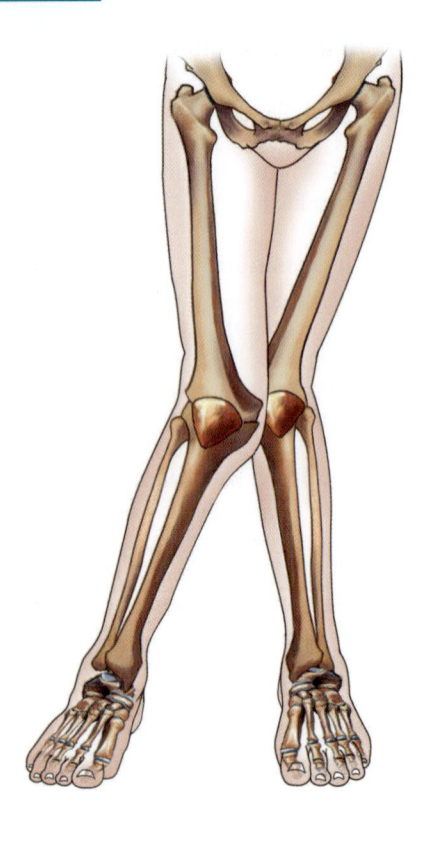

Figure 8.17 (cont.) (g) Genu valgum

corrected in athletes remains a source of controversy, with opinions ranging from 3 mm to 22 mm.[38] We recommend that clinicians take a 'treatment direction test' approach (see below) and adopt corrections if they substantially change symptoms.

Leg length can be measured in a variety of ways, including clinical measures using a tape measure in standing (anterior superior iliac spine or ASIS to floor) and in supine (ASIS to medial malleolus). However, these methods may be inaccurate, with reports of poor inter- and intra-rater reliability and errors of up to 20 mm compared to radiographic imaging.[38] There are a number of radiographic techniques to evaluate leg length differences, including magnetic resonance imaging (MRI), computed tomography (CT) 'scanograms' and standing full leg radiograph. Each of these methods has demonstrated high accuracy with average errors of less than 2 mm.[39]

Summary of static assessment
The 'static' biomechanical assessment of the foot, ankle and knee provides a substantial amount of valuable clinical information and can be completed within 5 minutes.

Possible mechanisms that underpin common clinical observations are shown in Table 8.2.

Functional lower limb tests
The next step is to assess simple functional movements. The patient should do these tests both with and without sporting footwear where appropriate. This will help the clinician determine whether the individual's footwear is detrimental, beneficial or has no effect on functional biomechanics.

Single-leg stance with progressions
The single-leg stance test begins to challenge lower limb balance and proprioception (Fig. 8.18a). Inability to maintain the single-leg stance position is likely to carry over to suboptimal biomechanics during sporting activity. The patient performs this test with (i) eyes open, (ii) eyes closed and (iii) challenged further by also performing a single heel raise. Depending on the balance requirements for the individual, once balance can be maintained in single-leg stance for at least 10 seconds, balance can be assessed using more challenging activities, including variations in surfaces and ability to adapt to internal and external perturbations.

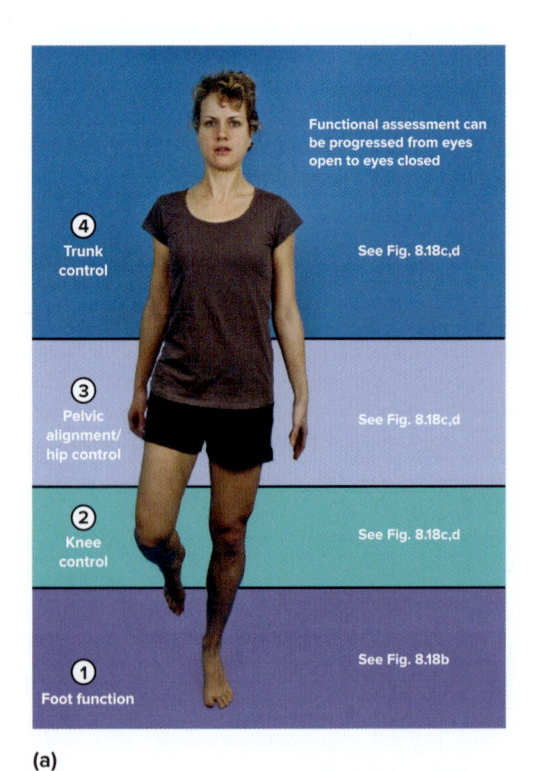

Figure 8.18 Functional assessment of the lower limb. (a) Single-leg stance to evaluate alignment and control

Introduction to clinical biomechanics   CHAPTER 8

Table 8.2 Common lower limb biomechanical observations, possible mechanisms and confirmatory assessments

Observations	Possible mechanisms	Confirmatory assessments
Excessive or asymmetrical pelvic or trunk movement (frontal, transverse, sagittal planes)	Inadequate ROM (hip)	Clinical ROM tests with inclinometer (Chapter 31); figure '4' test
	Inadequate strength (abdominals, lumbopelvic muscles, hip abductors)	Manual muscle tests
	Altered neuromotor control (hip abductors, lumbopelvic muscles)	Biofeedback
	Decreased muscle length (hamstrings, rectus abdominis, rectus femoris)	Muscle length tests
	Lumbar spine/sacroiliac joint stiffness/pain	Joint palpation
Increased hip adduction/femoral internal rotation	Structural (femoral anteversion)	Radiographic: MRI, X-ray; Clinical assessment
	Inadequate ROM (hip)	Clinical ROM tests with inclinometer (Chapter 31); figure '4' test
	Inadequate strength (hip external rotators, abductors)	Manual muscle test (Chapter 31) or hand-held dynamometry
	Altered neuromotor control (hip external rotators, hip abductors)	Biofeedback
Increased apparent knee valgus	Structural (genu varum, tibial varum, coxa varum)	Imaging: MRI, X-ray; Clinical assessment: goniometer, inclinometer
	Inadequate ROM (hip)	ROM tests: clinical (Chapter 31) inclinometer; figure '4' test
	Inadequate strength (hip external rotators, hip abductors, quadriceps, hamstrings)	Manual muscle test (Chapter 31) or hand-held dynamometry; Active gluteal and tensor fasciae latae trigger points
	Altered neuromotor control (hip external rotators, hip abductors, lumbopelvic muscles)	Biofeedback; Active gluteal and TFL trigger points
Ankle equinus	Inadequate ROM (ankle)	ROM tests
	Tight gastrocnemius or soleus	ROM tests with knee flexed and extended (Fig. 8.17c and d)
Excessive or prolonged foot pronation	Pronated foot type	FPI
	Impaired windlass mechanism	Jack's test (Fig. 8.17b)
	Tibialis posterior weakness	Single-leg heel raise; manual muscle test; inability to form arch
	Ankle equinus	Ankle dorsiflexion measures
	Leg length discrepancy (structural or functional)	Clinical measurement and radiographic imaging
Excessive or prolonged foot supination	Supinated foot type	FPI
	Chronic ankle instability	Ankle ligament integrity tests
	Leg length discrepancy (structural or functional)	Clinical measurement and radiographic imaging
Reduced propulsion	Impaired windlass mechanism	Jack's test (Fig. 8.17b)
	Tibialis posterior weakness	Single-leg heel raise; manual muscle test; inability to form arch
	Pronated foot type	FPI

ROM = range of motion; FPI = foot pronation index

PART A   Fundamental principles

Single-leg heel raise (with a focus on tibialis posterior function)

Tibialis posterior is an under-recognised contributor to normal lower limb biomechanics–it is particularly important for control of foot pronation and helps stabilise the plantar arch during activity. Through its attachments to the navicular, cuneiforms, cuboid and bases of the second to fourth metatarsals, tibialis posterior inverts the subtalar joint. It is a primary dynamic stabiliser of the foot against eversion forces and is also important for propulsion.

A simple functional test, the *single-leg heel raise*, tests the ability of tibialis posterior to re-supinate the foot during propulsion of gait (Fig. 8.18b). Tibialis posterior muscle weakness will manifest as an inability to rise up through the medial aspect of the foot and invert the rearfoot toward the end of the heel raise. (Note that the same procedure can be prescribed as a therapeutic exercise when deficits are observed–this may initially require the use of support or starting in bilateral stance).

If tibialis posterior problems or excessive dynamic foot pronation are suspected, the 'arch form' test can be used to evaluate the capacity of the intrinsic muscles of the foot and tibialis posterior to control the foot during stance in gait. The patient is instructed to gently lift up the inside arch while pushing the first metatarsophalangeal joint into the ground. The clinician can monitor performance by placing a finger underneath the joint to ensure sufficient downward pressure. The patient should be able to maintain this for 10 seconds. As above, the procedure provides a therapeutic exercise when deficits are observed. Note that the arch form test would not necessarily be part of a routine rapid biomechanical assessment–it provides additional information if this is warranted (e.g. if the patient demonstrates excessive or rapid foot pronation).

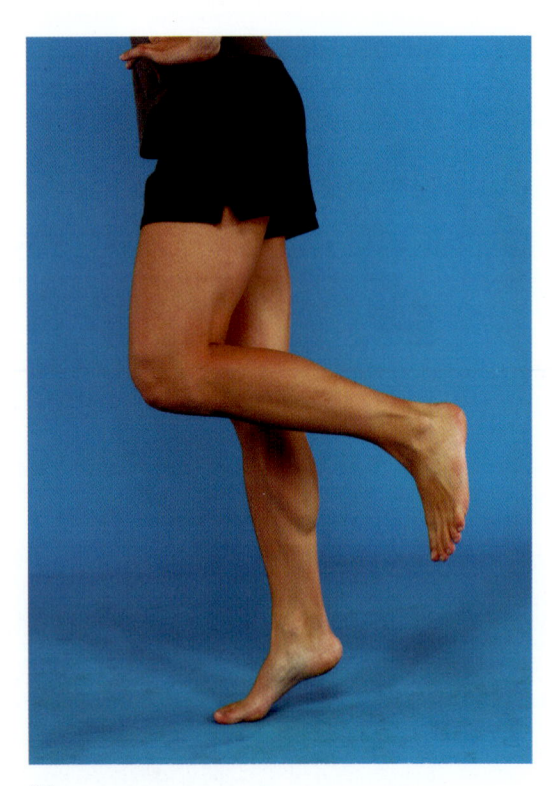

Single-leg squat to assess knee, hip and trunk muscle function

The continuum of activities from single-leg squat (at approximately 45° knee flexion), step down, hopping, to landing, provides a logical progression to the lower limb biomechanical assessment. There are many variations for performing a single-leg squat, including depth (knee flexion angle), arm position (crossed, hands on hips, no constraints) and posture of the unsupported leg (in front, behind) (Fig. 8.18c and d). Clinicians should ensure that they always use the same technique.

Assessment of hip and trunk function

Five main observations may indicate altered hip or trunk muscle function. The first four can be observed from in front of the athlete and the fifth is an overall assessment.[40]

Trunk

Trunk lean (and/or rotation) toward the stance leg may be an adaptation to altered control of hip abduction/rotation or trunk lateral flexion/rotation. This may be observed as a more lateral position of the shoulder, relative to the hip (Table 8.2, Fig. 8.18d).

Pelvis and hip

Altered control of hip abduction/rotation or trunk lateral flexion/rotation may present as either (a) inability to maintain a level pelvis or (b) ipsilateral shift of a level pelvis. Both presentations may be observed as a lateral hip (ASIS), relative to the knee (hip adduction) and may also be referred to as a 'Trendelenburg sign' (Table 8.2, Fig. 8.18d).

Knee

Does the centre of the knee remain over the centre of the foot? If the knee deviates toward a more medial position (relative to the foot), this is an indication of increased

Figure 8.18 (cont.) (b) Single-leg heel raise. Look for signs of tibialis posterior weakness, including (i) inability to rise through the medial arch or (ii) failure of the heel to invert

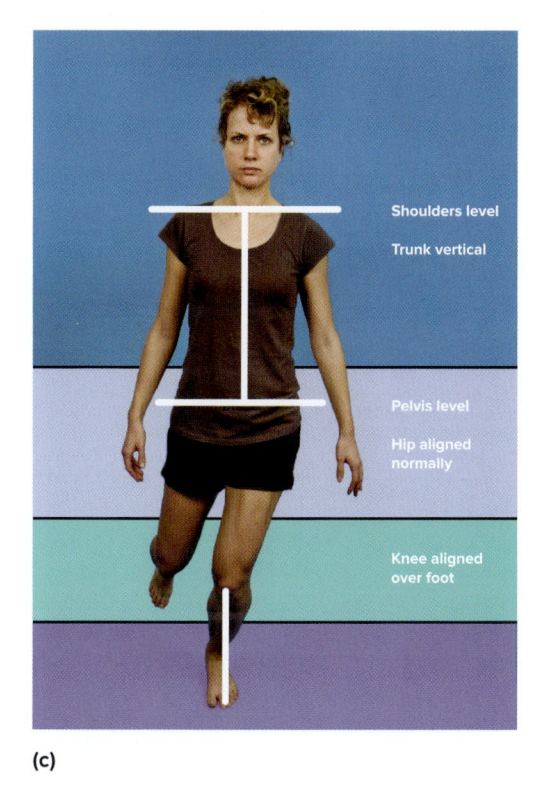

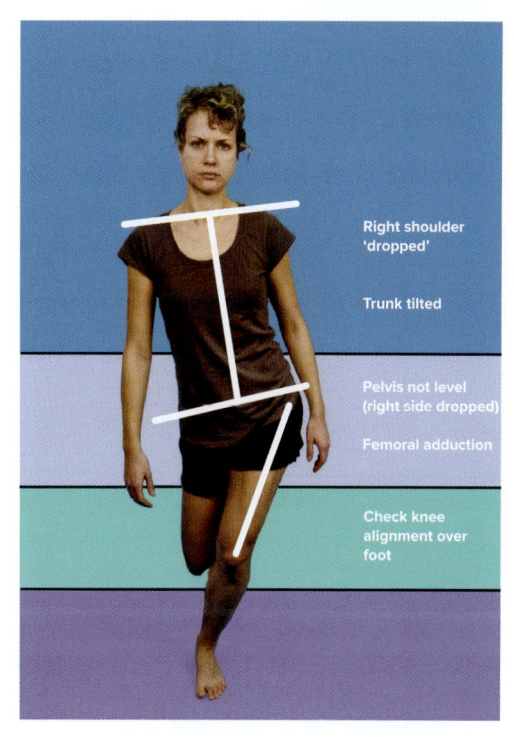

Figure 8.18 (cont.) Single-leg squat (c) Good form (d) Poor form

hip internal rotation and/or adduction and appears as an apparent knee valgus posture. Increased hip internal rotation/adduction may result from altered control of hip muscles (e.g. hip external rotators) (Table 8.2).

Overall impression
An individual with altered hip/trunk muscle function may exhibit global signs, such as poor quality of movement/coordination, inability to squat to the desired depth, or inability to control speed, depth and balance.

Landing—specific considerations
There are a number of ways to evaluate single-leg and double-leg landing biomechanics in the clinical setting. The clinician should determine what is appropriate taking into account the individual's sporting requirements and injury history. It may be more appropriate to evaluate single-leg landing if a higher-functioning athlete presents with a lower limb injury. The single-leg landing may be the best way to identify biomechanical deficiencies such as increased knee abduction, and decreased knee, hip and trunk flexion.

Conversely, in individuals recovering from injury and/or surgery, double-leg landing may be a more appropriate test so that healing tissue does not receive excessive stress. It may also be important to evaluate landing performance both pre- and post-exercise, since fatigue is associated with increased knee abduction and reduced knee flexion during landing.[41, 42]

We suggest evaluating both double-leg and single-leg landing using a drop landing assessment from a 30 cm high platform (Fig. 8.18e–g). The clinician should observe the landing pattern for signs of reduced knee and hip flexion and/or an abnormally erect landing posture. Apparent knee valgus is another movement to observe. Maximum knee valgus should reach approximately 10° for females and 5° for males for both tests from this height.[43] Excessive valgus and/or the presence of a heavy landing pattern involving minimal knee, hip and trunk flexion may increase the risk of future knee injury or re-injury, such as non-contact anterior cruciate ligament injuries.

As with running and squatting assessment, video footage can be used for more in-depth analysis of double-leg and single-leg landing. The clinician can use slow-motion replay and computer software packages to gain a more accurate picture of the degree of knee valgus during landing.

PART A   Fundamental principles

(e)

(f)

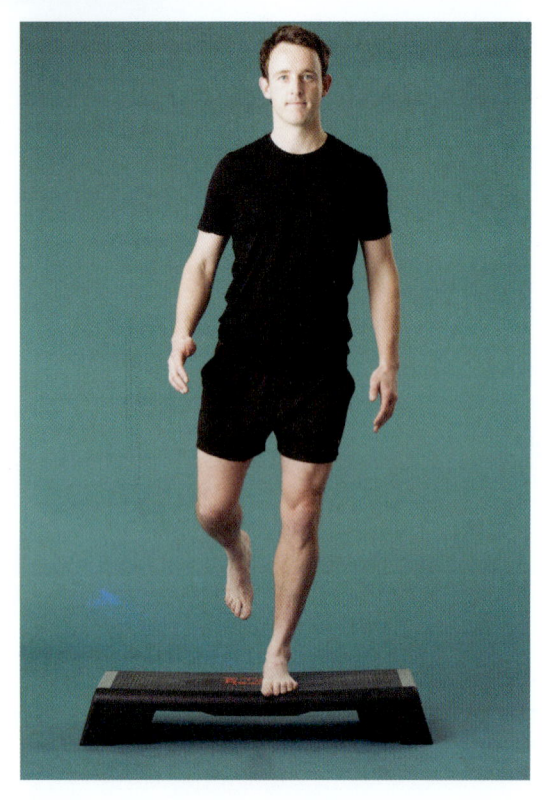

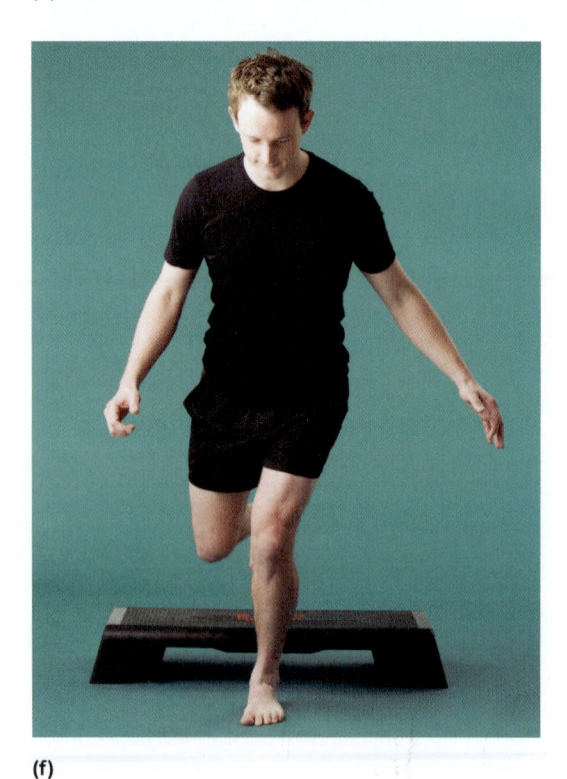

(g)

Dynamic movement assessment (e.g. running biomechanics)

A key to clinical biomechanical assessment is careful observation of functional movement. Running is a component of many sports and the clinician should have an effective method to assess for biomechanical problems associated with running. As a clinician, look for obvious deviations from the ideal running pattern, and use this to guide further assessment and treatment decisions. Common deviations and possible implications to injury are outlined in the 'ideal' biomechanics with movement–running' section. If possible, observe athletes participating in their sport. If necessary, sport-specific skills can be broken down into component movements to simplify observation in the clinic. Furthermore, functional clinical tests outlined in this chapter may provide insight into biomechanics during more sport-specific tasks when they cannot be evaluated in the clinical setting. For example, excessive

Figure 8.18 (cont.) (e) Starting position for single-leg landing (f) View from the front (g) View from the side

104

hip adduction during the completion of a single-leg squat may be indicative of excessive hip adduction during running and landing.

To detect sub-optimal biomechanics with the naked eye takes years of training and experience. Video analysis can provide valuable information from multiple views and assist the clinician greatly. This is usually done by having the patient run on a treadmill. Reflective markers can be added to identify anatomical landmarks and bony alignment. Video footage can then be slowed on a replay and this may reveal otherwise hidden abnormalities. A number of freely available computer software programs can also assist with this analysis. Examples include Hudl and Kinovea. The source of any biomechanical abnormalities may be further investigated by a thorough clinical assessment.

Sport-specific assessment

A detailed sport-specific assessment may help identify factors causing or contributing to injury. It is therefore important that clinicians understand the normal biomechanics of their patient's sport, as well as the normal range of variability between athletes. We encourage clinicians to collaborate closely with coaches and sport scientists when performing sport-specific assessments.

Sport-specific biomechanical issues thought to be associated with injury are examined in Chapter 9 for a range of different sports.

Summary of the lower limb biomechanical assessment

To iterate how we opened this section, there is no single way to perform the lower limb biomechanical assessment—it will vary by clinical specialty (e.g. physiotherapy, podiatry, medicine, exercise physiology). Also, the clinical problem will influence the order of the assessment and the relative emphasis on various elements. In this introductory chapter, we have focused on general lower limb biomechanics. This would apply, for example, to a patient with patellofemoral pain. The assessment may differ for other conditions.

CLINICAL ASSESSMENT OF FOOTWEAR—THE FOOTWEAR ASSESSMENT TOOL

Footwear assessment is a vital component of the lower limb biomechanical evaluation. The Footwear Assessment Tool is a freely available six item template to guide the clinician when assessing footwear.[44] The tool focuses on general structure and fit (Table 8.3), motion control properties and wear patterns.

Motion control is particularly important for excessive pronators. Footwear properties that influence motion control include heel counter stiffness, midfoot torsional and sagittal stability, and type of fixation (e.g. lacing). These properties can be quantified using the motion control properties scale outlined below (Table 8.4).[44] Scores range from 0 to 9, with 9 indicating the highest level of motion control.

The wear pattern of a shoe can provide insight into the biomechanics of gait. Medial tilt of the upper, medial compression of the midsole and greater medial than lateral wear of the outsole (Fig. 8.19) indicate excessive pronation. Lateral tilt of the upper, lateral compression of the midsole, and greater lateral than medial wear of the outsole reflect excessive supination.

Table 8.3 Footwear assessment—general structure and fit

Item	Measurement	Potential issues
Fit	Inadequate width or depth	Joint compression (e.g. Morton's neuroma) Restriction of normal foot function
Pitch	Difference between heel height and forefoot height (typical range 0–14 mm)	Small pitch may not be suitable for someone with ankle equinus Large pitch may increase likelihood of overstride and impair attempts to transition to midfoot or forefoot strike
Last	Straight last (0–5°) Curve last (>15°)	Accommodates a pronated foot Accommodates a supinated foot
Forefoot sole flexion point	Should line up with the first MTPJ	If too proximal, shoe stability may be impaired. If too distal, normal sagittal plane motion of the first MTPJ may be impaired, which can be problematic in the presence of poor intrinsic foot and tibialis posterior strength and function

PART A Fundamental principles

Table 8.4 Motion control properties scale[44]

Item	Score			
	0	1	2	3
Fixation (upper to foot)	None	Alternative to laces (e.g. strap, Velcro, zip)	Laces (at least 3 eyelets)	
Heel counter stiffness	No heel counter	Minimal	Moderate	Rigid
Midfoot sagittal stability	Minimal	Moderate	Rigid	
Midfoot torsional stability	Minimal	Moderate	Rigid	

Minimal = >45°; moderate = <45°; rigid = <10°

(a)

(b)

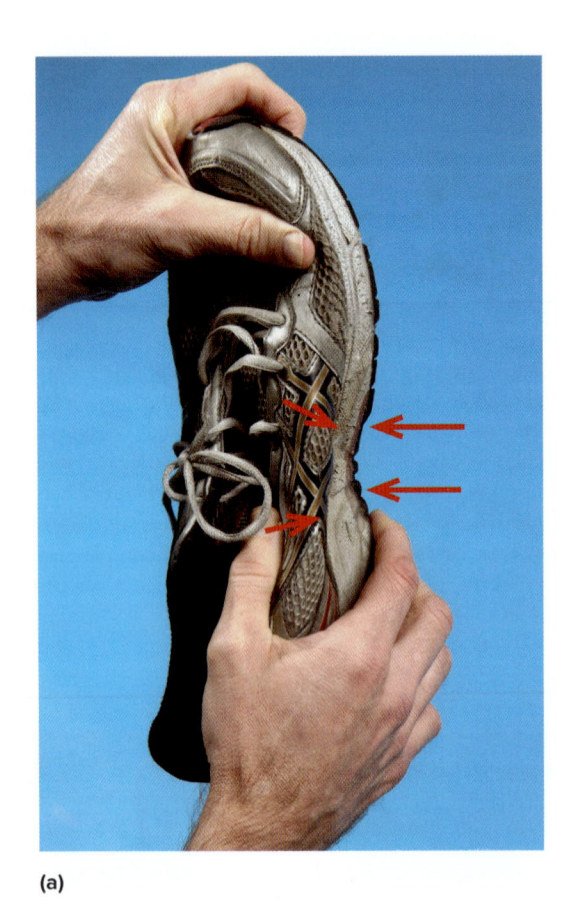

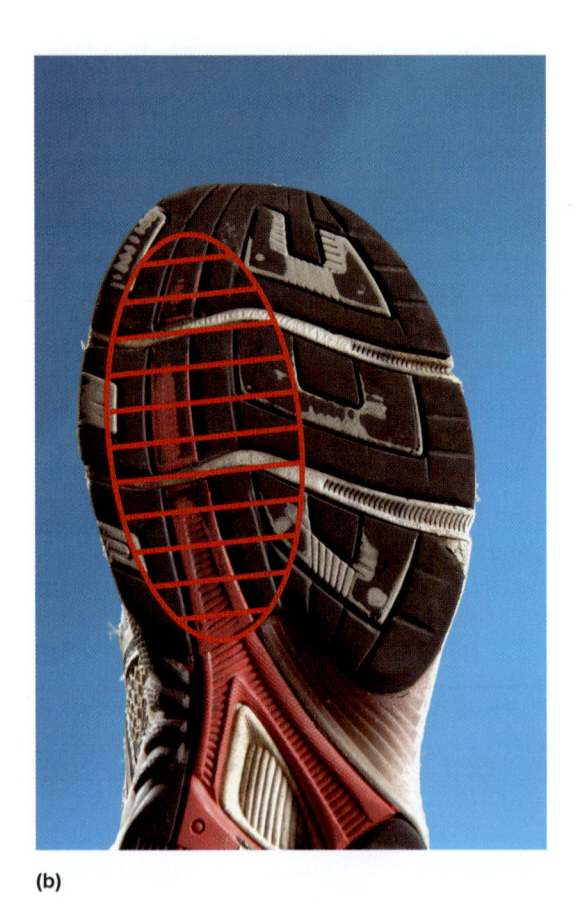

Figure 8.19 Shoe wear patterns—running shoe (a) with medial compression of the upper (b) With excessive pronation, there is greater wear on the medial than the lateral sole

CONDITIONS RELATED TO SUBOPTIMAL LOWER LIMB BIOMECHANICS

Conventional wisdom has linked suboptimal lower limb biomechanics with various injuries, but there is a lack of prospective empirical evidence to confirm that biomechanical factors increase risk for lower limb injuries.[45] Thus, for now, most biomechanical 'risk factors' have only level 3 to 5 evidence (Chapter 2).

Table 8.5 lists common lower limb injuries, common clinical considerations and evidence to support these considerations. It contains the 'best available evidence' at March 2016.

Introduction to clinical biomechanics — CHAPTER 8

Table 8.5 Best available evidence for the association between common lower limb overuse injuries and biomechanics (as at October 2016)

Injury/condition	Associated lower limb biomechanical risk factor
Sesamoiditis	Supinated foot type[46, 47] Pronated foot type Forefoot valgus, plantar flexed first ray[47] Decreased ankle DF/ankle equinus[47] Limited first ray range of motion
Plantar fasciopathy	Pronated foot type[48–50] Decreased ankle DF/ankle equinus[49, 51, 52] Increased ankle DF[48] Supinated foot type[53] Leg length difference[53]
Achilles tendinopathy	Increased subtalar joint inversion[54] Increased ankle DF[55] Decreased gastrocnemius length[54] Supinated foot type[56] Pronated foot type[56, 57]
Lateral ankle sprain, chronic ankle instability	Prolonged pronation[58] Decreased ankle DF[59] Increased first MTPJ extension[58, 60] Increased ankle inversion at heel strike[13, 14]
Peroneal tendinopathy	Supinated foot type[61]
Medial shin pain (medial tibial stress syndrome, shin splints)	Pronated foot type[62–64] Increased ankle PF[65] Supinated foot type[66] Decreased ankle DF/ankle equinus[67] Decreased hip IR[68]
Patellar tendinopathy	Decreased quadriceps and hamstrings flexibility[69] Anteriorly tilted patella[70] Pronated foot type Supinated foot type
Patellofemoral pain syndrome	Pronated foot type[71] Hypermobile patella[72] Decreased quadriceps flexibility[72] Increased hip IR (passive and dynamic)[71] Decreased knee flexion (dynamic, e.g. jump-landing)[71] Increased knee abduction moment[73, 74] Increased Q angle[75] Increased hip adduction (dynamic, e.g. running)[76] Decreased hamstrings flexibility[77]
Iliotibial band syndrome	Increased hip adduction (dynamic, e.g. running)[78] Increased knee IR (dynamic, e.g. running)[78] Increased knee flexion at heel strike[79] Increased velocity of knee IR (dynamic, e.g. running)[79] Increased maximal foot inversion[79]
Adductor tendinopathy	Decreased total hip rotation (IR, ER)[80]

continued

PART A Fundamental principles

Table 8.5 Cont.

Injury/condition	Associated lower limb biomechanical risk factor
Metatarsal stress fractures	Pronated foot type[12] Increased subtalar joint inversion[54] Supinated foot type
Tarsal stress fractures	Increased subtalar joint inversion[54]
Navicular stress fractures	Pronated foot type Ankle equinus
Fibular stress fractures	Supinated foot type Pronated foot type
Tibial stress fractures	Supinated foot type[12]
Femoral stress fractures	Supinated foot type[12] Decreased subtalar joint inversion[54]
Unspecified lower limb stress fractures	Pronated foot type[54] Supinated foot type[54] Increased hip ER[81] Leg length difference[82]

Evidence is included from the highest quality studies (i.e. if there is evidence from a prospective study, evidence from case-control studies are not included)
Blue = supported by prospective findings
Orange = supported by case-control or retrospective findings
Black = no/inconclusive evidence, clinical opinion
DF = dorsiflexion; PF = plantarflexion; IR = internal rotation; ER = external rotation

MANAGEMENT OF LOWER LIMB BIOMECHANICAL ABNORMALITIES

The next major theme of this chapter introduces management strategies to address biomechanical problems. There is increasing evidence about the role of therapies such as foot orthoses, footwear, taping, exercise and movement retraining to improve a patient's biomechanics. This section provides a background perspective and then chapters in Part B will address specific conditions. Here we focus mostly on interventions that affect the foot and lower leg.

Biofeedback and movement pattern retraining

In this chapter, we have described a number of suboptimal biomechanics or movement patterns which may be identified during assessment of an injured athlete. Of particular note, ideal running biomechanics and potential abnormalities have been described in some detail. In recent years, evidence supporting movement pattern retraining during running to manage lower limb injuries has begun to emerge.[83] This includes case series supporting visual and verbal biofeedback to reduce peak hip adduction in individuals with patellofemoral pain (PFP),[84, 85] and to transition from rearfoot to forefoot or midfoot strike pattern in individuals with anterior chronic exertional lower leg pain.[86, 87]

Recent evidence suggests that exercise interventions are unlikely to change actual running mechanics. This highlights the potential importance of using biofeedback to facilitate movement pattern retraining. For example, hip abductor strengthening does not appear to reduce peak hip adduction during running,[88-90] a variable linked to PFP[91] and iliotibial band syndrome[92] injury risk. Importantly, movement pattern retraining can also be used for other activities such as walking, stair negotiation, squatting and sit to stand; the key is to identify a potential movement pattern which may be increasing stress on the injured tissue, and implement biofeedback to alter the movement pattern and reduce stress. This should be guided by both clinical reasoning and reported changes in symptoms from the patient. A number of suggestions for common running injuries are provided in Table 8.6. When teaching your patients movement pattern changes, it is vitally important to consider the effect this may have on other structures. For example, transition from heel to forefoot strike will reduce load on the knee and hip, but will likely increase load on the foot and ankle.[83]

Simple clinical biofeedback methods can be divided into visual (mirror, video, etc.) and verbal (i.e. instructions). Visual biofeedback can be very important in the early stages of movement pattern retraining to ensure that the patient understands their faults and how to change them. Previously

Introduction to clinical biomechanics   CHAPTER 8

Table 8.6 Running retraining considerations for common lower limb injuries based on current evidence and expert opinion (from Barton et al.)[83]

Condition	Suggested retraining strategies to consider
Exertional lower leg pain	Increasing step rate, strategies to reduce overstride and land softer, and transition from rearfoot to forefoot or midfoot strike
Plantar fasciopathy	Increasing step rate, strategies to reduce overstride and land softer
Achilles tendinopathy and calf pain	Strategies to reduce overstride, increase lower limb stiffness (i.e. reduce ankle dorsiflexion) and increase hip extension
Medial tibial stress syndrome	Increasing step rate, strategies to reduce overstride and land softer, reduce hip adduction and scissoring and increase hip extension
Patellofemoral pain	Increasing step rate, strategies to reduce overstride and land softer, reduce hip adduction and internal rotation, transition from rearfoot to forefoot or midfoot strike
Iliotibial band syndrome	Reduce hip adduction and scissoring
Patellar tendinopathy	Strategies to reduce overstride and land softer, and transition from rearfoot to forefoot or midfoot strike
Hamstring injury, including proximal hamstring tendinopathy	Strategies to reduce overstride and land softer, and reduce anterior pelvic tilt and knee extension at foot strike
Gluteal tendinopathy	Increasing step rate, strategies to reduce overstride and land softer, reduce hip adduction and internal rotation, and reduce contralateral pelvic drop

published case series supporting the potential effectiveness of movement pattern retraining during running have all used some form of visual biofeedback. However, continued use in the field (e.g. using mirrors during over-ground running to reduce hip adduction) may be impractical, meaning we recommend concurrent use of verbal cues (e.g. instruction to run with knees pointing out) which can be used both in the early stages of rehabilitation and following progression into the field. Follow-up to ensure appropriate changes is essential in these circumstances, so that an athlete does not develop new maladaptive movement patterns or revert to their habitual pattern.

More complex biofeedback options are becoming easier to access in clinical practice. Clinicians can now access simple, small and affordable technologies to quantify movement analysis during assessment and provide feedback to patients during rehabilitation. One example of this is the ViMove™ (dorsaVi). This system has integrated movement and muscle sensors, and comes with software to allow the clinician to quickly analyse collected data and provide results to patients. Clinical electromyography (EMG) has been used clinically for many years to provide patients with real-time feedback regarding muscle activation patterns and magnitude. With technology in this area continuously and rapidly evolving, clinicians who are interested in incorporating more quantitative measures of biomechanics into their clinical practice should regularly review the literature and the internet for emerging technologies.

Foot orthoses

Foot orthoses (in-shoe devices) are used extensively in sports medicine to optimise lower limb function.[93] In this section we:

- review the various types of orthoses available
- introduce the debate about their mechanism of action
- highlight that there is high quality evidence for their effectiveness
- share three main approaches to deciding how to fit an orthosis for a specific patient.

Types of foot orthoses

Foot orthoses range in material from soft or flexible to semi-rigid devices, and may be prefabricated or custom-fabricated. Prefabricated or 'off the shelf' foot orthoses (Fig. 8.20a) are usually fabricated from materials such as EVA, polyurethane, cork or rubber. The devices' generic shape can be customised a little to the individual via heat moulding or the addition of wedges or heel raises. Prefabricated orthoses provide a quick and cheap intervention, but their limited potential for customisation and inability to achieve total plantar contact may restrict their use in some patients.

Custom-fabricated foot orthoses (Fig. 8.20b) are manufactured from a three-dimensional representation of the individual's foot using plaster impressions or laser-scanning devices. Custom foot orthoses may accommodate specific structural anomalies more effectively than prefabricated orthoses. Most often, custom foot orthoses are manufactured from polypropylene and carbon-fibre

109

PART A Fundamental principles

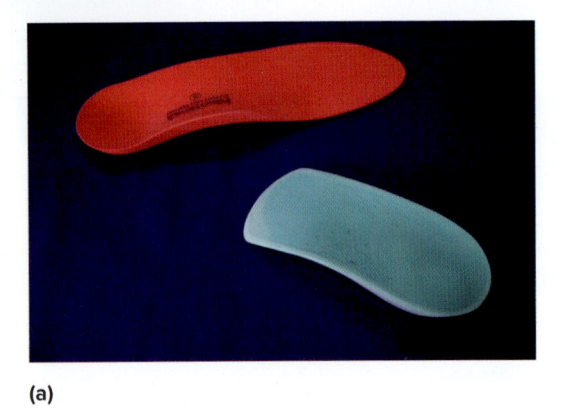

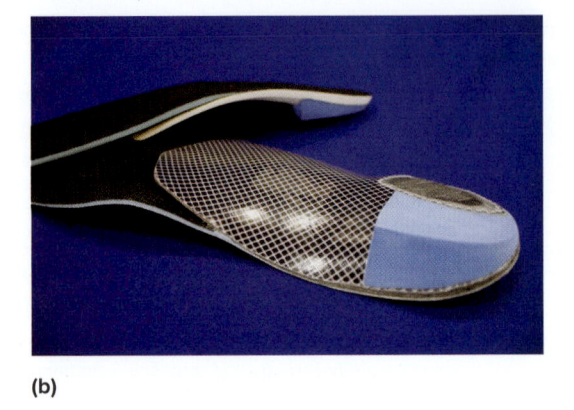

Figure 8.20 Orthoses (a) Prefabricated or 'off the shelf' orthoses (b) Custom-fabricated or casted orthoses

composites. As such, they are generally more rigid than prefabricated orthoses and are often perceived to provide more effective biomechanical control. Their prescription requires a higher level of expertise and specific equipment. In the sports and exercise medicine setting, a podiatrist will typically prescribe custom-fabricated foot orthoses, which will be manufactured in a laboratory. The prescription will typically contain information regarding materials to be used, extent of accommodative postings and shoe fit. In the laboratory, a solid model of the foot is manufactured from the three-dimensional representation. Additional material is added to provide the appropriate level (degrees) of control. The material of choice is then vacuum-pressed onto the model and covered to suit the individual.

To date, no study has identified an advantage for custom-fabricated devices over prefabricated orthoses when managing lower limb conditions.[93] The following factors should influence the recommendation for a particular type of orthosis.

- If the patient wears a wide range of footwear during training and competition, the custom-fabricated orthosis has an advantage as it can be designed to fit a wide range of footwear; prefabricated devices may need to be modified to fit in specific footwear.
- If the patient participates in sports that involve repetitive landing, a softer or more flexible device minimises the risk of arch discomfort or blistering. Furthermore, many athletes do not tolerate large degrees of arch support from orthoses. In these circumstances, it is often helpful to reduce the arch contour.
- The difference in cost may be an important determinant for some patients, although the more expensive custom orthosis also has greater durability. It is not unusual for a custom orthosis to last 5 years or more.
- There is generally a several-week interval between fitting and supply of custom orthoses, particularly when manufactured off site. Once the patient has the orthosis, there may be a further 'wearing-in' period to prevent adverse effects. This means that there may be a delay in attaining the full therapeutic benefits of the intervention. It may be appropriate to prescribe a prefabricated device for the interim period.
- Other considerations include the patient's body mass (a more rigid orthosis may be required for people with greater body weight, due to higher forces through the foot) and personal preference.

Mechanism of action—an unfinished story
Traditional dogma was that foot orthoses controlled foot motion, and thus improved biomechanical efficiency and balanced loads on structures more appropriately. However, this is now in dispute. Some studies indicate that foot orthoses can influence foot motion,[94-96] while others show that they impart no systematic effects on foot motion.[97, 98] It is important to keep in mind that the majority of studies on foot orthoses, mechanisms of action have been conducted on healthy, asymptomatic participants, and that people with pain or injury may have different biomechanical responses to foot orthoses.

Alternative paradigms relating to shock absorption and neuromuscular effects[99] include: (i) that the cushioning effect of orthoses attenuates the impact force that occurs when the foot hits the ground;[100-102] and (ii) that the input provided by foot orthoses through their total contact with the plantar surface of the foot stimulates the neuromuscular system, which may reduce muscle activity and fatigue, and optimise performance.[103-105] This is an exciting area of investigation which we will follow closely over the next few years.

Orthoses are effective—high quality evidence is accumulating
Irrespective of how foot orthoses exert their clinical effects, evidence from systematic reviews (level 1) and

controlled clinical trials (level 2) supports their use in a variety of conditions related to suboptimal lower limb biomechanics (Table 8.7). See Chapter 2 for a discussion of levels of evidence.

Three contemporary approaches for fitting an orthosis

Although evidence is accumulating that specific types of orthoses are effective in specific settings to treat specific clinical conditions, it is still difficult to recommend a 'gold standard' approach to prescribing orthoses. This part of our clinical approach remains an art based on limited science–as it is in many situations across healthcare. Thus, the clinician should integrate the research findings that provide support for some approaches (see below), and also take into account the clinical assessment findings, previous clinical experience with the condition and the type of patient, as well as the patient's preferred orthosis type.

The traditional approach—Root and the goal of 'subtalar joint neutral'

Merton Root developed the functional foot orthosis in the 1950s and 1960s.[124] He proposed that subtalar joint neutral served as a standard position to evaluate structural relationships in the foot[124] and that this position represented normal foot alignment during the midstance and heel-off phases of gait.[125] Unfortunately, the alignment measures proposed by Root are unreliable and the subtalar

Table 8.7 Best available evidence for the use of foot orthoses in the management of common lower limb conditions

Condition	Type of orthosis	Level of evidence	References
Prevention			
Lower limb overuse conditions (stress fractures, ankle sprains, foot and ankle problems)	Prefabricated, custom-fabricated	1	Collins[93]
Stress fractures (femoral, tibial, unspecified)	Custom-fabricated, shock-absorbing	1	Rome[106] Snyder[107]
Treatment			
Patellofemoral pain syndrome	Prefabricated	1	Barton[108]
Chronic musculoskeletal pain associated with pes cavus	Custom-fabricated	1	Burns[109]
Achilles tendinopathy	Custom-fabricated	2	Munteanu[110]
Plantar fasciopathy	Prefabricated	2	Baldassin[111]
	Custom-fabricated	2	Baldassin[111] Landorf[112] Lynch[114] Martin[113] Rome[115] Roos[116]
Tibialis posterior tendinopathy	Custom-fabricated	2	Kulig[117]
Lower limb overuse conditions (varied)	Custom-fabricated	2	Trotter[118]
Lateral ankle sprain/chronic ankle instability	Custom-fabricated	3	Guskiewicz[119] Orteza[120]
Medial shin pain (medial tibial stress syndrome, shin splints)	Prefabricated	3	Louden[121]
Sesamoiditis	Custom-fabricated	5	Sammarco[122] ACFAOM[123]
Peroneal tendinopathy	Custom-fabricated	5	ACFAOM[123]
Patellar tendinopathy	Custom-fabricated	5	ACFAOM[123]
Iliotibial band friction syndrome	Custom-fabricated	5	ACFAOM[123]

Blue = supported by systematic reviews or randomised controlled trials
Orange = supported by nonrandomised studies and case series
Black = expert opinion, clinical guidelines
Red = current evidence is contrary to common clinical consideration

joint is not in neutral during midstance.[125] Nevertheless, this approach to casting orthoses has been associated with many successful clinical outcomes and it remains one of the most common ways of prescribing orthoses.[126]

Treatment direction test

Professor Bill Vicenzino[127] proposed a 'treatment direction test' (TDT) to prescribe and apply foot orthoses for lower limb musculoskeletal disorders that have a biomechanical association. The TDT complements the 'tissue-stress model' of McPoil and Hunt,[125] in that it seeks to identify symptomatic tissues under excessive loads and reduce these loads using an external physical modality. This may consist of adhesive strapping tape, temporary felt orthoses, or prefabricated foot orthoses with or without add-on wedges. The modality is selected based on what the clinician identifies as an aberrant movement pattern such as excessive or prolonged pronation.

The quality and pain-free quantity of a patient-specific aggravating activity is assessed with and without the external modality. For example, the single-leg squat is suitable for patellofemoral pain, while a single- or double-leg heel raise test is more appropriate for Achilles tendinopathy. An improvement in the quality of movement or an increase in pain-free repetitions of at least 75% indicates a high likelihood of success with subsequent prescription of orthoses. The reliability and validity of the TDT is under review.

Comfort

Nigg et al.[104] proposed that comfortable devices (orthoses, footwear) that support the skeleton's preferred movement path could reduce muscle activity and resulting fatigue, and thus, improve performance. Vicenzino and colleagues[128] proposed a model of prescription for prefabricated foot orthoses based on patient comfort. Once the patient reports comfort, the clinician can further modify the device to improve pain-free performance of an aggravating functional task, while aiming to maintain comfort. The first clinical trial to utilise this method reported greater than 80% success with orthoses over a 1-year period.[129] Irrespective of the long-term outcome of this branch of research, comfort should always be an important consideration for all foot orthoses prescribed. If the device is not comfortable, there is a risk of skin blistering and/or new foot pain. Also, any device that is perceived to be uncomfortable is likely to lead to poor patient compliance.

Footwear as a therapy rather than as a cause of injury!

When considering any intervention addressing suboptimal lower limb biomechanics, the potential influence of footwear should be considered (see also 'Clinical assessment of footwear' earlier in this chapter). Consider how the current footwear influences the patient's condition, how footwear interacts with other treatment (e.g. foot orthoses) and whether altering footwear characteristics can help treat the condition.

Footwear fit is particularly important when prescribing orthoses. If an orthosis is added to a shoe that has inadequate room, it may result in forefoot pain or limit the time the orthosis is worn. Remember that athletes often wear a range of shoes in training and competition–check all of them!

If the patient's shoe has suboptimal motion control (e.g. minimal heel counter stiffness) leading to excessive foot pronation, shoe replacement may be the best treatment. Footwear with greater heel counter stiffness, midfoot sole rigidity, adequate lacing and possibly a multiple density sole (i.e. increased density on the medial aspect of the shoe) may reduce excessive foot motion. Footwear support can also be enhanced by education on how to complete loop lacing (Fig. 8.21). Such changes in relation to footwear may reduce the need for foot orthoses.

Taping

Adhesive strapping tape (Chapter 17) is a temporary intervention to address lower limb biomechanical issues. Anti-pronation tape is commonly used to treat plantar fasciopathy (Chapter 43) and patellofemoral pain (Chapter 36).

One of the most commonly used techniques for lower limb musculoskeletal pain is the Augmented low-Dye. This consists of the original low-Dye[130] (anchor running horizontally around the heel from the head of the fifth to the head of the first metatarsal, with strips of tape under

(a)

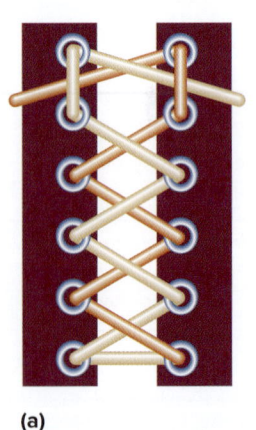

Figure 8.21 (a) Lock-lacing to prevent heel slippage. Lace the shoe normally until the second set of eyelets. Then feed the laces into the top eyelet on the same side. Now cross each lace over, and feed through the loop formed between the first and second eyelet on the opposite side. Laces should then be pulled and tied as normal

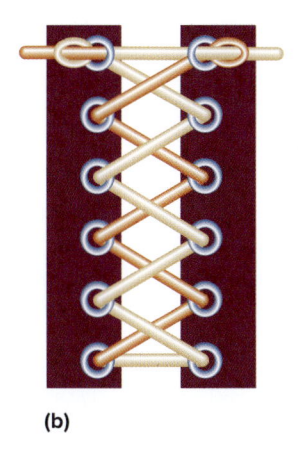

Introduction to clinical biomechanics   CHAPTER 8

Figure 8.21 (cont.) (b) Loop to create a snug fit. After lacing, put each lace end back through the last hole to create a small loop on the top side of the shoe. Then thread each loose end through the loop on the opposite side and tighten

the foot directed laterally to medially to support the arch, Fig. 8.22a), which is augmented with reverse sixes and calcaneal slings anchored to the lower leg[127] (Fig. 8.22b).

Anti-pronation tape has both biomechanical and neuromuscular effects during static and dynamic tasks.[131] Specifically, it increases navicular and medial longitudinal arch height, reduces tibial internal rotation and calcaneal eversion, alters patterns of plantar pressure, and reduces activity of particular leg muscles.[131]

Techniques such as patellar taping may also alleviate symptoms associated with PFJ biomechanics.[132, 133] It is important to be aware of skin breakdown associated with prolonged use of tape, particularly in athletes involved in vigorous activity and implement appropriate strategies to prevent this.

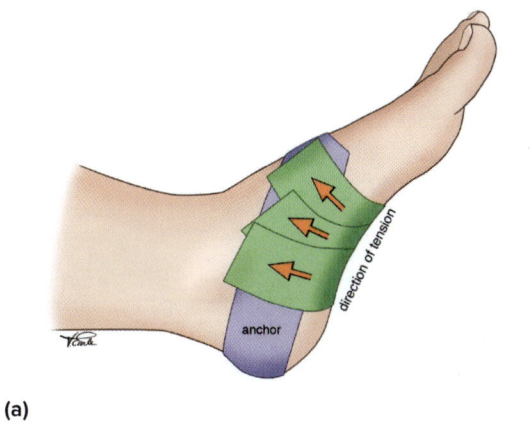

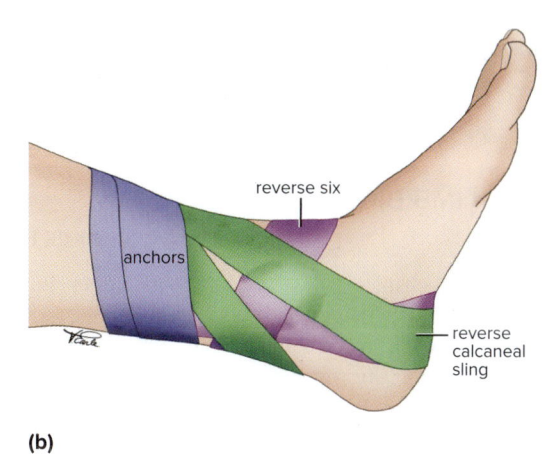

Figure 8.22 (a) Low-Dye taping can be used to restrict subtalar pronation (b) The addition of calcaneal slings and reverse sixes anchored to distal leg can augment low-Dye taping[127]

A team approach to biomechanical correction

In this box, we emphasise that clinicians working together can address biomechanical factors more effectively than one clinician working alone.

Exercises and functional retraining
Exercises and functional retraining should always be considered when managing lower limb biomechanical issues. All clinicians in sport and exercise medicine should appreciate the influence of muscle imbalance to biomechanical abnormalities. Thus, excessive tightness of muscles such as the psoas, tensor fascia latae, hip adductors, hamstrings and gastrocnemius can be addressed using exercises such as static and dynamic stretches, in conjunction with other modalities such as massage, heat or dry needling.

Muscle weakness or incoordination requires strengthening and retraining exercises, as follows.

- Dysfunction of the abdominals, gluteus medius and minimus, hip external rotators, vastus medialis obliquus and tibialis posterior should be considered in the patient with suboptimal lower limb biomechanics. While non weight-bearing exercises may be used initially, they should be progressed to functional weight-bearing positions as soon as possible.
- Once optimal static muscle activation has been achieved, exercises can be progressed by adding lower limb movements, resistance (e.g. dumbbells, resistance bands) or stability challenges (e.g. exercise balls, single-limb stance).

continued

PART A   Fundamental principles

- Motor control exercises of the hip and foot are useful to promote optimal alignment of the lower limb in the sagittal, frontal and transverse planes, as well as ideal muscle recruitment patterns.
- Exercises that incorporate the lower limb in its closed kinetic chain function include the single-leg squat, single-leg heel raise, single-leg stance and arch form.
- The next stage involves integration of this new control into functional activities, such as running, landing or sport-specific skills. Small components of the overall movement should be incorporated initially, along with specific instruction and feedback. These movements may need to be performed slowly to allow them to be integrated successfully into the functional activity (Chapter 18).

Attend to the entire kinetic chain

It is important to consider the potential causes and effects of suboptimal biomechanics on the entire neuromusculoskeletal system. For example:

- ankle joint stiffness may contribute to altered biomechanics during gait or occur as a consequence of calf muscle imbalance
- joint pain or stiffness can be addressed with active or passive mobilisation of peripheral or vertebral joints or 'mobilisation with movement'[134]
- increased neural mechanosensitivity can be managed with appropriate exercises, as well as correction of possible causes such as spinal hypomobility.

Other interventions aimed at reducing pain, such as pharmacotherapy, electrotherapy and dry needling may facilitate optimal performance of exercises (Chapter 17).

UPPER LIMB BIOMECHANICS

with W. BEN KIBLER

Correct biomechanics is as important in upper limb activities as it is in lower limb activities. For example, repeated throwing places tremendous stresses on the upper limb, especially the shoulder and elbow joints.[135] Throwing, however, is a 'whole body activity', involving the transfer of momentum from the body to the object being thrown. The following section uses baseball pitching as a model; however, the principles described are relevant to other overhead sports activities, such as the javelin throw, volleyball spike and tennis serve.

The biomechanics of throwing

Throwing is a whole body activity that commences with drive from the large leg muscles and rotation of the hips, and progresses through segmental rotation of the trunk and shoulder girdle. It continues with a 'whip-like' transfer of momentum through elbow extension and through the small muscles of the forearm and hand, transferring propulsive force to the ball.

The skilled clinician should assess both the scapulohumeral and the truncal mechanics in a throwing athlete. The role of the scapula in throwing is discussed in more detail below, and the back, trunk and hips serve as a centre of rotation and a transfer link from the legs to the shoulder.

Throwing can be divided into four phases:

1. Preparation/wind-up   ⎫
2. Cocking   ⎬ 80% time sequence
3. Acceleration   2% time sequence
4. Deceleration/follow-through   18% time sequence

Wind-up

Wind-up (Fig. 8.23) establishes the rhythm of the throw. During wind-up, the body rotates so that the hip and shoulders are at 90° to the target. The major forces arise in the lower half of the body and develop a forward-moving 'controlled fall.' In pitching, hip flexion of the lead leg raises the centre of gravity. The wind-up phase lasts 500–1000 milliseconds. During this phase, muscles of the shoulder are relatively inactive.

Cocking

The cocking movement (Fig. 8.24) positions the body to enable all body segments to contribute to ball propulsion. In cocking, the shoulder moves into abduction through full horizontal extension and then into maximal external rotation. When the scapula is maximally retracted, the acromion starts to elevate. With maximal external rotation, the shoulder is 'loaded', with the anterior capsule coiled tightly in the apprehension position storing elastic energy. The internal rotators are stretched.[136] At this stage, anterior joint forces are maximal and can exceed 350 newtons (N).

Toward the end of cocking, the static anterior restraints (anterior inferior glenohumeral ligament and anterior inferior capsule) are under the greatest strain. Because of the repetitive nature of throwing, these structures can become attenuated, leading to subtle instability.[137] In the trunk, tensile forces increase in the abdomen, hip extensors and spine, with the lead hip internally rotating just prior to ground contact.

The cocking phase ends with the planting of the lead leg, with the body positioned for energy transfer through the legs, trunk and arms to the ball. This phase also lasts 500–1000 milliseconds. The wind-up and cocking phases

114

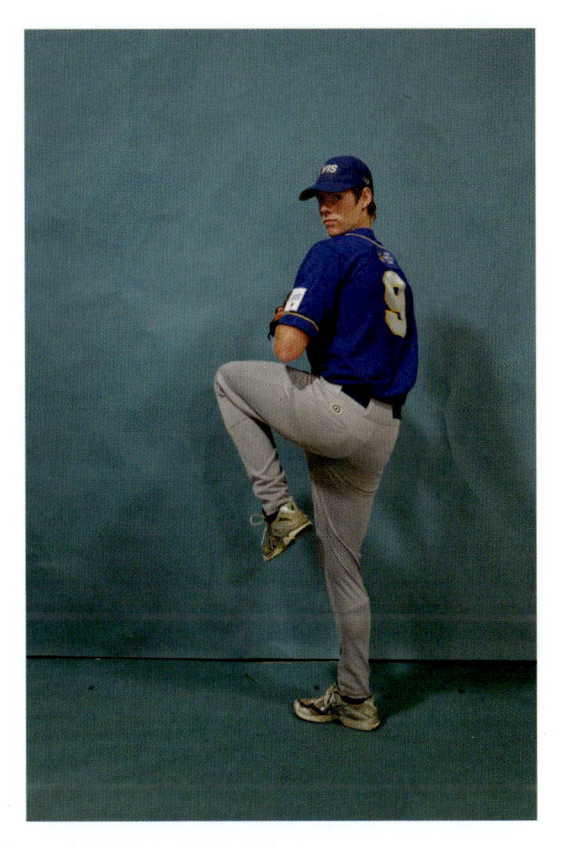

Figure 8.23 Throwing—wind-up

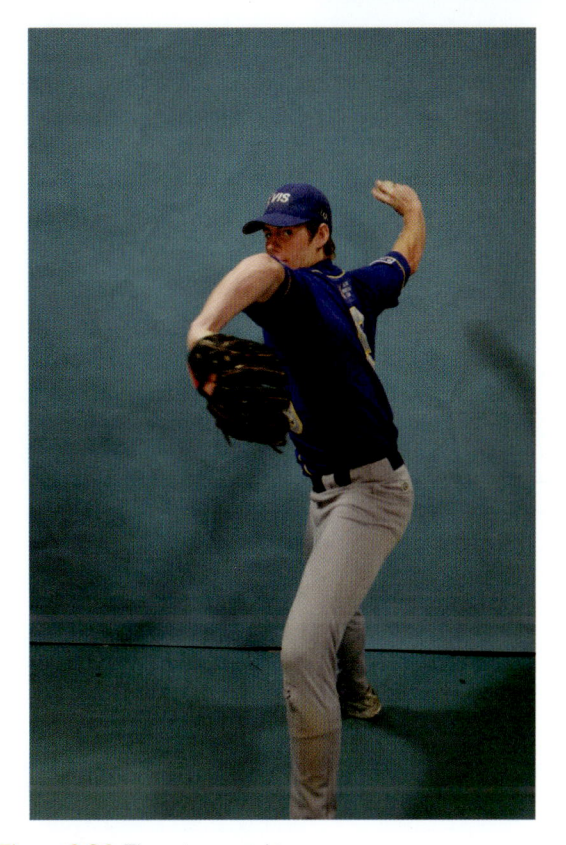

Figure 8.24 Throwing—cocking

together constitute 80% of the duration of the pitch (approximately 1500 milliseconds).

Shoulder cocking continues with the counterclockwise rotation of the pelvis and trunk (when a right-handed thrower is viewed from above), which abruptly places the arm behind the body in an externally rotated position.

Lateral trunk flexion determines the degree of arm abduction. When viewed in the frontal plane, the relative abduction of the humerus to the long axis of the trunk is a fairly constant 90-100°, regardless of style. The overhand athlete leans contralaterally, while the 'side-arm' or 'submarine' thrower actually leans toward the throwing arm. Rotation of the trunk also aids in abduction. Although the muscles of the shoulder produce little abduction during the early cocking phase of a well-executed throw, the periscapular muscles are quite active. The force couple between the upper trapezius and serratus initiates acromial elevation and the lower trapezius maintains elevation at abduction angles greater than 65°.

Acceleration

The acceleration phase (Fig. 8.25) is extremely explosive. It consists of the rapid release of two forces–the stored elastic force of the tightly bound fibrous tissue of the capsule, and forceful internal rotation from the internal rotators (subscapularis, pectoralis major, latissimus dorsi and teres major). This generates high forces at the glenohumeral articulation,[138] creating high demands on the cuff musculature to keep the humeral head located in the glenoid.

Large muscles outside the rotator cuff are responsible for the subsequent acceleration of the arm. This includes muscles of the anterior chest wall as well as the muscles and fascia that surround the spine. The critical role of the muscles controlling scapulothoracic motion–scapular positioning and stabilisation against the thorax–is discussed below.

At the shoulder, acceleration is the shortest phase of the throwing motion, lasting only 50 milliseconds (2% of the overall time). In both the acceleration and the late cocking phases, muscle fatigue (which is accelerated if there is mild instability due to attenuated static restraints) can lead to loss of coordinated rotator cuff motion and, thus, decreased anterior shoulder wall support.

The acceleration phase concludes with ball release, which occurs at approximately ear level. The movements involved in acceleration place enormous valgus forces on the elbow, which tends to lag behind the inwardly rotating shoulder.

PART A   Fundamental principles

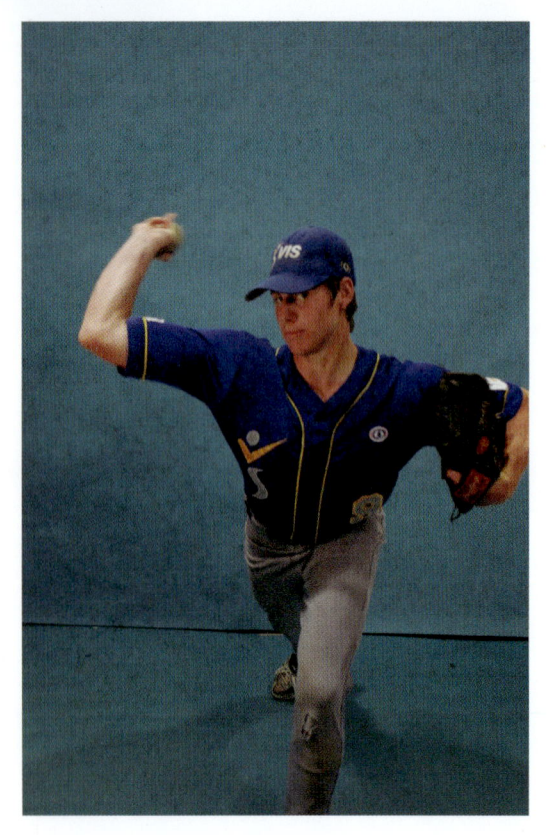

Figure 8.25 Throwing—acceleration

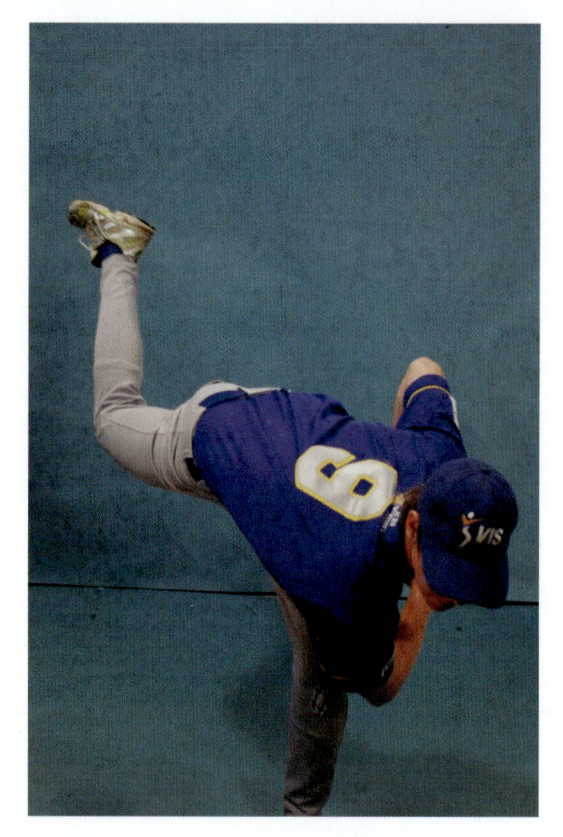

Figure 8.26 Throwing—deceleration/follow-through

Deceleration/follow-through
Not all the momentum of the throw is transferred to the ball. In the deceleration/follow-through phase (Fig. 8.26), large forces pull forward on the glenohumeral joint following ball release, which stresses the posterior shoulder structures. During this time both intrinsic and extrinsic shoulder muscles fire at significant percentages of their maximum, attempting to develop in excess of 500 N to slow the arm down. The force tending to pull the humerus out of the shoulder socket can exceed 500 N (roughly equivalent to 135 kg). The eccentric contraction of the rotator cuff external rotators decelerates the rapid internal rotation of the shoulder, as does eccentric contraction of the scapular stabilisers and posterior deltoid. In the properly thrown pitch, the spine and its associated musculature have a significant role as a force attenuator.

Toward the end of the pitching motion, the torso, having decelerated so the arm could acquire kinetic energy in the arm acceleration phase, begins to rotate forward. The forward rotation of this larger link segment helps to reacquire some of this energy. This theoretically reduces the burden on the serratus anterior and other stabilisers, which are attempting to eccentrically maintain the position of the scapula and maintain the humeral head within the glenoid.

In addition to the high stresses on the posterior shoulder structures, this phase places large stresses on the elbow flexors that act to limit rapid elbow extension. This phase lasts approximately 350 milliseconds and constitutes approximately 18% of the total time.

The role of the trunk in throwing is clear. When trunk motion is inhibited or the potential GRF reduced, throwing velocity is markedly lower. With a normal overhead throw rated at 100%, peak velocities dropped to 84% when a forward stride was not allowed and down to 63.5% and 53.1% when the lower body and lower body plus trunk were restricted, respectively.[139] Peak ball-release velocities attained by water polo players are approximately half the velocity that a thrown baseball might reach on land where a GRF can be generated.

The kinetic chain
The 'kinetic chain' is a term clinicians use to make the point that optimal function of a distal structure relies on well-functioning proximal elements. Consider the hand/fingers in throwing as a 'distal' structure. The kinetic chain that underpins successful throwing includes the

Introduction to clinical biomechanics   CHAPTER 8

lower limb (the very beginning of the 'chain'), the muscles that envelop the torso, the scapula and shoulder muscles and finally the upper arm and forearm that connect to the hand (Fig. 8.27). It does not require much imagination to see these elements (links) working like a 'whip' or a dynamic 'chain' to allow very speedy release of a baseball, cricket ball or tennis ball (with the racquet extending the chain even further).

Let us illustrate the concept more specifically using the scapula as a model. It links the proximal-to-distal sequencing of velocity, energy and forces that optimise shoulder function. For most shoulder activities this sequencing starts at the ground. Individual body segments, or links, move in a coordinated way to generate, summate and transfer force through various body segments to the terminal link. Large proximal body segments provide the bulk of the force.

Why is the kinetic chain concept important for clinicians? Because it highlights that treatment cannot merely address local symptoms. Right shoulder tendon pain in a right arm bowling/throwing athlete may arise because of calf muscle weakness, hip joint tightness and in coordination of the scapular movements. Clinicians must look for causes of symptoms along the entire kinetic chain and treat all contributing links.

Normal biomechanics of the scapula in throwing

In recent years, the importance of the scapula in normal throwing biomechanics has been increasingly recognised. For optimal shoulder function and to decrease injury risk, the scapula must move in a coordinated way (Fig. 8.28). This section outlines Ben Kibler's[140] description of the role of the scapula in throwing (Table 8.8). If the clinician understands the normal scapular biomechanics,

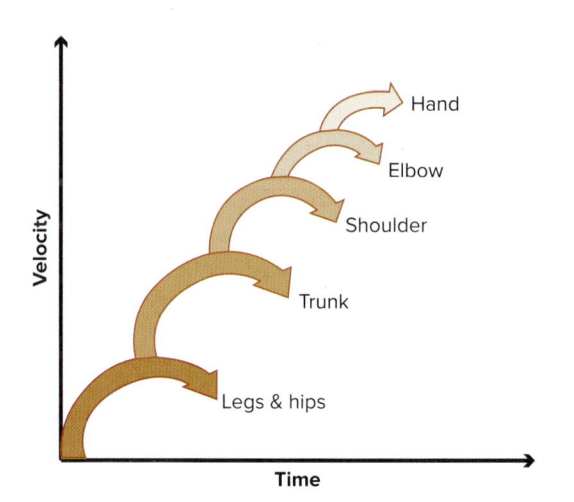

Figure 8.27 The kinetic chain in throwing

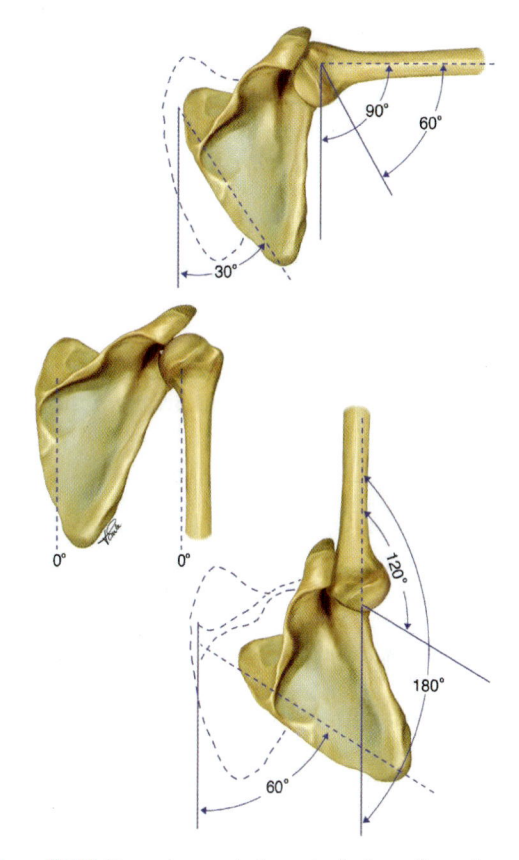

Figure 8.28 Normal scapulothoracic rhythm allows the scapula to rotate upwardly during abduction, bringing the glenoid fossa directly under the humeral head to lend stability to the glenohumeral joint

Table 8.8 Scapular function in normal shoulder mechanics

1. Provides a stable socket for the humerus
2. Retracts and protracts along the thoracic wall
3. Rotates to elevate the acromion
4. Provides a base for muscle attachment
5. Provides a key link in the kinetic chain

he or she will be then able to detect abnormal scapular biomechanics in patients with upper limb injuries.

The scapula provides a stable socket for the humerus

In normal shoulder function, the scapula forms a stable base for glenohumeral articulation. The glenoid is the socket of the ball-and-socket glenohumeral joint. Thus, the scapula must rotate as the humerus moves so that the centre of rotation of the glenohumeral joint remains optimal throughout the throwing or serving motion.

This coordinated movement keeps the angle between the glenoid and the humerus within the physiologically tolerable or 'safe zone', which extends about 30° of extension or flexion from neutral. In this range, there is maximal 'concavity/compression' of the glenohumeral joint, and the muscle constraints around the shoulder are also enhanced. The maximal concavity/compression results from the slightly negative intra-articular pressure of the normal joint, with optimal positioning of the glenoid in relation to the humerus and coordinated muscle activity.

The scapula must retract and protract along the thoracic wall

In the cocking phase of throwing (as well as in the tennis serve and swimming recovery), the scapula retracts (see above). Once acceleration begins, the scapula protracts smoothly laterally and then anteriorly around the thoracic wall to keep the scapula in a normal position relative to the humerus and also to dissipate some of the deceleration forces that occur in follow-through.

The scapula rotates to elevate the acromion

As almost all throwing and serving activities occur with a humerus-to-spine angle of between 85° and 100° of abduction, the scapula must tilt upwards to clear the acromion from the rotator cuff.

The scapula provides a base for muscle attachment

Stabilising muscles attach to the medial, superior and inferior borders of the scapula to control its position and motion. The extrinsic muscles (deltoid, biceps and triceps) attach along the lateral aspect of the scapula and perform gross motor activities of the glenohumeral joint. The intrinsic muscles of the rotator cuff attach along the entire surface of the scapula and work most efficiently with the arm between 70° and 100° of abduction. In this position, they form a 'compressor cuff' locating the humeral head into the socket.

The scapula provides a key link in the kinetic chain

The scapula is pivotal in transferring the large forces and high energy from the legs, back and trunk to the arm and the hand. Forces generated in the proximal segments are transferred efficiently and are regulated as they go through the funnel of the shoulder when the scapula provides a stable and controlled platform. The entire arm rotates as a unit around the stable base of the glenohumeral socket.

Thus, the scapula performs various interrelated functions to maintain the normal glenohumeral path and provide a stable base for muscular function. Abnormalities in scapular function that predispose to injury are discussed below.

Abnormal scapular biomechanics and physiology

The scapular roles can be altered by many anatomical factors to create abnormal biomechanics and physiology, both locally and in the kinetic chain (Table 8.9).

Clinical significance of scapular biomechanics in shoulder injuries

Abnormal shoulder biomechanics can compromise normal shoulder function. This observation has been given various descriptive titles, such as 'scapulothoracic dyskinesis', 'floating scapula' or 'lateral scapular slide'. It is important for the clinician to recognise that these are merely titles for the same phenomenon, that is, abnormal scapular function. We provide examples of how abnormal biomechanics can cause shoulder and elbow problems.

Lack of full retraction of the scapula on the thorax destabilises the cocking point and prevents acceleration out of a fully cocked position. Lack of full scapular protraction increases the deceleration forces on the shoulder and alters the normal safe zone between the glenoid and the humerus as the arm moves through the acceleration phase. Too much protraction because of tightness in the glenohumeral capsule causes impingement as the scapula rotates down and forward. These cumulatively lead to abnormalities in concavity/compression due to the changes in the safe zone of the glenohumeral angle.

Loss of coordinated retraction/protraction in throwing opens up the front of the glenohumeral joint and, thus, provides an insufficient anterior bony buttress to anterior translation of the humeral head. This increases shear stress on the rest of the anterior stabilising structure—the labrum and glenohumeral ligaments—which further decreases the stability of the glenoid for the rotating humerus.

Lack of acromial elevation leads to impingement in the cocking and follow-through phases. Impingement can also occur secondary to painful shoulder conditions that inhibit the function of the serratus and lower trapezius muscles. As these muscles normally act as a force couple to elevate the acromion, their inhibition commonly causes impingement. Thus, detecting and, if necessary, reversing serratus and trapezius inhibition is an important step in treating shoulder conditions.

If the scapula is unstable, the lack of an anchor affects the function of all scapula muscles. Muscles without a stable origin cannot develop appropriate or maximal torque and are predisposed to suffering muscular imbalance. If the scapula is truly unstable on the thoracic

Introduction to clinical biomechanics   CHAPTER 8

Table 8.9 Alterations to scapular function

Scapular function alteration	Effect on scapular function
Anatomical factors	
Cervical spine lordosis	Excessive scapular protraction—leads to impingement with elevation
Thoracic spine kyphosis	Excessive scapular protraction—leads to impingement with elevation
Shoulder asymmetry (i.e. drooping of the shoulder or 'tennis shoulder')	Impingement/muscle function and fatigue
Injuries of scapula, clavicle	Alters orientation of scapula, length of clavicular strut—painful conditions that inhibit muscle function
Abnormalities in muscle function	
Overuse, direct trauma, glenohumeral causes (instability, labral lesions, arthrosis)	Muscle weakness or force couple imbalances. Serratus anterior and lower trapezius particularly susceptible. Can be a non-specific response to a variety of glenohumeral pathologies (this can be seen as analogous to the knee in that weakness of the vastus medialis obliquus can result in patellofemoral syndrome)
Glenohumeral inflexibility, posterior (capsular or muscular)	Limits smooth glenohumeral joint motion and creates wind-up effect so that the glenoid and scapula get pulled forward and inferiorly by the moving arm. This leads to excessive protraction, which, in turn, holds the scapula and, importantly, the acromion inferiorly and, thus, makes it prone to impingement
Nerve injury (causes less than 5% of abnormal muscle function in shoulder problems)	Long thoracic nerve—serratus anterior function inhibited. Accessory nerve—trapezius function inhibited

wall, as in spinal accessory nerve palsies or in extremely inhibited muscles, then the muscle origins and insertions are effectively reversed, and the distal end of the muscle becomes the origin. The scapula is then pulled laterally by the muscle, which contracts from the more stable distal humeral end rather than from the proximal scapular end. A further problem of the unstable scapula is that it does not provide a stable base for glenohumeral rotation during link sequencing. Therefore, the arm works on an unstable platform and loses mechanical efficiency.

One of the most important scapular biomechanical abnormalities is the loss of the link function in the kinetic chain. The kinetic chain permits efficient transfer of energy and force to the hand. The scapula and shoulder funnel forces from the large segments, the legs and trunk, to the smaller, rapidly moving small segments of the arm.

Scapular dysfunction impairs force transmission from the lower to the upper extremity. This reduces the force delivered to the hand or creates a situation of 'catch up' in which the more distal links have to overwork to compensate for the loss of the proximally generated force. The distal links have neither the size, the muscle cross-sectional area, nor the time in which to develop these larger forces efficiently. For example, a 20% decrease in kinetic energy delivered from the hip and trunk to the arm necessitates an 80% increase in muscle mass or a 34% increase in rotational velocity at the shoulder to deliver the same amount of resultant force to the hand. Such an adaptation would predispose to overload problems.

This explains why injuries apparently unrelated to the upper limb, for example, decreased push off due to Achilles tendinopathy, decreased quadriceps drive after a muscle strain, or decreased segmental trunk rotation secondary to thoracic segmental hypomobility, can affect upper limb throwing mechanics and predispose to further or more serious, upper limb injury.

Changes in throwing arm with repeated throwing

Repeated throwing causes adaptive changes to gradually develop in the shoulder and elbow. Changes occur in flexibility, soft tissue/muscle strength and bony contour.

At the shoulder, long-term throwing athletes have increased range of external rotation. This arises because of the repeated stress to the anterior capsule in the cocking phase, and stretch or breakdown in the anterior static stabilisers of the shoulder joint (the inferior glenohumeral ligaments). This may compromise the dynamic balance that exists between shoulder function and stability. The combination of increased shoulder external rotation range of motion and breakdown of the static stabilisers may lead to anterior instability of the shoulder and secondary impingement.

The normal strength ratio of internal rotators to external rotators is approximately 3:2, but in throwers this imbalance is exaggerated and, over time, lack of external rotation strength may increase vulnerability to injury. These dynamic changes in the shoulder joint highlight the need for a structured exercise program to prevent or correct muscle imbalances.

Throwing also produces structural changes at the elbow. Due to the valgus stress applied in the throwing action, there is a breakdown of the medial stabilising structures (medial collateral ligament, joint capsule, flexor muscles). This leads to the development of an increased carrying angle at the elbow.

Less frequently, the eccentric overload on elbow structures causes anterior capsular strains, posterior impingement or forearm flexor strains and subsequently, a fixed flexion deformity.

Common biomechanical abnormalities specific to throwing

One of the most common biomechanical problems seen in throwing sports such as cricket, baseball and water polo is caused by the throwing athlete 'opening up too soon'. Normally the body rotates out of the cocking phase when the arm is fully cocked (externally rotated). If the body opens up too soon, the arm lags behind and is not fully externally rotated. This results in increased stress to the anterior shoulder structures and an increased eccentric load to the shoulder external rotators. It also results in increased valgus stress at the elbow.

The other common abnormality seen in throwing athletes is known as 'hanging', which is a characteristic sign of fatigue. Decreased shoulder abduction leads to dropping of the elbow and a reduction in velocity. There is an associated increase in the likelihood of injury, particularly to the rotator cuff as well as to the shoulder joint and the elbow. It is normally related to excessive intensity, frequency or duration of activity.

In baseball, the type of pitch is determined by the spin imparted onto the ball by the hands and fingers at ball release. The normal follow-through involves forearm pronation. In 'breaking' pitches, the forearm is relatively supinated at release and then pronates. 'Breaking' pitches are associated with an increased risk of injury. Some pitchers incorrectly forcefully supinate against the normal pronation of follow-through.

REFERENCES

References for this chapter can be found at www.mhhe.com/au/CSM5e

Chapter 9

Biomechanical aspects of injury in specific sports

with BEN CLARSEN

Nothing compares to the simple pleasure of riding a bike.
John F. Kennedy (1917-1963)

This chapter outlines the relationship between biomechanics and injury for a number of sports–cycling, cricket fast bowling, golf, rowing, swimming and tennis.

CYCLING

with PHIL BURT

The demands and injury risks differ greatly across the various disciplines of cycling. Traditional road cycling involves long-duration submaximal effort, and places stresses on the body due to monotonous loading and maintenance of static postures for extended periods. In contrast, BMX and track sprint cycling require maximal effort over a short duration. Riders from these disciplines are more likely to suffer injuries related to strength and power training, such as weightlifting and plyometrics. The various subdisciplines of mountain biking encompass a wide range of demands, and both acute and overuse injuries are common. This section focuses on the main overuse injury problems affecting cyclists across all disciplines–knee and low back pain.

Relationship between risk factors and loading

Overuse injuries in cycling are commonly blamed on extrinsic factors such as bike position or shoe and pedal setup, as well as intrinsic factors such as anatomical anomalies, poor cycling technique, or reduced neuromuscular control. These factors may certainly be important due to the repetitive, uniplanar nature of the sport. However, it is important to recognise that even among top professionals, a wide variation of anatomy, techniques, and bike setups is normally well-tolerated without injury occurring. In almost all cases of cycling-related overuse injury, symptom onset can be linked to a mismanagement of training and racing loads. Cyclists are most likely to develop injury following a rapid increase in load, such as when pre-season training is resumed after a winter break, as well as during intense periods of the season. When injuries are apparently 'caused' by a change in equipment, it is normally because the change was made at an inappropriate time of the season when the cyclist was already close to their limit of load tolerance.

The key to successful management of cycling injuries, therefore, is load management. The clinician, cyclist and coach should establish the volume, intensity and frequency of cycling that the rider can tolerate and create a systematic plan to increase these parameters over time. Wherever possible, loading should be quantified using a power meter and training software should be used to monitor the acute and chronic training load during rehabilitation (Chapter 12).

Once an appropriate training plan is established, intrinsic and extrinsic risk factors should be assessed. The following section covers biomechanical factors thought to be associated with the most common cycling injuries. It is important to note that there is little high-level evidence in the field of cycling injuries, with current practice largely based on indirect evidence and expert opinion. It is therefore necessary to take a trial-and-error approach; to be worthwhile, modification in technique or equipment should lead to an obvious improvement in symptoms.

Knee pain

The knee is the most common site of overuse injury among cyclists of all levels.[1-5] A majority of knee complaints are related to the patellofemoral joint.[6] However, there is a range of differential diagnoses including iliotibial band syndrome (ITBS), infrapatellar fat pad impingement, medial plica irritations and medial patellofemoral ligament

PART A Fundamental principles

strains.[6-8] Although tendinopathy is generally rare in cyclists, pain can also arise from the quadriceps tendon enthesis on the superolateral or superomedial patella.

Three biomechanical factors to assess in patellofemoral pain

Various biomechanical factors may play a role in the development of patellofemoral pain in cyclists, including patellofemoral joint compression forces, knee kinematics in the frontal plane and rotational torques in the lower limb.[9-12]

1. Saddle height

Patellofemoral joint contact pressure is inversely related to saddle height,[9] leading to the common belief that cycling with lower bicycle saddle heights increases the risk of patellofemoral pain development.[8, 11, 13] However, this remains to be confirmed in high-quality risk factor studies of competitive cyclists and one study found that altering the saddle height within the normal ranges used in rehabilitation led to negligible changes in patellofemoral joint contact pressure.[14] Nevertheless, it is advisable that cyclists with patellofemoral pain ride in a relatively high saddle position, with maximal knee extension of approximately 30° (Fig. 9.1).

2. Medial knee motion

Excessive medial motion of the knee in the frontal plane (Fig. 9.2a) may also be a risk factor for patellofemoral pain, as this position encourages lateralisation of the patella

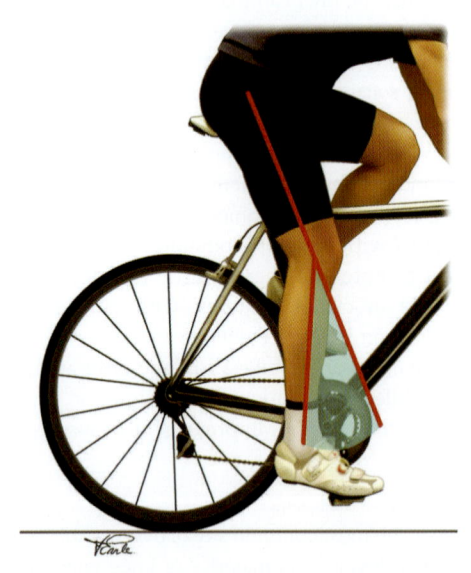

Figure 9.1 Maximum knee extension is a key bike fitting parameter, which typically ranges from 35–40° among professional riders. Patellofemoral joint contact pressures may be minimised by selecting a higher saddle position, with maximum knee extension between 30° and 35°.

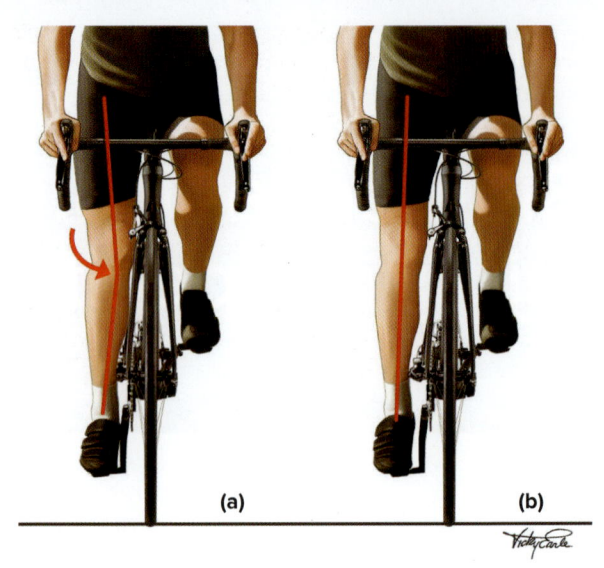

Figure 9.2 Frontal-plane knee motion in cycling (a) Excessive valgus motion of the knee is thought to contribute to a range of knee injuries (b) Improving the alignment of the hip, knee and ankle may lead to symptomatic improvement

in the femoral trochlea, increased lateral joint contact pressure and increased stress on medial soft tissues. This theory is supported by studies showing that cyclists with a history of knee pain adopt a more medial knee position compared to uninjured cyclists,[10] and that 'normalising' frontal plane motion (Fig. 9.2b) can lead to symptomatic improvement.[15] Knee motion may be altered by motor control training or through manipulation of the cyclist's shoes and pedals. For example, foot position can be adjusted using small angled wedges between the shoe and the pedal cleat or underneath the forefoot or by using custom-made insoles. However, manipulation of cycling shoes and pedals has an extremely unpredictable effect on knee motion.[16, 17] It is therefore important to test each individual's response, making sure that adjustments lead to symptomatic improvement.

3. Rotational torque

Rotational torque at the knee caused by the fixation of shoes to the pedals may also be a factor in patellofemoral pain in cycling. After the introduction of modern cleated pedals in the 1980s, there were anecdotal reports of an increase in the prevalence of knee injuries among cyclists.[6, 12] It was thought that the natural rotation of the lower limb during the pedalling cycle was constrained by fixing the shoe, leading to increased stress at the knee joint. Therefore, 'floating' pedals were designed that allowed a small degree of axial rotation, which attenuated the rotational torque at the knee.[12] Although there is no

Biomechanical aspects of injury in specific sports — CHAPTER 9

direct evidence that floating pedals reduce injury, their design has been widely accepted and they remain the most popular type used by cyclists today.[1]

Iliotibial band syndrome

ITBS, often called 'runner's knee', is also common among cyclists.[6, 18] Intrinsic factors thought to contribute to ITBS include large leg length discrepancies, external tibial torsion of greater than 20° and excessive subtalar pronation.[18] High saddle height, a *toe-in, heel-out* foot position and excessive medial knee motion also increase the stress on the ITB.[19]

> **PRACTICE PEARL**
>
> Therefore, cyclists with lateral knee pain should be instructed to ride with a relatively low saddle (maximum knee extension approximately 40°), keep their feet straight or pointed slightly outwards and avoid a knee-in position.

Low back pain

Although transient back discomfort is normal in cycling, studies have shown that performance-limiting low back pain is common among amateur[20] and elite cyclists.[1, 21]

Cyclists with low back pain typically present with non-specific symptoms provoked by the maintenance of sustained flexion positions and they can often be classified as having a flexion-pattern motor control dysfunction (Chapter 29).[22] Using a remote posture monitoring system, Van Hoof et al. showed that cyclists with low back pain adopt a more flexed position in their lumbar spine than do pain-free cyclists (Fig. 9.3).[23] This may be related to a number of pathomechanical mechanisms of low back pain,[22, 24] such as flexion/relaxation inhibition, or fatigue of the erector spinae muscles and mechanical creep of the spine's viscoelastic tissues. However, these theories remain largely untested in cyclists.

Encouraging a relaxed, anteriorly tilted pelvic position, with an even distribution of flexion throughout the spine, is often important in the overall management of cyclists with low back pain. A number of equipment modifications may help facilitate this, including lowering the saddle, raising the handlebars and shortening or lengthening the overall reach.

> **PRACTICE PEARL**
>
> Adjusting the saddle to a slightly nose-down position (2–4°) may also be helpful in achieving greater anterior pelvic tilt and reducing back pain.[25]

Excessive lateral flexion and/or rotation of the spine while cycling may also contribute to back pain, particularly if it is asymmetrical. This can be caused by a range of factors, such as large leg length differences, hip range of motion limitations and asymmetrical muscle activation patterns. These should be considered as a part of the comprehensive management of the cyclist with low back pain. Bike fit is a critical element in such a comprehensive assessment (see box).

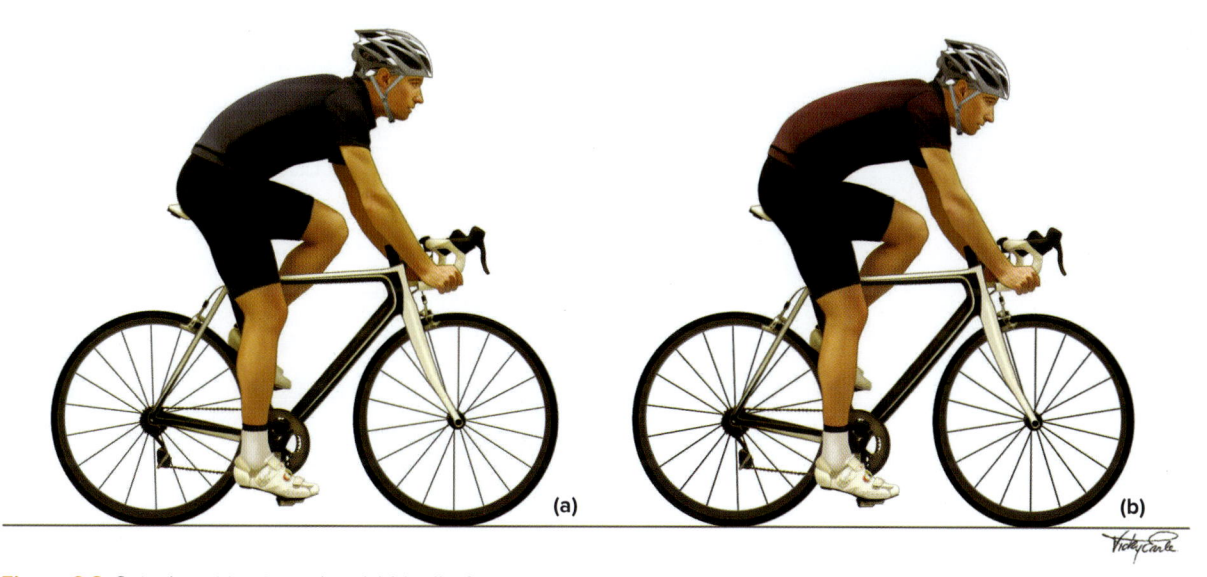

Figure 9.3 Spinal position in cycling (a) Ideally, forward bend should be achieved evenly (b) Cyclists with low back pain often adopt a more flexed lumbar spine, with less anterior pelvic tilt and a more extended thoracic spine

PART A Fundamental principles

Bike fitting

There are many approaches to bike fitting, ranging from simple anthropometry-based formulae to dynamic approaches utilising high-tech equipment (Table 9.1 and Fig 9.4).

As bike fitting involves the optimisation of a wide range of competing variables, such as aerodynamics, comfort and control, it always involves compromise. Despite the recent rapid pace of technological development in the cycling industry, there remains little research into bicycle equipment and injury, and bike fitting remains just as much an art as it is a science. We encourage clinicians to work closely with bike fitters who take a trial-and-error approach, considering the cyclist's previous and current injuries, cycling goals and physical limitations.

Table 9.1 Advantages and limitations of modern bike fitting methods

Formula-based approach	
Description	There are a number of formula-based approaches that convert anthropometric measurements (e.g. inseam height) to bicycle set-up parameters. The most well-known approach is named after two-time Tour de France winner, Greg LeMond.
Advantages	Quick and easy. Cyclists can perform measurements themselves.
Limitations	One-size-fits-all approach that does not consider the cyclist's physical limitations. Highly unreliable and variable results.[26]
Static angle-based approach	
Description	The cyclist's major joint angles are measured with a goniometer while he or she sits on the bike without cycling. The bike is adjusted to position each joint within a predetermined 'optimal' range of motion. Sometimes referred to as the Holmes method.
Advantages	Good reliability.[27]
Limitations	Does not consider dynamic cycling technique. 'Optimal' angles are not evidence-based.
Dynamic angle-based approach	
Description	Dynamic measure of joint angles collected with two-dimensional or three-dimensional motion analysis over a period of time and averaged as rider is actually riding.
Advantages	Good reliability.[27] Accounts for the rider's technique and physical limitations.
Limitations	Does not consider kinetic variables such as power distribution between legs.
Combined-input approach	
Description	Combination of data streams such as power, pedal forces, saddle pressure with motion analysis.
Advantages	Multiple sources of data can lead to more-informed clinical-reasoned decisions.
Limitations	More data does not always lead to better clinical decisions. Little research to assist data interpretation. Validity and reliability unknown.

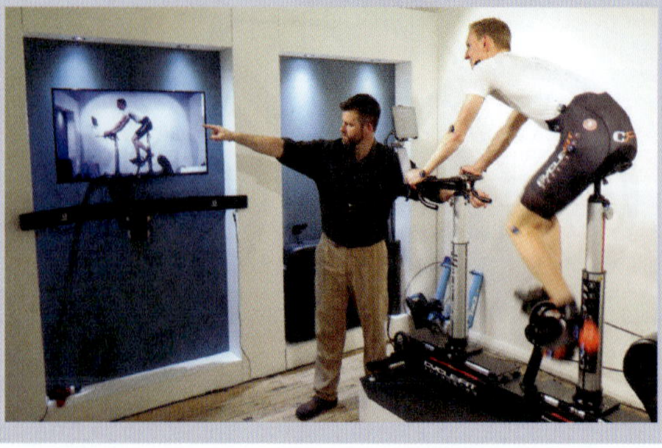

Figure 9.4 Modern bike fitting is an interactive process incorporating data from a variety of sources such as three-dimensional motion analysis, shoe and saddle pressure distribution, and pedal force application
IMAGE COURTESY OF CYCLEFIT UK

CRICKET FAST BOWLING

with ALEX KOUNTOURIS

Cricket fast bowling combines rapid near-end-range trunk movements (rotation, side flexion and extension), with high vertical and horizontal impact forces.[28-30] Elite fast bowlers bowl in excess of 300 deliveries in a single 4–5 day game, and have a higher rate of injury than any other players in cricket.[31]

Soft tissue and bone injuries are typically reported in injury surveillance studies of fast bowlers.[32] Lumbar spine injuries have received the most attention mainly because bone stress injuries of the posterior vertebral elements (pedicle, pars interarticularis and lamina) require lengthy recovery periods and are particularly common.[31]

> **PRACTICE PEARL**
>
> The most important risk factors are bowling biomechanics, age and workload.

Research into cricket fast bowling injuries has identified a number of possible modifiable and non-modifiable risk factors, particularly for lumbar spine injuries.[32, 33] It is likely that a combination of these factors determines the injury risk for fast bowlers, although a clear association between the three factors has not been established.

Age and risk of bowling injury

To highlight this important interplay between risk factors, younger fast bowlers, for example, are affected by biomechanical (technique) errors because they have an immature skeletal system that cannot cope with the high forces associated with fast bowling. As such, younger (adolescent) fast bowlers have a higher incidence of lumbar bone stress injuries than adult bowlers and have a disproportional high rate of lumbar spine radiological abnormalities and soft tissue injuries for their age.[34,35] Technique (biomechanical) faults that increase the amount of trunk rotation, extension and side flexion increase the load on the already susceptible musculoskeletal structures like the intervertebral disc and posterior vertebral arch.

Bowling workload and injury

Bowling workload is a modifiable factor associated with fast bowling injuries in both adolescent and adult fast bowlers. High bowling workloads in a single session, in a match or over a cricket season, have caused injuries in fast bowlers.[29, 36-38] More importantly, workload 'spikes' (a rapid increase in workload) have also been associated with fast bowling injuries and particularly lumbar spine injury.[39, 40]

The relationship between bowling technique and workload is not entirely clear, but it is likely that bowlers with a technique that is considered to be biomechanically sound may be able to tolerate higher workloads than those with other 'less safe' techniques because they are better equipped to dissipate forces. This relationship could be further complicated when considering age and that some structures may not have the resilience to absorb repetitive load (e.g. the posterior vertebral arch) until full maturity is reached. For example, in the lumbar spine, important geometric parameters that influence bone strength are not fully developed until the mid-twenties. In long bones, increases in bone mineral density (BMD) and bone mineral content (BMC) occur between pre-puberty and 18 years of age, but in the lumbar spine the increases in BMD, BMC, vertebral height and vertebral width continue to develop until 25 years of age.[41] This age (25 years) seems to be an important time in the development of lumbar bone stress and other lumbar spine injuries.

The relative impact of workload and age as risk factors needs to be considered along with bowling technique, because technical faults that result in exaggerated spinal positions and higher impact forces can magnify the impact of other risk factors.

> **PRACTICE PEARL**
>
> Biomechanical errors are arguably the most important risk factor for fast bowling injury.

Like other sporting activities, fast bowling technical faults are considered modifiable factors although making meaningful technical changes can be difficult.[42] To fully understand the biomechanical faults it is important to review the patterns of movement (kinematics) and forces (kinetics) that occur during the fast bowling action.

Fast bowling technique and injury

The simplest description of the fast bowling action is that it involves a combination of trunk rotation, and lateral flexion and extension during the delivery stride.[28-30] The sequence of movements and the associated ground reaction forces (GRF) during the fast bowling delivery stride are unique to every bowler, but can be broadly categorised into one of four bowling techniques: front-on, side-on, semi-open (semi-on) and mixed (Fig. 9.6).[43] These bowling techniques are defined by position of the feet, pelvis, trunk and shoulders at specific times during the delivery stride, and assessed using video (two-dimensional) or ideally, three-dimensional computer analysis.[43]

The fast bowling action can be broken down into three components that are interrelated and important for both performance and injury.[44] The main components are the run-up, the delivery stride and follow-through. The run-up is important as it allows bowlers to gain the momentum required to deliver the ball at a desired velocity and can pre-set the body position that occurs during the delivery stride. The delivery stride is the last ground contact of the back foot, known as back foot contact (BFC), and then the transition to front foot contact (FFC) and ends with ball release (Fig. 9.5). The highest GRF, between six to nine times body weight, occur during the period between FFC and ball release.[28, 29, 45] The follow-through begins at ball release and involves deceleration of the bowler until they come to a stop.

Importance of biomechanics of the delivery stride

Bowlers can be categorised into the four bowling techniques based on the positions and movements that occur during the delivery stride.[44] The four main bowling techniques are outlined in Figure 9.6.

Of the four bowling actions, the mixed technique has been identified as having the greatest association with lumbar spine injury and abnormal radiological features (Fig 9.6d).[35, 46] The maximum amount of shoulder–pelvis separation angle occurs just after FFC,[43] and possibly represents the period that places the bowler at greatest risk of injury, especially as it is also the time when the greatest ground impact forces are being absorbed.[29, 45] The mixed technique also typically involves higher rates of trunk contralateral side flexion and hyperextension compared to other bowling actions and therefore places greater stress through the lumbar spine.[47]

Another biomechanical aspect that has been associated with lumbar spine injuries in fast bowlers is shoulder counter-rotation (SCR), which is also closely associated with the mixed bowling technique. Bowlers with higher rates (greater than 30°) of SCR during the delivery stride have been associated with higher incidence of lumbar spine bone stress injuries and abnormal radiological features.[28, 29, 35, 44, 48] SCR (Fig. 9.7) is the change in shoulder alignment between BFC and FFC, from a more front-on to a more side-on alignment.[43, 44] The measurement of SCR is made using both two-dimensional and three-dimensional motion analysis and can vary slightly depending on the definition of BFC (first-foot contact with the ground versus foot flat on the ground).[43]

It is still unclear whether one particular bowling trunk position causes the most stress on the lumbar spine or if a combination of movements is required to exceed load tolerance. Cadaver studies indicated that lumbar extension was most likely to be associated

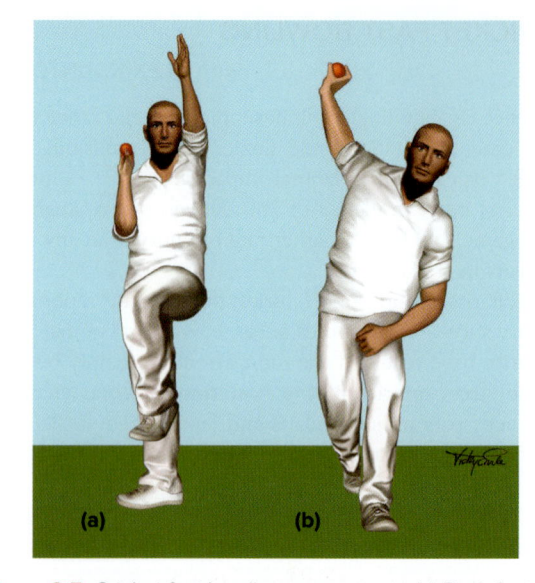

Figure 9.5 Cricket fast bowling components (a) Back foot contact (BFC) (b) Front foot contact (FFC)
DRAWING ADAPTED FROM PORTUS ET AL.[44]

with lumbar bone stress injury in fast bowlers, because of increased load on the posterior vertebral arch in a hyperextended position.[28, 49] Since then, the role of trunk side flexion and rotation has also received attention. Ranson et al. proposed that the amount of contralateral side flexion and ipsilateral rotation at FFC were important factors in the development of lumbar spine injury in fast bowlers.[50] They found that the greatest range of motion in the lower lumbar spine at FFC was contralateral lumbar side flexion and not lumbar extension as first thought. They concluded that the combination of high rates of contralateral side flexion, ipsilateral rotation and the large impact forces would be associated with lumbar spine bone stress in fast bowlers.[50] It is most likely that a combination of trunk positions is responsible for the high force required to develop lumbar spine injuries, in particular, bone stress injuries and the individual contribution of each movement to injury risk could be associated with the bowling technique used.

Apart from the spine and trunk positions adopted during the delivery stride, lower limb joint kinematics have also been linked with fast bowling injuries. The amount of knee extension at FFC influences the distribution of forces and influences the height at which the ball is released, so that a higher release height requires less knee flexion (straighter knee).[29, 51] The increase in front foot knee extension leads to a stiffer knee segment and greater impact forces.[44, 51]

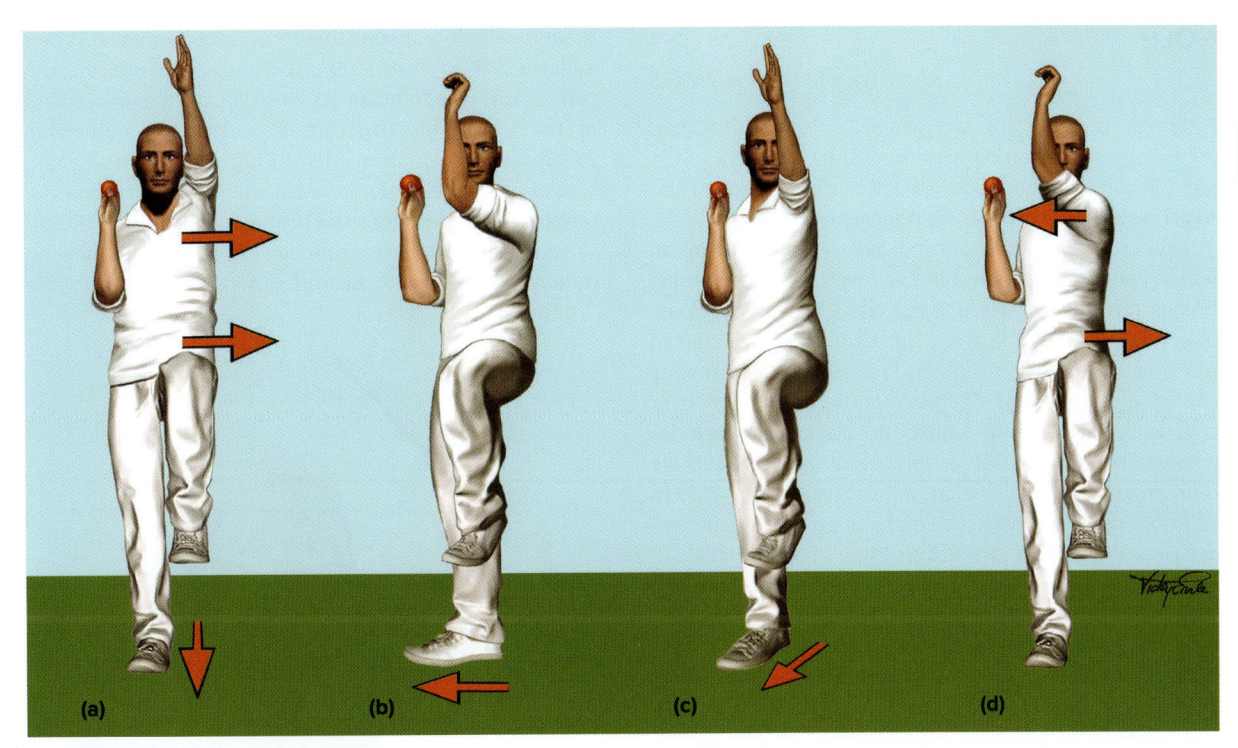

Biomechanical aspects of injury in specific sports   CHAPTER 9

Figure 9.6 Cricket fast bowling techniques
(a) *Front-on technique* involves the alignment of the pelvis and shoulders parallel to the batsman at back foot contact (BFC)
(b) *Side-on technique* involves the alignment of the bowler's shoulders and pelvis perpendicular to the batsman at BFC
(c) *Semi-on* or *semi-open technique* is defined as both shoulder and pelvis alignment somewhere between front-on and side-on positions at BFC
(d) *Mixed technique* involves dissociation between the shoulder and pelvis alignment at BFC, known as the shoulder–pelvis separation angle. For example, a front-on pelvis alignment and side-on shoulder alignment at BFC, or side-on pelvis position and front-on shoulder position at BFC. A shoulder–pelvis separation angle of 30° has been used to classify bowlers as having a mixed technique
DRAWING ADAPTED FROM PORTUS ET AL.[44]

Portus et al.[44] reported a relationship between a more extended front knee at FFC and ball release, and higher braking and vertical impact forces. They also demonstrated that bowlers with greater knee extension also reached peak forces more quickly than those with a more flexed knee at ball release. The higher forces associated with a more extended front knee may increase injury risk but also allow bowlers to deliver the ball at faster bowling speeds.[44] This is an important performance benefit and needs to be considered if technique modification is contemplated. It is therefore possible that there may be a trade-off between faster bowling speeds and higher injury risk.

In summary, it is important to consider bowling biomechanics as a critical risk factor for fast bowling injuries. The relative impact of biomechanical errors on injury risk should be considered along with bowling workload and the age of the fast bowler, as there is a delicate interplay between these key risk factors.

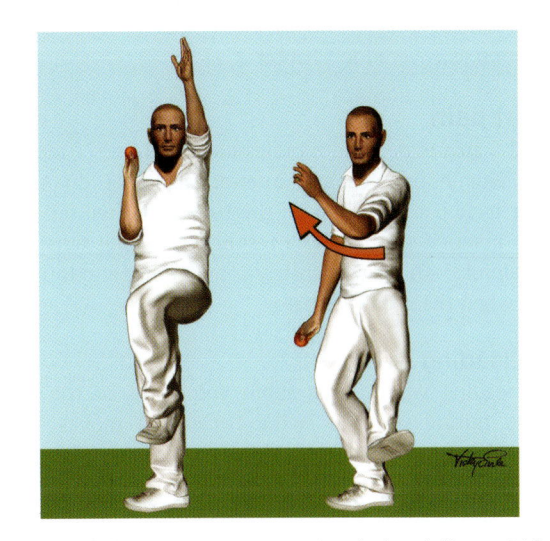

Figure 9.7 Shoulder counter-rotation during delivery stride
DRAWING ADAPTED FROM PORTUS ET AL.[44]

PART A Fundamental principles

GOLF

with ROGER HAWKES

Although injury rates are generally low, golf-related injuries are still common because of the popularity of the sport. It can be played into old age where the health and social benefits lead to increased longevity.[52]

Golf relies on a coordinated and repeated action in which energy is generated in the lower body and trunk. In long hitters, the force is transferred efficiently into the upper limbs and ultimately the club head, which can travel at speeds of 190 km/h. Professional tournaments are usually comprised of four rounds of 18 holes over a 4 day period during which the player also includes considerable practice. It is estimated that the average tour professional will hit around 200 shots per day. In addition, there has been an emphasis on hitting the ball as far as possible. It is not surprising therefore that, in spite of improving equipment and better conditioning, vulnerable tissues remain susceptible to injury. For instance, peroneal tendons in the leading ankle are used during the follow-through to prevent excessive inversion. Overuse can lead to tenosynovitis and lateral ankle pain and swelling. In addition, any deficiency in the kinetic chain may lead to compensation elsewhere and injury is more likely to occur. For instance, a player who is not able to rotate their thoracolumbar spine during the backswing may compensate by increasing the horizontal adduction of the leading shoulder in order to reach the top of the backswing. This may lead to shoulder injury.[53] Furthermore, fatigued players will have a reduced club head speed but an increased range of movement and this adds to injury risk.[54]

This chapter focuses on wrist, shoulder, hip and low back pain in golfers. Medial elbow pain, which is also common, is covered in Chapter 25.

Wrist pain

Good amateurs and professional players require considerable practice and intentionally take divots in order to impart backspin on the ball. In the winter they often practice on mats. As a result, the leading wrist can be painful.[55] This is particularly common in periods of the year when the ground is hard.

The leading wrist

The leading wrist is the more vulnerable of the two wrists during the golf swing because it moves from radial deviation at the top of the backswing (Fig. 9.8a) to ulnar deviation during follow-through. The trailing wrist follows a less stressful extension/flexion movement pattern (Fig. 9.8b). At impact, the ulnar side of the leading wrist is protected by the extensor carpi ulnaris tendon, which is susceptible to overuse synovitis. When a player hits an obstruction, the impact can rupture the sub-sheath which holds its position at the lower end of the ulna. This structure is particularly vulnerable in supination, which occurs during the golf swing and results in a large angle between the muscle axis and the tendon as it inserts into the fifth metacarpal.[56]

As a result of repetitive movement into ulnar deviation during the backswing, the leading wrist is also susceptible

(a)

(b)

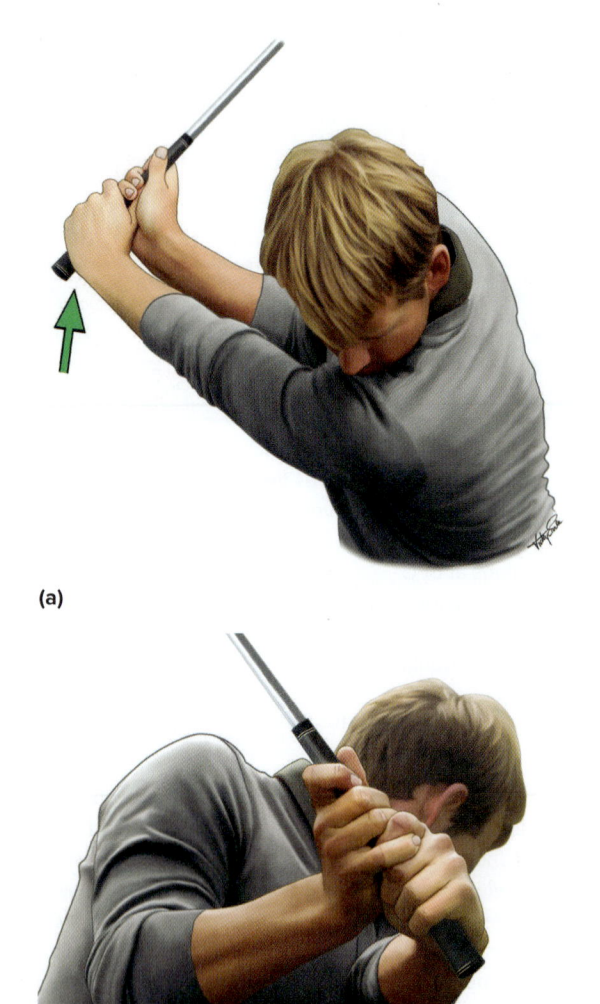

Figure 9.8 (a) The leading wrist (left) is in maximal radial deviation at the top of the backswing (shown) and moves into ulnar deviation during the follow-through (b) The trailing wrist (right) is in maximal extension at the top of the backswing (shown) and moves into flexion during the follow-through

to bone stress reactions, particularly of the hamate. Older players may develop osteoarthritic changes in the carpus, and players with long ulnas (either constitutionally or acquired after radial fracture) may be susceptible to ulnar-sided wrist pain as a result of impaction.

Fractures of the hook of hamate are rare, but 35% of them occur in golfers.[11] The hook of hamate is particularly vulnerable when a tall player uses standard length clubs. As a result, the end of the club may press onto the hook of hamate or piso-hamate ligament. Acute fractures can occur if the club hits the ground or an object, and with repetitive impacts the hook is also susceptible to bone stress injuries.

The trailing wrist

The trailing wrist extends during the backswing (Fig. 9.8b) and flexes during the follow-through. Players with dorsal rim impaction syndrome[57] pinpoint pain at the radial carpal joint in loaded extension, but often have no pain in passive extension. It is usually thought to occur as a result of nipping of the synovium, which can become chronically inflamed and hypertrophied. In some cases it can be due to loose bodies. Ultrasound is a good starting investigation but can be normal. Magnetic resonance imaging (MRI) can also show hypertrophy of the synovium (Fig. 9.9) and computed tomography (CT) scans can show loose bodies.

Players with tenosynovitis will need to reduce practice in order to reduce their symptoms. Amateur players may also choose a more forgiving shaft such as those made of graphite. They may improve the sweet spot by using hollow back clubs rather than blades. Other general treatments are covered in Chapter 26. Players who acutely sublux their extensor carpi ulnaris (ECU) tendons generally prefer to have operative repair of the subsheath, but conservative treatments have been used in tennis players with good results with no apparent increased time away from their sport. Some players have asymptomatic subluxing ECU tendons and do not require treatment.[55]

Players with dorsal rim impaction syndrome respond well to corticosteroid injection. However, the condition can return and arthroscopic resection of the thickened synovium can be indicated.

Finally, players who have had hook of hamate stress reactions or fractures will need to use longer clubs. If there is non-union of a fractured hook of hamate, resection is usually preferred in order to reduce the risk of injury to the ulnar nerve and artery injury, which can complicate pinning.[58]

Shoulder pain

The forces acting on the leading shoulder in golf are almost completely opposite to those involved in throwing (Chapter 8). The shoulder hyperadducts during the backswing, which can over stretch the posterior structures. During the follow-through, anterior structures work eccentrically to slow the shoulder down. The resultant combination of anterior capsular tightness and posterior laxity pushes the humeral head backwards, placing stress on the posterior labrum which can lead to posterior instability.[53] Players typically complain of pain or clunking at the top of the backswing. Clinical examination may show signs of posterior instability and MRI may show injury to the posterior labrum.

Players with a history of anterior instability in the leading shoulder may develop pain and apprehension toward the end of the follow-through when the shoulder is abducted and moving into external rotation. In the trailing shoulder, the movement (and injury) pattern is more similar to throwing sports.

Acromioclavicular joint pathology may occur in golfers. It is aggravated by joint compression, which occurs during the backswing for the leading shoulder and during the follow-through for the trailing shoulder.

In recent years there has been considerable interest in the phenomenon of glenohumeral internal rotation deficit (GIRD) in throwing athletes (Chapters 8 and 24). In golfers, however, the main focus is on identifying and addressing deficits in external rotation. Professional players are regularly screened for glenohumeral external rotation deficits (GERD) in an attempt to prevent posterior instability in the leading shoulder, although there is currently little research to show this as an effective prevention strategy.

Players with shoulder pathologies often need to limit golf participation in the early phases of rehabilitation. Resumption of practice should begin with putting and small chips with high irons, before gradually increasing the swing and playing with progressively longer clubs.

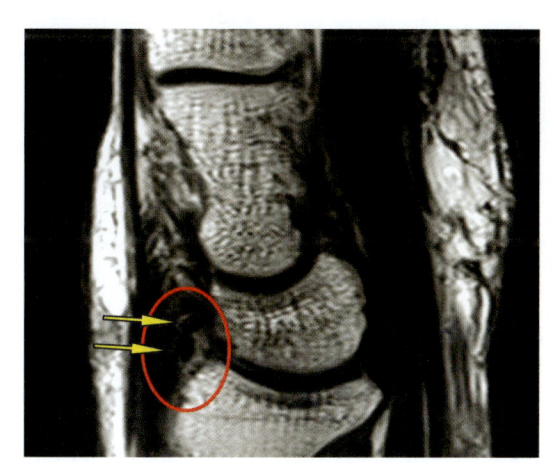

Figure 9.9 Dorsal rim impaction syndrome—Sagittal MR image showing synovial/capsular hypertrophy (arrows) of the dorsal aspect of the radiocarpal synovium. Normal capsule would be a thin low signal line

Hip pain

A recent survey of professional golfers found that 19% of players complained of current, significant hip and groin pain.[59] Common hip diagnoses in golfers include labrum pathology/femoroacetabular impingement and, in older players, osteoarthritis.

A majority of golf-related hip problems are located in the leading hip,[59] which undergoes higher rotational velocities and moves through a much greater range of motion than the trailing hip.[60, 61] However, both hips need to be able to move freely to facilitate an effective swing–particularly into internal rotation. The trailing hip goes into internal rotation at the top of the backswing and the leading hip is at maximum internal rotation at the end of the follow-through. Players with osteoarthritis and femoroacetabular impingement may present with 'hip pain' at either end of the swing.

Occasionally, players will present with reduced internal rotation in the leading hip without hip joint pathology. This may be due to tightness of the posterior structures that work eccentrically during the follow-through. Limited internal rotation of the leading hip can have a range of consequences on swing mechanics, such as causing the player to 'stand up' during the follow-through. Maximising hip internal rotation range of motion is therefore important for all golfers.

The effective internal rotation range of motion may also be increased by encouraging players to take a more externally rotated stance. This is recommended for players with femoroacetabular impingement and osteoarthritis, as well as for players who have had hip replacement surgery.

Low back pain

Younger players may be vulnerable to spondylolysis, especially if they end their swing with a 'reverse C' shaped thoracolumbar spine (Fig. 9.10). In addition, recent trends towards a more aggressive swing involving a larger separation between the hips and the shoulder may also lead to back injury. Both these technique factors should be reviewed in players with low back pain.

Reduced hip internal rotation in the leading hip increases stress on the thoracolumbar spine, as rotational demands of the follow-through are transferred higher up the kinetic chain. Tight hip flexors are also a risk factor because this leads to more anterior pelvic tilt and therefore more 'jamming' of the facets in the lumbar spine.[62]

ROWING

with FIONA WILSON

The biomechanics of rowing are complex with many variables contributing to the speed of the boat. Each of the three body segments contributes approximately one third of the stroke length. The legs execute their work when the force exertion is maximal in the first half of the stroke and produce nearly half the rowing power, with the trunk producing around one third and the arms only one fifth of the power output. Thus, contrary to common belief, the legs are the greatest source of power in rowing, increasing their contribution as the stroke rate increases.[63] High forces are generated at several specific points of loading on the rower's body. Due to the cyclical movement pattern and high volume of training, these forces are repeated hundreds of times during a typical training session. It is this combination of high forces acting on the rower, large training volume and type of training that places the rower at risk of injury.

This section will focus on three of the most common regions of rowing-related pain–the lower back, chest wall and wrist/forearm.

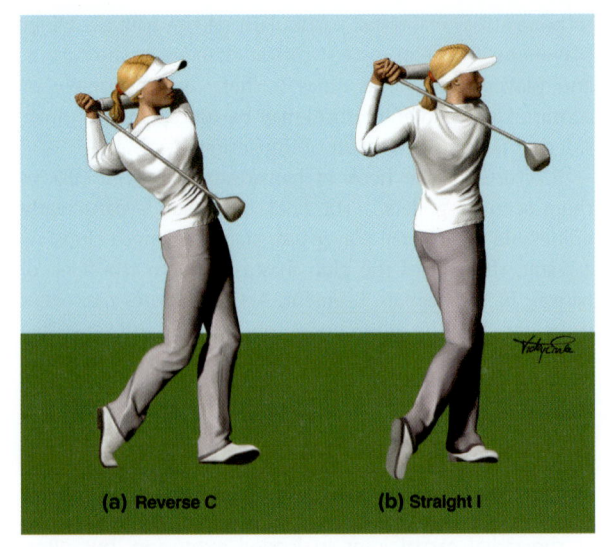

Figure 9.10 Follow-through position (a) Reverse C position increases stress on the lumbar spine, predisposing the player to spondylolysis (b) Ideal follow-through position for the lumbar spine. Note the large range of hip internal rotation in the leading hip

Low back pain

Between 32% and 50% of rowers experience rowing-related low back pain per year,[64, 65] and there are a number of biomechanical factors thought to contribute to the development of low back pain. The spine is maximally loaded at the front of the stroke–known as the 'catch' position–where the blade of the oar is placed in the water and force is applied through the trunk, arms and legs.

Biomechanical aspects of injury in specific sports — CHAPTER 9

Ideally, forward reach at the catch is achieved through maximal hip, knee and ankle flexion, with the lumbar spine in slight flexion and the pelvis in anterior rotation (Fig. 9.11a). However, inadequate lumbopelvic control or limitations in hip, knee or ankle range of motion may lead to a position of extreme lumbar flexion at the catch, with the pelvis in posterior rotation (Fig. 9.11b). In this position the intervertebral discs and posterior elements of the spine may be more vulnerable to injury.[66-68]

Good lumbopelvic control is also important in the finish position. Here, a neutral lumbar spine is ideal (Fig. 9.12a), whereas collapsing into lumbar flexion increases stress on the spine (Fig. 9.12b). Some rowers may also have inadequate posterior rotation of the pelvis, leading to hyperextension of the lumbar spine in the finish position.

Rowing technique deteriorates during continuous rowing leading to increased lumbar flexion and frontal plane motion, which is attributed to fatigue.[69-73] However, this could be dependent on rowing ability and experience. Novice rowers use high levels of lumbar flexion with limited pelvic rotation, deteriorating further with higher work intensities.[74] While similar changes are seen in elite rowers, these are of a much lower magnitude.[75] A number of factors have been identified as a predictor of lumbar spine injury in rowers. As with most cases of low back pain, a previous episode increases risk.[76] This is important to note at pre-season screening and those considering entry to the sport. Another factor is time spent ergometer training. Studies have shown that lumbar kinematics may be different in ergometer rowing compared to the boat, specifically that the increased lumbar flexion associated with prolonged rowing and fatigue is of greater magnitude in ergometer rowing.[72] Therefore, rowers with lower back pain should reduce their exposure to the ergometer and pay close attention to their lumbopelvic control while

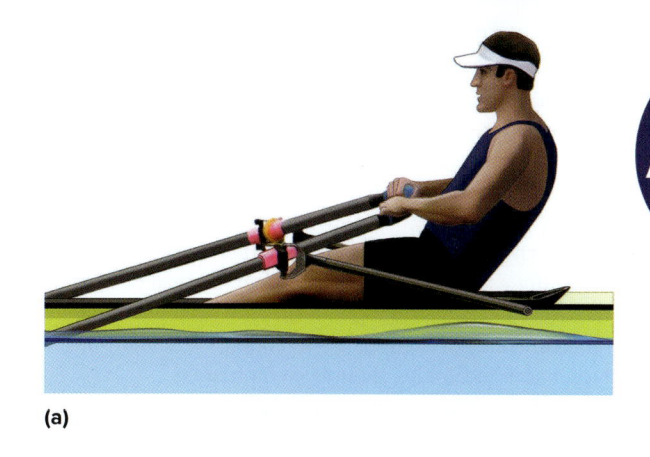

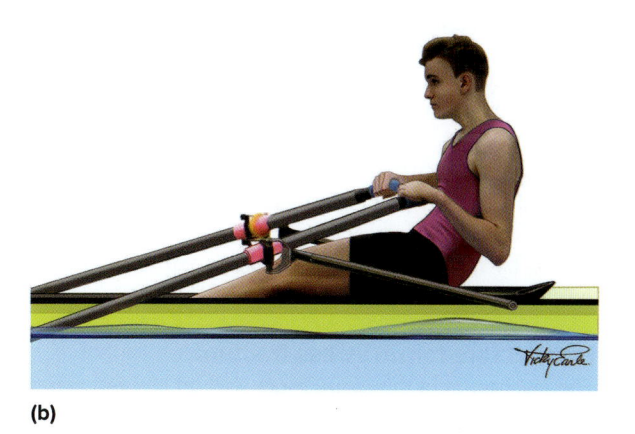

Figure 9.12 The finish position (a) Lumbar spine in a neutral position (b) Lumbar spine collapsed into flexion

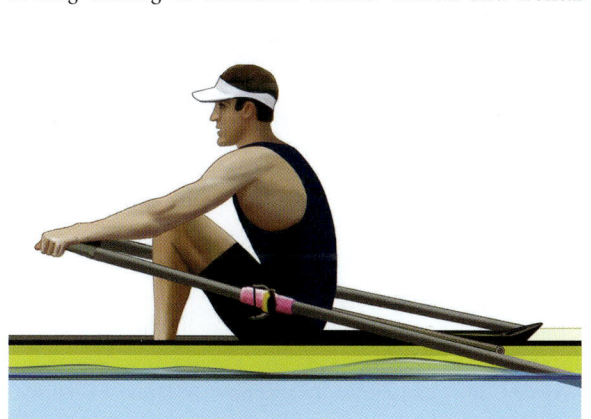

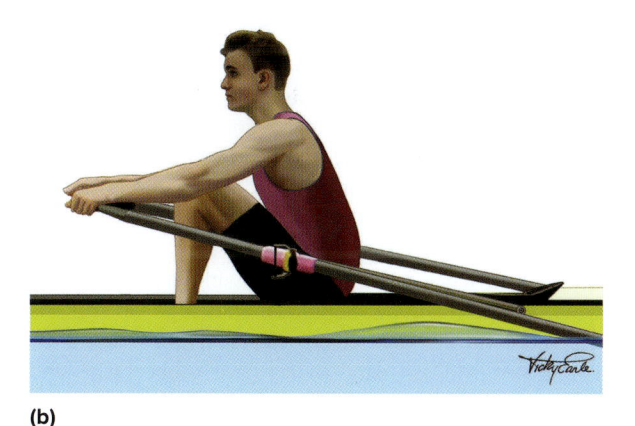

Figure 9.11 The catch position (a) Pelvis in relative anterior rotation with an even distribution of flexion throughout the spine (b) Pelvis in relative posterior rotation increases the stress on the lumbar spine

rowing, ideally using some form of biofeedback (mirror, video or electrogoniometer).

A majority of rowers with low back pain present with flexion-pattern motor control dysfunction.[77] As for other patient groups, a multi-dimensional cognitive functional approach (Chapter 28) has been shown to have the best efficacy in rowers.[78,79] However, a number of specific considerations should be applied to the rowing population. An exercise approach, which focuses on optimal position of the trunk and pelvis throughout the stroke, should underpin rehabilitation. Excellent range of motion, particularly at the hips, knees and ankles, should be emphasised.

A mistake made by many rehabilitating low back pain in rowing is poor specificity in exercise prescription, particularly overemphasis of isometric exercise in the trunk such as the 'plank' exercise. Rowing is a dynamic sport and rehabilitation exercises aimed at improving trunk endurance should allow fluid movement. The ability to hold static positions affords limited benefits.

Chest wall pain

Chest wall pain is particularly common in elite rowers,[80] but may occur in rowers of all levels. Most often it is caused by rib stress fractures (RSF), in particular in the anterolateral portion of the fourth to eighth ribs.

Risk factors for rib stress fracture

The mechanism of this injury is not well understood, but it is likely to include mechanical loading of the chest wall as well as individual intrinsic factors such as gender and bone mineral density.[81] A combination of force vectors acting on the ribs from scapula retractors, external obliques and rectus abdominis may initiate a stress response leading to RSF. Training volume (particularly a sharp load increase) and equipment issues such as blade size and type have also been implicated.[82] Thoracic hypomobility, particularly extension, is common in those sustaining RSF.

The incidence is higher in females and may be hormonally driven or may be associated with upper body strength differences from male rowers. As with any stress fractures, low energy availability is implicated in RSF pathogenesis. This may be particularly relevant in lightweight rowers. Emerging research has noted increased risk of RSF in paralympic rowing athletes.[83] This may reflect low thoracic bone mineral density in spinal-cord-injured athletes because of a reduced skeletal loading.

Clinical features

Rowers with RSF typically present with pain in the anterolateral chest wall that is initially aggravated by rowing. As the condition worsens, other activities become painful, point tenderness develops, and pain is aggravated by deep breathing, coughing, rolling over in bed and rising from supine. Examination may reveal a positive rib spring and reproduction of pain during movements mimicking the rowing stroke,[81] particularly on isometric resistance. Diagnosis is primarily from symptoms and examination and may be confirmed with a bone scan or MRI.

Management

Management is challenging and relative rest is the primary approach for 2-6 weeks. A symptom-dependent approach should be taken and the athlete should make a graduated return to training depending on pain. Many rowers report ongoing symptoms for many months (sometimes intermittently for longer) despite achieving good function. During rest, non-rowing exercise such as cycling can be maintained. Biomechanical factors such as poor thoracic extension or altered movement control should be corrected. Manual therapy of the thoracic spine can be very useful, although compression of the rib cage should be avoided. Taping for proprioceptive feedback may aid comfort. Liaison with the coach and video analysis can be very useful in identifying correctable faults such as 'over-reaching' or poor scapula control at the catch position.

The medical staff of the Great Britain rowing team have published clinical guidelines for the diagnosis and management of rib stress injuries in rowers.[84,85]

Wrist and forearm pain

Common wrist and forearm injuries in rowers include intersection syndrome (also known as 'oarsman's wrist'), de Quervain's tenosynovitis and exertional compartment syndrome (Chapters 25 and 26). All three conditions are related to excessive use of the forearm musculature, which is influenced by a variety of factors. Rowing requires the athlete to rotate the oar handle after taking it out of the water ('feathering the blade') and again prior to re-entering the water ('squaring the blade'). Ideally, the blade should be feathered and squared using a combination of wrist and metacarpophalangeal joint movement. However, a common technique fault, particularly among novice rowers, is to use wrist motion only during this action.

High grip pressure is also linked with forearm pain. This is a particular problem when rowing in poor weather conditions and among beginners, who tend to grip the oar more firmly. Oar handle size and grip should be considered. Modern oar handles have rubber grips and may be custom-fitted in different sizes; however, non-elite rowers are more likely to use older oars with wooden and 'one-size-fits-all' handles.

Sweep-oar rowers (i.e. those who row with only one oar), are more likely to suffer from intersection syndrome and de Quervain's tenosynovitis on their inside arm as that wrist is in a greater degree of ulnar deviation. Changing

Biomechanical aspects of injury in specific sports — CHAPTER 9

sides of the boat may help alleviate symptoms and allow for greater participation during rehabilitation.

Knee pain

Rowing-specific knee pain is rare. However, lateral knee pain may occur in rowers who steer coxless boats using a rotating shoe that is connected to a rudder wire. Tendinopathy of the distal biceps femoris tendon may also occur in rowers who actively use knee flexion to 'pull up the slide' rather than swing over from the hips with a stable trunk.

SWIMMING

with ELSBETH VAN DORSSEN

The clinical management of swimmers is a challenge. Swimmers begin their career earlier than many other athletes–typically between 8 and 12 years–and often train twice a day for a total of 3 to 6 hours. As elite swimmers perform a staggering 1.5 million strokes per arm every year, overuse injuries are common.

Swimming biomechanics

Swimmers use both the upper limbs and the lower limbs, but in freestyle, backstroke and butterfly the arms generate approximately 80% of the propulsion. Swimmers try to generate propulsive force while reducing the resistance to forward motion. Drag forces (friction drag, form drag and wave drag) are extremely important at all swimming speeds; when you double the speed in water, you quadruple the form drag force. Achieving a hydrodynamically efficient swimming position (long and lean body position, aligned with the direction of travel), while still being able to generate propulsive forces, requires specific strengths, flexibilities and skills. Swimmers will try to increase the length of the propulsive phase (when the arm is in the water), combined with a fast but 'relaxed' recovery phase (above the water).

Swimmers compete in four strokes: freestyle, butterfly, backstroke and breaststroke. However, irrespective of a swimmer's preferred stroke, more than 50% of their training will be spent doing freestyle.[86]

Freestyle technique

The freestyle stroke can be divided into four phases (Fig. 9.13):

1. hand entry
2. reach/glide
3. pull-through
4. recovery phase.

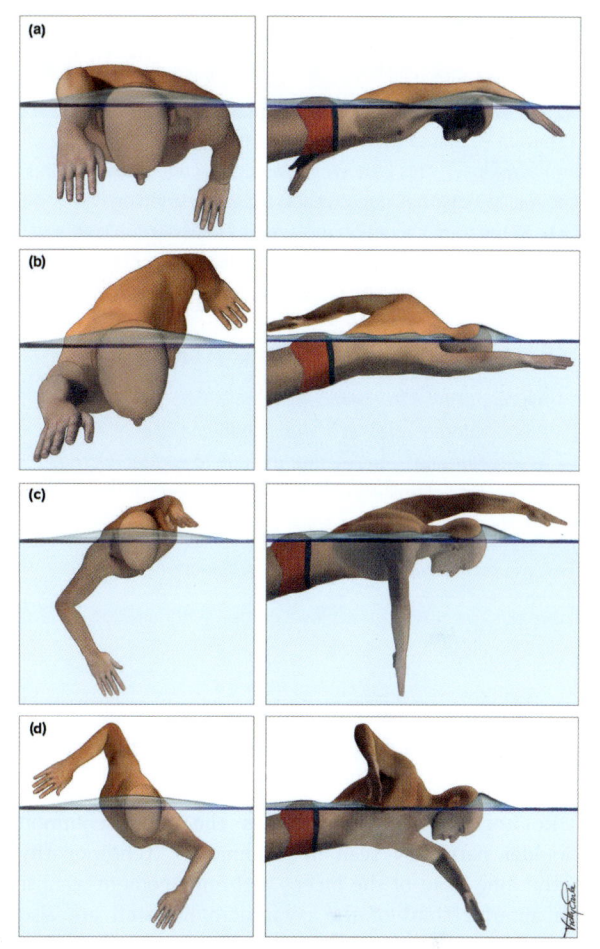

Figure 9.13 Phases of freestyle swimming (a) Hand entry (b) Reach/glide (c) Pull-through (d) Recovery

Shoulder pain

The shoulder region accounts for 31–39% of all swimming injuries.[87, 88] The prevalence of shoulder pain in elite swimmers has been found to be as high as 91%,[86] with 10–31% forced to stop training for some time during the year due to shoulder pain.[87–91]

There is a higher risk for shoulder injuries:

- after an abrupt increase of training volume or intensity[92]
- with training volume >35 km (or 15 h) per week[86]
- when a unilateral breathing pattern is used[93]
- after recent change of stroke technique; ask about any technical flaws that have been pointed out by the coach[94]
- when crossing the midline with the hand during pull-through (Fig. 9.13)
- with a history of shoulder injuries[90]
- with a recent change in coach (and therefore likely changed training loads)

PART A Fundamental principles

> ### Shoulder pain in swimmers—diagnostic labels
>
> The term 'swimmer's shoulder' was introduced by Kennedy and Hawkins.[96] This is, however, a nondescript and confusing catch-all which does not advance our understanding. We believe the term should be replaced by an individualised and more specific diagnosis, which accounts for the contributing factors (extrinsic and intrinsic) and suspected pathology of each injured swimmer.
>
> Instead we propose **Supraspinatus tendinopathy** with:
>
> - hypomobility of the cervicothoracic junction
> - loss of internal rotation of the glenohumeral joint
> - greater internal rotation strength due to sudden increase of intensity of training and possible overload in the use of hand paddles and drag suits.
>
> This will promote a patient-specific, problem-oriented approach to treatment.

93° of external rotation had a greater risk of shoulder impingement symptoms.[90] Internal rotation is the most important, as it allows the swimmer to have an early catch and high elbow. A measure between 40–50° seems to be necessary for freestyle, backstroke and butterfly. Breaststroke swimmers can have a little less.

Testing abduction with internal rotation gives important information about the swimmer's ability to achieve and maintain a high elbow. The swimmer sits on a bench, both arms are passively abducted, with the elbows maintained in 90° flexion (Fig. 9.14). The forearm must be perpendicular to the plane of abduction (causing internal rotation). The angle measured is the line of the humerus to the straight spine. An appropriate range for this measure is between 150° and 170°.[97]

The combined elevation test can give more information about the ability to achieve a high elbow position at the start of the stroke, recovery and streamline. The athlete lies in a prone position with both arms (with locked thumbs together and extended elbows) elevated above the head. The swimmer then elevates the arms as high as

- after increased use of hand paddles[89, 95]
- with the use of drag-increasing training devices (bags, elastic cords, drag suits, etc.).

Rotator cuff tendinopathy is the most common shoulder pathology seen in swimmers.[86] Tendinopathy of the long head of the biceps and impingement against the anterior third of the coracoacromial arch are also frequent diagnoses. However, a clear pathoanatomical diagnosis is often difficult to achieve; it is more important to diagnose and understand the underlying functional or pathomechanical reasons for the 'structural failure' and address these in the management plan.

A thorough clinical examination of the entire kinetic chain is important to assess the intrinsic contributing factors. Swimmers must be capable of extreme ranges of motion, especially in the shoulder girdle,[93] and they must be able to reach these positions easily. Mechanical cost to achieve this position will result in (i) unnecessary extra movements and drag, and (ii) suboptimal use and possible overload of musculoskeletal structures. Modelling studies suggest that, on average, the supraspinatus tendon is already in a position of potential mechanical impingement for nearly 25% of the freestyle arm stroke cycle.[93]

If swimmers are not flexible enough in the glenohumeral joint, they tend to pass this motion requirement to the scapulothoracic joint or the spine. On the other hand, hypermobility can also increase the potential for injury due to excessive translation of the humeral head. There might be a range of 'optimal motion' in swimmers. One study found that those with more than 100° or less than

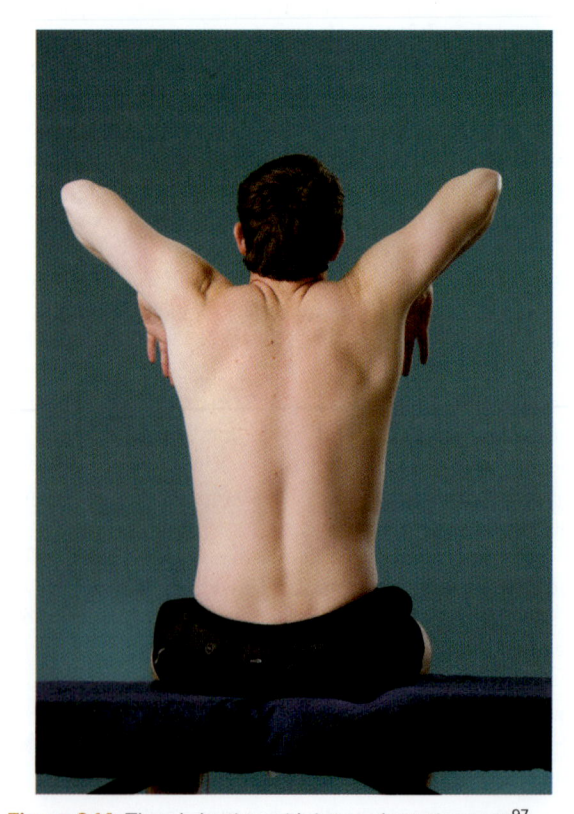

Figure 9.14 The abduction with internal rotation test.[97] The elbows should be kept in 90° flexion, and the upper arms should be prevented from moving forward as the shoulders are elevated. Swimmers should aim for 150–170° of abduction.

Biomechanical aspects of injury in specific sports **CHAPTER 9**

possible while keeping the head, chest and legs in contact with the bench (Fig. 9.15). An angle between the line of the humerus and the horizontal axis of between 5° and 15° is appropriate.[97]

To maintain a streamlined position, core stability is important. Swimmers need to transfer load efficiently between the arms and the legs under internally generated flexion torques.

Management of shoulder pain in swimmers

Individualised rehabilitation programs emphasising range of motion, flexibility, muscle balance, and motor control of the glenohumeral and scapulothoracic joints are the key features in the management of shoulder pain in swimmers (Chapter 24).[98] Modification of training load is often necessary.

Most commonly, the entire kinetic chain is involved, with multiple intrinsic and extrinsic contributing factors such as:

- reduced rotation and/or extension of the thoracic spine–important in relation to body roll
- tightness or improper motor control around the scapula
- muscular imbalance around the shoulder, in particular, internal and external rotators
- incorrect swimming technique (Table 9.2)
- too much training with hand paddles or drag-increasing devices
- improper land training, weight training or stretching
- suboptimal core strength and/or control.

A team approach: technical stroke analysis and adjustment with the coach, physiotherapist, doctor and sports scientists, keeping the clinical findings in mind.

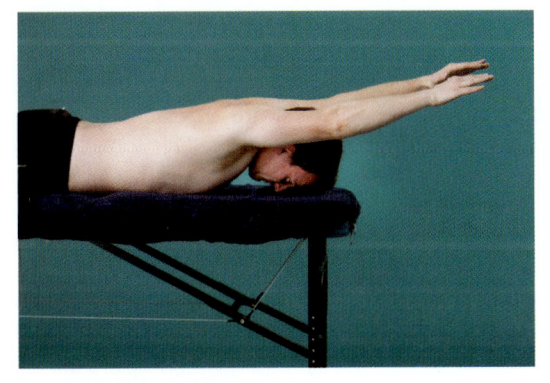

Figure 9.15 The combined elevation test—a test for thoracic extension, shoulder elevation and scapular retraction.[97] The swimmer lies in a prone position and is asked to lock their thumbs together, extend their elbows and elevate the arms as high as they can while keeping their head, chest and legs in contact with the bench. The humerus angle is measured relative to horizontal

Table 9.2 Technique factors related to shoulder pain in freestyle swimming

Presentation	Possible cause	Solution
Shoulder pain at hand entry	Thumb-first hand entry—excessive internal rotation in full elevation	• Palm-down hand entry • Ensure adequate abduction/internal rotation range of motion
	Crossing the midline with the hand at hand entry	• Avoid crossing the midline
	Lateral deviation of the trunk	• Improve mobility in the kinetic chain, improve core stability
	Insufficient upward rotation of the scapula	• Address scapulohumeral muscle flexibility • Train scapular upward rotation in overhead exercises
Shoulder pain during pull-through	Dropped elbow—elbow-first water entry or elbow below the level of shoulder and wrist during early pull-through	• Improve internal rotation ROM—sleeper's, stretch and cross-body stretch—check kinetic chain
	Crossing the midline with the hand during pull-through	• Avoid crossing the midline
	Insufficient or excessive body roll	• Body roll should be approximately 45°; this can be limited by thoracic rotation and core stability
Shoulder pain during recovery	Excessive horizontal abduction due to insufficient body roll—posterior cuff impingement	• Increase body roll • Optimise mobility of cervicothoracic spine
	Unilateral breathing pattern (pain on same side)	• Strive for a bilateral breathing pattern

135

PART A Fundamental principles

Swimmers with shoulder complaints should avoid the following drills:

- long leg drills with a kick board, as arms are maintained in maximum shoulder flexion; this can aggravate impingement symptoms
- hand paddles, as these increase the load on the shoulder during the pull-through
- pull buoy; the legs are held together without kicking, so 100% of the propulsion is generated by the arms.

Medial knee pain

Medial knee pain is common in breaststroke swimmers.[99] In one study, 75% of the surveyed breaststroke swimmers reported at least three episodes of knee pain per season and 47% of these swimmers reported weekly episodes of knee pain.[100]

Although the term 'breaststroker's knee' is nonspecific, it usually refers to overuse injury of the medial collateral ligament. However, the medial patellofemoral joint, pes anserine tendon, or bursa and adductor muscles may also be involved.[101]

The medial knee is highly loaded at the beginning of the breaststroke thrust phase, where the knee is flexed and externally rotated and the hips are flexed and internally rotated. The knee undergoes valgus loading throughout the leg thrust. A number of intrinsic factors and technique flaws can increase the valgus load and contribute to medial knee pain:

- valgus alignment of the lower limb
- inadequate or asymmetrical hip internal rotation or tibial external rotation
- large abduction angle of the hips during the kick (>30°)
- ineffective arm–leg coordination may increase loads on the lower limb
- sudden increase in amount or intensity of training
- hip extension and ability to achieve core and pelvic stability.

Clinical assessment of the lower back, hips, knees, and ankles is important, particularly the range of hip internal rotation and tibial external rotation. These two measures should add up to approximately 90°, so that at the beginning of the thrust phase the feet are square to the line of progression. This results in the biggest area to use to propel in the kick with the knees closer together, thus reducing form drag.[97]

As for shoulder injuries, the clinician should focus on both intrinsic and extrinsic factors during the rehabilitation process. Breaststroke training should be reduced, and exercises which place a valgus load on the knee should be avoided during land and weight training. Hip rotation range of motion should be optimised and the load capacity of the knee should be increased through progressive lower limb strengthening.

TENNIS

with BABETTE PLUIM

In a typical hour of tennis, players hit the ball between 150 and 250 times and run between 2.5 and 3.5 km in high-intensity 3-metre bursts. Due to the game's explosive, intermittent and repetitive nature, both acute and overuse injuries are common. Groups particularly at risk include elite players, who often train up to 5–6 hours per day, deconditioned players who suddenly increase their training loads and young players who play more than four matches per week.[102]

The main biomechanics-related tennis injuries are lateral elbow pain ('tennis elbow') and overuse shoulder injuries. These represent approximately 15–25% of all tennis injuries.[103]

Lateral elbow pain

Lateral elbow tendinopathy is colloquially referred to as 'tennis elbow' as it has been estimated to affect up to 50% of active tennis players at some point throughout their career.[104, 105] The prevalence among tennis players seems to be declining, which may be related to increasing use of the two-handed backhand across all levels of tennis. The condition is caused by a tendinopathy of the common extensor tendon, in particular the extensor carpi radialis brevis, at the insertion on the lateral humeral epicondyle. Here, forces are greatest during one-handed backhand shots, as the wrist extensors contract eccentrically on impact with the ball.

Lateral elbow pain is much more common in beginners and players over 40 years of age,[106] and is usually attributed to a combination of overuse and poor stroke biomechanics. Skilled players hit the ball with an extended wrist and extend the hand through impact (Fig. 9.16a), whereas novice players often hit the backhand with a flexed wrist, resulting in an eccentric contraction and less strength at impact (Fig. 9.16b).[107, 108] However, the relationship between this technique flaw and elbow injury remains unclear,[109] and other potential factors include hitting the ball off-centre and squeezing the grip too tightly during follow-through.[110] The topspin backhand usually provokes more complaints than the slice backhand.[111]

> **PRACTICE PEARL**
>
> Tennis elbow is very rare in players with a two-handed backhand.

Biomechanical aspects of injury in specific sports

CHAPTER 9

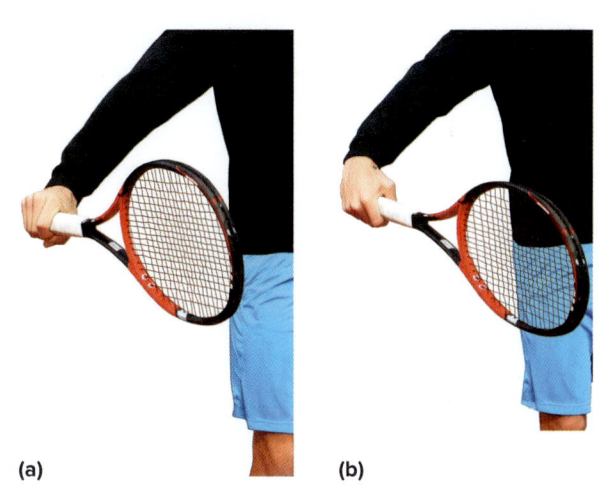

Figure 9.16 One-handed backhand technique (a) An extended wrist at impact reduces stress at the lateral epicondyle (b) A flexed wrist at impact increases stress at the lateral epicondyle

Tennis racquet grip size is traditionally considered to be a risk factor for lateral elbow pain, as grip sizes that are too small or too large may lead to extra strain on the forearm muscles. It is therefore important to optimise the racquet grip size to the player.[112] Other common recommendations to reduce load on the forearm muscles include using a larger racquet head, a flexible racquet, lower string tension (with high quality strings) and pressurised tennis balls. Playing with heavy, wet tennis balls, long hours of play, or a sudden increase in volume or intensity of play may lead to sudden overuse and the development of lateral elbow problems.

The general management principles for lateral elbow tendinopathy are detailed in Chapter 25. However, tennis-specific management should include developing muscular strength to better cope with the racquet-ball impact, and an analysis of backhand technique, with effort focused on using the right grip and achieving concentric wrist extension at the point of impact. Slow-motion video analysis may be a useful biofeedback tool to help players change technique. Low compression balls should also be considered during the early phase of treatment.

Shoulder injuries

The shoulder is subjected to high loads in tennis, particularly during the serve where the shoulder is abducted to 140–160° and rotates 160–180° at a rate of up to 2400° per second.[113] As a player serves approximately 100 times in an average match,[114] overuse shoulder injuries are common. Both the causes and the pathology of shoulder injuries in tennis are similar to other overhead and throwing sports (Chapter 8); common diagnoses include internal impingement, rotator cuff and biceps tendinopathy and glenoid labrum injuries.[115, 116]

During the cocking phase of the serve, the supraspinatus, infraspinatus and serratus anterior all contract concentrically to stabilise the scapula and glenohumeral joint. This is followed by a rapid eccentric contraction of the rotator cuff and serratus anterior to decelerate the arm during the follow-through. These repetitive concentric and eccentric demands, which occur during both serving and groundstrokes, may lead to muscular fatigue and so-called 'eccentric failure' of the tendons. Adding further stress, the supraspinatus and infraspinatus tendons can become compressed between the humeral head and the posterosuperior rim of the glenoid during the cocking phase of the serve, when the glenohumeral joint is in maximal external rotation and horizontal abduction. This is often referred to as *internal impingement*.

Local factors that contribute to internal impingement include muscular imbalances (external rotator weakness or dysfunction compared to the internal rotators), weakness or dysfunction of the scapular stabilisers (scapular dyskinesis) and tightness of the posterior capsule resulting in reduced internal rotation range of motion (GIRD). These factors should all be considered when treating shoulder injuries in tennis (Chapter 24).

Remote factors also play an important role in the development of shoulder injuries in tennis. To generate power during the serve, there should be coordinated activation of a number of body segments (legs, hips, trunk, shoulder, arm and hand)–the so-called 'kinetic chain'–to achieve a high racquet speed at impact.[117] Suboptimal kinetic chain mechanics may overload the upper limb as it tries to make up for lost energy production.[118] This is referred to as the 'catch-up phenomenon'.[116]

Common clues that point to poor kinetic chain mechanics during serving (Fig. 9.17) include:[119]

- insufficient knee bend–the front knee should flex more than 15° during the loading phase
- inadequate rotation–the player should be coiled enough that they show their back to the opponent
- inadequate shoulder and pelvis tilt during the loading phase.

PART A   Fundamental principles

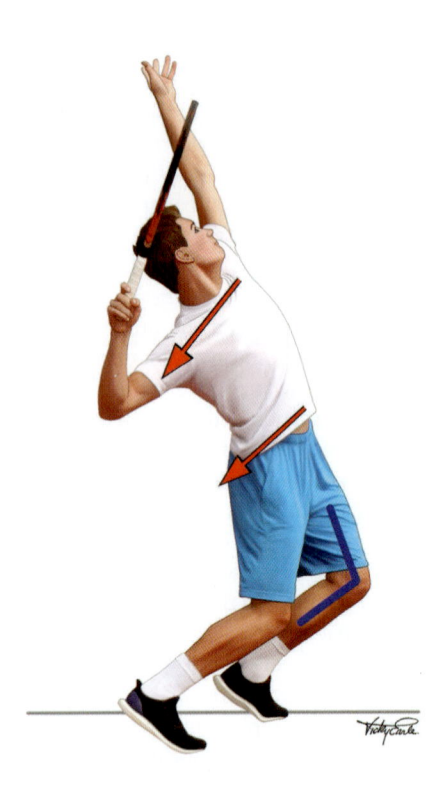

Figure 9.17 Tennis serve technique—loading phase. Look for a deep knee bend, rotated trunk, and tilted shoulders and pelvis

REFERENCES

References for this chapter can be found at www.mhhe.com/au/CSM5e

Chapter 10

Training programming and prescription

with DARREN BURGESS

In football as in watchmaking, talent and elegance mean nothing without rigour and precision.
Lionel Messi

The sports medicine clinician should understand the different elements of training and their possible relationship to injury. This facilitates the practitioner's obtaining a full training history from an injured athlete, learning about training strategy from a coach or fitness practitioner and enhances a clinician's understanding of the phases of rehabilitation outlined in Chapter 18. This chapter reviews the principles of training and outlines some more common training programming and assessment practices. The reader is directed to other sources for more detailed outlines of the various types of training.

PRINCIPLES OF TRAINING

'Training' is the pursuit of activity that will ultimately lead to an improved performance in a given sport. A number of general principles of training apply to all sports:

- periodisation
- overload
- specificity
- individuality.

Periodisation

Periodisation is an important component of all training programs, in both the long and short term. Training can be divided into three distinct phases: conditioning (preparation), pre-competition (transitional) and competition.

Generally, the conditioning phase emphasises developing aerobic and anaerobic fitness, strength and power. Often during this period, the athlete is training under fatigue and if required to compete would probably perform poorly. During the pre-competition phase of training, the emphasis switches from pure conditioning to more technical work. During the competition phase, the emphasis is on competitive performance while maintaining basic conditioning (Table 10.1).

In many sports (e.g. football, basketball, hockey), a 4–6-month competition season is usual. In some instances, an athlete is required to undertake two periods of competition in the one year. A suggested program for athletes in these two situations is outlined in Figure 10.1. In other instances, the competition period may last as long as 8–10 months and conditioning work can extend into the competitive season. However, in all of these scenarios the same principles of training periodisation apply.

To ensure complete recovery from the physical and mental stress of competition, adequate time should be allowed between the end of one season or competition phase and the start of the next season or phase. This period may last 4–6 weeks but is dependent on when the next competition begins.

In the intermediate time frame, it is important to introduce easy weeks into the training program; these give the athlete time to recover (Chapter 13) and diminish

Table 10.1 Different types of training are performed during the three phases of the yearly cycle

Training phase	Aerobic training	Anaerobic training	Plyometrics training	Weight training	Technique training
Preparation/conditioning	+++	++	++	+++	+
Transitional/pre-competition	++	+++	++	++	+++
Competition	+	+	–	+	++

PART A   Fundamental principles

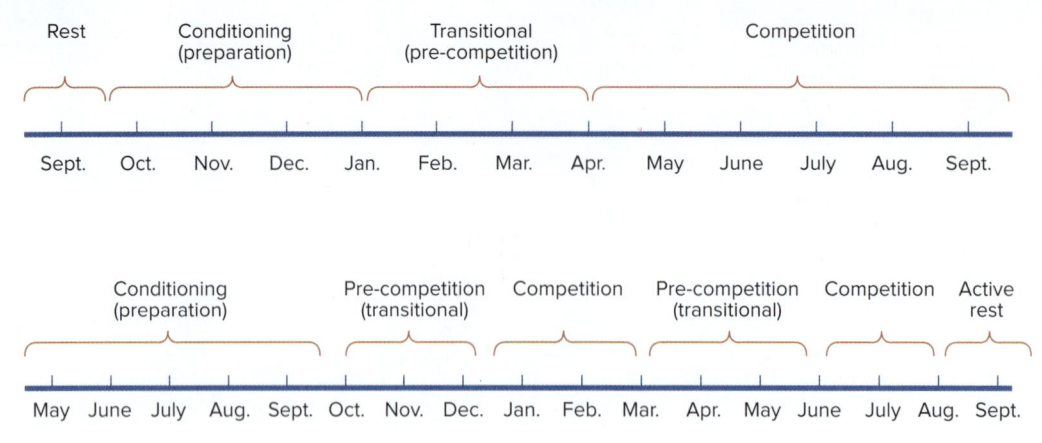

Figure 10.1 Periodisation of training showing a single cycle annual program (above) and a dual cycle annual program (below)

risk of injury. During these easy weeks, the volume of training is typically reduced; however, intensity should be maintained to prevent detraining.[1]

In the short term, the training program must allow for adequate recovery between training sessions. This ensures the athlete is able to train at appropriate intensities throughout the week and reduces the risk of injury.[1]

Overload

Overload is a variable that coaches manipulate to allow the athlete to perform work at a greater intensity or to perform a greater volume of work at a given intensity. Practically speaking, overloading an athlete involves applying stress to the body over and above that which is normally, or has been recently, encountered. If increased stress is not excessive and adequate adaptation time is allowed, the work capacity of the athlete will be increased ('supercompensation'). Athletes should be carefully monitored during periods of overload to prevent injury, overtraining and even poor performance from occurring.

Specificity

Specificity refers to the principle of directing training to performance in the athlete's given sport. It is important, therefore, to identify the most important components of fitness for each particular sport and to tailor the athlete's training toward improving these particular components. For example, there is no advantage for a strictly power athlete in doing large amounts of endurance training.

Specificity can refer to both training the specific fitness demands of a sport as well as training the direct movement patterns of the sport to improve the fitness of the athlete. Those choosing the latter method argue that specific training in this way has the advantage of training skills and decision making while improving fitness.[2] Most field sports (e.g. football) require a complex combination of both strength and endurance training and therefore specificity should include a combination of specific fitness training as well as training the specific movements of a sport.

Individualisation

As individual differences between athletes are great, training must be tailored to the individual's needs. Individuals differ in their tolerance of particular training loads, response to specific training stimuli, speed of recovery, psychological make-up, nutritional intake and lifestyle habits. Individual responses to training are influenced by previous training history, age, current state of fitness, genetic make-up and so on. Even in a team setting, it is vital that players are treated as individuals and trained accordingly.

The Central Governor Model (CGM) for the limits of performance and its relevance to interval training

The concept of maximum oxygen consumption (VO$_2$max) and lactic acidosis limiting athletic performance has undergone much critical evaluation. The 'classical' model of Hill,[3] which still enjoys support among a substantial number of exercise physiologists, suggests that:

- Progressive muscle hypoxia limits maximal exercise performance. As a result, the main determinant of exercise performance is the heart's ability to supply sufficient blood (and oxygen) to the exercising muscles.

Training programming and prescription — CHAPTER 10

- Anaerobiosis (lack of muscle oxygen) secondary to the inability further to increase the cardiac output (producing a 'plateau' in cardiac output) explains the onset of lactate production by skeletal muscle at the 'anaerobic threshold'.
- Mitochondrial adaptation in the exercising muscles, associated with an increased ability of the heart to pump a larger cardiac output, are the exclusive biological changes that explain changes in performance with endurance training.

This model has been challenged by the contemporary, but certainly not universally accepted, model of Professor Timothy Noakes. Noakes' data refute the classical model. Instead, he proposes that skeletal muscle recruitment and contractile function are regulated by a hierarchy of controls (conceptually 'the central governor') specifically to prevent damage to any number of different organs.[4–14] He, and subsequently others, argues that according to the Hill model in which a plateau in cardiac output precedes the development of skeletal muscle anaerobiosis and lactic acidosis, the first organ to be threatened by the plateau in cardiac output would be the heart, not skeletal muscle. The plateau in cardiac output would prevent any further increase in blood flow to the heart, leading to myocardial ischaemia, the onset of chest pain (angina pectoris) and heart failure.

He also provides evidence that this was, in fact, the belief of the early exercise physiologists, including Hill in England and Dill at the Harvard Fatigue Laboratory in the United States and was a central component of their teachings. Since Hill understood that the heart could not survive a prolonged period of ischaemia, he conceived the presence of a 'governor' in either the heart or the brain that would reduce heart function and spare the heart by causing a 'slowing of the circulation' as soon as myocardial ischaemia developed. Noakes and colleagues have extended this interpretation to suggest that the governor exists in the central nervous system, hence it is called the central governor and that it responds to multiple sensory inputs from all the organs in the body (Fig. 10.2). In response to those inputs, the central governor regulates the number of motor units that can be recruited in the exercising limbs on a moment-to-moment basis, reducing or limiting the number that can be recruited when their continued recruitment, necessary to maintain the work output or exercise intensity, threatens whole-body homeostasis.

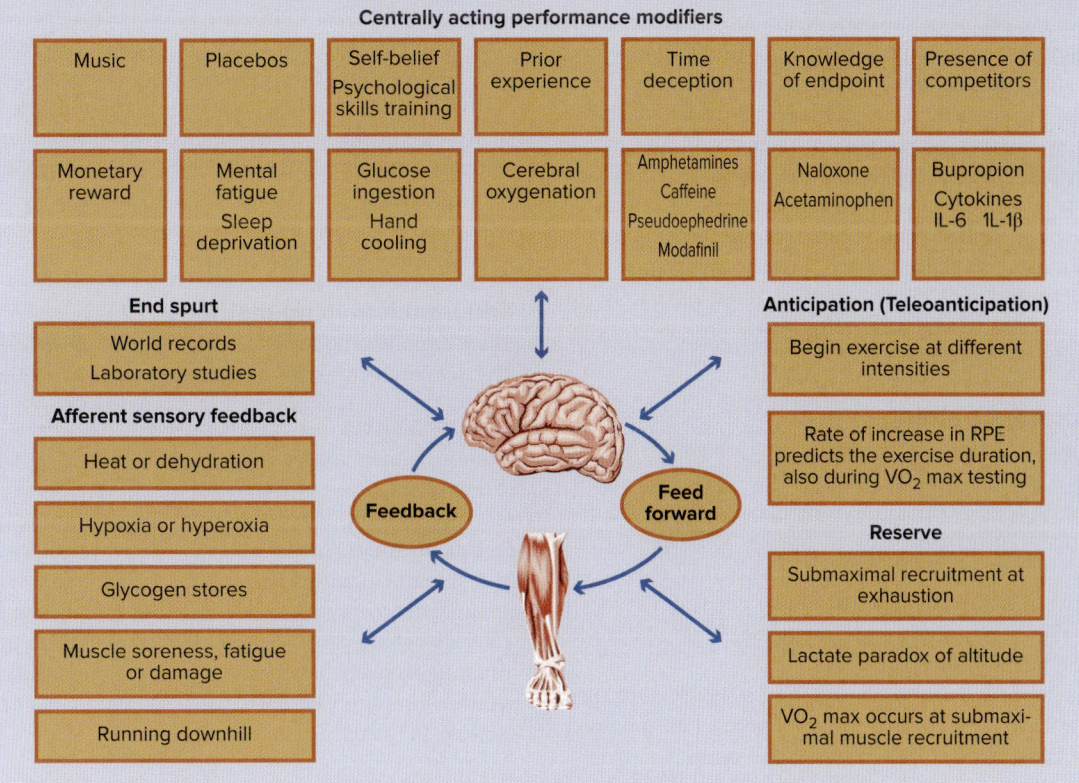

Centrally acting performance modifiers

| Music | Placebos | Self-belief / Psychological skills training | Prior experience | Time deception | Knowledge of endpoint | Presence of competitors |
| Monetary reward | Mental fatigue / Sleep deprivation | Glucose ingestion / Hand cooling | Cerebral oxygenation | Amphetamines / Caffeine / Pseudoephedrine / Modafinil | Naloxone / Acetaminophen | Bupropion / Cytokines / IL-6 1L-1β |

End spurt
- World records
- Laboratory studies

Afferent sensory feedback
- Heat or dehydration
- Hypoxia or hyperoxia
- Glycogen stores
- Muscle soreness, fatigue or damage
- Running downhill

Feedback — Feed forward

Anticipation (Teleoanticipation)
- Begin exercise at different intensities
- Rate of increase in RPE predicts the exercise duration, also during VO_2 max testing

Reserve
- Submaximal recruitment at exhaustion
- Lactate paradox of altitude
- VO_2 max occurs at submaximal muscle recruitment

Figure 10.2 The central governor responds to multiple sensory inputs from all organs of the body

continued

PART A Fundamental principles

> Hence, Noakes writes that 'during maximal exercise, progressive myocardial ischaemia preceding skeletal muscle anaerobiosis must be thwarted, so that neither the heart nor the skeletal muscle develop irreversible rigour and necrosis with fatal consequences'. The reader is directed to the publications that summarise this argument to date.[4, 7–14]
>
> ### Relevance to interval training
> Irrespective of the theoretical background that underpins the physiology, the most efficient method of increasing anaerobic fitness is a form of intermittent exercise or interval training. Interval training involves a number of bouts of exercise separated by periods of rest or recovery.
>
> The principle of such training is to achieve a level of lactic acidosis with one individual effort and then allow the body to recover from its effects before embarking on another bout of exercise. There is scope for enormous variation in the intensity and duration of the exercise bouts and the duration of the recovery period. Anaerobic training will also reset the central governor mechanism, perhaps teaching the governor that it can allow a slightly higher exercise intensity without risking a catastrophic bodily failure. In addition, interval training will also increase the ability of the skeletal muscle fibres to produce more force. There is some evidence suggesting that differences in skeletal muscle contractility may modify athletic performance by determining the shortest possible duration the foot is in contact with the ground. This is because faster running requires shorter foot contact times and hence greater skeletal muscle contractility and the recruitment of a greater number of muscle fibres.[15] In contrast, skeletal muscle contractility may be impaired in certain disease states.[16]

CONDITIONING TRAINING

The maintenance of fitness is not only crucial to sporting success and injury prevention it is also an essential component of the rehabilitation process. Regardless of the injury the athlete has sustained, exercises to maintain fitness should be incorporated as soon as possible. For example, with injuries to the lower limb, cardiovascular fitness may be maintained by performing activities such as swimming with a pool buoy or arm 'grinder' work. Depending on the athlete's particular sport, this may include a combination of endurance, interval, anaerobic and power work. It is important to maintain alternative training methods for cardiovascular fitness, to encourage motivation and compliance with general fitness goals.

We have divided conditioning into five separate types of training–endurance, speed, agility, resistance and flexibility–and will discuss each of these separately. In practice these methods are often combined for a more global conditioning effect.

Endurance training

Technically, endurance training aims to increase oxygen delivery to the working muscles and thereby increase aerobic capacity. Adaptations to endurance training include an increase in maximal oxygen uptake (VO_2max) and an increased ability of skeletal muscle to generate energy via oxidative metabolism.[17, 18] (For a more detailed discussion of the debate on VO_2max and the role of lactic acidosis in limiting training, see box below).

The long-term consequences of prolonged endurance training have been debated in recent years, with proposed cardiovascular risks associated with cardiac fatigue.[19, 20] However, a study of young Olympic athletes subjected to extreme uninterrupted endurance training over prolonged periods (up to 17 years) found that endurance training was not associated with significant changes in left ventricular morphology, deterioration in left ventricular function, or occurrence of cardiovascular symptoms or events.[21] Endurance sports include long-distance running (greater than 5 km), cross-country skiing, cycling, rowing and triathlon.

It is important here to be aware of the many benefits an increased aerobic capacity can have to a range of different sports. An enhanced aerobic capacity will not only improve the efficiency of oxygen delivery but will also improve the regeneration of anaerobic energy pathways. This means performance in intermittent sports such as ice hockey, soccer, American football and netball, all traditionally thought of as strictly anaerobic sports, will be improved with an enhanced aerobic capacity. This is important to remember when prescribing or reviewing rehabilitation programs for these sports.

Endurance training methods
There are numerous methods to train endurance capacity. This section focuses on the more popular techniques.

Interval training
Interval training involves numerous bouts of high intensity efforts of set times or distances. Both effort duration and recovery time in between efforts dictate the intensity of each bout. An endurance interval session might be 6 sets of 1 minute running efforts. For a high-intensity session, 2 minutes recovery could be prescribed in between efforts. To challenge the aerobic capacity to recover more quickly, 1 minute recovery between sets could be prescribed. These repeat-effort intervals have been shown to dramatically increase VO_2max.[22]

Fartlek training
'Fartlek', which means 'speed play' in Swedish, is a popular form of endurance training that involves high-intensity efforts

interspersed between constant paced exercise. A typical fartlek session on a bike might involve 30 seconds of high-intensity cycling every 2.5 minutes for 30 minutes. This example would provide the cyclist with 10 high-intensity efforts during a 30-minute ride. In some sports, athletes may be unaware of the duration and intensity of efforts and have to respond to the coach's feedback during the session.

Maximal aerobic speed (MAS) training
MAS training involves calculating an athlete's maximal aerobic speed and then prescribing a certain percentage of this within an interval training session.[23] Typically, the speed an athlete can complete a 2 km (or similar distance) time trial is used as that athlete's MAS. Precise distances and expected times can then be calculated for each athlete. The most common time periods for MAS are 15 seconds of work followed by 15 seconds of exercise (15:15).

Cross-training
To prevent injury, it may be beneficial to reduce the amount of weight-bearing exercise. Cross-training enables the athlete to maintain aerobic fitness while reducing stress on weight-bearing joints, muscles and tendons. In athletes with a chronic condition such as articular cartilage damage to a weight-bearing joint, cross-training may be used to reduce the impact load while maintaining adequate training volume. Similarly, in a patient returning to sport from an overuse injury (such as a stress fracture), cross-training can reduce the risk of recurrence. Runners may wish to introduce one to two sessions per week of activities such as cycling, swimming or water running. These alternative work-outs can mirror the athlete's usual training session (e.g. interval, fartlek).

Skill training as endurance
It is important to realise that a skill drill or indeed entire skill session can enhance endurance capacity. In particular, there are numerous ways to alter skill drills to emphasise endurance, while maintaining the important aspects of the skill (e.g. decision making, team combinations, specific skill execution). For example, a simple soccer game could be altered in any of the following ways to increase the aerobic requirements of the exercise:

- Increase the size of the field.
- Decrease the playing numbers.
- For a goal to be scored all players must be over the half-way line.
- Every 1 minute the coach blows a whistle and one player from each team must run to a specified marker outside of the field.

Speed training
Running speed, which is an important component of many sports, is a largely inherited ability. However, athletes can improve their speed by enhancing muscular power and strength, as well as by improving technique, which increases the efficiency of ground coverage. Therefore, running speed can be increased by undertaking resistance and power training as well as by performing technical running drills.

Speed training methods
There is much debate about how much speed can be developed or improved in the mature athlete. Speed can arguably be enhanced, or at the very least maintained, with an appropriate strength and power program– this will be discussed later in this chapter. However, debate remains about the extent to which speed can be improved through either technical modification or repeated exposure to a speed stimulus. Both of these will be discussed briefly below.

Technique training
Improving the technical aspect of speed requires significant time spent analysing athlete running mechanics and then performing extensive corrective exercises as required. Within most sports, time spent dedicated specifically to technical speed work might often be at the expense of other conditioning, strength training or even skill training. As a result, most speed technique work is often confined to small amounts of time with large groups of players and/or warm-up activities pre-training/strength sessions. This requires a fairly broad approach where emphasis is placed on high knee drive, exaggerated heel lift and horizontal foot position throughout the sprint motion. An ideal opportunity exists to improve speed technique during the rehabilitation process where a more individualised approach can be taken. Of course, in sports such as running and long jump, a large percentage of training time should be devoted to technical speed drills.

Speed intervals
Appropriate exposure to speed will not only maintain speed qualities but may also prevent soft tissue injury,[23] particularly in the hamstrings. These 'unpractised' movements that occur in games often cause muscle injury.

> **PRACTICE PEARL**
>
> Regular speed interval work, particularly during weekly competition cycles will ensure the muscles and tendons are not 'shocked' into unfamiliar explosive movements that may occur during games.

Practitioners should remember that absolute speed intervals should be performed while the athlete is fresh; however, speed exposure in training should also occur under fatigue to prepare the body to what it may encounter during competition.

143

PART A   Fundamental principles

Skill training as speed
In most sports, speed training can and should be integrated into skill training. This can be easily achieved by using execution of simple skills at the end of sprinting activities. Care should be taken in programming these drills as they can be quite physically and structurally demanding.

Agility training
Agility can be defined as the ability to alter direction to achieve a specific goal (e.g. evade/deceive/react to an opponent, create space). Agility and rapid reflexes are often inherited characteristics. However, like speed, they can be improved somewhat by training and, thus, are included in training programs of all sports. Agility training has also been implemented in seniors to prevent falls.[25]

Agility training methods
Agility is often incorrectly trained using stationary objects (e.g. cones, poles, ladders). This may allow the coach to teach the athlete the correct foot placement or stride mechanics; however, agility training requires a reaction and therefore a decision-making component.[26]

Technique training
Training agility technique may be appropriate in the initial stages of rehabilitation or perhaps within adolescent programs. The coach can spend some time on effective techniques to approach a known object. However, this type of training should be limited as it often leads to inappropriate habits such as a player keeping their head down to review foot placement.

Agility drills
A reaction component should always be included in agility drills. This can be reacting to a coach movement, coach command, opponent or teammate. Advanced agility drills should also include a decision-making element.

Skill training as agility
Most sports skill training could be counted as agility training. This is because the majority of field sports training involves reacting to opponents, the ball or teammates. This means any additional agility-specific training should be programmed carefully as repeated changes of direction could cause some overload issues to the pelvic region.

Resistance training
Resistance training can be used to enhance athletic performance, improve musculoskeletal health and correct muscle imbalances.[27] Resistance training is often used in rehabilitation when weakness compromises function and sports performance. This is particularly true following periods of immobilisation or injury and in pain presentations.

The primary goals of resistance training are normally to increase muscle size (hypertrophy), strength or power. Increases in muscle hypertrophy and strength are dependent on five biochemical and physiological factors that are all stimulated and enhanced by appropriate resistance training:

- increased glycogen and protein storage in muscle
- increased vascularisation
- biochemical changes affecting the enzymes of energy metabolism
- increased number of myofibrils
- recruitment of neighbouring motor units.

It is important that the athlete is provided with the correct environment in which to perform resistance training. The following factors will help maximise gains during resistance training:

- adequate warm-up to increase body temperature and metabolic efficiency
- good quality, controlled performance of the exercise
- pain-free performance of exercise
- use of slow, controlled exercise initially, with little or no resistance, to develop a good base for neural patterning to occur
- comprehensive stretching program to restore/maintain full range of motion
- muscle strengthening throughout the entire available range of motion.

Additionally, there is a training crossover effect— when one limb is trained, strength gains will also be recorded in the contralateral limb.[27, 28] This phenomenon is termed 'central adaptation' and reflects the important role the central nervous system plays in motor unit firing, as well as the bracing role the contralateral limb plays in most single-limb exercises.

Types of resistance exercises
The three main types of exercise used in resistance training are:

- isometric
- isotonic
- isokinetic.

Isometric exercise
An isometric exercise occurs when a muscle contracts without associated movement of the joint on which the muscle acts. Isometric exercises are often the first form of strengthening exercise used after injury, especially if the region is excessively painful or if the area is immobilised. These exercises are commenced as soon as the athlete can perform them without pain.

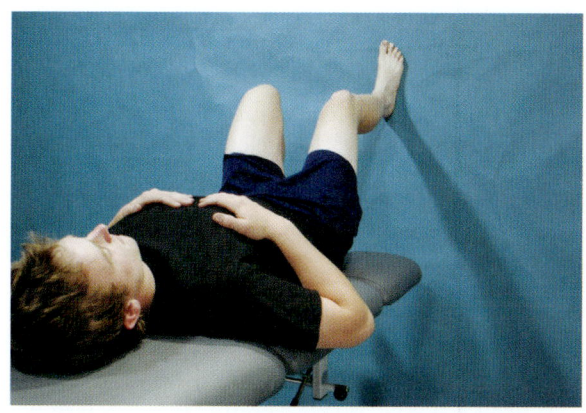

Training programming and prescription — CHAPTER 10

Figure 10.3 Isometric co-contraction of the hamstrings, gluteal and quadriceps muscles with the patient pushing foot into wall

Isometric exercises are used when a muscle is too weak to perform range of motion exercises, in conditions where other forms of exercise are not possible (such as patellar dislocation and shoulder dislocation) or when isometric contraction is required in activities (e.g. stabilising). Isometric exercises can minimise muscle atrophy associated with immobilisation and injury by maintaining or improving static strength, minimising swelling via the muscle pump action, and enhancing neural and proprioceptive inputs to the muscle.

Ideally, isometric exercises are initially held for 5 seconds with contraction time increasing as the athlete becomes more tolerant. They can be performed frequently during the day as pain permits. The number of sets will vary at different stages of the rehabilitation program. If an athlete has difficulty, exercises may be performed against resistance or against an immovable object. It is important to remember that the quality of exercise is more important than the quantity.

Isometric exercises should be carried out at multiple angles if possible, as strength gain can be specific to the angle of exercise. The athlete should progress from submaximal to maximal isometric exercise slowly within the limitations of pain and function.

Isometric exercises have demonstrated success in the rehabilitation of tendon injuries (see Chapter 4) and should form a large component of any musculotendinous rehabilitation program.[29]

When significant isometric effort is tolerated at multiple joint angles, dynamic exercises may begin. An example of an isometric exercise for the lower limb is shown in Figure 10.3.

Isotonic exercise

Isotonic exercises are performed when the joint moves through a range of motion against a constant resistance or weight. Isotonic exercises may be performed with free weights, such as dumbbells, pulleys or sandbags (Fig. 10.4).

Free weights encourage natural movement patterns and require muscle coordination and joint stability in all planes of movement and therefore may transfer strength gains more readily to the playing field.[30] With free weights it is possible to simulate athletic activities as the body position can be varied. Isotonic exercises may be:

- concentric–a shortening isotonic contraction in which the origin and insertion of the muscles approximate. Individual muscle fibres shorten during concentric contraction

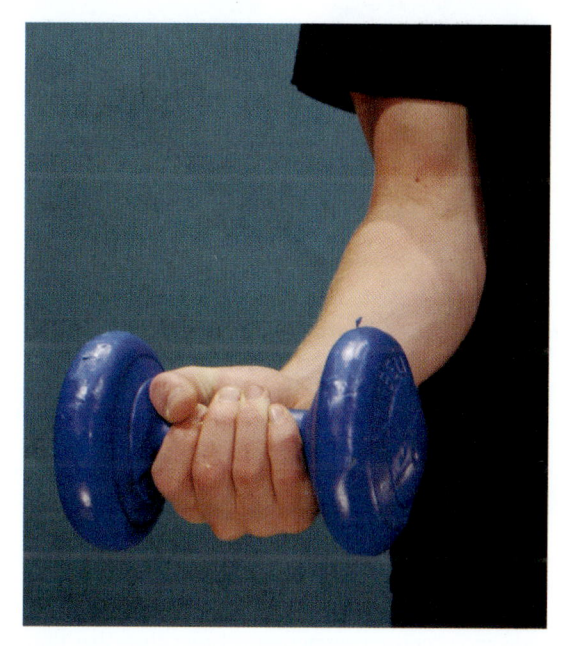

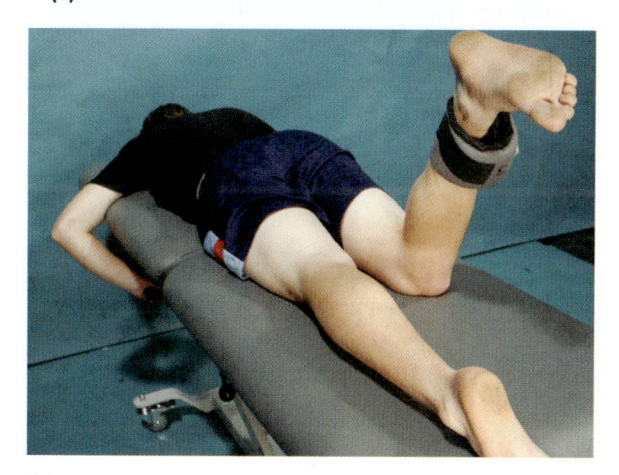

Figure 10.4 Isotonic exercises (a) Dumbbell (b) Sandbag

145

PART A Fundamental principles

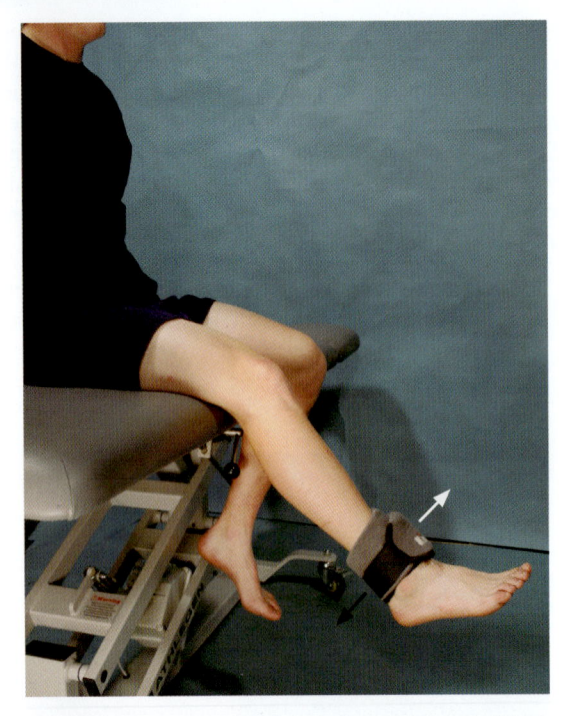

Figure 10.5 Concentric (white arrow) and eccentric (black arrow) quadriceps exercises

- eccentric—a lengthening isotonic contraction where the origin and insertion of the muscles separate. The individual muscle fibres lengthen during eccentric contraction.

Concentric and eccentric exercises for the quadriceps are shown in Figure 10.5.

The intramuscular force produced per motor unit during an eccentric contraction is larger than that during a concentric contraction.[28] Eccentric contractions may generate high tension within the series elastic component, which consists of connective tissue and the actin–myosin cross-bridges in muscles. It has been observed that eccentric exercise results in higher rates of delayed onset muscle soreness (DOMS) and even muscle damage if used inappropriately.[31, 32] Consequently, eccentric programs should commence at very low levels and progress gradually to higher intensity and volume. The use of eccentric exercise programs may help prevent recurrence of musculotendinous injuries.

Eccentric training has been advocated in the rehabilitation of tendon injuries, due to the proposed facilitation of tendon remodelling through promotion of collagen fibres within the injured tendon.[32-34] There is evidence that Achilles, patellar and lateral elbow tendinopathies respond well to an eccentric rehabilitation program.[31, 32, 34, 35]

However, not all tendon injuries benefit from eccentric exercises. Specifically, eccentric exercises have shown poor success rates for rotator cuff tendinopathy[36] and for insertional Achilles tendinopathy, compared to mid-tendon Achilles lesions.[32] Therefore, the site of tendon pathology should be considered when prescribing eccentric exercises.

Practically, there are some potential dangers of isotonic resistance training such as:

- Athletes require adequate supervision in the gymnasium.
- Athletes should never attempt to lift a maximal weight without a 'spotter' (an assistant who is able to help the athlete if problems arise).
- Isotonic machines such as Keiser® equipment may provide a safe alternative to free weights, but these machines limit the range of motion and are generally unable to provide truly constant resistance through the lift.

Isotonic exercises in which the body weight of the individual is used as resistance are also safer than free weights and are often more convenient to perform. Exercises such as sit-ups, push-ups and chin-ups can be done almost anywhere and require no supervision. However, it is difficult to increase the resistance of the exercise and the only way to increase the effort is to increase the number of repetitions performed.

Isokinetic exercises

Isokinetic exercises are performed on devices at a fixed speed with a variable resistance that is totally accommodative to the individual throughout the range of motion. The velocity is, therefore, constant at a preselected dynamic rate, while the resistance varies to match the force applied at every point in the range of motion. This enables the patient to perform more work than is possible with either constant or variable resistance isotonic exercise.

Isokinetic testing can highlight imbalances, such as scapular muscle imbalances in overhead athletes with chronic impingement signs.[37] A number of isokinetic devices are available and include the Ariel®, Biodex®, Cybex®, KinCom®, Lido and Merac® machines. However, these machines do come at a cost, which may explain why they are more commonplace in research than in clinical settings.

Classification of resistance exercises

Open chain and closed chain exercises

An open kinetic chain exercise often involves single joint movement performed in a non weight-bearing position where the distal extremity freely moves through space.[38] Closed kinetic chain exercises involve multiple joints and

146

Training programming and prescription — CHAPTER 10

Table 10.2 Advantages and disadvantages of open chain and closed chain exercises

	Advantages	Disadvantages
Open chain exercises	Decreased joint compression Can exercise in non weight-bearing positions Able to exercise through increased ROM Able to isolate individual muscles	Increased joint translation Decreased functionality
Closed chain exercises	Decreased joint forces in secondary joints (e.g. less patellofemoral force with squat) Decreased joint translation Increased functionality	Increased joint compression Not able to exercise through increased ROM Not able to isolate individual muscles

ROM = range of motion

are performed in weight-bearing positions with a fixed distal extremity. Closed kinetic exercises are thought to be more functional, provide more proprioceptive feedback and cause less shear joint forces than open kinetic chain exercises.[38]

Open and closed chain exercises in rehabilitation

Although some studies promote closed chain over open chain exercises,[38, 39] others advocate that both types of exercises play beneficial roles in rehabilitation, especially in regards to anterior cruciate rehabilitation and patellofemoral pain.[40, 41, 42] Proposed advantages and disadvantages of open and closed kinetic exercise are shown in Table 10.2.

Examples of these exercises are shown in Figure 10.6. Figure 10.6c shows an example of open (right arm) and closed (left arm) chain exercises for the shoulder girdle.

(a)

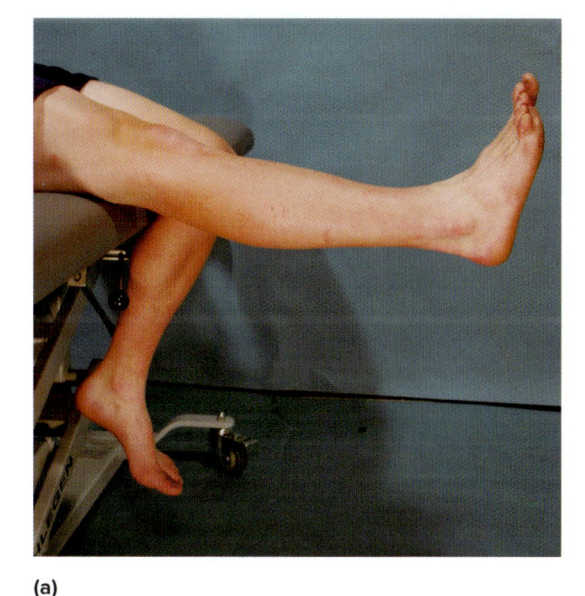

Figure 10.6 Open and closed chain exercises (a) Open chain knee extension with the foot moving freely

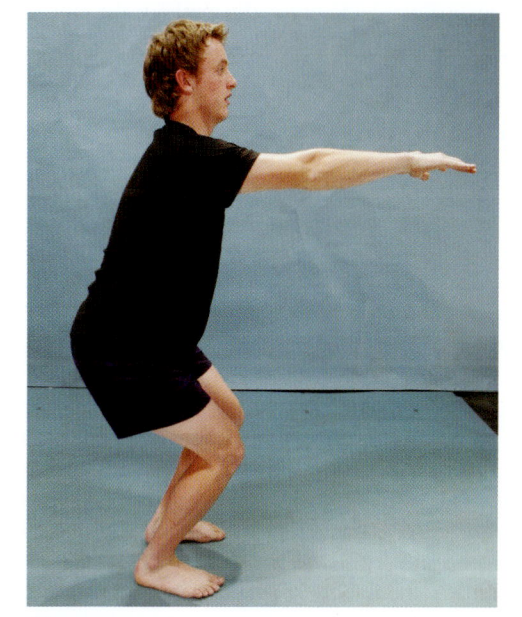

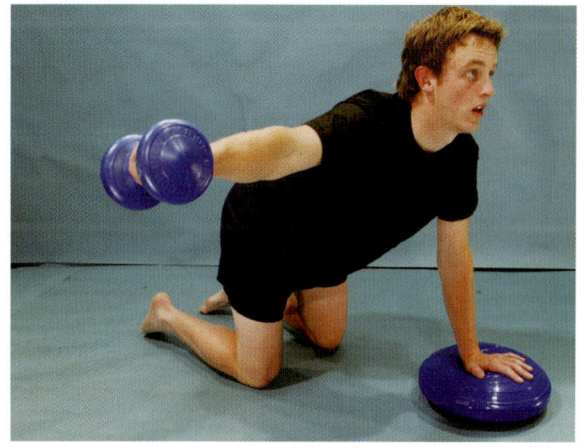

(b)

(c)

Figure 10.6 (cont.) (b) Closed chain knee extension with the feet immobile (c) Open chain (right arm) and closed chain (left arm) exercises on an unstable surface

Closed chain upper limb exercises are particularly useful during the early recovery period from shoulder surgery (Chapter 24). Excessive mobility and compromised static stability within the glenohumeral joint have been linked to capsular, labral and musculotendinous injuries in throwing athletes.[43] The positive benefits of closed kinetic chain exercises, performed under load-bearing positions, are thought to stimulate joint receptors and facilitate muscle co-contractions around the shoulder and therefore enhance joint stability.[37, 43]

Qualities of resistance training

This section will briefly describe the various resistance training qualities and outline the methods the clinician or coach may employ to train these qualities.

Strength

Muscle strength is the muscle's ability to exert force. Strength gains can be seen quickly, even before physiological hypertrophy occurs. The initial strength gain in response to exercise is thought to be related to increased neuromuscular facilitation (i.e. the nervous system enhances the motor pathways so that the muscle group becomes more neurologically efficient).[27, 28, 44] Neural adaptations facilitate changes in coordination and learning that enhance the recruitment and activation of muscles during a strength task.[27]

Typical loading patterns for strength training can be seen in Table 10.3. Most importantly the resistance needs to be at or near maximal levels with large rest periods in between sets. This enables the muscles to recuperate adequately in between sets.

Strength training is generally the base from which all other resistance training emanates and therefore it generally occurs at the beginning of pre-season training.

Power

Muscle power is the muscle's rate of doing work. Similar to strength training, the initial power gains observed with power training result from improvements in neuromuscular efficiency.[45] Specifically, initial improvements in power can be attributed to improved muscle coordination between agonist and antagonist muscles. Power exercises may include:

- fast-speed isotonic or isokinetic exercises (concentric and/or eccentric)
- increased speed of functional exercises (e.g. faster reverse calf raise, drop squat)
- plyometric exercises (e.g. hopping, bounding).

Power exercises often involve functional and sport-specific exercises. Exercises should be made appropriate to the athlete's sport to gain optimal benefits (e.g. bounding for a sprinter, jump and land for a basketballer).

Another technique of increasing power is plyometric training. Plyometric exercises (plyometrics) use the natural elastic recoil elements of human muscle and the neurological stretch reflex to produce a stronger, faster muscle response. Plyometrics combine a rapid eccentric muscle contraction with a rapid concentric contraction to produce a fast forceful movement. It must be performed in conjunction with a resistance training program, as athletes need to have minimum basic strength levels before commencing plyometrics.

> **PRACTICE PEARL**
>
> Because of their explosive nature, plyometrics have a great potential for injury. Therefore, an athlete's plyometrics program should be carefully supervised.

Plyometric exercises include hopping and bounding drills, jumps over hurdles and depth jumps. These activities emphasise spending as little time as possible in contact with the ground. This form of exercise can cause DOMS (Chapter 4). Plyometric training should only be performed when the athlete is fresh and the volume of work should be built up gradually. The training surface must be firm but forgiving, such as sprung basketball floors. When technique begins to deteriorate, the exercise should be stopped.

Olympic-type weightlifting is often used as part of a power training program. Olympic lifting involves explosively lifting a weight from the floor to a position above the ground using the entire body. Typical Olympic lifts include the power clean, snatch, and clean and jerk. These lifts exercise a greater number of muscle groups

Table 10.3 Resistance training loading patterns

	Sets	Reps	Rest (s)	%RM	Speed
Strength	3–5	3–6	90–120	90–100	Controlled
Power	3–4	8–12	45–60	40–60	Explosive
Hypertrophy	2–3	8–12	60–75	70–90	Slow on eccentric
Endurance	1–2	15–30	45–60	50–70	Sport-specific

than conventional weightlifting, exercising them both concentrically and eccentrically. The potential for injury is high and athletes must learn correct lifting techniques before attempting these lifts.

When injury has decreased muscle power or the athlete's sport includes periods of explosive power, the rehabilitation program should incorporate power exercises. Commonly, power-focused exercises are incorporated into the later stage of rehabilitation due to the potential for re-injury and explosive nature of this training.

Typical loading patterns for a power program can be seen in Table 10.3. The most important factor in a power development program is the speed of movement which must be as explosive as possible.

Muscular endurance

Muscle endurance is the muscle's ability to sustain contraction or perform repeated contractions. The aim of muscular endurance training is to increase the capacity to sustain repetitive, high-intensity, low-resistance exercise such as running, cycling and swimming.[17] Excessive bouts of muscular endurance training can result in fatigue and reduced sporting performance. Therefore, care should be taken in incorporating this type of training into a resistance training program, especially during prolonged pre-season training.

Typical loading patterns for muscular endurance training can be seen in Table 10.3. This type of training involves high repetitions with very little rest.

Hypertrophy training

Hypertrophy training aims to increase the muscle size. This quality is important particularly for combative sports where an increased muscle mass can be advantageous. Generally, hypertrophy occurs through an increase in the size or cross-sectional area of the muscle cells rather than an increase in the number of muscle cells.

Typical loading patterns for hypertrophy can be found in Table 10.3. As this table demonstrates, the eccentric or lowering component should be slower than the concentric component. This will create additional muscle damage and therefore take greater time for the muscle to repair and regenerate. As a result care must be taken when prescribing additional speed or resistance training around hypertrophy sessions.

Flexibility training

An athlete is susceptible to injury if they lack sufficient flexibility to meet their sport-specific demands. Stretching and range of motion exercises are performed to increase joint range of motion. The acute effects of stretching include:[46, 47]

- decreased muscle stiffness through viscoelastic deformation of the muscle tissue (this is likely to be extremely transient)
- increased muscle length through serial addition of sarcomeres
- altering sensation, thereby increasing stretch tolerance.

Traditionally, stretching has been widely promoted for injury prevention and performance enhancing for sporting activity. However, some authors have suggested stretching does not prevent injury in otherwise healthy individuals.[48] Others have noted that it is important to differentiate between pre-exercise stretching (where stretching does not appear to prevent injury)[49] and regular stretching outside periods of exercise (where there is some clinical and basic science evidence suggesting stretching may prevent injury).[50, 51] Additionally, stretching does not seem to reduce the effects of DOMS.[52]

Furthermore, the acute effects of stretching can cause temporary strength deficits and hence reduce sporting performance.[53] This deficit seems to be associated with stretches performed for more than 60 seconds, while stretches of shorter duration may have less significant deficits.[53] As traditional stretching routines are performed during warm-up sessions prior to playing sport, the amount of time athletes stretch should be taken into consideration.

Stretching is often promoted as having a number of beneficial effects,[54, 55] although not all of the following have been appropriately studied:

- increases muscle and joint flexibility
- increases muscle relaxation
- decreases muscle soreness
- improves circulation
- helps prevent excessive adhesion
- promotes a flexible, strong scar.

Types of stretching

There are three main types of stretching: static, dynamic and proprioceptive neuromuscular facilitation.

Static stretching

Static stretching involves moving the muscle or joint into an elongated position and holding the position for an extended period. Historically, this type of stretching has been used to prepare the muscle for exercise; however, research has consistently demonstrated a reduction in power immediately after static stretching.[56] As a result the more contemporary practice for athletic populations is to use static stretching both post training for recovery and away from training to improve flexibility.

PART A Fundamental principles

> ### Recommendations for effective stretching
>
> - A gentle warm-up before stretching increases tissue temperature and facilitates stretching. This may include activities such as jogging or cycling.
> - As with warm-up, superficial or deep heat modalities may be applied to the area prior to stretching to increase tissue temperature.
> - Cryotherapy may reduce pain and muscle spasm and thereby enhance the overall stretch of a muscle in the initial stages after an injury, even though the temperature is decreased (i.e. opposite to heat).
> - Athletes should be carefully instructed regarding the correct stretching position, as incorrect positioning may cause injury.
> - Different muscles seem to require different durations of stretch. In general, a slow sustained stretch should be held for a minimum of 10–15 seconds and progressed for 1 minute or longer. The athlete should feel stretch in the appropriate area.
> - As the athlete's flexibility improves, increases in intensity, duration, frequency and type of stretch can be considered.
> - Stretching should always be pain-free, that is, 'tightness' without pain.

Dynamic stretching

Dynamic or ballistic stretching is when the muscles and joints are taken through their range of motion during movement. This type of practice is more specific to preparation for exercise and sports in particular. During the rehabilitation process care should be taken to not 'bounce' the muscle that is recovering from injury. Dynamic stretches have been shown to significantly increase tendon flexibility and elasticity and have been promoted for end-stage rehabilitation for tendon injuries. However, ballistic stretching involves eccentric contractions during the stretch phase, which may result in soreness or injury and therefore care should be taken when incorporating such stretches.

Proprioceptive neuromuscular facilitation (PNF) stretching

PNF stretching involves the combination of contracting the antagonist (opposite) muscle and excessively stretching the agonist muscle. This type of stretching is quite aggressive but can result in rapid increases in flexibility. PNF flexibility sessions should not be performed more than 1–2 times per week and should be cycled into and out of training as it can cause some muscle damage.

Flexibility in the rehabilitation process

Regaining or maintaining full flexibility of joints and soft tissues is an essential component of the rehabilitation process. Following injury, musculotendinous flexibility often decreases as a result of spasm of surrounding muscles. Inflammation, pain and/or stiffness can limit joint range of motion and the normal extensibility of the musculotendinous unit can be compromised. This may result in dysfunction of adjacent joints and soft tissues.

For example, the lumbar spine may be restricted in range of motion and the paraspinal muscles may spasm following knee or hip surgery, especially after periods of restricted mobilisation. Adequate soft tissue extensibility after injury is essential to encourage pain-free range of movements. Stretching muscles and joints is one way of improving tissue and joint extensibility.

TRAINING LOAD MANAGEMENT FOR PERFORMANCE ENHANCEMENT

The ability to effectively periodise and manage training load will obviously have a large impact on athlete success. Long-term, gradually progressive training plans should be made, including periods of higher and lower loading to avoid improvement plateaus, injuries, illnesses or burn-out. This process, commonly referred to as *periodisation*, should consider time periods consisting of several months (macrocycles), weeks (mesocycles) and days (microcycles).

Load management not only comprises sound knowledge of training periodisation, but also an intimate awareness of when players are fatigued, undertrained, stressed or fresh. Typically, team-sport athletes have been advised to avoid strenuous mid-week training to 'freshen up' for the next game and/or avoid injury. However, recent evidence suggests that too little training can be a significant risk factor for injury.[57] This suggests a delicate balance exists between fitness, fatigue and freshness, with the ability to identify each state being crucial to performance enhancement and injury prevention.

To successfully manage load, it needs to be quantified. There are, of course, many influences on the total load placed upon an athlete, and the ability to identify these and alter training load accordingly is both an art and a science. Certainly, technology may assist the practitioner in quantifying load; however, just as important is the ability to 'sense' or 'feel' when players are fatigued or fresh. This 'sense', however, typically requires intimate knowledge of the players/athletes and much experience in this domain.

Training load is typically defined as either internal or external. Internal load refers to the impact the training has on the athlete and can be measured by subjective wellness questionnaires,[58, 59] as well as a range of objective metrics such as heart rate, blood markers (e.g. creatine kinase, testosterone, cortisol), RPE and heart rate variability.[59] External load refers to the estimation of the actual load the players are placed under and is usually measured using GPS devices, power meters or simply calculating training duration.[59]

Maximising training output (external load) while minimising training cost (internal load) is usually the goal of most training programs. Effectively estimating both of these, therefore, becomes a crucial element of the sports practitioner's role. RPE-load (also called session-RPE) has subsequently gained much popularity in both research[60] and practice as it represents both internal and external load and allows different forms of training (e.g. football and weightlifting) to be measured in the same units. RPE-load is calculated by multiplying player RPE (internal) with training or match duration (external) and has been shown to relate effectively to measures of internal load.[61]

The role of load monitoring in injury prevention is covered in Chapter 12.

REFERENCES

References for this chapter can be found at www.mhhe.com/au/CSM5e

Chapter 11

Core stability

by PAUL HODGES

Core strength and stability is very important to me. Tennis is all about rotation of the body and my ability to create power. I incorporate a lot of abdominal, back and glute exercises into my gym sessions.

Samantha Stosur

INTRODUCTION

'Core stability' refers to control of proximal regions of the body during movements and function. Although the concept appears straightforward, different interpretations or misconceptions of the term, and differences in applying this concept to the design of exercise programs for lumbopelvic pain, have led to substantial confusion and debate.

'Stability' has been interpreted to mean many things and, commonly, a simple objective to *restrict* motion. This has led to the development of many exercise programs that emphasise static maintenance of a specific lumbopelvic position during loading. Although this may be appropriate for some functions, restriction of motion does not necessarily assure stability of a system.

A stable system is one in which its intended *position* or *trajectory* (i.e. movement path) can be maintained, despite perturbation or disturbance.[1] This may be achieved by restricting motion in some tasks (e.g. restriction of spinal motion during lifting), but requires movement to manage, reduce or transfer internal and external forces in others (e.g. counter-rotation of the shoulders and pelvis during walking) (Fig. 11.1). Further, in a complex dynamic system such as the spine, the stability of many goals (e.g. spine control, breathing, balance) must be maintained concurrently.[2]

The 'core' refers to proximal regions of the body, which can include the spine, pelvis, scapulothoracic region and even the hips and shoulders. These regions are functionally distinct from the distal limbs, which have a critical role in fine controlled, goal-directed movements. The principal functions of the core are to provide a foundation for limb movements, a stable base for limb muscle contraction and a major contribution to overall postural control of the

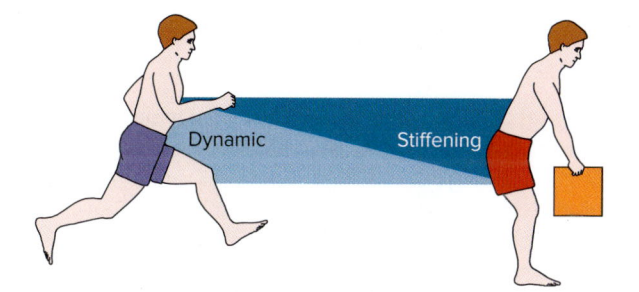

Figure 11.1 Optimal control of the spine depends on a balance between movement and stiffness. At one end of the spectrum are functions such as lifting that require high stiffness of the trunk; at the other are functions such as running and walking that demand movement to meet the demands of the task. Both too much and too little movement and stiffness could underlie suboptimal loading

body. This latter aspect is particularly important as the trunk contributes about 70% of body weight. The focus of this chapter is consideration of the lumbopelvic region, but clinical management must involve consideration of the adjacent regions, as they cannot act independently.

When the concepts of 'stability' and the 'core' are fully appreciated, it is clear that the design of exercise programs for lumbopelvic pain require the term 'core stability' to be applied in its broadest sense to encompass all features that might be necessary to ensure optimal control. This requires a motor control or learning approach, whereby muscle activation patterns, postures or alignments, and movements are trained, tuned or optimised to meet the demands of function[3] (Fig. 11.2). Although restriction of motion may be encouraged for some functions and some patients, this

PART A   Fundamental principles

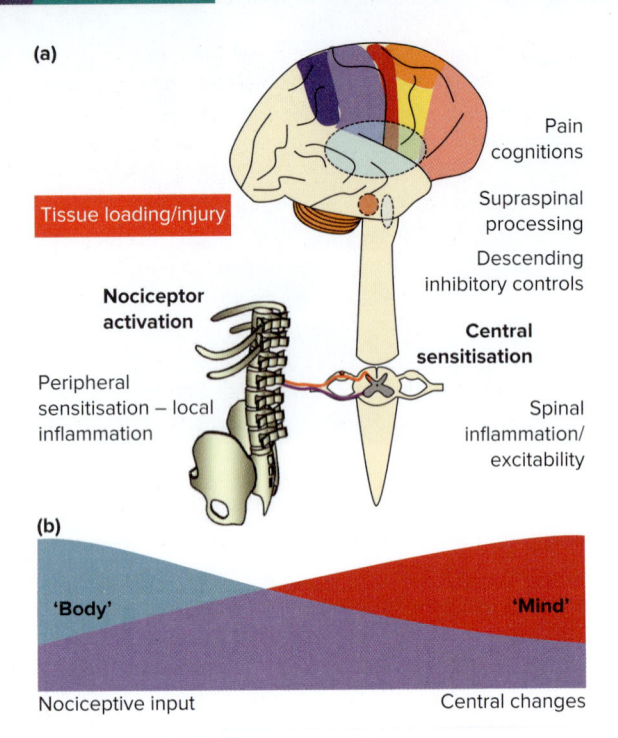

Figure 11.2 Contribution of body and mind to persistent pain. (a) The experience of pain involves peripheral and central components. Individual patients will vary in the relative contribution of peripheral and central contributions to their pain presentation. Some will maintain a major contribution of ongoing nociceptive input from suboptimal loading of tissues; others will have little input from tissues and major contribution from central processes. Motor control training is likely to be most effective for individuals with an ongoing contribution from peripheral afferents. (b) Different treatments will be required along the spectrum from treatments that target the body such as motor control training for core stability at one end, to psychologically grounded treatments for the mind at the other end

depends on the presentation of the individual patient, whereas for other functions and other patients the exercise may aim to increase motion. 'Motor control training' is a general term used to describe a comprehensive approach that uses a range of strategies (from low load training of precise control of muscles, posture and movement; progression of exercise with increasing load and complexity; and functional retraining; through to strength and endurance training, as required) in combination with education and behavioural strategies to promote pain management.

Training must:
- optimise the balance between movement and stiffness (which differs between tasks)
- consider the coordination of the multiple functions of the trunk and of the trunk muscles

- individualise the program to match the patient's unique presentation.

This chapter provides an overview of the rationale for motor control training to optimise core stability in the management of lumbopelvic pain, outlines key principles underlying this approach and discusses common misconceptions. It also describes the typical process for planning a motor control training program; from detailed assessment of motor control, formulation of the clinical hypothesis, development of an exercise program to optimise loading, and planning for progression of exercise.

RATIONALE FOR MOTOR CONTROL TRAINING FOR LUMBOPELVIC DYSFUNCTION

The premise underlying the effectiveness of motor control training to optimise core stability is that for many individuals with lumbopelvic pain, suboptimal loading of structures of the spine and pelvis (as a result of the muscle activation, posture or alignment, and movement typically adopted by an individual) places the tissues at risk of trauma or microtrauma, and drives peripheral nociceptive input which contributes to the development and persistence of pain (Fig. 11.2).

Motor control training of core stability aims to optimise tissue loading to prevent further injury and to reduce nociceptive afferent discharge.[3] Although it is acknowledged that symptoms may persist in the absence of ongoing nociceptive input, and it is widely agreed that central sensitisation will contribute to the pain experience for many[4] (Fig. 11.2), individuals who retain a peripheral component to their symptoms are likely to benefit from reduction of this input through optimisation of the manner in which the individual loads their tissues and body.

With the link between loading and pain in mind, it is clear that the exercise must be individualised to modify the features that are specific to the individual's unique presentation. Examples of suboptimal loading that could cause ongoing nociceptive input include reduced muscle activation leading to insufficient constraint or control of joint motion; sustained alignment of the pelvis and spine at the end of range of motion placing excess load on passive tissues;[5] excessive motion of the spine and pelvis rather than the hip during leg movement;[6] and excessive compressive load on the spine from augmented co-contraction of trunk muscles (e.g. during lifting[7]). Motor control training aims to change the suboptimal features of muscle activation, posture and movement to achieve optimal core stability with optimal tissue loading.

Although it would be impossible to test the validity of every permutation of suboptimal tissue loading, evidence is beginning to emerge that loading can be related to symptoms, and optimisation of loading may be necessary for recovery. For instance, training that aims to restore activation of the deep abdominal muscle, transversus abdominis, is more effective for individuals found to have poor activation of this muscle on clinical assessment at baseline, and recovery of symptoms is related to recovery of function of this muscle in those individuals.[8, 9] Further, low back symptoms are reduced when spine position is controlled during hip rotation in individuals who present with early and excessive lumbopelvic motion during this task.[10]

A thoughtful clinical reasoning approach is essential to:

- determine whether the patient's pain presentation includes a component that is maintained by peripheral nociceptive input
- identify any features of muscle activation, posture/alignment and movement that underpin the suboptimal tissue loading for the individual through detailed clinical assessments
- develop a clinical hypothesis to account for the relationship and inform treatment planning
- develop an exercise program to target the motor control changes to optimise tissue loading.

Of course it is critical to recognise that the presentation of lumbopelvic pain generally involves features within multiple domains of the biopsychosocial model (Chapters 15 and 23). In addition to peripheral nociceptive input from abnormal tissue loading, there may also be sensitisation of pain processing at multiple levels of the nervous system and some features of unhealthy pain cognitions and social features (Fig. 11.2). Depending on the individual patient's presentation, treatment is likely to be optimised when all factors relevant for the patient's presentation are considered in treatment design. This will include considering additional measures to manage attitudes and beliefs about pain, as well as other aspects such as pain-coping skills.

MOTOR CONTROL TRAINING TO OPTIMISE CORE STABILITY— KEY PRINCIPLES AND COMMON MISCONCEPTIONS

Key principles that underlie the application of motor control training to lumbopelvic pain are reviewed below to clarify the basis for clinical decisions when designing an exercise program to optimise core stability. A number of misconceptions regarding the approach also require clarification.

Optimal motor control requires a balance between movement and stiffness

The primary focus of many exercise programs for core stability has been to restrict motion (e.g. exercises that target maintenance of lumbar and pelvic position during limb movement or side-bridging). Although these strategies to brace the trunk are appropriate and necessary for some tasks (e.g. lifting a 100 kg weight from the floor, which requires high stiffness of the spine), they are not appropriate for other functions, such as walking and running, where movement is essential for optimal task performance. Most functions require a balance between movement and stiffness to optimise tissue loading; the optimal balance depends on the task being performed.

Sufficient stiffness is necessary to prevent collapse and maintain alignment. Movement is required to absorb impact, transfer load, minimise energy expenditure, allow some variation to share load between related structures, and to move along a trajectory. Even static tasks generally involve some movement (e.g. standing involves small movements to compensate for a range of challenges, including the cyclical postural disturbance from breathing[11]). A healthy system has the capacity to shift along a continuum from high stiffness at one end and high mobility at the other to match the balance between movement and stiffness required by task demands (Fig. 11.1). Individuals with lumbopelvic pain often present with inaccuracy in matching task demands.

> **PRACTICE PEARL**
>
> Evidence is emerging for poor control across this stiffness-mobility spectrum in people with lumbopelvic pain. This can present as excessive motion,[12] excessive stiffness[13] or elements of both.

A tennis player may use excessive lumbar rather than hip motion during a racket swing. A runner may brace the spine with excessive muscle co-contraction, and limit shock absorption and load transfer through the trunk. There may be a change in threshold, where a strategy normally reserved for a high load task is used at low load. All of these can lead to excessive tissue loading which is problematic for function, not only in terms of suboptimal lumbopelvic control, but also for the broader functions of the trunk. For instance, balance in standing is compromised if the trunk is stiffened.[14]

On this basis it would seem inappropriate to apply exercise universally to enhance stiffness (e.g. bracing co-contraction of abdominal and extensor muscles) for every patient or for every functional context. Such strategies should be reserved to enhance stiffness for moments of high demand. Other exercise is required to train appropriate movement.

Optimal lumbopelvic control involves three main neural strategies

The nervous system employs three basic strategies to optimise lumbopelvic control. The first is reactive control in which the nervous system activates a pattern of muscle activation in response to sensory input.[15] This class of response is involved in formulating the response when the system is unexpectedly disturbed (e.g. trip, slip, push) or to fine tune muscle activation.

The second is preparatory control when the muscle activation required to control the lumbopelvic region can be initiated in advance of a disturbance.[16] This type of adjustment can only be used when demands can be predicted (e.g. voluntary initiated stepping, catching a watched ball).

As reactions take time and not all disturbances can be predicted, the system relies on a third strategy of ongoing tonic muscle activation at a low percentage of contraction to maintain a state of preparedness, just in case the spine is perturbed.[17]

All muscles of the trunk can contribute to these three classes of motor control strategy. Dysfunctions may present in each and it may be necessary to consider all three in a treatment program (e.g. train reactive control through challenging the system with balance tasks; train preparatory control by pre-activating muscles in advance of a task; train sustained gentle tonic activation).

Optimal motor control requires a whole system, not a single muscle

A single muscle cannot be responsible for optimal motor control and core stability, and dysfunction would be unlikely to involve a single muscle. Instead control must depend on the integrated function of a whole system of muscles, and the muscles cannot be considered independently of the alignment of the spine and pelvis, and the pattern of movement.

All muscles of the lumbopelvic region contribute to optimal control of the region and this is influenced by muscles of adjacent regions (e.g. hip/thorax). But this does not mean that all muscles serve the same role. As a general principle, deeper muscles with attachments to individual vertebra and limited moment arms for torque generation can play a primary role in controlling intersegmental motion. The larger more superficial muscles with a greater moment arm for torque generation are more critical for stiffening the spine when co-contracting in antagonist muscle pairs, and for generation and control of movement when acting asymmetrically or in specific patterns of activation that promote torque in a specific direction.

> **PRACTICE PEARL**
>
> Research evidence universally shows that the transversus abdominis and multifidus muscles are not the only muscles required for lumbopelvic control and no function involves activation of these muscles in the absence of activation of other trunk muscles.

Both of these contributions are essential and deficits in either would lead to problems.

There has been considerable debate regarding the function and dysfunction of the transversus abdominis and multifidus muscles.[18, 19] Although always part of a more complex interplay of muscle activation, these muscles often act differently to other trunk muscles (e.g. less dependent on force direction, early and tonically),[16, 20] which is related to their distinct mechanical contribution to control.

Transversus abdominis acts primarily through generating intra-abdominal pressure and tension of fascial structures, both of which appear to control intersegmental and pelvic motion in multiple directions. Multifidus is situated close to the centre of rotation of the lumbar segments, suggesting limited role in torque generation. These muscles commonly have structural and functional changes in people with pain.[21-24]

Together these observations provide a foundation for detailed consideration of these muscles in the management of lumbopelvic dysfunction. Backed by biomechanical and modelling data of a contribution to optimal control, individuals with compromised activation of these muscles are likely to contribute to abnormal tissue loading. These patients would be likely to benefit from restoration of control as part of a comprehensive training program that includes considering other muscles, posture and movement.

Motor control training involves rehabilitation of whole system

Considering the breadth of features of motor function that can underpin suboptimal tissue loading, it is clear that a motor control training program must address multiple features, including muscle activation, posture, or alignment and movement (Fig. 11.3). The exact features addressed and the combination depends on the individual's presentation and function. Thus, to optimise core stability, planning a training program to optimise motor control requires detailed assessment to identify features related to abnormal loading.

In terms of muscle activation, motor control of core stability would be suboptimal if muscle activity was insufficient, excessive or lacked coordination in terms of timing, amplitude or pattern of activation. Insufficient activation (e.g. delayed activation of transversus abdominis[21]) may allow excessive motion or poor quality of motion within the normal range of motion, both of which would lead to increased tissue load.

Excessive activation (e.g. augmented activation of obliquus externus abdominis) could restrict motion (limiting shock absorption and compromising function); increase joint load; and reduce variation (reduce sharing of load between structures). Poor coordination of muscle

Core stability CHAPTER 11

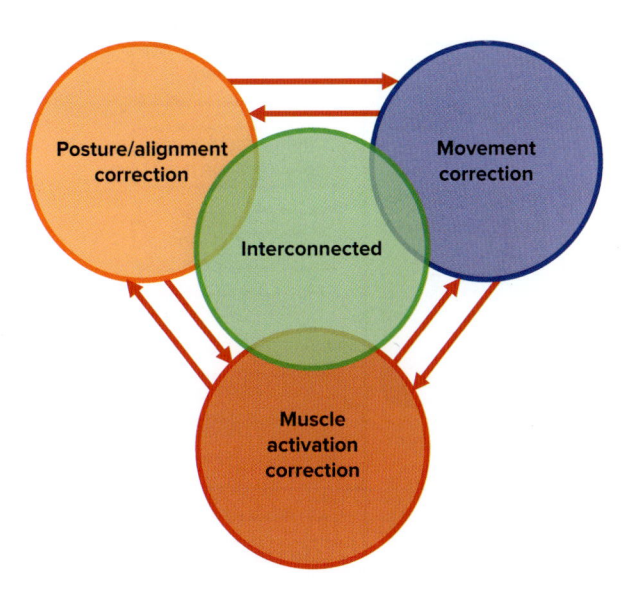

Figure 11.3 Suboptimal motor control generally involves features of posture or alignment, movement and muscle activation. The combination of features differs between individuals and each needs to be addressed, although there will be some interaction between them with exercise that targets one aspect having an effect on others

activation (e.g. *en bloc* activation of back muscles rather than differential activation) could change the location and amount of tissue load. None of these observations is universal and it would be illogical to target any change universally with exercise. The exercise program would involve the selection of techniques and strategies to change the pattern of activation.

A common clinical strategy that requires additional explanation is the common objective to isolate the activation of deeper muscles with specific exercises. It is important to clarify that this strategy does not aim to encourage a patient to activate *only* these muscles in function, but to train the *skill* of activating the muscles so that a patient can then integrate their activation into function, along with correcting any other suboptimal feature of motor control that is identified in the patient's presentation.

Like all elements of core stability, it is necessary to find a balance, and more muscle activity is not necessarily better. Although some degree of muscle activity, intra-abdominal pressure and fascial tension improves control,[25] if these are in excess of demands, this will lead to additional load or restriction of movement. It is necessary to tune muscle activity to meet, but not exceed, demands and to reduce it if the muscle is overactive.

Alignment or posture is also important. Although there is not one posture of the lumbopelvic region that is ideal for every patient, there is a range of features that clearly increase load on the lumbopelvic region.[5] Examples include resting at the end of range (e.g. sitting with posterior pelvic tilt with lumbar flexion); hanging on passive tissues (e.g. resting on an adducted hip in standing to tense the iliotibial band); and active holding of a posture by excessive muscle activation or asymmetrical postures. Changes to alignment or posture to reduce the resulting tissue loading may be necessary to optimise loading. This could be achieved with multiple techniques such as instruction, feedback, taping and manual therapy (see below).

It is critical to consider the pattern of movement. Like posture, there are features of movement that are likely to be suboptimal.[26] Every movement involves more or less ideal solutions and there are many ways that it can be suboptimal. Some examples include too little movement of a region or segment; too much movement; too little variation; and poor relationship between adjacent regions or segments. Again, selecting the strategy to change movement strategy in order to optimise load is required.

It is clear that motor control training for core stability requires an individualised approach. This is based on clinical and experimental data. When outcomes of randomised clinical trials are considered, there is a tendency for greater clinical effect size in trials that involve individualised training of specific subgroups of patients.[27] The least impressive outcomes are from trials that apply a generic treatment to a group of patients with non-specific back pain.

From an experimental perspective, there is clear evidence that exposure to pain induces adaptations that vary between individuals. For instance, if healthy individuals are provoked by a noxious stimulus to the back, all adapt to protect the spine, but no two participants achieve this with identical patterns of muscle activation.[28] Further, not all patients present with deficits in activation of the deep trunk muscles (transversus abdominis and multifidus muscles), and those that do have a deficit in these muscles have a better response to training that includes training of these components than do patients who do not have a deficit to start with.[9] Individualisation of training requires detailed assessment.

Motor control training involves a motor learning approach

When the objective of training is to modify specific features of motor control to optimise core stability, this can be targeted with a motor learning approach. Skill learning commences with identifying and then correcting the fault or suboptimal feature of a task. Once the modified skill is learnt, this can then be integrated into functions of increasing complexity. This applies to the learning of many skills.[29]

157

PART A   Fundamental principles

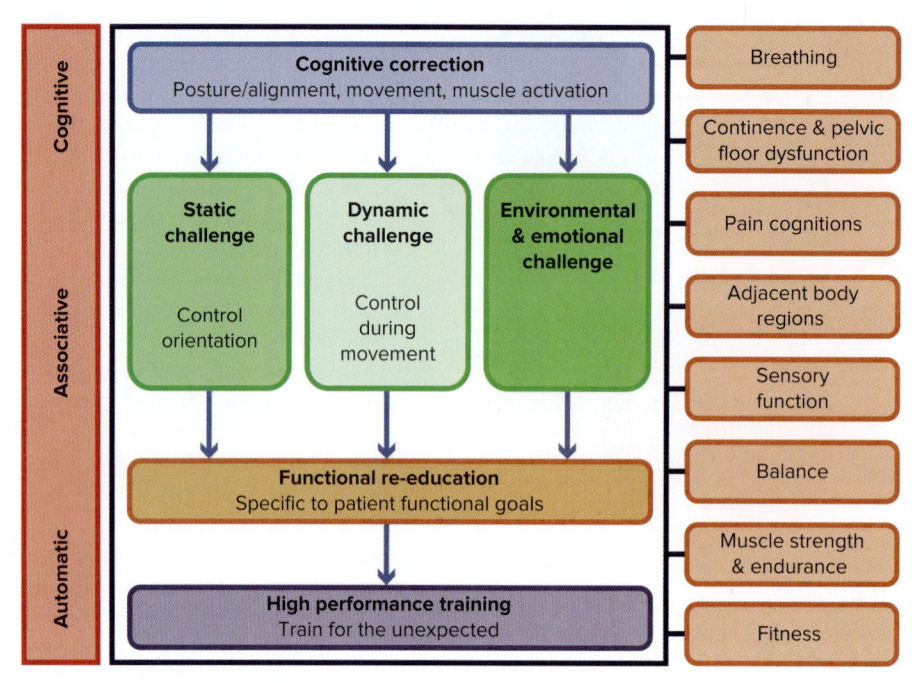

Figure 11.4 Motor control training for core stability. Training begins with detailed training of features of posture or alignment, movement and muscle activation that are considered to contribute to suboptimal tissue loading. Once these skills are learnt it is necessary to introduce static and dynamic challenges to encourage refinement and diversification of the skill. Functional training is necessary to ensure modified motor control strategies are introduced into functional tasks. Training then progresses to high performance for the unexpected. A range of issues, highlighted in boxes to the right, can be barriers to recovery and require consideration for individual patients if they are present

When applied to motor control training for core stability (Fig. 11.4), the initial stage would involve modifying and tuning the features of muscle activation, posture or alignment, and movement that are identified in the assessment. This can be achieved by conscious, cognitive correction of the feature, with feedback (visual, ultrasound imaging, palpation, electromyography), or the use of techniques such as taping and manual guidance (see below).

Skill learning can be enhanced by simplifying the task (e.g. non weight-bearing positions, slower speed) and segmenting a complex task into component parts (e.g. practice of correction of a muscle activation, practice of a specific alignment) prior to practice of a complete task. The selection of which features to address first depends on the individual. It is perhaps best guided by the features that are likely to achieve the greatest change in pain provocation or most able to be achieved by the patient.

As with any skill training, once the skill is learnt the patient can be progressed by challenging the patient with more complex tasks (e.g. increased load, more challenging postures and movements). This can involve progressive levels of increased demand and it is generally necessary to consider static control (of a specific alignment of the spine and pelvis) or dynamic control (of the lumbopelvic region as it moves) or control of the lumbopelvic region during whole body movement. Finally, the functions that a patient indicates are problematic can be practised with correction of the features of motor control.

Interplay between motor control and biology of pain

Motor control training would be expected to have a greater effect for patients with a nociceptive component. As highlighted above, but critical to reiterate, motor control training aims to optimise the load on the tissues and this is most likely to impact an individual's symptoms if they continue to have a nociceptive contribution to their symptoms (Fig. 11.2). Patients whose pain is maintained by central sensitisation may derive benefit from education of healthy movement, but this will impact their function through mechanisms other than reduction of peripheral nociceptive input, such as experience with healthy movement as a step towards fear-deconditioning.

It must be remembered that pain is not 'in' the tissues and is a result of interplay between nociceptive input, biological processes in the periphery and the nervous system that both inhibit and facilitate the pain experience, and cognitive and emotional aspects such as distress or fear (Fig. 11.2). Pain is a construct of the nervous system on the basis of each of those inputs and processes. Pain can be maintained by ongoing nociceptive input from the tissues and in its absence.

As highlighted above, the role of optimisation of tissue loading (through training of core stability) in the management of pain will be likely to be greatest in individuals with ongoing nociceptive contribution to pain. This type of pain is considered to have recognisable features such as a clear relationship with movement that is predictable and proportional, localised to an area, has clear aggravating and easing factors, and is localised on palpation.[30]

A recent clinical trial showed that motor control training and a graded activity general exercise approach were equally effective when the whole group of non-specific low back pain patients were considered together; however, motor control exercise was more effective for those who responded to a questionnaire that, although developed to identify instability (which may be considered too narrow a view of suboptimal motor control), also identifies characteristics that are consistent with nociceptive-type pain.[31]

Many patients also present with a host of biological changes (in addition to those that relate to suboptimal loading, such as modified inflammatory system activity[32]), and psychosocial features that also impact their pain presentation.[33] When present, these are likely to impact the efficacy of an exercise approach focused on motor control. For some, those processes are dominant and should be the primary target of intervention, for others, a combined approach may be helpful–restoration of function, but with attention to how people move.

An important consideration is that behavioural, psychologically informed treatments often encourage a patient to ignore pain, yet correction of motor control may demand consideration of when a movement is performed in a non-provocative manner. Care is required in selecting language to ensure the patient does not develop the belief that their spine is at risk and must be protected, which are concepts likely to reinforce unhealthy pain cognitions.

Implications of the role of trunk muscles in respiration and bladder and bowel function

In addition to their role in controlling the spine, trunk muscles, particularly those that surround the abdominal cavity, have critical roles in breathing and bladder and bowel function. These functions must be coordinated with the contribution of these muscles to lumbopelvic control. Yet in the present of disorders of continence (e.g. stress urinary incontinence), breathing (e.g. asthma) and back pain, the contribution to any or all of these functions may be disrupted.[34] Coordination of these functions is particularly critical for application to sport and more demanding physical activity.

Breathing requires modulation of pressure in the thorax–alternating activation of the diaphragm and other chest wall muscles in inspiration, and abdominal and internal intercostal muscles in expiration. These modulations of activity are coordinated with breathing in healthy individuals, but modified in those with respiratory disease and some with low back pain. Training to coordinate functions is likely to be required.

In terms of bladder and bowel function, continence is maintained if the pressure in the urethra or rectum exceeds that in the bladder/colon. Abdominal and diaphragm muscle activity increase intra-abdominal pressure, which concomitantly raises bladder and bowel pressure. Pelvic floor muscle activation is necessary to elevate intra-abdominal pressure. Thus, coordination between spine control and continence functions of the whole lumbopelvic system, including the abdominal wall, back, diaphragm and pelvic floor, requires consideration. This is particularly the case in the presence of pelvic floor muscle dysfunction, which may present as compromised or excessive muscle activation, both of which would have consequences for optimal control of the spine.

Is motor control training effective for everyone or is it more effective when targeted to specific individuals?

As highlighted above, there is emerging evidence that motor control training for core stability is more effective for some individuals, and more effective when tailored to the individual patient. Hypothetically, motor control training would be more effective for patients and athletes presenting with symptoms that are related to modified loading (including an ongoing nociceptive component). As highlighted above, recent work highlights that the treatment is most effective for patients with a high score on a questionnaire which purports to indicate signs of instability.[31] Further work is required to determine whether this questionnaire instead reflects signs of ongoing nociceptive contribution to pain. Further, training is more effective for patients who are identified to have a deficit in control of the deep trunk muscles at baseline.[8,9] It seems logical that this is not a treatment that can be applied in a blanket manner, but applied to the right patients and in a tailored manner.

PART A   Fundamental principles

PRINCIPLES OF THE CLINICAL APPLICATION OF MOTOR CONTROL TRAINING

As highlighted above, the basis of a motor control approach for core stability is to optimise the manner in which a person loads the tissue of the spine and pelvis by addressing any suboptimal features of muscle activation, posture or alignment, and movement. It follows then that the application of motor control training requires careful assessment to identify the suboptimal features, and then design a treatment or exercise program to target these features, before progressing into functions of increasing complexity. The basic stages of a program to optimise motor control of core stability are presented in Figure 11.4. A brief overview is provided below (for a detailed review see Hodges et al.[3]).

Assessment of motor control for core stability

Assessment involves a series of screening tests to identify key features of muscle activation, posture and movement that could imply suboptimal loading, combined with more detailed analysis to identify the specific nature of the loading issue (Fig. 11.5). Subjective assessment is essential to provide initial guidance of key functional demands and provocative or relieving postures, movements or functions. Physical tests of motor control are based on the premise that it is possible to identify features of posture, movement or muscle

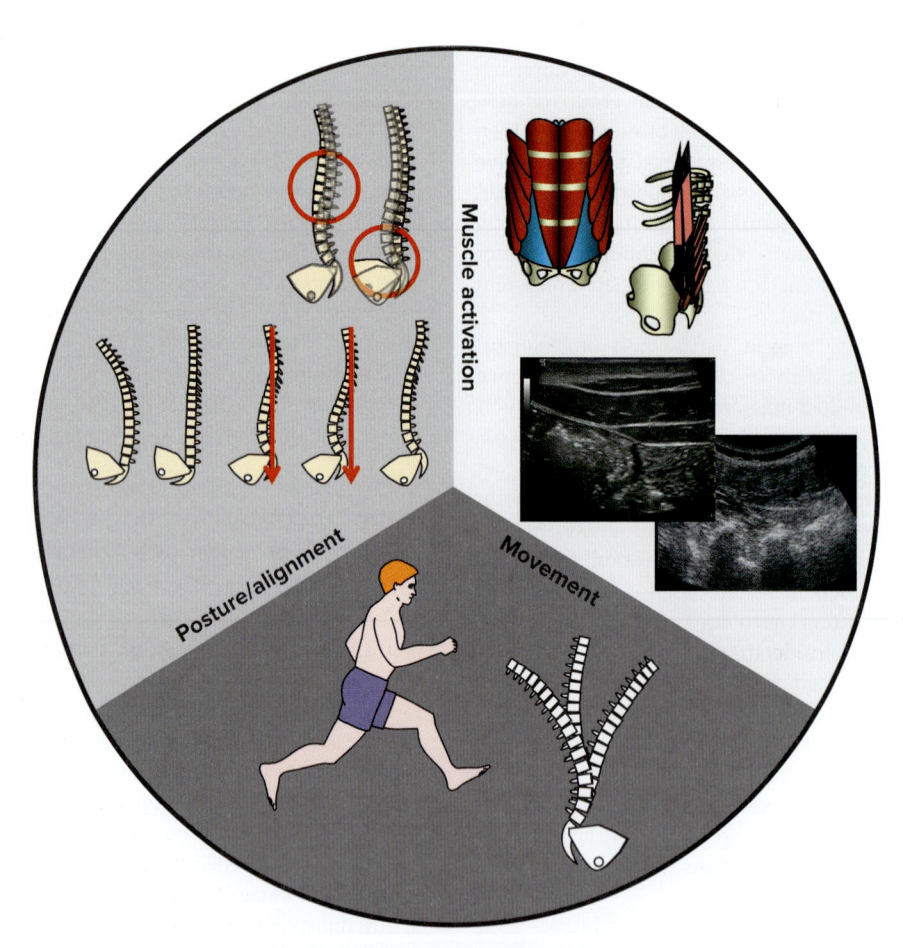

Figure 11.5 Assessment of motor control of core stability requires detailed assessment of posture or alignment, muscle activation and movement. Posture or alignment is compared against an ideal which is refined for consideration of the individual patient. Muscle activation involves assessment of underactivity, overactivity, threshold and asymmetry of the whole trunk muscle system. Assessment can be informed by evaluating the capacity to activate the deeper trunk muscles and concurrent substitution by the more superficial or global muscles. Movement assessment involves assessing the pattern of movement against an optimal strategy during physiological movements (e.g. trunk flexion), functional movements (e.g. sit-to-stand) and specific clinical movement tests (e.g. hip rotation in prone)

activation that deviate from a predicted ideal and, in many cases, provoke symptoms. Provocation or relief of symptoms does not always provide a perfect indicator of the relevance of a motor feature for a patient's presentation.

In some cases a clear relationship will be identified. But in others a highly inconsistent, unrepeatable relationship with motor features and disproportionate (area or intensity) pain provocation may be present. This may indicate a dominant central sensitisation, which might not be ideally managed with a motor control approach. For prevention of future symptoms of a patient in remission or for primary prevention, pain cannot be used as a guide, and the assessment depends on the clinician's understanding of ideal control.

Assessment of muscle activation

Assessment of muscle activation aims to identify evidence of overactivity or underactivity of any muscle(s). Observation of posture and movements can provide some indication of muscle activation (e.g. sitting with posterior tilt and extension at the thoracolumbar junction may suggest low activation of the multifidus and excessive activation of the thoracolumbar erector spinae).

A variety of clinical tests is available to analyse muscle activation. Some examples are described here. The common clinical tests of independent activation of the transversus abdominis and multifidus aim to assess both (i) the function of these deeper muscles (e.g. poor ability to activate the transversus abdominis independently is related to delayed activation in function[35]), and (ii) evidence of substitution or overactivity of the more superficial muscles. Clinical tools, observation, palpation, ultrasound imaging and electromyography can be used for the assessment. The capacity of the more superficial trunk muscles to control the lumbopelvic region can be derived from static tests that assess the capacity to control alignment when force is applied (e.g. load-applied limb movement). The threshold load that can be controlled, asymmetry in control and excessive bracing are assessed.

Assessment of posture or alignment

Assessment of posture or alignment begins with the identification of features that differ from the predicted optimal posture. Although not optimal for all, a starting point for evaluating sitting or standing posture is to identify features that differ from an ideal that includes a level or slightly anteriorly tilted pelvis, gentle lumbar lordosis with a smooth transition to a gentle thoracic kyphosis, cervical lordosis, symmetry in frontal plane and no rotation in the transverse plane. For many, this posture optimises load sharing and requires only gentle muscle activation to maintain.[36] This goal needs to be modified or refined when considering the individual patient as the same posture is not ideal for all.

Assessment involves identifying features that deviate from this ideal with confirmation of the relevance for the patient's presentation by evaluating the response of pain or discomfort and muscle activation. The ideal may feel unusual to the patient, but it should not be painful or require high muscle activation to hold. Analysis of alignment is generally necessary in a range of relevant functional postures to identify suboptimal features using a similar approach.

Assessment of movement

Assessment of movement involves a similar process to assessment of posture except that every movement pattern has its own ideal pattern of motion and muscle activation. For instance, forward flexion involves sharing motion between the hips, pelvis and spine with a specific sequence. Clear understanding of the requirements of movement is required. Movement tests typically involve assessment of physiological movements (e.g. trunk flexion), standardised functional movements (e.g. sit-to-stand) and specific movement tests (e.g. control of the spine and pelvis during hip rotation in prone). Several clinical approaches have been developed that include specific tests of movement to assist in identifying relevant features of movement (e.g. movement systems impairment[26]). In the case of the management of athletes, it is essential for the clinician to have a clear understanding of the features of optimal performance of the typical motor functions involved.

Consider subgrouping patients

Assessment can be facilitated by consideration of patient subgroups. Subgrouping based on motor control features has been developed by several groups and can help to simplify the process of identifying the cluster of features that may require attention with training.[26, 37] Subgrouping using this approach is based on the premise that there are groups of patients who present with a similar combination of motor control features that are related to their symptoms. When a clinician can identify the subgroup into which a patient belongs, then the task of selecting the combination of features that need to be prioritised and targeted with treatment can be simplified. For instance, if a patient is identified with a 'flexion' motor control impairment,[37] then the therapist can predict that relevant motor control features may include control of the lumbar lordosis, poor dissociation of motion of the pelvis and lumbar spine from the thoracolumbar junction, and compromised activation of the multifidus muscles. In this way subgrouping simplifies the clinical reasoning process by aiding the pattern recognition.

Training of motor control for core stability

At the conclusion of the assessment, a clinical hypothesis is formulated regarding the likelihood that suboptimal tissue loading is relevant for the patient's condition,

PART A   Fundamental principles

Table 11.1 Application of motor learning to skill training to lumbopelvic pain

1. Cognitive phase of learning

Learn and optimise features of basic motor skill, high degree of attention to:
- pattern of muscle activation
- alignment or posture
- movement strategy

2. Associative phase of learning

- challenge control with increasing demand
- diversify skill to different contexts
- refine skill:
  - static and dynamic challenges
  - different physical and mental contexts
  - enhance capacity for physical performance—endurance training or strength training for high-intensity control

3. Automatic phase of learning

- attention demand reduced
- enhance versatility of skill:
  - integrate learned features into function
  - high performance training for the unexpected

and the relationship between specific features of motor control and symptoms or potential symptoms. On this basis, an exercise program is tailored to modify the specific features of posture or alignment, movement and muscle activation to optimise tissue loading, with a plan for progression of exercise towards improved function.

Training applies the same principles of motor learning used to develop any new skill, and involves a sequence of steps from initial learning of the movement components followed by progressions of increasing complexity and load. The initial step involves modifying the target features of motor control that have been identified in the assessment to be relevant for the patient's symptoms. This is generally achieved with cognitive training using the principles of motor learning (see Table 11.1).[29] This process progresses from initial optimisation of the target features of motor control using a combination of exercise and clinical strategies that are tailored to the individual, followed by increasing the challenge to consolidate and diversify the control, and finally, integration into function.

There is substantial evidence that the initial step of training should be specific to the identified problem (e.g. control of a specific alignment or muscle activation) and that cognitive training with attention to the task (feedback and understanding of the goal) leads to greater cortical changes than unskilled practice with load. The principles of segmentation (practice of the specific elements of a task that require change prior to integration into the complete task) and simplification (practice with reduced load, demand or complexity to enable high-quality performance of the trained element) are applied. A range of clinical techniques can be tailored to the individual to achieve the required change in motor performance (Table 11.2). The basic objective of the first phase is to identify a strategy the patient or athlete can employ to modify the feature of motor control that requires improvement, followed by practice.

Once the patient or athlete has learnt to change the feature of motor control that underpins the suboptimal loading, it is then necessary to progress the individual to be able to control these features with progressively challenging tasks. This associative phase of motor learning[29] aims to *refine* the skill, *diversify* the skill and increase the physical capacity.

Progression should include both static and dynamic exercises. Static progressions are very common and there are many examples of exercise approaches that fit this domain. The basic premise is that the alignment of the pelvis and spine is optimised and then maintained statically while load is applied through either the limbs or an external force. Threshold loads and asymmetries are identified and targeted with training. Typical examples are pilates exercises (e.g. reformer exercise with the pelvis and spine maintained statically as the limbs move to slide the body), leg loading tasks in supine, side-bridging, etc. Exercise difficulty is progressed by increasing the load, speed or task instability (e.g. less stable surfaces), and the ability to maintain control of the alignment is the cue to determining the task difficulty that can be tolerated.

Dynamic progressions are less commonly applied in typical exercise programs, but they are no less critical for learning optimal control of the spine and pelvis. Dynamic training involves loading the corrected motor control

Core stability — CHAPTER 11

Table 11.2 Clinical techniques to aid motor learning

Technique	Purpose	Examples
Instructions	Verbal instructions to highlight how a task is to be performed differently	'Roll forwards on tailbone'; 'gently flatten the lower abdomen'
Imagery	Mental image to help a patient understand the modification that is required	'Lengthen spine'
Manual guidance	Therapist's hands on the patient to guide performance for patient to experience optimal performance	Therapist's hands on superior edge of sacrum to guide anterior rotation of pelvis
Manual cues	Patient's hands placed on specific landmarks to provide feedback of optimal alignment or movement	Patient's hands on manubriosternal junction and pubic symphysis to guide upright trunk alignment
Dissociation tasks	Change relative motion between adjacent regions of body	Separate motion of the lumbar spine and pelvis from the thorax
Feedback	Provide information regarding accurate or inaccurate performance of task. Used to provide information of movement strategy, alignment and muscle activation	Visual—mirror; ultrasound imaging (muscle activation) Kinaesthetic—tactile/palpation (finger and thumb on xiphoid and navel to provide feedback of thoracolumbar alignment), tape (applied to the lumbar spine for feedback of alignment) Auditory/visual—EMG biofeedback of obliquus externus abdominis to reduce overactivity
Muscle activation	Modification of muscle activity to enable change in posture or movement	Palpation, observation, EMG biofeedback
Cues/reminders	Technique to remind a patient to modify performance	Tape applied to the lumbar spine that provides input to skin when the lumbar spine flexes
Manual therapy and connective tissue techniques	Modification of joint mobility, muscle activation, muscle tension	Manual therapy to the thoracic spine to reduce thoracic paraspinal muscle activity

feature during movement. As for static training, load is applied while the patient maintains some objective, which in this case is a specific feature of movement. Dynamic training can involve control of the spine as it moves, control of the spine as the whole body moves, or control of spine while the patient is supported on an unstable surface. Examples might include control of the lumbar lordosis during rotation of the spine, and maintaining spine alignment while using movement to balance on a balance board.

Progression to functional exercise and functional tasks is essential. Transfer of improved motor control strategies to the patient's function is best achieved the closer to the function the person practices. This may require segmenting and simplifying a complex function initially to enable correct or optimal performance of the improved skill as a component of the complex task, but should progress to practice of the complete task. It is also necessary to provide challenges–physical (load,

endurance), emotional (stress, fatigue) and environmental (e.g. predictable, unpredictable) to ensure the skill is diversified to address all contexts (Fig. 11.4). Functional training requires that the patient or athlete has learnt to perceive (proprioceptive awareness) the correct performance in order to correct errors. A final phase is to challenge patients to prepare them for high performance with higher load and unexpected challenges.

All patients need to progress through the basic sequence from initial correction of the relevant features of motor control to function, but some also require consideration of other issues to ensure optimal performance is achieved and to overcome potential barriers. For an individual patient this might include management of issues of control of adjacent joints (e.g. foot control problems that modify leg, pelvis, spine movement; scapulothoracic control), continence, breathing, balance, muscle strength and endurance, cardiovascular fitness, unhealthy beliefs and cognitions about pain and injury and so on. Identification of these issues may be apparent from subjective questioning, observation of movement and specific tests or questionnaires. Treatments may need to be tailored for these aspects and draw on the expertise of other professionals.

Motor learning requires permanence of the learnt motor function. Through practice and diversification, it is a key objective for the improved motor control strategy to be automatically applied in function. In situations of high demand, reinforcement through additional cognitive attention to the correction may be necessary. Development of a versatile and robust motor strategy requires practice and challenge.

Training of motor control for core stability for prevention of pain and injury

Although there is not yet sufficient high-quality evidence to support the assumption that the application of principles of motor control training can prevent pain and injury, it is plausible that identifying suboptimal features of posture or alignment, muscle activation and movement in an individual, and modifying those features with training, will help to prevent future development of pain. This is a topic of considerable interest and programs have been developed and applied with this in mind. The challenge is to identify suboptimal features that may be relevant for future development of pain or injury when provocation of symptoms is not available for confirmation that relevant features are identified. This approach depends on theoretical models that predict which features may be relevant and how they can be recognised. For athletic and sports performance this requires detailed understanding of optimal motor control for the specific sporting tasks. The approach of screening motor control for risk is strongly advocated by some.[26]

Considerations for training of motor control for core stability in athletes

Motor control of core stability is particularly relevant for athletes at all levels. The major issues that require specific consideration are:

1. the features of motor control required to complete the task (e.g. the specific combination of movements, postures and muscle activation), which may be highly refined for the completion of the sport-specific function
2. the features of the task that may promote suboptimal control
3. training load and demands required to maintain sporting or athletic performance. This demands that the clinician has expert knowledge of the sport being considered.

Running is an ideal example to illustrate the breadth of goals that are inherent in optimal core stability for an athlete. When running, it is essential to maintain upright posture relative to gravity, to maintain the relative alignment between adjacent segments, both large (body regions–thorax relative to lumbar spine relative to pelvis) and small (intervertebral segments); while moving the spine to transfer load between body regions, absorb reactive moments from foot contact, minimise energy expenditre, achieve progression of the body through space; and maintaining respiration, continence, balance and cardiovascular function.

Any perturbation to this system can disrupt the stability of the system (e.g. landing on the outside of the foot, an unexpected increase in respiratory demand, a modified muscle activation or movement strategy to avoid pain) and lead to interference with other elements in this delicate balance. A holistic view that considers the interaction between elements is necessary. For instance, a runner with low back pain may have augmented co-contraction of trunk muscles to protect the spine from provocation of pain, but this may then compromise the efficiency of the spine for shock absorption, load transfer and use of the chest wall motion to breathe. Detailed understanding of the mechanics of running (Chapter 8) is critical to identifying features that are suboptimal.

CONCLUSION

This chapter aimed to discuss the rationale for motor control training for core stability, to dispel some common myths and to provide an overview of the comprehensive program required to optimise motor control. It is critical to remember that core stability does not imply stiffness with a sole objective to restrict motion. Optimal control depends on a balance between movement and stiffness that is matched to the demands of the task. Motor control training must be matched to the presentation of the patient and to his or her functional demands.

REFERENCES

References for this chapter can be found at www.mhhe.com/au/CSM5e

Chapter 12

Preventing injury

with ROALD BAHR, BEN CLARSEN and GRETHE MYKLEBUST

An ounce of prevention is worth a pound of cure.
Benjamin Franklin (1706–1790)

An important role for the sports medicine clinician is to minimise activity-related injury, that is, to improve the benefit:risk ratio associated with physical activity and sport. The 2000s saw a remarkable acceleration in the focus on sports injury prevention. Fortunately, athletes can now benefit from the knowledge that interventions can prevent many major injuries, such as acute knee, ankle and hamstring injuries.

Sports injury prevention can be characterised as being 'primary', 'secondary' or 'tertiary'. In this book, we use the term 'prevention' synonymously with what is technically known as 'primary prevention'.[1] Examples of primary prevention include health promotion and injury prevention (e.g. ankle braces being worn by an entire team, even those without previous ankle sprain). Secondary prevention can be defined as early diagnosis and intervention to limit the development of disability or reduce the risk of re-injury. We refer to this as 'treatment' in this book (e.g. early treatment of an ankle sprain; see Chapter 17). Finally, tertiary prevention is the focus on rehabilitation to reduce and/or correct an existing disability attributed to an underlying disease. We refer to this as 'rehabilitation' (Chapter 18); in the case of a patient who has had an ankle sprain, this would refer to balance exercises and graduated return to sport after the initial treatment for the sprain.

The proactive clinician will give prevention advice during consultations where treatment is being sought. Health professionals working with teams will initiate injury prevention strategies, whether engaged in a traditional team sport like football, or working with a team of individual athletes such as in athletics or swimming. To guide this process, this chapter will introduce the concept of risk management,[2] which includes systematic injury surveillance, pre- and in-season strategy planning sessions with coaches, regular screening of athletes (see also Chapter 46), and the development of specific prevention programs for the team and for the individual athlete.

From there, this chapter will cover specific topics in injury prevention, including:

- prevention of hamstring strains, ankle sprains and acute knee injuries
- prevention of overuse injuries
- managing load to prevent injury
- protective equipment
- appropriate surfaces.

A CONCEPTUAL APPROACH TO INJURY PREVENTION

Willem van Mechelen et al. introduced the now classic conceptual model for research on sports injury prevention (Fig. 12.1).[3] This model can be successfully applied by sports medicine clinicians as well. First, identify the magnitude of the problem and describe it in terms of the incidence and severity of sports injuries. If you are responsible for a team, this involves recording all injuries within the squad, as well as training and match exposure. Second, identify the risk factors and injury mechanisms that play a part in causing these sports injuries. For the clinician, this involves systematic steps to examine the athletes, and their training and competition program (see below). The third step is to introduce measures that are likely to reduce the future risk and/or severity of sports injuries, based on the aetiologic factors and injury mechanisms identified in the second step. Finally, the

PART A Fundamental principles

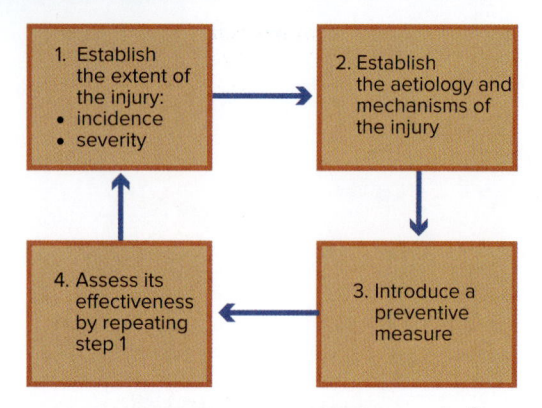

Figure 12.1 A conceptual model of injury causation[3]
FROM VAN MECHELEN ET AL

Diagram: 1. Establish the extent of the injury: incidence, severity → 2. Establish the aetiology and mechanisms of the injury → 3. Introduce a preventive measure → 4. Assess its effectiveness by repeating step 1 → (back to 1).

effect of the measures must be evaluated by repeating the first step. In the research setting, preventive programs are best evaluated using a randomised controlled trial design. For the clinician responsible for a team, continuous surveillance of the injury pattern within the team will reveal whether changes occur in the injury rate.

Clinicians wishing to prevent injuries in a systematic way could base their approach on the updated model by Meeuwisse et al. to describe the potential causative factors for injury.[4, 5] This conceptual model was also expanded by Bahr and Holme[6] and Bahr and Krosshaug[7] (Fig. 12.2). The model illustrates the multifactorial nature of sports injuries, emphasising the relationship of intrinsic and extrinsic risk factors to injury mechanisms.

First, it considers the intrinsic risk factors–factors which may predispose or protect the athlete from injury. This includes athlete characteristics such as age, maturation, gender, body composition and fitness level. One factor that consistently has been documented to be a significant predictor almost regardless of the injury type studied is previous injury. Intrinsic factors such as these interact to predispose to or protect from injury.

Intrinsic risk factors can be modifiable and non-modifiable, and both are important from a prevention point of view. Modifiable risk factors may be targeted for change (e.g. through specific training methods). Non-modifiable factors (such as sex) can be used to target intervention measures to those athletes who are at increased risk. An example of the clinical relevance of sex as a non-modifiable risk factor in sports injury prevention is the higher risk of injury to the anterior cruciate ligament (ACL) in female athletes compared with males. Female athletes are at up to six times greater risk for sustaining an ACL tear than their male counterparts in comparable team sports.[8]

The second group of risk factors is the extrinsic factors athletes are exposed to; for example, floor friction in indoor team sports, snow conditions in alpine skiing, a slippery surface (running track), very cold weather, or footwear. In the same way as intrinsic factors, extrinsic factors may increase risk (e.g. inappropriate footwear) or protect from injury (appropriate footwear). Exposure to such extrinsic risk factors may interact with the intrinsic factors to make the athlete more or less susceptible to injury.

When intrinsic and extrinsic risk factors act simultaneously, the athlete may be at far greater risk of injury than when risk factors are present in isolation. Note that risk factors–intrinsic (e.g. muscle strength) and extrinsic (e.g. weather conditions)–are usually not static, but change with time, and can even change during one training session (e.g. due to fatigue).

The inciting event

The final component in injury causation is the inciting event, which is usually referred to as the injury mechanism–what we see when watching an injury situation. Again, it may be helpful to use a comprehensive model to describe the inciting event, which accounts for the events leading to the injury situation (playing situation, player and opponent behaviour), as well as to include a description of whole body and joint biomechanics at the time of injury (Chapter 8).[7] Each injury type and each sport have their typical patterns, and for team medical staff it is important to consult the literature to reveal the typical injuries and their mechanisms for the sport in question. However, one limitation of the model is that it is not obvious how the team's training routine and competitive schedule can be taken into consideration as potential causes, and the model has therefore traditionally mainly been used to describe the causes of acute injuries. For overuse injuries, the inciting event is usually distant from the outcome. For example, for a stress fracture in a long-distance runner, the inciting event is not usually the single training session when pain became evident, but the training and competition program he or she has followed over the previous weeks or months.

RISK MANAGEMENT: APPLYING PREVENTION MODELS TO YOUR TEAM

For clinicians, the conceptual models can be adapted to identify potential causes of injury and develop a targeted prevention program. The key questions to ask are: What are the typical injuries? Who is at increased risk? Why? And how do injuries typically occur?

When caring for a defined group of athletes such as a football team or an alpine skiing team, this can be done using a systematic risk management approach.[2] This includes:

- reviewing the literature–what are the typical injuries patterns in the sport?

Preventing injury CHAPTER 12

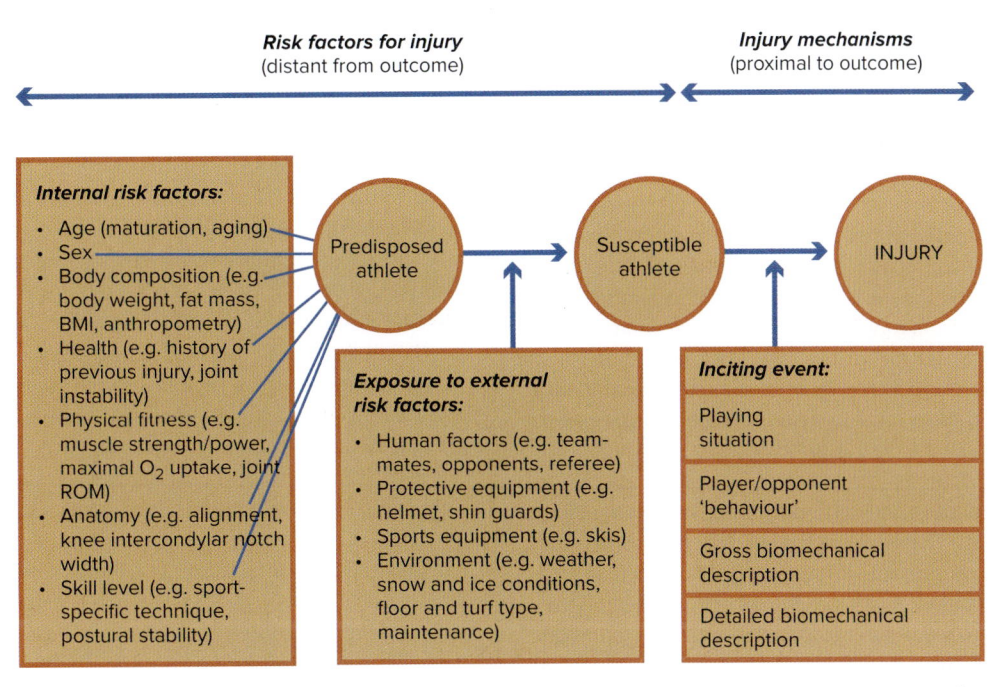

Figure 12.2 A comprehensive injury causation model based on the epidemiological model of Meeuwisse et al.[4] and modified by Bahr & Krosshaug.[7] BMI = body mass index; ROM = range of motion

- developing an injury surveillance program within the team—recording injury and participation data
- season analysis—risk profiling the training and competition program
- performing a periodic medical assessment—mapping current problems and intrinsic risk factors
- developing and initiating a targeted prevention program.

Reviewing the literature—risk identification and assessment

Each sport has its typical injury pattern. Just think of the names of some sports injuries: tennis elbow, runner's knee, jumper's knee. For most sports, there is ample data in the literature to identify and assess the risks. Note that injury risk is not just a question of injury frequency—the severity of injury must also be taken into account.

Injury data can be illustrated by a risk matrix that highlights risks in terms of likelihood and consequences. A risk matrix is a powerful tool for risk assessment. We derive the example shown in Figure 12.3 from soccer. It suggests that injury reductions in the areas of ACL, hamstring and ankle injuries are priorities. By further examining which factors contribute to the causation of these, we can formulate strategies to reduce injury rates. Therefore, in soccer it makes sense to target training programs to prevent ACL tears towards female athletes,

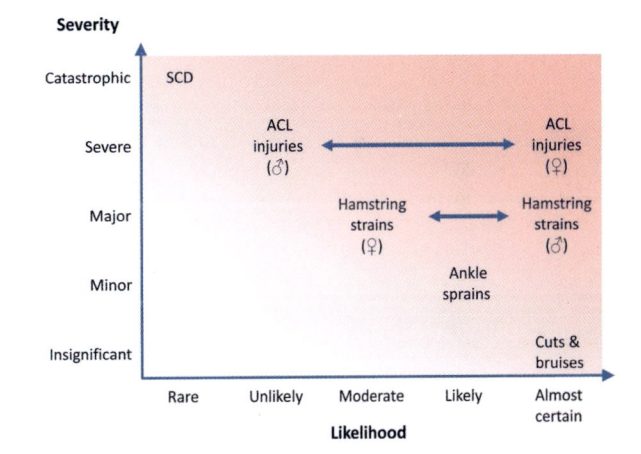

Figure 12.3 Qualitative risk matrix in elite soccer, illustrating the relationship between injury severity (consequence) and injury incidence (likelihood). The darker the colour, the greater the cross-product of severity and incidence, and the greater the priority should be given to prevention. The matrix also illustrates that risk differs between males and females. (SCD = sudden cardiac death)

while the lower risk among males may not justify such interventions. In contrast, a prevention program for male players should definitely focus on preventing hamstring strains.

167

Developing an injury surveillance program within the team

Although basing the risk assessment on data from the literature is valuable, it is necessary to establish a system to monitor injuries and exposure to assess risk within your own team. For medical staff, recording injuries is one of the easiest tasks in risk management as we are required to keep accurate records of all assessments and treatment provided to our patients. Thus, establishing a surveillance system simply involves analysing information that is already there. To make this task even easier, excellent electronic tools are available, with the necessary statistical tools integrated in software used to keep routine patient records.

Another task is to establish a system to record individual training and competition exposure within the team. This is a challenge for the medical team, since they are not always present during practices or on road trips. Therefore this task is often done by the coaching/fitness staff. Many of the injury-recording software programs also have the capability of recording exposure data, which can then be entered based on the coaching records. Exposure data is necessary to be able to calculate risk.

The standard method for calculating injury incidence typically used in team sports is the number of time-loss injuries per 1000 hours of exposure. For some sports and specific player positions (e.g. a baseball pitcher), injuries per pitch may be a more appropriate measure when identifying relationships between injury and exposure. It may also be relevant to record exposure in relation to extrinsic risk factors, such as turf type (e.g. training on grass, gravel, artificial turf), use of personal protective equipment, and whether the exposure is during competition or training.

Interpretation of injury data is difficult unless exposure data are collected. Consider the example where there is an increase of 30% in the number of match injuries from one season to the next. If the number of matches also increased by 30%, then there would be no increase in injury incidence.

A limitation with the standard methods for injury registration is that they substantially underestimate the true burden of overuse injuries due to a reliance on time-loss injury definitions. Overuse injuries represent the predominant injury type in sports that involve long, monotonous training sessions (e.g. cycling, swimming and long-distance running), as well as in technical sports that involve the repetition of similar movement patterns such as throwing or jumping. Symptoms such as pain or functional limitation most often appear gradually and may be transient in nature. Therefore it is likely that athletes will continue to train and compete despite the presence of overuse conditions, at least in the early phase. The same is the case for minor illness, such as the common cold.

Thus many health problems, especially overuse problems, do not lead to time loss from sport and are therefore not recorded in standard injury surveillance systems.[9] To address this limitation, Clarsen et al.[10,11] have developed the Oslo Sports Trauma Research Center (OSTRC) Questionnaire on Health Problems for prospective monitoring of all illness and injury, not just those leading to time loss from sports participation. This approach may be more appropriate for sports where overuse injuries and illnesses are expected to dominate.

Oslo Sports Trauma Research Center Questionnaire on Health Problems

The OSTRC Questionnaire on Health Problems is distributed to athletes once a week to record and monitor the consequences of any illnesses and injuries they have incurred, including those that do not lead to time loss from sport.[10] Ideally, it is delivered as an electronic questionnaire that directs athletes only to relevant questions, based on their responses.

The questionnaire begins with **four key questions** that all athletes should answer (Table 12.1). If they indicate a health problem in any of the questions (i.e. any response except the minimum value), they are then asked:

- whether they are referring to an illness or an injury
- to provide the location (for injuries) or the symptoms (for illnesses)
- to indicate the number of days of time loss the problem has caused in the past week
- whether they have received medical attention for the problem
- whether they have any more problems (in which case the questionnaire starts again).

In some teams and organisations, this weekly questionnaire can act as an important communication platform between athletes and sports medicine clinicians, particularly when athletes are geographically dispersed and/or have inconsistent contact with their team's medical staff. In these cases, it may be useful to add extra questions to the questionnaire such as 'who knows about this problem?' and 'do you have any comments for your team medical staff?'

Preventing injury CHAPTER 12

The severity of each reported problem is rated using the scoring system shown in Table 12.1. By adding the scores for Questions 1 to 4, a severity score out of 100 can be calculated. This score is tracked over time to give a reflection of the overall impact of the problem and of fluctuations in its severity (Fig. 12.4a). Summary data for the entire team can be collected (Fig. 12.4b).

Table 12.1 Oslo Sports Trauma Research Center Questionnaire on Health Problems

Participation	Severity score
Q1. Have you had any difficulties participating in normal training or competition due to injury, illness or other health problems during the past week?	
• Full participation without health problems	0
• Full participation, but with injury/illness	8
• Reduced participation due to injury/illness	17
• Cannot participate due to injury/illness	25
Training volume	
Q2. To what extent have you reduced your training volume due to injury, illness or other health problems during the past week?	
• No reduction	0
• To a minor extent	6
• To a moderate extent	13
• To a major extent	19
• Cannot participate at all	25
Performance	
Q3. To what extent has injury, illness or other health problems affected your sports performance during the past week?	
• No effect	0
• To a minor extent	6
• To a moderate extent	13
• To a major extent	19
• Cannot participate at all	25
Symptoms	
Q4. To what extent have you experienced symptoms/health complaints (e.g. pain, coughing, fever) during the past week?	
• No symptoms/health complaints	0
• To a minor extent	8
• To a moderate extent	17
• To a severe extent	25

continued

PART A   Fundamental principles

(a)

(b)

Figure 12.4 Example data from injury surveillance using the Oslo Sports Trauma Research Center (OSTRC) Questionnaire on Health Problems (a) Individual athlete data (b) Team data showing prevalence

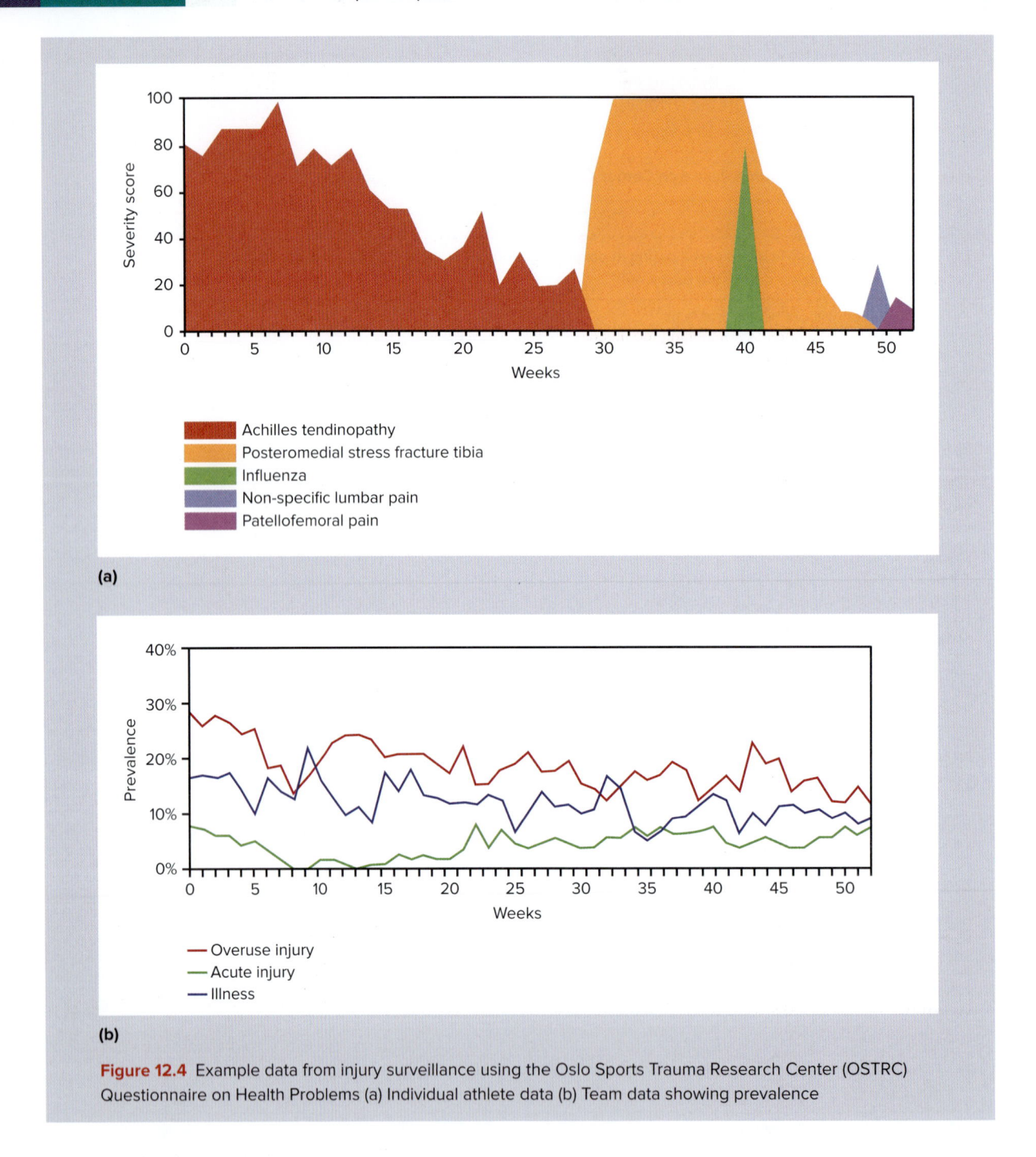

Season analysis—risk profiling the training and competition program

One helpful method to manage risk in sports is a pre-season review of the planned training and competition program to identify risks. The method of season analysis therefore is fundamentally different from injury surveillance, where data on injuries are collected as they happen. Season analysis represents an attempt to identify risks before they occur. Risks in the program can be related to the competition schedule, the training program, the possibilities for athlete recovery, travel or other issues.

Preventing injury   CHAPTER 12

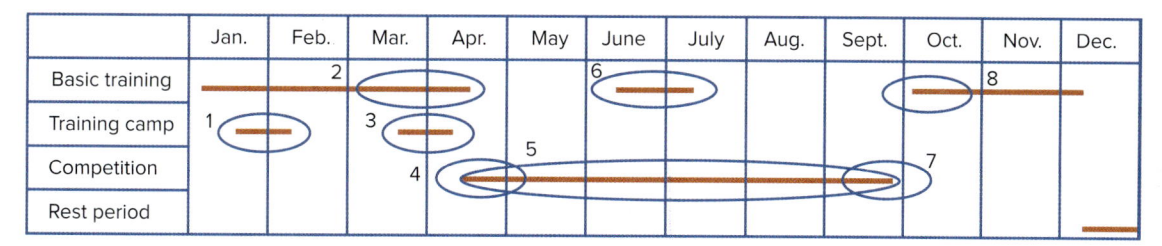

	Jan.	Feb.	Mar.	Apr.	May	June	July	Aug.	Sept.	Oct.	Nov.	Dec.
Basic training												
Training camp												
Competition												
Rest period												

Figure 12.5 Risk profile. Examples of periods of season when a college basketball team may be at particular risk of injury. The comments below concern the risk periods that are circled.

1. Change of time zone, off-court training surface, climate and altitude during training camp in Colorado. Emphasis on defensive stance training and quick lateral movements could lead to several groin injuries (Chapters 31 and 32). Athletes should not increase the amount or intensity of training too much.
2. Transition to greater amount of on-court training and intensity, combined with several practice games. Floor surface quite hard. Risk of lower limb injuries such as Achilles tendinopathy, medial tibial stress syndrome.
3. New training camp to fine-tune players before beginning the competitive season; practice games on unusually slippery courts. Competition to avoid being cut from the squad leads to increased intensity during training and competition.
4. The beginning of the competitive season. A higher tempo and a packed competitive schedule to which the athlete is unaccustomed. Risk of overuse injury (e.g. patellar tendinopathy, tibial stress fracture) compounded by heavy academic program leads to additional fatigue.
5. High risk of acute injuries during the competitive season, and a tough competition schedule at full intensity.
6. Interposed period of hard basic training, with strength exercises to which the athlete is not accustomed, and plyometric training increases risk of tendinopathy and muscle strain.
7. The end of the competitive season. Worn out and tired players? This is an important time to treat low-level 'grumbling' injuries aggressively. Waiting for the injury to heal with 'rest' alone is not recommended.
8. Transition to basic training period with running on trails.

The analysis is based on the idea that the risk of injuries is greater during transitional periods and that each stage has certain characteristics that may increase risk. Examples are when athletes switch from one training surface to another (e.g. from grass to gravel) or to new types of training (e.g. at the start of a strength training period). Figure 12.5 illustrates how a team may be at particular risk for different injury types at different stages of the season. Other examples of key events which could be correlated with increased injury risk include:

- poor sleep due to tight schedule or time differences
- changeover from heavy pre-season training to competition
- return to play after mid-season pause
- beginning of final rounds
- increased training and competition load associated with representative duties
- change of coach/manager with different training methods
- change in training volume
- change of climate (e.g. move from a training camp in a warm climate to a colder climate)
- selection time for important matches (e.g. representative schedule–a player may hide early symptoms of an injury, thinking this may prevent selection).

Although medical personnel responsible for teams or training groups may have to initiate this type of analysis, it is strongly recommended that the process be done in collaboration with the coaching team and, if at all possible, the athletes. Their inclusion will enable them to draw on their past experiences with the team, which is especially important if there are no injury surveillance data available from the past. If injury surveillance data are available, the season analysis is an opportunity to review past experiences formally, and discuss whether the injury patterns seen may be related to the training and competition program. For example, a surge in stress fractures in a soccer team may be attributed to a simultaneous increase in the volume of running and a change from a soft to a hard running surface. This type of analysis is an important basis for planning preventive measures, particularly to avoid overuse injuries. The risk profile usually varies from sport to sport, which underlines how important it is that medical staff be intimately familiar with the characteristics of the sport they cover.

The periodic medical assessment—mapping current problems and intrinsic risk factors

Periodic medical assessments (PMAs) are routinely performed on hundreds of thousands of athletes around the world every year, in some cases required by sports regulations or even by law.

PART A Fundamental principles

> **PRACTICE PEARL**
>
> The value of doing routine physical exams on athletes is questionable. If done properly, they can represent a key ingredient in the risk management program. If they are done simply to clear athletes for participation, their value in injury prevention is limited. Unfortunately, this is commonly the case.

Chapter 46 provides a detailed discussion of the many potential objectives of performing a PMA. In a prevention context, two of these are particularly relevant:

1. to identify current illnesses, injuries and chronic medical conditions
2. to identify factors that increase risk of future injury or illness.

While a PMA is often referred to as a pre-participation or pre-season examination, it is better performed at the end of the season, when there is still sufficient time for optimal treatment and rehabilitation of ongoing illness or injury and time to work on correcting any risk factors identified.

The factors included in the PMA should be tailored to the sport in question, by focusing on conditions known to be particularly prevalent (e.g. low back problems in rowers, eating disorders among female gymnasts, reduced pulmonary function among cross-country skiers), or where the physical requirements of the sport imply a higher risk of certain conditions (e.g. Marfan syndrome among basketball or volleyball players). However, if the purpose is to identify risk factors to predict future injury, the value of doing routine examinations alone is limited. For screening exams to serve a purpose in risk management, there are some additional requirements. First, the exam must be designed to identify athletes with risk factors relevant to the sport in question. Second, there must be a plan to follow up athletes with measures intended to reduce risk, if risk factors are identified. Third, the screening exam and follow-up must be planned and led by the medical and coaching staff of the team. Let us consider each of these requirements in turn.

1. Identify athletes with risk factors

The first requirement, that the exam be designed to identify athletes with risk factors relevant to the sport in question, is rarely met in current practice. In fact, in most cases the same screening exam is used across sports. This is inappropriate. There can be no single recipe for all sports, as injury patterns and risk factors differ significantly. To design a screening program for one particular sport, it is therefore necessary to define the key injury types (based on data from the literature on incidence and severity, and preferably also surveillance data as described earlier), and then to define the key risk factors (for these injuries). Based on this information, the screening exam can be tailored to the sport.

Even if the key risk factors have been defined, a key task remains–to select appropriate methods to screen for these risk factors. Screening methods should be valid, accurate, sensitive and specific. Valid means that the testing method measures the factor you wish to measure. For example, if low hamstring strength is a risk factor for muscle strains, what method should be used to measure this best? That the test is accurate (reliable), means that it will yield the same result each time. Finding valid and accurate tests to measure relevant risk factors is difficult.

However, to predict who may be at increased risk for injury is nearly impossible. A testing method with high sensitivity will identify all players with increased risk. A test with high specificity will identify only players with increased risk. Few, if any, tests exist which can clearly distinguish between athletes with high and low risk for a sports injury.[12] In fact, no tests exist which have high sensitivity *and* high specificity to predict future injury. Therefore, screening tests should be interpreted with caution.

2. Plan to follow up risk factors

The second requirement is that if the presence of a known injury risk factor is identified, an appropriate course of action can be taken to control the risk. If strength is inadequate, it should be followed up with a strength training program. If balance is poor, a training program should be designed and implemented to rectify this. This might be on an individual level, but in the absence of predictive screening tests, a team approach is probably more appropriate.

3. Medical and coaching staff of the team must be involved in screening and follow-up

In community-level sport, it may be tempting for a club or school to enlist the assistance of local sports medicine personnel to screen their athletes. This is only advisable if they can establish a mechanism to communicate the results to the team, and there are resources to follow up athletes with health problems or risk factors. Also, the specialist must be up to date with screening methods for the sport in question and their interpretation.

Developing and initiating a targeted prevention program

The final step in the risk management process is to assess the risks to the team and the individual athlete. The injuries (and illnesses) to be targeted are identified from the risk matrix (Fig. 12.3), the scientific literature and team injury surveillance data from past seasons. The season analysis may have identified specific risks associated with the training and competition program. Finally, the specific injury and risk profile for the individual athlete is mapped through the PMA. Based on this assessment, a prevention program targeting these risks should be developed for the team and for the individual athlete. The next sections provide examples of prevention programs targeting three acute sports injuries-hamstring strains, ankle sprains and acute knee injuries.

PREVENTING HAMSTRING STRAINS

Hamstring strains are frequent in sports involving maximal sprints and acceleration. Among sprinters, hamstring strains represent approximately one-third of all acute injuries.[13] In studies from professional sports, hamstring strains rank as the first or second most common injury in soccer,[14-17] Australian rules football,[18, 19] rugby union and league,[20, 21] and American football,[22, 23] accounting for one in every five to six injuries in most studies. There also seems to be a trend with a gradual increase in the proportion of hamstring strains compared to other injury types.[24, 25] Hamstring strain injuries are also common in dancing and waterskiing.[26]

Injury mechanisms

Hamstring strains most often occur during maximal sprints. It is difficult to document exactly at what time during the running cycle injuries occur.[27] However, since the net moment developed by the hamstrings is thought to be maximal in the late swing phase right before heel strike, this is thought to be a vulnerable position.[28, 29] In this instance, the hamstring muscles work eccentrically. Another suggestion is at push-off.

Risk factors

A number of risk factors have been proposed for hamstring strains, the most prominent being the following four intrinsic factors: age; previous injury; reduced hip range of motion (ROM); and poor hamstring strength.[6, 30] In theory, limited ROM for hip flexion could mean that muscle tension is at its maximum when the muscle is vulnerable close to maximum length. However, this hypothesis has yet to be confirmed, since there are several studies on soccer players suggesting that hamstring flexibility is not a risk factor for strains.[31, 32]

Low hamstring strength would mean that the forces necessary to resist knee flexion and initiate hip extension during maximal sprints could surpass the tolerance of the muscle-tendon unit. Hamstring strength is often expressed relative to quadriceps strength as the hamstrings:quadriceps ratio, since it is the relationship between the ability of the quadriceps to generate speed and the capacity of the hamstrings to resist the resulting forces that is believed to be critical. Several studies show that players with low hamstring strength or low hamstrings:quadriceps strength ratio or side-to-side strength imbalances may be at increased risk of injury.[6]

A history of previous hamstring strain greatly increases injury risk, as documented in numerous studies.[6, 33, 34] Injury can cause scar tissue to form in the musculature, resulting in a less compliant area with increased risk of injury. A previous injury can also lead to reduced ROM or reduced strength, thereby indirectly affecting injury risk. Soccer players with a history of previous hamstring injury have a 5-7 times higher risk of injury.

Older players are at increased risk for hamstring strains, and although older players will be more likely to have a previous injury, increased age is also an independent risk factor for injury.[32, 34]

Short fascicle length in the long head of the biceps femoris is an independent risk factor, especially when combined with low levels of eccentric knee flexor strength.[35] Notably, the greater risk of a future strain injury in older players or those with a previous hamstring injury is reduced when they have longer fascicles and high levels of eccentric strength.

It has been suggested that an indicator of susceptibility for the damage from eccentric exercise is the optimum angle for torque.[36] When this is at a short muscle length, the muscle is thought to be more prone to eccentric damage, but this theory has been challenged.[37]

Other risk factors, which have been suggested but are less well studied include race, sex, level of play, player position, improper running technique, superior running speed (peak performance), low back pain, increases or changes in the training program (particularly intense periods of training), insufficient warm-up and muscle fatigue. Players of African or Australian Aboriginal origin sustain significantly more hamstring strains than Caucasian players,[34] and it has been suggested that these players may be faster runners when compared to their Caucasian counterparts, possibly because of a higher proportion of type II muscle fibres. A faster running speed will generate higher hamstring torques, which may explain the increased injury risk.

Prevention programs

There are no intervention studies on elite athletes on the preventive effect of flexibility training on hamstring strains. However, one study on military basic trainees indicates a reduced number of lower limb overuse injuries after a period of hamstring stretching,[38] while another military-based study found no effect of stretching.[39] However, it should be noted that these studies were designed to examine the effect of general stretching on lower limb injuries in general, not a specific hamstring program on hamstring strain risk.

Questionnaire-based data on flexibility training methods collected from 30 English professional football clubs, where the stretching practices of the teams were correlated to their hamstring strain rates, indicate that using a standard stretching protocol reduces injury risk.[40] A study from Australian rules football has observed a

PART A Fundamental principles

reduction in the incidence of hamstring strains with a three-component prevention program, where stretching while fatigued was one of the components.[41] The other factors in the program were sport-specific training drills and high-intensity anaerobic interval training. Thus, it is not possible to determine which of these factors are responsible for the observed effect.

The best evidence for injury prevention is available for programs designed to increase hamstring strength, particularly eccentric hamstring strength. Some studies indicate that low hamstring strength may be a risk factor for sustaining hamstring strains,[31, 42, 43] particularly eccentric strength.[44, 45] EMG studies have shown that activity is highest late in the swing phase and during heel strike, when the hamstrings work eccentrically or transfer from eccentric to concentric muscle action.[29, 46] It is assumed that most hamstring strains occur during eccentric muscle actions, when the muscle activity is highest.[34, 35] It is well documented that strength training is mode specific.[47, 48] Based on this it may be argued that, to be specific, strength training for the hamstring muscles should be eccentric.

Recent studies from Scandinavia have shown that replacing the traditional hamstrings strength exercise used by teams–hamstring curls–with exercises to develop eccentric strength reduces the risk of hamstring strains.[14, 49] Traditional hamstring curls were ineffective in increasing eccentric hamstring strength among elite athletes.[50] In contrast, a simple partner exercise–the Nordic hamstring lower (Fig. 12.6)–improved eccentric strength.[50] A pilot study has also shown that using a special apparatus–the Yo-Yo™ flywheel ergometer–also increases eccentric hamstring strength.[51] Both of these methods prevented hamstring strains in studies on soccer players[14, 49-52] and rugby union players.[20]

Because it is easy to implement Nordic hamstring exercises in a team setting, we recommend this exercise as a specific tool to prevent hamstring injuries. However, to avoid delayed onset muscle soreness it is important to follow the recommended exercise prescription with

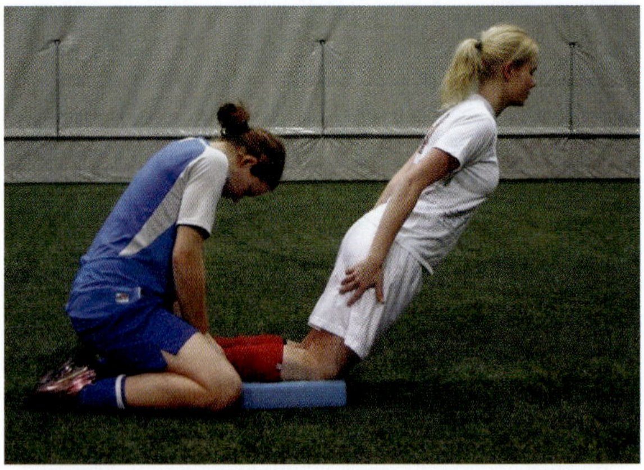

Figure 12.6 The Nordic hamstrings exercise. Subjects are instructed to let themselves fall forwards, and then resist the fall against the ground as long as possible by using their hamstrings

a gradual increase in training load when introducing a program of Nordic hamstring lowers (Table 12.2). By the end of a 10-week training period, many players are able to stop the downward motion completely before touching the ground (i.e. at about 30° of knee flexion), even after being pushed by their partners at a considerable speed. When a player can reach this stage, the characteristics of the Nordic hamstring lower exercise appear to resemble the typical injury situation: eccentric muscle action, high forces and near full-knee extension. The program has been implemented in several different sports and younger age groups, and injuries from the exercise itself have not been recorded.

PREVENTING ANKLE SPRAINS

with EVERT VERHAGEN

Ankle sprains are the most common injuries seen in sports and recreational activities. Nearly every fifth patient seen in the emergency room after sports-related injuries has

Table 12.2 Training protocol for Nordic hamstring exercises (see Fig. 12.6).[50] Load is increased as subject can withstand the forward fall longer. When managing to withstand the whole ROM for 12 reps, increase load by adding speed to the starting phase of the motion. The partner can also increase loading further by pushing at the back of shoulders

Week	Sessions per week	Sets and repetitions
1	1	2 × 5
2	2	2 × 6
3	3	3 × 6–8
4	3	3 × 8–10
5–10	3	3 × 12/10/8 reps

sustained an ankle sprain.[53] It has been estimated that there is one ankle sprain per 10 000 persons each day, which translates to approximately 10 million sprains every year in the United States alone.[54] It has been estimated that about 25% of all injuries across all sports are ankle injuries, and even more in some sports like volleyball, basketball and orienteering.[55-60]

Injury mechanisms

The typical injury mechanism is landing or stepping with the foot in an inverted position (i.e. plantarflexed, internally rotated and supinated). With the foot in this position, the ankle joint is inherently unstable. The posterior talar plafond is more narrow than the anterior portion, thereby reducing the bony stability of the ankle mortise when the foot is plantar flexed. Unless the dynamic musculotendinous ankle stabilisers can compensate for this reduced structural stability when the ankle joint is perturbed, the ligaments that statically stabilise the lateral ankle are acutely overloaded when the athlete puts weight on the inverted foot. In soccer, such perturbations often result from tackles, where the player receives a laterally directed hit on the medial side of the ankle or lower leg, whereupon landing in a supinated position leads to an inversion sprain.[55, 56] In volleyball and basketball, injuries often result from landing on the foot of an opponent or teammate.[57-59]

Risk factors

The most important risk factor that has been identified for ankle sprains is a previous ankle injury in the past 12–24 months. In fact, research has shown that among adult athletes, four out of five ankle sprains occur in previously injured ankles.[59, 61, 62] Compared to an ankle with no prior injury, the risk of injury is fourfold greater for an ankle that has been sprained one or more times.[57] Furthermore, the more recent the injury, the higher the risk. The injury rate during the first 6–12 months after an ankle sprain is nearly tenfold higher than for an ankle without previous injury. Following an ankle sprain, the proprioceptive system of the ankle is affected, hampering the stability and sense of movement of the ankle joint. This subsequently leads to more inverted positions upon landing from a jump or stride, as well as lesser control over the dynamic musculotendinous ankle stabilisers to counteract perturbations, leading up to a higher chance of subsequent injury in equal situations.[63, 64]

Postural sway is closely linked to a previous ankle sprain occurrence.[65] Postural sway is generally characterised in a practical approach that involves measurements of the duration of time that a subject can maintain a single-leg stance without touching down to recover balance. Athletes who are able to maintain a single-leg stance for at least 15 seconds are considered to have normal posture, while those that touchdown to regain balance within the 15-second test are considered to have abnormal posture. Athletes with abnormal posture are more likely to suffer ankle sprains.

A number of other risk factors have been suggested to be associated with an increased injury risk, such as sex, height and weight, limb dominance, foot type, foot size, anatomic alignment of the lower extremity, ankle ROM, ankle and generalised joint laxity, and muscle strength. However, the relationship between these factors and injury risk appears to be weak.[65]

Prevention programs

There is strong evidence that taping or bracing should be recommended for a period of up to 12 months after an ankle sprain, when risk of injury is increased several times.[66] The mechanism by which such ankle orthoses are thought to work is not known with certainty, but may involve simply enhancing the athlete's proprioceptive awareness of the ankle joint. This view is corroborated by the fact that the preventive effect of braces is limited to players with previous injury, where proprioceptive function is reduced.[67-70] In addition, orthoses do not seem to restrict ankle inversion enough to explain their prophylactic effect on ankle sprain incidence. If the protective effect were purely mechanical, one would expect an effect in healthy, previously uninjured ankles as well. The latter has been shown in basketball, but this finding remains to be confirmed in additional research.[71] Many different ankle supports are commercially available.

Ankle taping restricts inversion motion, although it appears that ankle supports are superior to ankle taping since ankle supports do not lose their ability to restrict inversion, while tape does 'loosen up' after several repeated cycles of vertical jumping. Unlike semi-rigid orthoses, the effectiveness of ankle taping has not been tested in randomised controlled trials, but if the effect is mainly through enhancement of proprioception, there is no reason to expect taping has less preventive effect than orthoses. Other factors, such as cost and skin care, should also be considered in the choice between tape and orthoses. Finally, there is no evidence that wearing an ankle orthosis increases the incidence of knee injuries, and most studies suggest that semi-rigid orthoses do not significantly impair athletic performance.[72]

Tropp et al.[68] and others[69, 70] have shown that proprioceptive function is reduced in athletes who complain of a feeling of persistent instability following an ankle sprain. Sensorimotor control of the affected ankle joint is impaired in the immediate recovery period following an acute sprain,[63, 64] but studies have shown that this function can

PART A Fundamental principles

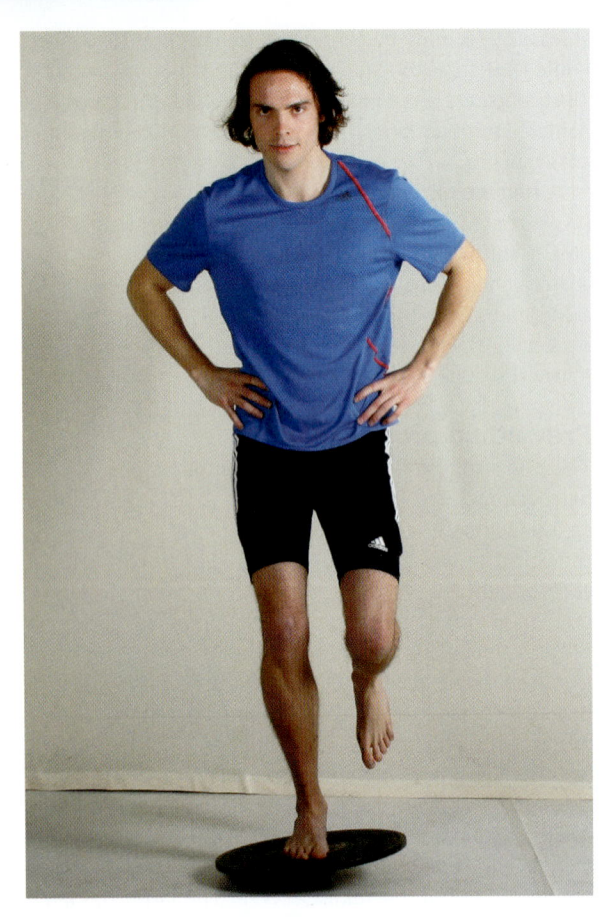

Figure 12.7 Balance board training

be restored through a balance board training program.[73-75] In these studies, proprioceptive function was quantified by measuring the reaction time to a sudden inversion strain, or the degree of postural sway during a one-legged balance test. It should be noted that the use of the term proprioceptive function, which is defined as the function of the afferent components only, may be inappropriate in this context. The ability to react to a sudden inversion stimulus or balance on one leg clearly depends on both sensory and motor function, and should perhaps therefore be termed sensori-motor control.

The preventive effect of balance and sensorimotor exercise has been well described in the literature.[66, 76] A balance board training program has been shown to reduce the risk of re-injury in functionally unstable ankles in soccer players.[68] This basic program consists of balance exercises on one leg on a disc (Fig. 12.7). Over the years, this basic program has evolved into a variety of sports-specific multifaceted sensorimotor training programs that involve more types of exercises than one-legged balance exercises alone. In a one-season randomised trial, for example, balance exercises were introduced as part of the regular warm-up

for high-level recreational volleyball players.[77] Ankle sprain incidence was reduced by 60% among players who reported a history of previous injury. Other effective examples can be found for other sports including soccer,[78] handball,[79] basketball[80] and American football.[81]

The specific preventive effect of sensorimotor training has also been studied as part of the rehabilitation process after an initial ankle sprain. This yielded positive results not only for the prevention of secondary injury,[82] but also for other complaints that may persist or develop after the initial ankle injury, such as pain and instability.[74] Consequently, clinical care guidelines advocate the application of sensorimotor training within or straight after the rehabilitation phase after an ankle sprain.[83]

The exact intensity and duration of the program depends on the individual patient and the severity of the initial ankle sprain.

> **PRACTICE PEARL**
>
> It appears reasonable to recommend a program of 10–20 minutes of balance board training five times a week over 10–12 weeks for all athletes with a history of ankle sprain (Fig. 12.7).

In other words, taping, bracing and neuromuscular training are all effective for the prevention of ankle sprain recurrences. Although preventive effects have been reported in a general athletic population, evidence suggests this overall effect is due to a strong preventive effect in previously injured athletes (tertiary prevention) and that any effect on fresh ankle sprains (primary prevention) is either non-existent or very low.

The next question is then: which measure should be preferred for the prevention of ankle sprain recurrences? Naturally, the answer is that the method the athlete prefers will achieve the best results. After all, this is the measure that the athlete is most likely to use. However, a combination of an extrinsic prophylactic measure (tape or brace) with neuromuscular training will probably achieve the best preventive outcomes with minimal burden for the athlete (Fig. 12.8).

The preventive potential of combining bracing/taping with balance training lies in the different pathways through which these measures achieve their preventive effect. Extrinsic measures provide immediate protection, but only when worn, as they only provide support for a previously injured ankle and do not target the underlying neuromuscular impairment. Neuromuscular training targets the underlying risk-increasing pathology, but it takes some time before a preventive effect is established. When extrinsic measures are employed during the period of neuromuscular training, the patient benefits

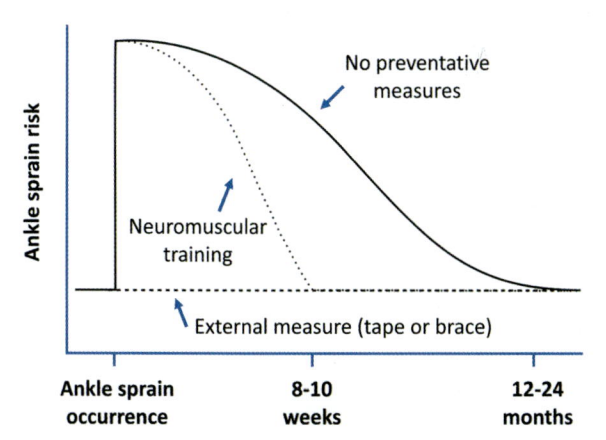

Figure 12.8 Conceptual illustration of optimal ankle re-injury prevention program[66]

from an immediate risk-reducing effect while targeting the underlying causes of an increased recurrence risk.

PREVENTING ACUTE KNEE INJURIES

Preventing major knee injuries such as ACL ruptures should be a priority in many sports, especially those characterised by pivoting movements, sudden changes of direction, and accelerations and decelerations. ACL ruptures are one of the most common types of serious sports injury. For example, a typical elite-level female soccer team can expect one ACL injury every season.[84] Due to the costly treatment, long rehabilitation time and increased risk of osteoarthritis associated with ACL injuries, they have received a great deal of attention in sports injury prevention research. Much of the research is also relevant to other types of traumatic knee injuries.

Injury mechanisms

Approximately 70% of ACL injuries occur in non-contact situations, often during a cutting manoeuvre or a single-leg landing after a jump.[85] Cutting or sidestep manoeuvres are associated with dramatic increases in the varus–valgus and internal rotation moments, as well as deceleration.

The typical ACL injury occurs with the knee externally rotated and in 10–30° of flexion when the knee is placed in a valgus position as the athlete takes off from the planted foot and rotates their upper body with the aim of suddenly changing direction. ACL injury mechanisms are discussed in detail in Chapter 35.

Risk factors

The most important intrinsic risk factor for ACL injury is sex, with studies in soccer, basketball, handball and wrestling showing that females have a 2–4 times increased risk compared to their male counterparts.[86, 87] The reasons for this are not completely clear. Various researchers have suggested differences in anatomy, and in hormonal and neuromuscular function as potential reasons for the higher injury risk in females. To date, however, there is little evidence linking all these potential intrinsic risk factors to non-contact ACL injuries, and a great deal of controversy exists on the relative importance of the different factors.[88] Recent studies also suggest that a history of knee ligament injury is a predominant risk factor for a subsequent injury, such as a re-rupture of the ACL graft, an ACL rupture to the contralateral knee, or another severe knee injury.[33, 89]

An extrinsic risk factor for ACL injury in handball and Australian rules football is high friction between shoes and the playing surface. This can cause the foot to stop abruptly during a cutting or turning manoeuvre, increasing stress on the knee.[90, 91] The relationship between playing surfaces and injury risk is discussed at the end of this chapter.

Prevention programs

There is strong evidence that acute knee injuries can be reduced by 25–50% using structured exercise programs targeting strength, balance and neuromuscular control.[92-96] A number of prevention programs are available, all of which are designed to be performed as a structured warm-up prior to training and matches aiming to:

- alter the quality of the movement in the lower limb
- increase core and lower limb stability
- raise awareness of knee position in relation to the foot
- emphasise alignment of the hip, knee and foot in all exercises.

The primary goal of this strategy is to engrain 'safe' movement patterns and discourage those believed to place the knee at high risk of injury (such as hip adduction/knee valgus).

A recent meta-analysis of nine randomised controlled trials investigating injury prevention programs in soccer players demonstrated an overall positive effect in reducing knee injuries in general (26% reduced risk) and a non-significant trend in reducing ACL injuries in particular.[97] Another meta-analysis, which included randomised and non-randomised trials in a range of sports, found a significant effect of prevention programs in reducing ACL injuries (17% reduced risk). This meta-analysis recommended that for best effect, programs should be aimed at younger athletes, performed for longer than 20 minutes duration, a minimum of twice per week, and include exercise variations and verbal feedback.[98]

Although the International Federation of Association Football (FIFA) 11+ was developed for soccer players, similar multifaceted warm-up programs exist for other sports such as floorball and handball and the same concept can be applied to other sports settings as well.[93, 100]

PART A Fundamental principles

11+ A complete warm-up program
with MARIO BIZZINI, ASTRID JUNGE and JIRI DVOŘÁK

The '11+' injury prevention program was developed by an international group of experts for the International Federation of Association Football (FIFA). It is a good example of a multifaceted 20-minute warm-up program that includes core stability, balance, strength and running exercises (Fig. 12.9). Youth football teams using 11+ as a standard warm-up had a significantly lower risk of injuries than teams who warmed up as usual. Teams that performed the 11+ at least twice per week had 37% fewer training injuries and 29% fewer match injuries.[95, 99]

The FIFA 11+ has three parts: Part 1 consists of running exercises at a slow speed combined with active stretching,

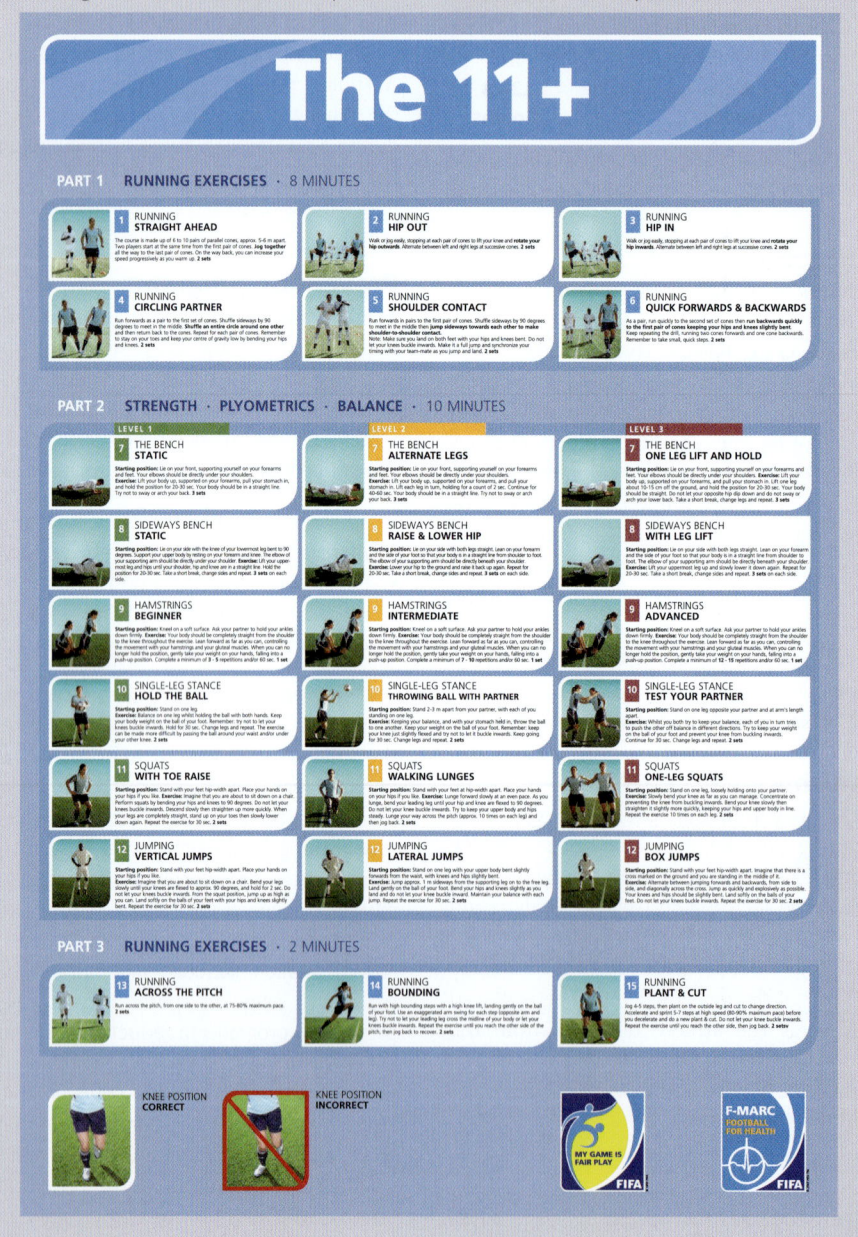

Figure 12.9 The FIFA 11+ poster can be downloaded for free from http://f-marc.com/fifa-11-plus/. It is available in nine languages and is provided to clubs free of charge

Preventing injury   CHAPTER 12

and controlled partner contacts; Part 2 consists of six sets of exercises, focusing on core and leg strength, balance and plyometrics/agility, each with three levels of increasing difficulty; and Part 3 consists of running exercises at moderate/high speed combined with planting/cutting movements.

The field set-up course is made up of six pairs of parallel cones, approximately 5–6 m apart. Two players start at the same time from the first pair of cones, jog along the inside of the cones and do the various exercises on the way. After the last cone, they run back along the outside. On the way back, speed can be increased progressively as players warm up.

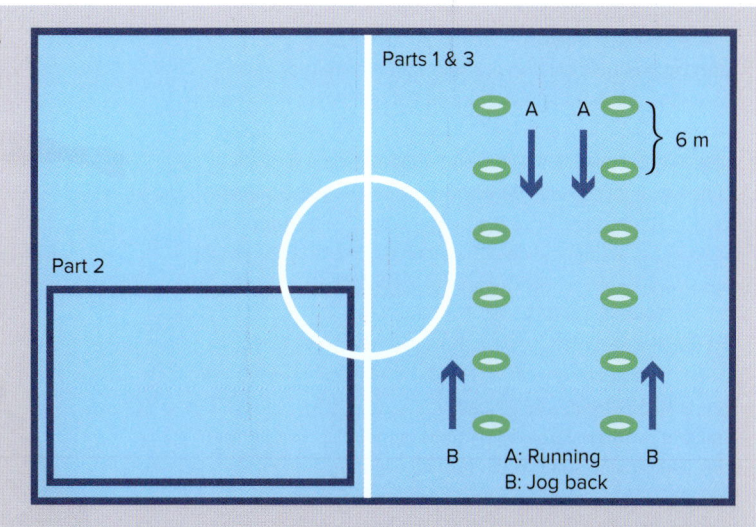

PART 1: RUNNING EXERCISES

1 RUNNING—STRAIGHT AHEAD
Jog straight to the last cone. Make sure you keep your upper body straight and your hip, knee and foot aligned. Do not let your knee buckle inwards. Run slightly more quickly on the way back. 2 sets.

2 RUNNING—HIP OUT
Jog to the first cone, stop and lift your knee forwards. Rotate your knee to the side and put your foot down. At the next cone repeat the exercise on the other leg. Repeat until you reach the other side of the pitch. 2 sets.

3 RUNNING—HIP IN
Jog to the first cone, stop and lift your knee to the side. Rotate your knee forwards and put your foot down. At the next cone repeat the exercise on the other leg. Repeat until you reach the other side of the pitch. 2 sets.

4 RUNNING—CIRCLING PARTNER
Jog to the first cone. Shuffle sideways towards your partner, shuffle an entire circle around one another (without changing the direction you are looking in), then shuffle back to the first cone. Repeat until you reach the other side of the pitch. 2 sets.

5 RUNNING—JUMPING WITH SHOULDER CONTACT
Jog to the first cone. Shuffle sideways towards your partner. In the middle, jump sideways towards each other to make shoulder-to-shoulder contact. Land on both feet with your hips and knees bent. Shuffle back to the first cone. Repeat until you reach the other side of the pitch. 2 sets.

6 RUNNING—QUICK FORWARD AND BACKWARD SPRINTS
Run quickly to the second cone then run backwards quickly to the first cone, keeping your hips and knees slightly bent. Repeat, running two cones forwards and one cone backwards until you reach the other side of the pitch. 2 sets.

PART 2: STRENGTH, PLYOMETRICS, BALANCE

All exercises have three levels of increasing difficulty.

Players should begin with level 1, which is presented here. Levels 2 and 3 of exercises 7–12 are presented on www.fifa.com/medical and videos are available in the free mobile application GET SET—Train Smarter.

Only when an exercise can be performed without difficulty for the specified duration and number of repetitions should the player progress to the next level.

7.1 THE BENCH—STATIC
Starting position: Lie on your front, support your upper body with your forearms, elbows directly under your shoulders.
Exercise: Lift up your upper body, pelvis and legs until your body is in a straight line from head to foot. Pull in stomach and gluteal muscles and hold the position for 20–30 seconds. 3 sets. **Important:** Do not sway or arch your back. Do not move your buttocks upwards.
7.2 ALTERNATE LEGS
7.3 ONE LEG LIFT AND HOLD

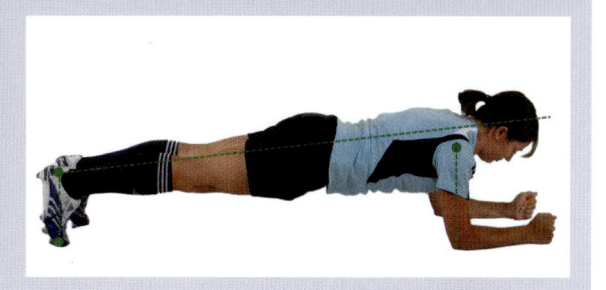

continued

179

PART A   Fundamental principles

8.1 SIDEWAYS BENCH—STATIC
Starting position: Lie on your side with the knee of your lowermost leg bent to 90°. Support yourself on your forearm and lowermost leg, elbow of supporting arm directly under shoulder. **Exercise:** Lift pelvis and uppermost leg until they form a straight line with your shoulder and hold the position for 20–30 seconds. Repeat on other side. 3 sets. **Important:** Keep pelvis stable and do not let it tilt downwards. Do not tilt shoulders, pelvis or leg forwards or backwards.
8.2 RAISE AND LOWER HIP
8.3 WITH LEG LIFT

9.1 HAMSTRINGS—BEGINNER
Starting position: Kneel with knees hip-width apart; partner pins your ankles firmly to the ground with both hands. **Exercise:** Slowly lean forwards, while keeping your body straight from the head to the knees. When you can no longer hold the position, gently take your weight on your hands, falling into a press-up position. 3–5 repetitions. **Important:** Do exercise slowly at first, but speed up once you feel more comfortable.
9.2 INTERMEDIATE
9.3 ADVANCED

10.1 SINGLE-LEG STANCE—HOLD THE BALL
Starting position: Stand on one leg, knee and hip slightly bent and hold the ball in both hands. **Exercise:** Hold balance and keep body weight on the ball of your foot. Hold for 30 seconds, repeat on the other leg. Exercise can be made more difficult by lifting the heel from the ground slightly or passing the ball around your waist and/or under your other knee. 2 sets on each leg. **Important:** Do not let your knee buckle inwards. Keep your pelvis horizontal and do not let it tilt to the side.
10.2 THROWING BALL WITH PARTNER
10.3 TEST YOUR PARTNER

11.1 SQUATS WITH TOE RAISE
Starting position: Stand with feet hip-width apart, hands on your hips. **Exercise:** Slowly bend hips, knees and ankles until your knees are flexed to 90°. Lean upper body forwards. Straighten upper body, hips and knees and stand up on your toes. Slowly lower down again, and straighten up slightly more quickly. Repeat for 30 seconds. 2 sets. **Important:** Do not let your knee buckle inwards. Lean upper body forwards with a straight back.
11.2 WALKING LUNGES
11.3 LEG SQUATS

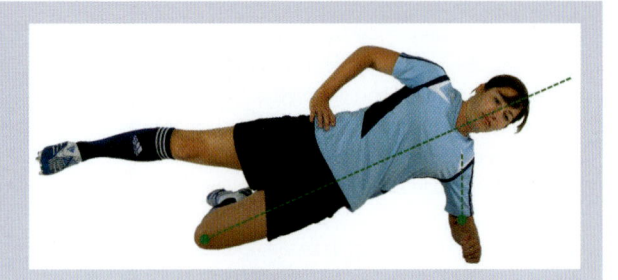

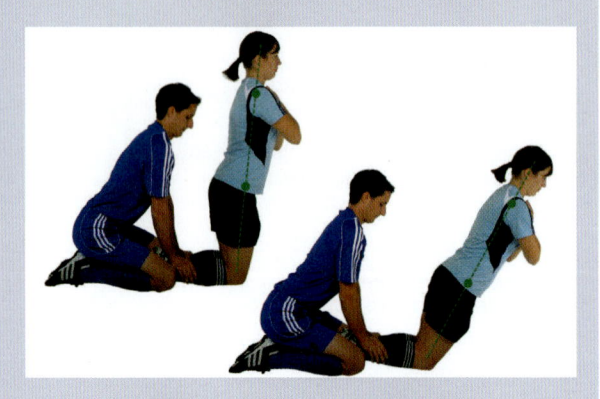

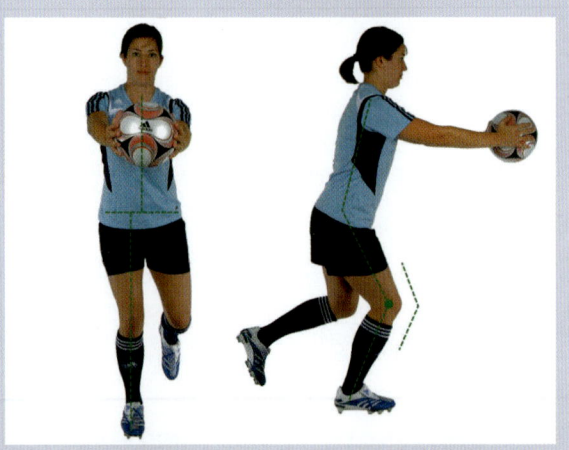

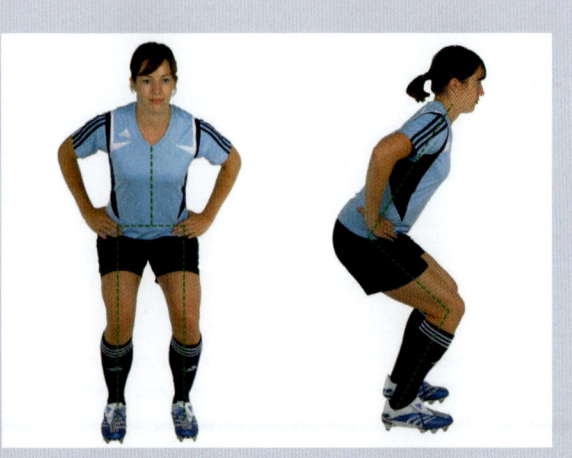

Preventing injury CHAPTER 12

12.1 JUMPING—VERTICAL JUMPS
Starting position: Stand with your feet hip-width apart, hands on your hips. **Exercise:** Slowly bend hips, knees and ankles until your knees are flexed to 90°. Lean upper body forwards. Hold this position for 1 second, then jump as high as you can, and straighten whole body. Land softly on the balls of your feet. Repeat for 30 seconds. 2 sets. **Important:** Jump off both feet. Land gently on the balls of both feet with your knees bent.

12.2 LATERAL JUMPS
12.3 BOX JUMPS

PART 3: RUNNING EXERCISES
13 RUNNING—ACROSS THE PITCH
Run approximately 40 m across the pitch at 75–80% of maximum pace, then jog the rest of the way. Keep your upper body straight. Your hip, knee and foot are aligned. Do not let your knees buckle inwards. Jog easily back. 2 sets.

14 RUNNING—BOUNDING
Take a few warm-up steps then take 6–8 high bounding steps with a high knee lift and then jog the rest of the way. Lift the knee of the leading leg as high as possible and swing the opposite arm across the body. Keep your upper body straight. Land on the ball of the foot with the knee bent and spring. Do not let your knee buckle inwards. Jog back easily to recover. 2 sets.

15 RUNNING—PLANT AND CUT
Jog 4–5 steps straight ahead. Then plant on the right leg and cut to change direction to the left and accelerate again. Sprint 5–7 steps (80–90% of maximum pace) before you decelerate and plant on the left foot and cut to change direction to the right. Do not let your knee buckle inwards. Repeat the exercise until you reach the other side of the pitch, then jog back. 2 sets.

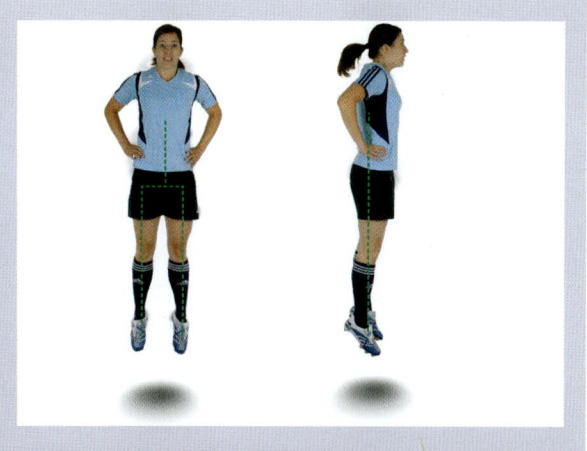

> **PRACTICE PEARL**
>
> The key point of the program is to use the proper technique during all exercises. Pay close attention to correct posture and body control, including straight-leg alignment, knee-over-toe position and soft landings. The FIFA 11+ should be completed as a complete warm-up at least 2–3 times per week; it should take approximately 20 minutes to complete.

See the instructional video of each exercise on http://f-marc.com/fifa-11-plus/. The FIFA 11+ poster can be downloaded for free. It is available in nine languages and is provided to clubs free of charge.

PREVENTING OVERUSE INJURIES
Overuse injuries are the predominant injury type in sports involving long, monotonous training sessions such as cycling, swimming and running, as well as in technical sports that involve the repetition of similar movement patterns such as throwing, jumping and kicking.[11] They occur among athletes of all levels, particularly in elite athletes and young, dedicated athletes whose total training and competition load increases rapidly.[101]

Although a majority of sports injury prevention research has focused on acute injuries, evidence for overuse injury prevention is increasing.[102] Similar to acute injuries, prevention strategies for overuse injuries can target modifiable intrinsic risk factors such as flexibility, strength and neuromuscular control, as well as extrinsic risk factors such as shoes or sports equipment. As the 'inciting event' for overuse injuries is cumulative tissue overload that occurs over time, close monitoring of athletes' training and competition loads may be a particularly effective prevention strategy. There is also an opportunity for secondary prevention of overuse injuries via early identification and rapid initiation of appropriate treatment.

Stretching
Although stretching has long been promoted as an injury prevention method, recent systematic reviews conclude that there is no evidence to support its efficacy.[103-105] However, targeted stretching of glenohumeral joint

internal rotation remains a popular prevention strategy in throwing athletes, and formed one part of a multimodal training program shown to reduce the rate of overuse shoulder injuries in elite handball players.[106]

Structured training programs

As discussed previously in this chapter, there is strong evidence that structured multimodal training programs targeting muscle strength and neuromuscular control (such as the FIFA 11+) are effective in preventing acute lower limb injuries in team sports. This approach has also been shown to be effective in preventing lower limb overuse injuries,[93, 95, 107] particularly among adolescent athletes whose risk of overuse injury is almost halved by completing injury prevention programs.[103]

> **PRACTICE PEARL**
>
> Structured warm-up programs consisting of strength and neuromuscular control exercises have been shown to halve the rate of lower limb overuse injuries among adolescent athletes.

These promising results have not been consistently replicated in adult populations. A number of studies have failed to show an effect of general or targeted prevention training on lower limb overuse injuries among amateur athletes, professional athletes and military recruits.[78, 108-112] For example, a study of 209 professional soccer players found that eccentric training programs commonly used to treat Achilles and patellar tendinopathy were ineffective when used as an across-the-board prevention strategy.[112] However, one randomised controlled trial found that patellofemoral pain could be prevented among military recruits using a daily exercise program consisting of gluteal and quadriceps strengthening exercises and lower limb stretching exercises.[113] Similarly, a recent randomised trial found that a 10-minute warm-up program consisting of glenohumeral internal rotation stretching, rotator cuff strengthening and scapular stability exercises reduced the prevalence of shoulder injuries among elite-level handball players.[106] Research in this field is ongoing.

Technique modification

Ensuring optimal sporting technique is likely to be an effective way of preventing overuse injuries, particularly in sports involving repetitive loading patterns. For example, runners should avoid excessive contralateral hip drop to prevent lower limb injuries and lower back pain (Chapter 8), and tennis players should aim for double-handed backhand shots to prevent 'tennis elbow' (Chapter 9). Further examples of sport-specific technique errors linked to injury are covered in Chapter 9.

Nutritional strategies to prevent stress fractures

Inadequate levels of calcium and vitamin D, which play an essential role in bone mineralisation, homeostasis and remodelling, are thought to be risk factors for stress fractures (Chapter 4).[114] This may be a particular problem in individuals with inadequate dietary intake or with limited sunlight exposure (due to geographical or cultural reasons), dark skin, or medical conditions that interfere with fat absorption (such as Crohn's disease).[115]

A randomised controlled trial involving female military recruits found that daily supplementation with 100 mg calcium and 800 IU vitamin D reduced the incidence of stress fractures by 20%.[116] This finding is supported by cohort studies of athletes which have shown that high dietary intake of calcium and of vitamin D are associated with lower stress fracture risk.[117, 118] For example, one study of female endurance runners found that for every cup of skim milk consumed per day, the risk of stress fractures was reduced by 63%.[117]

According to current recommendations, 1000 to 1200 mg of calcium per day is required for optimising bone health. Although there is debate regarding optimal vitamin D status, serum 25-hydroxy vitamin D levels should be at least 50 nmol/mL and should ideally be between 90 and 100 nmol/mL.[115] The current recommended daily intake of vitamin D is 600 to 800 IU; however, individual needs may vary according to many factors including sun exposure, and some suggest that up to 2000 IU is indicated in high-risk groups.[115]

It should be noted that bisphosphonates (osteoclast inhibitors), which are commonly used in the treatment of osteoporosis and which may be useful in the treatment of stress fractures,[114, 119] are not effective in preventing bone stress injuries.[120]

Modifying extrinsic risk factors

In certain sports, injuries are commonly attributed to extrinsic factors such as shoes, insoles and sporting equipment. The extent to which these factors play a role in injury prevention remains a source of much debate.

Shoe selection

Individual prescription of different shoe types (such as cushioning, motion control and stability shoes) based on static foot alignment is commonly promoted as an injury prevention method, particularly among shoe retailers.[121] However, a recent meta-analysis of randomised controlled trials suggests that this approach does little to prevent injuries.[122] In several large trials conducted on military recruits, individualised prescription of shoe type was compared to all subjects receiving a stability shoe.[123-125] No studies were able to demonstrate a difference in the incidence of overuse injuries between groups.

Barefoot/minimalist running

It has been proposed that running barefoot or in 'minimalist' shoes designed to replicate barefoot running may prevent lower limb overuse injuries.[126, 127] This is because several of the common biomechanical differences seen in barefoot running, such as reduced peak ground reaction forces and increased ankle plantarflexion and knee flexion at foot strike (Chapter 8),[128] are theoretically protective against some injury types. However, this may be an over-simplification of a complex relationship. Although the loads on some structures such as the knee and hip joints may be reduced in barefoot running, other structures such as the forefoot, ankle, Achilles tendon and calf muscles experience increased loading and may be at greater risk of injury. Also, certain individuals fail to adapt their running technique and experience *increased* vertical ground reaction forces when barefoot running.

There is currently no evidence that barefoot or minimalist-shoe running is an effective prevention intervention.[129] In fact, one study which randomly assigned normal (neutral), partial-minimalist and full-minimalist shoes to 103 runners found that the groups using minimalist shoes had injury rates up to three times higher than those in normal neutral shoes.[130] The use of barefoot or minimalist shoes is therefore likely to have more value as a targeted strategy in the management of certain types of running injuries (as discussed in Chapter 8) than as a generalised injury prevention intervention.

Orthotic insoles

The preventive effects of prefabricated and custom-made orthotic insoles have been investigated in 10 different studies of military personnel, including a total of 4788 subjects.[105] Seven studies found that insoles had a significant preventive effect for a range of lower limb overuse conditions, such as stress fractures, medial tibial stress syndrome, patellofemoral pain and Achilles tendinopathy. Based on these findings, several high-quality meta-analyses have supported the use of orthotic insoles for injury prevention.[104, 105, 131] However, the effects of orthotic insoles in athletes remain unknown, and the exact mechanism by which they prevent injury remains contentious.[131]

Sports equipment

Careful selection of sports equipment may play an important role in overuse injury prevention. Specific examples of equipment-related factors related to injury are discussed in Chapter 9.

MANAGING LOAD TO PREVENT INJURY
with TIM GABBETT

The concept of load management was introduced in Chapter 10 with a focus on athletic performance enhancement. Here, we revisit load management with greater focus on its increasingly recognised role in injury prevention. Of course, this is an artificial separation. In reality, injury prevention and performance enhancement are intimately linked.

The relationship between load and injury

High training and competition loads have been linked to increased injury risk in a wide variety of sports, including Australian rules football, baseball, basketball, cricket, rugby league, rugby union, rowing, soccer, swimming, volleyball and water polo.[132] This may not only be due to an increased rate of overuse injuries, but also of acute injuries, as overloaded athletes can have impaired neuromuscular control, reaction time and decision-making ability.

In some studies, high absolute loads have been shown to increase injury risk, which has led to certain sport-specific recommendations or regulations on the total amount of training and competition that athletes should perform. For example, in little league baseball there are specific age-based rules on the maximum number of pitches that players can perform per day and the minimum amount of rest required between matches.[133] The effects of these regulations remain undocumented. However, they have been well accepted by the sport and are often credited as having reduced the rate of injury among young baseball pitchers. Similar recommendations have been published by the English Cricket Board in an effort to prevent injuries in fast bowlers.

Although limiting the total amount of training and competition is likely to reduce injuries in many sports, that approach is unlikely to be accepted by elite-level athletes and coaches, whose primary concern is to train hard to maximise performance. The approach also fails to account for the large individual variation in load tolerance between athletes. Any given team will contain 'fragile' athletes as well as 'robust' ones who can tolerate very high loads. In fact, some studies have shown that high training loads may indeed be protective against injury, most probably due to enhanced physical resilience. This is the 'training-injury prevention paradox'.[134]

Rather than limiting the absolute amount of training and competition that athletes can perform, recent attention has focused on developing ways by which

PART A Fundamental principles

athletes can safely achieve and maintain high loads while minimising injury risk. These include:

1. managing the rate of load increase
2. managing the acute:chronic load ratio, and
3. adjusting training based on athletes' responses to external loads.

In order to monitor the loads athletes are subjected to, they must be quantified. The term 'external load' is often used to refer to loads placed upon the athlete, such as their training volume and intensity, the number of repetitions of certain movements (e.g. throws or jumps) or the number of impacts they are subjected to. Recent technological advances such as GPS, power monitors and wearable microsensors have greatly improved the ability to quantify external loads.[135]

The term 'internal load' is used to refer to the athlete's response to an external training or competition load. It can be measured using subjective measures such as the rate of perceived exertion (RPE) or standardised wellness questionnaires,[136, 137] or using objective measures such as heart rate, physical performance tests, blood markers and heart rate variability.[137]

Both external and internal loads, or indeed a combination of the two (e.g. training duration × RPE), can be used to monitor the rate of load increase and the acute:chronic load ratio.

Monitoring the rate of load increase

A number of studies have shown that large week-to-week differences in training load increase injury risk, irrespective of the total training load.[138-140] For example, a study of Australian Football League players by Piggott et al. showed that 40% of injuries were associated with a change in weekly training load of greater than 10%, compared to the preceding week.[138] Similarly, Gabbett found that when rugby league players' weekly training loads increased by less than 10%, their risk of injury was under 10%. However, when training load was increased by 15% or more, players' injury risk escalated to between 21% and 49% (Fig. 12.10).[134]

Of course, the rate at which week-to-week changes in load can be tolerated will vary between individual athletes and across sports. For example, Nielsen et al. found that novice runners could tolerate a weekly progression in training volume of between 20% and 25% in the first 10 weeks of a running program, without a dramatic increase in injury risk.[140] Nevertheless, based on the current evidence, limiting week-to-week training load increases to 10% seems to be a good rule of thumb.

Monitoring the acute:chronic load ratio

The acute:chronic load ratio reflects an athlete's training status at a given point in time, taking into account

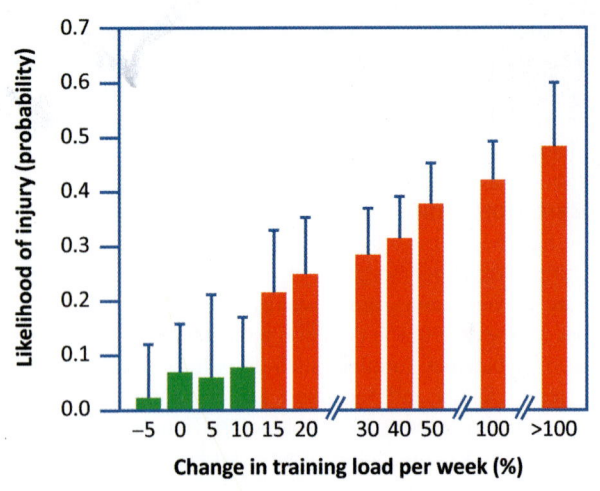

Figure 12.10 Likelihood of injury among professional rugby league players with different weekly changes in training load. Note the dramatic increase in risk when week-to-week loading increases by ≥15%. FIGURE ADAPTED FROM GABBETT[134]

their training completed over the previous week (their acute load, synonymous with 'fatigue') and their training completed over the previous 4 weeks (their chronic load, synonymous with 'fitness').

> **PRACTICE PEARL**
>
> The acute:chronic load ratio has been linked to both performance and injury risk. An athlete with a high chronic and low acute load will be fit, well rested and ready to perform. Conversely, an athlete with a low chronic and high acute load will be fatigued and have an increased risk of injury.

Studies in rugby league,[141, 142] cricket,[143] Australian rules football,[144] Gaelic football[145] and soccer[146] have demonstrated that athletes with high acute:chronic load ratios have an increased risk of injury. Modelling data from several of these studies, Gabbett showed that ratios exceeding 1.5 represented a 'danger zone' where injury risk was substantially increased.[134] In contrast, ratios between 0.8 and 1.3 represented a 'sweet spot' where injury risk was minimised (Fig. 12.11).

Although the exact thresholds may vary in other sports, the underlying concept is likely to remain the same. In order to minimise their injury risk, athletes should build up training loads gradually, closely monitoring their acute:chronic load ratio. This is especially relevant after a period of reduced training (e.g. due to illness or injury) or when resuming training after an off-season break.[147]

Preventing injury   CHAPTER 12

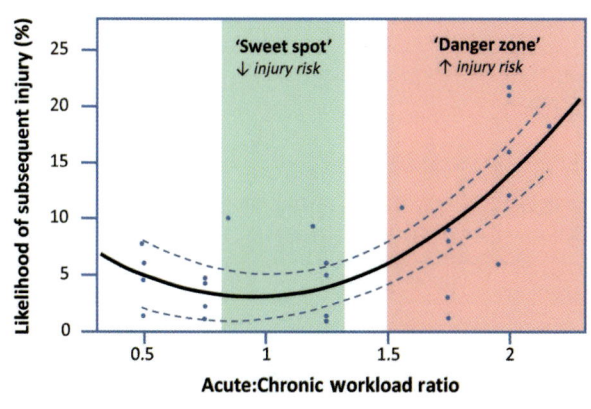

Figure 12.11 The relationship between the acute:chronic ratio and injury, modelled of using data from cricket, Australian rules football and rugby league
REPRODUCED WITH PERMISSION FROM *BRITISH JOURNAL OF SPORTS MEDICINE*[134]

The acute:chronic load ratio helps us understand how two athletes performing the same training session may have completely different injury risk, depending on the amount and consistency of training they have performed over the past month. Similarly, it provides athletes and coaches with a guide to what is an acceptable level of training progression to minimise injury risk.

Monitoring athletes' response to load—the traffic-light approach

Continuous monitoring of athletes' response to training is common practice in many high-level team sports, and may be useful in preventing overtraining, illness and injury. In this context, the goal of daily monitoring is to identify early signs of deleterious overtraining such that appropriate adjustments can be made to the athletes'

Calculating the acute:chronic load ratio

The acute:chronic load ratio can be calculated using a wide range of load measures, such as GPS and accelerometer-derived metrics,[146] throw counts,[143] and session RPE (training session duration multiplied by the athlete's rate of perceived exertion; see Chapter 10).

Table 12.3 shows an athlete's training data over 12 weeks. In this example, the acute load represents the cumulative session-RPE data for all training sessions completed by the athlete each week. The chronic load represents the rolling average of the previous 4 weeks' acute loads (i.e. in week 4, the chronic load is the average of weeks 1, 2, 3 and 4. In week 5, it is the average of weeks 2, 3, 4 and 5, and so on). The acute:chronic load ratio is calculated each week by dividing the acute load by the chronic load.

Table 12.3 An example of calculating the acute:chronic load ratio based on an athlete's session-RPE data over 12 weeks. Note that 4 weeks of data are necessary to calculate the chronic loads and acute:chronic load ratio

Week	Acute load (current week)	Chronic load (average of previous 4 weeks)	Acute:chronic load ratio
1	2750		
2	2250		
3	2500		
4	2750	2562.5	1.07
5	800	2075	0.39
6	1000	1762.5	0.57
7	1200	1437.5	0.83
8	2750	1437.5	1.91
9	2250	1800	1.25
10	2500	2175	1.15
11	2750	2562.5	1.07
12	2250	2437.5	0.92

continued

PART A Fundamental principles

In this example, the athlete had a period of reduced training in weeks 5, 6 and 7—perhaps due to a minor injury. The rapid resumption of normal training in week 8 leads to a spike in the acute:chronic load ratio into the 'danger zone' above 1.5 (Fig. 12.12), indicating an increased risk of subsequent injury.

Figure 12.12 Monitoring an athlete's acute:chronic load ratio, based on data presented in Table 12.3

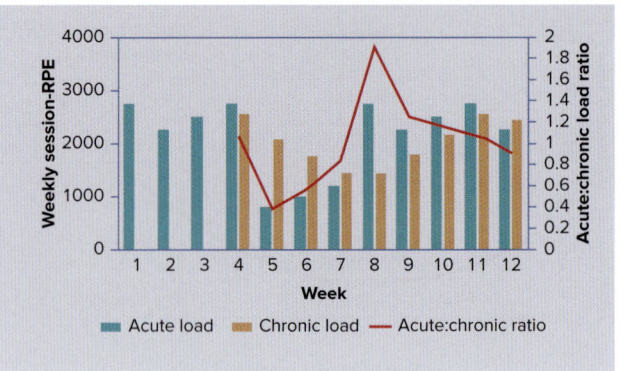

training program. We refer to this as the 'traffic light approach' as, based on their daily monitoring results, athletes are often categorised as: able to complete full training (green light); needing reduced training (orange light); or needing complete rest (red light).

Measures that have been used in efforts to detect overtraining can be broadly classified into objective and subjective measures (Table 12.4).

It is not easy for clinicians to decide on the best method of athlete monitoring. Each approach has its own strengths and limitations, and despite an increasing number of commercial claims to the contrary, there is no magic formula to predict which athletes will get sick or injured.

A recent systematic review found that subjective and objective measures generally did not correlate, with subjective measures being more responsive to changes in acute and chronic training loads.[136] As shown in Table 12.4, a number of validated questionnaires can be used to monitor athletes for signs of overtraining. However, these consist of 22-76 questions, making them too time consuming for daily administration.[158] Therefore, teams often use short questionnaires consisting of 5-7 Likert-scale questions for daily monitoring, with more comprehensive questionnaires administered less frequently.[159] The content of these short questionnaires varies; however, the following subscales have recently been identified as being responsive to acute changes in load:[136]

- non-training stress
- fatigue
- physical recovery
- general health/wellbeing
- being in shape.

Irrespective of the monitoring measures used, the main challenges facing the clinician include:

- establishing each athlete's baseline: their normal training response needs to be known before abnormal responses can be identified
- differentiating between intended and deleterious overtraining: coaches will often schedule hard training sessions to stimulate a training response (Chapter 10).

Due to these challenges, monitoring for overtraining remains as much art as science, and necessitates a close communication with athletes and coaching staff.

Table 12.4 Examples of measures used to monitor athletes for signs of deleterious overtraining

Objective measures
Heart rate (HR) measures (e.g. HR versus RPE,[148] HR recovery[149] and HR variability[150])
Biochemical, hormonal and immunological markers (from blood or saliva)[137, 151]
Physical performance tests (e.g. vertical jump height[152])
Psychomotor speed[153]

Subjective measures
Profile of mood states (POMS)[154, 155]
Recovery stress questionnaire for athletes (RESTQ-S)[156]
Daily analyses of life demands of athletes (DALDA)[157]

Preventing injury   CHAPTER 12

PROTECTIVE EQUIPMENT

Protective equipment has been designed to shield various parts of the body against injury without interfering with sporting activity. Protective equipment can also be used on return to activity after injury in situations where direct contact may aggravate the injury.

Helmets are mandatory in certain sports such as motor racing, motor cycling, cycling, ice hockey, horse-riding and American football. In other sports, the use of helmets is not universally accepted, such as in rugby and skateboarding.

Other protective equipment commonly worn includes: mouth guards in most collision sports; shoulder pads in American football and rugby; chest, forearm and groin protectors in ice hockey; knee pads when playing on artificial surfaces or while rollerblading; wrist guards in rollerblading and snowboarding; and shin pads in soccer and hockey. It is important that protective equipment fits correctly.

The use of protective equipment may increase an athlete's confidence. This may help prevent injuries, but may also lead the athlete to take bigger risks or play more aggressively.

APPROPRIATE SURFACES

with JOHN ORCHARD

Playing surfaces remain under the injury prevention spotlight, as differing traction and shock absorption properties have long been linked to injury risk. The association between playing surface and injury risk was first proposed in handball as early as 1990.[160] Later, a large epidemiological study compared the ACL injury rate between two different floor types—wooden floors (parquet, generally having lower friction) and artificial floors (generally having higher friction).[161] The results indicated that the risk of ACL injury among female handball players is higher on high-friction artificial floors than on wooden floors. However, other factors also play a significant role for shoe surface friction, principally shoe type and floor maintenance.

In Australian rules football, Orchard and colleagues noted the greater rate of ACL injuries in the northern (warmer) climates.[162] Although it was tempting to attribute this to drier weather, and thus ground hardness, that hypothesis was not supported by data from American football teams where games were played on natural grass.[163] Further analysis of both the Australian and US data suggested that the type of grass, and thus, the tightness of the thatch, may influence ACL risk; the more northern Australian rules football venues had grass types that permitted excessive shoe-surface traction (Fig. 12.13a-d).

According to turf authority McNitt, perennial rye grass is associated with lower shoe-surface traction than Kentucky blue grass or Bermuda grass because it creates less thatch.[164] These studies suggest that rye grass generally offers a safer surface with respect to ACL injuries for football than some other grasses.

Natural grass versus artificial turf

The link between artificial turf and injury risk has long been controversial. Early generations of turf, introduced in the 1960s, were linked to an increased risk due to their

(a)   (b)

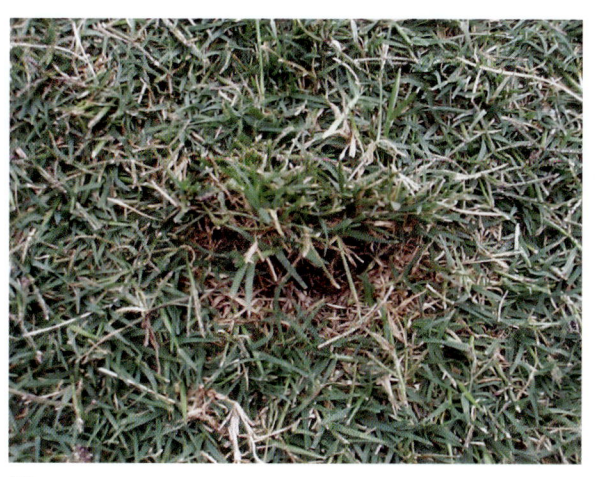

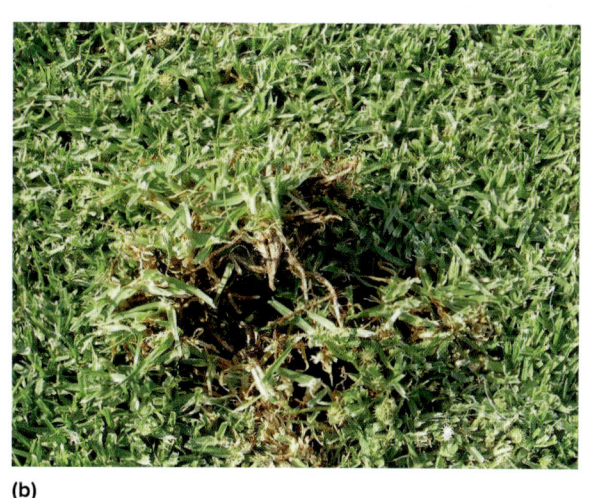

Figure 12.13 Four different types of grasses that provide the surface for Australian rules football and have been associated with different rates of ACL injury (a) Bermuda ('couch') grass surface, showing a thick thatch layer between grass leaves and soil (b) Kikuyu grass, also showing a thick thatch layer

187

PART A   Fundamental principles

(c)   (d)

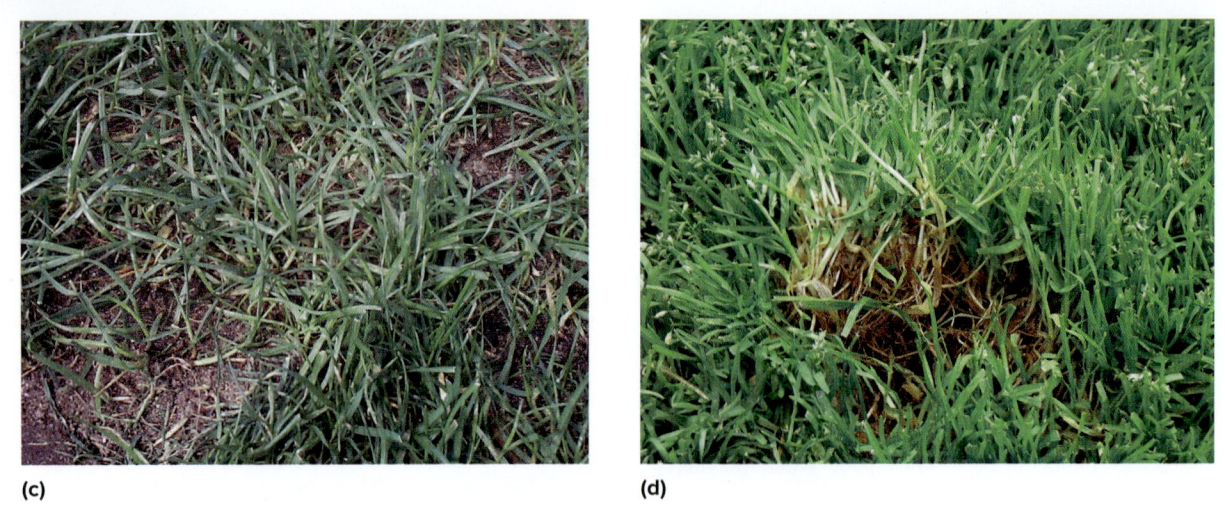

Figure 12.13 (cont.) (c) Rye grass surface, showing a minimal thatch layer. This is probably a safer surface than the others, as the blades or cleats of the football boot are less likely to be 'gripped' by the surface (d) Annual blue grass surface, showing a moderate thatch layer
REPRODUCED WITH PERMISSION FROM *BRITISH JOURNAL OF SPORTS MEDICINE*[162]

having minimal padding and high friction coefficients.[165] However, new turf types are continuously being developed, with newer types (third and fourth generation) having properties closer to natural grass.[166] Research into the injury risk of third- and fourth-generation turf is conflicting, and in some cases may have been biased by industry funding. Nevertheless, recent systematic reviews have concluded that there is little evidence of any difference in overall injury risk between natural and artificial turf.[165, 167]

REFERENCES

References for this chapter can be found at www.mhhe.com/au/CSM5e

Chapter 13

Recovery

with SHONA HALSON and PHIL GLASGOW

Paul Quantrill will never forget the feeling of pure exhaustion at the most important moment of his career. It was the fourth game of the 2004 American League Championship Series, at Fenway Park, with the Yankees trying to finish a sweep of the Boston Red Sox. The teams were tied, 4–4, heading into the bottom of the 12th. It was Quantrill's 100th relief inning of the season. 'We were done,' Quantrill said. 'We were wrecked. We battled, but we just weren't where we needed to be.'

www.nytimes.com, 31 March 2016

The concept of mechanotransduction (Chapter 17) recognises that when the body is exposed to mechanical stress, it adapts. In sport, careful manipulation of training parameters induces specific adaptations to enhance performance. Training-induced adaptations include improvements in strength, endurance, neuromuscular control and flexibility. Training to promote adaptation requires a delicate balance of overload and recovery. Strategies to expedite recovery are central to training and competition plans.

Effective recovery can permit greater levels and quality of training and thereby enhance performance. Conversely, inadequate recovery from training and competition impair performance and may eventually result in injury, illness or burnout. How performance changes in response to exercise depends on a complex interplay of factors that include peripheral muscle changes,[1] central neural drive[2] and psychological responses.[3] Effective recovery should seek to address the physiological, structural, neural and psychological limitations of performance.

A range of modalities have been purported to facilitate various aspects of recovery; the evidence for many of these modalities is scant and at times conflicting.

> **PRACTICE PEARL**
>
> As with many aspects of sports medicine, the most appropriate blend of recovery strategies depends on a detailed understanding of the sport and the athlete as well as the relative benefits of the choice of recovery modality.

ASSESSING RECOVERY

The traditional way to assess the effectiveness of interventions has been to test the athlete and investigate markers of the 'damage' associated with the test. The primary test models are (i) eccentric contraction induced delayed onset muscle soreness (DOMS); and (ii) sports-related training sessions. The variable nature of the exercise regimens used to induce damage and/or physiological stress make effective generalisation of findings challenging in some cases.

Following such a test, a typical test battery would include analysis of:

- general muscle function (peak torque maximum voluntary contractions: isometric and isokinetic)
- specific performance tasks (counter-movement jump (CMJ), squat jump, repeated sprint ability) which may be more meaningful in terms of direct impact on performance
- extent of tissue damage (creatine kinase, CK)
- level of metabolite removal (blood flow, blood lactate) and perception of soreness (pain on visual analogue scale, VAS)
- athlete's self-perception of recovery as well as psychological measures (e.g. profile of mood states, POMS).

ACTIVE RECOVERY

Active recovery refers to low-intensity work performed after exercise to facilitate better performance in a subsequent exercise bout. This is a common part of training; 81% of French professional soccer teams carry out some form of cool down after training.[4] Active recovery is therefore often the first form of recovery performed after exercise.

The type of active recovery performed will be heavily influenced by the duration, intensity and nature of the exercise from which the athlete is recovering. For example, the goals of recovery after a short maximal bout of exercise such as sprinting will be different to those following prolonged endurance events.

After high-intensity short-duration exercise

For recovery after short-duration high-intensity exercise, passive recovery appears to better promote resynthesis of phosphocreatine (PCr)–a rapidly mobilised reserve of high-energy phosphates in skeletal muscle–than does active recovery. Time to exhaustion was longer when intermittent exercise alternated with passive recovery (15s work: 15 s rest) than with active recovery.[5, 6] Similar observations were reported for short cycle sprints (4s duration) when followed by passive recovery of 21 seconds when compared to low-intensity active recovery (32% VO_2max).[7] Since recovery following repeated sprint activities involving the PCr system relies almost exclusively on aerobic factors,[8] the better outcomes with passive recovery may be due to greater availability of oxygen for PCr resynthesis in resting muscles than when muscles are still being contracted (active).[7, 9, 10] Passive rather than active recovery is therefore recommended following high-intensity short-duration exercise.

After longer-duration exercise—active recovery and metabolite clearance

Active recovery may have a greater role to play following longer duration activities. It may provide a benefit by increased removal of metabolites, particularly blood lactate. Muscle performance is impaired in the presence of high blood lactate levels,[11] so lactate level is widely considered to be important in determining the extent of recovery after high-intensity exercise. While the role of lactate in sports performance is still a subject of much debate, most studies consider it to be a useful indirect marker of cell and metabolic acidosis.[12]

Active recovery is the most effective way to increase blood flow and facilitate removal of metabolites following exercise.[13-15] Exercise intensity levels close to the anaerobic threshold have been identified as most effective for lactate clearance.[15-17] In a study of 10 moderately trained males, lactate levels were reduced most rapidly when participants ran at 80–100% of their lactate threshold.[17] Runners who self-regulated their speed tended to run at around 80% of threshold and experience comparable reductions in blood lactate. This suggests that moderately trained individuals may self-select the most appropriate exercise intensity. The physiological mechanism underpinning this observation is unclear.

Active recovery may be of greatest benefit in sports that involve a significant anaerobic contribution. It appears that active recovery is particularly effective if subsequent bouts of exercise are carried out within 10–20 minutes.[15, 18] Given that blood lactate levels return to baseline within one hour of passive recovery (Fig. 13.1),[16, 19] there is less convincing evidence for active recovery carried out several hours or days after exercise. In a series of studies investigating the effects of active recovery between games separated by 3 days in female soccer players, there was no influence on a wide range of measures of recovery including perceived muscle soreness, neuromuscular fatigue (CMJ, sprint performance, maximal isokinetic knee flexion and extension) or biochemical markers (inflammatory plasma cytokine response, plasma endogenous antioxidants, dietary antioxidants, oxidative stress markers, CK, urea).[20,21]

Similarly, in a study investigating self-selected recovery modalities in Australian Football League (AFL) players over a season, fewer players chose active recovery (pool or cycle) compared with cold-water immersion (CWI), compression garments or passive stretching.[22] There were no benefits on performance measures during a season for any of the recovery modalities. However, those players who used CWI, compression and floor stretching reported

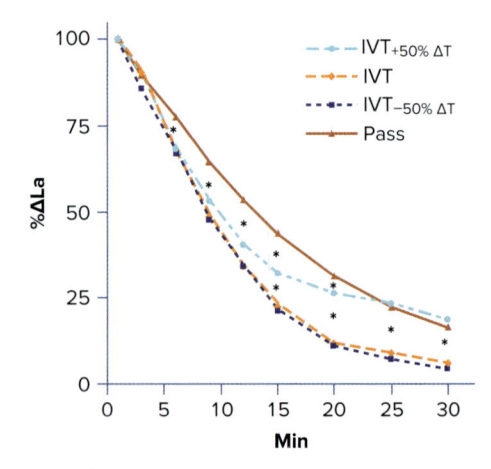

Figure 13.1 Blood lactate concentrations following exercise. Mean blood lactate (La) concentration during passive (Pass) and active recoveries at: (1) 50% of the difference (50%DT) between individual anaerobic threshold and individual ventilatory threshold (IVT) above the IVT (IVT+50%DT), (2) IVT recovery intensity and (3) 50%DT below the IVT (IVT50%DT). Comparison between recovery conditions within each time point for soccer players. *Significant difference versus IVT+50%DT recovery intensity
(FROM BALDARI ET AL. 2004[16])

greater perceived recovery. These findings highlight that players view recovery as an important part of their training and that AFL players tend not to select active recovery. The authors suggested that this may be due to players not wanting to expend further energy.

Psychological effects of active recovery

While metabolite elimination has been the primary focus of many studies, some authors have reported positive psychological effects of active recovery. Le Meur and Hausswirth have suggested that stimulation of metabosensitive type III and IV afferent nerves may facilitate better mental recovery.[23] In a study investigating the effect of active recovery following rugby matches, there were reductions in a measure of mental wellbeing, the POMS scores, in players who performed low-intensity water-based exercise when compared to passive recovery.[24] We cannot generalise these findings as the study measured only 15 players after one match.

In summary, active recovery most effectively reduces blood lactate levels at exercise intensity close to the lactate threshold; such reductions may improve performance for a subsequent exercise bout within 10–20 minutes. There is no strong evidence for the use of active recovery for exercise bouts that are several hours or days after the initial session. Note that active recovery has never been reported to impair performance.

MASSAGE

Massage has become ubiquitous in sports recovery. The effectiveness of massage has been attributed to increases in blood flow, mechanical effects on muscle tissue, reduced pain and psychological benefits.

Massage and blood flow

One of the postulated mechanisms by which massage may speed recovery is through increased local blood flow to remove metabolites and mobilise inflammatory markers. Studies that investigated the influence of massage on muscle blood flow and blood lactate removal reported no improvement in blood flow or blood lactate levels following either superficial or deep massage of the quadriceps after high-intensity cycling. They did, however, observe improved blood flow following active recovery.[12]

In the study by Wiltshire et al. of the effect of massage of the forearm after a fatiguing isometric grip protocol, massage *reduced* blood flow.[25] This may have been due to mechanical pressure on blood vessels. While no other studies have reported blood flow reductions with massage, many studies failed to detect any effect on either blood flow or lactate levels.[26-28] There is strong evidence that, when compared to active recovery, massage is no more effective in reducing blood lactate than passive control activity. As discussed earlier in this chapter, active recovery is well established as an effective way to facilitate blood flow. Therefore, if the goal of the recovery is to increase local blood flow, active recovery should be the modality of choice. Although some might argue that the lack of effect of massage on blood flow means massage does not assist recovery, massage may address other aspects of recovery.

Massage, muscle tone and viscoelasticity

Many recovery interventions, particularly the manual therapies, aim to influence the mechanical properties of soft tissues. Athletes and clinicians report reduced muscle tone and spasm following massage. The assumption is that this will reduce soreness, permit force production and enhance quality of movement. However, the influence of soft tissue mechanical properties on performance and recovery has not been well characterised. Massage may reduce tissue stiffness.[29, 30] Although a number of studies have considered the effect of compression on muscle viscoelastic behaviour, there are limited studies investigating the effects of massage on these factors.[30] Thus, the effect of massage on these factors following exercise and the potential performance benefits are not clear.

Massage and delayed onset muscle soreness (DOMS)

Massage in post-exercise recovery is often assessed using a delayed onset muscle soreness (DOMS) model to determine effects on soreness and measures of muscle performance. While there are challenges extrapolating findings from these studies due to the diverse exercise regimens and massage protocols employed, a few important trends emerge. A number of studies report that massage is effective in reducing post-exercise soreness; however, its effectiveness in improving measures of muscle function is less positive. Smith et al. observed significant reductions in soreness of the elbow flexors following eccentric exercise in participants who received a 30-minute massage 2 hours after exercise; reductions in pain were apparent from 24 to 96 hours post-exercise.[31] Similarly, Zainuddin et al. reported that massage applied for 10 minutes at 3 hours after exercise reduced pain, swelling and serum CK levels when compared to controls.[32] No such improvements were observed for recovery of muscle performance (maximum voluntary contraction). A positive effect on soreness but not muscle function was also observed for 20 minutes of massage administered to the hamstrings 2 hours after eccentric exercise when compared to sham massage.[33]

Positive effects for both muscle performance and soreness have been reported when massage is combined with other modalities. Jakeman, Byrne and Eston compared a control group with a combination of compression garments and a 30-minute massage administered immediately after exercise.[34] Athletes who received massage and wore compression garments reported less pain as well as improved CMJ, squat jump and isokinetic muscle strength, compared to control athletes. A further study in basketball players using a post-match recovery strategy of combined stretches and massage reported reduced soreness and increased CMJ in male players, while female players demonstrated improvements in sprint performance only.[35]

> **PRACTICE PEARL**
>
> The beneficial effects of massage on muscle recovery appear to be greatest when treatment is administered within two hours of exercise; there is no evidence to support the use of massage for recovery 24 hours after exercise has ceased.[36] This makes clinical sense: most recovery modalities discussed in this chapter should be administered as soon as possible after exercise.

Cellular and structural effects of massage

There is some evidence that massage may influence key cellular mediators. Rapaport et al. reported increases in circulating phenotypic lymphocyte markers and decreased mitogen-stimulated cytokine production following massage.[37] Similarly, Crane et al. observed a downregulation of pro-inflammatory cytokine expression following massage after eccentric exercise.[38] The authors also reported increased activity of mechanically sensitive proteins (FAK and ERK1/2). These observations suggest that the mechanical stimulus provided by massage may be capable of influencing mechanotransduction in the muscle (see Chapter 17). In a series of studies using a rabbit model, researchers from Ohio State University investigating the effects of massage-like compressive loading following eccentric exercise have demonstrated accelerated recovery of isometric torque production,[39] altered viscoelastic properties,[30] decreased number of torn muscle fibres and enhanced restoration of muscle function.[40] They have also identified a number of key variables that may be important to the use of massage in recovery. These have included timing,[41] magnitude and frequency of the applied force, and treatment duration.[39]

These findings provide a conceptual framework for some of the effects of massage; however, further studies are required to determine their clinical significance.

Psychological effects of massage

Consistent psychological benefits of massage are reported in the literature with positive effects reported for salivary IgA, POMS and perceived recovery of fatigue from exercise. Moraska observed that massage in non-athletic populations reduces psychological measures including anxiety, tension, stress and depression, while increasing mood and quality-of-life measures.[42] Arroyo-Morales et al. suggest that massage restores autonomic nervous system balance via its effects on the parasympathetic nervous system.[43] They observed that a 40-minute massage applied after three 30-second Wingate tests restored or maintained pre-exercise heart rate variability values when compared to sham ultrasound treatment. Massage also facilitates relaxation and has been demonstrated to improve scores on the General Wellbeing Scale (an 18-item scale with subscales measuring anxiety, depression, positive wellbeing, self-control, vitality and general health) and the Perceived Stress Scale in healthy adults.[44]

The type of massage used can influence the degree of relaxation. In one study comparing light, moderate and vibratory stimulation, moderate massage was demonstrated to offer greater reduction in stress with a concomitant decrease in heart rate and EEG.[45] Interestingly, the light and vibratory stimulation groups showed increased arousal as evidenced by increased heart rate and EEG activity. It is therefore important to consider the type of massage intervention used.

Massage is highly valued by athletes. Studies in both athletic and non-athletic populations have highlighted that one of the main reasons for using massage therapy is that it provides a personalised approach to care that enhances relaxation and creates a positive client–therapist relationship.[46] The 'culture' of a massage experience (how professional the setting, the relationship with the clinician) influences the athlete's perception of the massage. There is strong evidence that massage does not increase blood flow or aid metabolite removal, but it may influence various inflammatory and cellular responses. There is no evidence that massage is detrimental to recovery.

> **PRACTICE PEARL**
>
> Massage effectively modifies both perception of recovery and soreness. The effect of massage on correlates of performance is less clear and may be strongly influenced by the inclusion of other recovery strategies.

NEUROMUSCULAR ELECTRICAL STIMULATION

Neuromuscular electrical stimulation (NMES) is a modality commonly used to promote recovery in athletes. A review of NMES in post-exercise performance recovery highlighted the challenges associated with determining its effectiveness due to the wide variety of exercise types as well as stimulation protocols used.[47] In general, the application of electrical stimulation following exercise is proposed to have two primary effects:

1. increased blood flow and metabolite removal through muscle pump action
2. reduction in pain through stimulation of sensory nerve endings.

While attractive in its assumptions, the evidence regarding the ability of NMES to effectively increase local blood flow and reduce blood lactate levels is less convincing.

NMES and blood flow

The importance of the muscle pump to facilitate blood flow in the lower limb is well established. The calf muscle has been described as the second heart[48] and the effectiveness of low-level calf muscle activity to improve local blood flow has been identified.[49, 50] A number of studies have compared the effect of NMES with active recovery and have consistently shown that active recovery is more effective in increasing blood flow and reducing blood lactate levels. In a study comparing the effects of four modalities (active recovery, passive recovery, NMES and CWI) on the recovery of grip strength following a fatiguing rock-climbing protocol, Heyman et al. reported no difference in blood lactate levels between NMES and passive recovery while observing a significant increase in blood flow and a concomitant reduction in blood lactate following 20 minutes of gentle cycling.[18]

Some positive effects on lower limb blood flow for NMES have recently been reported using devices that focus on peroneal nerve stimulation. These studies derive from the use of electrical stimulation in angiology and highlight the importance of deep calf muscle activity. In two studies investigating peroneal nerve stimulation following a 90-minute shuttle test and a Yo-Yo intermittent recovery test,[51, 52] increases in local blood flow were reported. These observations suggest that NMES of this nature may enhance metabolite clearance following exercise when compared to passive recovery. However, it is not clear how these interventions compare with an active recovery protocol and whether they correspond to improvements in performance.

NMES and performance

The effect of NMES on correlates of sports performance such as strength, endurance and jump performance has been assessed following various types of exercise. While isolated studies have indicated that NMES may be slightly more effective than passive recovery for restoration of strength[53] and running performance,[52] the majority of authors conclude that NMES is no more effective than passive recovery for these parameters. Although the lack of consistent positive effects of NMES may be due to the wide range of methods of stimulation used following different exercise protocols, it is not possible to state whether NMES effectively restores performance following exercise.[47]

NMES and muscle soreness

As outlined above, reducing muscle soreness is a common aspect of sports recovery. A number of studies have investigated the effect of NMES on DOMS. Most studies have failed to observe any positive effect of NMES on soreness when compared to active or passive recovery.[47] A few studies have suggested that NMES may temporarily reduce pain,[54, 55] but these effects do not correlate with improved performance. Maffiuletti and DuPont make an interesting observation that NMES can effectively improve the subjective perception of recovery in athletes.[56] The authors highlight that athletes consistently report that they feel better recovered or have greater levels of perceived energy than those who do not use NMES despite displaying no associated improvements in sports performance. The role of altered pain perception and other psychological factors in this regard is unclear; however, as discussed below, the perception of recovery may have beneficial effects for performance.

In summary, there is some limited evidence that NMES can enhance blood flow and metabolite removal with certain types of electrical current applied over the peroneal nerve. There is no evidence that NMES can effectively enhance recovery of correlates of performance, but it may effectively enhance the perception of recovery through neuropsychological means. A pragmatic approach to the use of NMES in recovery is shown in Table 13.1.

STRETCHING

Athletes often stretch after exercise in an attempt to improve range of motion and reduce the perception of musculotendinous stiffness. While it is a regular component of post-exercise regimens, there is limited evidence of the effect of stretching on various aspects of recovery.

PART A Fundamental principles

Table 13.1 A pragmatic approach to the use of neuromuscular electrical stimulation (NMES) in recovery[56]

- NMES should be combined with submaximal voluntary dynamic contractions (such as toe curls) whenever possible, in order to maximise blood flow increase.
- NMES should be applied distally (to the calf or foot muscles and eventually to the common peroneal nerve) rather than proximally (to the quadriceps muscle belly) to maximise the muscle pump effect.
- NMES is most effective in weight-bearing and contact sports to reduce signs and symptoms of muscle damage.
- NMES should be delivered with low doses but for long durations (such as overnight), during travel or by means of electrostatically charged self-adhesive membranes.

Maffiuletti N, Dupont G. Electrostimulation-related recovery strategies. Aspetar Sports Medicine Journal 2015;4:64–70. Reproduced with permission.

Lund et al. suggested that stretching following bouts of eccentric exercise may delay recovery.[57] In a study investigating the effect of static stretching on DOMS following eccentric exercise in the quadriceps of seven untrained females, they reported that recovery of strength was impaired in the group who stretched their quadriceps for three repetitions of 30 seconds each day after exercise. The authors proposed that stretching after eccentric exercise caused further mechanical disruption and exacerbated muscle damage. In contrast, Torres et al. reported no effect of daily stretching on maximum voluntary contraction of the quadriceps following eccentric exercise in healthy untrained men.[58] They also reported no effect of static stretching on CK levels or soreness, but did observe improvements in muscle stiffness when compared to passive recovery. The authors suggest that the changes in muscle stiffness may have functional benefits in terms of normalising muscle tone and enhancing quality of movement. This is an interesting postulation and merits further research.

A few studies have reported positive effects of stretching on cycling performance; Dawson et al. noted improvements in a 6-second cycle sprint test 15 hours after an Australian rules football match with stretching when compared to a control.[59] Dynamic stretching also improved performance during a second exhaustive bout of cycling.[11] Given the isolated nature of these findings and the fact that they were only observed during cycling, it is not possible to state that stretching positively influences recovery of performance in other sport settings.

Most studies report no effect of stretching on recovery. A comparison of static stretching, CWI and passive recovery following strenuous stair climbing in rowers reported no differences between each of the interventions for strength or CK levels.[60] Similarly, no differences were observed for systemic markers of stress and inflammation, blood lactate, anaerobic performance or psychological mood states after an exhaustive bout of endurance exercise for static stretching or for active recovery using either an anti-gravity treadmill or cycle ergometer.[61] Reviews have consistently failed to detect any positive effect of stretching on correlates of recovery after exercise despite testing various different stretching protocols.[62] It is important to note that post-exercise stretching does not appear to have any detrimental effects on performance.

SLEEP

Optimal sleep quality and quantity is the single best recovery strategy available to athletes. In studies of performance following partial sleep deprivation, sustained exercise was more affected than single maximal efforts.[63] Thus, longer submaximal exercise tasks such as long-distance running may be affected following sleep deprivation.

Suboptimal sleep may have a range of consequences for athletes beyond reduced performance, such as impaired immunity and endocrine function. This can affect the recovery process and adaptations to training.[64] Sleep deprivation can also result in reduced cognitive function, increased pain perception, mood changes, altered metabolism and changes in inflammatory indicators.[64]

Athletes often rank sleep deprivation and poor sleep quality as prominent causes of fatigue and tiredness.[65] Many athletes often have difficulties sleeping prior to important competitions.[66,67] Juliff et al. questioned 283 elite Australian athletes and found that 64.0% of athletes indicated worse sleep on at least one occasion in the nights prior to an important competition over the past 12 months.[67] Athletes complained of difficulty falling asleep (82.1%) particularly because of thoughts about the competition (83.5%) and general nervousness (43.8%).

Activity monitors have recently been utilised to measure sleep in British[68] and Australian[69] athletes with quite similar results. The 47 elite British athletes spent a total of 8:40 ± 0:50 hours:minutes in bed, compared with 8:10 ± 0:20 in the control group. The athlete group had a longer sleep latency (time taken to fall asleep) (18 ± 17 vs. 5 ± 3 min) and a lower sleep efficiency (estimate of sleep quality) than controls (81 ± 6 vs 89 ± 4%), resulting in a similar time asleep (6:55 ± 0:43 vs 7:11 ± 0:25 hours:minutes; mean ± SD). Thus, athletes had a comparable quantity of sleep to controls, but inferior quality of sleep.

On average, the 124 Australian individual and team sport athletes went to bed at 23:59 ± 1.3, woke up at 07:15 ± 1.2 and obtained 6.8 ± 1.1 hours of sleep per night. Athletes from individual sports went to bed earlier,

Table 13.2 Sleep hygiene strategies. Adapted from Halson[64]

Bedroom	• The bedroom should be cool (19–21°C is best), dark and quiet. • A comfortable bed and pillows is important.
Electronics	• Avoid watching television in bed and using the computer or smartphone in bed. These can steal sleep time and form bad habits.
Food and fluid	• Avoid the use of caffeinated food and fluids later in the day. • Do not go to bed after consuming too much fluid; this may result in waking up to use the bathroom.
Behaviour	• Create a good sleep routine by going to bed at the same time and waking up at the same time. • Before bed routine can help the body prepare for sleep. The routine should start about 30 minutes before bedtime (i.e. clean teeth, read a book, etc.). • Avoid watching the clock. Many people who struggle with sleep tend to watch the clock too much. Frequently checking the clock during the night can wake you up (especially if you turn on the light to read the time) and may reinforce negative thoughts. • Be organised. Utilise a 'to-do' list or diary to ensure organisation and avoid unnecessary over-thinking while trying to sleep. • Investigate relaxation/breathing techniques. • If you haven't been able to get to sleep after about 20 minutes or more, get up and do something calming or boring until you feel sleepy, then return to bed and try again. Sit quietly on the couch with the lights off (bright light will tell your brain that it's time to wake up).

This is an open access article distributed under the terms of the Creative Commons Attribution License, which permits unrestricted use, distribution, and reproduction in any medium, provided the original work is properly cited.

woke up earlier and obtained less sleep (individual vs team; 6.5 vs 7.0 h) than athletes from team sports.[69]

Given the effects of sleep deprivation on performance and other important aspects of elite athlete physiology and psychology, athletes should be appropriately educated regarding the importance of sleep and potential strategies to enhance sleep. Sleep hygiene practices that may enhance sleep quantity and quality are outlined in Table 13.2.

WATER IMMERSION

Post-exercise water immersion of various types has become popular with elite athletes to accelerate recovery from training and competition. Three main forms of water immersion exist: cold water immersion (CWI), hot water immersion (HWI) and contrast water therapy (CWT). Several authors have conducted meta-analyses to help clarify and explore the effects of these modalities on performance. Poppendieck et al. examined effect sizes for a range of performance measures following various cooling strategies.[70] The largest average effect size was for sprint performance (2.6%, g=0.69), followed by endurance parameters (2.6%, g=0.19), jump performance (3.0%, g=0.15) and strength (1.8%, g=0.10). Similarly, Bieuzen et al. examined the effects of CWT on exercise-induced muscle damage and reported significantly greater improvements in CWT when compared to passive recovery.[71] Further, CWT reduced muscle strength loss compared to passive recovery. Studies that compare the different forms of water immersion typically report that CWI and CWT enhance recovery more than HWI when used appropriately following cycling[72,73] and resistance training.[74] Studies report accelerated performance recovery following CWI and CWT compared to HWI.[75]

> **PRACTICE PEARL**
>
> The results of recent meta-analyses suggest that on average CWI and CWT recovery interventions are beneficial for recovery of performance and perceptual parameters.

As a result, recent research has focused on possible underlying mechanisms to explain these improvements.

Cold water immersion and other forms of cryotherapy have traditionally been utilised to minimise inflammatory responses, and decrease oedema and pain. Physiologically, this has been shown to occur through reductions in limb blood flow, and reductions in skin, muscle and core temperature.[76] Further, hydrostatic pressure can limit swelling and fluid accumulation, increase central blood volume and facilitate removal of metabolic waste.[77] Positive cardiovascular effects have also been observed with CWI, including lower heart rate, increased cardiac output and/or stroke volume.[77]

The effects of CWI on both the brain and pacing strategies have also been examined as possible contributors to improved performance findings. De Pauw et al. used brain mapping via electroencephalography to demonstrate changes in brain electrical activity indicative of decreased arousal and increased somatosensory information processing.[78] The same research group also demonstrated different cycling time trial pacing strategies in the heat,[79] likely the result of decreased thermal strain.

For recovery techniques to be beneficial following training, they must not only accelerate recovery, but also allow adaptations to training to occur. Based on the improvements in performance observed in acute CWI studies, two adaptation theories have been proposed. The first is that hydrotherapy allows athletes to perform subsequent training sessions with a greater training load or quality, thus resulting in an enhanced stimulus for adaptation. Conversely, the second theory suggests that CWI may decrease adaptations to training due to minimisation of fatigue and inflammation occurring following training. Thus, some practitioners are questioning the use of chronic hydrotherapy treatment in elite athletes with respect to a potential negative influence on training adaptation.

Yamane et al. report that regular CWI resulted in an attenuation of cycling performance improvements when compared to a control condition over a training period of 4–6 weeks.[80] Similar findings were reported by Higgins et al. whereby repeat sprint test performance decreased with CWI when compared with control in amateur rugby union players.[81] Further, Frohlich et al. reported a small reduction in single-leg adaptation to strength training in trained male students when compared to cases where the leg was not immersed.[82]

In contrast, recent research using elite cyclists found that CWI had no effect on adaptation during 6 weeks of training.[83] CWI has also been shown to better maintain cycling performance over 5 days.[84,85] When examining submaximal performance, two recent studies have demonstrated an increase in submaximal cycling[86] and submaximal resistance exercise[87] suggesting that an athlete may be able to train at higher workloads, thereby increasing long-term training adaptation. This is an important new line of investigation as previous studies have focused almost entirely on maximal performance and not on the ability to enhance daily training.

Increasing evidence exists to support the use of CWI and CWT, particularly in acute settings such as that of a competition or event. Further research is needed to fully elucidate the longer-term effects of water immersion on adaptation to training.

COMPRESSION

Many recovery strategies for elite athletes are based on medical equipment or therapies originally used on patients. Compression clothing is one of these strategies as it has traditionally been used to treat various lymphatic and circulatory conditions.[88] Compression garments are thought to improve return of blood to the heart through application of graduated compression to the limbs from the ankle upwards. The external pressure created by compression garments may reduce swelling, inflammation and muscle soreness, and thereby enhance recovery.[89]

Research investigating compression in athletes typically focuses on wearing compression either during exercise or during recovery. Research examining performance while wearing compression is conflicting, mainly due to the heterogeneity in subjects, study design and type of compression worn. In a recent meta-analysis, Born et al reported small effect sizes for the application of compression clothing during exercise for short-duration sprints (10–60 m), vertical-jump height, extending time to exhaustion (such as running at VO_2max or during incremental tests) and time trial performance (3–60 min).[90]

From a specific recovery perspective, compression has been shown to improve performance between two 40 km time trials performed 24 hours apart.[91] In this case, the compression was worn for the full 24 hours, which may not be practical or comfortable for many athletes. Compression has also been shown to improve sprint performance, with a shorter recovery period. Maximal sprint performance was enhanced when using compression for 20 minutes between sprints.[92] Results of a meta-analysis suggest that when compression clothing was applied for recovery purposes after exercise, small to moderate effect sizes were observed in recovery of maximal strength and power, especially vertical-jump exercise; reductions in muscle swelling and perceived muscle pain; blood lactate removal; and increases in body temperature.[88] Research investigating a multifaceted approach to recovery (including the use of full-body compression garments, CWI and sleep) was shown to assist subsequent tennis performance as well as resulting in favourable physiological outcomes such as reduced blood lactate, heart rate and perceived muscle and joint soreness.[93]

From the research available, it appears that compression garments may be beneficial and do not appear to be harmful in any way. We recommend that compression garments be worn for at least 60 minutes after training or competition to maximise the recovery process.

NUTRITION

with GRAEME CLOSE

Nutrition is essential for complete recovery. Recovery eating and drinking should help meet the athlete's total nutritional goals in terms of energy needs, desire to manipulate physique and overall requirements for nutrients. It must also be manageable within the practical constraints that govern the athlete's food intake; for example, to be affordable, to fit in with the daily timetable and social commitments, and to involve foods and drinks that are acceptable and readily available. Three primary concerns are fluid replacement, restoring fuels (largely carbohydrate in competitive sport today) and repair (largely protein).

Replacing fluids

Substantial fluid loss should be replaced. The simplest way to determine the amount of fluid lost is by weighing the athlete pre- and post-event. Every 1 kilogram of weight loss equates to 1 litre of fluid loss. The athlete should consume (i.e. via drinks and meals) water and sodium at a modest rate that minimises diuresis/urinary losses.[94] Because sweat losses and obligatory urine losses continue during the post-exercise phase, effective rehydration requires the intake of about 125–150% of the final fluid deficit (e.g. 1.25–1.5 L fluid for every 1 kg of body weight lost).[95]

Dietary sodium/sodium chloride (from foods or fluids) helps to retain ingested fluids, especially extracellular fluids, including plasma volume. Therefore, athletes should include sodium in their post-exercise nutrition, particularly when large sodium losses have been incurred. The optimal sodium level in a rehydration drink appears to be close to the sodium content of sweat[96] and thus may be as high as 50–80 mmol/L; this is higher than the sodium concentration of typical sports drinks and is close to the level found in oral rehydration solutions manufactured for the treatment of diarrhoea. Fluid can be consumed with meals or snacks that include salt-rich foods (e.g. breads, breakfast cereals, crackers, cheese, preserved meats) or have been seasoned with added salt. Milk is a better sport drink for rehydration than many commercial products because of its sodium content as well as the protein and fat in it which may aid fluid retention.[97]

Alcohol, particularly strong beers and shots, is a diuretic and is thus discouraged in the recovery period. However, the previous warnings about caffeine as a diuretic appear to be overstated when it is habitually consumed in moderate amounts (e.g. <180 mg = 1–2 standard brewed cups).[95]

The athlete should start to consume fluids on finishing and aim to consume the target volume over the next 2–4 hours. Spreading fluid intake over a period of time promotes gastrointestinal comfort and maximises retention via smaller urine losses.[98] When the athlete's total energy needs are low, low-energy fluids such as water, low-energy soft drinks and mineral waters are recommended. When energy needs are higher, fluids can be combined with energy sources.

Replacing fuel

As most athletes use carbohydrates as their major fuel supply, glycogen restoration is one of the goals of post-exercise recovery, particularly between bouts of carbohydrate-dependent exercise where there is a priority on performance in the second session. Refuelling requires adequate carbohydrate intake and time. Provided that total energy intake is adequate,[99] increasing carbohydrate intake increases muscle glycogen storage until an upper limit for glycogen synthesis is reached.[100] The most recent guidelines for post-exercise glycogen storage recognise a scaling of requirements according to the fuel cost of training or competition and the athlete's body size.[101] (Figure 13.2)

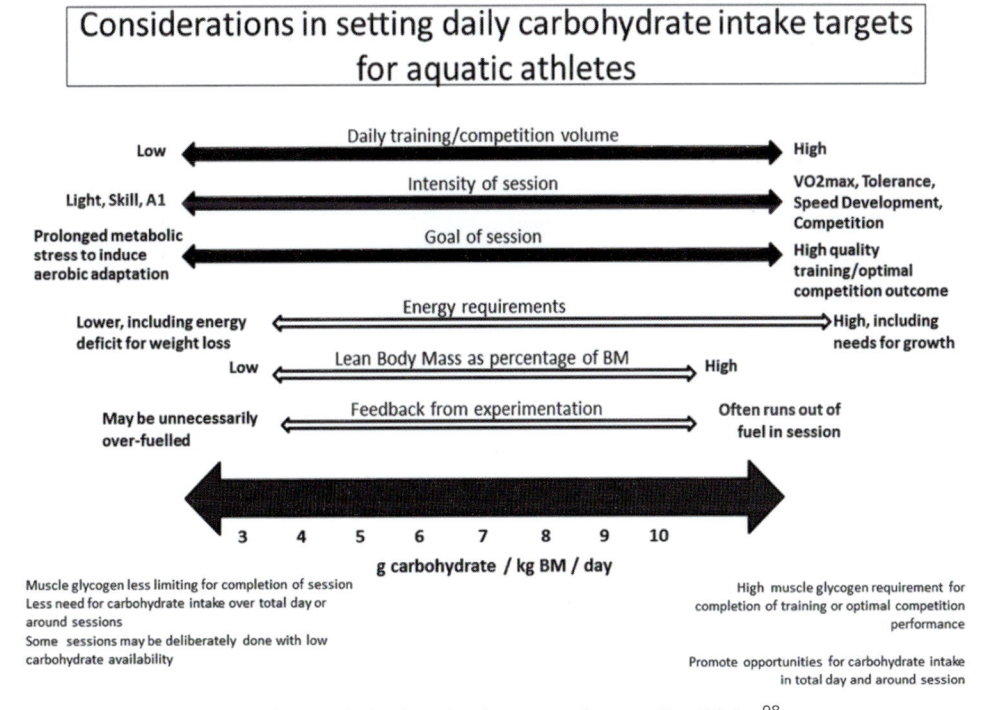

Figure 13.2 Considerations in setting daily carbohydrate intake targets for aquatic athletes[98]
REPRINTED WITH PERMISSION FROM L M BURKE AND I MUJIKA, 2014, 'NUTRITION FOR RECOVERY IN AQUATIC SPORTS', *INT J SPORTS NUTR EXERC METAB*

PART A Fundamental principles

Table 13.3 Carbohydrate-rich recovery snacks (50 g CHO portions)[104]

- 700–800 mL sports drink
- 2 sports gels
- 500 mL fruit juice or soft drink
- 300 mL carbohydrate loader drink
- 2 slices toast/bread with jam or honey or banana topping
- 2 cereal bars
- 1 cup thick vegetable soup + large bread roll
- 115 g (1 large or 2 small) cake-style muffins, fruit buns or scones
- 250 g baked potato with salsa filling
- 100 g pancakes (2 stack) + 30 g syrup

The mean hourly rate of glycogen restoration is about 2% of the total glycogen capacity per hour; the maximum rate is around 5%. Thus, it can take approximately 24 hours to normalise stores after substantial levels of depletion.[98] During the 2–4 hour period after exercise, there is a potential for high rates of muscle glycogen storage as a result of the depletion-activated stimulation of the glycogen synthase enzyme and exercise-induced increases in muscle membrane permeability and insulin sensitivity.[102] This potential can be realised only if carbohydrates are consumed during this period; if not, refuelling rates are very low.[103]

Meals and snacks can be chosen from a variety of foods and fluids according to personal preferences of type and timing of intake.[100, 101] The athlete should aim for recovery drinks, snacks or meals providing carbohydrate equal to approximately 1 g/kg/hour body mass for the first 4 hours post-exercise. Appropriate carbohydrate-rich foods are shown in Table 13.3.

Repair

The Australian Institute of Sport (AIS) provides the following information in its factsheet on recovery nutrition:

Prolonged and high-intensity exercise causes a substantial breakdown of muscle protein. During the recovery phase there is a reduction in catabolic (breakdown) processes and a gradual increase in anabolic (building) processes, which continues for at least 24 hours after exercise. Early intake after exercise (within the first hour) of essential amino acids from good quality protein foods helps to promote the increase in protein rebuilding. Consuming food sources of protein in meals and snacks after this 'window of opportunity' will further promote protein synthesis, though the rate at which it occurs is less.[104]

The maximal protein synthetic response to a resistance exercise bout is achieved with the intake of approximately 20–25 g of high-quality protein[105] or 0.3 g/kg body mass.

Protein consumed in excess of this threshold stimulates increased rates of irreversible protein oxidation and may be considered wasteful.[105] The pattern of intake over the rest of the day should probably involve a series of meals or snacks every 3–5 hours providing about 20–25 g of protein rather than frequent feedings of smaller protein doses or infrequent meals with larger protein doses.[106] Consuming protein just before bed may also be valuable because it can increase muscle protein synthesis at a time when it would otherwise be low.[107]

The important characteristics of protein-rich foods appear to be the digestibility of the food and its content of essential amino acids, especially leucine. High-quality protein-rich foods such as milk (or whey), eggs and meat are all associated with significant increases in muscle protein synthesis after exercise.[108] In the period immediately after exercise, at least, there is superior muscle protein synthesis with the intake of proteins that are rapidly digested to provide a rapid rise in plasma leucine concentrations; this includes whey protein (a rapidly digested, or 'fast', protein) and liquid protein forms.[109]

Adding a source of carbohydrate to the post-exercise protein will further enhance the training adaptation by reducing the degree of muscle protein breakdown. Chocolate milk is an excellent recovery drink combining carbohydrate and protein.[110] Table 13.4 provides a list of carbohydrate rich snacks that also provide at least 10 g of protein, while Table 13.5 lists a number of everyday foods that provide approximately 10 g of protein.[104]

According to the Australian Institute of Sport (AIS):

Some athletes finish sessions with a good appetite, so most foods are appealing to eat. On the other hand, a fatigued athlete may only feel like eating something that is compact and easy to chew. When snacks need to be kept or eaten at the training venue itself, foods and drinks that require minimal storage and preparation are useful. At other times, valuable features of recovery foods include being portable and able to travel interstate or overseas. Situations and challenges in sport change from day to day and between athletes, so recovery snacks need to be carefully chosen to meet these needs.[104]

Increasing numbers of athletes, especially endurance and ultra-endurance, are using fat rather than carbohydrate as their preferred primary fuel source.[111] Others are adopting the 'train low, compete high' regime which involves low carbohydrate intake during training with the aim of optimising use of fat as a fuel source, then using carbohydrates on the day of competition.[112, 113]

In those athletes using the low-carbohydrate high-fat method of fuelling, glycogen stores are not significantly depleted so restoration with a high-carbohydrate meal following exercise is not required. Most athletes on this

Recovery   CHAPTER 13

Table 13.4 Carbohydrate-protein recovery snacks (contain 50 g CHO plus valuable source of protein and micronutrients)[104]

- 250–300 mL liquid meal supplement
- 300 g creamed rice
- 250–300 mL milkshake or fruit smoothie
- 600 mL low-fat flavoured milk
- 1–2 sports bars (check labels for carbohydrate and protein content)
- 1 large bowl (2 cups) breakfast cereal with milk
- 1 large or 2 small cereal bars + 200 g fruit-flavoured yoghurt
- 220 g baked beans on 2 slices of toast
- 1 bread roll with cheese/meat filling + large banana
- 300 g (bowl) fruit salad with 200 g fruit-flavoured yoghurt
- 2 crumpets with thick spread peanut butter + 250 mL glass of milk
- 250 g baked potato + cottage cheese filling + glass of milk

Table 13.5 Foods providing approximately 10 g of protein[104]

- Animal foods
  - 40 g of cooked lean beef/pork/lamb
  - 40 g skinless cooked chicken
  - 50 g of canned tuna/salmon or cooked fish
  - 300 mL of milk/glass of Milo
  - 200 g tub of yoghurt
  - 300 mL flavoured milk
  - 1.5 slices (30 g) of cheese
  - 2 eggs
- Plant-based foods
  - 120 g of tofu
  - 4 slices of bread
  - 200 g of baked beans
  - 60 g of nuts
  - 2 cups of pasta/3 cups of rice
  - ¾ cup cooked lentils/kidney beans

regime find that simply having their normal meals is sufficient for nutritional recovery.

Before leaving the topic of fuel, we remind you that research funding influences which elements of sports medicine are addressed. Food companies have openly contributed to the advancement of science with research grant funding to quality scientists. Such funding helps to leverage national health research grants; for example, the National Institutes of Health (NIH) in the United States, the Medical Research Council (MRC) in the UK and the National Health and Medical Research Council (NHMRC) in Australia. Many of these grants were used to study the effects of carbohydrate on recovery and performance. Other industries, such as the dairy industry and the meat industry, contributed to scientific research but their funding has not matched that of companies whose profits derive largely from carbohydrate products.

PULLING THE DIFFERENT THREADS TOGETHER—PRACTICAL CONSIDERATIONS FOR THE CLINICIAN

As stated above, recovery modalities for athletes must not only accelerate recovery but also allow training adaptation. Different types of activities place different demands upon the system and as such may require distinct approaches. A sound understanding of the nature of the activity from which the athlete seeks to recover and the associated metabolic, neural, psychological and mechanical load is necessary to ensure that each aspect of recovery is maximised. Table 13.6 summarises some of the factors that influence decision making.

For example, reduced-impact or non weight-bearing exercise may be preferable following high-intensity exercise that involves lower limb mechanical loading. It is reasonable to consider that the tissue damage incurred during sports such as rugby may repair best with reduced mechanical loading; therefore, such strategies including cycling or water-based recovery may be more appropriate.

The perception of recovery appears to be important and has the potential to influence sports performance. Investigating the effect of the perception of soreness on vertical jump in male soccer players, Smith and Jackson reported an inverse relationship between perception of soreness and vertical jump performance.[114] This poses the interesting suggestion that performance during many of the tasks associated with recovery literature may be positively influenced by perception which, one would postulate, is related to central neuropsychological mechanisms rather than to local physiological effects. Given that many of the modalities commonly used as part of recovery have the potential to provide a strong psychological response, the positive effects reported by authors may include a large central effect. This should not be underestimated and specific strategies that maximise the complex interaction between perception, arousal and sports performance should be considered.

This is not without its challenges, as the ability to extrapolate these principles is limited and highly context-specific. For example, the increased stress associated with important matches or during a period of particularly high training load may have significant effects on the perception of fatigue and subsequent performance. It is reasonable to suggest that during periods such as these, various modalities that facilitate enhanced feelings of wellbeing and reduced pain may be preferable; such modalities may include massage, NMES and compression garments.

PART A — Fundamental principles

Table 13.6 Summary of the various recovery modalities

Modality	Systems influenced	Key recommendations
Active recovery	• Metabolic • Psychological	• Most effective when subsequent exercise bout is within 20 min • Exercise intensity close to lactate threshold
Massage	• Neural • Structural • Psychological	• Within 2 hours after exercise • Minimum 10 min duration • Moderate intensity
Neuromuscular electrical stimulation	• Neural • Psychological	• To increase blood flow, use distal application to initiate calf muscle pump • As soon as possible after exercise
Stretching	• Structural (muscle tone) • Psychological	• Static stretching immediately after exercise • Mild–moderate intensity
Cold-water immersion	• Psychological • Neural • Metabolic	• As soon as possible after exercise • A total duration of 10–15 min • Temperature range 10–15°C
Contrast water therapy	• Psychological • Neural • Metabolic	• As soon as possible after exercise • Cold: 10–15°C • Hot: 38–40°C • 5–7 rotations of 1–2 min
Compression	• Psychological • Neural	• Apply immediately after exercise for minimum of 60 min
Sleep	• All systems	• Use strategies outlined in Table 13.2 to enhance sleep quality
Nutrition	• Metabolic • Structural • Psychological	• Rehydrate to 1.5x the weighed fluid loss (to account for ongoing losses) • Refuel with appropriate carbohydrate (Tables 13.3 and 13.4) • Repair with protein (Tables 13.4 and 13.5)

Key considerations to aid decision making include the period of the annual training program (e.g. pre-season vs mid-season, high volume vs low volume), as well as the previous experience of the athlete and the culture of the specific sport. For example, CWI has become part of normal practice of many team sports and is now a usual part of the post-match recovery routine. Many such practices become embedded in preparation and scheduling; a recovery strategy that involves an alteration in the use of CWI has the potential to influence the perception of recovery as well as any associated psychological or physiological effects. Similarly, a decision to include specific interventions that are unfamiliar may place additional stress on the athlete. As such any changes (whether introduction or removal of specific practices) should be carried out at a time that minimises any secondary effects on the athlete.

SUMMARY

Sleep and good nutritional practices are the cornerstone of recovery and every effort should be made to maximise the benefits of these interventions. As outlined above, additional modalities may be used to augment recovery through the complex interaction of psychological, metabolic, structural and neurophysiological factors. The ability to influence recovery in the sporting environment relies on the intelligent application of these principles to meet the specific needs of the athlete.

REFERENCES

References for this chapter can be found at www.mhhe.com/au/CSM5e

Chapter 14

Clinical assessment: moving from rote to rigorous

by CHAD COOK

Listen: the patient is telling you the diagnosis.
Sir William Osler, Canadian physician (1849-1919)

Clinical assessment is every top clinician's foundation stone and it is a complex skill. Its three goals are to:

1. determine the diagnosis of the patient
2. identify appropriate treatment mechanisms specific to that condition, and
3. build a professional, interpersonal relationship with the patient to guide efficient management.

Differential diagnosis is used to identify the pertinent diagnosis (condition) of the patient and is the focus of this chapter. This chapter should be read together with Chapter 15.

Differential diagnosis is a systematic process used to identify the proper diagnosis from a competing set of possible diagnoses. The diagnostic process involves identifying or determining the aetiology of a disease or condition through evaluation of patient history, physical examination, and review of laboratory data or diagnostic imaging; and the subsequent descriptive title of that finding.[1]

WHY IS DIFFERENTIAL DIAGNOSIS IMPORTANT?

Failure to correctly identify an appropriate diagnosis can lead to negative patient-reported outcomes,[2] delays in appropriate treatment,[1] and unnecessary healthcare costs.[3]

What makes diagnostic tests inaccurate?

- failure to order appropriate tests (58% of instances)
- inadequate history/physical examination (42% of instances)
- incorrect test interpretations (37% of instances).[4]

With respect to medical errors, diagnostic errors are the most commonly recorded type (29% of all errors) and account for the highest proportion of total payments (35%).[5]

> **PRACTICE PEARL**
>
> Differential diagnostic errors result in death or disability almost twice as often as other error categories.

Although the exact prevalence of diagnostic error remains unknown, data from autopsy series spanning several decades conservatively and consistently reveal error rates of 10-15%.[6]

DIFFERENTIAL DIAGNOSIS: A THREE-STEP PROCESS

Regardless of treatment environment, most clinicians follow a three-step questioning process during diagnostic assessment.[7]

1. The first question of diagnosis involves the query of whether the patient's symptoms or emergent injury are reflective of a visceral disorder or a serious or potentially life-threatening illness. It is critical to be able to differentiate patients with symptoms that arise from a potentially life-threatening pathology or a non-mechanical disorder (i.e. referred pain).
2. The second question of diagnosis involves determining from where is the patient's pain arising? This step has three substeps that involve: a. ruling out a location; b. ruling in a location but not knowing the tissue-related structure; and c. confirming the tissue-related structure that is causal. Although it is assumed that one can make an accurate tissue-related diagnosis, it is well known that differentiating tissue in the low back, shoulder, abdomen and hip is very challenging and it is not uncommon to see clinicians treat these areas without full knowledge of the tissue of origin. We will discuss this further at the end of this chapter.

PART A Fundamental principles

3. The third question of diagnosis involves determining what has gone wrong with this person as a whole that would cause the pain experience to develop and persist.[7] This stage involves careful exploration of the social, psychosocial and socioeconomic contextual elements. This element is outlined in Chapter 17 (treatment) and given more detailed attention in Chapters 23 (neck pain) and 29 (low back pain).

HOW TO CALCULATE AN ACCURATE DIAGNOSIS

Diagnostic accuracy can be evaluated through a common set of metrics, metrics that are universally used regardless of testing type (e.g. imaging [Chapter 15], clinical testing, laboratory testing).

> **PRACTICE PEARL**
>
> Absolutely essential metrics that every clinician MUST understand include reliability, sensitivity and specificity, positive and negative predictive values, and positive and negative likelihood ratios (LR+ and LR−, respectively).

Reliability

In diagnostic terms, reliability involves the ability of a test to consistently identify a similar finding when retested (e.g. dynamometer testing for strength), or when used by a different clinician, or the level of consistent agreement among two or more clinicians when a particular test which requires interpretation is used (e.g. Lachman's test). Reliability is a required characteristic of diagnostic testing and is generally scored by 0–1 if one evaluates a numerically scored test such as a goniometer, or 0–1 if one assesses agreement among clinicians (higher scores reflecting greater agreement).

Sensitivity and specificity

Sensitivity and specificity are internal measures (meaning they are relatively independent of the sample) that are used in two distinct populations: 1. the disease of interest or injured population (sensitivity); and 2. a competing disease or non-injured population (specificity). Sensitivity is the percentage of people who test positive for a specific disease among a group of people who have the disease and this value is generally scored from 0%–100%. Higher values have a greater ability to accurately identify those *who have the disease of interest*. Specificity is the percentage of people who test negative for a specific disease among a group of people who do not have the disease and this value is also scored from 0%–100%. Higher values are more accurate at identifying those *who do not have the disease of interest*.

To recap, sensitivity and specificity capture values from two distinct populations: 1. the disease of interest or injured population (sensitivity); and 2. a competing disease or non-injured population (specificity). Figure 14.1 represents the conditions of interest for calculating sensitivity and specificity. Sensitivity only reflects those who have a 'true positive' and a 'false negative' test finding. Specificity only represents those who have a 'true negative' and a 'false positive' test finding. As one can see, each value only represents (potentially) one-half of the diagnostic story, and using these values independently is a mistake commonly made among clinicians.

> **PRACTICE PEARL**
>
> The assumptions of SP in ('high specificity rules in') and SN out ('high sensitivity rules out') are erroneously based on these assumptions.

Unfortunately, these outdated assumptions are misguided and cannot be advocated for clinical practice, primarily because routinely used tests have very high sensitivity and very low specificity (and vice versa), eliminating their capacity to discriminate conditions.

Positive and negative predictive values

Predictive values reflect the clinical setting. They are relevant when one asks the clinical question, 'The clinical screening test is positive. What is the likelihood that this patient truly has the condition?' Positive predictive value

	Has disease	Does not have disease
	True positive	False positive
	False negative	True negative

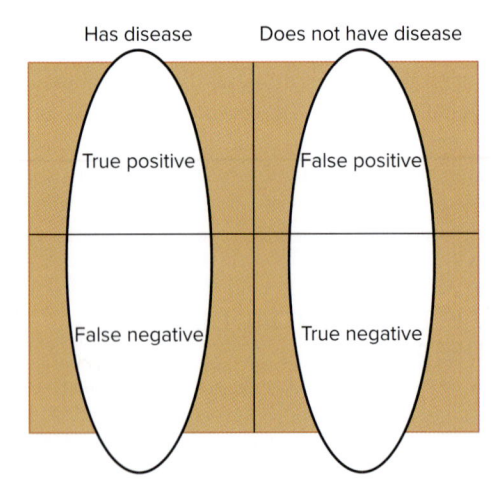

Figure 14.1 Sensitivity is measured among those individuals who have the disease. A great number of true positives and few false negatives lead to a high sensitivity (left ovoid). Specificity is measured among those who do not have the disease. In this case, a low number of false positives and a high number of true negatives generate a high specificity. Each of these numbers only represents half the diagnostic story.

Clinical assessment: moving from rote to rigorous CHAPTER 14

is the probability that subjects with a positive screening test truly have the disease. Negative predictive value is the probability that subjects with a negative screening test truly don't have the disease.

Like sensitivity and specificity, positive and negative predictive values only capture a portion of the population (Fig. 14.2) and should not be used exclusively in clinical practice because they fail to tell the full story of the test's utility. Positive predictive values include only true positives and false positives. Negative predictive values include only false and true negatives.

> **PRACTICE PEARL**
>
> Very importantly, positive and negative predictive values are markedly influenced by the prevalence of disease in the population that is being tested. If we test in a high-prevalence setting, it is more likely that persons who test positive truly have disease than if the test is performed in a population with low prevalence, thus artificially supporting the diagnostic value of a positive finding on a test.

Likelihood ratio

A high positive likelihood ratio (LR+) influences post-test probability with a positive finding. A value of >1 rules in a diagnosis. A low negative likelihood ratio (LR−) influences post-test probability with a negative finding. A value closer to 0 is best and rules out the condition. Although others have suggested thresholds for independent decision making, likelihood ratios should be evaluated within the context of pre-test prevalence and in each unique clinical setting.

Both sensitivity and specificity are used to determine positive and negative likelihood ratios. LR+ is calculated using the formula (sensitivity)/(100−specificity), whereas LR− is calculated using the formula (100−sensitivity)/(specificity). In LR+ and LR− the full population of interest, including those with and without the disease of interest, is factored into the decision-making metrics. This supports likelihood ratios as the most favourable metric for determining influence of post-test probability and for truly understanding the influence of a test on diagnosis accuracy. Further, likelihood ratios account for the prevalence, give further perspective, and allow for adjustments of test values in extreme cases of low or high prevalence. Some consistencies occur regardless of disease of interest. A higher pre-test probability will always improve the post-test probability. A lower pre-test probability will demand a strong LR+ (to rule in); conversely, a higher pre-test probability will require a lower LR− (to rule out) to notably alter the post-test probability.

Clinical utility

Clinical utility is a term used when evaluating the ability of the metrics to influence post-test probability (either in ruling out the condition or ruling it in) or just improving your likelihood of being correct. A nomogram is a routinely used mechanism to identify post-test probability. A nomogram has three scoring mechanisms, mounted vertically, left to right (Fig. 14.3).[8]

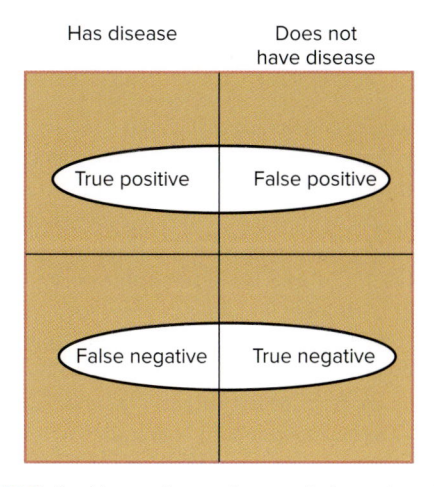

Figure 14.2 Positive and negative predictive values. These should be used when the clinician is trying to answer the question, 'The clinical screening test is positive. What is the likelihood that this patient truly has the condition?'

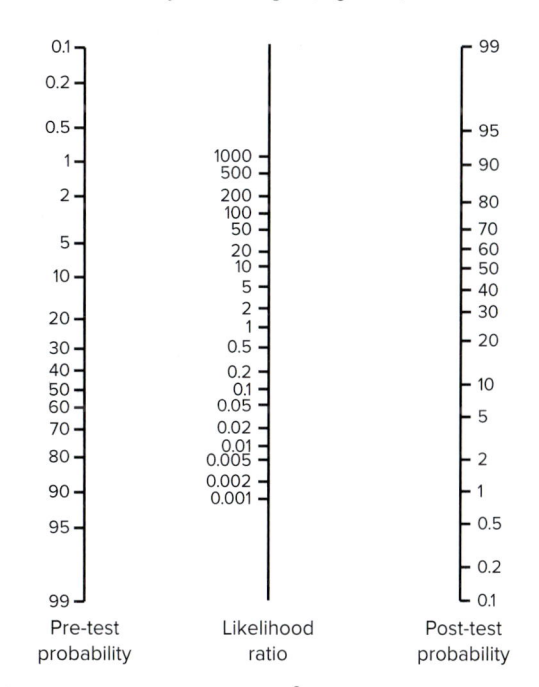

Figure 14.3 Fagan's nomogram[8]
REPRODUCED FROM FAGAN TJ. LETTER: NOMOGRAM FOR BAYES' THEOREM. N ENGL J MED. 1975;293(5):257

203

PART A   Fundamental principles

Applying Fagan's nomogram to the clinical setting: this tool is a key and underrated instrument for your career

Nomograms are an important learning mechanism to understand the interplay of pre-test probability, test metrics and post-test probability when differentially diagnosing. Consider the case of a patient with an anterior cruciate ligament (ACL) injury (Fig 14.4). Although ACL injuries are relatively uncommon per athlete exposure, the injuries make up a larger percentage of patients with knee problems in the sports medicine setting.[9]

If the percentage of individuals seen with an ACL injury in a busy sports medicine setting is 15%, one can assume that by chance, if the clinician 'guessed' ACL injury, he or she would be correct in 15% of cases. Since our goal is to improve post-test probability, the clinician may use a Lachman's test to further evaluate the likelihood of the condition. In a meta-analysis, the Lachman's test had an LR+ of 4.5 and LR− of 0.2.[10] Using the pre-test probability of 15% (based on numbers from the busy sports medicine setting) a positive Lachman's test would increase the post-test probability to 44% (green arrow, Fig. 14.4). In contrast, a negative finding on the Lachman's would result in a post-test probability of 4% (red arrow, Fig. 14.4).

Similar calculations can be performed for all conditions in all settings, with an understanding that pre-test prevalence will vary in different settings. Note that likelihood ratios are only as good as the influence they provide on post-test probability.

The left column represents the pre-test probability of the disease of interest with either no testing, based on the probability of occurrence in the practice environment of the clinician (i.e. anterior cruciate ligament tears are more common in a sports medicine specialist's environment), or based on the data used to evaluate the sample. This value is scored 0% (low prevalence) to 99% (high prevalence). The middle column represents the inherent likelihood ratio (positive in the upper column, negative in the lower column) and is generally combined with the pre-test probability to determine post-test probability.

The final column (on the right of the nomogram) represents the post-test probability. This value is determined by running a line from the pre-test probability, through the middle column (test metric) to the post-test probability value (Fig. 14.4).

> **PRACTICE PEARL**
>
> Differential diagnosis is case dependent and several rules of thumb are useful.

Tests will generally have high LR+ or a small LR− but rarely both. Consequently, the test metrics drive appropriate use: some should be used early to rule out a condition (those with small LR−) and some should be used later to confirm the presence of the condition (those with a large LR+). If the tests are used inappropriately, such as using a test with low LR− but also a low LR+, to rule in a condition, one is unlikely to accurately represent what the test is designed to do. Table 14.1 gives some examples of which tests are best for use early to 'rule out' a condition (small LR−) or late to 'rule in' a condition (large LR+).

For a comprehensive list of the best tests and measures, and each test's individual metrics, see the textbooks on physical examination by Professors Chad Cook and Eric Hegedus (Fig. 14.5)[11] and clinical assessment by Dr Michael Reiman (Fig. 14.5).[12] Both are essential resources.

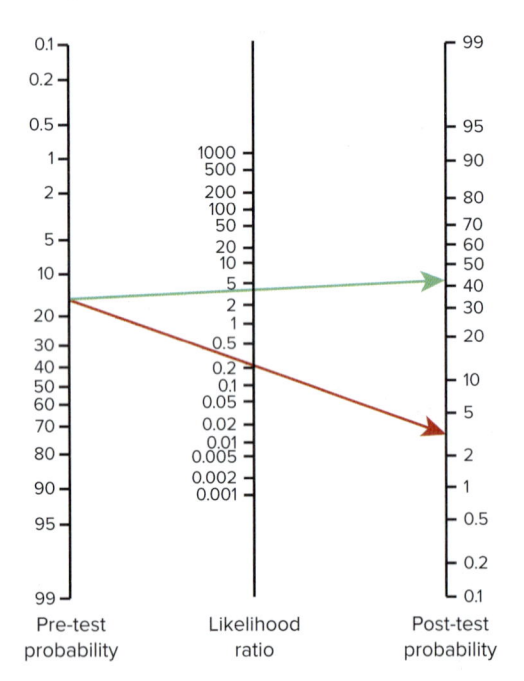

Figure 14.4 This illustrates the case where the pre-test probability (left) was 15%, LR+ (middle line) was 4.5 and the post-test probability (derived from those points if the test was positive, green arrow) was 44%. In practice, this means the clinician has increased his/her confidence about a diagnosis from 'relatively unlikely' to 'relatively likely'. This likely also affects the treatment plan and certainly the conversation with the patient as to treatment plan (see 'shared decision making' in Chapters 2 and 15.)
REPRODUCED WITH PERMISSION OF NEW ENGLAND JOURNAL OF MEDICINE

Clinical assessment: moving from rote to rigorous CHAPTER 14

Table 14.1 Common tests and measures and the test's ability to 'rule in' or 'rule out' a condition[11]

Test	Dominant test metric	Best use in clinical practice
Straight-leg raise for lumbar radiculopathy	A (negative) test has a small LR− and reduces to the post-test probability of lumbar radiculopathy	The test should be used early in the examination to rule out lumbar radiculopathy only
The External Rotation Lag sign for infraspinatus tears of the shoulder	A (positive) test has a high LR+ and increases the post-test probability of an infraspinatus tear	The test should be used near the end of the examination to rule in an infraspinatus tear of the shoulder
The Hawkins–Kennedy test for impingement of the shoulder	A (negative) test has a low LR− and reduces the post-test probability of shoulder impingement	The test should be used early in the examination to rule out impingement of the shoulder
The patellar-pubic percussion test for the hip (fractured femur)	The test has both a low LR− and a high LR+ and influences post-test probability with a negative and a positive	The test is a rare one that can rule in or rule out a hip fracture and can be used at all time points, respecting safety for the patient
The anterior drawer test for an ACL tear	A (positive) test has a high LR+ and increases the post-test probability of an ACL tear	The test should be used near the end of the examination to rule in an ACL tear
The squeeze test for a syndesmosis injury at the ankle	The test does not exhibit a high LR+ or a small LR−, thus it does not influence post-test probability	The test should not be used to rule in or rule out

Some adapted content from Cook C, Hegedus E. *Orthopedic Physical Examination Tests: An Evidence-Based Approach.* 2nd edn. Upper Saddle River NJ; Prentice Hall: 2013.

(a)

(b)

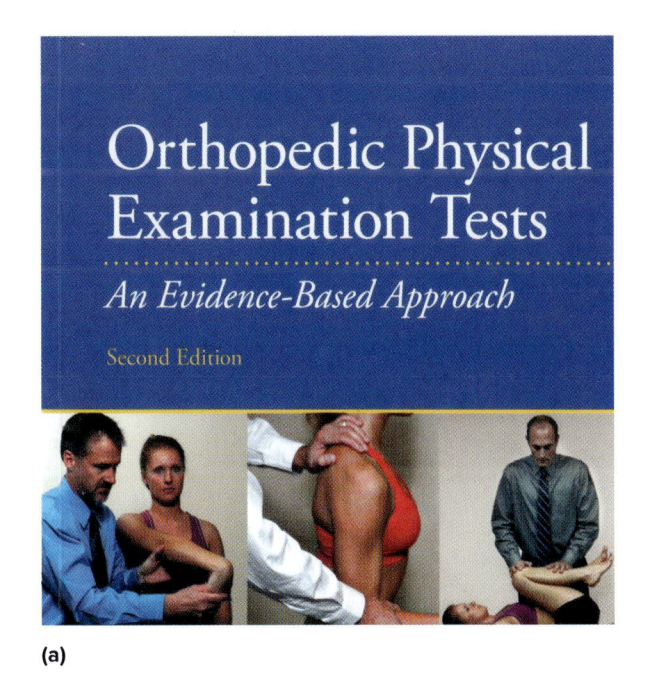

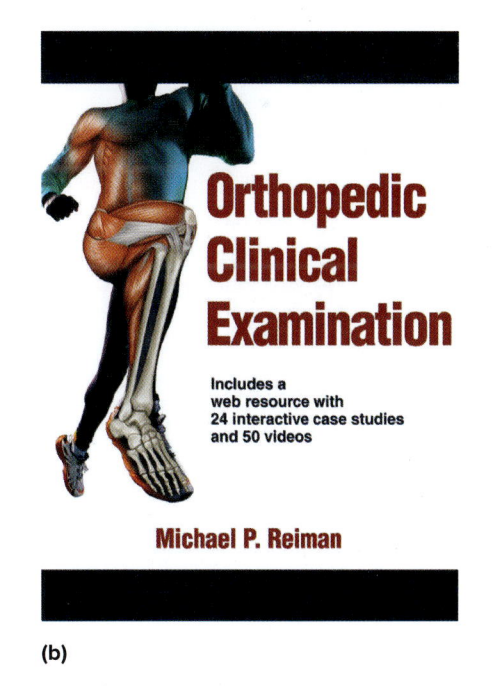

Figure 14.5 Two excellent resources to help you become a skilled clinician. (a) *Orthopedic Physical Examination Tests* by Professors Chad Cook and Eric Hegedus[11] (b) *Orthopedic Clinical Examination* by Dr Michael Reiman[12]
COOK, CHAD; HEGEDUS, ERIC, ORTHOPEDIC PHYSICAL EXAMINATION TESTS: AN EVIDENCE-BASED APPROACH, 2ND ED., ©2013. REPRINTED BY PERMISSION OF PEARSON EDUCATION, INC., NEW YORK, NEW YORK; REIMAN M.P., ORTHOPEDIC CLINICAL EXAMINATION, © 2016, REPRINTED BY PERMISSION OF HUMAN KINETICS, CHAMPAIGN, IL

PART A Fundamental principles

THE FORMAL DIAGNOSTIC ASSESSMENT

Diagnosis relies on taking a careful history, performing a thorough physical examination and using appropriate investigations. There is a tendency for clinicians to rely too heavily on sophisticated investigations and to neglect their clinical skills.[13] The goal of the clinical assessment when considering differential diagnosis is to improve post-test probability, thus providing the most appropriately aligned care to the athlete. During clinical assessment, all test findings have the capacity to influence post-test probability, including: 1. patient history and intake information; 2. observation; 3. the dedicated clinical (movement and performance) examination; and 4. special triage or confirmatory testing.

It is imperative to recognise that key features such as training history, nutrition, general health, work and leisure habits, past injury, equipment use, sports-specific demands, involvement in other sports and psychological features can markedly influence the diagnosis of a patient. These features paint a comprehensive picture of the state of the athlete's condition and the external factors that may drive future care needs.

It is well known that clinicians place too great a value on single testing mechanisms during differential diagnosis, and the tests do not have the capacity to discriminate in absence of these other important considerations. This includes ALL forms of tests, such as imaging, laboratory testing and so on. In essence, a good clinician evaluates all the information and places the test finding in context.

> **PRACTICE PEARL**
>
> Most clinicians overestimate the utility of special tests, assuming they provide more decision-making capacity than they do. Only use special tests in context to the rest of the clinical assessment.

The role of bias in influencing diagnostic metrics

Can you rely on published reports of test accuracy? Unfortunately not, because the design of a study can markedly influence its reported diagnostic accuracy. Recognising this, Whiting and colleagues created the Quality Assessment of Diagnostic Accuracy Studies tool (QUADAS) and subsequently QUADAS II.[14] A number of researchers have recognised the influence of bias through use of QUADAS and its impact on elevating test metrics. Each study should be carefully analysed for risk of bias before considering the test's use in clinical practice. Some biases can elevate the value of accuracy metrics by four times the realistic amount, suggesting far greater utility of a test that may provide very little in clinical practice.

> **PRACTICE PEARL**
>
> Diagnostic metrics from diagnostic accuracy studies that exhibit high risk of bias, regardless of where these studies were published, should not be incorporated into clinical practice. Bias markedly influences test metrics.

Challenges to making a diagnosis

Differential diagnosis is an imperfect science. For reasons beyond the limitations of testing, some diagnoses are extremely difficult to make. The following are examples of non-correctable challenges to diagnosis and deserve explanation.

- Verification bias occurs when the gold standard procedures (e.g. biopsy, surgery) are provided to only a select few (because of costs, effort and so on) and subsequently only reflect that select few. Unfortunately, the extra step needed to improve the accuracy limits the generalisability of the finding. Whether a more traditional population would yield the same result is unknown.[15]
- Syndromes refer only to the set of detectable (examination) characteristics (signs and symptoms) that are related to a defined diagnosis. Unlike diseases, which have hard imaging, clinical or laboratory findings, syndromes are purely based on numerous intangible features (e.g. thoracic outlet syndrome), increasing the likelihood that two individuals can be diagnosed with the same problem, despite exhibiting notably different clinical findings.
- Condition severity is a known mediator to diagnostic accuracy. For example, a superior labral anterior posterior (SLAP) lesion can be categorised into four distinct groups using Snyder's classification.[16] Type I and type II classifications exhibit clinical features that are strikingly similar to a rotator cuff tear, impingement, bursitis and so on, and these classifications are notably difficult to differentiate in clinical practice in comparison to the more severe classifications of type III and IV.
- Incorporation bias occurs when the test is part of the diagnosis. An example is patellofemoral pain syndrome which is a diagnosis based on anterior knee pain and challenges with functional activities. Often, the functional activities are testing for their predictability; despite that, these are part of the diagnosis itself. The main problem with incorporation bias is its overestimating diagnostic accuracy.

FINAL THOUGHTS AND GUIDANCE

There are a number of considerations one must make that go beyond diagnostic metrics and clinical tests and measures. First, as David Matcher implies, few tests markedly change clinical practice for the good of society.[17] One can argue that a minority of our clinical tests and measures are superfluous and do little in assisting in decision making for the long-term good of our athlete. This is likely why we have a proliferation of newly created clinical tests for diagnosis of the shoulder, the sacroiliac joint and other problematic regions.

It is imperative that differential diagnosis include a careful discussion with the athlete and the implications of the finding. Shared decision making is necessary for both parties to consider which treatment is appropriate for the condition. By being aware of the limitations highlighted in this chapter, clinical assessment and judicious use of imaging provides a great foundation for the treatment plan. In Chapter 15, we share some practical clinical approaches you can use to maximise your chances of arriving at the most likely diagnosis! The great clinician combines science and art.

REFERENCES

References for this chapter can be found at www.mhhe.com/au/CSM5e

Chapter 15

How to make the diagnosis

with ALI GUERMAZI, JON PATRICIOS and BRUCE FORSTER

Wherever the art of medicine is loved, there is also a love of humanity.
Hippocrates (c.460–370 BCE)

This chapter should be read in conjunction with Chapter 14. These chapters are very different from their fourth edition predecessors. In earlier editions of *Clinical Sports Medicine*, we argued for the importance of accurate pathological diagnosis. At times, this is realistic. A player falls on his or her wrist and sustains an acute scaphoid fracture. You can make a clinical diagnosis and confirm it with imaging. So far, so good. Accurate tissue diagnosis remains a foundation *where appropriate*.

In this fifth edition, we recognise that we previously overestimated the proportion of settings where *accurate, very specific* tissue diagnosis is possible. Consider patients who present with low back pain. Is the tissue diagnosis the facet joint, vertebra, fascia, muscle or disc? In these cases, can investigation, such as magnetic resonance imaging (MRI) provide the holy grail of tissue diagnosis? No, MRI cannot.

This chapter reinforces Chapter 14's key message– the art of diagnosis takes place against a backdrop of patient-based probabilities. Honest teachers will explain that the clinician is narrowing the odds from the 'pre-test probability' to a new 'post-test probability'. (See Likelihood ratios and Fagan's Nomogram, Chapter 14.)

DOES 'DIAGNOSIS' MEAN 'TISSUE DIAGNOSIS'?

Is there a difference between a diagnosis of: 1. 'swimmer's shoulder'; 2. 'rotator cuff tendinopathy'; and 3. 'shoulder pain related to training load errors and suboptimal biomechanics'? The first of these ('swimmer's shoulder') represents a 1970s advance in sports medicine. Alongside labels such as tennis elbow, goalie's elbow, hockey player's groin and footballer's ankle, 'diagnosis' consisted of the name of a sport paired with a commonly injured body part. This was an advance at the time, as many doctors were not aware of sports medicine conditions and sports physiotherapy had not yet emerged in many countries.

The major limitation of this type of label is lack of precision. Each of those labels (e.g. hockey groin) could apply to a number of pathological entities which may benefit from distinct treatment. Such labels have no place in 21st-century sports medicine.

What about 'rotator cuff tendinopathy'? Is that a valid diagnosis? The fourth edition of *Clinical Sports Medicine* asserted that accurate pathological diagnosis was essential for the following reasons.

- *It enabled the clinician to explain the problem and the natural history of the condition to the athlete, who will want to know precisely for how long he or she will be affected. A patient may present with an acute knee injury but the diagnosis of anterior cruciate ligament (ACL) tear has markedly different implications to the diagnosis of minor meniscal injury.*
- *It enabled optimum treatment. Numerous conditions have similar presentations but markedly different treatments. For example, consider the differences in treatment between: lateral ligament sprain of the ankle and osteochondral fracture of the talus; patellofemoral joint syndrome and meniscal tear; and hamstring tear and hamstring pain referred from the lumbar spine.*
- *It enabled optimum rehabilitation prescription. For example, rehabilitation after shin pain due to stress fracture will be more gradual than that after identical shin pain due to chronic compartment syndrome.*

PART A   Fundamental principles

In that edition, we acknowledged that 'occasionally' it can be impossible to make a precise pathological diagnosis as in the case of back pain mentioned above. In such cases, it is still possible to exclude certain causes of low back pain (e.g. spondylolysis) and identify abnormalities such as areas of focal tenderness, altered soft tissue consistency or abnormalities of range of motion. Treatment then aims to resolve the condition. How treatment affects symptoms and signs can help determine how each particular abnormality contributes to the overall picture. An important final step in management is to address the cause/s: intrinsic and extrinsic.

> **PRACTICE PEARL**
>
> Our current perspective is that we overestimated the number of cases where a 'tissue diagnosis' is accurate and we certainly underestimated the role of the psychosocial factors in the patient's perception of the injury.

The biopsychosocial model featured in the fourth edition of *Clinical Sports Medicine* but only in the chapter on neck pain, rather than in Part A: Fundamental Principles. We failed to feature the biopsychosocial model in the diagnosis or treatment chapters but amend that in this edition (Fig. 15.1).

It is widely appreciated that in many clinical settings 'accurate tissue diagnosis' is impossible. Despite that, the clinician can guide the patient by assessing impairments, documenting the patient's level of function, providing reassurance based on epidemiological evidence of clinical outcomes and natural history. In sum, the clinician contributes his/her knowledge of best evidence rehabilitation to the shared decision.[1, 2]

KEYS TO ACCURATE DIAGNOSIS

Diagnosis relies on taking a careful history, performing a thorough physical examination and using appropriate investigations. Today, patient-reported outcome measures (PROMs) may also be essential as part of the initial assessment and this is introduced in the next chapter (Chapter 16). Useful PROMs are also included in the regional injury chapters in Part B of this book. 'Over-reliance on sophisticated investigations and neglected clinical skills' has been a mantra of senior medical educators for decades and the problem may be worsening.

Keys to accurate diagnosis in patients presenting with apparent musculoskeletal pain include:

- the age of the patient
- the mechanism of injury

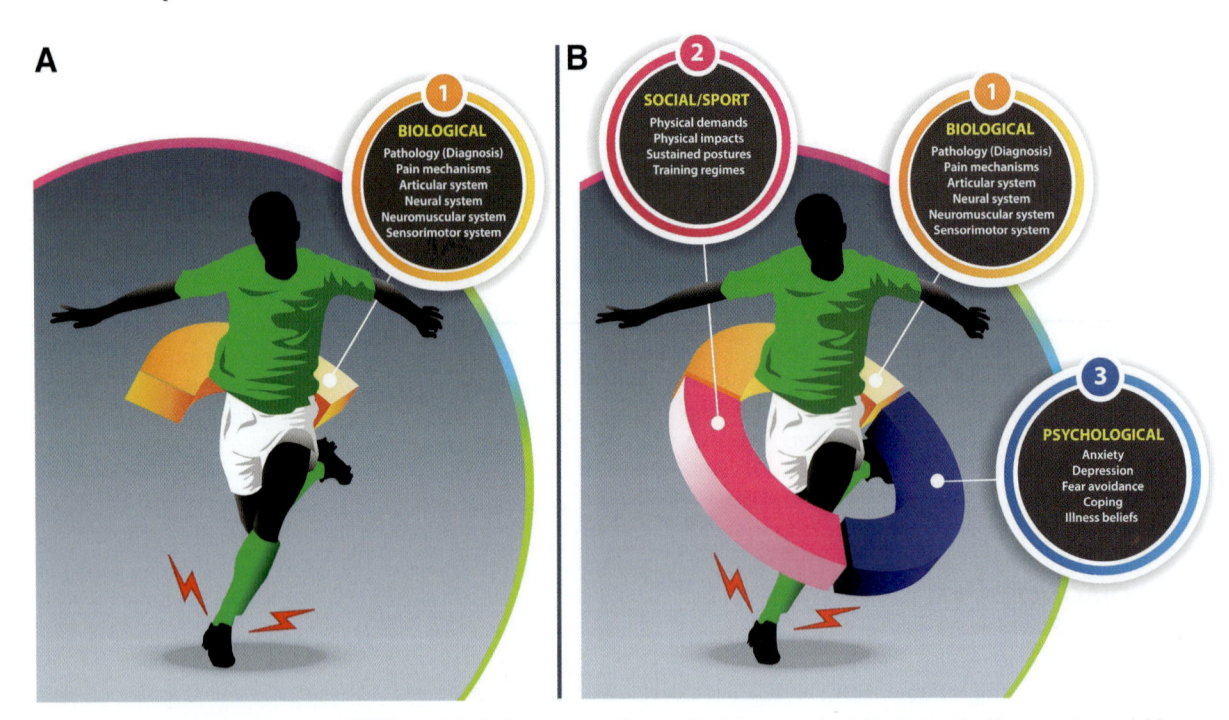

Figure 15.1 The biopsychosocial (BPS) model of disease provides an important context for the patient's experience (a) In a purely biomedical model, pathology explains the patient's pain experience and this is considered virtually equivalent to the patient's experience (b) The biopsychosocial model provides a holistic approach to diagnosis. Many factors, not only the tissue pathology, should be taken into account. Psychological and social/sport factors, depicted here, contribute to a more compete diagnosis. See also Chapters 5 and 6 that explain pain in sports injuries

How to make the diagnosis — CHAPTER 15

- whether the symptoms are of musculoskeletal origin (Chapter 7)
- possible local causes of the patient's symptoms
- sites that could be referring pain to the site of the symptoms (Chapters 5, 6)
- the relevant kinetic chain (e.g. the back and lower limb in a shoulder injury of a tennis player)
- biomechanics (Chapters 8 and 9)
- other possible causative factors (e.g. metabolic)
- patient expectations and understanding.

HISTORY

History remains the keystone of accurate diagnosis; it will provide the diagnosis in the majority of cases. Please consider the following principles when taking a history.

Allow enough time

The patient must feel that the clinician has time available to allow the story to unfold, otherwise important symptoms will not surface. In addition to the details of the injury, there must be time to take the history of the training program including details of training workload where this is available. Look into possible causes of injury. Diet history may be appropriate (i.e. contributing to stress fracture likelihood). As a minimum, 30 minutes is required to assess a patient with a new injury but in complex chronic cases up to one hour may be necessary.

Be a good listener

The clinician must let the story unravel. Appropriate body language and focus on the patient, and not the medical record or computer screen, will aid this. The sports clinician is in the fortunate position that many patients have good body awareness and are generally able to describe symptoms very well.

Know the sport

It is helpful to understand the technical demands of a sport when seeing an athlete as this engenders patient confidence. More importantly, knowledge of the biomechanics and techniques of a particular sport (see Chapter 9) can assist greatly in both making the primary diagnosis and uncovering the predisposing factors.

Discover the exact circumstances of the injury

The first task in history taking is to determine the exact context of the injury. The patient's age is the first clue: knee pain in an adolescent is more likely to be an apophysitis such as Osgood–Schlatter disease while in an elderly person degenerative causes are more likely; 'tennis elbow' in a child would be unusual but not in middle age. Next, the mechanism of injury warrants careful consideration. Most patients will be able to describe in considerable detail the mechanism of injury. In acute injuries, this is the single most important clue to diagnosis. For example, an inversion injury to the ankle strongly suggests a lateral ligament injury, a valgus strain to the knee may cause a medial collateral ligament injury, and a pivoting injury accompanied by a 'pop' in the knee and followed by rapid swelling suggests an ACL injury.

Obtain an accurate description of symptoms, both at the time of injury and at the initial consultation

Common musculoskeletal symptoms include pain, swelling, instability and loss of function.

Pain

Consider the characteristics of the patient's pain.

1. Location. Note the exact location of pain. Detailed knowledge of surface anatomy can be invaluable. If the pain is poorly localised or varies from site to site, consider the possibility of referred pain.
2. Onset. Speed of onset helps determine whether the pain is due to an acute or overuse injury. Was the onset of pain associated with a snap, crack, tear or other sensation?
3. Severity. Severity may be classified as mild, moderate or severe. Using a pain score (e.g. numerical rating scale [NRS]) or a specific outcome measure may be useful to gauge severity and monitor improvement. Another very helpful method is to have the patient detail the most important activity for them, and rate that with a score. Assess the severity of the pain immediately after the injury and subsequently. Was the patient able to continue the activity?
4. Irritability. This refers to the level of activity required to provoke pain and how long it subsequently takes to settle. The degree of irritability is especially important because it affects how vigorously the examination should be performed and how aggressive the treatment should be.
5. Nature. This refers to the quality of the pain. It is important to allow patients to describe pain in their own words. For example, 'burning pain' can suggest neural involvement.
6. Behaviour. Is the pain constant or intermittent? What is the time course of the pain? Is it worse on waking up or does it worsen during the day? Does it wake the patient at night?
7. Pain site and distribution. Does the pain radiate at all? If so, where?

8. Aggravating factors. Which activity or posture aggravates the pain?
9. Relieving factors. Is the pain relieved by rest or the adoption of certain postures? Do certain activities relieve the pain? Is the pain affected by climatic changes (e.g. cold weather)?
10. Associated features. These include swelling, instability, sensory symptoms (such as pins and needles, tingling or numbness) and motor symptoms (such as muscle weakness).
11. Previous treatment. What was the initial treatment of the injury? Was ice applied? Was firm compression applied? Was the injured part immobilised? If so, for how long? What treatment and rehabilitation has been performed and what effect did that treatment have on the pain? The latter is particularly important when you are providing a second or subsequent opinion in cases of long-standing problems.

Swelling

Immediate swelling following an injury may indicate a severe injury such as a fracture or major ligament tear accompanied by haemarthrosis. Record the degree of swelling (mild, moderate or severe) and subsequent changes in the amount of swelling.

Instability

Any history of giving way or feeling of instability is significant. Try to elicit the exact activity that causes this feeling. For example, in throwing, does the feeling of instability occur in the cocking phase or the follow-through?

Function

It is important to know whether the athlete was: 1. able to continue activity without any problems immediately after the injury happened; 2. able to continue with some restriction; or 3. unable to continue. Note subsequent changes in function with time. When patients present with chronic conditions, or have been receiving treatment already, see what level of function they have reached. Have they just failed to rehabilitate to the necessary level of function?[3] (See Chapter 18.)

History of a previous similar injury

If the athlete has had a previous similar injury, record full details of all treatment given, response to each type of treatment and whether any maintenance treatment or exercises have been performed following initial rehabilitation. Previous injury is the most important risk factor for recurrence.

Other injuries

Past injuries may have contributed to the current injury; for example, an inadequately rehabilitated muscle tear that has led to muscle imbalance and a subsequent overuse injury. Because of the importance of spinal abnormalities as a potential component of the athlete's pain (Chapter 5), the patient should always be questioned about spinal symptoms, especially pain and stiffness in the lower back or neck. Past or present injuries in body parts that may at first seem unrelated to the present injury may also be important. For example, a hamstring injury in a throwing athlete can impair the kinetic chain leading to the shoulder, alter throwing biomechanics and thus contribute to a rotator cuff injury.

General health

Is the patient otherwise healthy? Musculoskeletal symptoms are not always activity related (Chapter 7). Red flags for serious medical conditions masquerading as sports injuries include:

- no specific mechanism of injury
- pain unrelated to activity
- night pain
- associated symptoms and signs such as weight loss, fever, malaise, lymphadenopathy
- poor response to treatment.

Consider asking specifically about diabetes, possible undiagnosed inflammatory conditions (e.g. skin problems of psoriasis, bowel complaints associated with spondyloarthropathies) and familial conditions.

Work and leisure activities

Work and leisure activities can play a role in both the aetiology and subsequent management of an injury. For example, a patient whose job involves continual bending or who enjoys gardening may aggravate his or her low back pain. It is important to know about these activities and to ascertain whether they can be curtailed.

Consider why the problem has occurred

Predisposing factors should be considered not only in overuse injuries, but also in medical conditions and in acute injuries. In an athlete struggling to return to play after an ACL injury for example, there may be an underlying psychological component.

An athlete with an acute hamstring tear may have a history of low back problems or, alternatively, a history of a previous inadequately rehabilitated tear. Recurrence can only be prevented by eliminating the underlying cause.

Training/activity history

In any overuse injury, a comprehensive training history is required. This is best done as a weekly diary as most athletes train on a weekly cycle (Chapter 12). It should contain both the quantity and quality of training and describe any recent changes. Note the total amount of training (distance or hours depending on the sport) and training surfaces. Ideally, the patient will have a detailed training history that includes perception of how hard training was. Training can be measured as (i) 'internal load', such as measured by rating of perceived exertion (RPE), or (ii) 'external load', such as training volume in distance covered or balls pitched or bowled. Continual activity on hard surfaces or a recent change in surface may predispose to injury. In running sports, pay particular attention to footwear (Chapter 8). For both training and competition shoes, note the shoe type, age and wear pattern. Record recovery activities such as soft tissue therapy, spa/sauna and hours of sleep. Asking patients to bring a training diary or history to the consultation is a useful pre-emptive tactic.

Equipment

Inappropriate equipment may predispose to injury (Chapter 12). For example, a bicycle seat that is set too low may contribute to patellofemoral pain.

Technique

Patients should discuss technique problems that either they, or their coach, have noted. Faulty technique may contribute to injury. For example, a 'wristy' backhand drive may contribute to extensor tendinopathy at the elbow (Chapter 9).

Overtraining

Symptoms such as excessive fatigue, recurrent illness, reduced motivation, persistent soreness and stiffness may point to overtraining as an aetiologic factor.

Psychological factors

Injury can be caused or exacerbated by a number of psychological factors that may relate to sport (i.e. pressure of impending competition), or may concern personal or business life. The clinician needs to consider this possibility and approach it sensitively.

Nutritional factors

Inadequate nutrition can predispose to the overtraining syndrome and may play a role in the development of musculoskeletal injuries. Eating disorders may also inhibit healing. In an athlete presenting with excessive tiredness, a full dietary history is essential.

Drugs: prescription and others

As with all complete medical histories, a history of medication use may be appropriate. Fluoroquinolone antibiotics may be the cause of a patient's tendinopathy, while cold and influenza medications have been associated with arrhythmias. Athletes may take social drugs such as cocaine, and performance-enhancing anabolic steroids have a range of systemic side effects. Athletes are unlikely to volunteer this information, and direct questioning is not only appropriate but reveals a good clinical understanding of the context of injury in sport.

History of exercise-induced anaphylaxis

Exercise-induced anaphylaxis (EIA) and food-dependent, exercise-induced anaphylaxis (FDEIA) are rare, but potentially life-threatening clinical syndromes in which association with exercise is crucial. It is a clinical syndrome in which anaphylaxis occurs in conjunction with exercise. Given the rarity of the condition, our current understanding relies on case studies alone and is acknowledged as being very limited.[4]

Determine the importance of the sport to the athlete

The level of commitment to the sport, which will not necessarily correlate with the athlete's expertise, has a bearing on management decisions. Be aware of the athlete's short- and long-term future sporting commitments to schedule appropriate treatment and rehabilitation programs.

Differential diagnosis

At the conclusion of taking the history, it is important to consider the differential diagnosis and the possible aetiologic factors. Then proceed to a thorough focused examination.

PHYSICAL EXAMINATION

In this practical chapter, we share a number of general principles that might speed the novice clinician towards better physical examination. We acknowledge the limitations of physical examination (Chapter 14)[5] and of imaging (below), but they still provide valuable information that increases the likelihood of making the correct diagnosis and thus of choosing evidence-based treatment for a patient's complaints.

PART A Fundamental principles

Develop a routine
Use a specific routine for examining each joint, region or system as this forms a habit and allows you to concentrate on the findings and their significance rather than thinking of what to do next. In Part B we outline a routine for examining each body part.

Remember that in most sports the athlete functions in the upright position. Avoid the temptation to only examine the patient in a supine or prone position. Moreover, running sports involve supporting the body on one leg or the other most of the time. Simulate this in your examination. Consider starting the examination assessing posture and having the patient perform various stress tests on one leg (e.g. hopping, one-legged squat).

Where relevant, examine the other side
With some aspects of the examination (e.g. ligamentous laxity or muscle tightness), it is important to compare sides using the uninjured side as a control.

Consider possible causes of the injury
Try to ascertain the cause of the injury. It is not sufficient to examine the painful area only (e.g. the Achilles tendon). Acknowledge the importance of the kinetic chain. Examine joints, muscles and neural structures proximal and distal to the injured area, seeking predisposing factors (e.g. limited dorsiflexion of the ankle, tight gastrocnemius-soleus complex, lumbar facet joint dysfunction). A useful tip is to examine all the areas that may possibly contribute to the injury before honing in on the site of pain.

Attempt to reproduce the patient's symptoms
It is helpful to reproduce the patient's symptoms if possible. This can be achieved both by active and/or passive movements and by palpation either locally or, in the case of referred pain, at the site of referral. It may require you to send the patient for a run or some other test of function prior to examination (see below).

Assess local tissues
Assess the joints, muscles and neural structures at the site of pain for tenderness, tissue feel and range of motion.

Assess for referred pain
Assess the joints, muscles and neural structures that may refer to the site of pain (Chapter 4).

Assess neural mechanosensitivity
Neural mechanosensitivity (Chapters 5 and 6) should be assessed using one or more of the neurodynamic tests (see below).

Examine the spine
Many injuries have a spinal component to the pain or dysfunction. Abnormal neural mechanosensitivity suggests a possible spinal component. In lower limb injuries, examine the lumbar spine and the thoracolumbar junction. In upper limb injuries, examine the cervical and upper thoracic spines. Examine for hypomobility of isolated spinal segments as this may contribute to distant symptoms. See the routine for spinal examination later in this chapter.

Biomechanical examination
As biomechanical abnormalities are one of the major causes of overuse injuries, it is essential to include this examination in the assessment of overuse injuries (Chapters 8 and 9). The biomechanical examination of the lower limb is illustrated in Chapter 8. The mechanics of the lower limb may be relevant to an upper limb injury (e.g. weak hip stabilisers resulting in overload of the elbow in sports involving repetitive throwing).

Functional testing
If a particular manoeuvre reproduces the patient's pain, then have the patient perform that manoeuvre in an attempt to understand why the pain has occurred. This can sometimes be done in the office (e.g. a deep squat) or it may be necessary to watch the athlete perform the activity at a training venue (e.g. a long jumper taking off or a gymnast performing a backward walkover). Video analysis may be helpful.

The examination routine
Inspection
It is important to observe the individual walking into the office or walking off the field of play as well as inspecting the injured area. Note any evidence of deformity, asymmetry, bruising, swelling, skin changes and muscle wasting. There may, however, be a degree of asymmetry due to one side being dominant, such as the racquet arm in a tennis player.

Range of motion testing (active)
Ask the athlete to perform active range of motion exercises without assistance. Look carefully for restriction of range of motion, the onset of pain at a particular point in the range, and the presence of abnormal patterns of movement. In many conditions, such as shoulder impingement or patellofemoral pain, the pattern of movement is critical to making a correct diagnosis.

If a patient's pain is not elicited on normal plane movement testing, examine 'combined movements' (i.e. movements in two or more planes). By combining movements and evaluating symptom response, additional information is gained to help predict the site of the lesion. Other movements, such as repeated, quick or sustained movements, may be required to elicit the patient's pain.

Range of motion testing (passive)

Passive range of motion testing is used to elicit joint and muscle stiffness. Injury may be the cause of joint stiffness. Alternatively, stiffness may already have been present and predispose to injury by placing excessive stress on other structures (e.g. a stiff ankle joint can predispose to Achilles tendinopathy). Range of motion testing should include all directions of movement appropriate to a particular joint, and should be compared both with normal range and the unaffected side. Overpressure may be used at the end of range to elicit the patient's symptoms.

Palpation

Palpation is a vital component of examination and precise knowledge of anatomy, especially surface anatomy, optimises its value. At times it is essential to determine the exact site of maximal tenderness (e.g. in differentiating between bony tenderness and ligament attachment tenderness after a sprained ankle). When palpating soft tissues, properties of the soft tissue that need to be assessed include:

- resistance
- muscle spasm
- tenderness.

Palpate carefully and try to visualise the structures being palpated. Commence with the skin, feeling for any changes in temperature or amount of sweating, infection or increased sympathetic activity. When palpating muscle, assess tone, focal areas of thickening or trigger points, muscle length and imbalance.

It is important not only to palpate the precise area of pain (e.g. the supraspinatus tendon attachment), but also the regions proximal and distal to the painful area, such as the muscle belly of the trapezius muscle. Determine whether tenderness is focal or diffuse. This may help differentiate between, for example, a stress fracture (focal tenderness) and periostitis (diffuse tenderness).

To palpate joints correctly, it is important to understand the two different types of movement present at a joint. Physiological movements are movements that patients can perform themselves. However, in order to achieve a full range of physiological movement, accessory movements are required. Accessory movements are the involuntary, interarticular movements, including glides, rotations and tilts that occur in both spinal and peripheral joints during normal physiological movements. Loss of these normal accessory movements may cause pain, altered range or abnormal quality of physiological joint movement. Palpation of the spinal and peripheral joints is based on these principles. An example of palpation of accessory movements involves posteroanterior pressure over the spinous process of the vertebra, producing a glide between that vertebra and the ones above and below.

Ligament testing

Ligaments are examined for laxity and pain. Specific tests have been devised for all the major ligaments of the body. These involve moving the joint to stress a particular ligament. This may cause pain or reveal laxity in the joint. Laxity is graded into +1 (mild), +2 (moderate) and +3 (severe). Pain on stressing the ligament is also significant and may indicate, in the absence of laxity, a mild injury or grade I ligament sprain. A number of different tests may assess a single ligament; for example, the anterior drawer, Lachman's and pivot shift tests all test ACL laxity.

Strength testing

Muscles or groups of muscles should be tested for strength and compared with the unaffected side. Muscle weakness may occur as a result of an injury (e.g. secondary to a chronic joint effusion) or may be a predisposing factor towards injury. Muscle strength can be assessed manually or with the use of a hand-held dynamometer.

Testing neural mechanosensitivity

Advances in the understanding of neural mechanosensitivity have improved our awareness of why pain occurs in chronic overuse injuries and pain syndromes. Changes in neural mechanosensitivity are an important component of these disorders; see Chapter 4 (overuse) and Chapters 5 and 6 (pain).

Just as restrictions of the normal mechanics of joints and muscles may contribute to symptoms, restriction of the normal mechanics of the nervous system may also produce pain. Certain movements require considerable variations in nerve length. Neurodynamic testing (formerly known as 'neural tension tests') examines restriction of these normal mechanics and their effect on the patient's symptoms. Treatment aims to restore normal nerve mechanics.

Neurodynamic tests use movement to systematically increase neural mechanosensitivity. The tests may provoke the presenting symptoms or, alternatively, other symptoms such as pins and needles or numbness. The amount of resistance encountered during the test is also significant, especially when compared with the uninjured side. The assessment of symptom production and resistance may be affected by each step in the neurodynamic test (see Figs 15.2 to 15.5). This may give an indication of the location of the abnormality.

The main neurodynamic tests are:

- straight-leg raise (SLR) (Fig. 15.2a and b)
- slump test (Fig. 15.3a–e)
- neural Thomas test (Fig. 15.4a and b)
- upper limb neurodynamic test (Fig. 15.5a–e).

PART A   Fundamental principles

(a)

(b)

Figure 15.2 Straight leg raise (a) Patient lies supine. The examiner places one hand under the Achilles tendon and the other above the knee. The leg is lifted perpendicular to the bed with the hand above the knee, preventing any knee flexion (b) Dorsiflexion of the ankle is added. Eversion and toe extension may sensitise this test further. Other variations can be added (Table 15.1)

(a)

(b)

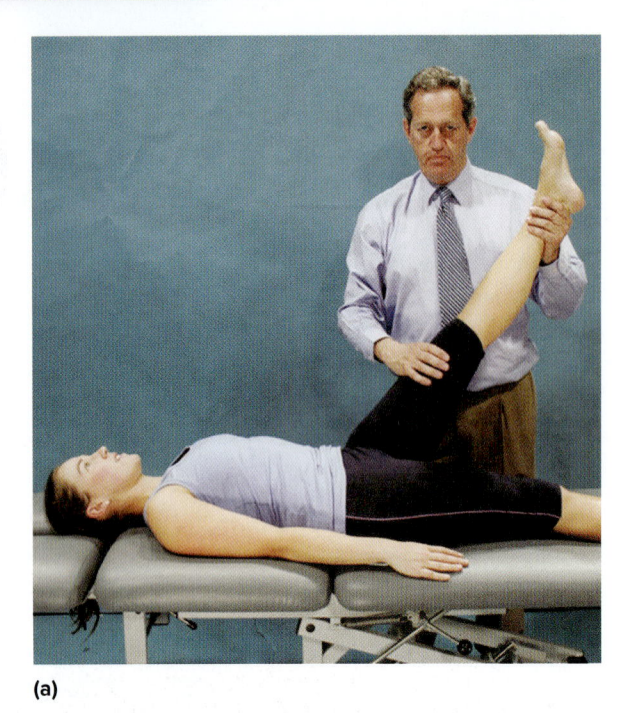

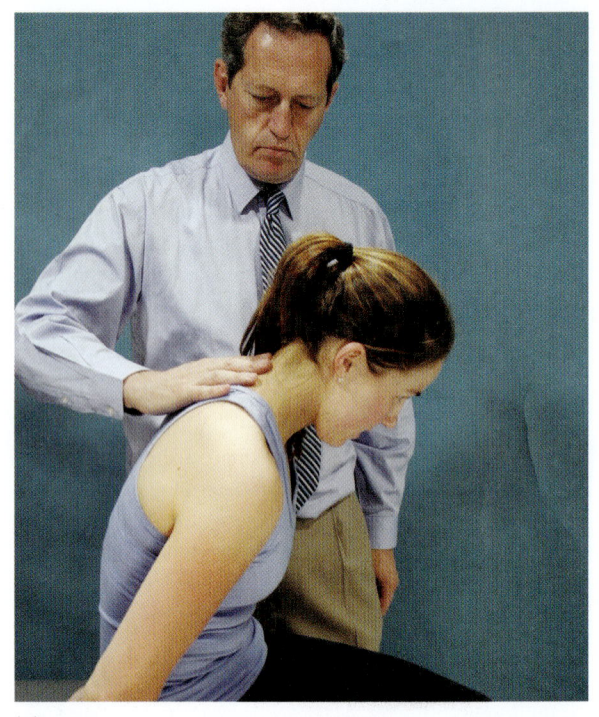

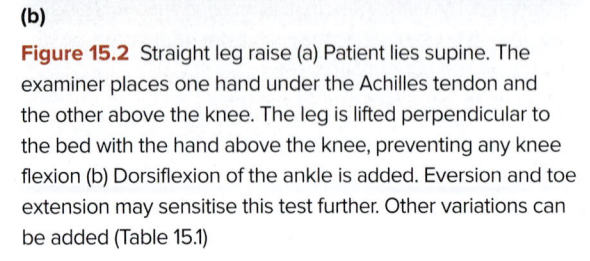

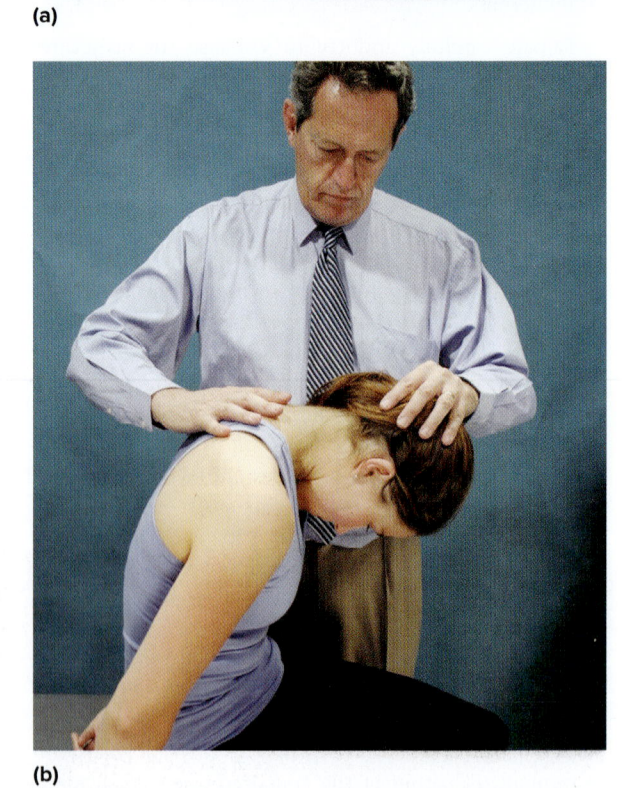

Figure 15.3 Slump test (a) Patient slumps forward and overpressure is applied. The sacrum should remain vertical (b) Patient is asked to put chin on chest and overpressure is applied

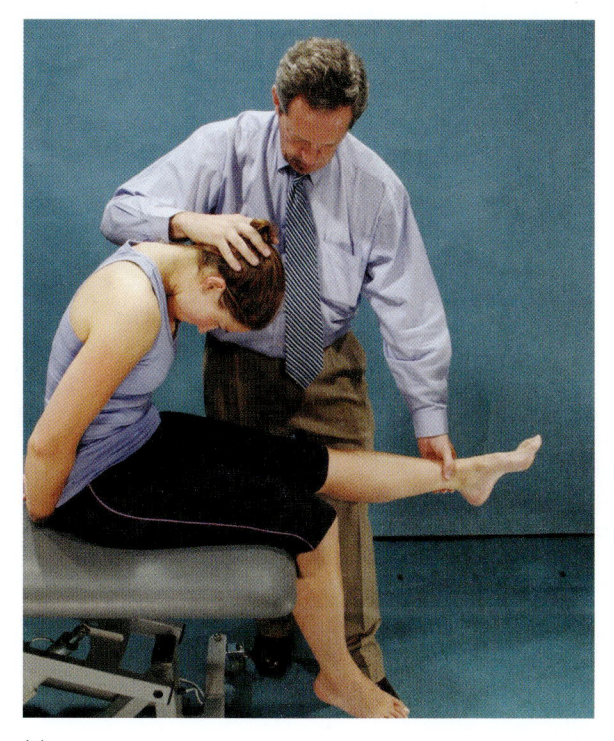

How to make the diagnosis CHAPTER 15

(c)

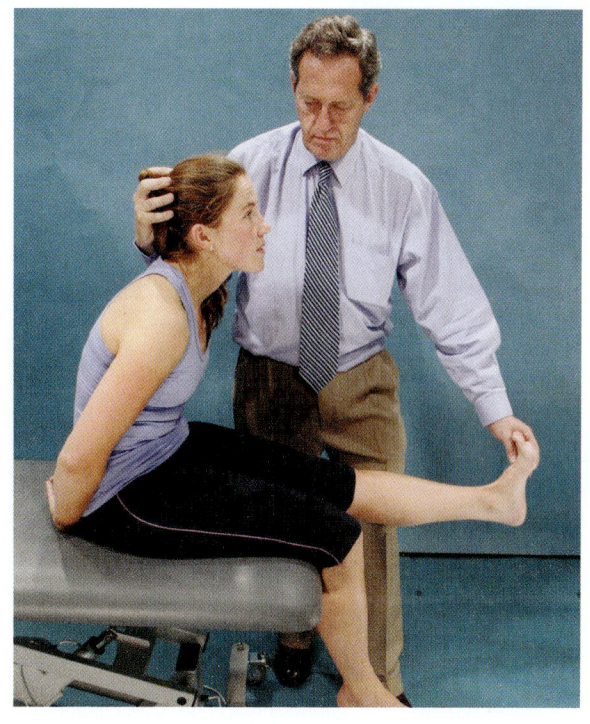

(e)

Figure 15.3 (cont.) (c) Patient actively extends one knee (d) Patient actively dorsiflexes the ankle and overpressure may be applied (e) Neck flexion is slowly released. Steps (d), (e) and (f) are repeated with the other knee. Other variations can be added (Table 15.1)

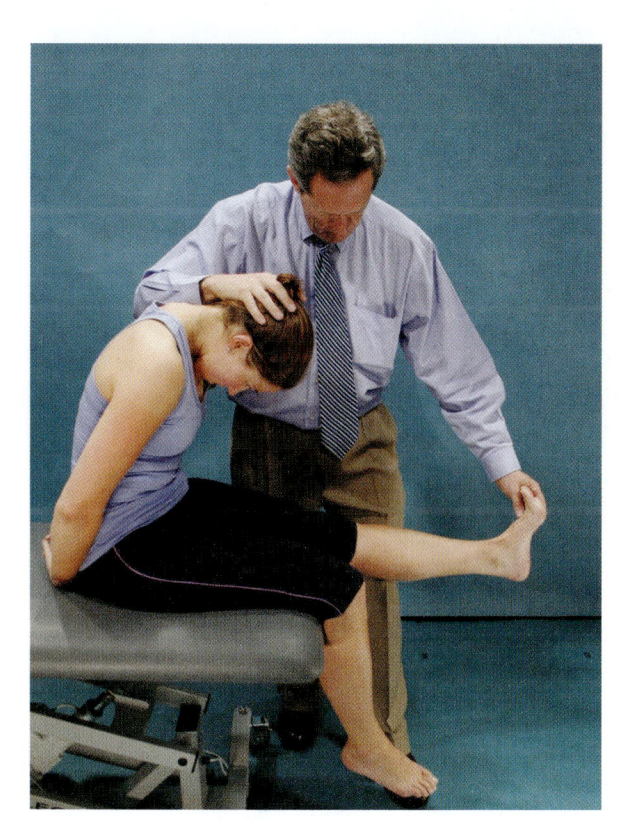

(d)

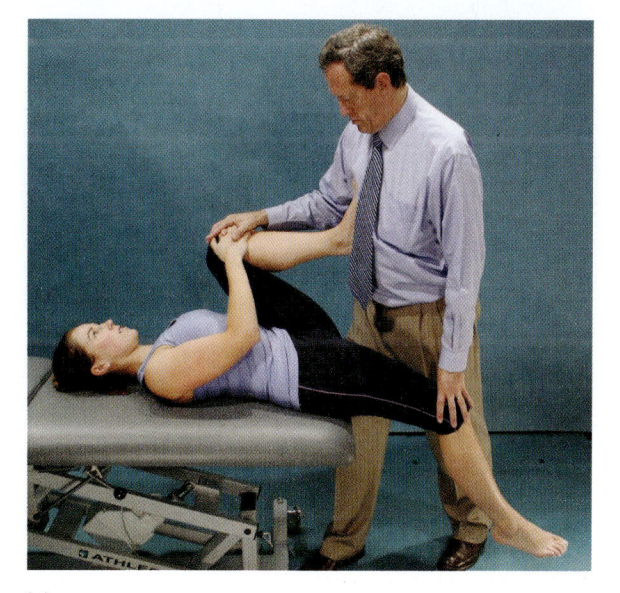

(a)

Figure 15.4 Neural Thomas test (a) Patient lies supine over the end of the couch in the Thomas position

217

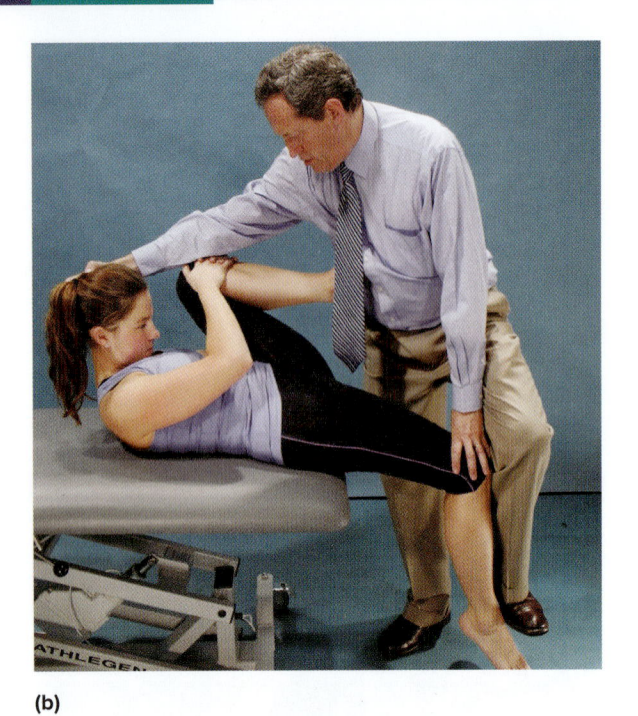

PART A   Fundamental principles

(b)

Figure 15.4 (cont.) (b) Patient's neck is passively flexed by the examiner, then the examiner passively flexes the patient's (right) knee with his leg

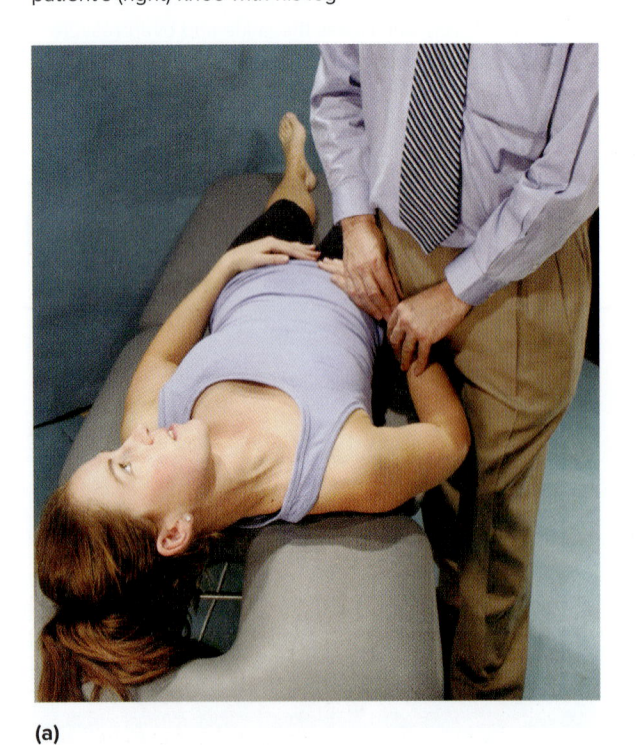

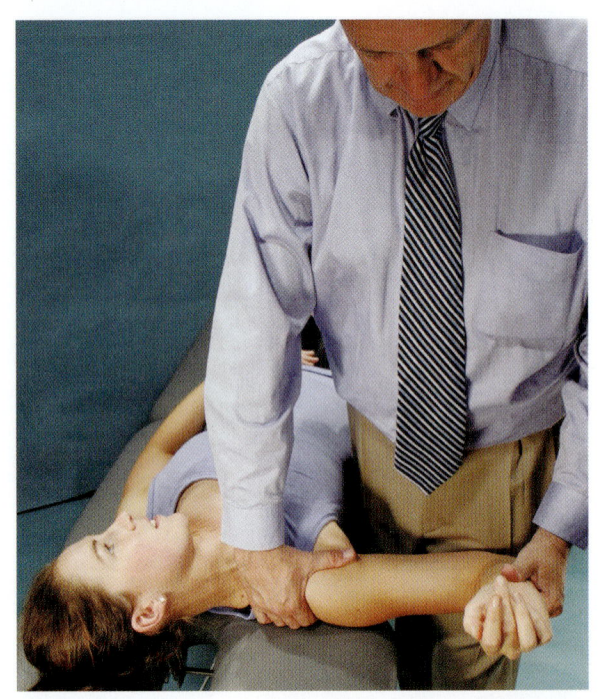

(b)

(a)

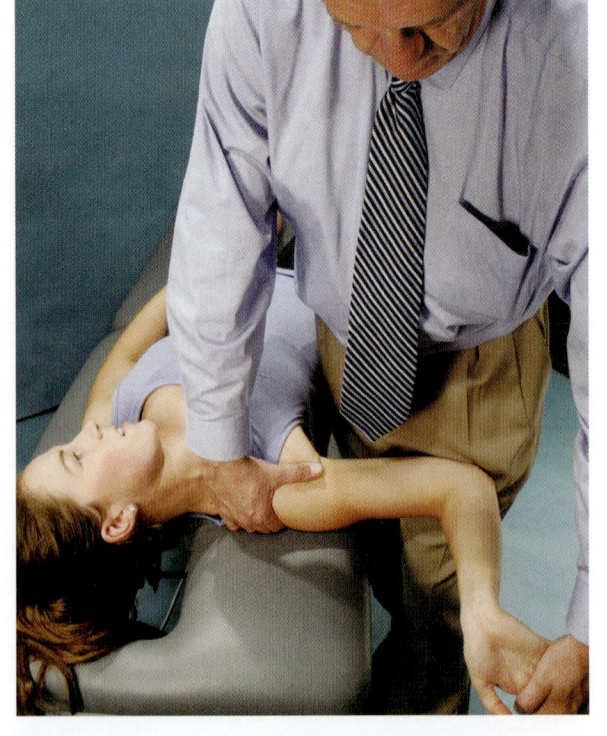

(c)

Figure 15.5 Upper limb neurodynamic test (a) Patient lies supine close to the edge of the couch. Neck is laterally flexed away from the side to be tested (b) The shoulder is depressed by the examiner's hand (left) and the arm abducted to approximately 110° and externally rotated (c) The forearm is supinated and the wrist and fingers extended

(d) (e)

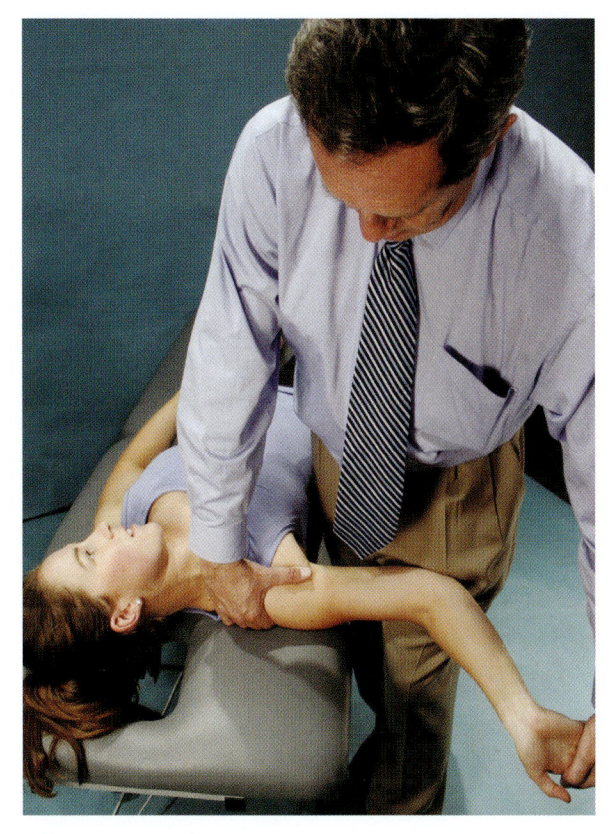

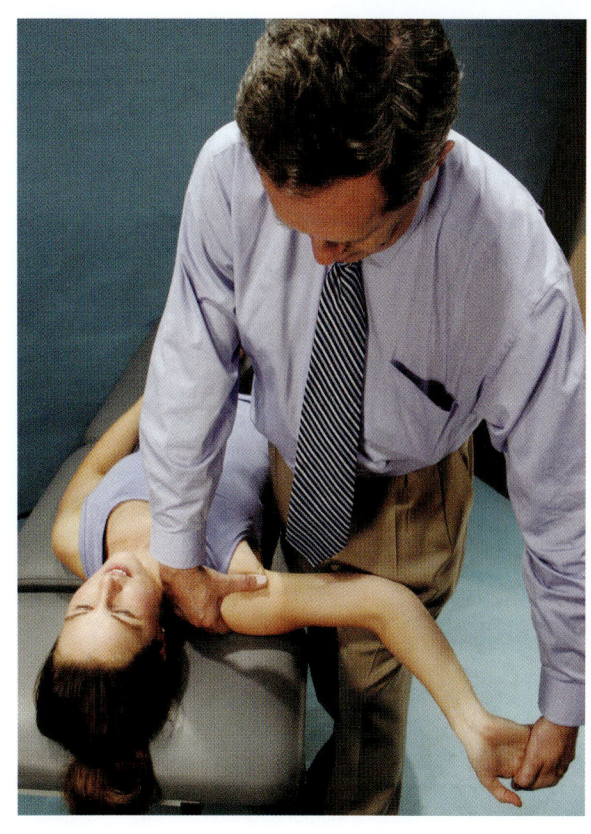

Figure 15.5 (cont.) (d) The elbow is extended to the point of onset of symptoms (e) The neck position returns to neutral and is then laterally flexed towards the side of the test. Any change in symptoms is noted. Other variations can be added (Table 15.1)

A summary of the tests, the methods, user guidance, normal responses and variations of each test is shown in Table 15.1.

A neurodynamic test can be considered positive if:

- it reproduces the patient's symptoms
- the test response can be altered by movements of different body parts that alter the neural mechanosensitivity
- differences in the test occur from side to side and from what is considered normal.

Neurodynamic tests are non-specific but form an extremely useful part of the examination. Abnormalities of neural mechanosensitivity should lead the clinician to examine possible sites of abnormality, especially the spine. The techniques used in neurodynamic tests can also be used as a treatment procedure. This is discussed in Chapter 17.

Spinal examination

Clinical experience suggests that spinal abnormality (e.g. hypomobility) can present in various ways. The presentation may be as pain or injury, and this may occur either locally (at the spine) or distantly. Examples for both upper limb and lower limb spinal abnormalities are given in Table 15.2. The pathophysiology underlying these concepts has been discussed in Chapters 5 and 6.

In patients presenting with upper limb pain, examine the cervical and upper thoracic spines. Examine the lumbar spine (including the thoracolumbar junction) in any patient presenting with lower limb pain. An abnormal neurodynamic test strongly indicates a spinal component to the pain. However, a negative neurodynamic test does not rule out the possibility of a spinal component.

Begin examining the relevant area of the spine by assessing range of movement with the patient standing. The patient should then lie prone on a firm examination table so the examiner can palpate the vertebrae centrally over the spinous processes and laterally over the apophyseal joints to detect any hypomobility and/or tenderness. Hypomobility or tenderness at a level appropriate to that of the patient's symptoms indicate the site is a possible source of referred pain (Chapters 5 and 6).

PART A Fundamental principles

Table 15.1 Neurodynamic tests

Test	Method	Indications	Normal response	Variations
Straight leg raise (Fig. 15.2)	Patient lies supine Leg extended Clinician lifts leg	Leg pain Back pain Headache	Tightness and/or pain in posterior knee, thigh and calf	Ankle dorsiflexion Ankle plantarflexion/inversion Hip adduction Hip medial rotation Passive neck flexion
Slump test (Fig. 15.3)	Patient sitting Slumps Neck flexion Knee extension Ankle dorsiflexion Release neck flexion	Back pain Buttock pain Leg pain	Upper thoracic pain Posterior knee pain Hamstring pain	Leg abduction (obturator nerve) Hip adduction Hip medial rotation Ankle and foot alterations
Neural Thomas test (Fig. 15.4)	Patient lies supine Hip extension Neck flexion Knee flexion	Groin pain Anterior thigh pain	Quadriceps pain and/or tightness	Hip abduction/adduction Hip medial/lateral rotation
Upper limb neurodynamics test (Fig. 15.5)	Patient supine towards side of couch Cervical contralateral flexion Shoulder girdle depression Shoulder abducted to 110° and externally rotated Forearm supination Wrist/fingers extended Elbow extended	Arm pain Neck/upper thoracic pain Headache	Ache in cubital fossa Tingling in thumb and fingers	Forearm pronation Wrist deviation Shoulder flexion/extension Add straight leg raise

Table 15.2 Examples of how spinal abnormality can manifest locally or distantly, with either pain or injury in the upper limb and lower limb

Presentation	Local manifestation	Distant manifestation
Upper limb		
Pain	Hypomobility of C5–C6 joint presenting as neck pain	Hypomobility of C5–C6 joint presents as elbow pain
Injury		Hypomobility of C5–C6 joint predisposing to lateral elbow tendinopathy in a tennis player
Lower limb		
Pain	Hypomobility of L5–S1 joint presenting as lumbosacral pain	Hypomobility of L5–S1 joint presents as buttock and hamstring pain
Injury		Hypomobility of L5–S1 joint predisposing to a hamstring tear in a sprinter

After detecting spinal abnormality on examination, perform a trial treatment (Chapter 17) and then reassess the patient's symptoms and signs. If there is a change in the pain and/or range of movement, then this strongly suggests that the spine is contributing to the symptoms.

Occasionally, palpation of a particular site in the spine will actually reproduce the patient's symptoms distant from the spine. It is important to understand, however, that even if the symptoms are not produced by palpation of the spine, this does not rule out the possibility of a spinal component.

Biomechanical examination

The role of abnormal biomechanics in the production of injuries, especially overuse injuries, is discussed in Chapters 8 and 9. Because abnormal biomechanics can contribute to any overuse injury, all clinicians need to perform a biomechanical examination. As with other components of the examination, it is important to develop a routine for the assessment of biomechanical abnormalities. A routine for the assessment of lower limb biomechanics is illustrated in Chapter 8.

Technique

Faulty technique is another common cause of injury. Technique faults associated with particular injuries are discussed in Chapter 9. While the clinician cannot be aware of all techniques in various sports, he or she should be able to identify the common technique faults in popular activities (e.g. pelvic instability while running or faulty backhand drive in tennis). Clinicians should seek biomechanical advice and assistance with assessment from the athlete's coach or a colleague with expertise in the particular area. Video analysis with slow motion or freeze frame may be helpful.

Equipment

Inappropriate equipment predisposes to injury (Chapter 12). Inspect the athlete's equipment, such as running shoes, football boots, tennis racquet, bicycle or helmet.

Differential diagnosis

At the conclusion of the examination, consider the differential diagnosis and possible predisposing factors. If the clinician is certain of the diagnosis and of the predisposing factors, then counselling and treatment can begin. However, in many cases, further information may be required and the clinician must decide what, if any, investigations may be needed.

DIAGNOSTIC IMAGING

This section introduces imaging–which has provided dramatic advances for sports medicine, and is widely used in clinical medicine. As well as providing remarkable insight to sports medicine pathologies, superior imaging capability has brought with it new challenges for clinicians: 'Yes, that bright signal is abnormal most of the time but what does that mean in this patient?'. But before we tackle that difficult question, we begin with what we know to be true–the five habits of highly effective clinicians, with respect to imaging. Every top sports clinician is highly skilled at interpreting sports imaging and he or she works closely with top musculoskeletal radiologists to perform at the level that champions expect, and every patient who sees a specialist deserves.[6]

The five imaging-related habits of highly effective sports medicine clinicians

In certain clinical settings, appropriate investigations can confirm or exclude a diagnosis suggested by the history and physical examination. A conventional radiograph can confirm that a cyclist has fractured her clavicle. Computed tomography (CT) with multiplanar reformat and three-dimensional volumetric rendering can provide the precise configuration of that fracture. MRI can rule out a stress fracture in a dancer's foot if there is no sign of any abnormal signal.

> **PRACTICE PEARL**
>
> In many clinical contexts imaging does not identify a single structure that is the source of pain. Imaging the patient with back pain is the historical example used to illustrate that point but there are many more examples.

As an example, MRI of a professional baseball player's painful shoulder or elbow illustrates the point clearly.[7-9] Most baseball players have structural changes visible on MRI of their shoulder and elbow (e.g. thickening of their ulnar collateral ligament); one needs to consider if this appearance is 'normal' for that player or not. Other very prominent regions where structural changes are often evident on MRI but which may or may not be symptomatic include the tennis player's elbow, the football player's ankle, the fast bowler's back in cricket. The take-home message is that imaging alone cannot substitute for careful history taking and a comprehensive examination (Chapter 14). Because diagnosis is complex, the leading clinicians in our field have embraced the following behaviours.

PART A Fundamental principles

1. Understand imaging results

The sport and exercise medicine physician must be able to interpret investigation results him or herself. Learn imaging anatomy of the musculoskeletal system–it is only a fraction of what radiologists have to know.[10] It is unwise to rely blindly on imaging reports. A competent sports clinician knows that about 25% of asymptomatic elite jumping athletes have ultrasound appearances of structural change in their patellar tendons (hypoechoic regions, Fig. 15.6a and b).[11, 12] This is critical knowledge as the patient may have no pain there; in fact, the extremity may have been scanned as the asymptomatic contralateral knee for comparison with the symptomatic side. Without requisite clinical awareness, the clinician could let the test guide him or her to a potentially 'false positive' result (depending on the criteria for 'positive', see below). Management must be guided by clinical assessment, not by imaging appearance.

- *Timing of imaging tests.* Imaging may be performed too early to detect a pathology. That radiography can be performed too early to detect a stress fracture is widely known and therefore a 'negative' result does not exclude this diagnosis (high or moderate negative likelihood ratio, so not good for ruling out that pathology).
- *A 'true' finding may be age-related.* For example, triangular fibrocartilage tears of the wrist seen on MRI can be a normal finding, even in a non-athlete, for patients over 50 years of age. Clinical correlation with the patient's symptoms and the physical examination is crucial.
- *The wrong test can give false positive or false negative information.* For example, a routine MRI of the shoulder in a 26-year-old baseball pitcher will miss most labral tears; an MR arthrogram is needed to make the diagnosis. Radiologists are not only 'image interpreters', they are also consultants who can advise on the choice of imaging tests to best demonstrate pathology. Indeed, the most accurate imaging test for a given musculoskeletal pathology may not necessarily be the most sophisticated or complicated test.
- *Be able to judge the adequacy of the quality of obtained images for diagnostic purposes.* Be alert so as not to draw conclusions from imaging tests that may be incomplete or are limited by image degradations. Also, one needs to understand that each imaging test may be specifically obtained to evaluate for one type of pathology but not others. For example, two-view radiographs of the shoulder in internal and external rotation to evaluate for calcific tendinopathy should not be used to exclude glenohumeral dislocation.
- *Intravenous contrast is usually reserved for CT or MRI cases in which the diagnosis of neoplasm or tumour is being considered.* It is very important to indicate as such on the requisition if these need to be ruled out.
- *It is important to minimise ionising radiation, especially in children and adults aged under 30 years.* The dose is especially significant in nuclear medicine bone scans, positron emission tomography (PET) scans and CT scans. If any of these tests are truly indicated, the principle of ALARA (as low as reasonably achievable) with respect to dose should be respected by the imaging department. Note that there is no ionising radiation in MRI, and the dose is negligible in routine conventional radiographs.

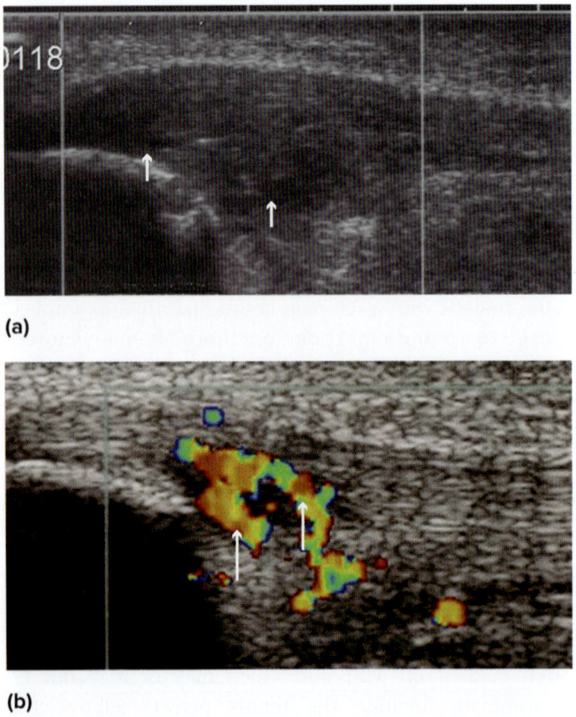

Why do we share these detailed examples about clinicians needing to understand tests? Because the days of thinking that 'imaging reveals X, therefore treatment is Y' are essentially over. Imaging fits into the treatment algorithm and helps update the clinician's thinking of the likelihood of a diagnosis (See Likelihood ratios, Chapter 14). The clinician must understand imaging because it is a tool, not a solution, and far from a panacea.

Figure 15.6 Variations from 'normal' imaging are common among athletes who place great loads on tissue. (a) Grey-scale and (b) Doppler ultrasound appearances of the patellar tendon in a volleyball player, demonstrating hypoechoic regions (arrows in a) and hyperaemia (arrows in b). Clinical reasoning needs to consider the high prevalence of these findings in asymptomatic players[12]

2. Only order imaging that will influence management

It is inappropriate to perform imaging to confirm an already obvious diagnosis, or a diagnosis for which the investigation result will not influence management. Most concussions are diagnosed clinically and do not need brain CT or MRI. Most cases of back pain in sport are not helped by adding low back imaging (radiography, CT or MRI). If an ankle sprain does not appear to have caused a fracture (and there are clinical guidelines to help with the assessment), initial management does not include any imaging. Players/athletes can put clinicians under pressure to order tests; in theory this should always be resisted. In real life, it can be difficult to resist such pressure in the professional sport setting so we will not pretend that ideal management is always followed. But understanding the usefulness of tests and test metrics (Chapter 14) as well as normal patterns of imaging in sport (principle 1, above), allows the clinician to have a valuable conversation with the patient/athlete, and the patient to make an informed decision (see also Figure 2.1 in Chapter 2).

3. Explain the imaging to the patient

Give the patient an understanding of the rationale behind each imaging test. An athlete who complains of persistent ankle pain and swelling several months after an ankle sprain may need a radiograph and MRI. If the patient is merely told that radiography is necessary to exclude bony damage, he or she might become confused when told that the radiograph is normal, but that further investigations are required to exclude bony or osteochondral damage. Also, be sure to alert patients undergoing a procedure that involves contrast (e.g. MR arthrogram) that there will be an injection. It is helpful to provide the patient with resources (either as printed material or as weblinks to videos) explaining the investigation. Follow-up plans should be made explicit in the clinical consultation.

4. Provide relevant clinical findings on the requisition

Accurate and complete clinical information on requisition forms helps to avoid imaging and reporting errors. When particular radiographic views are required, they should be specified. If you cannot remember the names of certain views, write that down on the request forms–the radiographer will generally know them and, if not, the radiologist will. If there is uncertainty, it is always helpful to call the radiologist in advance to discuss the best way to image a patient. Do not assume that radiographers are familiar with the specific views required for sports-related musculoskeletal conditions (e.g. correct anteroposterior [AP], 'frog' and Dunn views for hip femoroacetabular impingement [FAI], skyline views for patellofemoral joint evaluation, the Bernageau view

for shoulder instability). Remember that weight-bearing views are important to assess suspected osteoarthritis at the hip, knee and ankle. 'Functional' views (with the patient placing the joint in the position of pain) are useful for anterior and posterior impingement of the ankle (Chapter 42).

5. Develop a close working relationship with investigators

Optimising communication between colleagues improves the quality of the service.[6] Discuss optimal imaging sequences with radiographers, and view the images together with radiologists providing clinical input. Regular clinical-radiological rounds or case presentations should be encouraged. Digital imaging and telemedicine has made this much easier.

SPECIFIC IMAGING MODALITIES

In this overview of imaging modalities commonly used in sports medicine, our goal is to highlight some key principles that junior clinicians have told us they would have liked to have known earlier in their careers. Read this together with other resources such as the comprehensive, authoritative and beautifully illustrated text in this field: *Imaging in Sports-Specific Musculoskeletal Injuries* (Fig. 15.7).[10]

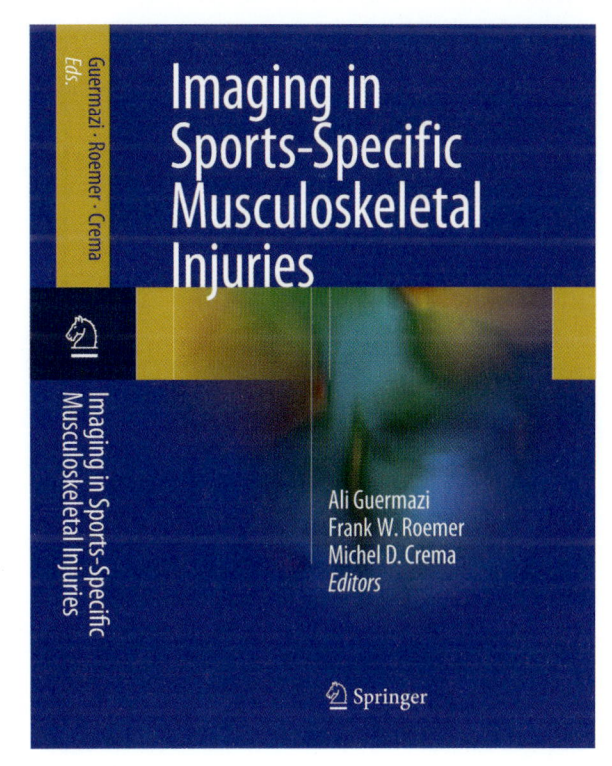

Figure 15.7 A great resource for specialists who work in sports medicine.
REPRODUCED WITH PERMISSION FROM GUERMAZI A, ROEMER F, CREMA M. *IMAGING IN SPORTS SPECIFIC MUSCULOSKELETAL INJURIES*. SPRINGER, 2015.

PART A   Fundamental principles

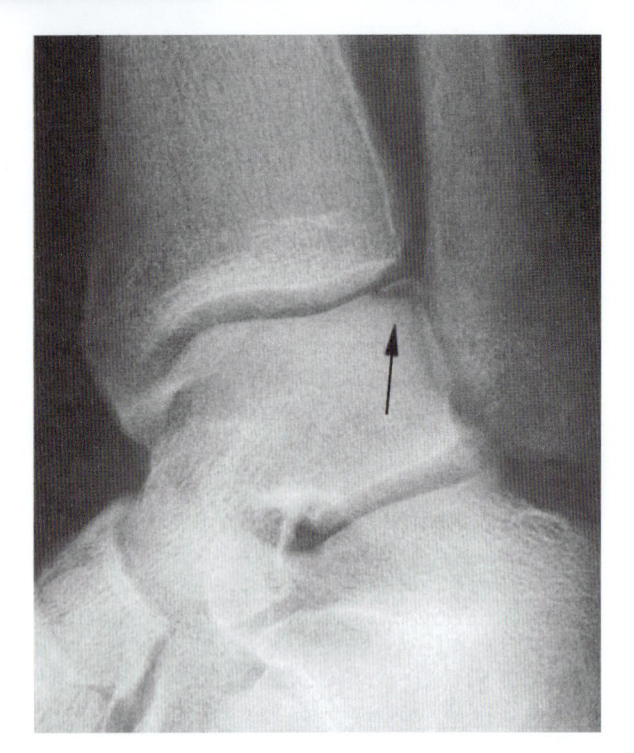

Figure 15.8 Plain radiograph showing an osteochondral fracture of the lateral talar dome COURTESY OF IF ANDERSON

MRI allows clinicians to appreciate fairly dynamic processes such as bone and cartilage turnover, changes in tendon structure even in the absence of rupture, and recovery of ligament after acute sprain.

The physics that underpins MRI is well beyond the scope of this book. At a most superficial level, MRI can be understood to rely on the biology that free water protons exist within a tissue sample. Those protons align with the external magnetic field of the magnet. When a series of radiofrequency (RF) pulses are applied to the tissue sample in the magnet, protons change their alignment relative to the external magnetic field and release energy which creates the MR image.

Unparalleled sensitivity to detect deviation in structure from anatomical norms does not, however, equal unparalleled accuracy in diagnosis for the patient (Chapter 14). Erroneous interpretation of an MRI can have serious clinical consequences. For example, if a 50-year-old person's knee MRI is misinterpreted, a patient who in reality has patellofemoral pain may be inappropriately slated for arthroscopic meniscal surgery (Fig. 15.9).

Conventional radiography

Even as we approach 2020, radiography still provides diagnostic information about bony abnormalities, such as fractures, dislocations, dysplasia and calcification (Fig. 15.8), and is highly cost-effective. Correctly positioning the patient is vital for obtaining radiographic images that are meaningfully interpretable. A minimum of two orthogonal views is required to evaluate any bone adequately. Complex joints such as the ankle, wrist or elbow may require additional or specialised views. Weight-bearing or 'stress' views may give further information for weight-bearing structures and joints.

MRI: massive blessing for active patients

The 2003 Nobel Prize was awarded to the inventors of MRI. This imaging method has revolutionised sports medicine by providing clinicians with remarkably detailed information about structure, especially soft tissues, and helpful information about dynamic pathophysiology. Because of MRI's unparalleled contrast resolution, commonly injured musculoskeletal tissues such as the menisci in the knee, the labrum in the shoulder and hip, spinal discs and joint surfaces can be visualised non-invasively and without ionising radiation.

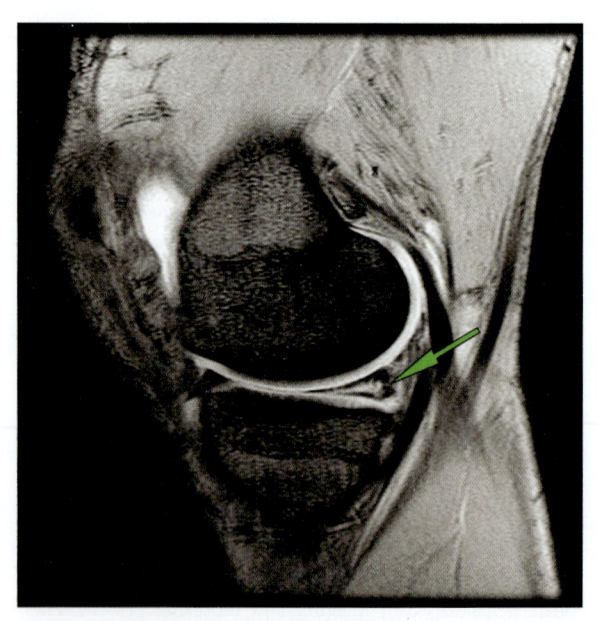

Figure 15.9 Incidental MRI-detected meniscal pathology occur in 19% of women aged 50–59 years[13]. The figure shows a horizontal cleavage tear of the posterior horn of the medial meniscus (arrow). Whether or not this MRI-detected lesion is clinically relevant in a patient presenting with knee pain depends on the entire clinical picture, including detailed history and physical examination findings. The take-home message is that a clinician cannot, and should not, make a diagnosis and decide how to treat the patient solely based on MRI findings

How to make the diagnosis   CHAPTER 15

What does this MRI tell me? Tips for clinicians

The four most common sequences a clinician will see are outlined below and shown in Figure 15.10.

15.10a T1-weighted image showing bone marrow oedema (also called bone marrow lesion (BML) (Chapter 35) after full-thickness ACL tear. Arrows to high signal fat, (yellow arrow), very low signal normal lateral menisci (green arrows), low signal oedema (blue arrow).

15.10b Proton density-weighted image showing normal anterior and posterior horns of the lateral menisci (green arrows).

15.10c T2-weighted image showing full thickness ACL tear (white arrow). Note bright joint fluid (blue arrow).

15.10d STIR image (fat suppressed) showing the same patient as in part (a). Bone marrow oedema (high signal, blue arrow) as a result of the acute knee giving way episode and ACL rupture. Note additional bone marrow oedema (high signal, blue arrowheads) in the fibular styloid process as a result of a concomitant torn arcuate ligament.

1. **T1-weighted** provides sharp anatomical detail, shows bone marrow and is good for meniscal pathology. It lacks the sensitivity to detect soft tissue injury (Fig. 15.10a). MRI signal key: fat = bright; muscle = intermediate; water, tendons and fibrocartilage all dark.

2. **Proton density-weighted** is good for imaging menisci and ligaments (Fig. 15.10b). MRI signal key: fat = bright or intermediate signal, calcium, tendons and fibrocartilage, all dark; water = intermediate.

3. **T2-weighted** is highly sensitive for most soft tissue injury, especially tendons. Abnormal tendons have high signal intensity (bright) which contrasts with normal tendons black (arrowhead) (Fig. 15.10c). MRI signal key: water = bright; fat = intermediate muscle, hyaline and fibrocartilage all dark.

4. **STIR** highlights excess water (blue arrow and blue arrowheads) which can occur due to bone stress and bone marrow oedema (shown), joint fluid and soft tissue pathology. This is the sequence of choice for bone stress injuries or subtle, radiographically occult fractures (Fig. 15.10d). MRI signal key: water = very bright; fat, muscle, menisci all dark.

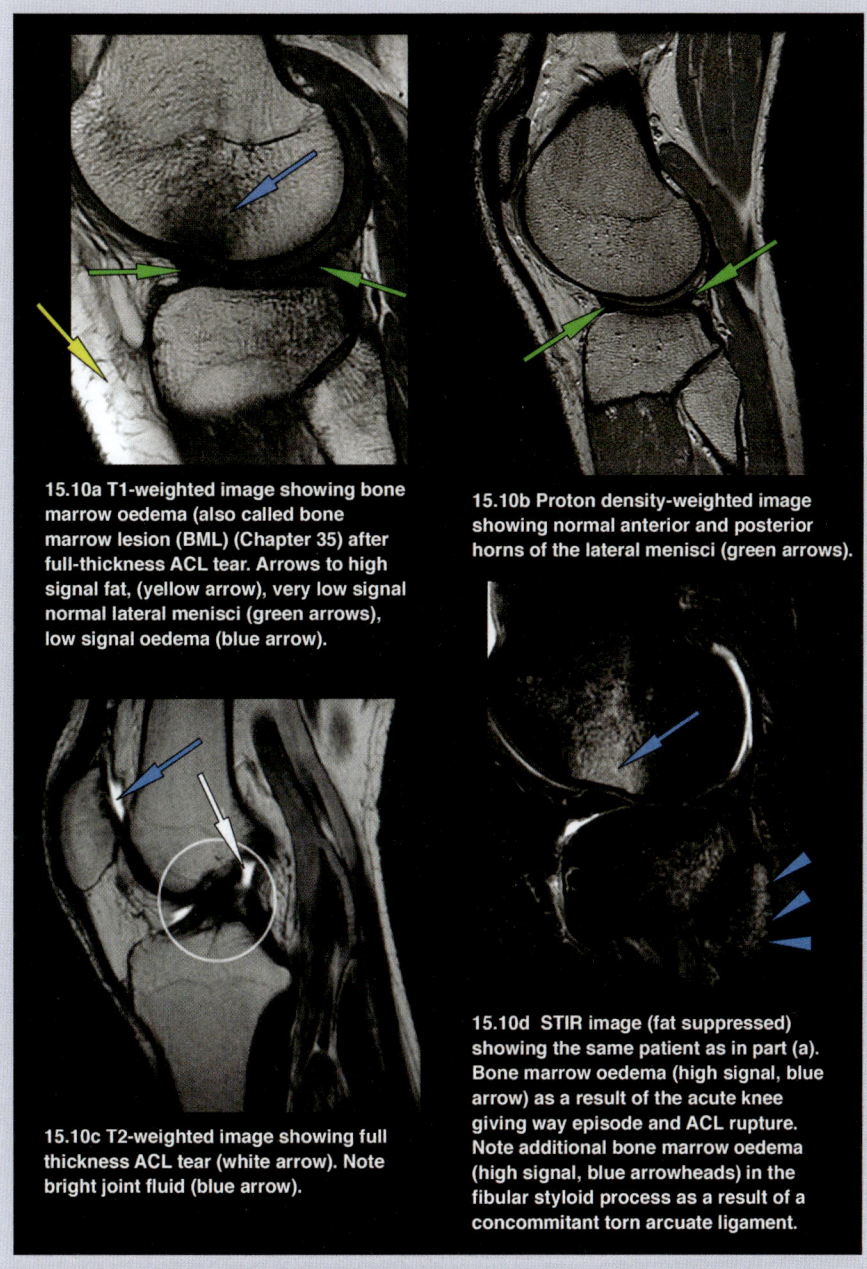

Figure 15.10 The legend for the arrows/arrowheads to structures in the four MRI sequences is as follows: fat = yellow; tendon and ligament = off-white; water = blue; menisci = green

The price of additional medical data is that the clinician who cares for the patient needs to determine how heavily to weigh the imaging information. Specifically, the clinician must arrive at a post-test probability of a diagnosis based on how much the MRI result (positive or negative) changes the pre-test probability of the diagnosis. (See Fagan's nomogram, Chapter 14.)

Specific features and patient benefits of MRI

MRI is now a routine part of the medical landscape the world over, although access to MRI for sports medicine imaging is limited in some regions. The tide is heading powerfully in one direction towards greater and greater utilisation of MRI in sports medicine. Paradoxically, in developed countries that have private medicine (radiology), too much imaging and overdiagnosis, associated with overtreatment (particularly arthroscopic surgery) has a deleterious effect on health. So the challenge for both policy makers and skilled clinicians is to choose imaging wisely. Towards that aim, we first review the features of MRI as a tool for clinicians working in sport and promoting physical activity.

MRI has the following features which translate into patient and clinician benefits.

- MRI is non-invasive, so it has dramatically reduced the need for diagnostic arthroscopy.
- It can provide images in multiple planes. Need a sagittal view of the knee to image the patellar tendon? Sure! How about a coronal to assess joint surfaces and menisci? No problem!
- MRI does not involve ionising radiation. This is particularly important in the age group often treated by clinicians in sports medicine: adolescents, as well as for professional athletes who may have many clinical encounters and thus need many scans.
- MRI has superb contrast resolution for soft tissues, allowing accurate assessment of most ligaments, tendons and hyaline and fibrocartilage. Note that although bones are also well-assessed, if the clinical concern is one of primarily bony pathology (e.g. lumbar spondylolysis), CT may be more appropriate, bearing in mind radiation dose.
- It is ideal to assess patients who have had soft tissue trauma (e.g. contact injuries) and it complements the use of CT in high-velocity injuries.
- MRI has an emerging role in helping clinicians evaluate overuse injuries. Anatomy in patients in the sports medicine setting is markedly affected by microtrauma/adaptation to load and this is increasingly being well characterised. In the late 1980s, journals commonly carried treatment recommendations from 'experts' based on false premises of what was 'normal' in athletes.[14] The problem was that 'normal' for an elite athlete had not been well documented. The subspecialty of sports radiology and greater experience of musculoskeletal radiologists with sport is addressing that challenge.[6] As with all research, knowledge translation remains a challenge; getting the key messages to the community of clinicians who will apply it.

Difference added by MRI sequences

Spin echo (SE), gradient echo (GRE) and inversion recovery (IR) sequences are the basic categories of sequences used in musculoskeletal imaging.[3] T1-weighted, T2-weighted, proton density-weighted and short tau inversion recovery (STIR) sequences are often utilised (Figure 15.10). Fat-suppressed fast spin echo sequences are used in almost every musculoskeletal protocol to demonstrate bone marrow oedema, focal cartilage defects and tendon/ligament pathology with the highest conspicuity.

Other clinical points about MRI

The clinical workhorse for sports MRI is the 1.5 T (Tesla) MRI platform. For almost all clinical indications, MRI at this field strength is generally sufficient. The 3 T magnets, which are more expensive to purchase, offer higher spatial resolution, and therefore may offer advantages in evaluating small structures, such as tendon pulley injuries in rock climbers (although there are currently no trials to support this). Advanced applications in 3 T may prove useful in the future in dedicated cartilage imaging.

The contrast agent for MRI is gadolinium, which has an excellent safety profile, even more so than the safe iodinated contrast agents used in CT. It is used intravenously for musculoskeletal imaging in cases in which tumour or neoplasm are being considered, and in an intra-articular fashion to optimally evaluate hyaline cartilage, such as shoulder and hip labra.

A less common architecture for MRI is so-called 'open' units, which do offer advantages in allowing patients with claustrophobia to be scanned; this occurs at the expense of image quality. The weight-bearing and kinematic options that these units provide are still investigational in nature (Fig. 15.11).

Physiologic (also called compositional) imaging of cartilage can be performed at 1.5 T and 3 T, but not accurately at lower field strengths. Special sequences can assess for loss of cartilage proteoglycan content (T1-rho mapping and dGEMRIC) and for collagen degradation (T2 mapping). These techniques hold great promise in biochemical, pre-morphologic chondral assessment in early osteoarthritis, and for follow-up of interventions (e.g. chondral surgery and, one day, biologics that can block the progression of osteoarthritis). However, currently their clinical role is undefined.

How to make the diagnosis CHAPTER 15

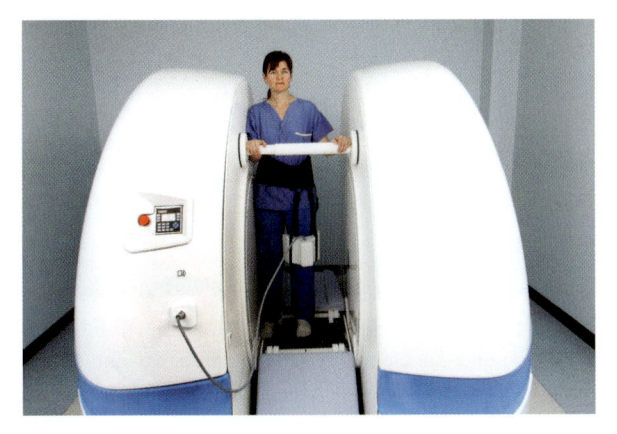

Figure 15.11 The 'open' MRI instrument allows the patient to be weight-bearing. In this figure the model is wearing a knee coil
IMAGE COURTESY OF CENTRE FOR HIP HEALTH AND MOBILITY, UNIVERSITY OF BRITISH COLUMBIA HTTP://WWW.HIPHEALTH.CA/

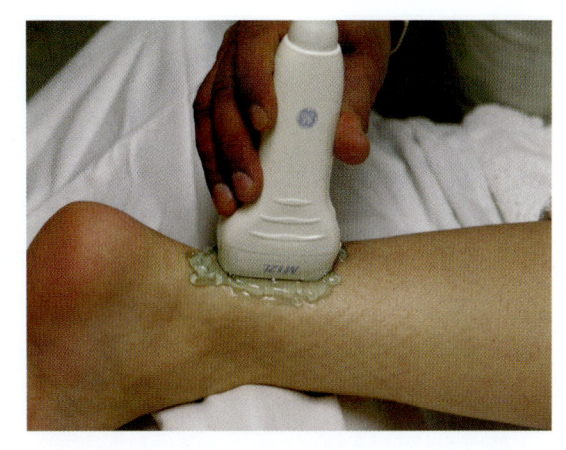

Figure 15.12 High-resolution ultrasound scanning with 10–12 megahertz (MHz) probes is a painless method of imaging tendons, muscles and other soft tissues without exposing the patient to any radiation

There are a few strict contraindications to MRI (e.g. certain brain aneurysm clips, neurostimulators and cardiac pacemakers) but, contrary to popular medical opinion, patients with metallic orthopaedic hardware and metallic surgical clips outside the brain, in place for more than 6 weeks, can be safely scanned.

MRI can be overly sensitive to abnormal tissue signals and, thus, provide false positive results. In asymptomatic athletes in numerous studies, MRI revealed structural appearances consistent with significant injury but the athletes were asymptomatic and high functioning.[12, 13] This emphasises the need for the appropriate selection of patients for investigation and careful clinical–imaging correlation.[1] As with any medical investigation, diagnostic errors can occur; ideally, images should be read by an experienced musculoskeletal MRI radiologist.

Ultrasound scan (for diagnosis)

High-resolution ultrasound scanning (Fig. 15.12) with 10–12 MHz probes is a painless method of imaging tendons, muscles and other soft tissues without exposing the patient to any radiation.[15] It allows clinical correlation–imaging with the patient reproducing his or her pain and providing feedback to the radiologist. Adding to its diagnostic utility, both sides can be readily imaged for comparison. Other advantages include its dynamic nature (the patient can move the part and/or reproduce pain during the examination), short examination time and ability to guide therapeutic aspiration or injection under real time.

Ultrasound is the imaging instrument of choice 'in clinic'.[16, 17] As it is an excellent way to visualise tendon and muscle, it can be the workhorse in a sports clinician's office where patients present with injuries of these tissues.

Units are priced to be affordable in the clinic because the unit cost, installation and service are of the order of 100 times cheaper than MRI.

> **PRACTICE PEARL**
>
> Ultrasound has been referred to as the sports physician's stethoscope and the analogy applies to the portability of ultrasound—small units can be used on the sideline.[18] Laptop-sized portable units have a different level of image quality to the larger units that are designed to stay in the clinic.

Clinicians in sport might consider ultrasound equipment as having three different levels.

1. The most expensive, best quality equipment would be located at a specialist radiology clinic. The radiologist and his/her team with the full battery of complementary imaging modalities provides the tertiary resource as well as continuing professional education (formal and informal) and research partnerships as appropriate.
2. Leading specialised clinical practices often choose to have quality ultrasound imaging capacity at the clinic to assist with speed of diagnosis, for injections with ultrasound imaging and because having ultrasound skills advances those clinicians understanding of anatomy.
3. Portable sideline equipment (laptop scanner shown in Fig. 15.13) still provides quality images but the users appreciate the limitation compared with that outlined in point 1.

Disadvantages of ultrasound include the less graphic images, the fact that it is more operator-dependent with

PART A Fundamental principles

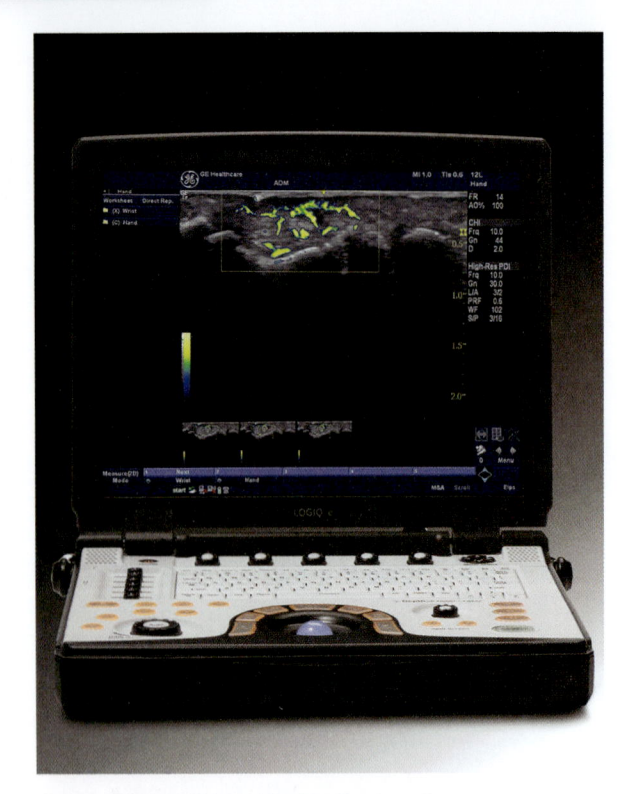

Figure 15.13 Portable sideline ultrasound unit
REPRODUCED WITH PERMISSION OF GE HEALTHCARE

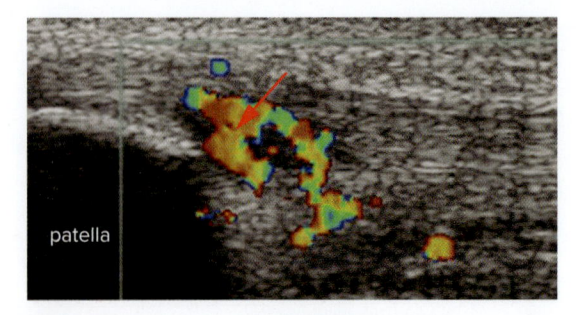

Figure 15.14 Sagittal colour Doppler ultrasound scan showing abnormal blood flow (arrow) at the mid- and deep surface of the patellar tendon near the patellar attachment

respect to image quality than any other modality, and the fact that it cannot penetrate tissues to show deeper structures, such as shoulder/hip labra or anterior cruciate ligaments/menisci. The most commonly examined areas are large tendons, (e.g. the Achilles, patellar and rotator cuff tendons) and the muscles of the thigh and calf. Ultrasound can also demonstrate muscle tear, haematoma formation or early calcification, and may be useful in localising foreign bodies.

Ultrasound scanning is able to distinguish complete tendon rupture from other tendon abnormalities (e.g. tendinopathy). As with MRI, ultrasound imaging of elite athletes reveals morphological 'abnormalities' that are not symptomatic and do not appear to predict imminent tendon pain.

Real-time ultrasound examination during active movement (dynamic ultrasound) is particularly helpful in the evaluation of shoulder impingement. The use of ultrasound to help guide injection is discussed in Chapter 17.

The role of colour Doppler

Colour Doppler ultrasound gained popularity in sports medicine for the assessment of tendons in the early 2000s, as it was hoped that abnormal tendon flow detected using the colour Doppler feature would provide a better guide as to whether or not tendons were painful (Fig. 15.14). Longitudinal studies failed to show that colour Doppler ultrasound findings of vascularity predicted changes in symptoms.[19] Also, exercise affects the level of vascularity, which adds a challenge to the clinical utility of this method. This modality is proving useful in certain areas of medicine but has dropped off the 'hot topics' list in sports medicine. To return to a theme from early in this chapter, there appears to be no substitute for careful clinical examination and patient monitoring to track patients' current progress and to predict outcomes.

The role of ultrasound tissue characterisation

In the 2010s, a novel ultrasound modality, called ultrasound tissue characterisation (UTC), was introduced to evaluate human tendons (Fig. 15.15).[20] The innovation aims to provide a three-dimensional image of the tendon where structure is quantified (in contrast to conventional greyscale ultrasound which provides no numerical data). Data are obtained from the stability of pixel attributes (brightness) over a set scan length to a maximum of 25 scan slices at present. UTC has high reproducibility with excellent intra-observer and interobserver reliability.[20] Detailed descriptions of the use of this emerging technology are reported in various clinical research reports.[20, 21]

Is this method ready for general use in 2017? No. Ultrasound tissue characterisation is currently a research instrument with potential that marketers would say is at the early stage of the 'product life cycle'.[22] As with any new technology, there will be extreme claims as to its potential capacity; over time a body of evidence will emerge as to the best ways for clinicians and patients to benefit from the technological advance.[21] At the time of writing, there is only one manufacturer of this patented technology (UTC imaging, Stein, The Netherlands) and the cost of an instrument is in the range of US$40 000 to US$ 60 000, depending on service costs and the options that the user chooses for elements such as probes.

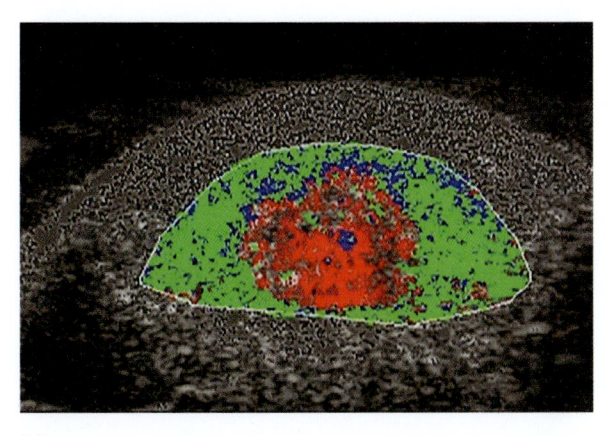

How to make the diagnosis CHAPTER 15

(a)

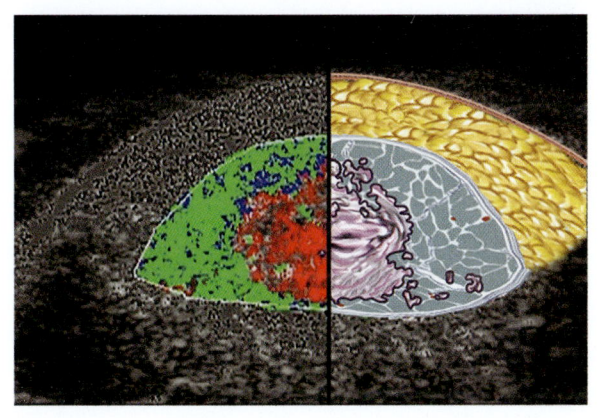

(b)

Figure 15.15 Ultrasound tissue characterisation (UTC) of the Achilles tendon. Standard image (axial plane) in (a), and put in context in (b) with yellow being subcutaneous tissue. The tendon tissue would all be green in a normal tendon. This tendon has collagen pathology which is seen as blue, red and black signal. Green = echo-type I (normal tendon); blue = echo-type II; red = echo-type III; black = echo-type IV. Echo-types II–IV are abnormal

CT scanning

CT scanning (Fig. 15.16) allows cross-sectional imaging of soft tissue, calcific deposits and bone. CT scanning is particularly useful in evaluation of the spine, fractures in small bones and fractures in anatomically complex regions, such as the ankle, foot or pelvis. CT scanners provide high-resolution reconstructions of the imaging

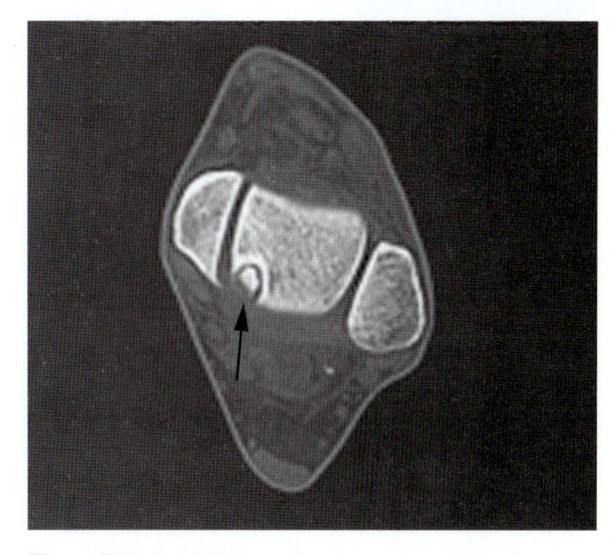

Figure 15.16 Axial CT scan showing cross-section of osteochondral lesion of the posteromedial talar dome (arrow)

data in any plane. Remember that CT defines bone details and can detect small areas of calcification better than MRI can, even though the latter will reveal occult bony abnormalities. Advances in multidetector CT technology allow rapid image acquisition and superb multiplanar reconstruction. The disadvantage of CT scanning is the significant radiation dose, especially in children.

Radioisotopic bone scan

Radioisotopic bone scan (scintigraphy) has fallen out of favour in sports medicine practice because of the availability of MRI with appropriate pulse sequences (e.g. STIR) which can often provide similar information about bone while adding anatomical localisation that was limited with bone scan. The high sensitivity and low negative likelihood if negative for stress fracture meant that the test was useful for ruling out stress fractures. Does radioisotopic bone scanning still have a role? Very rarely. Expert and experienced radiologists may use it at times to seek a tibial or a metatarsal stress fracture but it has essentially been superseded by MRI and CT.

Single photon emission computed tomography (SPECT) techniques are also used in sports medicine, particularly in the detection of stress fractures of the pars interarticularis of the lumbar spine, although the correct MRI sequence should be able to detect these changes.

PART A Fundamental principles

REFERENCES

References for this chapter can be found at www.mhhe.com/au/CSM5e

Chapter 16

Patient-reported outcome measures in sports medicine

with NATALIE COLLINS, KAY CROSSLEY and EWA M ROOS

The operation was entirely successful, but the patient succumbed.
Manual of Operative Surgery, published 1887

Sports medicine clinicians likely had their first encounter with patient-reported outcome measures (PROMs) in the research setting, as PROMs are commonly used to capture treatment response. However, PROMs can also be useful in clinical practice. This chapter outlines what PROMs are, why they are important to use in clinical practice and what constitutes a 'good' PROM. It also provides examples of generic PROMs to use in sports medicine patients, which can be used to complement more specific measures outlined in the regional chapters. We emphasise that the key letters in the term 'PROMs' are the first two–P and R–for 'patient-reported.' That is what differentiates PROMs from 'objective' clinical measures such as range of motion or strength.

WHAT ARE PROMS?

PROMs are measures in which the patient provides his or her own perspective of a health condition or treatment. This is particularly useful when the aspect of interest is either impossible or impractical to observe directly, such as pain or high-level sporting function.[1] PROMs can be specific for the region (e.g. knee), condition (e.g. tendinopathy) or intervention (e.g. anterior cruciate ligament reconstruction or exercise). The clinician may be familiar with measures such as the IKDC (International Knee Documentation Committee) for knee function, the Western Ontario and McMaster Universities Arthritis Index (WOMAC) score for osteoarthritis, and the Victorian Institute of Sport Assessment (VISA) score which rates patients who have tendinopathy. All of these are examples of various types of PROMs.

A type of PROM can also provide a generic measure of overall health status (i.e. not 'disease-specific').[2] PROMs can measure a variety of constructs, such as pain, symptoms, physical function and quality of life. An example of a very simple, commonly used PROM in clinical practice is asking the patient to rate their pain severity on a scale from zero to ten–a visual analogue scale (VAS). Contemporary PROMs provide more comprehensive insight into a number of aspects that are important to consider in the patient's condition.

WHY IS IT IMPORTANT TO USE APPROPRIATE PROMS IN SPORTS MEDICINE?

Clinicians who work in sports and exercise often use standard clinical tests to evaluate physical aspects, such as joint range of motion, ligament integrity and functional performance. While these provide important information about particular aspects of the patient's condition, they are unable to measure how the patient feels and performs. PROMs complement clinical tests to evaluate the patient's overall health and performance status more comprehensively.

In sports medicine, PROMs are mostly used to evaluate the effectiveness of treatment. However, they may also:

- focus the clinical appointment toward aspects that most concern the patient (i.e. by asking the patient to complete the PROM prior to the appointment)
- build a profile of the patient's health condition over time and quickly identify those who have experienced improvement or deterioration and may require refinements to their training or management[3]
- identify dimensions that the patient deems to be important in their treatment planning and goal setting

PART A   Fundamental principles

- predict which patients are likely to have a good prognosis or respond to a particular treatment
- decide a patient's readiness for return to activity[3]
- empower the patient to monitor his or her own health profile over time, by providing benchmarks for the ideal health state (vs peers, normative cohorts)
- screen patients for injury risk
- provide a method of standardising health status reporting, to allow pooling of data from international cohorts (e.g. ACL registries) and detect clinical patterns that may influence prognosis and response to treatment.

CONSIDERATIONS FOR WHAT CONSTITUTES A 'GOOD' PROM FOR USE IN SPORTS MEDICINE

Several factors should be considered before integrating PROMs into clinical practice. This will ensure that implementing the PROM is feasible and it will help to ensure that the PROMs provide relevant, reliable and valid information about the patient and can measure change in the patient's condition over time. Clinicians can obtain this information from a variety of sources, including the PROM's original publication (e.g. journal article, book), online resources (e.g. specific PROM websites such as www.koos.nu) and systematic reviews of PROMs. It is also important to recognise that measurement properties are often population-specific. This means that clinicians should confirm that the PROM has been evaluated in the specific patient cohort relevant to their patient (e.g. ACL-reconstruction versus knee osteoarthritis).

Is the PROM easy to use in a sports medicine setting?

One of the perceived barriers to integrating PROMs into clinical practice is the burden on patients and clinicians, and how this will affect sports medicine services in the clinic, clubrooms, or during competition and travel. At the elite level, patients are accustomed to completing regular log-books to track factors such as their training load, dietary intake and sleep patterns. As such, the inclusion of appropriate PROMs is unlikely to be too burdensome, especially if it provides information that they see to be relevant to their injury or health condition and goals, and is delivered in the same format as their regular log-books (i.e. mobile device or paper diary).

By definition, PROMs should be patient-administered, without input from the clinician or others, as this captures the patient's impression of their health condition and minimises the potential for bias introduced with clinician-completed measures. This is also likely to minimise the burden on clinicians, as patients can complete the PROMs prior to their appointment or in the waiting room.

Another consideration regarding patient burden is the format and layout of the PROM. Are the items logical and easy to interpret, or does the patient need to read each item carefully to ensure that they provide the correct response? For example, some PROMs reverse the wording or responses to some items and then invert the scoring (e.g. items 4, 8, 12 and 16 of the Tampa Scale for Kinesiophobia).

Although it may be preferable in clinical practice to use PROMs with the shortest completion time, this needs to be considered along with the information that the PROM provides. Some PROMs that take longer to complete may provide substantially more information about different aspects of the patient's condition (e.g. PROMs such as the Knee Injury and Osteoarthritis Outcome Score (KOOS) and Copenhagen Hip And Groin Outcome Score (HAGOS) that provide separate subscales for pain, function and quality of life take 5–10 minutes to complete) than shorter PROMs that only measure one construct (e.g. numerical rating scale for pain taking seconds to complete). The completion time is also important to consider in the context of how frequently the PROM will be administered. If the frequency is at least 3 months apart, longer PROMs are feasible, while shorter PROMs are more feasible if daily, weekly or monthly administration is desired.

The clinician should also consider how burdensome the PROM is to score and interpret in the sports medicine setting. To minimise clinician burden, we recommend that electronic or online data collection platforms be used where possible. This allows clinicians to receive scores in real time using computer algorithms, which enhances their clinical utility.[3] Electronic questionnaires have high agreement with their paper-based predecessors.[4] Furthermore, information needs to be made available to clinicians regarding how to interpret PROM scores, relate them to the patient's condition and use them to make decisions about treatment.[3] The availability of a user guide for the PROM will facilitate ease of administration and scoring.

Finally, the accessibility of the PROM should be considered. Many PROMS are open access and freely available for clinical use (e.g. KOOS). However, some PROMs have licensing requirements and fees associated with their use, even in clinical practice (e.g. WOMAC). Given that sports medicine clinicians can manage patients of various cultural and language backgrounds, they should also consider whether a particular PROM is available in languages other than English and whether non-English versions have undergone cross-cultural validation. This ensures that the same meaning of the items and stability of measurement properties (e.g. reliability, validity, responsiveness) is retained when the PROM is translated into another language.

Does the PROM evaluate dimensions that are relevant for the patient?

In selecting a PROM for use in sports medicine, it is vital that it evaluates specific dimensions, subscales, items or questions that are relevant for the particular patient. The first step in determining relevance of dimensions is to obtain information regarding the patient group that the PROM was intended for. This is generally available in the PROM's original publication. For example, the iHOT-33 was intended for young active patients with hip disorders,[5] which would be suitable for use in athletic populations. In comparison, the KOOS was intended for use in young, middle-aged and elderly patients with knee injuries and/ or osteoarthritis.[6] Thus, items in the subscale pertaining to function during sport and recreational activities (e.g. running, jumping, twisting/pivoting) may be more relevant to younger active patients than function in activities of daily living (e.g. putting on socks/stockings).

Validity refers to the degree to which a PROM measures the constructs that it intends to measure.[7] This is an important consideration when making inferences based on PROM scores.[1]

Content validity is the degree to which the content of the PROM adequately reflects the constructs to be measured, with respect to their relevance and comprehensiveness.[1, 7] A PROM has adequate content validity if the developers provide a clear description of the measurement aim, the target population, concepts to be measured and item selection.[8] Importantly, patients from the target population should have been involved in the development or selection of included items.[8] Face validity is a component of content validity that is useful for clinicians. This refers to the degree to which, on face value, the items of a PROM look as though they adequately reflect the construct to be measured.[7] Clinicians should ensure that PROMs demonstrate content validity and that they do not overrule dimensions that patients deem to be important–it is the patient who is the expert in this scenario.

Construct validity refers to how well the PROM measures its intended constructs.[2] This is typically evaluated by testing hypotheses regarding the expected relationship between the PROM and other instruments. Evidence for convergent construct validity is provided when higher correlations are found between the PROM and existing measures that evaluate similar constructs.[8] Evidence for divergent construct validity is provided when lower correlations are observed between the PROM and existing measures that evaluate dissimilar constructs.[8] For example, in patients who had undergone hip arthroscopy, the pain subscale of the Copenhagen Hip And Groyne Outcome Score (HAGOS) demonstrated larger correlations with the SF-36 bodily pain subscale and smaller correlations with the mental health subscale.[9]

Clinicians may also see reference to another form of validity in the literature, termed criterion validity. This refers to how well the scores of an instrument reflect a 'gold standard.'[7] Because there is no gold standard measure of patient-reported outcome,[10] criterion validity is not applicable to PROMs.

Do all items within a PROM measure the same construct?

For scoring and interpretation purposes, it is important that all items within a PROM or individual subscales reflect the same dimension.[11] The internal consistency measures how well all items within a PROM are correlated and thus measure the same construct.[8] This is an important consideration for PROMs that use multiple items to measure a single construct (e.g. Tampa Scale for Kinesiophobia), to ensure that all items are likely to respond in a similar way to a change in the patient's condition.

The first step in determining the internal consistency of a PROM is to examine the structural validity. During the development phase of the PROM, specific analyses (principal component analysis or exploratory factor analysis) are used to determine whether the items form one overall dimension (unidimensionality) or more than one dimension (multidimensionality).[8] For PROMs that consist of a single overall score (e.g. VISA Score), all items should reflect a single construct.[1] For PROMs that consist of several subscales that are scored individually (e.g. HAGOS), several dimensions should be demonstrated.[1] Clinicians should confirm that all items within an overall score or subscale score, as appropriate, reflect only one dimension.

Once the unidimensionality of the PROM or its subscales has been established, Cronbach's alpha can be used to measure the interrelatedness of all items within a (sub)scale.[7, 8] Cronbach's alpha is considered adequate if it falls between 0.7 and 0.95. A low Cronbach's alpha (<0.7) indicates that the items are not well correlated and that a single summary score is not appropriate.[8] A very high Cronbach's alpha (>0.95) is also not ideal and suggests that one or more items within the (sub)scale are redundant.[8]

Can the PROM be trusted to detect true change in the patient and be free from error?

To be able to trust and interpret PROM scores, it is important to establish the error associated with the PROM.

This gives clinicians an idea as to whether any change observed in the PROM between repeated administrations reflects a true change in the patient's condition or is due to error inherent in the measure.

The test-retest reliability of a PROM indicates how stable the results are when you measure a patient's unchanged condition on two separate occasions.[2] For PROMs that are patient-completed, reliability is considered to be intra-rater, as the same person (the patient) completes the PROM on different occasions.[7] Typically, test-retest reliability is reported using intraclass correlation coefficients (ICC). This indicates the strength of the relationship between the two administrations, from 0 (no relationship) to 1 (the relationship between the repeated administrations can be predicted without error).[1] Interpretation of ICCs differs depending on whether clinicians intend to use the PROM in individual patients or in groups of patients (e.g. sporting teams).

> **PRACTICE PEARL**
>
> Test-retest reliability is considered adequate for use in individual patients if the ICC is greater than 0.9,[12] and for use in groups if the ICC is greater than 0.7.[8]

The absolute measurement error or agreement can also be determined. This provides clinicians with a value, expressed in the measurement unit of the specific PROM, which can be used to determine whether a PROM change score is greater than the error of the measure. The standard error of measurement (SEM) estimates one standard deviation of the error associated with one measurement.[1] This is then used to calculate the minimal detectable change (MDC), also known as the smallest detectable change (SDC). The MDC can be determined for individuals ($MDC_{ind} = 1.96 \times \sqrt{2} \times SEM$), reflecting the smallest change occurring within a patient that can be interpreted as 'real' change (at the 0.05 significance level).[8] It can also be determined for groups (MDC_{group}), by dividing the MDC_{ind} by $\sqrt{n}$ (where n is the number of participants).[8] In clinical practice, if a patient's change score on a PROM is greater than the MDC_{ind}, clinicians can interpret this as a true change in the patient's condition.

Is the PROM sensitive enough to detect real change in the patient's condition?

Because PROMs are frequently used to evaluate a patient's response to treatment or monitor their condition over time, they must be sufficiently sensitive to be able to detect real changes in a patient's condition. Responsiveness refers to the ability of a PROM to detect change over time in the measured construct.[7] This is arguably the most important measurement property, as it gives an indication of how robust the PROM is on all other measurement properties (e.g. validity, reliability). Responsiveness is specific to the population and treatment of interest, so clinicians should seek evidence from studies that test responsiveness in cohorts that have similar characteristics to the specific patient (e.g. age, injury/condition/treatment).

The difficulty for clinicians is the lack of consensus regarding the optimal method of evaluating responsiveness for PROMs. Earlier studies frequently present effect sizes as a measure of responsiveness. However, this is more a reflection of treatment effects (i.e. the magnitude of the change score), rather than whether the PROM can detect change over time (i.e. validity of the change score).[11] More recently, the COSMIN group recommended that responsiveness should be evaluated in a similar way to construct validity, by testing predefined hypotheses regarding the expected correlation between change scores of two PROMs that are administered simultaneously or expected differences in changes between 'known' groups.[13] PROMs may be compared to a 'global rating of change' (GROC) scale, which is an adequate estimate of the magnitude and direction of health status change,[14] or to other measures of the same construct.[15] Thus, responsiveness can be viewed as longitudinal validity.[8] Clinicians can gain evidence of PROM responsiveness from studies where predefined hypotheses regarding change scores (e.g. effect sizes) are supported. Effect sizes are also useful when comparing PROMs head to head, or when comparing groups that are better, unchanged or worse.

The other component of responsiveness relates to whether the PROM can distinguish clinically important change from measurement error.[13] This is particularly important for clinical practice, as clinicians need to be confident that changes they are observing in their patient, measured using PROMs, represent meaningful change in the patient's condition. The minimal clinically important difference (MCID), also known as the minimal important change (MIC), is the smallest change in a PROM score that patients consider to be important.[11] The MCID provides clinicians with an estimate of the average amount of change in PROM score that patients would typically consider to represent a meaningful improvement.[1]

> **PRACTICE PEARL**
>
> When interpreting MCIDs, clinicians should ensure that the MCID is larger than the MDC, indicating that the magnitude of important change is greater than the error associated with the PROM.[8]

Patient-reported outcome measures in sports medicine — CHAPTER 16

One consideration with the ability of a PROM to detect change is whether it demonstrates any floor or ceiling effects when used in particular patient groups. Floor effects occur when patients score the lowest possible value on the (sub)scale at baseline measurement, meaning that there is no room for the PROM to detect further deterioration. Ceiling effects occur when patients score the highest possible value, meaning that the PROM is unable to detect improvements in the condition.

Athletic patients may demonstrate ceiling effects on PROMs that were originally designed for use in older, more inactive cohorts. For example, the KOOS subscale for activities of daily living often demonstrates ceiling effects when used in young ACL-injured[16] and reconstructed patients,[17] as the items in this subscale relate to low-level daily activities such as putting on socks. Also, older patients with osteoarthritis may demonstrate floor effects on PROMs designed for younger, more active cohorts. For example, the KOOS subscale for sport and recreation may demonstrate floor effects when used in older patients who have moderate to severe knee osteoarthritis after ACL reconstruction, because they have extreme difficulty participating in running, jumping and twisting activities.

For PROMS that have multiple subscales, it is up to the clinician to decide whether all subscales are relevant to the patient of interest. Since scores are calculated and presented per subscale, individual subscales can be omitted in the population of interest or at specific time points. For example, it may not be relevant to evaluate the KOOS sport/rec subscale 2 weeks after ACL reconstruction. Floor and ceiling effects are considered acceptable if less than 15% of patients score the lowest or highest score, respectively.[8]

SUMMARY

PROMs measure items that matter to patients. They can add valuable information to the assessment and management of patients. Selected PROMs are easy to integrate into the sports medicine setting, evaluate patient-relevant constructs, represent single dimensions and can detect real changes in the patient's condition (beyond a defined measurement error). The reader is directed to Part B chapters for recommendations regarding PROMs for specific body regions, conditions and interventions.

Table 16.1 gives some examples of commonly used generic PROMs, while an example of the clinical use of a PROM is shown in the box below.

Examples of generic PROMs appropriate for use in clinical sports medicine

A number of generic PROMS can be applied across a variety of patient groups (i.e. different conditions or injuries) and interventions. Table 16.1 lists some commonly used generic PROMs that measure constructs that are applicable for sports medicine patients.

Table 16.1 Commonly used generic PROMs

Pain

Pain Numerical Rating Scale (NRS)[18]
- Single item
- Most commonly 11-point scale, anchored with 'no pain' (0) and 'worst imaginable pain' (10)
- Patient selects the number that represents their pain severity over the nominated time period (e.g. last 24 hours, past week)
- Manual scoring, score range 0–10
- Freely available

Function

Patient-specific Functional Scale[19]
- 3–5 items, single aggregate score
- Patient nominates up to 5 activities that are difficult because of their injury/condition, then rates the difficulty for each activity on an 11-point NRS (0 = 'unable to perform activity'; 10 = 'able to perform activity at same level as before injury or problem')
- Manual scoring (average of all scores), score range 0–10
- Freely available

continued

Health-related quality of life

SF-36[20]
- 36 items across domains of physical functioning, physical role, bodily pain, general health, vitality, social functioning, emotional role and mental health; can also derive two aggregate summary measures: physical component summary and mental component summary
- Scored by recording some items, summing responses and transforming scores to a 0–100 scale (higher score = better health state). Computer scoring algorithms are necessary and freely available
- Normative data available in multiple populations[21]
- Original version available in English and Arabic, free of charge (www.rand.org). Most recent version (developed in 1998) requires licence and is available in more than 170 languages (www.optum.com/optum-outcomes/what-we-do/health-surveys/sf-36v2-health-survey.html)

AQoL-6D[22]
- 20 items across 6 domains (independent living, mental health, relationships, senses, coping, pain)
- Scoring algorithms and an online scoring service are available (www.aqol.com.au). Score range −0.04 (health state worse than death) to 0.0 (death) and 1.00 (full health)
- Available in 6 languages
- Normative data available
- Freely available; requires registration for use in studies, but not clinical practice

Psychological impairments

Pain Catastrophising Scale[23]
- 13 items across 3 subscales (rumination, magnification, helplessness)
- Manual scoring by summing items. Single aggregate score can be calculated (0–52), as well as individual subscale scores. Higher scores represent higher degree of catastrophising
- Freely available in 21 languages (http://sullivan-painresearch.mcgill.ca/pcs.php)

Tampa Scale for Kinesiophobia[24]
- 17 items evaluating kinesiophobia
- Manual scoring by summing all items (after converting individual scores of 4 items). Total score ranges from 17 to 68, where a high score indicates a high degree of kinesiophobia
- Freely available[25]

Case study: Measuring knee symptoms, function and quality of life after ACL reconstruction

David is a 34-year-old man who underwent an ACL reconstruction (ACL) (hamstring tendon autograft) of his right knee 7 years ago. He returned to social soccer 18 months after surgery. He has recently been experiencing pain and stiffness in his right knee, and has stopped playing soccer and running as he fears that this may increase his pain and any damage in his knee. His family physician ordered X-rays, which revealed mild to moderate osteoarthritis in his right patellofemoral and tibiofemoral joint compartments. David was then referred for physiotherapy management.

In addition to performing his usual clinical assessment, David's physiotherapist administered the KOOS to better understand David's knee condition. The KOOS was developed for patients with knee injuries and/or osteoarthritis. It consists of five individually scored subscales: pain, symptoms, function in activities of daily living (ADL), function in sport and recreation activities and knee-related quality of life (QoL). The KOOS is reliable and valid in patients with ACL injury and/or knee osteoarthritis.[26] The minimal detectable change (MDC), for individuals in adults with mild OA after ACL reconstruction is: pain 20; symptoms 24.9; ADL 14.4; sport/rec 24.9; QoL 20.5 (calculated from SEM data [27].)

Figure 16.1a shows David's KOOS scores at baseline (at his first physiotherapy session) compared to population normative data.[28] There are marked differences in scores

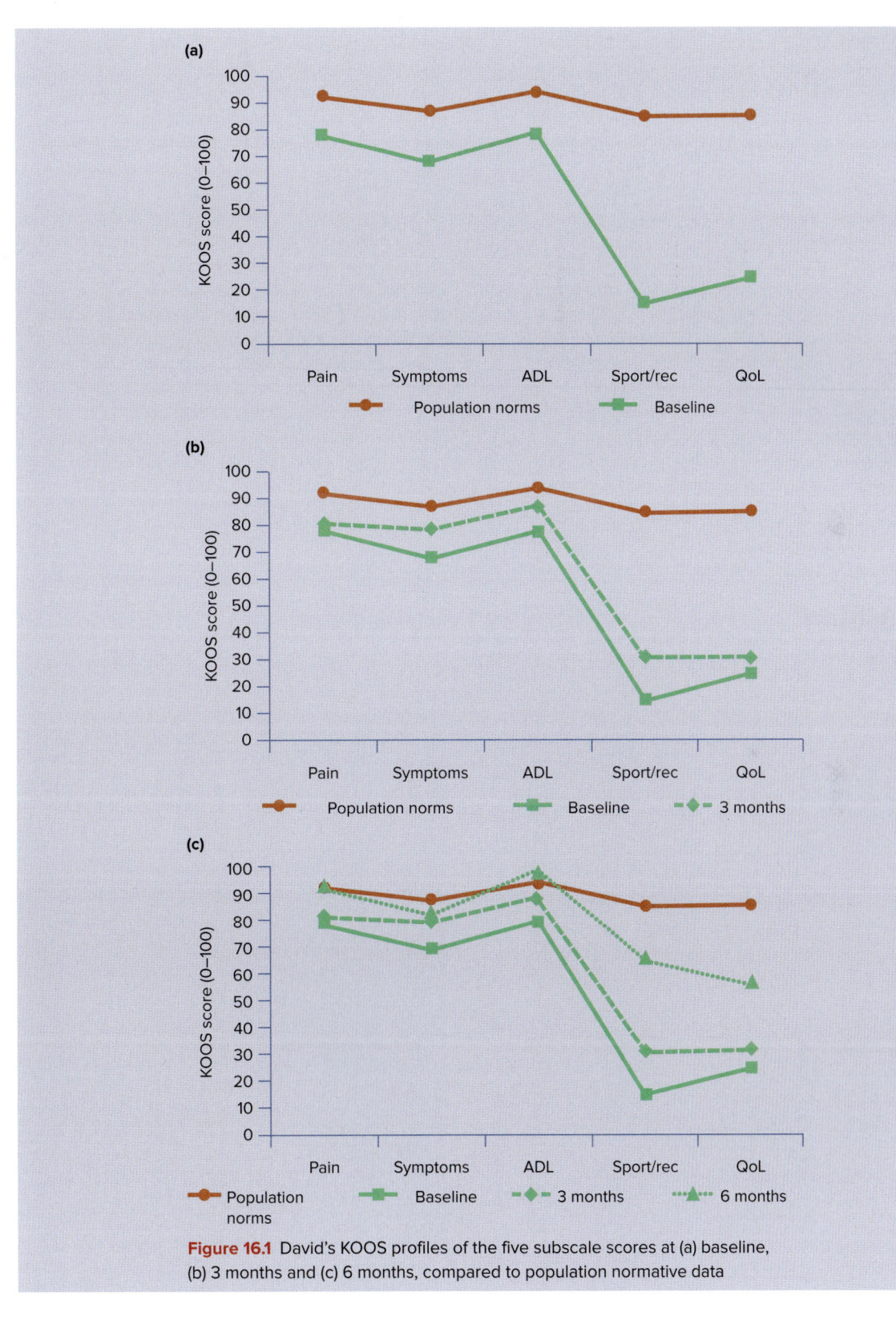

Figure 16.1 David's KOOS profiles of the five subscale scores at (a) baseline, (b) 3 months and (c) 6 months, compared to population normative data

continued

for the sport/rec and QoL subscales. In comparison, the differences in scores for the pain, symptoms and ADL subscales are smaller. This may be because younger patients who undergo ACL reconstruction are more concerned with sport/rec function and QoL and it may reflect ceiling effects observed in this population. However, the difference between David's scores and population norms for the ADL, sport/rec and QoL subscales are greater than the MDC_{ind}, indicating that real differences are present.

The physiotherapist implements a rehabilitation program of lower limb strengthening and neuromuscular control exercises, combined with manual therapy and patella taping to address pain and symptoms.

David's KOOS scores after 3 months are presented in Figure 16.1b. Although his scores are better on the symptoms, ADL and sport/rec subscales, the change scores from baseline are within the error of the measure and therefore may not represent real change. Furthermore, while his scores on the pain, symptoms and ADL subscales are approaching population norms, the sport/rec and QoL scores remain substantially lower.

Based on these outcomes, the physiotherapist decides to integrate some interventions to address QoL into David's rehabilitation program. Specifically, she uses some graded exercises, combined with education, to improve David's confidence in his knee (assessed by KOOS QoL item 3) and reduce any fear-avoidance of potentially damaging activities (KOOS QoL item 2). She continues to progress his strength and neuromuscular exercises, in preparation for return to sport.

From Figure 16.1c you can see that David's pain, symptoms and ADL scores are almost identical to population norms. His sport/rec and QoL scores have also increased by an amount that exceeds the MDC_{ind}. The physiotherapist interprets these findings as representing a true change in David's knee condition. At the last appointment, the physiotherapist hands over the KOOS profiles to David and asks him to score himself from time to time to keep track of his status.

REFERENCES

References for this chapter can be found at www.mhhe.com/au/CSM5e

Chapter 17

Treatment of sports injuries

with BEN CLARSEN

Healing is a matter of time, but is sometimes also a matter of opportunity.
Hippocrates (c.460–370 BCE)

This chapter is integrally linked to the following chapter on the principles of injury rehabilitation. While the terms *treatment* and *rehabilitation* are often used synonymously, we define *treatment* as specific interventions aimed at tissue pathology, impairments or symptoms. Examples of treatments include targeted tendon loading (therapeutic exercise), mobilisation of a cervical spine facet joint (manual therapy), extra-corporal shockwave therapy (electrotherapy) and non-steroidal anti-inflammatory drugs (therapeutic medications). In contrast, we define *rehabilitation* as a holistic process aimed at restoring the athlete to his or her pre-injury function–a part of which involves the application of the right treatments at the right time.

This chapter provides essential background for the treatments detailed in Part B: Regional Problems. Evidence for treatment effectiveness is continually changing. However, remember that our craft remains as much art as science. Level 1 evidence is not always available (see box) and the decision to use (or not to use) certain treatments is also influenced by our experience, professional training and patient's expectations (see 'A cautionary tale' below and Chapters 1 and 2). Nevertheless, clinicians should have a solid understanding of the theoretic rationale for the treatments they provide, as well as up-to-date knowledge of the evidence of their effectiveness.

The effect of each treatment should be evaluated by objectively comparing symptoms and signs before and after the treatment, and at the next visit. Functional testing and patient-reported outcome measures (PROMs–Chapter 16) should also be used regularly throughout the course of treatment. This enables the clinician to choose the most appropriate mode of treatment for the specific injury and individual. In presentations that fail to improve, this also allows the clinician to change modalities or pursue further investigations.

High-level evidence is not always available

There are no randomised controlled studies to demonstrate that jumping out of a plane with a parachute leads to superior outcomes than jumping without one.[1] The best evidence for the effectiveness of parachutes comes from retrospective case series (level 4 evidence; Fig. 17.1). Would this stop you from recommending their use?

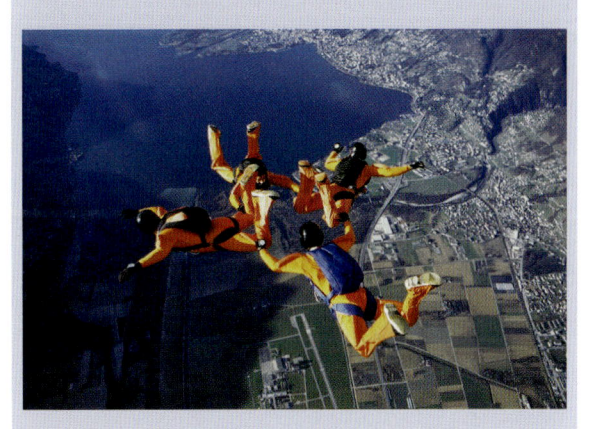

Figure 17.1 The level of research evidence supporting the use of parachutes is low CORBIS

PART A Fundamental principles

A cautionary tale
with KIERAN O'SULLIVAN

Before we launch into specific treatments and the evidence that underpins them, we need to share a cautionary tale. Just as Chad Cook (Chapter 14) alerted us that clinical assessment is not as accurate as the 1990s textbooks made out, treatment is not what a glitzy pharmaceutical video might suggest it is.

Unfortunately, several very important factors—that are unrelated to the pathology of a condition itself—can influence treatment outcomes. You have seen patients who are positive in their outlook and others who seem to live in a world of gloom and doom. You probably suspect that this might affect the outcome of treatment, and evidence indicates it most certainly does.

Patients' response to treatment is greatly influenced by *cognitive* (e.g. thoughts, self-efficacy, hypervigilance), *psychological* (e.g. depression, stress, anxiety, perceived injustice), *social* (e.g. work, family, financial, cultural, social support, life events) and *lifestyle* (e.g. poor sleep, sedentary behaviours, physical activity levels, diet, smoking) factors (Fig. 17.2). These systemic factors are widely acknowledged as being key in the onset and maintenance of pain[2–4] among non-sporting populations reporting pain or injury (e.g. chronic low back pain, hip and knee osteoarthritis). Sports medicine is just beginning to embrace this undeniably important concept.

> **PRACTICE PEARL**
>
> Psychosocial, cognitive and lifestyle factors are related to (i) the onset of symptoms,[5, 6] (ii) treatment response[7, 8] and (iii) return to sport.[9, 10]

While these systemic factors are often perceived as difficult to modify, they are likely to be at least as modifiable as many physical factors (e.g. posture, muscle thickness), which are often the main targets for treatment, but which often do not objectively change as the athlete recovers.[11, 12] Successful clinical outcomes after treatments typically considered to be 'physical', such as exercise, are often mediated by changes in cognitive and psychological factors.[13] Critically, there is evidence that these systemic factors are related to more traditional physical factors (e.g. fear affects movement patterns and, thus, can slow the athlete's return to sport).[14, 15]

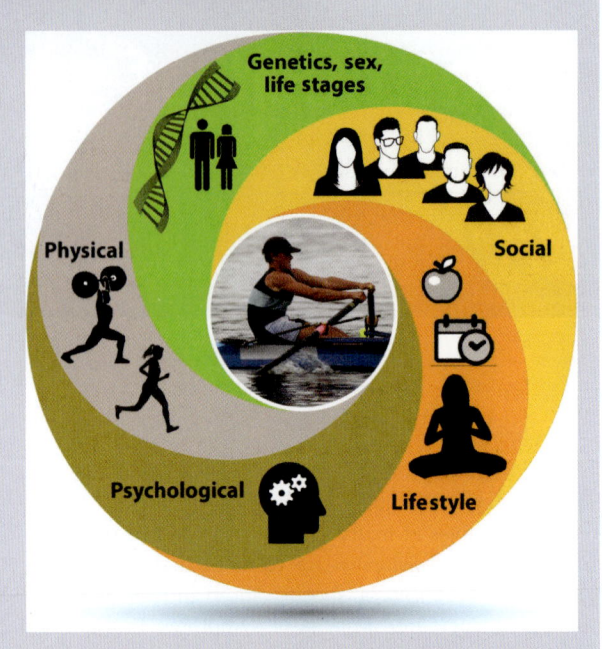

Figure 17.2 A wide range of factors influence patients' response to treatment

> **PRACTICE PEARL**
>
> Rather than considering rehabilitation from injury as physical or psychological, rehabilitation might often need to combine these aspects in a manner that best matches the individual needs of each athlete.

For example, as discussed below, exercise is a core component of injury rehabilitation. Since exercise can enhance a range of systemic factors (e.g. sleep, mood, catastrophising, fear, self-efficacy), there may be occasions when athletes benefit more from the health-enhancing systemic effects of exercise (e.g. it aids relaxation and sleep) than from local loading tissue effects (e.g. an athlete whose pain or injury is not explained by the typical tissue injury model). In situations such as this, clear communication with athletes regarding the mechanism of effect of exercise, and the context in which that exercise is completed, is critical. Furthermore, traditional rehabilitation can then evolve to incorporate additional treatment components (e.g. relaxation, cognitive behavioural therapy, sleep hygiene, dietary advice) to influence several of these wellness factors as required with each athlete.

Treatment of sports injuries CHAPTER 17

THERAPEUTIC EXERCISE

The health benefits of regular physical activity have been recognised since before the time of Hippocrates and proven more and more convincingly since Jeremy Morris' London bus study in the 1950s. The slogan 'exercise is medicine' has been adopted by many public health groups aiming to prevent non-communicable diseases such as cardiac disease, type 2 diabetes and cancer.

'Exercise is medicine' also applies to the treatment of musculoskeletal injury. There is abundant evidence for exercised-based therapy as treatment of a wide range of conditions including tendinopathy,[16] osteoarthritis[17, 18] and lower back pain.[19]

The following section will review a number of mechanisms that may explain the benefits of therapeutic exercise, such as stimulation of tissue repair and remodelling, altering biomechanics and exercise-induced hypoalgesia.

> **PRACTICE PEARL**
>
> Abundant high-level evidence supports therapeutic exercise as a first-line treatment across a wide range of conditions. It should be considered as a first-line treatment for almost any musculoskeletal condition.

Stimulation of repair and remodelling: mechanotherapy

The prescription of therapeutic exercise to promote beneficial tissue adaptations has been called 'mechanotherapy'.[20] This refers to the employment of mechanotransduction–the process by which cells convert physiological mechanical stimuli into biochemical responses–to promote repair and remodelling of injured tissue (see boxed text).

Mechanotransduction: how loading tissue can stimulate repair and remodelling

The process of mechanotransduction is integral to the homeostatic maintenance of the musculoskeletal system in the absence of injury. It also explains how therapeutic exercise can strongly influence injured tissue.

Mechanotransduction consists of three steps: (i) mechanocoupling, (ii) cell–cell communication and (iii) the effector response. Here we use tendon tissue to illustrate this process, but the fundamental principles also apply to other musculoskeletal tissues such as bone, muscle, ligament and articular cartilage.

Mechanocoupling—the loading trigger

Mechanocoupling refers to physical load (often shear or compression) causing a physical perturbation to cells that make up a tissue. For example, with every step, the Achilles tendon receives tensile loads generated by the three elements of the gastrocnemius–soleus complex and, thus, the cells that make up the tendon (Fig 17.3a) experience tensile and shearing forces (Fig. 17.3b). Tendon cells can also experience compression forces (Fig. 17.3c). These forces elicit a deformation of the cell that can trigger a wide array of responses depending on the type, magnitude and duration of loading.[21] The key to mechanocoupling, as the name suggests, is the direct or indirect physical perturbation of the cell, which is transformed into a variety of chemical signals both within and among cells.

Cell–cell communication—distributing the loading message

The previous paragraph illustrated mechanocoupling by focusing on a single cell, but let us draw back to examine a larger tissue area that contains thousands of cells embedded

(a)

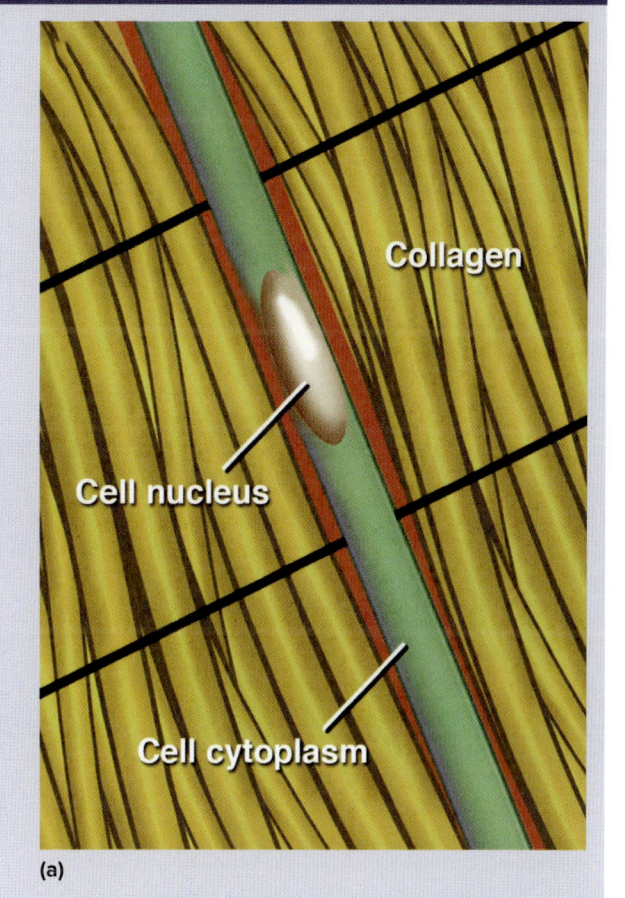

Figure 17.3 The various elements of the tendon cell (a)

continued

241

PART A   Fundamental principles

(b)

(c)

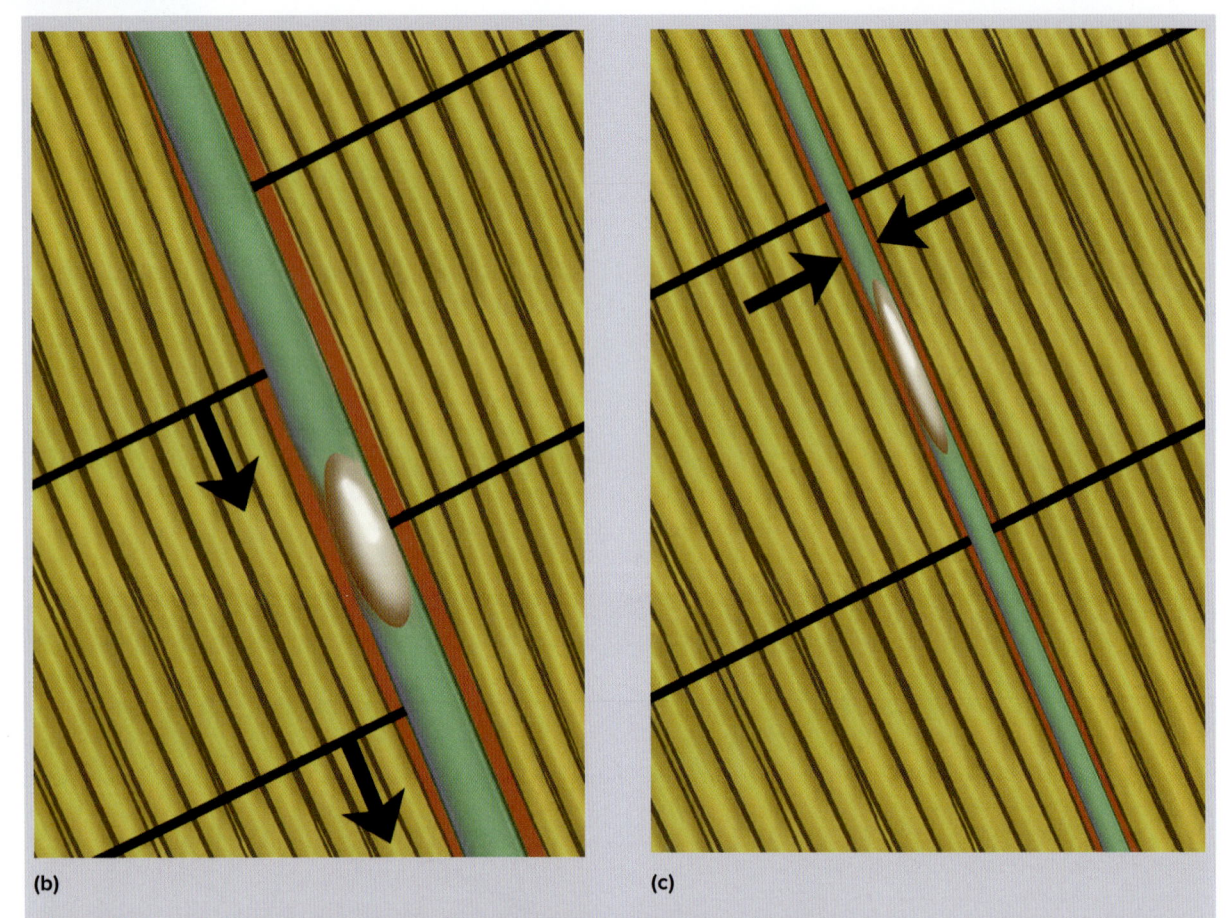

Figure 17.3 (cont.)   The various elements of the tendon cell undergo shear (b) and compression (c) during a loading cycle

within an extracellular matrix (Fig. 17.4). The signalling proteins for this step include calcium and inositol triphosphate (IP$_3$). The process of cell–cell communication is best understood by illustration (Fig. 17.4). The critical point is that stimulus in one location (location 1 in Fig. 17.4c) leads to a distant cell registering a new signal (location 2 in Fig. 17.4e) even though the distant cell does not receive a mechanical stimulus.[21]

Effector cell response
To illustrate the third part of mechanotransduction (effector cell response), we focus on a single cell at the boundary of the extracellular matrix (Fig. 17.5). With movement, integrin proteins located in the cell membrane activate at least two distinct pathways that influence the cell nucleus to initiate the production of new proteins. These pathways include physical and biochemical signals (Fig. 17.5d).

Figure 17.4 Tendon tissue provides an example of cell–cell communication (a) The intact tendon consists of extracellular matrix (including collagen) and specialised tendon cells (arrowheads)

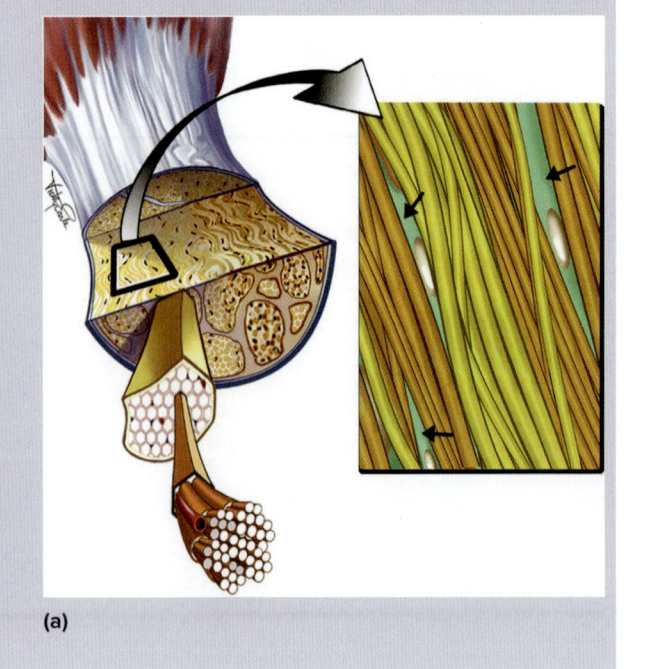

(a)

Treatment of sports injuries   CHAPTER 17

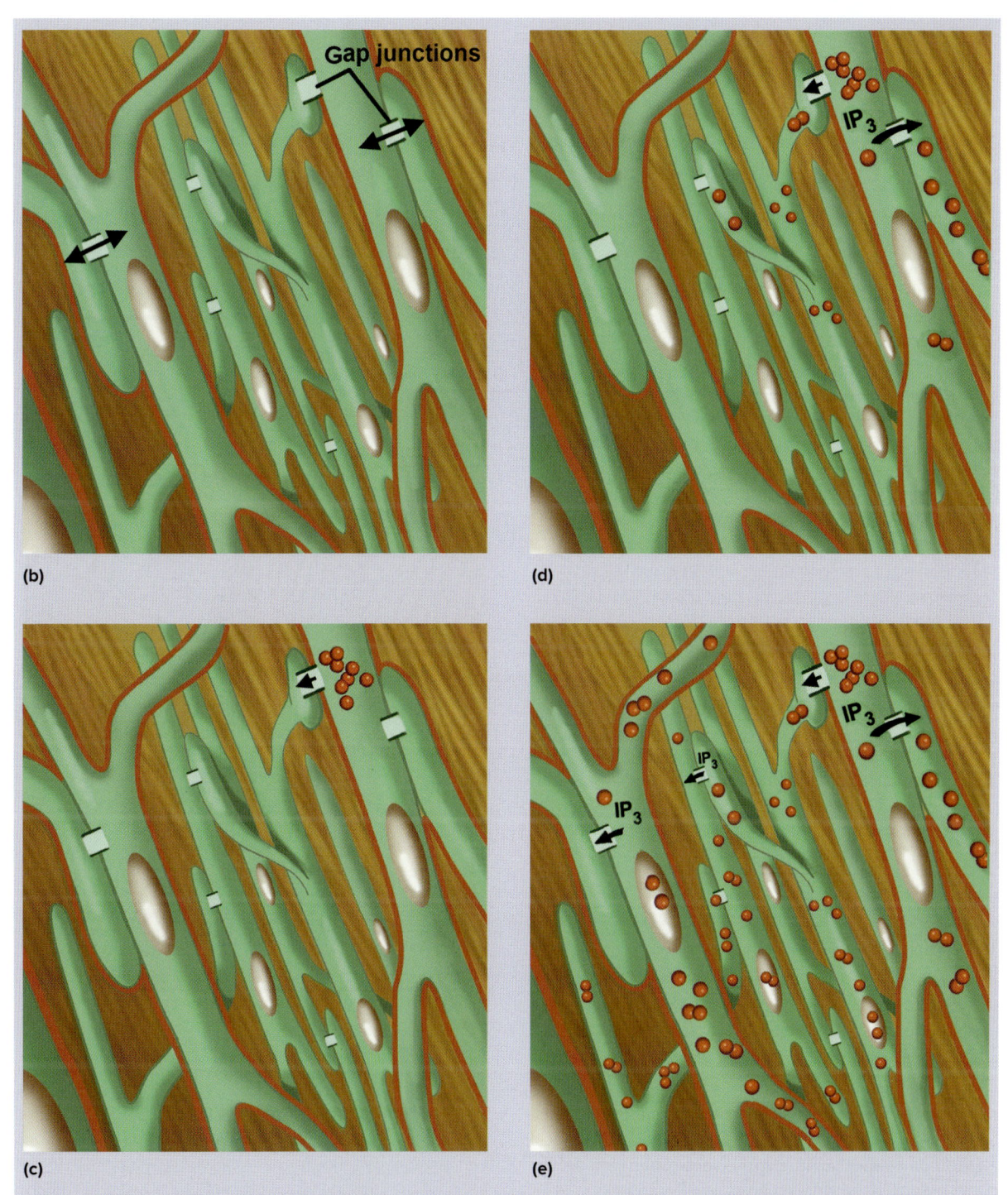

(b) (c) (d) (e)

Figure 17.4 (cont.) (b) Tendon with collagen removed to reveal the interconnecting cell network. Cells are physically in contact throughout the tendon, facilitating cell–cell communication. Gap junctions are the specialised regions where cells connect and communicate small charged particles. They can be identified by their specific protein, connexin 43. Time course of cell–cell communication from (c) the beginning, through (d) the midpoint to (e) the end. The signalling proteins for this step include calcium (red spheres) and inositol triphosphate (IP_3)

continued

PART A   Fundamental principles

Figure 17.5 Mechanical loading stimulates cells to synthesise protein (a) A larger-scale image of the tendon cell network for orientation. We focus on one very small region (b) Zooming in on this region reveals the cell membrane, the integrin proteins that bridge the intracellular and extracellular regions, and the cytoskeleton, which functions to maintain cell integrity and distribute mechanical load. The cell nucleus and the DNA are also illustrated (c) With movement (shearing is illustrated), the integrin proteins activate at least two distinct pathways (d) One pathway involves the cytoskeleton that is in direct physical communication with the nucleus (yellow arrow) (i.e. tugging the cytoskeleton sends a physical signal to the cell nucleus). Another pathway is triggered by integrins activating a series of biochemical signalling agents, which are illustrated schematically (green lever). After a series of intermediate steps, those biochemical signals also influence gene expression in the nucleus (e) Once the cell nucleus receives the appropriate signals, normal cellular processes are engaged. mRNA is transcribed and shuttled to the endoplasmic reticulum in the cell cytoplasm, where it is translated into protein. The protein is secreted and incorporated into the extracellular matrix (f) In sum, the mechanical stimulus on the outside of the cell promotes intracellular processes leading to matrix remodelling

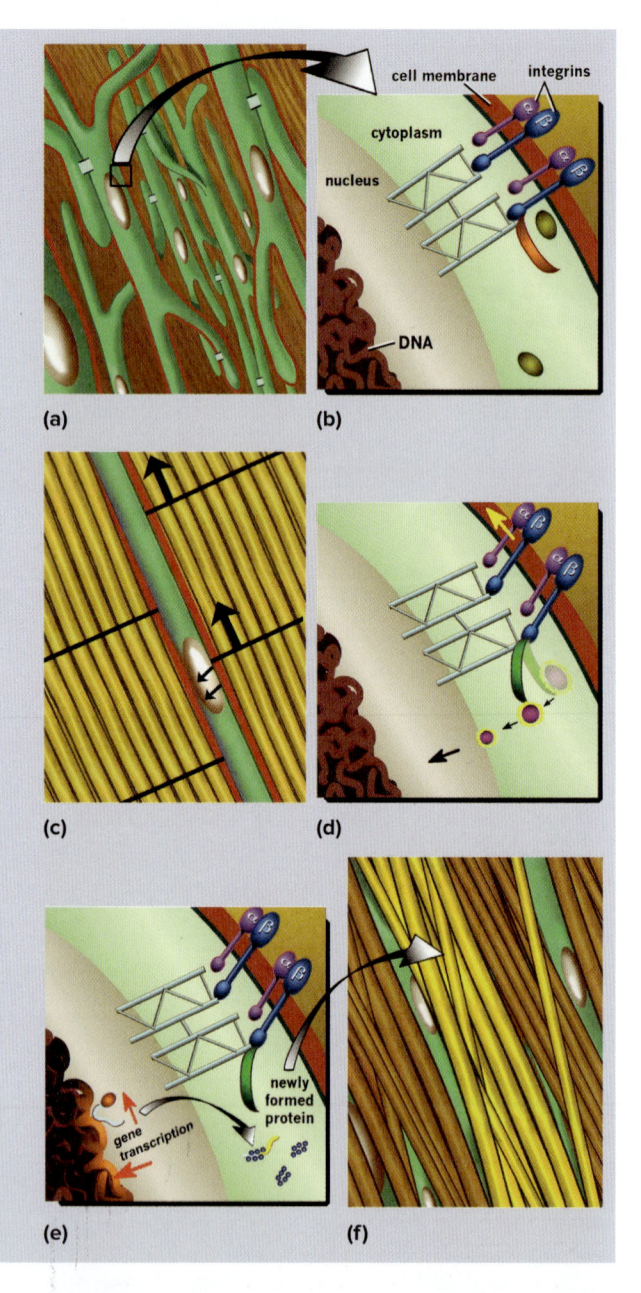

A range of studies have shown or implied a potential for mechanotherapy to promote healing of muscle, tendon, ligament, cartilage and bone. The key to successful clinical application of mechanotherapy is most often finding the correct dosage (and thus progression of exercises).

In some cases, such as patellar and Achilles tendinopathy, literature exists to guide the clinician's exercise prescription. 'Research-proven' treatment regimens, such as tendon training protocols (Chapter 40) or 'heavy slow resistance training'[22] have considerable clinical popularity and are often applied to a variety of other injury types. However, we warn against taking a 'one size fits all' approach. General training principles of progressive overload, periodisation and specificity should be followed (Chapter 10), and exercise prescription should be individualised according to each patient's functional capacity, sport-specific demands and treatment response.

The following section reviews the specific mechanisms and clinical application of mechanotherapy for muscle, tendon, cartilage and bone.

Muscle

Muscle offers one of the best opportunities to exploit and study the effects of mechanotherapy as muscle is highly responsive to changes in loading. Increasing load on muscle leads to the immediate, local upregulation of mechanogrowth factor (MGF), which in turn stimulates muscle hypertrophy via activation of satellite cells.[23] The opposite mechanism is at play in cases where athletes are forced to rest a body part (immobilise or greatly reduce muscle load), such as after a fracture or surgery. In such cases, mechanotransduction causes catabolism of tissue–the tissue adapts to the load it senses.

The benefits of loading include improved alignment of regenerating myotubes, faster and more complete regeneration, and minimisation of atrophy of surrounding myotubes.[24] We revisit this topic later in the section on acute injury management.

Tendon

Tendon is a dynamic, mechanoresponsive tissue. One of the major load-induced responses in tendon, which has been shown both *in vitro*[25] and *in vivo*,[26-28] is an upregulation of insulin-like growth factor (IGF-I). This upregulation of IGF-I is associated with cellular proliferation and matrix remodelling within the tendon. However, other growth factors and cytokines in addition to IGF-I are also likely to play a role.[29]

Recent studies show a significant increase in stiffness, Young's modulus and cross-sectional area in human tendons subjected to mechanical loading programmes.[30] However, the extent of tissue adaptation appears to be highly dependent on the applied loading parameters. In particular, several studies indicate that high-intensity muscle contractions (70–90% of maximum) are necessary to increase tendon stiffness,[31-34] and that interventions longer than 12 weeks are necessary to achieve optimal adaptations.[35, 36] The mechanical, material and morphological properties of tendons respond similarly to high-intensity loading programmes involving eccentric, concentric–eccentric and isometric muscle contractions.[16, 30, 37] However, plyometric training may not lead to optimal adaptations.[30]

Articular cartilage

Like other musculoskeletal tissues, articular cartilage is populated by mechanosensitive cells (chondrocytes), which signal via pathways highly comparable to those described for tendon. Animal studies have shown that immobilisation leads to cartilage atrophy and loss of stiffness, whereas cartilage subjected to high loads has a higher proteoglycan content and higher cell volume, and is stiffer.[38]

Recent advances in magnetic resonance imaging (MRI) technology, in particular the ability to estimate cartilage glycosaminoglycan (GAG) content,[39] have improved our understanding of loading on human articular cartilage. A 16-week moderate loading program increased the GAG content of articular cartilage among patients at high risk of developing tibiofemoral osteoarthritis.[40] Vigorous loading programs have provided mixed results. Some led to improved cartilage quality among people with[41] and without[42] osteoarthritic changes, whereas others were detrimental in people with pre-existing bone marrow lesions.[43]

There is little high-level evidence to guide loading dosage for articular cartilage injuries–the dose-response curves are still being determined. However, there was clinical improvement among 48 patients with full-thickness femoral condyle lesions who utilised a 3-month progressive exercise program consisting of moderate resistance training (3–4 sets of 8–10 repetitions at 40–60% of maximum), as well as neuromuscular and cardiovascular training.[44] A key clinical principle of loading articular cartilage lesions is to avoid pain and swelling during or after training.[44, 45]

Bone

The process of mechanotransduction has been well described in human bone.[46] Appropriate loading of osteocytes, which are believed to be the primary mechanosensors, activates a number of extracellular and intracellular signalling pathways which stimulate osteoblast proliferation and new bone formation. However, both insufficient and excessive loading of bone stimulates osteoclast activity, which leads to a loss of bone tissue.[46]

There is growing evidence that mechanotransduction can be exploited to improve fracture healing, through either active load bearing (e.g. partial weight-bearing mobilisation), pneumatic compression or electrophysical agents.[47] There are no definitive guidelines on the amount of loading required to optimise bone formation, particularly as many factors influence each case, such as the loading type, the site and size of the fracture, and the patient's age and hormonal status. However, studies agree that dynamically applied loads are more effective than static loads in stimulating bone remodelling.[47]

Altering biomechanics: motor-control training

In addition to stimulating repair and remodelling of injured tissues, clinicians also prescribe therapeutic exercise to influence the way a patient moves his or her body. We often refer to this as 'neuromuscular' or 'motor-control' training.

Clinicians usually prescribe motor-control training in an attempt to:

1. Directly or indirectly unload injured or sensitised tissue. For example, overhead athletes with rotator cuff tendinopathy are often prescribed scapular retraction and upward rotation exercises to reduce posterior impingement of their cuff tendons during throwing (Chapter 24).
2. Reduce the risk of injury or re-injury by improving strength, balance, coordination and/or sensorimotor control. For example, patients recovering from anterior cruciate ligament injury are prescribed a wide range of neuromuscular exercises throughout the entire rehabilitation process to optimise their functional outcome and reduce the risk of re-injury (Chapter 35).

There are no definitive guidelines for the dosage of motor control training. However, neuromuscular 'perturbation' programs performed three times per week over a period of 3-4 weeks have been shown to alter motor control patterns in uninjured[48] and ACL-injured athletes,[49] and to improve ACL rehabilitation outcomes.[50] Similarly, training programmes aiming to improve neuromuscular control during standing, cutting, jumping and landing have been shown to prevent injuries in female handball and football players when performed for 15 minutes, three times per week (Chapter 12).[51, 52] As for all types of skill acquisition, regular high-quality practice is necessary to learn and engrain new motor patterns.

> **PRACTICE PEARL**
>
> Effective motor control training programmes focus on movement quality and are sport-specific. Athletes need to concentrate hard throughout the training session and should understand what they are trying to achieve and why it is important. When introducing a new exercise, the clinician should provide a lot of feedback; however, athletes should always be encouraged to assess their own performance.

Motor control training programmes should target specific deficits identified during the clinical assessment. Complex movements should first be broken down into separate components, before the whole task is trained. As pain (or the distraction caused by pain) may interfere with the normal neuroplastic changes that occur with skill training,[53] motor-control training should be pain-free.

Exercise-induced hypoalgesia

In addition to stimulating local repair and remodelling and altering biomechanics, clinicians may prescribe therapeutic exercise due to its hypoalgesic effects. There is a large body of evidence demonstrating that in healthy adults and a range of patient populations, exercise attenuates experimentally-induced pain.[54] This is achieved by elevating pain thresholds and pain tolerance, as well as by reducing pain intensities during and after exercise.[55, 56]

Exercise-induced hypoalgesia is likely to be caused by a combination of factors, including the release of endogenous opioids and other non-opioid substances affecting pain perception such as endocannabinoids, serotonin and norepinephrine (noradrenaline),[56, 57] as well as activation of spinal or supraspinal mechanisms of pain inhibition.[58, 59] Different exercise parameters may alter the predominant mechanism.[56, 60]

Exercise type and dose to maximise hypoalgesia

Aerobic exercise, isometric muscle contractions and traditional resistance training have all been shown to reduce pain, with isometric exercise having the largest effect.[54] Although a recent meta-analysis was unable to calculate the exact dosage required to maximise exercise-induced analgesia, the dose-response relationship favours moderate to high intensities for both aerobic and isometric exercise.[54] Current recommendations, therefore, are that aerobic exercise be performed at intensities above 75% of maximal aerobic capacity (VO$_2$max) for at least 10 minutes,[54] and isometric contractions should be above 50% of maximum voluntary contraction (MVC) held for long durations or until task failure.[61, 62] Recent studies of athletes with patellar tendinopathy have found that five 45-second isometric contractions at 70% of MVC with two minutes' rest between contractions significantly reduced pain for at least 45 minutes after training.[63] Based on these findings, isometric training is currently recommended in the early management of tendinopathy (Chapter 4).

In certain groups of patients with generalised chronic pain such as fibromyalgia syndrome, vigorous-intensity exercise has been shown to increase pain. However, low- to moderate-intensity aerobic and isometric exercise has an effective hypoalgesic effect in this group.[54]

> **PRACTICE PEARL**
>
> As the hypoalgesic effects of exercise are transient, regular exercise is necessary to reduce pain effectively. For example, isometric contractions for the treatment of painful tendinopathy should be performed several times every day.

Treatment of sports injuries — CHAPTER 17

ACUTE INJURY MANAGEMENT

Acute soft tissue injury causes an immediate inflammatory response that manifests clinically as pain, redness, swelling and loss of function. Inflammation is an essential process that initiates tissue regeneration and repair. However, excessive bleeding and oedema can delay recovery and may cause secondary ischaemic damage to nearby tissues.[64] The goal of acute injury management, therefore, is to prevent excessive bleeding and oedema, reduce pain and promote faster return to function.

The principles of acute injury management are based largely on expert opinion and laboratory studies (level 4–5 evidence), and there are few randomised controlled trials upon which to base recommendations.[65, 66] Traditionally, treatment is guided by one of the most commonly known acronyms in sports medicine: PRICE (**P**rotection, **R**est, **I**ce, **C**ompression and **E**levation). Recently, however, a call has been made to change the acronym to POLICE:[67]

- **P**   Protection
- **OL**   Optimal loading
- **I**   Ice
- **C**   Compression
- **E**   Elevation

Protection

A brief period of complete immobilisation is necessary to prevent excessive distention at the injury site, reduce the size of the haematoma and thus minimise the size of the connective tissue scar.[68] During this period, the clinician may consider the use of casts, splints or rigid braces to protect the injured body part, as well as crutches for severe lower-limb injuries.

Although protection is important in the period immediately following trauma, prolonged immobilisation has a detrimental effect on healing in a range of soft tissues, including ligament, tendon and muscle.[68-71] Immobilisation also affects surrounding structures, leading to joint stiffness, degenerative changes in articular cartilage, osteopenia, muscle atrophy and loss of strength. It is therefore important that tissues remain completely unloaded for as short a period as possible. This will vary depending on the extent and nature of the injury and the tissue involved. For most muscle injuries, two days is sufficient before the forming scar has adequate tensile strength to withstand gentle stress.[24] Severe ligament sprains (grades II and III) may require up to ten days of immobilisation before the patient can begin controlled loading.[72, 73]

Optimal loading

Optimal loading replaces *rest* in the acute management acronym due to concerns that the word *rest* may encourage an overly conservative approach that fails to harness the benefits of early tissue loading through exercise.[67, 74]

In comparison to immobilisation, early loading has been shown to have a range of beneficial strength, morphological and functional effects on regenerating tissue, and on the wider neuromusculoskeletal system.[67, 75] For example, early mobilisation of lateral ankle sprains has been shown to improve subjective function, patient satisfaction, swelling, and return to activity, work and sports participation (level 1 evidence).[76, 77] Basic science studies also support early loading compared to immobilisation for a range of soft tissue injuries.[68-71] For example, early mobilisation of muscle injuries improves capillarisation and muscle fibre regeneration, and leads to a more parallel orientation of the regenerating myofibres compared to immobilisation (Fig. 17.6).[68] Muscle injuries demonstrate persisting weakness when treated with prolonged immobilisation (Fig. 17.7).[68]

A major challenge facing the clinician is to determine the 'optimal' loading for each individual at each phase of healing. This should be driven by the tissue type and pathological presentation, as well as the tissue adaptation required; for example, increased tensile strength, collagen reorganisation, increased muscle–tendon unit stiffness or neural reorganisation.[74]

The clinician needs to consider a range of variables when attempting to achieve optimal loading, such as the magnitude, duration, frequency, direction, intensity and direction of load. Manipulation of these variables will not only affect local tissue healing processes, but also stimulate central nervous system adaptations leading to improved motor learning and movement efficiency.

Variable loading offers a range of potential benefits. First, small variations in the magnitude, direction and rate of loading may provide injured tissues with a degree of stress shielding from overload. Second, load variability

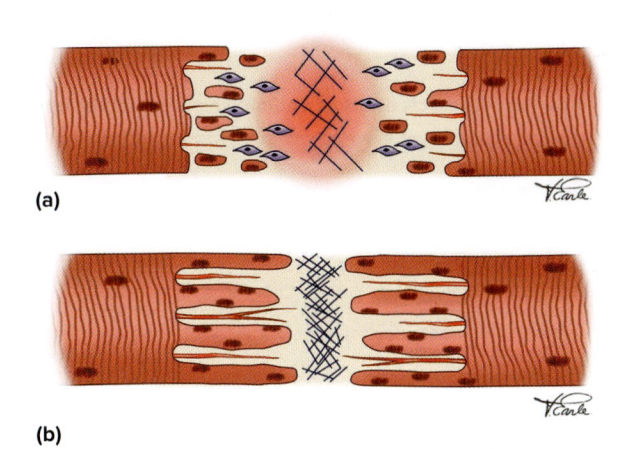

Figure 17.6 Muscle injury treated with (a) immobilisation and (b) early mobilisation. ADAPTED FROM JÄRVINEN ET AL.[68]

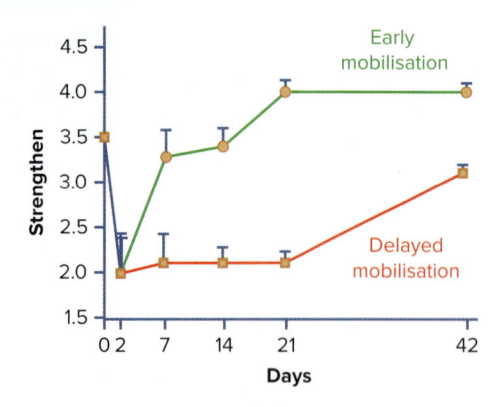

Figure 17.7 Strength improvements in rat skeletal muscle injuries treated with a progressive exercise protocol after two days of immobilisation (shown in green) and in injuries treated with the same protocol after 21 days of immobilisation (shown in red). Note that strength did not naturally return during the immobilisation period. ADAPTED FROM JÄRVINEN ET AL.[68]

may provide a better mechanotransductive effect through broader stimulation of mechanoreceptors and prevention of accommodation. Finally, variable tensile, compressive and torsional forces may promote the creation of a stronger biological scaffold that is better able to withstand a range of loading types.[74]

The characteristics of optimal and suboptimal loading are outlined in Table 17.1.

Ice

Ice (or other forms of cryotherapy) is one of the most common treatment modalities used in the initial management of acute musculoskeletal injuries.[65] Cryotherapy aims to decrease oedema through vasoconstriction and reduce secondary hypoxic injury by lowering the metabolic demand of injured tissues.[65, 68] Local analgesia is thought to occur when the skin temperature drops below 15°C because of decreasing nerve conduction velocity.[78, 79]

Laboratory studies show that cooling injured tissue to between 5°C and 15°C reduces cellular metabolism, white blood cell activity, necrosis and apoptosis.[64, 80] However, this amount of cooling is difficult to achieve in practice, with human studies showing that intensive cooling leads to tissue temperatures of between 21°C and 25°C. The actual metabolic effects of cryotherapy may therefore be questionable, particularly for deep injuries or in patients with higher levels of adipose tissue.[80]

Nevertheless, the analgesic effects of cryotherapy are well established and icing remains a part of current acute injury management guidelines.[81] Ice is typically applied for 20 minutes every two hours for the first 48–72 hours following injury. Intermittent application–for example, 10 minutes on, 10 minutes off–may enhance analgesia and reduce the risk of adverse reactions such as skin burns and nerve damage.[78, 81] Ice should not be applied where local tissue circulation is impaired (e.g. in Raynaud's phenomenon or peripheral vascular disease), or to patients who suffer from a cold allergy.

Although there are many commercial cryotherapy products available, in most situations a plastic bag containing crushed ice and water remains the modality of choice.[82] A wet towel should be placed between the ice pack and the skin. Cryotherapy modalities are summarised in Table 17.2.

Compression

Compression is often used following acute soft tissue injury in order to increase pressure gradients in the venous and lymphatic systems, thereby counteracting oedema. Combining compression with ice may also help reduce tissue temperatures.[83] Although there are a number of specific products commercially available, such as cold compression wraps and devices, a standard elastic bandage is a cheap, versatile and effective solution. Compression can be focussed on certain tissues by applying ice packs underneath the elastic bandage. Similarly, pressure peaks

Table 17.1 Characteristics of optimal and suboptimal loading[74]

Optimal loading	Suboptimal loading
Directed to appropriate tissues	Non-specific generalised loading
Loading through functional ranges	Loading through limited ranges of movement
Appropriate blend of compressive, tensile and shear loading	Loading exclusively in a single manner
Variability in magnitude, direction, duration and intensity	Constant, unidirectional load
Include neural overload	Minimal neural stimulus
Tailored to individual characteristics	Generic, non-individualised
Functional	Non-functional, isolated segmental loading

Reproduced with permission from *British Journal of Sports Medicine*

Treatment of sports injuries — CHAPTER 17

Table 17.2 Cryotherapy modalities used to treat sports injuries

Modality	Description	Special concerns	Surface temperature	Duration	Exercise during application	Expense
Reusable cold packs	Durable plastic packs containing silica gel that are available in many sizes and shapes	Apply a towel between the bag and skin to avoid nerve damage or frostbite	≤15°C (59°F)	20–30 min	No	Inexpensive
Endothermal cold packs	Packets are squeezed or crushed to activate: convenient for emergency use	Single use only	20°C (68°F)	15–20 min	No	Expensive
Crushed ice bags	Crushed ice moulds easily to body parts	Apply a towel between the bag and skin to avoid nerve damage or frostbite	0°C (32°F)	5–15 min	No	Inexpensive
Vapocoolant sprays	Easily portable therapy for regional myofascial pain syndrome, acute injuries, pain relief, and in rehabilitation with spray and stretch techniques	Intermittently spray the area for <6 sec to avoid frostbite	Varies depending on duration of treatment	Multiple brief sprays	Spray <6 sec and stretch to increase range of motion	Expensive
Ice water immersion	An athlete's body part is submerged in cold water	Carries the most risk of hypersensitivity reactions; restrict amount of extremity immersion	0°C (32°F)	5–10 min	Allows motion of the extremity during treatment	Inexpensive
Ice massage	Used to produce analgesia: freeze water in a foam cup, then peel back cup to expose the ice; massage area as often as needed	Apply for short intervals to avoid frostbite; avoid excess pressure	0°C (32°F)	5–10 min	Can allow supervised, gentle, stretching during analgesia	Inexpensive
Refrigerant inflatable bladders	When cold and compression are needed	Avoid excess compression	10–25°C (50–77°F)	Depends on temperature	No	Expensive
Thermal cooling blankets	To provide constant temperature, such as after surgery	Scrutinise temperature settings	10–25°C (50–77°F)	Depends on temperature	No	Expensive
Contrast baths	Transition treatment between cold and heat for a subacute injury, sympathetic mediated pain, stiff joints	Do not use in acute setting due to potential to increase blood flow	Hot bath 40.5°C (105°F) Cold bath 15.5°C (60°F)	4 min hot, 1 min cold	Allows motion of the extremity during treatment	Inexpensive

Reproduced with permission from *British Journal of Sports Medicine*

PART A   Fundamental principles

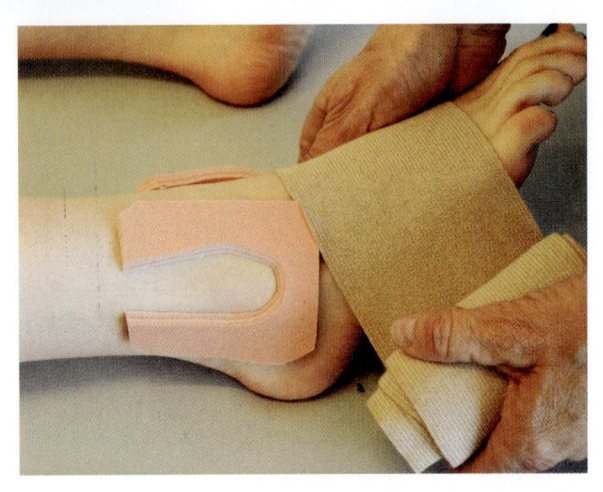

Figure 17.8 Applying compression to a lateral ankle sprain: horseshoe-shaped felt around the ankle malleolus may help distribute compression pressures more evenly

around bony prominences can be avoided by applying felt or other material to fill gaps (Fig. 17.8).

Despite a lack of consensus on the optimal compression pressures, there is some evidence that high pressures (80 mmHg) are ineffective.[81] Standard protocols often recommend light to moderate pressures of 15–35 mmHg. Bandaging should start just distal to the injury site, with each layer of bandage overlapping the underlying layer by one-half. It should extend to at least a hand's breadth proximal to the injury margin.

Elevation

The rationale for elevation stems from the fundamental principles of physiology and traumatology. Elevation of an injured extremity above the level of the heart results in a decrease in hydrostatic pressure and, subsequently, reduces the accumulation of interstitial fluid.[24] Elevation can be achieved by using a sling for upper limb injuries and by resting lower limbs on a chair, pillows or bucket. It is important to ensure that the lower limb is above the level of the pelvis. A graduated return to standing after elevation is likely to minimise rebound swelling and discomfort.[81]

Do no HARM!

In the 72 hours following injury, **HARM**-ful factors should be avoided:

H *Heat and heat rubs*
   Heat may increase the bleeding at the injured site. Avoid hot baths, showers, saunas, heat packs and heat rubs.

A *Alcohol*
   A moderate consumption of alcohol after eccentric-based leg exercises has shown to significantly increase the loss of dynamic and static quadricep strength.[84] Alcohol may mask pain and severity of injury and therefore increase the risk of re-injury.[85] To minimise exercise-related losses in muscle function and to accelerate recovery, avoidance of alcohol post injury is paramount.

R *Running/moderate activity*
   Running or any form of moderate activity can cause further damage at the injury site.

M *Massage/vigorous soft tissue therapy*
   Vigorous massage should be avoided in the first 24–48 hours. It could cause further bleeding and swelling to the injury site.

MANUAL TREATMENTS

In this section, we refer to 'hands-on' treatments, including techniques targeting joints (mobilisation and manipulation), soft tissues (massage/myofascial release techniques) and nerves (neurodynamic techniques). There is a substantial body of evidence demonstrating immediate effects of manual treatments, such as altered pain sensation, muscle activation and joint range of motion.[86-91] However, these effects are unlikely to be maintained over time, or to change the natural history of a disorder. Therefore, clinicians should regard manual treatments as an adjunct to addressing the underlying causes of injury.

Manual treatments are typically directed at specific tissues or structures identified as being abnormal on physical examination, such as stiff joints, tight muscles or restricted nerves (Chapter 15). Traditionally, the rationale for using manual treatments is their proposed local biomechanical and physiological effects; for example, to reduce joint stiffness, increase intramuscular temperature and circulation, or break up adhesions in connective tissue. However, the following factors suggest that local tissue changes are unlikely to explain the clinical benefits of manual treatments:

- Spinal manipulations are only associated with transient increase in joint mobility; there is no evidence of lasting changes in mobility[92] or joint position.[93]
- There is no evidence that massage affects passive or active muscle stiffness, and the effect on global range of motion and muscle blood flow is marginal.[94]
- Clinical methods for assessing joint position, joint motion and soft tissue qualities have poor reliability.[95-98] Different clinicians are therefore unlikely to agree upon which structures require treatment.
- The effect of manual treatments may be distant from the area treated. For example, treatment of the thoracic and cervical spine may affect lateral elbow pain (Chapter 25).[99,100]

Treatment of sports injuries — CHAPTER 17

The actual mechanism of manual treatment is thought to be a complex neurophysiological response from the peripheral and central nervous system, initiated by a local biomechanical stimulus.[95] Mechanical stimulation of afferent neurones located in skin, joints and muscle can activate a number of responses such as pain inhibition[86, 101-103] and neuromuscular inhibition or facilitation.[100, 104-106] Manual treatments also have been shown to have autonomic,[107-109] endocrine,[110, 111] immunologic[112] and psychological effects,[113] which may further explain their potential clinical efficacy.

Joint techniques: mobilisation and manipulation

There are a number of different philosophical approaches towards manual treatment of joints, such as those of Cyriax, Kaltenborn, Maitland, McKenzie and Mulligan.[114-117] Each philosophy differs in its approach to patient assessment and in their justification for treatment selection. The Cyriax and Kaltenborn approaches, for example, base their examination and treatment selection on arthrokinematic and biomechanical theories such as capsular patterns, coupled motions and concave–convex rules. In contrast, the Maitland, McKenzie and Mulligan approaches place more emphasis on patient response during assessment and treatment (symptom provocation and resolution) rather than rigid biomechanical theories.[118]

Irrespective of the clinical reasoning paradigm, the most common manual techniques applied to joints include mobilisations and manipulations. Mobilisations are rhythmic, low-velocity, oscillatory movement techniques applied to spinal or peripheral joints. They are usually passive techniques performed within the patient's tolerance (Fig. 17.9) and may involve physiological joint motion (movements that patients could perform themselves) and/or accessory motions (movements that patients cannot actively control, such as distraction, compression, sliding, spinning and rolling).

The aim of mobilisation is often to restore full, pain-free range of motion to a joint found to be stiff or painful on clinical examination. Treatment parameters such as the location, direction and magnitude of applied force, and the duration of loading, will vary based on patient presentation, clinical examination findings and response to treatment. In general, however, highly irritable joints should initially be treated with low-grade mobilisations (grades I-II, see Table 17.3), whereas higher grades (III-IV) can be used for stiff, non-irritable joints.

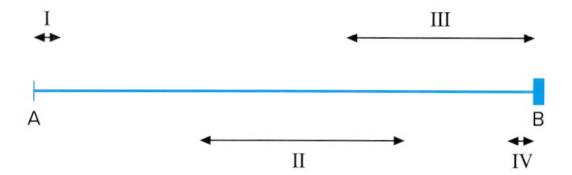

Figure 17.9 Grades of mobilisation: (a) beginning of range of movement; (b) end of range of movement

Mobilisations may also be combined with active movements (mobilisation with movement, see Fig. 17.10), and in some cases patients may be able to perform mobilisations themselves (self-mobilisation, see Fig. 17.11).

Joint manipulations are high-velocity thrust techniques exerted at the end of joint range, using either a long or a short lever arm. Long-lever techniques move many joints simultaneously, such as rotatory manipulations of the cervical spine. Short-lever techniques involve a low-amplitude thrust aimed at a specific joint or spinal segment. This is achieved through careful positioning of the patient, using arthrokinematic principles to isolate movement in the target joint and 'lock' surrounding joints. Manipulation differs from mobilisation due to the velocity of the technique; patients can theoretically prevent the movement during mobilisation but with manipulation they cannot.

Manipulations are usually associated with an audible 'pop' sound, which is thought to be caused by an event called cavitation (Fig 17.12). This refers to the formation of bubbles (or cavities) within synovial fluid due to reductions in hydrostatic joint pressure. Cavitation is traditionally viewed as the sign of a successful manipulation.[119] However, a number of studies have shown that there is little association between an audible pop and the clinical outcomes of spinal manipulation techniques.[120-123]

Safety of manipulation techniques

Manipulation has been associated with a variety of adverse effects, ranging from minor short-term reactions

Table 17.3 Maitland's grades of mobilisation[117]

Grade	Degree of mobilisation
I	Small amplitude movement performed at the beginning of range
II	Large amplitude movement performed within the free range but not moving into any resistance or stiffness
III	Large amplitude movement performed up to the limit of range
IV	Small amplitude movement performed at the limit of range

Reproduced with permission of Elsevier

PART A Fundamental principles

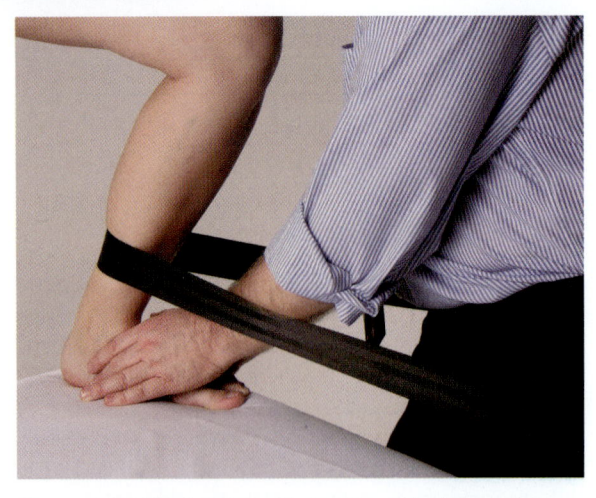

Figure 17.10 Mobilisation with movement technique for ankle dorsiflexion

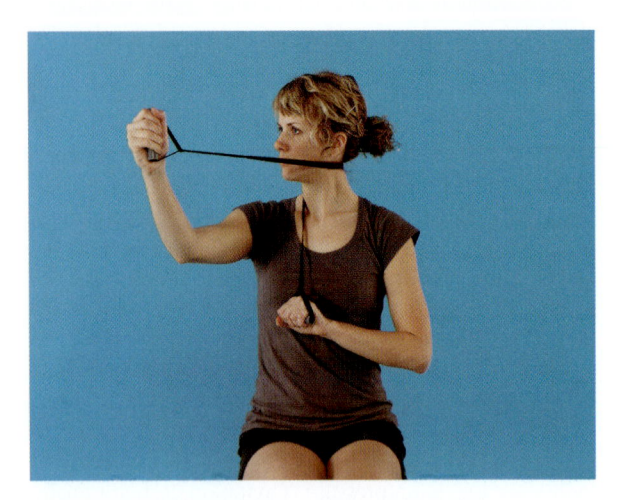

Figure 17.11 Self-mobilisation of cervical rotation

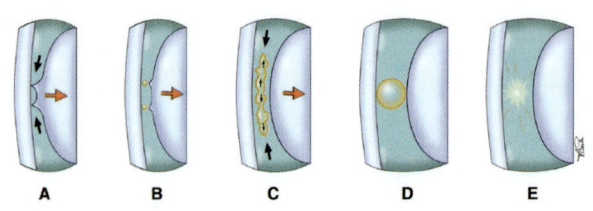

Figure 17.12 The principle of cavitation explains the audible popping sound made during joint manipulation (a) During separation of the joint surfaces, the outer regions of the circular contact zone become pointed. This deformation occurs because at high speeds, the central region of the contact zone separates before the outer region moves, creating a circular rim (b) Joint surfaces snap back at the circular rim where the cavity initially forms, forming small bubbles (c) Small bubbles collect to form a single large bubble (d) The newly formed spherical bubble reaches its maximum size (e) Because of its instability, the single bubble collapses to form a 'cloud' of many smaller bubbles (demonstrable by radiography as a radiolucent region), which later shrink as the gas and vapour dissolve. IMAGE ADAPTED, WITH PERMISSION, FROM EVANS.[119]

such as headache, stiffness and local discomfort, to severe catastrophic events including stroke and death. Minor reactions can be surprisingly common, with one study finding that more than 60% of patients experienced a mild adverse reaction in the 24 hours after receiving a spinal manipulation.[124] While a vast majority of side effects are benign, self-limiting problems, clinicians should inform patients of their likelihood prior to treatment.

Fortunately, severe injuries caused by spinal manipulations are extremely rare. While the actual risk is unknown, estimates range from one case in fifty thousand manipulations to one in five million.[124] A majority of catastrophic injuries caused by cervical spine manipulation are due to the proximity of the vertebral artery to the lateral vertebral joints. However, thoracic and lumbar spine manipulations may also cause serious injury, such as rib fractures and cauda-equina syndrome.[125–128]

Manipulations should only be performed by practitioners with formal training in manipulative skills. Cervical artery function should be tested prior to manipulation of the cervical spine (see Chapter 23), and short-lever techniques should be used in preference to long-lever techniques.

Clinicians also need to be aware of the contraindications to the use of mobilisation and manipulation techniques (Table 17.4).[118]

Soft tissue therapy

with ROBERT GRANTER

Direct treatment of soft tissues, using hands or treatment tools, to treat specific pain or injury is commonly referred to as soft tissue (or massage) therapy (see Chapter 13 for the use of soft tissue massage techniques in post-exercise recovery). As with other manual treatments, soft tissue therapy is traditionally directed at subjective clinical examination findings such as reduced quantity and quality of joint movement, muscles with increased tone, soft tissue thickening, or muscles containing taut, sensitive bands that may refer pain in distinct patterns, often referred to as myofascial trigger points (Chapter 4).

This section provides an overview of several key techniques that clinicians can use to treat muscular pain, and alert the reader to some self-treatment options.

Treatment position

For successful soft tissue therapy, the clinician should place the target tissue in a position of either tension or laxity.

Treatment of sports injuries — CHAPTER 17

Table 17.4 Absolute and relative contraindications for mobilisation and manipulation techniques

Absolute contraindications—high risk of a deleterious consequence	Mobilisation	Manipulation
Malignancy or tumour in the targeted region	×	×
Cauda equine lesion producing bladder or bowel disturbance	×	×
Fractures	×	×
Local bony infection (e.g. osteomyelitis, tuberculosis)	×	×
Systemic disturbance	×	×
Rheumatoid collagen necrosis	×	×
Unstable upper cervical spine	×	×
Signs of coronary or vertebral artery dysfunction	×	×
Practitioner lack of ability		×
Spondylolisthesis (symptomatic)		×
Gross foraminal encroachment		×
Children/adolescents with open epiphyseal plates		×
Pregnancy (last trimester)		×
Joint fusions		×
Psychogenic disorders		×
Immediately postpartum		×

Relative contraindications—possibility of deleterious consequences	Mobilisation	Manipulation
Active inflammatory conditions	×	×
Significant segmental stiffness	×	×
Systemic diseases	×	×
Neurological deterioration	×	×
Irritability	×	×
Osteoporosis	×	×
Condition worsening with present treatment	×	×
Acute radiculopathy	×	×
History and examination do not add up	×	×
Use of oral contraceptives (cervical spine)	×	×
Long-term corticosteroid use (cervical spine)	×	×
Blood clotting disorder	×	×

Treating soft tissue in an elongated position can make focal sites of abnormality more easily palpable, and may enhance referral patterns from myofascial trigger points. Treating in a position of laxity enhances the ability to access and assess deeper layers of soft tissue.

Digital ischaemic pressure

Digital ischaemic pressure describes the application of direct pressure perpendicular to the skin towards the centre of a muscle with sufficient pressure to evoke a temporary ischaemic reaction (Fig. 17.13).

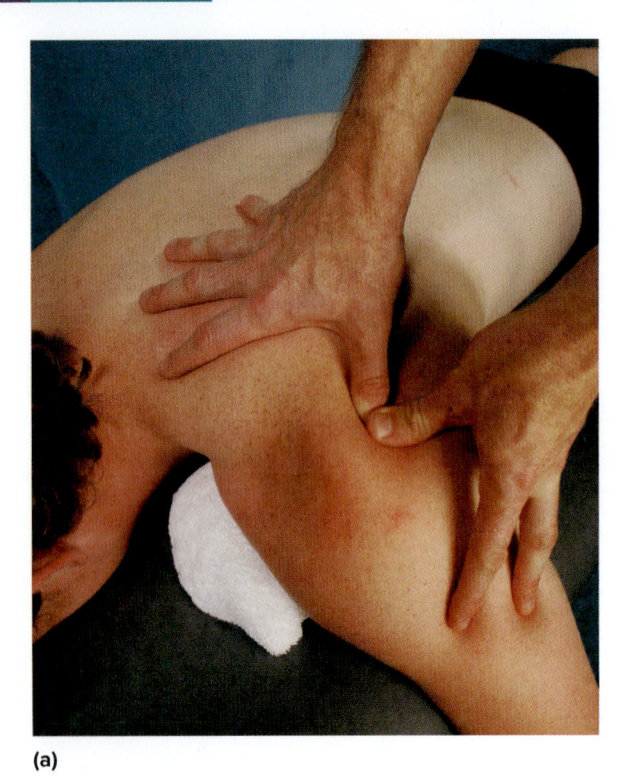

PART A   Fundamental principles

(a)

Figure 17.13 (a) Digital ischaemic pressure to the infraspinatus trigger point using the clinician's thumb (b) Digital ischaemic pressure to the gluteus medius trigger point using the clinician's elbow

(b)

The aims of this technique are to stimulate the mechanoreceptors within muscle and fascia to reduce resting muscle tone, to provide an analgesic response in soft tissue by eliciting a release of pain-mediating substances, and to deactivate symptomatic trigger points which may optimise muscle activation patterns.[129]

The clinician can apply digital ischaemic pressure using the thumb (Fig.17.13a), elbow (Fig. 17.13b) or a hand-held device such as a T-shaped bar.

Sustained myofascial tension

Sustained myofascial tension is performed by applying a tensile force with the thumb, braced digits, or forearm (Fig. 17.14) to an assessed site of fascial thickening or reduced fascial glide in the direction of greatest restriction, or in the direction of elongation necessary for normal function. Tension is developed in the tissue by application of compression to the appropriate fascial layer, then moving the thumb, braced digit or forearm through the target tissue to impart a shear force. Greater shear force can be imparted using passive through-range movement or active movement in the direction of assessed restriction in conjunction with the local tissue contact.

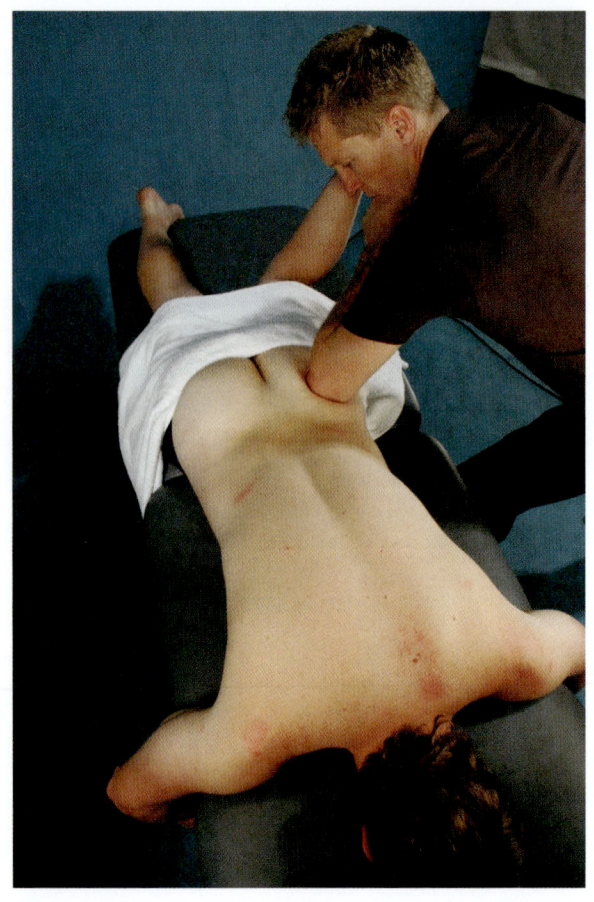

Friction

Friction massage is applied selectively to a localised area palpated as an abnormal tissue thickening; for example, due to excessive intramuscular scar formation following acute muscle injury. It is essential to assess pain and restrictions in muscle length and/or neural mobility before, during and at the end of each treatment session to monitor its effectiveness.

Sufficient pressure must be applied so that the clinician's finger/thumb and the patient's skin move as one, and the friction must work deeply enough and be of sufficient sweep to impart a friction movement to the target tissue. The friction is normally applied at 90° (perpendicular) or at 45° to the target structure, and must be applied at a level that maintains contact with the target tissue and is within the patient's pain tolerance.

It is vital to ensure that the region being treated is totally relaxed. Pressure should be increased gradually to reach the required treatment level within the

Treatment of sports injuries   CHAPTER 17

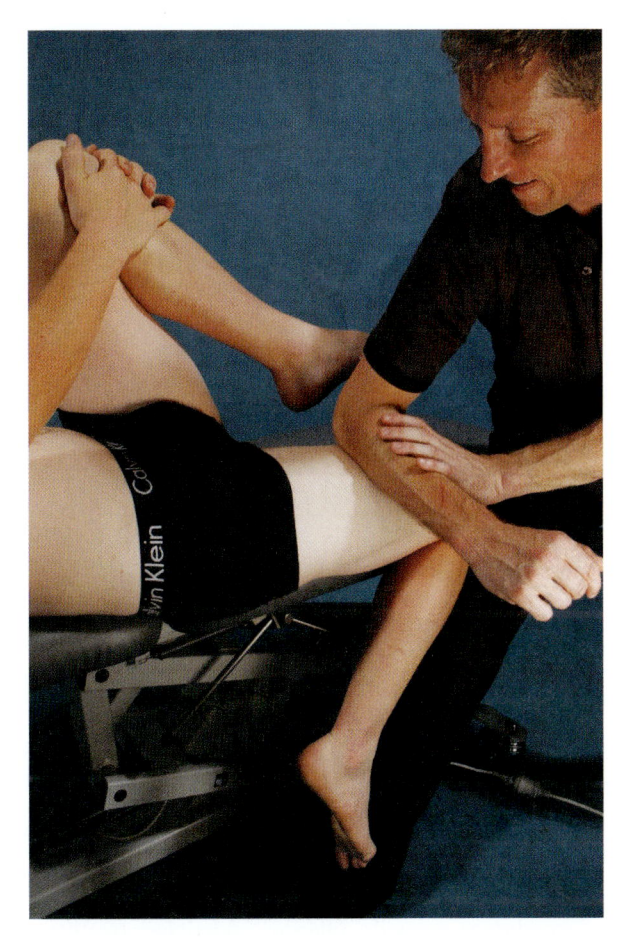

Figure 17.14 Sustained myofascial tension

Table 17.5 Granter–King scale for grading the depth of soft tissue therapy

Pain grade (P)	Patient's perception of pain
I	No pain perceived
II	Commencement of pain
III	Moderate level of pain
IV	Severe level of pain (seldom used)
Resistance grade (R)	**Clinician's perception of tissue resistance**
A	No sense of base tissue resistance
B	Onset of base tissue resistance
C	Moderate level of base tissue resistance

Lubricants
Many soft tissue techniques require a lubricant applied to the skin to aid both patient comfort and the clinician's ability to palpate the tissue for abnormalities. There should be sufficient lubricant particularly when palpating areas with large amounts of hair, as irritation of hair follicles may result in contact dermatitis.

With techniques such as sustained myofascial tension, skin contact should be maximal. Therefore, no lubricant is required. As there are fewer repetitive movements used in this technique, there is less risk of irritation to hair follicles.

Vacuum cupping
The aim of vacuum cupping is to restore optimal length and mobility of soft tissues, with changes most likely achieved through neurophysiological responses. Oil is applied to the skin to contain the negative pressure created in the cup by a vacuum pump. Within the vacuum cup, the soft tissue is 'drawn' upwards in a unique perpendicular direction, thereby stretching the soft tissue in a regulated, sustained stretch. The cup contains a one-way valve that allows the pump to be removed.

Cupping can cause significant capillary rupture and damage to the periosteum if used with excessive vacuum pressure or with incorrect placement. The skin colour should be monitored closely and the cup removed if the skin becomes more deeply rose-coloured than normal reactive hyperaemia. Generally, the longer a cup is left *in situ* or the more vacuum force is applied, the more bruising can develop. This is unnecessary and can be avoided by diligent observation during application. The cup should not be applied to vulnerable regions of the body, such as cubital and popliteal fossae and soft tissue attachment sites to bone.

patient's pain tolerance. Ice can be applied to the region post-treatment in a position of pain-free stretch for 5–10 minutes, particularly for the initial application, to minimise post-treatment tenderness.

Depth of treatment
Granter and King developed a grading system for depth of soft tissue therapy as a guide for clinicians and researchers to adopt consistency in describing treatment dosage (Table 17.5).

The scale of treatment depth is based on two factors: first, the patient's perceived level of pain during the treatment (grade I–IV); and second, the clinician's sense of soft tissue resistance to palpation (A–C).

Combination treatment
If soft tissue techniques are aimed at restoring joint range of motion, they can be followed by static, contract/relax or dynamic stretching to maximise the effect.

255

PART A   Fundamental principles

Self-treatment

In recent years, there has been an increase in the popularity of using devices such as spiky balls, tennis balls and foam rollers for self-treatment of soft tissues (Fig. 17.15). A number of studies have found that this approach leads to a short-term increase in range of motion, without any detriment in sports performance.[130-133] Self-treatment may also be aimed at treating myofascial trigger points.

Self-treatment can be undertaken daily and should not cause excessive or lasting pain that adversely affects training or increases symptoms. Typically, self-treatment involves the application of a sustained force to the identified sites, with a sustained pressure until tone/tension reduces and pain or referred symptoms resolve. Functional re-assessment should be carried out after an initial trial period, for example 1-2 minutes, to ensure that positive changes are occurring. As initial presenting symptoms, soft tissue characteristics and patient responses vary, clinicians and patients need to individualise dosage in relation to time and repetitions to achieve optimal results.

Dry needling

The terms 'acupuncture' and 'dry needling' are often used interchangeably in sports medicine to describe treatments using thin monofilament needles without injectate.[134] However, *acupuncture* denotes the use of the modality within a traditional Chinese medical paradigm, in which needles are used to unblock the flow of vital energy, 'qi', along meridians or channels,[135] whereas *dry needling* implies the use of a modern biomedical paradigm.

Dry needling is thought to have a range of neural and biochemical effects that can contribute to pain relief.[135] Insertion of needles stimulates free nerve endings, sensory receptors and autonomic fibres in skin, muscle and connective tissue. It also causes the release of a range of neuroactive mediators, including endogenous opioids, which can inhibit transmission of nociceptive signals in the peripheral and central nervous system and alter pain perception.[135, 136] Local tissue injury caused by needle insertion is also thought to cause 'positive' inflammatory and immune responses, which can contribute to analgesia.[134, 135]

Dry needling is most commonly used to treat intramuscular trigger points, but techniques targeting joints, tendons, ligaments, bone and scar tissue are also described.[134] Trigger point techniques often aim to produce a local muscular twitch response, thought to be caused by stimulation of a spinal reflex loop.[137] This has been linked to an immediate reduction in extracellular neurotransmitter concentration in muscle tissue surrounding a trigger point,[138] and a twitch response is anecdotally associated with an improved treatment effect.[139]

There is a vast amount of research on the effects of dry needling and acupuncture. However, interpretation of the literature is complicated by the wide variety of conditions treated, differing underlying treatment paradigms (traditional Chinese medicine versus a modern biomedical model), as well as a large variation in treatment protocols and methodological quality. It is particularly difficult to blind patients and clinicians in RCTs which is problematic as needling is associated with a potent placebo effect.

Nevertheless, a substantial body of level 1 evidence suggests needling is more effective than placebo or sham treatments for a range of musculoskeletal conditions such as chronic lower back, neck and shoulder pain, chronic muscular pain, headache, and knee osteoarthritis.[140-144]

Clinicians should consider the following points when using dry-needling techniques.

- The patient is comfortably positioned with the target region well-supported.
- The target tissue is clearly identified, a taut band is palpated within the muscle and symptoms are reproduced by palpation. This site is 'marked' by compressing a used guide-tube onto the skin above the identified site (Fig. 17.16a).
- The correct equipment is prepared. Sterile, single-use needles must be used. Tubed needles are recommended

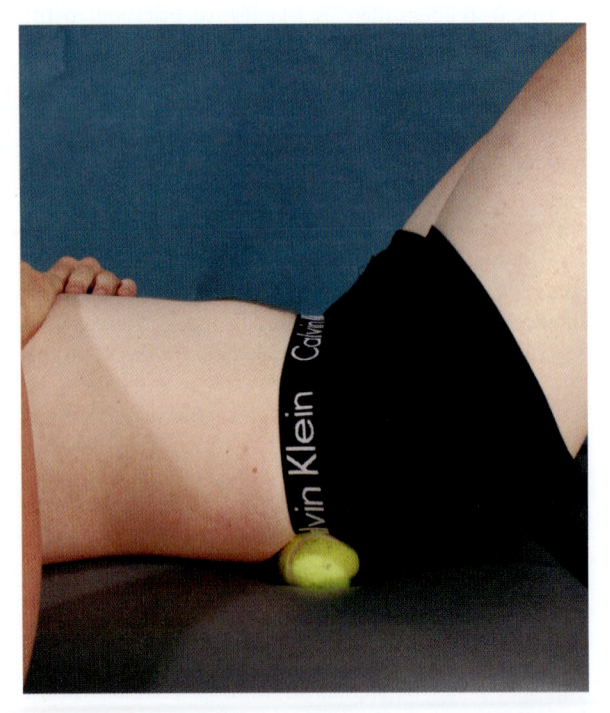

Figure 17.15 Self-treatment: treating the gluteus medius with a tennis ball

Treatment of sports injuries   CHAPTER 17

to expedite placement and reduce the risk of touching the needle shaft. Cotton swabs and a sharps container should be within easy reach.
- A hygiene protocol is followed. The patient's skin is cleaned and disinfected with an alcohol swab. The clinician should wash his or her hands and wear latex gloves (at least on the palpating hand most likely to be exposed to blood).

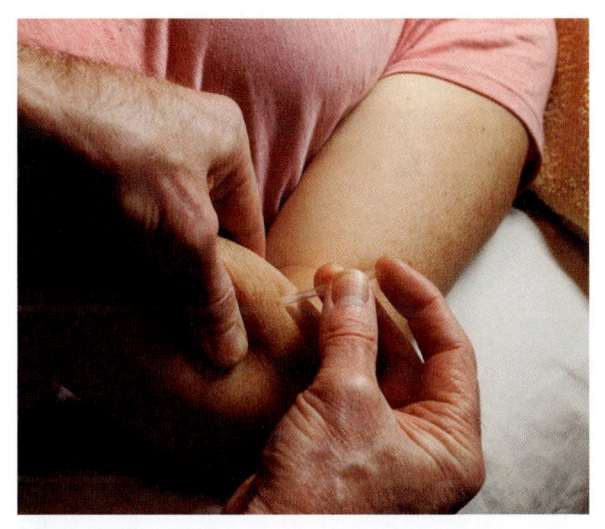

(a)

(b)

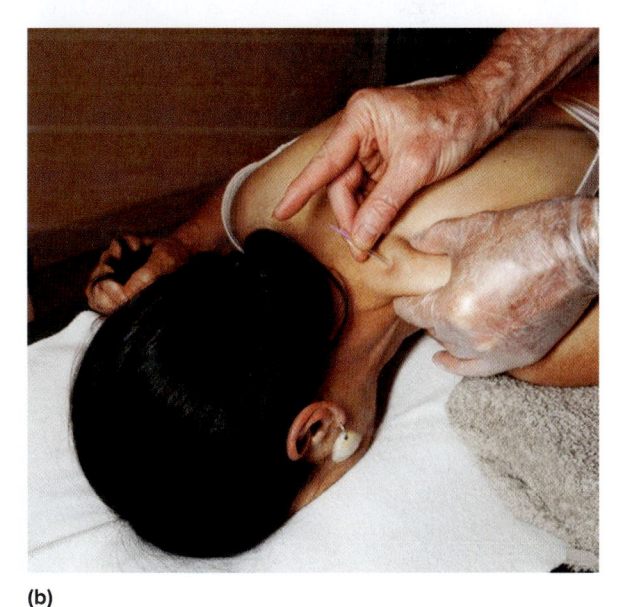

Figure 17.16 Dry needling (a) A needle tube can be pressed into the skin to temporarily mark the injection site (b) The target muscle should be supported by one hand while the other hand focuses on accurate insertion of the needle

- The target muscle is supported to maximise accurate needle penetration. For example, when treating the upper trapezius, the muscle should be held anteriorly and posteriorly between the fingers and thumbs of one hand while the other hand focuses on accurate insertion of the needle (Fig. 17.16b).
- The needle and guide tube are placed perpendicular to the skin on the marked site and the needle is inserted with a short, sharp tap to the top of its handle.
- The guide tube is removed and the needle is fully inserted to the appropriate depth by only touching the needle handle, never the shaft.
- Various dry needling techniques can be utilised (see below).
- The needle is removed and local compression is applied over the site via a cotton swab for approximately 30 seconds.
- The joints associated with the muscle treated should be moved passively through their full comfortable range of motion after treatment.
- Needles and equipment are disposed of by correct medical waste disposal protocols.

The most commonly used dry needling technique involves inserting the needle into focal trigger points within a palpable taut band and leaving it in place for a few minutes. There is no clear consensus on the time left in situ–some authors have suggested time ranges from 10–30 minutes.[134] This will vary according to patients' experience with dry needling, as well as their emotional and physiological responses and the degree of presenting symptoms.

Some clinicians also apply electrical stimulation to the inserted needles. However, there are no clear guidelines for treatment parameters and no evidence that electrostimulation improves the treatment effect.

Alternatively, the clinician can insert the needle into the muscle and then repeatedly move the needle in and out (such that it still remains in the sub-dermal region), constantly trying to find specific points that reproduce the patent's local or referred pain, or produce a 'twitch' response. Initially, the needle may be 'grasped' by the muscle, followed by a gradual relaxation.

Clinicians can apply needles to a number of trigger points during each treatment session. Usually, pain relief lasts 3–4 days after the first treatment session. The duration of the pain relief may be longer following subsequent sessions. Up to three or four treatments may be required initially to eliminate a trigger point, and no single trigger point should be needled more than twice in a week.

Various research studies have compared dry needling to injection of local anaesthetic and various other substances. There is some evidence that dry needling can be just as effective.[145, 146]

257

PART A Fundamental principles

Risks of adverse events during dry needling
The most common adverse effect associated with dry needling is soreness in the first 24 hours post treatment.[147] Application of heat and stretching exercises may minimise this,[147] and aggressive treatment should be avoided until the patient's reaction to dry needling is known. High quality needles, which are sharper and thinner, may also reduce pain during and after treatment. If there is excessive resistance to needle removal, the needle should be removed more slowly.

In patients unfamiliar with or apprehensive about dry needling, it is possible to induce an episode of vasovagal syncope. The risk of this occurring can be minimised by careful patient selection–it is especially important to identify those with needle phobias. Clinicians should avoid excessive stimulation of specific sites until the patient learns to tolerate this new treatment. The patient's response should be closely monitored during treatment, with constant communication to ensure patient comfort. If at any stage the patient becomes distressed with the treatment, needles should be removed. Contraindications to dry needling include bleeding disorders, active infection, blood-borne diseases, allergies to metal, unstable epilepsy and the third trimester of pregnancy. Additionally, extreme care should be taken when dry needling near the lungs as there is a risk of causing a pneumothorax.

Neurodynamic techniques
The nervous system needs to adapt to mechanical loads. It can do this through elongation, sliding, cross-section change, angulation and compression.[148] However, when the nervous system cannot cope under loads, it can lead to neural oedema, ischaemia, fibrosis and hypoxia–all of which can alter neurodynamics.[148] This change in neurodynamics may make a significant contribution to the patient's symptoms and signs in certain injuries. Unless these abnormalities are addressed in addition to other soft tissue abnormalities associated with the injury, full recovery as indicated by full pain-free range of motion may not occur.

Neural tension was a term used in the past to describe peripheral nervous system dysfunction, but was thought to only address the mechanical aspects of the dysfunction.[148] Nowadays the term *neurodynamics* is employed to describe the biomechanical, physiological and structural dysfunction of the nervous system.[148]

Neural stretching (mobilisation) is a treatment modality that addresses neurodynamics. Neural stretches aim to restore dynamic balance of the nervous system.[148] Proposed benefits include facilitation of nerve gliding, decrease in nerve adherence, dispersion of noxious fluids, increased neural vascularity and improved axoplasmic flow.[148]

These stretches are adaptations of the neural tension tests (Chapter 15). The two most commonly used neural stretches are adaptations of the upper limb tension test (Fig. 17.17a) and the slump test (Fig. 17.17b).

A systematic review[148] evaluated the effectiveness of neural mobilisations and found that even though the identified studies did report positive effects, low methodological quality and limited number of studies suggest that currently there is limited evidence for their use. However, these stretches can often be helpful in the treatment of conditions in which neurodynamics are

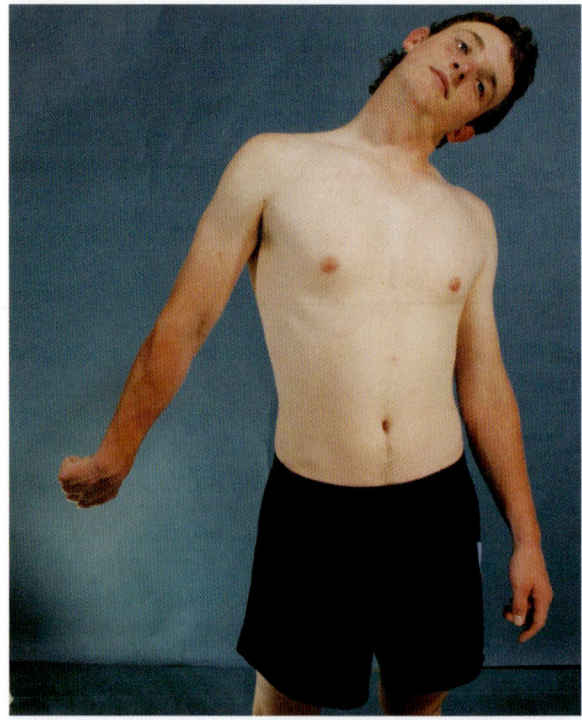

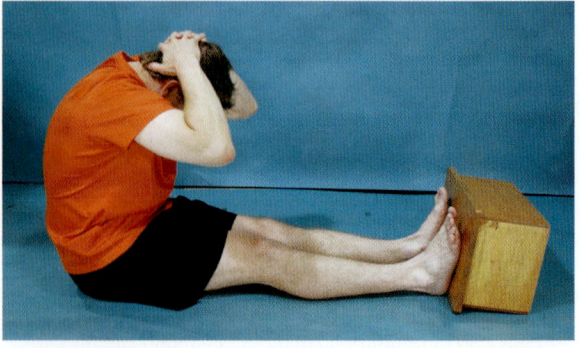

(a)

(b)

Figure 17.17 Common neurodynamic techniques (a) Upper limb neurodynamics stretch test (b) Slump stretch

Treatment of sports injuries — CHAPTER 17

abnormal, and variations of these tests may be used for both diagnosis and treatment.

Clinicians should take particular care when considering neural mobilisation exercises for acute or irritable conditions, as they may aggravate the patient's symptoms. Stretches should always begin gently, and gradually increase under the close supervision of an experienced clinician. As with other methods of treatment, neural stretches alone are rarely sufficient to correct all abnormalities present. They can be particularly effective in long-standing, chronic conditions where neural hypersensitivity is common.

TAPING

with SAM BLANCHARD

Taping was the third-most utilised intervention at the London 2012 Olympic Games polyclinic,[149] reflecting its current popularity as a treatment modality and injury prevention intervention. However, research into both the mechanisms and effects of taping is limited and marked by heterogeneous results,[150, 151] making it difficult for clinicians to draw firm evidence-based conclusions on its benefits and application.

Proposed mechanisms of taping

Taping is proposed to have a range of effects depending on the application method and the type of tape used. Traditionally, clinicians have applied rigid strapping tape in an attempt to restrict patients' range of motion or to alter their anatomical alignment; for example, to realign the patella within the femoral trochlea (Fig. 17.18).[152] More recently, the use of flexible cloth tape, often referred to as kinesiology tape, has also gained popularity.

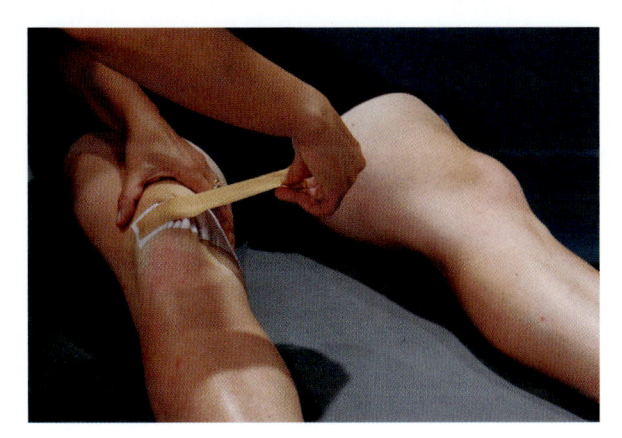

Figure 17.18 Taping is often used to relieve patellofemoral pain

Taping also appears to have a range of neurophysiological effects.

- Cutaneous stimulation by tape may inhibit afferent nociceptive signals at the spinal level (pain-gate theory).[153]
- Tape application has been shown to alter brain activity in a variety of areas, including the motor cortex, sensory cortex, thalamus, basal ganglia and cerebellum.[154] This may have a wide range of effects, including improved proprioception[155] and motor coordination, and explain how taping influences factors such as muscle activation timing[156] and concentric/eccentric control.[157]
- Restriction of the range and amplitude of joint motion may enable increased reaction time of surrounding musculature during high-velocity injury situations.[150, 157-159]
- Patients' conscious and subconscious expectations of the effects of taping may relieve pain (i.e. placebo effect).[153] Once thought to be a 'purely psychological' phenomenon, it is now considered to be at least partly caused by the secretion of endogenous opioids in response to treatment.[58]

However, the proposed mechanisms of taping remain largely speculative or controversial. For example, tape intended to limit range of motion has been shown to loosen after 10–30 minutes,[160, 161] and recent systematic reviews disagree on whether patellofemoral joint taping influences VMO onset timing and knee extensor moments.[156, 162] Research in this area is ongoing.

Evidence of efficacy

Although taping is used for a wide range of conditions across the body, high-level evidence of its efficacy is scant. The available evidence is of varying quality–one of the main challenges when studying taping is the inability to blind patients or practitioners.[156, 166]

Patellofemoral pain

A number of systematic reviews have investigated the use of patellar realignment taping (often referred to as McConnell taping–see Chapter 36) in patients with patellofemoral pain syndrome.[156, 166, 167] Although their results are somewhat conflicting, there is moderate evidence that taping provides an immediate reduction in pain,[156, 167] particularly when an individualised taping technique is used.[156] However, its benefit seems to be limited to the short term, and prolonged use is not supported. The effect of kinesiology tape on patellofemoral pain remains unclear; one randomised crossover trial found that McConnell and kinesiology taping were equally effective in immediately reducing pain,[168] whereas two

PART A Fundamental principles

Kinesiology tape: valuable tool for athletes or fashion statement?

Kinesiology tape has gained considerable popularity in recent years, as demonstrated by the large number of athletes using it at the Olympic Games and other major sporting events (Fig. 17.19). The approach was developed in Japan in the 1970s and is claimed to permit unrestricted range of movement while supporting the fascia, muscles and joints.[163] Kinesiology tape has been proposed to improve pain and blood flow via dermal lifting, which decreases the pressure on cutaneous nerve receptors and capillaries, decreasing nociceptive input and increasing afferent feedback.[163] However, these effects last less than 24 hours and may be trivial, and the actual benefits for injured athletes are yet to be established in high-quality studies.[164] The use of kinesiology tape remains controversial among clinicians, with some even claiming it may provide a psychological crutch for athletes.[165]

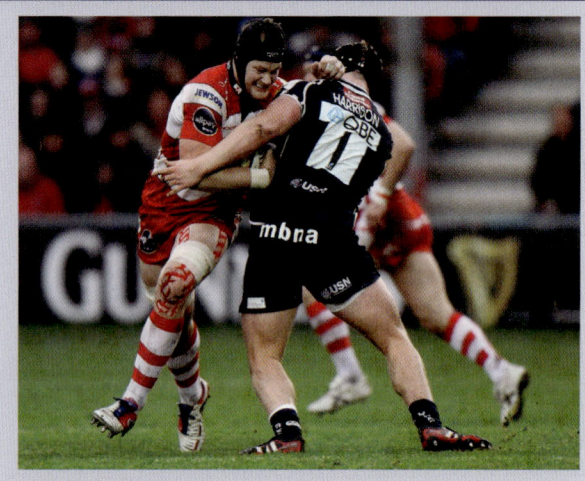

Figure 17.19 Kinesiology tape has gained popularity among athletes in recent years (note player on left, tape on knee and thigh) IMAGE COURTESY OF ROCKTAPE UK

---

randomised controlled trials found kinesiology tape was ineffective in reducing pain.[169, 170]

Ankle sprains

Three studies have suggested that taping is effective in prevention of ankle sprains.[171-173] However, the highest-quality prevention research has focussed on the effects of rigid or semi-rigid prefabricated braces, and it is unclear whether taping is equally effective.[174] Irrespective of the form of support used, any preventive effect of taping and bracing seems to be limited to athletes with a history of ankle sprain. As the risk of re-injury is increased sevenfold in the year following an initial sprain,[174] taping or bracing could be used in that time (Chapter 12).

Other conditions

There is some evidence that taping may be effective in treating pain and strength with lateral epicondylalgia,[175] de Quervain's tenosynovitis,[176] plantar fasciopathy pain[153, 177, 178] and shoulder pain.[153, 163, 179] However, many of these studies are of low quality with a moderate to high risk of publication bias. These conditions are covered in Part B.

Practical considerations

In practice, taping is applied across a far wider range of conditions than there exists evidence for, and should be considered just as much an art as a science.[174] Clinicians should consider not only the available literature, but also the diagnosis, the scenario (e.g. competition, acute management, rehabilitation), and the patient's preference and expectations.

We recommend the use of a trial-and-error approach. A 'treatment direction test', first proposed by Professor Bill Vicenzino for the prescription of orthotic insoles,[180] can be applied whenever tape is used to relieve pain. In order for the intervention to be judged worthwhile, it should lead to a substantial reduction in symptoms (at least 50% on a visual analogue scale) during a relevant functional task.

Much like any exercise program should be progressive, the use of taping should be gradually reduced over time.[72] When taping is successful in alleviating a chronic condition such as patellofemoral pain, clinicians should make a plan to wean the patient off the use of tape to avoid creating a dependence on a passive treatment. Following an acute injury, taping may provide immediate pain relief and restrict excessive movement.[181] Controlled stress (optimal loading) can then be facilitated by gradually reducing the amount of support taping provides over subsequent days and weeks.

> **PRACTICE PEARL**
>
> For long-term application of tape, consider teaching the athlete to tape him- or herself. This will increase the sense of control over his or her own management, decrease dependency on the clinician and save valuable time in a busy treatment clinic.

In order to protect the patient's skin from irritation, hypoallergenic tape can be applied under rigid sports tape. This is particularly important when tape containing zinc oxide is used for longer durations. In some situations, such as prophylactic ankle taping, pre-wrap may be applied under the tape. This does not alter the amount of motion restriction, the time to maximum range or the velocity of range;[159] however, it may reduce the cutaneous stimulus.

> **PRACTICE PEARL**
>
> Where possible, new taping techniques should be introduced to athletes in a controlled environment prior to competition.

Despite the limited and conflicting evidence base, taping continues to play an important role in clinical sports medicine practice. Clinicians should consider the available literature, retain a healthy scepticism towards commercial claims and trends, and take a trial-and-error approach. Clinical experience and athlete preference should not be discredited.

ELECTROPHYSICAL AGENTS

with NICK GARDINER, ADAM GLEDHILL, LAWRENCE MAYHEW and VASILEIOS KORAKAKIS

Electrophysical agents (electrotherapy) have been used to treat musculoskeletal conditions for over 70 years.[182] Although their popularity appears to be waning in favour of active treatments, traditional modalities such as ultrasound and interferential stimulation, and newer ones such as extracorporeal shockwave therapy remain highly used in clinical practice. In this section, we review the proposed mechanisms and evidence of effect of the most common electrophysical agents currently used in sports medicine.

The decision of whether to use electrotherapy will be individual and influenced by factors such as time and resource availability, patient expectation and clinician preference. However, it should be stressed that electrophysical agents should never be used in isolation. If they are to be used at all, it should be as an adjunct to other forms of treatment, advice and education.

Therapeutic ultrasound

Therapeutic ultrasound has traditionally played a large role in physiotherapy practice around the world,[183-188] and remains a popular treatment modality among physiotherapists and other health professionals such as osteopaths, chiropractors and sports therapists.[183, 189]

A range of proposed effects of ultrasound form the biological rationale for its therapeutic use. These include thermal effects such as increased local blood flow, metabolic activity and collagen extensibility, as well as non-thermal effects such as stimulation of fibroblast activity, mast cell degranulation, growth factor production and angiogenesis.[190] Although these effects have largely only been demonstrated *in vitro*,[183, 190] they are commonly cited to justify the clinical use of ultrasound to treat a wide variety of musculoskeletal conditions, with the belief that it can reduce pain, inflammation and oedema, and enhance scar tissue remodelling, tissue extensibility and soft tissue healing.[189] Treatment is traditionally directed towards collagen-rich tissues such as ligament, tendon, fascia, joint capsule and scar tissue, as these are thought to absorb the greatest amount of energy.[183]

Despite the theoretical appeal of ultrasound, however, there is little high-quality evidence to support its clinical effectiveness.[182, 191, 192] For example, a recent systematic review of the effect of ultrasound on a range of lower-limb soft tissue conditions found that no placebo-controlled trials were able to demonstrate a significant difference between true and sham ultrasound therapy.[191]

Although some argue that this may be due to heterogeneous study populations, conditions treated and dosage parameters,[183] the current lack of research evidence supporting therapeutic ultrasound for soft tissue conditions should be taken into account by clinicians considering its use.

Ultrasound as a stimulator of bone repair

In recent years, ultrasound has been increasingly used in the treatment of acute bone fractures. Although this was traditionally thought to be contraindicated, recent meta-analyses suggest that daily administration of low-intensity pulsed ultrasound (LIPUS) can accelerate the healing of fractures by approximately 35%.[193-195]

LIPUS appears to be most effective for conservatively managed diaphyseal fractures, reducing the time to clinical union by approximately 18 days.[195] The evidence is strongest for upper limb fractures, whereas it is conflicting for metaphyseal and operatively managed acute fractures.[193, 195]

LIPUS is typically applied for 20 minutes every day, which may be an excessive treatment regimen for many patients. However, in elite sports environments a faster return to training and competition might be very important. LIPUS may also be valuable in cases that fail conservative management (non-union) after bone-graft surgery is performed.[193]

Few studies have investigated LIPUS for the treatment of stress fractures; however, the available results are not encouraging[196, 197] and its use cannot currently be recommended for this purpose. Similarly, there is currently no evidence that LIPUS is effective for soft tissue injuries.

PART A Fundamental principles

Transcutaneous electrical nerve stimulation

Transcutaneous electrical nerve stimulation (TENS) delivers biphasic electrical current with the use of electrodes applied to the skin.[198] There are several mechanisms by which TENS can provide short-term pain relief, including stimulation of opioid and noradrenergic receptors at the site of application, and opioid, serotonin and muscarinic receptors in the spinal cord and brainstem.[199]

Although there is no evidence that TENS improves long-term outcomes,[200] it may play an adjunct role in pain management in certain patient groups. It is reported to provide effective short-term pain relief in patients with spinal cord injuries,[201, 202] lumbar disc disease,[203] and chronic neck and lower back pain.[204] There is currently little evidence to support its use for knee osteoarthritis[198, 205] and it is not widely used in the athletic population.

TENS can be used in combination with exercise and medication.[201, 206] Potential adverse effects include mild erythema and itching underneath the electrodes.[206]

Neuromuscular stimulators

Neuromuscular electrical stimulation (NMES) is purported to have a range of effects on healthy athletes, including enhanced recovery, improved sports performance and reduced muscle soreness. However, as discussed in Chapter 13, commercial claims regarding the benefits of NMES for athletes often go well beyond the existing evidence.[207] In a clinical setting, NMES may be valuable to enhance muscle strengthening after a major injury such as anterior cruciate ligament rupture.[208]

Traditionally, it has been thought that NMES improves muscle performance because it reverses the normal motor unit recruitment order, preferentially activating larger motor units composed primarily of fast-twitch fibres.[209] However, this theory has recently been challenged, with evidence suggesting that the normal clinical methods for applying NMES cause random, non-selective motor unit activation.[210] Nevertheless, there is high-level evidence that combining NMES with traditional exercise training is more effective than training alone in improving quadriceps strength following anterior cruciate ligament reconstruction.[208]

The decision of whether or not to use NMES in rehabilitation is dependent on a number of factors. Effective therapeutic intensity may be uncomfortable, so a high degree of patient motivation is necessary. Clinicians should also remember that, for many patients, traditional strength training produces the desired results. However, a subset of patients experience persistent weakness following major joint injury due to arthrogenic muscle inhibition.[211] In this group, the use of NMES in combination with heavy strength training may be recommended.[212]

The recommended parameters to enhance muscle strengthening in rehabilitation are shown in Table 17.6.

Interferential stimulation

Like therapeutic ultrasound, interferential stimulation has long played a role in traditional physiotherapy practice and remains widely used in some areas of the world.[215, 216] It is characterised by the interference of two medium-frequency currents passed through the tissues, causing analgesic effects. The analgesic effect may be due to stimulation of cutaneous receptors that inhibit c-fibre nociceptive transmission,[217] motor stimulation increasing the removal of pain-inducing substances[218] and the release of endogenous opioids.[219]

The pain-relieving effects of interferential stimulation are transient and there is little evidence to support its use in athletic populations. However, its efficacy in the management of knee osteoarthritis[198, 217] suggests potential benefits for athletes following major knee surgery such as ACL reconstruction.

Laser

Low-level laser therapy (LLLT) is a non-invasive treatment in which non-thermal laser irradiation is applied to the site of pain using light generated by high-intensity electrical stimulation of a medium. It modulates cell and tissue

Table 17.6 Recommended treatment parameters to maximise muscle strength gains using NMES[210, 213, 214]

Stimulation intensity	The intensity should be as high as the patient can tolerate, and at least 50% of MVC
Pulse frequency	High-frequency stimulation (50–80 Hz) leads to higher force production, smoother contractions and greater muscle fatigue. Frequencies over 80 Hz may be more painful
Pulse duration (width)	A longer pulse duration (up to 600 µs) maximises force production for a given stimulation intensity. The currently recommended duration is 200–400 µs
Training regimen	3–10 s 'on-time' followed by 10–40 s recovery; 10–15 min per session
Program parameters	1–3 sessions per week for 4–6 weeks

Treatment of sports injuries   CHAPTER 17

physiology to obtain therapeutic effects,[220] including promotion of tissue repair,[221, 222] and inflammatory effects,[223, 224] thereby providing pain relief in common musculoskeletal disorders.[220, 225, 226]

LLLT may assist in pain relief following acute sports injury[227] and has been found to reduce pain and improve function in patients with rotator cuff tendinopathy, both as a stand-alone treatment and when used in combination with therapeutic exercise.[228] It may also improve outcomes for patients with chronic midportion Achilles tendinopathy when combined with an eccentric loading programme (Chapter 40).[229] Although there is some evidence that LLLT is an effective treatment in certain conditions, there is little knowledge of dose–response and no consensus on optimal treatment parameters for specific pathologies. Further research utilising large, homogenous samples of similar pathologies would clarify the efficacy of LLLT in sports injury management.[227]

Electromagnetic therapy

Low-frequency pulsed electromagnetic field therapy (PEMF) is purported to have a wide range of local cellular and systemic effects affecting the healing process. Its use is recommended in wound care,[230, 231] and there is some evidence supporting the use of PEMF in the treatment of certain sports injuries.

Laboratory studies suggest that it may be valuable in the treatment of tendon, bone and cartilage pathology.[232-235] For example, when applied to human tendon cells, PEMF may cause cellular proliferation, tendon-specific gene expression, the release of growth factors, and the release of pro- and anti-inflammatory cytokines.[234, 235] Similarly, when applied to articular hyaline cartilage, PEMF can stimulate chondrocyte proliferation and the stimulation of proteoglycans and extra-cellular matrix.[232]

The results of clinical studies of PEMF in athletic populations are mixed.

- In athletes who underwent arthroscopic treatment of osteochondral defects of the talus, PEMF did not lead to earlier return to play than did a placebo treatment.[236]
- Compared to a placebo, patients who received PEMF after arthroscopic knee surgery had improved functional outcomes at 45 and 90 days and at a 3-year follow-up.[237]
- PEMF may have short-term functional, analgesic and anti-inflammatory benefits in shoulder and elbow tendon conditions.[238, 239] However, there is little evidence of any long-term benefits.[239, 240]
- A systematic review of the effects of PEMF and LIPUS on bone injuries found a reduction in healing time following acute diaphyseal fractures.[195] However, due to the small number of studies investigating PEMF, no conclusions on its specific effects could be made.

Extracorporeal shockwave therapy

In 1980, extracorporeal shockwaves were first used in medicine to destroy kidney stones.[241, 242] Subsequent animal research on extracorporeal shockwave therapy (ECSWT) demonstrated dose-dependent destructive (high-energy) and regenerative (lower-energy) effects on a range of tissues, including bone and tendon.[243, 244] Since then, ECSWT has been used extensively in clinical practice to treat superficial musculoskeletal conditions (Fig. 17.20).[245, 246]

Several RCTs and case-control studies have shown ECSWT, either alone or in combination with exercises, to be beneficial for a number of musculoskeletal disorders including plantar fasciopathy,[247, 248] midportion and insertional Achilles tendinopathy,[249-253] medial tibial stress syndrome,[254, 255] patellar tendinopathy,[256, 257] proximal hamstring tendinopathy,[258] greater trochanteric pain syndrome,[259] medial and lateral epicondylitis,[260, 261] and calcific supraspinatus tendinopathy.[262, 263]

There is a growing body of evidence supporting the clinical use of shock wave therapy. However, even though level 1 and level 2 studies are available for data pooling and meta-analyses, clinicians should interpret the results of systematic reviews with caution. This is because the included studies are often marked by methodological flaws, biases and low reporting quality.[264-266] Furthermore, there is inconsistent reporting of the type of shock wave used (extracorporeal, radial, focused), the intensity (high, medium, low) and the method of application (focal, local, area of pain distribution).

Clinicians should consider the following when using ECSWT in clinical practice.

- ECSWT is not a panacea–its efficacy varies considerably for individual pathologies, and careful selection of patients is essential.[267, 268] For example, it is only effective in treating supraspinatus tendinopathy when

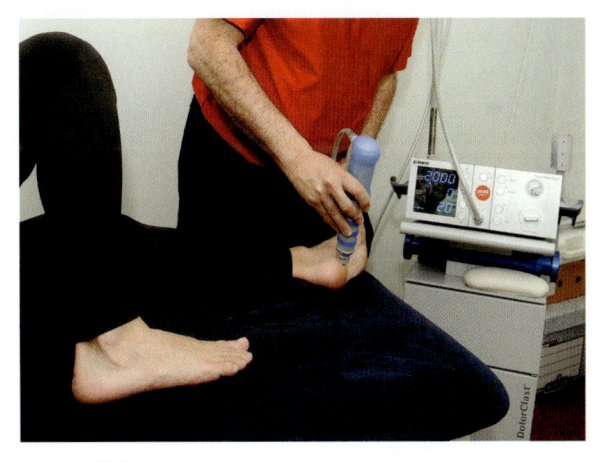

Figure 17.20 Extracorporeal shock wave therapy

263

calcification is present. For normal (non-calcified) supraspinatus tendinopathy, it has no effect.[245]
- There is no universal agreement regarding the definition of low-, medium- and high-energy flux density.[244, 263] Resulting energy is dependent on the device and applicator and should be calculated.
- There is evidence of a dose-related ECSWT effect, with lower-energy flux densities requiring more sessions to obtain the same result.[269]
- Although there is no consensus on treatment parameters, successful RCTs have used 1–3 sessions of 1500–2000 impulses at weekly intervals,[246] regardless of the underlying pathology.[241]
- Treatment parameters should be individualised based on the patient's presentation. For example, the pre-treatment symptom duration was significantly correlated with the number of ECSWT sessions applied.[270]
- As for all electrophysical agents, ECSWT should not be used in isolation. Prescribing therapeutic exercise in addition to shock waves can lead to better results.[250, 254]

THERAPEUTIC MEDICATION IN MUSCULOSKELETAL INJURY

with NOEL POLLOCK

Therapeutic drugs can be helpful in the management of musculoskeletal injury by treating pain, modulating inflammation and augmenting recovery. The use of therapeutic drugs should be aligned with the overall management plan and support the particular goals of that management phase. This section will discuss a range of oral and injectable therapeutic drugs used in the management of musculoskeletal injury.

Doctors prescribing medications to athletes should be fully aware of the current anti-doping regulations for the sport in which their patient is participating. This is updated annually by the World Anti-Doping Agency (WADA) and the current list can be found on the WADA website. There is also an online anti-doping resource for athletes and clinicians for products sold in Canada, USA, UK, Japan and Australia accessible at www.globaldro.com where medication can be checked. The site also contains links for other nationalities.

Analgesics

Analgesic medication is used to relieve and modulate pain, and is often prescribed in the acute phase after injury to reduce pain in conjunction with ice, compression or splinting. Analgesia may also facilitate early movement, although the medical team should decide the optimal initial load based on the diagnosis. Analgesic medication may also have a role in other management phases to treat central sensitisation or to facilitate desired movements in rehabilitation.

Paracetamol

Paracetamol (acetaminophen) has an analgesic and antipyretic effect without affecting the inflammatory process. The mechanism of action is probably through the modulation of cannabinoid receptors. Adult oral doses are 1000 mg every 4–6 hours to a maximum daily dose of 4 g. At these doses, paracetamol is well tolerated and can be an excellent choice in acute sports injuries. Soluble paracetamol is more quickly absorbed and may be an effective choice in athletes who need a quicker onset of analgesia. At higher doses, paracetamol is hepatotoxic and it may be fatal in overdose.

Codeine

Codeine is a more potent opiate analgesic and may be considered in the initial treatment of painful acute injury. However, codeine preparations are commonly associated with side effects such as nausea, dizziness and constipation, which limits prolonged use in the treatment of athletes.

Emergency analgesia

In severe acute musculoskeletal injury, stronger and parenteral analgesia may be required. Clinicians that provide event cover should be familiar with the indications and risks of these medications and have access to appropriate emergency analgesia. This may include opiate-based medication, ketamine and Entonox®.

Non-steroidal anti-inflammatory drugs (NSAIDs)

NSAIDs are drugs with analgesic and anti-inflammatory properties. The term non-steroidal is used to distinguish these drugs from corticosteroids that also produce anti-inflammatory effects. NSAIDs' mechanism of action is to inhibit the cyclo-oxygenase (COX) system. Cyclo-oxygenase has a key role in the inflammatory cascade that occurs at the site of acute injury. It converts arachidonic acid to prostaglandins and thromboxane which are key mediators of inflammation.[271] There are two cyclooxygenase iso-enzymes, COX-1 and COX-2, with different physiological roles (Fig. 17.21).

COX-1 is associated with the maintenance of the gastric mucosa and COX-1 inhibition with traditional NSAIDs can result in gastritis and ulceration. Selective COX-2 inhibitors have been available since 1999 with similar efficacy, but fewer gastro-intestinal side effects. The most commonly prescribed NSAIDs include aspirin, ibuprofen, diclofenac and naproxen, and the COX-2 selective NSAIDs, celecoxib and etoricoxib. The normally recommended dosage and frequency of administration varies between the different drugs (Table 17.7).

Treatment of sports injuries — CHAPTER 17

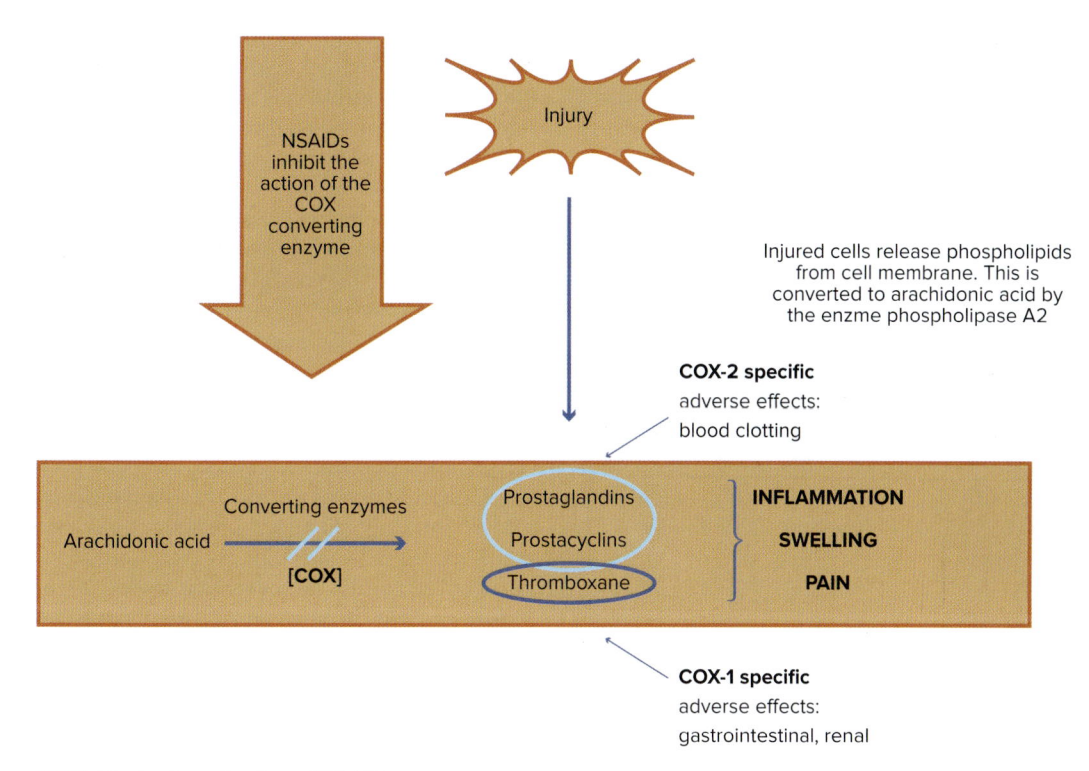

Figure 17.21 Mechanism of action of NSAIDs

Table 17.7 Commonly used NSAIDs

Drug	Some trade names	Usual dose (mg)	Half-life	Daily doses
Acetylsalicylic acid (ASA)	Aspirin®	650	30 mins	3–4
Celecoxib	Celebrex®	100–200	11–12 hours	1–2
Diclofenac	Voltaren®, Voltarol®	25–50	1–2 hours	2–3
Ibuprofen	Brufen®, Motrin®, Advil®	400	1–2.5 hours	3–4
Meloxicam	Mobic®	7.5–15	20–24 hours	1
Naproxen	Naprosyn, Anaprox®	250–1000	12–15 hours	1–2

Topical anti-inflammatory preparations are also available in creams and prolonged-release patches. These are effective delivery methods for superficial injuries, with less risk of side effects than orally administered NSAIDs.[272] Overnight patches or wraps may be particularly useful in limiting early morning stiffness that may be associated with excessive inflammation.

There is high-level evidence that topical NSAIDs are effective in relieving pain associated with acute musculoskeletal injuries such as sprain, strains and contusions,[272, 273] as well as with osteoarthritis.[274] Some of the pain relief they provide can be explained by a powerful placebo effect, which is greater with topical NSAID administration than with oral.

NSAID use in sport

NSAIDs are widely used in competitive sport, with more than a third of all athletes at Olympic Games,[275] half of all players at recent soccer World Cups[276] and about a quarter of athletes in international track and field athletics[277] reporting in-competition NSAID use. They are commonly used in the treatment of injury, but also prior to competition in an attempt to reduce discomfort of potential future injury or post-exercise soreness in both elite and non-elite athletes.[278-280] This practice should be discouraged, as there is no evidence of a reduction in delayed onset muscle soreness (DOMS) or improved performance with prophylactic NSAIDs. However, player perception and the placebo effect can make behaviour

265

change challenging for team clinicians. Regular NSAID use causes significant health risks for the cardiovascular, renal and gastrointestinal systems. Clinicians should educate their athletes about these risks and seek safer alternatives, perhaps from nutraceutical products.

NSAID use in the treatment of musculoskeletal injury

NSAIDs are usually an excellent choice in the short-term treatment of inflammatory conditions, such as bursitis or synovitis. However, the impact of NSAIDs on cellular metabolism and the tissues of the musculoskeletal system should be considered by athletes and clinicians using these medications in the treatment or prevention of injury. With this knowledge, NSAIDs may be prescribed for particular injuries or in stages of healing determined by the overall goals of the current rehabilitation and management phase.

NSAID and muscle

At a cellular level, NSAIDs probably have a negative effect on both muscle healing following injury and muscle hypertrophy after athletic training.[281] NSAIDs can inhibit protein synthesis[282] and reduce satellite cell activation, which is an essential step in muscle repair and regeneration.[283, 284] Inhibition of protein synthesis after resistance exercise may be limited to COX-1 NSAIDs, as selective COX-2 inhibitors have not been shown to induce similar reductions in protein synthesis.[285]

NSAIDs are often used by athletes in the treatment and prevention of DOMS, but scientific trials demonstrate very little evidence for a positive effect.

NSAIDs have been recommended for use in deep muscle contusions at risk of developing myositis ossificans.[286] Regular indomethacin for more than seven days is widely used by clinicians in this condition.

NSAIDs are not effective in the treatment of acute muscle tears and cannot be routinely recommended.[287, 288] They may have a short-term role to modulate an excessive early inflammatory response, but as this phase is necessary for appropriate satellite cell activation and initiation of regeneration, their use at this time may be detrimental to overall muscle repair.

NSAID and tendon

Basic science and animal-model studies of tendon tearing or surgical repair have consistently shown that NSAIDs reduce tenocyte proliferation and collagen formation, and therefore negatively affect tendon healing. However, in clinical studies of acute reactive tendinopathy, NSAIDs may facilitate short-term improvements in pain.[289] One small study also demonstrated improvements in leg stiffness and tendon function following treatment with a COX-2 inhibitor.[290]

It has been suggested that they may be useful in acute tendon overload despite (or perhaps because of) the potential negative effects on tenocyte activation.[268] However, clinicians should remember that basic science and clinical studies have shown that NSAIDs blunt exercise-induced collagen synthesis within tendon tissue.[291] Therefore, the prescribing of NSAIDs should, as with all medication, be considered within the overall treatment goals of the current rehabilitation phase. In Cook and Purdam's model of a continuum of tendon pathology (Chapter 4),[268] NSAIDs may be considered in the reactive tendinopathy phase, but are not recommended in the dysrepair or degenerative phases.

NSAID and ligament

NSAIDs have been shown to have a negative impact on collagen formation, fibroblast proliferation and healing in animal models of ligament injury.[292-295] Clinical studies of ligament injuries also do not support their use. One study of patients who underwent ACL reconstruction found increased joint laxity at six weeks in an NSAID-treated group compared with a group that had not been prescribed NSAIDs.[296] Another study demonstrated similar analgesic efficacy for paracetamol and NSAID (diclofenac) following acute ankle ligament injuries, but found increased oedema at day three in the NSAID group.[297]

NSAID and bone

Prostaglandins have an important role in bone metabolism, simulating both osteoblasts and osteoclasts.[298] Numerous animal studies have reported a delay in bone healing with NSAID treatment.[299] It appears that COX-2 inhibition has the most negative impact due to inhibition of endochondral ossification.[300-302] Although high-quality clinical studies are lacking, a number of studies suggest a delay in bone healing with NSAID use.[303, 304]

> **PRACTICE PEARL**
>
> NSAIDs could be considered a risk factor for fracture healing and cannot be recommended in fracture management.

Adverse effects of NSAIDs

Adverse effects of NSAIDs may be associated with the gastrointestinal, cardiovascular and renal systems, and susceptibility increases with prolonged use and patient age.[305] The most common adverse effects are gastrointestinal with epigastric pain, nausea or reflux symptoms. The risk of experiencing these dyspeptic adverse effects can be lowered by using the minimum effective dose, taking the medication with food, using gastroprotective formulations or the concomitant use of proton pump inhibitors (such as omeprazole or lansoprazole) or H2 antagonists (such as ranitidine). Occult gastrointestinal bleeding may contribute to iron depletion and therefore clinicians should enquire about NSAID self-prescribing in iron-deficient athletes.

Selective COX-2 inhibitors with reduced gastrointestinal side effects have been available since 1999. In 2004, a number of COX-2 inhibitors (valdecoxib and rofecoxib) were taken off the market, as they were specifically associated with a high number of adverse vascular events. COX-2 inhibitors, and some non-selective NSAIDs such as diclofenac, are associated with an increased risk of thrombotic events, and are contraindicated in ischaemic heart and cerebrovascular disease. They should be used with caution in patients with risk factors for cardiovascular events. However, they are often used in athletes with musculoskeletal injury due to their effective analgesic properties and low adverse effect profile.

Medications for neuropathic pain and central sensitisation

Neuropathic pain is defined as pain arising from a lesion or disease affecting the somatosensory nervous system (Chapter 6).[306, 307] It is often characterised clinically by amplified pain responses following noxious or non-noxious stimuli and may be present in combination with true nociceptive pain arising from tissue damage. In patients with neuropathic pain, both peripheral and central neural sensitising mechanisms may be present.

Recent research has suggested that central sensitisation is a potentially important feature of a number of musculoskeletal presentations, including shoulder pain, lateral epicondylalgia and patellar tendinopathy.[308, 309] Central sensitisation is defined as 'an amplification of neural signalling within the central nervous system (CNS) that elicits pain sensitivity'.[310] It is an important feature for clinicians to detect and treat within the overall rehabilitation plan.

The management of neuropathic pain or central sensitisation in musculoskeletal injury should have a number of interdisciplinary elements and may incorporate therapeutic medication. In addition to the analgesic medication previously discussed, a number of other pharmaceuticals may have a therapeutic role. However, although these medications have demonstrated efficacy in RCTs and meta-analyses, there have been no clear predictors of treatment success in patients with neuropathic pain. The therapeutic approach is therefore usually a stepwise trial approach to identify which medication or combination provides the greatest pain relief with the fewest side effects.

Tricyclic antidepressants

Tricyclic antidepressants inhibit serotonin and noradrenaline neurotransmitter re-uptake and block sodium channels. Nortriptyline is most widely used and is the active metabolite of amitriptyline. It is recommended in UK, European, US and Australian guidelines for the treatment of neuropathic pain, although not as a first-line treatment.[311] A dose of 10–25 mg is usually prescribed at night to avoid sedative effects during the day. A recent Cochrane review concluded that there was little evidence to support the use of nortriptyline in neuropathic pain, particularly when compared with duloxetine and pregabalin.[311]

Serotonin reuptake inhibitors

Duloxetine is a serotonin re-uptake inhibitor with moderate to strong evidence for efficacy in the treatment of neuropathic pain.[312, 313] A starting dose of 30 mg is often increased to an efficacious treatment dose of 60 mg. Similar to other medications for neuropathic pain, fatigue may be a side effect.

Gabapentin and pregabalin

Gabapentin and pregabalin are gamma-aminobutyric acid analogues that bind to calcium channels on afferent nociceptors and subsequently reduce neurotransmitter release. Pregabalin has a half-life of around six hours.[314] Starting dose of pregabalin is usually 75 mg twice daily and this may be titrated to a total daily dose of 300 mg over the course of one week. The most common adverse effect of these medications is fatigue or a mild sedative effect, and they are often not appropriate to take before training sessions. Gabapentin is also available in an extended-release preparation that may be more effective for neuropathic pain, but is more likely to impact on athlete's training programs.

Local anaesthetic patches

Topical lignocaine (lidocaine) patches have demonstrated positive effects in short-term studies on neuropathic pain[312] and may be helpful as a second-line treatment, although the quality of the evidence is weak.

Counterirritants

Topical heat rubs are often used by athletes and mainly act as counterirritants. Their mechanism of action is probably related to their effect on transient receptor potential (TRP) channels (Fig. 17.22). These channels are sensitive to heat and initiate a local inflammatory response. Prolonged activation of the nociceptors may result in a depletion of local neurotransmitters, which may result in a reduction in pain and nociceptor transmission from the site of the more long-standing injury. Counterirritants, such as

PART A Fundamental principles

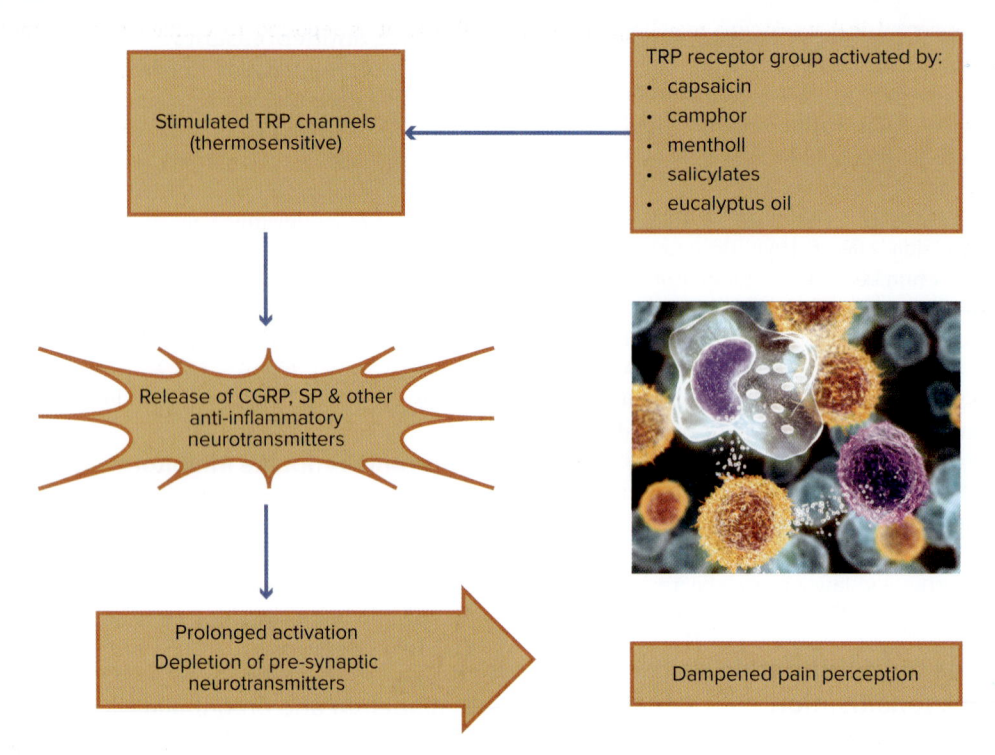

Figure 17.22 Mechanisms of action of counterirritants

Flow diagram:
- Stimulated TRP channels (thermosensitive) ← TRP receptor group activated by:
  - capsaicin
  - camphor
  - mentholl
  - salicylates
  - eucalyptus oil
- ↓ Release of CGRP, SP & other anti-inflammatory neurotransmitters
- ↓ Prolonged activation / Depletion of pre-synaptic neurotransmitters → Dampened pain perception

---

Injection therapy: should injections be performed under ultrasound guidance?

There is consistent high-quality evidence that ultrasound-guided injections are more accurate than landmark-guided injections.[315] There is moderate limited-quality evidence that ultrasound-guided injections are more efficacious than landmark-guided injections, particularly in large joints, subacromial bursal injections,[316] carpal tunnel and inflamed joints.[317] The interpretation of the research in this area is challenging, as corticosteroid injection is often studied. Not only may this be an inappropriate therapeutic choice for the particular pathology,[318, 319] but there are known systemic effects of corticosteroid injections that may affect outcome measures. It is also reasonable to assume that with the development of injectable therapeutic agents without systemic effects, such as hyaluronic acid, these would be unlikely to demonstrate maximal therapeutic efficacy unless accurately positioned. Therefore, we recommend that clinicians who regularly perform musculoskeletal injections undertake training in ultrasonography and perform injection therapy under ultrasound guidance.

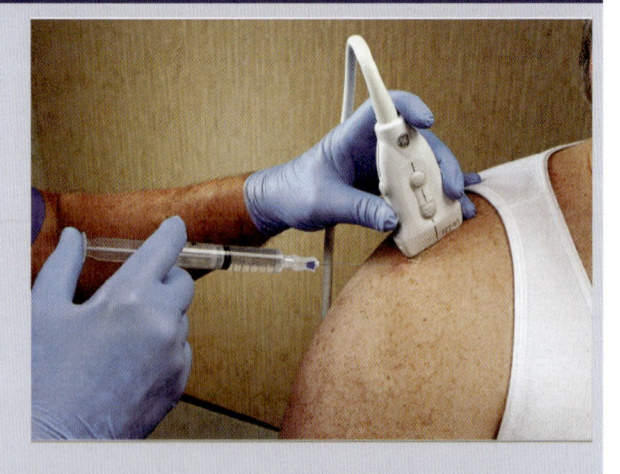

Figure 17.23 Ultrasound-guided injection
USED WITH PERMISSION OF GE HEALTHCARE

---

capsaicin or camphor, may therefore have a use for mild analgesia before activity, but also potentially in a chronic injury that demonstrates increased neural sensitisation or elements of neuropathic pain.[312]

Local anaesthetic injections

Local anaesthetic injections may be used in sports medicine for a number of reasons. They can be used in the treatment of musculoskeletal injury to reduce pain or facilitate movement. Local anaesthesia may be performed on competition day to enable athletes to participate in sport despite injury. Local anaesthetic injections are also frequently used in conjunction with a corticosteroid injection to reduce needle pain.

Local anaesthetics cause a reversible block to conduction along nerve fibres by inhibiting sodium channels, particularly in small neurones. There is a wide variation in speed of onset, duration of action and potency. Lignocaine (lidocaine) and bupivacaine are the most commonly used preparations for musculoskeletal injection. Lignocaine 1% is a quick-acting local anaesthetic that is effectively absorbed from mucous membranes. The duration of anaesthesia is usually 60–120 minutes. Bupivacaine has a slower onset, taking up to 30 minutes for effect, and a longer duration of action, lasting for several hours.

Local anaesthetic in competition

Anaesthetic injections are sometimes used to enable participation in elite sport despite the presence of AC joint injuries, finger and rib injuries, and iliac crest haematomas.[320] These injections appear to be relatively safe in the short and long term. We do not recommended intra-articular injections in weight-bearing joints or around tendons of the lower limb, due to the significant risk of further injury to these structures.

Local anaesthetic in routine musculoskeletal injections

Clinicians have traditionally used local anaesthetic in most musculoskeletal injection protocols to reduce the pain of the procedure. However, as local anaesthetic has been shown to be myotoxic,[321] chondrotoxic[322] and tendon toxic,[323, 324] clinicians should reconsider their use of local anaesthesia during routine injection protocols.

Traumeel

Traumeel is a herbal preparation of arnica, belladonna, calendula, heparin and echinacea that is reported to have an antioxidant and anti-inflammatory action. Some clinicians inject it in the treatment of muscle injuries[325] and it is also available as a topical anti-inflammatory. The topical application of traumeel has been demonstrated to be as efficacious as topical diclofenac for pain relief in low-grade acute ankle ligament injuries.[326] There are no clinical studies that evaluate its efficacy in the treatment of muscle injuries.

Actovegin

Actovegin is a deproteinised ultrafiltrate of calf serum produced in Austria, a bovine spongiform encephalopathy-free country,[327] and a licensed drug in Europe, China and Russia. It is reported to contain trace elements, amino acids, electrolytes, and carbohydrate and fat metabolites. The active ingredients have not been identified. Some basic science studies suggest Actovegin has a role in modulation of inflammatory processes, but no quality clinical evidence exists to support its use in muscle injury.

Sclerosant

Early studies reported positive effects of sclerosing injections of polidocanol to areas of neovascularisation, just outside the Achilles tendon.[328, 329] However, more recent studies have not demonstrated positive effects[330] and it is currently not widely used in clinical practice.

Prolotherapy

Prolotherapy is a collective term for the injection of an irritant, usually hyperosmolar dextrose, in the treatment of chronic painful musculoskeletal conditions.[331] The mechanisms of action are not fully understood, but it is claimed that prolotherapy stimulates inflammation and growth factor release, initiates a proliferative response and results in desensitisation through a denervating effect. There is conflicting evidence regarding its efficacy.[332]

Mechanical and high-volume injections

The pain and pathological processes involved in tendinopathy are not fully understood. Some theories suggest that tendon adherence to the adjacent fat pad or neurovascular in-growth from the fat pad are implicated in the pain and pathogenesis of Achilles and patellar tendinopathy. An injection protocol that infiltrates a high volume (up to 40 ml) of normal saline (with a small amount of local anaesthetic, hydrocortisone or aprotinin) to the interface between the tendon and the fat pad has been described.[333-335] While case series have demonstrated positive effects, further high-quality studies are needed.

Hyaluronic acid

Chondrocytes and synovial cells produce hyaluronic acid, which is the major constituent of synovial fluid and a component of the extracellular matrix of cartilage. Hyaluronic acid maintains the structural integrity of cartilage and assists with joint mobility and shock absorption. It can also modulate the inflammatory response through inhibition of pro-inflammatory factors, such as arachidonic acid and Interleukin-1 (IL-1), which have a degradative effect on the cartilage matrix.

Hyaluronic injection can be useful in the treatment of chondropathy and may cause an initial reduction in pain due to this anti-inflammatory effect. However, it is generally most effective in the medium and long term,[336] probably through its stimulation of synovial cells to synthesise endogenous hyaluronic acid (Fig. 17.24). A meta-analysis

PART A Fundamental principles

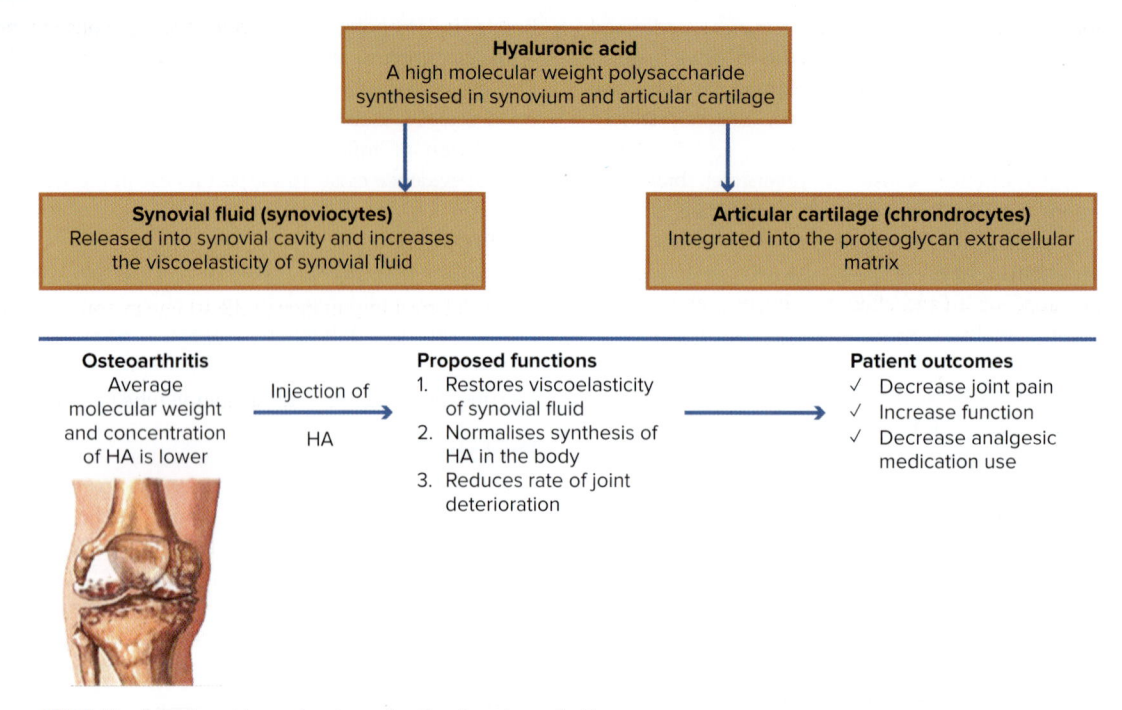

Figure 17.24 Hyaluronic acid: mechanism of action in osteoarthritis

comparing hyaluronic acid injections to corticosteroid injections suggested greater pain relief following corticosteroid at two weeks but not at four weeks, and greater benefit of hyaluronic acid at 8–26 weeks.[337]

Hyaluronic acid in tendons

Hyaluronic acid has been used in the field of hand surgery for several years to provide surface lubrication and enhance postoperative tendon mobility. With emerging evidence suggesting the importance of the Achilles or patellar tendon-fat pad interface in the development of tendon pathology, there have been some proposals for a role for hyaluronic acid injection in this interface[338]. Although there have been a number of case series publications,[339, 340] no high-level evidence currently exists to support this therapeutic approach.

Corticosteroids

Corticosteroids are strong anti-inflammatory agents that reduce vascular permeability and leucocyte activation, and block inflammatory mediators. The proposed aim of corticosteroid injection is to reduce pain and inflammation to facilitate normal movement and allow therapeutic exercise. However, there are significant detrimental effects associated with the injection of corticosteroids. Therefore, clinicians should consider their use carefully in each case with specific regard to the current evidence, injured tissue, and the stage and goals of rehabilitation.

Peritendinous injection of corticosteroids is generally not recommended. Corticosteroids inhibit collagen synthesis and are detrimental to tendon healing. Biopsy studies have demonstrated an increase in the glutamate NMDA receptor following corticosteroid injection.[341] This receptor has been associated with chronic pain and tendinopathy.

Recent studies have demonstrated negative medium- and long-term outcomes from corticosteroid injection around elbow common extensor origin tendinopathy (tennis elbow) even compared with a 'wait and see' approach.[318] However, there is no doubt that they can provide effective pain relief in the short term and, in certain cases after informed discussions with the athlete and coach, this may be the main priority. Corticosteroid injection may be of value in inflammatory bursitis with healthy local tendon tissue. However, even in apparently isolated retrocalcaneal bursitis, caution is advised in elite athletes who place high demands on their Achilles tendons.

Intra-articular injections of corticosteroid for joint disease will reduce synovial inflammation and catabolic enzymes that are probably implicated in cartilage breakdown. However, there are negative joint consequences to be considered with respect to intra-articular corticosteroid injection. Cartilage matrix degradation and reduction in elasticity has been observed following intra-articular injections of corticosteroids to weight bearing joints.

Corticosteroid, particularly if combined with local anaesthetic, is known to be toxic to chondrocytes,[342, 343] and repeated injections may limit cartilage repair and regeneration. The injection of corticosteroid followed by a quick return to running is thought to be more detrimental to the articular cartilage. Injection directed to the inflamed synovial tissue rather than the joint fluid may be considered to limit negative impact on the cartilage. In summary, corticosteroid injection into weight-bearing joints should be approached with caution and considered only in the presence of excessive inflammation. There may be a more appropriate and effective role for corticosteroid injection into smaller, nonweight-bearing joints or spinal, apophyseal joints or epidural injections.

Other adverse effects of corticosteroids

The adverse effects of corticosteroids on tendons and cartilage have been presented above. However, there are other side effects that should be considered and discussed with the patient. Corticosteroid injection can commonly result in skin depigmentation, which may be permanent. Fat atrophy is also a possible effect, particularly in superficial injections. The risk of this can be minimised by accurate guided-needle placement and care to avoid steroid placement along the needle track during withdrawal.

Intra-articular injection may result in pericapsular calcification and severe adverse events such as avascular necrosis have been reported, usually following several injections within a short time frame. Joint infection is another significant serious adverse effect and appropriate sterilisation measures with a good injection technique are essential for these injections. The presence of an overlying skin infection is a contraindication to injection.

Corticosteroid injections commonly cause a short-term exacerbation in symptoms for several days after the injection. Patients are recommended to have a short period of rest and to modify athletic activity after a corticosteroid injection.

Choice of corticosteroid

The most commonly used corticosteroids are triamcinolone, methylprednisolone, hydrocortisone and dexamethasone. They each have a different duration of action and solubility that should be considered when choosing an appropriate steroid for injection.

Triamcinolone and methylprednisolone are hydrophobic preparations and therefore form microcrystalline suspensions. As a result, they should have a longer duration of action than hydrophilic preparations, such as dexamethasone or hydrocortisone, which have a quicker onset of action but reduced duration of effect. Triamcinolone and methylprednisolone are particulate steroids that, according to recent guidelines in the USA, should be avoided in spinal injections. This is due to the risk of inadvertent arterial puncture and subsequent particulate injection with severe vascular consequences. The debate on particulate versus non-particulate spinal injections continues, but there is some evidence to suggest that non-particulate steroids, such as dexamethasone, have an equivalent effect. Therefore, it may be prudent to choose this form of steroid for spinal injections.[344, 345]

Other medications
Sleep medication

Sleep is of great importance to the athlete in normal training to enable adaptation and recovery (Chapter 13). A lack of sleep is associated with an increased injury risk and impaired sporting performance. During injury rehabilitation, sleep can be disrupted due to pain and anxiety. For the injured athlete, good quality sleep is essential for many reasons, but particularly to enable optimal protein synthesis, for soft tissue healing and strengthening, and neuromotor learning to achieve the gait, running or skill re-education required during rehabilitation. The sleep strategy for an athlete in rehabilitation is a broad remit for the multidisciplinary team, but medication may have a useful short-term role.

There are several medications that can assist with sleep. The clinician should be aware of the dependence and tolerance that can occur with the use of hypnotics and should therefore reserve their use for short courses (of several days only). The use of sleep medication should be carefully documented in the patient's notes, particularly if there are a number of team physicians. Generally, short-acting hypnotics are the most appropriate for athletes with sleep disturbance associated with acute injury. These will assist with sleep onset and not have a sedative effect the following day.

Temazepam is a short acting benzodiazepine with little 'hangover' effect, although tolerance can develop quickly. Diazepam is a long-acting benzodiazepine that also reduces muscle spasm and can be of use if this is also a therapeutic goal, most commonly in the treatment of acute low back pain with muscle spasm. Non-benzodiazepine hypnotics, such as zolpidem or zopiclone, have a short duration of action without hangover effects.

> **PRACTICE PEARL**
>
> Clinicians, as well as athletes, should always be aware of the dangers involved with the abuse of sleep medications. There have been multiple high-profile cases of such abuse across a multitude of sports. When athletes are prescribed sleep medications, they should always be warned of interactions with other drugs, including alcohol, which if taken in combination can cause enhanced central nervous system depression and lead to catastrophic consequences.

Quinolone antibiotics

Unless there is no suitable antibiotic alternative, quinolone antibiotics (e.g. ciprofloxacin, ofloxacin) should not be prescribed to athletes. There is clear evidence linking quinolones with both acute tendon rupture and increased lifetime risk of tendon disease.[346, 347]

Glyceryl trinitrate patches

Glyceryl trinitrate (GTN) patches have been proposed to modulate tendon healing by providing nitric oxide, which may stimulate collagen synthesis. There were some early studies that demonstrated improvements in tendon pain and function in patients with non-insertional Achilles, supraspinatus and elbow common extensor origin tendinopathies.[348-350] However, more recent RCTs fail to demonstrate clinical improvements compared with, or as an adjunct to, exercise rehabilitation.[351-354] There is a notable incidence of headache associated with initiation of treatment. Current evidence suggests that GTN patches do not appear to have an important therapeutic role in the management of tendinopathy.

Bisphosphonates

Bisphosphonates inhibit osteoclastic function and therefore increase bone mass. They have been used for many years in the treatment of osteoporosis and decrease fracture risk in this population. The use of bisphosphonates in the prevention or treatment of stress fractures and one-off intravenous injections to reduce bone pain from pubic bone stress (osteitis pubis)[355] in athletes has been proposed.

One study found that bisphosphonates had no effect on stress fracture prevention in military recruits.[356] In stress fracture treatment, a small study suggested bisphosphonates could result in accelerated and safe return to sport.[357] Some clinicians also recommend the use of bisphosphonates for the treatment of athletes with osteitis pubis.

However, there are several significant concerns regarding the rationale and use for bisphosphonate treatment in athletes. Bisphosphonates have a half-life of 1-10 years, limit normal microdamage repair and suppress bone remodelling. This may be detrimental to an athlete in the long term, after recovery from the current injury, as normal bone remodelling is essential for adaptation and resilience to normal athletic training. Indeed, their short- and long-term use in an elderly osteoporotic population has demonstrated an increased risk of fatigue fractures.[358, 359] High-quality studies of the short- and long-term impact of bisphosphonate prescription in athletes are required.

The safety of bisphosphonates in women who may subsequently become pregnant has not been established. Animal studies have shown that bisphosphonates can cross the placenta and therefore affect foetal bone mineralisation. While there have been no case reports of teratogenic effects in humans, it would seem prudent to avoid the use of bisphosphonates in female athletes.

In addition to the potential adverse effects above, there are side effects of bisphosphonates that should be recognised. Nausea, arthralgia and myalgia for 48 hours after intravenous treatment are common. Oral bisphosphonates can induce oesophageal inflammation and erosion. Osteonecrosis of the jaw has also been reported, usually in patients over 60 years with significant dental pathology. However, this risk should be discussed and a dental examination performed prior to bisphosphonate administration.

NUTRACEUTICALS IN INJURY MANAGEMENT

with NOEL POLLOCK

In recent years there has been an increased focus on the potential role of dietary supplements and herbal products—often collectively referred to as neutraceuticals—in the treatment of sports injuries.

Glucosamine, chondroitin and omega-3 fatty acids

Glucosamine has been advocated as a treatment for cartilage injury. The availability of glucosamine is a rate-limiting step in proteoglycan production.[360] Proteoglycans are large complex molecules which provide elasticity and integrity to cartilage tissue. There are numerous basic science studies that provide evidence for the important role of glucosamine in supporting joint health. In addition to its role in proteoglycan production, it may also have an anti-inflammatory role and limit chondrocyte apoptosis.

Some meta-analyses have concluded that long-term treatment with glucosamine can reduce pain and disease progression, and improve joint function and mobility in patients with osteoarthritis.[361, 362] Supplementation is often recommended in European and international guidelines on the treatment of osteoarthritis; however, while there is some rationale for its use in chondropathic conditions, the evidence is conflicting.[363] A daily oral dose of 1500 mg is most consistently recommended.

Chondroitin sulphate is a natural glycosaminoglycan and an important component of the extracellular matrix. Similarly to glucosamine, its use has been recommended in the treatment of inflammatory arthropathy including osteoarthritis and chondropathy.[364]

The role of glucosamine and chondroitin in the synthesis of large proteoglycans, such as aggrecan, has led some clinicians to consider their use in patients with tendinopathy.[268] Early tendon overload is characterised by tendon swelling and aggrecan production,[365] and therefore further increase in large molecule proteoglycan synthesis may be detrimental. The role of glucosamine and chondroitin in proteoglycan synthesis suggest that it may be appropriate to avoid the use of these products in early, reactive tendinopathy.

Omega-3 polyunsaturated fatty acids have been used as dietary supplements in musculoskeletal injury, particularly joint injury, due to their anti-inflammatory and anti-oxidant effects. Reactive oxygen species are increased in arthritis and associated with cartilage degradation. Some low-level evidence suggests that omega-3 fatty acids may be helpful at reducing morning stiffness in patients with osteoarthritis.[366]

Vitamin D

Vitamin D is a secosteroid hormone with a wide range of important physiological effects for health and athletic performance. Regarding musculoskeletal injury, Vitamin D has an essential role in the maintenance of muscle strength and mass, particularly for type II muscle fibres and in optimal bone health. Correction of vitamin D deficiency can improve muscle strength and reduce the risk of stress fractures.[367, 368] Vitamin D deficiency is prevalent in elite athletes, and screening and treatment of deficiency is recommended.[369]

Green tea/polyphenols

Green tea and other polyphenol-rich foods such as cherry juice may have an important future role in the management of musculoskeletal injury. There have been some basic science and animal studies demonstrating a positive impact on tendon and cartilage healing.[370, 371] Clinical studies are required to determine the clinical impact of polyphenol supplements and nutrition.

AUTOLOGOUS BLOOD, BLOOD PRODUCTS AND CELL THERAPY

with ROBERT-JAN DE VOS

Autologous blood, specific blood products, and cells are increasingly used in clinical trials in the field of musculoskeletal medicine. These autologous products secrete many growth factors that are thought to have a positive effect on healing of bone, cartilage, ligament, tendon and muscle injuries. This has been based on laboratory studies showing increased cell proliferation and collagen synthesis, and stimulation of a well-ordered angiogenesis.[372-374] The rationale, applications and efficacy of these treatments are summarised below.

Autologous blood injections

The main rationale behind treatment with autologous blood injections is the presence of various growth factors in blood with a potential healing effect. Blood is usually drawn from an arm vein and injected directly into the injured part. Ultrasound guidance can be helpful for improving delivery of autologous blood to the injury site, but in superficial injuries or in presence of clear anatomical landmarks, this is not always necessary. The amount of blood injected depends on the location and type of injury, but 3 mL or 6 mL are the most commonly used volumes.[375]

This procedure has been used mainly in tendinopathies; however, a systematic review did not show efficacy of this treatment for these injuries.[375] More recent randomised trials show efficacy of autologous blood injections in comparison with detrimental corticosteroid injections,[376-378] but not compared with placebo or standard physical therapy.[379, 380]

Platelet-rich plasma

Platelet-rich plasma (PRP) is the product derived when autologous whole blood is centrifuged to separate out a preparation with a very high platelet content. The preparation is rich in both plasmatic and platelet α-granule derived growth factors, as well as many thousands of other substances.[372]

With the preparation of a PRP injection, a larger amount of blood is withdrawn. The blood is then placed into a tube, which in turn is placed into a centrifuge, which spins many thousand times a minute, for various lengths of time depending on the protocol. At this point, the platelets have separated from the other blood components and can be aspirated for injection. Many different versions of PRP are described depending on the duration, force and number of spins. Several sub-classifications of PRP have been made, which can serve as a basis for evaluation of efficacy in clinical studies.[381]

Initially, many case series showed benefit of PRP injections in several clinical conditions.[382] In comparison with detrimental corticosteroid injections, it was found efficacious.[383] However, systematic reviews and more recent randomised studies with appropriate control groups receiving placebo injection therapies (e.g. saline) did not show efficacy of PRP in patients with Achilles tendon ruptures,[384] anterior cruciate ligament reconstruction,[385] arthroscopic rotator cuff repair,[386] Achilles tendinopathy,[387] lateral epicondylar tendinopathy,[388] patellar tendinopathy,[389] plantar fasciopathy[390] or acute hamstring injuries.[391] PRP injections showed limited to moderate evidence in a systematic review on efficacy in patients with knee osteoarthritis.[392] More high-quality randomised studies with low risk of bias are needed for this indication.

In conclusion, there is currently insufficient evidence to advise PRP injections as a routine part of management for musculoskeletal injuries.

PART A   Fundamental principles

Cell therapy

Preclinical studies have shown the potential for cellular therapies to regenerate rather than repair the tissues. The cells can be harvested from embryos (embryonic stem cells–ESCs), bone marrow, adipose tissue (mesenchymal stem cells–MSCs) or differentiated cells from the preferred tissue (e.g. tenocytes or chondrocytes).[393] Cell lines such as ESCs have superior potency and proliferative properties, but their main disadvantages are ethical considerations and potential complications including tumorogenesis. MSCs offer promise in tissue engineering due to their proliferative capacity and the secretion of growth factors. Autologous cells can be harvested from the preferred tissue and expanded, prior to re-implantation. For example, healthy tendon cells (tenocytes) can be harvested from the patellar tendon (Fig. 17.25), expanded in a laboratory and injected into a tendinopathic tendon (e.g. Achilles). A disadvantage of this technique could be the donor site morbidity.

Clinical studies using cell therapy for the treatment of musculoskeletal conditions are currently increasing. Small case series in patients with lateral epicondylitis and rotator cuff tendinopathy treated with autologous tenocytes, bone-marrow-derived cells and skin-derived fibroblasts showed functional and structural improvement.[394-396] A recent randomised study in patients with patellar tendinopathy and Achilles tendinopathy showed efficacy of a local skin-derived fibroblast injection.[397] These conclusions are, however, hampered by several major shortcomings.

Effectiveness of cell therapy is also evaluated more frequently in cartilage defects. One systematic review did not demonstrate sufficient evidence for the use of bone-marrow-derived MSCs.[398] There is currently also insufficient evidence for surgical autologous chondrocyte implantation (ACI), the surgical implantation of healthy cartilage cells into the damaged areas.[399] While ACI has been suggested to provide better results in tissue quality and is increasingly performed in clinical practice, more high-quality studies with long-term follow-up are needed in this field.

There are no high-quality clinical studies available to support the use of cell therapy. We expect high-quality randomised clinical trials will be published in the coming years.

In conclusion, there is currently insufficient evidence to advise autologous blood injections, PRP or autologous tendon cell injections as a routine part of management for musculoskeletal injuries.

SURGERY

Despite the many advances in the non-operative management of sports injuries, surgery has a major role to play in the management of both acute and overuse injuries. Surgery is used to remove, repair, reconstruct or realign damaged tissue. Sports surgery can be classified as arthroscopic surgery or open surgery.

Arthroscopic surgery

Arthroscopy involves the introduction of a fibre-optic telescope into a joint space to provide diagnostic information and afford the opportunity to undertake minimally invasive surgery. It is a well-established procedure for the knee, shoulder, elbow, ankle and hip, and, more recently, the wrist.

Arthroscopy utilises a light source to illuminate the joint and a video camera to capture the image, which is then displayed on one or more screens. The arthroscope is introduced through a standard portal, while another portal or portals are used to introduce operating instruments. The location of portals is important to minimise the risk

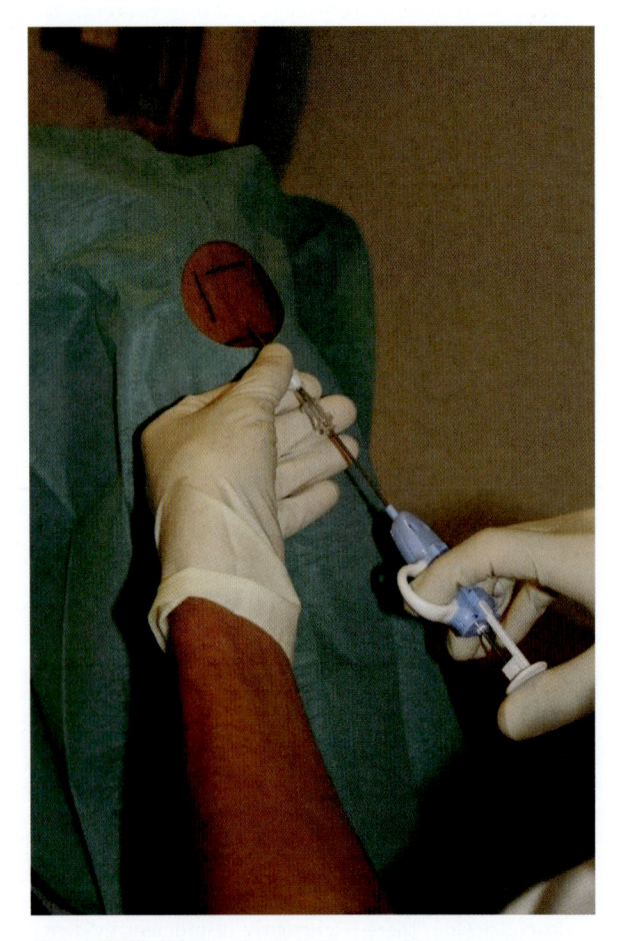

Figure 17.25 Biopsy of patellar tendon for tenocyte harvesting

of damage to vessels and nerves. A number of instruments are available for use in arthroscopic procedures.

Arthroscopy can be carried out under local, regional or, often, general anaesthesia as a day procedure. The main areas of interest to be viewed through the arthroscope are the articular surfaces, the synovium and intra-articular structures such as the meniscus and cruciate ligaments of the knee, the glenoid labrum and rotator cuff tendons of the shoulder, and the acetabular labrum of the hip. In most joints, the majority of the articular surfaces can be viewed. Assessment of stability can be aided by combining a direct view of the joint with manoeuvres that place the joint under stress.

Common procedures performed through the arthroscope include removal of loose bodies within the joint, separation of and removal of the torn part of a meniscus, repair of a torn structure such as a peripheral tear of the meniscus or a labral detachment in the shoulder, or dividing a tight structure such as the glenohumeral joint capsule in the shoulder or scar tissue in the knee. More complex reconstructive joint procedures (ACL reconstruction, rotator cuff repair) can be performed with the aid of an arthroscope.

Arthroscopy has a low complication rate. There is a small incidence of infection and delayed portal healing. Occasionally, arthroscopy can produce a persistent joint reaction manifesting as prolonged joint effusion, persistent pain and muscle wasting. Whether this is due to the arthroscopy itself or to the underlying joint pathology is sometimes difficult to determine. Complex regional pain syndrome type 1 may occasionally develop after arthroscopy.

Open surgery

The open surgical treatment of sports-related problems includes surgery related to acute trauma and surgery for the treatment of overuse injuries. Surgery after an acute injury aims to recreate the pre-injury anatomy by the repair of damaged tissues. This may require internal bone fixation for an unstable fracture, or repair of torn ligaments or tendons. If repair of the damaged tissue is not possible, a reconstructive procedure may be performed; for example, ACL reconstruction.

Following an acute injury, the athlete may develop chronic problems, such as instability, that may require surgical repair or reconstruction. Chronic ligamentous or capsular inadequacy may develop following an injury or as a gradual process. Surgery may be required to tighten the stretched tissue, either by moving the attachment of the tissue or by a shortening procedure, such as plication, reefing or shifting.

Overuse injuries that have failed to respond to conservative measures are sometimes managed by surgical tissue release, division or excision. Excision may be performed if impingement is present or if degenerative change has led to tissue necrosis. In nerve compression, decompression or transposition of the nerve may be required. Stress fractures that fail to heal (non-union) are treated by fixation or bone graft.

With all surgical procedures, arthroscopic or open, the surgery must be considered as only a part of the treatment. Adequate post-surgical rehabilitation is as important as the procedure itself. Rehabilitation following injury and surgery is discussed in Chapter 18.

REFERENCES

References for this chapter can be found at www.mhhe.com/au/CSM5e

Chapter 18

Principles of sports injury rehabilitation

with HÅVARD MOKSNES and PHIL GLASGOW

The pearl of long-term rehabilitation is to build a small team of core people who collaborate with other professions. Never walk alone!
Kjetil Jansrud, alpine skiing gold medallist at the 2014 Sochi Winter Olympic Games,
13 months after rupturing his anterior cruciate ligament

Sports injury rehabilitation is a dynamic, structured process that aims to:

- restore the injured athlete's function and performance level
- return the athlete to sports participation in a safe and timely manner
- minimise the risk of re-injury.

As previous injury is a prominent risk factor for future injury,[1-3] rehabilitation is a critical aspect of our professions. In most cases, the goal should be to improve the athlete's physical function to above their pre-injury level.

The foundation of sports injury rehabilitation is a targeted exercise program that is progressed gradually. As outlined in previous chapters (including 6 and 17), exercise therapy acts at the local tissue level and in the central nervous system. It may be used as a direct injury treatment (mechanotherapy)[4] or to unload injured tissue via altered movement and muscle activation patterns. It is also important to maintain the athlete's condition as much as possible throughout the rehabilitation process. A model of the parallel priorities of exercise prescription during the rehabilitation process is shown in Figure 18.1.

Exercise prescription, progress and supervision is often performed by a physiotherapist (or similar health professional, for example sports rehabilitator, trainer, therapist). However, where possible, a broader multidisciplinary team including the sport and exercise medicine physician, orthopaedic surgeon and other sport scientists (such as strength and conditioning specialists) should collaborate in rehabilitation planning. It is also critical to engage coaches in all phases of rehabilitation. In the early phases, coaches need to understand the plan and appreciate the functional milestones. In the later phases they should take an increasingly active role in implementing the program (Fig. 18.1).

Active rehabilitation is often supplemented with medical and manual therapies that may enhance the effects of exercise through pain management and improved tissue adaptations (Chapter 17). The success of rehabilitation depends on introducing the most effective intervention at the right time in an adequate dosage.[5]

Modern sports injury rehabilitation is progressed through phases based on sound clinical reasoning, sequenced functional achievements and the completion of functional milestones. At the same time, knowledge of tissue-specific biological healing processes should be respected and will guide the rehabilitation timeline. Exercise prescription, communication and clinical reasoning are core skills for clinicians involved in rehabilitation of sports injuries. Although most experienced clinicians are probably subconsciously following a progression model through rehabilitation, few theoretical models have been published.[5]

This chapter outlines the general principles of sports injury rehabilitation and provides a framework for progression through phases.

GENERAL PRINCIPLES

The primary aim of rehabilitation is to return the athlete to sport with appropriate function and fitness to participate at the desired level with a low risk of re-injury.

PART A   Fundamental principles

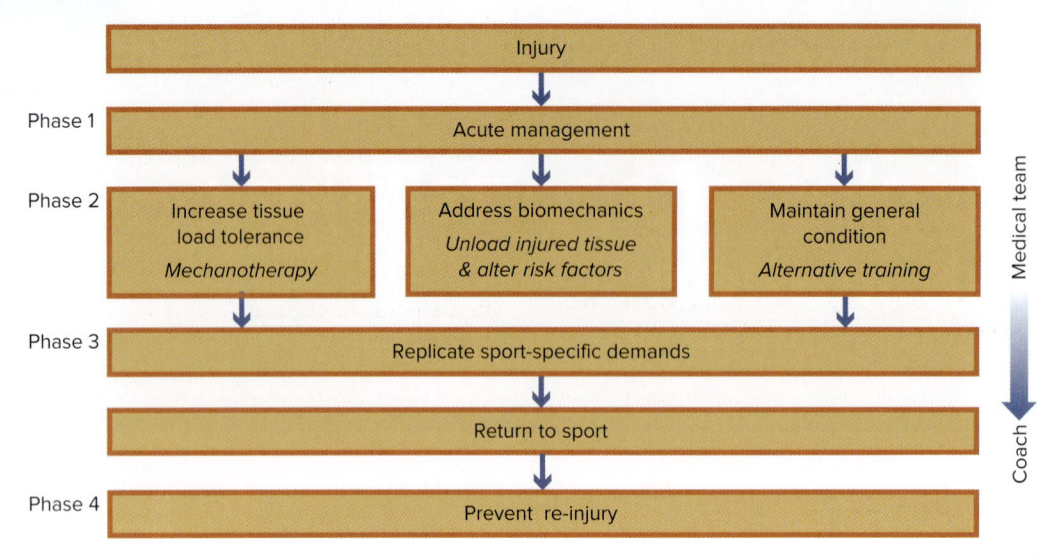

Figure 18.1 A model of the parallel priorities of exercise prescription during sports injury rehabilitation. The responsibility for implementation of the program should be gradually transferred from the medical team to the coach throughout the later phases of rehabilitation

However, this is sometimes challenging due to the desire of the athlete, coach, parents, management and others to return athletes to competition prematurely. Regardless of the circumstance, the medical team is obliged to ensure that the athlete's long-term health is not compromised by a premature return to sport which may have serious consequences. Thus, all rehabilitation protocols should include a predefined sport-specific functional battery of tests to ensure that the athlete is fit to return to sport with minimal risk of re-injury.

The rehabilitation principles described in this chapter primarily apply to the treatment of acute sports injuries and post-operative musculoskeletal rehabilitation. These rehabilitation processes are usually relatively linear and, for the most part, predictable. The principles can also be applied to overuse injuries. However, because the symptoms of overuse injuries often fluctuate and athletes often continue to train and compete with pain/impaired function, athletes may present at different stages of the rehabilitation continuum.

Rehabilitation plans following sports injury are usually separated into distinct phases and include active interventions aimed at addressing body impairments and functional limitations, with the aim of facilitating the athlete's participation in his or her desired physical activity and sport.[6]

An essential element—effective planning

Effective detailed planning is one of the most important aspects of rehabilitation. The plan should integrate accurate anatomical, pathophysiological, biomechanical and sport-specific knowledge with physical training principles.

> **PRACTICE PEARL**
>
> When designing a rehabilitation program, the clinician should identify specifically how the injury affects or impairs the athlete's function—taking into account the sport and the player's role within it (e.g. their event, discipline or position).

For example, a professional athlete can devote more time to rehabilitation and to rest between exercise bouts than an amateur athlete with a demanding work schedule. This will influence the total volume of training that can be tolerated. Top athletes with day-to-day follow-up can usually progress more rapidly than recreational athletes who have less frequent encounters with their clinician. Hence, the clinician has to create a larger safety buffer when designing rehabilitation programs for non-professionals. Furthermore, physiological responses to rehabilitation stimuli vary between individuals, making the prediction of recuperation following an exercise more uncertain. Thus, the expected time to recovery differs depending on the injury, intrinsic personal and contextual factors, and the amount of stimuli that can be applied to facilitate tissue healing and recovery.

Principles of sports injury rehabilitation CHAPTER 18

GOAL SETTING AND TARGETED INTERVENTIONS

Early goal setting and an outline of the rehabilitation plan are important elements that should be addressed in collaboration with the athlete, coach, physiotherapist and other members of the clinical team.[7] In the first meeting between the medical team and the athlete, the key steps should include:

1. obtaining a thorough history, including the current injury, previous injuries and available resources
2. setting long-term goals
3. striving for an accurate diagnosis, which may be provisional and subject to supplementary investigations
4. identifying key impairments in body structure and function
5. raising potential physiological, psychological and logistical barriers
6. drafting a realistic progress plan that includes functional and measurable short-term goals.

Identifying the athlete's ultimate goal is usually straightforward–most athletes want to return to participation in sport as quickly as possible. However, the expectations of a rapid return may sometimes be unrealistic, and misconceptions can undermine the collaboration and focus of the rehabilitation. Thus, giving the athlete an early outline of the expected progress with specific short-term goals accompanied by specific tasks will usually build a bond of confidence. Communicating the expected progress plan to coaches, team members, family and sometimes the media usually fosters a collaborative environment for focused rehabilitation.

Physical impairments and limitations are commonly subdivided into the areas of restricted range of motion (ROM), motor control and muscle strength. Different injuries will, in combination with previous injuries and fitness status, result in different impairments and limitations (Fig 18.2). The medical team should analyse the status of the injury and decide to what extent each of the impairments or limitations should be targeted during rehabilitation. The skill of prioritising exercise interventions throughout the rehabilitation has been designated as the 'X factor' in Figure 18.2. Prioritising rehabilitation interventions relies on the ability of the clinician and the broader team to effectively synthesise complex information (via skilled clinical assessment) and identify key limitations to performance as well as barriers to progression. While a large part of the 'X factor' will be based on sound clinical reasoning, it also involves the clinician's ability to relate to the athlete, to collaborate with other professions, to motivate and guide the athlete, and to educate key persons.

> **PRACTICE PEARL**
>
> The clinician must clearly indicate that the rehabilitation plan is dynamic—the focus will change depending on the patient's response to the program.

Endurance and its specific subcomponents may also have to be integrated throughout the phases of rehabilitation. Examples are strength endurance for alpine skiers and speed endurance for footballers. The ability to

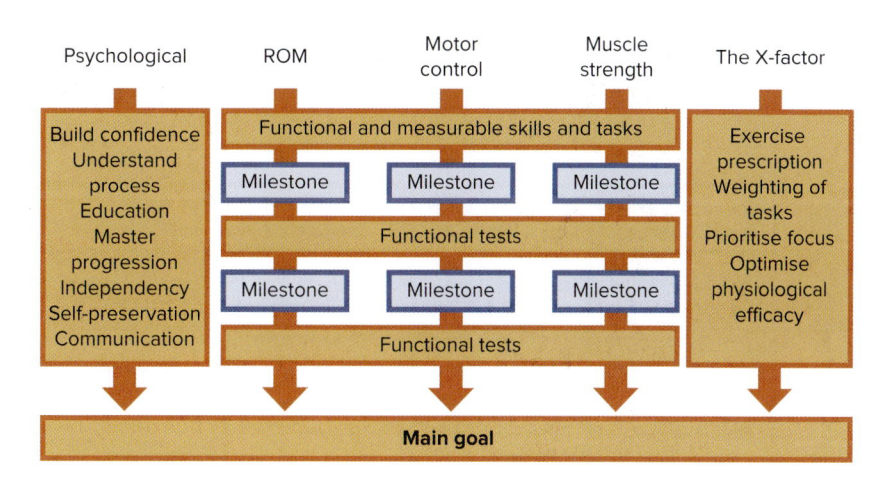

Figure 18.2 A theoretical model of clinical focus throughout the sports injury rehabilitation process

279

PART A Fundamental principles

continue to carry out a specific task or exercise for an extended period of time without a reduction in the quality or effort of the task is also an important component of the rehabilitation process. Fatigue has been identified as a risk factor for injury,[8] therefore, ensuring that the athlete is able to maintain good technique under fatigue is essential. Particular attention should be given to enhancing specific sub-qualities of endurance, such as skill execution under fatigue, as well as other strength and mobility parameters.

PHASES OF REHABILITATION

A four-phase structure can guide the aims and content of the rehabilitation process (Fig. 18.3). Specific functional milestones and achievement goals are identified within each phase. Some goals will be primary in each phase; for example, achieving full knee extension and quadriceps activation after knee surgery in Phase 1. At the same time, preservation of gluteal muscle activation and ankle mobility will be important secondary areas of focus. Therapists with different backgrounds, knowledge and experience will choose different exercises and treatments to achieve rehabilitation aims. Although there is now consensus regarding the importance of individually tailored rehabilitation after injuries,[9] well-documented rehabilitation guidelines are scarce for most conditions in sports medicine. Also, treatment algorithms differ between cultures, countries and institutions.

Due to the multidimensional nature of sports rehabilitation, the clinician should be able to manage several parallel focus areas throughout the various phases of rehabilitation, each with different goals and milestones. The relative importance of each focus area will change throughout the rehabilitation process (Fig. 18.3). Progressing active rehabilitation requires continuous evaluation, which is necessary to guarantee a confident and timely return to training and competition.

Phase 1: Acute

In line with the increased focus on active rehabilitation strategies, the traditional acronym PRICE (Protection, Rest, Ice, Compression and Elevation) for treatment of acute soft tissue injuries is increasingly replaced with POLICE (Protection, Optimal Loading, Ice, Compression and Elevation).[10] Optimal loading refers to the clinician evaluating the ability of the tissue to withstand and adapt to mechanical load.[11] The clinical challenge is not only to choose the most effective and safe exercise interventions, but also to apply the intervention in the appropriate dose. Immediate protection and relative rest after an acute injury still plays a role, but because of the detrimental effect of inactivity on biological tissues, leading clinicians look to have the athlete begin active movement (optimal loading) as soon as possible. For example, a player may begin hamstring activation exercises (loading) within 24 hours of a hamstring muscle strain depending on the severity of the injury and other factors.

Goal setting in the acute phase should be unidimensional and targeted toward impairments and limitations. For example, after knee ligament surgery the acute phase goals are for the athlete to regain voluntary quadriceps activation toward end-range extension (impairment) and to perform a straight-leg raise without extension lag (limitation). The combination of these two comprises the functional milestone of controlled active terminal knee extension, which allows the athlete to progress to walking without crutches for short distances.

The next goal could then be for the athlete to perform a step-up exercise with proper alignment and controlled loaded terminal extension (Fig. 18.4). When adequate step-up quality of movement is achieved, the use of crutches can be terminated for all distances. Blanchard and Glasgow have depicted the process for how to progress single exercises and this can be adapted to the rehabilitation process in general (Fig. 18.5).[5] The model describes how the clinician can build and manipulate the

	ROM	Motor control	Muscle strength	Exercise prescription
Phase 1	Regain active & passive range	Proprioception & motor output	Voluntary activation	Controlled
Phase 2	Cyclic, full-range loading	Joint stability	Hypertrophy	Extrinsic stimuli
Phase 3	Manual therapies if necessary	Speed & agility	Generate strength	Complex movements
Phase 4	Maintenance & recovery	Ingrain new patterns	Power & endurance	Sport-specific

Figure 18.3 Model of rehabilitation through phases. Box outlines represent primary (green), secondary (orange) and tertiary (red) focus

Principles of sports injury rehabilitation CHAPTER 18

exercises to gradually increase the demands on the athlete, while at the same time allow the healing tissue to adapt to the increase in mechanical load.

A variety of interventions are available to the clinician in Phase 1. Traditional low-load controlled exercises are at the core of interventions. However, adjunct modalities such as neuromuscular electrical stimulation (NMES) can help the athlete regain voluntary muscular control.[12, 13] Furthermore, manual therapies can be effective in the recovery of impairments during this phase (Chapter 17).

Phase 2: Restore activities of daily living

The aim of the second phase of rehabilitation is to allow the athlete to return to daily activities and basic sport-specific technical movements. The clinician should gradually increase the complexity of movements from single joint controlled actions to more complex tasks including movements through several biomechanical planes. For example, the overhead athlete who has regained pain-free external rotation in the scapular plane with adequate scapular control in Phase 1 will typically progress to mimic the throwing motion at low velocity in Phase 2. While the throwing motion will be the primary focus of the rehabilitation program, the clinician must ensure that secondary functions such as contralateral hip stability and ankle range of motion are maintained.

Exercises can be progressed by increasing the number of repetitions, the velocity of the movement, or the frequency (rate) of the exercises. Further, adding external loads and increasing the complexity of movement will stimulate muscle strength and motor control. Thus, Phase 2 challenges the clinician to prioritise exercises successfully. Skilled clinicians are able to keep their eye on several parallel processes at the same time (the X-factor).

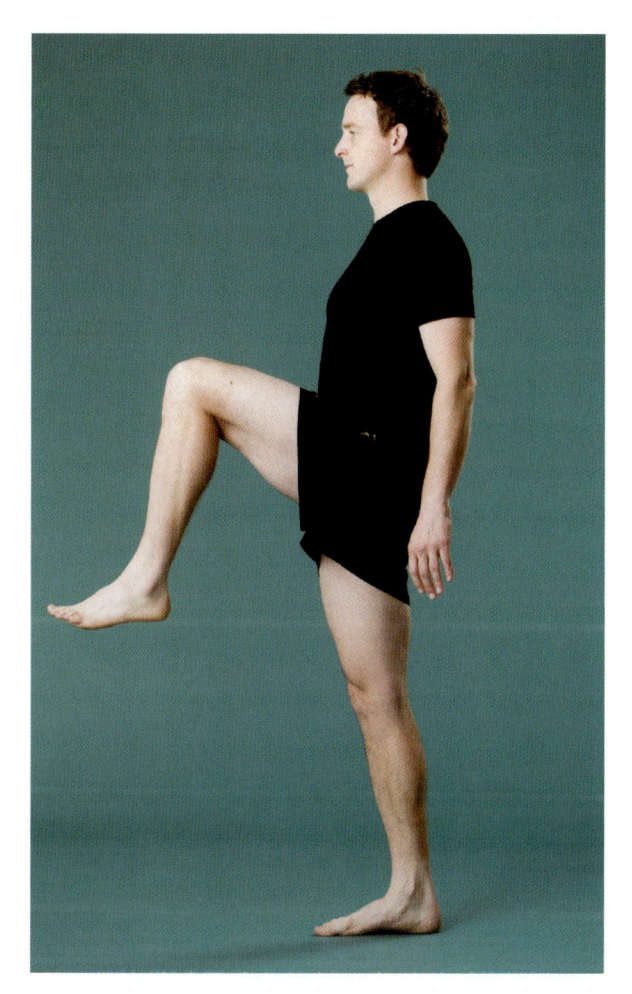

Figure 18.4 The ability to perform a high step-up with good control of terminal knee extension is a common functional goal during Phase 1 rehabilitation of acute knee injuries

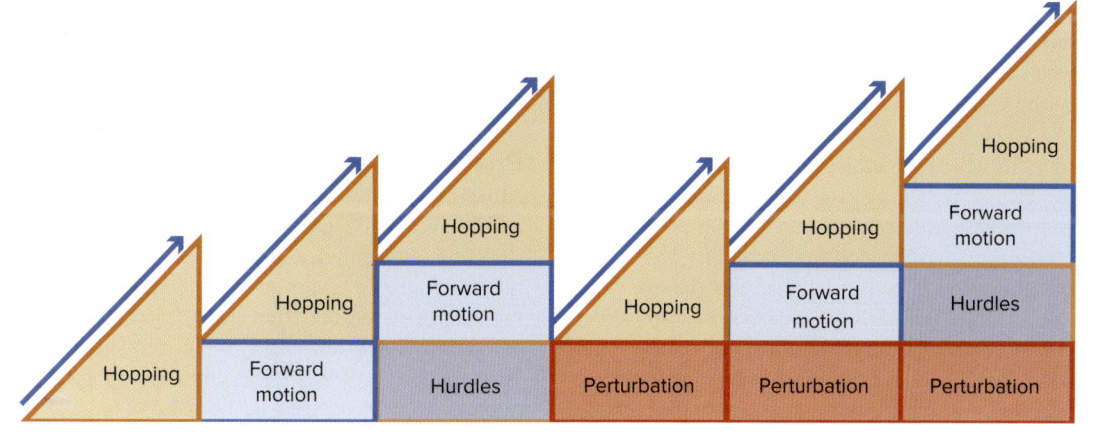

Figure 18.5 Visual aid to demonstrate a complex rehabilitation progression with undulating tiers using lower limb injury as an example[5]. The horizontal axis represents time and the vertical axis represents difficulty. The clinician adds and subtracts elements of the rehabilitation to progressively challenge the athlete while keeping the overall workload appropriate

REPRODUCED FROM FIGURE 2 IN BLANCHARD S, GLASGOW P. A THEORETICAL MODEL TO DESCRIBE PROGRESSIONS AND REGRESSIONS FOR EXERCISE REHABILITATION. *PHYS THER SPORT.* 2014 AUG;15(3):131–5

Goal setting in the second phase will still focus on the remaining impairments, although the main goals are related to addressing functional limitations in activity and improving performance of semi-complex sport-specific movement patterns. Examples of Phase 2 functional milestones for an ACL-injured athlete can be jogging with good form, and the ability to perform single leg hops with full knee extension at take-off and high degrees of knee and hip flexion during landing.

The primary intervention throughout Phase 2 is to continue progressing the therapeutic exercise program. The program will mainly incorporate elements to improve motor control and muscle strength, with additional sessions of cardiovascular training. When determining the exact nature of cardiovascular training in rehabilitation, the clinician should ensure that the correct energy system is being trained and that adequate time is allowed for recovery and physiological adaptation. For athletes who are rehabilitating over longer periods of time (i.e. months after ACL reconstruction), the acute:chronic workload ratio should be considered (Chapter 12). The nature of training used should minimise stress on the injured tissues while simultaneously exercising muscle groups involved in the athlete's sport. Aerobic and anaerobic endurance can be effectively trained using pool-based conditioning or cardiovascular equipment such as a bicycle ergometer, cross-trainer, rowing ergometer and step machine.

> **PRACTICE PEARL**
>
> The nature, intensity, duration and work:rest ratio of individual training sessions should reflect sporting demands.

An example of a weekly schedule may consist of two muscle strength sessions, two motor control sessions, two cardiovascular sessions and one recovery day. The precise nature of the sessions and the order in which exercises are carried out will be dictated by the clinician's understanding of the sport to which the athlete must return, the effects of the specific impairments and an appreciation of how the prescribed exercise will influence restoration of function. The clinician must have a good understanding and ability to appropriately modify load and difficulty of the exercises, while still guarding the healing tissue from abrupt forces and overload. Efficient communication with specific cues that facilitate a move from an internal focus of attention to an external focus, in combination with careful explanation and involvement of the athlete can greatly increase the efficacy and adherence to interventions.[14, 15]

Phase 3: Returning to sports activities

In the third phase of rehabilitation the clinician guides the athlete towards returning to participation in sports. More traditional strength and conditioning training can be incorporated in the weekly rehabilitation plan with increased focus on more complexity and velocity. Emphasis should be on a higher rate of force development and introduction of on-field sessions to bring in environmental adaptation. An athlete recovering from a knee injury can be brought to the field to perform sessions focused on higher speed running, cutting and turning tasks, and the inclusion of relevant equipment (ball, racquet, skis, etc.). Physical conditioning in the gym will be similar to pre-season training for the specific sport, although a majority of exercises should still be unilaterally focused to stimulate adaptation and reverse any remaining impairments.

Goal setting in Phase 3 will relate to all levels of function. Typically, muscle strength measurements (impairment) and single-leg hop tests (activity) are compared with the goal of 90% of the uninjured side.[16, 17] Participation goals can include completing specific parts of the team training sessions without symptoms during or after training. An important task for the clinician will be to monitor the overall load on the healing structures, which again calls for close collaboration and clear communication with coaches and strength and conditioning professionals.

Return-to-play decisions are perennially challenging and require a team approach that focuses on ensuring that function has been adequately restored. To facilitate safe return to sport, it is paramount that functional testing with valid and reliable outcome measures be performed. (See Chapter 16 for more on relevant outcome measures.) Multidimensional sets of tests that evaluate the different layers of function are best.[18-21] However, the scientific backing regarding content and cut-off limits for the test batteries are still lacking for most injuries. The return-to-play process is discussed in Chapter 19.

Phase 4: Prevention of re-injury

All sports injuries with tissue disruption will render the athlete more susceptible to re-injury even though tissue structure and physical function may be restored after rehabilitation. In spite of the increased attention and knowledge on rehabilitation of sports injuries, the incidence of re-injury remains high in professional sports.[22, 23] The classical model on the aetiology of sports injuries published by Meeuwisse in 1994 (see Fig.12.1) points to the importance of recognising internal risk factors such as previous injuries in the prevention of sports injuries.[24]

Principles of sports injury rehabilitation CHAPTER 18

> **PRACTICE PEARL**
>
> Every clinician involved in the rehabilitation of sports injuries must work diligently with the athlete, coach and conditioning professionals to continue targeted individualised prevention training after the athlete has returned to the competitive level.[25]

Interventions should be aimed at impairments and functional limitations known to exist as a result of injury such as altered muscle activation patterns and inadequate landing and cutting strategies.[26-28]

WHEN REHABILITATION DOES NOT GO ACCORDING TO PLAN

Sports injury rehabilitation seems like a straightforward linear process when presented in this chapter (Fig. 18.6a). However, as every clinician has experienced, progression does not always go according to plan (Fig. 18.6b). Longstanding pain, recurrent effusion, persistent range of motion deficits and muscle inhibition are a few of the most common obstacles. What to do when progression fails?

A thorough look at the content and volume of the rehabilitation program is usually indicated. Are the interventions targeting the impairments they were intended to target? It is often prudent to follow the athlete through a full session to ensure proper technique and understanding is present. Experienced clinicians will often state that 'less is more' and that splitting the original rehabilitation program into two parts is often a wise decision.

> **PRACTICE PEARL**
>
> It may be necessary to revisit the diagnosis and the functional assessment.

Symptoms tend to change over time–and not always in a predictable fashion. A step back to address the basic functional impairments is often necessary.

Sit down with the athlete and analyse the total load during the week. Is there enough time to recover between sessions? How much load is placed on the healing structures between training sessions? Are there any environmental challenges related to family, friends, facilities or motivation? Collaborate with the athlete to resolve underlying challenges. Ask open questions and probe their psychological status. A few days off rehabilitation may be a relief to many athletes.

Ask a colleague! A referral back to the physician or orthopaedic surgeon may be indicated. A second opinion from another clinician within the field can often open new doors. Additionally, a multidisciplinary meeting with all involved parties can adjust and streamline the expectations and responsibilities of each member of the rehabilitation team.

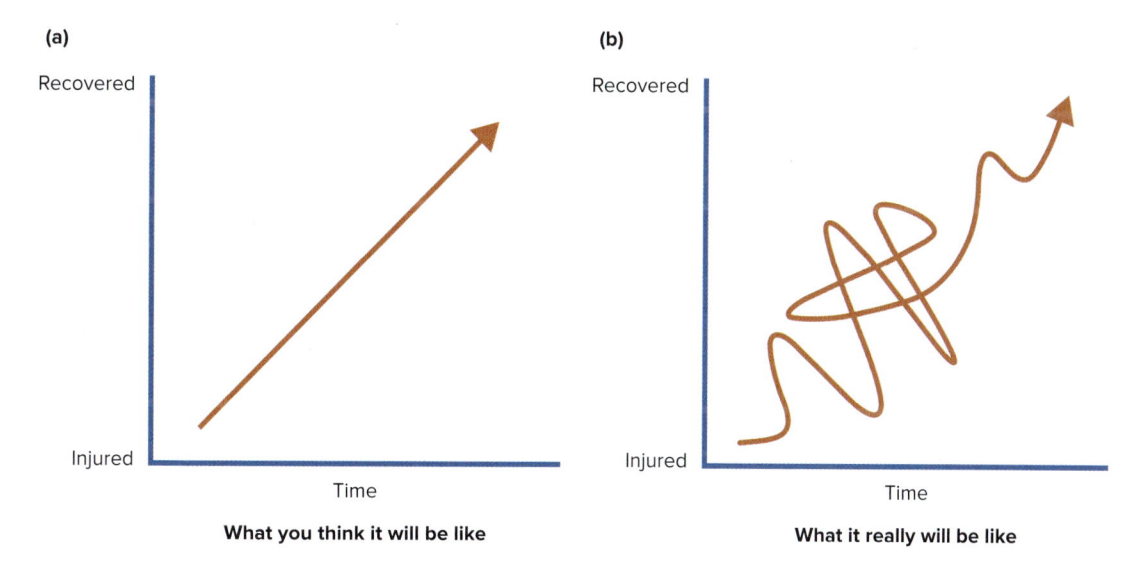

Figure 18.6 It can be helpful to share a map of the rehabilitation journey with your patient (a) Most patients believe rehabilitation should be straightforward and speedy (b) Sports physiotherapist Adam Meakins has added his own take to the traditional 'winding road'. Patients can feel they are travelling backwards in time on occasions. The expert clinician anticipates this in his or her discussion while planning rehabilitation

REFERENCES

References for this chapter can be found at www.mhhe.com/au/CSM5e

Chapter 19

Return to play

with IAN SHRIER

Perhaps the most common question for every active but injured patient is
'When can I return to play?'

Return-to-play (RTP) decisions can be difficult and complex.[1] The clinician is expected to provide an opinion based on a large number of factors including the history of the injury, physical examination, type of injury, rehabilitation, type of activity, psychological state, competitive level and ability to protect the injury. Further, these decisions do not occur in a vacuum. The athlete may receive advice from family, friends, coaches, other clinicians and, in the case of elite athletes, agents.

Because determining prognosis is difficult and frequently subjective, some disagreements regarding RTP will always occur.[2] Differing sociocultural and clinical perspectives of the medical doctor, coach, athlete and others lead to a high potential for conflict. Apart from being challenging and an unpleasant experience, such conflicts are believed to lead to a number of negative scenarios including:

1. miscommunication
2. loss of trust
3. potential litigation
4. declines in sport participation rates–some individuals never 'get back in the game' due to fear of re-injury (despite acceptable levels of risk)
5. serious medical complications–some athletes return to activity while still at unacceptable levels of risk for subsequent sport-related injury.[3-6]

Two important factors may minimise development of such conflict: a formal structure or process outlining how an actual RTP decision should be made and a formal process to guide the interactions between individuals who contribute in any way to the RTP process. It is important to note that in some cultures the clinician is expected to determine the reasonable course of action for a seemingly independent third party–the athlete–who is otherwise capable of making autonomous decisions. In other cultures shared decision making may be promoted by the medical community in general, but the clinician is usually still considered legally responsible for any consequences of the decision. Regardless of the cultural context in which one is situated, having a transparent framework for arriving at RTP decisions should help minimise any conflict that might arise.

The purpose of this chapter is to provide such a framework. In 2010, we published a 3-Step framework[7] developed specifically for RTP decision making. The framework is consistent with clinicians' beliefs independent of country of practice or clinician specialty,[8] and represents a framework to help organise complex information; it should not be interpreted as proscriptive. After feedback from clinicians, this has now evolved into a revised framework called the Strategic Assessment of Risk and Risk Tolerance (StARRT).[9]

The StARRT framework is based on causal relationships and considers that differences in RTP decisions are partly due to differences in (1) risk assessment and (2) risk tolerance. Differences in risk assessment could be decreased through the application of research and knowledge dissemination leading to improved evidence-based practice. Differences in risk tolerance are based on societal and personal values, which are independent of research and evidence-based practice. This may be part of the reason why different participants presented with the same information come to different RTP decisions.[10] Finally, the framework's general approach means that it can be applied by whoever represents the decision-making

PART A Fundamental principles

authority: a clinician, non-clinician or a multidisciplinary team.

STRATEGIC ASSESSMENT OF RISK AND RISK TOLERANCE FRAMEWORK FOR RTP DECISION MAKING

The StARRT framework for RTP decisions is illustrated in Figure 19.1. Rational decision making requires weighing the benefits and risks of different alternatives.[11-13] For RTP decisions, the clinician is generally concerned with managing risk of re-injury, but may at times be concerned with risk of any injury, death or illness.

The foundation of the framework is that an injury or re-injury will occur whenever the stress applied to a tissue is greater than the stress the tissue can absorb (tissue health).

Step 1—Tissue health

The first step in the StARRT framework is to assess the stress the tissue can absorb before becoming damaged. This is a function of the health of the tissue. For the same level of activity, the risk of re-injury increases with increasing damage to the tissue that is generally evaluated through the presence of symptoms (e.g. pain), signs

StARRT Framework

Strategic assessment of risk & risk tolerance

Step 1 – Assessment of health risk — *Tissue health*
- Patient demographics (e.g. age, sex)
- Symptoms (e.g. pain, giving way)
- Personal medical history (e.g. recurrent injury)
- Signs (physical exam) (e.g. swelling, weakness)
- Special tests (e.g. pain with function, X-ray, MRI)

Step 2 – Assessment of activity risk — *Tissue stresses*
- Type of sport (e.g. collision, non-contact)
- Position played (e.g. goalie, forward)
- Limb dominance (e.g. MSK alignment)
- Competitive level (e.g. professional, playoffs)
- Ability to protect (e.g. padding)
- Functional tests (e.g. diagonal hop test)
- Psychological readiness (e.g. affecting play)

Step 3 – Assessment of risk tolerance — *Risk tolerance modifiers*
- Stage of the season (e.g. playoffs)
- Pressure from athlete (e.g. desire to compete)
- External pressure (e.g. coach, athlete family)
- Masking the injury (e.g. effective analgesia)
- Conflict of interest (e.g. financial)
- Fear of litigation (e.g. if restricted or permitted)

Return-to-play decision

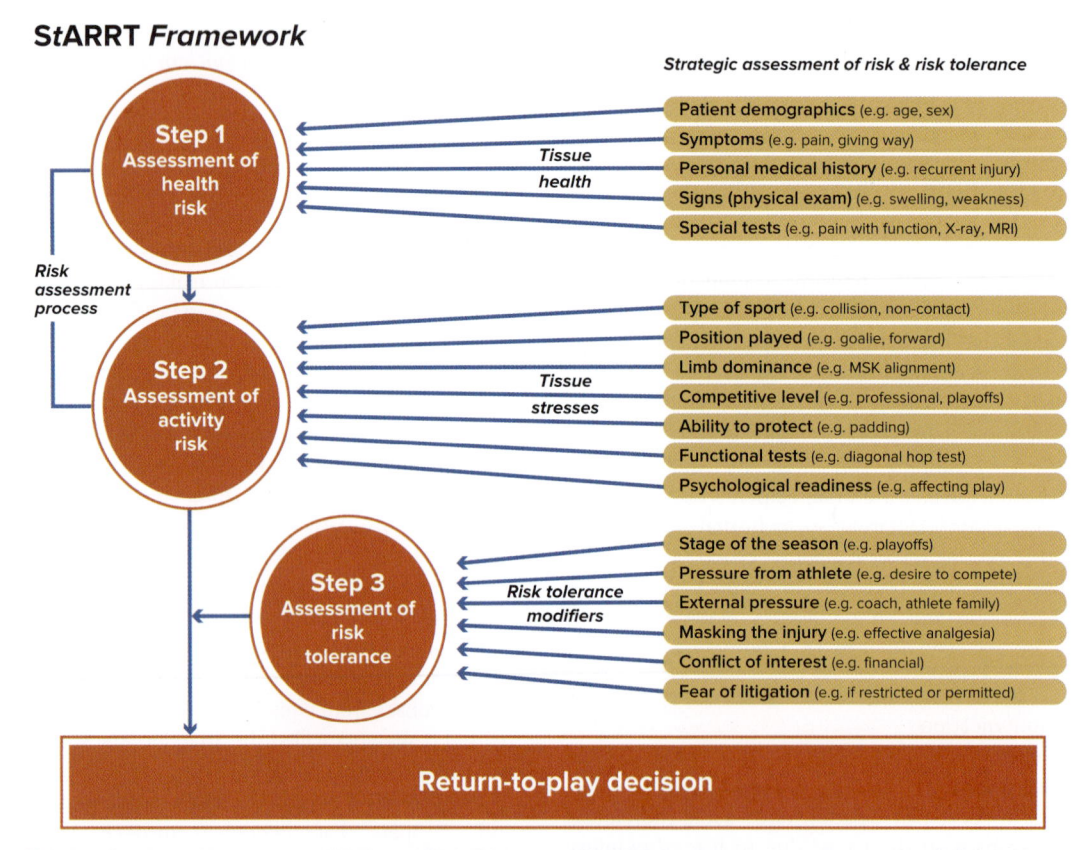

Figure 19.1 The Strategic Assessment of Risk and Risk Tolerance (StARRT) framework for return-to-play (RTP) decisions. This framework illustrates that athletes should be allowed to return to play when the risk assessment (Steps 1 and 2) is below the acceptable risk tolerance threshold (Step 3) and not allowed to return to play if the risk assessment is above the threshold. The StARRT framework groups factors according to their causal relationships with the two components of risk assessment (tissue health, stresses applied to tissue) and risk tolerance, as opposed to the 3-Step framework that groups factors according to the sociological source (medical culture, sport culture, decision maker) of the information. In some cases, an apparently single factor can have more than one causal connection and would be repeated. For example, playoffs will increase the competitive level of play and therefore increase tissue stresses and increase risk. However, playoffs are also expected to affect an athlete's desire to compete (i.e. mood, risk of depression if not allowed to RTP) and could affect financial benefit as well. These causal effects would lead to increased risk tolerance. In this framework, each outcome is evaluated for RTP, and the overall decision is based on the most restricted activity across all outcomes (see text and Table 19.1).

(e.g. swelling) and diagnostic tests (e.g. muscle strength). As this information comes from health professionals, the factors were originally considered 'medical'.

Step 2—Tissue stresses

The second step of the framework is to assess the stress that will be applied to the tissue. This is directly related to the planned activity, as opposed to the status of the original injury and is therefore considered sport-related. Using the frequency, intensity, time and type (FITT) training principle, one can modify activity through frequency (e.g. 3 days per week), intensity (e.g. running fast or climbing hills), timing (e.g. 20 minutes per session) and type. For the type of activity, one can think in general terms such as running or swimming.

However, for re-injury risk, the most salient detail is the required biomechanics that increase stress (i.e. the causes of injury), and the categories 'type of sport' and 'position played' are meant to capture this information. For example, the biomechanics of freestyle swimming are very different from those of breaststroke (analogous to different positions in other sports). Therefore, trying to assess the risk of re-injury in 'swimming' is likely not the best clinical approach. Rather, clinicians should focus on the activities that cause the underlying stresses on the musculoskeletal system to increase. If these can be modified to reduce stress to the injured area (e.g. switch from crawl to breaststroke for some types of shoulder injuries or from whip kick to flutter kick for some types of knee injuries), then the injury risk is decreased.

Psychological factors are listed in Step 2 because, as noted above, they affect risk of re-injury via the way the athlete plays the game and therefore the potential stresses applied to the body. Similarly, functional capacity such as endurance, range of motion and proprioception also describe factors that increase or decrease stresses applied to the injured area and are included here. For example, tight hamstrings mean that forward flexion must come more from the back, which increases lumbar and thoracic stress. Limitations in scapular rotation lead to a decrease in the subacromial space during abduction (increasing the risk of impingement syndrome) as more motion must come from the glenohumeral joint.

Step 3—Risk tolerance modifiers

Step 3 is designed to account for the reasons why two clinicians (or two athletes) presented with the same risk assessment, may come to different RTP decisions. Because the risk is the same, the different RTP decisions reflect differences in risk tolerance. If the competition is the Olympics, a clinician's risk tolerance for the worsening of a sprained ankle may be greater than if the athlete is a 14-year-old male playing high school basketball. A factor is included as a risk tolerance modifier if there is any context where changing the factor would change one's threshold of an acceptable risk (e.g. for the Olympian) even if it does not affect the decision under other contexts (e.g. high school basketball player).

Return-to-play decision making—beyond risk for injury

The StARRT framework is about arriving at a decision based on whether the assessment of risk exceeds one's risk tolerance. Most clinicians likely think that the framework is about risk for re-injury. Although we are certainly concerned about the risk of re-injury, our focus should be on the overall health or wellbeing of the athlete.[14] How do we define wellbeing or health? Should this be restricted to pathology of muscle, tendon or bone (as for re-injury)? Should we also consider mental health or socioeconomic health?

In a series of studies, we found that sports and exercise medicine clinicians from various fields and regions considered many factors unrelated to risk as important factors in their decisions.[8] These included several psychological-related factors (desire to compete, psychological impact of not returning to play, loss of competitive standing) as well as potential financial loss, timing of the season, competitive level and fear of litigation. Most interesting was that the pattern of responses in one study that included both clinicians and non-clinicians found very little difference between these two groups.[14]

In summary, the StARRT framework organises the information available into risk assessment (Steps 1 and 2) for a particular outcome and information related to other factors that affect one's risk tolerance for that outcome (Step 3) because they may affect other aspects of the athlete's overall wellbeing. In the next section, we discuss how the framework can be applied in some challenging situations.

APPLYING THE StARRT FRAMEWORK

The application of the framework to most clinical situations is straightforward. Consider a case that we used in one of our validation studies where a collegiate American football linebacker (lots of contact at high speed) injured his acromioclavicular joint (Fig. 19.2).[10]

As the severity of signs and symptoms increases (from Example 1 through Example 6 in Fig. 19.2), most would agree that the stress the tissue could absorb prior to re-injury would decrease. In our study, as the health of the tissue decreased in the vignettes, clinicians became

PART A Fundamental principles

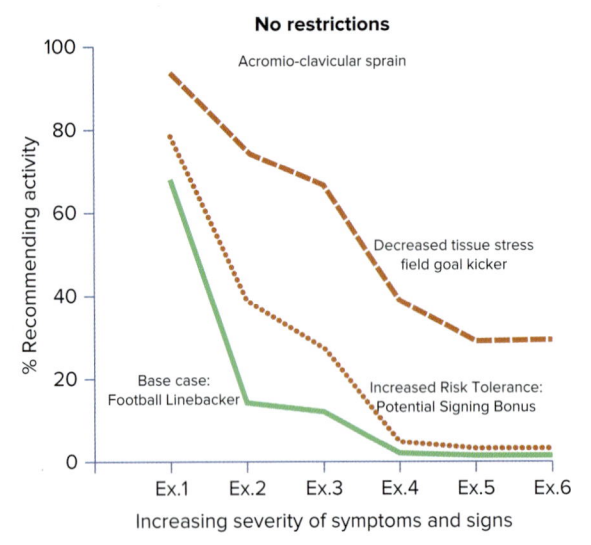

Figure 19.2 The proportion of respondents who would allow activity without restriction is plotted for the different acromioclavicular injury severity levels (increasing severity from Example 1 to 6) described in clinical vignettes.[10] The solid line presents the results for the base case when the athlete is an American football linebacker. The dashed line presents the results when we decreased the likelihood of excessive stress by considering the player to be a field goal kicker instead of a linebacker (tissue stresses). The dotted line presents the results when the linebacker (base case) was being evaluated for a multi-million dollar bonus (risk tolerance modifiers)[9]
REPRODUCED WITH PERMISSION FROM BRITISH JOURNAL OF SPORTS MEDICINE[9]

less likely to allow the athlete to full RTP. We then changed the scenario so that the athlete was a field goal kicker (very low risk of contact) instead of a linebacker. By decreasing the risk of applying excessive stress to the tissue (i.e. contact), the risk of re-injury decreases and this explains why more clinicians allowed full RTP than when the athlete had been a linebacker. Finally, returning to the context of a linebacker, we changed the vignette and said the athlete was being evaluated for a million dollar signing bonus. Given the potential benefit to his economic condition and overall wellbeing, the risk tolerance of many clinicians changed and these clinicians now allowed the athlete to RTP even though the risk of re-injury remained unchanged.

The StARRT framework may appear to discuss RTP decisions as if they are all or none. In clinical practice, RTP may refer to 'full return without restrictions', 'partial return', 'allowed to practice' and so forth. In fact, StARRT is a general framework for any decision-making process and will work equally well when one is trying to decide about return to training, return to practice or any level of activity.

Assessing across outcomes and probabilities

Steps 1 and 2 of StARRT evaluate only a single risk at a time. Yet, RTP decisions usually need to account for many outcomes (e.g. both in the short and long term) simultaneously. In the short term, clinicians and athletes might focus on risk of re-injury or decreased performance (leading to decreased competitive standing). With respect to long-term outcomes, one might focus on risk of osteoarthritis from joint injuries or long-term cognitive deficits following concussions. Each of these represents a different outcome that could be assessed through StARRT. An example of the process for a hypothetical case is shown in Table 19.1. For simplicity, Table 19.1 shows only the overall risk tolerance and omits the particular factors that affect it.

In Table 19.1, Clinician A is the decision maker and evaluates the risk for each outcome. In this hypothetical example, Clinician A considered the risks acceptable and allowed RTP for 6/7 outcomes (column 3), but unacceptable for short-term disability. The *overall RTP decision* must represent the most restricted decision in the table and the athlete is not allowed to RTP. The process is in fact, the same as that which occurs when there is more than one injury (e.g. assessing overall restrictions for an athlete with a knee injury and an ankle injury).

An ankle injury might result in an athlete only partially participating, but a concurrent knee injury might cause the clinician to restrict the athlete's activity to only weight training. The decision-making process for considering five outcomes on one injury in an athlete is the same as that for two outcomes on two injuries in an athlete: evaluate

Table 19.1 Applying the StARRT framework for RTP across different short-term and long-term outcomes. The final decision is the one that imposes the most limiting restrictions of all the outcomes (no RTP in this example)[9]

Outcome	Risk assessment	Risk tolerance	Decision
Short term			
Re-injury	<10%	Acceptable	RTP
Pain	50–70%	Acceptable	RTP
Work disability	20–30%	Not acceptable	No RTP
Performance	20–40%	Acceptable	RTP
Long term			
Osteoarthritis	2%	Acceptable	RTP
Disability	2%	Acceptable	RTP
Cost prohibitive	1%	Acceptable	RTP

across all outcomes and the highest level of restriction becomes the overall restriction.

Risk tolerance modifiers reflect contexts where risk tolerance is affected. These modifiers themselves have particular values (e.g. yes/no or a numerical value if a continuous scale) but are not necessarily risks themselves. For example, timing of the season is pre-season, regular season, finals/playoffs, off-season. In the finals/playoffs, athletes are often playing at higher intensities and more aggressively, leading to increased risk of injury. This is captured in Step 2 under 'competitive level'. In addition, finals/playoffs also have effects on financial compensation, ego and prestige, which are likely to affect risk tolerance in many contexts. Therefore, there may be contexts where timing of the season has minimal effect on risk assessment (Table 19.1, column 2), but large effects on risk tolerance (Table 19.1, column 3) or vice versa.

Baseline risk tolerance simply refers to one's risk tolerance under some arbitrary set of values for the risk tolerance modifying factors. In the case of a knee injury, we might consider a 15% increased risk of re-injury (compared to the uninjured knee) as acceptable. If we believe an athlete's mental health state might be affected by not playing, we might raise the acceptable risk for a knee injury from 15% to 25%. Risk tolerance modifiers are defined by this interaction. Contrast this with the risk of osteoarthritis. If the risk of osteoarthritis is high (or low), we might prevent (or allow) RTP because of the risk of knee osteoarthritis, but it does not change our risk tolerance for the risk of knee re-injury *per se*.

Additional perspectives

The StARRT framework is a simplified version of a more complex process that can lead to decision-tree analysis. When evaluating any action, there must be a comparison with a different action, which may or may not be 'no action'. Table 19.2 illustrates the process for comparing action A (Allow RTP) with action B (Do not allow RTP).

In making a decision, we are hoping for a particular outcome.

Let us consider re-injury as our outcome of interest. If we allow RTP, the athlete may get injured or not get injured. The mental health of the athlete will likely be healthy because they are doing what they want to do. If we do not allow RTP, they cannot get injured. In this context, the mental health of the athlete may be unhealthy (if we are correct that preventing RTP is damaging to the psyche) or may be healthy (if we are not correct that preventing RTP is damaging to the psyche).

In a full decision-tree analysis, one attaches probabilities to the results defined in each row of Table 19.2 (i.e. combination of physical and mental health). Preferably, the probabilities would be based on actual risk scores developed from surveillance or intervention studies (similar to Framingham risk score for cardiovascular disease[15]). One could also include the severity of the outcome in terms of disability or decreased capacity. If we assume equal probabilities for each row (25%), one still has to make a value judgment whether being injured with a healthy mental state is better or worse than being uninjured with an unhealthy mental state.

This is a value judgment and there are no algorithms or statistical analyses that can provide the best answer for an individual athlete. Statistically, one multiplies the probability by the value, but this calculation is based on several assumptions that may or may not be true. Regardless, the optimal choice will obviously depend on the disability and long-term consequences of the injury, the disability and long-term consequences associated with the poor mental health and the personal values of whoever is the decision maker.

In reality, the probabilities will not be equal. But the question remains the same and only the proportions change. Is a 20% risk of injury with 10% risk of poor mental health a better choice than 0% chance of being injured with an 80% risk of poor mental health?

Table 19.2 Hypothetical example for an RTP decision-tree analysis approach to RTP. Each action leads to a particular physical state and cognitive state. The probability for the combined physical and cognitive state is estimated, and the 'value' associated with the combined state is given a number between 0 (no value) and 100 (maximum value). The value associated with the state is multiplied by its probability of occurring to provide a total score. The total scores for each row associated with a particular action are summed and the decision is the action that provides the highest decision value

Action	Physical state	Mental state	Probability	Value	Total score (prob*value)	Decision value
Allow RTP	Not injured	Healthy	25%	100	25	37.5
Allow RTP	Injured	Healthy	25%	50	12.5	
No RTP	Not injured	Healthy	25%	60	15	22.5
No RTP	Not injured	Unhealthy	25%	30	7.5	

PART A Fundamental principles

WHO SHOULD BE THE DECISION MAKER?

Within society at large, most people have the authority to make decisions about their own risks for health unless otherwise restricted by law (e.g. helmets while driving motorcycles in many countries). In the context of returning to play or work after an injury, the decision-making power is often shifted from the individual athlete to the healthcare clinician. For many people, this loss of autonomy can be challenging.

In this section, we discuss different approaches to deciding who should have the authority to make the decision and when and why. A fairly complete list of possible options are: the athlete (or designated representative such as parent or power of attorney), any one of the clinicians (e.g. medical doctor, physiotherapist, athletic trainer, chiropractor, nurse, nutritionist), coach, management (e.g. sport association, team employer), athlete's family, agent or some multidisciplinary team made up of a combination of the above stakeholders. Some of these may be clearly inappropriate in some contexts, but the list is provided to highlight the different factors that need to be considered.

Although power relationships within society are commonly studied in medical sociology,[16] this has not occurred within the context of RTP decisions. The interactions between the athlete, family, friends, agents, coaches, clinicians, and institutional or corporate managers are often complex and confusing. Although clinicians and athletes may 'negotiate' approaches to treatment,[17] the clinician usually has ultimate decision-making power. When athletes avoid interaction with clinicians,[17] they retain power over the decision-making process by default except where the clinician's approval is expressly required.

The first two steps of the StARRT framework require the capacity to evaluate risk. To our knowledge, there is no evidence examining if clinicians are actually better than non-clinicians at evaluating risk of sport injury or whether certain types of clinicians (e.g. medical doctors) are better at evaluating risk compared to other types of clinicians (e.g. physiotherapists).

In one study,[14] we asked members of different Canadian sports medicine professional groups as well as athletes, coaches and sport associations to rank which professional group members might be best to answer such questions. First, most participants felt that medical doctors were the most capable of assessing the health of the tissue. However, when asked who was best to assess the risk of re-injury, short-term and long-term consequences, the members of each of the main clinical professions (medical doctors, physiotherapists, athletic therapists, chiropractors) generally felt that their own professional members had the greatest capacity to evaluate these risks (e.g. physiotherapists believed physiotherapists were best, chiropractors believed chiropractors were best).

On the other hand, official sport association members generally believed medical doctors were best, athletes believed physiotherapists were often equal to or better than medical doctors, and coaches believed physiotherapists and medical doctors were generally equal but medical doctors were better at assessing long-term consequences. When the same respondents were asked which group had the greatest capacity to assess the importance of risk tolerance modifiers, the athletes and coaches were generally considered the best.

Although these results do not directly speak to who should have the authority to make the RTP decision, they do suggest that an informed decision requires information from several sources. Most importantly, the decision maker needs to act in the best interests of the athlete, which means they have to understand the best interests of the athlete. A coach might have the athlete's best interests at heart, but may not have the experience of watching people suffer with severe osteoarthritis and cannot evaluate the magnitude of disability. A medical doctor may have only limited contact with an athlete and not understand their wishes, dreams or psychological stability.

In addition, as we have seen, there may be differences in opinion about how to weigh all the benefits and risks, but factors that benefit or harm others (i.e. not the athlete) should generally not be included in the decision-making process. Such factors can occur when there are power imbalances. For example, if a clinician is worried about losing his or her status as team doctor or physiotherapist as a result of restricting a player from playing, there may be an unconscious or conscious bias to allow the athlete to RTP even though the risk assessment suggests a risk higher than the decision maker's risk tolerance level in the absence of this fear. Similarly, a coach's performance is based on winning, which might (inappropriately) affect the risk tolerance level even though it is unrelated to the athlete's wellbeing. Table 19.3 summarises some major strengths and weaknesses of each of the stakeholders. The rest of this section discusses some particular points in more detail.

Clinicians

In the workers' compensation injury context, a medical doctor's opinion is generally required to return to work following an injury. This is to protect the worker from unreasonable pressure by the employer. Because the medical doctor is independent, the assumption is that the medical doctor's opinion will be free of bias. This is also the current framework model for most of sports medicine.

However, the external pressures in sport are different from the traditional work environment. In sport, the medical

Return to play   CHAPTER 19

Table 19.3 Strengths and weaknesses when the decision maker is a particular stakeholder

Stakeholder	Strengths	Weaknesses
Clinicians		
Medical doctor	Knowledge about injury risk and consequences of injury. More often not an employee of management so lower probability of coercion	Less personal contact with individual athletes and may not understand them as well
Team therapist*	Knowledge about injury risk and consequences of injury. Generally know athletes better than medical doctors	Usually an employee of management and may have less perceived power than medical doctor. This might mean more likely subject to coercion
Other (e.g. nutritionist, psychologist)	Similar to medical doctors and usually knowledgeable about injury/illness risk and consequences of injury/illness within their field of expertise	Usually a paid consultant to management. If perceived power is less than that of a medical doctor, then more subject to coercion
Non-clinicians		
Athlete	Knowledge of the athlete's global needs is near complete (but not complete). By definition, provides the best source for information about athlete's needs and values	Only has personal experience about injuries incurred so knowledge base is limited. Difficulty assessing risk. During heightened emotion of competition, may not be able to weigh the risks and benefits properly, even if given information. For injuries affecting cognition (e.g. concussion), informed consent is not possible
Coach	Often aware of athletes' strengths, desires and values. On occasion, will have a more complete view of athlete's benefits such as sport career potential	Limited experience to evaluate risk. During heightened emotion of competition, may be difficult to evaluate risks properly. Potential conflict if athlete may be important to win the game
Family / friends	Often strong knowledge of athlete's global needs, desires and values	Least experience to evaluate risk. On occasion, could be motivated by own personal gains if athlete RTP
Management (sport association / team)	Often aware of career potential and the benefits (or lack thereof) that can occur with RTP	Objective to win may increase risk tolerance even though athlete would not benefit

* The term 'team therapist' is used to refer to a professional who is not a medical doctor and has clinical training to evaluate and treat sport injuries and illnesses. In some cases, the term used to represent a recognised clinical profession in one country represents a completely different (and unrecognised) profession in another country. Team therapists include physiotherapists, athletic therapists, sports therapists, sports rehabilitators, athletic trainers, chiropractors and massage therapists

doctor is usually hired by the team and experiences dual allegiances. Although professional athletes may have access to non-team medical doctors when major conflicts arise, the team medical doctor usually retains the final decision-making power unless legal proceedings ensue. Therefore, unlike the workers' compensation context, medical doctors may indeed be subject to coercion. The same principle is true for all clinicians working for a team. Although financial remuneration will differ with each individual profession, team and region, one should not underestimate the power of social status even when clinical staff are unpaid.

When several health professionals are involved in caring for an athlete, the lines of communication and authority must be clearly defined.[1] Otherwise, what is already a complex situation for RTP is likely to become even more problematic. According to one consensus document, the essential elements for RTP decisions are the safety of the injured athlete and other athletes, as well as compliance with any rules or regulations.[1] Although some have mentioned that social and economic factors may create pressure for the clinician, the role such factors play in RTP has not been explicitly studied.[18] Because of the absence of clear recommendations, individual treating clinicians have been described as using their own value and belief systems which often include issues other than safety.[17]

Athletes

Making RTP decisions requires informed consent. The short-term and long-term consequences of any decision must be evaluated. Therefore, when an athlete's mental status is impaired, he or she would not normally be able to process the information. Although this is obviously the case in certain injuries like concussion, one could also argue that it is the norm in any game or competition context. Simply put, the lack of time available during a competition, accompanied by the emotions that occur during the event, would be expected to affect the ability of almost anyone to process the complex interactions of factors and possible consequences of RTP. However, outside the context of a competition or game, the athlete would normally have the time available to become informed and to evaluate the different consequences with respect to all aspects of health.

What motivates an athlete to want to RTP as soon as possible? In general, the internal factors include (1) that injury may represent a form of body-betrayal and a source of self-resentment,[19] and (2) psychological needs such as the desire to compete or 'love of the game '.[20] In addition, the external factors[21] include sociocultural influences, as well as greater status among peers and fans.[2, 19] Not playing when injured can lead to identity crises, feelings of guilt and shame, or experiences of alienation from the team.[20-22] All of these factors can lead to low self-esteem and depression.[2]

In some countries, there is a push towards medical care based on shared decision making for medical conditions.[23] The general concept is that clinicians are sources of information, and help patients through the maze of complex issues and values to achieve greater insight, and therefore participate in the decision-making process. This is in contrast to the traditional model where medical doctors are the authority and patients simply comply. Although some athletes would like to be more involved in RTP decisions themselves,[20] others indicate they have learned to trust medical doctors and trainers to make decisions for them,[22] and believe it is important for medical personnel to prevent them from returning to sport prematurely.[21] Conversely, some athletes have reported being pressured into returning to sport too early by the medical doctor, trainer or coach.[21]

The coach

The primary role of the coach is to maximise athletic performance. Some coaches believe athletes can be caught in a 'risk-pain-injury paradox' and that one of the coach's functions is to push athletes to their limits without taking excessive risks.[24] This may include competing while injured. Further, some coaches have suggested that medical personnel do not appreciate a need for an individualised approach or that delaying RTP can harm the athlete psychologically. Coaches also see their role as managing unrealistic athlete expectations about progress following an injury and return to sport.[21]

Family, friends, agents

Family, friends, agents, and institutional or corporate managers all have interests in RTP decisions and their interactions are often complex and confusing. Although it is often believed these persons will place 'non-health issues' above 'health issues', it is apparent that when 'health' is defined very narrowly, it may not represent the best interests of the athlete.

Management

It is clear that management's objective is to win and there is a strong possibility of conflict of interest. That said, management may have important information and perspectives to offer with respect to career potential.

A multidisciplinary approach

If we assume that the RTP decision should be based on the best interests of the athlete, then each of the stakeholders represents a source of information about a different aspect of the athlete. With different personal and societal values, there is clearly not going to be one 'correct' answer for the vast majority of injuries in the vast majority of athletes. In this framework, the key component is to ensure the decision is being based on some combination of the athletes' needs, desires and interests, and that there is no coercion or misrepresentation of information. Could a multidisciplinary model achieve this?

All stakeholders have a potential conflict of interest. Whether this manifests as a real conflict of interest depends on the individuals involved. Although a team approach does not eliminate this risk, its strength is that each team member can help ensure that others' (and their own) potential conflicts of interest are made transparent and documented. This may temper the enthusiasm of some to inappropriately argue in favour of a decision that is mostly for their own self-benefit, as opposed to the wellbeing of the athlete.

There remain significant challenges with a team approach. First, when decisions have to be made very quickly (e.g. during competition), a team approach is not always feasible. Second, a team approach does not eliminate contradicting values, but only brings them together in a transparent fashion. Decisions about risk assessment and risk tolerance can elicit strong emotions and there is a risk that systematising such decisions within a team approach may create interpersonal conflicts that would otherwise be avoided when there is one clear decision maker. Third, when there are conflicting opinions, a mechanism must be available to resolve the issue and come to a decision:

either the athlete returns to activity or does not return to activity.

Should there be a democratic vote with each member having one vote, or should some members' votes have greater weight than others to account for their different capacities and potential conflict of interests? Such a method seems difficult to operationalise, but would have the advantage of providing a significant voice to aspects of athletes' wellbeing that may otherwise go ignored. Exploring solutions to these challenges could be helpful in transforming the current model into one that maximises the chances for athletes' wellbeing to be the focus of the decision.

SUMMARY

In this chapter, we describe the StARRT framework for RTP decision making. The first two steps focus on risk assessment and the third step focuses on factors that alter the decision maker's risk tolerance. If the risk of the outcome is less than the risk tolerance after all factors are considered, the decision should be to RTP. Otherwise, the decision should be not to RTP.

The current decision-making process is embedded within a social context reflected principally by the values, beliefs and attitudes of a single decision maker. The steps in the process are not always transparent and can lead to confusion and unnecessary conflict. Although the medical doctor is often the ultimate decision maker, many organised sports do not have team doctors and other clinicians make these decisions. Theoretically, each of the stakeholders has information that might be helpful in understanding the best interests of the athlete, and each of the stakeholders is in a potential conflict of interest where their own interests may benefit from one decision or the other.

Finding a solution is likely to be difficult. To borrow a thought from Winston Churchill, at the current time, our current process seems to be the worst form of decision making, 'except for all those other forms that have been tried from time to time'.[25] But that doesn't mean we should stop trying yet.

REFERENCES

References for this chapter can be found at www.mhhe.com/au/CSM5e

PART B

Regional problems

Chapter 20

Sports concussion

with PAUL McCRORY, MICHAEL MAKDISSI, GAVIN DAVIS and MICHAEL TURNER

I've been knocked out a few times in there, but I have no idea how many concussions I've ever had.

Hulk Hogan

Although head injuries are common in all contact sports, the vast majority are minor. Sports in which minor head injuries are commonly observed include equestrian sports, various codes of football, boxing, gymnastics and martial arts. The incidence ranges from 0.25-9 per 1000 player hours of exposure in professional team sports. Amateur point-to-point (cross-country) jockeys have the highest concussion rate of any sport (95 concussions per 1000 player hours of exposure), followed by professional jumps and flat jockeys. With increasing media awareness, more concussions are being reported; however, direct epidemiological comparisons between sports are limited by methodological issues.

Head injuries of all levels are a medical emergency because they can prove fatal if misdiagnosed or incorrectly managed. The clinician's role in the management of acute head injuries is to (i) recognise the problem, (ii) ensure immediate resuscitation (if required) and (iii) transfer the injured athlete to the appropriate facility.

In this chapter we cover the following topics:

- definition
- prevention of concussion
- clinically relevant pathophysiology
- management of the concussed athlete
- complications of concussion
- return to play issues.

The chapter helps the reader to learn to diagnose and manage concussions in sport using the Sport Concussion Assessment Tool 3 (SCAT3™)[1] (Fig. 20.2), the Pocket Concussion Recognition Tool™ (Pocket CRT)[2] (Fig. 20.3) and Child SCAT3™ (Fig. 20.6).

We emphasise that the SCAT3 tools and the Pocket CRT are critical aspects of concussion management, as they are the result of more than 10 years of global collaboration and development by experts, at the 4th International Consensus Conference on Concussion in Sport held in Zurich in November 2012 (Fig. 20.1). These tools are designed to standardise the medical assessment and create a framework for the diagnosis of an acute concussion.

> **PRACTICE PEARL**
>
> The SCAT3, (Fig. 20.2) Child SCAT3 (Fig. 20.6) and Pocket CRT (Fig. 20.3) are derived from international conferences on concussion in sport and have been used internationally to assist clinicians and athletes reach 'quality decisions' about return to play (RTP) following concussion.

DEFINITION

'Concussion' is the term commonly used to describe a subtype of head injury. It is worth noting that the terms concussion and 'mild traumatic brain injury' (MTBI) refer to entirely different injury constructs and the terms cannot be used interchangeably. While concussion is a subset of mild traumatic brain injury, the converse is not true. A term often used in Europe is *commotiço cerebri*, which has the same meaning as *concussion* in this setting.

Some publications on concussion refer to the Glasgow Coma Scale (GCS) as a means of classifying traumatic brain

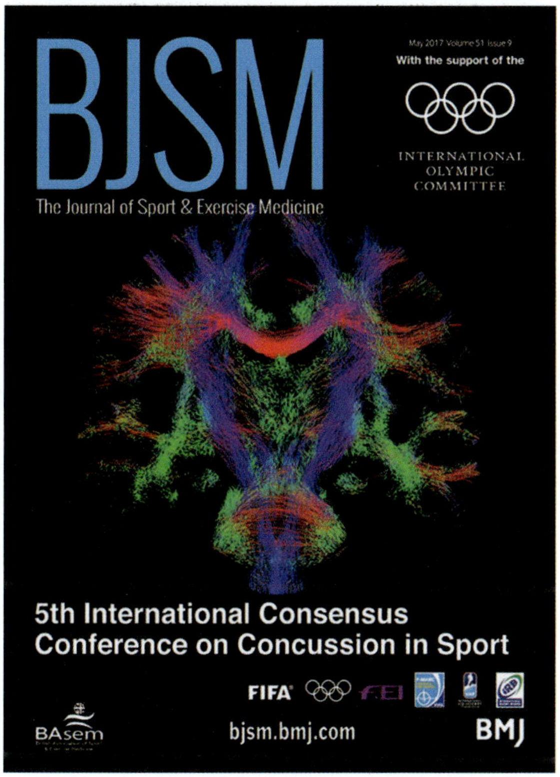

Sports concussion — CHAPTER 20

injury (TBI). This is a validated and widely used measure of conscious state used in the assessment of TBI. Its primary role is in the monitoring of serial change in neurological status post-injury, which is critical in determining the need for further intervention. It also has a secondary role in determining the prognosis of TBI by subdividing the spectrum of injury into mild, moderate and severe TBI based on an assessment at 6 hours post injury. The scale, however, does not encompass sport concussion due to the mild nature of the symptoms involved and the fact that many concussion symptoms affecting the conscious state are well and truly resolved by 6 hours.

The 4th International Consensus Conference on Concussion in Sport re-affirmed the clinical definition of sports concussion reached previously by experts at earlier meetings (see box below).[3-6]

PREVENTION OF CONCUSSION

There is no good clinical evidence that currently available protective equipment will prevent concussion, although mouth guards have a clear role in preventing dental and oro-facial injury.[7-10] Biomechanical studies have shown a small reduction in impact forces to the brain with the use of commercially available helmets, but these findings have not been translated to show a reduction in concussion incidence in published RCTs. For skiing and snowboarding there are a number of studies to suggest that helmets provide protection against head and facial injury and hence should be recommended for participants in alpine sports. In specific sports such as cycling, motor and equestrian sports, protective helmets may prevent other forms of head injury (e.g. skull fracture) that are related to falling on hard road surfaces and these may be an important injury prevention issue for those sports.[7]

Figure 20.1 The Concussion in Sport Group met in Berlin in October 2016. Their updated consensus statement and systematic reviews will be available in peer-reviewed journals including the *British Journal of Sports Medicine* (BJSM) by May 2017
COVER REPRODUCED WITH PERMISSION FROM BMJ GROUP AND CONCUSSION IN SPORT GROUP

Definition of concussion

Concussion is defined as a complex pathophysiological process affecting the brain, induced by traumatic biomechanical forces. Several common features that incorporate clinical, pathologic and biomechanical injury constructs that may be utilised in defining the nature of a concussive head injury include:

1. Concussion may be caused either by a direct blow to the head, face, neck, or elsewhere on the body with an 'impulsive' force transmitted to the head.
2. Concussion typically results in the rapid onset of short-lived impairment of neurologic function that resolves spontaneously. However, in some cases symptoms and signs may evolve over a number of minutes to hours.
3. Concussion may result in neuropathological changes, but the acute clinical symptoms largely reflect a functional disturbance rather than a structural injury and, as such, no abnormality is seen on standard structural neuroimaging studies.
4. Concussion results in a graded set of clinical symptoms that may or may not involve loss of consciousness. Resolution of the clinical and cognitive symptoms typically follows a sequential course. However, it is important to note that in some cases symptoms may be prolonged.

It is expected that future evolution of the definition of concussion will encompass clinical features, imaging changes, biomarkers, proteomics, epigenetic changes and genotype in a more comprehensive matrix of post-injury changes.

The major concern with the recommendation for helmet use in sport is the phenomenon known as 'risk compensation', whereby helmeted athletes change their playing behaviour in the misguided belief that the protective equipment will stop all injury. This is where the use of protective equipment results in behavioural change such as the adoption of more dangerous playing techniques, which can result in a paradoxical increase in injury rates. This may be a particular concern in child and adolescent athletes where head injury rates are often higher than in adult athletes.[11]

Consideration of rule changes to reduce the head injury incidence or severity may be appropriate where a definite mechanism is implicated in a particular sport. An example of this is in soccer where research studies demonstrated that upper limb to head contact in heading contests accounted for approximately 50% of concussions.[12] Rule changes have recently been introduced in certain sports (e.g. rugby) to allow an effective off-field medical assessment to occur without compromising the athlete's welfare, affecting the flow of the game or unduly penalising the player's team. It is important to note that rule enforcement is a critical aspect of modifying injury risk in these settings and referees play an important role in this regard.

The competitive/aggressive nature of sport, which makes it fun to play and watch, should not be discouraged. However, sporting organisations should be encouraged to address violent conduct that may increase concussion risk. Fair play and respect should be supported as key elements of sport.[13]

THE INITIAL IMPACT: APPLIED PATHOPHYSIOLOGY

In a concussion, the athlete has sustained a significant impact to the brain. Although the pathophysiology of concussion remains poorly understood, the current consensus is that it reflects a disturbance of brain function rather than a structural injury. The impact sets in train a number of physiological mechanisms including a neurochemical metabolic cascade, lipid peroxidation, tau phosphorylation and amyloid folding, in addition to membrane gene-expression changes. Unlike more severe brain injury, these changes are not related to structural or neuropathological damage.

The concussed athlete, although conscious and without obvious focal neurological signs, may have impaired higher cortical function, for example, impaired short-term memory and speed of information processes. These subtle cognitive changes may only be detected by neuropsychological testing (discussed later in this chapter). While there are no gross structural changes on traditional imaging, newer imaging techniques (such as functional MRI or connectomics) demonstrate transient alterations in brain function following concussion. The clinical significance of these results remains unclear. Subtle functional deficits are also suggested by recent work on eye movement abnormalities in the setting of TBI. These have been used as markers in other neurological diseases (e.g. Huntington's disease) and can be measured relatively easily.

Following a blow to the head, the athlete's conscious state may be altered. This may vary from simply being stunned to a significant loss of consciousness. Memory is typically affected in a concussive episode. A period of retrograde amnesia, that is, loss of memory of events prior to the incident, or anterograde amnesia, that is, loss of memory of events after the incident, may follow minor head injury.

The ability to think clearly, concentrate on tasks and process information may also be affected. Concussive symptoms such as headache, dizziness, blurred vision and nausea, as well as reduced reaction times, may place the athlete at risk of injury if they return to sport before symptoms have resolved.

Frequently, in episodes of mild concussion ('bell ringers'), the athlete will be dazed or stunned for a period of seconds only and continue playing. The other players and coaches may be unaware that a concussive episode has occurred. Any visual clues or signs and symptoms, as highlighted on the Pocket CRT, can be indicative of concussive injury. As such, it is recommended that alert medical and training staff should closely observe the actions of a player who has received a knock to the head for signs or symptoms of concussion.

It is a key aspect of concussion management that athletes are educated regarding the significance of concussion injuries and the importance of reporting symptoms to medical staff. While athletes may try to minimise problems to avoid removal from play, they may increase their risk of short and long-term problems related to the concussion.

MANAGEMENT OF THE CONCUSSED ATHLETE

Patient management is discussed in the on-field setting and with respect to return to play.

On-field management

Every athlete who sustains a head injury is at risk of having a structural brain or neck injury (e.g. brain contusion or cervical spine fracture). One of the critical roles of the initial medical assessment is to examine the player neurologically for such injuries. Having said that, it is not possible on the sidelines to absolutely exclude structural brain injury especially when a player may have ongoing cognitive impairment that limits examination or where structural injury (e.g. subdural haematomas) may take time to develop post injury.

Clinical features that may raise concerns of structural injury include:

- the mechanism of injury, particularly if there is a high velocity of impact or collision with an unyielding body part (e.g. head to knee impact) or where the injury involves a vertical fall (e.g. fall from a horse, spear tackle in rugby)
- immediate and/or prolonged loss of consciousness
- evidence of a skull fracture and/or bleeding or cerebrospinal fluid (CSF) leak from ears/nose
- examination finding of a focal neurological deficit
- seizure
- progression of any clinical features over time.

Any deterioration in clinical state, in particular worsening headache, nausea or vomiting, or deterioration in conscious state, should raise suspicion of a structural head injury and warrant urgent investigation. Similarly, structural head injury should be kept in mind in any case where symptoms persist beyond 10 days.

A player with a suspected structural head injury requires immediate transport to a hospital with a neurosurgical unit and urgent computerised tomography (CT) brain scan to exclude intracranial pathology (e.g. haemorrhage, swelling) and to exclude/manage any associated cervical spine injury.

It is essential that all team physicians who have an on-field injury management role in their sport have formal training and certification in both first aid and trauma management. Depending upon the country concerned, there may be regional differences in certification and accreditation courses; some of the best known include Advanced Trauma Life Support (ATLS); Emergency Management of Severe Trauma (EMST); Pre-Hospital Emergency Care Course (PHECC); Pre-Hospital Trauma Life Support (PHTLS) and the British Association of Immediate Care Course (BASICS). This list is not exhaustive; all these courses deliver the skill-set required to appropriately and safely manage acute injuries. A medical degree alone is insufficient training in this regard.

The initial priorities when confronted by an acutely injured athlete are the basic principles of first aid. The simple mnemonic DRABC may be a useful aide-memoire.

D	Danger	Ensure that there are no immediate environmental dangers that may potentially injure the patient or treatment team. This may involve stopping play in a football match or marshalling cars on a motor racetrack.
R	Response	Is the patient conscious? Can he/she talk?
A	Airway	Ensure a clear and unobstructed airway. Remove any mouth guard or dental device that may be present.
B	Breathing	Ensure the patient is breathing adequately.
C	Circulation	Ensure an adequate circulation.

Once the basic first aid aspects of care have been achieved and the patient is stabilised, consideration of removal of the patient from the field to an appropriate facility for further assessment is necessary. At this time, careful assessment for the presence of a cervical spinal cord or other injury is necessary. If an alert patient complains of neck pain, has evidence of neck tenderness or deformity, or has neurological signs suggestive of a spinal injury, then neck bracing and transport on a suitable spinal frame is required. If the patient is unconscious, then a cervical injury should be assumed until proven otherwise. Airway protection takes precedence over any potential spinal injury. In this situation, the removal of helmets or other head protectors should only be performed by individuals trained in this aspect of trauma management.

The clinical management of a concussed athlete may involve the treatment of a disorientated, confused, unconscious, uncooperative or convulsing patient (see Table 20.1 for other symptoms and signs of concussion). The immediate treatment priorities remain the basic first aid principles outlined above. Once this has been established and the patient stabilised, a full medical and neurological assessment exam should follow. On site physicians are in an ideal position to initiate the critical early steps in an athlete's care to ensure optimal recovery from a head injury. Typically, with a medical doctor present on the sidelines the more detailed assessment of the injured athlete would occur in the medical rooms where a quiet and unhurried environment exists. This would be the normal situation in the case of an athlete that is conscious and without a spinal cord injury. In some situations, where no doctor is present, safe removal to a hospital emergency department is the correct approach.

When examining a concussed athlete, a full neurological examination is important. Because the major management priorities at this stage are to establish an accurate diagnosis and exclude a potentially catastrophic intracranial injury, this part of the examination should be particularly thorough. Having determined the presence of a concussive injury, the patient needs to be serially monitored until full recovery ensues. In the acute situation following a traumatic brain injury of any severity,

PART B   Regional problems

Table 20.1 **Symptoms and signs of concussion**

Symptoms	Signs
• Headache	• Loss of consciousness or impaired conscious state
• Dizziness	• Poor coordination or balance
• Nausea or vomiting	• Concussive convulsion or impact seizure
• Unsteadiness or loss of balance	• Unsteady gait or loss of balance
• Confusion	• Slow to answer questions or follow directions
• Unaware of period, opposition, score of game	• Easily distracted, poor concentration
• Feeling 'dinged', stunned or 'dazed'	• Displaying unusual or inappropriate emotions
• Seeing stars or flashing lights	• Vacant stare or glassy eyed
• Ringing in the ears	• Slurred speech
• Double vision or blurred vision	• Personality changes
	• Inappropriate playing behaviour
	• Significantly decreased playing ability
	• Double vision or blurred vision

conscious state is the key element to assess initially. This is measured in the GCS which is included in the SCAT3.

Once severe brain or cervical spine injury has been excluded, the most important components of concussion management include:

- confirming the diagnosis (includes differentiating from other pathologies, e.g. post-traumatic headaches)
- determining when the player has fully recovered so that he/she can safely return to competition.

Confirming the diagnosis

Common symptoms of concussion include headache, nausea, dizziness and balance problems, blurred vision or other visual disturbance, confusion, memory loss and a feeling of slowness or fatigue (Table 20.1). Many of these symptoms are not specific to concussion. Nevertheless, concussion should be suspected in any player who presents with any of these symptoms following a collision or direct trauma to the head. When performing an on-field assessment it is suggested that the CRT (Fig. 20.3) be utilised as a rapid means of making such assessment.

Clinical features that are more likely to suggest a diagnosis of concussion include loss of consciousness (LOC), concussive convulsions, confusion or attention deficit, memory disturbance and balance disturbance.

> **PRACTICE PEARL**
>
> If a concussion is suspected, the player should be removed from the playing environment, with appropriate care of the cervical spine and evaluated in a place free from distraction (e.g. medical room).

These may not be present in all cases and in some cases may present in a delayed fashion. The assessment as per the SCAT3 (Fig 20.2) form should be used and focus on:

- symptom checklist
- tests of cognitive function (e.g. Maddocks' questions, Standardised Assessment of Concussion [SAC])
- tests of balance function
- neurological examination.

One of the critical aspects of the SCAT3 is that it should be used after 10 minutes have passed following the injury. In that time, the clinician should ensure that the first aid priorities have been completed, a GCS recorded, spinal and other injuries excluded and the opportunity to review any video of the incident (if available) completed. This delay in the concussion assessment is important as, in many cases, the concussion injury is an evolving one and many athletes only begin to exhibit symptoms and signs several minutes after injury. If the SCAT3 is done too early following the injury, then the critical concussion features may be missed.

Any player with symptoms and/or evidence of a disturbance of cognitive function (e.g. LOC, balance disturbance, disorientation or cognitive deficit) can be considered to have a concussive injury. Once concussion is medically diagnosed then the player should be removed from the game or training and not return to play on that day (Fig 20.4). As a general rule, even in cases where the diagnosis is not entirely clear, a conservative approach should be adopted ('*If in doubt sit them out*').

For practical purposes, the CRT (Fig. 20.3) can be utilised on-field or on the sideline to screen for concussion and once concussion is diagnosed, the player removed to the medical room and the full SCAT3

Sports concussion   CHAPTER 20

SCAT3™

Sport Concussion Assessment Tool – 3rd Edition
For use by medical professionals only

B

Name _____ Date/Time of Injury: _____ Examiner: _____
                              Date of Assessment:

What is the SCAT3?[1]

The SCAT3 is a standardized tool for evaluating injured athletes for concussion and can be used in athletes aged from 13 years and older. It supersedes the original SCAT and the SCAT2 published in 2005 and 2009, respectively[2]. For younger persons, ages 12 and under, please use the Child SCAT3. The SCAT3 is designed for use by medical professionals. If you are not qualified, please use the Sport Concussion Recognition Tool[1]. Preseason baseline testing with the SCAT3 can be helpful for interpreting post-injury test scores.

Specific instructions for use of the SCAT3 are provided on page 3. If you are not familiar with the SCAT3, please read through these instructions carefully. This tool may be freely copied in its current form for distribution to individuals, teams, groups and organizations. Any revision or any reproduction in a digital form requires approval by the Concussion in Sport Group.
NOTE: The diagnosis of a concussion is a clinical judgment, ideally made by a medical professional. The SCAT3 should not be used solely to make, or exclude, the diagnosis of concussion in the absence of clinical judgement. An athlete may have a concussion even if their SCAT3 is "normal".

What is a concussion?

A concussion is a disturbance in brain function caused by a direct or indirect force to the head. It results in a variety of non-specific signs and/or symptoms (some examples listed below) and most often does not involve loss of consciousness. Concussion should be suspected in the presence of **any one or more** of the following:

- Symptoms (e.g., headache), or
- Physical signs (e.g., unsteadiness), or
- Impaired brain function (e.g. confusion) or
- Abnormal behaviour (e.g., change in personality).

SIDELINE ASSESSMENT

Indications for Emergency Management

NOTE: A hit to the head can sometimes be associated with a more serious brain injury. Any of the following warrants consideration of activating emergency procedures and urgent transportation to the nearest hospital:

- Glasgow Coma score less than 15
- Deteriorating mental status
- Potential spinal injury
- Progressive, worsening symptoms or new neurologic signs

Potential signs of concussion?

If any of the following signs are observed after a direct or indirect blow to the head, the athlete should stop participation, be evaluated by a medical professional and **should not be permitted to return to sport the same day** if a concussion is suspected.

Any loss of consciousness?	Y	N
"If so, how long?" _____		
Balance or motor incoordination (stumbles, slow/laboured movements, etc.)?	Y	N
Disorientation or confusion (inability to respond appropriately to questions)?	Y	N
Loss of memory:	Y	N
"If so, how long?" _____		
"Before or after the injury?" _____		
Blank or vacant look:	Y	N
Visible facial injury in combination with any of the above:	Y	N

1 Glasgow coma scale (GCS)

Best eye response (E)
No eye opening	1
Eye opening in response to pain	2
Eye opening to speech	3
Eyes opening spontaneously	4

Best verbal response (V)
No verbal response	1
Incomprehensible sounds	2
Inappropriate words	3
Confused	4
Oriented	5

Best motor response (M)
No motor response	1
Extension to pain	2
Abnormal flexion to pain	3
Flexion/Withdrawal to pain	4
Localizes to pain	5
Obeys commands	6

Glasgow Coma score (E + V + M)   of 15

GCS should be recorded for all athletes in case of subsequent deterioration.

2 Maddocks Score[3]

"I am going to ask you a few questions, please listen carefully and give your best effort."
Modified Maddocks questions (1 point for each correct answer)

What venue are we at today?	0	1
Which half is it now?	0	1
Who scored last in this match?	0	1
What team did you play last week/game?	0	1
Did your team win the last game?	0	1

Maddocks score   of 5

Maddocks score is validated for sideline diagnosis of concussion only and is not used for serial testing.

Notes: Mechanism of Injury ("tell me what happened"?):
_____
_____
_____
_____

Any athlete with a suspected concussion should be REMOVED FROM PLAY, medically assessed, monitored for deterioration (i.e., should not be left alone) and should not drive a motor vehicle until cleared to do so by a medical professional. No athlete diagnosed with concussion should be returned to sports participation on the day of Injury.

(a)

Figure 20.2 SCAT3™
REPRODUCED WITH PERMISSION FROM *BRITISH JOURNAL OF SPORTS MEDICINE*

PART B Regional problems

BACKGROUND

Name: _____ Date: _____
Examiner: _____
Sport/team/school: _____ Date/time of injury: _____
Age: _____ Gender: ☐ M ☐ F
Years of education completed: _____
Dominant hand: ☐ right ☐ left ☐ neither
How many concussions do you think you have had in the past? _____
When was the most recent concussion? _____
How long was your recovery from the most recent concussion? _____
Have you ever been hospitalized or had medical imaging done for a head injury? ☐ Y ☐ N
Have you ever been diagnosed with headaches or migraines? ☐ Y ☐ N
Do you have a learning disability, dyslexia, ADD/ADHD? ☐ Y ☐ N
Have you ever been diagnosed with depression, anxiety or other psychiatric disorder? ☐ Y ☐ N
Has anyone in your family ever been diagnosed with any of these problems? ☐ Y ☐ N
Are you on any medications? If yes, please list: ☐ Y ☐ N

SCAT3 to be done in resting state. Best done 10 or more minutes post excercise.

SYMPTOM EVALUATION

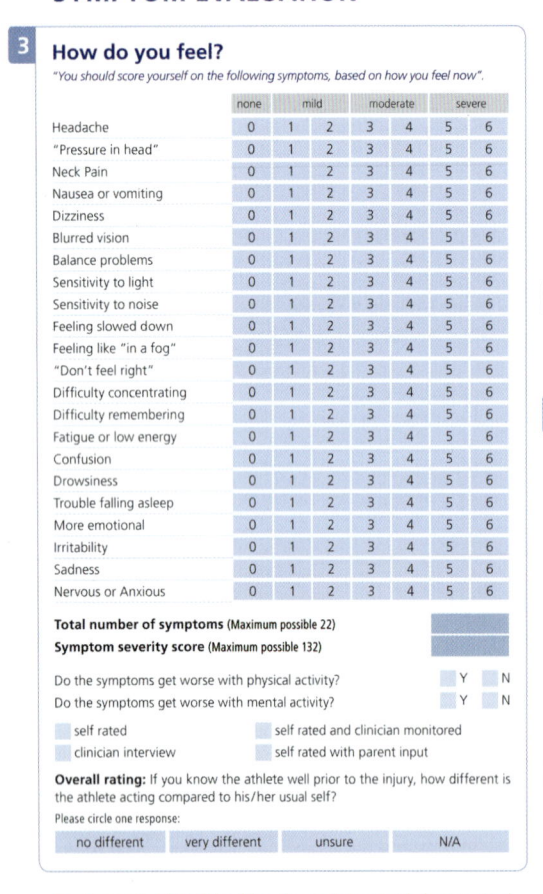

3 How do you feel?
"You should score yourself on the following symptoms, based on how you feel now".

	none		mild		moderate		severe
Headache	0	1	2	3	4	5	6
"Pressure in head"	0	1	2	3	4	5	6
Neck Pain	0	1	2	3	4	5	6
Nausea or vomiting	0	1	2	3	4	5	6
Dizziness	0	1	2	3	4	5	6
Blurred vision	0	1	2	3	4	5	6
Balance problems	0	1	2	3	4	5	6
Sensitivity to light	0	1	2	3	4	5	6
Sensitivity to noise	0	1	2	3	4	5	6
Feeling slowed down	0	1	2	3	4	5	6
Feeling like "in a fog"	0	1	2	3	4	5	6
"Don't feel right"	0	1	2	3	4	5	6
Difficulty concentrating	0	1	2	3	4	5	6
Difficulty remembering	0	1	2	3	4	5	6
Fatigue or low energy	0	1	2	3	4	5	6
Confusion	0	1	2	3	4	5	6
Drowsiness	0	1	2	3	4	5	6
Trouble falling asleep	0	1	2	3	4	5	6
More emotional	0	1	2	3	4	5	6
Irritability	0	1	2	3	4	5	6
Sadness	0	1	2	3	4	5	6
Nervous or Anxious	0	1	2	3	4	5	6

Total number of symptoms (Maximum possible 22) _____
Symptom severity score (Maximum possible 132) _____

Do the symptoms get worse with physical activity? ☐ Y ☐ N
Do the symptoms get worse with mental activity? ☐ Y ☐ N

☐ self rated ☐ self rated and clinician monitored
☐ clinician interview ☐ self rated with parent input

Overall rating: If you know the athlete well prior to the injury, how different is the athlete acting compared to his/her usual self?
Please circle one response:
no different | very different | unsure | N/A

Scoring on the SCAT3 should not be used as a stand alone method to diagnose concussion measure recovery or make decisions about an athlete s readiness to return to competition after concussion. Since signs and symptoms may evolve over time it is important to consider repeat evaluation in the acute assessment of concussion.

(b)

Figure 20.2 (cont.) SCAT3™

COGNITIVE & PHYSICAL EVALUATION

4 Cognitive assessment
Standardized Assessment of Concussion (SAC)[4]

Orientation (1 point for each correct answer)
What month is it?	0	1
What is the date today?	0	1
What is the day of the week?	0	1
What year is it?	0	1
What time is it right now? (within 1 hour)	0	1
Orientation score		of 5

Immediate memory

List	Trial 1	Trial 2	Trial 3	Alternative word list		
elbow	0 1	0 1	0 1	candle	baby	finger
apple	0 1	0 1	0 1	paper	monkey	penny
carpet	0 1	0 1	0 1	sugar	perfume	blanket
saddle	0 1	0 1	0 1	sandwich	sunset	lemon
bubble	0 1	0 1	0 1	wagon	iron	insect
Total						

Immediate memory score total _____ of 15

Concentration: Digits Backward

List	Trial 1	Alternative digit list		
4-9-3	0 1	6-2-9	5-2-6	4-1-5
3-8-1-4	0 1	3-2-7-9	1-7-9-5	4-9-6-8
6-2-9-7-1	0 1	1-5-2-8-6	3-8-5-2-7	6-1-8-4-3
7-1-8-4-6-2	0 1	5-3-9-1-4-8	8-3-1-9-6-4	7-2-4-8-5-6

Total of 4 _____

Concentration: Month in Reverse Order (1 pt. for entire sequence correct)
Dec-Nov-Oct-Sept-Aug-Jul-Jun-May-Apr-Mar-Feb-Jan 0 1

Concentration score _____ of 5

5 Neck Examination:
Range of motion   Tenderness   Upper and lower limb sensation   strength
indings: _____

Balance examination
Do one or both of the following tests.
Footwear (shoes, barefoot, braces, tape, etc.) _____

Modified Balance Error Scoring System (BESS) testing[5]
Which foot was tested (i.e. which is the non-dominant foot)   ☐ Left ☐ Right
Testing surface (hard floor, field, etc.) _____
Condition
Double leg stance: _____ Errors
Single leg stance (non-dominant foot): _____ Errors
Tandem stance (non-dominant foot at back): _____ Errors

And/Or

Tandem gait
Time (best of trials): _____ seconds

Coordination examination
Upper limb coordination
Which arm was tested: ☐ Left ☐ Right
Coordination score _____ of 1

8 SAC Delayed Recall[4]
Delayed recall score _____ of 5

INSTRUCTIONS

Words in *Italics* throughout the SCAT3 are the instructions given to the athlete by the tester.

Symptom Scale

"You should score yourself on the following symptoms, based on how you feel now".

To be completed by the athlete. In situations where the symptom scale is being completed after exercise, it should still be done in a resting state, at least 10 minutes post exercise.
For total number of symptoms, maximum possible is 22.
For Symptom severity score, add all scores in table, maximum possible is 22 x 6 = 132.

SAC[4]
Immediate Memory

"I am going to test your memory. I will read you a list of words and when I am done, repeat back as many words as you can remember, in any order."

Trials 2 & 3:

"I am going to repeat the same list again. Repeat back as many words as you can remember in any order, even if you said the word before."

Complete all 3 trials regardless of score on trial 1 & 2. Read the words at a rate of one per second. **Score 1 pt. for each correct response.** Total score equals sum across all 3 trials. Do not inform the athlete that delayed recall will be tested.

Concentration
Digits backward

"I am going to read you a string of numbers and when I am done, you repeat them back to me backwards, in reverse order of how I read them to you. For example, if I say 7-1-9, you would say 9-1-7."

If correct, go to next string length. If incorrect, read trial 2. **One point possible for each string length**. Stop after incorrect on both trials. The digits should be read at the rate of one per second.

Months in reverse order

"Now tell me the months of the year in reverse order. Start with the last month and go backward. So you'll say December, November ... Go ahead"

1 pt. for entire sequence correct

Delayed Recall

The delayed recall should be performed after completion of the Balance and Coordination Examination.

"Do you remember that list of words I read a few times earlier? Tell me as many words from the list as you can remember in any order."

Score 1 pt. for each correct response

Balance Examination

Modified Balance Error Scoring System (BESS) testing[5]

This balance testing is based on a modified version of the Balance Error Scoring System (BESS)[5]. A stopwatch or watch with a second hand is required for this testing.

"I am now going to test your balance. Please take your shoes off, roll up your pant legs above ankle (if applicable), and remove any ankle taping (if applicable). This test will consist of three twenty second tests with different stances."

(a) Double leg stance:

"The first stance is standing with your feet together with your hands on your hips and with your eyes closed. You should try to maintain stability in that position for 20 seconds. I will be counting the number of times you move out of this position. I will start timing when you are set and have closed your eyes."

(b) Single leg stance:

"If you were to kick a ball, which foot would you use? [This will be the dominant foot] Now stand on your non-dominant foot. The dominant leg should be held in approximately 30 degrees of hip flexion and 45 degrees of knee flexion. Again, you should try to maintain stability for 20 seconds with your hands on your hips and your eyes closed. I will be counting the number of times you move out of this position. If you stumble out of this position, open your eyes and return to the start position and continue balancing. I will start timing when you are set and have closed your eyes."

(c) Tandem stance:

"Now stand heel-to-toe with your non-dominant foot in back. Your weight should be evenly distributed across both feet. Again, you should try to maintain stability for 20 seconds with your hands on your hips and your eyes closed. I will be counting the number of times you move out of this position. If you stumble out of this position, open your eyes and return to the start position and continue balancing. I will start timing when you are set and have closed your eyes."

(c)

Figure 20.2 (cont.) SCAT3™

Balance testing – types of errors

1. Hands lifted off iliac crest
2. Opening eyes
3. Step, stumble, or fall
4. Moving hip into > 30 degrees abduction
5. Lifting forefoot or heel
6. Remaining out of test position > 5 sec

Each of the 20-second trials is scored by counting the errors, or deviations from the proper stance, accumulated by the athlete. The examiner will begin counting errors only after the individual has assumed the proper start position. **The modified BESS is calculated by adding one error point for each error during the three 20-second tests. The maximum total number of errors for any single condition is 10.** If a athlete commits multiple errors simultaneously, only one error is recorded but the athlete should quickly return to the testing position, and counting should resume once subject is set. Subjects that are unable to maintain the testing procedure for a minimum of **five seconds** at the start are assigned the highest possible score, ten, for that testing condition.

OPTION: For further assessment, the same 3 stances can be performed on a surface of medium density foam (e.g., approximately 50 cm x 40 cm x 6 cm).

Tandem Gait[6,7]

Participants are instructed to stand with their feet together behind a starting line (the test is best done with footwear removed). Then, they walk in a forward direction as quickly and as accurately as possible along a 38mm wide (sports tape), 3 meter line with an alternate foot heel-to-toe gait ensuring that they approximate their heel and toe on each step. Once they cross the end of the 3m line, they turn 180 degrees and return to the starting point using the same gait. A total of 4 trials are done and the best time is retained. Athletes should complete the test in 14 seconds. Athletes fail the test if they step off the line, have a separation between their heel and toe, or if they touch or grab the examiner or an object. In this case, the time is not recorded and the trial repeated, if appropriate.

Coordination Examination

Upper limb coordination
Finger-to-nose (FTN) task:

"I am going to test your coordination now. Please sit comfortably on the chair with your eyes open and your arm (either right or left) outstretched (shoulder flexed to 90 degrees and elbow and fingers extended), pointing in front of you. When I give a start signal, I would like you to perform five successive finger to nose repetitions using your index finger to touch the tip of the nose, and then return to the starting position, as quickly and as accurately as possible."

Scoring: 5 correct repetitions in < 4 seconds = 1
Note for testers: Athletes fail the test if they do not touch their nose, do not fully extend their elbow or do not perform five repetitions. **Failure should be scored as 0.**

References & Footnotes

1. This tool has been developed by a group of international experts at the 4th International Consensus meeting on Concussion in Sport held in Zurich, Switzerland in November 2012. The full details of the conference outcomes and the authors of the tool are published in The BJSM Injury Prevention and Health Protection, 2013, Volume 47, Issue 5. The outcome paper will also be simultaneously co-published in other leading biomedical journals with the copyright held by the Concussion in Sport Group, to allow unrestricted distribution, providing no alterations are made.

2. McCrory P et al., Consensus Statement on Concussion in Sport – the 3rd International Conference on Concussion in Sport held in Zurich, November 2008. British Journal of Sports Medicine 2009; 43: i76-89.

3. Maddocks, DL; Dicker, GD; Saling, MM. The assessment of orientation following concussion in athletes. Clinical Journal of Sport Medicine. 1995; 5(1): 32 – 3.

4. McCrea M. Standardized mental status testing of acute concussion. Clinical Journal of Sport Medicine. 2001; 11: 176 – 181.

5. Guskiewicz KM. Assessment of postural stability following sport-related concussion. Current Sports Medicine Reports. 2003; 2: 24 – 30.

6. Schneiders, A.G., Sullivan, S.J., Gray, A., Hammond-Tooke, G. & McCrory, P. Normative values for 16-37 year old subjects for three clinical measures of motor performance used in the assessment of sports concussions. Journal of Science and Medicine in Sport. 2010; 13(2): 196 – 201.

7. Schneiders, A.G., Sullivan, S.J., Kvarnstrom. J.K., Olsson, M., Yden. T. & Marshall, S.W. The effect of footwear and sports-surface on dynamic neurological screening in sport-related concussion. Journal of Science and Medicine in Sport. 2010; 13(4): 382 – 386

PART B Regional problems

ATHLETE INFORMATION

Any athlete suspected of having a concussion should be removed from play, and then seek medical evaluation.

Signs to watch for

Problems could arise over the first 24–48 hours. The athlete should not be left alone and must go to a hospital at once if they:

- Have a headache that gets worse
- Are very drowsy or can't be awakened
- Can't recognize people or places
- Have repeated vomiting
- Behave unusually or seem confused; are very irritable
- Have seizures (arms and legs jerk uncontrollably)
- Have weak or numb arms or legs
- Are unsteady on their feet; have slurred speech

Remember, it is better to be safe.
Consult your doctor after a suspected concussion.

Scoring Summary:

Test Domain	Score
	Date: ____ Date: ____ Date: ____
Number of Symptoms of 22	
Symptom Severity Score of 132	
Orientation of 5	
Immediate Memory of 15	
Concentration of 5	
Delayed Recall of 5	
SAC Total	
BESS (total errors)	
Tandem Gait (seconds)	
Coordination of 1	

Return to play

Athletes should not be returned to play the same day of injury.
When returning athletes to play, they should be **medically cleared and then follow a stepwise supervised program,** with stages of progression.

For example:

Rehabilitation stage	Functional exercise at each stage of rehabilitation	Objective of each stage
No activity	Physical and cognitive rest	Recovery
Light aerobic exercise	Walking, swimming or stationary cycling keeping intensity, 70% maximum predicted heart rate. No resistance training	Increase heart rate
Sport-specific exercise	Skating drills in ice hockey, running drills in soccer. No head impact activities	Add movement
Non-contact training drills	Progression to more complex training drills, eg passing drills in football and ice hockey. May start progressive resistance training	Exercise, coordination, and cognitive load
Full contact practice	Following medical clearance participate in normal training activities	Restore confidence and assess functional skills by coaching staff
Return to play	Normal game play	

There should be at least 24 hours (or longer) for each stage and if symptoms recur the athlete should rest until they resolve once again and then resume the program at the previous asymptomatic stage. Resistance training should only be added in the later stages.

If the athlete is symptomatic for more than 10 days, then consultation by a medical practitioner who is expert in the management of concussion, is recommended.

Medical clearance should be given before return to play.

Notes:

CONCUSSION INJURY ADVICE

(To be given to the **person monitoring** the concussed athlete)

This patient has received an injury to the head. A careful medical examination has been carried out and no sign of any serious complications has been found. Recovery time is variable across individuals and the patient will need monitoring for a further period by a responsible adult. Your treating physician will provide guidance as to this timeframe.

If you notice any change in behaviour, vomiting, dizziness, worsening headache, double vision or excessive drowsiness, please contact your doctor or the nearest hospital emergency department immediately.

Other important points:

- Rest (physically and mentally), including training or playing sports until symptoms resolve and you are medically cleared
- No alcohol
- No prescription or non-prescription drugs without medical supervision.
  Specifically:
  · No sleeping tablets
  · Do not use aspirin, anti-inflammatory medication or sedating pain killers
- Do not drive until medically cleared
- Do not train or play sport until medically cleared

Clinic phone number _____

Patient's name _____
Date/time of injury _____
Date/time of medical review _____
Treating physician _____

Contact details or stamp

(d)

Figure 20.2 (cont.) SCAT3™

Sports concussion — CHAPTER 20

Figure 20.3 Pocket Concussion Recognition Tool™ (CRT)[2]
REPRODUCED WITH PERMISSION FROM *BRITISH JOURNAL OF SPORTS MEDICINE*

Pocket CONCUSSION RECOGNITION TOOL™
To help identify concussion in children, youth and adults

RECOGNIZE & REMOVE
Concussion should be suspected **if one or more** of the following visible clues, signs, symptoms or errors in memory questions are present.

1. Visible clues of suspected concussion
Any one or more of the following visual clues can indicate a possible concussion:

- Loss of consciousness or responsiveness
- Lying motionless on ground / Slow to get up
- Unsteady on feet / Balance problems or falling over / Incoordination
- Grabbing / Clutching of head
- Dazed, blank or vacant look
- Confused / Not aware of plays or events

2. Signs and symptoms of suspected concussion
Presence of any one or more of the following signs & symptoms may suggest a concussion:

- Loss of consciousness
- Seizure or convulsion
- Balance problems
- Nausea or vomiting
- Drowsiness
- More emotional
- Irritability
- Sadness
- Fatigue or low energy
- Nervous or anxious
- "Don't feel right"
- Difficulty remembering
- Headache
- Dizziness
- Confusion
- Feeling slowed down
- "Pressure in head"
- Blurred vision
- Sensitivity to light
- Amnesia
- Feeling like "in a fog"
- Neck Pain
- Sensitivity to noise
- Difficulty concentrating

3. Memory function
Failure to answer any of these questions correctly may suggest a concussion.

- "What venue are we at today?"
- "Which half is it now?"
- "Who scored last in this game?"
- "What team did you play last week / game?"
- "Did your team win the last game?"

Any athlete with a suspected concussion should be IMMEDIATELY REMOVED FROM PLAY, and should not be returned to activity until they are assessed medically. Athletes with a suspected concussion should not be left alone and should not drive a motor vehicle.

It is recommended that, in all cases of suspected concussion, the player is referred to a medical professional for diagnosis and guidance as well as return to play decisions, even if the symptoms resolve.

RED FLAGS
If ANY of the following are reported then the player should be safely and immediately removed from the field. If no qualified medical professional is available, consider transporting by ambulance for urgent medical assessment:

- Athlete complains of neck pain
- Increasing confusion or irritability
- Repeated vomiting
- Seizure or convulsion
- Weakness or tingling / burning in arms or legs
- Deteriorating conscious state
- Severe or increasing headache
- Unusual behaviour change
- Double vision

Remember:
- In all cases, the basic principles of first aid (danger, response, airway, breathing, circulation) should be followed.
- Do not attempt to move the player (other than required for airway support) unless trained to so do
- Do not remove helmet (if present) unless trained to do so.

from McCrory et. al, Consensus Statement on Concussion in Sport. Br J Sports Med 47 (5), 2013
© 2013 Concussion in Sport Group

---

assessment tool used by the attending physician. If the diagnosis of concussion is confirmed following the medical assessment, the player should not be returned to play on the day and serial monitoring should be commenced immediately. New portable technologies are continually being incorporated into acute sports concussion assessment; however, research is yet to establish how effective and clinically applicable these new methods are.[14]

In addition to post-injury assessment, it is recommended that the SCAT3 be used by medical staff for pre-season baseline testing. This may be helpful for interpreting post-concussion test scores as it provides an objective record of possible change. More importantly, it provides an educative opportunity for the physician to highlight the importance of reporting all concussive injuries.

Does amnesia associate with injury severity?

There is renewed interest in post-traumatic amnesia and its role as a surrogate measure of injury severity.

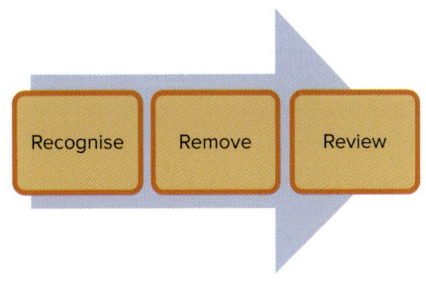

Figure 20.4 Recognition of concussion, removal from play, and review and assessment of the athlete are the key steps in management

Post-traumatic amnesia can be separated into retrograde amnesia (loss of memory prior to injury) and anterograde amnesia (loss of memory post injury). Virtually all concussed athletes will have periods of amnesia, however brief, whether they were unconscious or not.

> **PRACTICE PEARL**
>
> In broad terms, the duration of post-traumatic amnesia does not reflect the severity of concussion or mild TBI. This contrasts with moderate to severe traumatic brain injury where post-traumatic amnesia is a prognostic factor and should be assessed in all cases.

Note that retrograde amnesia varies depending on when it is measured after injury; thus, it is a particularly poor indicator of injury severity.

The number and duration of the clinical post-concussive symptoms may be more important than the presence or duration of amnesia alone. The overall clinical management and return to play depends on the presence and recovery of all symptoms and signs.

Does an acutely concussed athlete need to go to hospital or have urgent neuroimaging?

The treating clinician may face the decision of whether the athlete should be referred on to a hospital emergency facility or for urgent neuroimaging. In general terms, an uncomplicated concussion does not need routine neuroimaging. Imaging, however, has a role in the exclusion of suspected intracranial injury and the indications are listed in the box. Apart from 'cookbook' type approaches, referral to such a centre depends on the experience, ability and competency of the physician at hand. If the team physician happens to be an SEM physician, neurologist or neurosurgeon experienced in concussion management, the clinical referral pathways will be different to a family practitioner called to assist at a football match after an injury has occurred.

> **PRACTICE PEARL**
>
> The overall approach should be 'when in doubt, refer'.

Other diagnostic tests such as biomarkers, EEG and functional MRI brain scanning do not have a role in the early diagnosis and management of a concussion injury, except in an experimental or research context.[15] Structural neuroimaging such as CT and MRI does not clinically add to a diagnosis of concussion; however, these have an important role in excluding more significant injuries.

How should acute concussion be graded?

There is no reliable or scientifically validated system of grading the severity of sports-related concussion. At the present time, there are at least 45 published anecdotal

> **Indications for urgent imaging or hospital referral**
>
> Any player who has or develops the following:
> - fractured skull
> - penetrating skull trauma
> - deterioration in conscious state following injury
> - focal neurological signs
> - confusion or impairment of consciousness >30 minutes
> - loss of consciousness >1 minute
> - persistent vomiting or increasing headache post injury
> - any convulsive movements
> - more than one episode of concussive injury in a match or training session
> - where there is assessment difficulty (e.g. an intoxicated patient)
> - all children with head injuries
> - high-risk patients (e.g. haemophilia, anticoagulant use)
> - inadequate post injury supervision
> - high-risk injury mechanism (e.g. high velocity impact, missile injury).

severity scales. The danger is that athletes and/or their coaches may 'shop around' for a scale that is not in their best medical interests. At the end of the day, good clinical judgment should prevail over written guidelines. At all four international conferences on concussion in sport to date, the expert committee has strongly recommended that combined measures of recovery should be used to assess injury severity and guide individual decisions on return to play.[5] Individual assessment was strongly re-endorsed at the 2012 Zurich meeting.[6]

Determining when the player can return safely to competition

Return-to-play decisions remain difficult. Expert consensus guidelines recommend that players should **not** return to competition until they have recovered **completely** from their concussive injury. The majority (80-90%) of clinical symptoms and cognitive deficits resolve in a relatively short 7–10 day period. MRI diffusion or connectomic radiological changes may still be present for longer; however, the significance of such changes is unknown.[16-18] Children and adolescents may take longer to recover from concussive injuries.[19]

Currently, there is no single gold standard measure of brain disturbance and recovery following concussion. It should be noted that most athletes wanting to return to play will report 'feeling fine'. Therefore, clinicians should incorporate both subjective and objective measures to determine readiness to return to play (RTP). In practical terms, this can involve a multifaceted and multidisciplinary clinical approach, which includes assessment of symptoms, signs (such as balance) and cognitive function.

Return to play on the day of injury

> **PRACTICE PEARL**
>
> The Zurich consensus group reaffirmed the previous general management principle that no return to play on the day should be contemplated for a concussed athlete.

There is published evidence in high school and college athletes that RTP on the day of injury resulted in delayed and prolonged cognitive deterioration. It is not within the scope or expertise of a physiotherapist, trainer or other non-medical person to manage a concussive injury or determine the timing of return to play. A player should never RTP while symptomatic: 'When in doubt, sit them out!'

Return to play during the subsequent week(s)

Whether or not to allow the concussed athlete to return to training and then competition is one of the most difficult decisions the SEM physician must make. In minor cases of concussion, where all symptoms resolve quickly and there is no sign of cortical dysfunction, or evidence of impairment of short-term memory or information processing, the player may be allowed to return once recovered. Neuropsychological testing may be used to confirm full recovery. A player permitted to return to play should be closely observed for any signs of impaired function. A multifaceted clinical approach is used to manage players following injury (Fig. 20.5). In practical terms, this involves five sequential steps:

1. a brief period of cognitive and physical rest to facilitate recovery
2. monitoring for recovery of post-concussion symptoms and signs
3. the use of neuropsychological tests to estimate recovery of cognitive function
4. a graduated return to activity with monitoring for recurrence of symptoms
5. a final medical clearance before resuming full contact training and/or playing.

Period of cognitive and physical rest to facilitate recovery

Early rest is important to allow recovery following a concussive injury; however, prolonged rest may be counterproductive.[20, 21] In the immediate post-concussion stage (24–48 hours), physical activity, physiological stress (e.g. altitude and flying) and cognitive loads (e.g. studying, video games or computer work) can all worsen symptoms and possibly delay recovery. Players should be advised to rest from these activities in the early stages after a concussive injury, especially while symptomatic (see 'Concussion injury advice', p. 4 of the SCAT3). Similarly, the use of alcohol, narcotic analgesics, anti-inflammatory medication or sedatives can exacerbate symptoms following head trauma, delay recovery or mask deterioration, and should also be avoided. Specific advice should also be given on avoidance of activities that place the individual at risk of further injury (e.g. driving).

The recovery and outcome of concussion may be modified by a number of factors that may require more sophisticated management strategies. The Zurich consensus panel agreed that a range of 'modifying' factors may influence the investigation and management of concussion and, in some cases, may predict the potential for prolonged or persistent symptoms.[6, 22] These modifiers would also be important to consider in a detailed concussion history and are outlined in Table 20.2.

When these modifying influences are present, simple RTP advice may be inappropriate. It may be wise to consider additional investigations including: formal neuropsychological testing, balance assessment and neuroimaging. It is envisioned that athletes with such modifying features would be managed in a multidisciplinary manner coordinated by a physician with specific expertise in the management of concussive injury.

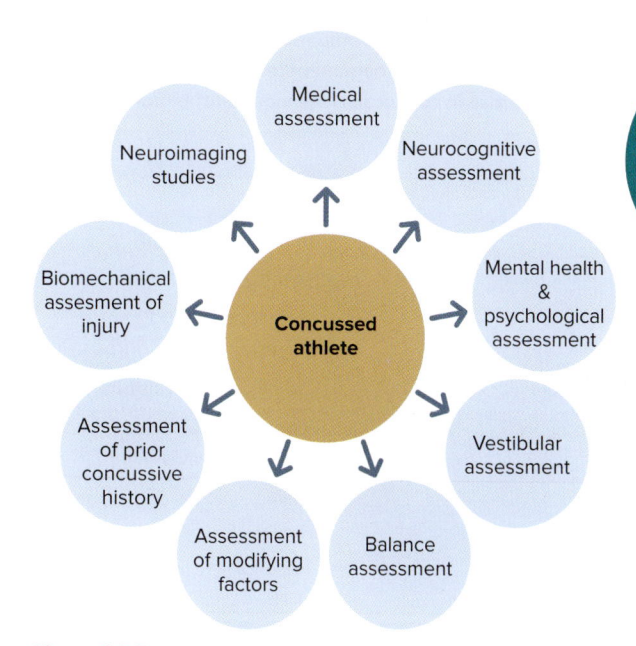

Figure 20.5 Multimodality concussion assessment

PART B Regional problems

Table 20.2 Factors that influence whether investigation or more sophisticated management (e.g. referral to a physician with expertise in concussion management) is indicated

Factors	Modifier
Symptoms	Number
	Duration (>10 days)
	Severity
Signs	Prolonged LOC (>1 min), amnesia
Sequelae	Concussive convulsions
Temporal	Frequency—repeated concussions over time
	Timing—injuries close together in time
	'Recency'—recent concussion or TBI
Threshold	Repeated concussions occurring with progressively less impact force or slower recovery after each successive concussion.
Age	Child and adolescent (<18 years old)
Co- and pre-morbidities	Migraine, depression or other mental health disorders, attention deficit hyperactivity disorder (ADHD), learning disabilities (LD), sleep disorders
Medication	Psychoactive drugs, anticoagulants
Behaviour	Dangerous style of play
Sport	High-risk activity, contact and collision sport, high sporting level

Monitoring for recovery of post-concussion symptoms and signs

The symptoms of concussion are dynamic and evolve over time. It is important that players who are suspected of having a concussion be monitored over time to assess for delayed symptom onset. Monitoring of post-concussion symptoms and signs can be facilitated by the use of the SCAT3.

Use of neuropsychological tests to estimate recovery of cognitive function

Cognitive deficits associated with concussion are typically subtle and may exist in a number of domains. Common deficits that follow concussion in sport include reduced attention and ability to process information, slowed reaction times and impaired memory.

The use of neuropsychological tests in the management of concussion overcomes the reliance on subjective symptoms, which are known to be poorly recognised and variably reported. It allows detection of cognitive deficits, which have been observed to outlast symptoms in many cases of concussion.

There are a number of levels of complexity of cognitive testing, including:

- formal neuropsychological testing
- screening computerised cognitive test batteries
- basic paper-and-pencil evaluation (i.e. SCAT3).

Formal neuropsychological testing performed by trained neuropsychologists remains the clinical best practice standard for the assessment of cognitive function.[23] Formal testing is logistically impractical for routine use following all concussive injuries, but is recommended in any case where there is uncertainty about recovery or in difficult cases (e.g. prolonged recovery).

Screening computerised cognitive tests provide a practical alternative for the assessment of cognitive recovery. Ideally, the tests should be compared to the individual's own pre-injury baseline. A number of screening computerised cognitive test batteries have been validated for use following concussion in sport and are readily available. These include test platforms such as CogState Sport/Axon Sports (www.cogstate.com/go/Sport), ImPACT (www.impacttest.com) and the US military-developed tool Automated Neuropsychological Assessment Metrics (ANAM) (www.armymedicine.army.mil/prr/anam.html).

Computerised tests provide a quick, valid and reliable measure of cognitive recovery following a concussive injury. Furthermore, routine use of computerised screening tests in the pre-season facilitates screening of players for cognitive deterioration over time.

Basic paper-and-pencil cognitive tests (e.g. SCAT3, Fig. 20.2) are the quickest and simplest of the cognitive screening tests; however, they are the least sensitive to subtle cognitive changes that accompany concussion. In cases where the concussion has resulted in brief symptoms and clinically the player has recovered well, basic paper-and-pencil cognitive tests can be used to provide an estimate of cognitive function. The use of a basic paper-and-pencil evaluation should be combined with a conservative return to play approach and careful monitoring of symptoms as the player progresses through a graduated RTP program.

Overall, it is important to remember that neuropsychological testing is only one component of assessment and therefore should not be the sole basis of management decisions. Neuropsychological testing

Sports concussion — CHAPTER 20

does not replace the need for a full history and clinical/neurological assessment.

Graduated return to activity

Following a concussive injury, players should be returned to play in a graduated fashion once clinical features have resolved and cognitive function returned to 'baseline'. When considering RTP the athlete should be off any medications prescribed in the management of the concussion at the time of considering commencement of the rehabilitation phase or at the final medical assessment.

In accordance with current consensus guidelines, there is no mandatory period of time that a player must be withheld from play following a concussion. However, at minimum, a player must be symptom free at rest and with exertion and determined to have returned to baseline level of cognitive performance.

The Zurich consensus statement recommends a stepwise Graduated Return to Play Protocol (Table 20.3). If a player remains asymptomatic for 24 hours at level 1, they may progress to level 2. They are allowed to advance provided that they remain asymptomatic. Using this protocol, an athlete should take approximately 1 week before returning to normal game play. If any symptoms surface during the progression, players should drop back to the previous level in which they were asymptomatic for a further 24 hours before attempting to progress again.

A final medical clearance before resuming full contact training and/or playing

A player who has suffered from a concussive injury must not be allowed to return to play before having a medical clearance. In every case, the decision regarding the timing of return to training should be made by a medical doctor with experience in concussive injuries. This assessment is multidimensional and based on evidence of resolution of the athlete's symptoms, physical signs and cognitive deficit. Ideally, concussed players should be examined by an experienced medical practitioner with the decision about RTP based on the clinical findings and, if possible, neuropsychological testing. In general, a more conservative approach (i.e. longer time to return to sport) is used in cases where there is any uncertainty about the player's recovery ('If in doubt, sit them out').

In a number of contact sports, such as boxing and rugby (previously), authorities have legislated for a mandatory exclusion period from competition for concussed players. While the intent of such a policy is praiseworthy, an arbitrary exclusion period is hard to justify scientifically as each episode of concussion requires individual evaluation. For some players, the period of exclusion will be too long and for other players not long enough. More importantly, the assumption that a player has recovered simply because a prescribed period of time has passed has the potential to lead to premature return to play and resultant problems.

The risk of premature return to play and concussion sequelae

There are several risks associated with premature RTP.

Risk of further injury

The principal concern of premature RTP of a concussed athlete is that due to the impaired cognitive function (e.g. slowed information processing, reduced attention) the

Table 20.3 Graduated Return to Play Protocol

Rehabilitation stage	Functional exercise at each stage of rehabilitation	Objective at each stage
1. No activity	Complete physical (no training, playing, exercise, weights etc.) and cognitive rest (no television, extensive reading, video games etc.)	Recovery* Beware of exertion with activities of daily living and caution regarding daytime sleep
2. Light aerobic exercise	Walking, swimming or stationary cycling keeping intensity <70% HR max. No resistance training	Increase heart rate
3. Sport-specific exercise	Skating drills in ice hockey, running drills in soccer. No head-impact activities	Add movement
4. Non-contact training drills	Progression to more complex training drills, e.g. passing drills in hockey and football	Exercise, coordination and cognitive load
5. Full contact practice	Following medical clearance participate in normal training activities	Restore confidence and assess functional skills by coaching staff
6. Return to play	Normal game play	

Reproduced with permission from Table 1: Zurich consensus statement in BJSM[3]

athlete will sustain further injury (both concussive and other) when returning to a dangerous playing environment.

Second impact syndrome
Second impact syndrome (SIS) is frequently mentioned in the concussion literature, but surprisingly, has little scientific evidence for its existence. It is a term used to describe the potential catastrophic consequences resulting from a second concussive blow to the head before an individual has fully recovered from the symptoms of a previous concussion. The second head injury is believed to result in loss of cerebrovascular auto-regulation, which in turn leads to brain swelling secondary to increased cerebral blood flow. Mortality in this condition approaches 100%. The evidence that repeated concussion was a risk factor for SIS has been critically reviewed and published cases of SIS were classified as definite, probable, possible or not SIS according to four criteria.[24]

Seventeen published cases of SIS were identified from the literature. None were classified as 'definite' SIS, five were considered to be 'probable' SIS cases and 12 were classified as 'not' SIS primarily because there was an absence of a witnessed second impact. In addition, the veracity of teammate recall of concussive episodes, which is often the basis of a 'first impact' in such cases, was shown to be unreliable. Based on these results, the investigators concluded that there is a lack of evidence to support the claim that the second impact is a risk factor for diffuse cerebral swelling.

In the review paper,[24] the central issue is whether repeated concussion was a risk factor for cerebral swelling which is the putative definition of SIS. There is published evidence that acute (and delayed) brain swelling may occur following a single blow to the head, in association with a structural injury such as a subdural haematoma and in disorders of calcium channels, suggesting a possible genetic basis for some of these cases. Such events are virtually only seen in children and adolescents.

Concussive convulsions
A variety of immediate motor phenomena (e.g. tonic posturing) or convulsive movements may accompany a concussion. Although dramatic, these clinical features are generally benign and require no specific management beyond the standard treatment of the underlying concussive injury. These dramatic phenomena are a non-epileptic manifestation of concussion.[25]

Prolongation of symptoms
If a player recommences playing while symptomatic, post-concussive symptoms may be prolonged. It is important to be aware that studies have demonstrated measurable cognitive deficits in individuals even after the symptoms have resolved, which argues for an increasingly conservative RTP strategy.[17] Premature RTP may also increase the chance of developing the 'post-concussive syndrome', in which fatigue, difficulty in concentration and headaches persist for some time, often months, following the original injury. This syndrome is uncommon in sport. These patients should undergo formal neuropsychological testing as well as an MRI brain scan and be evaluated by a physician experienced in concussion management. Other potential contributing factors should be assessed and treated where appropriate, for example vestibular system disturbance.

Chronic traumatic encephalopathy (CTE)
Recent publications have suggested that US footballers may suffer similar neuropathological risks to boxers. Pathological case reports and cross-sectional studies have suggested that retired NFL footballers, who have had recurrent concussions during their sporting careers, disproportionately suffer from mild cognitive impairment, depression and other mental health problems. What is becoming increasingly clear from a number of diverse lines of research is that a percentage of footballers seem to suffer chronic or long-term sequelae.[26] While there has been an association demonstrated between recurrent head trauma and appearance of abnormal Tau protein in post-mortem assessment of brains, whether this is a consequence of head injury, the effect of brain injury on ageing, or the development of neurodegenerative disease unrelated to sports participation is unclear. At this time, very little is known about what type, frequency or amount of trauma is necessary to induce the accumulation of pathological proteins in the brain and more importantly why only a small number of athletes are at risk of CTE.[18] Nevertheless, until these issues are resolved, it is recommended that conservative management strategies are used to ensure player welfare.

Mental health issues
Mental health issues (e.g. depression) have been reported as a long-term consequence of traumatic brain injury including sports-related concussion. Neuroimaging studies using functional MRI (fMRI) suggest that a depressed mood following concussion may reflect an underlying pathophysiological abnormality consistent with a limbic-frontal model of depression. All players with ongoing symptoms or a prolonged clinical course should be screened for depression.

THE 'DIFFICULT' CONCUSSION
A 'difficult' concussion can be defined as one in which clinical recovery falls outside the expected window (i.e. 10–14 days).[17] The incidence of persistent symptoms

following sports-related concussion varies from about 10-30% depending on the cohort being investigated and definitions used.

Clinical assessment

Common persistent symptoms include headache, dizziness, mood changes (e.g. depression/anxiety), 'difficulty concentrating', irritability, 'fatigue or low energy', 'difficulty sleeping' or 'feeling not quite right, in a fog or slowed down'. The symptoms are non-specific and overlap with other conditions such as structural head injury, cervicogenic headaches and anxiety/depression. Clinical assessment, therefore, requires careful history and a detailed, multimodal examination (including neurological, cognitive function, cervical spine, balance and vestibular function).

Role of investigations

Formal neuropsychological testing is useful to identify persistent cognitive deficits, monitor recovery and help guide return to school or work plans.

Conventional neuroimaging (CT or MRI) should be considered in any athlete with persistent symptoms where there is any suspicion of an underlying structural brain injury. Advanced neuroimaging and other investigation techniques (e.g. diffusion tensor imaging, fMRI, magnetic resonance spectroscopy, electroencephalography) have demonstrated changes in cohorts of patients with persistent symptoms. Changes have also been observed in subjects well after clinical recovery following sports-related concussion. At present, the clinical significance of these changes remains unclear. Consequently, the use of advanced investigation techniques is currently not recommended in the routine management of athletes with concussion.

Treatment

A brief period of rest is important in the acute period following sports-related concussion. There is no evidence, however, that prolonged rest is beneficial for athletes with persistent symptoms. Preliminary studies demonstrate that an active rehabilitation program ('sub-symptom threshold activity') may be useful for the management of cases where symptoms are prolonged.[27-28] Cervicovestibular rehabilitation may also be useful to facilitate recovery in cases with persistent symptoms.[29]

Other treatments may be used to manage specific symptoms. For example, manual or physical therapy may be used to treat myofascial pain or neck trigger points contributing to headaches; cognitive therapy may be useful for some patients with persistent cognitive symptoms; and meditation, biofeedback or psychological therapy may benefit those who have problems with psychological symptoms.

Medications are often used to treat specific symptoms (e.g. analgesics for headache, anti-depressants), although there is limited evidence for their use in the setting of persistent post-concussive symptoms.

Overall, the difficult concussion should be managed in a multi-disciplinary manner. Ideally, this is in the setting of a concussion clinic with access to expertise in a wide range of areas.

CHILDREN AND CONCUSSION IN SPORT

The CRT (Fig. 20.3) aims to identify concussion in children, youth and adults. It is simple to use and is designed so that anyone can use it. This tool is particularly useful at children's sports events that may not have a recognised health professional present. If a concussive injury is suspected, the child should be removed from play and sent urgently for medical evaluation.[16] It is never appropriate for a child or adolescent athlete with concussion to return to play on the same day as the injury regardless of the level of athletic performance.

For medical assessments in this setting, the SCAT3 (Fig. 20.2) is appropriate for use in children and adolescents older than 13 years of age and the Child SCAT3 (Fig. 20.6) for 12 years and under. An additional consideration in assessing the child or adolescent athlete with a concussion is the need to include parent input as well as teacher and school input when appropriate.

The decision to use neuropsychological testing is broadly the same as the adult assessment paradigm. However, timing of testing may differ in order to assist planning in school and home management (and may be performed while the child is still symptomatic). If cognitive testing is performed then it must be developmentally sensitive until late teen years due to the ongoing cognitive maturation that occurs during this period which, in turn, makes the utility of comparison to either the person's own baseline or to population norms limited. In this age group it is more important to consider the use of trained neuropsychologists to interpret assessment data, particularly in children with learning disorders and/or ADHD who may need more sophisticated assessment strategies.

Children should not be returned to practice or play until clinically completely symptom free, which may require a longer time frame than for adults. In addition, the concept of 'cognitive rest' is highlighted with special reference to a child's need to limit exertion with activities of daily living and to limit scholastic and other cognitive stressors (e.g. text messaging, video games) while symptomatic.

PART B Regional problems

Child-SCAT3™
Sport Concussion Assessment Tool for children ages 5 to 12 years
For use by medical professionals only

What is childSCAT3?[1]

The ChildSCAT3 is a standardized tool for evaluating injured children for concussion and can be used in children aged from 5 to 12 years. It supersedes the original SCAT and the SCAT2 published in 2005 and 2009, respectively[2]. For older persons, ages 13 years and over, please use the SCAT3. The ChildSCAT3 is designed for use by medical professionals. If you are not qualified, please use the Sport Concussion Recognition Tool[3]. Preseason baseline testing with the ChildSCAT3 can be helpful for interpreting post-injury test scores.

Specific instructions for use of the ChildSCAT3 are provided on page 3. If you are not familiar with the ChildSCAT3, please read through these instructions carefully. This tool may be freely copied in its current form for distribution to individuals, teams, groups and organizations. Any revision and any reproduction in a digital form require approval by the Concussion in Sport Group.

NOTE: The diagnosis of a concussion is a clinical judgment, ideally made by a medical professional. The ChildSCAT3 should not be used solely to make, or exclude, the diagnosis of concussion in the absence of clinical judgement. An athlete may have a concussion even if their ChildSCAT3 is "normal".

What is a concussion?

A concussion is a disturbance in brain function caused by a direct or indirect force to the head. It results in a variety of non-specific signs and/or symptoms (like those listed below) and most often does not involve loss of consciousness. Concussion should be suspected in the presence of any one or more of the following:
- Symptoms (e.g., headache), or
- Physical signs (e.g., unsteadiness), or
- Impaired brain function (e.g. confusion) or
- Abnormal behaviour (e.g., change in personality).

SIDELINE ASSESSMENT

Indications for Emergency Management

NOTE: A hit to the head can sometimes be associated with a more severe brain injury. If the concussed child displays any of the following, then do not proceed with the ChildSCAT3; instead activate emergency procedures and urgent transportation to the nearest hospital:

- Glasgow Coma score less than 15
- Deteriorating mental status
- Potential spinal injury
- Progressive, worsening symptoms or new neurologic signs
- Persistent vomiting
- Evidence of skull fracture
- Post traumatic seizures
- Coagulopathy
- History of Neurosurgery (eg Shunt)
- Multiple injuries

1 Glasgow coma scale (GCS)

Best eye response (E)	
No eye opening	1
Eye opening in response to pain	2
Eye opening to speech	3
Eyes opening spontaneously	4

Best verbal response (V)	
No verbal response	1
Incomprehensible sounds	2
Inappropriate words	3
Confused	4
Oriented	5

Best motor response (M)	
No motor response	1
Extension to pain	2
Abnormal flexion to pain	3
Flexion/Withdrawal to pain	4
Localizes to pain	5
Obeys commands	6

Glasgow Coma score (E + V + M)	of 15

GCS should be recorded for all athletes in case of subsequent deterioration.

Potential signs of concussion?

If any of the following signs are observed after a direct or indirect blow to the head, the child should stop participation, be evaluated by a medical professional and **should not be permitted to return to sport the same day** if a concussion is suspected.

Any loss of consciousness?	Y	N
"If so, how long?"		
Balance or motor incoordination (stumbles, slow/laboured movements, etc.)?	Y	N
Disorientation or confusion (inability to respond appropriately to questions)?	Y	N
Loss of memory:	Y	N
"If so, how long?"		
"Before or after the injury?"		
Blank or vacant look:	Y	N
Visible facial injury in combination with any of the above:	Y	N

2 Sideline Assessment – child-Maddocks Score[3]

"I am going to ask you a few questions, please listen carefully and give your best effort."

Modified Maddocks questions (1 point for each correct answer)

Where are we at now?	0	1
Is it before or after lunch?	0	1
What did you have last lesson/class?	0	1
What is your teacher's name?	0	1
child-Maddocks score		of 4

Child-Maddocks score is for sideline diagnosis of concussion only and is not used for serial testing.

Any child with a suspected concussion should be REMOVED FROM PLAY, medically assessed and monitored for deterioration (i.e., should not be left alone). No child diagnosed with concussion should be returned to sports participation on the day of Injury.

BACKGROUND

Name: _____   Date/Time of Injury: _____
Examiner: _____   Date of Assessment: _____
Sport/team/school: _____
Age: _____   Gender: M   F
Current school year/grade: _____
Dominant hand: right   left   neither
Mechanism of Injury ("tell me what happened"?): _____

For Parent/carer to complete:

How many concussions has the child had in the past?		
When was the most recent concussion?		
How long was the recovery from the most recent concussion?		
Has the child ever been hospitalized or had medical imaging done (CT or MRI) for a head injury?	Y	N
Has the child ever been diagnosed with headaches or migraines?	Y	N
Does the child have a learning disability, dyslexia, ADD/ADHD, seizure disorder?	Y	N
Has the child ever been diagnosed with depression, anxiety or other psychiatric disorder?	Y	N
Has anyone in the family ever been diagnosed with any of these problems?	Y	N
Is the child on any medications? If yes, please list:	Y	N

(a)

Figure 20.6 Child SCAT3™
REPRODUCED WITH PERMISSION FROM *BRITISH JOURNAL OF SPORTS MEDICINE*

Sports concussion — CHAPTER 20

SYMPTOM EVALUATION

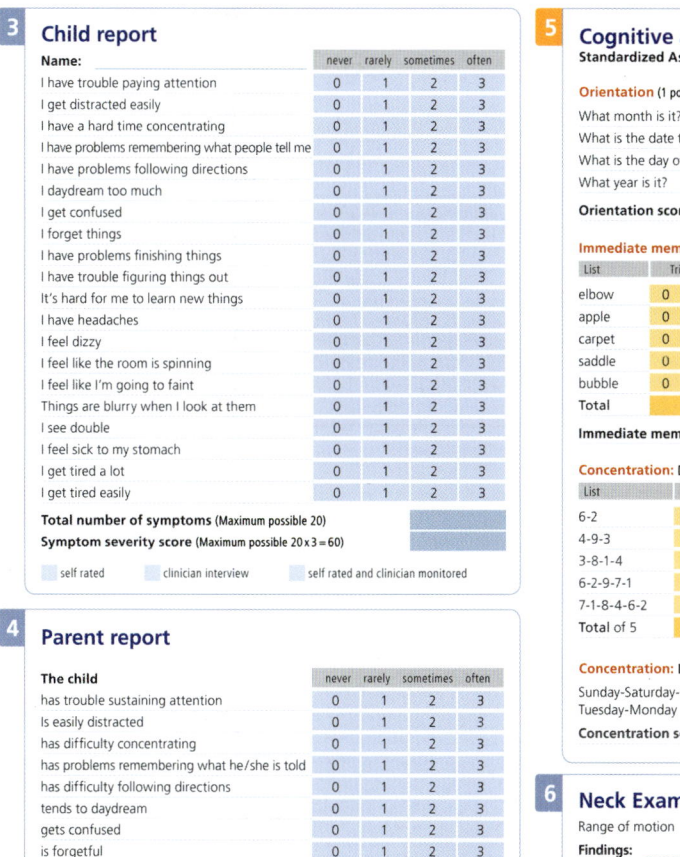

3 Child report

Name: _____

	never	rarely	sometimes	often
I have trouble paying attention	0	1	2	3
I get distracted easily	0	1	2	3
I have a hard time concentrating	0	1	2	3
I have problems remembering what people tell me	0	1	2	3
I have problems following directions	0	1	2	3
I daydream too much	0	1	2	3
I get confused	0	1	2	3
I forget things	0	1	2	3
I have problems finishing things	0	1	2	3
I have trouble figuring things out	0	1	2	3
It's hard for me to learn new things	0	1	2	3
I have headaches	0	1	2	3
I feel dizzy	0	1	2	3
I feel like the room is spinning	0	1	2	3
I feel like I'm going to faint	0	1	2	3
Things are blurry when I look at them	0	1	2	3
I see double	0	1	2	3
I feel sick to my stomach	0	1	2	3
I get tired a lot	0	1	2	3
I get tired easily	0	1	2	3

Total number of symptoms (Maximum possible 20) _____
Symptom severity score (Maximum possible 20 x 3 = 60) _____

☐ self rated ☐ clinician interview ☐ self rated and clinician monitored

4 Parent report

The child	never	rarely	sometimes	often
has trouble sustaining attention	0	1	2	3
is easily distracted	0	1	2	3
has difficulty concentrating	0	1	2	3
has problems remembering what he/she is told	0	1	2	3
has difficulty following directions	0	1	2	3
tends to daydream	0	1	2	3
gets confused	0	1	2	3
is forgetful	0	1	2	3
has difficulty completeing tasks	0	1	2	3
has poor problem solving skills	0	1	2	3
has problems learning	0	1	2	3
has headaches	0	1	2	3
feels dizzy	0	1	2	3
has a feeling that the room is spinning	0	1	2	3
feels faint	0	1	2	3
has blurred vision	0	1	2	3
has double vision	0	1	2	3
experiences nausea	0	1	2	3
gets tired a lot	0	1	2	3
gets tired easily	0	1	2	3

Total number of symptoms (Maximum possible 20) _____
Symptom severity score (Maximum possible 20 x 3 = 60) _____

Do the symptoms get worse with physical activity? ☐ Y ☐ N
Do the symptoms get worse with mental activity? ☐ Y ☐ N

☐ parent self rated ☐ clinician interview ☐ parent self rated and clinician monitored

Overall rating for parent/teacher/coach/carer to answer.
How different is the child acting compared to his/her usual self?
Please circle one response:

| no different | very different | unsure | N/A |

Name of person completing Parent-report: _____
Relationship to child of person completing Parent-report: _____

Scoring on the ChildSCAT3 should not be used as a stand-alone method to diagnose concussion, measure recovery or make decisions about an athlete's readiness to return to competition after concussion.

(b)

Figure 20.6 (cont.) Child SCAT3™

COGNITIVE & PHYSICAL EVALUATION

5 Cognitive assessment
Standardized Assessment of Concussion – Child Version (SAC-C)[4]

Orientation (1 point for each correct answer)

What month is it?	0	1
What is the date today?	0	1
What is the day of the week?	0	1
What year is it?	0	1
Orientation score		of 4

Immediate memory

List	Trial 1	Trial 2	Trial 3	Alternative word list
elbow	0 1	0 1	0 1	candle baby finger
apple	0 1	0 1	0 1	paper monkey penny
carpet	0 1	0 1	0 1	sugar perfume blanket
saddle	0 1	0 1	0 1	sandwich sunset lemon
bubble	0 1	0 1	0 1	wagon iron insect
Total				

Immediate memory score total _____ of 15

Concentration: Digits Backward

List	Trial 1	Alternative digit list		
6-2	0 1	5-2	4-1	4-9
4-9-3	0 1	6-2-9	5-2-6	4-1-5
3-8-1-4	0 1	3-2-7-9	1-7-9-5	4-9-6-8
6-2-9-7-1	0 1	1-5-2-8-6	3-8-5-2-7	6-1-8-4-3
7-1-8-4-6-2	0 1	5-3-9-1-4-8	8-3-1-9-6-4	7-2-4-8-5-6
Total of 5				

Concentration: Days in Reverse Order (1 pt. for entire sequence correct)

Sunday-Saturday-Friday-Thursday-Wednesday-Tuesday-Monday   0   1

Concentration score _____ of 6

6 Neck Examination:
Range of motion   Tenderness   Upper and lower limb sensation & strength
Findings: _____

7 Balance examination
Do one or both of the following tests.
Footwear (shoes, barefoot, braces, tape, etc.) _____

Modified Balance Error Scoring System (BESS) testing[5]
Which foot was tested (i.e. which is the non-dominant foot)   ☐ Left ☐ Right
Testing surface (hard floor, field, etc.) _____
Condition
Double leg stance: _____ Errors
Tandem stance (non-dominant foot at back): _____ Errors

Tandem gait[6,7]
Time taken to complete (best of 4 trials): _____ seconds
If child attempted, but unable to complete tandem gait, mark here ☐

8 Coordination examination
Upper limb coordination
Which arm was tested: ☐ Left ☐ Right
Coordination score _____ of 1

9 SAC Delayed Recall[4]
Delayed recall score _____ of 5

Since signs and symptoms may evolve over time, it is important to consider repeat evaluation in the acute assessment of concussion.

PART B   Regional problems

INSTRUCTIONS

Words in *Italics* throughout the ChildSCAT3 are the instructions given to the child by the tester.

Sideline Assessment – child-Maddocks Score

To be completed on the sideline/in the playground, immediately following concussion. There is no requirement to repeat these questions at follow-up.

Symptom Scale[8]

In situations where the symptom scale is being completed after exercise, it should still be done in a resting state, at least 10 minutes post exercise.

On the day of injury
- the child is to complete the Child Report, according to how he/she feels now.

On all subsequent days
- the child is to complete the Child Report, according to how he/she feels today, **and**
- the parent/carer is to complete the Parent Report according to how the child has been over the previous 24 hours.

Standardized Assessment of Concussion – Child Version (SAC-C)[4]

Orientation
Ask each question on the score sheet. A correct answer for **each question scores 1 point.** If the child does not understand the question, gives an incorrect answer, or no answer, then the score for that question is 0 points.

Immediate memory
"I am going to test your memory. I will read you a list of words and when I am done, repeat back as many words as you can remember, in any order."

Trials 2 & 3:
"I am going to repeat the same list again. Repeat back as many words as you can remember in any order, even if you said the word before."

Complete all 3 trials regardless of score on trial 1 & 2. Read the words at a rate of one per second. **Score 1 pt. for each correct response.** Total score equals sum across all 3 trials. Do not inform the child that delayed recall will be tested.

Concentration
Digits Backward:
"I am going to read you a string of numbers and when I am done, you repeat them back to me backwards, in reverse order of how I read them to you. For example, if I say 7-1, you would say 1-7."

If correct, go to next string length. If incorrect, read trial 2. **One point possible for each string length.** Stop after incorrect on both trials. The digits should be read at the rate of one per second.

Days in Reverse Order:
"Now tell me the days of the week in reverse order. Start with Sunday and go backward. So you'll say Sunday, Saturday ... Go ahead"

1 pt. for entire sequence correct

Delayed recall
The delayed recall should be performed after completion of the Balance and Coordination Examination.
"Do you remember that list of words I read a few times earlier? Tell me as many words from the list as you can remember in any order."

Circle each word correctly recalled. **Total score equals number of words recalled.**

Balance examination

These instructions are to be read by the person administering the childSCAT3, and each balance task **should be demonstrated to the child.** The child should then be asked to copy what the examiner demonstrated.

Modified Balance Error Scoring System (BESS) testing[5]

This balance testing is based on a modified version of the Balance Error Scoring System (BESS)[5]. A stopwatch or watch with a second hand is required for this testing.

"I am now going to test your balance. Please take your shoes off, roll up your pant legs above ankle (if applicable), and remove any ankle taping (if applicable). This test will consist of two different parts."

(a) Double leg stance:
The first stance is standing with the feet together with hands on hips and with eyes closed. The child should try to maintain stability in that position for 20 seconds. You should inform the child that you will be counting the number of times the child moves out of this position. You should start timing when the child is set and the eyes are closed.

(b) Tandem stance:
Instruct the child to stand heel-to-toe with the non-dominant foot in the back. Weight should be evenly distributed across both feet. Again, the child should try to maintain stability for 20 seconds with hands on hips and eyes closed. You should inform the child that you will be counting the number of times the child moves out of this position. If the child stumbles out of this position, instruct him/her to open the eyes and return to the start position and continue balancing. You should start timing when the child is set and the eyes are closed.

(c)

Balance testing – types of errors - Parts (a) and (b)

1. Hands lifted off iliac crest
2. Opening eyes
3. Step, stumble, or fall
4. Moving hip into > 30 degrees abduction
5. Lifting forefoot or heel
6. Remaining out of test position > 5 sec

Each of the 20-second trials is scored by counting the errors, or deviations from the proper stance, accumulated by the child. The examiner will begin counting errors only after the child has assumed the proper start position. **The modified BESS is calculated by adding one error point for each error during the two 20-second tests. The maximum total number of errors for any single condition is 10.** If a child commits multiple errors simultaneously, only one error is recorded but the child should quickly return to the testing position, and counting should resume once subject is set. Children who are unable to maintain the testing procedure for a minimum of **five seconds** at the start are assigned the highest possible score, ten, for that testing condition.

OPTION: For further assessment, the same 2 stances can be performed on a surface of medium density foam (e.g., approximately 50cm x 40cm x 6cm).

Tandem Gait[6,7]
Use a clock (with a second hand) or stopwatch to measure the time taken to complete this task. Instruction for the examiner – **Demonstrate the following to the child:**

*The child is instructed to stand with their feet together behind a starting line (the test is best done with footwear removed). Then, they walk in a forward direction as quickly and as accurately as possible along a 38mm wide (sports tape), 3 meter line with an alternate foot heel-to-toe gait ensuring that they approximate their heel and toe on each step. Once they cross the end of the 3m line, they turn 180 degrees and return to the starting point using the same gait. **A total of 4 trials are done and the best time is retained.** Children fail the test if they step off the line, have a separation between their heel and toe, or if they touch or grab the examiner or an object. In this case, the time is not recorded and the trial repeated, if appropriate.*

Explain to the child that you will time how long it takes them to walk to the end of the line and back.

Coordination examination

Upper limb coordination
Finger-to-nose (FTN) task:
The tester should **demonstrate it to the child.**

"I am going to test your coordination now. Please sit comfortably on the chair with your eyes open and your arm (either right or left) outstretched (shoulder flexed to 90 degrees and elbow and fingers extended). When I give a start signal, I would like you to perform five successive finger to nose repetitions using your index finger to touch the tip of the nose as quickly and as accurately as possible."

Scoring: 5 correct repetitions in < 4 seconds = 1
Note for testers: Children fail the test if they do not touch their nose, do not fully extend their elbow or do not perform five repetitions. **Failure should be scored as 0.**

References & Footnotes

1. This tool has been developed by a group of international experts at the 4th International Consensus meeting on Concussion in Sport held in Zurich, Switzerland in November 2012. The full details of the conference outcomes and the authors of the tool are published in The BJSM Injury Prevention and Health Protection, 2013, Volume 47, Issue 5. The outcome paper will also be simultaneously co-published in other leading biomedical journals with the copyright held by the Concussion in Sport Group, to allow unrestricted distribution, providing no alterations are made.

2. McCrory P et al., Consensus Statement on Concussion in Sport – the 3rd International Conference on Concussion in Sport held in Zurich, November 2008. British Journal of Sports Medicine 2009; 43: i76-89.

3. Maddocks, DL; Dicker, GD; Saling, MM. The assessment of orientation following concussion in athletes. Clinical Journal of Sport Medicine. 1995; 5(1): 32–3.

4. McCrea M. Standardized mental status testing of acute concussion. Clinical Journal of Sport Medicine. 2001; 11: 176–181.

5. Guskiewicz KM. Assessment of postural stability following sport-related concussion. Current Sports Medicine Reports. 2003; 2: 24–30.

6. Schneiders, A.G., Sullivan, S.J., Gray, A., Hammond-Tooke, G. & McCrory, P. Normative values for 16-37 year old subjects for three clinical measures of motor performance used in the assessment of sports concussions. Journal of Science and Medicine in Sport. 2010; 13(2): 196–201.

7. Schneiders, A.G., Sullivan, S.J., Kvarnstrom. J.K., Olsson, M., Yden. T. & Marshall, S.W. The effect of footwear and sports-surface on dynamic neurological screening in sport-related concussion. Journal of Science and Medicine in Sport. 2010; 13(4): 382–386

8. Ayr, L.K., Yeates, K.O., Taylor, H.G., & Brown, M. Dimensions of post-concussive symptoms in children with mild traumatic brain injuries. Journal of the International Neuropsychological Society. 2009; 15:19–30.

Figure 20.6 (cont.) Child SCAT3™

Sports concussion CHAPTER 20

CHILD ATHLETE INFORMATION

Any child suspected of having a concussion should be removed from play, and then seek medical evaluation. The child must NOT return to play or sport on the same day as the suspected concussion.

Signs to watch for

Problems could arise over the first 24–48 hours. The child should not be left alone and must go to a hospital at once if they develop any of the following:

- New Headache, or Headache gets worse
- Persistent or increasing neck pain
- Becomes drowsy or can't be woken up
- Can not recognise people or places
- Has Nausea or Vomiting
- Behaves unusually, seems confused, or is irritable
- Has any seizures (arms and/or legs jerk uncontrollably)
- Has weakness, numbness or tingling (arms, legs or face)
- Is unsteady walking or standing
- Has slurred speech
- Has difficulty understanding speech or directions

Remember, it is better to be safe.
Always consult your doctor after a suspected concussion.

Return to school

Concussion may impact on the child's cognitive ability to learn at school. This must be considered, and medical clearance is required before the child may return to school. **It is reasonable for a child to miss a day or two of school after concussion, but extended absence is uncommon.** In some children, a graduated return to school program will need to be developed for the child. The child will progress through the return to school program provided that there is no worsening of symptoms. If any particular activity worsens symptoms, the child will abstain from that activity until it no longer causes symptom worsening. Use of computers and internet should follow a similar graduated program, provided that it does not worsen symptoms. This program should include communication between the parents, teachers, and health professionals and will vary from child to child. The return to school program should consider:

- Extra time to complete assignments/tests
- Quiet room to complete assignments/tests
- Avoidance of noisy areas such as cafeterias, assembly halls, sporting events, music class, shop class, etc
- Frequent breaks during class, homework, tests
- No more than one exam/day
- Shorter assignments
- Repetition/memory cues
- Use of peer helper/tutor
- Reassurance from teachers that student will be supported through recovery through accommodations, workload reduction, alternate forms of testing
- Later start times, half days, only certain classes

The child is not to return to play or sport until he/she has successfully returned to school/learning, without worsening of symptoms. Medical clearance should be given before return to play.

If there are any doubts, management should be referred to a qualified health practitioner, expert in the management of concussion in children.

Return to sport

There should be no return to play until the child has successfully returned to school/learning, without worsening of symptoms.
Children must not be returned to play the same day of injury.
When returning children to play, they should **medically cleared and then follow a stepwise supervised program**, with stages of progression.

For example:

Rehabilitation stage	Functional exercise at each stage of rehabilitation	Objective of each stage
No activity	Physical and cognitive rest	Recovery
Light aerobic exercise	Walking, swimming or stationary cycling keeping intensity, 70% maximum predicted heart rate. No resistance training	Increase heart rate
Sport-specific exercise	Skating drills in ice hockey, running drills in soccer. No head impact activities	Add movement
Non-contact training drills	Progression to more complex training drills, eg passing drills in football and ice hockey. May start progressive resistance training	Exercise, coordination, and cognitive load
Full contact practice	Following medical clearance participate in normal training activities	Restore confidence and assess functional skills by coaching staff
Return to play	Normal game play	

There should be approximately 24 hours (or longer) for each stage and the child should drop back to the previous asymptomatic level if any post-concussive symptoms recur. Resistance training should only be added in the later stages.
If the child is symptomatic for more than 10 days, then review by a health practitioner, expert in the management of concussion, is recommended.
Medical clearance should be given before return to play.

Notes:

CONCUSSION INJURY ADVICE FOR THE CHILD AND PARENTS/CARERS
(To be given to the **person monitoring** the concussed child)

This child has received an injury to the head. A careful medical examination has been carried out and no sign of any serious complications has been found. It is expected that recovery will be rapid, but the child will need monitoring for the next 24 hours by a responsible adult.

If you notice any change in behavior, vomiting, dizziness, worsening headache, double vision or excessive drowsiness, please call an ambulance to transport the child to hospital immediately.

Other important points:

- Following concussion, the child should rest for at least 24 hours.
- The child should avoid any computer, internet or electronic gaming activity if these activities make symptoms worse.
- The child should not be given any medications, including pain killers, unless prescribed by a medical practitioner.
- The child must not return to school until medically cleared.
- The child must not return to sport or play until medically cleared.

Patient's name
Date/time of injury
Date/time of medical review
Treating physician

Contact details or stamp

Clinic phone number

(d)

Figure 20.6 (cont.) Child SCAT3™

315

PART B Regional problems

School attendance and activities should be considered and modified as appropriate to avoid provocation of symptoms.

Due to the different physiological response and longer recovery after concussion, and specific risks (e.g. diffuse cerebral swelling) related to head impact during childhood and adolescence, a more conservative RTP approach is recommended.[22] It is appropriate to extend the amount of time of asymptomatic rest and/or the length of the graded exertion in children and adolescents. In the management paradigm of children post concussion, return to school should be achieved prior to consideration of return to sport.

REFERENCES

References for this chapter can be found at www.mhhe.com/au/CSM5e

Chapter 21

Headache

with TOBY HALL

In the beginner's mind there are many possibilities, in the expert's mind there are few.
Shunryu Suzuki, *Zen Mind, Beginner's Mind*

Headache is one of the most prevalent pain conditions present at all stages of life. It affects the majority of the global population and is among the top 10 causes of disability.[1] Despite this, the burden of headache has been largely underestimated, with headache disorders often dismissed as minor and undeserving of medical care.[1, 2] Although athletes suffer from the same causes of headache as non-athletes, there are several key causes of headache that relate directly to exercise or to the sport itself. An additional factor to consider is that headache can impair both training and sports performance.

The International Headache Society (IHS) classifies headache into a range of disorders comprising three broad categories with more than 300 underlying headache forms.[3] The majority of these disorders are not particularly relevant to an athletic population or the IHS definitions do not adequately cover the symptoms experienced by athletes.[4] Figure 21.1 lists the broad classification according to the IHS and the common headache disorders seen in sport.

HEADACHE IN SPORT

The prevalence of headache directly related to sport has been poorly investigated or reported, although there is increasing attention in contact sport on concussion or trauma-related headache.[5] In a New Zealand university setting, 35% of athletes surveyed reported headaches, both traumatic and non-traumatic.[6] Importantly, 54% of people who reported headache associated with sport or exercise gave up their activity.[7] In some codes of football, more than 50% of athletes experience regular headaches from matches and training.[4]

While the latest edition of the IHS headache classification is comprehensive, it is not aimed specifically at a sporting setting. Williams and Nukada proposed a simple framework for specific sporting headaches.[8] This included:

- effort-exertional headache
- effort migraine
- trauma-triggered migraine
- post-traumatic headache.

An alternative sports-specific headache organisational framework has been proposed that incorporates the non-sporting as well as sporting headaches.[9] Headaches are categorised as follows:

- a recognised headache syndrome (migraine, tension-type headache, cluster headache) coincidental to sporting activity

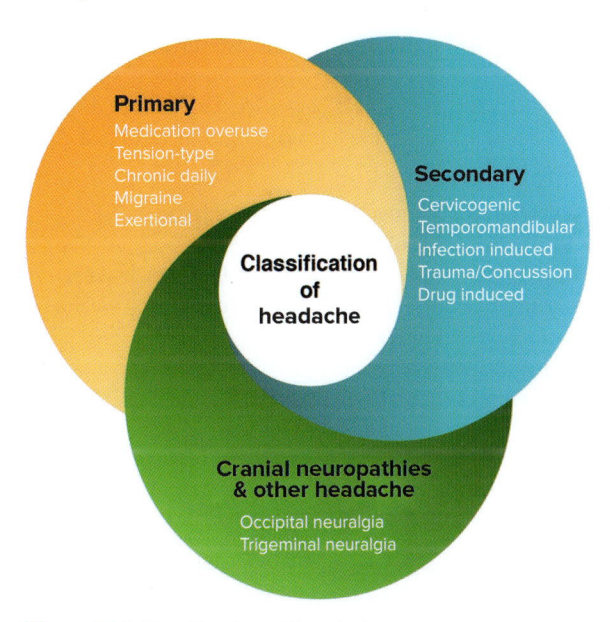

Figure 21.1 Classification of headache

Primary
Medication overuse
Tension-type
Chronic daily
Migraine
Exertional

Secondary
Cervicogenic
Temporomandibular
Infection induced
Trauma/Concussion
Drug induced

Cranial neuropathies & other headache
Occipital neuralgia
Trigeminal neuralgia

Classification of headache

- headache arising from mechanisms that occur during exertion; these can be primary (mechanism unknown) or secondary where a causal factor can be demonstrated, such as a headache:
  - related to changes in cardiovascular parameters
  - related to trauma
  - arising from structures in the neck
  - arising from mechanisms that are specific to an individual sport.

CLINICAL APPROACH TO THE PATIENT WITH HEADACHE

Headache is an unusual condition being both a symptom and a disease, which can make diagnosis and management challenging. Of primary importance is identifying when headache is a symptom of serious pathology such as a tumour, aneurysm, meningitis, subdural haemorrhage or space-occupying lesion. These are life-threatening events that the clinician must be vigilant for, and if suspected require urgent medical evaluation. Hence, a good knowledge of the following warning signals, or red flags, is essential:

- new, unaccustomed or atypical headache
- stiff neck or meningeal signs
- systemic symptoms (e.g. fever, weight loss, malaise)
- neurological symptoms (e.g. drowsiness, weakness, numbness of limbs)
- local extracranial symptoms (e.g. ear, sinus, teeth)
- changes in the pattern of headache
- headache increasing over a few days
- sudden onset of severe headache or headaches that wake the patient
- headache triggered by cough or Valsalva.

The majority of headaches are benign and do not require such intensive medical assessment.

> **PRACTICE PEARL**
>
> In each case, the clinician should seek a potential underlying cause for the headache, as this will influence management.

Common illnesses that may provoke headache include respiratory tract infection, sinusitis and influenza. Drug-induced headaches are also common. The most common are alcohol and caffeine, but many other commonly used drugs can also provoke headache including analgesics, antibiotics, antifungals and antihypertensives. Of particular importance is the frequency of analgesic use. Analgesic medication used on more than 15 days per month may sensitise the trigeminocervical nucleus, and is defined as medication overuse headache.[10] A thorough knowledge of the patient's drug history is therefore important.

Following the exclusion of headaches associated with red flags, drugs and infections, the clinician aims to differentiate between the more common headache categories: either primary or secondary headache. Primary headache includes migraine, exertional headache and tension-type headache. Secondary headache includes cervicogenic headache, temporomandibular dysfunction headache and concussion headache arising from musculoskeletal dysfunction around the neck and orofacial region.

Exertional headache follows exercise, and concussion post-traumatic headache follows a history of trauma. Tension-type headache typically presents without features of migraine or cervicogenic headache, and tends to be of a low-grade frequent bilateral headache described as pressing or squeezing. In contrast, differentiating cervicogenic headache from migraine is more challenging.

Although a comprehensive large-scale survey of people with 'pure' migraine and cervicogenic headache found that each has distinctive features (Table 21.1),[11, 12] in many cases features coexist, which makes a definitive diagnosis difficult.

History

Headache location is unilateral in cervicogenic headache,[13] but is less so in migraine, often starting on one side of the head and spreading to the opposite side during a migraine attack. The presence of associated neck and arm symptoms should also be noted. Cervicogenic headache usually starts in the neck before spreading to the head, whereas migraine starts in the head and spreads to the neck.

The nature of onset can be informative. A sudden onset of severe, unfamiliar headache, with altered consciousness or cognition, may indicate a cerebral haemorrhage or other intracerebral pathology.[14] Cervicogenic headache typically has a more gradual onset. A recent history of a head and neck trauma, with or without concussion, is also relevant.

The intensity and temporal pattern is helpful in diagnosis. Migraine is episodic and more severe than cervicogenic headache, building up to a crescendo in a set time period (24–48 hours), unless early preventive analgesic medication is taken. Cervicogenic headache is typically less severe, does not have a set time period and does not progressively increase in intensity unless the provocative stimulus is maintained.

The relationship between exercise and headache onset is informative. Although exercise usually aggravates headaches of all types, brief episodes of headache brought

Table 21.1 Summary of subjective diagnostic criteria contrasting migraine and cervicogenic headache[9, 10]

	Migraine	Cervicogenic headache
Gender ratio	1.7 female/male	0.7 female/male
Age at onset	18 years	33 years
Headache onset	Anterior head	Posterior head/neck
Pain area	50% unilateral	Predominantly unilateral
Nausea	Frequent	Infrequent
Photo/phonophobia	Very frequent	Infrequent
Throbbing pain	Frequent	Infrequent
Pain on trunk forward bend	Very frequent	Infrequent
Migraine medication	Usually helpful	Not helpful
Neck position pain	Rare	Universal

on by exercise may indicate exertional headache. More prolonged headache brought on by exercise might indicate cervicogenic headache or exertional migraine. Hence, a cyclist who develops headache while riding could have exertional headache, but equally if they have an inadequately set-up bike and associated poor posture this might be causing stress on the neck and hence cervicogenic headache. Once migraine has started, exercise is usually provocative. Conversely, aerobic exercise may be helpful in reducing the frequency of headache attacks.[15]

> **PRACTICE PEARL**
>
> Headache aggravated by specific neck movements or postures in sport may indicate cervicogenic headache, and identifying provocative movement is usually helpful for planning manual therapy.

Rest usually helps alleviate all headache forms during an attack. For example, migraine is usually relieved by sleep, but this might not always be the case for cervicogenic headache, particularly if the sleeping position, mattress or pillow is not suitable.

Prior to the onset of migraine headache, there may be associated visual or sensory symptoms (migraine with aura). Photophobia, phonophobia, nausea and vomiting are also commonly associated with migraine headache and usually occur concurrently with the headache episode. The presence of neurological symptoms or systemic symptoms such as weight loss and malaise is a 'red flag' and may indicate a more serious cause of headache (e.g. tumour).

Common forms of secondary headache are associated with symptoms in the upper or lower respiratory tract, sinuses and temporomandibular joints (jaw clicking or painful limitation of mouth opening), or influenza-like symptoms. These features should be looked for to enable differentiation from primary headache.

A past history of head trauma, even if relatively minor, may be significant as subdural heamatoma may present well after the trauma, even weeks later. Previous problems such as encephalitis or major systemic illnesses should also be recorded.

Psychological comorbidities are factors in cases where headache becomes long lasting, such as in chronic migraine where headache persists for more than 3 months.[16] An assessment of life stresses is an important part of the history. These include personal relationships, work pressures and problems related to the athlete's sporting activity. Identified problems require management as part of an overall care package.

Clinical measurement of headache

Headache is a complex multidimensional problem, which needs to be assessed using a range of different measurement tools including diaries and questionnaires. There are specific instruments that measure headache burden and severity.[17] Primary measures of headache include attack frequency or headache days per month, which can be combined with headache severity and duration to form an index.[18] Additional parameters include measures of disability and quality of life such as the headache disability inventory,[19] as well as medication consumption, psychiatric symptoms, stress and coping, and treatment satisfaction. Simply measuring headache frequency, intensity and duration as an outcome measure may be problematic as people tend

PART B   Regional problems

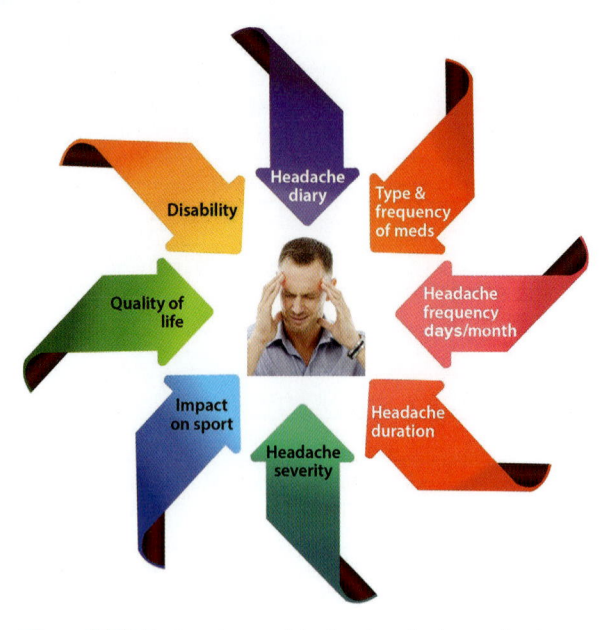

Figure 21.2 Factors to consider in a headache evaluation

to either underestimate or overestimate their symptoms depending on how they feel at the time they are asked.[17] Hence evaluating a range of headache parameters is likely to give a clearer, bias-free estimate of change. Figure 21.2 illustrates typical measurements taken during evaluation.

Examination

In all patients presenting with headache, a full neurological examination is required, and the skull, cervical spine and orofacial region must always be carefully examined. The examination should consist of some or all of the following components depending on the presence or absence of specific symptoms in the history:

- general appearance
- mental state
- speech
- skull examination
- cervical spine examination
- temporomandibular joint
- gait and stance
- pupils and fundi
- special senses (e.g. smell, vision, hearing)
- other cranial nerves
- motor system
- sensory system
- general examination.

PRIMARY HEADACHE

Primary headache includes migraine, tension-type headache, medication overuse headache, exercise-related headache and some types of post-traumatic headache.

In the general population, the 1-year prevalence rate for primary headache is 62%.[20] By survey, approximately 40% of migraine sufferers experience migraine precipitated by exercise, and 34% of Australian rules football players suffered migraine according to IHS criteria, a rate higher than population controls.[7] In that study, almost 60% of subjects experienced regular headaches related to sport.[4]

Migraine

Previously primary headache, in particular migraine, was thought to be a vascular disorder, or due to cortical spreading depression. More recent evidence points to abnormality of brain function leading to a chain of events in the periphery.[21-23] In simple terms, migraine pain can be thought of as an altered perception of normality, such that normal sensory input is misinterpreted as pain.[24] This concept of the variable modulation of sensory input is explained in Lorimer Moseley's YouTube video 'Why things hurt' (http://ow.ly/S9n0h). (See also Chapters 5 and 6.)

The neuroanatomical basis for migraine is the trigeminocervical nucleus. The migraine pain process is likely to be a combination of direct factors, that is, activation of the trigeminal nociceptors, in concert with a reduction in the normal functioning of the centrally mediated endogenous pain control pathways that normally gate that pain.[25] Thus there are both central and peripheral mechanisms involved.

Migraine is broadly categorised into migraine with and without aura. An aura is a specific set of neurological symptoms that typically precede the headache which include visual disturbances (e.g. scotomas), paraesthesia, vertigo, hemiplegia and ophthalmoplegia. Although most people think of migraine as headache alone, the true migraine sufferer usually notices a spectrum of symptoms, including nausea, vomiting, diarrhoea and weight gain. The important point for sports clinicians is that there does not have to be an aura. The IHS criteria for the diagnosis of migraine without aura are shown in Table 21.2.[3]

Clinical features

The typical features of migraine are precipitation by a change in homeostasis such as tiredness, temperature, altitude, thirst, hunger or stress. Ensuing headache pain is described as sharp and intense, throbbing or beating in time with their pulse. Commonly, it begins in the temple or forehead on both sides. When it starts on one side, it may spread to the other side. Occasionally, the headache begins at the back of the head and moves forwards.

The common neurological accompaniments to migraine with aura are visual. Patients speak of bright or dark objects often to one side of the visual field. These objects may shine or flicker and typically move across the visual field. The visual symptoms usually last about 20 minutes

Headache CHAPTER 21

Table 21.2 Diagnostic criteria for migraine without aura[3]

A. At least five attacks fulfilling criteria B–D below
B. Headache attacks lasting 4–72 hours
C. Headache has at least two of the following four characteristics:
  1. unilateral location
  2. pulsating quality
  3. moderate or severe pain intensity
  4. aggravation by or causing avoidance of routine physical activity (e.g. walking or climbing stairs)
D. During headache at least one of the following:
  1. nausea and/or vomiting
  2. photophobia and phonophobia
E. Not better accounted for by another diagnosis

and most often clear before the sensory, cognitive or headache symptoms begin. Sensory symptoms are usually described as tingling, pricking or pins and needles. These commonly commence in the face or fingers and gradually spread up the limb or over the same side of the body. Nausea, vomiting and dizziness are common during or after the attack.

Precipitating factors in migraine

A number of precipitating factors in addition to a change in homeostasis are commonly found in association with migraine headaches. These are:

- endocrine changes (e.g. premenstrual or menstrual, oral contraceptive pills, pregnancy, puberty, menopause, hyperthyroidism)
- metabolic changes (e.g. anaemia, thyroid disease)
- infective causes (e.g. fever, rhinitis)
- change in activity including extreme exercise
- alcohol
- drugs (e.g. glyceryl trinitrate [nitroglycerine], nitrates, indometacin).

Chocolate and cheese are anecdotally reported triggers of migraine, but this is not confirmed in trials.[26]

Treatment

Although sleep and resting quietly in a dark room often helps alleviate a migraine attack, the primary method of active treatment is typically pharmacological. High-dose aspirin (ASA) (900 to 1200 mg), often combined with an antiemetic, is the drug of choice in the acute phase. Other acute agents such oral, intranasal or parenteral triptans may be used as rescue medications if the initial therapy is unsuccessful. Determining the best drug option depends on a number of patient factors as well as the nature of the headache and timing of treatment. This is best done by a medical practitioner experienced in this area. A person experiencing frequent or disabling migraine episodes,

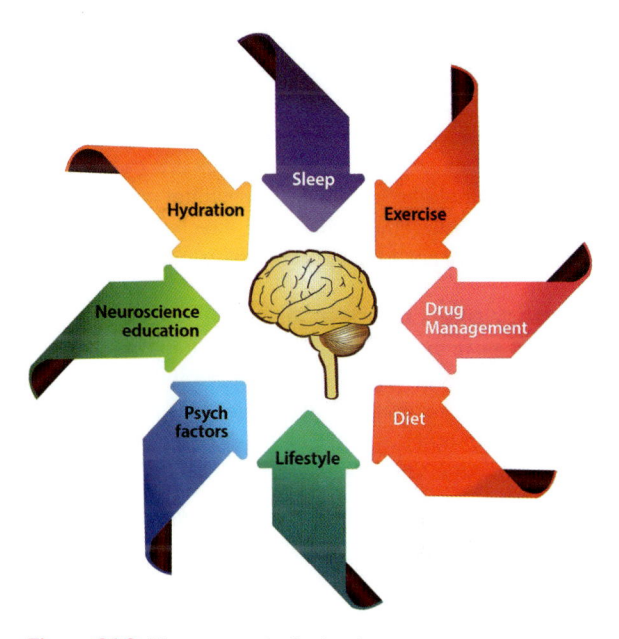

Figure 21.3 Management of migraine

especially when he or she is losing considerable time off work or school, may find prophylactic therapy necessary.

The long-term management of migraine should be multifactorial (Fig. 21.3). An important part of this plan is to identify and avoid precipitating factors. Central to this is the patient's understanding of homeostasis, maintaining equilibrium through adequate diet, hydration and sleep, as well as reducing stress and anxiety.[27] Neuroscience education may also be valuable in this regard, and involves the careful explanation of pain mechanisms and central sensitisation. Other options include traditional herbal remedies such as 'feverfew'.

Exercise can induce and exacerbate migraine, but exercise can also activate a pain modulatory mechanism, ideal in the management of migraine.[28] The prophylactic effects of exercise in migraine were shown in a randomised controlled trial.[29] Intervention comprised three arms: home relaxation; controlled aerobic exercise on a static bike; or the oral medication topiramate. The study included an extended follow-up period. Exercise was equally effective as medication in reducing episodes of migraine. A second pilot study evaluated the effects of an 8-week running program and also found positive benefits compared to a control group.[15]

It is critical in the management of migraine and other forms of headache that the use of repeated doses of analgesia alone be avoided. One of the consequences of the overuse of analgesic medication is medication overuse headache, which becomes a self-generating headache. The underlying mechanisms of medication overuse headache appear similar to migraine with alteration in cortical neuronal excitability and central sensitisation. The diagnosis is based on the presence of chronic headache on 15 days per month for 3 months, with simple analgesic medication taken on 15 days per month.[3] The condition can be managed with variable success with a structured management program.[30] For this reason, the use of simple analgesics in headache treatment should be limited to a maximum of 3 days per week. Drug management should be directed at the cause of the problem, not simply short-term pain relief.

Primary exercise headache

Primary exercise headache is precipitated by exercise in the absence of any intracranial disorder. It has been reported in association with weightlifting, cycling, running and other sporting activities. The IHS criteria include that the headache:

- is specifically brought on by sustained strenuous physical exercise
- has a pulsating quality that lasts from 5 minutes to 48 hours
- is prevented by avoiding excessive exertion
- occurs particularly in hot weather or at high altitude.[3]

The onset of the headache can be with straining and Valsalva manoeuvres such as those seen in weightlifting and competitive swimming. The prevalence may be high, as headache consistent with primary exercise headache was reported in 26% of 4000 competitors in a tough cycling event in Holland, and was particularly associated with extreme exertion, low fluid intake and warm weather.[31] In the Vaga study in Norway, 12% of a sample of 1646 people were reported to have primary exercise headache.[32] Patients with this form of headache have significantly higher prevalence of internal jugular venous valve incompetence, which suggests that intracranial venous congestion caused by retrograde jugular venous flow may play a role in the pathophysiology of this disorder.[33] The major differential diagnoses are subarachnoid haemorrhage, cervical arterial dissection and reversible cerebral vasoconstriction syndrome, which need to be excluded by the appropriate investigations.

It has been postulated that primary exercise headache is due to dilatation of the pain-sensitive venous sinuses at the base of the brain as a result of increased cerebral arterial pressure due to exertion.[34] In weight lifters, systolic blood pressure may reach levels above 400 mmHg and diastolic pressures above 300 mmHg with maximal lifts.

The management of this condition involves either avoiding the precipitating activity or drug treatment, for example, indomethacin (25 mg three times a day). In practice, the headaches tend to recur over weeks to months and then slowly resolve, although in some cases they may be lifelong.

Exertion may also be a triggering factor in migraine. In this case, the presentation shows the typical pattern of migraine with exertion as the precipitating factor. Most patients with this condition describe the migraine beginning immediately after exercise, more frequently when the exercise has been vigorous. Exertional migraine is often severe and like primary exercise headache may be worse in hot weather. Modulation of exercise programs including adequate warm up, particularly prior to intense periods of exercise or before a game, is important. Where this does not help, migraine prophylactic medication may be required.

SECONDARY HEADACHE
Cervicogenic headache

A large survey of the general population revealed that people who suffer from headache seek physical treatment from physiotherapists and other complementary medical practitioners.[35] These people believe that their headache may be a referred phenomenon from a disorder affecting structures in their cervical spine. While not all patients with headache respond to these varied treatments, many do and there is now substantial evidence of a distinct subgroup of headache, termed cervicogenic headache, where treatment to the cervical spine has a substantial lasting effect.[36]

Mechanism

The underlying pathophysiology of cervicogenic headache is one of convergence, whereby afferents from the upper three cervical nerve roots converge in the same brain region as trigeminal afferents.[37] Hence, in the presence of sensitisation of this complex, cervical afferent input is misinterpreted, and as well as perceiving neck pain, headache is also felt. Evidence of such sensitisation in cervicogenic headache was shown in a study comparing trigeminocervical sensory processing in patients with cervical facet joint pain with and without headache.[38]

Sensitisation of the trigeminocervical nucleus is an important factor in many different forms of headache.[38-40] To explain this, it has been postulated that primary headaches form a spectrum, with shared common pathophysiological mechanisms,[41] and with cervicogenic headache one part of this spectrum,[42] despite being a secondary headache. Notwithstanding this shared pathophysiology among different headache forms, it is apparent from systematic reviews that different headache forms respond to different forms of intervention; for example, in the long-term, migraine does not respond to physical intervention.[43] Knowledge of the underlying mechanisms of headache may provide insight into potential management and will be discussed later.

Clinical features

A thorough history and comprehensive examination is required.

History

The subjective features of cervicogenic headache contrast to those reported by people with migraine and other headache forms. Table 21.3 identifies the characteristics of cervicogenic headache and Table 21.1 illustrates the difference in presentation between migraine and cervicogenic headache based on a survey of all people with chronic headache evaluated in a small town in Norway.[9, 10] Despite this, it can still be difficult to distinguish migraine from cervicogenic headache and an incorrect diagnosis is made in up to 50% of cases.[44, 45]

A good example might be a cyclist who develops headache during training after a specific time period on his or her bike. This could be exercise-induced migraine or cervicogenic headache from neck stress as a consequence of an incorrectly adjusted bike or poor posture and associated altered muscle function. In this case, the physical examination becomes increasingly important in differential diagnosis. A further difficulty is that patients more often than not present with multiple rather than single headache forms, making definitive diagnosis more challenging. Amiri et al. reported that 55% of subjects in a sample of 196 people had multiple forms of headache, with up to four different types.[46]

Table 21.3 Classification of cervicogenic headache

	International Headache Study Group[47]	International Headache Society[3]
Symptoms	• Unilateral headache without side shift • Ipsilateral neck, shoulder and arm pain of a rather vague, non-radicular nature • Pain episodes of varying duration or fluctuating, continuous pain • Moderate, non-excruciating pain, usually of a non-throbbing nature • Pain starting in the neck, eventually spreading to head, where the maximum pain is often located • Pain triggered by neck movement and/or sustained awkward position • Sustained neck trauma prior to the onset • Autonomic symptoms and signs (e.g. nausea, vomiting, dizziness, photo- and phonophobia, blurred vision)	A. Any headache fulfilling criterion C

Physical examination	• Reduced cervical spine range of motion
	• Symptoms on palpation of the cranium or neck
	• Anaesthetic blockades abolish the pain transiently
		B. Clinical, laboratory and/or imaging evidence of a neck disorder, known to be able to cause headache
		C. Evidence of causation demonstrated by at least two of the following:
		  1. Headache has developed in temporal relation to the onset of the neck disorder
		  2. Headache has significantly improved in parallel with improvement in the neck disorder
		  3. Cervical range of motion is reduced and headache made worse by provocative manoeuvres
		  4. Headache is abolished following cervical diagnostic anaesthetic blockade

Other		D. Not better accounted for by another headache diagnosis

PART B   Regional problems

Examination

Any structure innervated by the upper three cervical nerve roots is a potential contributing factor to sensitisation of the trigeminocervical nucleus and a factor in cervicogenic headache, hence a thorough clinical examination is required of these structures including the cervical articulations C0–1, C1–2 and C2–3, as well as cervical myofascial and neural structures. Caution is required as abnormalities found do not necessarily indicate the involvement of the cervical spine in headache and need to be considered in a diagnostic framework. For example, cervical movement impairments[48] and abnormal neurodynamic tests[49] have been reported in people with migraine.

There are a number of classification systems described to aid in identifying cervicogenic headache. These include those published by the IHS[3] and the International Headache Study Group[13] and are shown in Tables 21.1 and 21.3. Using the criteria in Table 21.1, it is possible to gain a level of confidence regarding the diagnosis of cervicogenic headache, with five criteria required for diagnosis.[47] Successful management from treatment directed to the cervical spine would be confirmatory evidence based on the IHS criteria.[3] In the absence of these criteria, further clinical evaluation should be undertaken.

> **PRACTICE PEARL**
>
> Examination of the patient with suspected cervicogenic headache involves a systematic examination of the articular, myofascial and neural structures of the cervical and orofacial region, including temporomandibular joints.

As with any musculoskeletal examination, one of the aims of the examination is to reproduce the patient's symptoms, but this by itself does not indicate a musculoskeletal cause for pain. In a recent study, headache was reproduced on palpation of the cervical spine in all but one patient with migraine and tension-type headache.[42] If headache can be provoked and, importantly, then relieved by manual techniques to the cervical spine then there is greater confidence of a cervical musculoskeletal cause and the potential for such treatment to be effective in the management.

Articular function can be determined by examining range of motion of the cervical spine, either in single cardinal planes or combined. Combining movements

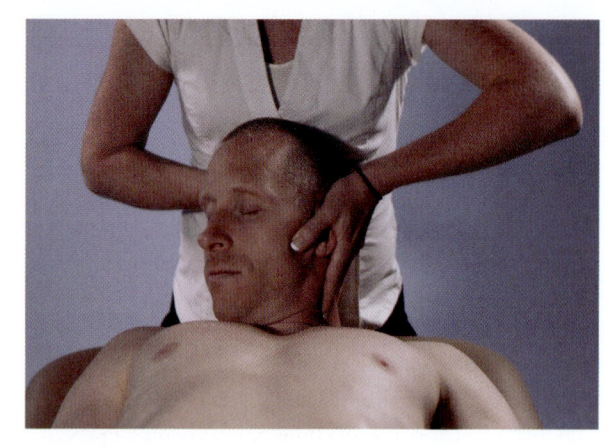

Figure 21.4 The cervical flexion–rotation test

increases the potential to identify movement impairment at the segmental levels between the occiput and C3. One example is the flexion–rotation test (Fig. 21.4), which can be used to isolate impairment of movement in the upper cervical spine. The neck is placed in end-range flexion and range of rotation to each side recorded. Normal range is 44° to each side.[50] The minimum cut-off value for a positive test is approximately 33° and there is a close relationship between headache severity and restricted range of movement (ROM) on a positive test.[51-54] This test has also been shown to be helpful, with good diagnostic accuracy, in distinguishing people with migraine from those with cervicogenic headache.[52]

A positive test is not universal in cervicogenic headache, but is found in as many as 72%.[53] While the test has been shown to be a valid marker of C1–2 segmental movement in normal people,[55] potentially unilateral altered suboccipital muscle tone (obliquus capitis inferior) associated with any painful articulation above C3, may give a positive flexion–rotation test. With further careful examination of the articular structures by palpation and segmental motion tests, it is possible to determine the spinal level of involvement.[56]

Temporomandibular disorder (TMD) is a common accompaniment to different headache forms, not specifically cervicogenic headache.[57] Evidence for the relationship between impairment of the cervical spine and TMD is shown in the significant correlation (r = 0.82) between jaw disability and neck disability.[58] Upper cervical movement impairment identified by the flexion–rotation test is found in people with TMD,[59] and in people with TMD and cervicogenic headache.[60] Careful examination of the temporomandibular joints and

Headache CHAPTER 21

orofacial muscles should be performed according to recommended guidelines.[61]

Identification of impairment of cervical motor control and myofascial system is important in cervicogenic headache evaluation,[62-65] as illustrated by evidence of long-term improvement in cervicogenic headache symptoms following retraining cervical and scapular motor control.[66] Impairment includes loss of postural alignment (forward head posture) and neuromuscular control as well as muscle weakness, endurance and extensibility.[67]

Impairments of craniocervical flexion control are some of the defining features of neck-related headache.[62, 63, 68] This test evaluates the deep neck flexor muscles, which typically become substituted by the superficial flexors sternocleidomastoid, hyoids and platysma. Similar impairments in craniocervical flexion control have not been found in migraine or tension-type headache according to one study,[62] but were in tension-type headache in another.[69] Other changes to the muscle system in cervicogenic headache include evidence of muscle tightness[65] and trigger points.[70] See Chapter 23 for more details of evaluation of cervical muscle control.

Sensitisation of the upper cervical neural tissue is found in approximately 10% of cases with cervicogenic headache, less commonly when compared to the cervicobrachial region.[65, 71] Identification is important, as the presence of such sensitisation is likely to lead to treatment failure unless addressed. Typically, the patient will adopt an antalgic forward head posture with retraction and upper cervical flexion will be provocative and limited in range. Suboccipital muscle tone may be raised as a protective measure. Neurodynamic tests (Chapter 15), such as in Figure 21.5 involving upper cervical spine flexion with the arms in a neural provocative position, should reproduce head pain. The upper cervical neural tissue (e.g. greater occipital nerve) is likely to be sensitive to palpation in positive cases (Fig. 21.6).

In this section, various aspects of examination have been described to aid in the identification of cervicogenic headache. While the individual items of assessment may be of importance, consideration of multiple physical examination criteria is likely to increase the accuracy of diagnosis. This is supported by one study which revealed that collectively, impairment in motor control identified by the craniocervical flexion test and restricted neck movement, in association with evidence on manual examination of upper cervical joint dysfunction had 100% sensitivity and 94% specificity to identify cervicogenic headache.[62]

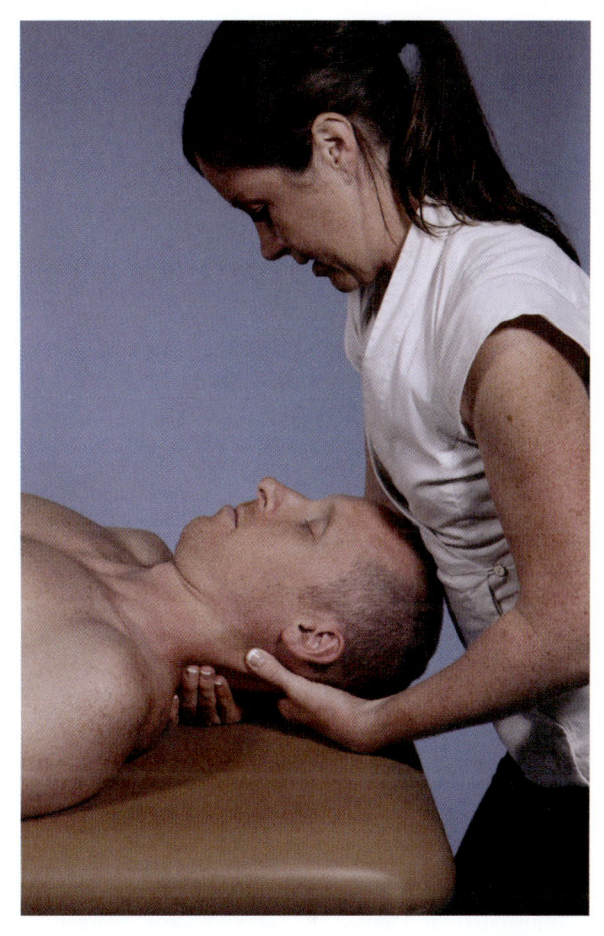

Figure 21.5 Upper cervical neurodynamic test involving upper cervical spine flexion with the arms in various neural provocative positions, with an aim to reproduce head pain

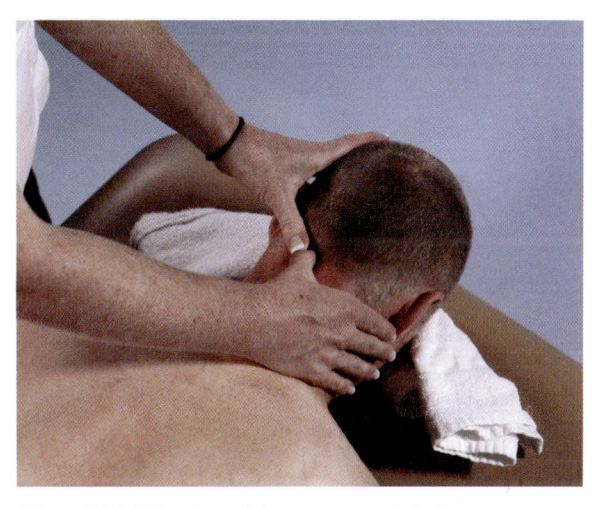

Figure 21.6 Palpation of the greater occipital nerve

325

PART B   Regional problems

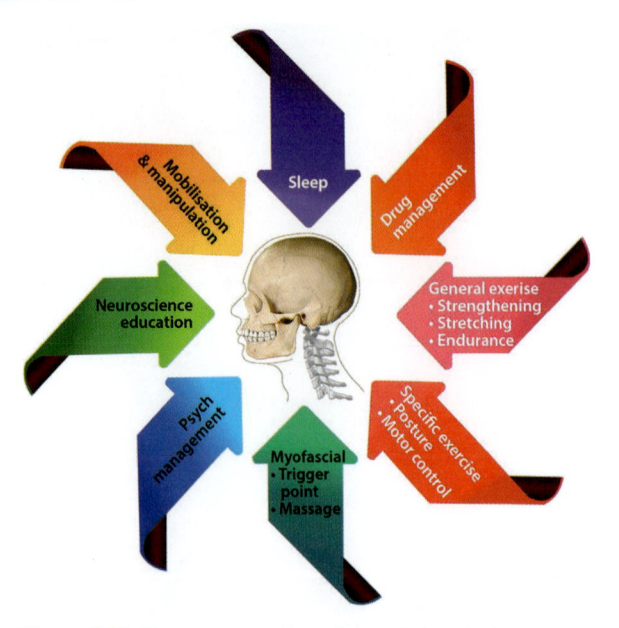

Figure 21.7 Management of cervicogenic headache

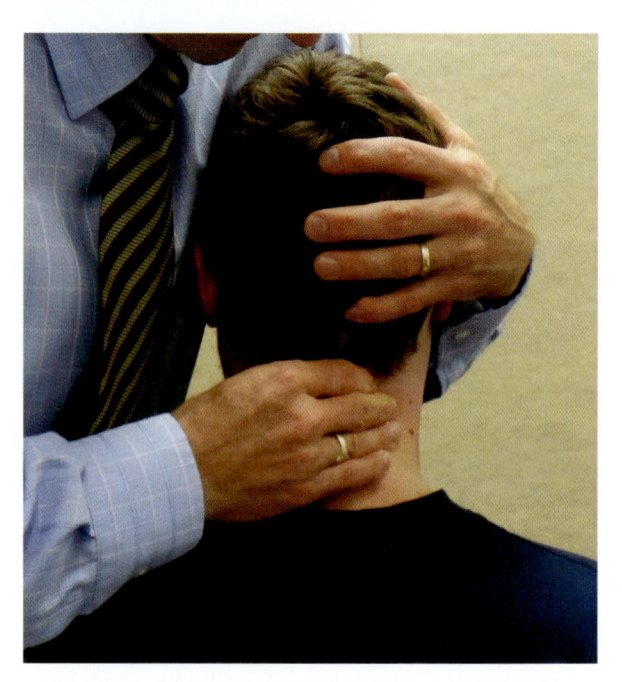

Figure 21.8 Passive upper cervical rotation mobilisation technique
COURTESY OF TOBY HALL

Treatment

The clinician's confidence in diagnosis of cervicogenic headache, and thus potential for response to physical interventions, are improved by combining information from all aspects of the examination, as currently there is no consensus as to which examination criteria predict success for cervicogenic headache.[72, 73] Hence treatment, as illustrated in Figure 21.7, should ideally target all factors identified during the examination as contributing to the athlete's problem. An important factor associated with recovery from neck pain is sleep quality,[74] hence physical factors (articular, neural and muscle function) are not the only ones to consider in management. Since cervicogenic headache is associated with sensitisation of the trigeminocervical nucleus, factors that might reduce this, such as neuroscience education and lifestyle management, as well as reducing stress and anxiety, should also be considered.

Evidence for a multisystem approach to management was shown in a multicentre randomised controlled trial.[66] While manipulation/mobilisation and, separately, motor control re-education were found to be effective in the long-term, combining both these approaches was found to be more effective.

There is evidence for a range of different manual therapy techniques in management of cervicogenic headache. Manipulation of the cervical spine may be effective,[75] but is potentially more hazardous and has been found to be no more effective than more gentle, potentially less dangerous forms of treatment including joint mobilisation or Mulligan mobilisation with movement.[76] Joint mobilisation might include Maitland passive accessory mobilisation or physiological mobilisation techniques in appropriate cervical positions (based on assessment) to stretch the impaired joints to restore normal movement (Fig. 21.8). Such techniques should include exercise to maintain improved mobility.

Mobilisation with movement is a combination of pain-free passive accessory joint glide applied together with active movement (Fig. 21.9) and can be used to improve segmental joint mobility at any level in the cervical spine.[77] The aim of this approach is to restore normal segmental movement in a painless way by encouraging normal biomechanics. For example, a cyclist may develop cervicogenic headache due to abnormal movement at the C2–3 segment, which might provoke headache during prolonged cycling activity. Improving C2–3 segmental motion with a mobilisation with movement technique together with a self-mobilisation home exercise, postural control exercise and muscle re-education typically eliminates the problem.

Another common clinical situation in athletes with chronic cervicogenic headache is a positive flexion–rotation test (Fig 21.4). This usually responds in a rapid and sustained way to a simple Mulligan self-mobilisation technique (Fig. 21.10) directed to the upper cervical spine.[78] In this case, treatment is aimed at the impaired cervical articulations in an attempt to increase mobility specifically in the upper

Headache **CHAPTER 21**

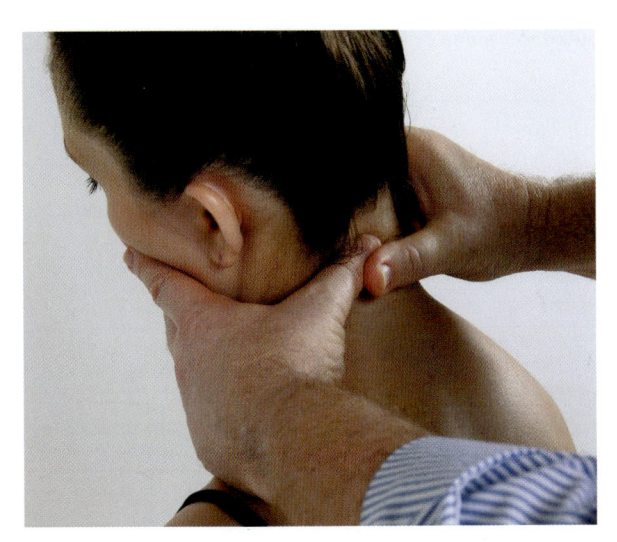

Figure 21.9 Mobilisation with movement into flexion at C2–3
COURTESY OF TOBY HALL

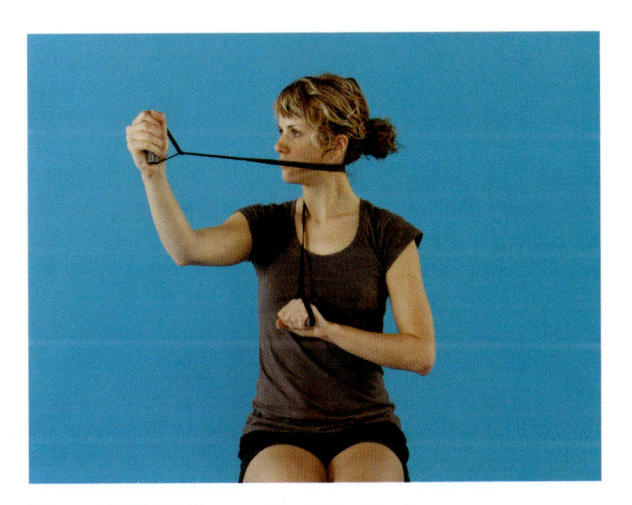

Figure 21.10 Mulligan self-mobilisation for upper cervical rotation impairment identified by the flexion–rotation test

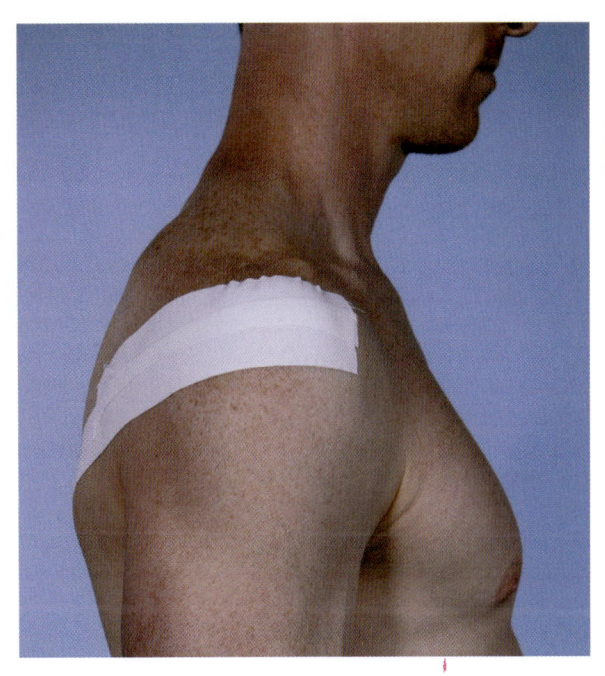

Figure 21.11 Tape to improve scapula control

> **PRACTICE PEARL**
>
> A comprehensive exercise program should include motor control exercises including postural control, particularly in the functional complaint activity/position.

cervical spine. The positive sustained long-term improvement following this intervention goes some way to validate the use of mobilisation in cervicogenic headache.[78]

Dosage of mobilisation and manipulation is important. For example, a single session of manipulation is not effective in the long term,[79] but eight sessions are effective, as are 16.[75] Specific trigger point and other soft tissue techniques may be used if these have been found to be involved in the disorder. There is some evidence to show that simple soft tissue therapy techniques can improve the flexion–rotation test, thus helping headache symptoms.[80]

For example, cervical and scapular postural control needs to be addressed while riding a bike in the patient with cycling-induced cervicogenic headache, but to achieve this may also require attention to lumbopelvic posture and bike set-up. Postural faults may develop through repetitive sporting activity. For example, an increased thoracic kyphosis, cervical protrusion and scapula anterior tilt and protraction may develop in a swimmer, cyclist or body builder through uncorrected muscle activity. This position may abnormally stress the upper cervical spine, inducing headache. Correcting these faults may require joint mobilisation as well as postural and motor control re-education. Sports tape may be used to facilitate postural correction of the scapula (Fig. 21.11) until the athlete learns to correct his or her posture independently.

Exercise may also include stretching of any muscles found to be short, together with strengthening of the shoulder girdle and neck muscles. Important muscles for stretching include pectoralis minor, upper trapezius, levator scapula and suboccipitals, among others.[65] Neck strengthening combined with stretching exercises were found to be more effective compared to endurance training

PART B   Regional problems

Table 21.4 The IHS criteria for the diagnosis of headache attributed to trauma or injury to the head and/or neck (IHS 5.1 and 5.2)[3]

A. Any headache fulfilling C and D
B. Traumatic injury to the head
C. Headache is reported <7 days after:
   1. injury to the head
   2. regaining consciousness following head injury
   3. discontinuing medication that impairs ability to sense headache following injury to the head
D. Headache disappears within 3 months after trauma (acute) or headache persists for greater than 3 months (persistent)

or stretching alone in the management of cervicogenic headache.[81]

Recent evidence suggests a close interaction between the upper cervical spine, temporomandibular dysfunction and cervicogenic headache.[59, 82] This might explain why combining manual therapy techniques to the temporomandibular joint and orofascial muscles with cervical manual therapy was found to be more effective in the management of cervicogenic headache than cervical manual therapy alone.[83] The clinician should consider incorporating management of temporomandibular dysfunction when this is evident in examination.

Post-traumatic headache

Trauma to the head and neck in sport may lead to the development of headache. The initiating traumatic event may not necessarily be severe and could involve repetitive minor blows as in boxing. The IHS diagnostic criteria for post-traumatic headache are shown in Table 21.4.[3]

Most often these forms of headache resemble cervicogenic headache, tension-type or migraine. Not surprisingly, trauma to the head affects the neck and could lead to cervicogenic headache. Indeed, the presence of neck pain appears important in post-traumatic headache sufferers without premorbid headache.[84] Hence the diagnosis is made on the close temporal relationship between the traumatic event and the onset of headache, but should also require careful examination of the cervical spine and the potential for cervicogenic headache.

The presence of migraine-like headache after concussion correlates with more severe injuries and identifies athletes at risk of prolonged recovery to baseline.[85] Headache may occur in isolation or may be part of a range of symptoms including dizziness, sleep disturbance, balance disturbance and loss of cognition. This is dealt with in more detail in Chapter 20 on concussion.

Evidence for the management of post-traumatic headache is not well established. Generally, treatment should be provided according to the category the particular headache most resembles.[4] The clinician should be aware of the potential for medication overuse headache, a known factor in the development of persistent symptoms, unless analgesic medication is carefully monitored.[86]

Post-traumatic migraine

Headache may follow repetitive relatively minor traumatic events to the head and neck. This may be seen in sports such as soccer, where repetitive heading of the ball gives rise to the term 'footballer's migraine'.[87, 88] Boxing and similar sports also lead to problems like these. Even mild head trauma can induce migraine. One particular syndrome that is recognised in the setting of minor head blows is migrainous cortical blindness. This disturbing condition often raises fear of serious cerebral injury but tends to resolve over 1–2 hours.

External compression headache

External compression headache (IHS 4.2), formerly known as 'swim goggle headache,' presents with pain in the facial and temporal areas produced from wearing excessively tight face masks or swimming goggles. It is commonly seen in swimmers and divers. In divers, this may be referred to as 'mask squeeze', and is seen on descent to depth as the effects of pressure reduce the air space inside the mask. The aetiology is believed to be due to continuous stimulation of cutaneous nerves by the application of pressure.

High-altitude headache

High-altitude headache (IHS 10.1.1) is a well-recognised accompaniment of acute mountain sickness (although it can occur on its own), which occurs within 24 hours of ascent to altitudes above 3000 m.[89] The headaches are vascular in nature and are seen in unacclimatised individuals. Typically, these are associated with other physiological effects of altitude or may be an early manifestation of acute mountain sickness. The treatment is to descend to lower altitude, although pharmacological interventions such as ibuprofen, acetaminophen/paracetamol and acetazolamide may be used.

Hypercapnia headache

Headache in divers, while uncommon and generally benign, can occasionally signify serious consequences of hyperbaric exposure such as arterial gas embolism, decompression sickness, and otic or paranasal sinus barotrauma. Inadequate ventilation of compressed gases can lead to carbon dioxide accumulation, cerebral vasodilatation and headache.[90]

Since carbon dioxide (CO_2) relaxes cerebrovascular smooth muscle, hypercapnia leads to cerebral vasodilatation and increased intracranial pressure. Carbon dioxide can accumulate insidiously in the diver who intentionally holds the breath intermittently (skip breathing) in a mistaken attempt to conserve air, or takes shallow breaths to minimise buoyancy variations in the narrow passages of a wreck or cave. The diver may hypoventilate unintentionally if a tight wetsuit or buoyancy compensator jacket restricts chest wall expansion, or if ventilation is inadequate in response to physical exertion when swimming against a strong current.

The headache associated with CO_2 retention develops gradually and affects the bifrontal, bitemporal or bioccipital head regions. Throbbing pain ranging from mild to severe in intensity typically lasts from 10 to 30 minutes, yet in some may persist for several hours along with nausea and malaise. Onset accompanies a slow buildup or may follow a reduction in sharply rising CO_2 tension. Pain typically worsens during the decompression phase of the dive or upon surfacing, possibly because of the disparity between increased intracranial pressure and more rapidly decreasing ambient pressure. Non-steroidal anti-inflammatory and ergotamine preparations have been reported to be ineffective.[90]

Other types of headache encountered in divers include exertional headache, cold stimulus headache, migraine, tension-type headache, acute traumatic headache, cervicogenic headache, carbon monoxide poisoning headache and headache associated with envenomation.

REFERENCES

References for this chapter can be found at www.mhhe.com/au/CSM5e

Chapter 22

Face, eyes and teeth

with RODNEY FRENCH, GEOFFREY ST GEORGE, IAN NEEDLEMAN and STEFFAN GRIFFIN

> *Having looked at it on YouTube, I don't like to look at it too much because it freaks me out a bit. The bail hit me in the eye and went two centimetres back.*
> South African cricket player Mark Boucher on his career-ending eye injury

Injuries to the face in sport usually result from direct trauma. After reviewing clinical assessment and soft tissue injury management, we outline management of injuries to the nose, ear, eye, teeth and facial bones.

FUNCTIONAL ANATOMY

The bones of the face are shown in Figure 22.1. As most of these bones are subcutaneous, they are easily examined. Examination should include palpation of the forehead and supraorbital rims for irregularities and contour deformities.

The orbit is a cone-shaped cavity, with a margin that consists of the supraorbital ridge above, the infraorbital margin below, the zygomatic arch laterally and the nasal bone medially. The recess formed protects the eye from a blow from a large object. A smaller, deformable object such as a squash ball may, nevertheless, compress the globe and orbital contents, leading to a 'blow-out' fracture in the orbital floor that orbital content can herniate through.

The zygomatic arch of the malar bone creates the prominence of the cheek. Fractures in this region may cause flattening of the cheek and a palpable irregularity in the inferior orbital margin.

The maxilla forms the upper jaw. Its superior surface helps create the floor of the orbit and the inferior surface forms the major part of the hard palate. Mobility of the hard palate, determined by grasping the central incisors, may indicate a maxillary fracture.

The lower jaw consists of the horseshoe-shaped mandible. The mandible is made up of body, angle and ramus, which are easily palpated. The coronoid process can be palpated by a direct intraoral approach. The gingiva overlying the alveolar ridge may be lacerated in mandibular body fractures.

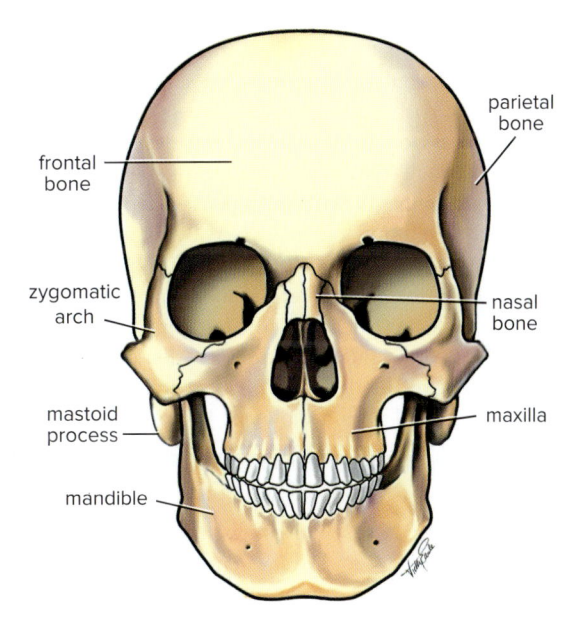

Figure 22.1 Facial bones

CLINICAL ASSESSMENT

Facial injuries[1] are frequently associated with profuse bleeding. While it is important to control the bleeding, it is also vital to fully assess the underlying structures. All head and neck injuries should be considered closed head injuries. Cervical spine precautions should be taken if the patient is unconscious, has neurological deficits or cervical spine tenderness, or if cervical spine injury is feasible considering the mechanism of injury. The airway is particularly vulnerable to obstruction because

PART B Regional problems

of bleeding, structural compromise of bony structures (e.g. mandible), or dislodged teeth, tooth fragments or dental appliances. The practical steps to assess facial injuries are:

- ascertain the mechanism of injury and locate the source of the patient's pain
- check for blurred vision, diplopia (double vision), concussion or cerebrospinal fluid leakage
- inspect the nasal septum and external ear for haematomas and nasal obstruction
- observe facial asymmetry or structural depressions
- look for a sunken eye globe suggestive of a blow-out fracture
- observe lacerations or deep abrasions overlying suspected fractures.

Palpate facial bones (orbital rims, nasal bones, temporomandibular joints) for significant tenderness, crepitus, numbness or contour irregularities. Midface instability or crepitus may be demonstrated by stabilising the forehead with one hand while gently pulling on the maxillary incisors with the other gloved hand. Bimanual palpation along the mandible and maxilla (one gloved hand palpating intraorally) will uncover instability, irregularity or tenderness.

Assess extraocular eye movements and cranial nerves III, IV and VI by having the patient keep his or her chin in a fixed position while tracking the examiner's finger movements in all four quadrants. If the patient is able to track the movements without reporting diplopia, acute extraocular nerve entrapment caused by an orbital blow-out fracture can be ruled out. An inability to raise the eyebrow or wrinkle the forehead following laceration to the eyebrow suggests injury to the temporal branch of the facial nerve on that side. Reduced sensation over the skin below the eye in the distribution of the infraorbital nerve may be associated with a blow-out fracture of the orbit. The nerve distribution includes the upper gum and lip.

> **PRACTICE PEARL**
>
> If the patient is unable to open his or her mouth or exhibits severe pain along the lateral aspect of the cheek or jaw when attempting to open, a fracture of the mandible or zygoma must be considered.

With the mouth open, the oral cavity should be assessed to rule out damage to the teeth and lacerations in the intraoral mucosa or tongue. Locate fractured or missing teeth, when possible, to avoid accidental aspiration. When asked to close the mouth, the patient's sense of malocclusion suggests a significant fracture of the mandible, maxilla or palate.

Leakage of cerebrospinal fluid (CSF) following a blow to the nose (CSF rhinorrhea) may indicate a fracture of the base of the anterior cranial fossa. CSF is a clear discharge and the patient may report a salty taste in the mouth. If there is doubt about the origin of a nasal discharge associated with trauma, the discharge should be tested with a urinary dipstick for glucose. CSF is positive for glucose.

A list of common conditions and conditions not to be missed is shown in Table 22.1.

LACERATIONS AND CONTUSIONS

Lacerations and contusions to the face and scalp are prevalent in sports such as football, ice hockey, martial arts and racquet sports.[1] Examination should include palpation of the underlying bone to detect bony tenderness. Neurological examination is required if there is a history of loss of consciousness or suspected skull fracture.

Immediate management of lacerations

Begin immediate management with ice and pressure to reduce local swelling. Control bleeding with direct pressure over the wound using sterile gauze. A player with a bleeding wound must be removed from the field of play immediately as there is concern that the presence of blood may increase the risk of hepatitis B or human immunodeficiency virus (HIV) infection for other players.

After removing the athlete from the field of play, examine the laceration closely under good light. Further cleaning and removal of foreign bodies may be required. If necessary, infiltrate a local anaesthetic agent to adequately clean the wound. The local anaesthetic used should be 1% or 2% lignocaine (lidocaine) containing adrenalin (epinephrine) 1:100 000 to provide some vasoconstriction as well as analgesia.

Management of larger lacerations

Lacerations greater than 0.25–0.5 cm long should be closed if they appear clean. Closure may be obtained by suturing or by taping with adhesive strips (Steristrips®). Steristrips are ideal for small wounds; however, persistent bleeding or excessive sweating may prevent adhesion. To overcome this, tincture of benzoin (friar's balsam) may be applied to increase adhesiveness. Adequate dressings will be required to keep the adhesive strips in place, especially if the player is returning to the field. Scalp wounds often bleed profusely. Small wounds can be controlled with local pressure, but larger ones require suturing.

If facial lacerations require suturing, use 5/0 or 6/0 nylon. It is important that the skin edges are healthy. Pieces of devitalised skin should be debrided. Take care to approximate the skin edges carefully while suturing. Remove sutures after 5 days and place adhesive strips over the wound for a further week. The wound should be kept dry for at least 48 hours.

An alternative to suturing is skin staples. These must be covered if the player is returning to the field to prevent them from being accidentally torn out or from injuring

Face, eye and teeth — CHAPTER 22

Table 22.1 Facial injuries in sport

Category	Common	Less common	Not to be missed
Facial soft tissue	Contusion Laceration		Associated underlying fracture/nerve injury
Nose	Fracture of nasal bones Epistaxis	Fracture of nasal septum	Septal haematoma
Ear	Contusion ('cauliflower ear') Otitis media Otitis externa	Laceration Ruptured tympanic membrane	Fractured petrous temporal bone Torn auditory nerve
Eye	Corneal abrasion Corneal foreign body Conjunctival foreign body Subconjunctival haemorrhage Eyelid laceration	Chemical burns Vitreous haemorrhage Retinal haemorrhage Retinal oedema Hyphaema	Corneal laceration Retinal detachment Lens dislocation Blow-out fracture of the orbit Optic nerve injury Injury to lacrimal system
Teeth	Enamel chip fracture Luxated tooth Avulsed tooth	Crown fracture	Impacted tooth
Facial bones	Temporomandibular joint sprain or malalignment Zygoma fracture Orbital blow-out fracture	Fractured maxilla Fractured mandible	

Table 22.2 Management of specific lacerations

Laceration type	Management considerations
Deep lacerations (e.g. to galea aponeurotica in forehead)	Interrupted 5/0 absorbable sutures (prior to skin closure)
Eyebrow laceration	Do not shave eyebrow hair. Strict anatomical approximation required
Partial-thickness lip laceration at vermilion border	Place first suture at mucocutaneous junction to ensure accurate alignment
Full-thickness lip laceration	Three layer closure required (preferably by plastic surgeon) consisting of: oral mucosa first; orbicularis oris second; skin last
Deep intraoral laceration	Use 3/0 silk sutures and keep in place for 1 week

another player in a collision. Another alternative is the use of histoacryl glue.

Additional considerations

All patients with potentially contaminated wounds should receive tetanus prophylaxis and a short course of oral antibiotic therapy, for example, cephalexin (250–500 mg, 6 hourly) or flucloxacillin (250–500 mg, 6 hourly). Wounds that may be contaminated by another player's saliva, such as bite wounds, should not be closed but should be cleaned meticulously. The player should be treated with oral metronidazole (400 mg, 8 hourly) in addition to penicillin and observed very closely for the development of cellulitis. If signs of infection appear, treat with intravenous antibiotics.

NOSE

The three main conditions that affect the nose in sports medicine are epistaxis (bleeds), fractures and septal haematomas.

Epistaxis (nosebleed)

Nasal haemorrhage occurs frequently in association with nasal injuries. It usually arises from the nasal septum, which receives its blood supply from branches of the internal and external carotid arteries. In most non-traumatic cases, the bleeding arises from a rich plexus of vessels in the anterior part of the septum, known as Little's or Kiesselbach's area (Fig. 22.2), whilst bleeding will originate from the vessels local to the affected area in traumatic cases.

PART B   Regional problems

Epistaxis 'game-day' management flowchart

Proceed to next stage of flowchart if epistaxis not controlled
↓
Apply prolonged digital pressure on the lower nose for up to 20 minutes (with patient sat upright)
↓
Apply cotton wool soaked in adrenalin (epinephrine) 1:1000 to nasal septum
↓
Cauterise bleeding site with silver nitrate applicators (only if bleeding site visualised)
↓
Refer to specialist for further management.

Initial management consists of prolonged direct digital pressure on the lower nose for up to 20 minutes, compressing the vessels on the nasal septum with the patient sitting upright. Cold compresses over the bridge of the nose promote vasoconstriction. If bleeding continues, apply cotton wool soaked in adrenalin (epinephrine) 1:1000 to the nasal septum. If the bleeding site can be located, it may be cauterised with silver nitrate applicators (cotton swabs soaked in 4% trichloracetic acid).

If bleeding persists, specialist referral is indicated. The nose will usually be packed with 1 cm ribbon gauze impregnated with bismuth iodoform petroleum paste (BIPP) and left for 48 hours. Post-nasal packing may be required if the bleeding originates from the back of the nose. In the rare cases that bleeding persists despite these local measures, maxillary artery or anterior ethmoidal artery ligation may be indicated.

Nasal fractures

Fractures of the nose are usually caused by a direct blow. Symptoms and signs of nasal fracture include pain, epistaxis, swelling, crepitus, deformity and mobility of the nose. Nasal distortion may not be obvious once soft tissue swelling develops. Initial management is directed towards controlling the nasal haemorrhage. An associated laceration should be sutured with 6/0 nylon and requires prophylactic antibiotic therapy. The nasal passages should be examined to exclude a septal haematoma and patients should be advised to return if they notice increased pain or develop a fever (see below).

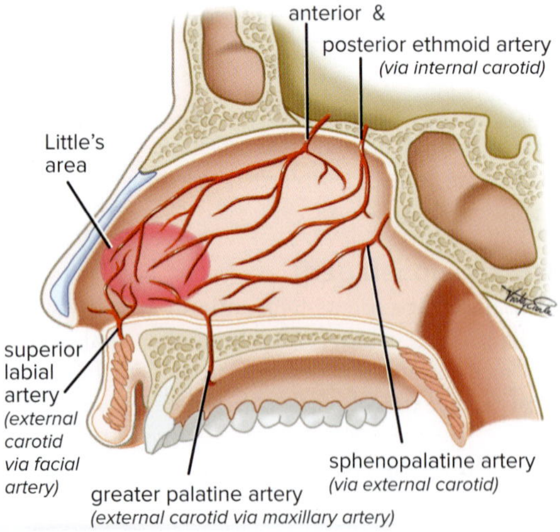

Radiographs are probably not required as undisplaced fractures require no treatment and displaced fractures are clinically obvious. Displaced nasal fractures may require reduction. There are two indications for reduction of fractures. The first is obstruction of the nasal passages and the second is cosmetic deformity.

In young athletes, displaced fractures are almost always reduced because of a tendency towards increased sinus infections and a decrease in the size of the nasal passage. Attempts at immediate reduction of nasal fractures are associated with a risk of arterial damage and severe acute haemorrhage. It is preferable to delay fracture reduction and refer the patient to a surgeon within 7 days of the injury. When the soft tissue swelling has settled sufficiently, reduction, if necessary, can be carried out under general anaesthesia.

Septal haematoma

This important condition can complicate what seems to be a trivial nosebleed. A septal haematoma is caused by haemorrhage between the two layers of mucosa covering the septum (Fig. 22.3). The presenting complaint is either nasal obstruction or nasal pain. The patient may be febrile and nasal examination reveals a cherry-like structure (the dull, red swollen septum) that occludes the nasal passages. Treatment of a large septal haematoma involves evacuation of the clot using a wide-bore needle or through a small incision followed by nasal packing to prevent recurrence of the haematoma. Antibiotic prophylaxis should be given to prevent development of a septal abscess and subsequent cartilage necrosis.

Figure 22.2 Little's (Kiesselbach's) area

Face, eye and teeth CHAPTER 22

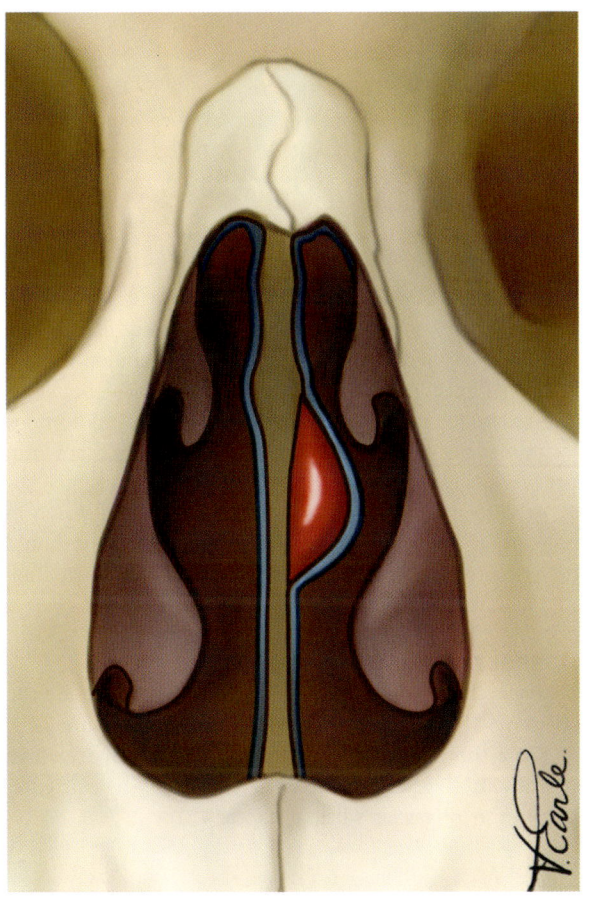

Figure 22.3 Septal haematoma

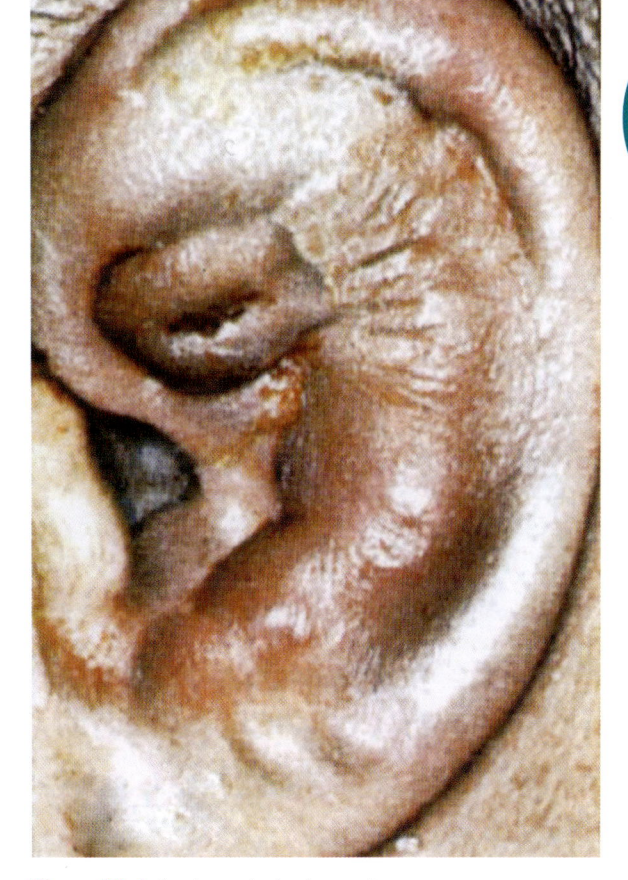

Figure 22.4 Acute auricular haematoma

EAR
Ear injuries in most sports are not common. Nonetheless, they can pose a clinical challenge to sports physicians working in sports such as rugby and wrestling. The most frequent injury is a contusion to the ear known as an auricular haematoma.

Auricular haematoma
This injury occurs mainly in rugby scrums, boxing or wrestling as a result of a shearing blow. Recurrent contusions result in haemorrhage between the perichondrium and the cartilage. This may eventually develop into a chronic swelling, commonly known as 'cauliflower ear'. An acute haematoma (Fig. 22.4) should be treated initially with ice and firm compression, but may need to be drained by aspiration under strict aseptic conditions. A pressure dressing (cotton wool soaked in collodion) is then applied and is carefully packed against the ear to follow the contours of the outer ear. This is bandaged firmly. The ear must be examined daily to assess progress. Return to non-contact sports can be immediate, but headgear or a helmet is required for return to contact sport. Rugby forwards frequently wear headgear which protects their ears as a preventive measure.

Lacerations to the ear require careful cleansing and suture. As lacerations located between the scalp and the ear are easily missed, this area should always be examined, especially if there is a history of the ear being pulled forwards. If the auricular cartilage is torn, the overlying skin should be carefully aligned and sutured with absorbable 5/0 sutures; however, the cartilage itself has natural physical 'memory' properties, leading to natural alignment without the need for sutures. The perichondrium should be closed as a separate layer. Prophylactic oral antibiotic therapy is recommended.

Perforated eardrum
A blow across the side of the head may occasionally injure the eardrum. Pain, bleeding from the ear or impaired hearing suggest tympanic membrane rupture.

PART B Regional problems

These ruptures usually heal spontaneously. Prophylactic antibiotic therapy (amoxycillin 250–500 mg, 8 hourly if not allergic to penicillin) should be administered. It is important to keep the ear dry while a perforation is present. In sports where significant pressure changes occur, such as platform diving, scuba diving and high-altitude mountain climbing, athletes should not return to play until the tympanic membrane has healed. Athletes participating in water sports, such as swimming and water polo, should use custom-fabricated ear plugs to maintain a dry ear canal. Dry land athletes may return to play as soon as any vertigo has resolved.[1]

Athletes will often ask whether it is safe to fly with a perforated eardrum. It is generally considered safe to do so, unless they have had surgery to repair the perforation (myringoplasty), in which case guidance should be sought from the surgeon.

A severe blow across the head may fracture the skull and cause inner ear bleeding. Discharge from the ear (otorrhoea) may signal a neurosurgical emergency and, thus, patients should be referred immediately for specialist treatment.

Otitis externa

Otitis externa is the most common ear condition affecting competitive swimmers. It is generally caused by bacteria, although fungal infection can also contribute. Symptoms include earache, pruritus, discharge and impaired hearing. On examination, there may be discharge in the ear and local redness along the external auditory meatus. There may be tragal tenderness and pain on tragal pull.

Management involves careful aural toilet combined with topical antibiotic and corticosteroid ear drops. The patient should, preferably, abstain from swimming until fully recovered and avoid rubbing or drying the ear until after the infection has cleared. The use of earplugs in this condition is controversial. They may traumatise the ear canal and predispose the swimmer to infection.

> **PRACTICE PEARL**
>
> Recurrent attacks of otitis externa may be prevented by instillation of alcohol ear drops, for example, 5% acetic acid in isopropyl alcohol (aqua ear®), after each swimming session.

EYES

Eye injuries occur most commonly in stick sports, racquet sports, especially squash, and contact sports.[2] All eye injuries, even those that appear to be minor, require thorough examination. All serious eye injuries should be referred immediately to an ophthalmologist. The indications for immediate referral to an ophthalmologist are shown in the box below.

Athletes with a previous history of impaired vision in one or both eyes or previous eye trauma or surgery should be evaluated by an ophthalmologist prior to participating in a high-risk sport.

Assessment of the injured eye

To assess the injured eye, it is important to understand the anatomy. The anatomy of the eye is shown in Figure 22.5.

For a thorough assessment of the injured eye, an 'eye injuries kit' (Fig. 22.6) is very useful and can be carried as part of the 'physician's bag' (Chapter 47).

History

The history of the eye injury provides useful diagnostic information. Seek to discover the history of the mechanism of injury. Were glasses, contact lenses or a protective device being worn at the time of injury? Note any previous eye injury or problems. Ask about symptoms such as pain, blurred vision, loss of vision, flashing lights and diplopia.

Examination

Test the visual acuity of each eye using a Snellen chart, with and without glasses or contact lenses. If a Snellen chart is not available, use pages of a newspaper with

Clinical indications for immediate referral to a specialist ophthalmologist

Symptoms	Signs
Severe eye pain	Suspected penetrating injury (corneal laceration, pear-shaped pupil)
Persistent blurred or double vision	Hyphaema
Persistent photophobia	Embedded foreign body
	No view of fundus (suspected vitreous haemorrhage or retinal detachment)
	Markedly impaired visual acuity: 6/12 or less
	Loss of part of visual field

Face, eye and teeth CHAPTER 22

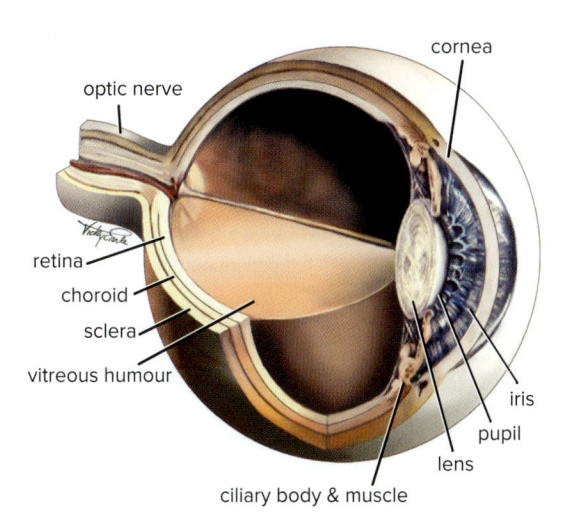

Figure 22.5 Anatomy of the eye

Eye injuries kit

Small mirror
Pencil torch
Ophthalmoscope
Snellen chart
Sterile solution for irrigation
Local anaesthetic eye drops
Fluorescein
Antibiotic drops and ointments
Cotton buds
Contact lens lubricant and case(s)
Eye patches
Tape

Inspect the eyelids for bruising, swelling or laceration. Note any obvious foreign body, haemorrhage or change in pupil size.

If there is pain or photophobia due to the injury prevent examination of the eye, instil a drop of a sterile topical anaesthetic agent, such as amethocaine, to assist examination.

> **PRACTICE PEARL**
>
> Inspect the cornea for foreign material and abrasions. Fluorescein staining under cobalt blue light will help reveal areas of corneal ulceration or foreign bodies. Evert the upper lid to exclude the presence of a subtarsal foreign body.

Test eye movements in all directions. A restriction in any direction or the presence of diplopia may indicate orbital fracture. Compare the size, shape and light reaction of the pupil with the uninjured eye. An enlarged, poorly reacting pupil may be present after injury to the iris. A pear-shaped pupil suggests the presence of a full thickness corneal or scleral laceration (penetrating injury).

Inspect the anterior chamber for the presence of blood. Blood in the anterior chamber is known as hyphaema (Fig. 22.7).

> **PRACTICE PEARL**
>
> Ophthalmoscopic examination should routinely be performed to inspect the lens, vitreous humour and retina.

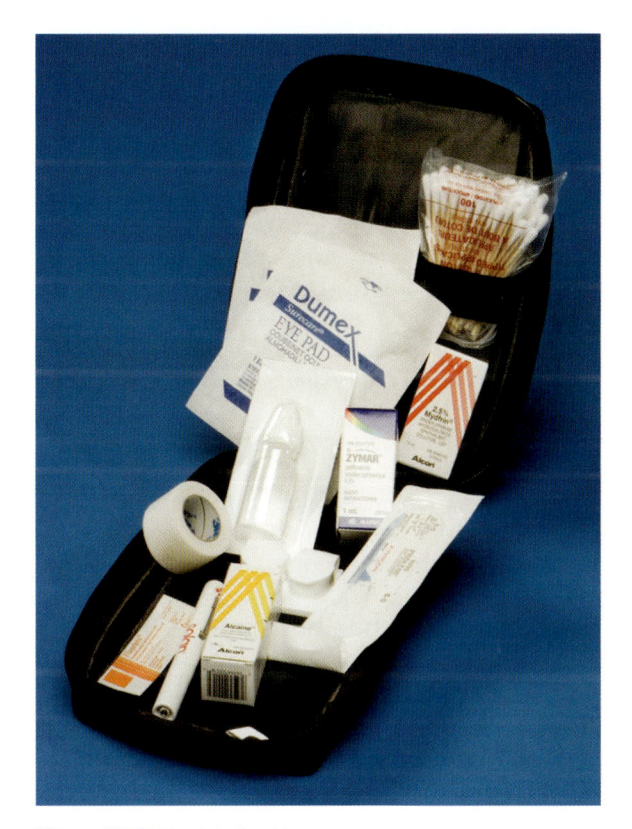

Figure 22.6 Eye injuries kit

variable print sizes as an approximate assessment of visual acuity. On the sporting arena, a scoreboard can be used to test distant vision.

The absence of a red reflex on ophthalmoscopic examination may be due to a corneal opacity, a lens opacity (cataract), intraocular bleeding or a retinal detachment. Failure to visualise the fundus may be a sign of vitreous

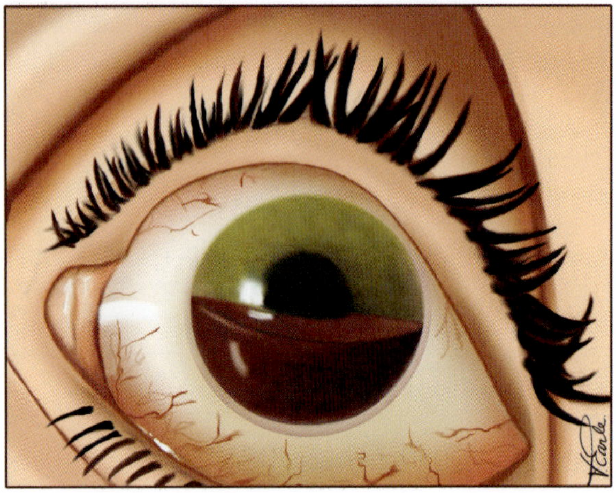

PART B   Regional problems

Figure 22.7 Hyphaema—note the fluid level in the anterior chamber

haemorrhage, which can result from a retinal tear. Contusion of the retina may produce retinal oedema, seen as areas of pallor (and thickening) as well as retinal haemorrhage.

> **PRACTICE PEARL**
>
> Radiological examination of the orbit is indicated in all cases of traumatic eye injury with diplopia and in cases where an intraocular or intraorbital foreign body is suspected.

Corneal injuries: abrasions and foreign body

Corneal injuries in sport include abrasion, foreign body and, less commonly, alkali burn. Corneal abrasion, one of the most frequent injuries to the eye during sport, occurs as a result of a scratch from either a fingernail or foreign body. The patient complains of pain, a sensation of a foreign body being present in the eye and blurred vision if the central cornea is involved.

A topical anaesthetic drop should be instilled to assist corneal examination. Fluorescein staining under cobalt blue light will help locate corneal abrasions or foreign bodies. Evert the upper lid to exclude a subtarsal foreign body.

Treatment of corneal abrasions includes the instillation of antibiotic eye drops, for example, chloramphenicol and padding of the eye (Fig. 22.8). If pain and photophobia are severe, add a topical mydriatic (e.g. 2% homatropine). A local anaesthetic agent should never be used for pain relief as it can delay healing and result in further damage.

Eye-injury 'game-day' assessment

1. Test the visual acuity of each eye using a Snellen chart, with and without glasses or contact lenses (use newspaper pages or a scoreboard if unavailable)
2. Inspect the eyelids for bruising, swelling or laceration. Note any obvious foreign body, haemorrhage or change in pupil size (instil a drop of sterile topical anaesthetic agent to assist examination if pain or photophobia prevent examination)
3. Evert the upper lid to exclude the presence of a subtarsal foreign body
4. Inspect the cornea for foreign material and abrasions (fluorescein staining under cobalt blue light will assist greatly)
5. Test eye movements in all directions
6. Compare the size, shape and light reaction of the pupil with the uninjured eye
7. Inspect the anterior chamber for the presence of blood
8. Ophthalmoscopic examination should be performed to inspect the lens, vitreous humour and retina.

Corneal foreign bodies can be removed with a cotton tip applicator by a trained clinician. If foreign bodies are more deeply embedded, patients should be referred to an ophthalmologist. Rust rings, which occasionally remain after metallic foreign bodies have been embedded in the cornea, require removal by an ophthalmologist. Antibiotic eye ointment should be administered following foreign body removal and the eye padded for 24 hours until the corneal epithelium has healed.

If an athlete has sustained an alkali burn (from line markings), irrigate the eye copiously for 20 minutes with sterile saline or tap water and instil a local anaesthetic agent to assist this. The athlete should be seen as soon as possible by an ophthalmologist.

Subconjunctival haemorrhage

Trauma to the conjunctiva may cause subconjunctival haemorrhage—a bright red area in the white conjunctiva. Unless the haemorrhage is extensive or visual symptoms or photophobia are present, it is not clinically important.

> **PRACTICE PEARL**
>
> Subconjunctival haemorrhage is a classic finding with periorbital fractures, which need to be ruled out if the athlete participates in a sport where facial trauma is possible.

Face, eye and teeth **CHAPTER 22**

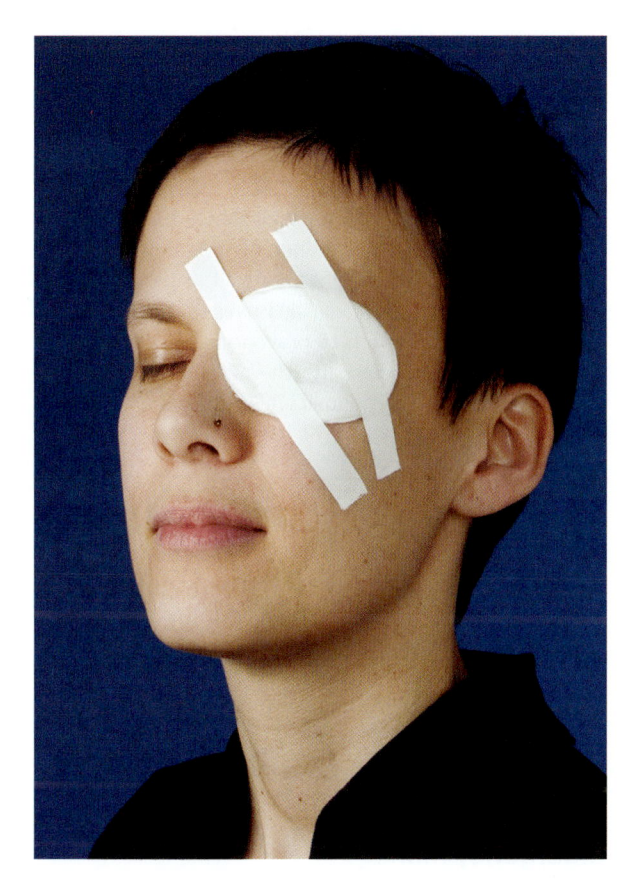

Figure 22.8 Eye padding

> **PRACTICE PEARL**
>
> In all injuries to the eyelids, the eye also needs to be examined to exclude ocular injury.

Hyphaema
Bleeding into the anterior chamber of the eye results from ruptured iris vessels and may only be visible with slit lamp examination. More significant bleeds will present with a bloody layer in the anterior chamber (Fig. 22.7). In hyphaemas of small volume, visual acuity may be unaffected. Associated injuries may occur and all patients with a hyphaema should be referred to an ophthalmologist.

The aim of treatment of this condition is to prevent further bleeding, which may, in turn, result in uncontrollable glaucoma or blood staining of the cornea. The patient needs to rest in bed while the haemorrhage clears, usually over 3–5 days. Aspirin and other anti-inflammatory medications should be avoided as these may provoke further bleeding.

Lens dislocation
Blunt trauma may result in varying degrees of lens displacement. Partial dislocation causes few symptoms. Complete lens dislocation results in blurred vision. A common sign of lens dislocation is a quivering of the iris when the patient moves the eye. Iritis and glaucoma are possible sequelae of lens dislocation. Immediate ophthalmological referral is required. Surgical removal of the displaced lens may be indicated.

Vitreous haemorrhage
Bleeding into the vitreous humour signifies damage to the retina, choroid or ciliary body. Ophthalmoscopic examination reveals loss of the red reflex and a hazy appearance. Treatment generally consists of bed rest, but more severe cases may require specialist referral for removal of the blood and vitreous humour.

Retinal haemorrhage
Injury to the retina can result from a direct blow to the eye or a blow to the back of the head. Valsalva manoeuvres (e.g. in weightlifting) may also produce retinal oedema and haemorrhage. The patient may remain asymptomatic if peripheral areas of the retina are affected. Central retinal damage, however, blurs vision. On ophthalmoscopic examination, central retinal oedema appears as a white opacity that partially obscures the retinal vessels. Boxers may develop atrophic macular holes and loss of central vision as a result of recurrent contusive injuries. This condition requires specialist management.

Blood pressure should be measured to rule out hypertension. Subconjunctival haemorrhage may obscure a perforation of the globe. If this is suspected, the patient should be referred to an ophthalmologist. In most cases, however, the athlete merely requires reassurance.

Eyelid injuries
Direct trauma to the eyelids may cause a large amount of bruising, which should be treated with cold compresses in the first 24 hours. Haemorrhage may spread subcutaneously across the midline to the other eye. A coexisting orbital fracture needs to be excluded in these patients.

Lacerations of the eyelid require meticulous primary repair. Each anatomical layer (conjunctiva, tarsal plate and skin) should be repaired separately by an ophthalmic or plastic surgeon.

Trauma near the medial canthus may lacerate the upper or lower lacrimal canaliculus (tear duct). If this is not repaired, the patient may have permanent watering of the eye. Such injuries require ophthalmological referral for microscopic suturing of the cut ends of the canaliculus.

PART B Regional problems

Retinal detachment
Retinal detachment is more common in those with extreme myopia and may result from any blunt or perforating trauma. The patient complains of flashes of light or the appearance of a 'curtain' spreading across the field of vision, which can present months or even years after the initial injury. Ophthalmoscopic examination reveals elevation and folding of the detached retina, which trembles with each eye movement. Immediate referral for surgical treatment is indicated. An unusual case of retinal detachment in sport occurred in a swimmer who received an accidental blow to the goggles.[3]

Prevention of eye injuries
Athletes with certain eye problems should avoid contact sports altogether. These problems include:

- functionally only one eye
- severe myopia
- Marfan syndrome
- previous retinal detachment.

For squash, protective eyewear must be worn by people who have either only one good eye, amblyopia (lazy eye), recent eye surgery, history of pre-retinal detachment conditions or diabetic retinopathy. Protective eyewear should meet the Australian Standard AS4066 1992 or the US Standard ASTM F803.

Contact lenses offer no protection against eye trauma. Hard contact lenses are not suitable for sporting activity and should never be used in contact sport. Soft lenses appear to be reasonably safe in contact sport. One of the most common 'crises' in injury management is a lost contact lens. The athlete will complain that the contact lens is no longer in its correct position and cannot be located. Usually the lens has been displaced and with careful examination can be located elsewhere on the eye, often at the lower lid. Occasionally, the lens is displaced completely from the eye and lost on the playing surface. Those who wear contact lenses during sport should always carry a spare pair of contact lenses or a pair of protective spectacles as a back-up.

Those athletes who cannot or do not like to wear contact lenses can use protective goggles made of polycarbonate, which are available for most prescriptions. These polycarbonate goggles are also used as eye protection in sports with a high risk for eye injuries. The most obvious examples of these are squash and racquetball, where the size of the ball enables it to enter the orbit and compress the globe. The routine use of closed goggles is strongly recommended.

Certain sports require protection not only of the eye, but of the other facial structures. In sports such as American football, ice hockey, cricket and lacrosse, protective helmets and faceguards should also provide adequate eye protection. Because of the profound effect of major eye injury, we encourage athletes and sport governing bodies to be proactive in promoting and enforcing the use of eye protection where indicated out of order.[4]

TEETH
Trauma to the teeth and dental tissues is a relatively common occurrence in certain sports. A large study, from over 70 000 episodes of basketball, showed mouth guard wearers had a reduced number of dental injuries and referrals to the dentist when compared to those who did not wear mouth guards.[5] This illustrates the importance of the team doctor or coach in preventing injuries through education of athletes and also the requirement to know how to manage dental trauma, when it occurs.

Nature of injuries
Within the mouth are a number of tissues which can be traumatised as seen in the image below (Fig. 22.9).

Trauma results in tissues being crushed, stretched or torn, as seen in the image of a dento-alveolar fracture (Fig. 22.10). The damage caused to teeth and their supporting tissues following trauma is dependent on a number of factors, such as the energy of the impact, the direction of the blow, the tissues traumatised, the resilience or elasticity of the striking object, and the local anatomy. Therefore, dental trauma may present in a number of different ways despite apparently similar causes.

Emergency management
Options for treatment of dental injuries at a sporting event may be limited, due to lack of equipment and facilities. Some injuries may not be visible and may require further special investigations to diagnose. However, many injuries do not need immediate treatment and the most common injuries seen are detailed in Table 22.3 below.

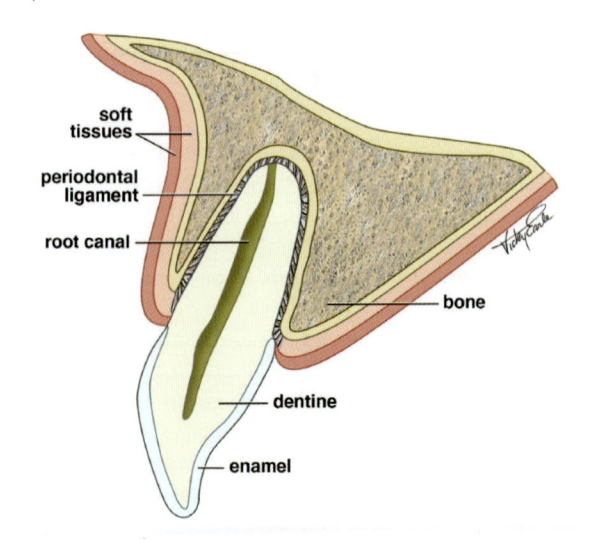

Figure 22.9 Sagittal view showing the jaw and a tooth in the maxillary incisor region identifying the tissues that may be damaged following dental trauma

Face, eye and teeth   CHAPTER 22

can be complex and complications of healing are common. Therefore, athletes who experience trauma should be informed they need close follow-up at regular intervals over a number of years.

Prevention
Although prevention of injuries is often thought to just include the wearing of protective mouth or headguards, an important aspect is education. Athletes should be individually assessed to determine if guards should be worn, for example when engaging in high-risk contact sports, and if prominent upper incisor teeth are present. All efforts should be made to encourage their use.

The two most common types of protection are listed below.

Faceguards:
- are pre-formed cages that attach to a helmet
- provide protection from blows to the front of the head
- often fail to prevent similar blows to the chin, therefore mouth guards also may need to be worn
- significantly reduce injuries in certain sports such as hockey[6] and baseball.[7]

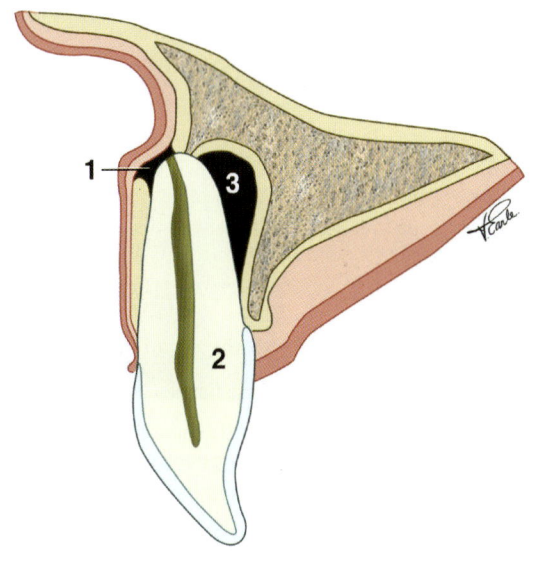

Figure 22.10 Dento-alveolar fracture showing fracture (1) and displacement of a tooth (2) from its socket (3)

Certain situations require special consideration in dental trauma:

- Mouth guard in situ–in general, leave a mouth guard in place as removal might further damage traumatised teeth. If mouth guard must be removed, ensure the patient is seated upright and check the mouth and mouth guard following its removal for teeth and teeth fragments. The mouth guard should not be used to splint teeth due to the problems of oral hygiene.
- Dentures, crowns and bridges–if loose, then remove if possible as they present a choking hazard.
- Unconscious patients–store avulsed teeth in a suitable storage medium and pass to the Emergency Department.

Mouth guards:
- use has also reduced the frequency of dental trauma-related injuries[8]
- prevent damage to teeth, soft tissues and mandible, by cushioning against the opposing teeth following a direct blow
- can also prevent teeth from being lost from the mouth, swallowed or inhaled
- do not appear to prevent concussion injuries.[9]

Three types of mouth guard exist (Fig. 22.11):

1. Stock mouth guard (Fig 22.11a)–loose fitting, made of plastic or rubber and should be avoided as they provide none of the protective functions already discussed.

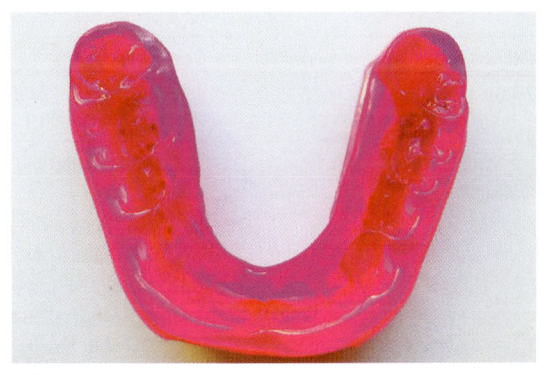

Dental management and follow-up
Injured athletes must be examined by a dentist as soon as possible, with a referral letter if time permits. Treatment

(a)   (b)

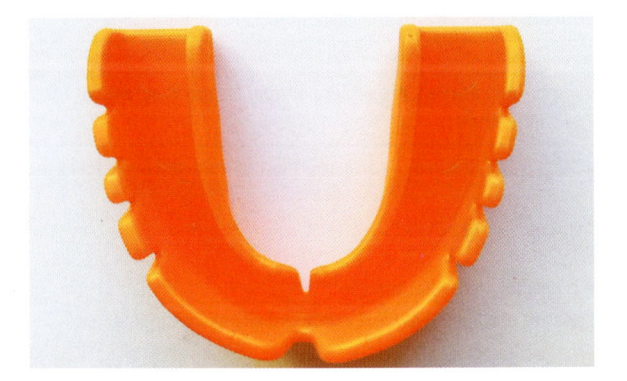

Figure 22.11 (a) Stock mouth guard (b) Mouth-formed mouth guards

341

PART B   Regional problems

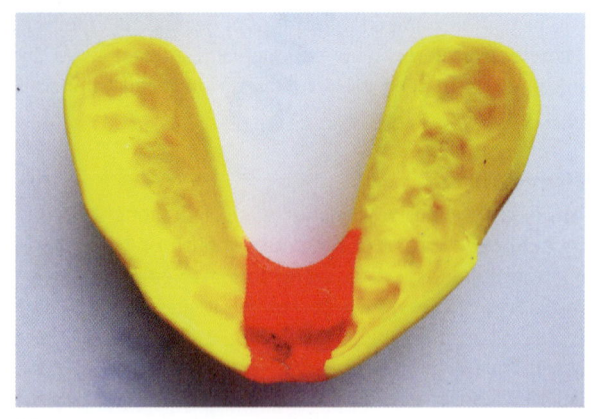

(c)

Figure 22.11 (cont.) (c) Custom-made mouth guard

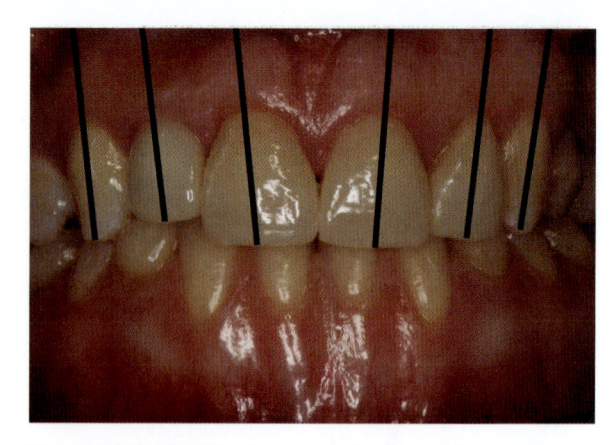

Figure 22.12 Maxillary incisors and canines showing how tooth/root axes are inclined towards the back of the mouth to guide tooth replantation if avulsed

Table 22.3 Emergency dental treatment

Injury	Treatment required
Fractured teeth	• Collect tooth fragments and store in milk or saline • Fragments can be re-attached to teeth in the dental surgery • Assume lost fragments have been swallowed or inhaled. These must be located with chest or abdominal radiographs as the consequences of inhaling infected tooth fragments are serious • Attached fragments should be left unless they can be easily detached
Avulsed tooth	• Reposition in socket as soon as possible (within 5 minutes[10]) • Hold avulsed tooth up by its crown, not root • Wash with saline or water for 10 seconds only, until the root looks clean • Re-implant the tooth in its socket • Check it is correctly aligned and the athlete can bite together • Bite on clean gauze • Visit general doctor for a tetanus booster if needed
Multiple avulsed teeth	• Teeth are unique in shape and their sockets closely replicate their contour • Gently insert into their sockets, one at a time • If teeth do not fit in their sockets, try another socket • Do not force teeth into their sockets • Upper central incisors are larger than lateral incisors • Lower incisors are difficult to tell apart • As a guide, the root tips of teeth are tilted towards the back of the mouth (Fig 22.12)
Displaced teeth	• Gently reposition • If any resistance to repositioning or pain are felt, the athlete should attend their dentist for this to be performed under local anaesthetic

Avulsed teeth that cannot be reimplanted	• Teeth must be kept in a suitable storage medium for transport to the dentist. Never store in water
	• Type of storage medium depends on storage time:
	  – <10 minutes—physiological saline
	  – Up to several hours[11]—fresh milk (cold, low fat is best)[12]
	  – Up to 24 hours[13]—special culture medium, available commercially as Dentosafe® or EMT™ Tooth Saver
	• If no medium is available, store in athlete's saliva

Face, eye and teeth   CHAPTER 22

2. Mouth-formed mouth guards (Fig. 22.11b)–two types:
   a. a shell filled with a plastic or rubber to improve fit
   b. pre-formed plastic mouth guard softened in hot water and moulded to the shape of the teeth and soft tissues

   Both types can be tight fitting, but can be bulky, less comfortable and therefore less likely to be used.

3. Custom made (Fig. 22.11c)–constructed on accurate models of the athlete's teeth. They are well retained and less bulky than other designs, but are more expensive to purchase. Due to their size and fit, they are more comfortable to wear than other types of mouth guards, and as a result more likely to be used in sport.

Mouth guards should be kept clean using standard mouthwashes to rinse. They should be kept away from extreme heat, such as hot water, which will cause distortion of fit.

Therefore a custom-made mouth guard from a dentist is advised, as this will be the most comfortable, least bulky and best fitting. If not available, consider using one that can be moulded in the mouth.

FRACTURES OF FACIAL BONES

In sport, facial fractures may result from blows by implements such as bats or sticks, equipment such as skis[14] and from collision injuries. Mountain biking is a sport that causes a significant proportion of facial injuries. Eye wear[15] and face shields[16] can protect against facial injuries.

Symptoms and signs range from pain, swelling, ipsilateral epistaxis, laceration and bruising to gross deformity. Examination may reveal facial asymmetry, crepitus, discoloration or obvious deformity. Most facial fractures are not overly painful and so there should be little objection to firm palpation, which aids in the diagnostic process. Objectively, the bite should be examined for malocclusion while the patient should also be subjectively asked whether their bite 'feels' out of alignment. Bimanual examination of the facial bones may show areas of discontinuity and mobility. If maxillary fracture is suspected, the upper teeth can be grasped to determine evidence of excessive movement of the upper jaw and midface. Opening and closing the jaw may reveal pain, limitation or deviation with mandibular injuries.

Initial management of facial fractures is directed towards maintenance of the patient's airway. In mandibular body fractures or maxillary fractures, this may require emergency manual reduction. Associated head and cervical spine injuries should be excluded. The oral cavity requires inspection for bleeding or dental damage. CT scans have supplanted plain radiographs as the imaging modality of choice.

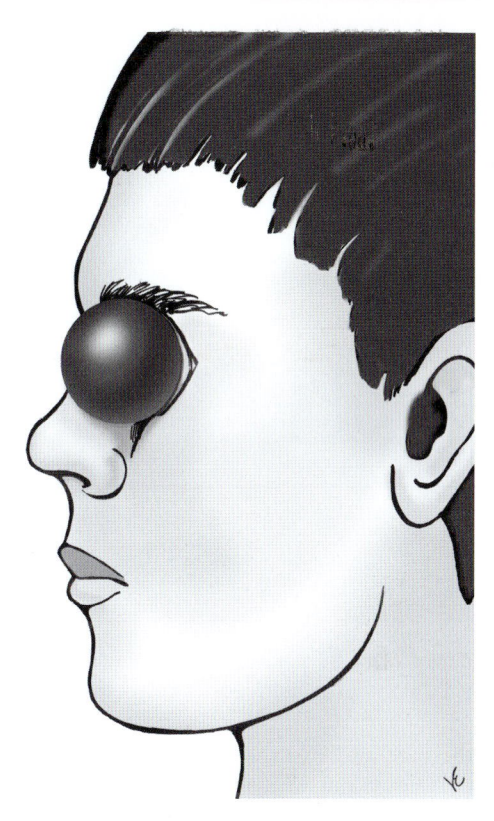

Figure 22.13 A squash ball fits precisely into the eye socket

Orbital fracture with and without globe trauma

'Blow-out' fracture of the orbit results from direct trauma such as a fist, cricket ball, baseball[17] or squash ball (Fig. 22.13). Compression of the globe and orbital contents produces a fracture in the weakest part of the orbit, the orbital floor. Contents of the orbit may herniate through the defect. The patient typically presents with a periorbital haematoma, protruding or sunken eye, double vision on upward gaze and numbness of the cheek. Double vision on upward gaze is due to the entrapment of the inferior rectus muscle in the fracture.

A detailed examination of the eye must be performed to exclude intraocular injuries such as hyphaema, lens dislocation or ruptured globe. If an orbital fracture is suspected, a birds-eye plain radiograph should be performed. The radiograph may not show the fracture, but may demonstrate some clouding of the maxillary sinus. CT examination is used to confirm the fracture. Children require early surgery and as such should be investigated with high clinical suspicion.

Antibiotic therapy should be commenced immediately and the patient referred to an ophthalmologist. Surgery may be required to release the trapped muscle and repair

PART B Regional problems

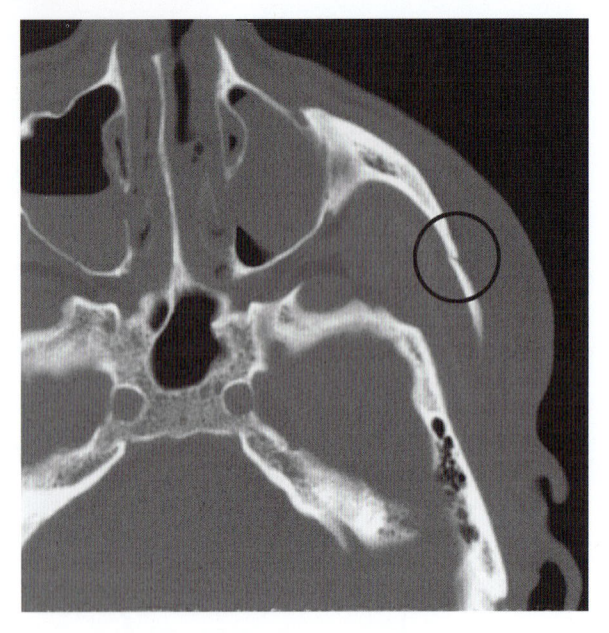

Figure 22.14 CT scan confirming a fractured zygomatic arch; plain radiography did not detect the fracture

the bony defect. Athletes who undergo surgery should be warned not to blow their nose, due to the risk of displacing the fracture and further haemorrhage.

Fractures of the zygomaticomaxillary complex

Zygomaticomaxillary complex fractures (Fig. 22.14) occur from a direct blow to the cheek such as from a fist, hockey stick or baseball. Signs include swelling and bruising, flatness of the cheek and mandibular function disturbance. If associated with an orbital fracture, there may be concomitant diplopia, limitation of ocular movement and asymmetry of the eyes, as well as numbness of the affected cheek, nose, upper lips and upper teeth.

Surgical treatment consists of closed or open reduction under general anaesthesia. Unstable fractures require fixation. Associated orbital fractures are treated by open reduction and reconstruction of the orbital floor.

Maxillary fractures

Maxillary fractures usually result from a direct high-velocity crushing blow to the middle portion of the face, and are extremely rare in sports other than motor sports. They are classified as Le Fort I, II and III fractures (Fig. 22.15) depending on whether the nasal or cheek bones are involved. Le Fort I fractures result in the separation of the maxilla from the nasal–septal structures and the pterygoid plates. Clinically, Le Fort I fractures are identified when the entire maxilla moves as a separate unit. Le Fort II fractures separate the maxilla and the nasal complex from the orbital–zygomatic structures. On clinical examination the maxilla and nose move together as one unit. Le Fort III fractures separate the maxillary, zygomatic, nasal and orbital structures from the cranial base (Fig. 22.16).[18]

Maxillary fractures are often accompanied by cranial damage, obstruction of the nasal airway, oedema of the soft palate, haemorrhage into the sinuses and disturbance of the contents of the orbit. CSF rhinorrhoea may occur, indicating fracture of the cribriform plate. Reduced sensation in the infraorbital region is common.

Examination findings include lengthening of the face, midface mobility, malocclusion of the bite and periorbital bruising. Initial treatment is aimed at protecting the airway–the conscious patient should sit leaning forward. This should be followed by rapid transfer for definitive diagnosis and treatment. Surgical treatment involves reduction and fixation with plates and screws.

Mandibular fractures

Fracture of the mandible is one of the most common facial fractures in sport and usually results from a direct blow. The most common fracture sites are the mandibular angle and the condyle. The mandible usually breaks in more than one place as a result of the trauma and these

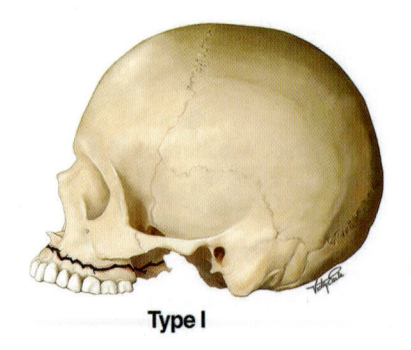

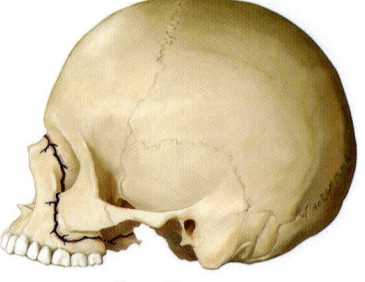

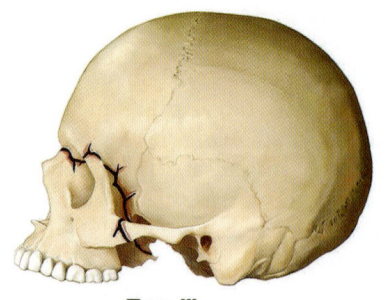

Figure 22.15 Le Fort I, II and III fractures

Face, eye and teeth — CHAPTER 22

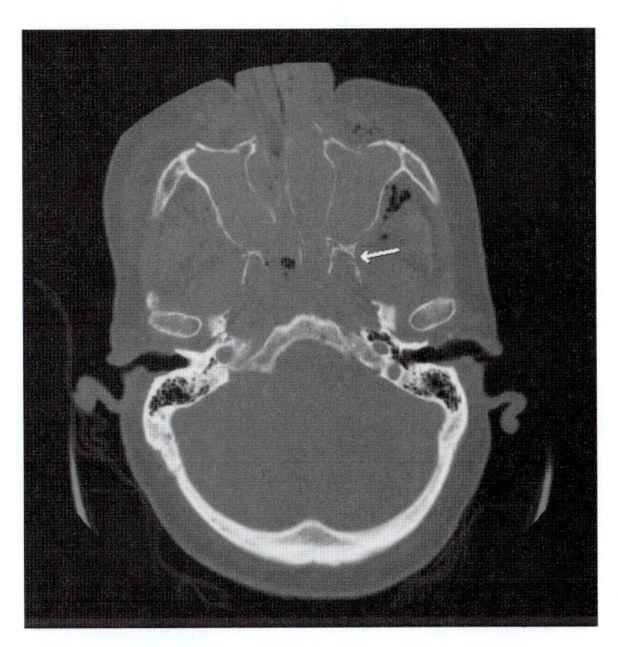

Figure 22.16 CT scan of Le Fort III fracture (arrow)

fractures usually occur on opposite sides of the midline. Fractures may be undisplaced or displaced.

Undisplaced fractures
Minor mandibular fractures are painful, tender and swollen. These are managed conservatively with analgesia and rest. The patient should eat soft food only for up to 4 weeks as symptoms resolve.

Displaced mandibular fractures
Displaced mandibular fractures are severe injuries that result from considerable force. Alveolar (tooth-bearing) fractures are the most common type. These fractures range from single tooth fractures or avulsions to complete segment mobility. The clinical diagnosis is obvious when two or more teeth move as a unit.

Inspection may reveal malalignment of teeth and bruising to the floor of the mouth. Palpation reveals malocclusion, tenderness and defects along the lower border of the mandible. Paraesthesia or anaesthesia of the lower lip and chin suggest damage to the inferior alveolar nerve.

Initial treatment includes maintenance of the airway in a forward sitting position with the patient's hands supporting the lower jaw. A jaw bandage can be used in comminuted or badly displaced fractures, although this is generally not used due to the increased associated risk of compromising the airway by causing backward displacement of the mandible. A cervical collar can be used as an alternative. A concussed or unconscious patient should be placed in a lateral position with head tilt and jaw support after the mouth has been cleared of any dislodged teeth or tooth fragments. Occasionally, the tongue may need to be held forward to maintain an open airway.

Most displaced mandibular fractures require closed reduction and intermaxillary fixation for 4–6 weeks. If adequate closed reduction cannot be achieved, then open reduction and internal fixation is required. A fracture of one condyle usually does not require immobilisation except to control pain. Active jaw exercises should be commenced as soon as pain permits.

During the period of intermaxillary fixation, the athlete may perform mild exercises such as stationary bike riding and light weightlifting. Resumption of contact sport should be delayed until at least 1–2 months after the jaws are unwired. Earlier resumption is possible when internal fixation has been used. The use of a protective polycarbonate facial shield may offer some protection if early return to play is contemplated.

Patients with mandibular fractures who are eating soft food or have their jaws wired can be referred to a dietitian for advice on suitable liquid meals and foods suitable for vitamising.

Temporomandibular injuries
Blows to the mandible can produce a variety of temporomandibular joint (TMJ) injuries. Trauma to the jaw while the mouth is open occasionally produces TMJ dislocation. Other injuries include haemarthrosis, meniscal displacement and intracapsular fracture of the head of the condyle.

Examination of the injured TMJ may reveal limitation of opening, pain and malocclusion. Dislocation of the TMJ causes inability to close the mouth. A dislocated TMJ may be reduced by placing both thumbs along the line of the lower teeth as far posteriorly as possible and applying downward and backward pressure. Longstanding dislocations may require general anaesthesia for reduction. Management of TMJ dislocation includes rest with limitation of mouth opening for up to 7–10 days, a soft diet and analgesics such as aspirin. Contact sport should be avoided for up to 2 weeks depending on the symptoms. Boxers should not attempt sparring for at least 6 weeks.

Chronic temporomandibular pain
Chronic TMJ problems are sometimes referred to as 'temporomandibular joint dysfunction' or 'myofascial pain dysfunction syndrome'. This syndrome appears to affect males more than females with a peak incidence in the early twenties. Patients complain of pain, limitation of movement, clicking and locking of the TMJ. Treatment should include assessment by a dentist to exclude any

malocclusion problem. Physiotherapy evaluation with a view to manual therapy and exercise therapy can be invaluable.

PREVENTION OF FACIAL INJURIES

Protective equipment has been designed for sports where facial injury is a risk (Chapter 9). Properly designed helmets have reduced the incidence of faciomaxillary injuries. Helmets are designed for a single impact or multiple impacts, and should be individually fitted for each athlete. Single-impact helmets such as most pushbike and motorbike helmets must be discarded after the user has had a fall.

Facial protective equipment is constantly developing, with items such as face shields, cages and eyeglasses often used in high-risk sports such as ice-hockey and baseball. Such equipment may also be a useful adjunct to minimise any re-injury risk in the return-to-play process. The legality of the equipment should always be checked with the sport's governing body.

REFERENCES

References for this chapter can be found at www.mhhe.com/au/CSM5e

Chapter 23

Neck pain

by GWENDOLEN JULL and DEBORAH FALLA

It makes your arm very hot, heavy and difficult to move. Stingers don't tend to last too long: you get pins and needles down your arm as the heaviness goes away. Sometimes it's 10 seconds, sometimes maybe a minute.

England Rugby star Jonny Wilkinson, who required neck surgery after recurrent injuries

This chapter focuses on the assessment and management of non-catastrophic painful neck conditions in the athlete. While there is much attention on prevention and acute management of catastrophic neck injuries, these injuries occur predominantly, but not exclusively, in contact sports.[1, 2] Yet, many athletes suffer from debilitating non-traumatic neck pain that can affect both their participation in sport and their quality of life. Such conditions range across a spectrum from acute muscle injury to chronic repetitive strains to cervical degenerative joint disease.[3-5]

ANATOMICAL CONSIDERATIONS

It is usually not possible to make a definitive patho-anatomical diagnosis in most neck pain conditions. Lesions can be identified on imaging with injuries such as cervical fractures or dislocations, or disc disruption (linked with symptoms of a radiculopathy), as can anatomical abnormalities which may predispose the athlete to neck pain or injury.[6] However, for the majority of neck pain presentations in both the athletic and the general population, radiological imaging is unable to identify the pathoanatomical pain source with any certainty. As a result, the majority of disorders are generically classified as non-specific or mechanical neck pain. Despite having one label, the presentation of neck pain conditions is highly variable. Thus, the clinical examination assumes primary importance in identifying the symptom sources and any sensory, neuromuscular and sensorimotor abnormalities associated with the individual athlete's neck pain. The clinical examination relies on a foundation of anatomical knowledge.

The cervical spine is designed for movement, in contrast to the lumbar spine that is designed to carry load. As the most mobile region of the spine, its movements ensure a wide visual field. The functional cervical spine extends from the atlanto-occipital (C0-1) segment to the upper thoracic region (approximately T3-4 segment).

There are many key features to note when performing a clinical evaluation. Movement occurs independently and interdependently between the cranio-cervical, cervical and cervicothoracic regions. The atlanto-axial (C1-2) segment contributes about half the total rotation of the cervical region and this head movement can be performed relatively independently. Most of the remaining rotation occurs at the cervical segments (C2-7), but the head will not rotate to its full excursion unless the upper thoracic region provides the necessary 10° of this movement.[7] From a postural perspective, there is interdependence of the lumbar, thoracic and cervical spinal curves.[8] Evaluation must be both local and regional.

The neck muscles have many diverse roles given the broad functional requirements of the cervical region. For example, an ice hockey player needs fast movements to locate an opponent or puck, a target shooter requires fine movement adjustments for clear vision and head alignment, and a soccer player requires good stability of the neck to head a ball. To perform these tasks there must be fine muscle coordination for movement and adequate kinaesthetic awareness, as well as muscle strength.

There are 44 muscles in the neck, topographically arranged to provide these functional requirements (Fig. 23.1). Some act exclusively over the cranio-cervical

PART B   Regional problems

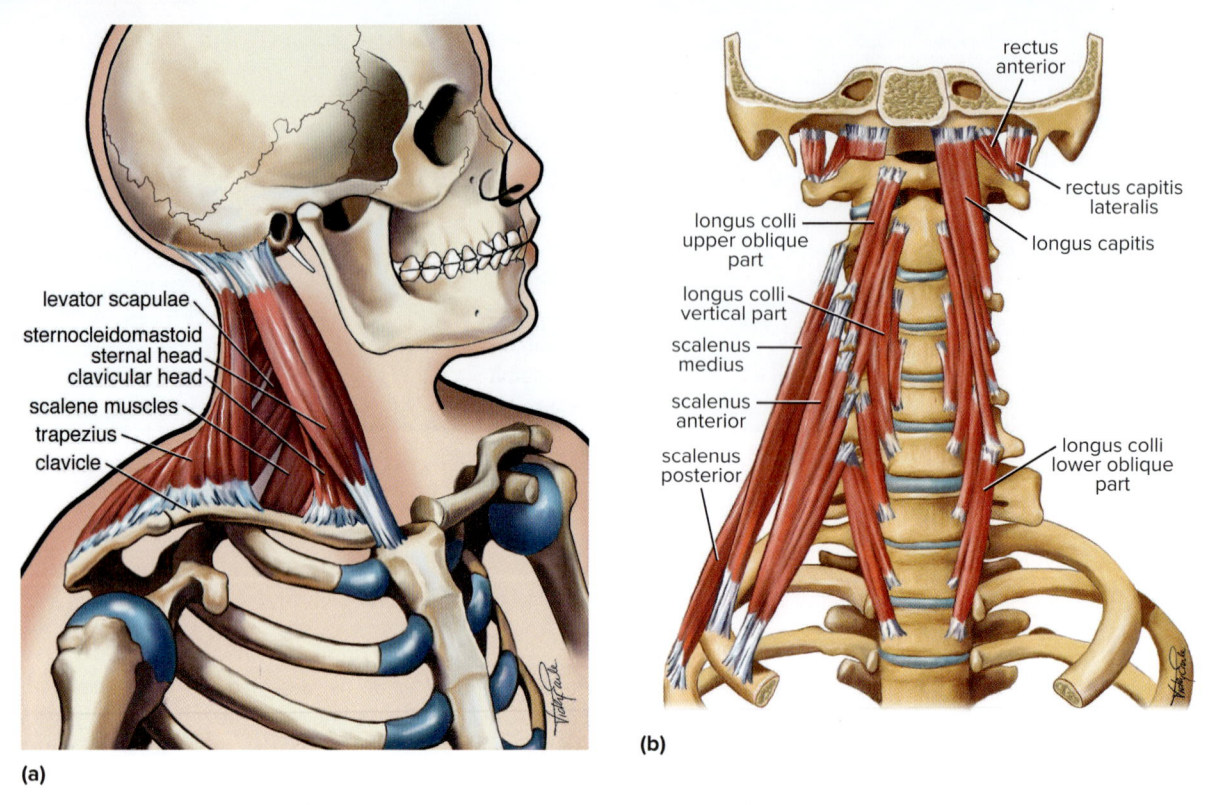

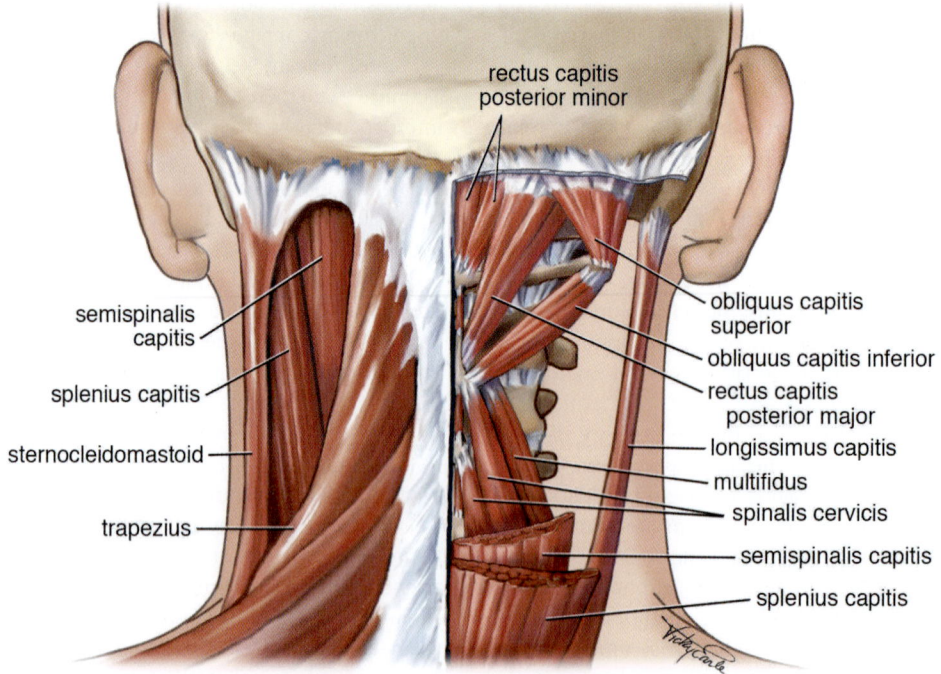

Figure 23.1 Anatomy of the neck (a) Anatomy of the anterior neck—superficial musculature (b) Anatomy of the anterior neck—deep musculature (c) Anatomy of the posterior neck—deep and superficial musculature

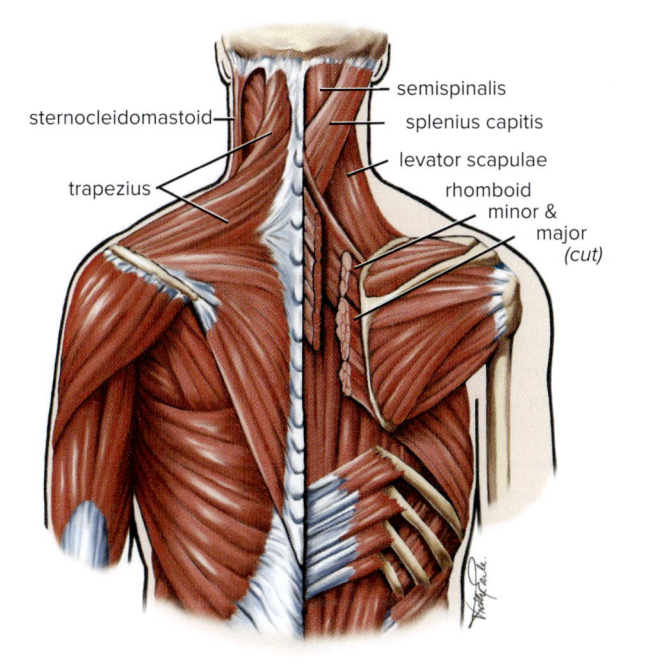

Neck pain CHAPTER 23

(d) Anatomy of the posterior neck and scapulothoracic region showing sternocleidomastoid, trapezius, semispinalis, splenius capitis, levator scapulae, and rhomboid minor & major (cut).

Figure 23.1 (cont.) (d) Anatomy of the posterior neck and scapulothoracic region

region (e.g. suboccipital muscles), others act mainly on the cervical region (e.g. semispinalis cervicis), and still others span the cranio-cervical and cervical regions with attachments from the upper thoracic region (e.g. splenius capitis). The mobile structural design of the cervical spine also relies on the vital role of the muscle system to provide stability.[9] For stability, there is some functional specificity between the layers of both the neck flexor and the extensor muscles.

Broadly, the superficial muscles have larger lever arms and cross-sectional areas with a greater capacity to exert torque than the deep muscles.[10] In contrast, the deeper muscles are more segmentally arranged with segment-to-segment attachments, larger spindle densities and muscle fibre compositions that enable them to guide and support the cervical motion segments.[11]

Coordination between the deep and superficial muscles is required for normal neck function as the deep muscles cannot support the load of the head and the superficial muscles are not placed to support the cervical segments.[12] The cervical region also provides a point of attachment for muscles of the shoulder girdle (Fig. 23.1d) and must bear the load and absorb the forces induced on the cervical segments during upper limb function.[13, 14]

All structures of the cervical region are innervated and thus any could be a source of nociception. These may include the zygapophysial joints, discs, ligaments, muscles and nerves. Pain may be perceived in the neck, upper thoracic region, upper limb or head (cervicogenic headache). Various studies have mapped pain areas when discs or zygapophysial joints have been stimulated.[15, 16]

The overlap between pain patterns of both the zygapophysial joints and discs challenges the ability to make a structural diagnosis from pain distribution alone. Furthermore, the pain distribution from symptomatic joints is more extensive than that of experimentally stimulated asymptomatic joints.[17] Importantly, the suboccipital and deep cervical muscles in the neck region (multifidus and longus colli) have the highest density of muscle spindles of all muscles in the body.[11, 18, 19] There are reflex connections between the neck and the vestibular and ocular systems (for review, see Röijezon and Treleaven).[20] Thus, when cervical afferentation is altered, these interconnections can underlie symptoms of unsteadiness, light-headedness or visual disturbances when associated with neck pain.

CLINICAL PERSPECTIVE

Neck pain is considered within a biopsychosocial framework that embraces biological, psychological (e.g. anxiety, fear) and social (e.g. sports or training requirements) features and their interactions that may contribute to the athlete's disorder and recovery (Fig. 23.2). Neck pain can be a recurrent condition with repeated episodes over a lifetime, with variable degrees of recovery between bouts.[21, 22]

The Global Burden of Disease 2010 study ranked the burden of neck pain as the 4th highest in terms of years lived with disability and ranked it 21st of 291 conditions in terms of overall burden.[23] The lifetime impact of neck conditions should not be underestimated in planning rehabilitation programs for athletes. The challenge is not only to resolve an acute episode of pain to meet an immediate goal of return to sport, but to also prevent or limit recurrence for future quality of life.

Effective management of individuals with neck pain is based on good communication, a thorough history and physical examination, and sound clinical reasoning in a patient-centred approach (Fig. 23.3). The clinician carefully elicits information from the athlete and interprets it on several levels for the purposes of: ensuring patient safety (red flag conditions); making a provisional pathoanatomical diagnosis; making a definitive physical diagnosis in terms of pain mechanisms, movement, neuromuscular and sensorimotor impairments to inform a treatment plan; identifying social (sport) factors which might be driving or causing the disorder; identifying psychological features (e.g. fear of movement, anxiety)

PART B   Regional problems

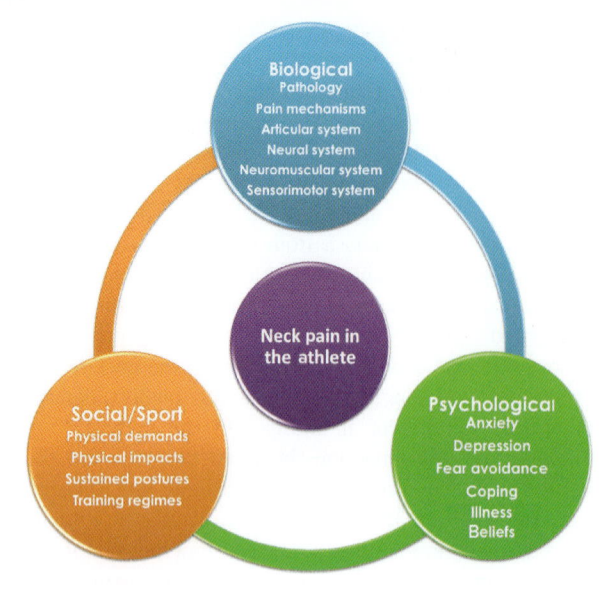

Figure 23.2 The biopsychosocial model for neck pain in sport. The biological, psychological and social components are artificially equally weighted in this diagram. The relationship is fluid. Weighting of biological, psychological and social features differ within and among domains, and within and between individuals. They also change at various time points within the course of an athlete's recovery

History

There are four key areas of information to elucidate when taking an athlete's history. First, establish the athlete's sport and understand its requirements and implications for loads and strains on the neck region. Second, ascertain whether this is an initial onset or a recurrent neck pain condition. Third, determine the duration of neck symptoms in this current presentation (i.e. whether acute, subacute or longstanding in nature). Fourth, clarify how the neck condition began: whether symptoms arose from trauma, either direct or indirect forces (and their direction), or was insidious; and whether the onset was rapid or gradual in nature.

Identifying red flags is a vital aspect in managing athletes with cervical conditions, and the history often raises first suspicions. Except for catastrophic trauma, there are fortunately relatively few serious or life-threatening conditions that present as acute neck pain. Nevertheless, there are two conditions in particular that require clinicians' vigilance in younger to middle-aged athletes: cervical arterial dissection (CAD) and cranio-cervical ligament injury (Table 23.1). CAD can initially be misdiagnosed as a cervical musculoskeletal disorder, and the history and presentation are central to recognition of the condition. Immediate referral for medical investigation and management is essential if suspicions are raised.[26, 27] It is unknown how frequently the alar or transverse ligaments are non-catastrophically injured. Magnetic resonance imaging (MRI) studies have found no convincing evidence of alar or transverse ligament involvement in the common motor vehicle collision and resultant 'whiplash' injury.[28, 29] Immediate referral for medical investigation and management is essential if suspicions are raised.

In more benign cervical conditions, a detailed history can provide valuable information on adverse repetitive that might moderate recovery; and identifying possible prognostic indicators.[24, 25] There is more certainty in decision making when the assessment reveals a clinical pattern that aligns with current knowledge of painful cervical conditions. This pattern should reflect the relationships within and between biological, psychological and social features.

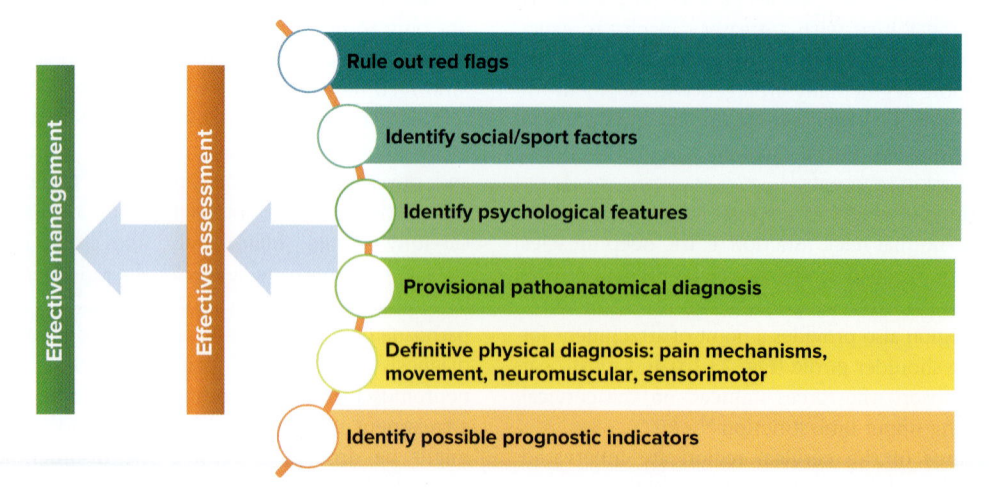

Figure 23.3 Decisions made from effective assessments will inform safe, individualised and effective management plans

350

Neck pain CHAPTER 23

Table 23.1 Red flags in acute neck pain presentations

Condition	Presentation
Cervical arterial dissection	• Acute onset 'unusual' neck pain or headache, increasing in severity over hours or days • Neurological or ischaemic signs • Recent infection or minor trauma
Cranio-cervical ligament injury	• Head or neck trauma • Acute neck pain with perioral paraesthesia, tinnitus, 'lump in the throat' or nausea

movements or prolonged abnormal postures relating to the athlete's sport or training which may be underlying the condition. If the neck pain is recurrent, determine the original time and nature of the onset and the pattern of recurrence, and track the progression of the condition.

Symptoms and their behaviour

Clinicians should obtain information about the area, nature and intensity of pain. The area of pain will give some idea of the likely segmental level that is the source of the pain. Nociception from the C0–4 segments is usually perceived in the upper cervical and possibly the head region, C4–5 in the mid to lower neck, and C5–7 in the lower neck, upper thoracic region and shoulder/arm. Identification of a particular zygapophysial or disc disorder by area of pain is not possible due to overlap of their referral patterns.[15-17] If the athlete pinpoints the pain more posterolaterally, there is an increased possibility that a zygapophysial joint is the source of pain, as these joints are relatively superficial. Pain from irritation of nerve structures can refer into the back of the head (upper cervical nerves) or down into the shoulder and arm (C4–T2), often in a fairly typical dermatomal pattern.

The nature and intensity of the pain can give some indication of pain mechanisms. As a very basic statement, neck pain may reflect a peripheral nociceptive source (e.g. from the joints, ligaments, muscles). When there is an injury or irritation of nerves, it is termed a neuropathic pain. The former is the more common in neck pain conditions and often manifests as an ache or catching pain of mild to moderate intensity. A neuropathic pain is usually a more severe, well-delineated pain that may have lancinating and burning qualities (e.g. a 'stinger' or 'burner' caused by traction to the brachial plexus during a tackle in rugby). Pain from either source may be associated with peripheral or central nervous system sensitisation. In instances of neuropathic pain, the clinician should question the patient regarding more widespread sensitivity to touch or sensitivity to cold.[30, 31] Pain neuroscience has advanced remarkably over the past decades. Chapters 5 and 6 provide a more comprehensive overview of pain physiology.

The presence of other symptoms should be investigated. If the athlete has a 'stinger' or a cervical radiculopathy, there may be paraesthesia or anaesthesia in the upper limb and feelings of weakness. Other symptoms such as unsteadiness, light-headedness or visual disturbances may accompany neck pain as manifestations of cervical sensorimotor disturbances. These symptoms may also be associated with concussion, a vestibular disorder or, more often in the older patient, a vascular disorder. Thus their temporal relationship with neck pain and movement should be explored. If the athlete reports headache in association with neck pain, additional information is necessary to determine whether it is cervicogenic in nature or if it is a primary headache, such as migraine or tension-type headache. Cervicogenic headaches are typically unilateral, side-consistent headaches, associated with neck pain, and pain usually begins in the neck, later developing into a headache.[32] Refer to Chapter 21 for a fuller discussion on headache.

Understanding the behaviour of symptoms as well as which activities, postures or movements provoke and ease symptoms, and how they respond to rest/sleep, can confirm the mechanical nature of the condition and inform the clinician on the possible pain source. If local neck movements are the main aggravator of symptoms, the pain source may be a segmental joint dysfunction. If lifting is the primary aggravating activity, then how the axioscapular muscles are transferring the loads to the cervical segments should be examined. If the cocking phase of throwing is the main aggravator, then any link with mechanosensitivity in the upper quadrant nervous system should be investigated. The reported aggravating activities and positions should be confirmed in the physical examination, as they can direct treatment and guide re-education of appropriate postures and movements/skills pertaining to the athlete's sport or work.

Irritability of the pain and condition is also evaluated (i.e. how easily the pain is aggravated and how long it takes an acute exacerbation to settle). Sleep disturbance is also an important indicator of pain severity. High pain intensity, irritability and acuteness of the condition will limit the extent of the physical examination and the intensity of early treatment.

Psychological features

Psychological reactions to pain such as anxiety and fear of re-injury are normal responses.[33] It is important for the clinician to listen to how the athlete describes his or her pain, how he or she is dealing with it and how it has affected his or her training or sports participation to gain an impression of whether the athlete seems to be unduly anxious or is expressing any fear of movement or activity because of the neck condition. This informs the nature and extent of the assurance and education required in their management. Mild depression could be expected if the neck injury has prevented the athlete from competing in his or her sport; however, moderate or marked depression is a psychopathology requiring expert assessment and care. The clinician can also gain an impression of the athlete's pain-coping strategies (e.g. high reliance on medication or passive treatment modalities versus continuing with activities and actively coping with the pain).

Social/sport factors

It is vital for the clinician to explore and understand the requirements of the athlete's sport, training regimens and occupational activities, and their relationship to the neck pain. A formal analysis of provocative activities is mandatory (e.g. analysis of a tennis serve which aggravates/causes neck pain, analysis of the heading skill in football, analysis of cycling and bike fit, or analysis of weight-training regimens). It is also important to assess the effects of correcting the skill on the athlete's immediate neck pain, to provide some proof of the relationship between the action and pain. This is convincing evidence for the athlete on the need to modify the skill. If the 'driver' of the pain can be removed, this increases the chances of preventing neck pain recurrences. However, the nature of certain sports makes it difficult to remove the 'driver'. For example, modifications of spinal postures and head positions may be limited in road cycling. It will be important to determine tissue tolerance to these postures and develop a program that relieves the strain on these structures before this threshold for pain is reached. This analysis of the symptom-provoking aspects of the sport is crucial for any long-term solutions for the athlete's neck pain.

Patient-reported outcome measures

There are numerous patient-reported outcome measures (PROMs) recommended for the assessment of neck pain. Three common measures are the Numeric Pain Rating Scale (NPRS),[34] the Neck Disability Index (NDI)[35] and the Patient Specific Functional Scale (PSFS).[36] They are described in detail in Table 23.2. PROMs allow the clinician to understand the pain and disability level of the athlete in relation to all individuals with neck pain (NPRS and NDI), as well as to understand the specific functional concerns of the individual (PSFS). PROMs are essential to evaluate the course of recovery throughout treatment.

Table 23.2 Patient-reported outcome measures (PROMs) in neck pain

Measure	Description	Minimum clinically important difference (MCID)[37]	Minimal detectable change (MDC)[38]
Numeric Pain Rating Scale	Quantifies self-reported pain levels and measures pain changes over time. Athletes rate their pain on a scale from 0 and 10; 0='no pain'; 10='the worst pain imaginable'	1.3 points[39]	3 points[40]
Neck Disability Index	Ten items on functional abilities and symptoms. Each item has a 5-point scale and the score is summed and converted to a percentage	9.5 points (19%)[39]	10.2 points (20%)[41]
Patient Specific Functional Scale	Athletes nominate at least 3 activities where they are experiencing difficulty as a result of their condition. For each activity, they rate their ability to perform it, with 0='completely unable' and 10='able to complete the task at full, pre-injury level'	2.0 points[41]	2.1 points[41]

MCID: The smallest difference that patients perceive as beneficial
MDC: The amount of change that must be observed before the change can be considered to exceed the measurement error

Imaging

When the neck pain has resulted from trauma (e.g. collisions, crashes, falls), imaging (plain radiography, computed tomography [CT] scans) is indicated to identify or rule out such lesions as fractures or subluxations/dislocations. There are clear protocols (Canadian C-Spine Rule; NEXUS Criteria) to guide the need for imaging after trauma which have proven sensitive, although their specificity has been challenged.[42, 43] This can affect adherence to these guidelines, as clinicians and athletes want to ensure that serious pathology is not missed. Imaging is also indicated when, on clinical grounds, there is any suspicion of a lesion or fracture.

There is long-standing debate about the need for routine imaging of people presenting with neck pain because the majority of routine imaging provides no additional or certain information to assist structural diagnosis. Even recent studies using MRI have failed to detect and define differences between the non-pathological age-related changes of the cervical spine in people without neck pain and the cervical spines of people with neck pain conditions.[28, 44, 45] Thus routine diagnostic imaging is not indicated for most people with neck pain. The decision to order imaging for the athlete with a neck pain condition should be based on clinical grounds to confirm a clinical diagnosis or clinical suspicion.

Physical examination

The clinical reasoning process commenced in the history continues throughout the physical examination. The physical examination further defines the condition and has three principal aims:

1. to gain a clear picture of the immediate source(s) of pain and the nature of the dysfunction (e.g. a painful cervical segment, protected by local muscle spasm that is restricting segmental and regional motion)
2. to detect and document the effect of pain and injury on the sensory, neuromuscular and sensorimotor systems, and gain an understanding of the interactions between these systems
3. to develop a management program directed by the findings of the physical examination; this management program may be moderated by knowledge of history of onset and pain intensity/mechanisms.

No single test will provide the answer; rather, the clinician seeks a pattern of test responses from the various systems. Two clinical examples illustrate this important point.

The first is the athlete who reports that neck and right arm pain is provoked in the early cocking phase of throwing. Nothing abnormal was detected in the glenohumeral complex. It was reasoned that a cause of this pain could be mechanosensitivity of nerve tissue of the upper quadrant. The pattern of signs that would fit this hypothesis[46] is shown in the box below. If such a pattern of physical impairment and pain responses was not elicited, the clinician would need to reflect on his or her provisional diagnosis and propose an alternative hypothesis to test.

The second is an athlete who presents reporting headaches that are increasing in frequency and who believes they are caused by his or her neck (the athlete has neck pain and tenderness with the headache). The clinical confounder is that most primary frequent intermittent headaches (migraine and tension-type headache) have some neck pain and tenderness in association with headache.[47] This reflects the bi-directional pathway of the trigeminocervical nucleus.[48] A cervicogenic headache is classified as a secondary headache (i.e. secondary to a primary cervical musculoskeletal dysfunction). If the athlete's headache is cervicogenic, then it would be expected to be associated with a pattern of cervical musculoskeletal dysfunction: cervical movement impairment, segmental joint dysfunction (C0-4 which refers pain into the head) and muscle function impairment.[49] Neck tenderness as a single sign has no diagnostic significance. Failure to find this pattern of cervical musculoskeletal dysfunction would rule out a cervical cause of headache. This chapter does not cover the temporomandibular joint complex. Nevertheless, the clinician is reminded of the role that craniomandibular dysfunction may play in head, face and neck pain.

There are many tests that may be employed in the physical examination to evaluate the function and integrity of articular, neural, neuromuscular and sensorimotor systems of the cervical region. The tests used will depend on the individual athlete. For example, there is no indication to use the upper limb neurodynamic tests or Spurling's test in an athlete presenting with right upper cervical pain aggravated by looking upwards. Likewise, in acute injury or pain, examination will be curtailed to those tests absolutely necessary to gauge severity and to inform initial management. The order in which tests are conducted in the physical examination usually considers the athlete's position and comfort. However, for ease of description here, tests will be described in groups rather than the ideal order of application.

The physical examination involves the following.

1. Postural analysis
    a. dynamic postures (symptom provoking positions or relevant sports/activity-related positions)
    b. static posture of the spine and axioscapular region in sitting and standing in all three planes
    c. axioscapular posture.

PART B Regional problems

> **An example of clinical reasoning in the physical examination to confirm the hypothesis that an athlete's neck and arm pain while throwing was related to mechanosensitivity of nerve tissue of the upper quadrant**
>
> **Functional complaint:** Neck and (R) arm pain provoked in the early cocking phase of throwing
> **Shoulder joint:** No abnormality detected in any test
> **Reasoning:** Pain from mechanosensitivity of nerve tissue of the upper quadrant
> *Physical examination confirmation*
> **Posture:** Slightly elevated (R) shoulder
>   Scapular depression reproduced slight arm pain (stress on brachial plexus)
> **Active/passive movement dysfunction:** Cervical lateral flexion (LF) to the left most provocative of arm pain (strain on right nerves)
>   Range of lateral flexion is restricted (compared to normal) and right arm pain is present when the nerves are pre-tensioned
>   Arm pain ↓ when arm passively supported in 90° abduction and external rotation with elbow flexed (nerves off tension)
> **Adverse responses to neurodynamic tests:**
>   Upper limb neurodynamic test
>   – lacks 30° elbow extension and neck and arm pain reproduced
>   – cervical LF (L) increases pain; LF (R) decreases arm pain
> **Evidence of a local area of pathology:** Manual examination: painful segmental joint dysfunction C5–6

2. Active movement tests–each assessed for cranio-cervical (C0–2), cervical (C2–7) and cervicothoracic (C7–T4) regions
   a. flexion
   b. extension (Fig. 23.4)
   c. lateral flexion
   d. rotation
   e. flexion/rotation (Fig. 23.5).
3. Quantitative sensory testing (e.g. pressure pain threshold, thermal pain threshold)
4. Manual examination of segmental dysfunction (e.g. posterior-anterior glides [Fig. 23.6], PPIVMs)
5. Tests of the nervous system
   a. clinical neurological examination (if indicated)
   b. upper limb neurodynamic tests (movement and mechanosensitivity of nerves)–Chapter 15.
6. Tests of muscle function
   a. cervical flexors
      i. cranio-cervical flexion test (Fig. 23.7)
      ii. cervical flexor strength and endurance.
   b. cervical extensors
      i. cranio-cervical extension test (Fig. 23.8a)
      ii. cranio-cervical rotation test (Fig. 23.8b)
      iii. cervical extensors (biased towards the deep cervical extensors) (Fig. 23.8c)
      iv. modified Biering–Sorensen test.
   c. axioscapular
      i. dynamic scapular control (Fig. 23.9)
      ii. lower trapezius, serratus anterior in prone and quadruped
      iii. muscle length tests (e.g. levator scapulae, pectoralis major/minor).
7. Tests of cervical sensorimotor function
   a. test of joint position sense (Fig. 23.10)
   b. test of movement sense (Fig. 23.11)
   c. static and dynamic balance
   d. ocular motor tests (gaze stability, smooth pursuit neck torsion test [SPNTT] and evaluation of rapid eye movements).
8. Additional tests (if indicated)
   a. cervical arterial dysfunction
   b. additional passive movement tests when indicated (e.g. Spurling's)
   c. cranio-cervical ligament tests (e.g, Sharp–Purser test; alar ligament tests).

Postural analysis

One of the most important assessments is the analysis of the relevant sports/work or activity-related postures and movements that aggravate the athlete's pain. The athlete demonstrates the activity or position that is pain provoking. The clinician analyses the movement and its control from local and regional perspectives. The clinician should facilitate correction of the posture, movement or technique to gauge the effect on pain or performance. This will accurately and relevantly inform the management approach.

Posture is then formally examined in standing and sitting. The regions of the spine are interdependent, and assessment of head and neck orientation can only be made in relation to orientation of the lumbopelvic region and thoracic spine. The most common poor sitting posture is the slumped 'flexed' posture which facilitates a forward head posture. Some persons have an extended spinal

Neck pain CHAPTER 23

posture in sitting (e.g. some ballet dances and gymnasts) while others have a good 'neutral' posture. It is necessary to determine whether the person's 'non-ideal' posture is contributing to their neck pain.

An answer can be gained by a simple test–retest approach. Test cervical rotation in the person's natural posture and note any movement restriction or reproduction of their neck pain. Correct posture to the ideal upright neutral position and retest cervical rotation. If the range and pain response improve significantly, this suggests that poor posture is one driver of the neck pain or loss of function and indicates that postural re-education will be an important strategy in management.

At the other extreme, if there is no change in rotation range or pain with postural correction, then the clinician can reason that posture is not a major contributor. In this case, postural correction will not be taught with a rationale that it is a driver of pain. As will be discussed in the management section, postural correction will be taught, but with the intent of facilitating the postural supporting muscles.

A similar process is undertaken in the evaluation of scapular orientation and this is described more fully in the later section on axioscapular muscles.

Active movement tests

The observation of reduced cervical range of movement is valuable in the diagnosis of cervicogenic headache, cervical radiculopathy and cervical spine injuries.[50] Movement is an impairment in most neck pain conditions. Movements of flexion, extension, lateral flexion and rotation should be assessed in the three functional regions of the cervical spine: cervical (C2-7), cranio-cervical (C0-2) and cervicothoracic (C7-T4) regions. The information gained from this movement analysis includes range of motion, pain with motion and the ability to control motion. Movements can be affected by articular, muscular or neural tissue, and differentiation of the source of restriction or pain will inform treatment planning.

In the examination of cervical flexion, ensure that the chin stays in a neutral position since anatomically, full

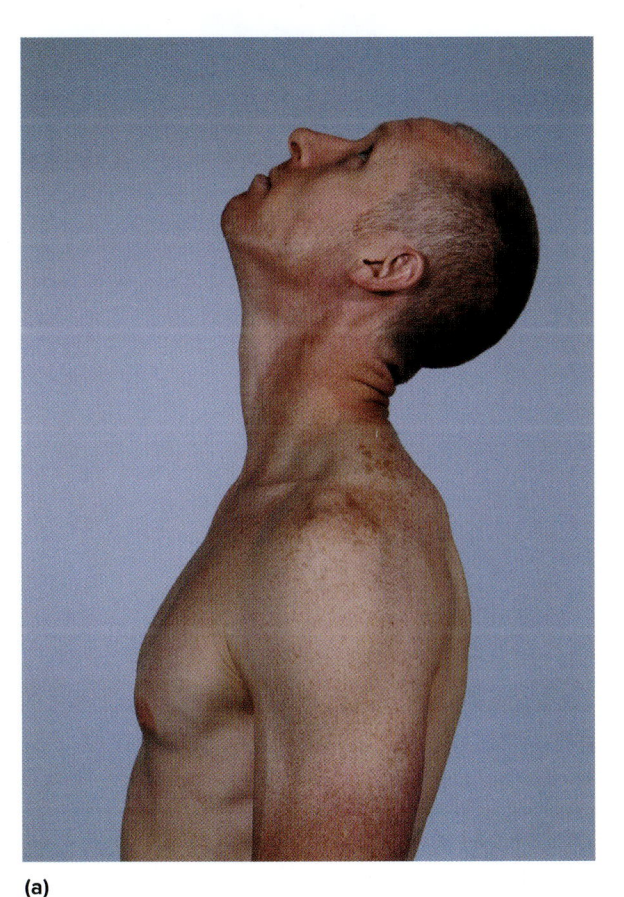

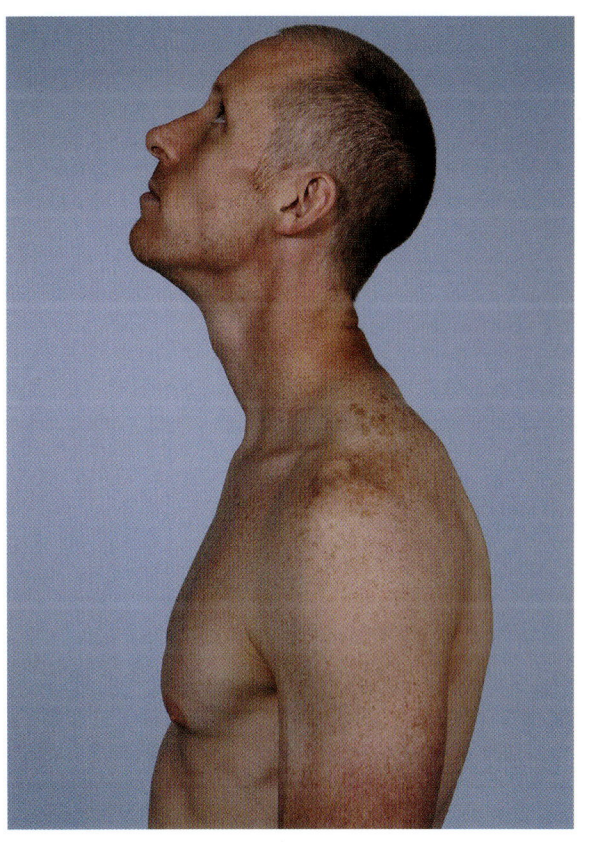

Figure 23.4 (a) Cervical extension. Note the displacement of the head behind the line of the shoulders (b) Cervical extension. If movement is only occurring in the upper cervical region, there is no posterior displacement of the mid to lower cervical segments

355

cervical flexion cannot be performed with simultaneous full upper cervical flexion. Extension is informative in detecting both articular and motor control problems. Normally, the head should displace behind the line of the shoulders in full extension. While the person's face may be directed to the ceiling (upper cervical extension), it is often observed that the mass of the head is not displaced posteriorly to a sufficient extent (Fig. 23.4). This may be a protective strategy for a painful cervical joint, or masking poor muscle control of the region (or both). Encouragement is given to perform the movement correctly and the response noted. If pain limits the movement, the movement usually stops at the segmental source of the pain. If the problem is poor control (i.e. poor eccentric control of the deep cervical flexors), a 'give' in the mid-cervical region may be observed as the neck extends, or the patient may protrude their chin as the initiating action on return from extension to the upright position (due to poor concentric control of the deep cervical flexors).

Assessment of axial rotation gives a clear indication of the contribution of the cranio-cervical, cervical and cervicothoracic regions to total head rotation. Cranio-cervical rotation can be tested in relative isolation from the remainder of the cervical region with the flexion–rotation test (Fig. 23.5a).[51, 52] The contribution of the cervicothoracic region[7] to total rotation can be assessed through observation, and the segmental contribution to the movement can be determined by palpation of the movement at each spinous process as the patient repeatedly rotates his or her head (Fig. 23.5b). The clinician can detect segments that are hypomobile and not contributing to the movement.

Lateral flexion is probably the most useful movement to differentiate between an articular, neural or muscular restriction to movement (see box above).

Despite difficulties in imaging relevant pathoanatomy, selected movement tests can identify facet joint dysfunction. The flexion–rotation test has been proven to be a reliable test with content and discriminant validity.[51-55] It can be used with confidence to locate C1–2 joint dysfunction, especially in the diagnosis of cervicogenic headache. The extension-rotation test,[56] when used in combination with a palpation and manual

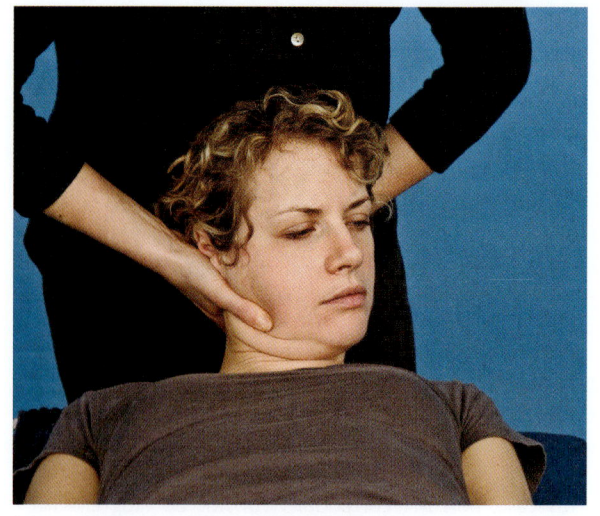

(a)

(b)

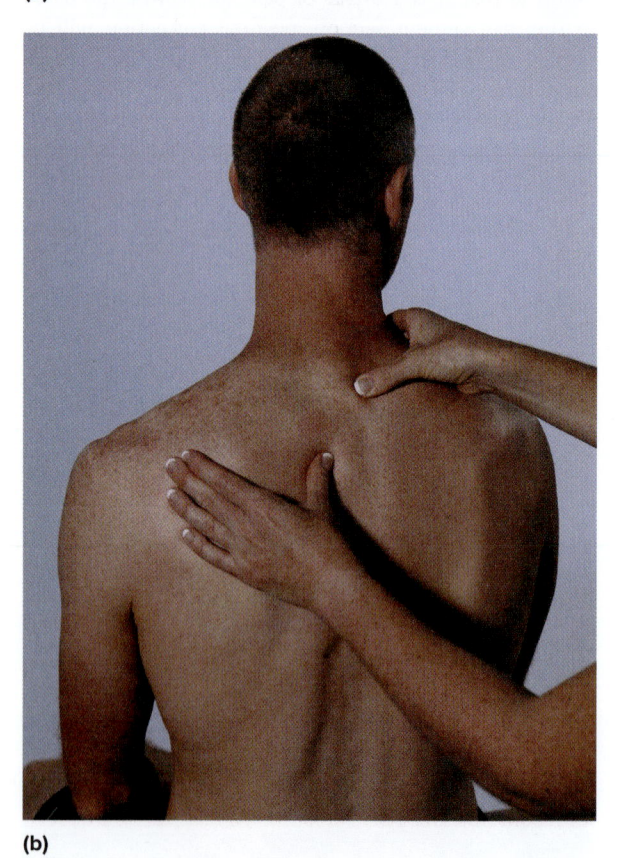

Figure 23.5 (a) The cervical flexion rotation test (C1–2 rotation). The athlete is positioned in supine and the head is supported by the clinician. The athlete is asked to look down at his/her toes (cervical flexion) and simultaneously the clinician moves the athlete's neck into full flexion. The head is then rotated to the left and right and the clinician is assured of performance of a correct test when there is a definite end to the movement. There should be at least 30° of rotation, and a side-to-side difference of 10° is considered a positive test result[53] (b) Assessment of cervicothoracic rotation. The athlete actively and repeatedly rotates his/her head. Using a gentle lateral glide on the spinous process in time with the active movement, the clinician perceives the presence (or not) of rotation of each thoracic vertebra to approximately the T4 level

examination, is able to detect the painful zygapophysial joint–as tested against facet anaesthetic blocks.

Quantitative sensory testing

Many neck pain conditions involve peripheral nociception with or without peripheral sensitisation. Of particular concern are athletes who present with central nervous system sensitisation. Care must be taken in both the examination and management approach for these individuals as overzealous examination and management may easily aggravate their condition. Examination and management techniques should cause no further pain. Conditions in which central sensitisation may occur include cervical radiculopathy,[30] cervicogenic headache[57] and whiplash-associated disorders (WAD).[58] Such individuals may present with many sensory disturbances including widespread mechanical hyperalgesia and cold hyperalgesia. Pressure pain thresholds may be tested with an algometer or the clinician could determine if the athlete seems oversensitive to touch, not only over the neck but also more distally in the arms and legs. A simple clinical test can test cold hyperalgesia.[59] If patients report pain >5/10 on a NPRS after a 10-second application of an ice pack to the neck region, the clinician could be suspicious of the presence of cold hyperalgesia.

Passive tests

Manual examination of segmental dysfunction

Manual examination is used to detect the painful segment(s), and to qualitatively assess segmental motion and tissue resistance to the manually induced movement ('end feel'). The segments from C0-1 to the upper thoracic region are examined. Posterior-anterior glides (Fig. 23.6) can be regarded as a gentle provocative test to locate the symptomatic facet joint or cervical segment. Passive physiological intervertebral movements (PPIVMs) are used to both confirm the segment(s) with altered mobility and to understand the nature of the movement impairment. Although not without historical controversy, manual examination is proving to be an accurate method to locate the symptomatic segment(s). Manual examination with and without other physical tests accurately identifies segmental levels of dysfunction and assists in differential diagnosis of disorders such as cervicogenic headache.[49, 56, 60]

Other passive movement tests (when indicated)

There are several additional testing procedures that can be employed when necessary in the examination of an athlete with a neck pain condition. Some clinicians extend the examination to direct a particular treatment approach; for example, examining movements in combination or gauging the effect of repeated movements.[61, 62] Other

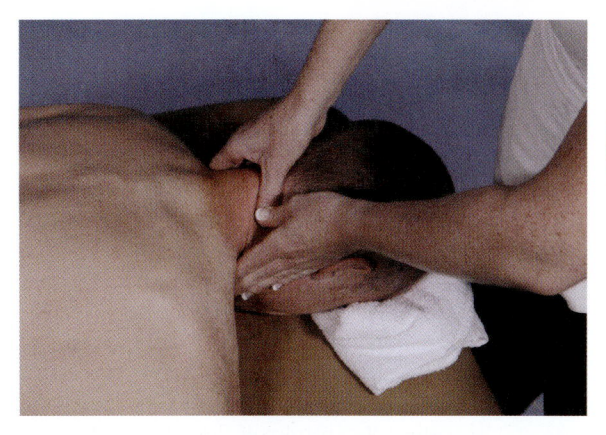

Figure 23.6 Posteroanterior glides on the C2–3 zygapophysial joint. Gentle manual forces are applied over the lamina of the zygapophysial joints of all segments as well as over the spinous processes to determine which is the painful segment associated with the athlete's neck pain disorder. Good technique is required and the posteroanterior glides must be applied painlessly to avoid false positive results

tests seek a particular pathoanatomical compromise, such as Spurling's test. This test, a combination of cervical extension and lateral flexion, narrows the intervertebral foramen and is used to determine if arm symptoms are related to a sensitive and/or compromised cervical nerve root.[63] There are clinical tests for the cranio-cervical ligaments, specifically the transverse ligament, tectorial membrane and alar ligament, as well as the integrity of the cervical segments. Such tests would be indicated after trauma. A variety of symptoms are proposed that might arouse suspicion, such as feeling unable to hold the head up or a desire for support either by a collar or hands.[64] The test for the transverse ligament (Sharp–Purser test) has been validated in a population with rheumatoid arthritis.[65] MRI has established the construct validity of both the side-bending and rotation clinical stress tests for alar ligament integrity.[66] However, clinicians should consider that the true clinical utility of these tests has yet to be proven and the true incidence of non-catastrophic cranio-cervical ligament injury is yet to be established.[28, 29]

Tests of the nervous system

Clinical neurological examination

A clinical neurological examination (sensation, muscle strength and reflexes) is indicated when there is suspicion of a cervical radiculopathy and compromised nerve conduction (i.e. athlete presents with referred arm pain or has suffered a 'stinger' due to traction of the brachial plexus or compression of the cervical nerve roots).

Tests of movement and mechanosensitivity of nerve structures

Nerves and their surrounding structures are pain sensitive and can contribute to neck pain conditions. The classic upper limb neurodynamic test (see Chapter 15) is a valid and reliable test of brachial plexus mechanosensitivity.[46, 67-69] The test is considered positive when there is at least partial reproduction of symptoms and these symptoms can be altered via structural differentiation.[67] Further, there is usually a side-to-side difference in the range of movement in the final test component (usually elbow extension) with increased muscle resistance to limit the provocative movement. As illustrated earlier (see Box earlier in the chapter), there is usually a pattern of clinical symptoms and signs that nerve tissue mechanosensitivity is a pain source.

Tests of muscle function

There are potential changes in control and structure of neck and axioscapular muscles in the presence of neck pain and injury. Changes in motor control include altered coordination between deep and superficial neck muscles, which may compromise the deep muscles' capacity to support the cervical segments in posture and movement.[12] Evidence of this impairment is strong for the flexor muscles[70-72] and is emerging for the extensor muscles.[73, 74]

Altered muscle coordination has been found in persons with neck pain of both insidious and traumatic onset,[70-72, 75] indicating that it is common motor dysfunction (analogous to the inevitable quadriceps muscle dysfunction that occurs with knee conditions regardless of cause). Muscles lose directional specificity,[76] and increased co-activation of the neck flexor and extensor muscles during isometric and functional tasks has been found.[75-77] Onsets of muscle activity are delayed, as demonstrated by an increased latency between the onset of the deltoid muscle and onset of the neck muscles with rapid arm movement,[78, 79] and by delayed activation of the neck muscles in response to full-body perturbations.[80] This has implications for unprotected loading on cervical segments during sport and functional activities. People with neck pain also display reduced strength and endurance at various contraction intensities, and their neck muscles may demonstrate increased muscle fatigability.[81-83]

Muscle biopsies reveal changes in fibre type within the neck flexors and extensors in people with longstanding neck pain.[84] Specifically, there is an increased proportion of type IIC transitional fibres, consistent with a transformation of slow-twitch oxidative type I fibres to fast-twitch glycolytic type IIB fibres, which aligns with the cervical muscles' decreased endurance capacity. Muscle atrophy has been documented in individuals with chronic neck pain conditions[85-87] and widespread fatty infiltrate has been identified in the flexor and extensor muscles, particularly in the deep muscles of those with moderate to severe chronic WAD.[88] It appears that fatty infiltrate may be a feature of chronic whiplash, but not of chronic, insidious-onset neck pain,[89, 90] which suggests there might be differences in pathophysiological mechanisms between these two neck pain groups.

The axioscapular muscles are commonly tender to palpation but more importantly, poor muscle function of the shoulder girdle may overload cervical structures and contribute significantly to pain. The upper trapezius attaches to the cranium and ligamentum nuchae, and the levator scapulae attaches directly to the upper four cervical segments. Normal upper limb function induces both compressive loads and movement in the cervical segments.[13, 14] Poor scapular muscle control may adversely increase these loads and strains.

Electromyographic studies have revealed greater fatigability of the upper trapezius[91] and altered patterns of trapezius muscle function in functional tasks in individuals with neck pain disorders.[75, 92] Moreover, the spatial distribution of upper trapezius muscle activity changes in the presence of pain.[93, 94] Evidence for serratus anterior dysfunction in neck pain patients is also emerging.[95] A link between neck pain and altered axioscapular muscle function has recently been established in an experimental pain study, where the neck pain resulted in some reorganisation in axioscapular muscle activity.[96]

Assessment of cervical flexors

The cranio-cervical flexion test (CCFT) assesses the activation and holding capacity of the deep longus capitis and colli muscles (for review see Jull et al.).[97] It is a low load test performed in supine. The test is conducted in two stages (Fig. 23.7).

The first stage evaluates motor control. The athlete performs five progressive stages of increasing cranio-cervical flexion range and is guided to each stage by feedback from a pressure sensor (such as the Stabilizer Pressure Biofeedback unit) placed behind the upper neck. The pressure sensor indirectly monitors the slight flattening of the cervical curve that occurs with longus colli contraction. The displacement, registered by the pressure sensor, permits some quantification of deep cervical flexor muscle performance.[98] The assessment determines the pressure level that the athlete can achieve in the test when asked to target each of the five stages of 2 mmHg pressure increments from a baseline of 20 mmHg to a maximum 30 mmHg. A 'correct' performance is when the athlete performs a slow and controlled cranio-cervical flexion action (rather than retraction) and no excessive activity of the sternocleidomastoid (SCM) or anterior

Neck pain   CHAPTER 23

(a)

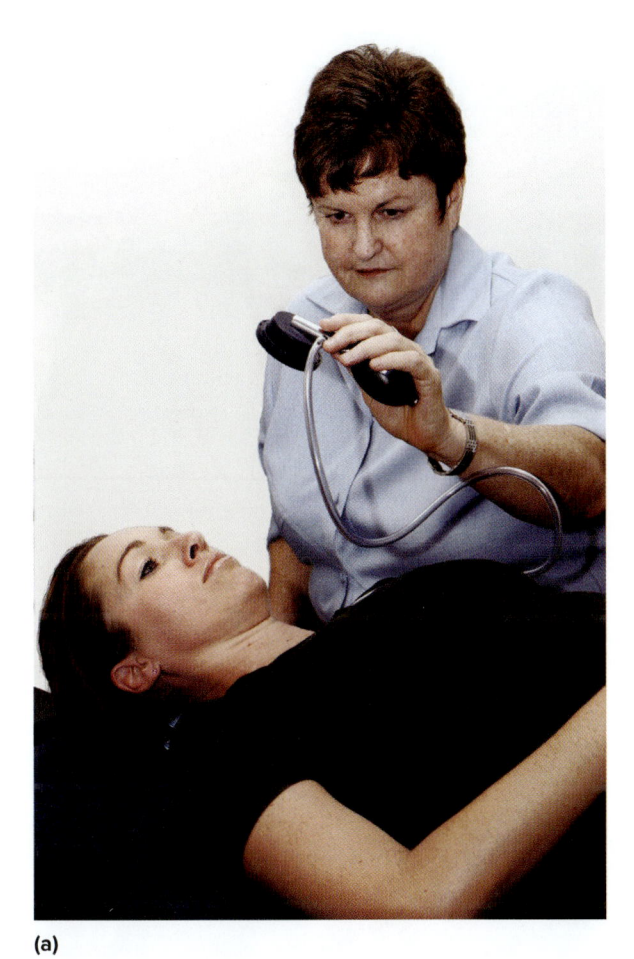

Figure 23.7 (a) The cranio-cervical flexion test (CCFT). The pressure sensor is placed suboccipitally and inflated until a stable baseline of 20 mmHg is gained. In stage 1 of the test, the athlete is instructed to feel the back of his or her head slide up the bed to nod his or her chin. The athlete repeats the action five times, progressively targeting increasing increments of 2 mmHg from 22–30 mmHg, holding each pressure target for 1–2 seconds and relaxing between each. The clinician analyses the quality of cranio-cervical flexion movement at each point. Each pressure target should be achieved with increasing ranges of flexion, which will not be observed if the patient substitutes with a retraction action. Any excessive use of the superficial flexors should be observed and palpated. In stage 2 of the test, the athlete nods to the target pressure and holds the contraction. In an acceptable performance, the athlete uses the correct cranio-cervical flexion action and can hold the pressure steady. Inadequate performance is judged when the patient cannot hold the pressure steady (the pressure drops off target), it is held with a jerky action, or dominant activity of the superficial flexors is observed
COURTESY OF GWENDOLEN JULL

(b)

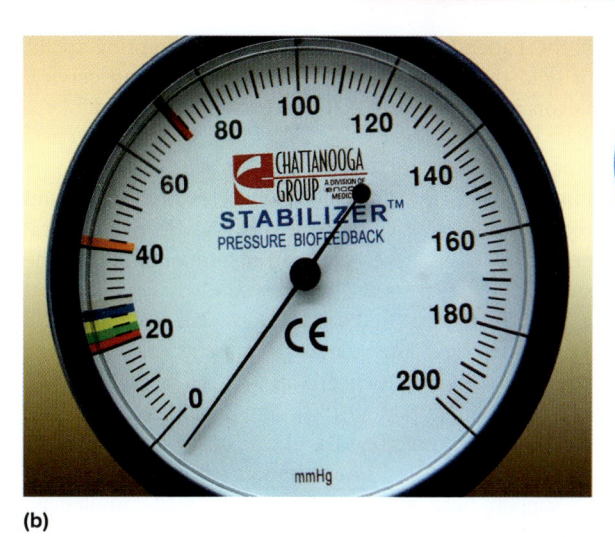

Figure 23.7 (b) The face of the pressure sensor showing the marked 2 mmHg increments that the patient targets in the CCFT

scalene (AS) muscles is observed. Note the SCM and AS muscles flex the neck but not the head, so they should not be excessively active during cranio-cervical flexion.

Stage 2 tests the endurance of the deep cervical flexors at functionally relevant low contractile intensities. Stage 2 is performed when the patient can correctly perform the cranio-cervical flexion action; thus, this stage may be tested at the second treatment session, once the athlete has mastered the action.[97] In a formal assessment of the endurance capacity, the athlete performs 10 repetitions of 10-second holds at each progressive pressure level from 22 mmHg until failure. Most asymptomatic individuals perform well to at least 26 or 28 mmHg whereas individuals with neck pain can usually only achieve stages 22 or 24 mmHg.[97] As a clinical note, the formal assessment of endurance can take up to 5 minutes or more to perform, which is a long time in a busy practice. The clinician can take a shortcut and use the test to determine at which pressure level the athlete can commence training. In this case, the clinician judges the athlete's performance on approximately three repetitions of 5-second contractions at 22 mmHg. If performance is satisfactory, the test is quickly progressed to 24 mmHg and so forth, until the patient shows difficulty in maintaining a steady contraction. Training commences at the level below the stage of failure.

Strength and endurance of the neck flexors (both superficial and deep flexors) are tested at a time only when the patient's pain and muscle performance level permits. These are tested with a head lift task while maintaining a cranio-cervical flexion position. This is a test predominantly of the SCM and AS muscles, which provide more than 80% of the cervical flexion torque.[10,99]

PART B Regional problems

If the patient's chin protrudes when attempting to lift or hold the head position, this means the deep cervical flexors are too weak to cope with the level of load.[100]

Assessment of cervical extensors

Impairment in the suboccipital muscles is common and recent research is suggesting that the deeper cervical extensors may have greater impairments than the superficial extensors.[73, 74] Hence, these muscles are of particular interest in clinical tests. The topographical arrangement of the extensor muscles allows some targeting of these muscle groups.

The athlete is positioned in four-point kneeling or lies prone, propped on elbows, with the cranio-cervical region in a neutral position.[101] All extensors work in this position to support head mass, but the suboccipital muscles are targeted with a test of cranio-cervical extension (chin lift and lower, rectus capitis posterior major and minor) and cranio-cervical (C1–2) rotation (rotate 30–40°, obliquus capitis superior and inferior) (Fig. 23.8a & b). Often no obvious impairment is observed due to the low load nature of the test. However, in athletes with an upper cervical disorder, it is not uncommon to observe that the athlete has difficulty in actually performing rotation at C1–2, and rotates through the mid and lower cervical region. This deficit should be remediated in the exercise program.

The deeper cervical extensors, semispinalis cervicis and multifidus, are targeted by testing cervical extension with the cranio-cervical region maintained in a neutral position.[102, 103] The superficial extensors attach to the cranium and the neutral head position takes away some of their mechanical advantage. The axis of motion for cervical extension passes through the lower cervical region.

To test cervical extension of the deeper muscles, the athlete flexes his or her head and neck to look at the knees and then curls the head and neck back into extension (Fig. 23.8c). The neutral cranio-cervical region is maintained with eye facilitation. The athlete pretends that there is a book between his or her hands, keeping his or her eyes on the book while curling the head into extension. Neck extension should be around 30°. An inadequate performance occurs when the athlete can only extend to the neutral position, reports fatigue after a few repetitions, or cannot extend without use of cranio-cervical extension (i.e. the superficial extensors).

The second phase of strength and endurance testing for the neck extensors is performed once the athlete can perform multiple repetitions of cervical extension in the four-point kneeling position, and only as their pain permits. The modified Biering-Sorensen test can be used.[104] The athlete lies prone with his or her head supported over the end of the couch such that the cranio-cervical and cervical regions are in a neutral position.

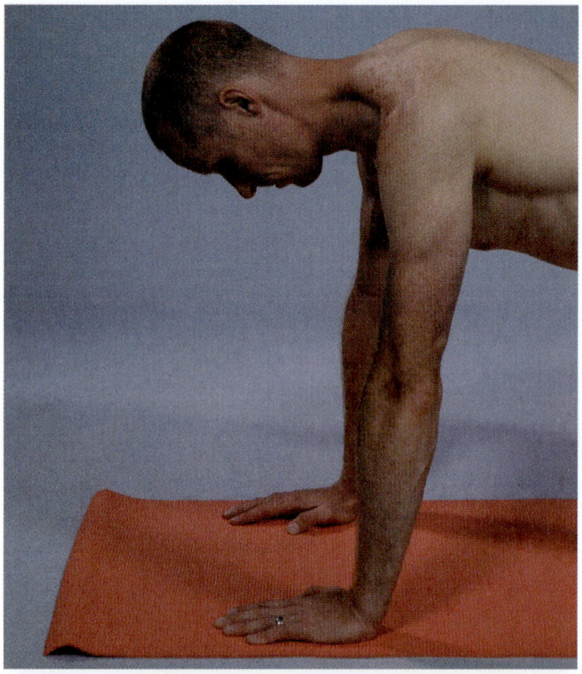

(a-i)

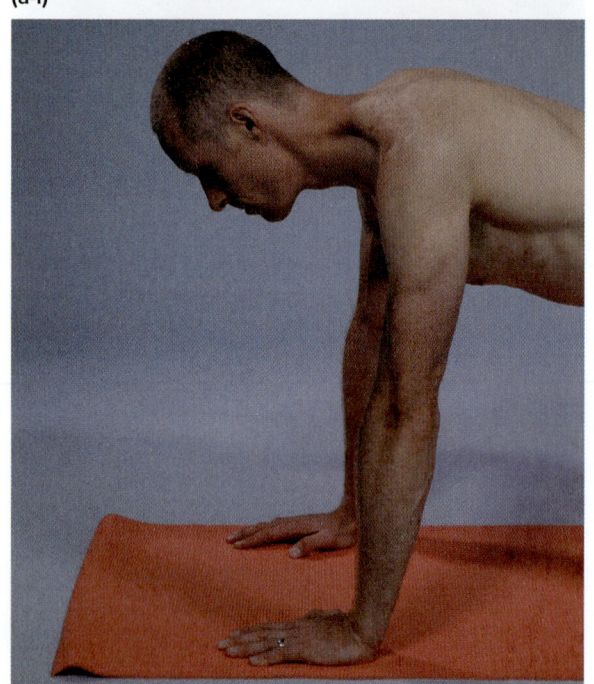

(a-ii)

Figure 23.8 (a) The suboccipital extensors are tested with the movement of head extension (a 'yes' nodding action). The cervical spine should remain in neutral and the athlete should be able to perform discrete cranio-cervical extension. The neutral starting position is shown in (i), the cranio-cervical extension position in (ii).

Neck pain　CHAPTER 23

Support is released and the time for which the athlete can hold the head/neck position without deviation is recorded. The test can be made more time-efficient if a light weight (e.g. 1 kg) is placed on the head and baseline values recorded. The test can be extended to evaluate the thoracic extensors by having the athlete raising their shoulders from the supporting surface.

Axioscapular muscles

It is the interaction of several muscles that control the movement of the scapulae. Clinical assessment of scapular muscle function involves analysis of scapular posture at

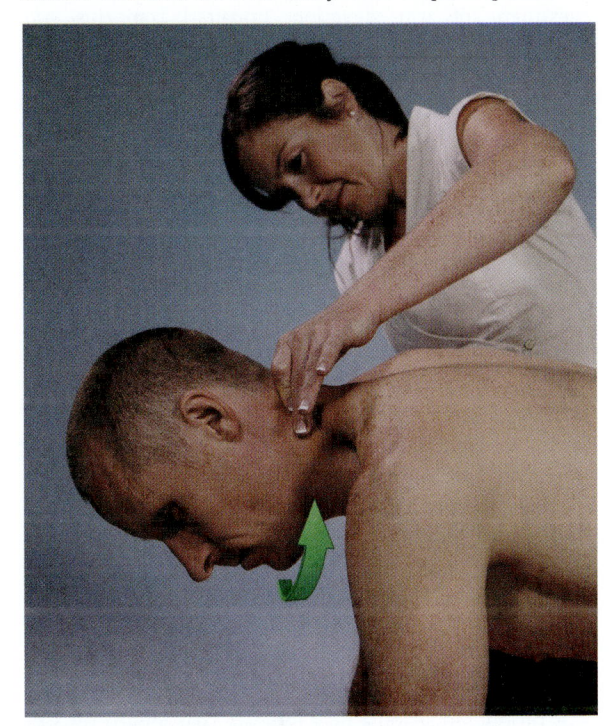

(b)

(c-i)

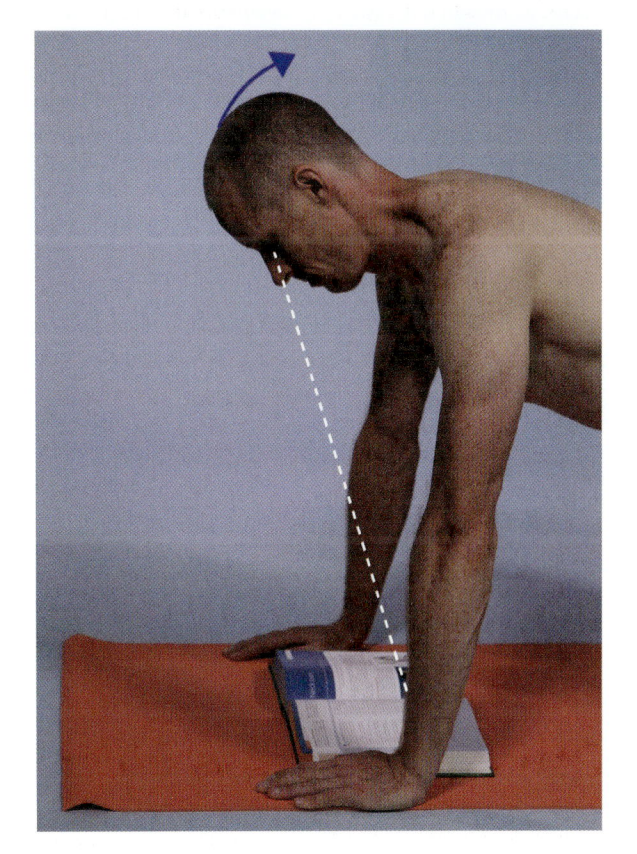

(c-ii)

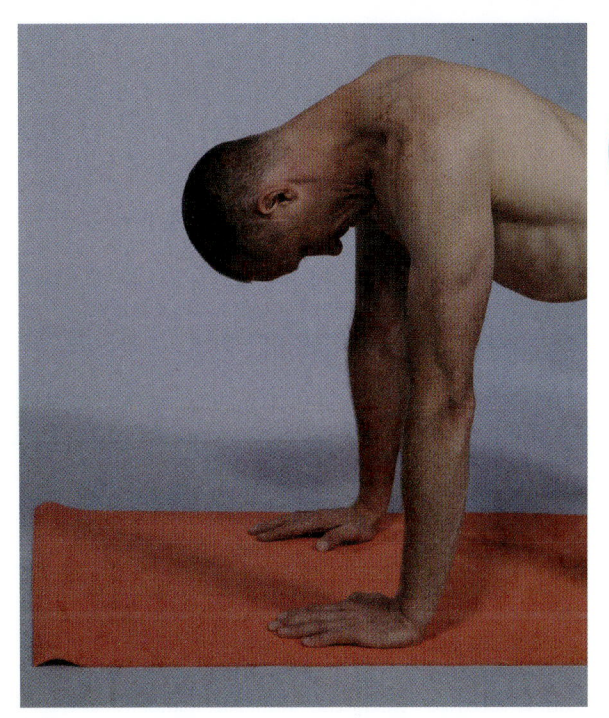

Figure 23.8 (cont.) (b) The suboccipital rotators are tested with the movement of head rotation (a 'no' action). The cervical spine should remain in neutral. Movement should occur as a head rotation only, without rotation in the mid lower cervical spine. The clinician may gently fix C2 to help the patient localise the C1–2 rotation (c) The cervical extensors are tested by performing cervical extension while maintaining the cranio-cervical region in a neutral position. This neutral position is attained and maintained through eye facilitation. The athlete first curls his/her head down to look towards the knees (i). As the athlete curls the head and neck in extension, the eyes are kept fixed on an imaginary book located between the hands, which will encourage the cranio-cervical neutral position (ii). Good cervical extension is demonstrated here, but many athletes cannot extend past the neutral position

rest, under light load with arm movement, as well as by using formal tests of the muscles' contractile abilities and extensibility.

Variation in scapular orientation is common and examination is necessary to disentangle normal variations from scapular dysfunction contributing to the athlete's neck pain. There are several common scapular positional faults.[105]

A downwardly rotated scapula ('ski slope' appearance of line of the nape of the neck) may be due to poor function of the three portions of the trapezius and overactivity or tightness of the levator scapulae muscle. Medial border winging of the scapula may be caused by weakness of serratus anterior muscle, and prominence of the inferior scapular border because of excessive anterior scapular tilt may be due to weakness of the lower trapezius muscle. There may be increased resting tone and tenderness to palpation of the levator scapulae and rhomboid muscles if they are compensating for poor upper trapezius function.

An indication of a direct relationship between scapular posture, poor axioscapular muscle function and the neck pain can be assessed with a simple test (Fig 23.9).[101, 106] First, the athlete's baseline cervical range of motion and pain is assessed. Next, the clinician manually corrects scapular position and the athlete repeats the cervical rotation movement. An improvement in range and/or pain signals that poor scapular posture and muscle dysfunction is likely contributing to the cervical pain or restricted movement and warrants attention in treatment.

There is minimal scapular motion within the first 30–40° of arm elevation.[107] An initial impression of dynamic scapular control in this neutral posture can be gained by applying very light isometric resistance to shoulder flexion, abduction and external rotation while observing any subtle movement of the scapula. With resisted flexion, an inability to maintain posterior tilt of the scapula would suggest weakness in the lower trapezius and serratus anterior muscles. With resisted abduction, an inability to maintain an upward rotation of the scapula (i.e. there is a slight depression of the acromion) suggests weakness of the upper trapezius muscle. With resisted external rotation, an inability to maintain external rotation of the scapula suggests weakness in the serratus anterior and lower trapezius muscle. In summary, with assessment of arm elevation, impaired trapezius and serratus anterior muscle function is revealed by a reduced ability to posteriorly tilt, upwardly rotate and externally rotate the scapula during full arm elevation as well as by poor eccentric control with arm lowering.

Control and endurance of the axioscapular muscles relevant to their postural function is tested in prone lying under low load, using a modified grade 3 muscle test for the lower trapezius[108] (i.e. the arms rest on the bed by the side with the elbow in 90° flexion). One side is tested at a time. The athlete's scapula is passively placed in a neutral position on the thorax and the athlete holds the position. Muscle activity to hold the scapula is analysed by observation and palpation. Signs of compensation for poor axioscapular muscle activation are noted such as adduction and extension of the arm via compensation by the latissimus dorsi. Signs of fatigue (tremor or loss of position) are also noted. The capacity of the axioscapular muscles to fix the scapula to the thorax in a neutral position is also tested under load in the quadruped position. Substantial winging of the medial border of the scapula is an indication of poor axioscapular muscle control, particularly of the serratus anterior muscle.

A protracted scapula may indicate that length tests of levator scapulae or pectoralis major and minor muscles are warranted. Muscle length tests should not be performed when the neck pain is acute or in the presence of mechanosensitive neural tissue. Testing may aggravate the neck condition in these circumstances, as the upper trapezius and the scalene muscles provide protection to sensitive nerve structures. The upper trapezius muscle is a common sight of pain and tender points; however, the muscle is often in a lengthened position (in association with a downwardly rotated scapula). Stretching is not indicated in these circumstances; rather, rehabilitation should target its contractile capacity, along with the other portions of trapezius and serratus anterior muscle.

Tests of cervical sensorimotor function

The cervical sensorimotor system is one of three systems contributing to postural control (i.e. the control of both

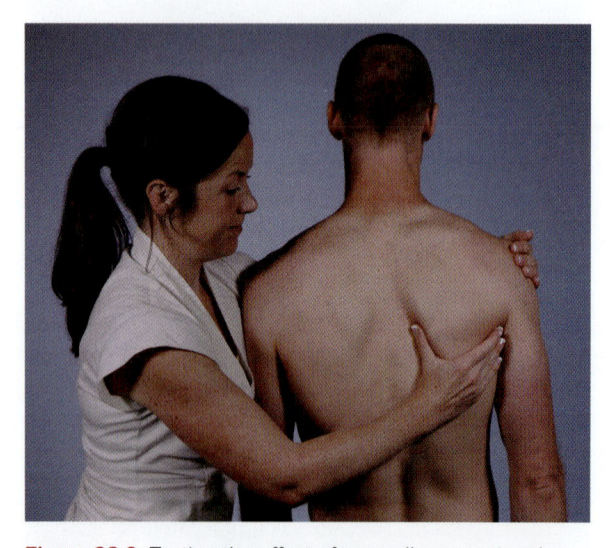

Figure 23.9 Testing the effect of manually correcting the scapula to a neutral position on range and pain in cervical rotation. Improved range and reduced pain indicates a role for aberrant scapular posture in the neck pain condition

Neck pain CHAPTER 23

static and dynamic postural equilibrium). The others are the vestibular and visual systems. The cervical muscles, and especially the suboccipital muscles, contain a high percentage of muscle spindles per gram of muscle and these relay sensorimotor information to the central nervous system.[11, 18, 19] These afferent signals are important for the control of head and neck position and coordination.

Cervicogenic dizziness is caused by altered afferent input from cervical structures in the presence of pain, inflammation, morphological changes or altered muscle activity. Typical symptoms include a vague unsteadiness, light-headedness, nausea and an array of visual symptoms such as blurred vision, the need to concentrate to read, visual fatigue, difficulty judging distances and sensitivity to light.[109] Symptoms are thought to result from conflicting input from the altered cervical afferentation and normal afferent input from the visual and vestibular systems (for reviews, see Clark et al.[110] and Röijezon et al.[111]).

It should be noted that these symptoms may also arise from concussion or vestibular dysfunction, or possibly a combination of both. In a blow to the head sufficient to concuss an athlete, the neck and particularly the upper cervical region will also absorb the force and could be injured. Some clinical tests have some differential diagnostic potential[112, 113] but often it is difficult to differentiate the source unequivocally.

Cervical sensorimotor function may be impaired in any neck pain condition, but is most frequent when the neck pain is a result of trauma or when the athlete complains of such symptoms as light-headedness, unsteadiness or visual symptoms.[114–117] Three functions are tested: joint position and movement sense, standing balance and oculomotor control.

Joint position sense is measured clinically by assessing the accuracy with which an athlete returns to their natural head posture following movement. Tests of relocation accuracy using rotation in each direction and extension are most common. The athlete sits in a chair positioned 90 cm from a wall to which a pre-calibrated target is attached.[118] A laser fastened to a headband is mounted on the athlete's head. The target is positioned on the wall, the centre of which corresponds to the athlete's natural starting position. Following a familiarisation session, the athlete closes his or her eyes, rotates the head as far as possible to the left (at least 45° for a valid test), then returns as closely as possible to the starting position (Fig. 23.10). The test is repeated at least 3–5 times and the mean measurement recorded. Relocation with more than 4.5° of error (the outer red circle and beyond) is outside normal limits.

Movement sense may also be tested by having the athlete follow a moving object with the laser pointer.[119] Patterns of movement with increasing difficulty are tested, and normative values have been established for each

(a)

(b)

(c)

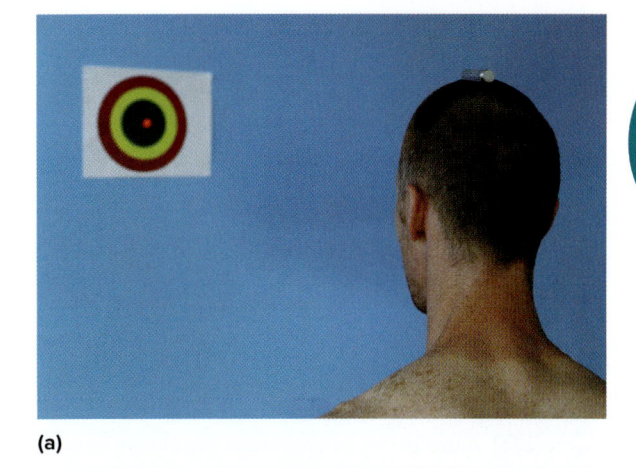

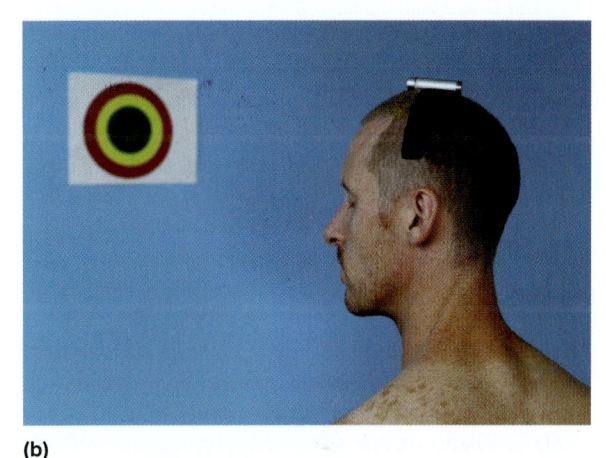

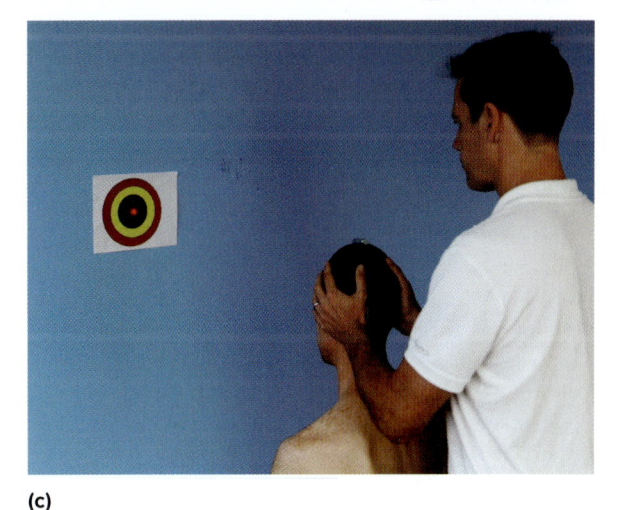

Figure 23.10 Testing joint reposition sense from rotation (a) The athlete should sit in a supported position with eyes closed throughout the test (b) Each movement direction is tested three times (c) The clinician repositions the head on target between each repetition

363

PART B Regional problems

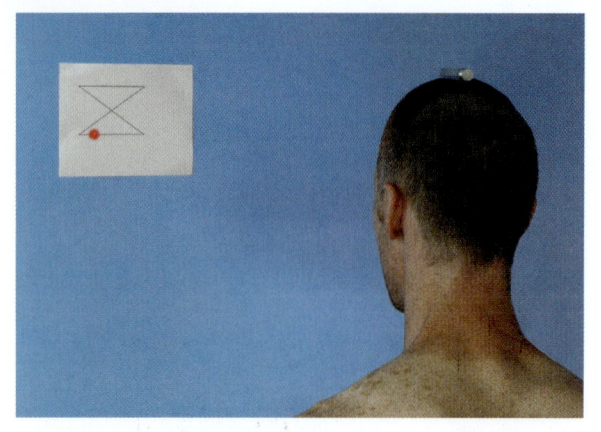

Figure 23.11 A test of movement sense. The athlete must trace the shape with the laser as accurately and as fast as possible. Emphasis is placed on accuracy and the patient must keep the laser on the marked lines

scenario.[120] Alternatively, the athlete can be requested to trace a static target with a laser, with irregular trajectories being assessed (Fig. 23.11).[121]

Balance can be measured both statically and dynamically. The cervical sensorimotor system is best challenged with higher-level balance tests than those that may be initially used for a sprained ankle. This is especially so for the athletic population, where balance problems may be overlooked if tests are not challenging enough to detect high-level balance deficits.

Static balance is first assessed by testing the athlete's ability to stand in tandem stance with eyes open for 30 seconds. The test is progressed from eyes open to eyes closed, or from standing on a firm surface to a soft surface (e.g. 10 cm thick dense foam). Further testing progression includes single leg stance or placing the head in a rotated position while in the different stance positions.[122]

Dynamic balance tests include the conventional Dynamic Gait Index, a 10-metre walk with head turns, or a step test.[123, 124] These tests could also be progressed to include sport-specific positions and performing multiple tasks. For example, a fencing athlete could be asked to perform an 'advance lunge' while accurately targeting the sword tip. A more dynamic task could be practice of 'balestra', which demands holding a steady end position.

Oculomotor control is tested qualitatively using three tests: gaze stability, the smooth pursuit neck torsion test (SPNTT) and evaluation of rapid eye movements.

Gaze stability is tested by requesting that the athlete fix his or her gaze on an object (e.g. a pen) while comfortably rotating the head to the left and right. The clinician holds a pen about 1 metre away in line with the athlete's nose and observes whether he or she can easily dissociate eye movement from head movement.

The SPNTT evaluates eye follow ability. Impairments in eye follow can be a normal phenomenon or due to neck pain, concussion or a vestibular disorder. The SPNTT was designed to differentiate a probable cervical cause.[125] In the test, the clinician moves a finger or pen back and forth, crossing the athlete's midline, and assesses eye movement control by watching the athlete's eyes follow the target, noting any saccadic movements (rapid 'catch-up' movements). The test is then repeated with the trunk rotated 45° (the head remaining in neutral position). This targets the neck, but has no effect if the underlying cause is vestibular or due to a concussion. The cervical spine is implicated if eye saccades increase in the turned position compared to the neutral position.[116] It is not uncommon for one side only to be compromised. Finally, quickly alternating gaze between two targets (saccadic movements) can also be tested.

Additional tests
Cervical arterial dysfunction
Clinicians who use cervical manual therapy as a treatment modality are very mindful of cervical arterial dysfunction, inclusive of vertebral artery insufficiency and cervical arterial dissections (see Table 23.1). This is reflected in a recently developed international framework that provides safety guidelines for vascular screening prior to hands-on orthopaedic intervention.[126] Any suspicion of a cervical arterial dissection in progress requires immediate referral to an emergency department.

While any age group could present with symptoms of vertebral artery insufficiency, the risk increases with age due to increased atherosclerosis. Tests are indicated when the athlete complains of symptoms such as dizziness (vertigo), visual disturbances, unsteadiness or other neurological signs. Testing arterial integrity is also recommended as routine before any high-velocity manipulation is performed.

However, clinical provocative tests for the vertebral artery have been shown to have poor validity with low sensitivity.[127, 128] The sustained rotation and extension tests probably more generally assess the adequacy of collateral flow to the brain rather than the competency of one artery. Yet, they still may have a place to identify the few persons with abnormal vessels in whom collateral compensation is insufficient.[129] As mentioned previously, of greater concern in the sport context is recognition of CAD (vertebral or carotid) which can be triggered by even minor trauma in the susceptible young to middle-aged athlete.[129] This history of trauma is a warning signal.

Performance-based outcome measures
Measurements of pain, function and participation levels are important patient-reported outcomes, but equally

important are performance-based outcome measures. These physical measures serve several purposes including testing the immediate effectiveness of a treatment technique, guiding treatment progression, and ensuring that physical impairment associated with the pain and injury has been rectified and the sporting performance skill restored. In addition, showing athletes the results of their individual performance-based outcome measures, in conjunction with objective evidence of improvement over time, can provide powerful incentives for treatment compliance.

A combination of performance-based outcome measures is used for an athlete who has a painful neck condition. An outcome measure should be documented for each impaired system in the athlete's presentation. This could include, for example, a measure of cervical range of motion; a measurement of the upper limb neurodynamic test (range of elbow extension); a measure of motor control (e.g. the cranio-cervical flexion test: stage 1–pressure level achieved with correct movement, and stage 2–pressure level which was achieved and on which training commences); and relocation error in the test of joint position sense. Equally important are performance-based outcome measures of functional skills specific to the athlete's sport. All outcome measures will need to be revisited and upgraded as the athlete progresses in treatment.

MANAGEMENT OF MECHANICAL NECK PAIN

It is usually not possible to make a definitive patho-anatomical diagnosis in most people presenting with a neck pain condition, but this should not compromise conservative management. After red-flag pathologies have been eliminated, the athlete's presenting complaint, the physical examination and any other athlete- or sport-specific issues will direct the treatment approach. In some cases, definitive pathology can be identified, such as a cervical radiculopathy. Alternatively, various syndromes such as a 'stinger', an acute wry neck or a whiplash-associated disorder can provide a label for the neck pain condition. These labels may suggest a certain lesion or underlying structural cause, but the treatment approach should be directed by the examination findings and the athlete's needs. Reference will be made to these syndromes later in this section.

Most athletes fall under the broad diagnosis of mechanical neck pain. The inadequacy of this single classification is that it belies the heterogeneity of neck pain conditions. There are no recipe approaches for mechanical neck pain and each athlete should be regarded as an individual, with management programs designed and tailored to meet their own needs. This section will mention many different treatment approaches. Not all are needed for every athlete. Specific treatment strategies should be selected based on the current research, the sound clinical reasoning and experience of the clinician, and the unique presentations and goals of the athlete.

Systematic reviews have synthesised and scrutinised the effectiveness of treatment strategies that can be used to reduce pain and disability in the conservative management of neck pain.[130-136] Of these various treatments, exercise and manual therapy as single modalities show greatest effect, albeit with modest effect sizes. Used together as a multi-model approach, there is a larger effect.[132, 133, 136] Other methods of management (e.g. education),[130] when used as a single-treatment approach, have not been found to be effective. This is hardly surprising considering the nature and extent of all of the impairments or features that may present within biological, psychological and social domains in neck pain conditions, as well as the potential interactions between these domains.

No single modality or method can address such a spectrum. A multimodal approach is essential when neck pain is considered within the biopsychosocial framework. A multimodal approach is summarised in Figure 23.12.

Sport and functional modifications

A comprehensive understanding of the physical requirements of the athlete's sport and training demands, as well as his or her occupational or other recreational activities, is essential to understanding possible provocative factors in order to meet the goals of rehabilitation. If an athlete is performing a task (during sport or work) that is producing or aggravating neck pain, long-term pain relief and prevention of recurrence will not be achieved until this potential 'driver' of the condition is addressed.

For example, an athlete's weight-training regimen is causing neck pain and analysis reveals that when the athlete does a certain lift, his/her head subtly drifts forward. This posture unnecessarily places the upper cervical joints into extension and increases the activity in the neck extensors,[137] with a net result of added, unnecessary compressive load on the cervical joints. Management must include correction of neck posture to maintain the cervical and cranio-cervical regions in a neutral position during weight training. This may require a temporary reduction in resistance/weight for the lift to allow the neck joints to settle, and rehabilitation of the deep and superficial neck muscles to be effective so that there is adequate muscular support of the cervical region.

As a second example, throwing is aggravating an athlete's neck pain. It is important to consider that there is normal movement of the cervical segments during arm movements.[14] In the presence of neck pain, irregular movements may occur at the cervical segments with throwing and catching actions.[138] The posture and muscle control of the neck, as well as any deficiency in throwing

PART B Regional problems

Sport and functional modifications
- Review of sport and training techniques
- Appreciate possible provocative factors
- Possible change/correction of technique

Education
- Ensure the athlete understands the nature of their disorder
- Allay any fear or anxiety
- Pain education
- Empower the athlete with knowledge and understanding as a basis for appropriate goal setting

Pain management
- Pharmacotherapies in circumstances of moderate to severe pain or neuropathic pain
- Manual therapy and exercise used for their pain-modulating effects
- Acupuncture, dry needing and trigger point therapy may be useful adjuncts

Manual therapy
- Articular dysfunction is managed using a combination of manual therapy and segmentally directed active excercise
- Techniques may include passive mobilisation, mobilisation with movement and/or manipulation
- Gains from manuel therapy must be reinforced with active exercise

Neural tissue mobilisation
- Progress from mobilising the nerve and nerve bed to techniques which tension the nerve and nerve bed
- Manual therapy and active exercise are employed to facilitate the management of sensitised nerve tissue

Training motor function
- Exercise should be prescribed according to the neuromuscular impairments revealed during the clinical assessment
- Exercise are prescribed in two stages. Stage 1 is training to enhance motor control and stage 2 involves resistance training

Training sensorimotor control
- Several physical therapies can improve cervicogenic dizziness
- However, targeted exercises, including proprioception training, balance excercises and oculomotor control exercises, may be superior in reducing measurable impairments

Figure 23.12 Components of a multimodal approach for the management of neck pain disorders. The findings of the assessment will direct precisely the components of management for the individual athlete

---

technique, should be assessed and addressed in this athlete to eliminate this potential 'motor performance' driver.

A third example involves cycling, which can be provocative for neck pain.[3] Despite an ideal bike fit, the neck will inevitably be subjected to non-ideal postures and susceptible to strains in road racing. The athlete is encouraged to reverse the pain-provoking forward-head, upper cervical extension posture as regularly as possible during the ride. Adjusting his postures slightly out of an end-range position may help. In addition, there should be follow-up to ensure that in all other daily activities, the athlete avoids the pain-provoking posture as much as possible.

A final example involves a rugby player with neck pain. Contact sports can be challenging for prevention of neck injury. While rules, equipment and technique may protect the neck to some extent, it will still be placed under unpredictable forces.[4, 139-141] A review of the player's rugby tackling techniques or scrum techniques should be a part of the management to lessen the risk, to treat the painful neck condition and to prevent recurrences.

Education

While education alone might not be sufficient for the management of neck pain,[130] effective multi-modal rehabilitation cannot be delivered without education to ensure the athlete understands the nature of his or her condition. The clinician must demonstrate appropriate interest and empathy, provide assurance and understand the athlete's beliefs about his or her condition as well as his or her coping style, to develop an effective partnership. Good communication skills are essential and all explanations about the condition should be provided in non-mystical, non-alarmist language.

Pain education is proving to be an important aspect of management. It is also important that the athlete understand what is causing and moderating the condition and how it will be addressed by the management approach. Discuss the evidence for the effectiveness of the proposed management program with the athlete. Education aims to empower the athlete with knowledge and understanding as a basis for appropriate goal setting and stimulates the athlete's participation and compliance with the management program.

Pain management

Pain relief is usually a first priority in people with neck pain and thus most clinical trials have pain as a primary outcome measure, regardless of what treatment is investigated. Pain is an individual, multidimensional sensory and emotional experience, and clinical trials reveal that there are many ways in which the pain experience can be modulated, albeit some more effective than others.

Pharmacotherapies are indicated in circumstances of moderate to severe pain or neuropathic pain. In these circumstances, conservative management or rehabilitation strategies must be limited and not provoke pain, and management can be very challenging for all health professionals. Conservative therapies alone are often not successful for these severe pain states,[142, 143] and multi-disciplinary management is necessary. Fortunately, most people with neck pain do not have these severe or neuropathic pain states, and conservative management is the typical first-line approach.

Physical modalities including manipulative therapy, exercise and electrophysical agents can modulate pain. Research indicates that a major effect of manual therapy is pain relief through neurophysiological mechanisms.[144] In addition, both low-load and high-load exercises can relieve pain.[132] Manual therapy and exercise will be discussed in some detail in subsequent sections for, in addition to their effects on pain, they are used for improving motion and enhancing neuromuscular function. Electrophysical agents have little evidence of added benefit,[145] but clinical experience would suggest that they can be quite soothing when part of a multi-modal treatment regimen. There is some evidence for acupuncture, dry needling and trigger-point therapy for immediate and short-term effects on pain.[135, 146-148] Thus these modalities may also be useful adjuncts to a rehabilitation program.

It is quite normal for some level of anxiety and depression to accompany pain of any origin[33] and this could be especially so if the athlete has had to withdraw from competition. Psychological features can moderate the pain state. Thus appropriate assurance and information to address such features is an important part of pain management. A decrease in pain parallels a decrease in anxiety and general distress.[142]

Manual therapy

Restriction of neck movement is pathognomonic of painful cervical conditions.[50] The cervical facet joints and discs are common sources of nociception and movement dysfunction. Articular dysfunction can be managed using a combination of manual therapy (also termed 'manipulative therapy') and segmentally directed active exercise.

Manual therapy techniques generally fall under three categories. The first is passive mobilisation, or rhythmically applied, segmentally directed passive movements. The second is mobilisation with movement, and the third is manipulation, a single high-velocity thrust technique.

There is always concern about cervical manipulation because of the rare possibility of a vertebral or carotid arterial dissection and the associated catastrophic outcomes of stroke or even death.[126, 129] In response, there has been a recent shift away from the use of purportedly riskier end-of-range cervical rotation techniques.[149]

If a clinician has any reservation about the use of cervical manipulation, the evidence suggests that outcomes achieved with cervical mobilisation and manipulation are similar.[133] One randomised controlled trial compared outcomes of mobilisation versus manipulation for subacute neck pain. Patients were randomised to manipulation or mobilisation only after the clinician had decided that the patient would benefit from a manipulation.[150] The results showed that even when manipulation was considered to be clinically indicated, but the patient received mobilisation, the outcomes for these patients were the same as those patients who received cervical manipulation. There is no doubt that cervical manipulation can be very effective, but if there is a perceived risk, or the clinician lacks skills to manipulate safely, then the evidence suggests the patient will respond equally well to passive mobilisation.

There are many different theoretical models and clinical approaches to guide specific treatment techniques for the cervical spine, both within and between the different healthcare professionals who use manipulative therapy.[151-153] Evidence continues to emerge that outcomes are similar regardless of the approach used.[154, 155]

Selection of technique should be based on the examination findings including: the direction(s) of movement restriction; segmental level of pain and dysfunction; pain severity; the nature of resistance to segmental motion (e.g. muscle spasm); and the provisional diagnosis. The athlete must be informed about the approach to be used and consent to the treatment, especially in relation to high-velocity procedures. For the latter, pre-manipulative protocols should be utilised as required by the relevant discipline.[126]

PART B Regional problems

Once an initial technique has been selected, it should be trialled for its effectiveness by assessing its immediate effect on pain and range of motion. Positive within-session changes have been shown to be good predictors of between-session improvements.[156] As indicated previously, mobilisation techniques can be applied passively only, or they can be applied in conjunction with active movement (mobilisation with movement).[151-153]

The upper thoracic area should not be neglected as full head rotation is reliant on an approximately 10° contribution from the upper thoracic area.[7] There is early evidence of improvement in neck pain and range of motion when upper thoracic manipulation is included in the management of neck conditions.[157, 158]

Manual therapy should be progressed as the patient improves. This can be done in a variety of ways such as increasing the duration of the technique, changing the neck position while the technique is performed using the principles of a combined movement approach,[159, 160] using a combination of techniques in a single session or, where indicated, adding a high-velocity thrust technique.

Range of motion exercises to accompany manual therapy

Any gains in range of movement from manual therapy[50] must be reinforced and maintained with a program of active exercise. Active exercises can be performed in any plane of movement and it is logical to prescribe exercises to target the segment(s) that are hypomobile and that have just been treated. As an example, Figure 23.13 illustrates two self-guided ways that active (a) or assisted active (b) exercise can target (albeit not strictly localise)

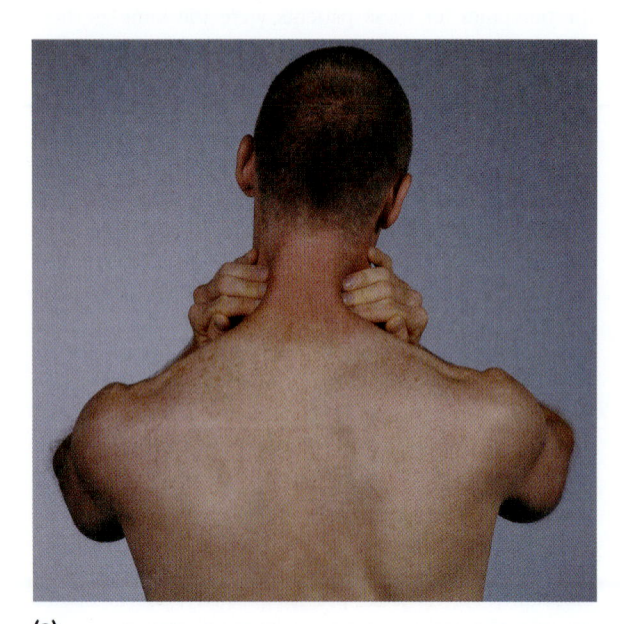

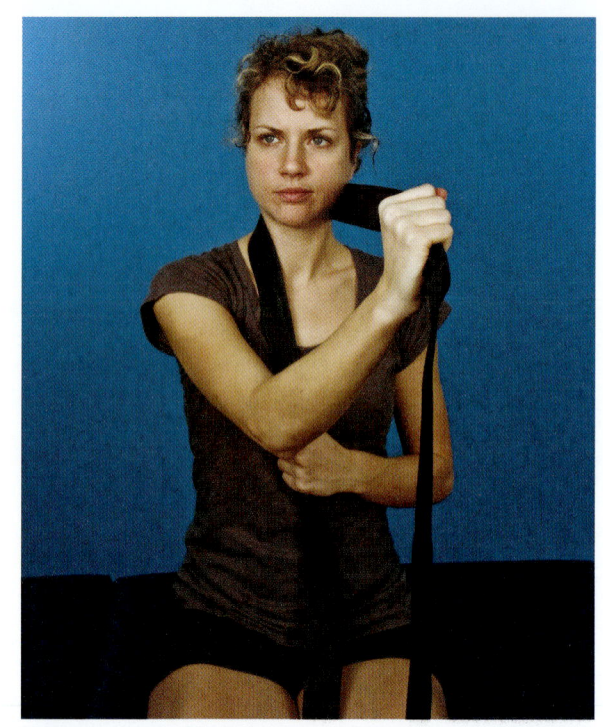

(b-i)

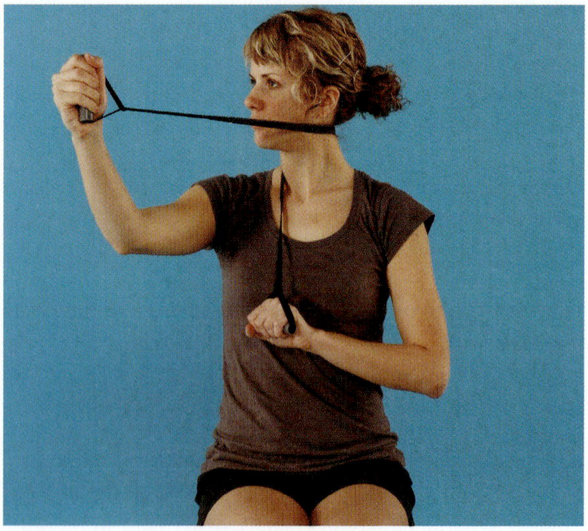

(b-ii)

Figure 23.13 Range of motion exercises (a) Active exercise for lateral flexion. The athlete is taught to localise the segment of interest with his or her fingertip (e.g. if the segment is C2–3, the fingertip is placed on the lamina of C3). The athlete then laterally flexes down to the fingertip to ensure that the segment is moved into lateral flexion (b) The patient uses an assistive strap to localise segmental rotation. For rotation at C1–2, the strap is placed on C1. These techniques are part of the mobilisation with movement regimen[151]

(a)

Neck pain | CHAPTER 23

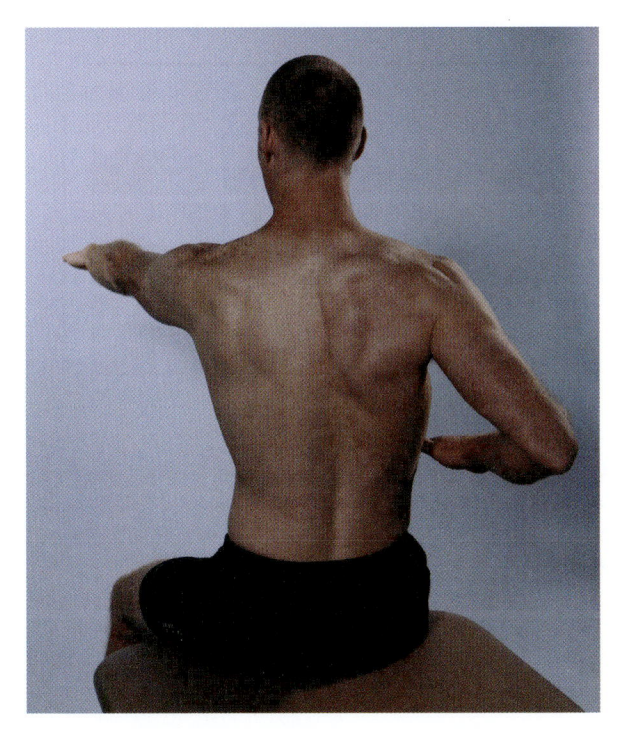

Figure 23.14 An active exercise which will mobilise rotation throughout the functional cervical spine (C0–1 to T3–4). The athlete imagines shooting a bow and arrow (holding the bow in alternate hands). The athlete must focus on rotation through the upper thoracic region, keeping the mid and lower thoracic regions relatively still

movement to a segmental level. In the acute stage, exercise should be gentle and can be performed three or four times throughout the day as tolerated. It can be progressed in repetitions and intensity as the athlete improves.

Figure 23.14 illustrates an exercise that focuses on mobilising the cervicothoracic region into rotation. It would be an appropriate exercise to prescribe once any acute pain has settled. It is an easy exercise that an athlete can practise throughout the day, which encourages compliance. Alternatively, the combined movements of arm elevation and ipsilateral cervical rotation can also be used to help mobilise the cervicothoracic region.

Neural tissue mobilisation

Treatment of neural tissue mechanosensitivity is a priority when the physical examination confirms that it is contributing to the athlete's neck and arm pain. Some exercises, such as cranio-cervical flexor training, scapular postural correction and certain neck and arm movement exercises, can stress sensitive nerve structures and thereby aggravate pain. Such exercises should not be commenced until the nerve tissue has been addressed.

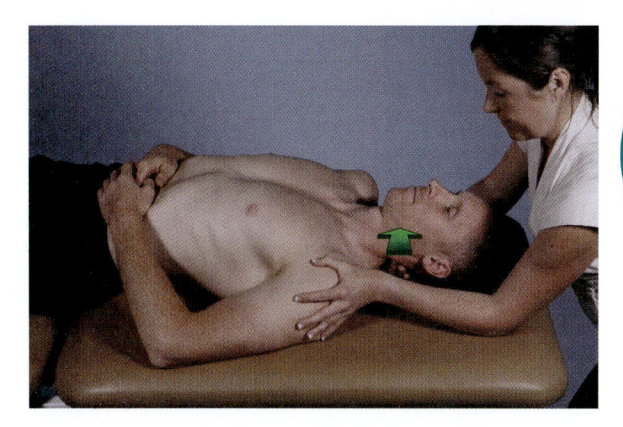

Figure 23.15 Cervical lateral glide technique. If the (L) C6 nerve and brachial plexus are mechanosensitive, the clinician gently maintains the scapular position, grips C6 and glides the head and neck down to C6 to the right. The movement should be gentle and rhythmical. The athlete can contribute to the techniques by gently moving their arm in sequence with the passive technique to enhance the sliding of the nerve and nerve bed

Nerve tissue pain (neuropathic pain) should always be respected, regardless of the presenting pain intensity and the acuteness or chronicity of the condition. Restriction in motion during the upper limb neurodynamic tests is principally due to protective muscle guarding.[161, 162] The emphasis in contemporary management of neural tissue mechanosensitivity is on mobilising the nerve and nerve bed, with final progression–as the athlete improves–to techniques that tension the nerve and nerve bed.[163] Both manual therapy and active exercise can be employed in the management of nerve tissue mechanosensitivity.

The cervical lateral glide technique is one efficacious technique (Fig. 23.15).[164-167] The sliding of the nerve and nerve bed can be enhanced by using combinations of movements to lengthen a nerve bed across one joint while shortening the nerve bed of an adjacent joint. This results in greater nerve excursion with minimal nerve strain and is achieved by the athlete performing the active arm movement while the clinician performs the cervical lateral glide.[163, 168] For example, in an acute state, the athlete's arm could be positioned by his or her side. As the clinician glides the neck away from this side (lengthens the nerve bed), the patient flexes his or her wrist (shortens the nerve bed). When the clinician returns the neck to neutral (shortens), the patient extends the wrist (lengthens). Progression is achieved by increasing the angle of arm abduction, as well as by flexing or extending the elbow, wrist and hand. A further progression could be to slowly convert the sliding technique to a tensioning technique (i.e. when the neck is glided away, the athlete extends the wrist and hand).

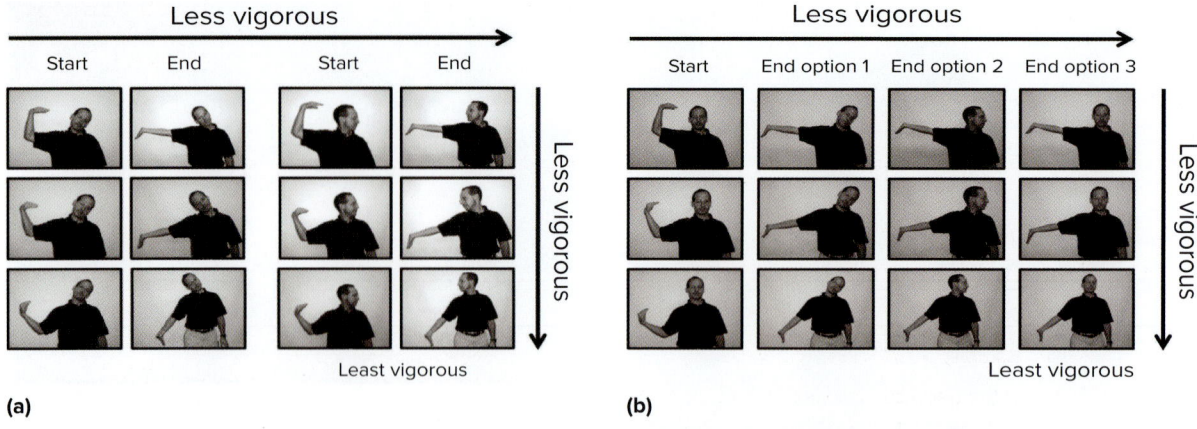

Figure 23.16 (a) Active exercise is used in addition to clinician-delivered technique. The progression for the 'sliding' nerve gliding exercise is illustrated and the level chosen is one that does not provoke the patient's symptoms. The most gentle sliding technique combines neck rotation with elbow and wrist movements while the arm is in 30° abduction. The most vigorous (and the ultimate goal) is to perform the sliding technique in 90° abduction with cervical lateral (top left). The figure illustrates the various transitions from least to most vigorous.[169] (b) The progression for the 'tensioning' nerve gliding exercise. The level chosen is one that does not provoke the patient's symptoms. The most gentle tensioning technique uses elbow and wrist movements with the neck in neutral and the arm in 30° abduction. The most vigorous (and the ultimate goal) is the tensioning exercise in 90° abduction and contralateral lateral flexion (top left). The figure illustrates the various transitions from least to most vigorous.[169]

REPRINTED FROM NEE RJ, VICENZINO B, JULL GA, CLELAND JA, COPPIETERS MW. A NOVEL PROTOCOL TO DEVELOP A PREDICTION MODEL THAT IDENTIFIES PATIENTS WITH NERVE-RELATED NECK AND ARM PAIN WHO BENEFIT FROM THE EARLY INTRODUCTION OF NEURAL TISSUE MANAGEMENT. *CONTEMP CLIN TRIALS*. 2011;32(5):760–70 WITH PERMISSION FROM ELSEVIER

This treatment should be supplemented with a home program of active exercise (Fig. 23.16).[169] These exercises are designed to replicate the precise stage of the cervical lateral glide. In relation to dosage, it is prudent to start with low repetitions (e.g. 5 repetitions) two or three times a day to evaluate the athlete's response. Treatment can be progressed by increasing the number of repetitions or altering the arm and neck position, or changing the intention (slide or tension).

Training motor function

A research-informed exercise protocol is used to address the changes identified in the neuromuscular system of the athlete with neck pain (see section on muscle tests above). The neuromuscular and functional changes induced by training are specific to the mode of exercise performed.[79, 170-173] People with neck pain present with an array of deficits ranging from subtle changes in muscle coordination through to reduced neck strength. Different forms of exercise must be considered and prescribed to address the specific neuromuscular impairments revealed during the clinical assessment. Exercises are prescribed in two stages. Stage 1 is training to enhance motor control. This stage includes exercises to: increase the activation and endurance of the deep cervical postural muscles; improve coordination between the deep and superficial layers of the neck flexor and extensor muscles and the axioscapular muscles; and train muscle coordination within functional and work activities. Stage 2 involves resistance training and commences once adequate motor control of the region is achieved. As the goal of therapeutic exercise is to restore normal motor control, function and quality of movement, the exercises should be challenging, yet be performed with correct technique and without aggravation of symptoms. Pain can inhibit the motor learning process.[174] For convenience, the rehabilitation of each muscle group is outlined separately, but rehabilitation is concurrent and prescribed based on assessment findings.

Stage 1. Motor control
Neck flexors
Based on assessment findings, any altered coordination between the deep and superficial cervical muscles or decreased endurance capacity of the deep neck flexors must be addressed. Often, athletes must first learn the correct movement of cranio-cervical flexion. They practise a large extension-to-flexion excursion head movement in the supine position, gaining feedback of correct movement by feeling the back of their head sliding up and down the bed. The movement is facilitated with eye movement

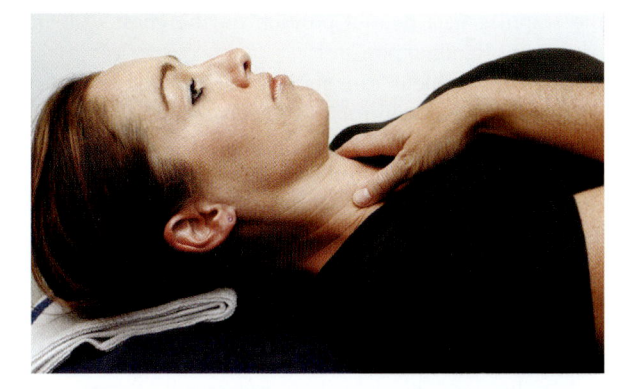

Figure 23.17 Training the deep cervical flexors in stage 1. The patient concentrates on performing the correct craniocervical flexion movement and palpates to ensure that there is no dominant activity of the superficial flexors. Inner-range contractions are held to improve endurance capacity of these muscles at contraction intensities in line with those required in sitting and standing postures. The pressure biofeedback is used only to teach the patient the holding contraction and to monitor progression of the exercise

and the athlete can palpate his or her sternocleidomastoid and anterior scalene muscles to ensure they are relaxed throughout the entire range of movement (Fig. 23.17). Once the correct movement is attained, endurance of the deep cervical flexors can be trained.

Feedback on performance is necessary so that the athlete knows he or she is performing the task correctly. A pressure sensor can be placed behind the athlete's neck to indicate his or her ability to perform and hold a contraction of the deep cervical flexors (Fig. 23.7). The athlete can practise with the feedback under the clinician's supervision, while learning the sensation of the movement and holding contraction in order to be able to practise at home without the external feedback.[101] Training commences at the pressure level that the athlete can control. The athlete practices to achieve 10 repetitions of 10-second holds at that level, twice per day.

Posture
Postural re-education training for spinal and scapular posture commences immediately. The physical examination may have directly linked the athlete's spinal posture to his or her pain state and, importantly for a training effect, the correction of posture facilitates the activity of the deep cervical flexors.[175, 176] The motor learning process requires multiple repetitions within a day, and postural correction allows the patient to perform multiple repetitions of the muscle contraction during the day with convenience. Furthermore, training the deep cervical flexors in this exercise will help remediate the altered behaviour between

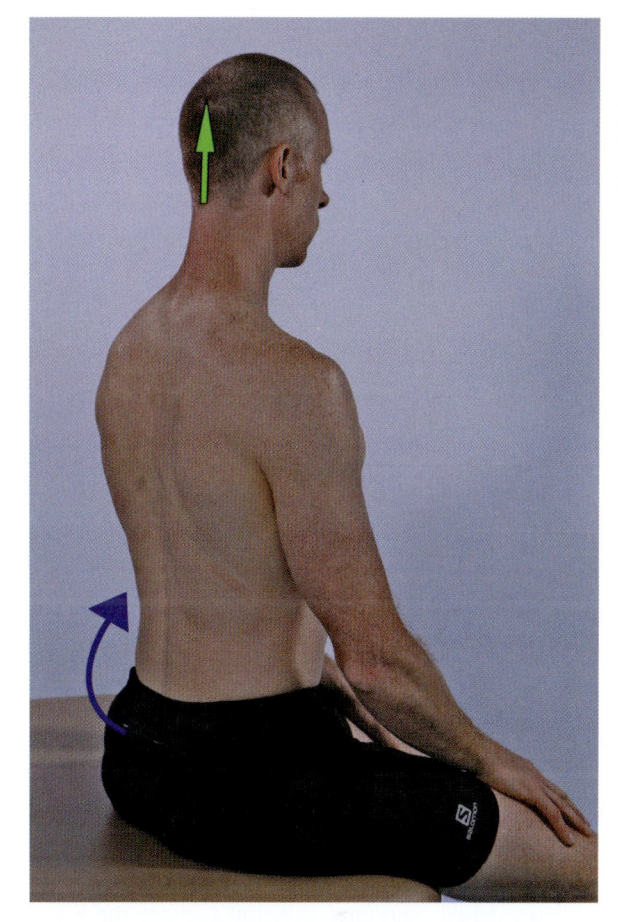

Figure 23.18 Spinal posture correction is facilitated by first correcting the lumbopelvic region into a neutral upright posture. Correct the thoracic posture if necessary, and correct head position by asking the patient to gently lengthen the back of the neck. Once spinal posture has been addressed, the patient will be taught to correct scapular posture as is necessary

the deep and superficial flexors demonstrated in the CCFT.[177] An upright posture is facilitated by first moving the lumbopelvic region into a neutral position (Fig. 23.18). This will usually correct thoracic posture, although a slight correction of excessive thoracic flexion or extension may be necessary. As a final correction, the athlete should gently lengthen the back of the neck, which will not only facilitate the longus colli further,[176] but will correct the cervical and cranio-cervical position.

The athlete is advised to perform this posture correction exercise ideally 2–3 times per hour. They should hold the position for 10 seconds. The exercise can be incorporated into daily activities while sitting, standing and walking. Repetition is the key and the athlete must identify or develop 'cues' as reminders for the exercise.

Formal training of cranio-cervical flexion continues until the patient can perform 10 repetitions of 10-second holds at each of the five pressure increments on the CCFT from the baseline of 20 mmHg to the maximum of 30 mmHg. Once this goal for the deep cervical flexors is achieved, the program is progressed and the interaction between the deep and superficial flexor muscles is trained during movement. One of the movements to train is control of neck extension. This movement is initiated with cranio-cervical extension and return to the upright position from extension is initiated by cranio-cervical flexion. Concomitantly as required, control of neck position in any sport-specific position is trained.

Neck extensors

Stage 1 training for the neck extensors commences in inclined sitting, prone on elbows or, most commonly, in a quadruped position, depending on the athlete's ability to control scapular and trunk posture. The athlete can train the movements of cranio-cervical extension and rotation and cervical extension (C2-7) (Fig. 23.8a and b). Instructing the athlete to read an imaginary book (eyes focused down between hands) while curling the head and neck backwards maintains the cranio-cervical region in a neutral position, facilitating the desired cervical extension (Fig. 23.8c). Manual resistance can be applied by the clinician in extension over the vertebral arch to emphasise the activation of the deep extensor muscles while familiarising the athlete with the exercise.[178] Athletes should train until they can perform three sets of 10 repetitions through a full excursion of movement without fatigue.

Axioscapular muscles

Stage 1 training focuses initially on improving the activation and endurance capacity of the trapezius and serratus anterior muscles as well as re-educating the axioscapular muscles functionally to provide adequate scapular stability in posture and during arm movements.

In this motor relearning phase, the lower portion of trapezius can initially be targeted with the athlete in a side-lying (gravity-eliminated) position with the arm supported on pillows at approximately 140° of elevation. The athlete practises drawing the scapula diagonally across the thoracic wall and holding the position for 10 seconds (10 repetitions). Serratus anterior is formally trained with a scapular protraction exercise which can be progressed as indicated from a side-lying position, to standing against a wall, to a prone position on elbows, to a four-point kneeling position. The exercises in the latter two positions can be combined with neck extension exercises. The scapular muscles are also trained concurrently in the postural correction exercise and the athlete learns to hold the scapulae in a neutral position on the chest wall in sitting and standing postures.

Once the athlete can control 'ideal' static scapular posture, scapular control is re-educated for functions requiring less than 30° of arm elevation (control of the scapula in a neutral position), during arm movement throughout range and, importantly, in sport- or occupation-specific arm postures and movements.

Stage 2. Resistance training

Stage 2 addresses any deficits in muscle strength and demands greater levels of endurance. Neck flexor strength and endurance are trained at progressive contraction intensities by increasing the gravitational load using a head lift exercise.

Initially, the athlete sits on a chair close to a wall with his or her head resting on the wall in a neutral position. Cranio-cervical flexion is performed by sliding the back of the head up the wall, and then the head weight is lifted just off the wall (Fig. 23.19). Cranio-cervical control is essential in this exercise. If the patient loses cranio-cervical flexion when the head is lifted, this means that the exercise load is too high. The load is increased by progressively moving the chair further from the wall and ultimately moving to crook-lying and supine positions. The exercise can be further progressed in supine from having support of two pillows to no pillows to performing the exercise with weighted sandbags on the forehead.

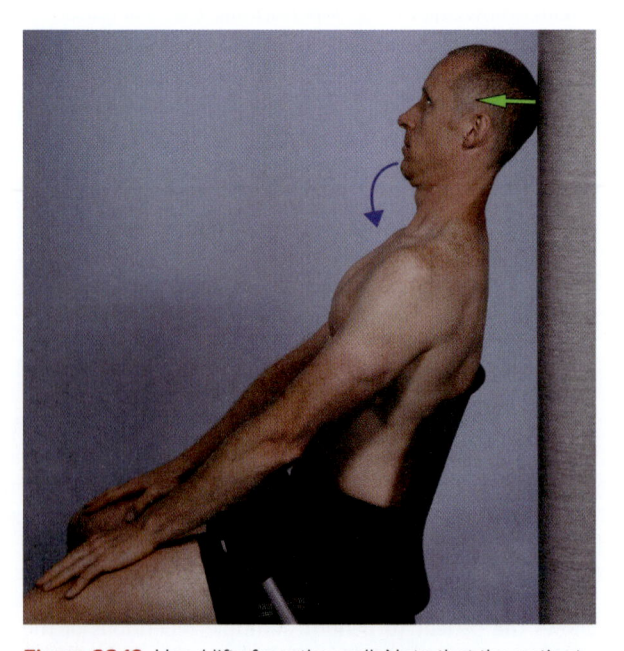

Figure 23.19 Head lifts from the wall. Note that the patient must control the cranio-cervical flexion position in this initial strengthening exercise in stage 2 training

For the cervical extensors, the athlete can perform repeated cervical extension or sustained neck extension holds in a prone or quadruped position. Progressive weights (commencing with 0.5 kg) can be attached to headgear (e.g. a bike helmet) if neck-specific resistance equipment is not available. For the axioscapular muscles, free-weight or machine-based exercises can be performed. Strengthening exercises should commence with light loads concentrating on spinal and scapular control with both concentric and eccentric arm loading. Strengthening exercises should be task-specific with a focus on upper limb movements that are relevant to the athlete's sport. Load is progressed, but the emphasis is always placed on control of scapular and spinal posture, and indeed all body segments. Resistance training for each muscle group is advanced as appropriate to the individual athlete's requirement (e.g. neck strength requirements for pistol shooting versus wrestling or rugby).

When the aim is to enhance strength, high loads should be prescribed for a low number of repetitions, whereas a large number of repetitions at low intensity will enhance endurance. A key principle in resistance training is that of overload.[179] This principle states that a greater-than-normal stress or load on the body is required to induce training adaptation. As performance improves with training, the intensity or volume of exercise must be increased to continue to put adequate demand on the athlete to stimulate muscle development.

Training sensorimotor control

There are several treatment options that can improve symptoms of dizziness, lightheadedness and unsteadiness of cervical origin. These include specific and targeted exercises as described below which directly address the impairments,[180-183] as well as treatments such as manual therapy, exercise and acupuncture.[154, 183] There is some evidence that the targeted exercises may be best at making a measurable improvement in these impairments.[180]

Joint relocation sense can be trained with eyes open, progressing to eyes closed with use of a laser and target for feedback. Similarly, a target can be traced with a laser to train movement sense progressing from simple to complex patterns (Fig. 23.20). Following a moving target is another treatment strategy, and various computerised applications such as training with virtual reality are being developed to train cervical movement sense.[120, 182, 184] The task difficulty can be progressed in the training of both position and movement sense by changing the size or stability of the base of support (i.e. sitting to standing to tandem stance to one-foot stance).

When training balance in an athlete with neck pain, it is usually necessary to commence training at a fairly high level; for example, in tandem stance. This can be progressed

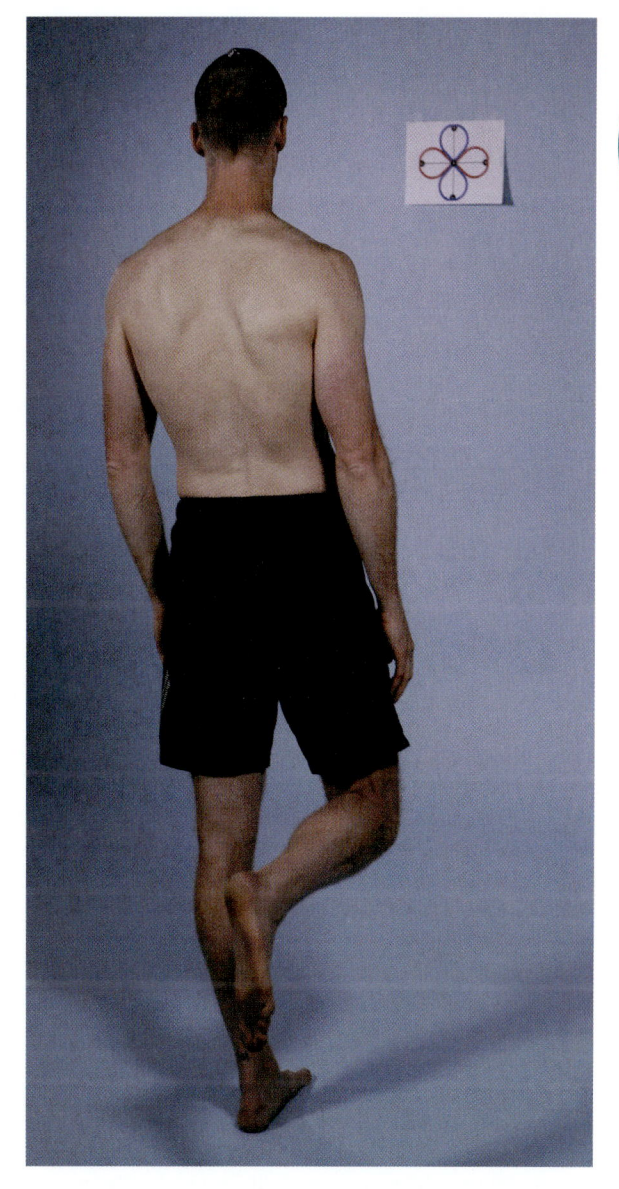

Figure 23.20 Movement sense is trained with the athlete tracing simple to complex patterns with a laser light mounted on the head. The exercise can also be progressed by advancing the position in which the exercise is performed (e.g. from sitting to standing to one-foot standing)

to one-leg standing and performed on hard, then soft and then unstable surfaces. Ensure that training is progressed to the functional demands of the athlete's sport.

Training eye movement control could include any of the following strategies: gaze stability, eye follow and eye follow of rapid movements; it should be based on the impairments detected in the physical examination. The tests described above can be converted to training exercises, with the clinician ensuring that the athlete can dissociate head and eye movement in all exercises. The exercises are usually commenced at a speed over which the athlete has control and they are progressed by increasing exercise speed or performing the exercises in more challenging postures (e.g. sitting to standing to tandem stance) as done when training joint relocation sense. Athletes with neck pain often need more advanced exercises, and combining training of two aspects of the cervical sensorimotor system (e.g. eye follow and balance) will produce a greater challenge to the cervical sensorimotor system.

Maintenance program

Specific self-management and maintenance programs should be included within the athlete's training regimen. A self-management program developed during treatment should incorporate motor relearning, resistance and sensorimotor exercises as indicated. As previously mentioned, repetition and adequate dosage are vital components to the success of any training program. Neck pain is a recurrent condition. With the possibility of re-injury during sport or the potentially continuing influence of arthogenous inhibition,[185] it is necessary for the athlete to continue to perform a simple maintenance program after formal management has ceased. For long-term compliance, this should consist of two or three key exercises aimed at reducing the probability of recurrent neck pain episodes.

NECK PAIN CONDITIONS

The majority of neck pain conditions are grouped under the broad term 'mechanical neck pain' and then qualified by a description of duration as being acute, subacute, persistent or recurrent acute episodes. Management is based on examination findings, as discussed throughout this chapter. Certain neck pain conditions are further characterised in relation to a specific clinical presentation, injury mechanism, identifiable pain mechanism or pathology. Management will again be based on examination findings, but some additional notes are relevant from a diagnostic or treatment perspective.

Cervicogenic headache

Cervicogenic headache is classified as a secondary headache (Chapter 21): it is secondary to a cervical musculoskeletal condition.[186] Pain sources are usually located in one or more of the upper three cervical segments and headache results from physiological convergence between cervical and trigeminal afferents in the trigeminocervical nucleus.[187] There is symptomatic overlap between migraine without aura headaches, tension-type headaches and cervicogenic headaches, and thus differential diagnosis is critical for proper management.

Research has sought to determine which physical tests characterise cervicogenic headache to differentiate it from migraine and tension-type headaches. In cervicogenic headaches, the athlete should present with a combination of cervical movement dysfunction, muscle function impairments and upper cervical joint dysfunction.[49, 55, 188] The clinical findings in the articular and neuromuscular systems are consistent with mechanical neck pain, and any reported unsteadiness or lightheadedness is consistent with sensorimotor disturbances. Management generally follows that described earlier in this chapter for mechanical neck pain, but care should be taken to ensure that treatments are non-pain provocative. This is because sensitisation of the trigeminocervical nucleus appears to be a factor in the development of cervicogenic headache.[57] If treatments are painful, the added peripheral nociception is likely to produce or worsen a headache.

Acute wry neck

Acute wry neck is characterised by an acute onset of neck pain with protective deformity (contralateral lateral flexion position) and limitation of movement. It typically occurs after a sudden, quick movement or on waking. There may have been an unguarded movement or prolonged abnormal posture prior to the onset of pain. It is hypothesised that the zygapophysial joint or disc may be the source of symptoms. When of zygapophysial origin, there may be entrapment or extrapment of the meniscus.[189] If the disc is suspected to be the source of symptoms, treatment is more conservative (i.e. gentle mobilisation; manipulation is not recommended). The differentiation between a zygapophysial joint or disc origin of symptoms is principally made collectively from historical features, presenting symptoms and manual detection of a pain source either over the zygapophysial joint or centrally through the spinous process, which is interpreted as a discal origin.

Although relatively rare, the clinician should be alert for atlanto-axial rotary fixation, a fixed rotary subluxation of C1 on C2.[190, 191] It is principally observed in young children and may occur spontaneously or can be secondary to congenital anomalies of the upper cervical spine and arthritides (e.g. juvenile onset rheumatoid arthritis). It may be associated with trauma and there may be instability. Medical and radiological diagnosis is required.

Cervical nerve injury
Cervical radiculopathy

Cervical radiculopathy usually presents as neck and arm pain or, occasionally, arm pain only, and may be accompanied by sensory disturbances and weakness in the upper limb. This neuropathic pain can often be intense and athletes require appropriate pharmacological pain management. The cervical nerve root can be compromised in the intervertebral canal by a disc lesion, or by zygapophysial or uncovertebral osteophytes. Inflammation also plays a significant role. Sensitisation of nerve tissue will be present. Surgery may be indicated in some instances, but conservative treatments should always be trialled in the first instance.[192]

Brachial plexus injuries ('stingers/burners')
Brachial plexus injuries occur in contact sports such as rugby union and rugby league, and can vary from severe injuries with avulsion or rupture[192,3] to less catastrophic traction injuries, often referred to as 'stingers' or 'burners' due to their characteristic symptoms.[194]

Assessment of an acute stinger involves first ruling out more serious injury such as spinal cord or brain involvement, fracture or vascular injury.[195] The athlete should be removed from the field if there are any such indications. In a stinger or burner, the athlete experiences transient neuropraxia characterised by upper extremity burning-type pain that may also be accompanied by paraesthesia and/or weakness. Tensile or compressive forces are the most likely underlying mechanism of this neuropraxia. Downward displacement of the shoulder with concomitant contralateral side flexion of the neck can cause a traction injury to either the cervical nerve root (most likely C5 or C6) or the brachial plexus. Alternatively, compression injuries can be caused by combined cervical extension and ipsilateral side flexion or a direct blow to the brachial plexus.[194]

Symptoms are usually transient, resolving over a varying period of time from minutes to days, but persistent neurological dysfunction and recurrent stingers may occur. A gentle exercise program that does not provoke typical symptoms may be started early in treatment, with care to avoid aggravating positions. As in all cases of nerve damage, there will be an element of the recovery that is time- and rest-dependent, and treatment cannot speed this process.

Acceleration/deceleration injury ('whiplash')
Acute acceleration/deceleration injury to the cervical spine is an injury commonly caused by a motor vehicle collision and it is commonly termed a whiplash-associated disorder (WAD). Theoretically, such an injury could also occur in sports when the cervical spine is subject to a sudden acceleration force. However, direct extrapolation from injuries sustained in motor vehicle collisions to a sporting injury may be unwise, and more comparative research is required. Management of most athletes with WAD will be similar to mechanical neck pain, but there is a small proportion of those with WAD who may not respond well to any treatments (medical, physical or psychological) and who generally have a poor prognosis.[25, 196-198]

CONCLUSION
Mechanical neck pain conditions can be troublesome for any athlete, but most can be managed well with conservative therapies. Nevertheless, neck pain is characteristically recurrent and its lifetime impact should not be underestimated. Management must aim to first address the presenting condition and resolve the acute episode of neck pain. The challenge is the second stage of treatment that aims to prevent or limit the recurrence of neck pain to improve future quality of life and sports performance. This broader aspect of effective secondary prevention should be a focus of both clinical practice and research.

REFERENCES
References for this chapter can be found at www.mhhe.com/au/CSM5e

Chapter 24

Shoulder pain

by ANN MJ COOLS*

When I dislocated my shoulder back in 2005 and (went through) rehab throughout 2006, I was told by Dr Andrews 'you're always going to have to stay on top of that shoulder. You're always going to have to do a little bit extra to keep it at the level you want to keep it at'. In a lot of ways it was the best thing that ever happened to me because I started doing things that I'd never done before. So I learned so much about my shoulder and how to manage my shoulder.

Drew Brees, NFL quarterback

Shoulder pain and dysfunction are a significant health issue, in the general population as well as in an athletic population. Whilst acute shoulder injuries occur mainly in collision sports or as a result of a sports accident like falling in skiing or biking, athletes performing overhead sports such as tennis, baseball, swimming and gymnastics are also prone to chronic shoulder pain, due to the high demands on their shoulders during their sports performance. In this chapter, the following topics regarding assessment and treatment of shoulder pain are discussed:

- functional anatomy and biomechanics
- overview of most common, less common, and not-to-miss causes of shoulder pain
- clinical examination: from history and basic clinical exam to special tests and outcome scores
- investigation
- general treatment and specific rehabilitation guidelines for the most common shoulder injuries in athletes
- less common causes of shoulder pain: overview of treatment guidelines
- special considerations for the overhead athlete: the thrower's program, sport-specific kinetic chain principles and return to play after injury.

FUNCTIONAL ANATOMY AND BIOMECHANICS

The glenohumeral joint is an inherently unstable shallow ball and socket joint, often described as the equivalent of a golf ball (head of humerus) on a tee (glenoid). In fact, the relationship between the humeral head and the glenoid cavity more accurately parallels a sea lion balancing a ball on its nose. Thus, effective shoulder function and stability requires both static constraints–the glenohumeral ligaments, glenoid labrum and capsule–and dynamic constraints, predominantly the rotator cuff and scapular stabilising muscles (Fig. 24.1).

Static stabilisers

In the neutral position, the coracohumeral ligament and the superior glenohumeral ligament control inferior translation of the humeral head. In an abducted position, all parts of the inferior glenohumeral ligament prevent excessive inferior translation. During external rotation in slight elevation (0–45°), the medial glenohumeral ligament prevents anterior translation. The main static stabilisers of the shoulder in the functional position (abducted) are the anterior and posterior bands of the inferior glenohumeral ligament. Together with the axillary pouch, these three parts of the inferior glenohumeral ligament (IGHL) are the thickest of all glenohumeral ligaments (Fig. 24.1d). They are attached to the labrum, which, in turn, attaches directly to the margin of the glenoid fossa. The anterior band of the inferior glenohumeral ligament prevents anterior translation and the posterior band prevents posterior translation of the humeral head. The superior margin of the anterior band of this ligament attaches to the

---
* 4th edition authors: W Ben Kibler, George AC Murrell and Babette Pluim

PART B   Regional problems

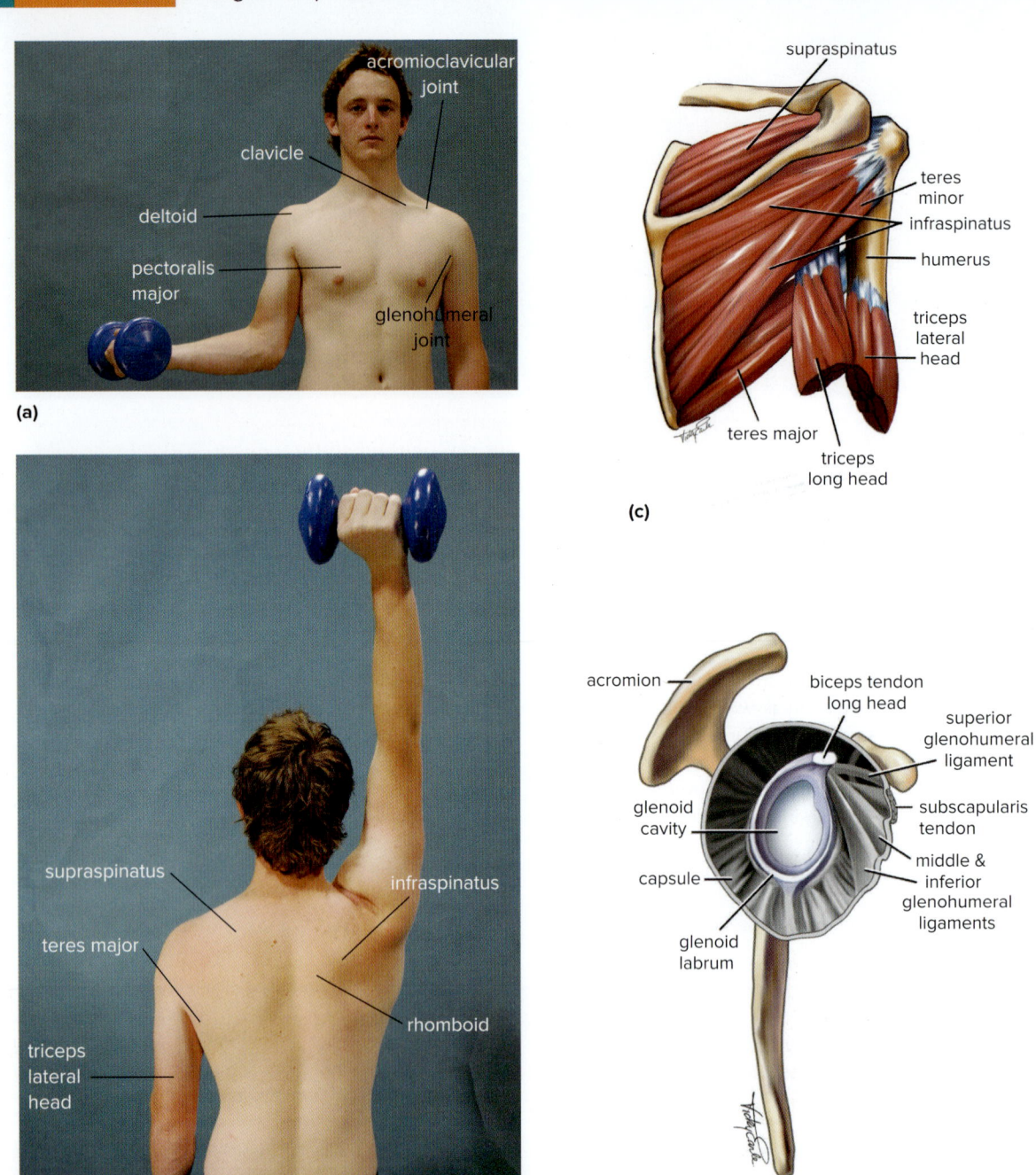

Figure 24.1 Anatomy of the shoulder region (a) Surface anatomy from the front (b) Surface anatomy from behind (c) Rotator cuff musculature from behind (d) Ligaments and muscles around the glenohumeral joint

glenoid fossa anteriorly at the two o'clock position. When the arm is placed into abduction and external rotation, this broad ligamentous band of the IGHL rotates anteriorly to prevent subluxation of the joint.[1] In addition, the IGHL seems to have a dual role–it also forms a substantial posterior barrier when the arm is internally rotated in the abducted or forward flexed position. Shoulder stability is also enhanced by the glenoid labrum, a ring of fibrous tissue attached to the rim of the glenoid, which expands the size and depth of the glenoid cavity. It increases the superior-inferior diameter of the glenoid by 75% and the anterior-posterior diameter by 50%. Moreover, the plasticity of the glenoid allows expanding the size of the glenoid fossa without losing range of motion, and is an attachment site for ligaments and the biceps tendon.

Dynamic stabilisers

The dynamic stabilisers of the glenohumeral joint are the rotator cuff muscles, consisting of the supraspinatus, infraspinatus, subscapularis and teres minor, which act in co-contraction to seat the humeral head in the glenoid (Fig. 24.1c). Since the tendons splay out and interdigitate to form a common, continuous insertion to the humerus, their roles are highly interrelated. The specific roles of the different tendons are debated in literature. The most recent studies attribute similar stabilising roles to infraspinatus and supraspinatus performing external rotation, and avoiding anterior translation of the humeral head, whereas subscapularis is contracting to avoid posterior translation.[2] In addition, the rotator cuff muscles counteract the action of the deltoid (which elevates the humeral head) by preventing the head of the humerus from moving superiorly when the arm is raised. The key issue in this force couple concept of the rotator cuff, is muscular balance between the different components of the rotator cuff, in particular between the internal and external rotators (ER/IR ratio). Overhead athletes often exhibit stronger internal rotators, with subsequently relative weak external rotators,[3] resulting in a lower ER/IR ratio, and thus increasing the risk for chronic shoulder pain.

The role of the scapula in normal shoulder function

The scapular stabilisers also play an important role in shoulder joint movement. Normal shoulder function requires smooth integration of movement not only at the glenohumeral joint but also at the scapulothoracic, acromioclavicular (AC) and sternoclavicular (SC) joints. This integrated movement is referred to as 'scapulohumeral rhythm'. Scapulohumeral rhythm should be smooth, coordinated and symmetrical. Full upper limb elevation requires three-dimensional rotation of the scapula and the clavicle as coupled movements into upward rotation, posterior tilting and adequate internal or external rotation, depending on the plane of the moving humerus, which ensures that the coracoacromial arch is removed from the path of the greater tuberosity of the elevating humerus, thus avoiding potential impingement.

Scapular control also enhances joint stability at greater than 90° of abduction by placing the glenoid fossa under the humeral head, where stability is assisted by the action of the deltoid muscle. The muscles controlling the scapula are the trapezius (all three portions), serratus anterior (upper and lower portions), rhomboids, levator scapulae and pectoralis minor. These muscles work in coordinated patterns called force couples to control three-dimensional scapular motion.

The main upward rotation force couple involves the upper trapezius/lower part of the serratus anterior, with a stabilising role for the middle and lower trapezius. The rhomboids and levator scapulae are supposed to lengthen in order to allow sufficient scapular upward rotation. Anterior/posterior tilt involves the lower trapezius/lower part of the serratus anterior force couple, and requires relative relaxation of the pectoralis minor. Together with the levator scapulae and the rhomboid, pectoralis minor is considered to have a rather postural function, keeping the scapula steady on the thoracic wall in rest and during movement. Interestingly, these muscles (pectoralis minor, levator scapulae and rhomboid) are very often tight rather than weak in patients with shoulder pain, and need to be addressed aiming at relaxation rather than strengthening.

The third scapular movement, internal and external rotation, is controlled by a complex force couple consisting of both parts of the serratus anterior versus all three parts of the trapezius. All three movements, and their working force couples are summarised in Figure 24.2. A stable scapula provides a base for the muscles arising from the scapula and acting on the humerus, allowing them to maintain their optimal length-tension relationship.

There is a body of evidence suggesting altered scapular rhythm or scapular dyskinesis, consisting of abnormal scapular positioning and/or movement patterns in patients suffering from shoulder pain, although the cause-consequence relationship is still under debate. Scapular dyskinesis has been found to be related to shoulder instability, impingement and stiff shoulders in a variety of patient populations, and is identified as a primary risk

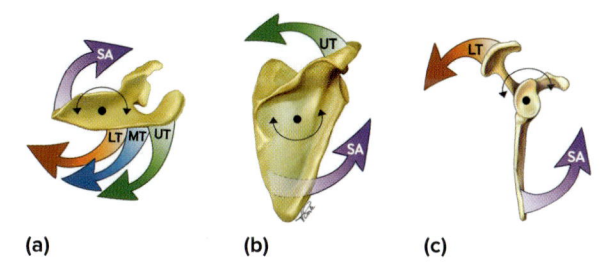

Figure 24.2 Force couples controlling scapular motions
(a) Internal/external rotation (b) Upward/downward rotation
(c) Anterior/posterior tilting

SA = serratus anterior, UT = upper trapezius, MT = middle trapezius, LT = lower trapezius factor for shoulder injury in handball[3] and rugby players.[4] Scapular malpositioning and abnormal muscle patterning have been associated with experimentally induced shoulder pain, thus suggesting scapular dyskinesis might be secondary to shoulder pain.[5] Abnormalities of scapulohumeral rhythm are most commonly due to shortening of the scapulohumeral or glenohumeral muscles, or weakness and/or poor motor control of the scapular stabilisers (with or without weakness of the rotator cuff muscles).

CAUSES OF SHOULDER PAIN—OVERVIEW

Most athletic shoulder injuries are the result of one of two mechanisms: (1) an acute external force applied on the shoulder complex (macrotrauma) or (2) repetitive overhead activity and overuse (microtrauma).

Acute versus overuse shoulder pain

The shoulder is susceptible to traumatic injuries such as dislocations, subluxations, acromioclavicular joint sprains, and soft tissue injuries, in particular in collision and contact sports. However, most injuries result from repetitive overuse mechanisms, due to overload, aberrant overhead throwing biomechanics and dysfunctional adaptations to the sport, leading to chronic symptoms like impingement and bursitis.[6] Moreover, the shoulder is predisposed to athletic injury because of the large amount of mobility of the glenohumeral joint, allowing powerful throwing and smashing, but putting the shoulder at risk for injury due to the inherently poor glenohumeral stability.

A list of possible causes of shoulder pain is presented in Table 24.1

Impingement

Impingement is one of the most frequently described pathologic shoulder conditions in general practice and in sports medicine. Early literature described impingement as a pathology or a diagnosis but today impingement is considered to be a cluster of symptoms, rather than a pathology itself. Various investigations have confirmed the association between impingement symptoms and a variety of underlying pathologic mechanisms. Rotator cuff pathology, scapular dyskinesis, shoulder instability, biceps pathology and superior labrum anterior to posterior (SLAP) lesions, and glenohumeral internal rotation deficit (GIRD) or posterior shoulder stiffness have been suggested to cause shoulder impingement symptoms. In addition, thoracic posture and mobility are considered to be key factors in the development of shoulder pain.

The literature describes two types of impingement: subacromial and internal. Subacromial or external impingement is the mechanical encroachment of the soft tissue (bursa, rotator cuff tendons) in the subacromial space between the humeral head and the acromial arch (Fig. 24.3). This encroachment particularly takes place in the midrange of motion, often causing a 'painful arc' during active abduction.

Internal impingement comprises encroachment of the rotator cuff tendons between the humeral head and the glenoid rim. Based on the location of the impingement, anterosuperior and posterosuperior glenoid impingement have been described. Posterosuperior glenoid impingement involves mechanical encroachment of the rotator cuff tendons, particularly the supraspinatus and infraspinatus, between the greater tubercle of the humerus and the

Table 24.1 Causes of shoulder pain

Common	Less common	Not to be missed causes outside the shoulder girdle
Rotator cuff pathology (strain, tear, tendinopathy)	Other muscle tear (pectoralis major, long head of biceps (LHB))	Somatic referred pain (cervical and thoracic spine, myofascial structures)
Glenohumeral instability (traumatic, atraumatic, congenital)	Adhesive capsulitis	Tumour (bone tumours in proximal humerus)
Biceps related pathology (SLAP labral tears, biceps tendinopathy, tenosynovitis)	Neurovascular entrapment or traction injury (suprascapular nerve, long thoracic nerve, axillary nerve, axillary vein compression, thoracic outlet syndrome)	Visceral referred pain (e.g. diaphragm, gall bladder, heart, spleen, apex of lungs)
Posterior shoulder stiffness (GIRD)	Fractures (scapula, humerus, stress fracture of coracoid process)	
Scapular pathology and dysfunction, including AC and SC joint pathology (sprain, fracture, dislocation, clavicular fracture)	Snapping scapula	

SLAP = superior labrum anterior to posterior; GIRD = glenohumeral internal rotation deficit; AC = acromioclavicular; SC = sternoclavicular

Shoulder pain CHAPTER 24

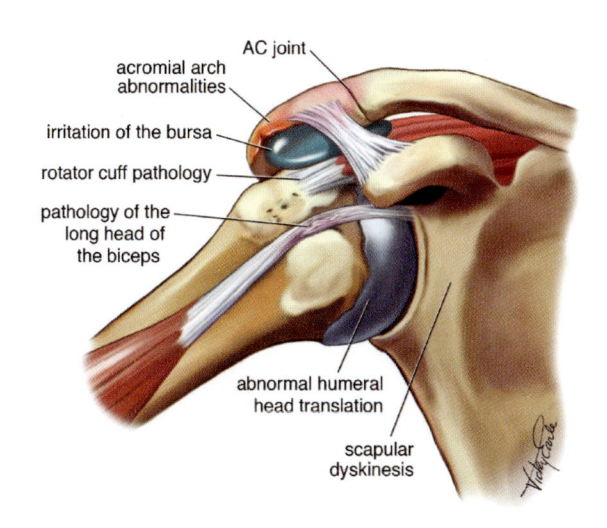

Figure 24.3 Subacromial impingement

posterosuperior rim of the glenoid (Fig. 24.4a). This occurs during the late cocking position of throwing, which is maximal external rotation, horizontal abduction, and depending on the specific sport discipline, a certain amount of elevation. Because of the specific position of this internal impingement, it is considered to be the primary cause of chronic shoulder pain in the overhead athlete. Internal impingement particularly occurs when the humeral shaft goes beyond the plane of the body of the scapula during the cocking position of throwing. Under normal circumstances, the scapula goes into retraction simultaneously with the horizontal abduction movement of the humerus. When the body of the scapula and the humeral shaft fail to remain in the same plane of movement during the cocking phase of throwing, encroachment of the rotator cuff tendons between the humeral head and the glenoid rim may cause internal impingement symptoms. This phenomenon is called 'hyperangulation' (Fig. 24.4b).[7]

Besides the classification of impingement based on the site of encroachment, impingement is also classified based on the cause of the problem, dividing it into primary versus secondary impingement. In primary impingement, a structural narrowing of the subacromial space causes pain and dysfunction, such as acromioclavicular arthropathy, type II or III acromion, subacromial bone spurs, or swelling of the soft tissue in the subacromial space, for instance the subacromial bursa. The bony subacromial abnormalities result from either a congenital abnormality (os acromiale) or osteophyte formation. In addition, the under surface of the acromion may be abnormally beaked, curved or hooked (Fig. 24.5). However, abnormalities are not necessarily associated with clinical symptoms.[8]

In secondary impingement, there are no structural obstructions causing the encroachment, but rather functional problems occurring only in specific positions. Rotator cuff weakness, instability and scapular dyskinesis are possible underlying functional deficits, leading to secondary impingement symptoms. Secondary impingement may occur in the subacromial space as well as internal in the glenohumeral joint.

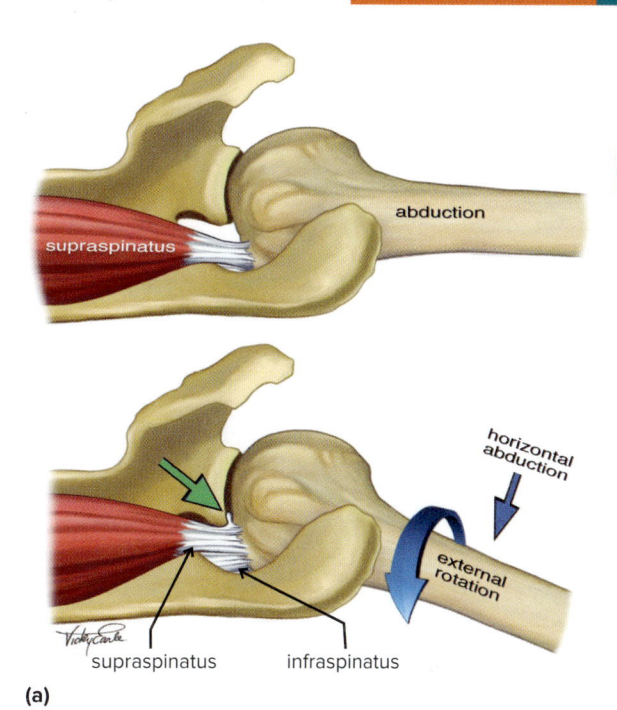

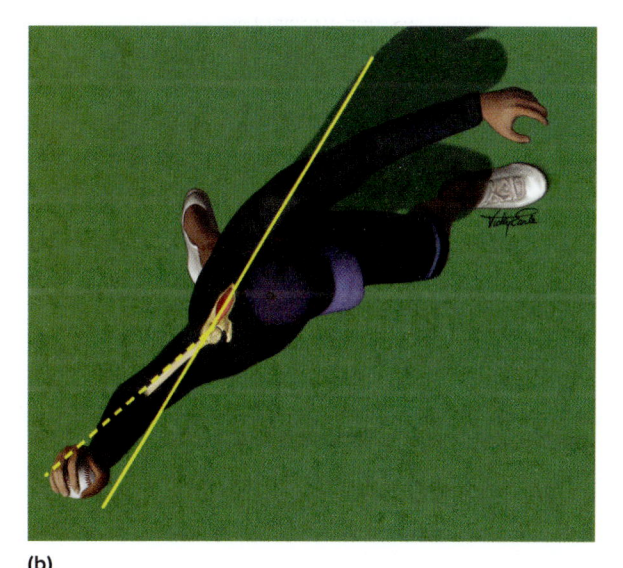

Figure 24.4 Internal impingement in overhead athletes (a) Posterosuperior impingement of the supraspinatus and infraspinatus tendons (b) Hyperangulation of the humerus in the late cocking phase of throwing is a common mechanism of internal impingement

PART B   Regional problems

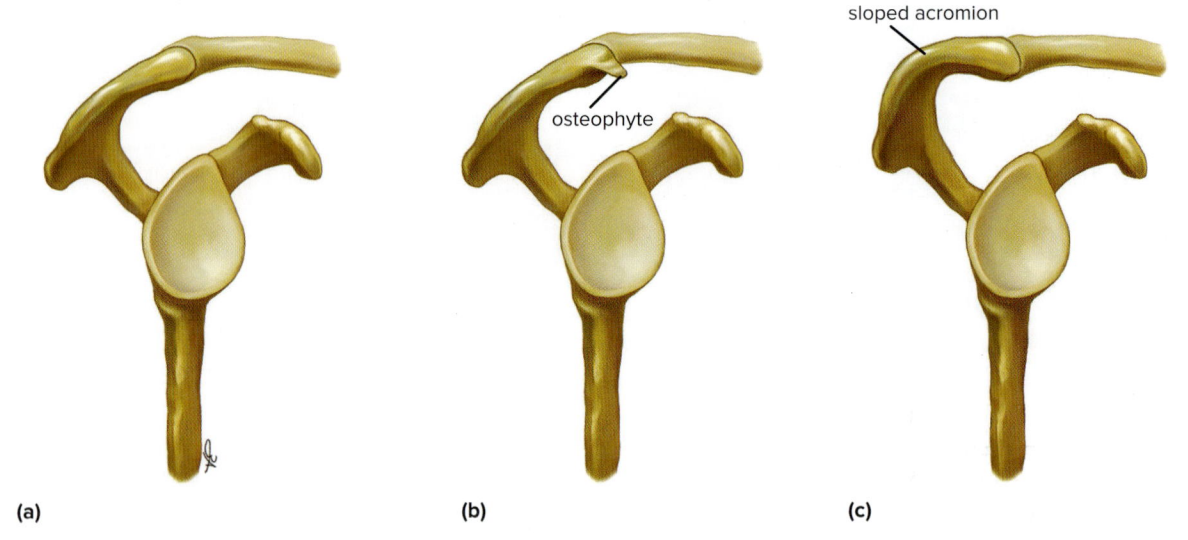

Figure 24.5 Acromial shapes. Abnormalities are not necessarily associated with clinical symptoms (a) Normal acromion (b) Acromion with anterior osteophyte (c) Congenital sloped acromion

> **PRACTICE PEARL**
>
> Primary impingement might be considered as structural impingement, whereas secondary impingement is in most cases functional impingement.

In view of the assumption that impingement symptoms may be the result of various underlying pathologies, it is important to describe the biomechanical relationship between these symptoms and shoulder diagnoses. Rotator cuff pathology may be associated with impingement symptoms in primary as well as secondary impingement. In primary impingement, swelling of the injured rotator cuff tendons causes the narrowing of the subacromial space; in secondary impingement, dysfunction of the rotator cuff (whose function is amongst others performing a caudal glide of the humeral head during elevation in order to avoid impingement) results in more cranial migration of the humeral head, thus causing secondary impingement.

Scapular dyskinesis has also been described in relation to impingement symptoms. The rationale behind this association is that during arm elevation, impingement may occur if the scapula insufficiently follows the humeral head movements because of a lack of upward rotation, posterior tilting and external rotation, thus clearing the acromial arch or the glenoid rim from impinging the soft tissue.

The association between impingement symptoms and shoulder instability is well established. Excessive humeral head translation, based on capsular laxity and instability, cause temporal narrowing of the subacromial space, thus leading to impingement symptoms and pain.

Since the biceps plays an important role in shoulder stability and function, biceps pathology may cause secondary impingement symptoms. Indeed, biceps tendon problems (tendinopathy or tenosynovitis) as well as SLAP lesions (labral lesions at the site of origin of the long head of the biceps) compromise optimal shoulder function, and may result in impingement.

Glenohumeral internal rotation deficit, often referred to as GIRD, is a sport-specific adaptation of posterior shoulder structures to chronic excessive overload of these structures during frequent throwing. There are several theories concerning the occurrence and development of GIRD. A first hypothesis is that GIRD results from contracture or shortening of the posterior capsule. Other researchers believe that GIRD begins in the early years of overhead throwing with a bony adaptation of the humerus, resulting in altered humeral torsion. A third hypothesis regarding the cause of GIRD is muscle hypertonicity in the external rotators due to frequent eccentric loading. GIRD may cause aberrant glenohumeral kinematics and thus result in impingement symptoms.

CLINICAL APPROACH

A complete clinical assessment involves:

1. history
2. observation and pre-examination palpation
3. basic clinical exam (BCE) and tissue-specific palpation
4. special tests: diagnostic testing and symptom modification tests
5. screening of the kinetic chain
6. objective measurements and outcome scores.

History

Endeavour to determine the exact site of the patient's pain; this can be difficult. Although acromioclavicular (AC) joint pain (C4 dermatome) and bicipital pain (along the bicipital groove and the line of the muscle belly) are well localised, the pain of most other shoulder pathologies is more diffuse. The onset of shoulder pain may be either acute, for example, a dislocation, subluxation or rotator cuff tear, or insidious, such as rotator cuff tendinopathy. Although most patients with chronic impingement-related shoulder pain report pain distribution in the deltoid area (and the C5 dermatome), overhead athletes with internal impingement and tissue involvement of the infraspinatus accentuate posterior shoulder pain in their history.

For acute injuries, identify the position of the shoulder at the time of injury. If the arm was wrenched backwards while in a vulnerable position, it suggests anterior dislocation or subluxation. A fall onto the point of the shoulder can cause AC joint injury. In chronic shoulder pain, the activity or position that precipitates the patient's pain should be noted, such as the cocking phase of throwing or the pull-through phase of swimming.

Note the severity of the pain, aggravating and easing factors, and the effect of the pain on activities of daily living and sporting activity. Night pain is very common in rotator cuff dysfunction and adhesive capsulitis. In order to identify the actual irritability of the injured tissue, ask (a) if the patient can sleep on the injured shoulder, (b) if the pain is only at the shoulder region, and not referring into the upper arm or elbow, and (c) if there is no pain at rest. If the answer is yes on all three questions, irritability is low, and controlled loading of the structures will be allowed. However, if the answer to one or two of the three questions is no, high irritability is present, meaning initial treatment will mainly have to focus on pain control and tissue protection.[9]

> **PRACTICE PEARL**
>
> Shoulder pain should be considered irritable if the patient cannot sleep on the painful shoulder, if their pain extends into the upper arm or elbow, or if they have resting pain. Initial treatment should then focus on pain control and tissue protection.

Sensory symptoms such as numbness or pins and needles should be noted as well as any episodes of 'dead arm'. In a baseball pitcher this suggests a labral injury. He or she may report catching and locking, or inability to develop normal speed in the action.

Inquire as to past or present problems elsewhere in the kinetic chain such as knee or ankle sprains or lower back pain. Also, clarify the exact treatment for previous local or distant problems. Look for predisposing factors. For example, a training diary may reveal excessive load on the region.

Physical examination

Examination should begin with observation of the patient from the front, from behind, and from the side. Check for asymmetry in muscle bulk, scapular position, shoulder height, spinal curves, head position, general posture, and AC and sternoclavicular (SC) joint protuberances. Next, a pre-examination palpation should be performed, checking for muscle atrophy, swelling, temperature and general trophic condition of skin. Tissue-specific palpation should be avoided prior to the examination, as this might influence the results of the clinical examination.

A basic clinical examination should then be performed, consisting of active and passive movements and resistance tests.

Active movements

These consist of forward flexion in the sagittal plane, abduction in the frontal plane, elevation in the scapular plane, functional external rotation (hand to neck) and functional internal rotation (hand behind back) (Fig. 24.6). Check for range of motion (ROM), pain and quality of

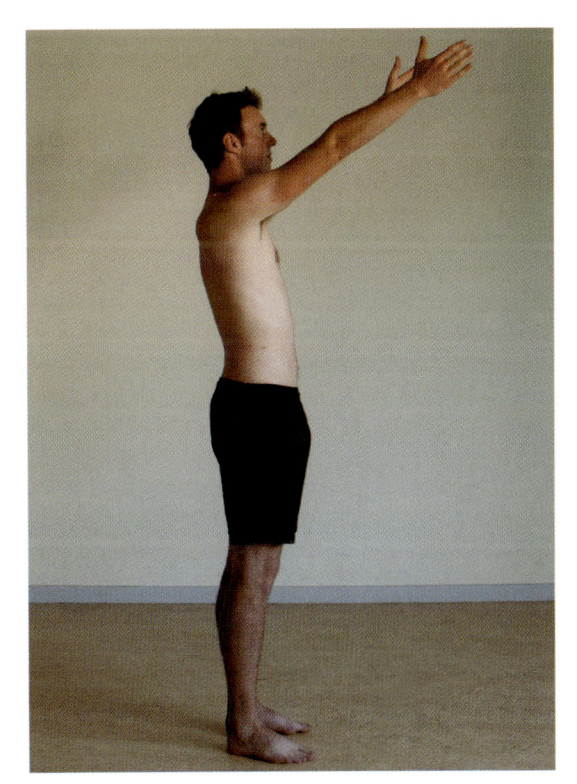

(a)

Figure 24.6 Basic clinical examination—active movements
(a) Forward flexion

PART B   Regional problems

(b)

(c)

(d)

(e)

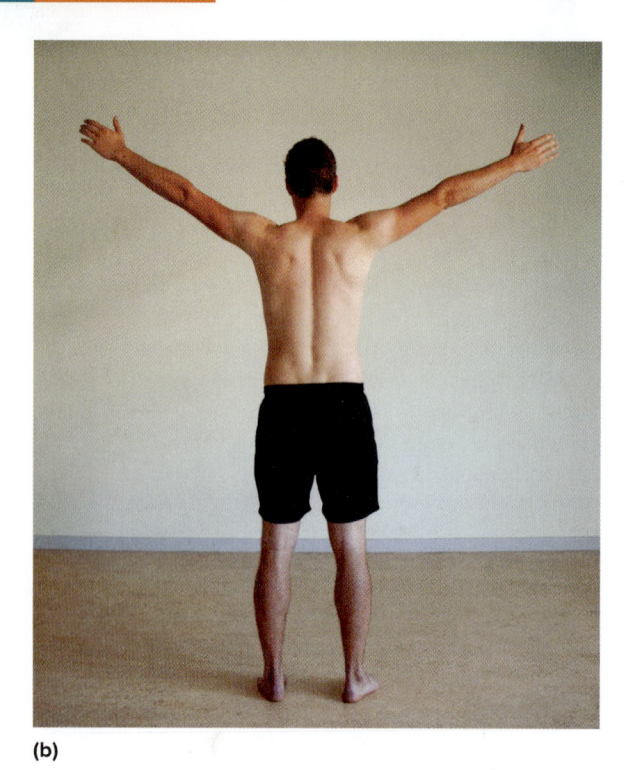

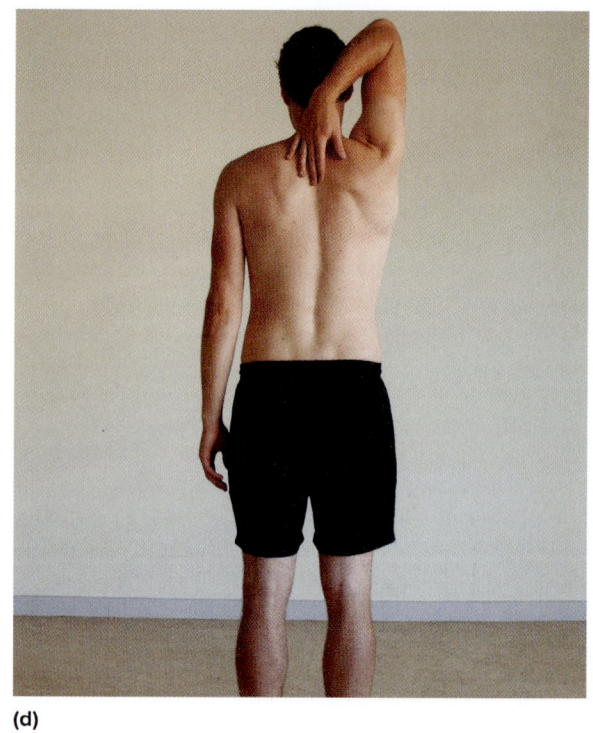

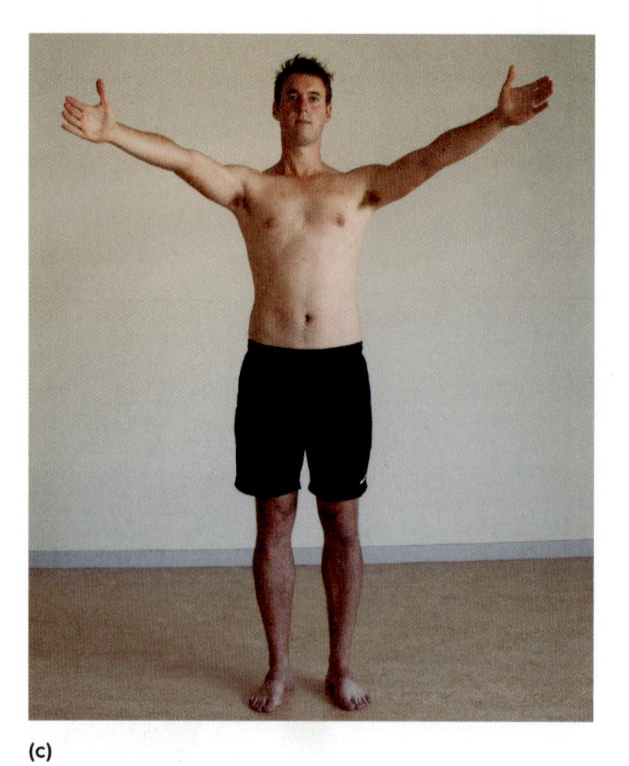

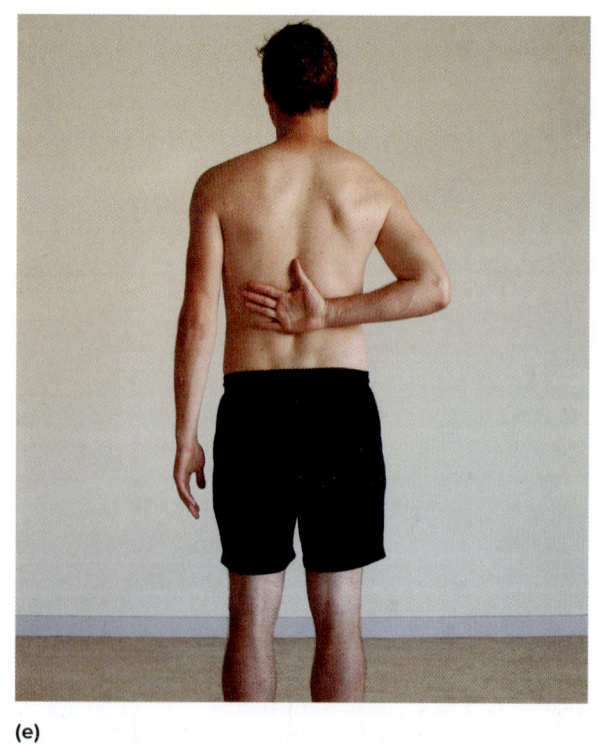

Figure 24.6 (cont.) (b) Abduction (c) Elevation in the scapular plane (d) Functional external rotation—hand to neck (e) Functional internal rotation—hand behind back

Shoulder pain CHAPTER 24

movement. A specific pain pattern can be found in the painful arc, in which the patient experiences pain in the midrange of motion, and not in the extremes. Specifically observe scapular movements. Scapular dyskinesis may be observed during all active movements. Depending on the specific kind of dyskinesis, they may be divided into type I (prominent inferior angle of the scapula), type II (prominent medial border of the scapula), and type III (prominent superior medial angle of the scapula). In addition, check for a possible protracted scapular position and rounded shoulder posture.

Passive examination
This consists of forward flexion, abduction, external rotation in neutral position, internal rotation from neutral, and horizontal adduction (Fig. 24.7). Check for ROM, pain and end feel. Be aware of the specific pattern in case of adhesive capsulitis: both rotations limited, as well as abduction in the frontal plane, and a stiff end feel. Loss of ROM and/or pain during passive examination indicate articular, capsular or ligamentous injury or stiffness in the surrounding muscles.

Resistance examination
In this stage, isometric resistance is given against forward flexion, extension, abduction and adduction, external and internal rotation, elbow flexion and extension, all with

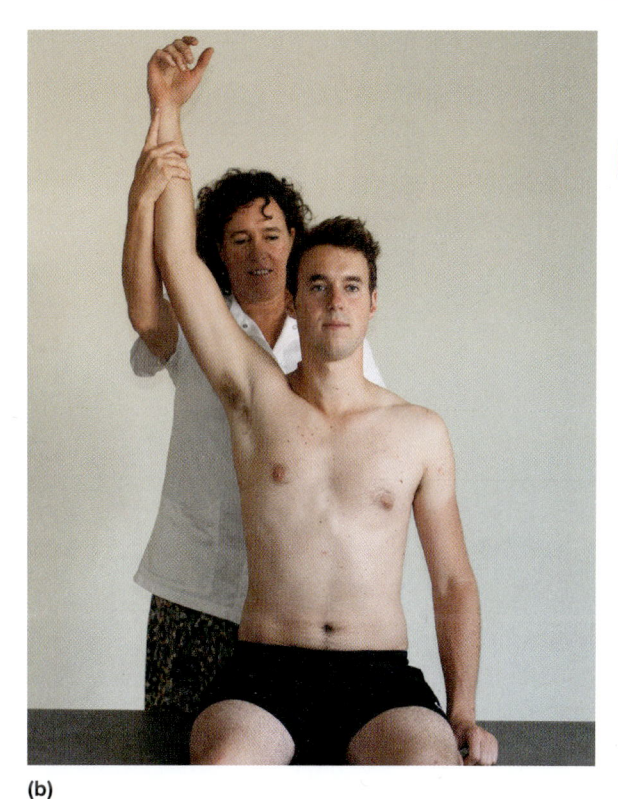

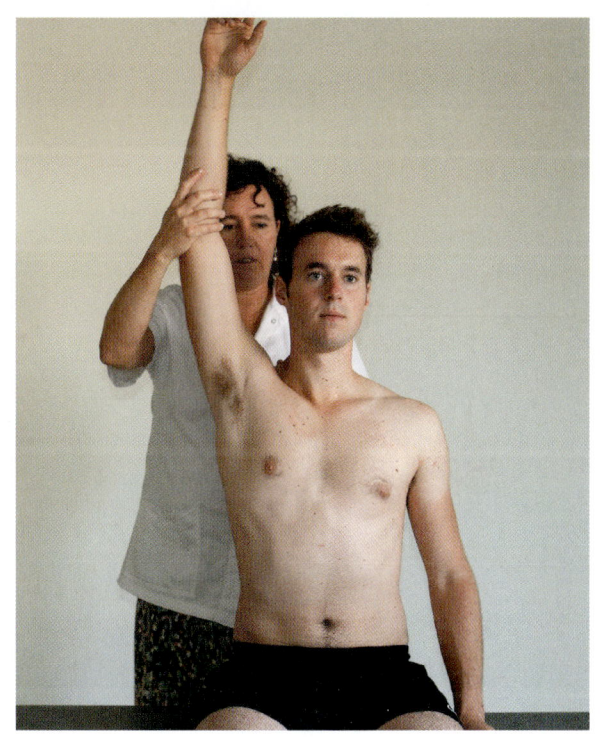

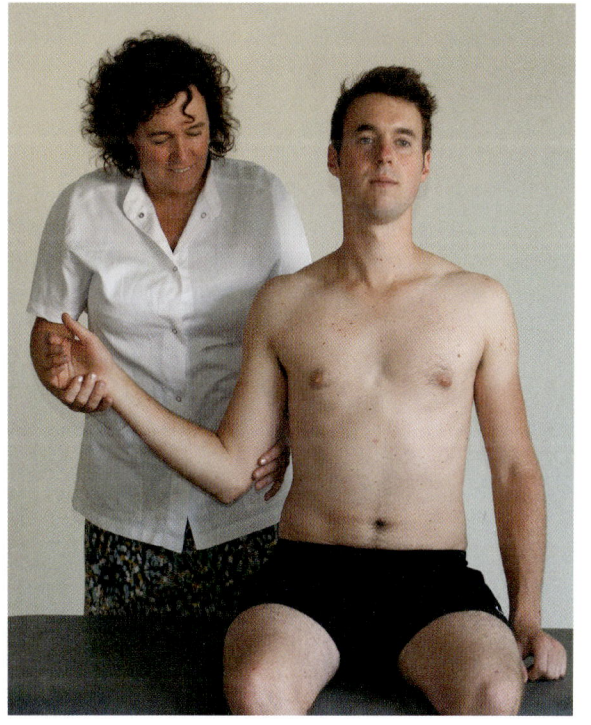

Figure 24.7 Basic clinical examination—passive movements (a) Forward flexion (b) Abduction (c) External rotation

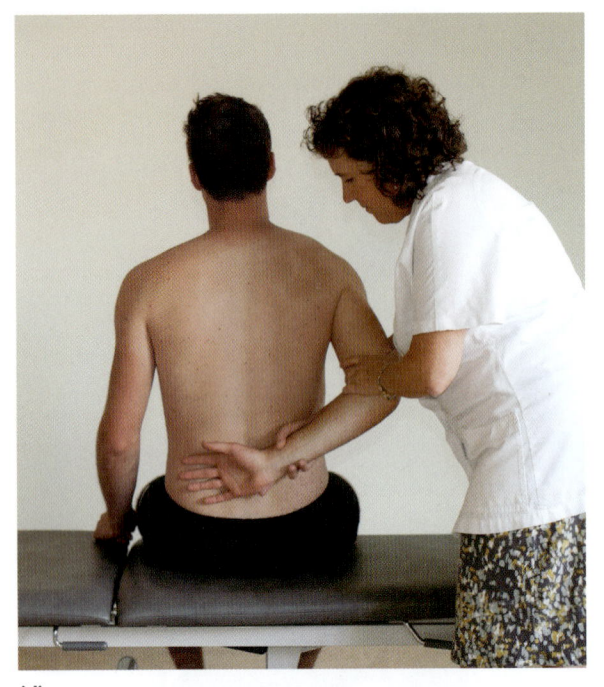

PART B   Regional problems

the shoulder in the neutral positions (Fig. 24.8). Pain and/or weakness are noticed, and might reflect injury to the musculotendinous system. Pain without weakness often is the result of tendinopathy, whereas weakness is the result of muscle tears. However, be aware that the patient might exhibit protective muscle inhibition in case of an injury with high irritability, possibly leading to a false diagnosis of muscle tear. In that case, resistance tests will be weak and painful. Weakness without pain might be the result of a complete but asymptomatic tear (e.g. external rotation

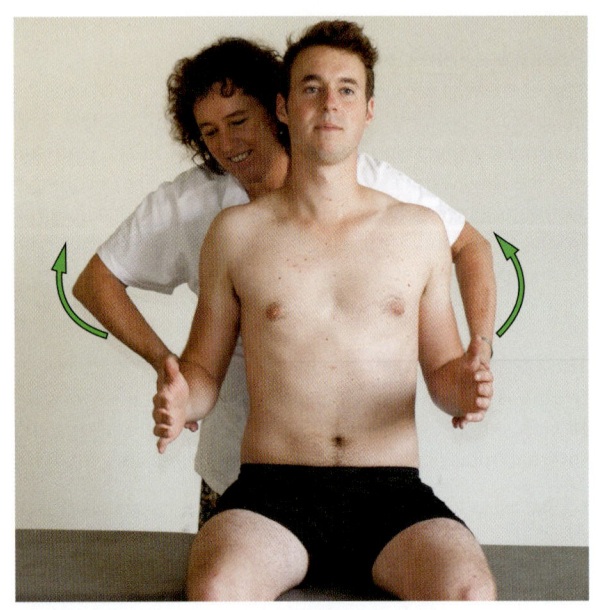

(d)

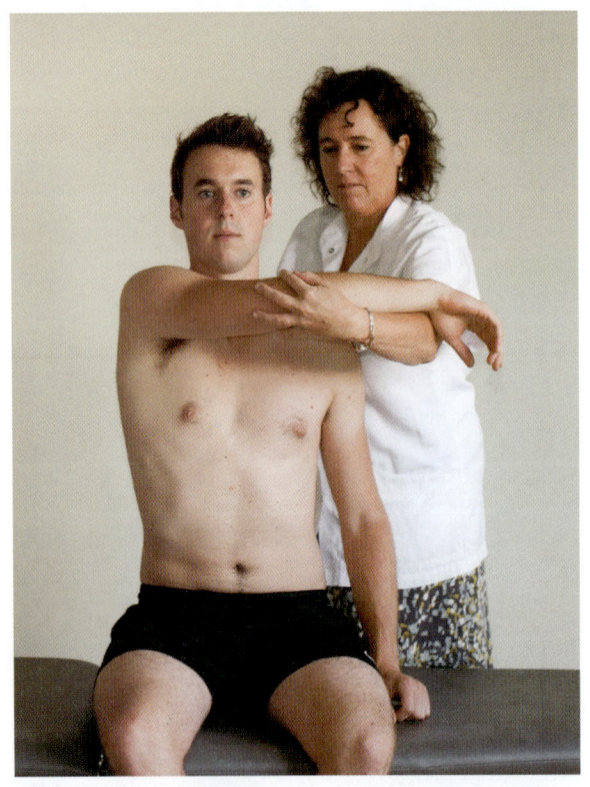

(e)

Figure 24.7 (cont.) (d) Internal rotation (e) Horizontal adduction

(a)

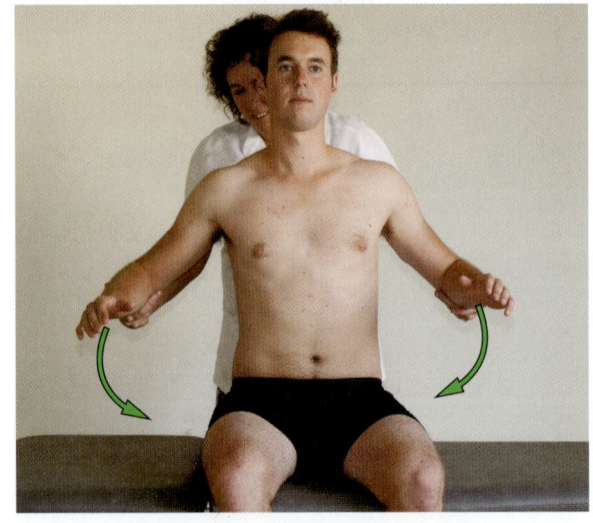

(b)

Figure 24.8 Basic clinical examination—resistance (a) Abduction (b) Adduction

Shoulder pain CHAPTER 24

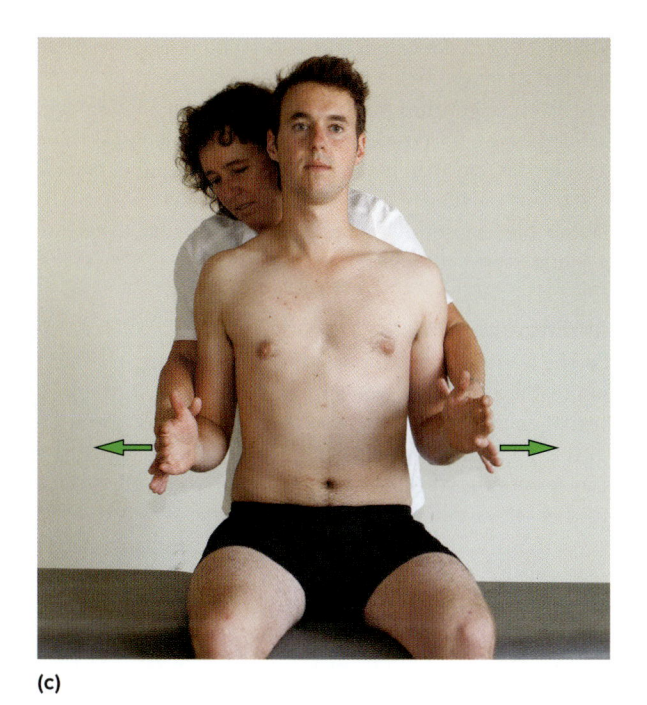

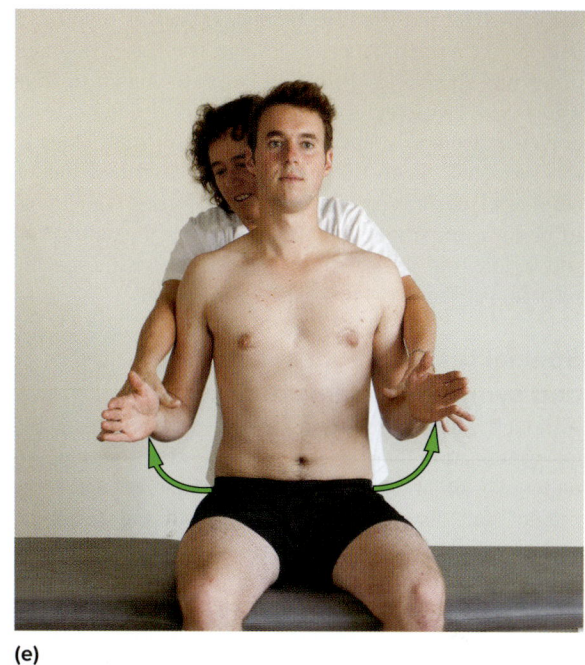

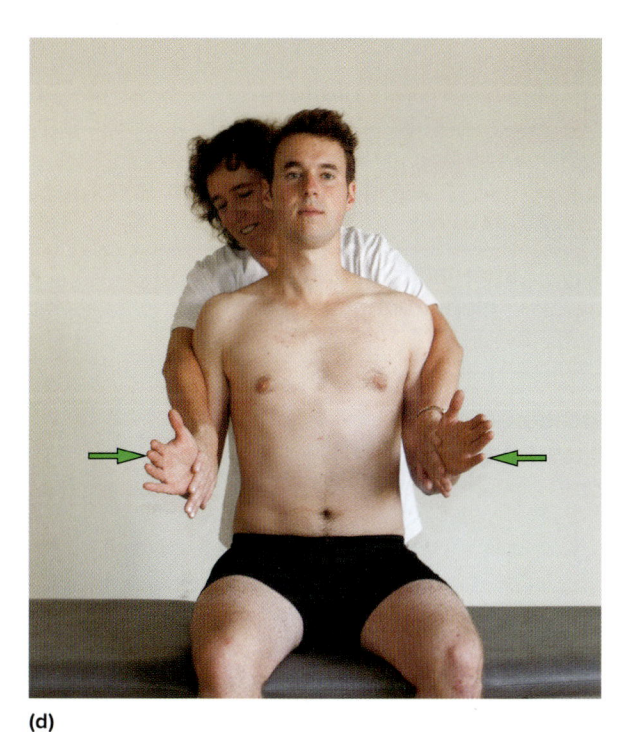

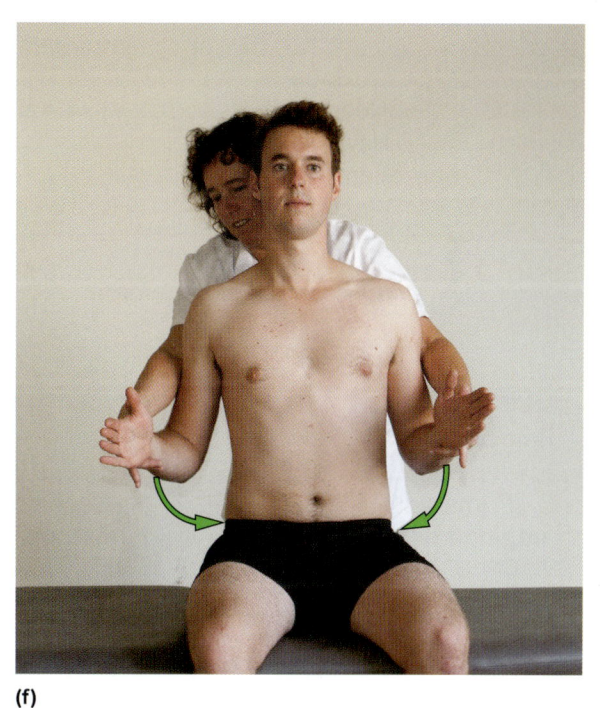

Figure 24.8 (cont.) (c) External rotation (d) Internal rotation (e) Elbow flexion (f) Elbow extension

in a total tear of the infraspinatus), sport-specific weakness of the antagonist (e.g. external rotators in overhead athletes) or a neurological problem (e.g. weak abduction due to an axillary nerve injury).

After the basic clinical examination, and based on the hypothesis of tissue injury, tissue-specific palpation may be performed. In overhead athletes, check routinely for tenderness of the supraspinatus, infraspinatus, subscapularis,

AC joint line, and the LHB tendon, as well as myofascial pain in the upper trapezius, levator scapulae, pectoralis minor and rhomboids. Palpation has been shown to have similar sensitivity and specificity as to some clinical tests; however, accuracy depends upon the palpation skills of the examiner. Since the special tests, described below, often tend to irritate or impinge the tendons, it is advisable to perform palpation after the basic clinical examination and before the special tests. Repeat the tissue-specific palpation at the very end of the examination.

Special tests—diagnostic testing and symptom modification tests

Although a large number of special tests are described for examination of the shoulder, it is not feasible to undertake all of them in every examination. Here we present and discuss an algorithm for clinical reasoning and physical examination testing to assist the clinician in the assessment of impingement-related shoulder pain (Fig. 24.9).[10] Clinical tests are selected based on the available evidence regarding their diagnostic accuracy (Table 24.2); however, given the large number of available clinical tests, also based on the examiner's preference. Any test in the algorithm may be substituted by another one, as long as the purpose of the test and its diagnostic value are comparable. In general, in the interpretation of clinical tests, latest evidence and systematic reviews suggest it is favourable to interpret a 'best-test combination' instead of a solitary test.

Impingement tests

Of the various provocative impingement tests, the most popular are the Jobe, Hawkins and Neer tests. In the Jobe test or empty can test, the shoulder is put in 90° elevation in the scapular plane in maximal internal rotation (empty can position) and manual resistance is given against further elevation (Fig. 24.10a). The test is positive for subacromial impingement if the patient reports pain. The test will be negative if the patient has posterosuperior glenoid impingement.

In the Hawkins test, passive internal rotation is performed with the shoulder in 90° of forward flexion (Fig. 24.10b).

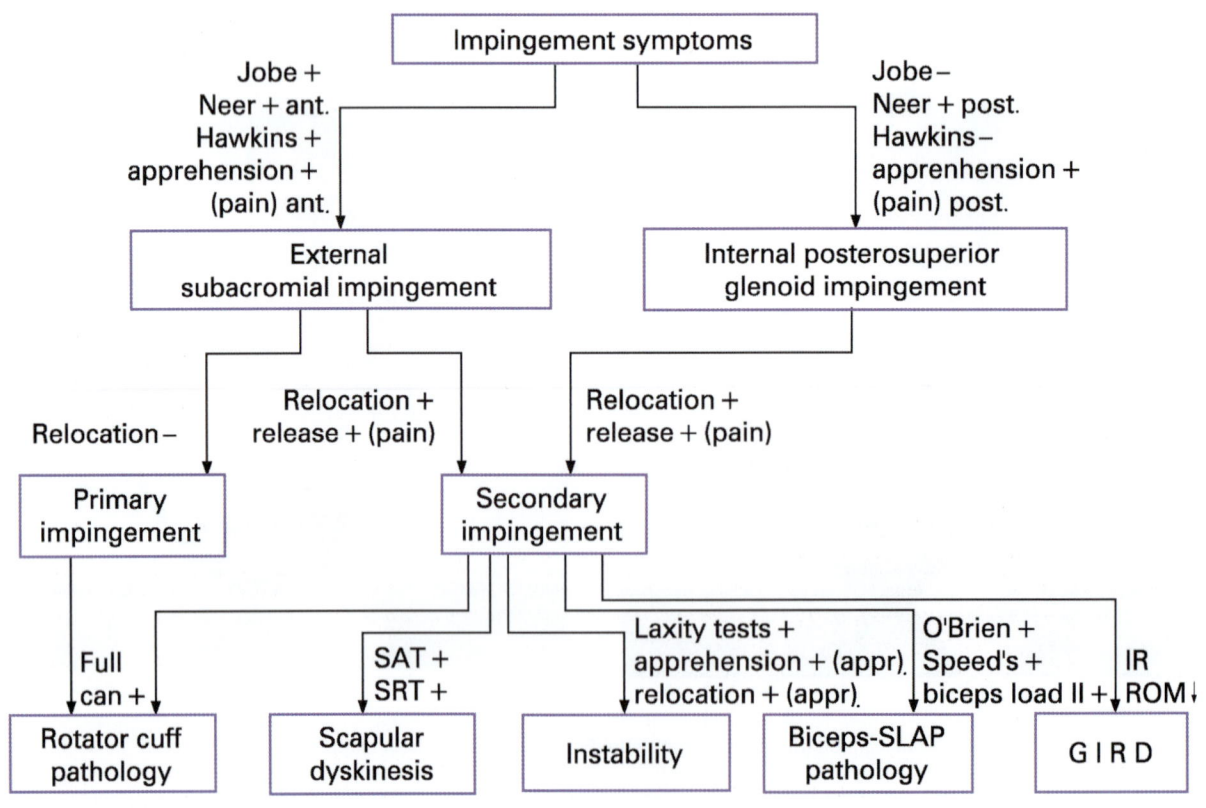

Figure 24.9 Clinical reasoning and physical examination algorithm for impingement-related shoulder pain[10]
+ = positive test; − = negative test; ant = anterior; post = posterior; SAT = scapular assistance test; SRT = scapular retraction test; SLAP = superior labrum anterior to posterior; GIRD = glenohumeral internal rotation deficit; IR = internal rotation; ROM = range of motion; appr = apprehension REPRODUCED WITH PERMISSION FROM BRITISH JOURNAL OF SPORTS MEDICINE

Table 24.2 Clinical utility of selected assessment findings for shoulder pain

Assessment finding	What is a positive finding?	Sensitivity	Specificity	LR−	LR +	Accuracy
Impingement						
Subacromial: Jobe + Hawkins + Neer + Painful arc + resistance ER	Pain, cut off 3/5 +	75	74	0.34	2.93	79
Internal: posterior impingement sign ('apprehension position')	Posterior pain	75.5	85	0.39	3.34	78
Rotator cuff pathology						
Full can test	Weakness and pain: tendinopathy/ tear supraspinatus	59–89	54–82	0.2–0.5	1.6–3.2	65–74
Lift-off test (Gerber) + resistance IR	Weakness: tear subscapularis	50	88	0.56	4.1	97
ER lag sign	Weakness: tear infraspinatus	36	95	0.67	7.2	74
Scapular dyskinesis						
Scapular assistance test (SAT)	Decreased pain	21–24	71–72	1.07–1.10	0.75–0.83	
Scapular resistance test (SRT)	Increased strength or decreased pain	26–100	33–70	0–1.06	0.87–1.49	
Instability						
Apprehension	Apprehensive feeling	98.3	71.6	0.02	3.46	81.7
Relocation	Relief of apprehension	96.7	78	0.04	4.39	85.2
Release	Sudden (surprise) apprehension	91.7	83.5	0.10	5.55	86.4
Load and shift	↑ translation humeral head anteriorly	71.7	89.9	0.32	7.10	83.4
Sulcus	↑ translation humeral head inferiorly	28–72	86–97			
Posterior subluxation test	↑ translation humeral head posteriorly	50–91	85–100			
Slap and biceps related pathology						
Apprehension AND Speed AND O'Brien	Pain	25	92	0.82	3.13	
Speed	Pain: LHB pathology	54	81	0.58	2.77	72
O'Brien	Pain: SLAP	61	84	0.47	3.83	72
Biceps load test	Pain: SLAP	29	78	0.9	1.4	55.5
Passive compression test	Pain: SLAP	82	86	0.21	5.1	83.6

+ = positive test; ER = external rotation; IR = internal rotation; SAT = scapular assistance test; SRT = scapular resistance test; SLAP = superior labrum anterior to posterior; LR− = negative likelihood ratio; LR+ = positive likelihood ratio; LHB = long head of biceps
Table based on Hegedus et al.[11] and Hanchard et al.[12]

A painful test is an indication for subacromial impingement; the test will be negative in case of internal impingement.

The Neer test consists of forced maximal forward flexion in internal rotation with the scapula fixed into depression (Fig. 24.10c). Pain at the front of the shoulder is an indication for subacromial impingement, whereas patients with internal impingement will exhibit pain at the posterior aspect of the shoulder (slightly change testing position into neutral rotational position/external rotation and fixing the scapula to front).

It is suggested that interpretation for subacromial impingement should be based on five tests: the three impingement tests described above, painful and/or weak external rotation against resistance, and a painful arc during active elevation. Sensitivity and specificity are the highest when a cut-off value of three positive tests on five is used (Table 24.2).

Besides these impingement tests, instability tests are often used as provocation tests for impingement. In the apprehension position, the shoulder is placed passively in maximal external rotation and horizontal abduction (Fig. 24.10d). Pain at the anterior aspect of the shoulder suggests subacromial impingement; pain at the posterior aspect implies posterosuperior glenoid impingement. It might be necessary to change the position into more or less elevation to elicit subtle symptoms in the overhead athlete. In the relocation test, the investigator manually performs a dorsal glide on the humeral head in the apprehension position (Fig. 24.10e). The test is positive if the pain exhibited during the apprehension test disappears. The relocation test allows us to identify primary versus secondary impingement. If the test is positive, this means that the impingement pain is secondary, based on excessive anterior translation of the humeral head. A negative test suggests primary impingement, not dependent on the position of the humeral head.

Rotator cuff tests

To define the involvement of rotator cuff pathology in the impingement symptoms, the full can test is a valuable tool. The test consists of resisted elevation in the scapular plane with the thumbs up (Fig. 24.10f). Research has indicated that rotator cuff muscles are also highly active in this position, like in the empty can (or Jobe) test. If both tests are painful, rotator cuff pathology is present. If only the empty can test is painful, and the full can test is negative, the patient probably suffers from impingement symptoms, but not primarily related to rotator cuff pathology.

In the presence of rotator cuff pathology, the examiner can perform a number of specific tests for the supraspinatus, subscapularis and infraspinatus to find out whether one of more tendons are ruptured. Although recent research indicates isolation of rotator cuff muscles in a clinical setting is very difficult,[13] the Gerber lift-off test, and the belly press test may be useful for subscapular tears, and the lag sign is often used to detect infraspinatus tears. In the Gerber lift-off test, the patient is asked to lift their hand from their back in a maximally internally rotated position (Fig. 24.10g); during the belly press test, the quality of movement is observed when the patient pushes his hand into his stomach (Fig. 24.10h). A positive external rotation lag sign occurs when the patient is unable to maintain the position of external rotation in a slightly abducted position and the shoulder rotates internally (Fig. 24.10i).

Scapular involvement tests

Scapular involvement in impingement-related shoulder pain may be examined by the scapular assistance test (SAT) and the scapular retraction test (SRT). The SAT, in which scapular movement quality is examined, consists of manual assistance of correct scapular movement during elevation of the arm (Fig. 24.10j). Reduction of pain during this movement compared to non-assistance confirms scapular involvement in the shoulder complaints.

In the SRT, in which scapular stability is examined, the empty can test is performed while the examiner stabilises the patient's scapula and shoulder in a position of retraction by placing the forearm along the medial border of the scapula (Fig. 24.10k). The test is positive for scapular involvement when the initial pain, present in the empty can position disappears during the SRT. Since the diagnostic value of these tests for shoulder pathology is low, they should be considered as symptom modification tests (see below) rather than diagnostic tests.

Instability tests

The clinical tests to examine shoulder instability can be divided into provocative tests and laxity tests. Commonly used provocative tests for instability are the apprehension and relocation tests, described earlier (Fig. 24.10d, e). In case of instability, patients will exhibit symptoms, such as apprehensive muscle tension and subluxation, rather than pain.

Distinct from the provocative tests, the laxity tests assess humeral translation with respect to the glenoid fossa. For anterior laxity, the load and shift test may be used (Fig. 24.10l). In this test, the humeral head is loaded in such a way as to centre it congruently within the glenoid fossa. Subsequently, the humeral head is manually shifted anteriorly, relative to the glenoid fossa, and the amount of translation is graded from 1 (translation up to, but not beyond the glenoid rim), over grade 2 (translation beyond the glenoid rim with spontaneous reduction after releasing the humeral head) to grade 3 (subluxation without spontaneous reduction). The sulcus sign allows examination of inferior laxity. In this test, inferior subluxation is produced by downward traction on the arm (Fig. 24.10m).

For posterior laxity, the posterior subluxation test is described. This test is performed by placing the patient's arm in adduction, internal rotation and 70–90° flexion. The examiner applies a posteriorly directed force along the arm, and then slowly moves the shoulder to horizontal abduction and external rotation (Fig. 24.10n). The test is considered to be positive if a clunk is felt during the latter movement, indicating the humeral head is relocated in the glenoid after being subluxed posteriorly.

Shoulder pain CHAPTER 24

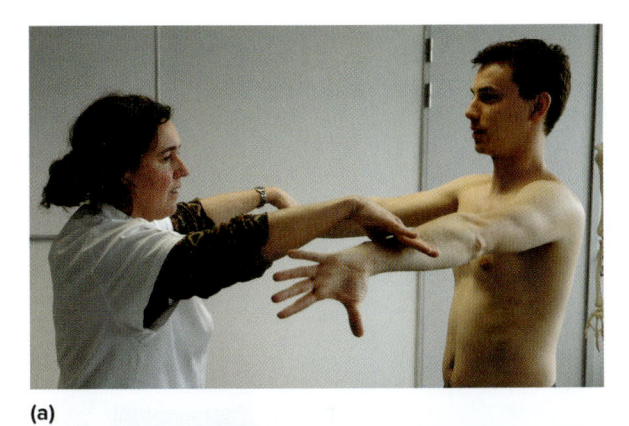

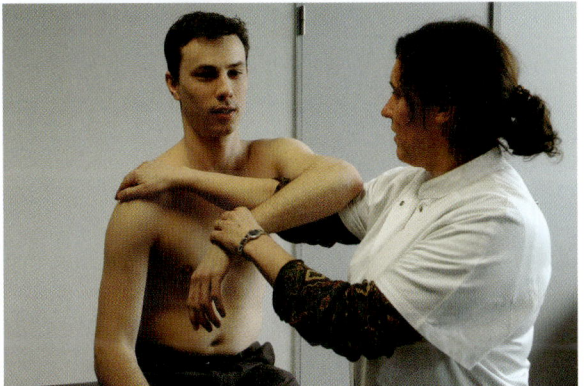

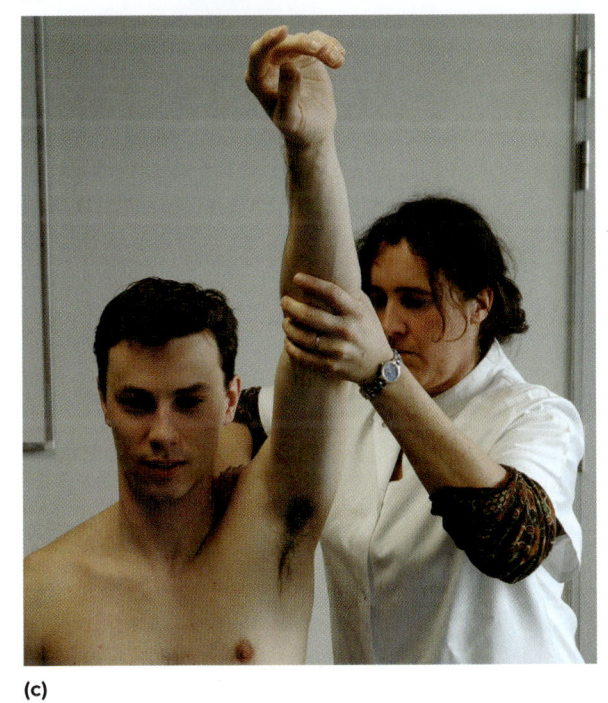

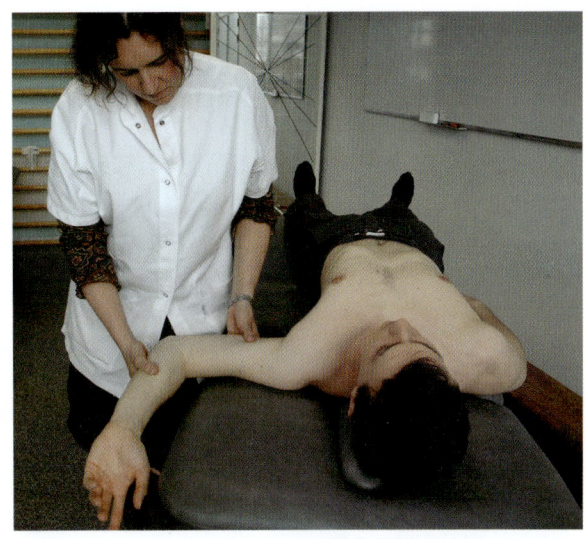

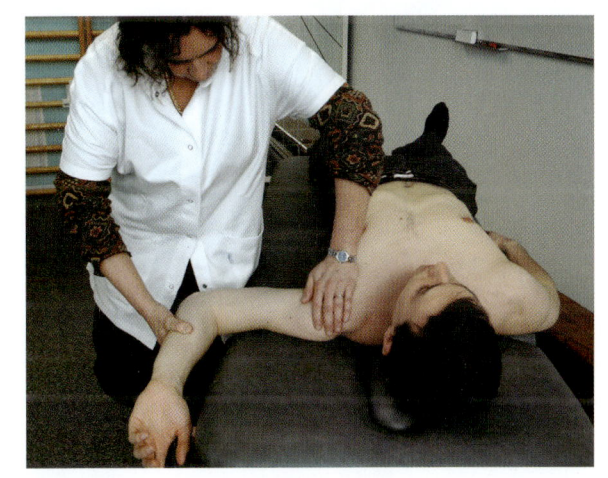

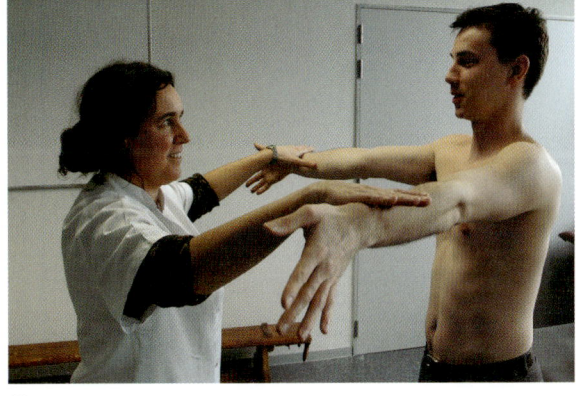

Figure 24.10 Special tests for the shoulder (a) Jobe test (b) Hawkins test (c) Neer test (d) Apprehension test (e) Relocation test (f) Full can test

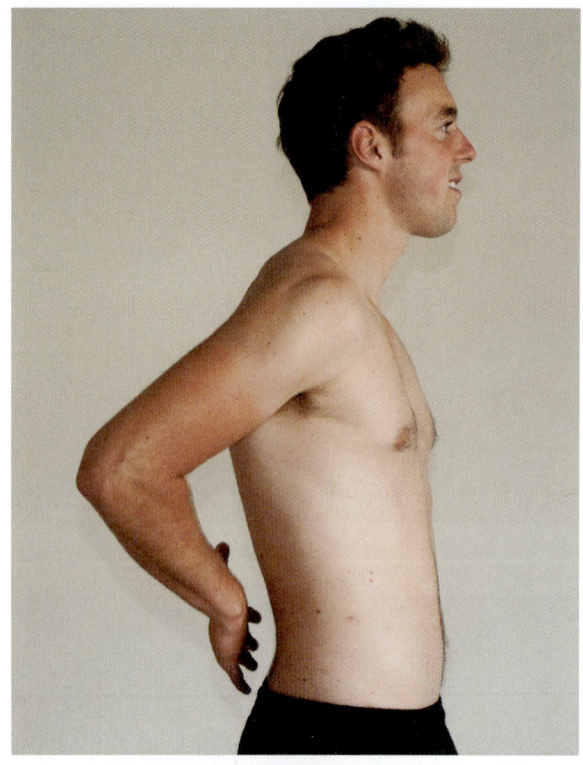

PART B   Regional problems

(g)

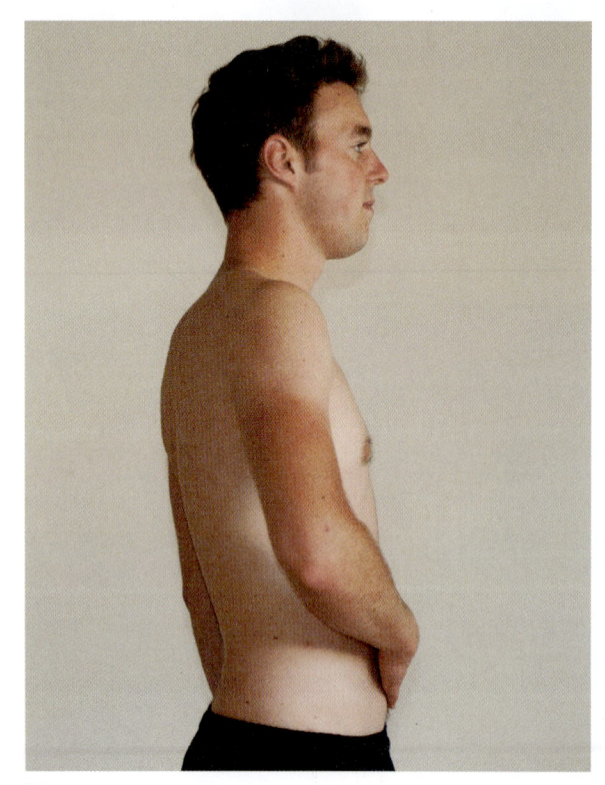

(h)

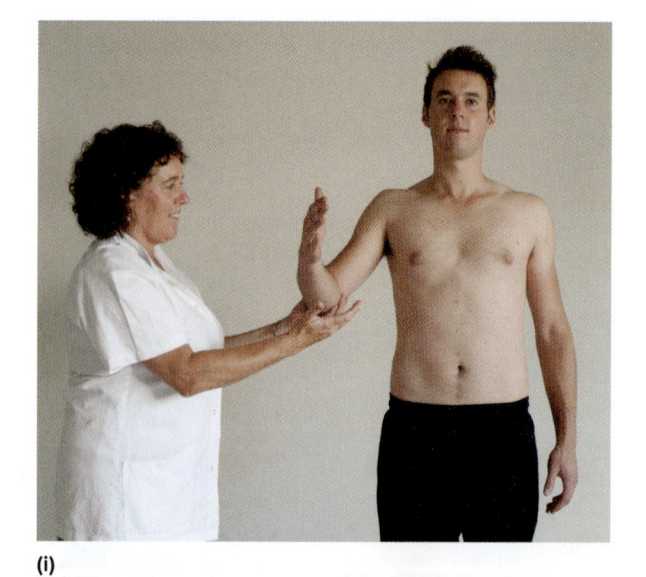

(i)

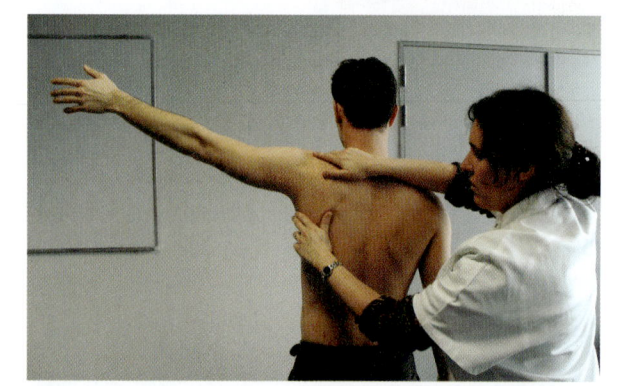

(j)

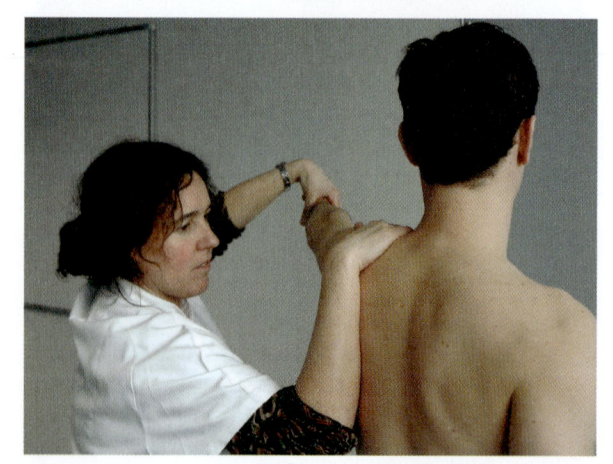

(k)

Figure 24.10 (cont.) (g) Gerber lift-off test (h) Belly press test (i) External rotation lag sign (j) Scapular assistance test (k) Scapular retraction test

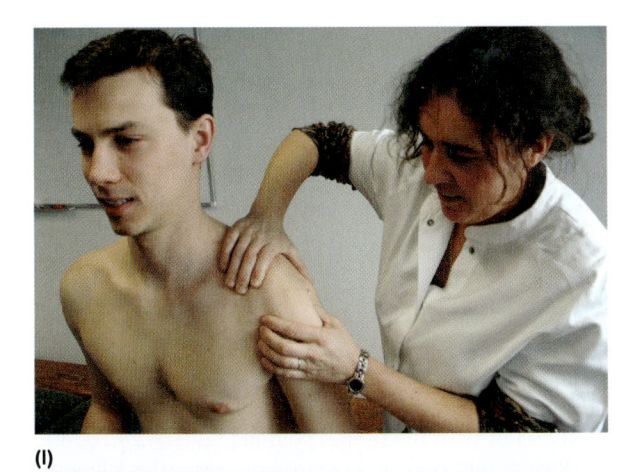

Shoulder pain — CHAPTER 24

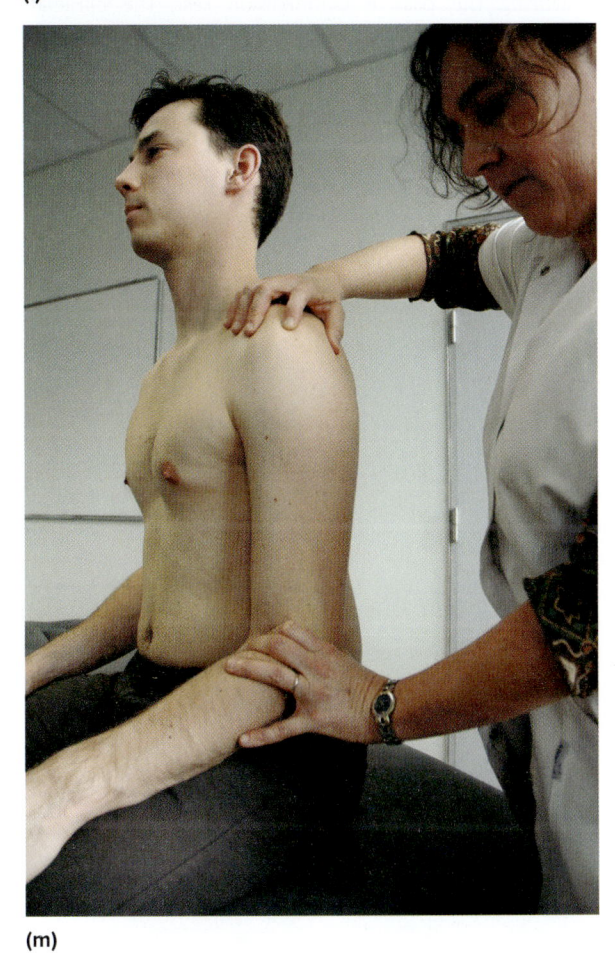

Figure 24.10 (cont.) (l) Load and shift test (m) Sulcus sign (n) Posterior subluxation test (o) O'Brien test (i) thumb pointing down, (ii) thumb pointing up

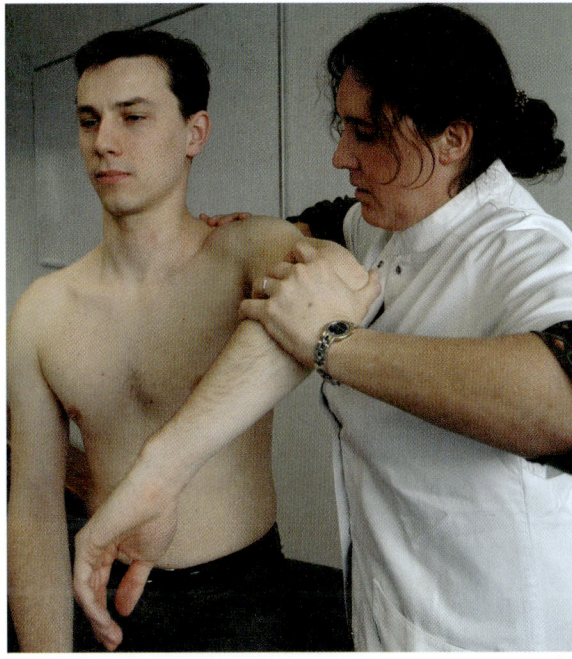

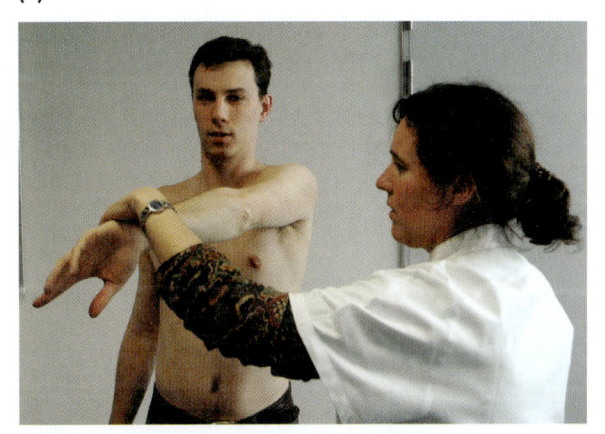

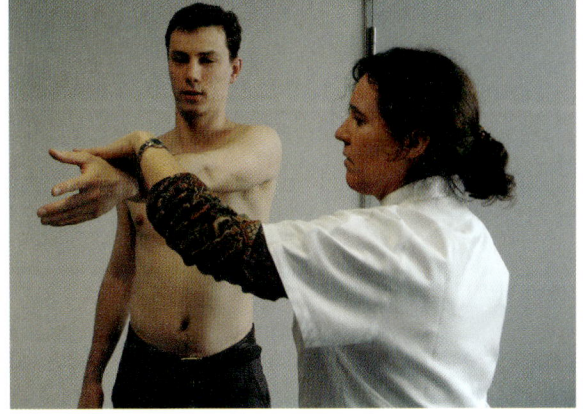

393

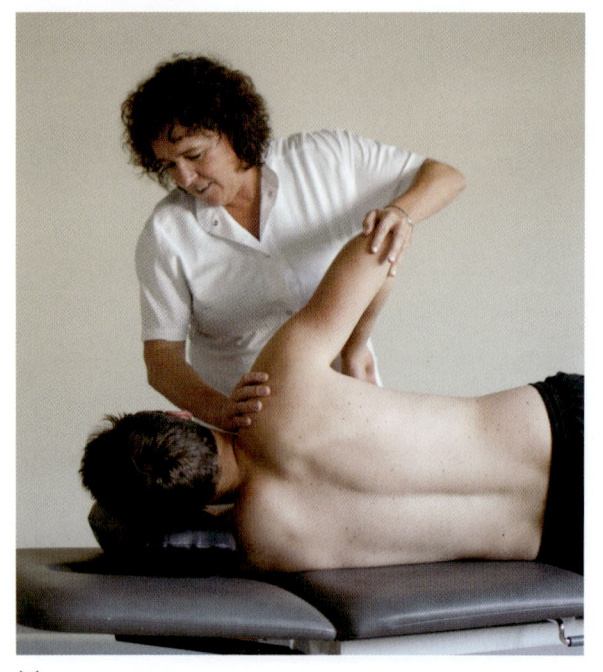

PART B Regional problems

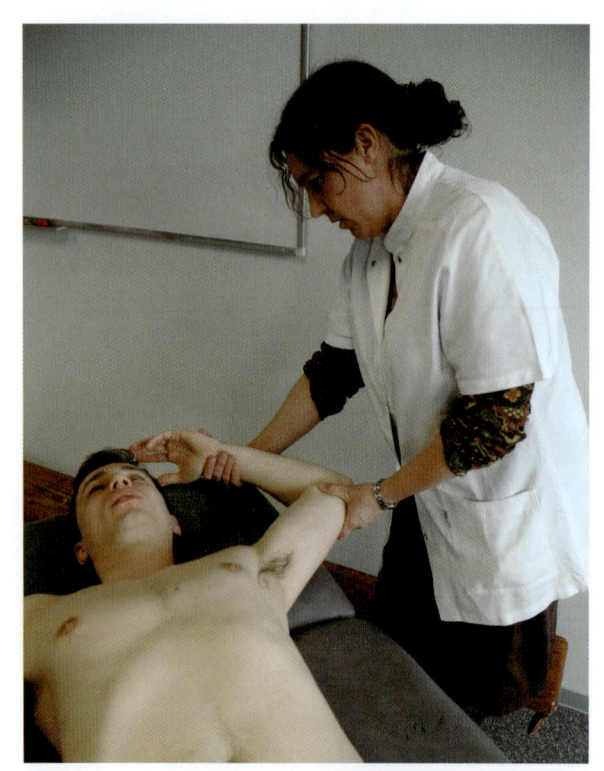

Biceps pathology and SLAP lesion tests

Numerous SLAP and biceps tests exist in the literature. However, we prefer the Speed test, the O'Brien test, the passive compression, and the biceps load II tests. The Speed test is performed by resisting downwardly applied pressure to the arm when the shoulder is positioned in 90° of forward flexion with the elbow extended, and forearm supinated; a positive test result should produce pain into the biceps region.

In the O'Brien test, resistance is tested with the arm forward flexed to 90° and adducted 10° with the thumb pointing down (Fig. 24.10o–i). Pain is lessened or disappears when the test is repeated in the same shoulder position but with the thumb pointing up (Fig. 24.10o–ii).

During the passive compression test, the clinician rotates the patient's arm externally with 30° of abduction and then pushes the arm proximally while extending the shoulder, which results in the passive compression of the superior labrum onto the glenoid (Fig. 24.10p).

The biceps load II test consists of applying resistance against elbow flexion with the shoulder in 120° of abduction and the elbow in 90° flexion (Fig. 24.10q). The test result is considered positive if the patient complains of pain during the resisted elbow flexion.

A best-test combination consisting of three tests (two sensitive and one more specific test) has been recommended for the interpretation (Table 24.2).[11]

Clinical evaluation of GIRD

The assessment of glenohumeral internal rotation deficit (GIRD) is performed by measuring glenohumeral internal rotation range of motion, preferably in the supine position with the shoulder abducted 90° and the scapula stabilised against the table (Fig. 24.11). Goniometric/inclinometric

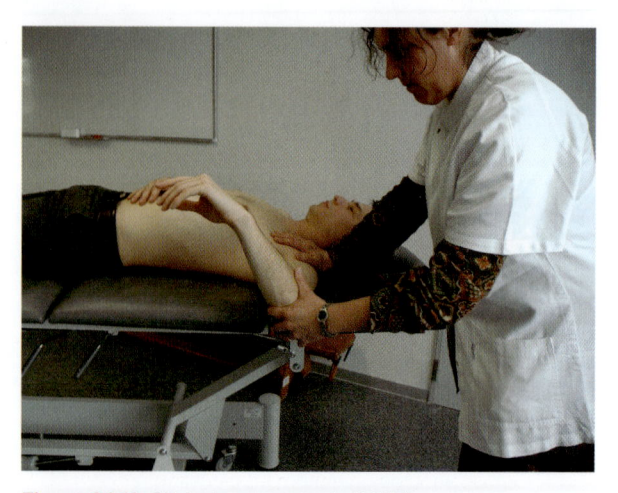

Figure 24.10 (cont.) (p) Passive compression test (q) Biceps load II test

Figure 24.11 Clinical assessment of GIRD

assessment as well as interpretation of the 'end feel' is described as criteria for GIRD evaluation. A side difference of 20° is considered to be positive for GIRD. However, in view of a possible shift in rotational range of motion due to bony adaptations, GIRD may be associated with a gain in external rotation ROM. Therefore it is imperative to measure internal as well as external rotation, interpreting the total range of motion (TROM). Besides the measurement in an abducted position, additional evaluation of GIRD with the shoulder in 90° forward flexion may even give the clinician a better impression of the posterior stiffness, since there is more stretch on the posterior aspect of the shoulder.

Shoulder symptom modification procedure

In view of the limited diagnostic accuracy of the existing clinical tests (Table 24.2), as well as the relevance of the rest of the kinetic chain, it is important to perform symptom modification tests. Once the movement or activity that reproduces the shoulder symptoms has been agreed upon (and assessed during the clinical examination), the shoulder symptom modification procedure (SSMP) is applied.

The SSMP is a series of mechanical techniques that are applied while the patient performs the activity or movement that most closely reproduces the symptoms experienced by the patient (Fig. 24.12). These techniques may be applied on different levels of the kinetic chain, starting with the shoulder locally, going to the scapula (see scapular tests), thoracic and cervical spine and posture, lumbar spine and the lower extremities. Modifications may include correcting posture (for instance sitting versus standing or correcting thoracic kyphosis), ensuring correct muscle contraction (for instance scapular correction, core stability) or mechanically correct kinematics (for instance posterior glide humeral head).

The basic principles, however, are always similar: (a) define a position or movement that causes the

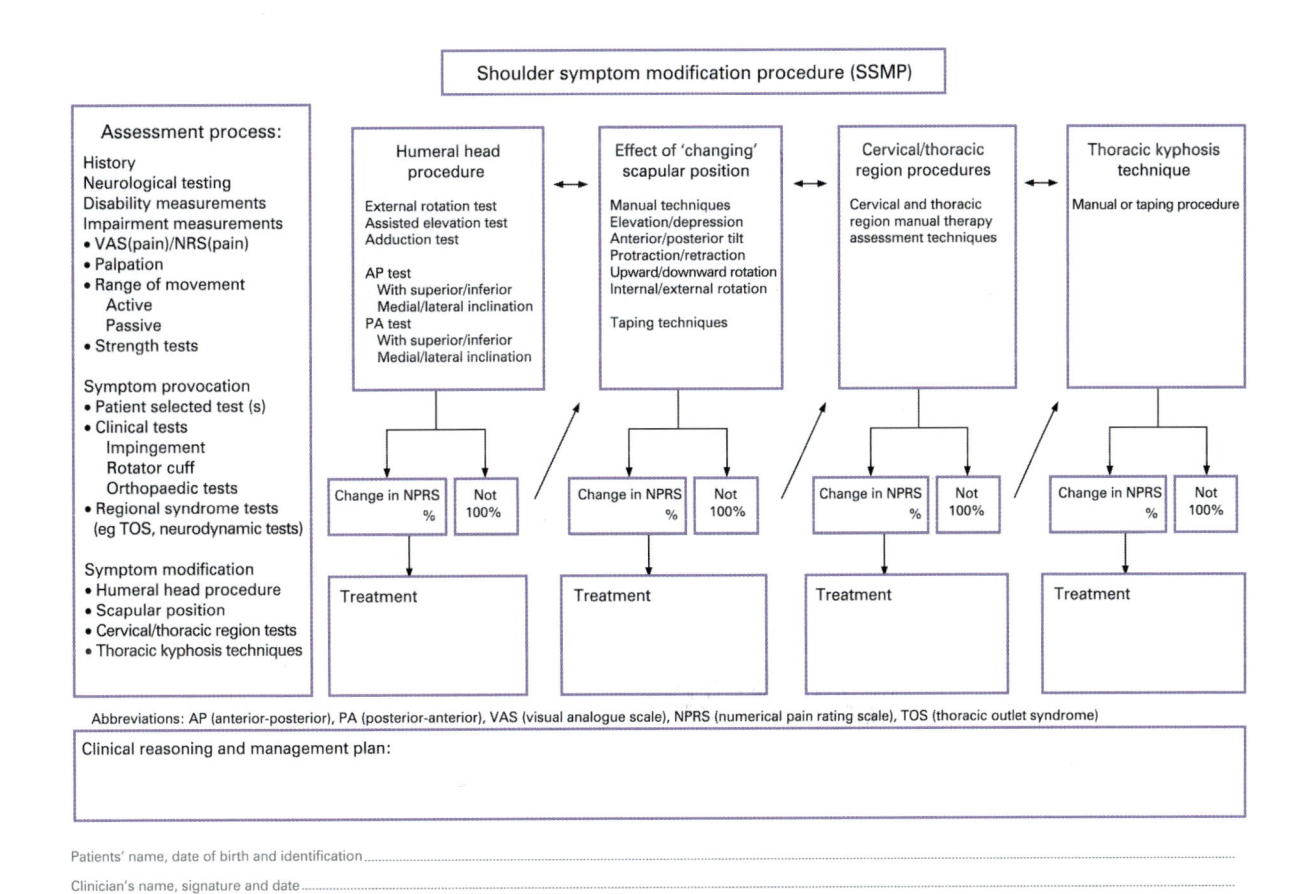

Figure 24.12 Shoulder symptom modification procedure (SSMP)
FROM LEWIS 2009.[16] REPRODUCED WITH PERMISSION FROM *BRITISH JOURNAL OF SPORTS MEDICINE*

symptoms, based on the clinical exam, (b) correct the possible cause of the symptoms, based on biomechanics or arthrokinematics, and (c) observe possible change in symptoms. Based on this procedure the clinician will know the key points in the rehabilitation program and advise the patient. As stated by the authors, the SSMP is not meant as a replacement for current clinical practice but as an adjunct to help support the clinical decision-making process by identifying factors that alleviate the patient's shoulder symptoms.[14-16]

Additional shoulder tests

Depending on the history and the results of the basic clinical examination, the clinician may need to perform additional special tests to those described in the previous section. In particular, neurologic, neurodynamic and/or vascular examination might be necessary in case of a suspicion of for instance thoracic outlet syndrome (TOS) or neurodynamic upper limb pathology. The Roos test (Fig. 24.13a) is a very sensitive and specific test for TOS and easy to perform: ask the patient to open and close their hands for at least 60 seconds with the shoulders abducted and externally rotated and the shoulder girdle in depression. Motor deficits, change of colour of the hands, numbness, and slowing down of the movement are considered to be signs of TOS. For the neurodynamic examination, the basic upper limb neurodynamic tests (ULNT) may be performed, evaluating the mechanosensitivity of the nervous system in the upper quarter (Fig. 24.13b). The tests are considered positive if they provoke or reproduce the symptoms, or are in a relevant distribution to the nerve being tested. The second feature of a positive test is that the response received (sensory symptoms, ROM or resistance perceived by the examiner) is different from the asymptomatic limb, and different from what is known to be a normal response. Cervicogenic shoulder involvement needs to be assessed by a cervical spine screening and differential diagnostic tests such as the Spurling test (Chapter 23).

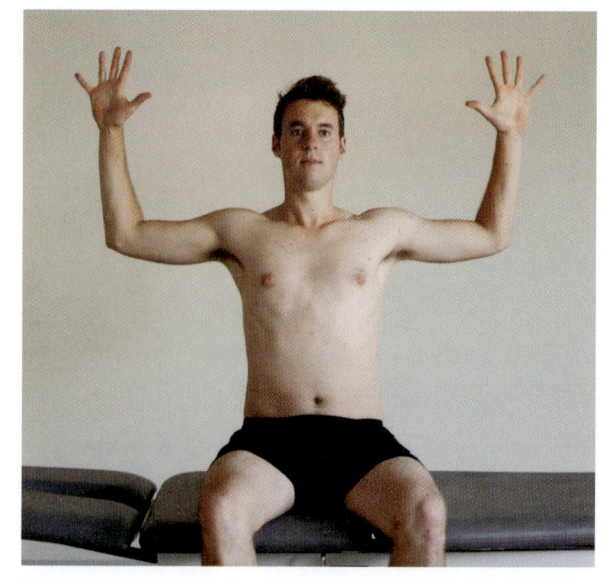

Screening of the kinetic chain

Regardless of the SSMP, screening of the kinetic chain is imperative in overhead athletes. Quick screening of kinetic chain variables consists of:

- observation of spinal curves and general posture (forward head posture, hyperlordosis cervical spine, hyperkyphosis and protracted shoulders, sway back, hyperlordosis or hypolordosis, flexed position of the hips, knee position into valgus or varus, foot position)
- single-leg/double-leg squat observe hip and core stability

(a)

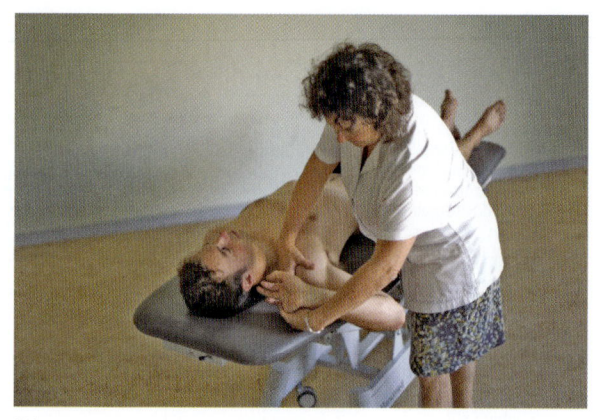

(b)

Figure 24.13 Additional tests for shoulder pain (a) Roos test for thoracic outlet syndrome (b) Upper limb neurodynamic tests

- bilateral deep squat: observe quality of movement, repetitive movements to evaluate lower limb strength and endurance
- trunk ROM into rotation, flexion and extension
- ROM of the hips, in particular into extension and rotation.

The clinician may use some specific testing protocols, such as the functional movement screen or the 9+[17] (Chapter 46) or a similar standardised screening program, looking at ROM as well as strength and stability, and at the trunk as well as the extremities.

Shoulder pain CHAPTER 24

Key outcome measures

There are numerous patient-reported outcome measures to assess functional status, treatment effect and return-to-play criteria for people with shoulder pain. The clinician's selection should be based on the specific clinical outcome to be measured (body structures, function, activity, participation), the specific pathology (instability, rotator cuff pathology) and whether disease-specific, region-specific or generic outcome is required. Table 24.3 summarises the most commonly used outcome scales for shoulder pain patients.

INVESTIGATIONS

We discuss the principles of shoulder investigations (including diagnostic arthroscopy) as it is a critical element of efficient management of the patient with shoulder pain.

Objective measurements of the shoulder

The assessment of the ROM into rotation of the shoulder can be measured with a goniometer or an inclinometer, and in many positions of the body and the shoulder. A comprehensive reliability study showed good to excellent inter- and intra-tester reliability for a variety of test positions and equipment.[18] Based on the results of this study, no specific procedure can be acknowledged as superior to another. However, the clinician has to take into account that large variability exists in literature regarding shoulder position (for instance scapular or frontal plane) and the specific method of scapular stabilisation (none, hand on shoulder top, or specific fixation of coracoid), and therefore be consequent in repeated measurements. Based on the above-mentioned reliability study and in view of optimal standardisation of body and shoulder position, the authors advise the procedure supine, arm 90° in frontal plane, palpation of the coracoid process, performed with digital inclinometer (Fig. 24.11).

Regarding rotator cuff strength, isokinetic (Fig. 24.14a) as well as isometric (Fig. 24.14b) and eccentric (Fig. 24.14c) strength measurements may be performed. Absolute side differences as well as muscle balance ratio between external and internal rotators are to be interpreted. In general, with respect to cut-off values distinguishing a healthy shoulder from a shoulder at risk, an isokinetic ER/IR ratio of 66% or an isometric ER/IR ratio of 75% (when measured in neutral or in abduction 90° and external rotation 90°), or +/− 100% (when measured in 90° abduction and 0° rotation) and 60–80% (when measured in 90° abduction and 90° external rotation) is advised, with a general rotator cuff strength increase of 10% of the dominant throwing side[19] compared to the non-dominant side. The preferential functional eccentric/concentric ratio (eccER/concIR) depends on the speed and specific procedure tested. For the eccentric test with the hand-held dynamometer (HHD), values slightly higher than 100% (114–121%) were found in a sample of 201 adult overhead athletes from volleyball, tennis and handball.[19] All procedures have been found to show high to excellent reliability.

Scapular performance or behaviour can be evaluated by measuring scapular inclination (upward rotation), scapular muscle strength (isokinetic or isometric testing) and muscle length (pectoralis minor).

Scapular inclination may be measured using an inclinometer in several arm elevation positions (Fig. 24.15). In

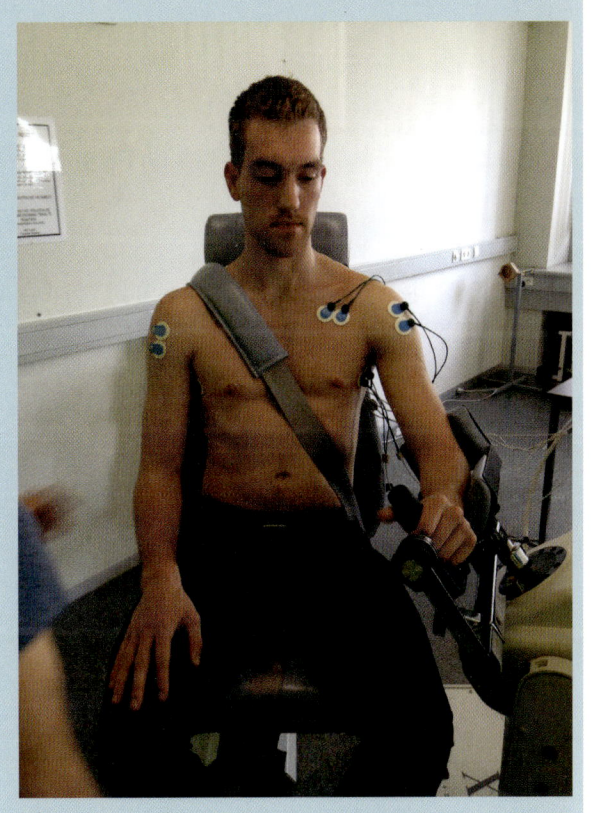

(a)

Figure 24.14 Rotator cuff strength testing (a) Isokinetic testing

continued

397

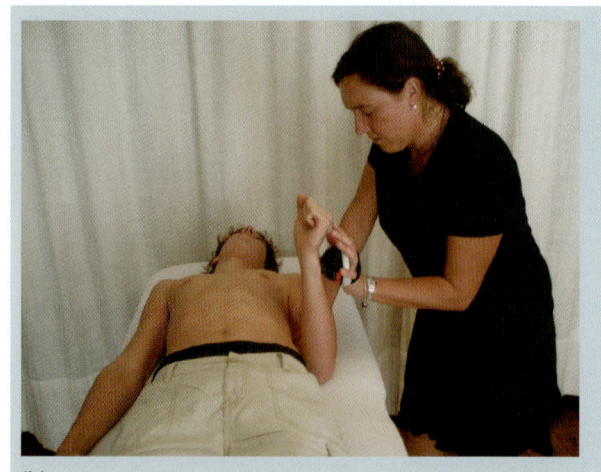

PART B Regional problems

(b)

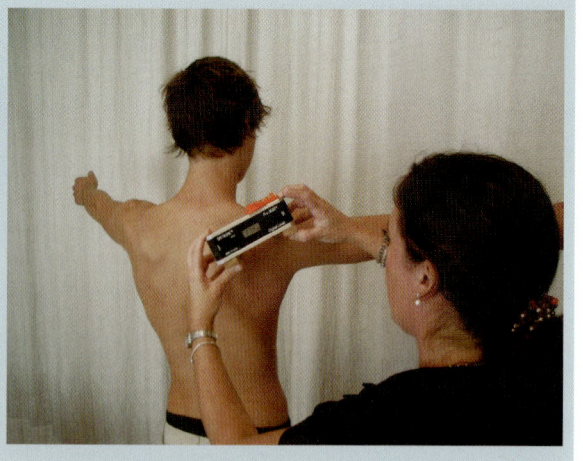

Figure 24.15 Measurement of scapular inclination using an inclinometer along the spine of the scapula

general, an upward inclination of approximately 60° should be reached at full active arm elevation.

For the scapular muscles proper intermuscular and intramuscular balance should be assessed. Isokinetic protraction/retraction ratio (Fig. 24.16) should be 100% in a healthy population, with slight changes in overhead athletes who have slightly stronger protractors. When measured isometrically with an HHD, it is advisable to use standardised positions[20] and to be consistent doing a make or a break test, since results might differ significantly. In bilateral sports (swimming, rowing, gymnastics) there should be no side

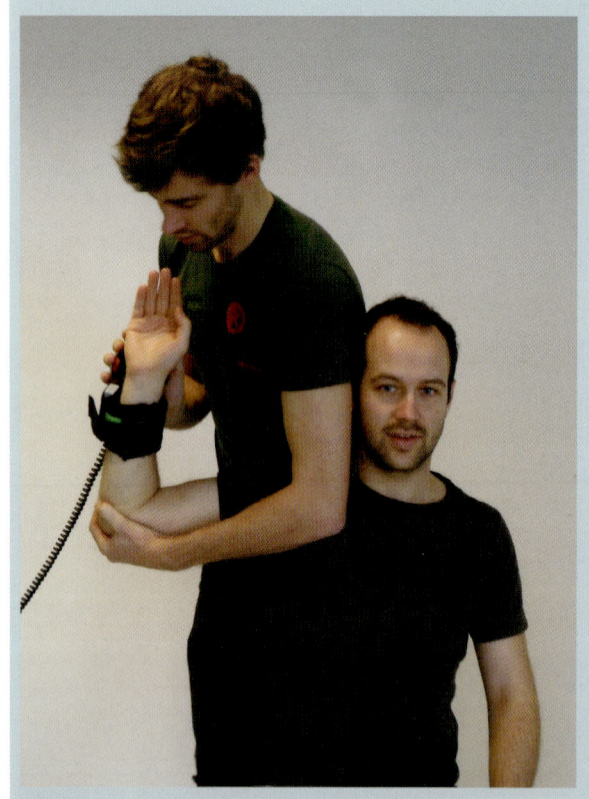

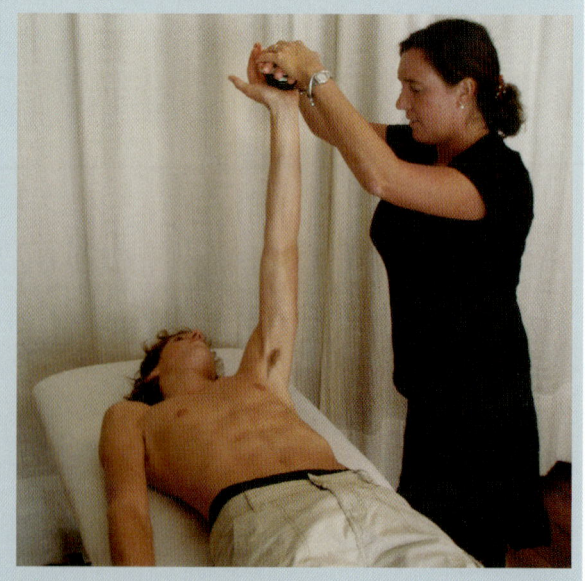

(c)

Figure 24.14 (cont.) (b) Isometric testing with a hand-held dynamometer (c) Eccentric testing with a hand-held dynamometer—the assessor performs an internal rotation of the shoulder while the patient maximally resists against this pressure

(a)

Figure 24.16 Isometric strength testing of the scapular muscles (a) Protraction

398

Shoulder pain CHAPTER 24

(b)

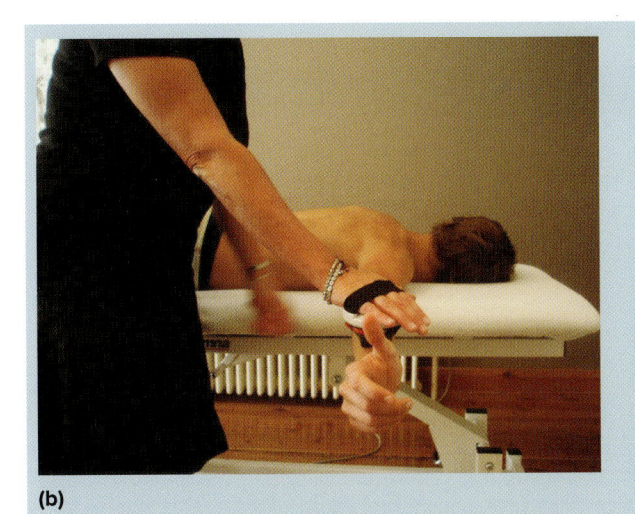

Figure 24.16 (cont.) (b) Retraction

differences in scapular muscle strength, in one-handed overhead sports an increase of scapular muscle strength of 10% is advised on the dominant side. In particular, the lower trapezius and serratus anterior should receive special attention, since these muscles are shown to be susceptible to weakness in injured athletes. However, a statement saying that scapular behaviour should be symmetrical in overhead athletes is not supported by data. On the contrary, in volleyball, as well as in handball players, asymmetry in resting scapular posture is often found. Therefore clinicians should be aware that some degree of asymmetry in resting scapular posture is often found. It should not be considered automatically as a pathological sign but rather an adaptation to sports practice and extensive use of the upper limb.

Tightness of the pectoralis minor may be clinically observed by evaluating shoulder position with the patient supine (with more protracted shoulder position in case of short pectoralis minor) and objectively measured by determining the distance between the coracoid process and the fourth rib at the sternum (Fig. 24.17a). When normalised to body height (pectoralis minor index (PMI) = pectoralis length/body height), the PMI should not be below 7.65, indicating a short pectoralis minor.[21]

Functional performance tests for shoulder function are gaining interest, although not yet fully explored in clinical practice. The seated medicine ball throw (SMBT) (Fig. 24.17b) and the Y-balance test for the upper extremity (Fig. 24.17c) have been described for evaluation of the front chest throwing performance and static weight-bearing shoulder stability, respectively. However, normative data and cut-off values for injury prevention and return to play are lacking. Recently, it was shown that the SMBT and isokinetic shoulder, and elbow strength correlate highly, whereas no significant correlation between the Y-balance test and these isokinetic strength measures was found.[22]

(a)

(b)

(c)

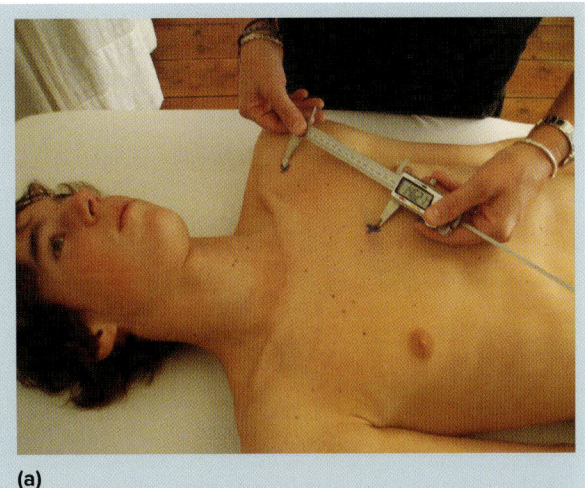

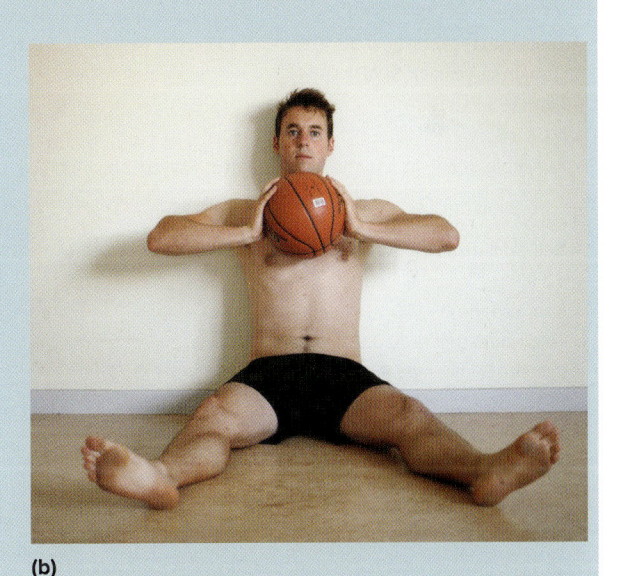

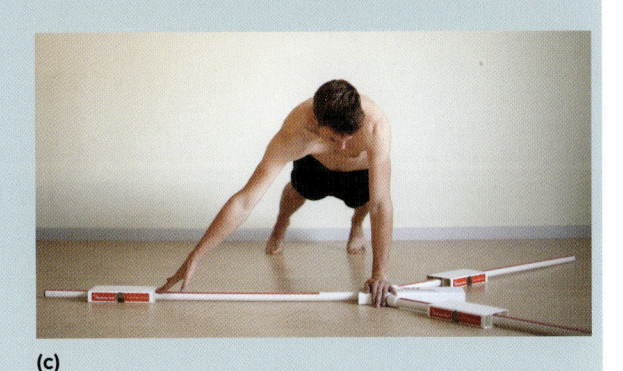

Figure 24.17 (a) Measurement of pectoralis minor length (b) Seated medicine ball throw (c) Y-balance test for the upper extremity

PART B Regional problems

Table 24.3 Patient-reported outcome measures for shoulder pain

Generic shoulder pain

Disabilities of the Arm, Shoulder and Hand questionnaire (DASH)

- Self-administered questionnaire evaluating symptoms and function of the entire upper extremity
- 30 items
- Two optional additional modules available for work and sports/performing arts
- Score range 0–100
- Test-retest reliability: 0.93–0.98[23–27]
- Construct validity: shoulder Pain and Disability Index (SPADI) 0.55–0.93[24, 28, 29]
- MDC95%: 7.9–14.8[24, 26, 30]
- MCID: 10.2[26]
- Available online in a range of languages: www.dash.iwh.on.ca

QuickDASH

- Self-administered questionnaire evaluating symptoms and function of the entire upper extremity[23]
- 11 items
- Test-retest reliability: 0.90–0.94[31–33]
- Construct validity: SPADI: 0.84[34]
- MDC95%: 13.3[33]
- MCID: 8[33]
- Available online in a range of languages: www.dash.iwh.on.ca

Simple Shoulder Test (SST)

- Self-administered questionnaire that evaluates functional disability of the shoulder
- 12 items[35]
- Score range 0–100
- Test-retest reliability 0.97[36]–0.99[37]
- Construct validity: SPADI 0.74[35]–0.80[38]/DASH: 0.72[39]
- MDC95%: 32.3[38]
- MCID: 17.1–25[40]
- Available online in a range of languages: www.orthop.washington.edu

Shoulder Pain and Disability Index (SPADI)

- Self-administered questionnaire evaluating symptoms and function of the shoulder
- 13 items
- Two optional additional modules available for work and sports/performing arts
- Test-retest reliability 0.84–0.95[26, 30, 36, 41, 42]
- Construct validity: DASH 0.93,[28] 0.55[29] and 0.88[41]
- MDC95%: 13.2–21.5[26, 38, 41, 42]
- MCID: 13.2–23.1[26, 38, 43]
- Available online: www.workcover.com

Rotator cuff pathology

Western Ontario Rotator Cuff Index (WORC)

- Self-administered, condition-specific questionnaire evaluating quality of life
- 21 items
- Score range 0–2100
- Test-retest reliability 0.84–0.96[44–46]
- Construct validity: DASH 0.49[45] and 0.63[46]
- MDC95%: 19.1[45]
- MCID: 245.26[47]
- Available online: www.secec.org/pages/r-d/assessments-scores.php

Shoulder instability

Western Ontario Shoulder Instability Index (WOSI)

- Self-administered questionnaire evaluating quality of life of patients with symptomatic shoulder instability
- 21 items
- Score range 0–2100
- Test-retest reliability: 0.87–0.98[48–51]
- Construct validity: 0.77[48]
- MDC95%: 483[52]
- MCID: NA
- Available online: www.secec.org/pages/r-d/assessments-scores.php

Injuries in overhead athletes

Kerlan–Jobe Orthopaedic Clinic Shoulder and Elbow Score

- Self-administered 10 item questionnaire that evaluates throwing specific symptoms and function in throwing athletes
- 10 items (five on symptoms and five on shoulder function)
- Test-retest reliability: 0.88[53]
- Construct validity: NA
- MCD95% NA
- MCID: NA

NA = not available

Radiography

Plain X-rays are important in the diagnosis of shoulder abnormalities. Routine views (AP with internal and external rotation and axillary lateral) provide a good overview of the region. A 'true' AP view is useful for assessing joint space narrowing, (i.e. arthritis). In cases of trauma, an adequate axillary view may not be possible and a true lateral film must be obtained to exclude dislocation. The following can be identified on plain films: calcific tendinopathy, glenohumeral joint arthritis, impingement (sclerosis of anterior and/or lateral acromion, sclerosis of greater tuberosity), proximal humeral head migration (severe rotator cuff dysfunction) and fractures.

Special views have been described to evaluate instability and impingement. Supraspinatus outlet views and down-tilted acromial films are obtained to evaluate impingement. In cases of instability, special views such as the West Point view or the Stryker notch view are used to better detect Bankart and Hill-Sachs' lesions.

Arthrography

Detailed anatomical information is obtained when arthrography (joint injected with dye) is combined with CT of the shoulder (CT arthrogram) or MR arthrography (see below). This examination gives excellent detail of capsular attachments and of the labrum. Small avulsion fractures of the glenoid rim (Bankart lesion) and the humeral head (Hill-Sachs' lesion) are clearly defined.

Ultrasound

High-resolution ultrasound, in the hands of an experienced operator, is a reliable non-invasive technique for imaging the rotator cuff and adjacent muscles, the bursae and the long head of the biceps muscle. The examination may be performed as a static or dynamic investigation. Tendon swelling, thickening of the bursa, abnormal fluid collection or calcific tendonitis may be detected, as may a partial or complete rotator cuff tear. It is important to define the size and location of the tear, and if there is any supraspinatus muscle atrophy (indicating a chronic and usually irreparable rotator cuff tear). If there is a partial thickness tear it is important to determine the thickness of the tear—as a percentage of the thickness of the tendon—as tears over 50% usually progress and are less likely to respond to non-operative treatment. It is also important to determine if the partial thickness tear is on the bursal side, under surface or intrasubstance. A dynamic examination performed while the patient is actively abducting the shoulder may confirm the presence of impingement (see tendinopathy management).

Magnetic resonance imaging

MRI allows multiplanar, non-invasive examination of the shoulder and is used to detect a rotator cuff tear. Bone detail is not defined as well as with CT and examination with shoulder movement is not possible. MR arthrogram with contrast is well suited to evaluate labral tears or instability.

PART B   Regional problems

Diagnostic arthroscopy

Arthroscopy of the shoulder, as well as being therapeutic, can provide useful diagnostic information. Shoulder arthroscopy permits inspection of the glenohumeral joint and the subacromial space in turn. Arthroscopy of the glenohumeral joint cavity is particularly useful as it:

- enables inspection of the glenoid labrum for evidence of a Bankart lesion or a SLAP lesion
- permits assessment of the state of the articular cartilage
- will demonstrate the presence of a Hill-Sachs' lesion
- allows inspection of the shoulder capsule and synovium (a red synovium and thickened capsule are characteristic of adhesive capsulitis)
- will identify a drive-through sign for laxity
- permits inspection of the under surface of the rotator cuff tendons, the biceps tendon and the subacromial bursa
- enables inspection and probing of the bursal surface of the rotator cuff.

Arthroscopy of the subacromial space allows assessment of:

- bursitis
- coracoacromial ligament ossification (spur formation)
- lateral spurs
- os acromiale
- bursal side rotator cuff tears
- full thickness rotator cuff tears.

The examination under anaesthesia (EUA) performed in conjunction with arthroscopy may sometimes be helpful to assess the presence, direction and severity of shoulder laxity, and to assess shoulder range of motion.

It is important to remember that these sophisticated investigations are only an adjunct to the clinical findings. In many cases of shoulder pain, the clinical findings provide sufficient information to diagnose the cause of the shoulder pain.

GENERAL TREATMENT AND REHABILITATION GUIDELINES FOR THE MOST COMMON SHOULDER INJURIES IN ATHLETES

It is important to note that shoulder pain may have several underlying causing factors, structural and functional. The treatment approach must be based on the results of the clinical examination and the diagnostic imaging, and may comprise several of the treatment strategies described below. In case several factors are identified within the kinetic chain, it is imperative to start the treatment dealing with correcting the most proximal parts in the kinetic chain.

In general, four phases can be recognised in the rehabilitation of the overhead athlete:[54] (1) acute phase, (2) intermediate phase, (3) advanced strengthening phase, and (4) return-to-play phase. In the acute phase, the goals are to diminish pain and inflammation, normalise motion, delay muscle atrophy and restore dynamic stability. Strengthening exercises focus on rotator cuff and scapular retractors. Functional loading is limited until full range of motion is restored. During the intermediate phase strengthening exercises progress into isotonic training of the shoulder girdle and the core, and flexibility is controlled by intensive stretching exercises, in particular of the posterior shoulder structures. The advanced strengthening phase consists of more aggressive strength training, including power and endurance enhancement. A plyometric program, endurance drills and controlled throwing are initiated. In the return-to-play phase, the athlete progressively increases the throwing program, continues flexibility drills and prepares to return to competitive throwing.

ROTATOR CUFF INJURIES

Rotator cuff injuries consist of tendinopathy and tears (complete or partial), often associated with an underlying tendinopathy.

Rotator cuff tendinopathy

The aetiology of rotator cuff tendinopathy (Fig. 24.18a) is multifactorial, and has been attributed to both extrinsic and intrinsic mechanisms. Extrinsic factors that encroach upon the subacromial space (subacromial impingement) or against the posterosuperior rim of the glenoid (internal

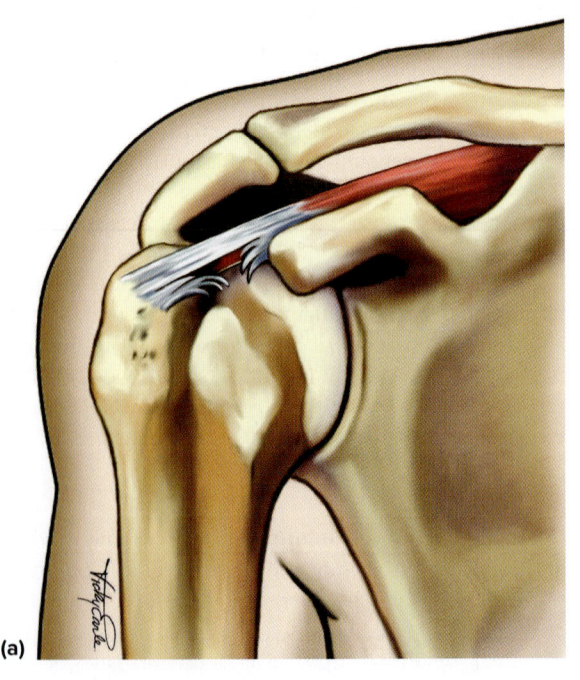

Figure 24.18 Rotator cuff tendinopathy (a) Pathology generally begins on the inferior (articular) surface of the tendon and may be associated with a partial tear

Shoulder pain   CHAPTER 24

(b)

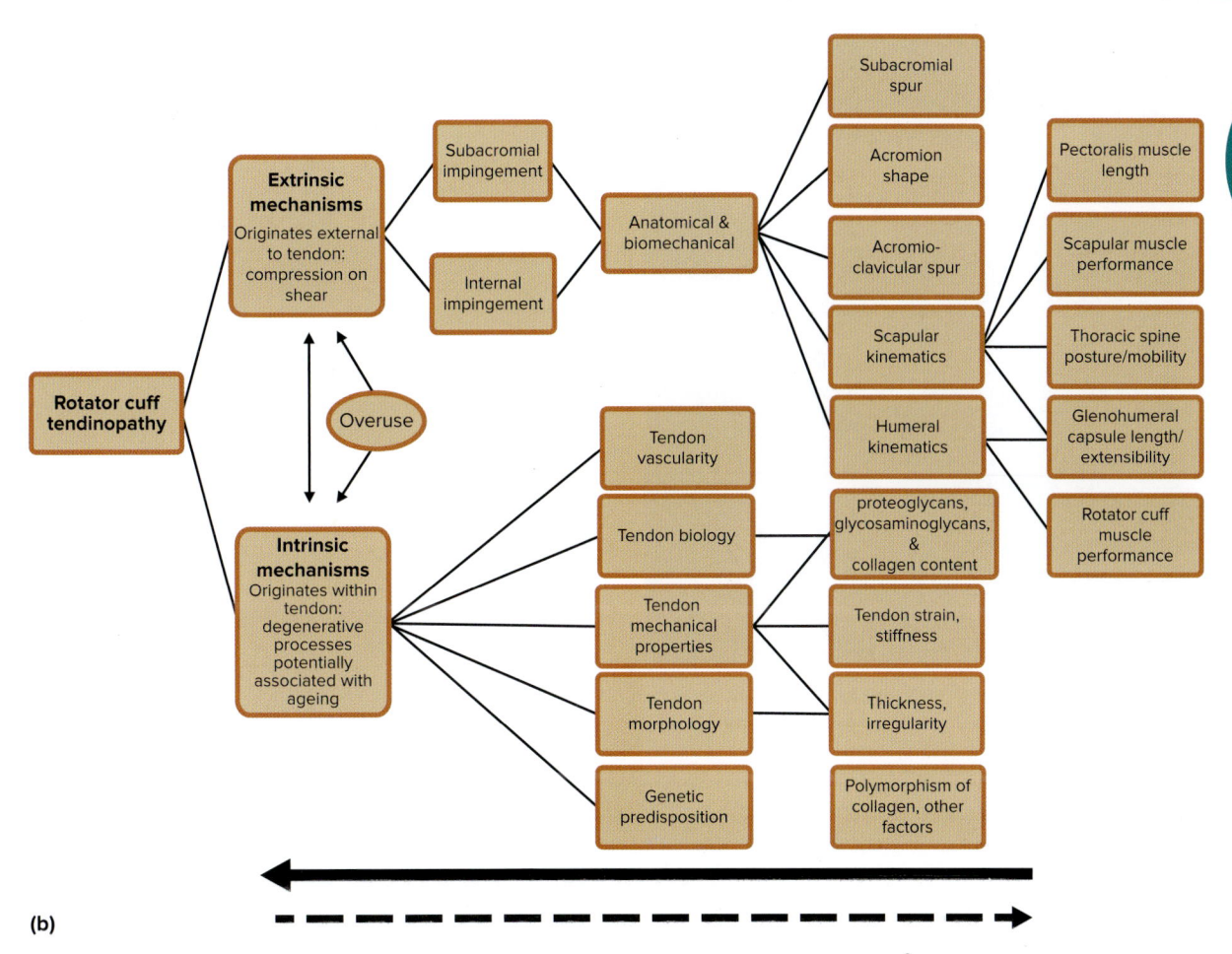

Figure 24.18 (cont.) (b) Intrinsic and extrinsic factors contributing to rotator cuff tendinopathy[6]
PG = proteoglycans; GAG = glycosaminoglycans

impingement), include anatomical variants of the acromion, alterations in scapular or humeral kinematics, postural abnormalities, rotator cuff and scapular muscle performance deficits, and decreased extensibility of the pectoralis minor or posterior shoulder. Intrinsic factors that contribute to rotator cuff tendon degradation with tensile/shear overload include alterations in biology, mechanical properties, morphology and vascularity. An overview of extrinsic and intrinsic mechanisms contributing to rotator cuff tendinopathy is given in Figure 24.18b.

Clinical features

The athlete with rotator cuff tendinopathy complains of pain with overhead activity such as throwing, swimming and overhead shots in racquet sports. Activities undertaken at less than 90° of abduction are usually pain-free. On examination, there may be tenderness over the supraspinatus tendon proximal to or at its insertion into the greater tuberosity of the humerus. If the infraspinatus is involved, there is also tenderness on the insertion dorsally on the greater tuberosity. Active movement may reveal a painful arc on abduction between approximately 70° and 120°. Symptoms can be reproduced with impingement tests and in the apprehension position, and also the full can test and external rotation against resistance may be painful. The investigation of choice in rotator cuff tendinopathy is MRI arthrogram (Fig. 24.19). This may also identify a partial tear of the rotator cuff. Ultrasound can rule out a full thickness tear; define a partial thickness tear; identify a thickened subacromial bursa and rule in or out 'impingement' of the bursa under the lateral acromion as the arm is abducted.

Treatment of rotator cuff tendinopathy

Treatment should be considered in two parts. The first part is to treat the tendinopathy symptomatically. The patient should avoid the aggravating activity and apply ice locally. There is no level 2 evidence (Chapter 2) to support NSAIDs, ultrasound, interferential stimulation, laser, magnetic field therapy or local massage.

PART B   Regional problems

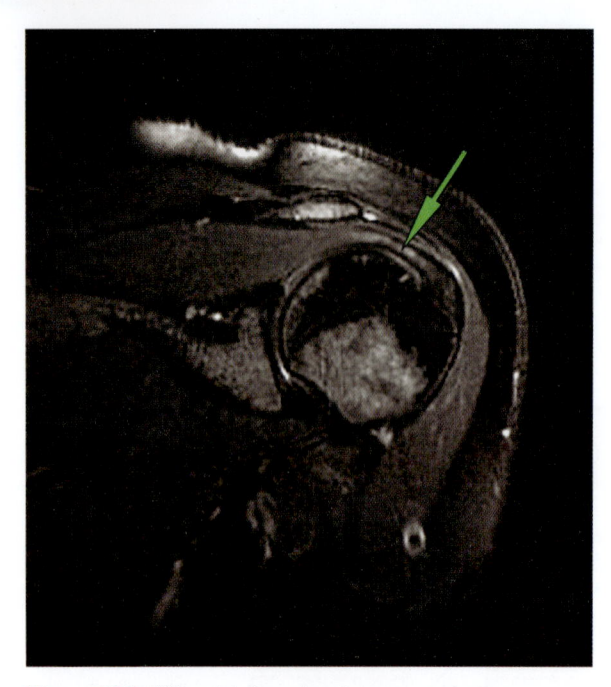

Figure 24.19 MR axial view showing supraspinatus tendinopathy (green arrow), with non-focal T2 signal increase not equal to that of fluid

with external rotation (infraspinatus) (Fig. 24.20d). In overhead athletes special attention needs to go to the external rotators, since weakness of this muscle group is often present as a sport-specific adaptation.
- Eccentric training of the rotator cuff: evidence on structural changes in the rotator cuff tendons after eccentric training is currently lacking but clinical improvement was established.[59, 60] Moreover, it needs to be recognised that the rotator cuff functions very much in an eccentric mode during sports activity, which strengthens the argument to include eccentric training in rehabilitation of the overhead athlete with rotator cuff tendinopathy. Exercises may be performed in a controlled slow manner, avoiding the concentric phase to allow maximal loading of the eccentric phase (Fig. 24.21), in a more plyometric way (Fig. 24.22), or accentuating the stretch-shortening cycle (Fig. 24.23).

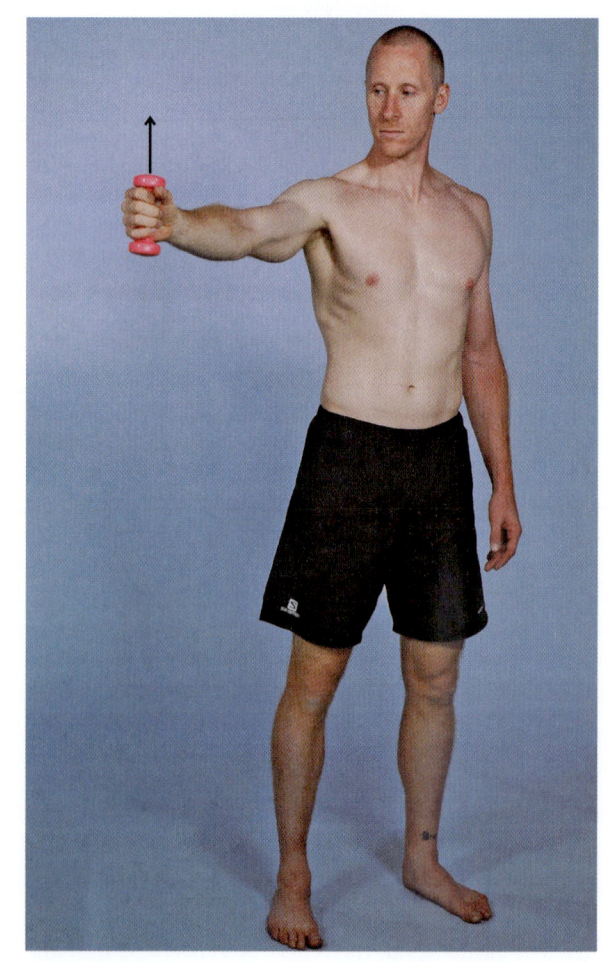

Clinical dogma has suggested a corticosteroid injection into the subacromial space may reduce a patient's symptoms and allow him or her to begin shoulder rehabilitation. However, randomised trials have failed to support this position. The body of evidence in sports medicine is that corticosteroid injection provides short-term pain relief but impairs long-term recovery for tendinopathies[55] (Chapter 17).

In choosing a management plan, clinicians should consider patient preference, availability of practitioners and other health care use. If a patient prefers a more active or self-management approach, manual physical therapy, exercise and referral to a physiotherapist should be discussed. There is systematic review evidence for the benefits of exercise therapy.[56]

The second part of treatment should consist of rehabilitation exercises of the rotator cuff itself. Several kinds of exercises can be applied, the selection depends upon the irritability of the tendons, the goal of the program, and the specific sport the athlete is involved in.

- Strengthening the rotator cuff (Fig. 24.20): based on EMG studies the following exercises are advised to strengthen the rotator cuff:[57, 58] elevation in the scapular plane (supraspinatus, infraspinatus and subscapularis) (Fig. 24.20a), external rotation (supraspinatus, infraspinatus and teres minor) (Fig. 24.20b), internal rotation (subscapularis) (Fig. 24.20c), horizontal abduction

(a)

Figure 24.20 Exercises for the rotator cuff (a) Elevation in the scapular plane

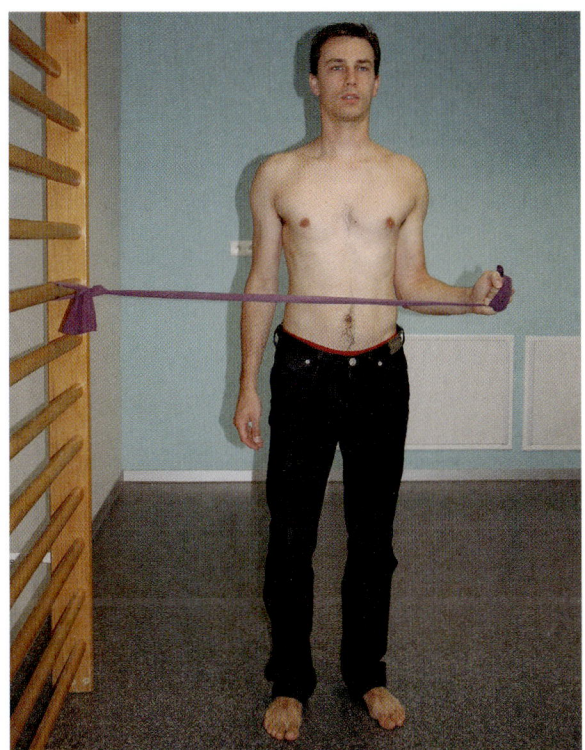

Shoulder pain CHAPTER 24

(b)

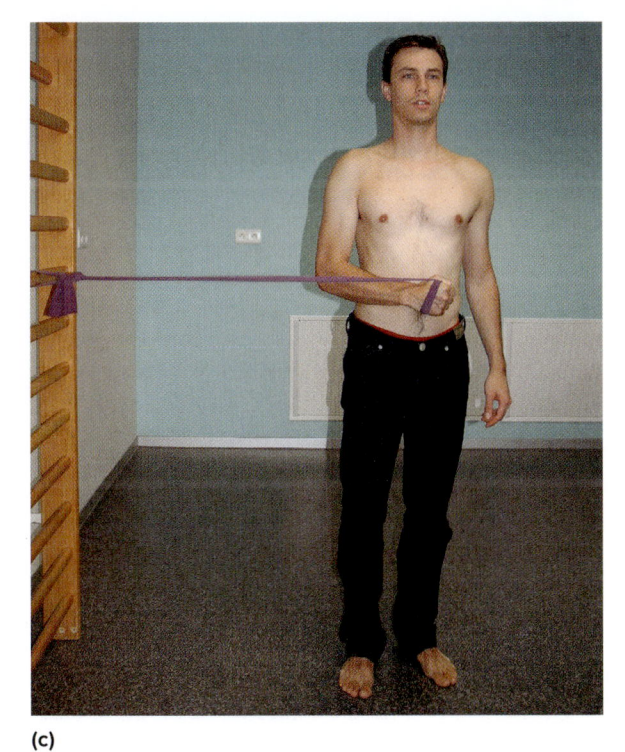

(c)

Figure 24.20 (cont.) (b) External rotation against resistance
(c) Internal rotation against resistance

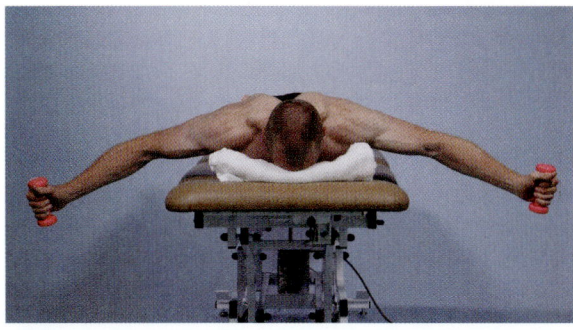

(d)

Figure 24.20 (cont.) (d) Horizontal abduction with external rotation

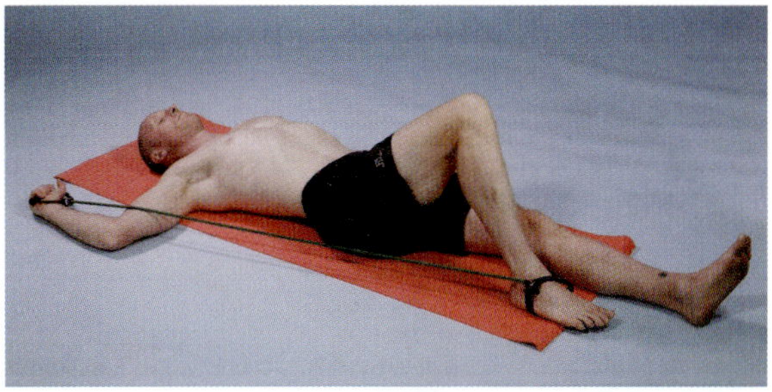

(a)

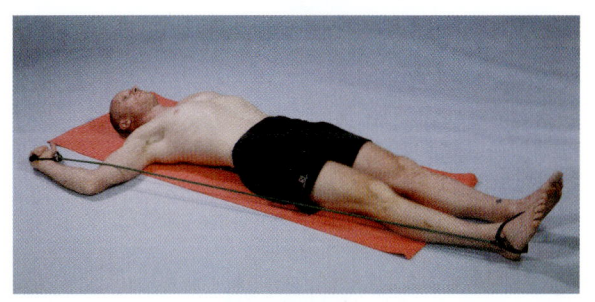

(b)

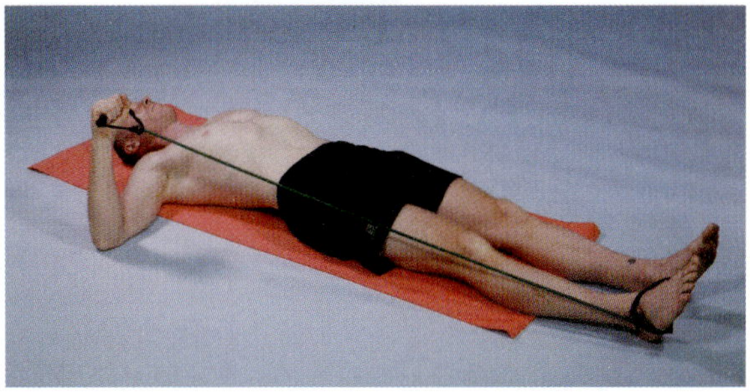

(c)

Figure 24.21 Eccentric exercise for the external rotators
(a) Starting position (b) Increasing load (c) Ending position

PART B   Regional problems

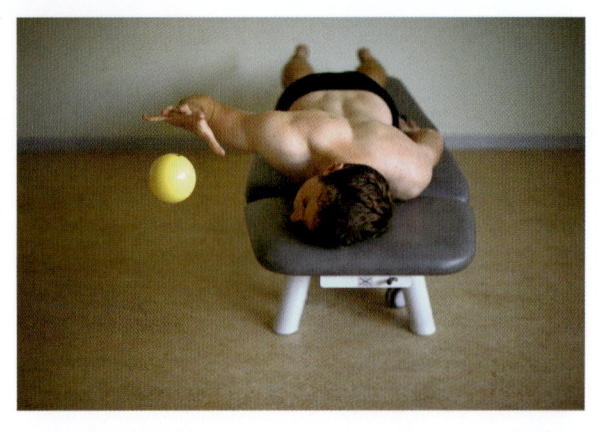

Figure 24.22 Plyometric catching exercise

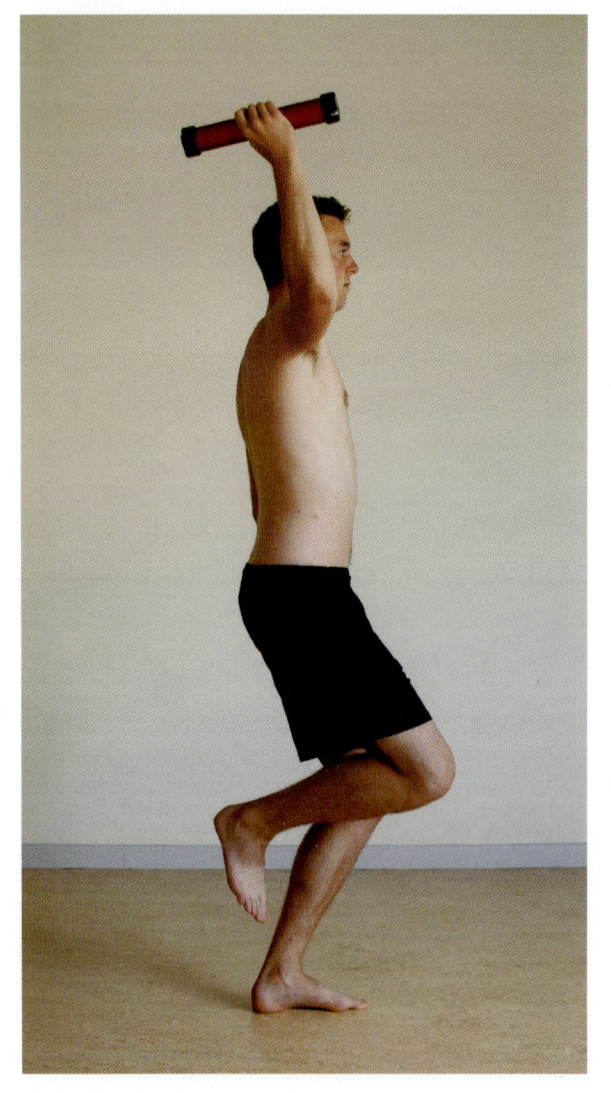

Figure 24.23 XCO-Trainer® exercise

Management of calcific tendinopathy can be difficult. In general the presence of calcifications in the rotator cuff is not always associated with symptoms of impingement. The aetiology is unclear, and seems to be rather a biochemical intratendinous process in particular in the supraspinatus tendon. Calcifications are not related to rotator cuff tears or glenohumeral arthritis. In some cases ESWT (extracorporeal shock wave therapy) may be indicated, supported by evidence; however, evidence regarding the effects in non-calcific rotator cuff disease is inconclusive.[61] In some cases, chronic symptomatic calcific tendinopathy is treated arthroscopically.

Rotator cuff tears

Complete and partial tears of the rotator cuff tendon are commonly seen in older athletes who present with shoulder pain during activity. These patients often complain of an inability to sleep on the affected shoulder. Examination reveals positive impingement signs and sometimes weakness on supraspinatus testing. Diagnosis is confirmed on MRI (Fig. 24.24) or ultrasound.

If the tear is small and of partial thickness, treatment may be conservative. Full thickness rotator cuff tears in young athletes require surgical repair; however, athletic performance often does not return to preoperative levels.[62]

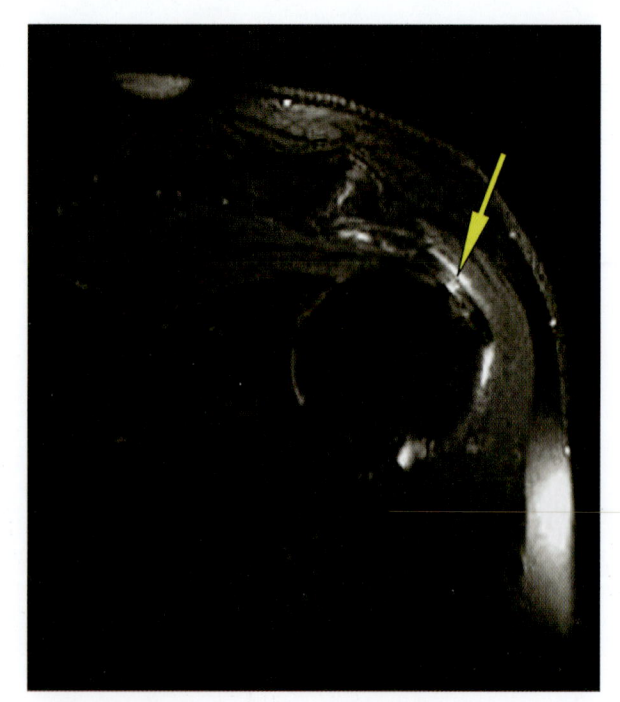

Figure 24.24 MR axial view showing partial thickness intra-substance supraspinatus tear (yellow arrow), with focal T2 signal equal to that of fluid

Shoulder pain CHAPTER 24

In older patients, still active in overhead sports, the choice for surgery or conservative treatment depends upon the degree of discomfort and pain during daily and sports activities as a result of the shoulder pain, and the expectations of the patient. Given the increasing age of people performing (overhead) sports at a recreational but also at a senior competitive level, the management of rotator cuff tears including return to sports in older athletes gains interest. Analysing the definition of a master athlete as: 'Active individual aged 50 years or older, who desires optimal levels of performance or wishes to exercise for general health and has high expectations for sports medicine care, including return to sport or activity after injury', achieving these goals is a huge challenge for all healthcare professionals involved with older athletes.

Although there is no general consensus on the approach of rotator cuff tears, there seems to be a shift towards conservative treatment.[63, 64] Although not proven to be efficient, we advise to perform exercises with minimal load on the rotator cuff, and maximally aim to restore function, in order to postpone the 'final match'. Exercises improving function (elevation) with minimal load on the rotator cuff are:

- semi-closed chain exercises with increasing gravity impact and increasing resistance[65] (Fig. 24.25)
- shoulder balance exercises in increasing elevation[66] (Fig. 24.26).

SHOULDER INSTABILITY

Based on the cause, direction and typical clinical presentation of instability, patients may be divided into three groups: the TUBS (traumatic unidirectional instability with Bankart lesion, for which surgery is often needed), AIOS (acquired instability due to overstress syndrome), and AMBRI (atraumatic multidirectional instability with bilateral laxity, in which rehabilitation is mandatory, but in case of failure inferior capsular shift surgery is performed). On the field these types may be combined, for instance a gymnast with general laxity (AMBRI) may develop overuse instability (AIOS), or a volleyball player with sports-specific minor instability (AIOS) may experience an acute trauma and dislocation (TUBS).

Traumatic shoulder instability—TUBS

One of the most common traumatic sports injuries is acute dislocation of the glenohumeral joint (Fig. 24.27a, b). In almost all cases, this is an anterior dislocation and it results from the arm being forced into excessive abduction and external rotation. Most anterior dislocations damage the attachment of the labrum to the anterior glenoid margin (Bankart lesion) as shown on MRI (Fig. 24.27c).

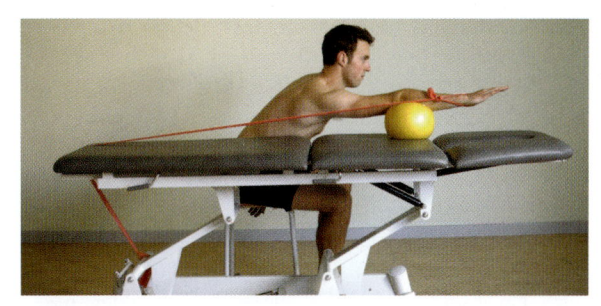

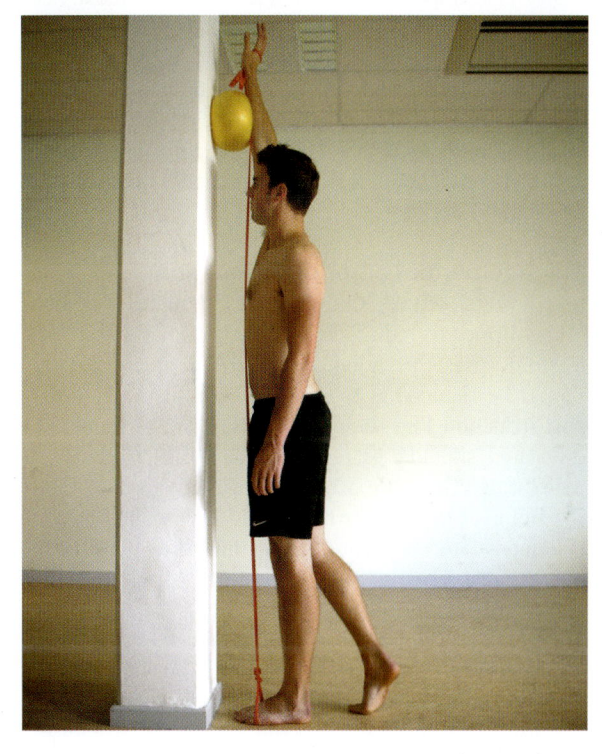

Figure 24.25 Semi-closed chain exercises against external resistance (a) Without gravity (b) Against gravity

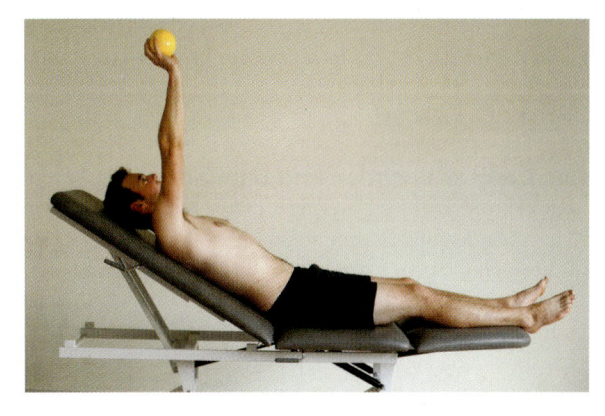

Figure 24.26 Shoulder balance exercise

An associated fracture of the anterior glenoid rim, a bony Bankart lesion (Fig. 24.27d) may be demonstrated on X-ray (Fig. 24.27e) or CT scan (Fig. 24.27f).

A compression fracture of the humeral head posteriorly (Hill-Sachs' lesion) (Fig. 24.27g) or tearing of the posterior or superior labrum may also be present. The history is usually one of acute trauma, either direct or indirect, associated with sudden onset of acute shoulder pain. A patient may describe a feeling of the shoulder 'popping out'. On examination, the dislocated shoulder has a characteristic appearance with a prominent humeral head and a hollow below the acromion. There is a loss of the normal smooth contour compared with the uninjured side. Anterior dislocations of the glenohumeral joint are occasionally associated with damage to the axillary nerve, resulting in impaired sensation on the lateral aspect of the shoulder and deltoid weakness. This should be assessed in any acute dislocation.

Management of anterior dislocation

In a hospital setting, the dislocated shoulder should be X-rayed prior to reduction as a fracture may be present. In most cases this is not practical and the dislocation should be reduced as soon as possible. In these cases, a post-reduction film should be obtained. The sooner the dislocated shoulder is reduced, the easier it usually is to relocate. There are a number of methods to relocate the humeral head onto the glenoid cavity. One method is demonstrated in Figure 24.27h. Injection of 10–15 mL of xylocaine into the joint can reduce pain and muscle spasm and aid reduction.

Once the shoulder has been reduced, it is usually stable unless placed in gross abduction and external rotation. A traditional sling should not be used—when the arm is internally rotated, the Bankart lesion worsens by becoming detached from bone. It is better to position the arm in 30° external rotation (i.e. an external rotation pillow or splint). Non-operative treatment in such a brace for 3 weeks, day and night, reduced the incidence of recurrent dislocation. However, we acknowledge it is awkward for patients to have the arm in external rotation for several weeks and many surgeons do not insist on this rehabilitation method.

Recurrent dislocation and Bankart repair

Shoulder dislocations in young athletes have a high rate of recurrence, leading to chronic shoulder instability. Because of this high incidence of recurrent dislocation, arthroscopy should be considered after shoulder dislocation in the younger athlete. If a Bankart lesion is found at arthroscopy, this should be repaired, either arthroscopically or as an open surgical procedure. Arthroscopic repair of a Bankart lesion can reduce the rate of redislocation to <5%.

Following a Bankart repair, the patient may commence pendular movements with the arm within 24 hours, and maintain the arm in a sling for 3–4 weeks. Once the initial pain from the procedure has subsided, active external rotation movements, to just short of the limit of rotation achieved on the operating table, are commenced. It may be helpful to place the arm in a splint in some abduction and external rotation to limit the amount of anterior capsular shortening. Active rotation exercises and stabilisation exercises can be gradually introduced as pain subsides. By 6 weeks, active strengthening can commence. Return to full sport is often achieved at 3–4 months.

The Latarjet procedure, or a bone block augmentation, is a frequently performed surgical procedure (Fig. 24.28). The choice between a Bankart repair or a Latarjet depends particularly upon the extent of bony damage to the shoulder, the type of sport and the surgeon's preference. The post-operative rehabilitation after a Latarjet procedure is similar to a Bankart repair; however, progression may be slightly quicker. Because the Latarjet procedure involves a bone block procedure it is characterised by faster tissue healing (bone to bone) than the healing of the labrum on the glenoid in the Bankart repair. After an immobilisation period of 3 weeks, gentle mobilisations are allowed, with full recovery of ROM after 8 weeks. Strengthening and stabilisation exercises can start 4–6 weeks after surgery, and return to sports, depending on the specific type of sport, from 12 weeks.

Posterior dislocation of the glenohumeral joint

Acute traumatic posterior dislocation is far less common than anterior dislocation. It occurs either as a result of direct trauma or due to a fall on the outstretched arm that is in some degree of internal rotation or adduction. It may also be caused by a seizure of any cause (e.g. electric shock or epileptic fit). The cardinal sign of posterior dislocation is limited external rotation. Suspicion of this diagnosis should be based on the mechanism of injury and the presence of pain and impaired function. Posterior dislocation can easily be overlooked in the AP X-ray. X-ray must include a true lateral or, if possible, axillary view.

Acquired sport-specific instability—AIOS

Overhead athletes very often exhibit acquired glenohumeral instability, characterised by laxity of the anterior capsule, as a result of the extreme use of their shoulder during overhead throwing or smashing activities. This type of acquired instability is often referred to as acquired instability overuse syndrome (AIOS). This kind of 'minor' instability may induce the hyperangulation phenomenon during throwing by excessive anterior translation of the humeral head, causing posterosuperior

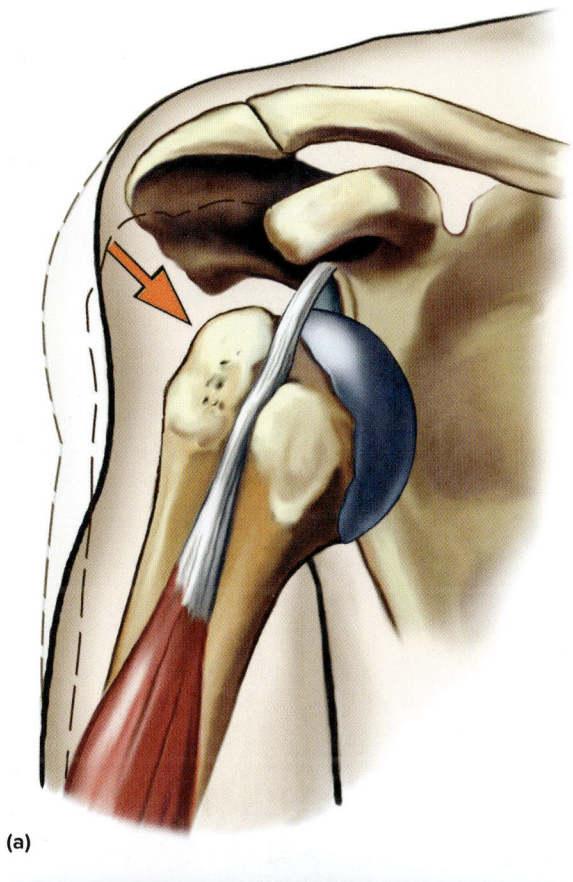

Shoulder pain   CHAPTER 24

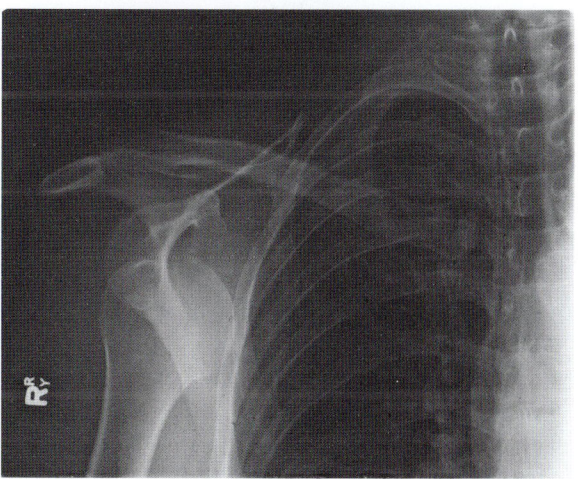

Figure 24.27 Dislocation of the shoulder (a) Anterior dislocation of the shoulder disrupts the joint capsule +/− the stabilising ligaments (b) Typical radiographic appearance—the humeral head sits medially over the scapula (c) MR arthrogram axial view showing detachment of the anterior glenoid labrum (yellow arrow), Bankart lesion (d) Bankart lesion showing a fragment of bone separated from the glenoid rim

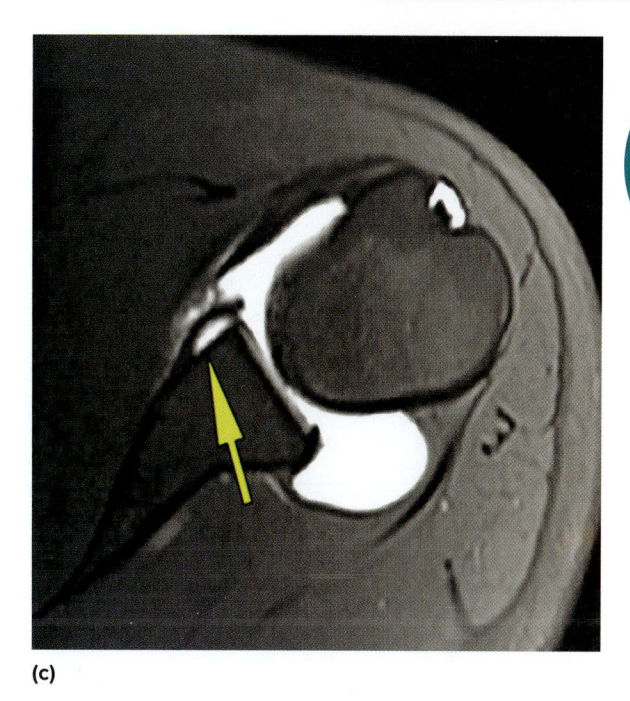

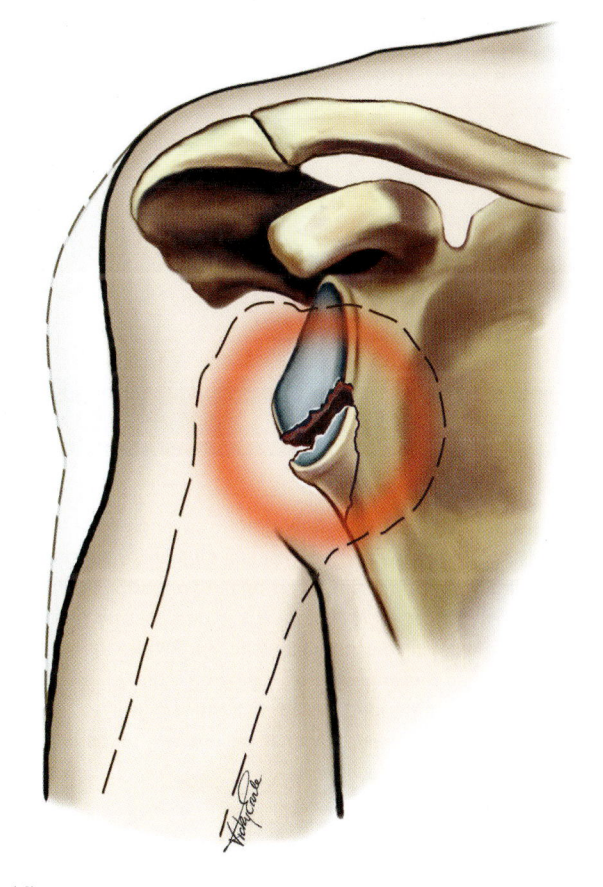

PART B   Regional problems

(e)

(f)

(g)

(h)

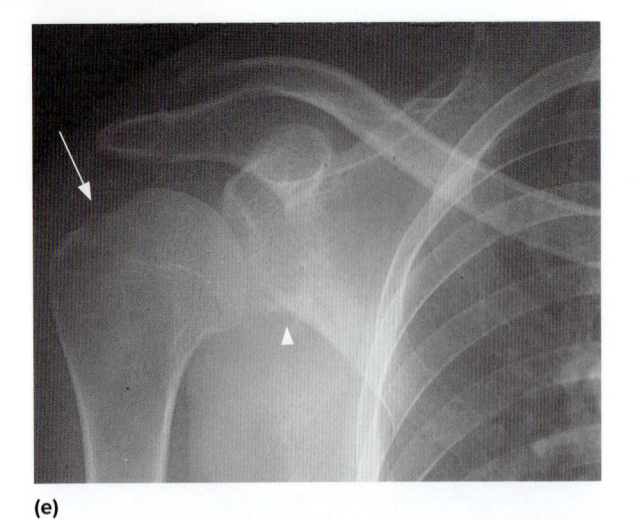

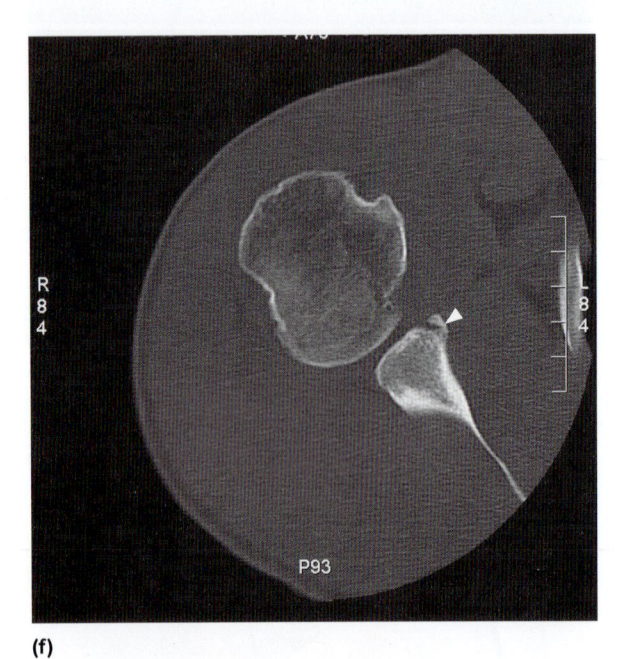

Figure 24.27 (cont.) (e) A radiograph showing a Hill-Sachs' lesion (arrow) and bony Bankart lesion (arrowhead) (f) CT scan of a bony Bankart lesion (arrowhead). CT scan may show this pathology where it is undetected by plain radiography (g) Hill-Sachs' lesion showing where the humeral head has impacted on the glenoid rim (h) Position of patient with anterior dislocation of the shoulder to allow reduction of the shoulder. A small weight may be held in the hand to facilitate reduction

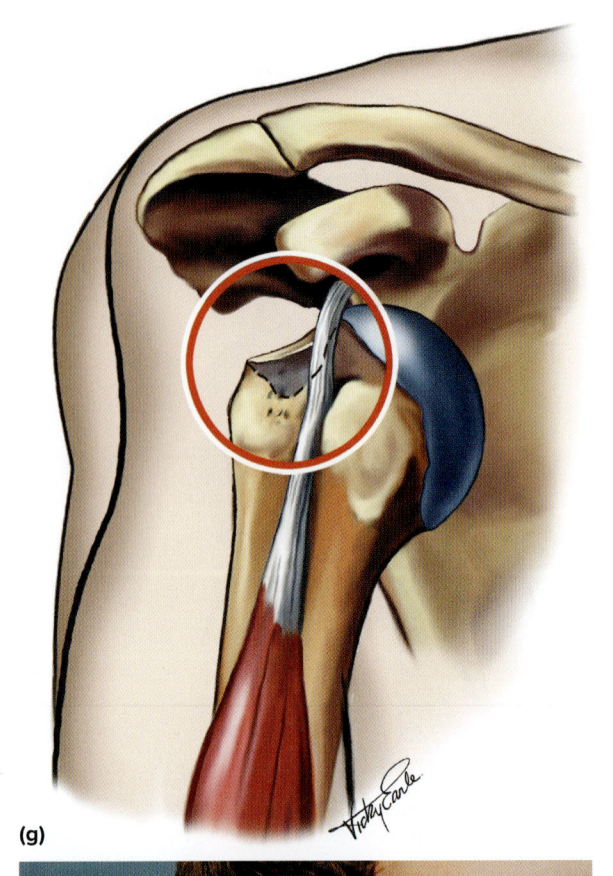

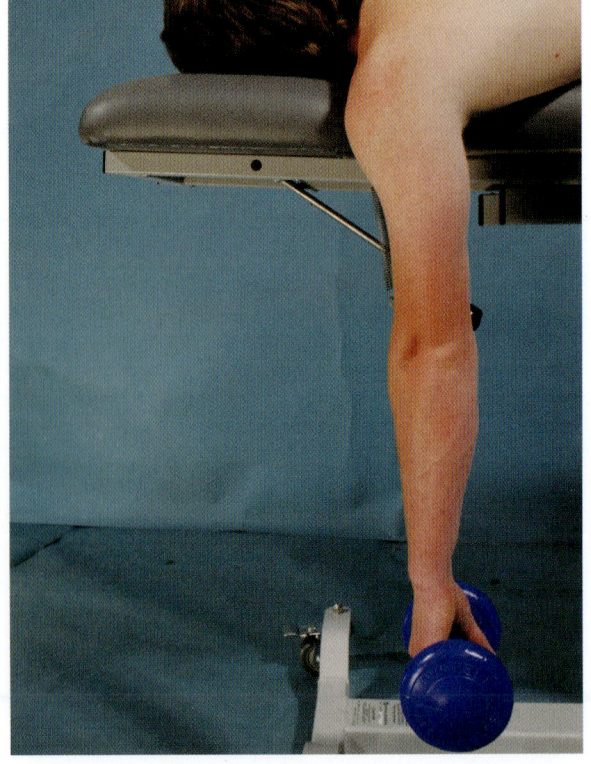

Shoulder pain CHAPTER 24

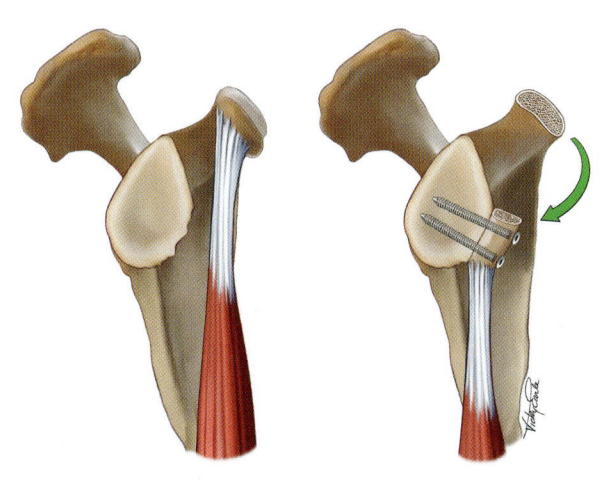

Figure 24.28 Latarjet procedure—one important element of the Latarjet procedure is repositioning the horizontal part of the coracoid to restore bone at the previously damaged anterior inferior margin of the glenoid

impingement. The clinical features comprise recurrent shoulder pain during throwing, possible but not always recurrent subluxations, 'dead arm' syndrome, meaning the athlete reports a sudden inability to throw or smash and a feeling of a 'dead arm'. Chronic pain usually arises from impingement of the rotator cuff tendons, as a result of abnormal humeral head translations, leading to subacromial as well as internal impingement. These recurrent episodes of functional impingement lead to rotator cuff tendinopathy. Apprehension and relocation tests might be painful and/or causing subluxations. These athletes very often show in addition some scapular dyskinesis, GIRD and clinical signs of labral pathology (SLAP lesion).

Atraumatic multidirectional instability—AMBRI

Multidirectional instability of the glenohumeral joint involves a combination of two or three instabilities–anterior, posterior or inferior. Most commonly, multidirectional instability is an atraumatic type of instability, often associated with generalised ligamentous laxity throughout the body. However, it may also result from repetitive trauma, especially at the extremes of motion or, rarely, from a direct blow.

Generalised ligamentous laxity can be assessed by examination of the wrists, thumbs, elbows and knees to determine the presence of hyperextensibility, or obtaining the Beighton score for general laxity.[67] On examination of the shoulder, besides the functional deficits during active movements and hypermobility during passive movements, two or three laxity tests will be positive. During the basic clinical examination, one might also find external rotation up to 90° and glenohumeral abduction >90° (Fig. 24.29).[68]

One of the major characteristics of multidirectional instability is that pain in translation occurs in the mid ranges of motion. This indicates a prominent role of altered muscle activation. Lower trapezius and serratus anterior activity is decreased, while pectoralis minor and major and lattissimus dorsi increase, creating a position of scapular protraction and glenoid tilting. Frequently the symptoms and pain can be alleviated by placing the scapula in a corrected and stabilised position. Relief of symptoms and decreased translation will point to the need for a therapeutic exercise program for the scapular and shoulder stabilisers. Stretching of the muscles around the shoulder joint should be avoided. If multidirectional instability fails to respond to conservative measures, then surgical treatment may be attempted. However, the results of surgical treatment, particularly in those patients with generalised ligamentous laxity, are not as good as in post-traumatic instability.

A special kind of multidirectional instability is the posterior voluntary subluxation, frequently seen in gymnasts or swimmers with hyperlaxity. Their shoulder 'pumps out' during forward flexion posteriorly, and often the patient is able to perform this subluxation voluntarily. These patients exhibit a marked scapular dyskinesis, characterised by anterior tilting and downward rotation during arm elevation. The posterior subluxation test is positive, and they often exhibit weak external rotation strength.

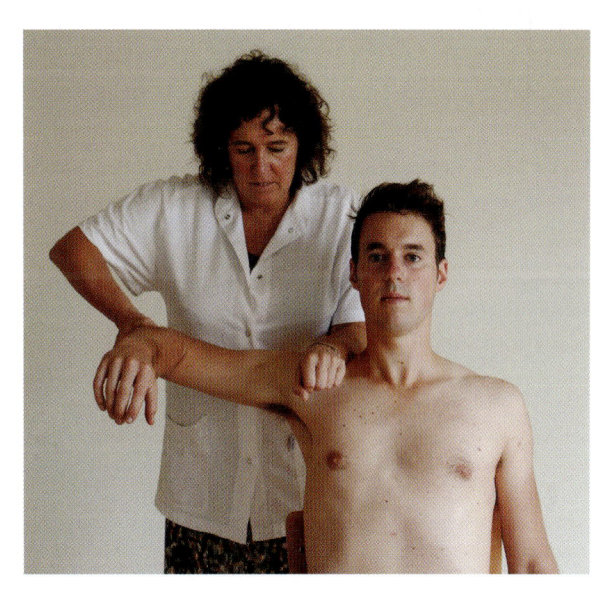

Figure 24.29 The hyperabduction test

411

PART B Regional problems

Rehabilitation guidelines for shoulder instability—overview

The rehabilitation guidelines for shoulder instability depend greatly upon the kind of instability the patient exhibits, and the degree or severity of the symptoms. In general, the three kinds of instabilities described need a different rehabilitation approach, described in Table 24.4. The guidelines are aimed to increase local glenohumeral stability as well as to correct aberrant muscle patterning around the shoulder.

The main differences in therapeutic approach are based on the actual best knowledge and best practice regarding muscle patterning and local neuromuscular control in the unstable shoulder, the benefits and the pitfalls of open versus closed chain exercises, and the value of kinetic chain exercises.

Open versus closed chain shoulder exercises

In closed chain exercises, the final link of the chain, in the case of the upper limb, the hand, is supported on a surface, which is fixed or moveable. As a result of the compressive forces in the joint, the patient feels safer to preserve the local glenohumeral stability. In addition, closed chain exercises stimulate normal proprioceptive pathways, enhance local co-contraction in the stabilising muscles, and minimise translations in the midway of motion. However, in view of the functional demands of the upper extremity in daily life, in particular in overhead athletes, requiring functional stability during open chain overhead throwing or smashing, the limitation of the closed chain exercises is that they do not prepare the athlete for full return to sport, and do not load the tissues around the shoulder in the most functional way, thus jeopardising tissue-specific adaptation to training.

In open chain exercises, the hand is free to move in space (with or without an additional resistance) and shear and translational forces are caused in the glenohumeral joint, increasing the challenge for shoulder stability. It is imperative these exercises are implemented in the rehabilitation program of anterior instability (traumatic or acquired); however, only in later stages (for instance after a dislocation), or on the condition that the athlete feels safe performing the exercise (for instance in acquired instability). However, in multidirectional instability, often the only way to initiate and pursue an effective rehabilitation program is to implement mostly closed chain exercises.

Local neuromuscular control of stabilising muscles

Several studies confirm the lack of adequate muscle activity of the local stabilisers. In anterior instability mainly the rotator cuff shows deficiencies in strength, accurate muscle activity and timing of muscle activation. Therefore the first stage in anterior shoulder instability rehabilitation should be to encourage local conscious muscle control in the rotator cuff by teaching the patient how to consciously contract the rotator cuff (with palpation, EMG feedback, local proprioceptive feedback) or by stimulating cuff activity by putting the shoulder in a controlled manner in positions challenging the cuff (Fig. 24.30). However, in AMBRI patients, it is mainly the deltoid, in particular the posterior part, that has recruitment problems. For that reason, deltoid activation should be the main focus in the first stage of the rehabilitation of AMBRI. In addition, since closed chain exercises increase glenohumeral compression, these exercises should be performed in a closed chain (Fig. 24.31). If needed, local taping techniques might facilitate deltoid activation and promote superior translation of the humeral head (Fig. 24.32).

Table 24.4 Rehabilitation guidelines for shoulder instability

TUBS	AIOS	AMBRI
Scapular rehabilitation (below)	Scapular rehabilitation	Scapular rehabilitation
Control of the rotator cuff, followed by rotator cuff strengthening	Control of the rotator cuff, focus on external rotators, followed by external rotator strengthening	Control of the deltoid—posterior cuff
From closed to open chain exercises	From closed to open chain exercises	Mainly closed chain exercises, except if in progression open chain is needed for return to sport
Stretching is not primary goal, but can be added if necessary	Stretching of the posterior shoulder (GIRD) (below)	No stretching
Kinetic chain exercises (below)	Kinetic chain exercises	Kinetic chain exercises

Shoulder pain CHAPTER 24

(a)

(b)

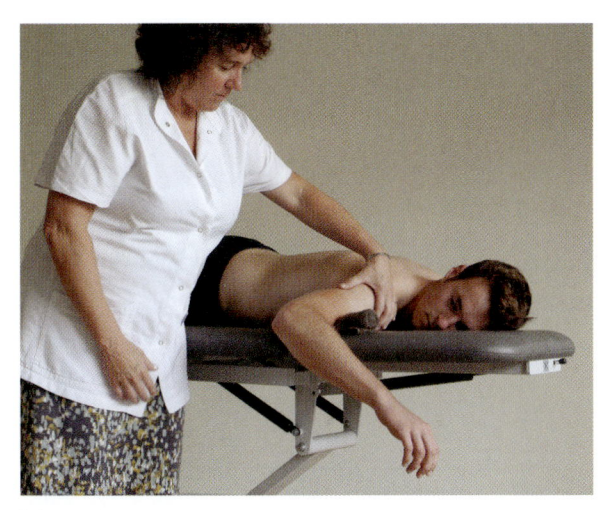

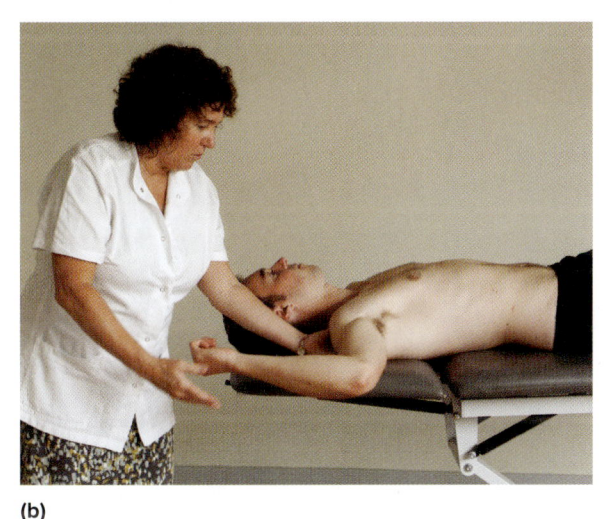

Figure 24.30 Exercises stimulating local control of the rotator cuff (a) Prone (b) Supine

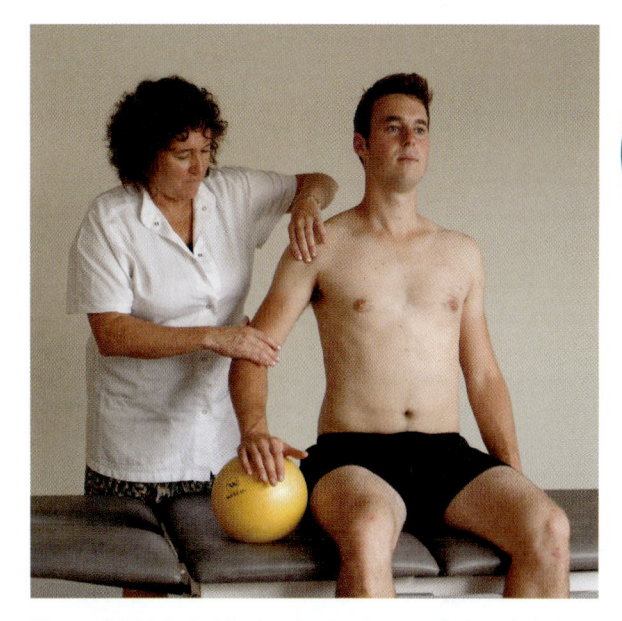

Figure 24.31 Deltoid co-activation in a semi-closed chain

Progression in closed chain exercise program—practice

During closed chain exercises, progression is determined by the load (from low or no body weight, over moderate body weight, to full body weight) and whether the exercises are static or dynamic. In static exercises, the shoulder is loaded, but no shoulder movement is required, whereas in dynamic exercises the shoulder moves (from low to high elevation grades). Theoretic progression is shown in Table 24.5 and illustrated in Figure 24.33. It is the therapist's responsibility to find the appropriate progression, based on the specific capacity and instability problems of the patient.

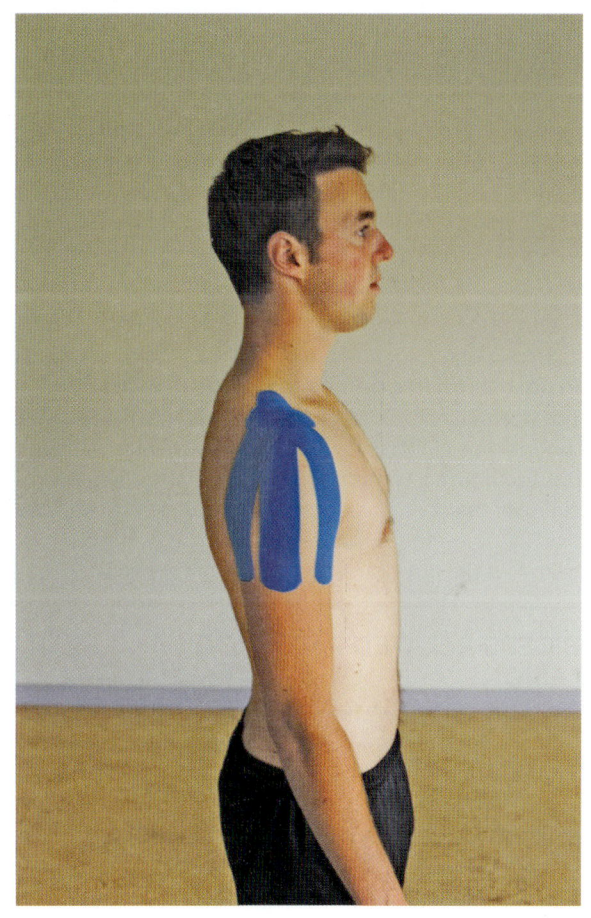

Figure 24.32 Local taping technique for a patient with AMBRI

413

PART B Regional problems

Table 24.5 Progression in closed chain exercises

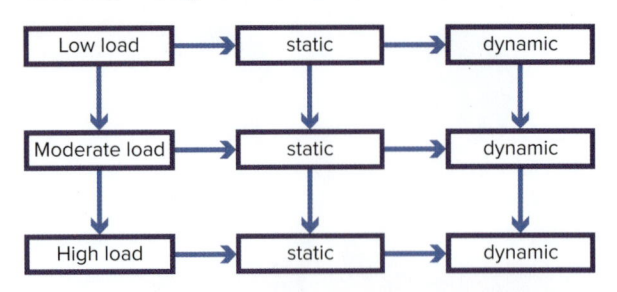

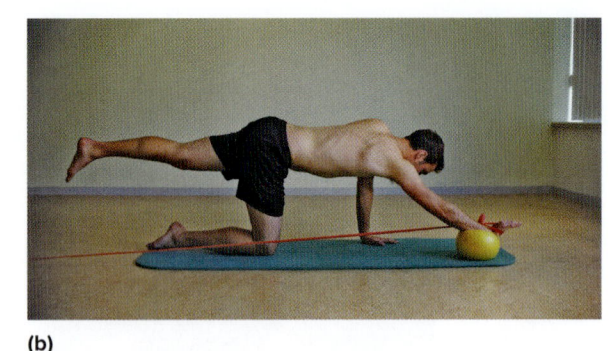

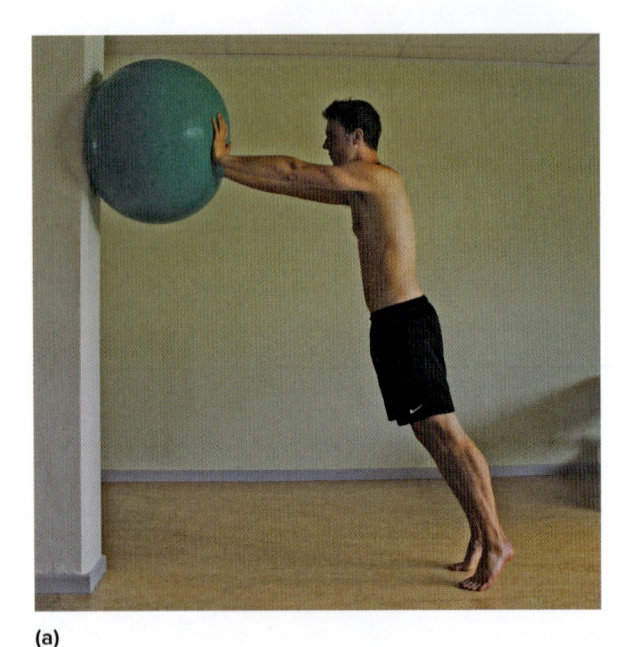

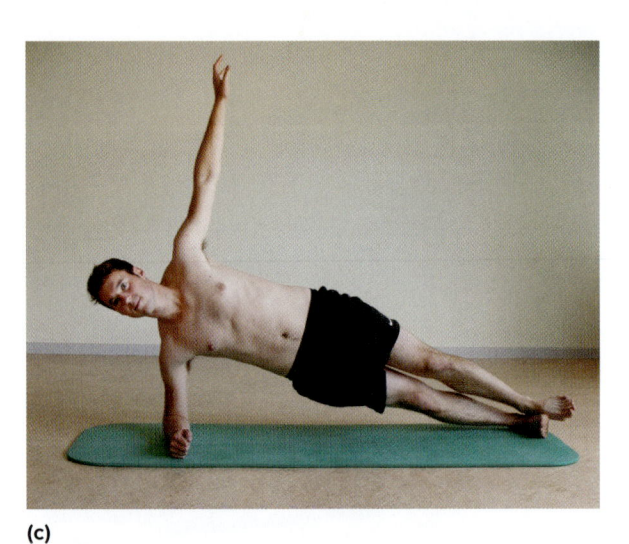

Figure 24.33 Progressively more difficult closed chain exercises (a) Low load (b) Moderate load (c) High load

Progression in open chain program—practice

The open kinetic chain program should commence with basic rotator cuff training (see above); however, it should proceed into more functional exercises, challenging rotator cuff load, functional positions and include eccentric and plyometric exercises. We refer to the thrower's program below for the practical aspect of this progression.

BICEPS-RELATED PATHOLOGY AND SLAP LESIONS

Biceps-related pathologies are a common cause of shoulder pain and disability, and can result in limited work or athletic performance.[69]

Pathomechanics of biceps-related shoulder pain

Pathologic disorders can be divided into three categories: (1) inflammatory/degenerative conditions and partial tears of the long head of the biceps, (2) instability of the biceps tendon into the bicipital groove, and (3) superior labrum anterior to posterior (SLAP) lesions.[70] The three categories of disorders may all present with shoulder pain, and although they differ widely in patient populations and pathogenesis, there is significant overlap among the pathologies.

The labrum is the primary attachment site for the shoulder capsule and glenohumeral ligaments. The superior aspect of the glenoid labrum also serves as the attachment site for the tendon of the long head of the biceps muscle (Fig. 24.34). Injuries to the glenoid labrum are divided into SLAP or non-SLAP lesions, and further into stable or unstable lesions. SLAP lesions are injuries to the labrum that extend from anterior to the biceps tendon to posterior to the tendon. They are divided into four types based on the severity and the instability of the biceps tendon (Fig. 24.35).

SLAP lesions are either stable or unstable depending on whether the majority of the superior labrum and the biceps

Shoulder pain CHAPTER 24

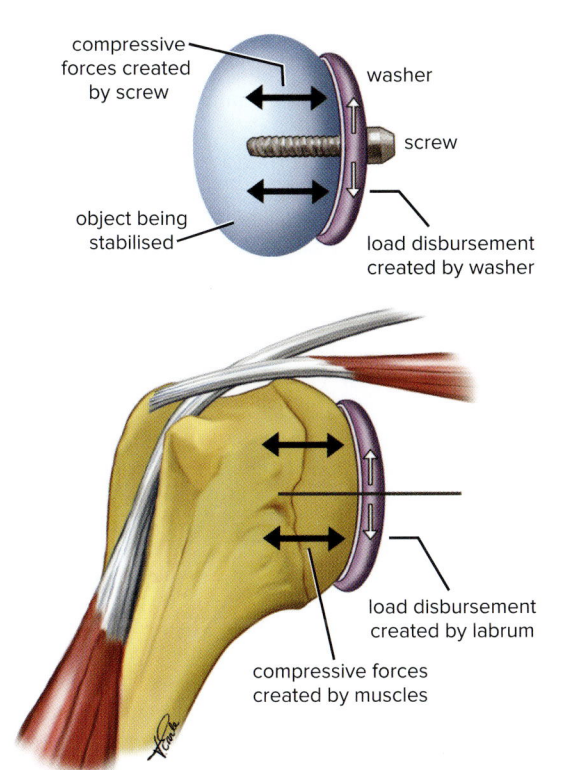

Figure 24.34 The glenoid labrum contributes to proprioception and stability. Dr Ben Kibler compares the stability role with that of a washer (top panel). Like a washer, the deformable labrum (bottom panel), expands the depth and increases the size of the glenoid to increase stability of the interface. The labrum helps to spread load over the glenohumeral joint

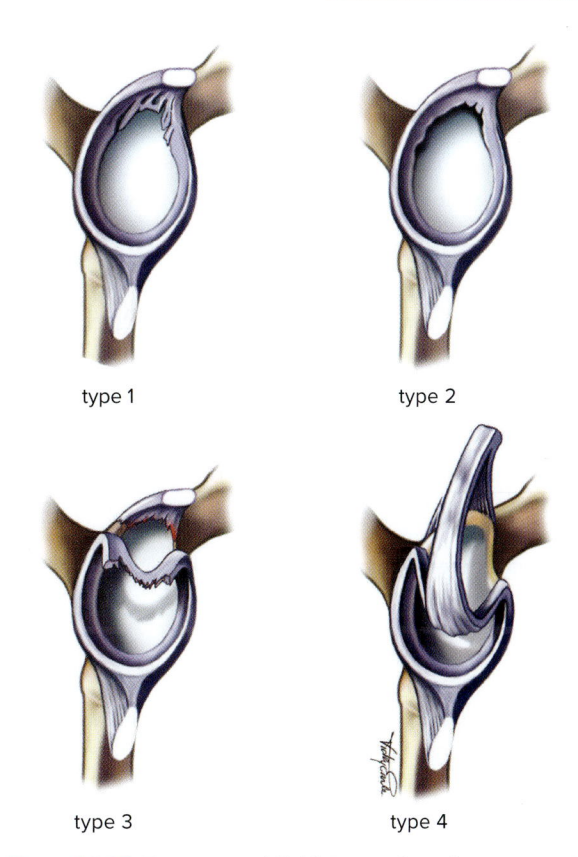

Figure 24.35 Four types of SLAP lesions have been described. In type 1, the attachment of the labrum to the glenoid is intact but there is evidence of fraying and degeneration. Type 2 lesions involve detachment of the superior labrum and tendon of the long head of biceps from the glenoid rim. In type 3 injuries, the meniscoid superior labrum is torn away and displaced into the joint but the tendon and its labral rim attachment are intact. In type 4 lesions, the tear of the superior labrum extends into the tendon, part of which is displaced into the joint along with the superior labrum

tendon are firmly attached to the glenoid margin. Non-SLAP lesions include degenerative, flap and vertical labral tears, as well as unstable lesions such as Bankart lesions.

In general, repetitive overhead activity has been hypothesised as a common mechanism for producing biceps-related shoulder pathology.[69, 70] Although the pathomechanics are debated, the torsional compressive force on the base of the biceps during the cocking position, as well as the high eccentric activity of the biceps muscle during the follow-through phase of throwing and the impingement of the biceps tendon underneath the acromial arch during overhead activities are believed to possibly cause irritation, dysfunction and failure of the superior labral and biceps tendon complex.[69]

Clinical features
The diagnosis of a glenoid labral tear relies on eliciting a history of an appropriate mechanism of injury, clinical assessment and appropriate investigation. The most common mechanisms of injury to the superior glenoid labrum are excessive traction on the labrum through the long head of biceps (e.g. carrying or dropping and catching a heavy object). Throwing injuries occur due to a combination of peel-back traction of the biceps on the labrum in shoulder cocking, abnormal posterosuperior humeral head translation in cocking due to glenohumeral internal rotation deficit, and excessive scapular protraction. Patients complain of pain localised to the posterior or posterosuperior joint line, especially in abduction. Pain in the shoulder is exacerbated by overhead and behind-the-back arm motions. Popping, catching or grinding may also be present.

415

On examination, there may be tenderness over the anterior aspect of the shoulder and pain on resisted biceps contraction. No current SLAP lesion test is able to guarantee sufficient diagnostic value when used alone, in general an interpretation of 'best-test combinations' is advised in the diagnosis of SLAP lesions (Table 24.2).

Plain radiography is usually unremarkable. MR arthrography, a further refinement of MRI by injection of contrast agent into the shoulder, yields greater detail of intra-articular shoulder structures than does conventional MRI (Fig. 24.36). MR arthrography is particularly useful for the detection and assessment of not only glenoid labral tears, but also small loose bodies, or cartilage flaps. Interpretation of MR arthrograms of the shoulder is best performed by a radiologist with particular expertise in the area, as interpretation is complicated by a wide range of normal anatomical variants. The static MRI is well complemented by dynamic tests which provide a context for interpreting the clinical importance of the MRI.

Treatment of SLAP lesions

In recent clinical guidelines, it is suggested that the vast majority of overhead athletes with shoulder pain should be initially treated with non-operative methods.[70] Only certain diagnoses, such as traumatic injuries with documented structural damage such as unstable labral tears, dislocations or rotator cuff tears, may warrant earlier and more aggressive operative intervention.[70]

Only a few studies examined the results of conservative treatment in SLAP lesions. Edwards et al.[71] showed that 50% of the conservatively treated athletes returned to play, with similar return to sports as those who had surgery. Fedoriw et al.[72] concluded from their case series that non-surgical treatment correcting scapular dyskinesia and GIRD had a reasonable success rate in professional baseball players with documented SLAP lesions.

Arthroscopic repair of SLAP lesions results in good to excellent results in patients who are not involved in sports. However, results of surgery in overhead athletes are much less predictable, with a return to previous level of play ranging between 20% and 94%.[72, 73] In particular, the rate of return to previous performance levels seems to be rather low among specialist throwing athletes such as baseball pitchers.

Rehabilitation of biceps-related shoulder pain and SLAP lesions (conservative and postoperative) should follow the general guidelines containing a phased progression of rotator cuff exercises, scapular exercises and stretching. However, tension on the long head of the biceps should be implemented carefully and increased gradually, with early protection of the site of the injury. In addition, in post-operative rehabilitation programs after SLAP repair, biceps activity needs to be controlled during the first 12 weeks following surgery, with no resisted biceps activity during the first 8 weeks to protect the healing of the biceps anchor, and no aggressive strengthening of the biceps for 12 weeks following surgery.[74]

A progressive program consisting of selected rotator cuff and scapular exercises with low to moderate load on the biceps (based on EMG analysis) was proposed, giving the clinician the opportunity to select the appropriate exercises based on the goal and the load on the biceps.[75] In this continuum of exercises with an increasing level of EMG activity in the biceps, exercises targeting the trapezius resulted in less load on the biceps compared with exercises for the serratus anterior. In addition, exercises with an internal rotation component showed low activity in the biceps, and exercises meant to target the biceps–such as the uppercut exercise (Fig. 24.37a) or resisted forward flexion in supination (Fig. 24.37b)–showed the highest levels of activity in the biceps.

In the advanced stages of rehabilitation, higher load on the biceps is needed to increase its strength in order to prepare the athlete to return to sport, by performing eccentric exercises in throwers or pull-up exercises in gymnasts or pole jumpers.

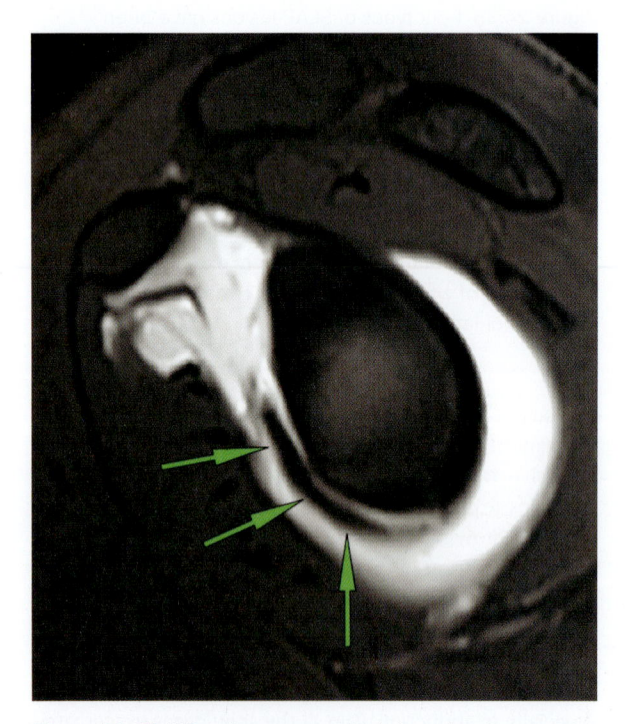

Figure 24.36 MR arthrogram sagittal view showing anterior glenoid labral tear (arrows)

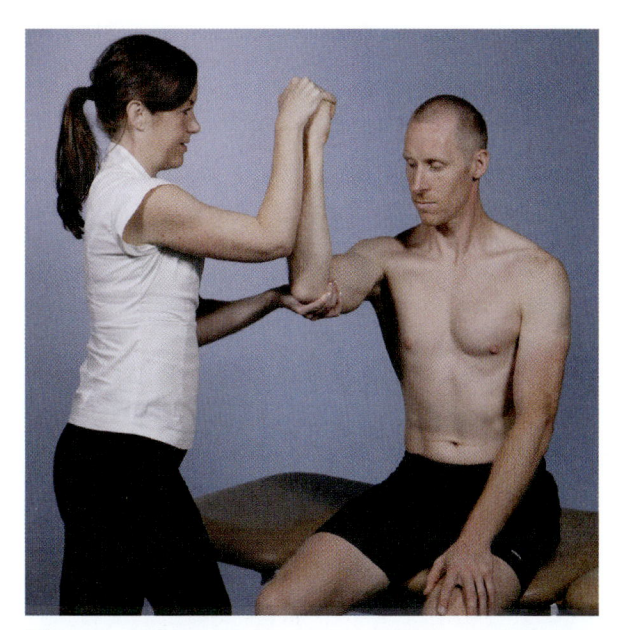

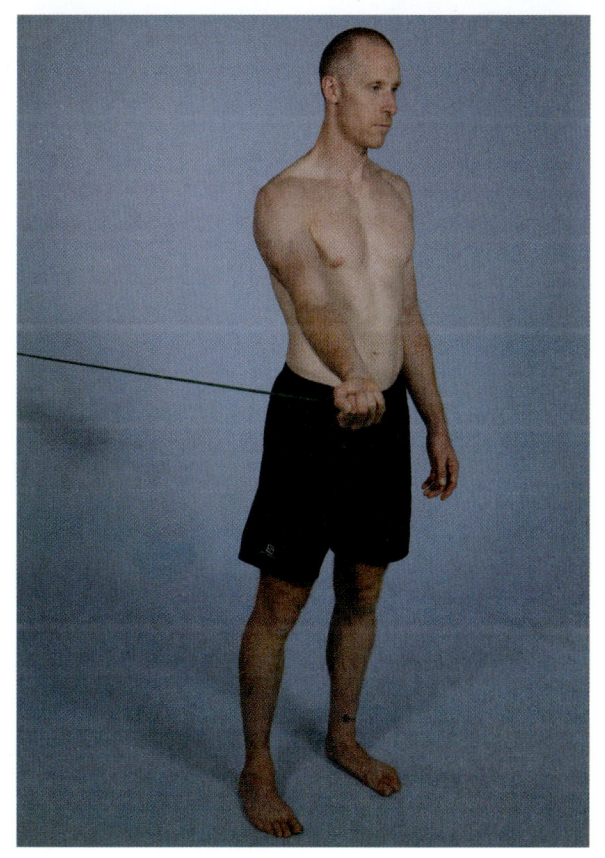

Shoulder pain   CHAPTER 24

PATHOLOGICAL GLENOHUMERAL INTERNAL ROTATION DEFICIT

Pathomechanics of GIRD

Posterior shoulder stiffness is the most common adaptation seen at the dominant side of overhead athletes of multiple sports disciplines.[76] This manifests clinically as decreased glenohumeral cross-body adduction and internal rotation mobility and is believed to be the result of both capsular tightness and muscular contracture. It is hypothesised that the cumulative loads onto the posterior shoulder during the deceleration phase of the throwing motion cause microtrauma and scarring of these soft tissues.

Posterior shoulder stiffness therefore has been suggested to be a causative or perpetuating factor in shoulder impingement and labral pathology.[3,54,77] Abnormal humeral head translations, caused by selective tightening of the posterior-inferior capsule may decrease the width of the subacromial space, thus causing subacromial impingement. Other studies suggest a posterior and superior translation of the humeral head during cocking with a tight posterior capsule, possibly leading to an encroachment of the rotator cuff tendons against the posterosuperior rim of the glenoid.[78]

In addition, posterior shoulder tightness seems to affect kinematics of the scapula and the humeral head and is associated with a decreased acromiohumeral distance.[79] As a result, posterior capsule shortness possibly increases the risk for internal as well as subacromial impingement in the overhead athlete.[19,23,26] A study of elite handball players found that for every 5° increase in total rotational motion, the odds of shoulder injury were reduced by 23%.[3]

Treatment of GIRD

Given the evidenced impact of posterior shoulder tightness on shoulder kinematics, increasing posterior shoulder flexibility is advisory when mobility deficits exceed the limits associated with increased injury risk. In baseball, reduced internal rotation ROM of 18–25° and reduced total range of motion of 5° are considered to increase the risk for shoulder injury.[80,81] Both the cross-body stretch (Fig. 24.38a) and the sleeper stretch (Fig. 24.38b) can be recommended to decrease posterior shoulder tightness.[81,82] It was shown that a 6-week daily sleeper stretch program (three reps of 30 seconds) is able to significantly increase the acromiohumeral distance in the dominant shoulder of healthy overhead athletes with GIRD.[79] Additional joint mobilisation performed by a physiotherapist has a small but non-significant advantage over a home stretching program alone.[83] No difference in mobility gain was seen after angular (sleeper stretch and horizontal adduction stretch) and non-angular (Fig. 24.39) joint mobilisation by a physiotherapist.[84] Muscle energy techniques (hold-relax) during the sleeper stretch and

Figure 24.37 (a) The uppercut exercise (b) Forward flexion in external rotation

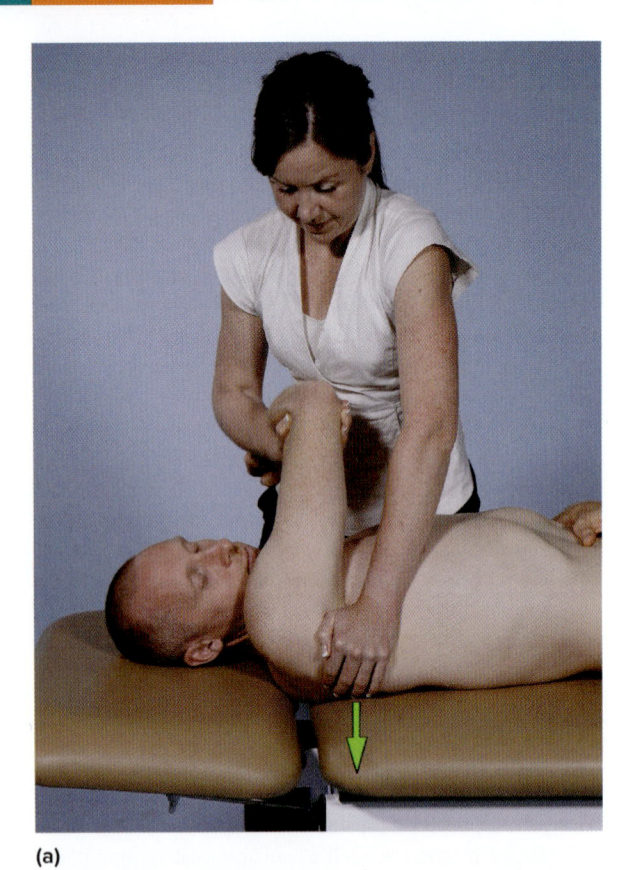

PART B Regional problems

(a)

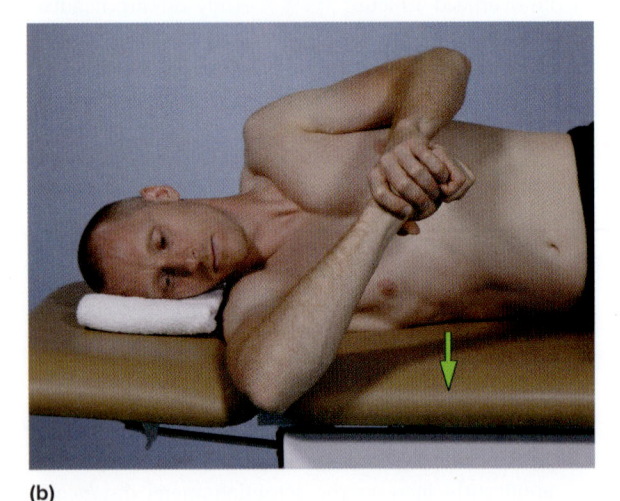

(b)

Figure 24.38 (a) The cross-body stretch (b) The sleeper stretch

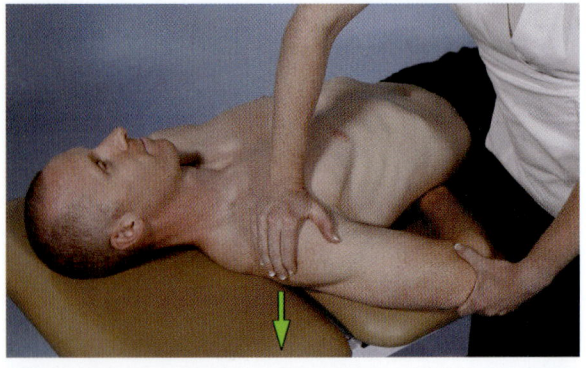

(a)

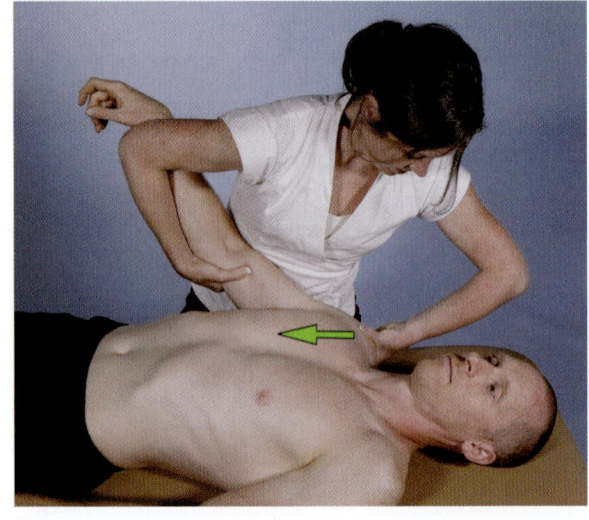

(b)

Figure 24.39 (a) Dorsal and (b) Caudal glides

the horizontal adduction stretch have proven useful to immediately increase internal rotation range of motion.[85] Two studies[84, 86] showed symptom relief after a stretching program in a population of overhead athletes with impingement-related shoulder pain.

GIRD in the overhead athlete is often associated with acquired instability (AIOS), both leading to imbalances in shoulder kinematics and hyperangulation during cocking. Therefore, in most athletes stretching exercises of the posterior shoulder should be combined with rotator cuff strengthening.

A valuable treatment tool in the mobilisation of the shoulder joint, however, until now, not fully explored or investigated in scientific literature, is mobilisation with movement (MWM). In these techniques, active or passive angular shoulder movements are performed, accompanied by a translational mobilisation of the glenohumeral joint. In view of the arthrokinematic characteristics of impingement, with abnormal anterior and superior translation of the humeral head, in particular dorsal (Fig. 24.40a) and inferior (Fig. 24.40b) glides during active movements are of interest in the treatment of these patients.

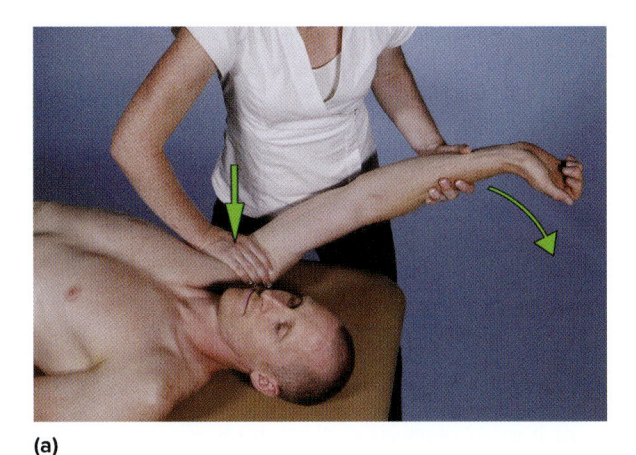

Shoulder pain CHAPTER 24

help restore ROM. Home exercises may include using a foam roller (Fig. 24.41d). After resolution of symptoms, the athlete should continue the home stretching program, together with external rotator strength training.

SCAPULAR DYSKINESIS

Most of the studies investigating scapular dyskinesis in relation to shoulder pain have been performed in patients with impingement symptoms and rotator cuff pathology. In general, the identified deviations can be summarised as a lack of scapular upward rotation, posterior tilting and external rotation, increased clavicular elevation and retraction, or characterised by scapular asymmetry in rest or during movement (abnormal scapulohumeral rhythm).

Several authors have demonstrated altered muscle activity patterns in the scapular muscles in patients with shoulder impingement. In particular, researchers consistently demonstrated decreased strength in the serratus anterior, hyperactivity and early activation of

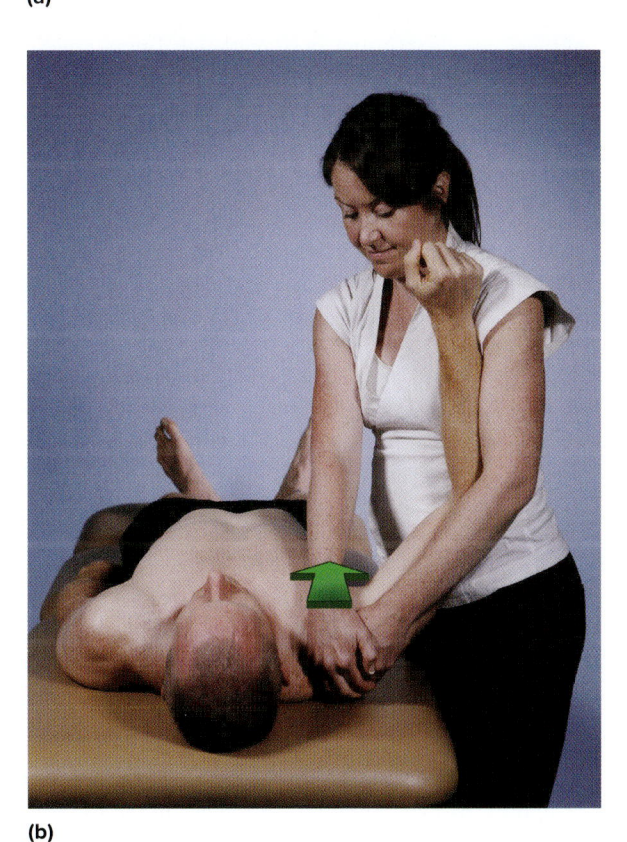

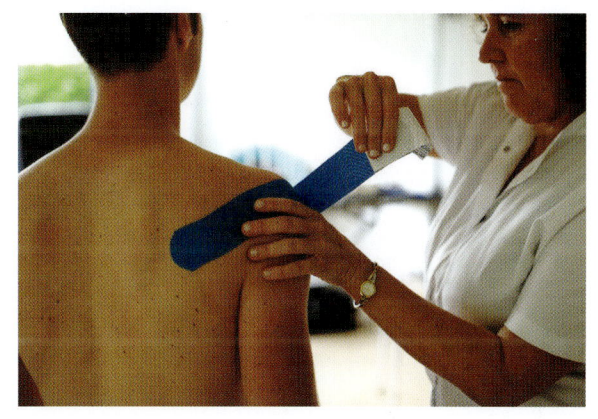

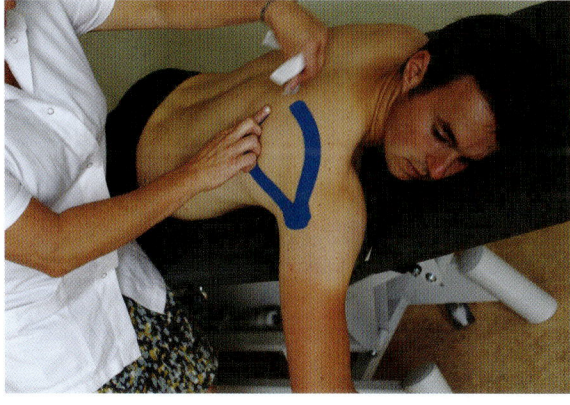

Figure 24.40 (a) Mobilisation with movement—dorsal glides during forward flexion (b) Inferior glides during scapular elevation

Additional taping to correct humeral head position, as described by McConnell,[87] might be useful (Fig. 24.41a). However, this should result in immediate symptom relief. In addition, in case of hypertonicity in the infraspinatus, taping with elastic tape (Fig. 24.41b) and dry needling of the infraspinatus (Fig. 24.41c) may relax muscle and

Figure 24.41 (a) Shoulder taping to correct humeral head position (b) Elastic tape on the infraspinatus

419

PART B   Regional problems

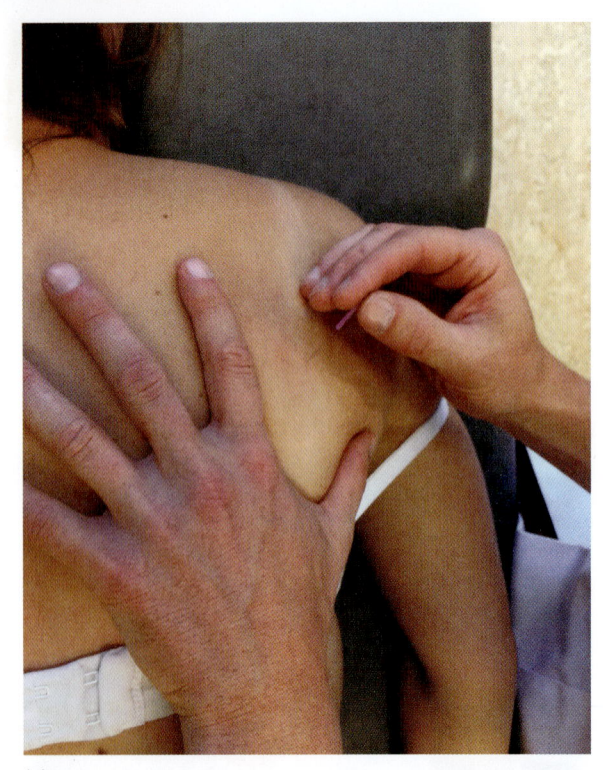

(c)

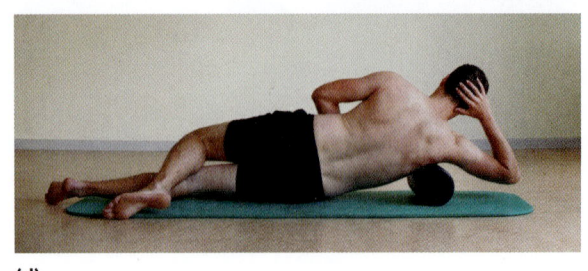

(d)

Figure 24.41 (cont.) (c) Dry needling of the infraspinatus (d) Foam roll exercise for the latissimus dorsi

the upper trapezius (resulting in a shrug–excessive elevation of the shoulder girdle during arm elevation), and decreased activity and late activation of the middle and lower trapezius muscle part. Although some of these studies were performed on non-athletic populations, many of the possible causes for scapular dyskinesis have been established in overhead athletes, and have been suggested to be a contributing and perpetuating factor in the development of impingement symptoms in athletes performing overhead sports.

With respect to soft tissue inflexibility, tightness of the pectoralis minor and posterior glenohumeral capsular stiffness have been established in relation to abnormal scapular position. Increased scapular internal rotation, as well as increased anterior tilting, has been demonstrated in subjects with a short pectoralis minor or posterior shoulder stiffness. These alterations in scapular position are similar to the scapular deviations established in patients with impingement symptoms, and possibly put the shoulder at more risk for developing shoulder pain.

> **PRACTICE PEARL**
>
> There is no consensus about the cause–consequence relationship between scapular dyskinesis and shoulder pain.

At least six biomechanical mechanisms can potentially alter scapular kinematics. These include pain, soft tissue tightness, muscle activation or strength imbalances, muscle fatigue and thoracic posture. It is unclear whether the alterations found in scapular kinematics are compensatory or contributory to shoulder impingement symptoms and rotator cuff pathology. Regardless of whether the scapular dyskinesis is the cause or the result of painful shoulder conditions, the clinician should focus on scapular evaluation and rehabilitation prior to the treatment of the shoulder. Scapular dyskinesis tends to change the relationship between the glenoid and humerus, to decrease the width of the subacromial space, to jeopardise the fulcrum of the humeral head into the glenoid fossa, and to alter the length–tension relationship of the rotator cuff muscles, hence possibly leading to glenohumeral instability. Moreover, scapular dyskinesis may interrupt the kinetic chain, in particular during overhead throwing and athletic activities.

During overhead movements, the scapula plays a very important role as a link between the trunk and the arm, transferring and increasing the energy and power from the lower extremities and the trunk into the rapidly moving arm. To fulfil this task, the scapula has to be in the correct position and all scapular muscles should be activated at the right time and sufficiently to allow the ground reaction forces to transfer into the shoulder, and finally into the most distal link of the chain, the hand.

Rehabilitation of scapular dyskinesis—a scapular rehabilitation algorithm

The algorithm presented in Figure 24.42 guides the progression of exercises for rehabilitation of scapular dyskinesis.[88] The upper part of the algorithm summarises the possible causes of scapular dyskinesis, divided in flexibility and muscle performance deficits. The lower part of the algorithm offers guidelines for progressive rehabilitation. Since scapular dyskinesis nearly always is caused by both kind of deficits, the rehabilitation program

Shoulder pain — CHAPTER 24

Dr Ann Cools' Scapular Rehabilitation Algorithm

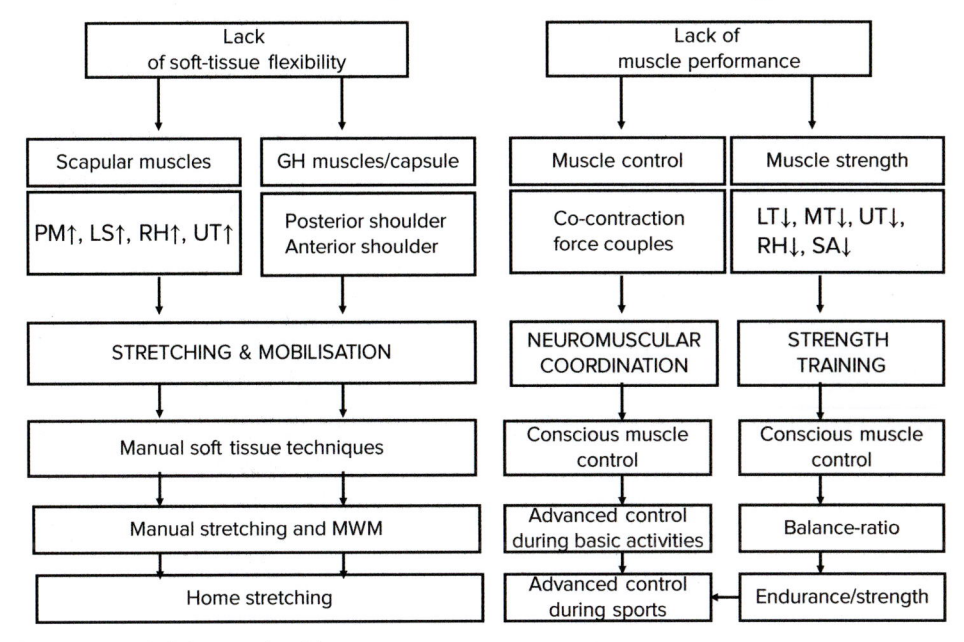

```
                Lack                                    Lack of
        of soft-tissue flexibility              muscle performance
               │                                         │
      ┌────────┴────────┐                     ┌──────────┴──────────┐
 Scapular muscles   GH muscles/capsule    Muscle control      Muscle strength
 PM↑, LS↑, RH↑, UT↑  Posterior shoulder   Co-contraction    LT↓, MT↓, UT↓,
                     Anterior shoulder    force couples       RH↓, SA↓
      └────────┬────────┘                     │                    │
   STRETCHING & MOBILISATION            NEUROMUSCULAR          STRENGTH
                │                        COORDINATION          TRAINING
   Manual soft tissue techniques       Conscious muscle    Conscious muscle
                │                           control             control
   Manual stretching and MWM          Advanced control        Balance-ratio
                │                    during basic activities
        Home stretching               Advanced control      Endurance/strength
                                         during sports
```

Figure 24.42 Scapular rehabilitation algorithm
PM = pectoralis minor, LS = levator scapulae, RH = rhomboid, UT = upper trapezius, MT = middle trapezius, LT = lower trapezius, SA = serratus anterior, GH = glenohumeral
COOLS ET AL.[88] REPRODUCED WITH PERMISSION FROM *BRITISH JOURNAL OF SPORTS MEDICINE*

is multifactorial, including stretching as well as muscle recruitment and strengthening exercises.

Rehabilitation of flexibility deficits

Several stretching techniques have been described to increase pectoralis minor length. Superior effects of the 'unilateral corner stretch' (performing passive horizontal abduction with the shoulder in 90° of abduction and external rotation) over 'sitting manual stretching' (in which the therapist performs scapular retraction with the shoulder in a neutral position) and 'supine manual stretch' (similar to the unilateral corner stretch, but performed by the therapist with the patient in a supine position) were established in a study on healthy subjects.[89] However, from a clinical perspective, these stretches (with the exception of the 'sitting manual stretching') put the athlete's shoulder into a position, possibly causing pain in the case of subacromial or internal impingement.

Therefore in clinical practice, the pectoralis minor might be stretched by performing passive retraction and posterior tilting of the scapula with the shoulder in a neutral or small elevation position and slight external rotation. In particular, direct pressure on the coracoid process provides an intense stretching effect on the pectoralis minor (Fig. 24.43a). In healthy athletes, the corner stretch might be advised, taking care not to stretch the anterior shoulder capsule too much. An alternative self-stretch exercise, resulting in scapular retraction and posterior tilt is given in Figure 24.43b.

With respect to stretching techniques of the posterior capsule, we refer to the previous section.

Rehabilitation of muscle performance deficits

In view of the new insights and research findings on the role of the scapula in shoulder pathology, current exercise protocols emphasise scapular muscle training as an essential component of shoulder rehabilitation. In the early stage of scapular training, conscious muscle control of the scapular muscles may be necessary to improve proprioception and to normalise scapular resting position. To selectively activate the scapular stabilisers, the 'scapular orientation exercise' has been described.[90] Prior to high-intensity strength training, the clinician should focus on facilitating correct timing and control of muscle recruitment. Strength training in the presence of faulty scapular control probably might reinforce poor kinematics and fail to reduce pain or improve function.

PART B   Regional problems

(a)   (b)

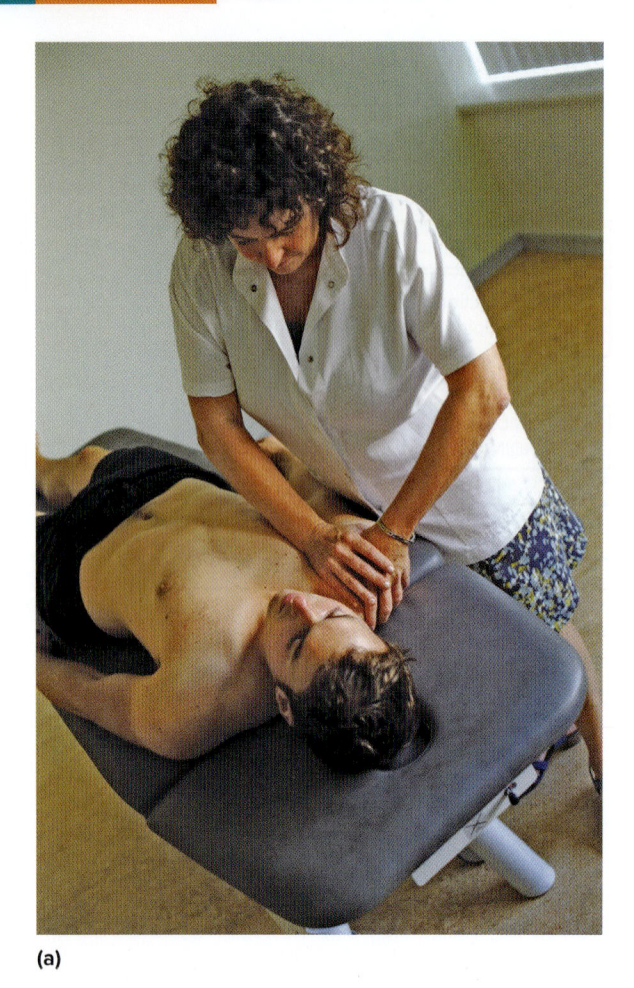

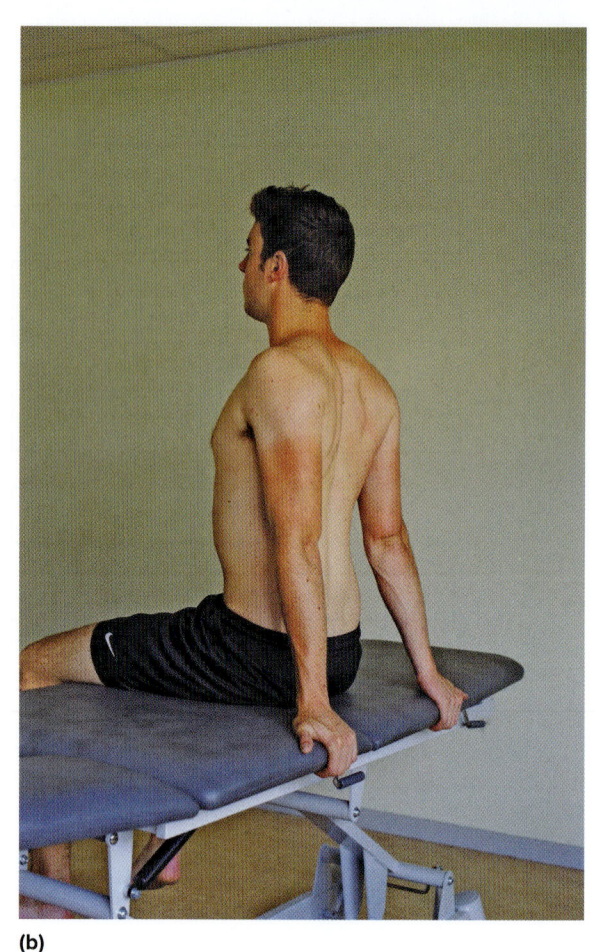

Figure 24.43 (a) Direct manual stretching of the pectoralis minor—therapist performs a posterior tilt of the scapula with direct pressure on the coracoid process (b) Home stretching for the pectoralis minor

Depending on the results of the clinical examination, the therapist may decide in the second stage of scapular muscle training to focus more on muscle control (appropriate co-activation of the scapular force couples) or muscle strength (in case of isolated strength deficit in one or more scapular muscles).

Following the scapular orientation exercises, scapular co-contraction may be trained in basic positions, movements and exercises, activating the key scapular-stabilising muscles without putting high demands on the shoulder joint. In this stage of scapular rehabilitation, very often closed chain exercises are used. They are believed to improve dynamic glenohumeral stability through stimulation of the intra- and periarticular proprioceptors, and enhance co-contraction of the rotator cuff, thus being beneficial in case of shoulder instability. However, open chain functional exercises are also imperative in this stage. Exercises with an external rotation component tend to improve proper scapular muscle recruitment (Fig. 24.44).

For patients with a strength deficit and muscle imbalance in the scapular muscles, selective activation of the weaker muscle parts with minimal activity of the hyperactive muscles is an important component in the second stage of scapular muscle rehabilitation. Because of relative inactivity in lower trapezius (LT) and serratus anterior (SA), often combined with excessive use of upper trapezius (UT), exercises with a low UT/LT, UT/MT and UT/SA ratio are particularly important (Figs 24.45, 24.46).[91] Several studies have examined the effectiveness of a scapula-based rehabilitation program.[60,92,93] Although there are those who advocate for the primacy of treating scapular mechanics, there is no evidence to suggest this has clinical benefits over a comprehensive shoulder treatment program as outlined in this chapter.

In the third stage of scapular rehabilitation, in which the treatment goal is to exercise advanced scapular muscle control and strength during sport-specific movements,

Shoulder pain   CHAPTER 24

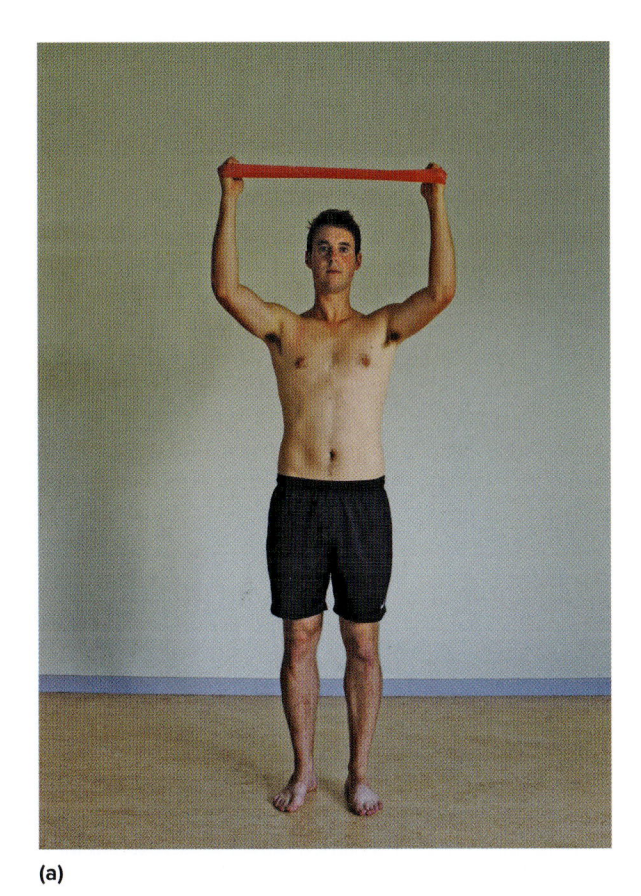

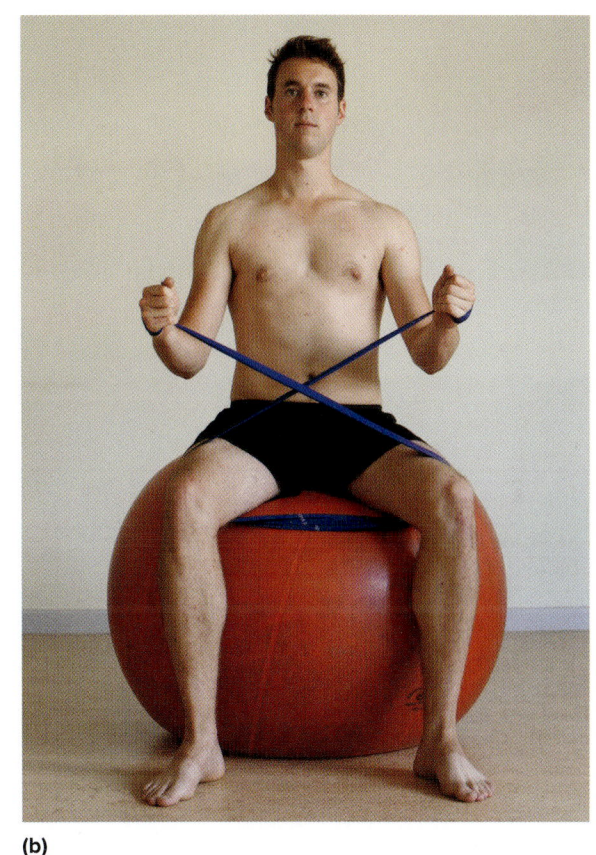

Figure 24.44 Examples of exercises with glenohumeral external rotation component (a) During elevation, (b) Combined with core stability and hip abductor training

special attention is given to integration of the kinetic chain into the exercise program, implementation of sport-specific demands by performing plyometric exercises and eccentric exercises. Scapular control should be automatic and integrated into all sport-specific exercises. Throwing athletes should perform exercises in which the external rotators are eccentrically loaded (see thrower's program in Chapter 8).

On the other hand, swimmers should not focus on plyometrics, but rather train in sport-specific positions such as lying prone or supine in situations demanding a lot of core stability and demanding a large number of repetitions. Gymnasts and athletes performing climbing sports should perform high-level closed chain exercises, such as side- and prone-bridging, and sling exercises might

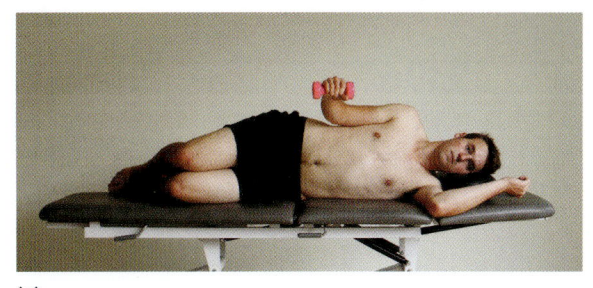

Figure 24.45 Four exercises to improve UT/MT and UT/LT ratio (a) Side-lying external rotation, (b) Side-lying forward flexion

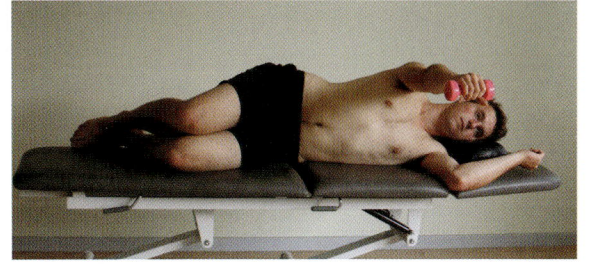

423

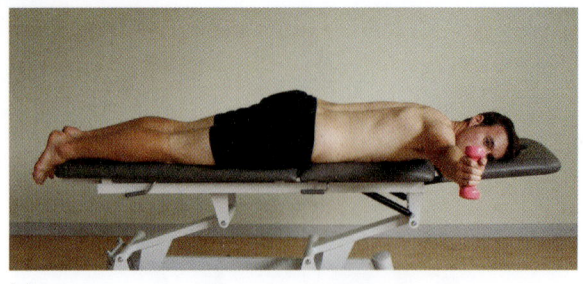

PART B Regional problems

(c)

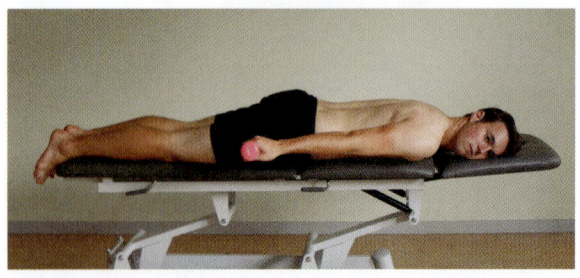

(d)

Figure 24.45 (cont.) (c) Prone horizontal abduction with external rotation (d) Prone extension

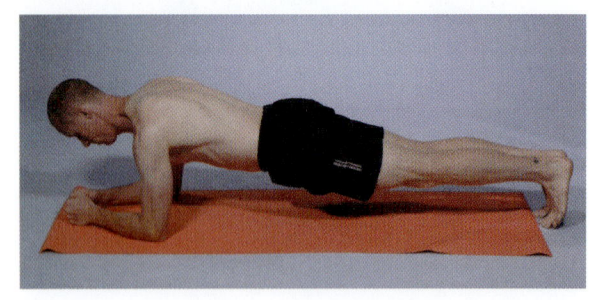

(a)

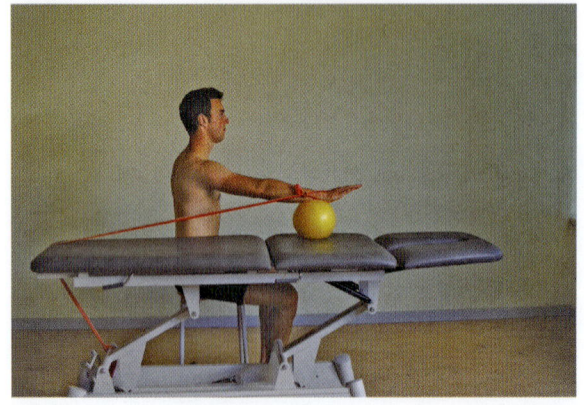

(b)

Figure 24.46 Two exercises to improve UT/SA ratio (a) Elbow push-up, (b) Serratus push-in closed chain

be added to their program. These exercises have been shown to highly activate the large glenohumeral muscles compared to exercises on a stable surface.[92]

Throughout the rehabilitation program, and given the evidence that scapular dyskinesis is often related to thoracic kyphosis or flexed thoracic postures, thoracic posture should also be addressed in the rehabilitation of patients with shoulder pain and related scapular dyskinesis. This includes correction of posture into extension, and also mobilisation exercises into extension (Fig. 24.47a) and rotation (Fig.24.47b), and core-stability training and muscle training of the trunk muscles. The use of therapeutic tape (Fig. 24.48) can be helpful in this stage of the rehabilitation, since it has been shown that taping the thoracic spine and the scapula into extension, posterior tilting and retraction improves trunk posture and shoulder range of motion.

FRACTURES OF THE CLAVICLE

Clavicle fractures are usually caused by either a fall onto the point of the shoulder, for example in horse riding or cycling, or by direct contact with opponents in sports such as football.

The clavicle usually fractures in its middle third with the outer fragment displacing inferiorly and the medial fragment superiorly. It is extremely painful. On examination, there is localised tenderness and swelling and the bony deformity may be palpated. With clavicular shortening or angulation, the scapula will assume a protracted position.

Radiography reveals the fracture. There has been a change in perspective about imaging clavicle fractures as it is sometimes difficult to assess true clavicle position using radiographs. Thus, overlap and shortening need to be carefully monitored for the first 3–4 weeks of non-operative management because significant deformity can occur.

The principles of treatment are to provide pain relief. Clavicle fractures almost always heal in 4–6 weeks. However, often the ends overlap and the clavicle is foreshortened. A foreshortened clavicle is associated with significant functional deficits. A figure-of-eight bandage is designed to prevent foreshortening and has significant advantages over a sling or collar and cuff. During this time the patient should perform self-assisted shoulder flexion to a maximum of 90° to prevent stiffness of the glenohumeral joint.

These fractures[94] are best managed conservatively and usually heal well. Early surgical fixation is indicated if there is compromise of the skin by bony fragments or foreshortening of greater than 1–2 cm. Occasionally, non-union of a fracture of the clavicle may occur with a fibrous pseudoarthrosis forming. This is treated surgically by open reduction and internal fixation with a dynamic

Shoulder pain CHAPTER 24

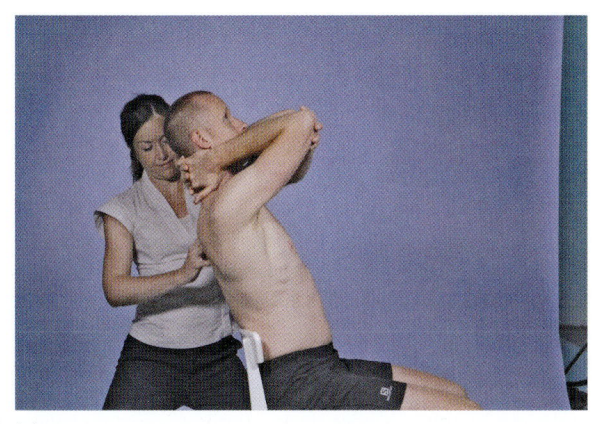

(a)

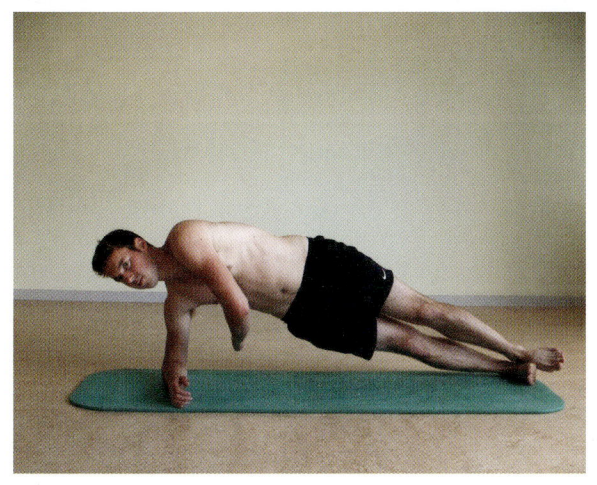

(b–i)

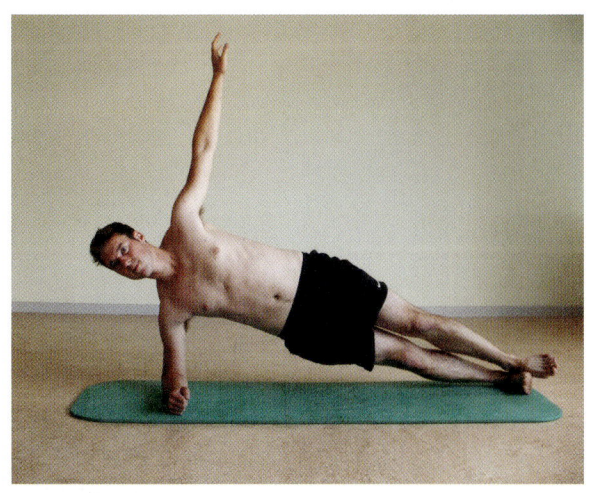

(b–ii)

Figure 24.47 (a) and (b–i, ii) Exercises promoting trunk rotation

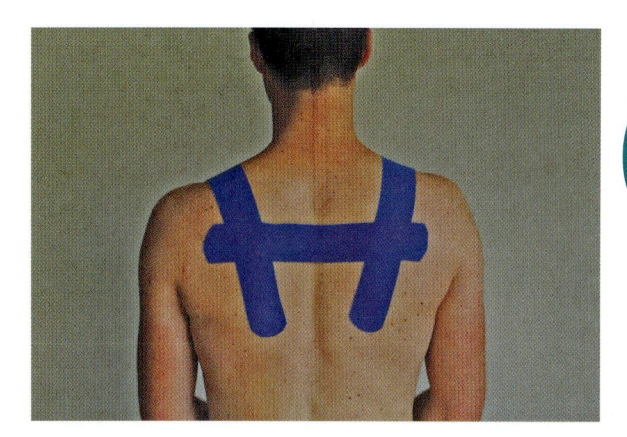

Figure 24.48 Taping technique to promote scapular posterior tilt and retraction

compression plate and bone chips to ensure the length of the clavicle is maintained.[94]

Distal clavicle fractures comprise 12–15% of all clavicle fractures. Many of these fractures involve disruption of the AC joint and/or coracoclavicular ligaments. These fractures are more prone to non-union and delayed union. Classification for these fractures is shown in Table 24.6

Generally, fractures medial to the ligament attachments have greater displacement of fracture fragments and this is associated with increased risk of delayed or non-union if treated non-operatively.[94]

Minimally displaced fractures distal to the coracoclavicular ligament attachments (type I) may be treated with a sling for comfort and early range of motion and isometric strengthening exercises. If displacement is present, then rehabilitation should progress slowly, with active range of motion exercises only introduced when pain resolves and healing has begun radiographically.

Treatment of the more medial (type II) fractures is more controversial.[94] As there is a high rate of non-union, surgical treatment is often recommended. Distal intra-articular fractures (type III), if stable, should be treated non-surgically as they tend to heal with minimal dysfunction.

Table 24.6 The American Shoulder and Elbow Society classification of distal clavicle fractures

Type	Pathology
I	Fracture distal to coracoclavicular ligaments with little displacement
IIa	Fracture medial to coracoclavicular ligaments
IIb	Fracture between coracoclavicular ligaments
III	Intra-articular fracture without ligament disruption

425

PART B Regional problems

Special note—immature skeleton
The treatment of distal clavicle fractures in the immature adult is different from that in the adult. Even fractures that present with significant displacement are stable and will eventually heal in an anatomical position. This is due to the fact that, although the fracture is medial to the coracoclavicular ligament attachment, the periosteal envelope remains attached to the coracoclavicular ligaments. The haematoma and subsequent new bone formation stimulated by the periosteum results in remodelling and complete union.

ACROMIOCLAVICULAR JOINT INJURIES
The AC joint is another common site of injury in athletes who fall onto the point of the shoulder. Stability of the AC joint is provided by a number of structures. In order of increasing importance, these are the joint capsule, the AC ligaments and the coracoclavicular ligament comprising the conoid and trapezoid ligaments (Fig. 24.49).

Acute acromioclavicular joint injuries
A modified classification system by Rockwood describes six different types of AC joint injuries (Fig. 24.50). Type I injury corresponds to sprain of the capsule of the joint and is characterised clinically by localised tenderness and pain on movement, especially horizontal flexion. Type II injuries correspond to a complete tear of the AC ligaments with sprain of the coracoclavicular ligaments. On examination, as well as localised tenderness, there is a small palpable step deformity. Type III and V injuries consist of complete tears of the coracoclavicular ligaments, the conoid and trapezoid. In type III and V injuries, a marked step deformity is present (Fig. 24.51).

Type V injuries can be distinguished from type III injuries radiographically by the amount of displacement. A type V injury has between three and five times greater coracoclavicular space than normal, whereas a type III injury has 25–100% greater coracoclavicular distance than the uninjured side. Type V injury typically involves much greater soft tissue injury and includes damage to the muscle fascia and occasionally the skin. Type IV injuries are characterised by posterior displacement of the clavicle and type VI injuries have an inferiorly displaced clavicle into either a subacromial or subcoracoid position. Type IV, V and VI injuries also have complete rupture of all the ligament complexes and are much rarer injuries than types I, II and III.

Management is based on the general principles of management of ligamentous injuries. Initially, ice is applied to minimise the degree of damage and the injured part is immobilised in a sling for pain relief. This may be for 2–3 days in the case of type I injuries or up to 6 weeks in severe type II or type III injuries. Isometric strengthening exercises should be commenced once pain permits. Return to sport is possible when there is no further localised tenderness and full range of pain-free movement has been regained. The athlete may feel more comfortable on return to sport by taping the AC joint (Fig. 24.52).

The major functional problems in a high grade (III-IV) injury result from loss of strut function to stabilise the scapula, glenohumeral joint and arm. Most type III AC separations showed an alteration of scapular mechanics.[95, 96] Thus, much more consideration should be given to reconstruction in those patients exhibiting altered scapular mechanics.

> **PRACTICE PEARL**
>
> The treatment of type III injuries is controversial. Historically, most of these injuries have been treated surgically. However, most clinicians now consider conservative management to be equally effective.

Surgery is clearly indicated for type IV, V and VI injuries and those type III injuries that fail to respond adequately to conservative management.[97]

Chronic acromioclavicular joint pain
Chronic AC joint pain may occur as a result of repeated minor injuries to the AC joint or following a type II or

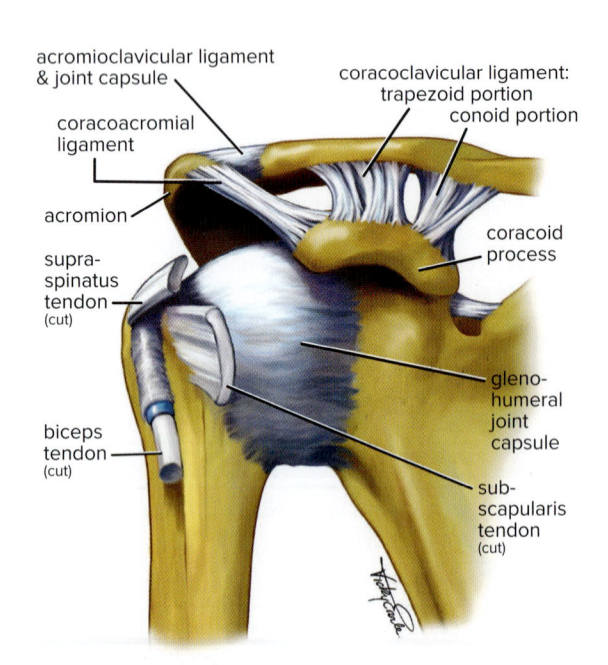

Figure 24.49 The acromioclavicular joint

Shoulder pain   CHAPTER 24

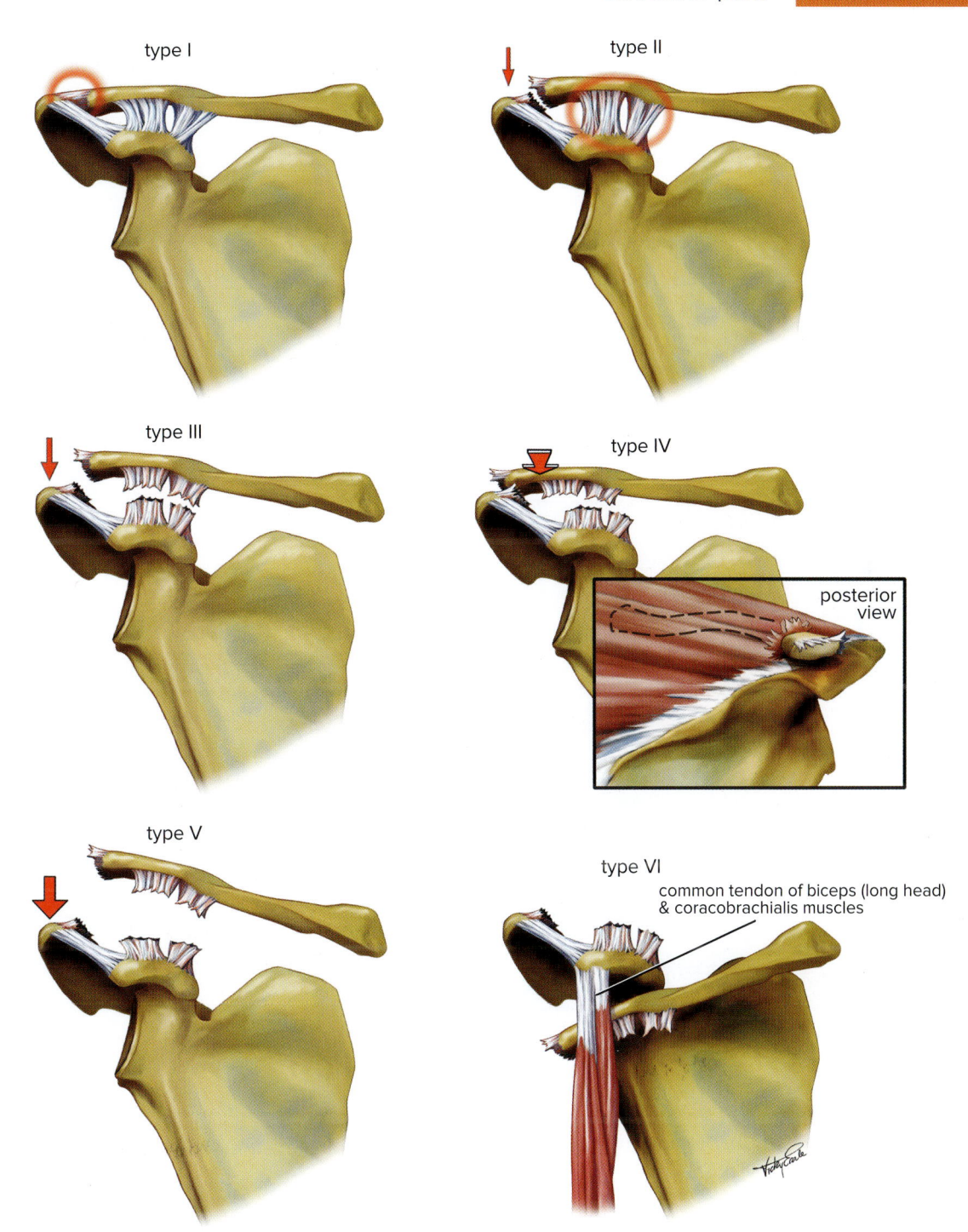

Figure 24.50 Classification of acromioclavicular joint injuries

type III injury. This can damage the fibrocartilaginous meniscus situated within the AC joint.

Another cause of chronic AC joint pain, osteolysis of the outer end of the clavicle, is seen occasionally, especially in weightlifters performing large numbers of bench presses. X-ray in this condition shows a 'moth-eaten' appearance of the distal end of the clavicle (Fig. 24.53). Horizontal flexion is painful. Rotator cuff impingement may occur due to the abnormal scapular position that results from loss of the clavicle strut. Treatment consists

427

PART B   Regional problems

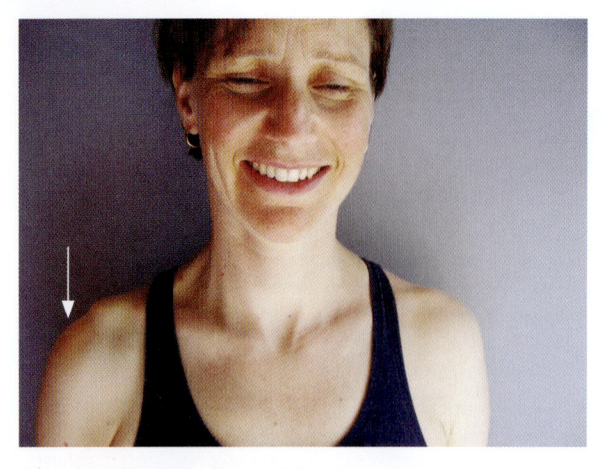

Figure 24.51 Marked step deformity at the acromioclavicular joint in type III injury

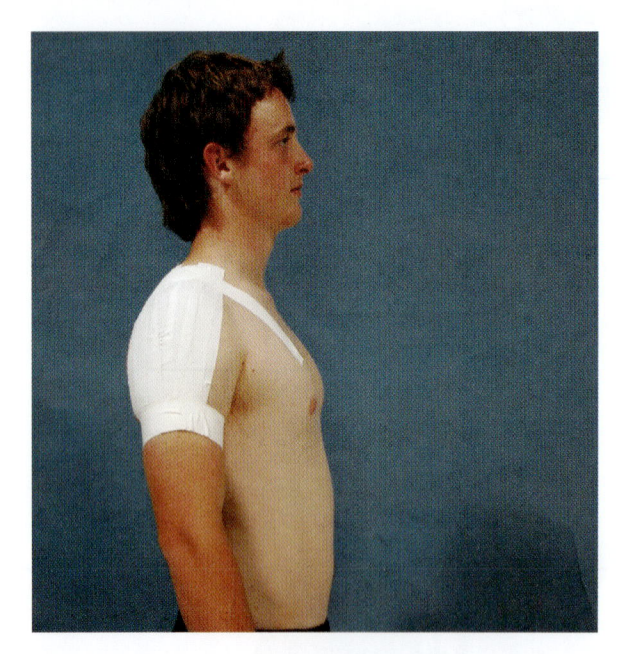

Figure 24.52 Taping after acromioclavicular joint injury

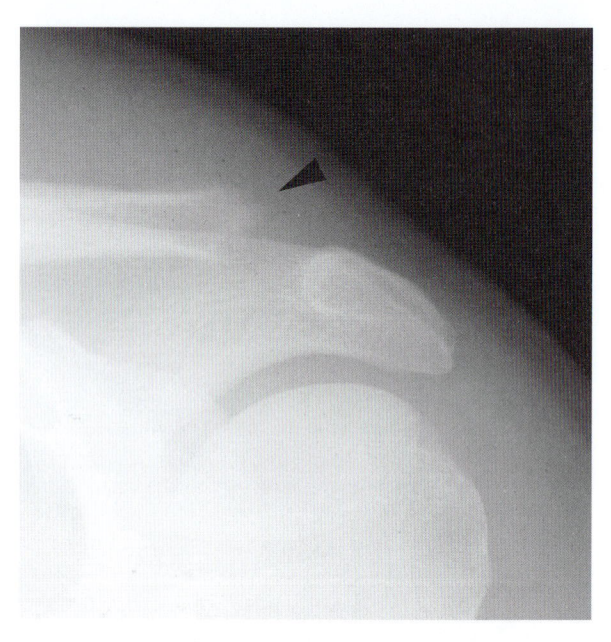

Figure 24.53 Osteolysis of the outer end of the clavicle, showing a 'moth-eaten' appearance

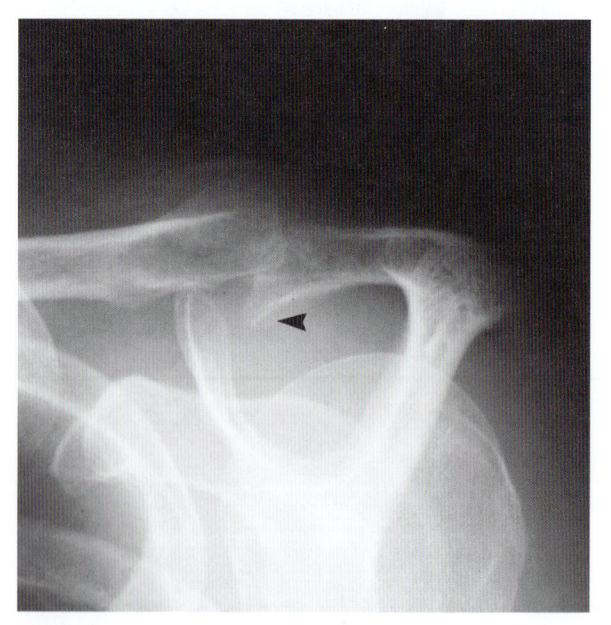

Figure 24.54 Post-traumatic osteoarthritis of the acromioclavicular joint showing a spur and bony irregularity on the acromion

of physiotherapy, including pain relieving modalities and mobilisation, combined with muscle strengthening.

Osteoarthritis of the AC joint may occur as a result of recurrent injuries. This is characterised by a typical radiographic appearance with sclerosis and osteophyte formation (Fig. 24.54).

AC joint pain is usually localised over the joint. Symptoms may be reproduced by AC joint compression using O'Brien's test (with both test positions giving symptoms) or cross-arm adduction. An injection of local anaesthetic and corticosteroid into the AC joint can confirm the diagnosis and provide effective symptom relief.

Persistent AC joint pain may require arthroscopic distal clavicle excision.[98] The surgeon must take care not to disrupt the ligamentous attachments to the distal clavicle. More than 5 mm resection alters the joint loads and removes the bony attachments.[98]

Shoulder pain CHAPTER 24

LESS COMMON CAUSES OF SHOULDER PAIN

As shown in Table 24.1, there are a number of less common causes of shoulder pain. These include other muscle tears, adhesive capsulitis, neurovascular injuries, other fractures and the 'snapping scapula'.

Other muscle tears around the shoulder

Other muscle tears around the shoulder include the long head of biceps, pectoralis major and subscapularis.

Rupture of the long head of the biceps

Rupture of the loaded long head of the biceps muscle may occur in the older athlete and is usually accompanied by immediate sharp pain and a tearing sensation.

The deformity is obvious—the muscle is detached from its proximal attachment and bunches up in the distal arm. The deformity is accentuated by contraction of the biceps. Often there is little ongoing pain. Surprisingly, biceps strength is almost fully maintained. Imaging is via MRI or ultrasound. Those who do not rely on their upper arm in sport are generally satisfied with reassurance and require no definitive treatment. In those who perform power sports, surgery may be indicated.

Pectoralis major tears

Pectoralis major tears may be partial ruptures (grades I–II) or complete (grade III).[99] Complete rupture occurs at the site of its insertion to the humerus. This is usually seen in weight training, especially when performing a bench press. The typical history is of sudden onset of pain on the medial aspect of the upper arm. Examination reveals localised tenderness and swelling. Resisted contraction of the pectoralis major is weak and may be painful.

A partial tear is treated conservatively with ice and a strengthening program over a period of 4–6 weeks. A complete tear of the pectoralis major should be treated by surgical repair.[100] It is usually possible to differentiate between a partial and a complete tear clinically. Ultrasound or MRI examination may assist in this differentiation.

Subscapularis muscle tears

Tears of the subscapularis muscle can occur with sudden forceful external rotation or extension applied to the abducted arm. There is usually no associated instability. The main complaint is pain, and range of motion may be maintained or even increased. On examination, the patient will have increased passive external rotation with the shoulder adducted at the side, weakness of internal rotation and a positive lift-off sign (Fig. 21.2h). MRI and ultrasound will confirm the diagnosis. Treatment should be immediate surgical repair.

Adhesive capsulitis—'frozen shoulder'

Glenohumeral joint stiffness is not uncommon after significant trauma, for instance, a fracture or surgery. It may also follow an injury to the neural structures in the neck or it may occur spontaneously.

The age group in which spontaneous shoulder stiffness, commonly referred to as adhesive capsulitis, occurs is between 40 and 60 years of age. Idiopathic adhesive capsulitis more commonly affects the non-dominant shoulder and is more prevalent in women than men (1.3:1). Adhesive capsulitis is more common in patients with diabetes and there is an association with thyroid disorders and drugs that involve inhibition of matrix degradation.

The diagnosis of shoulder stiffness is relatively easy to make by evaluating passive external rotation with the elbow at the side. Care should be taken to stabilise the scapula when examining for shoulder stiffness as significant range of motion can occur at the scapulothoracic articulation. Surgical or post-traumatic scapular stiffness usually resolves within 12 months and further surgical intervention is rarely necessary. Physiotherapy may be valuable.

Idiopathic adhesive capsulitis is a self-limiting condition that resolves, on average, over 1.5 years.[101] There is no evidence that intensive physiotherapy, injections[102] or drugs change the outcome of idiopathic adhesive capsulitis. However, pain-relieving techniques and modalities, as well as patient education during the painful phase are useful and appreciated by the patient. During the resolving phase, graded mobilisation and a home stretching and strengthening program assist the patient in the natural recovery process.

Arthroscopic capsular release to divide the thickened shoulder capsule and an early aggressive supervised range of motion program are not effective at restoring motion and relieving pain in patients with idiopathic adhesive capsulitis.[103, 104]

Neurovascular injuries

Suprascapular nerve entrapment

The most common entrapment is of the suprascapular nerve.[105] The suprascapular nerve is derived from the upper trunk of the brachial plexus formed by the roots of the C5 and C6 nerves. The course of the nerve is shown in Figure 24.55. The nerve passes downwards beneath the trapezius to the superior border of the scapula. Here it passes through the suprascapular notch. The roof of this notch is formed by the transverse scapular ligament. After passing through the notch, the nerve supplies the supraspinatus muscle as well as articular branches to both the glenohumeral and AC joints. The nerve then turns around the lateral edge of the base of the spine of

429

PART B Regional problems

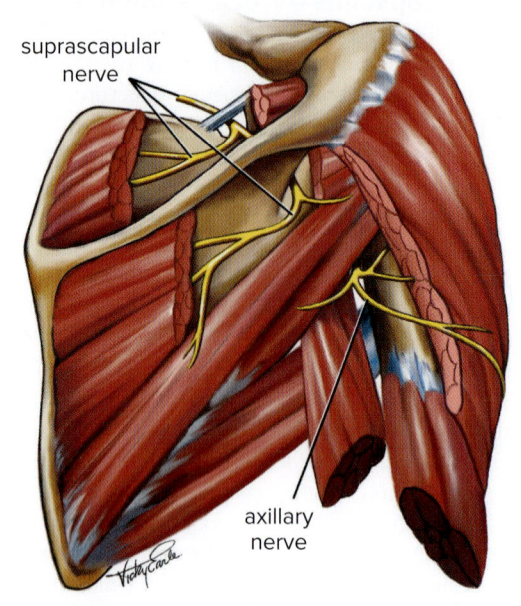

Figure 24.55 Course of the suprascapular nerve

the scapula (the spinoglenoid notch) to innervate the infraspinatus muscle. Entrapment of the suprascapular nerve may occur at either the suprascapular notch or the spinoglenoid notch.

The patient usually complains of pain that is deep and poorly localised. It is often felt posteriorly and laterally in the shoulder, or referred to the arm, neck or upper anterior chest wall. The patient may describe shoulder weakness. On examination, there may be wasting of the supraspinatus and/or infraspinatus muscles accompanied by weakness on abduction and external rotation. Tenderness over the suprascapular notch may also be present.

The site of entrapment in cases of combined supraspinatus and infraspinatus weakness is the suprascapular notch. The nerve may be stretched and kinked in this position by extremes of scapular motion associated with the throwing action. It may also occur in tennis players who complain of weakness and lack of control over backhand volleys. Diagnosis is made on the clinical symptoms and confirmed by an abnormal electromyogram. Surgical decompression of the nerve at the site of entrapment is occasionally required.

Isolated infraspinatus weakness and wasting may occur when the suprascapular nerve is trapped at the spinoglenoid notch. This condition has been seen in volleyball players who use the 'float' serve[106, 107] and in weight lifters. It can also arise due to a cyst that results from superior glenoid labral tears compressing the nerve. Treatment should be directed to repairing the labral tear.

The main task of the coach and sports physician is to monitor external rotation strength on a regular basis (for instance using a hand-held dynamometer) in an athletic population known to be at risk for suprascapular nerve pathology such as volleyball players, and to give an external rotator strengthening program in the injury prevention program. In particular, focusing on external rotation strength training in several positions (neutral, abduction, forward flexion) guarantees sufficient training of all external rotators, infraspinatus as well as teres minor.[108]

Long thoracic nerve injury

The long thoracic nerve is formed from the roots of the C5, C6 and C7 nerves. The nerve passes behind the brachial plexus to perforate the fascia of the proximal serratus anterior, passing medial to the coracoid with branches throughout the length of the serratus anterior. Long thoracic nerve palsy causes paralysis of the serratus anterior, with winging of the scapula. The nerve may be injured by traction on the neck or shoulder or by blunt trauma. Isolated long thoracic nerve palsy may also follow viral illnesses.

Clinical features include pain and limited shoulder elevation. Patients may complain of difficulty in lifting weights or an uncomfortable feeling of pressure from a chair against a winged scapula while sitting. They may also develop secondary impingement due to poor scapular control. The most striking feature on examination is winging of the scapula when pushing against a wall with both hands. Electromyographic studies will confirm the diagnosis. Initial treatment is conservative and most patients will recover fully. During the rehabilitation period, it is extremely important to give the patient exercises in which the winging is minimally present or suppressed. Very often, this is only possible with low load closed chain exercises. Surgical tendon transfer may occasionally be required.

Axillary nerve injury

Axillary nerve compression or quadrilateral space syndrome is an uncommon condition caused by compression of the posterior humeral circumflex artery and axillary nerve or one of its major branches in the quadrilateral space.[109] The quadrilateral or quadrangular space is located over the posterior scapula in the subdeltoid region and consists of the teres minor superiorly, teres major inferiorly, the long head of triceps medially and the surgical neck of the humerus laterally. The axillary nerve and the posterior humeral circumflex artery pass through the space at a level inferior to the glenohumeral joint capsule.

Quadrilateral space syndrome is seen in throwing athletes and is characterised by poorly localised posterior shoulder pain, paraesthesia over the lateral aspect of the shoulder and arm, and deltoid and teres minor weakness. The condition may occur secondary to abnormal fibrous

Shoulder pain   CHAPTER 24

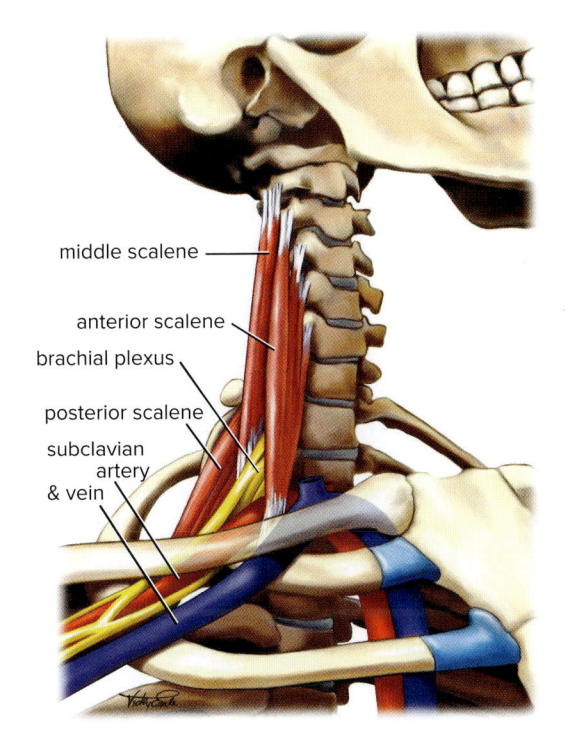

Figure 24.56 Anatomy of the thoracic outlet

bands, although traumatic causes have been described. Diagnosis is by electromyography or subclavian arteriogram, although this is associated with some risk. Treatment is initially conservative. Occasionally, surgical exploration is required.

Axillary nerve injuries can also occur with anterior dislocation of the shoulder and by blunt trauma to the anterior lateral deltoid muscle.[110]

Thoracic outlet syndrome

The term thoracic outlet syndrome (TOS) refers to a group of conditions that result from compression of the neurovascular structures that course from the neck to the axilla through the thoracic outlet (Fig. 24.56). The brachial plexus and subclavian vessels are especially susceptible to compression because of their proximity to one another in the thoracic outlet. The most common site of compression is the costoclavicular space between the clavicle and the first rib (costoclavicular syndrome).[111] Other sites of compression are the triangle between the anterior scalene muscle, the middle scalene muscle and the upper border of the first rib (anterior scalene syndrome); and the angle between the coracoid process and the pectoralis minor insertion (hyperabduction syndrome or pectoralis minor syndrome).

This condition may occur in overhead athletes. Poor posture with drooping shoulders and scapular protraction can decrease the diameter of the cervicoaxillary canal, causing TOS symptoms.

Congenital anatomical abnormalities including complete cervical rib, incomplete cervical ribs with fibrous bands, fibrous bands from the transverse process of C7, and clavicular abnormalities, can all compress the neurovascular structures. Complete cervical ribs are rare but, if present, are often bilateral. However, only 10% of patients with cervical ribs have TOS symptoms.

Traumatic structural changes that can cause TOS include fractures of the clavicle and/or first rib, pseudoarthrosis of the clavicle, mal-union of clavicle fractures, exuberant callus formation or a crush injury of the upper thorax. TOS symptoms are common in patients with chronic scapular dyskinesis. They have tight pectoralis minor, scalene and upper trapezius muscles, with weak serratus anterior and lower trapezius muscles; this causes excessive anterior tilt and protraction.

Clinical features

While patients with TOS occasionally present with a pure arterial, venous or neurogenic picture, most often the picture is mixed. The patient with TOS may complain of pain in the neck or shoulder, or numbness or tingling involving either the entire upper limb or the forearm and hand. The patient may state that the arm feels weak or easily fatigued. There may be venous engorgement or coolness of the involved arm.

Physical signs may be absent. A patient with arterial compression may have a positive Adson's test. The patient begins the test with the head laterally rotated to the side of the symptoms and extended. The patient then abducts the involved arm and inspires deeply. A positive test obliterates the radial pulse and reproduces symptoms. The sensitivity of this test can be greatly increased by the use of Doppler flow patterns during the manoeuvre. The most sensitive provocation test is the Roos hyperabduction/external rotation test (Fig 24.13a), in which the patient opens and closes his or her hands for 1–3 minutes with elbows bent and arms abducted to 90° and externally rotated in an attempt to reproduce the symptoms. Evaluation of scapular motion and position can help to rule scapular dyskinesis in or out.

Treatment

Treatment for any subset of TOS focuses on the specific area compromised. However, certain treatments apply to all forms of TOS. Correction of drooping shoulders, poor posture and poor body mechanics is vital. The patient should be taught proper positioning while sitting, standing and lying down. Physiotherapy should include pectoral and scalene stretching and trigger point treatment, and soft tissue mobilisation of restricted tissues, as well as scapular and scapulothoracic mobilisation. Joint mobilisation of the first rib can restore accessory motion of the sternoclavicular and AC joints. Therapeutic exercise, education and manual therapy can correct forward head posture. Thoracic extension and brachial plexus neuromobility exercises are added as tolerated.

Surgical consultation and treatment is warranted for patients who have neurogenic TOS that does not respond to aggressive conservative management and for patients who have vascular compromise or thrombus formation.[112] Arterial compression caused by a complete cervical rib is usually treated by first rib resection.

Axillary vein thrombosis ('effort' thrombosis)

Axillary vein thrombosis is also known as 'effort' thrombosis because of its frequent association with repetitive, vigorous activities or with blunt trauma that results in direct or indirect injury to the vein. The axillary vein can be compressed at various sites along its path, most significantly in the costoclavicular space. Compression most often occurs when the patient hyperextends the neck and hyperabducts the arm simultaneously, or when the patient assumes a military brace position with a backward thrust of the shoulders. Compression can also occur between the clavicle and the first rib, the costocoracoid ligament and first rib, or the subclavian muscles and first rib.

Patients complain of dull, aching pain, numbness or tightness, and heaviness of the upper arm and shoulder, along with fatigue after activities involving the extremity. In axillary vein thrombosis, the entire upper extremity will be swollen, the skin may be mottled and cold, and superficial veins may be prominent. The diagnosis is confirmed on venography.

Treatment involves immediate anticoagulant therapy. Most patients make a full recovery and are able to resume sporting activities.[113]

Less common fractures around the shoulder

Stress fractures around the shoulder joint are uncommon. Stress fracture of the coracoid process is associated with the sport of trapshooting. Patients with this stress fracture have localised tenderness over the coracoid process and a focal area of abnormality on MRI or isotopic bone scan. Another specific site of stress fractures is anterolateral rib fractures in rowers, probably due to excessive activation of the serratus anterior (see Chapter 9).

Scapular fractures are usually due to a crushing force, either a fall on the shoulder or direct violence. Examination reveals marked tenderness and swelling. X-rays should be taken to exclude other associated injuries, such as a rib fracture, dislocated shoulder or dislocated sternoclavicular joint. Scapular fractures usually heal well, even if displaced. A broad arm sling is worn for comfort and active movements are commenced as soon as pain permits.

Fracture of the neck of the humerus is caused by a fall on the outstretched hand or direct violence.[114] It is seen in adolescents, young adults and the elderly. Fractures involving more than two fragments displaced by more than 1 cm or associated with shoulder dislocation require surgical assessment. Minimally displaced or angulated fractures may be treated conservatively. Impacted fractures heal rapidly and can be supported in a broad arm sling. Displaced fractures are best treated in a collar and cuff that allows gravity to correct any angulation. For the first 2 weeks the arm should be kept in a sling under a shirt. After 2 weeks, pendular movement exercises of the shoulder joint should be commenced. From 4 weeks, a collar and cuff may be worn outside the clothes and gradually removed in stages over the following 2 weeks.

An unusual fracture is seen among throwing athletes. These athletes sustain a closed external rotation spiral fracture of their humerus immediately below the insertion of the deltoid muscle at the junction of the middle and lower thirds of the humerus or along the radial groove. Many, but not all, patients with this fracture give a history of pain at the site of the fracture so it may be regarded as a rapid-onset stress fracture. The fracture heals well in a cast or functional brace.

Snapping scapula

The scapula is surrounded by a number of scapular bursae to allow smooth movement over the thoracic wall. Snapping scapula syndrome or scapulothoracic bursitis is a condition characterised by periscapular crepitus and pain during arm movements. While some patients are mildly symptomatic, others may complain of severe pain and poor shoulder function even with simple tasks.

Snapping scapula is the result of a lack of congruence between the concave scapula and the convex thoracic wall, which can occur from anatomic predisposition, space-occupying skeletal lesions, fibrotic bursae, poor thoracic posture or scapular muscle control.[115] Often the scapulothoracic bursitis is the result of combined structural (fibrotic bursae, elastofibroma) and functional (tightness of surrounding musculature, for instance pectoralis minor) deficits.

Regardless of the aetiology, current data support initial conservative treatment in patients with symptomatic snapping scapula. Non-operative treatment consists of non-steroidal anti-inflammatory medications, therapeutic injections of steroids and local anaesthetics into the inflamed bursa, activity modification and physiotherapy. Surgical treatment, bursectomy, is indicated after failure of conservative management. However, if anatomical lesions or deformities capable of producing scapular snapping are identified on imaging, primary surgical intervention is the favourable treatment option. Radiographic evaluation of the snapping scapula is important to rule out osseous deformity, tumours or other bony causes of the patient's pain. Three-dimensional CT and MRI aid in detecting muscle, bony and soft tissue abnormalities.[116]

SPECIAL CONSIDERATIONS FOR THE OVERHEAD ATHLETE

In any overhead athlete with a shoulder injury, the role of the kinetic chain (Chapter 8) must be considered.

Kinetic chain integration

It is important to re-establish the kinetic chain early in the rehabilitation process. While the shoulder is recovering from the injury or surgery, leg and trunk exercises can be prescribed so that when the shoulder is ready for rehabilitation, the base of the kinetic chain is also ready for linked activity. After the shoulder is ready for rehabilitation, sport-specific activation of the kinetic chain patterns restores the force-dependent motor activation patterns and normal biomechanical positions. This then allows normal link sequencing to generate velocity and force.

The athlete's kinetic chain is highly sport-specific, and varies for every athlete. In ground-based sports, like baseball, tennis or cricket, all of the activities of the shoulder work within a kinetic chain linkage from the ground through to the trunk, mostly in a diagonal pattern. These athletes benefit from diagonal pattern exercises in a closed chain for the lower extremities. In addition, performing shoulder exercises standing on the contralateral leg enhances scapular muscle activity[117] (Fig. 24.57a). However, sports like volleyball, gymnastics and swimming have totally different movement patterns, and thus different demands from their kinetic chain. Volleyball players load their shoulder the most

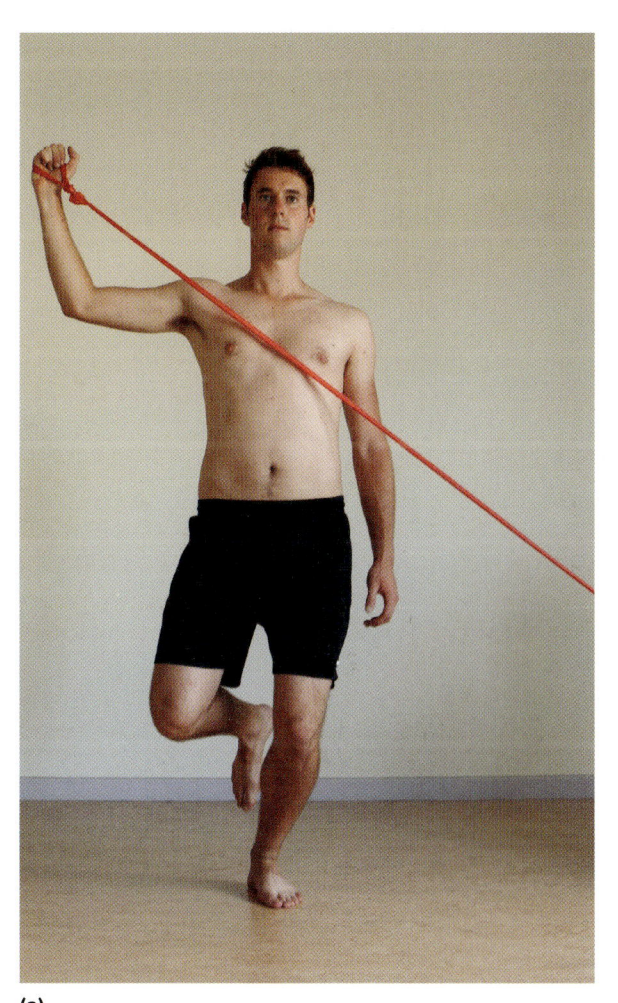

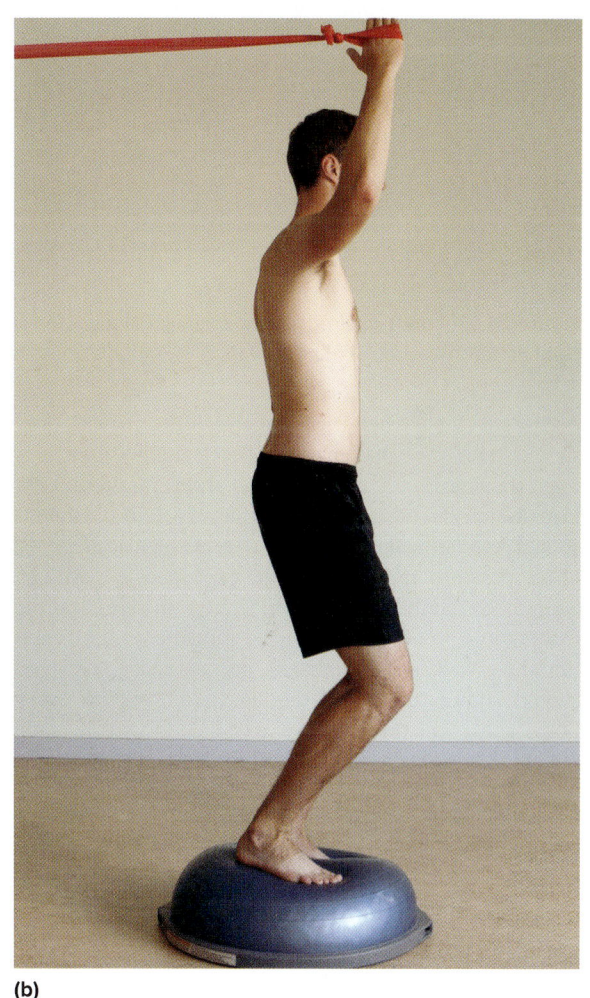

(a)   (b)

Figure 24.57 (a) Diagonal external rotation exercise standing on the contralateral leg (b) Throwing exercise on an unstable surface

PART B Regional problems

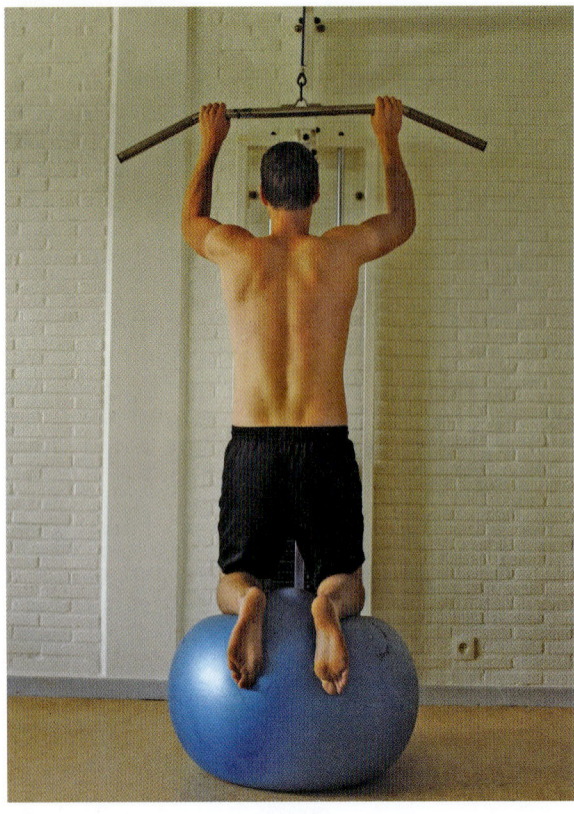

(c)

Figure 24.57 (cont.) (c) Progressive 'training hanging' for gymnasts

during smashing, when their feet are off the ground. They should train the smashing and decelerating capacity of their shoulders with minimal input from the ground, for instance on an unstable surface (Fig. 24.57b). Gymnasts should train in hanging (Fig. 24.57c) or high load closed chain positions mimicking their sport-specific positions. Swimmers should focus on endurance in a concentric manner in a prone (Fig. 24.58) and supine position. Tennis (for the two-handed backhand), hockey and golf players should additionally pay attention to movements using both hands. Athletes who have to be able to 'fall' (diving in volleyball, goal keepers in soccer) should be trained to do so, for instance using sliding boards (Fig. 24.59).

> **PRACTICE PEARL**
>
> It is important to correct any inflexibilities of the hamstrings, hip and trunk; weakness or imbalances of the rotators of the trunk, flexors and extensors of the trunk and hip; and any subclinical adaptations of stance patterns or gait pattern.

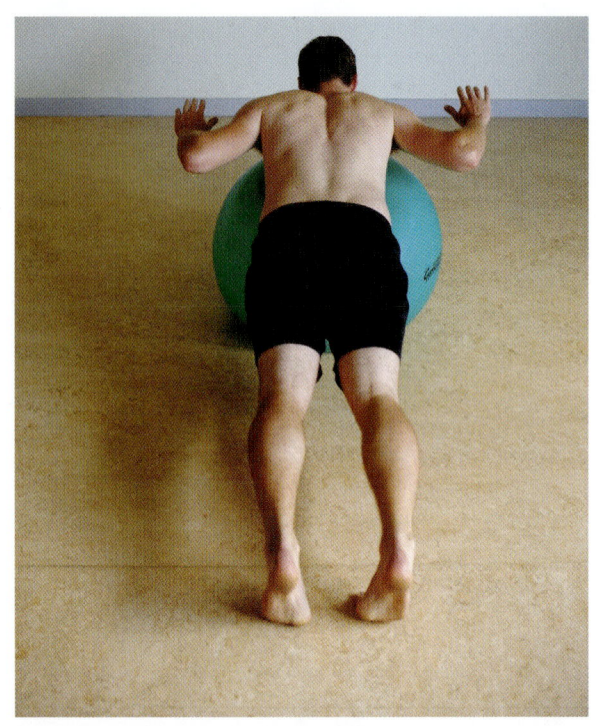

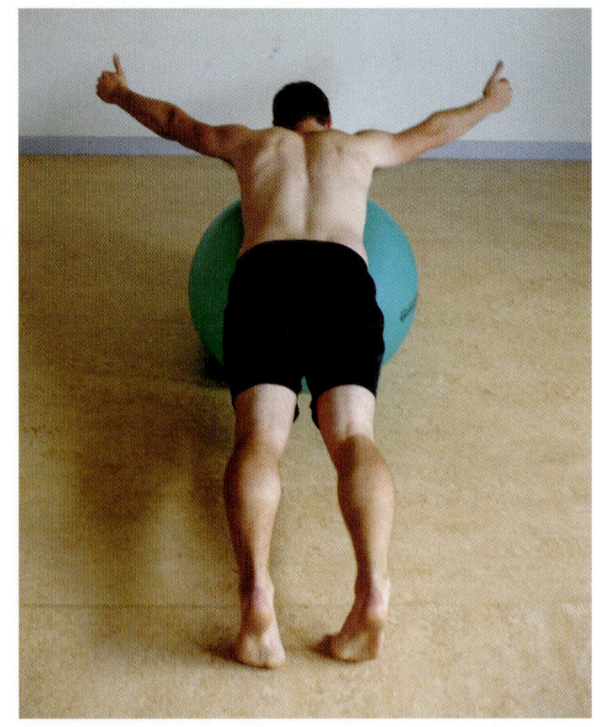

(a)

(b)

Figure 24.58 Prone exercise W-V—patient moves the arms from (a) Elbow in the back pockets (W) up to (b) High elevation (V)

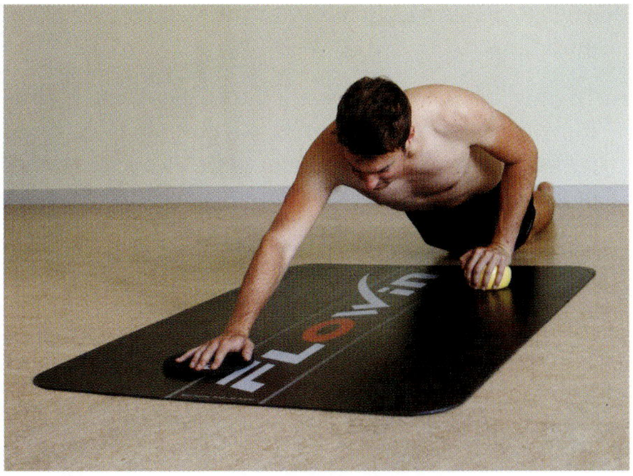

Shoulder pain CHAPTER 24

Figure 24.59 Exercise training for impact on a gliding surface

In ground-based sports, rehabilitation of the legs and hips should be concerned with generating appropriate sport-specific force and velocity from the lower extremity and should be done in a closed chain. This pattern, which is done with the foot on the ground, simulates the patterns that exist in the throwing or hitting activities. Eccentric patterns should also be emphasised to absorb the load from jumping forward movement or stopping of the plant leg in the baseball throw. Combined patterns of hip and trunk rotation in both directions, hip and shoulder diagonal patterns should also be emphasised. Integration of the scapular retraction muscles to the hip is very important because these reactions tend to be coupled in the cocking phases of throwing. Hip extension and trunk stability should be trained performing squatting exercises.

Endurance activities in the legs should also be emphasised, as should aerobic endurance for recovery from exercise bouts and anaerobic endurance for agility and power work. Examples include mini-trampoline exercises, agility drills with running and jumping, jumping jacks and slider or fitter boards.

When working in closed chain, the kinetic chain activity also benefits from diagonal patterns. Research has shown that lower trapezius activity is increased when, during the four-point kneeling position, the contralateral leg is extended.[118]

The thrower's program

Various thrower's programs are published, all aiming at progressively training the shoulder in order to prepare the athlete to throw in baseball, serve in tennis, smash in volleyball.[74] The main goal is to increase the challenge versus throwing by (a) changing shoulder position from neutral to full abduction/external rotation (ABER), (b) gradually increasing speed of movement, (c) implementing sport-specific kinetic chain skills, such as diagonals and core stability, into the shoulder exercises. For the latter we refer to the previous paragraph. All the following exercises should be considered to be functional, meaning adding kinetic chain principles where appropriate, depending on the specific sports; they are described below in view of shoulder loading only.

The goals and types of exercises are summarised in Table 24.7.

Table 24.7 Which exercises to prescribe depends on the clinician's goal

Goal	Type of exercise
Basic RC training	ER and IR in neutral
From neutral to functional ABER	ER and IR diagonal with limited load in ABER
Increasing load in ABER	'Throwing' movement slow with high load in ABER
increasing speed in ABER—low load	Quick low-load ER and IR movements in ABER
Functional throwing and decelerating	'Throwing' movement fast with high load in ABER
Focus on eccentric strength of the external rotators	Slow high-resistance eccentric exercise (avoid or limit concentric phase to enhance eccentric loading)
Focus on deceleration of the posterior shoulder muscles	'Catching' exercises
Focus on stretch-shortening phase of throwing	Use material that challenges plyometric cycle of throwing

RC = rotator cuff; ER = external rotation; IR = internal rotation; ABER = abduction external rotation

PART B Regional problems

The program starts with IR and ER exercises with the shoulder in neutral position (Fig. 24.21b and c) or in slight elevation in the scapular plane. These positions put no strain on the shoulder capsule and allow strengthening in a safe position; however, they should be considered as non-functional from a sport-specific point of view. ER may also be performed with the athlete side-lying, to enhance proper UT/LT muscle balance (Fig 24.45a). If allowed (depending on the injury), eccentric drills in neutral may be performed, with side-lying catching exercises (Fig. 24.60). This exercise can be performed in the early stage, for instance in labral injury or instability, however, in case of muscle or tendon strain or overload injury, it should be postponed to a later stage.

The next stage of exercises brings the athlete's shoulder from neutral position to higher elevation angles and towards the throwing position; however, with limited load in that position. Examples are IR and ER diagonals towards or starting at the contralateral hip, standing sideways to the point of resistance (Fig. 24.61a and b). In addition, side-lying forward flexion and prone horizontal abduction with external rotation may be performed (see scapular rehabilitation). Eccentric exercises for the infraspinatus/trapezius may be implemented performing side-lying catching exercises with the shoulder in 90° of forward flexion.

- To increase the challenge of the shoulder towards throwing positions, the load in this position is increased by facing the point of resistance (for ER) (Fig. 24.62a), or standing backwards towards it (for IR) (Fig. 24.62b), and performing slow throwing movements.
- After these rather slow exercises, speed is implemented in two steps: first, quick movements are performed in the ABER (abduction-external rotation) position into

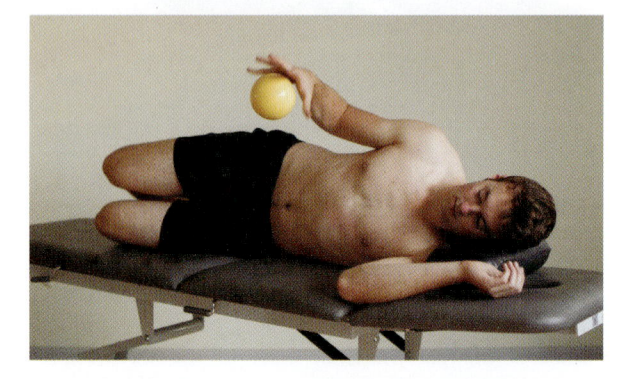

Figure 24.60 Side-lying plyometric catching exercise

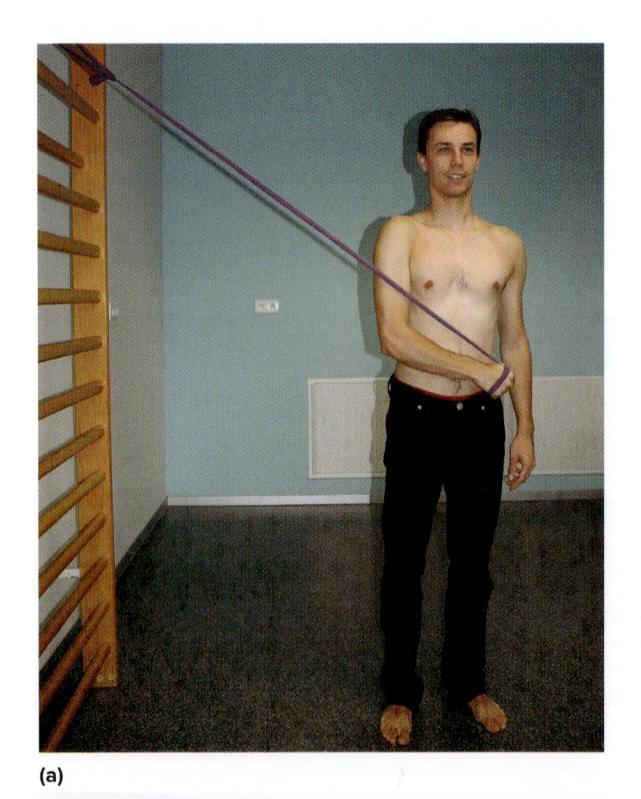

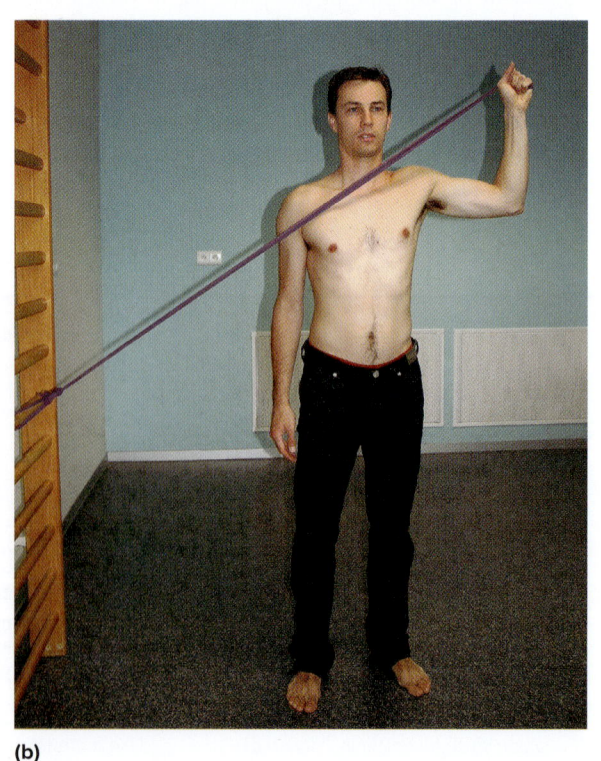

Figure 24.61 Diagonal (a) Internal and (b) External rotation with moderate load

Shoulder pain   CHAPTER 24

(a)   (b)

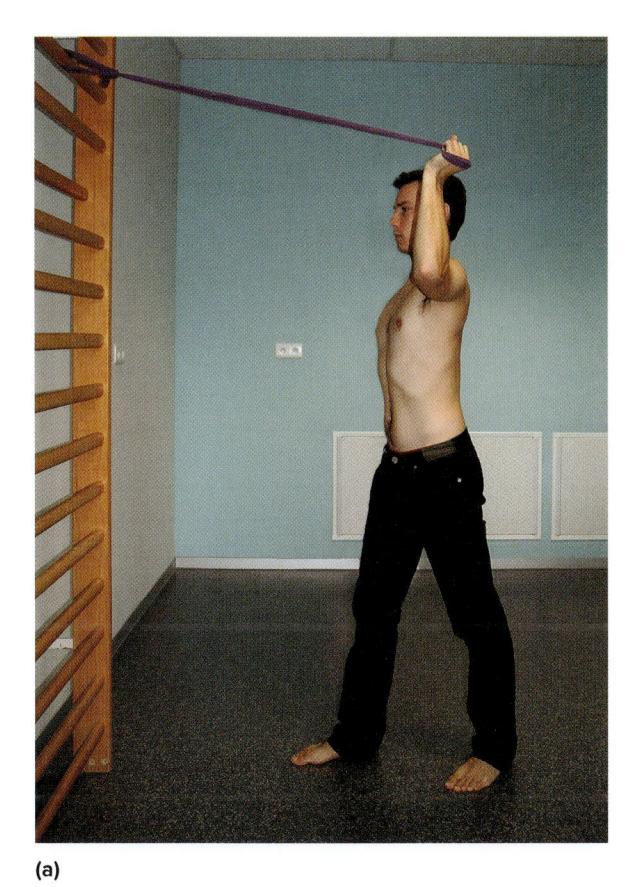

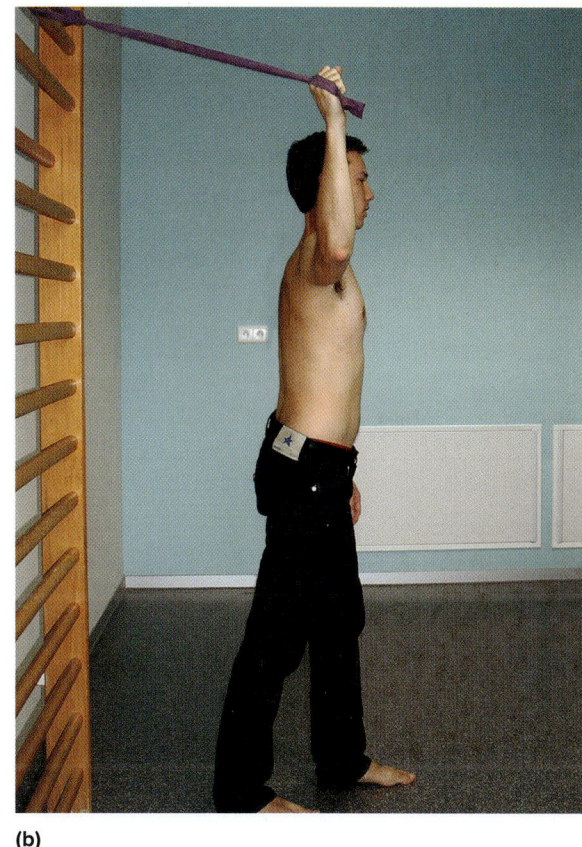

Figure 24.62 The load is increased by facing the point of resistance (a) For ER or (b) Standing backwards towards it for IR

IR and ER without explosive strength, later on more explosive exercises, challenging the stretch-shortening cycle and plyometric nature of throwing are performed. During the first step, endurance is the exercise goal, and the athlete is encouraged to perform the exercise at two or more reps per second for 30 to 60 seconds consecutively. At the end of this stage, the athlete should also be able to perform catching exercises prone with the shoulder in ABER (Fig. 24.22).

- In the final stage of basic throwing exercises, the patient performs quick throwing movements against resistance to train the acceleration as well as the deceleration mechanism. In addition, the stretch-shortening cycle may be trained by the use of equipment that 'decelerates' the turning point between IR and ER (Fig. 24.23).
- In line with specific shoulder training, the therapist should not forget to pay additional attention to the elbow and the wrist and grip strength muscles.

Return to play following shoulder injury

According to the decision-based return-to-play model[119] (Chapter 19), three steps need to be taken prior to full return to sports. In the first step, the health status of the athlete is evaluated, including assessment of symptoms and a battery of analytical and functional tests, for instance strength and flexibility, and throwing performance. Then the clinician evaluates the participation risk, based on the type of sport, level of competition and ability to protect the shoulder. Finally, some factors might modify the decision such as the timing in the season, pressure from the athlete or the environment. However, little evidence exists regarding the physical return-to-play criteria of the shoulder after injury. In particular, for each of the described risk factors, from a clinical perspective, there is a need for cut-off values to be used as criteria for return to train and return to play. In addition, the clinician needs objective and valid assessment tools applicable on the field or the

PART B   Regional problems

training area of the athlete, and finally, once deficits are assessed, there is a need for science-based training programs to restore normal values.

The following return-to-play criteria (Table 24.8), although not extensively supported by scientific evidence, may be used.[120, 121]

Table 24.8 Return-to-play (RTP) criteria for the overhead throwing athlete following shoulder injury

Return-to-play criterion	Specific details
No/little pain	Self-report
Full ROM	Side difference GIRD <20°, TROM <5°
Normal strength	Dominant side 10% stronger in throwers, equal in strength in symmetric sports ER/IR ratio 66% (isokinetic), 75% (HHD in neutral), 95% (HHD in 90° abduction)
Normal scapular function	Slight scapular asymmetry allowed in resting position Scapular upward rotation +/− 60° in full elevation Dominant side 10% stronger in throwers, equal in strength in symmetric sports
Normal functional ability	Seated medicine ball throw Y-balance test Endurance test rotator cuff (elastic band, X-CO Trainer®)
Normal sport-specific skills	Having completed the thrower's program or another sport-specific program (non-throwing sports)

ROM = range of motion; GIRD = glenohumeral internal rotation deficit; TROM = total range of motion

REFERENCES

References for this chapter can be found at www.mhhe.com/au/CSM5e

Chapter 25

Elbow and arm pain

with BILL VICENZINO, ALEX SCOTT, SIMON BELL and NEBOJSA POPOVIC

Throwing warmup pitches to start the bottom of the second inning, Hudson felt some tightness around his elbow. On the second pitch that inning, he felt that something was seriously wrong. His fastball dipped to about 85 mph, and he became hittable. He stayed in the game and completed the inning . . . but that . . . would be Hudson's last pitch for another year.
Report on Major League Baseball pitcher Daniel Hudson's return from two ulnar collateral ligament surgeries

A well-functioning elbow is essential for upper limb use in sports. Elbow injuries may even interfere with an athlete's everyday activities. Tennis was the classic cause of elbow pain, but the double-handed backhand has reduced the prevalence of 'tennis elbow' dramatically. Elbow pain remains a problem in golf and in sports such as volleyball and handball, which involve forceful elbow hyperextension.

To approach elbow pain in clinical practice, consider which of the following categories describes your patient's elbow pain:

- lateral elbow pain, with a particular focus on extensor tendinopathy
- medial elbow pain
- posterior elbow pain
- acute elbow injuries
- forearm pain
- upper arm pain.

ANATOMY

The elbow is situated between two highly mobile joints, the shoulder and the wrist, and comprises three distinct articulations–the ulna-humeral, radio-capitellar and proximal radio-ulnar joints. The first two provide flexion (150°) and extension (0°) of the elbow and the third provides pronation/supination (85°/85°) of the forearm. The proximal radio-ulnar joint works in conjunction with the distal radio-ulnar joint at the wrist to achieve forearm pronation-supination. With the forearm in full extension and supination there will be a physiological valgus (carrying angle) of 9–14° in men or 12–17° in women. Any increase or loss of this physiological angle is a sign of pathology (instability, mal-union or overuse). Elbow stability is provided by the osseous anatomy, capsuloligamentous structure and musculotendinous units that cross the elbow.

Ligaments

The ligaments of the elbow are divided into lateral and medial collateral ligament complexes. The medial collateral ligament complex is composed of discrete bands; the lateral collateral ligament complex consists of complex ligament fibres.

The medial collateral ligament complex (MCLC) is composed of the anterior oblique, posterior and transverse bands. The anterior band is the primary constraint against valgus stress, contributing 55 to 70% of valgus stability of the elbow. There are two elements of the anterior band: the anterior non-isometric and posterior isometric bundles. There is sequential tightening of these bundles proceeding from anterior to posterior when the elbow is flexed from full extension. The fan-shaped posterior band of the MCLC is a thickening of the capsule that is best defined with the elbow flexed at 90°. The posterior band does not contribute significantly to valgus stability of the elbow except in near terminal flexion. The transverse band

(TB) does not cross the joint, but exists as a thickening of the most caudal portion of the joint capsule. The TB contributes little to elbow stability because it originates from and inserts on the ulna.

The lateral collateral ligament complex (LCLC) consists of four components–the annular ligament, radial collateral ligament, lateral ulnar collateral ligament and accessory lateral collateral ligament–as well as the anconeus muscle (which acts as a dynamic stabiliser). These ligaments provide varus and external rotation stability to the elbow. This ligament complex is isometric throughout the normal range of flexion and extension with little change in the distance between ligament origin and insertion as the ligament complex is near the axis of rotation. There is controversy about the function of the different components of the LCLC.

Muscles

Four muscle groups control elbow dynamic stability: the flexors and extensors of the elbow and the pronators and supinators of the proximal radio-ulnar joint. The flexor and extensor muscles provide some compression across the joint, increasing the inherent stability provided by the congruent articular surfaces.

The brachialis and triceps muscles have broad cross-sectional areas and their insertions are close to the axis of elbow joint rotation, providing a bulk effect to gain further stability of the joint. The overall effect of these muscle contractions on the stability of the elbow is likely to be important, but the magnitude of these effects has yet to be determined.

The muscles that cross the medial side of the elbow joint have an alignment favouring dynamic protection of the MCLC. On the medial side of the elbow the flexor carpi ulnaris (FCU) is the most important dynamic stabiliser, with the flexor digitorum superficialis (FDS) being less important. The FCU and FDS are optimally positioned to provide secondary valgus stability of the medial side of the elbow, especially at between 90 and 120° of elbow flexion (the position of cocking in throwing).

LATERAL ELBOW PAIN

The lateral side is the most common site of elbow pain (Fig. 25.1). Some diagnoses that should be considered are lateral elbow tendinopathy, referred pain from the cervical and upper thoracic spine, synovitis of the radiohumeral joint, radiohumeral bursitis, osteochondritis dissecans of the capitellum and radius, posterolateral elbow instability and combinations of these problems (Table 25.1).

If your patient is between 30 and 60 years of age with local lateral elbow pain with or without some spread into the forearm, but no pain in the neck, arm and beyond the wrist, then lateral elbow tendinopathy is the likely diagnosis. Although evocative, the term 'tennis elbow' is unsatisfactory as it gives little indication of pathology; in fact, sports medicine clinicians are more likely to see this condition in non-tennis players than in tennis players. The term 'lateral epicondylitis' is not accurate as the primary pathology is not inflammatory as implied by the suffix 'itis'. The term epicondylosis is also problematic, as not all patients will present with degenerative changes implied by the suffix 'osis' (Chapter 4). Lateral elbow tendinopathy or lateral elbow pain are more general terms that do not assume a given pathology or an exact source of symptoms and thus better reflect the clinical situation.

History

Begin by eliciting the characteristics of the patient's lateral elbow pain. The pain of lateral extensor tendinopathy is typically located around the lateral epicondyle and proximal forearm. Occasionally the pain may radiate into the forearm extensor muscle mass, but it never extends into the hand and fingers or proximally into the upper arm. The onset of pain is often insidious but may be acute.

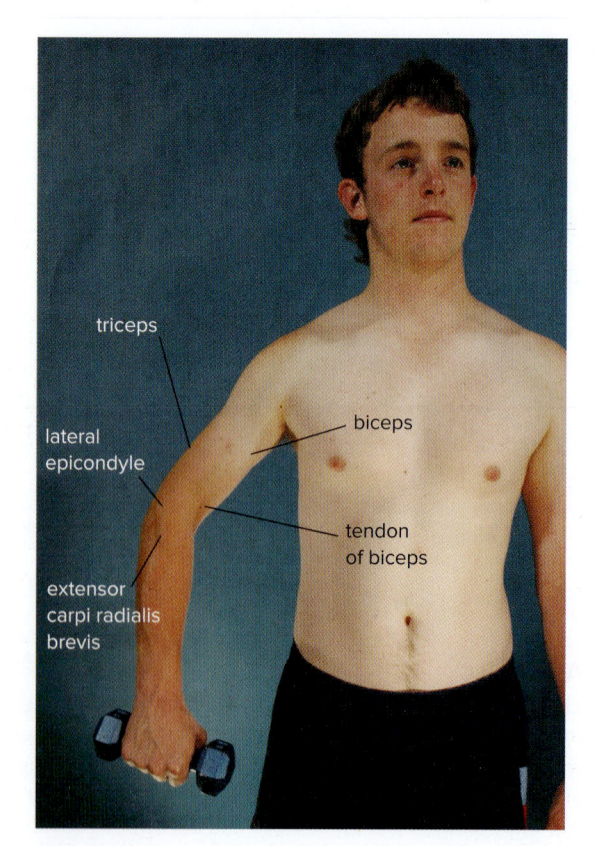

Figure 25.1 Anatomy of the lateral elbow (a) Surface anatomy of the lateral elbow

Elbow and arm pain CHAPTER 25

by light everyday activities, such as picking up a cup, or requires repeated heavy activity to become painful.

Pain in the lateral aspect of the forearm may also implicate entrapment of the posterior interosseous nerve or irritation of other nerves. If pain is closely related to the activity level, it is more likely to be of a mechanical origin. If pain is persistent, unpredictable or related to posture, consider a source of pain from other anatomical structures, non-musculoskeletal pathologies or abnormal central nervous system functioning (e.g. complex regional pain or neuropathic pain states). Lateral elbow tendinopathy is typically painful with gripping or wrist extension, whereas referred pain may be provoked by prolonged postures such as in lengthy periods seated at a desk or in a car. Associated sensory symptoms, such as pins and needles, also suggest a neural component. Presence of neck, upper thoracic or shoulder pain should be noted, especially when symptoms extend beyond the lateral elbow and forearm.

Often patients presenting to sports medicine clinicians will have undergone a variety of treatments. It is important to note the response to each of these.

An activity history should also be taken, noting any recent change in the level of activity. In tennis players, note any change in racquet size, grip size or string tension and whether or not any comment has been made regarding the patient's technique. This is also relevant to occupations involving manual tool handling tasks.

Examination

Examination involves:

1. Observation from the front
2. Active movements
    a. elbow flexion/extension
    b. supination/pronation
    c. wrist flexion (forearm pronated) (Fig. 25.2a)
    d. wrist extension
3. Passive movements
    a. as above
4. Resisted movements
    a. wrist extension (Fig. 25.2b)

(b)

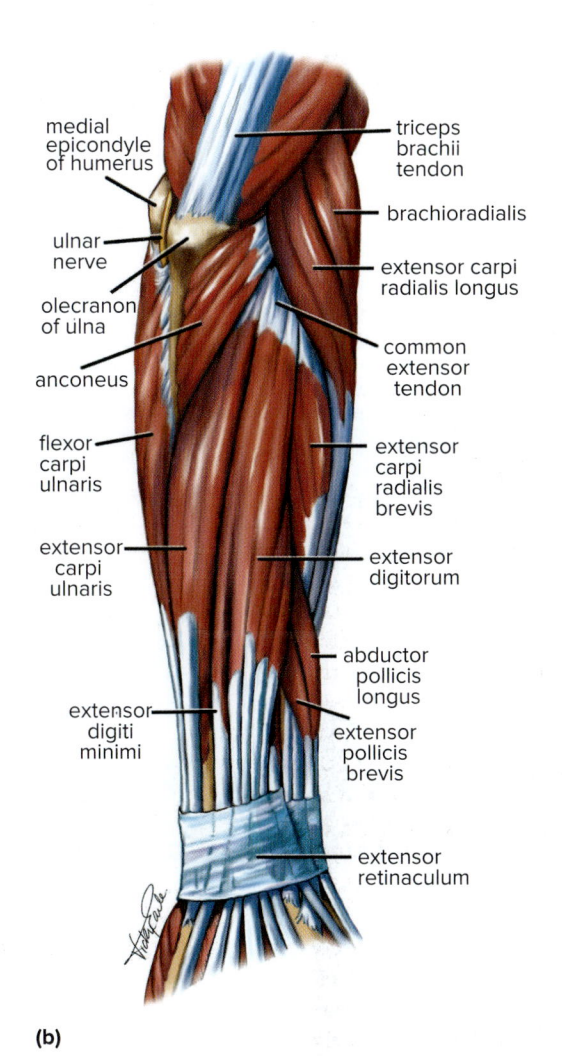

Figure 25.1 (cont.) (b) Anatomy of the lateral elbow from behind

There may have been recent changes in training load, technique, duties or equipment used in sports or work.

The severity of pain ranges from relatively trivial to almost incapacitating, keeping the patient awake at night. It is important to note whether the pain is aggravated

Table 25.1 Causes of lateral elbow pain

Common	Less common	Not to be missed
Extensor tendinopathy	Synovitis of the radiohumeral joint	Osteochondritis dissecans (in adolescents)
Referred pain	Radiohumeral bursitis	
• Cervical spine	Posterior interosseous nerve entrapment (radial tunnel syndrome)	• Capitellum
• Upper thoracic spine		• Radius
• Myofascial		

PART B   Regional problems

      b. extension at the third metacarpophalangeal joint (Fig. 25.2c)
      c. grip test (Fig. 25.2d)
5. Palpation
      a. lateral epicondyle (Fig. 25.2e)
      b. extensor muscles (Fig. 25.2f)
6. Special tests
      a. neurodynamic tests
      b. cervical spine examination (Chapter 23)
      c. thoracic spine examination (Chapter 28)
      d. periscapular soft tissues (Fig. 25.2g).

Investigations

Investigations are usually not performed in a straightforward case of lateral elbow pain. However, in longstanding cases, plain radiograph (AP and lateral views) of the elbow may show osteochondritis dissecans, degenerative joint changes or evidence of heterotopic calcification.

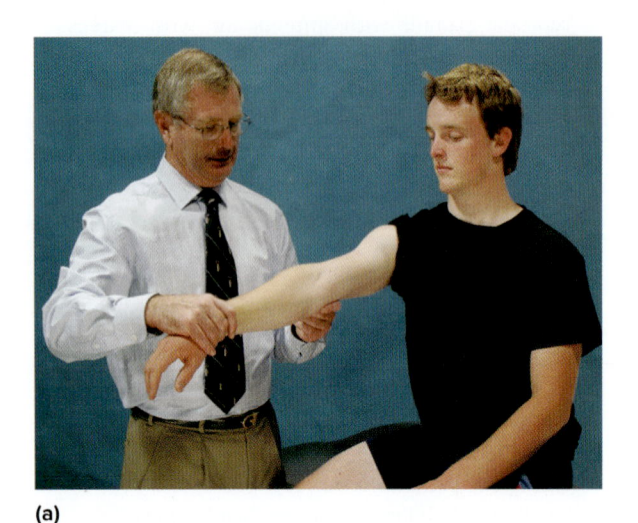

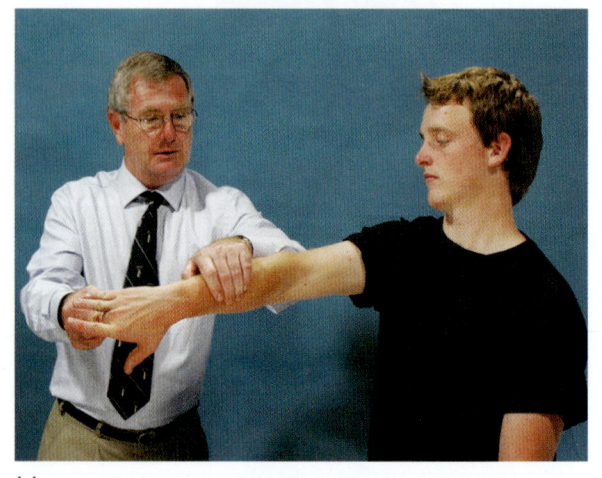

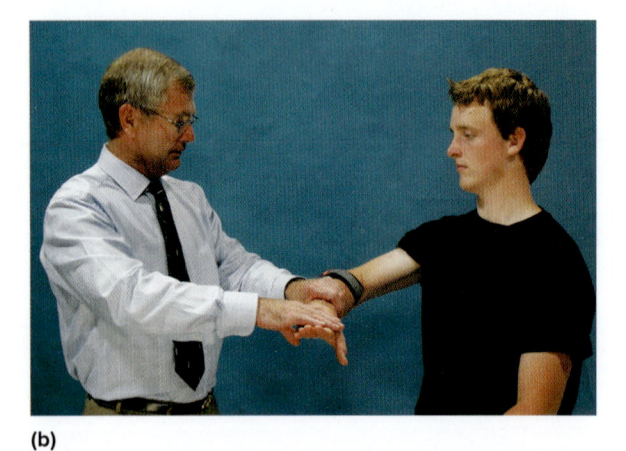

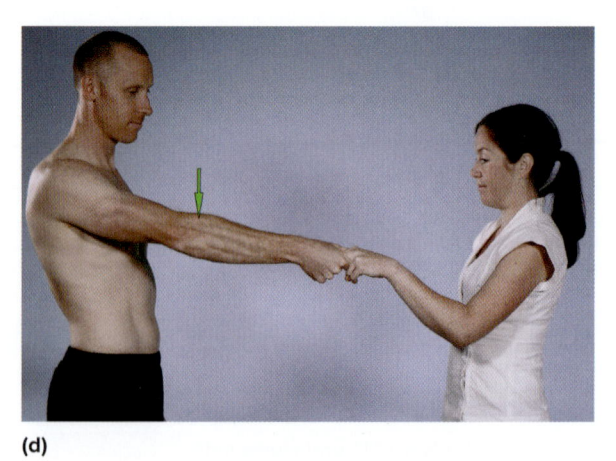

Figure 25.2 Examination of the patient with lateral elbow pain (a) Active movement—wrist flexion with forearm fully pronated (b) Resisted muscle testing—patient resists the clinician's pressure by extension of the wrist (c) Resisted muscle testing—extension at third metacarpophalangeal joint (d) The patient (in sitting or standing position) raises his or her arms up to horizontal, keeping the elbows extended and the palms facing down to the floor, then grips the examiner's two radial fingers as firmly as possible with the unaffected side, followed by the affected side until painful. A positive test is indicated by markedly reduced force to pain onset

Elbow and arm pain **CHAPTER 25**

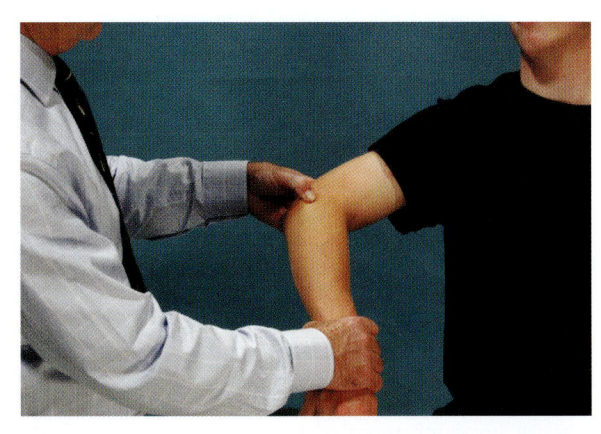

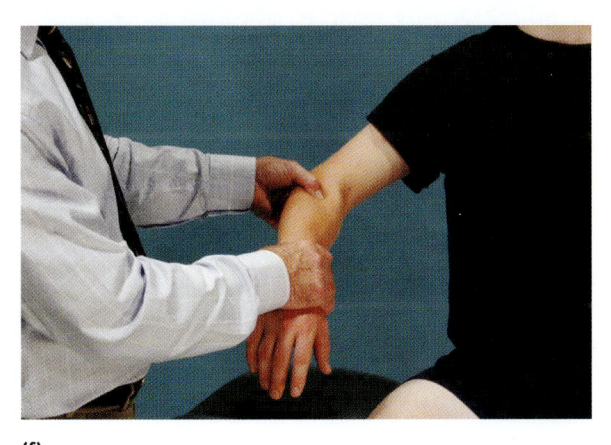

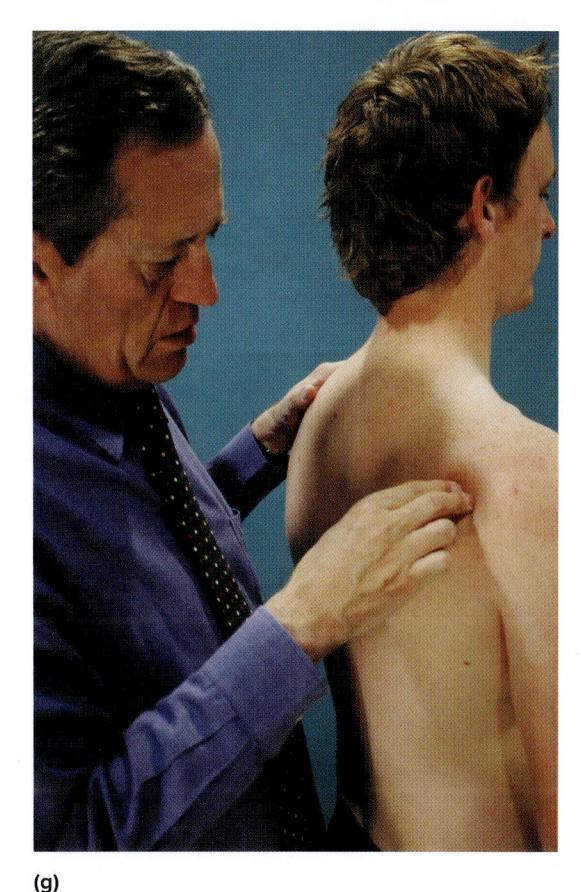

Figure 25.2 (cont.) (e) Palpation—lateral epicondyle. Attempt to locate painful site distal to lateral epicondyle (f) Palpation—extensor muscles. Pincer grip is used with passive flexion and extension to provide exact feel of damaged tissue (g) Periscapular soft tissues—palpation of active trigger points and changes in muscle tone and length in the periscapular soft tissues

Ultrasound examination may be helpful.[1] It may demonstrate the degree of tendon or ligament damage[2] as well as the presence of a bursa; MRI identifies tendinopathy[3] but is not indicated routinely. It may provide valuable anatomic detail when the diagnosis is challenging.

Lateral elbow tendinopathy

For this major sports medicine condition, we review the pathology, outline the clinical presentation and then discuss evidence-informed and clinically-reasoned treatment.

Clinically relevant pathology

The extensor carpi radialis brevis (ECRB) tendon is the most common tendon to become problematic, but the extensor digitorum (or extensor carpi ulnaris) may be implicated if the middle finger extension test is more provocative than the wrist extension test.[4] In addition to locating which muscle is involved, the tendon may be affected at its origin[5] or mid-substance. The latter is characterised on light microscopy as an excess of both fibroblasts and blood vessels.[6-8] The vessels appear consistent with what Alfredson calls 'neovessels',[9] pathologists call 'angiogenesis' and Nirschl called 'angiofibroblastic hyperplasia'.[7] With continued use, the lesions may extend into microscopic partial tears.[10] Conversely, a tear may be the primary abnormality, with degenerative changes being secondary. A summary of the processes leading to extensor tendinopathy is shown in Figure 25.3.

Manual tasks that require wrist stabilisation, such as gripping, or that require wrist extension movements,

443

PART B Regional problems

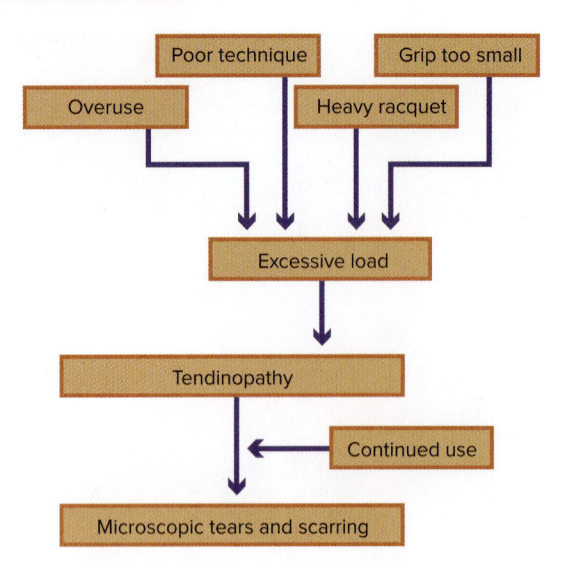

Figure 25.3 Processes leading to the development of lateral elbow tendinopathy

place considerable load on the ECRB tendon. The highest stresses occur in the ECRB tendon when the elbow is extended and the forearm pronated–the most provocative position to reproduce a patient's pain and test grip force.

Pain-free grip force is reduced in lateral elbow tendinopathy and there is altered motor control of the gripping action. In lateral elbow tendinopathy during a low force gripping action, there is a relatively lower activation of the ECRB and a relatively greater activation of the long finger flexors and extensors.[11] Associated with this, the wrist is held in a more flexed position.[12] The only muscle that is not weaker in this condition is the extensor digitorum longus.[13] Taken together, this evidence points to altered control mechanisms of the wrist in lateral elbow tendinopathy.

This abnormal gripping action was also present on the unaffected elbow side in unilateral tendinopathy, suggesting central neural mechanisms at play.[14] Consistent with these findings are impaired reaction time and speed of movement that are bilaterally present in unilateral tendinopathy.[12,15] Most intriguingly, tendinosis-like tissue changes can also be triggered bilaterally in response to unilateral overuse as documented in a recent animal model.[14] These discoveries provide a basis for the clinician to be alert to potential central mechanisms and to carefully evaluate, and possibly treat, both sides even when the presentation is unilateral.

Clinical features

Lateral elbow tendinopathy occurs in association with repeated gripping and/or wrist extension actions and activities. These tasks includes sports, such as tennis, squash and badminton, as well as occupational and leisure pursuits, such as carpentry, bricklaying, sewing and knitting. Keyboard use is also associated with the condition.[16] The peak incidence is between the ages of 40 and 60 years, but the condition may affect any age group, in which case careful attention to differential causes of the symptoms is imperative.

History

There are two distinct clinical presentations of lateral elbow tendinopathy. The most common is an insidious onset of pain, which occurs 24–72 hours after unaccustomed activity involving repeated wrist extension. This occurs typically after a person spends the weekend engaged in manual activity such as laying bricks or using a screwdriver, or after prolonged sessions of sewing or knitting. In the tennis player, it may occur following the use of a new racquet; playing with wet, heavy balls; or overhitting, especially when hitting into the wind. It also occurs when the player is hitting 'late' (getting into position slowly), so that body weight is not transferred correctly and the player relies excessively on the forearm muscles for power (see also discussion of specific tennis biomechanics in Chapter 9).

The other clinical presentation is a sudden onset of lateral elbow pain associated with a single instance of exertion involving the wrist extensors, for example lifting a heavy object, or in tennis players attempting a very forceful single-handed backhand with too much reliance on the forearm and not enough on the trunk and legs. The insidious onset is thought to correspond to microscopic tears within the tendon, whereas the acute onset may correspond to larger macroscopic tendon tears.

Physical examination

On examination, insertional versus mid-substance lesions will be differentiated by the site of maximal tenderness, with the latter being approximately 1–2 cm distal to the lateral epicondyle. Palpation of the entire tendon and the associated muscle(s) will provide valuable information on tissue tightness or hypersensitivity, which is useful in guiding treatment.

Typically, the pain is reproduced by resisted wrist extension, especially with the elbow extended and forearm pronated. Resisted extension of the middle finger is also painful (Fig. 25.2c). It is thought that the ECRB tendon is preferentially stressed in this position as it contracts synergistically to anchor the third metacarpal to allow extension to take place at the digits.

The upper limb neurodynamic or neural provocation test (Chapter 15), especially with radial nerve bias, may

444

reproduce lateral elbow pain or show restriction of movement compared with the other side. In either situation, this may implicate a neural component to the pain.

Examination of the cervical spine will frequently detect decreased range of movement, especially lateral flexion. The cervical and upper thoracic spine may be stiff to palpation and tender both centrally and over the painful apophyseal joint, usually around the C5-6 level.[17] Active trigger points can occur in the periscapular soft tissues (Fig. 25.2g). In chronic cases, it is not uncommon to find decreased joint play in the elbow joints.

Treatment

No single treatment is totally effective and it is most likely that the patient will be best served through a combination of different treatments selected on the basis of the patient's clinical presentation[18] and preferences, and informed by current best evidence.

The basic principles of treating soft tissue injuries apply, with a specific focus on addressing the grip strength deficit and coordination impairments of the upper limb and specifically at the wrist. These deficits are best addressed through exercise. There must be control of pain (e.g. ice, analgesic medications, relative rest, electrotherapy), encouragement of the healing process, restoration of any flexibility deficit, correction of any predisposing factors and a gradual return to activity.

Treatment of any spinal or neural dysfunctions often speeds up resolution[19] and is highly recommended if there is concomitant neck pain.[20, 21]

> **PRACTICE PEARL**
>
> Exercise is the key to managing lateral elbow tendinopathy. Other treatments are adjunctive, mainly to resolve pain and facilitate tissue healing.

Exercises for strengthening and coordination

We recommend the following exercises:

- Progressively graduated exercise to improve strength and endurance capacity (Fig. 25.4) as well as normalise flexibility of the forearm muscles (Fig. 25.5).
- Exercises geared at improving coordination (Fig. 25.6) should also be considered.[22]

It is unknown how much pain should be experienced during exercise without compromising resolution, but experience indicates that it should be minimised through careful selection of load and type of exercise. For example, in very painful elbows, isometric low load exercise with taping, and/or mobilisation with movements (Fig. 25.7)

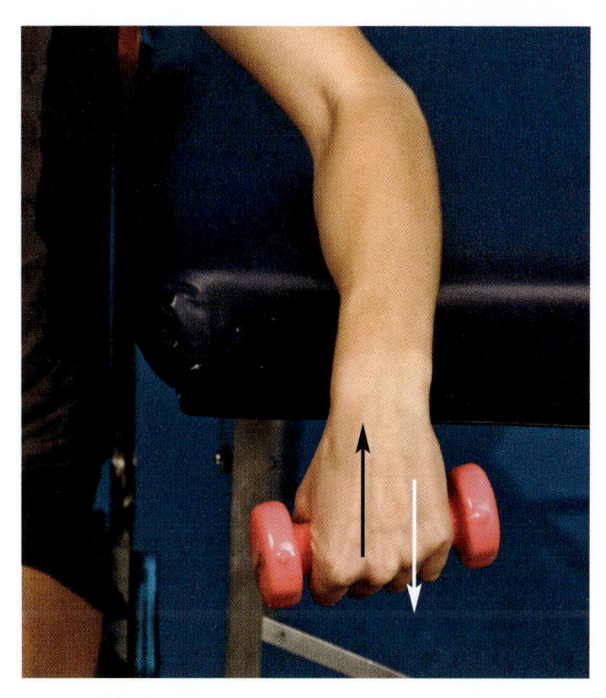

Figure 25.4 Strengthening exercises for wrist extensors. Exercises can be isometric, concentric (raising the weight, black arrow), eccentric (lowering the weight, white arrow) or functional

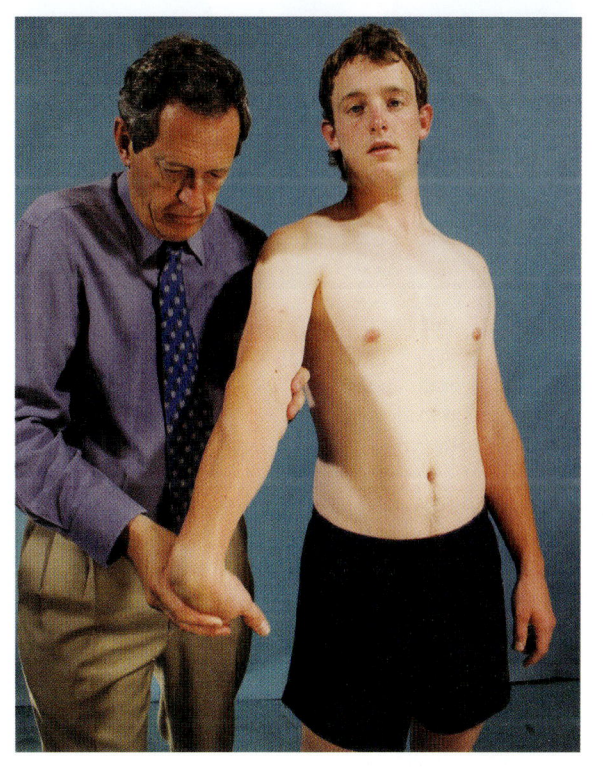

Figure 25.5 Stretching the extensor carpi radialis brevis tendon

PART B Regional problems

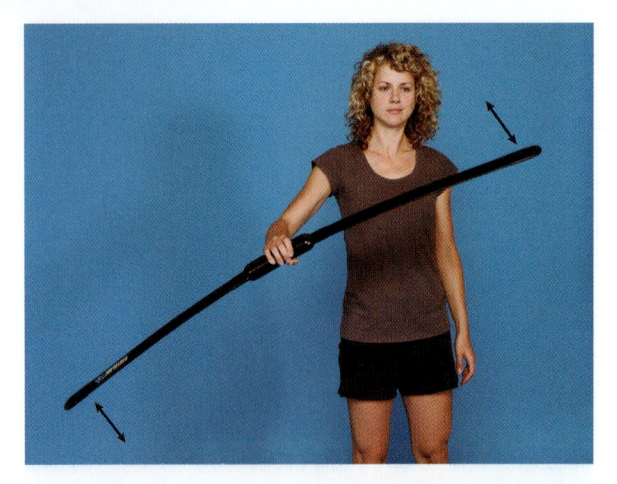

Figure 25.6 Coordination exercise focusing on supination/pronation at an early stage in rehabilitation of lateral elbow tendinopathy. The patient oscillates the body blade with the shoulder in a position that approximates the scapular plane

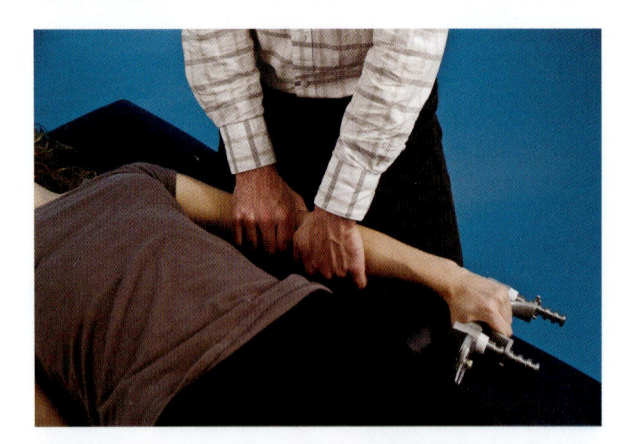

Figure 25.7 Mobilisation with movement

to improve endurance should be favoured initially, with progression in load and complexity (concentric, eccentric) as pain subsides to emphasise strengthening.

Exercise is supported by clinical trials[23, 24] and in one particular study,[21] long-term benefits and prevention of recurrence were seen in patients who had previously failed common treatments such as corticosteroid injections and oral medications.

Electrotherapeutic modalities

Electrotherapeutic modalities such as laser, extracorporeal shockwave therapy (ESWT), TENS and ultrasound are often used in practice for these conditions despite mixed evidence on their effectiveness. In some part related to this mixed evidence is the fundamental issue of what constitutes an appropriate dosage, which can be challenging to the practitioner. For example, laser administered at a wavelength of 904 nm (but not 820 and 1064 nm) offers short-term pain relief and a reduction in disability, applied either in isolation or in combination with exercise.[25]

A modality where a perplexing situation arises is ESWT, which is effective at some sites of tendinopathy but not for lateral elbow tendinopathy,[26] though the issue of dose for this modality has perhaps not been adequately explored. Interestingly, TENS, which is a scientifically developed modality for the reduction of pain, has only recently been considered in clinical trials of tennis elbow.[27] Practitioners should be aware that dosage plays an important role in delivering beneficial outcomes;[28] high frequencies (e.g. 85–110 Hz) and pulse durations of approximately 200 μs delivered at a strong but sub-noxious intensity are recommended.

Therapeutic ultrasound (i.e. not diagnostic ultrasound), which tends to be widely used in clinics for many musculoskeletal conditions, has very little evidence to support its use.[29] A recent clinical trial showed that while therapeutic ultrasound reduced pain over time, as did the comparator laser treatment, the patients did not rate their condition as being sufficiently improved.[30]

Manual therapy

Specific manual therapy applied to the joints or soft tissues of the elbow and forearm is beneficial for lateral elbow tendinopathy.

There is evidence of benefit with elbow mobilisation with movement[31] (Fig. 25.7), in combination with exercise,[32] and with the addition of cervical and thoracic spine treatment to elbow treatment.[33]

Cervical mobilisation (Fig. 25.8), thoracic mobilisation and neural stretching (Fig. 25.9) are commonly used as adjuncts to other forms of treatment.

Transverse frictions are frequently advocated at the site of the lesion; however, there is little evidence that these are beneficial. There is some evidence that they are less effective than supervised exercise, when frictions are combined with Mill's manipulation, which is a small-amplitude, high-velocity thrust performed at end of elbow extension while the wrist and hand are flexed.[33-35]

There is little evidence to support the use of digital ischaemic pressures and myofascial massage, though it may be trialled to judge whether the individual patient will benefit from its application. A critical aspect of such soft tissue manual therapy techniques is targeting them to areas exhibiting increased resistance, tightness

Elbow and arm pain CHAPTER 25

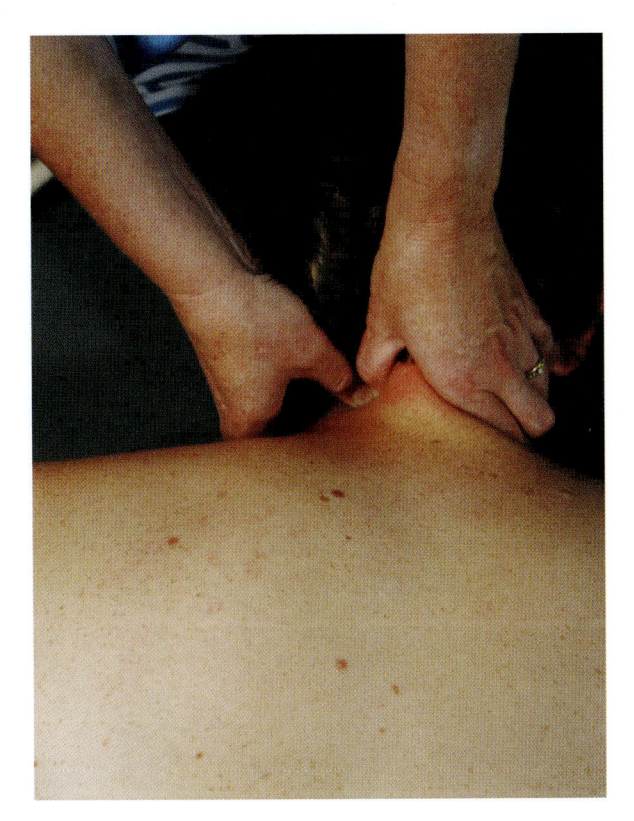

Figure 25.8 Cervical mobilisation

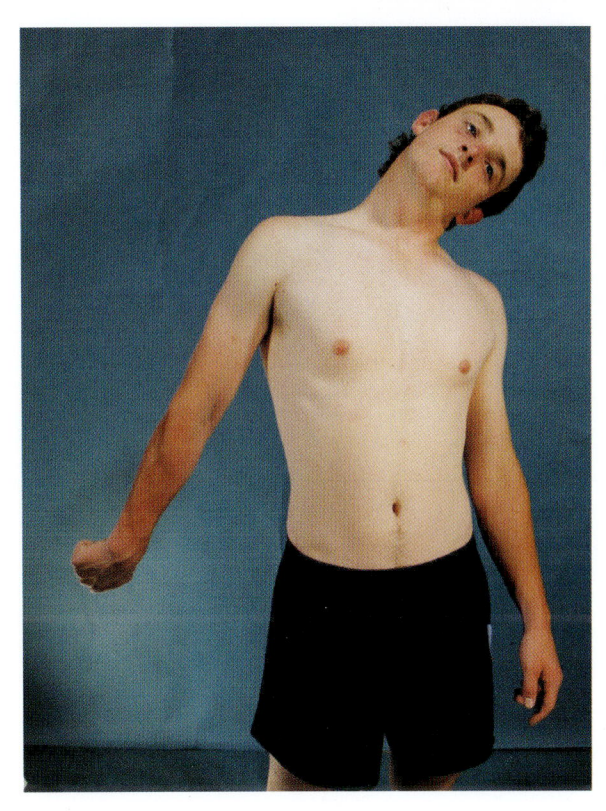

Figure 25.9 Neural tissue mobilisation positioned at end of range

or thickening to digital pressure in the absence of severe pain. In this situation the tissues are usually placed under various conditions of stretch while digital pressure is applied, either sustained (Fig. 25.10a) or longitudinally directed in motion (Fig. 25.10b).

These techniques usually produce pain during application, but this pain should be within the patient's tolerance, not be severe and not outlast the treatment. The presence of severe pain and very little or no resistance, tightness or thickening are contraindications to high force/load soft tissue techniques.

Trigger points
In patients with lateral elbow pain, active trigger points associated with muscle shortening are frequently found in the forearm extensor muscles–brachioradialis, extensor carpi radialis longus, ECRB, extensor digitorum, extensor carpi ulnaris, extensor digiti minimi and anconeus, as well as the periscapular area.[36] Digital ischaemic pressure or dry needling of these trigger points may help in the treatment.

Acupuncture
There is some evidence of short-term (2–8 weeks) benefit with the use of acupuncture for lateral elbow pain.[37]

Bracing and taping
Counterforce bracing (Fig. 25.11) increases forearm extensors' stretching pain tolerance, but it does not appear to influence neuromuscular parameters such as strength or proprioception of these muscles.[38] If a brace is to be used, it should demonstrably reduce pain on gripping or on resisted tests of wrist and middle finger extension. In these cases, the brace should be worn during the performance of pain provocative tasks, such as on returning to an aggravating activity like tennis. The brace should be correctly applied approximately 10 cm below the elbow joint. Tensioning the brace up to 50 N has been found to be beneficial.[38]

A deloading taping technique has been shown to initially improve pain-free gripping[39] and to reduce tissue stress within the taped area. Our clinical experience

447

PART B   Regional problems

(a)   (b)

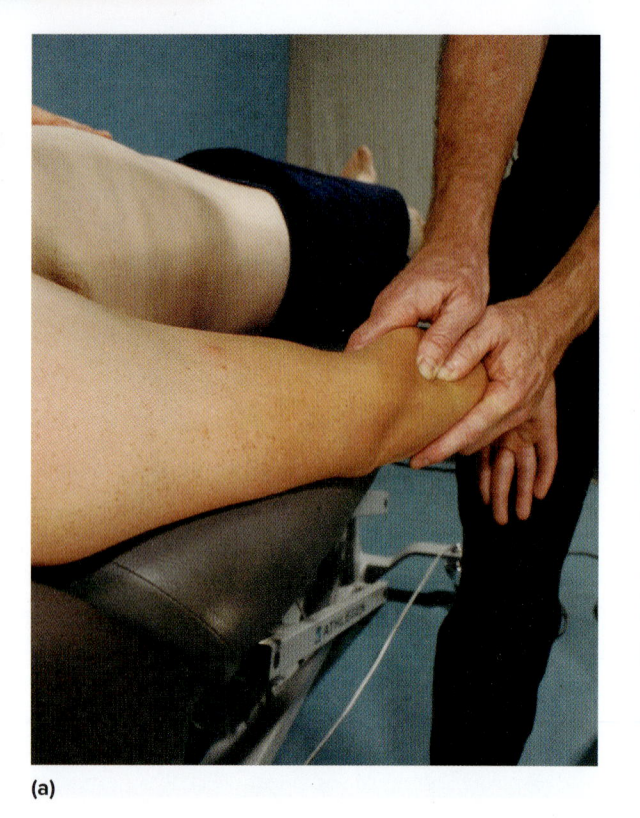

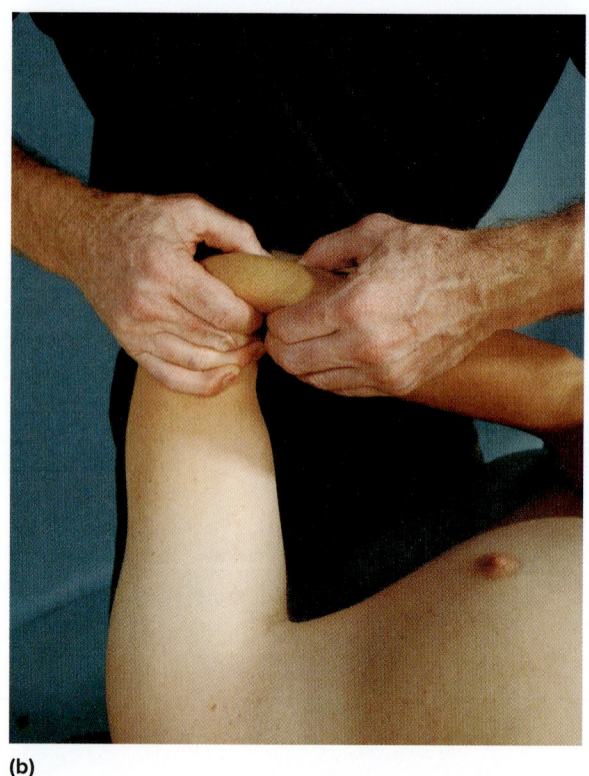

Figure 25.10 Soft tissue techniques (a) Sustained longitudinal pressure to the extensor carpi radialis brevis muscle in the position of maximum elbow extension and wrist flexion (b) Digital ischaemic pressure to deep muscle fibres in the shortened position

indicates that it is very useful in patients who have severe pain and pain at night (Fig. 25.12).

Iontophoresis

There is insufficient evidence from clinical trials to support or refute the use of corticosteroids delivered by iontophoresis.

Corticosteroid injection

> **PRACTICE PEARL**
>
> The use of corticosteroid injection in the treatment of this condition requires careful consideration because the best evidence to date indicates that while it is very effective in the short term (i.e. >80% success rate), there are unfavourable consequences later (i.e. >6–12 months), such as delayed recovery and a 62% greater recurrence rate than if the patient were advised to adopt a wait and see approach.[40]

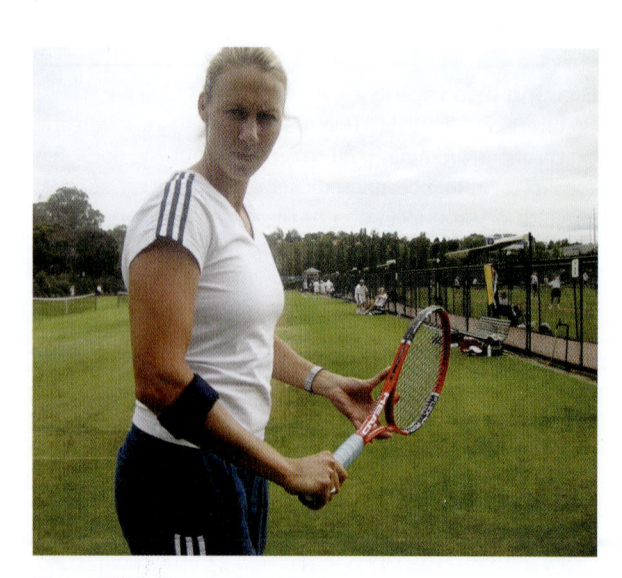

Figure 25.11 Counterforce brace

448

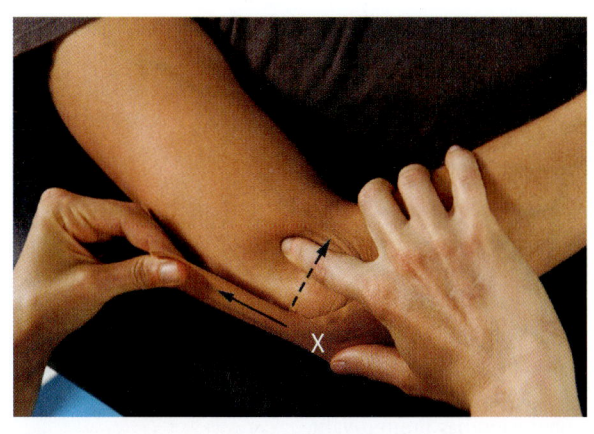

Elbow and arm pain CHAPTER 25

(a)

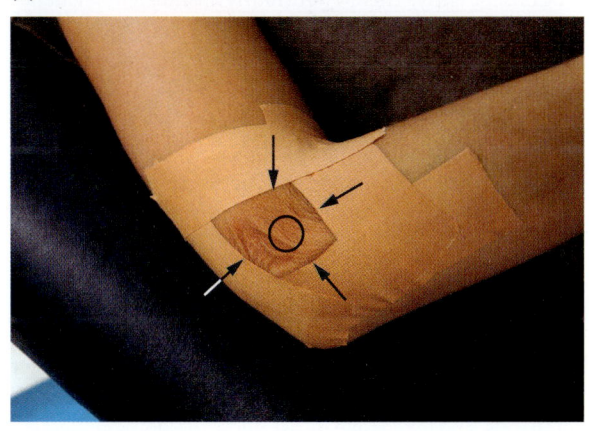

(b)

Figure 25.12 The diamond tape technique
(a) The anchor point X marks the site from which the tape is tensioned longitudinally (along the solid-line arrow) and laid onto the skin. The skin should be pulled towards the site of pain (dotted-line arrow)
(b) Note the overlapping ends of the tape and the orange-peel effect on the skin with the diamond tape, resulting in a translation of skin away from the tape towards the site of pain (O) as shown by the arrows
FROM VICENZINO ET AL[39]

Combining physiotherapy with an injection does not seem to improve this situation.[41] Thus, it is prudent to consider using this injection within a more comprehensive management framework as illustrated (Fig. 25.13).

Prior to any injection, the clinician should fully inform the patient of likely short- and long-term outcomes, as adopting a wait and see policy will result in approximately 80% success rate at 12 months, with much lower risk of recurrences.[42] When corticosteroid and local anaesthetic agents are injected, the aim should be around the ECRB tendon, directly over the point of maximal tenderness but not into the tendon substance itself.

> **PRACTICE PEARL**
>
> A comprehensive program for the management of lateral elbow pain (Fig. 25.13) would include implementing a graduated progressive exercise program over 8 weeks, pain relief if required, ergonomic advice and activity modification.[42]

Nitric oxide donor therapy

Initial studies of lateral elbow, Achilles and supraspinatus tendinopathies provided level 2 evidence that nitric oxide donor therapy (glyceryl trinitrate [GTN] patches applied locally, 1.25 mg/day) improved outcomes within

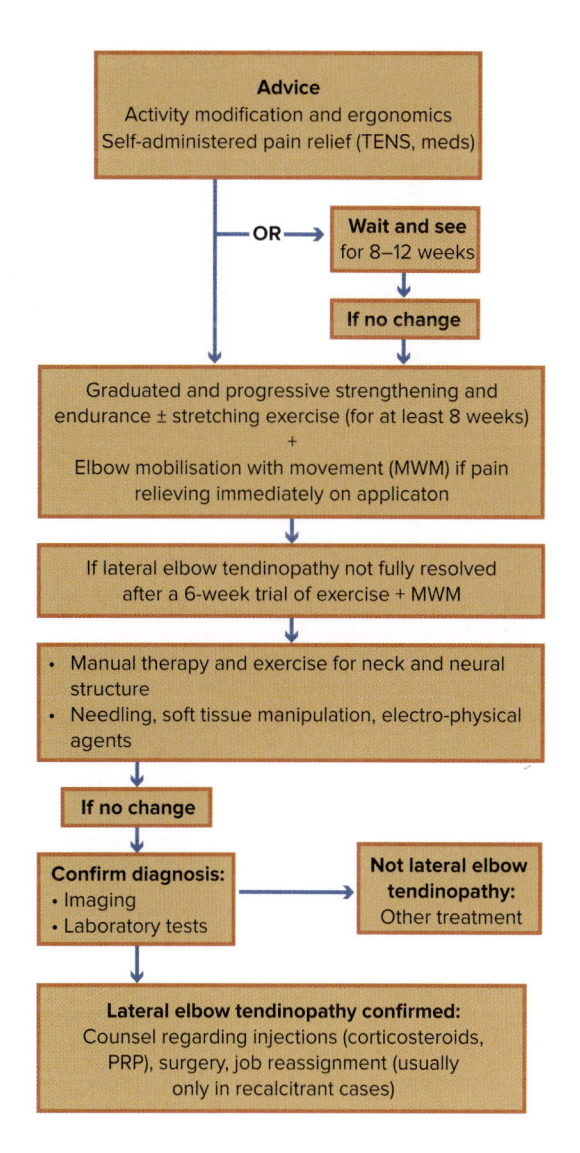

Figure 25.13 Treatment algorithm

449

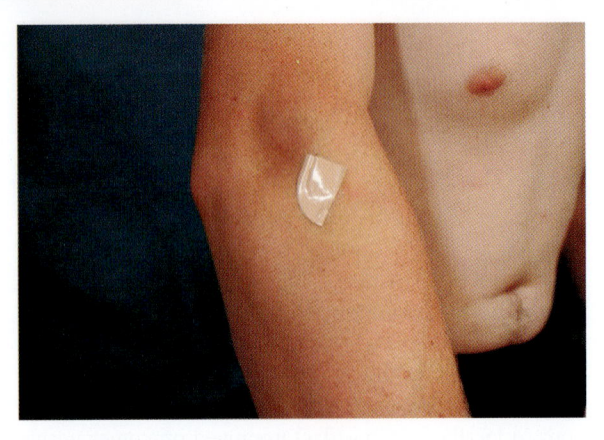

Figure 25.14 Nitric oxide donor therapy—one quarter of a 0.5 mg/24 h glyceryl trinitrate (GTN) patch in place over the most tender site of extensor tendinopathy

3-6 months[43] (Fig. 25.14). One mechanism by which this treatment might work is through enhanced collagen synthesis. However, a recent dose-ranging clinical trial for lateral elbow tendinopathy failed to confirm the initial findings, but highlighted that the type of exercise (strengthening as opposed to stretching) is a significant consideration.[44]

Pragmatically, the practitioner and patient need to be aware that 4-5% of patients will develop headaches or skin rash that are severe enough to discontinue treatment with GTN and that this seems to be dose dependent. Thus it is important to carefully meter the dose and monitor response.

Botulinum toxin

Historically used for neuromuscular conditions, botulinum toxin (Botox®) injection is a new and unproven treatment of tendinopathy. There is evidence that it produces short-term improvement in pain when compared to placebo,[40, 45] though it is important to counsel the patient prior to the treatment that there will be a high likelihood (92% at 8 weeks post injection)[46] of an extensor muscle lag. This treatment-induced extensor weakness is an important consideration for athletes who need good grip strength.

Autologous blood, platelet-rich plasma and autologous cell injections

with ROBERT-JAN DE VOS

Autologous blood and platelet-rich plasma (PRP) are increasingly proposed as treatment for lateral elbow tendinopathy.[47] The rationale behind these treatments is improvement of tendon healing though delivery of growth factors and cytokines present in blood.[48, 49] There are various protocols for preparation and injection of these blood products.

A relatively high number of clinical trials have been performed on patients with longstanding lateral elbow tendinopathy. One recent qualitative systematic review, concluded that there is strong evidence against the use of PRP.[50] Also after pooling of data in a Cochrane review, there was no significant improvement after PRP treatment compared to other treatments for this condition.[51] There is a lot of discussion about the interpretation of these results; nonetheless, the data are clearly not in favour of PRP treatment.[52] One case series showed pain reduction and functional improvement after an injection with autologous tenocytes for longstanding lateral elbow tendinopathy.[53, 54] However, due to the study design, this conclusion has limited value.

Consequently, there is currently insufficient evidence to recommend injections with autologous blood, PRP or autologous tenocytes in patients with chronic lateral elbow tendinopathy.

Correct predisposing factors

Probably the most important factor to be avoided is exposure to activity levels for which there is inadequate preparation (e.g. inappropriate training load, poor technique). In tennis players, a major cause is a faulty backhand technique with the elbow leading (Fig. 25.15). Other technique faults that may predispose to the development of extensor tendinopathy include excessive forearm pronation while attempting to hit topspin forehands and excessive wrist flick (flexion) movement while serving. Correction of these faults requires the assistance of a qualified tennis coach. Other factors, such as racquet type, grip size, string tension, court surface and ball weight, may influence the amount of shock imparted to the elbow (Chapter 9). A mid-sized racquet with a large 'sweet spot' and a grip size that feels comfortable should be used. Care should be taken to avoid using racquets with excessively large or, especially, small grips.

Surgery

Surgery might be considered occasionally in cases with a long history (e.g. >18 months) of lateral elbow pain that is recalcitrant to the treatment strategies outlined above. Surgery is varied, but most recent approaches involve ECRB tendon release from the lateral epicondyle with or without some degree of excision of the degenerative tissue within the common extensor tendon. A recent systematic review concluded that there is a lack of quality evidence to recommend one surgical approach over others.[55]

Graduated return to activity

As with all soft tissue injuries, it is important to return gradually to activity following treatment. The tennis

Elbow and arm pain CHAPTER 25

length of the rehabilitation program, this graduated return should take place over a period of at least 3–6 weeks.

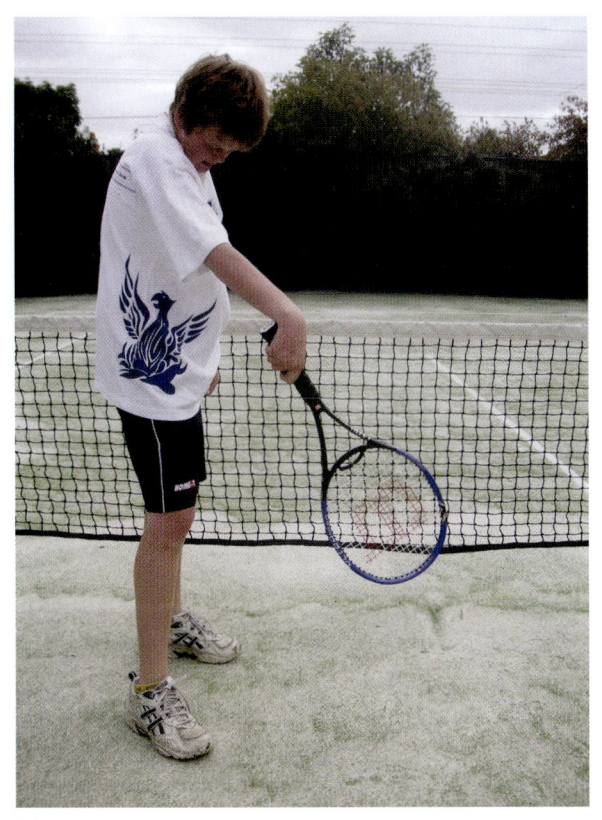

Other causes of lateral elbow pain

Other causes of lateral elbow pain may occur in isolation or in conjunction with the previously mentioned conditions. Radiohumeral bursitis is occasionally seen in athletes. This may be distinguished from extensor tendinopathy by the site of tenderness that is over the radiohumeral joint and distal to the lateral epicondyle, maximally over the anterolateral aspect of the head of the radius. The presence of this bursitis may be confirmed on ultrasound examination. Injection with a corticosteroid agent is the most effective form of treatment.

Osteochondritis of the capitellum or radial head may occur in younger athletes (Chapter 44) involved in throwing sports. This is a significant condition as it can cause an enlarged, deformed capitellum that may predispose to the development of osteoarthritis. The treatment of this condition involves avoidance of aggravating activities.

The lateral elbow is a common site of referred pain, especially from the cervical and upper thoracic spine and periscapular soft tissues. Most patients with chronic lateral elbow pain are likely to have some component of their pain emanating from the cervical and thoracic spine (Chapters 23 and 28). Any associated abnormalities of the cervical and thoracic spine should be treated and the patient's signs reassessed immediately after treatment. If there is a noticeable difference, this may indicate a significant component of referred pain.

MEDIAL ELBOW PAIN

Patients who present with medial elbow pain can be considered in two main groups. One group has pain associated with excessive activity of the wrist flexors. This is the medial equivalent of lateral elbow tendinopathy, with a similar pathological process occurring in the tendons of pronator teres and the flexor group. This condition will be referred to as 'flexor/pronator tendinopathy'.

The second group of patients has medial elbow pain related to excessive throwing activities. Throwing produces a valgus elbow stress that is resisted primarily by the anterior oblique portion of the medial collateral ligament (MCL) and secondarily by the stability of the radiocapitellar joint. Repetitive throwing, especially if throwing technique is poor (Chapter 8), leads to stretching of the MCL and a degree of valgus instability. A fixed flexion deformity of the elbow may develop as a result of scarring of the MCL. Subsequently, there may be some secondary impingement of the medial tip of the olecranon onto the olecranon fossa, producing a synovitis or loose

(a)

(b)

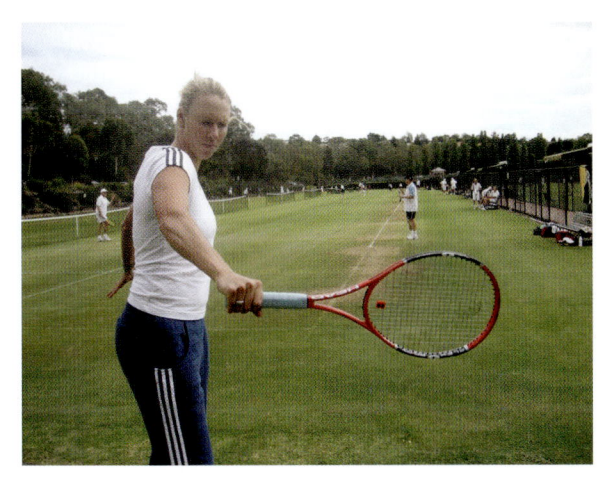

Figure 25.15 Backhand technique (a) Incorrect (b) Correct

player should initially practice backhand technique without a ball, then progress slowly from gentle hitting from the service line to eventually hitting full length shots. Depending on the severity of the condition and the

451

PART B   Regional problems

body formation. With valgus stress, the compressive forces may also damage the radiocapitellar joint. Several of these pathological entities may be present in combination.

In children, repetitive valgus stress may result in damage to the medial epicondylar epiphysis with pain and tenderness in this region. This usually responds to a period of rest followed by a gradual return to throwing activity, but may progress to avulsion with continued activity. This condition, commonly known as 'little leaguer's elbow', is considered in Chapter 44. The causes of medial elbow pain are shown in Table 25.2.

Flexor/pronator tendinopathy

This condition is not as common as its lateral equivalent, accounting for 9–20% of all epicondylalgia diagnoses.[56] It is seen especially in golfers ('golfer's elbow') and in tennis players who use a lot of topspin on their forehand. The primary pathology exists in the tendinous origin of the forearm flexor muscles, particularly in the pronator teres tendon.[57] Ultrasound is sensitive and specific for detecting clinically defined medial epicondylitis, with focal hypoechoic areas of tendinosis being the most common finding, followed by partial tears–that is, identical to lateral tendinopathy ultrasound findings.

On examination, there is usually localised tenderness just at or below the medial epicondyle with pain on resisted wrist flexion and resisted forearm pronation (Fig. 25.16).

Treatment is along the same lines as treatment of lateral elbow tendinopathy (Fig. 25.13). Particular attention should be paid to the tennis forehand or the golf swing technique. Due to its close proximity to the medial epicondyle, the ulnar nerve may become irritated or trapped in scar tissue. This should be treated with neural mobilisation.

Medial collateral ligament sprain

Sprain of the MCL of the elbow may occur as an acute injury, which is discussed below, or as the result of chronic excessive valgus stress due to throwing. This occurs particularly in baseball pitchers, javelin throwers, and water polo, handball, tennis and cricket players.

Throwing is a highly dynamic activity (see Chapter 8) where body segments move through long arcs of motion at high speed. Large joint forces and torques are generated at the medial side of the elbow. In general, the throwing motion is similar among various sports and the overuse pathology of the medial side of the elbow is similar.

Medial elbow stability between 20 and 120° of elbow flexion is provided primarily by the MCL. The static function of the MCL is to serve as the primary restraint to valgus strains in this functional range of motion. During each throw the elbow is subject to tremendous forces and functional demands. The elbow is designed for planar motion whereas the act of throwing relies on a peak rotatory power to propel the ball.

Biomechanical studies of pitching have shown arm rotation speeds of >7000°/second and arm extension velocity of 2300°/second. The anterior bundle of the MCL is the primary static restraint against valgus stress at 30 to 90° of flexion with an average load to failure of 260 N. Muscle contraction during throwing can reduce the stress on the MCL by compressing the joint and adding some stability. Because of the intensity of activity in these athletes with high numbers of repetitions (in some sports, up to 60 000 throwing motions per year), the abnormal forces over time can lead to subtle microscopic tearing within the soft tissues of the medial side of the elbow with imperfect healing. This chronic attenuation of the MCL with repeated high valgus stress can result in acute rupture of the MCL.

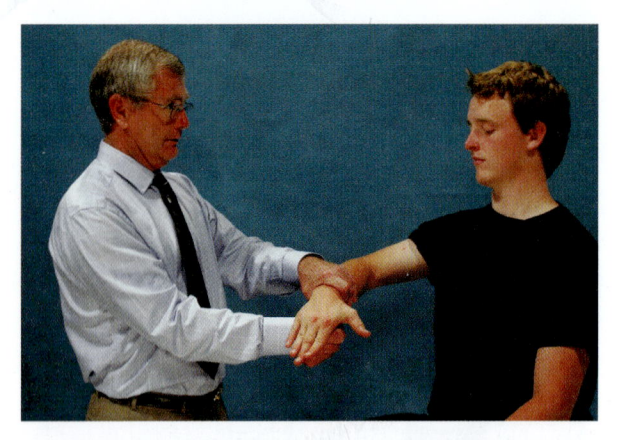

Figure 25.16 Medial elbow pain reproduced with resisted wrist flexion and forearm pronation

Table 25.2   Causes of medial elbow pain

Common	Less common	Not to be missed
Flexor/pronator tendinopathy	Ulnar nerve compression	Referred pain
Medial collateral ligament sprain	Avulsion fracture of the medial epicondyle (adolescents)	
• Acute	Apophysitis–'Little Leaguer's elbow' (adolescents)	
• Chronic		

Elbow and arm pain CHAPTER 25

The athlete with an acute MCL injury typically describes the sudden onset of pain with throwing. In approximately 50% of cases the patient will report hearing or feeling a 'pop' and is typically unable to continue throwing. More chronic injuries may not present as obviously.

They will likely be described as a gradual onset of pain localised to the medial elbow that worsens in the late cocking or early acceleration phase of throwing. A decrease in maximum velocity is also typically reported in chronic cases. Local inflammation of the unstable ligamentous complex can lead to other common elbow complaints such as ulnar nerve symptoms secondary to irritation of the nerve within the cubital tunnel (see below), flexor-pronator mass strain or medial epicondylitis.[58]

On examination, there will be localised tenderness over the ligament *just distal to the medial epicondyle* and mild pain/instability on valgus stress (Fig. 25.17a). The *milking manoeuvre* or the moving valgus stress test is a useful test to access partial tear of MCL. The milking manoeuvre is performed by pulling on the patient's thumb in order to apply valgus stress while the patient's shoulder is forward elevated to 90° and elbow flexed beyond 90°.[59]

There will often be associated abnormalities such as a flexion contracture of the forearm muscles, synovitis and loose body formation around the tip of the olecranon, as well as damage to the radio-capitellar joint. However, many throwers demonstrate a flexion contracture without concurrent MCL pathology.[60] Ultrasound and MRI are the preferred imaging modalities in these athletes.

Treatment in the early stages of the injury involves modification of activity, correction of faulty technique, local electrotherapeutic modalities (just as with lateral elbow tendinopathy, little research exists) and soft tissue therapy to the medial ligament. Medial strapping of the elbow may offer additional protection (Fig. 25.17b). Specific muscle strengthening should be commenced, concentrating on the forearm flexors and pronators (Fig. 25.18).

> **PRACTICE PEARL**
>
> Surgery is indicated for the throwing athlete with elbow pain associated with medial dynamic valgus instability that precludes participation in sport at the pre-injury level.

The first successful UCL reconstruction surgery was performed in 1974 by Dr Frank Jobe on Los Angeles Dodgers pitcher, Tommy John. Prior to this surgery, a UCL tear was considered to be a career-ending injury. Tommy John's return to baseball in 1976 changed the way this injury was viewed and sparked an evolution of surgical techniques that would take place over the next 40 years.

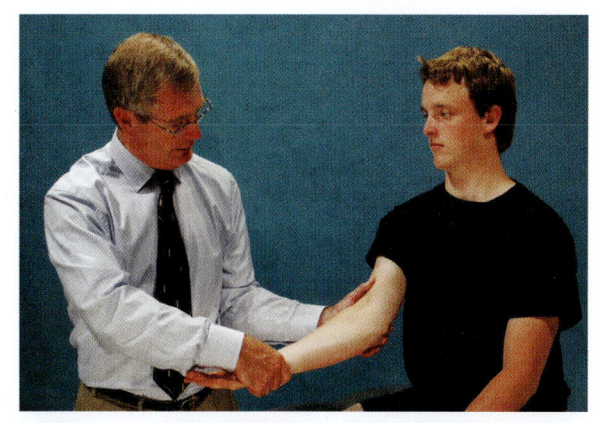

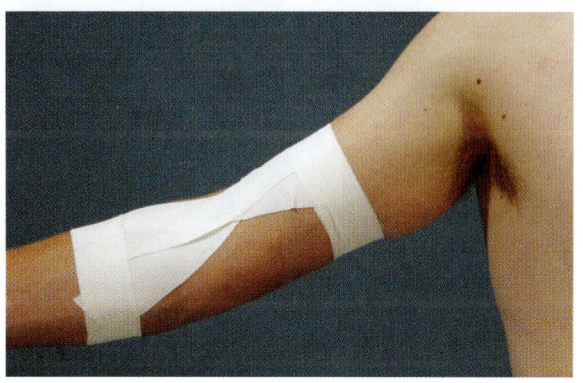

Figure 25.17 (a) Assessment of integrity of the medial collateral ligament with humerus fully internally rotated and controlled for pro/supination. Laxity should not exceed 5° (b) Elbow stability tape

Most MCL reconstruction techniques ('Tommy John surgery') use a free autograft tendon (e.g. palmaris longus) placed in ulnar and humeral bone tunnels. Transmuscular splitting approach to the medial elbow is used to expose the MCL. Time to return to throwing is about 1 year for full competition. Current techniques allow competitive throwing athletes to return to their previous levels of sport in more than 80% of cases.[61]

Ulnar nerve entrapment/neuritis

The ulnar nerve pierces the intermuscular septum in the middle of the arm and then passes deep to the medial head of the triceps muscle into a superficial groove (ulnar sulcus) between the olecranon and medial epicondyle. It enters the forearm between the humerus and the ulnar heads of the flexor carpi ulnaris muscle.

PART B Regional problems

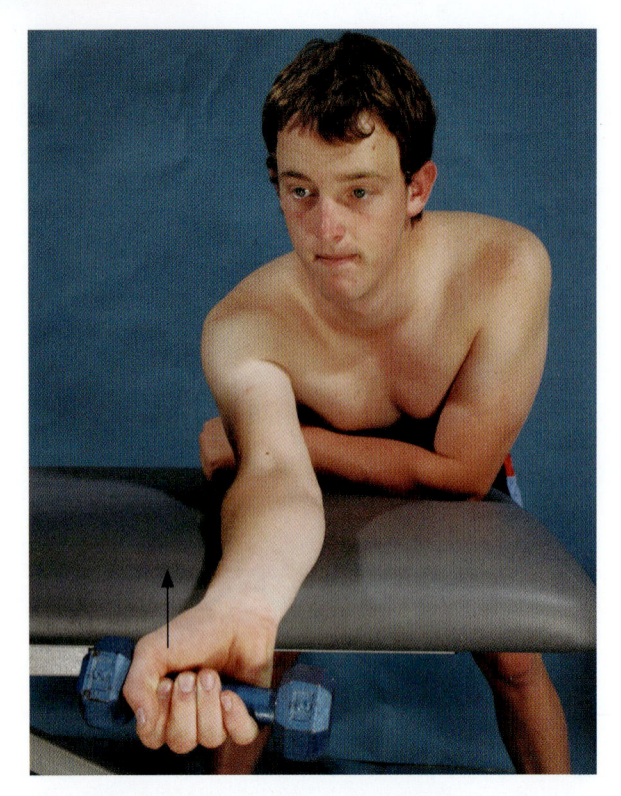

Figure 25.18 Strengthening exercises for the forearm flexors and pronators

Inflammation of the ulnar nerve can occur as a result of a combination of any of four factors:[62]

1. Traction injuries to the nerve may occur because of the dynamic valgus forces of throwing, especially when combined with valgus instability of the elbow.
2. Progressive compression can occur at the cubital tunnel secondary to inflammation and adhesions from repetitive stresses, or where the nerve passes between the two heads of the flexor carpi ulnaris due to muscle overdevelopment secondary to resistance weight-training exercises.
3. Recurrent subluxation of the nerve due to acquired laxity from repetitive stress or direct trauma. A subluxing ulnar nerve is present in about 8% of the population. Can be an important differential diagnosis—the athlete feels a 'click' and might have some pain at the same time.
4. Irregularities within the ulnar groove, such as spurs commonly seen from overuse injuries in older throwers.

The patient presents with posteromedial elbow pain and sensory symptoms such as pins and needles or numbness along the ulnar nerve distribution—the ulnar border of the forearm and the ulnar one and a half fingers. The nerve may be tender behind the medial epicondyle (Fig. 25.19) and tapping over the nerve may

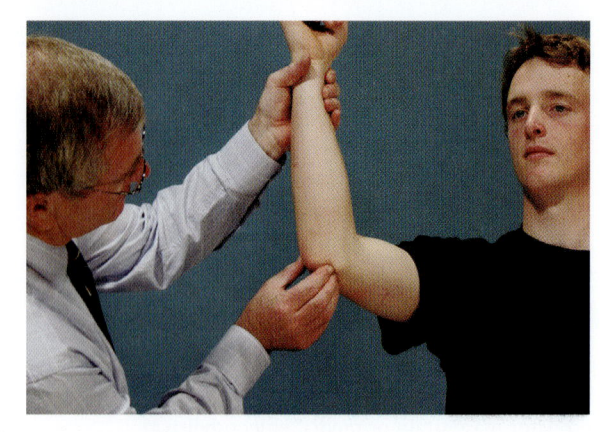

Figure 25.19 Palpation of the ulnar nerve

reproduce symptoms in some cases. Placing the elbow in maximum flexion, the forearm in pronation and the wrist in full extension for one minute may reproduce medial elbow pain and tingling/numbness in the ring and little finger if ulnar neuritis is present. Patients with clinical features of ulnar nerve involvement should undergo nerve conduction studies.[56] Reports of snapping sensation should lead one to suspect ulnar nerve subluxation, which can be confirmed with dynamic ultrasound examination.[63]

Treatment of this condition depends on the initiating factor.

1. Traction injuries related to valgus instability from throwing are best served by treating the instability to reduce the ongoing nerve irritation.
2. If adhesions are felt to be present, treatment may include local soft tissue therapy to the nerve in the ulnar groove to mobilise soft tissue that may be compressing or tethering the nerve. Neural mobilisation is often beneficial.
3. Recurrent subluxation of the ulnar nerve should be referred to a neurologist or surgeon experienced in managing this condition in active individuals. Management will depend on the degree of symptoms, electrophysiological evidence of nerve injury and local management expertise (in relation to nerve transposition surgery).
4. Bony irregularities may be amenable to arthroscopic debridement.

POSTERIOR ELBOW PAIN

The main causes of posterior elbow pain are olecranon bursitis, triceps tendinopathy and posterior impingement. Gout should always be considered.

Olecranon bursitis

Olecranon bursitis may present after a single episode of trauma or, more commonly, after repeated trauma, such as

Elbow and arm pain CHAPTER 25

falls onto a hard surface affecting the posterior aspect of the elbow. This is commonly seen in football goalkeepers and in basketball players 'taking a charge'. It is also seen in individuals who rest their elbow on a hard surface for long periods of time and is known as 'student's elbow'. The olecranon bursa is a subcutaneous bursa that may become filled with blood and serous fluid (Fig. 25.20).

Treatment in acute traumatic cases consists initially of ice, rest, firm compression and NSAIDs. If this fails, then aspiration of the contents of the bursa and injection with a mixture of corticosteroid and local anaesthetic agents will usually be effective. The needle should be inserted at an oblique angle to reduce the risk of sinus formation.

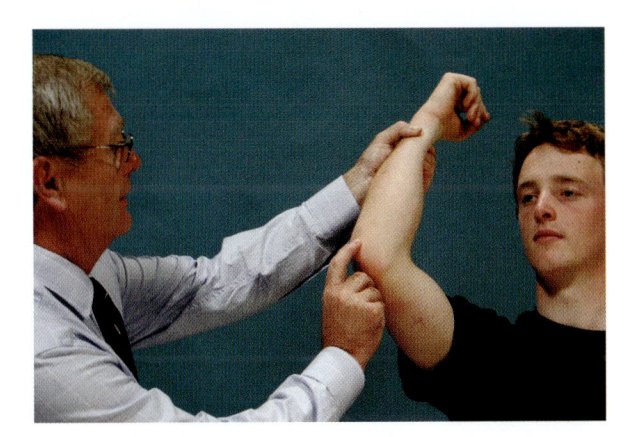

(a)

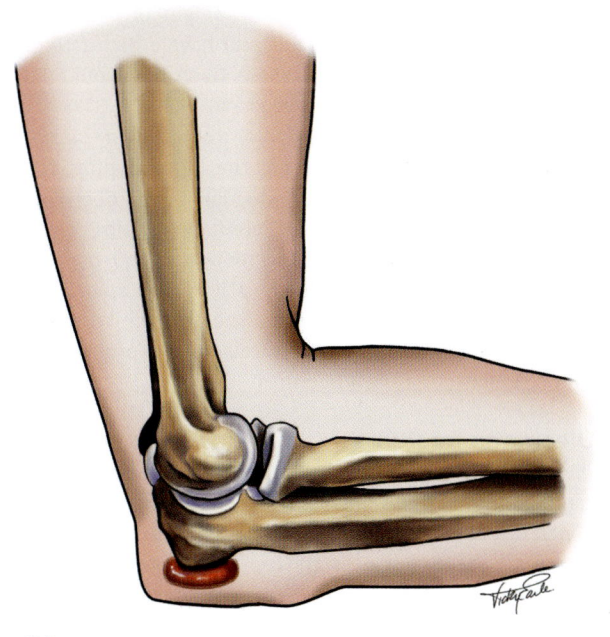

(b)

Figure 25.20 Olecranon bursa (a) Palpation site of bursa (b) Olecranon bursitis

Although this is considered a straightforward procedure among experienced clinicians, there is a trend to do this with ultrasound imaging support to increase the accuracy of needle insertion. If recurrent bursitis does not respond to aspiration and injection, surgical excision of the bursa should be considered.

Occasionally, olecranon bursitis can become infected. This is a serious complication that requires immediate drainage, immobilisation and antibiotic therapy. Osteomyelitis and septic arthritis can follow. Excision of the bursa is occasionally required.

Triceps tendinopathy

Tendinopathy at the insertion of the triceps onto the olecranon is occasionally seen. Standard conservative measures for treatment of tendinopathy should be used. Soft tissue therapy including self-massage with a Styrofoam™ roll and dry needling to reduce excessive tightness of the triceps musculotendinous complex may be helpful.

Posterior impingement

Posterior impingement is probably the most common cause of posterior elbow pain. It occurs in three situations. In the younger athlete there is the 'hyperextension valgus overload syndrome'. Repetitive hyperextension valgus stress to the elbow results in impingement of the posterior medial corner of the olecranon tip on the olecranon fossa. Over time this causes osteophyte formation, exacerbating the impingement and leading to a fixed flexion deformity. Valgus instability can be a primary driver of posterior impingement as the olecranon will then no longer be fitting into the olecranon fossa, but will impact more medially.

In the older patient the most common cause is early osteoarthritis, which often predominantly affects the radiocapitellar joint. Generalised osteophytes form through the elbow. Impingement of these osteophytes posteriorly results in posterior pain. The main clinical feature in athletes with posterior impingement is a fixed flexion deformity of some degree and posterior pain with forced extension (Fig. 25.21).

Treatment may include strategies to minimise hyperextension forces such as taping or bracing, along with a strength and flexibility program and graduated return to sport or activity. If lost range is the only problem, surgery is rarely indicated.

If conservative measures fail, then arthroscopic removal of the impinging posterior bone and anterior capsule release is very effective in relieving symptoms and improving extension especially in elderly patients. Acute painful locking however is an indication for surgery. The patient must be counselled that sometimes the loose bodies can be hard to find in the elbow, and the surgeon may miss one or more.

PART B   Regional problems

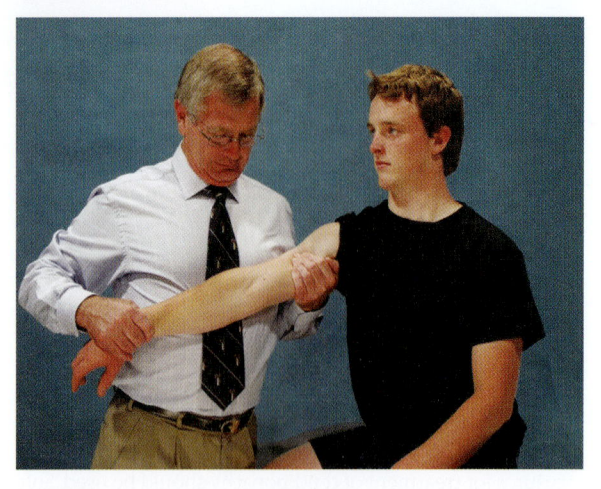

Figure 25.21 Posterior impingement. The elbow is forced into end-range extension. If posterior pain is produced then posterior impingement is present

ACUTE ELBOW INJURIES

Acute elbow injuries include fractures, dislocations and ligament or tendon ruptures. Elbow dislocation associated with fracture can lead to long-term instability and must be recognised early.

Fractures

As the complication rate for elbow fractures is higher than with fractures near other joints, it is essential that fractures in this region be recognised and treated early and aggressively. Those who are fully able to extend the elbow are unlikely to have a fracture, though they should be followed up in 7-10 days if symptoms have not resolved. A clinical protocol has been proposed to detect the presence of a fracture.[64] Plain radiography is the first line of investigation.

> **PRACTICE PEARL**
>
> Patients who cannot fully extend their elbow after injury should be referred for plain radiography because there is a 50% chance of fracture.

Unstable fractures, usually those associated with displacement, should be referred early for orthopaedic management. When the articular or cortical surface has less than 2 mm of vertical or horizontal displacement, the fracture can be regarded as stable and treated conservatively.[65]

The most common complication of elbow fractures is stiffness, particularly loss of terminal extension. Prompt diagnosis and treatment that includes an early rehabilitation program can help avoid loss of extension. Thus, treatment of elbow fractures must be aggressive. Surgically stabilising a displaced adult elbow fracture allows early commencement of a post-operative range of motion program.

A stable fracture that involves no significant comminution, displacement or angulation may be treated conservatively. In adults, immobilising the arm for a few days, even up to a week, is generally well tolerated. Then the arm should be placed in a removable splint and early motion commenced. The fracture should then be protected for 6-8 weeks, with early and frequent radiographic checks to ensure the reduction stays anatomical.

Heterotopic ossification is the other main complication of elbow fractures, particularly in high energy injuries. This usually appears within the first month after surgery and plateaus after 4-6 months. Traumatised elbows that are forcefully or passively manipulated may also be at greater risk of this complication.[66] Therefore, gentle, active assisted range of motion and pain-free stretching exercises are preferred. Mobilisation with movements, applied correctly in a pain-free manner, may be helpful in restoring motion.[31] Heterotopic bone formation has also been associated with elbow fracture-dislocation treated surgically 1-5 days after injury or treated with multiple surgical procedures. Thus, surgery should be performed in the first 24 hours after injury or after 5-7 days.

Supracondylar fractures

Supracondylar fractures are more common around the age of 12 than in adults. They often occur from a fall on an outstretched arm, either from a height or a bicycle. As they are rotationally unstable and have a high rate of neurovascular complications, these fractures should be regarded as an orthopaedic emergency.

For fractures that are unstable, displaced or cannot be reduced without jeopardising the blood supply, the treatment of choice is closed reduction in the operating room under general anaesthesia. Percutaneous pins placed across the fracture maintain the reduction and prevent late slippage. The arm is initially placed in a splint and then several days later in a cast. The pins are removed after 4-6 weeks. Stiffness is typically not a problem in children recovering from fractures.

Olecranon fractures

Olecranon fractures occur from a fall onto an outstretched hand or from direct trauma to the elbow. If the fracture is non-displaced and stable, the patient should be able to extend the arm against gravity. Treatment consists of immobilising the arm for 2-3 weeks in a posterior splint and then in a removable splint, and commencing a range of motion program. If the patient is unable to extend the elbow against gravity or if radiographs show significant displacement, open reduction with internal fixation by tension-band wiring is preferred.[67] Early motion is started within one week of surgery.

Radial head fracture

The most common fracture around the elbow in athletes is the radial head fracture, almost always resulting from a fall onto an outstretched hand. The radial head can be considered a multifunctional stabiliser of the elbow. In the frontal plane its contribution to valgus stability may be as high as 30% even with the intact MCL. In disruption of the MCL, the radial head becomes a critical secondary stabiliser of the elbow with up to 70% of resistance to valgus stress. In the sagittal plane, the radial head contributes to preventing posterior elbow dislocation in association with the coronoid process, lateral and medial ligament complex. In the longitudinal plane, the radial head prevents proximal migration of the radial shaft along with the interosseous membrane.

The main mechanism of injury in contact sports is a fall onto the outstretched hand–the radial head may fail under compressive axial or valgus loads. If there is a rotatory component it may cause a marginal shearing fracture. High energy injuries are more likely to provoke an associated fracture (capitellum, coronoid or even olecranon). MCL ligament injuries are very frequently associated.

AP, lateral and oblique elbow radiographs usually provide sufficient information for diagnosis and deciding on treatment. CT scan of the elbow in some cases can be very useful if surgery is needed, or in doubtful cases after plain radiography (for more complex cases).

Radial head fractures have been classified by Mason.[68]

- Type I–undisplaced
- Type II–displaced wedge fragment
- Type III–comminuted fracture
- Type IV–fracture associated with elbow dislocation.

Most radial head fractures are minimally displaced or non-displaced (type I) and are very difficult to see on radiographs. Sometimes the only clue is the fat pad sign, which appears as a triangular radiolucency just in front of the elbow joint. Early aspiration, splinting with an easily removable device and early commencement of a range of motion program will yield excellent results. Complete healing can be expected within 6-8 weeks.

Open reduction and internal fixation of displaced type II radial head fractures should only be attempted when anatomic reduction, restoration of articular congruity and initiation of early motion can be achieved. If these goals are not obtainable, open reduction and internal fixation may lead to early fixation failure, non-union, and loss of elbow and forearm motion and stability.

Comminuted radial head fractures are frequently associated with elbow dislocation and other destabilising injuries.[69] The scarce literature on the subject is of little help in defining optimal treatment.[70] Radial head excision in young or adult athletes with comminuted fracture of the radial head, associated with medial, lateral or interosseous ligament injury, has a poor clinical outcome. There is currently more emphasis on preservation or replacement of the radial head, attempting to avoid radial head excision if at all possible.[70, 71]

Coronoid fractures

The coronoid process provides an anterior bony buttress to resist the posteriorly directed forces that occur from the flexor/extensor muscles. Regan and Morrey in their study[72] showed a correlation between coronoid fragment size and a tendency for elbow dislocation.

Coronoid fracture can be isolated, but most commonly occurs in association with radial head fracture and elbow dislocation ('terrible triad'). The injury pattern is determined by the position at the time of injury and the loading pattern across the elbow. A common mistake is to misidentify a coronoid fragment as a radial head fragment. Coronoid fractures have been classified on the base of anatomic location of the primary fracture:

- tip (anteromedial facet)
- body.

Plain AP, lateral and oblique lateral radiograph views can be helpful and CT scan is highly useful.

> **PRACTICE PEARL**
>
> Dislocated elbow with radial head fracture usually has an associated coronoid fracture. The coronoid fragment is always bigger than it appears on the radiograph because of the articular cartilage cup on the fragment.

Caution is required when treating isolated coronoid fractures as they appear benign, but usually are fracture subluxations with ligament avulsion. Many of these fractures require some form of surgical treatment by specialised elbow surgeons.

Posterior dislocation

The most serious acute elbow injury is a posterior dislocation. This can occur either in contact sports or when falling from a height such as while pole vaulting. There is often an associated fracture of the coronoid process or radial head. The usual mechanism is a posterolateral rotatory force resulting from a fall on an outstretched hand with the shoulder abducted, axial compression, forearm in supination and then forced flexion of the elbow.[73]

There are three grades of elbow dislocation:[73]

1. subluxation of the elbow in the posterolateral direction
2. incomplete elbow dislocation with the coronoid perched on the trochlea
3. complete posterior dislocation of the elbow, so that the coronoid rests behind the trochlear
   a. where the anterior band of the MCL is intact and the elbow is stable to valgus stress following reduction
   b. where the MCL is completely disrupted so the elbow is unstable in all directions after reduction. This pattern of dislocation is associated with progressive soft tissue disruption that commences laterally and progresses around anteriorly, medially and posteriorly, termed the Horii circle described by O'Driscoll.[74]

The major complication of elbow dislocation is impairment of the vascular supply to the forearm. Assessment of pulses distal to the dislocation is essential. If pulses are absent, reduction of the dislocation is required urgently. Reduction is usually relatively easy. With the elbow held at 45°, the clinician stabilises the humerus by gripping the anterior aspect of the distal humerus and traction is placed longitudinally along the forearm with the other hand (Fig. 25.22). The elbow usually reduces with a pronounced clunk. If vascular impairment persists after reduction, urgent surgical intervention is required.

Following reduction, the stability of the collateral ligaments should be assessed (Fig. 25.17a). A post-reduction radiograph should also be performed. Small fractures of the coronoid process or undisplaced fractures of the radial head only require conservative treatment with support in a sling for 2-3 weeks. Large coronoid fractures, however, may result in chronic instability and should be reduced and fixed surgically. Large fractures of the radial head may be difficult to manage, but in most cases can be internally fixed. Occasionally, a large fracture of the capitellum may occur. This also requires internal fixation. Sometimes a piece of bone becomes trapped in the joint after reduction. This needs to be excluded with good quality post-reduction radiographs.

Acute injuries at the elbow after subluxation or dislocation are best treated non-surgically, with brace or splint keeping the forearm in pronation to allow the lateral ligament complex to heal. Long-term loss of terminal extension is frequently a problem following elbow dislocation. Immediate active mobilisation under supervision has been shown to result in less restriction of elbow extension with no apparent increase in instability.[75] Professional athletes with a simple dislocation with no associated fracture or instability are able to return to sports relatively quickly after an appropriate rehabilitation program. Verrall described three cases of stable dislocations in professional footballers who returned to sport after 7, 13 and 21 days with no further complications.[76] Joint mobilisation (Fig. 25.23) may be required as part of the treatment.[31] The surrounding muscles should also be strengthened. Elbow stability taping should be applied on return to the sport (Fig. 25.17b).

Heterotopic ossification occasionally occurs following elbow dislocation. The use of NSAIDs for a period of three months following the injury may reduce the incidence of this complication.

Elbow dislocations in directions other than posterior occur occasionally. These are often associated with severe ligamentous disruption and patients should be referred to an orthopaedic surgeon immediately.

Instability post-dislocation

When the competency of the soft tissue restraints after elbow dislocation or injury is inadequate, it can lead to recurrent elbow instability. The condition is more common in some sports than has previously been recognised. On the lateral side, instability is posterolateral and rotatory. On the medial side it is valgus.

Athletes with posterolateral rotatory instability (PLRI) usually present with the symptoms after an elbow subluxation or dislocation. Less commonly there is a history of previous lateral elbow surgery (iatrogenic) for tennis elbow. Recurrent lateral instability is always rotatory.[77] PLRI is defined as a posterior radial head subluxation relative to the humerus while maintaining normal relationship at the proximal RU joint. O'Driscoll et al. identified the ulnar part of the lateral collateral ligament as the key lateral soft tissue restraint preventing posterolateral rotatory instability;[77] however, the radial collateral ligament also contributes to both varus and posterolateral stability.

The patient with PLRI presents with recurrent painful clicking, snapping, clunking or locking of the elbow occurring in extension of the arm with the forearm in

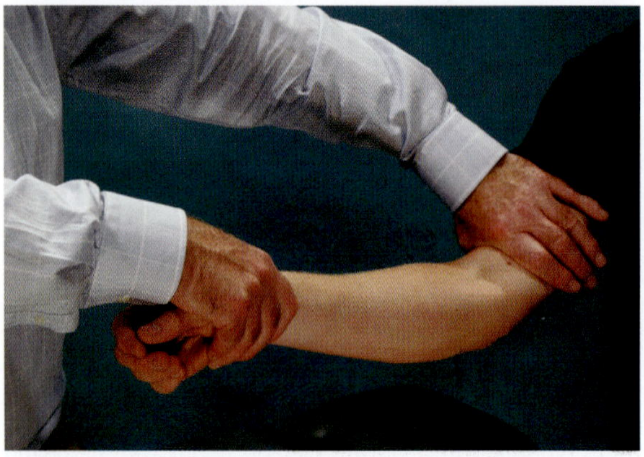

Figure 25.22 Technique for reduction of posterior dislocation of the elbow

Elbow and arm pain   CHAPTER 25

(a)

(b)

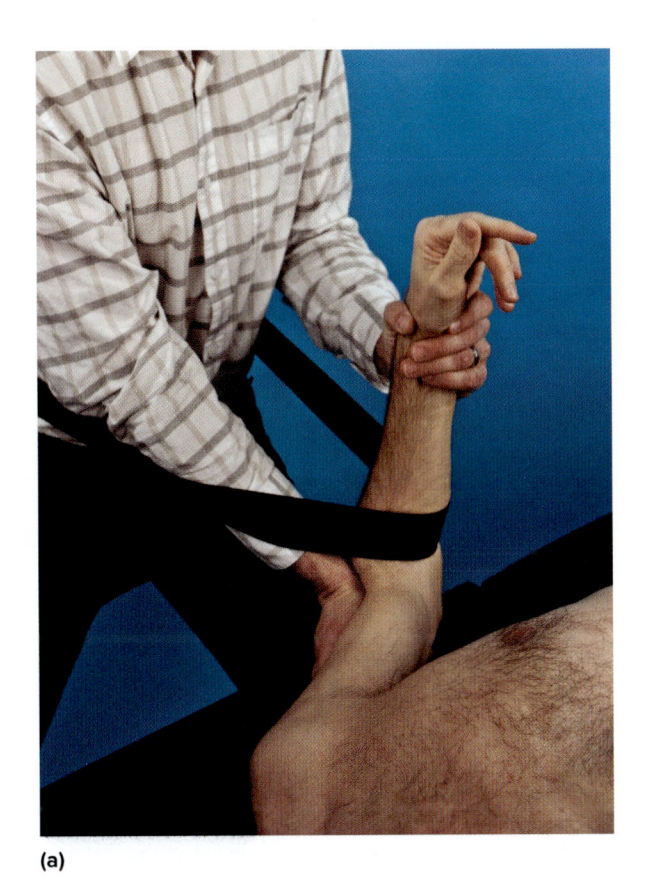

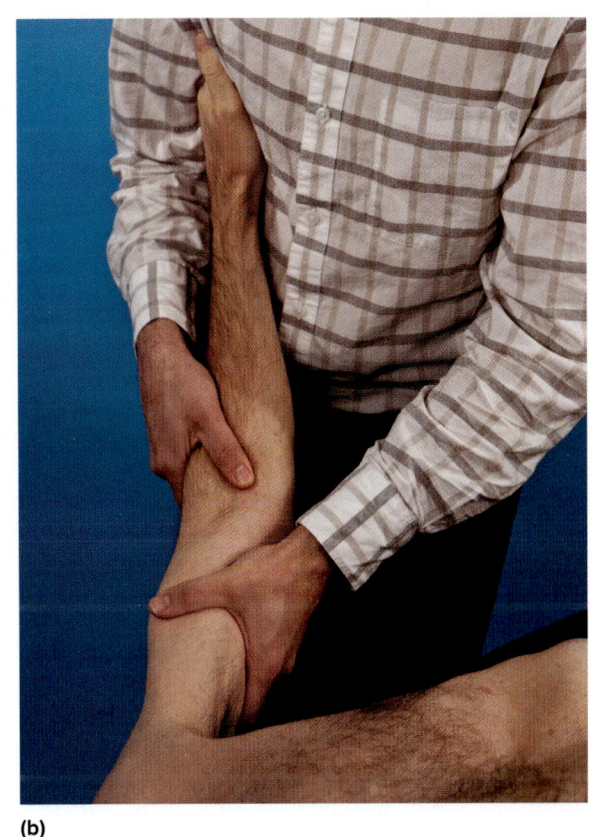

Figure 25.23 Examples of mobilisation with movement techniques that use a glide out of the plane of extension to improve extension (a) Sustained lateral glide applied through a belt while assisted active extension is performed (b) Sustained internal rotation

supination. Typically these symptoms are more prominent with loading of the joint in the supinated and slightly flexed position. Several provocative manoeuvres have been described, including the posterolateral rotatory apprehension test (or lateral pivot shift test)[77] and the chair and push-up tests.[78]

Chronic PLRI does not respond well to conservative treatment and usually requires ligament reconstruction with a free ligament autograft (ipsilateral palmaris longus, gracilis, semintendinosis, triceps). Published studies on the clinical outcome after surgical treatment of chronic PLRI demonstrate mostly good and excellent outcomes.[79, 80]

Acute rupture of the medial collateral ligament

Acute rupture of the MCL may occur in a previously damaged ligament or in a normal ligament subjected to extreme valgus stress, for example elbow dislocation. In a study of 14 MCL injuries in American National Football League (NFL) gridiron players,[81] the two most common mechanisms of injury were blocking at the line of scrimmage (50%) and the application of a valgus force with the hand planted on the playing surface (29%). The degree of laxity should be assessed by applying valgus stress to the elbow at 30° of flexion (Fig. 25.17a). If complete disruption is present with associated instability, surgical repair of the ligament is required. Incomplete tears should be treated with protection in a brace and muscle strengthening exercises for a period of 3–6 weeks, followed by graduated return to sports.

Tendon ruptures

Acute avulsion of the biceps or triceps tendons from their insertions is a rare condition. Rupture of the distal biceps tendon insertion occurs predominantly in young or middle-aged men engaged in strength activities (e.g. weightlifting). Partial ruptures are more painful than complete ruptures, due to mechanical irritation of the remaining intact tendon. Early surgical repair of complete ruptures would be expected to lead to better outcomes, as complete rupture of tendons leads to degenerative processes due to the loss of mechanical load. Rupture of the triceps tendon occurs

459

PART B Regional problems

most commonly with excessive deceleration force, such as occurs during a fall or by a direct blow to the posterior aspect of the elbow. Partial and complete triceps ruptures are seen in NFL linemen.[34] Partial tears tend to heal well without surgery. Acute complete ruptures at the insertion of either of these tendons should be treated surgically.

Hyperextension injuries

Hyperextension injuries caused by direct force to the forearm pushing the elbow into hyperextension may be acute, in which case the athlete is usually unable to continue activity, or repetitive, when the athlete feels sudden pain but is able to continue. These injuries are probably more common than previously thought.

Kenter et al. reported that hyperextension was the most common (56%) cause of acute elbow sprain in NFL players.[81] Hyperextension injuries are common (75%) in goalies in handball.[82, 83] Hyperextension of the elbow is caused by the ball hitting the fully extended distal part of the forearm when blocking a shot. This injury is frequently bilateral. Most handball goalkeepers could usually remember their first elbow accident. The goalies routinely minimise their symptoms in an attempt to continue to play, despite the fact that the injury affects their performance. Their first symptoms (pain) usually began acutely but developed into chronic elbow pain, with intermittent pain as the chief complaint. There are reports of similar mechanisms of injuries in other sports such as water polo players, soccer goalkeepers, volleyball players, wrestlers and judo practitioners.

The force of the blow of the ball to the forearm produces a valgus load on the elbow, applying stress to the anterior band of the MCLC. Specific injuries include (i) lesions of the anterior capsule including rupture, (ii) L-shaped rupture of the flexor/pronator origin with elongation of the anterior part of the MCL, (iii) occasional incomplete rupture of the LCL and, rarely, (iv) detachment of small fragments of cartilage near the posterior edge of the olecranon. Imaging studies (ultrasound/MRI) can confirm the diagnosis.

FOREARM PAIN
Fracture of the radius and ulna

The bones of the forearm are commonly injured by a fall on the back or front of the outstretched hand. It is usual for both bones to break, although a single bone may be fractured in cases of direct violence or in fractures of the distal third where there is no shortening.

A displaced fracture is usually clinically obvious. Plain radiographs should be taken for post-reduction comparison and for exclusion of a concurrent dislocation. Two types of dislocation occur–the Monteggia injury (fractured ulna with dislocated head of the radius at the elbow joint) and the Galeazzi injury (fractured radius with dislocated head of the ulna at the wrist joint).

In the child, angulation of less than 10° is acceptable. Other fractures should be reduced under local or general anaesthesia depending on the age of the child. The usual position for immobilisation is in pronation, although in proximal radial fractures and in Smith's fracture at the wrist, the forearm should be held in supination. The plaster should extend above the elbow and leave the metacarpophalangeal joints free. Depending on the age of the child, immobilisation should last 4–6 weeks. The position should be checked by radiography every 1–2 weeks depending on stability.

In the adult, perfect reduction of radial and ulnar fractures is necessary to ensure future sporting function. Most of these fractures are significantly displaced and require anatomical internal fixation with a plate and screws. Depending on the accuracy of reduction, either a cast or a crepe bandage support is required post-operatively for 8–10 weeks. Isolated fractures of the ulna are treated conservatively by an above-elbow cast in mid-pronation for 8 weeks. Monteggia and Galeazzi injuries are usually displaced and should be referred to an orthopaedic surgeon for reduction.

Stress fractures

Stress fractures of the forearm bones occur occasionally in athletes involved in upper limb sports, such as baseball, tennis or swimming. Treatment involves rest and correction of the possible predisposing factors, such as faulty technique.

Entrapment of the posterior interosseous nerve (radial tunnel syndrome)

The radial nerve divides into the superficial radial and the posterior interosseous nerve at the level of the radiocapitellar joint (Fig. 25.24). The posterior interosseous nerve (PIN) passes distal to the origin of the ECRB and enters the arcade of Frohse. Prior to entering the arcade of Frohse, it gives off branches to the ECRB and supinator muscles. The arcade is a semicircular fibrous arch at the proximal head of the supinator muscle, which begins at the tip of the lateral epicondyle and extends downwards, attaching to the medial aspect of the lateral epicondyle. The PIN then emerges from the supinator muscle distally, where it divides into terminal branches that innervate the medial extensors. Compression of the PIN may occur at one of four sites:[84]

- fibrous bands anterior to the radial head
- recurrent radial vessels
- arcade of Frohse
- tendinous margin of the extensor carpi radialis brevis muscle.

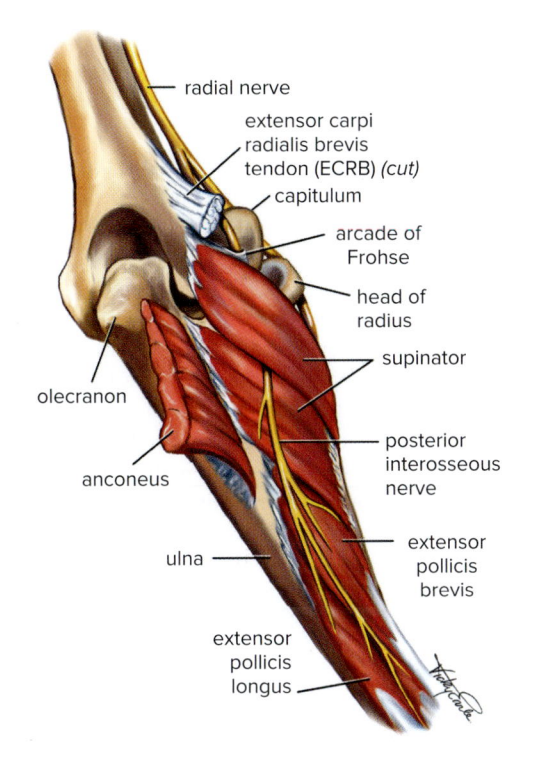

Figure 25.24 Anatomy of the posterior interosseous nerve

It may be difficult to differentiate between lateral elbow tendinopathy and the early stages of PIN entrapment. PIN entrapment is seen in patients who repetitively pronate and supinate the forearm, whereas lateral elbow tendinopathy is more frequently associated with repetitive wrist extension. Symptoms of PIN entrapment include paraesthesia in the hand and lateral forearm, pain over the forearm extensor mass, aching wrist and middle or upper third humeral pain. It is these symptoms that critically differentiate this condition from lateral elbow tendinopathy.

Maximal tenderness is over the supinator muscle, four finger breadths below the lateral epicondyle (distal to the area of maximal tenderness in extensor tendinopathy). Reproduction of symptoms by manual palpation of these local structures and the relief of such palpation-induced symptoms by injection of local anaesthetic should be considered as part of the physical examination.[85] Nerve entrapment also causes marked pain on resisted supination of the forearm with the elbow flexed to 90° and the forearm fully pronated. Neurodynamic tests (with radial nerve bias) may reproduce the patient's symptoms, and nerve conduction studies may be performed to confirm the diagnosis.

Treatment consists of soft tissue therapy over the supinator muscle at the site of entrapment and neural tissue mobilisation, along with exercises targeting strength and endurance deficits in the forearm muscles. If this is unsuccessful, decompression surgery may be required.

Pronator teres syndrome (median nerve entrapment)

The median nerve can become entrapped as it passes between the two heads of the pronator teres muscle. Median nerve entrapment presents as diffuse anterior elbow pain that radiates distally into the forearm with paraesthesia in the median nerve distribution distally and weakness of the thenar muscles. The most common cause in athletes is forceful pronation, for example throwing or racquet sports.

A similar clinical picture can be produced by cervical radiculopathy at C6–7 level, compression of the median nerve underneath the lacertus fibrosis or by the ligament of Struthers. The diagnosis can be confirmed on nerve conduction studies.

Activity modification is the first line of treatment. Surgical resection of the humeral head of pronator teres is occasionally required.

Forearm compartment pressure syndrome

Forearm compartment pressure syndromes have been described in kayakers, canoeists, motorcyclists (popularly termed 'arm pump' in motorcross) and weight-training athletes. The flexor compartment is most usually affected. Symptoms include activity-related pain that is relieved by rest. Diagnosis requires compartment pressure testing. Treatment consists of local soft tissue therapy. Surgical fasciotomy may be required.

UPPER ARM PAIN

An aching pain in the upper arm is a common complaint, especially among manual workers (e.g. bricklayers, carpenters) and athletes. The most common cause is myofascial pain, but stress fracture of the humerus needs to be considered.

Myofascial pain

A dull non-specific pain in the upper arm is most likely to be myofascial in nature. The most common source of the upper arm pain is trigger points in the infraspinatus muscle (Fig. 25.25). Firm palpation of these trigger points will often reproduce the patient's pain. The cervical spine and glenohumeral joint need to be assessed for their possible involvement and treatment directed accordingly.

Treatment consists of digital ischaemic pressure or dry needling to the trigger points. Attention should also be paid to the lower cervical and upper to mid-thoracic spine. Increased muscle tone and trigger points may be found in the paraspinal muscles, and hypomobility of the intervertebral segments may be present. These abnormalities must also be treated with soft tissue techniques.

PART B   Regional problems

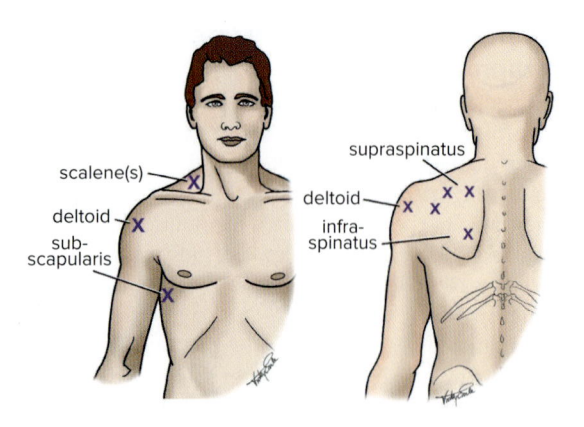

Figure 25.25 Myofascial trigger points around the shoulder region that refer pain to the upper arm

Stress reaction of the humerus

Stress reactions and fractures of the humerus have been described in tennis players, javelin throwers, baseball pitchers, bodybuilders and weightlifters. In a group of symptomatic elite tennis players, MRI of the humerus demonstrated bone marrow oedema and/or periostitis, and the extent of imaging changes was related to the severity and duration of symptoms.[86] Most of the fractures occurred in adolescents and were associated with a recent increase in activity. In a number of cases the diagnosis was made retrospectively when an acute fracture occurred and the patient admitted symptoms leading up to the acute episode.

Recommended treatment follows the general principles of management of simple stress fractures: avoidance of the aggravating activity until symptom-free with no local tenderness, then gradual resumption of the activity.

REFERENCES

References for this chapter can be found at www.mhhe.com/au/CSM5e

Chapter 26

Wrist pain

with GREGORY HOY and HAMISH ANDERSON*

> *Laura Robson admits she will have to start her career all over again after she recovers from major wrist surgery. Robson said she 'felt like a child again' in the aftermath of her operation, struggling to dress herself and cut her own food. Itching to return to action, Robson said she has been reduced to tears, at times frustrated with rehabilitation while her peers train and compete.*
>
> Sky Sports, 20 June 2014

The wrist is frequently injured during sport.[1] Distal radial fractures are common, as are scaphoid fractures and tendon problems. Carpal instabilities are less frequent but often career threatening.

Men are more likely to sustain a hand or wrist injury and children/adolescents are more likely to have a wrist injury compared with adults.[3] Injuries to the wrist range from acute traumatic fractures, such as occur during football, hockey and snowboarding, to overuse conditions, which occur more commonly in racquet sports, golf and gymnastics. If wrist injuries are not treated appropriately at the time of injury, they can lead to future impairments that may affect not only sporting endeavours, but also activities of daily living.[4]

In this chapter, we will assess wrist injuries from an anatomical viewpoint, based on the site of pain. They are:

- radial-sided wrist pain, both acute and chronic
- central wrist pain, including volar and dorsal
- ulnar-sided wrist pain.

The differential diagnoses of wrist pain are listed in Table 26.1.

CLINICAL APPROACH

The wrist joint has multiple axes of movement: flexion/extension and radial/ulnar deviation occur at the radiocarpal and midcarpal joints, and pronation/supination occurs at the distal and proximal radio-ulnar joints. These movements provide mobility for hand function.

The anatomy of the wrist is complex (Fig. 26.1). It is helpful to know the surface anatomy of the scaphoid tubercle, hook of hamate, pisiform, Lister's tubercle and anatomical snuffbox. The bony anatomy consists of a proximal row (lunate, triquetrum, pisiform) and a distal row (trapezium, trapezoid, capitate, hamate), which are bridged by the scaphoid bone. Normally, the distal carpal row should be stable; thus, a ligamentous injury here can greatly impair the integrity of the wrist. The proximal row permits more intercarpal movement to allow wrist flexion/extension and radial and ulnar deviation. Here, a ligamentous injury disrupts important kinematics that have been recently labelled the 'dart thrower's motion' between the radius, scaphoid, lunate and the capitate in the central column, resulting in carpal instability with potential weakness and impairment of hand function. Recognising these ligamentous injuries early is not just important for athletic performance, but also for minimisation of any subsequent post-traumatic arthritis.

History

It is essential to determine the mechanism of the injury (if there is one) causing wrist pain. A fall on the outstretched hand may be severe enough to fracture the scaphoid or distal radius, or damage the intercarpal ligaments and/or triangular fibrocartilage complex. These injuries are commonly encountered in high-velocity activities such as snowboarding,[5] rollerblading[6,7] or falling off a bike. A patient may fracture the hook of hamate while swinging a golf club,[8] tennis racquet or bat and while striking a hard object (e.g. the ground). Rotational stress to the distal radio-ulnar joint and forced ulnar deviation and rotation may tear the triangular fibrocartilage complex.

PART B   Regional problems

Table 26.1 Causes of wrist pain divided into regions

Zone	Common	Less common	Not to be missed
Dorsal wrist			
Radial zone	Extensor carpi radialis tenosynovitis De Quervain's tenosynovitis (volleyball) Scaphoid fracture Distal radius fracture (often intra-articular in the athlete)	Intersection syndrome (rowing/paddling) Anterior interosseous nerve compression Radial sensory nerve compression (volleyball) Extensor pollicis longus impingement on Lister's tubercle with occasional rupture (gymnastics)	Carpal dislocation Radial epyphyseal stress reaction (gymnastics)
Central zone	Posterior interosseous nerve/radial nerve entrapment Ganglion cyst Scapholunate ligament sprain (football)	Impingement syndromes: lunate (gymnastics); capitate (weightlifting); triquetrohamate (racquet sports); radial styloid (golf)	Scapholunate dissociation Perilunar dislocation Kienböck's disease
Ulnar zone	Extensor carpi ulnaris tenosynovitis (golf/tennis) Triangular fibrocartilage complex tear (water skiing) Ulnar styloid fracture Triquetral fracture (boxing)	Distal radioulnar joint instability Luno-triquetral ligament sprain Ulnar fracture Extensor carpi ulnaris subluxation (cricket)	Lunotriquetral dissociation
Volar wrist			
Radial zone	Carpo-metacarpal osteoarthritis	Flexor carpi radialis tendinopathy	Carpal instability
Central zone	Carpal tunnel syndrome (motorcycling)	Pisotriquetral degenerative joint disease	
Ulnar zone	Thoracic outlet syndrome Lunotriquetral ganglion	Hook of hamate fracture (golf) Ulnar nerve compression at Guyon's canal (cycling, baseball) Flexor carpi ulnaris tendinopathy	Anterior dislocation of lunate Traumatic ulnar artery aneurysm or thrombosis (karate)

When a patient presents with gradual-onset or chronic wrist pain, the clinician should consider whether the pain may be a manifestation of a systemic condition (e.g. metabolic disorder or spondyloarthopathy, see Chapter 7). Also, the clinician should rule out an uncommon presentation of radiating pain from a more proximal problem such as a herniated cervical disc.

A detailed history will reveal whether the problem stems from an overuse condition (e.g. tenosynovitis), or from an acute injury that has not been correctly diagnosed or treated. Some patients suffer only minor discomfort at the time of an initial injury and fail to seek attention at that time. Factors that aggravate the pain provide useful information as to which structures are involved in chronic wrist pain.

Pain after repeated movement, with stiffness after a period of rest, suggests an inflammatory condition such as tenosynovitis. Pain aggravated by weight-bearing activities, such as gymnastics or diving, suggests bone or joint involvement. A history of joint clicking may be

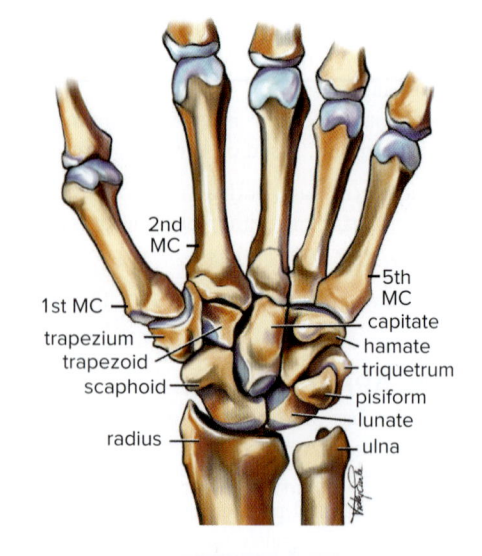

(a)

Figure 26.1 Anatomy of the wrist (a) Carpal bones (MC = metacarpal)

Wrist pain CHAPTER 26

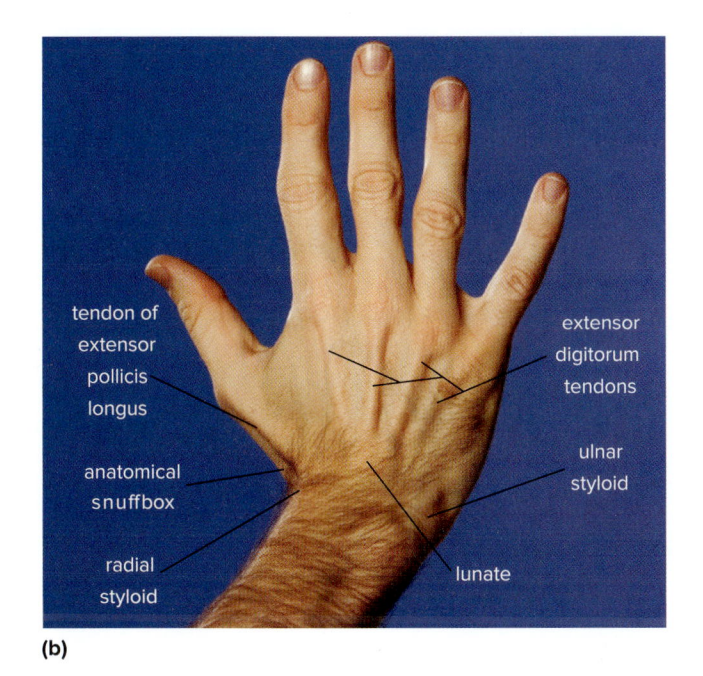

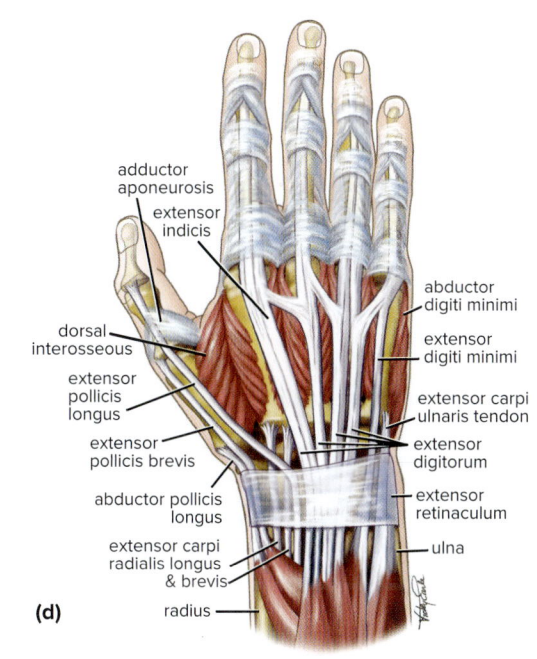

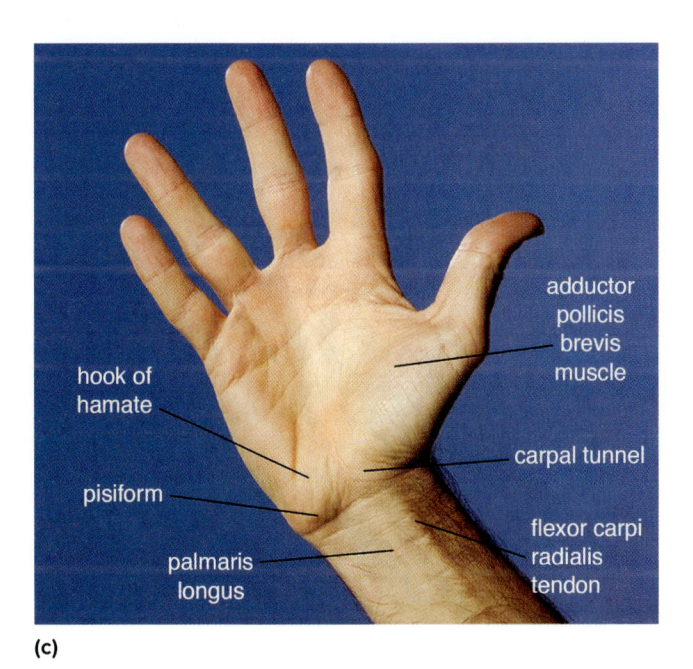

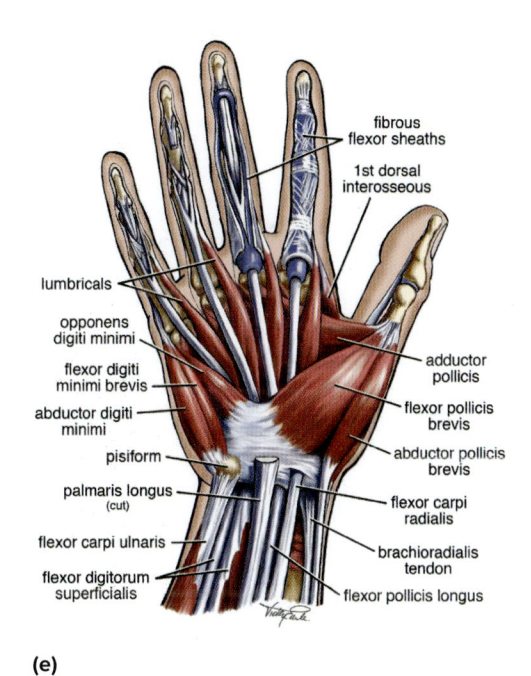

Figure 26.1 (cont.) (b) Surface anatomy, dorsal view (c) Surface anatomy, volar view (d) Dorsal aspect (e) Volar aspect

associated with carpal instability, triangular fibrocartilage tears or extensor carpi ulnaris subluxation. Characteristic night pain, with or without paraesthesia, is found in carpal tunnel syndrome. Associated neck or elbow symptoms suggest referred pain.

Other important aspects of the history may include:

- hand dominance
- occupation (e.g. computer-related, manual labour, food service industry)

PART B Regional problems

- degree of reliance upon hands in occupation/recreation
- musician (number of years playing, hours of practice per week, change in playing, complex piece, etc.)
- gardening, crafts, hobbies.
- history of past upper extremity fractures including childhood fractures/injuries
- history of osteoarthritis, rheumatoid arthritis, thyroid dysfunction, diabetes
- any unusual sounds (e.g. clicks, clunks, snaps, etc.)
- recurrent wrist swelling raises the suspicion of wrist instability

Physical examination
Examination involves:

1. Observation (Fig. 26.2a)
   Inspection may reveal a ganglion on the dorsum of the wrist. Swelling over the radial styloid may indicate de Quervain's tenosynovitis. Muscle wasting of the thenar or hypothenar eminence is found in the late stages of median or ulnar nerve compression, respectively.
2. Active movements
   a. flexion/extension
   b. supination/pronation
   c. radial/ulnar deviation (Fig. 26.2b)
3. Passive movements
   a. extension (Fig. 26.2c)
   b. flexion (Fig. 26.2d)
4. Palpation
   Palpate the wrist to detect tenderness and to determine whether the pathology appears to be extra-articular (i.e. soft tissue) or articular.
   a. distal forearm (Fig. 26.2e)
   b. radial snuffbox (Fig. 26.2f)
   c. base of metacarpals
   d. lunate (Fig. 26.2g)
   e. head of ulna (Fig. 26.2h)
   f. radio-ulnar joint
   g. hamate/pisiform (Fig. 26.2i)
   h. tuberosity of trapezium
   On the volar aspect of the wrist, palpate the tuberosity of the trapezium as a bony prominence at the base of the thenar eminence.
5. Special tests
   a. Watson's test for scapholunate injury (Fig. 26.2j)
   b. stress of triangular fibrocartilage complex (Fig. 26.2k)
   c. ulnar fovea sign for foveal disruption and ulnar triquetral ligament injury (Fig. 26.2l)
   d. press test for triangular fibrocartilage complex pain (Fig. 26.2m)
   e. Finkelstein's test (Fig. 26.2n)
   f. Tinel's sign for nerve entrapment (Fig. 26.2o)
   g. Phalen's test for carpal tunnel syndrome
   h. two point discrimination (Fig. 26.2p).

The clinical utility of selected assessment findings is shown in Table 26.2.

Key outcome measures
Several valid and reliable assessment scales can quantify function of the wrist specifically or the upper extremity after an injury. These include the Patient Rated Wrist Evaluation (PRWE),[15, 16] the Disability of the Arm, Shoulder and Hand (DASH and QuickDASH)[17, 18] and the Mayo Wrist Score[19] (Table 26.3).

Investigations
Plain radiography
Plain radiographs taken should include a posteroanterior (PA) view and a PA with both radial and ulnar deviation. If ligament injury is suspected, also obtain a PA view with clenched fist. A straight lateral, with the dorsum of the distal forearm and the third metacarpal forming a straight line, permits assessment of the distal radius, the lunate (or 'intercalated segment'), the scaphoid and the capitate, and may reveal subtle instability called DISI (dorsal intercalated segment instability) or VISI (volar intercalated segment instability). Undisplaced distal radial and scaphoid fractures, however, may be difficult to see on initial radiographs; clinical suspicion warrants use of other modalities (see 'Special imaging studies', below).

The normal PA view is shown in Figure 26.3a. Inspect each bone in turn. Note the line joining the proximal ends of the proximal row of the carpus and the C shape of the midcarpal joint (Gilula's arcs). If these lines are not smooth, a major abnormality is present. Assess the size of the scapholunate gap and look for scaphoid flexion (the signet ring sign) as these are signs of scapholunate instability.

The lateral radiograph of the normal wrist can be seen in Figure 26.3b. The proximal pole of the lunate fits into the concavity of the distal radius and the convex head of the capitate fits into the distal concavity of the lunate. These bones should be aligned with each other and with the base of the third metacarpal.

A clenched fist PA view should be taken if scapholunate instability is suspected. This is indicated by a widened gap of 3 mm or greater between the scaphoid and lunate on the PA view, but this may not present until some time after a scapholunate tear.

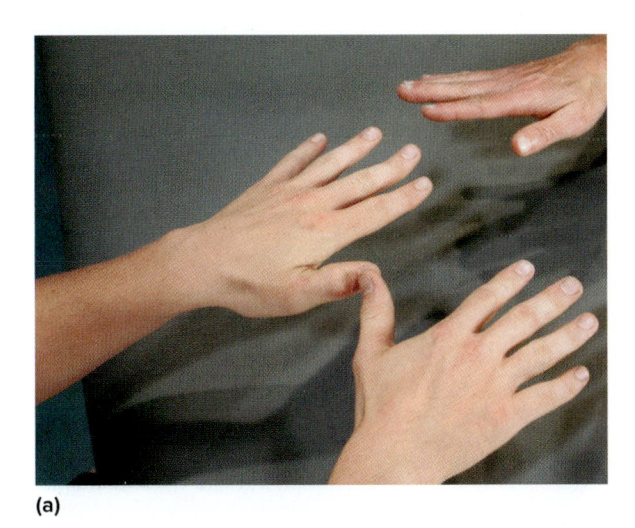

Wrist pain   CHAPTER 26

(a)

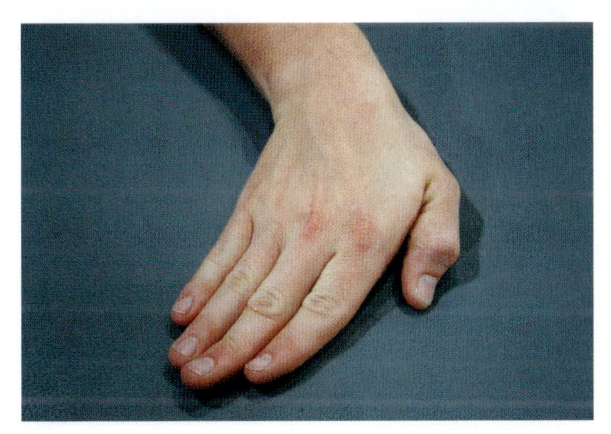

(b)

(c)

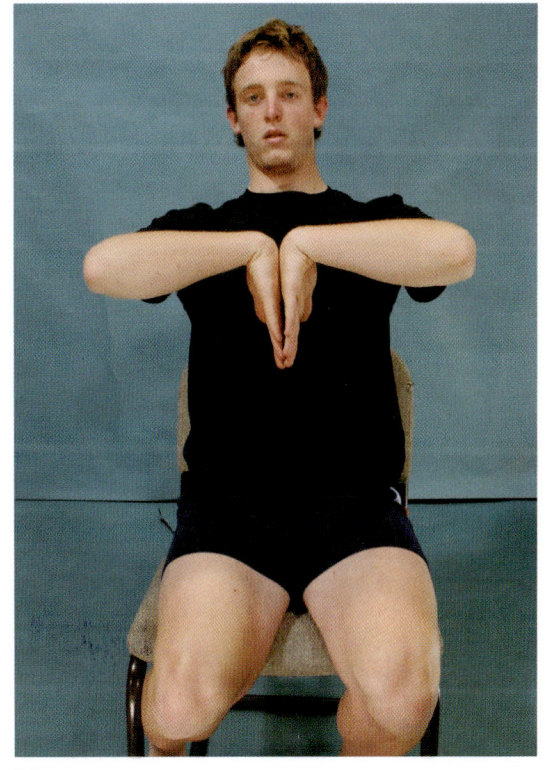

(d)

Figure 26.2 Examination of the patient with an acute wrist injury (a) Observation—inspect the wrist for obvious deformity suggesting a distal radial fracture. Swelling in the region of the radial snuffbox may indicate a scaphoid fracture. Inspect the hand and wrist posture, temperature, colour, muscular wasting, scars, normal arches of the hand (b) Active movement—radial/ulnar deviation. Normal range is radial 20° and ulnar 60°. Pain and restriction of movement should be noted. Always compare motion with that of the other hand (c) Range of motion—extension (the 'prayer position'). Normal range of motion in wrist extension is 70° (d) Range of motion—flexion (the 'reverse prayer position'). Normal range of motion in wrist flexion is 80–90°

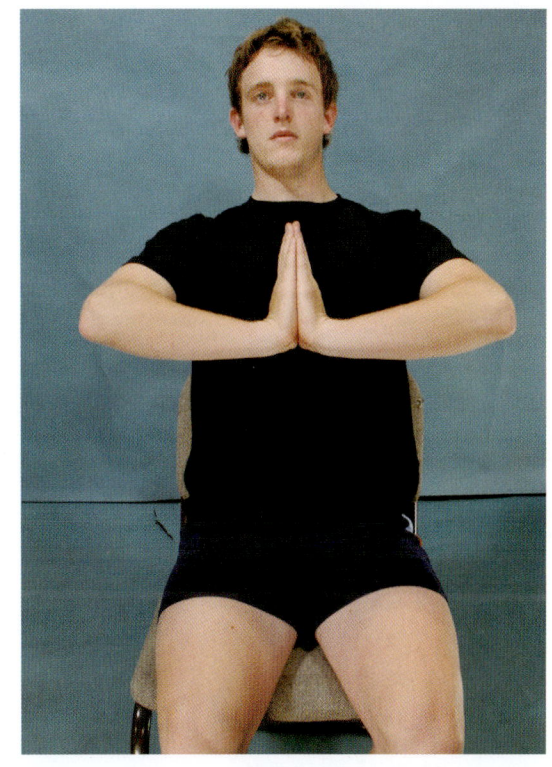

PART B   Regional problems

(e)

(g)

(f)

(h)

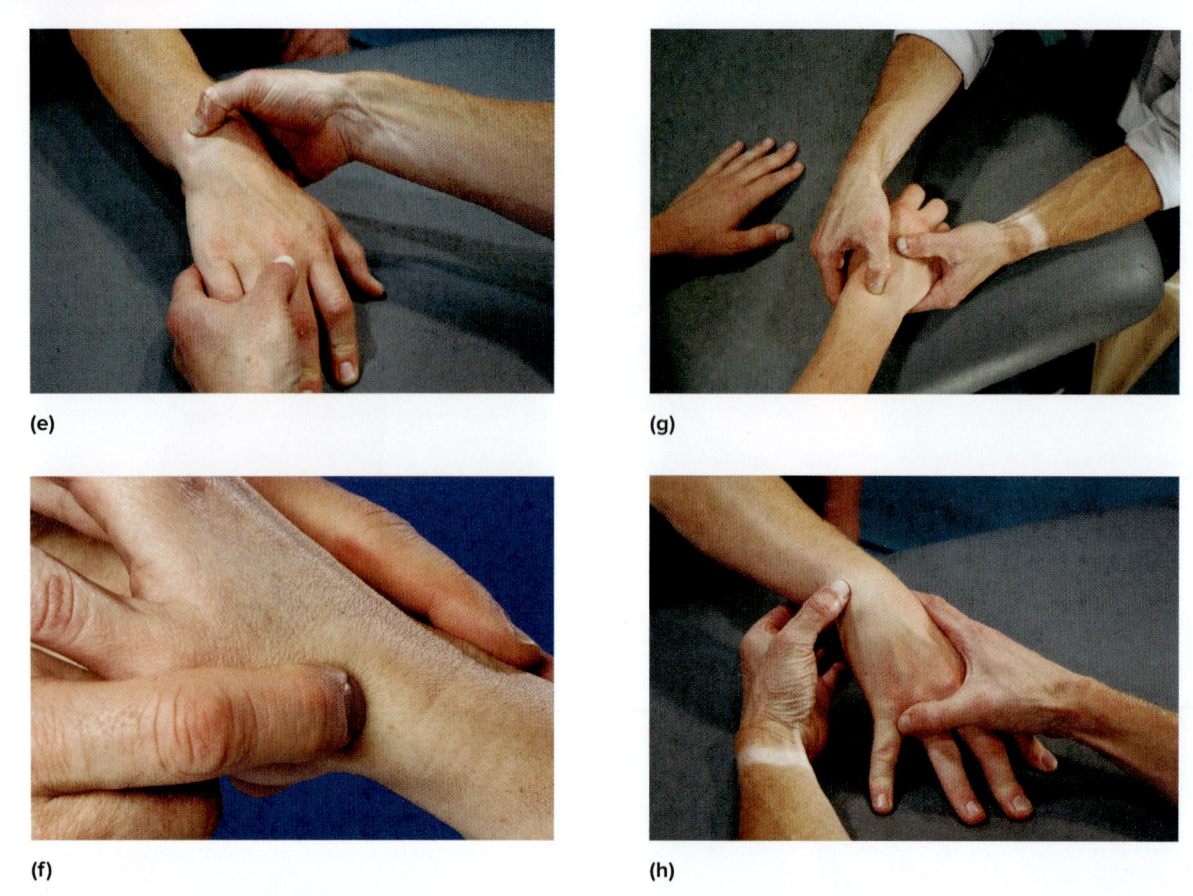

Figure 26.2 (cont.) (e) Palpation—the distal forearm is palpated for bony tenderness or deformity (f) Palpation—radial snuffbox. The proximal snuffbox is the site of the radial styloid, the middle snuffbox is the site of the scaphoid bone, while the distal snuffbox is over the scaphotrapezial joint (g) Palpation—the lunate is palpated as a bony prominence proximal to the capitate sulcus. Lunate tenderness may correspond to a fracture. On the radial side of the lunate lies the scapholunate joint, which may be tender in scapholunate ligament sprain. This is a site of ganglion formation. On the ulnar side of the lunate lies the triquetrolunate ligament. Tenderness and an associated click on radial and ulnar deviation of the wrist may occur with partial or complete tears of this ligament (h) Palpation—head of ulna and ulnar snuffbox. Swelling and tenderness over the dorsal ulnar aspect of the wrist is present with fractures of the ulnar styloid. Distal to the ulnar head is the ulnar snuffbox. The triquetrum lies in this sulcus and can be palpated with the wrist in radial deviation. Tenderness may indicate triquetral fracture or triquetrolunate injury. The triquetrohamate joint is located more distally. Pain here may represent triquetrohamate ligament injury

> **PRACTICE PEARL**
>
> Scapholunate instability cannot be excluded on a normal plain radiograph as the instability is initially dynamic, occurring only with grip.

Special imaging studies

The combination of the complex anatomy of the wrist and subtle wrist injuries that can cause substantial morbidity has led to development of specialised wrist imaging techniques. Scaphoid views should be requested if a scaphoid fracture is suspected. A carpal tunnel view with the wrist in dorsiflexion allows inspection of the hook of hamate and the ridge of the trapezium. For suspected mechanical pathology, such as an occult ganglion, an occult fracture, non-union or bone necrosis, several modalities are useful (e.g. ultrasonography, radionuclide bone scan, computed tomography (CT) scan or magnetic resonance imaging (MRI) scan).

Wrist pain   CHAPTER 26

(i)

(k)

ulnar deviation   radial deviation

(j)

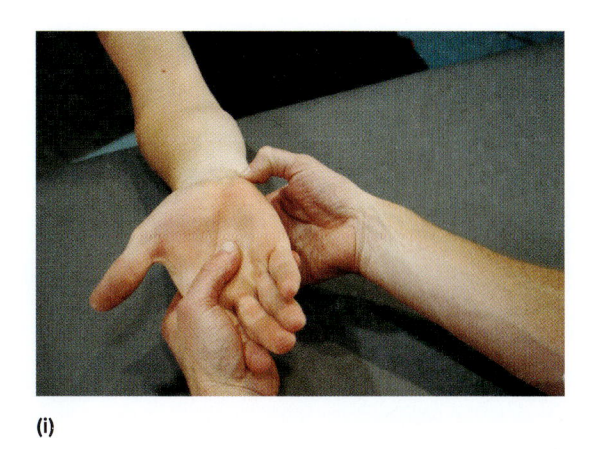

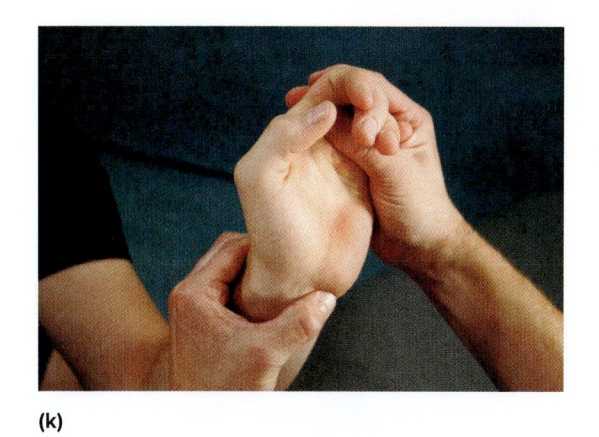

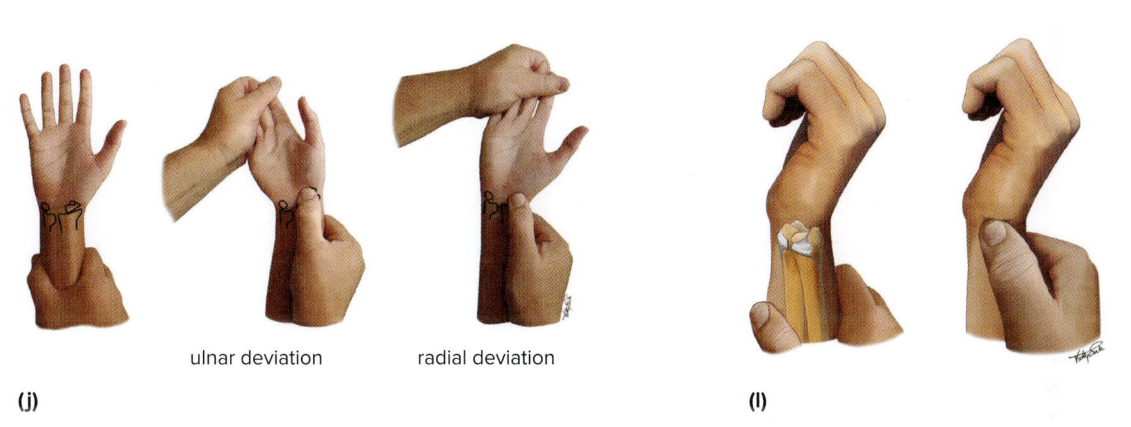

(l)

Figure 26.2 (cont.) (i) Palpation—the pisiform is palpated at the flexor crease of the wrist on the ulnar side. Tenderness in this region may occur with pisiform or triquetral fracture. The hook of hamate is 1 cm (0.5 in.) distal and radial to the pisiform. Examination may show tenderness over the hook or on the dorsal ulnar surface (j) Special test—Watson's test for scapholunate instability. The examiner places the thumb on the scaphoid tuberosity as shown, with the wrist in ulnar deviation. The wrist is then deviated radially with the examiner placing pressure on the scaphoid. If the athlete feels pain dorsally (over the scapholunate ligament) or the examiner feels the scaphoid move dorsally, then scapholunate dissociation is present (k) Special test—triangular fibrocartilage complex integrity. The wrist is placed into dorsiflexion and ulnar deviation and then rotated. Overpressure causes pain and occasionally clicking in patients with a tear of the triangular fibrocartilage complex (l) Special test—ulnar fovea sign for foveal disruption and ulnar triquetral ligament injury

Ultrasonography is a quick and accessible way to assess soft tissue abnormalities such as tendon injury, synovial thickening, ganglions and synovial cysts. Bone scans have high sensitivity but low specificity; thus, they can effectively rule out stress fractures, although MRI may be equally sensitive and more specific than a bone scan.

CT scanning is particularly useful for evaluating fractures that are difficult to assess fully on plain radiography, but MRI can also provide information about soft tissue injuries. Thus, a complete scapholunate ligament tear is more effectively identified with MRI than with CT.

Arthrography of the wrist is no longer used as an investigative tool except in combination with MRI–MR arthrogram or MRA. If all imaging results are negative but clinically significant wrist pain persists, the clinician should refer the patient to a specialist for further evaluation.

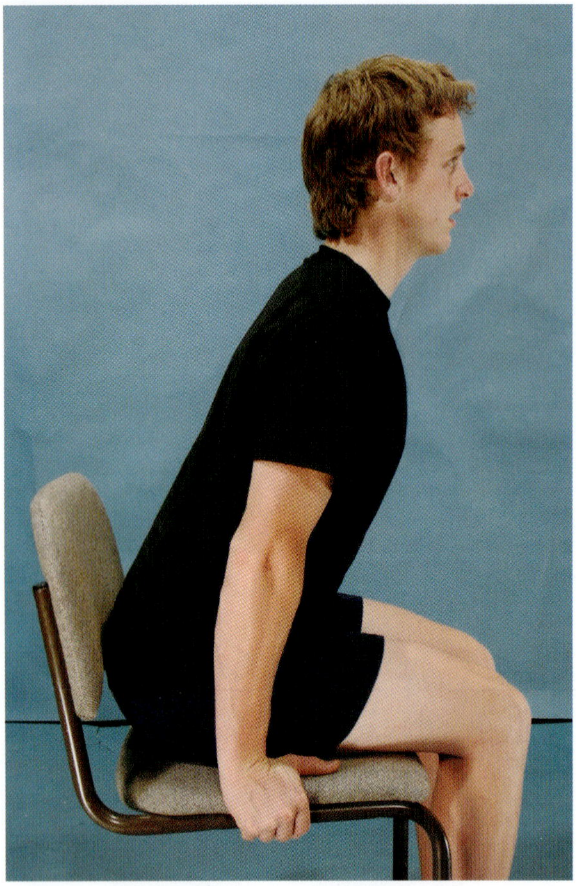

PART B   Regional problems

(m)

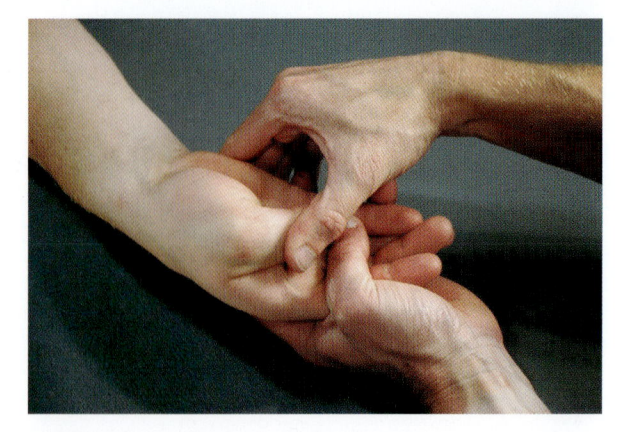

(n)

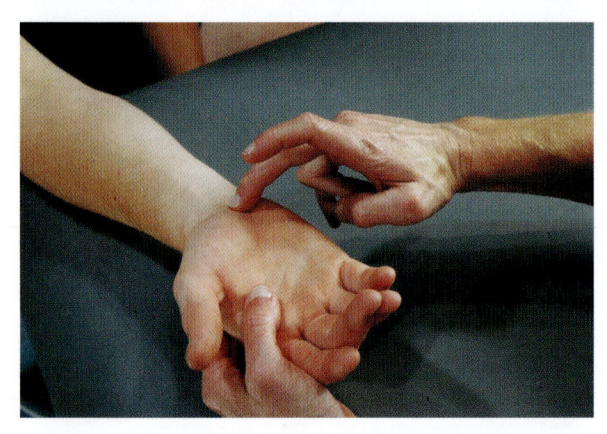

(o)

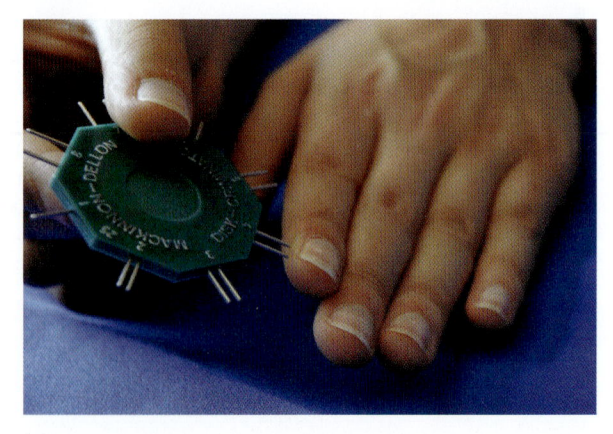

(p)

Figure 26.2 (cont.) (m) Special test—press test (or 'sitting hands' test). Attempting to raise body weight from a chair reproduces the pain of the triangular fibrocartilage complex injury (n) Special test—Finkelstein's test to detect de Quervain's disease. The thumb is placed in the palm of the hand with flexion of the metacarpophalangeal and interphalangeal joints while the examiner deviates the wrist in the ulnar direction (o) Special test—Tinel's sign. Tapping over the median nerve at the wrist produces tingling and altered sensation in the distribution of the median nerve in carpal tunnel syndrome (p) Special test—two point discrimination. Assessment of fine sensory ability. Apply the two points with even pressure horizontally over the medial and lateral aspects of the distal phalanx, starting wide and becoming narrower, with single point comparison

RADIAL COLUMN PRESENTATIONS

Fracture of the distal radius

Distal radius fractures are very common peripheral fractures.[23] As the force required to fracture young adults' bones is great, athletes may simultaneously incur an intra-articular fracture and ligamentous strain or rupture. The higher the forces involved (e.g. in high-velocity sports), the greater the likelihood of a complex injury involving articular structures (Fig. 26.4). Thus, thorough assessment of ligamentous injury is essential when fractures occur.

Wrist pain CHAPTER 26

Table 26.2 Clinical utility of selected assessment findings for wrist pain

Test	What is a positive finding?	Sensitivity	Specificity	LR+	LR−
Carpal tunnel syndrome					
Phalen's test[9]	Reproduction of symptoms	0.92	0.88	2.68	0.54[10]
Tinel's sign[9]	Paraesthesia in median nerve distribution or electric shock-like sensation	0.97	0.91	2.95	0.57[10]
Scapholunate injury					
Watson's scaphoid shift[11]	Reproduction of pain with or without hypermobility	69	66	1.78	0.55[12]
Triangular fibrocartilage complex disruption					
Ulna foveal sign[13]	Exquisite tenderness that replicates pain	95.2	86.5	7.06	0.05
Press test[14]	Axial ulnar load that replicates symptoms	100	NA	NA	NA

LR+ = positive likelihood ratio; LR− = negative likelihood ratio; NA = not available; see Chapter 14 for a guide to interpreting test sensitivity, specificity and likelihood ratios

Table 26.3 Patient-reported outcome measures for wrist pain

Patient Rated Wrist Evaluation (PRWE)
- Measures pain and disability in persons with wrist pathology with reference to functional activity
- 15 items
- Score range: 0 (no impairment)–100 (worst score)
- Test–retest reliability: >0.90[16]
- Validity established[16]
- MDC95% (minimal detectable change): 11.0[20]
- MCID (minimal clinically important difference): 11.5[20]
- Available online: www.physio-pedia.com/PRWE_Score
Disability of the Arm, Shoulder and Hand (DASH and QuickDASH) questionnaires
- Measure physical function, symptoms and quality of life in people with musculoskeletal disorders of the upper limb
- DASH 30 items; QuickDASH 11 items
- Score range: 0 (no impairment)–100 (worst score)
- Test–retest reliability: DASH >0.96[17]; QuickDASH >0.91[21]
- Validity: DASH Pearson Realize >0.70[17]; QuickDASH Pearson Realize >0.70[22]
- MDC95%: DASH 12.75%[17]; QuickDASH 11.2%[21]
- MCID: 8%[21] to 10.83%[17]
- Available online: www.physio-pedia.com/DASH_Outcome_Measure
Mayo Wrist Score
- Widely used but not validated, brief, objective and subjective assessment of pain/function/range of movement and strength
- 5 items
- Score range: 0 (worst score)–100 (no impairment)
- Available online: www.orthopaedicscore.com

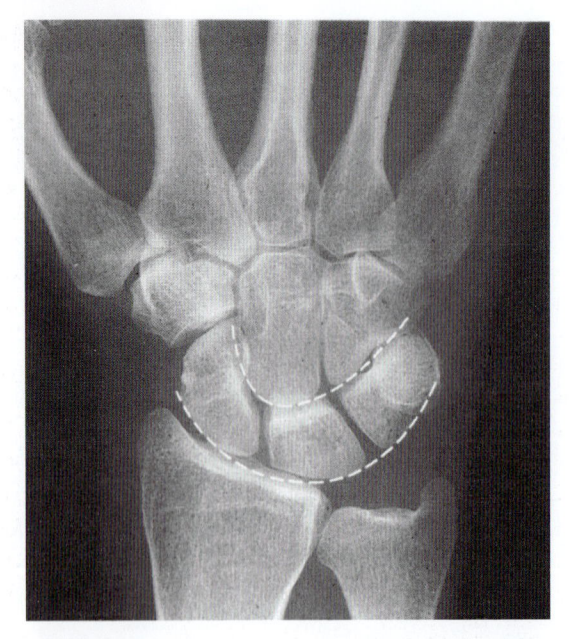

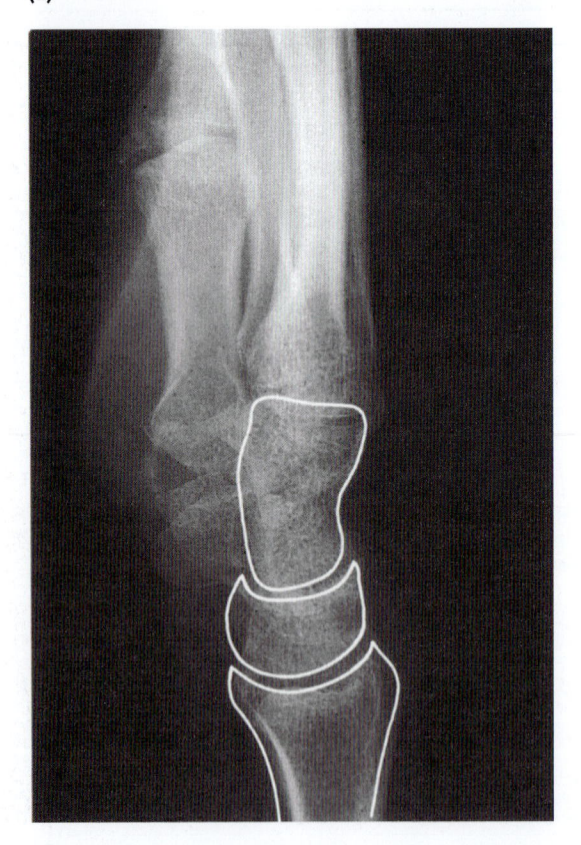

PART B   Regional problems

Initial treatment of the fracture is anatomical reduction, which should be done even if later internal fixation is contemplated, thus reducing swelling and making later anatomical alignment more likely.

Conservative management by reduction and casting with radiological follow-up at 3 and 6 weeks is appropriate for stable fractures post-reduction with minimal risk of displacement. Casts should be moulded with the wrist flexed to no more than 20° and slight ulnar deviation, and permit full finger motion. As oedema reduces, the cast should be changed. There is no evidence to support the use of thermoplastic splints or braces for acute distal radius fracture.[24]

Surgical intervention with early mobilisation for distal radius fracture has become the norm, with a particular emphasis on volar, locked plating. In spite of Cochrane reviews not being able to prioritise one surgical method over another, volar plating is being increasingly adopted.[25] Volar plating avoids the complications associated with external fixation and the surgical experience demands of fragment-specific fixation, as well as reducing the risk of extensor tendon rupture associated with dorsal plates.[25] Indications for open reduction are dorsal comminution, intra-articular involvement, instability on reduction, dorsal angulation of more than 20°, an articular surface step of greater than 1 mm, or radial shortening of greater than 5 mm, with anatomical alignment a necessity to avoid ongoing functional impairment.[26, 27]

Post-operatively, there is little published evidence for early mobilisation with reference to long-term results;[24, 28] however, a stable fixation, control of oedema and a controlled early mobilisation program in the athlete is crucial to an early return to sport, accompanied by suitable brace protection if appropriate. Inaccurate reduction, articular surface angulation, radial inclination or inadequate restoration of length all require early internal fixation with fixed angle-volar plating, although relative indications such as return-to-sport timelines and career goals are now just as important to the athlete.[29, 30] Overall, there is a trend to more aggressive treatment using volar plating and this has led to improved functional outcomes, especially in the young active adult.

Fracture of the scaphoid

The most common carpal fracture involves the scaphoid[4] and the usual mechanism is a fall on the outstretched hand. As pain may settle soon after the fall, presentation may be late after injury. The key examination finding is tenderness in the anatomical snuffbox. This may be accompanied by swelling and loss of grip strength. A more specific clinical test for scaphoid fracture is pain on axial compression of

Figure 26.3 Radiograph of the wrist (a) PA view—Gilula's arcs (b) Lateral view

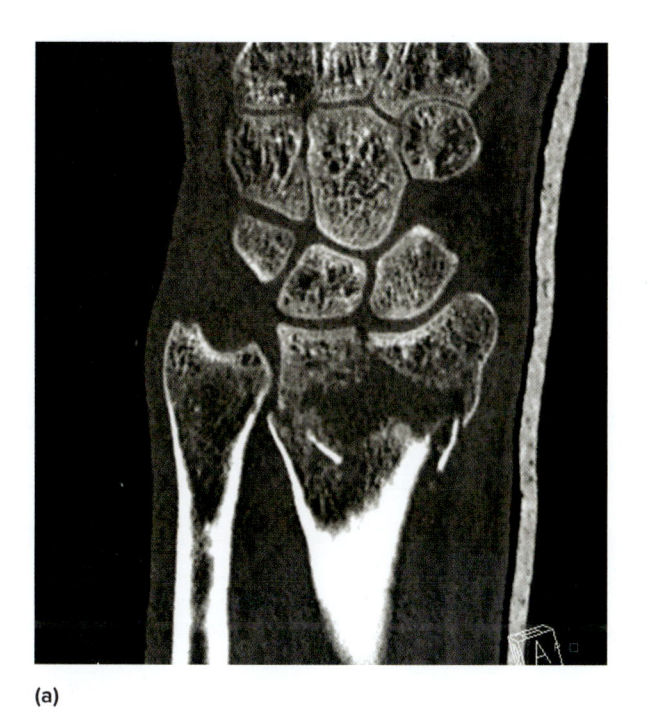

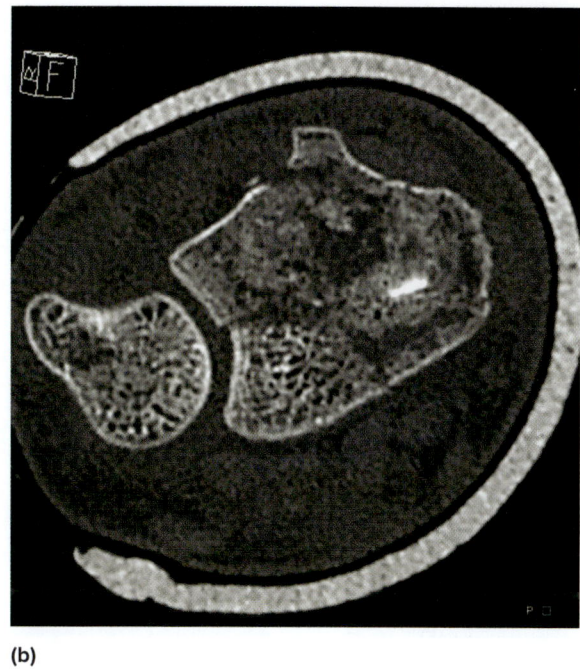

Figure 26.4 Fracture of radius (a) Coronal CT of comminuted fracture of radius (b) Axial CT of comminuted fracture of radius

the thumb towards the radius or direct pressure on the scaphoid tuberosity with radial deviation of the wrist. Plain radiographs with special scaphoid views will usually demonstrate the fracture (Fig. 26.5a), but CT scan may be required to detect more subtle fractures (Fig. 26.5b).

Scaphoid fracture is the most commonly missed fracture leading to litigation. If there is no bony damage, scapholunate instability should also be considered (see below).

> **PRACTICE PEARL**
>
> If a scaphoid fracture is suspected clinically but the radiograph is normal, a fracture cannot be ruled out. CT is an ideal diagnostic test for an acute injury that may be cost-saving in some settings. Note that it can take 24 hours for the injury to be revealed on MRI.

Traditional treatment of stable and unstable scaphoid fractures

A stable scaphoid fracture (including stress fractures of the scaphoid, which occur in high-board divers and gymnasts[31]) may be immobilised for eight weeks in

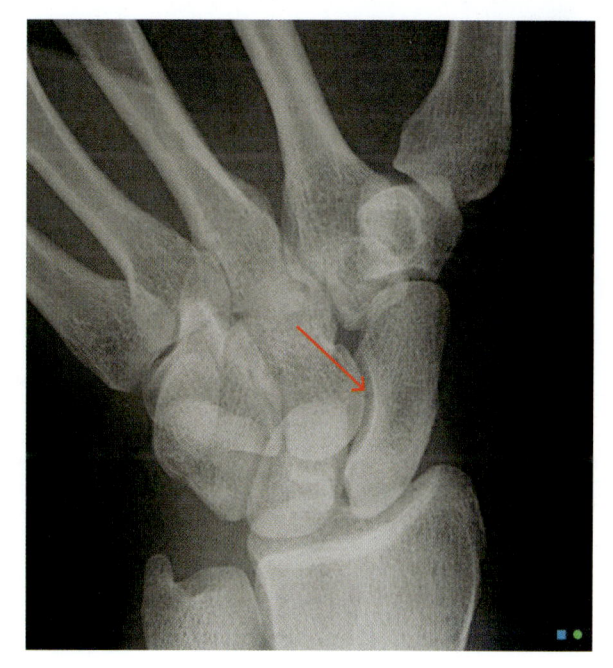

Figure 26.5 Scaphoid fracture (a) Plain radiograph of subtle scaphoid fracture (arrow)

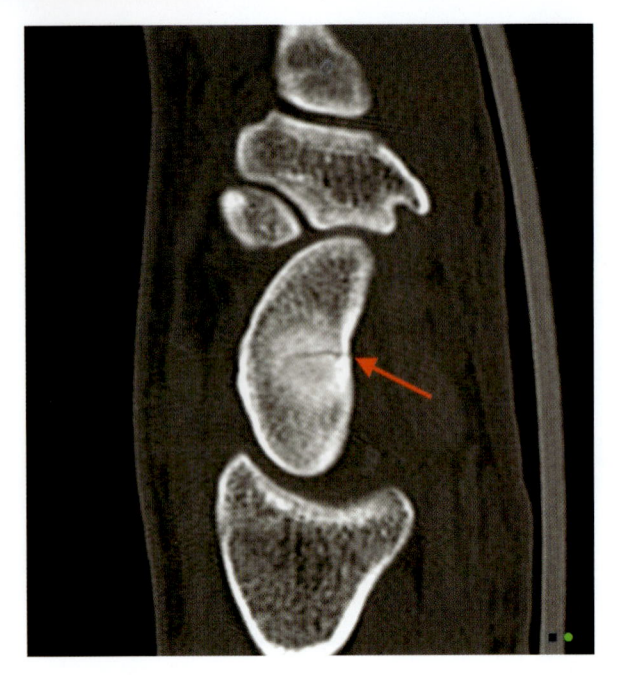

PART B   Regional problems

(b)

Figure 26.5 (cont.) (b) CT requested in plane of scaphoid shows scaphoid fracture (arrow)

a scaphoid cast extending from the proximal forearm to, but not including, the interphalangeal joint of the thumb (Fig. 26.6a). Upon removing the cast, re-evaluate the fracture clinically and radiologically. Unstable, angulated (>15–20°) or significantly displaced fractures (diastasis in the fracture gap >1.5 mm) require immediate percutaneous fixation (Fig. 26.6b) or open reduction and internal fixation. There are initial reports of using scaphoid plates but no long-term follow-up.

> **PRACTICE PEARL**
>
> **Current treatment of scaphoid fractures**
>
> The most reliable method of achieving scaphoid union with anatomic position is with internal fixation using mixed threaded (or graduated thread) screws which compress the scaphoid.

Complications of scaphoid fracture

The blood supply to the scaphoid originates distally (Fig. 26.7a), so the flow to the proximal pole can be diminished, which can then be at risk of necrosis after a fracture (Fig. 26.7b). Scaphoid fractures also have a risk of delayed union or non-union. Non-union and osteonecrosis can occur on their own or can occur in combination.[32]

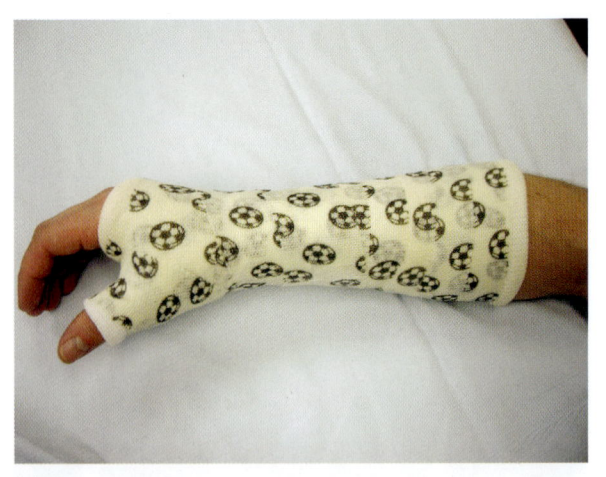

If there is clinical evidence of incomplete union when the cast is removed, the fracture should be immobilised for a further four to six weeks. Further immobilisation beyond this time is unlikely to prove beneficial. CT scan is the investigation of choice to detect non-union, but MRI can be used if CT is not available.

(a)

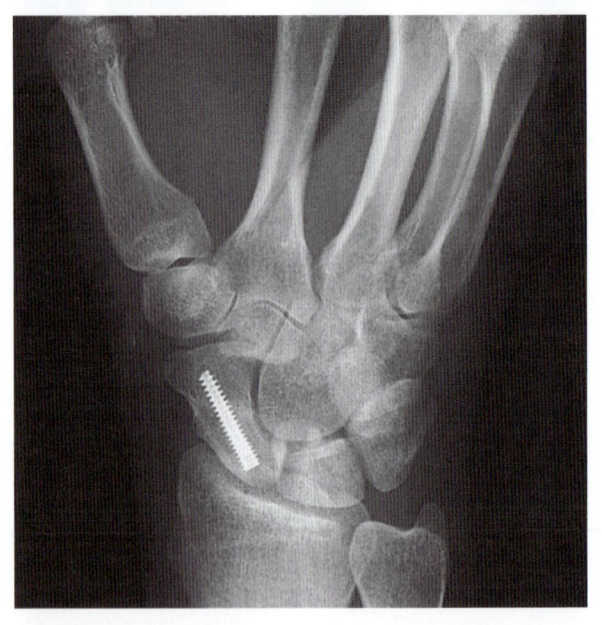

(b)

Figure 26.6 Treatment of scaphoid fractures (a) Cast immobilisation (b) Surgical fixation is now first-line treatment for scaphoid fracture

Wrist pain **CHAPTER 26**

(a)

(b)

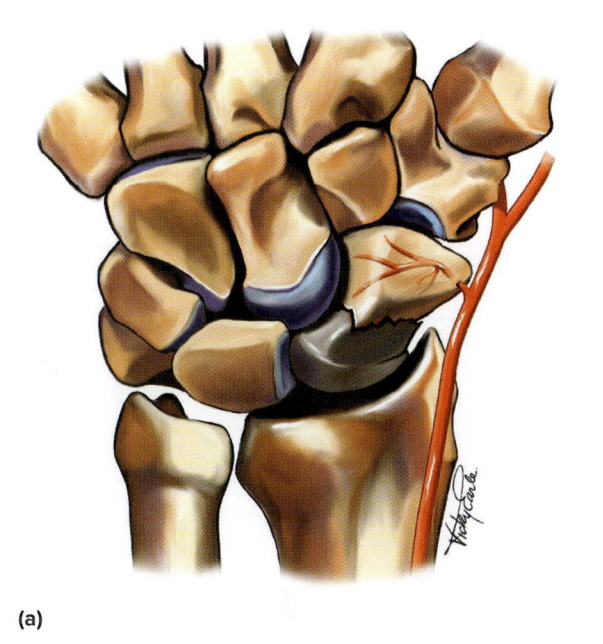

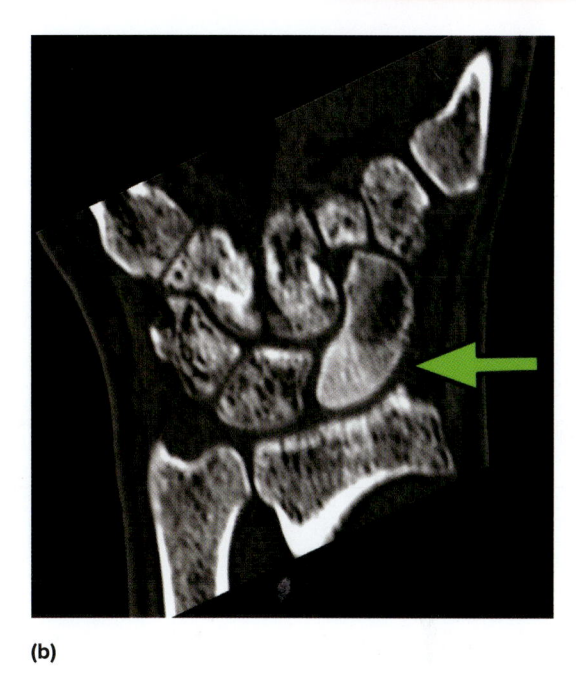

Figure 26.7 (a) The artery to the scaphoid enters via the distal pole, so a fracture at the waist of the scaphoid compromises the proximal fragment (b) MRI showing the characteristic hypointense appearance of avascular necrosis (arrow) in the proximal pole of the scaphoid

Contemporary management of scaphoid non-union
Contemporary treatment of non-union requires specialist hand surgeon management. Simple non-unions may be treated with fixation with bone graft (if there is a deformity or there has been bone resorption), while osteonecrosis with or without non-union may require a vascularised bone graft.[33]

Post-immobilisation wrist rehabilitation
Following successful treatment of a scaphoid fracture, the athlete can gradually return to activity using a protective device. Compression tubing worn under the protective splint reduces oedema and improves comfort. Different sports have different rules about what constitutes an 'allowable' protective cast (Fig. 26.8).

Fracture of the trapezium
Fractures of the trapezium make up 1–5% of carpal fractures. The most common pattern is a vertical, intra-articular fracture associated with axial compression from the thumb metacarpal. Rarely occurring in isolation, it often accompanies a Bennett's fracture. Presentation will be point tenderness and localised swelling, with the fracture itself best confirmed on CT scan (Fig. 26.9). Examination should be thorough because of the high risk of associated fracture dislocation and/or fractures of neighbouring carpals.[34]

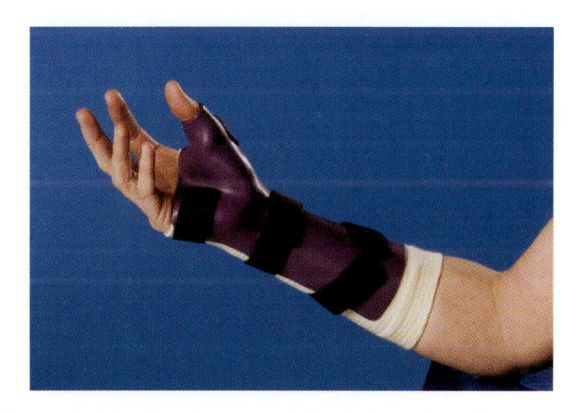

Figure 26.8 Following a scaphoid fracture, the athlete may wear a protective cast

Intervention will be determined by the amount of displacement of the fracture. The risk of degenerative arthritis at the trapezial articulations is high for a displaced fracture in a young, active individual, and can lead to reduced carpometacarpal motion, with a painful pinch and grip. Surgery can involve percutaneous pinning or open reduction with screw fixation. Non-displaced fractures do well with thumb spica casting.

PART B Regional problems

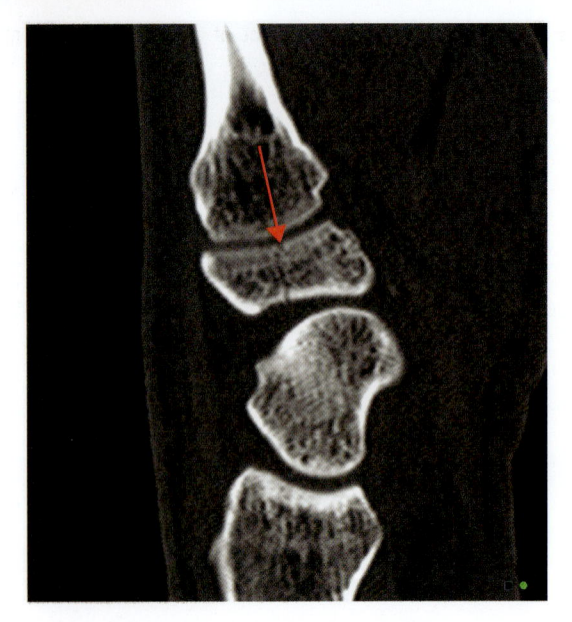

Figure 26.9 CT scan of fracture of trapezium

Radial epiphyseal injury (gymnast's wrist)
Skeletally immature athletes may place substantial compressive and shear forces across the distal radial physes, making them prone to growth arrest. Gymnasts, both elite and recreational, are particularly at risk of this injury, which occurs due to repetitive loading through a dorsiflexed wrist. It has been frequently hypothesised that this injury then puts them at risk of developing a positive ulnar variance; however, no definitive relationship has been established.[35]

The patient will present with dorsal wrist pain that is directly associated with activity. Radiographic changes in order of severity are haziness around the physis, cystic changes and/or metaphyseal sclerosis and widening of the physis itself (Fig. 26.10). Salter Harris V stress fracture should be considered if the growth plate is narrowed. The adolescent (ages 10–14) is more at risk than the younger athlete.[36]

Recovery can take several months and is activity dependent. Both athlete and family need to be aware of the long-term consequences of poor management. Treatment includes rest, adaptation of technique and forearm strengthening, particularly the flexors. Bracing to reduce hyperextension of the wrist has been shown in biomechanical studies to reduce load, and should be considered along with alternating swinging and loading skills during training.[37]

De Quervain's tenosynovitis
De Quervain's tenosynovitis affects the synovium of the abductor pollicis longus and extensor pollicis brevis tendons as they pass in their synovial sheath in a fibro-osseous tunnel at the level of the radial styloid (Fig. 26.11). This is a common radial-sided tendinopathy in athletes and occurs particularly with racquet sports, ten-pin bowlers, rowers and canoeists.

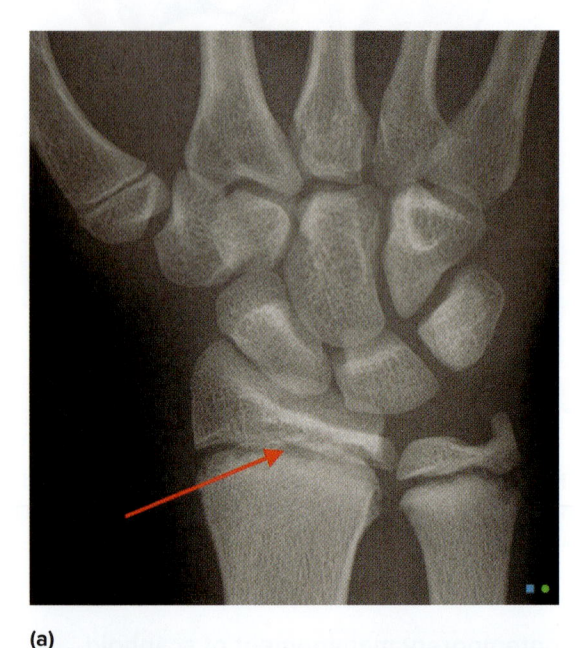

(a)

(b)

Figure 26.10 Radial epiphyseal injury in gymnast showing widening of the radial growth plate indicating stress reaction (a) Anteroposterior wrist X-ray (b) Lateral wrist X-ray

Wrist pain CHAPTER 26

arise from compartment syndrome of the thumb extensors, causing a tight band over the wrist extensors. Tenderness is found dorsally on the radial side, with swelling and crepitus a short distance proximal to the site of maximal tenderness in de Quervain's disease (Fig. 26.11). This condition is sometimes called 'oarsman's wrist' because of its common occurrence in rowers,[39] but it is also seen in canoeists and in weight training and racquet sports.

Treatment involves early intervention with corticosteroid injection into the junction. Acute surgical

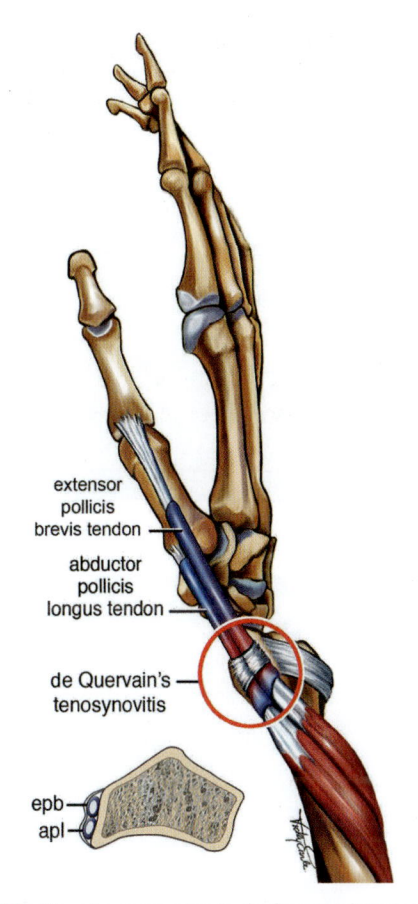

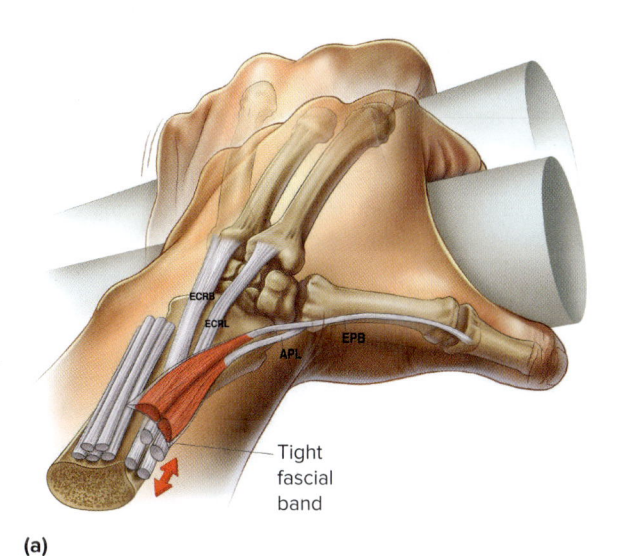

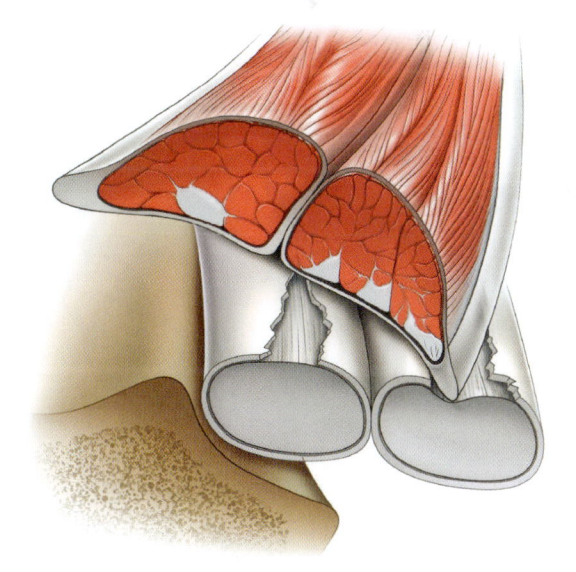

Figure 26.11 Site of compression in de Quervain's tenosynovitis

The left thumb of a right-handed golfer is particularly at risk because of the hyperabduction required during a golf swing. There will be local tenderness and swelling, which may extend proximally and distally along the course of the tendons. In severe cases, crepitus may be felt. A positive Finkelstein's test (Fig. 26.2n) is suggestive of the diagnosis; however, flexor carpi radialis tendinopathy also causes a positive test.

Treatment includes splinting, local electrotherapeutic modalities, stretches and graduated strengthening. Patients often find a pen build up (a rubber addition to enlarge the diameter of the pen) or golf grip widener useful as this reduces the stretch on the extensor tendons. An injection of corticosteroid and local anaesthetic into the tendon sheath will usually prove helpful.[38] In rare cases, surgical release is necessary.

Intersection syndrome

Intersection syndrome is a true tendinitis that occurs between the first and second dorsal wrist tendon compartments (Fig. 26.12), just proximal to the extensor retinaculum. It may be due to friction at the site of crossing or it may also

Figure 26.12 Intersection syndrome (a) Tight fascial band rubbing on tendons COURTESY OF DR GREG HOY (b) Close up of pathology COURTESY OF DR GREG HOY

477

decompression[40] and immediate return to training and events for rowers is very effective, and removes the need for changing rowing technique.[39]

Radial sensory nerve compression

As the dorsal radial sensory nerve exits brachioradialis 5–7 cm proximal to the wrist, it becomes superficial and subject to damage. Compression can occur following radial styloid fracture, be caused by a tight cast or by repetitive trauma in sports like volleyball. It can also be compressed more proximally when squeezed between brachioradialis and extensor carpi radialis longus tendons during rapid, repeated pronation and supination.

It is differentiated from de Quervain's tenosynovitis by the presence of sensory changes over the radiodorsal aspect of the hand. Treatment is initially conservative with corticosteroid injection, splinting and addressing of potential causes of entrapment. Surgical decompression has good results in chronic conditions.[41]

CENTRAL COLUMN PRESENTATIONS

Ganglions

Ganglions occur in athletes of any age. They are a synovial cyst communicating with the joint space (Fig. 26.13a). They most often present as a relatively painless swelling. They occur in several common sites on both the dorsal and volar aspects of the wrist, most commonly the scapholunate space, due to the poorly named 'mucinous degeneration' of the scapholunate ligament. They may also be intracapsular or even intra-osseous.

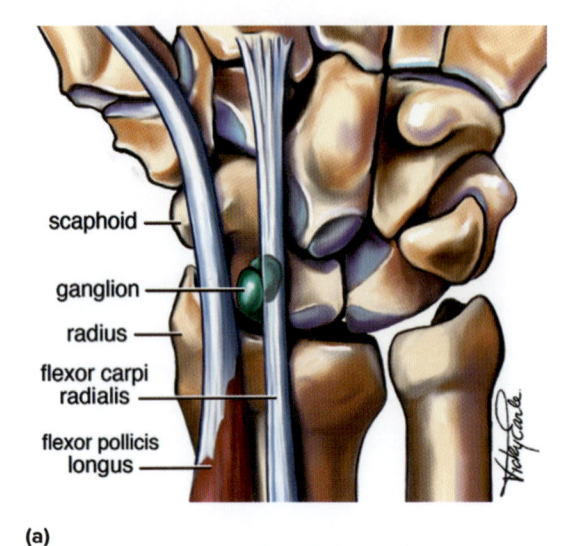

Figure 26.13 Ganglion cyst (a) Graphic view of the dorsum of the wrist showing the ganglion arising from the joint

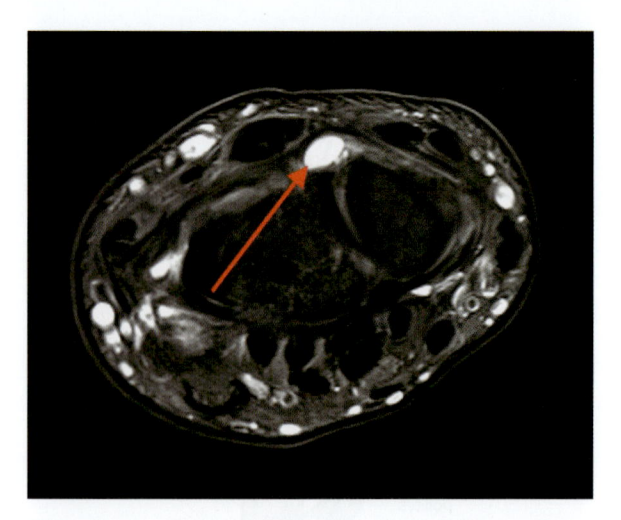

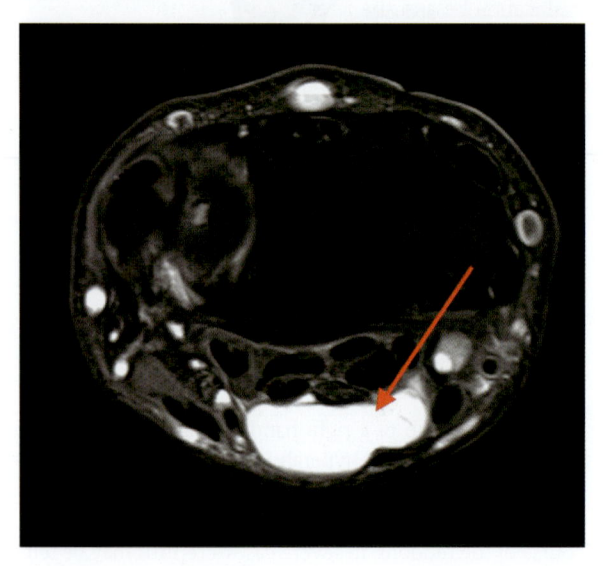

Figure 26.13 (cont.) (b) MRI axial view of dorsal scapholunate ganglion (c) MRI axial view of volar wrist ganglion

The patient's main complaint is of intermittent wrist pain and reduced movement. Swelling may be visible intermittently or not at all, and so should not be relied upon to make the diagnosis. Ultrasonography is a useful investigation, however, T2-weighted MRI highlights ganglion cysts (Fig. 26.13b & c) and is the investigation of choice. The athlete must be reassured that the ganglion is benign, and that the average number in normal people is approximately two per wrist.[42]

Treatment is only indicated for a symptomatic ganglion. When symptoms persist, aspiration and/or corticosteroid infiltration are at least temporarily effective and can be performed under ultrasound guidance where this is feasible. Some persistent symptomatic ganglions require surgery, in which the neck of the ganglion must be removed to prevent recurrence.

Dislocation of the carpal bones

There are a number of different types of dislocation of the carpal bones, mostly involving the lunate. They are the uncommon end stage of severe ligament disruption. Failure to recognise them generally results in disastrous consequences.

Anterior dislocation of the lunate

In rare cases, the lunate may dislocate anteriorly as the end point of a perilunar injury. Pain is usually severe and deformity obvious. Plain radiography reveals the dislocation best in the lateral view with the lunate tilted volarly and not articulating with the capitate.[43] Treatment is URGENT open reduction and primary ligament repair, followed by eight weeks of cast immobilisation. Anterior lunate dislocation is often associated with severe median nerve compression and numbness in the radial three and a half digits.[44] This requires urgent surgical decompression.

Perilunar dislocation of the lunate

Perilunar dislocation is occasionally associated with a fractured waist of the scaphoid (so-called 'trans-scaphoid perilunate dislocation') when the lunate remains with the radius and the capitate is dislocated dorsally. This complex injury is often overlooked if the deformity is moderate, but the sequelae are catastrophic for the wrist, and this is a common cause of litigation when missed. It requires treatment by a hand and wrist surgeon, as long-term instability and radiographic wrist arthritis can occur.[45, 46]

Scapholunate dissociation

Scapholunate dissociation is due to a complex injury involving dorsal scapholunate ligament tear and loss of secondary restraints (Fig. 26.14a). Rotatory subluxation (mainly flexion) of the scaphoid may occur as a result of disruption of its ligamentous attachments due to acute trauma (e.g. a fall on the dorsiflexed hand). Examination reveals tenderness 2 cm distal to Lister's tubercle on the radial side of the lunate. There may be little or no swelling. The key examination manoeuvre is Watson's test (Fig. 26.2j). If the test causes pain or reveals dorsal movement of the scaphoid, scapholunate instability is likely.

Conventional radiographic views may not show any abnormality, but stress films (clenched fist postero-anterior view) may reveal a scapholunate gap (Fig. 26.14b). A lateral radiograph may show an increased volar flexion of the distal pole of the scaphoid and dorsiflexion of the lunate. If these tests are negative but the injury is suspected clinically, MRI is indicated (Fig. 26.14c).

Treatment of scapholunate dissociation is open reduction and reconstruction of the ligaments with temporary internal fixation. Many techniques are published[47, 48] and the main aim in athletes is return of grip strength and pain relief. Prevention of future arthritis (scapholunate advanced collapse (SLAC) wrist) is the ideal, although there is currently no significant evidence that this is achieved.

Kienböck's disease

Kienböck's disease is otherwise known as avascular necrosis of the lunate. It is associated with repetitive microtrauma and negative ulnar variance, and it is most commonly diagnosed in adult males. However, there is a published case report of it occurring in a 14-year-old female gymnast.[49]

The patient will report a gradually worsening history of wrist pain. There may be swelling over the lunate which will be painful to palpate, and wrist motion will be affected. Imaging confirmation is increasingly using MRI. Interpretation of what is currently classified as Lichtman's stage 1 on MRI is controversial, with some authors arguing that this is an example of lunate overload and not Kienböck's disease.[50]

Surgical treatment will depend on the stage of the disease and the patient's level of function. Radial

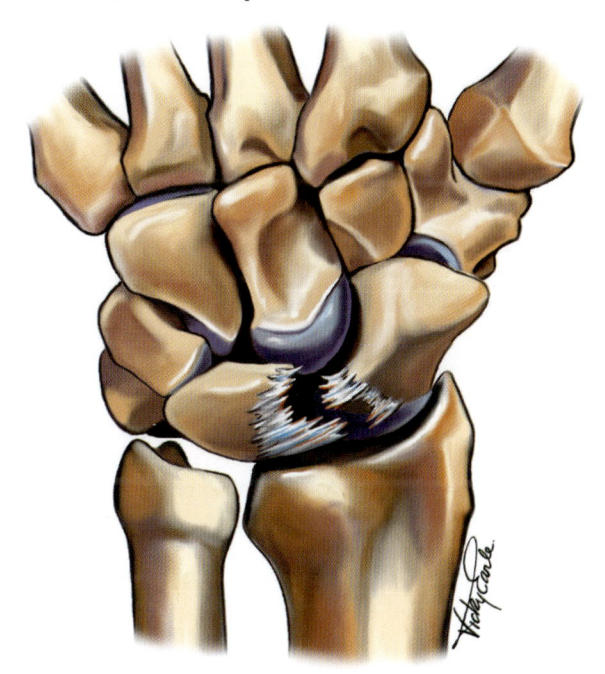

(a)

Figure 26.14 Scapholunate dissociation (a) Coronal graphic shows a tear of the dorsal component of the scapholunate ligament

PART B   Regional problems

(b)

(c)

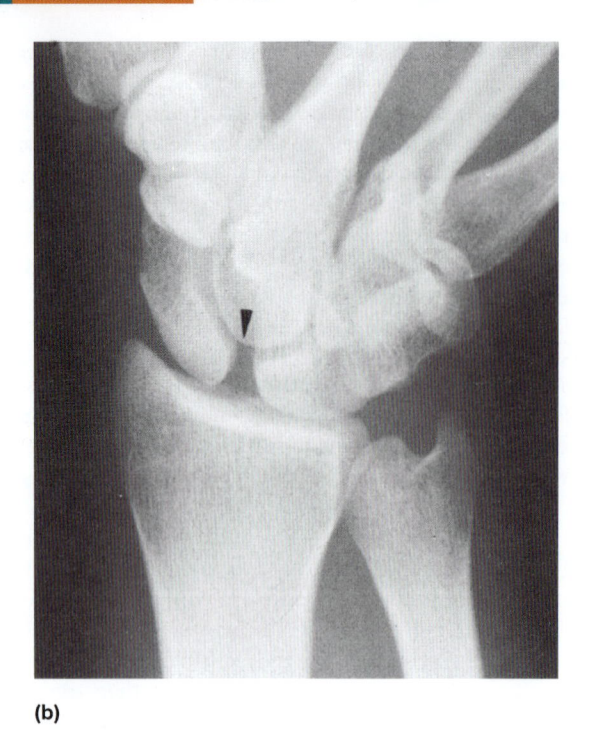

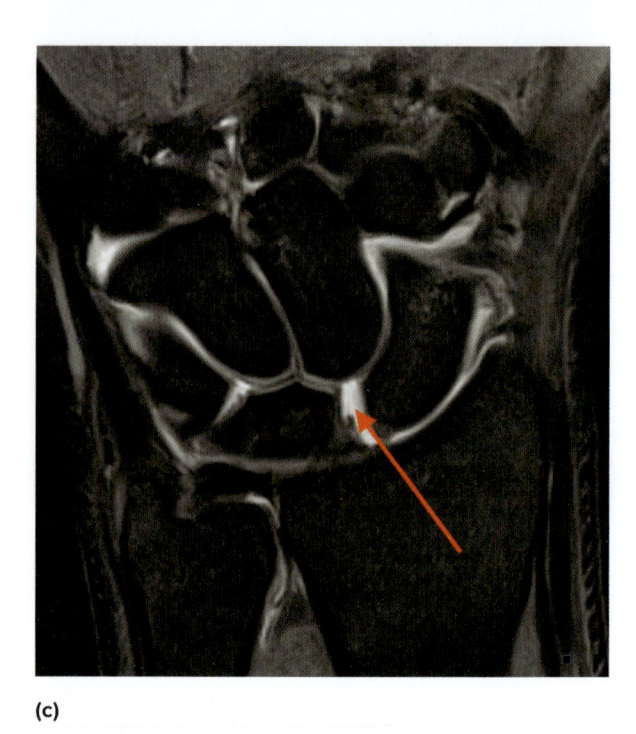

Figure 26.14 (cont.) (b) In a classic case, radiograph reveals separation of the scaphoid and lunate. This can be a late sign, so normal radiography does not rule out this condition (c) Coronal MRI T2 image of scapholunate instability (arrow)

shortening osteotomy has been shown to have had good long-term results, with only slight loss of grip strength.[51] Salvage procedures are required for advanced cases due to the presence of carpal collapse.[52]

Conservative management of prolonged casting with consistent radiological follow-up has been shown not to be sufficient to stop progression of the disease once accurately diagnosed. Reported success of casting is possibly an indication that what was thought to be early-stage Kienböck's was in fact something else.[53] For this reason, it is important to differentiate between a stress reaction of the lunate and Kienböck's disease. Tennis players and other high-use athletes presenting with overuse syndromes in the wrist require exclusion of bony stress reactions including MRI scanning of good quality.

Diagnostic criteria for MRI for stage 1 Kienböck's disease have not been defined in the literature. We do not consider the use of proton density (PD) and T2 MRI images alone as sufficiently reliable for the diagnosis of Kienböck's disease. We recommend that T1 images must be obtained to exclude Kienböck's disease, and stress reactions must be considered in the differential diagnosis of these patients (Fig. 26.15).

Conservative treatment with restriction of high-level impact loading is excellent for the relief of these bony

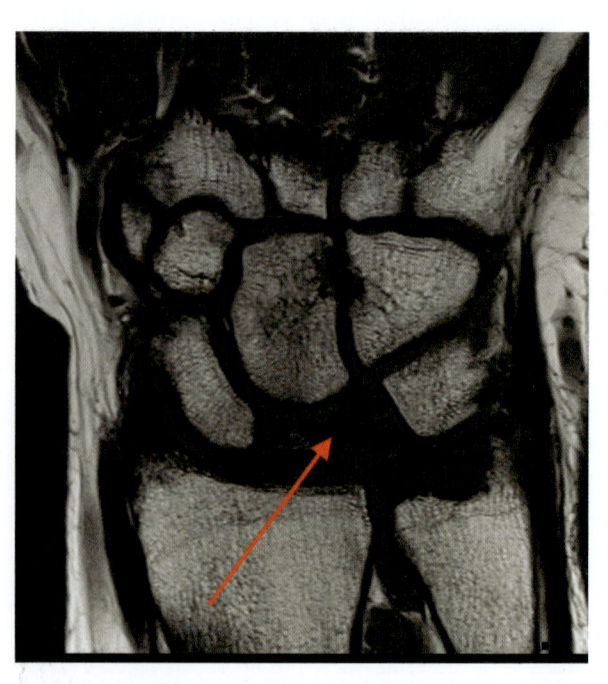

Figure 26.15 MRI coronal view of Kienböck's disease of lunate

480

stress injuries when diagnosed in the first three months of symptoms. Alteration of technique deficits may prevent recurrence, but little is known of the possible cause-and-effect relationship with completed fractures. The evidence base regarding treatment of this condition is controversial.[54]

Impingement syndromes

A number of impingement syndromes may cause wrist pain. Scaphoid impaction syndrome may occur because of repetitive hyperextension stresses (e.g. in weightlifting or gymnastics). This mechanism is also responsible for avascular necrosis of the capitate in weightlifters. Impaction of the dorsal pole of the lunate on the distal radius is seen in gymnasts. The extensor pollicis longus may impinge on Lister's tubercle and it occasionally ruptures. Triquetrohamate impingement syndrome may result from forced wrist extension and ulnar deviation (e.g. in racquet sports and gymnastics).

Radial styloid impaction syndrome can result from repeated forced radial deviation, especially among golfers (Chapter 9). Patients with these syndromes present with localised tenderness and are treated with rest and a protective brace. Occasionally, corticosteroid injection or surgical exploration may be helpful.

ULNAR COLUMN PRESENTATIONS

Ulnar styloid fracture

Ulnar styloid fractures are present in over 50% of distal radius fractures, with 25% of them never uniting. There is no benefit in fixation of an ulnar styloid fracture unless it can be demonstrated that it is associated with distal radio-ulnar joint (DRUJ) instability.[55] Its presence should alert the clinician to assess for triangular fibrocartilage complex injury and monitor for ulnar instability through the rehabilitative period. If the fracture requires addressing, options include small k-wires with a tension band or, when DRUJ instability is present, volar plating of the radius and supination splinting.[56] A recent study did demonstrate that patients with distal radius fractures who had an associated ulnar styloid fracture had decreased function and reported more pain initially; however, by 12 months these differences were no longer significant.[57]

Fracture of the hook of hamate

Fracture of the hook of hamate may occur while swinging a golf club,[8, 58, 59] tennis racquet or baseball bat. The fracture is especially likely to occur when the golf club strikes the ground instead of the ball, forcing the top of the handle of the club against the hook of the hamate of the top hand (Fig. 26.16a). This mechanism may compress the superficial and deep terminal branches of the ulnar nerve, producing both sensory and motor changes. Symptoms include reduced grip strength and ulnar wrist pain. Examination reveals volar wrist tenderness over the hook of hamate. Routine radiographs of the wrist do not image the fracture and even the classic 'carpal tunnel view' with the wrist in dorsiflexion is an insensitive test. CT scan (Fig. 26.16b) and MRI are the best imaging tools.

This fracture often fails to heal with immobilisation; most sports medicine cases of the fracture are actually stress fractures that present late. In some athletes (e.g. baseball players), the hook of hamate fracture is likely to be a completed stress fracture not due to acute trauma. If diagnosis is delayed, or the fracture fails to heal clinically within four weeks of immobilisation, current surgical

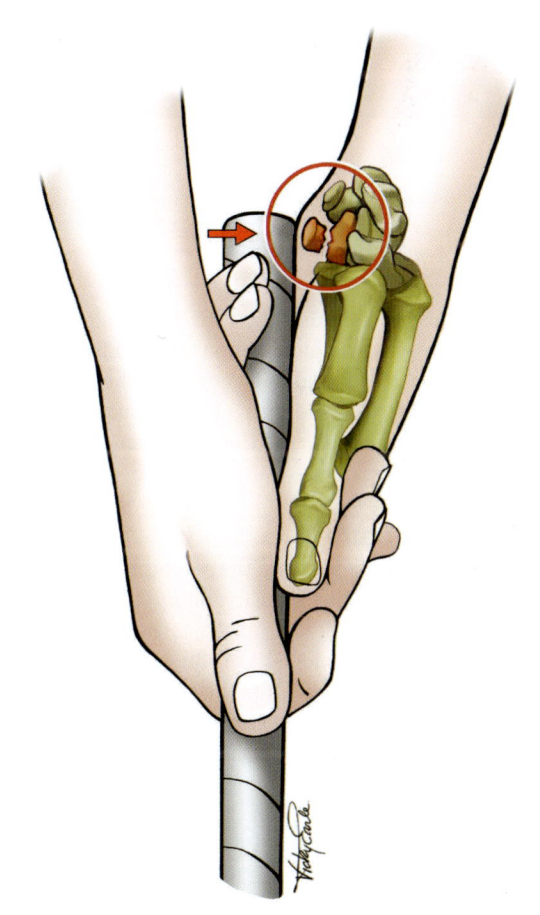

(a)

Figure 26.16 Fracture of the hook of hamate (a) Possible mechanism—when the golf club is suddenly decelerated (e.g. hitting the ground), the grip is forced against the hook of hamate

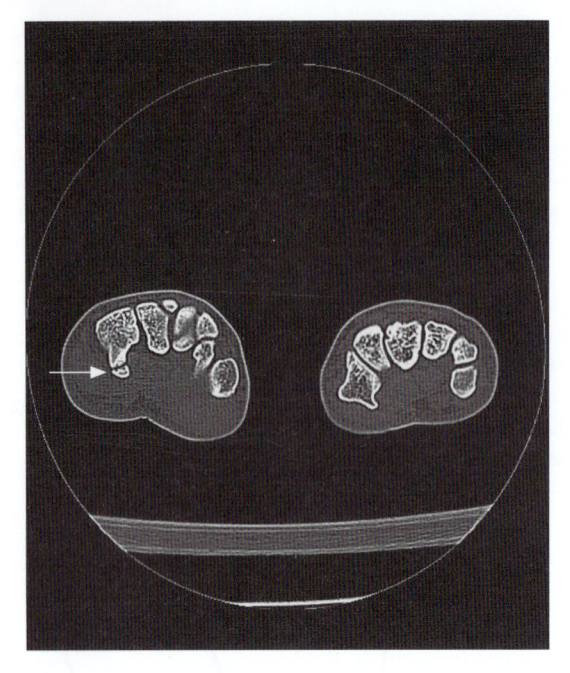

(b)

Figure 26.16 (cont.) (b) CT scan of a fracture of the hook of hamate

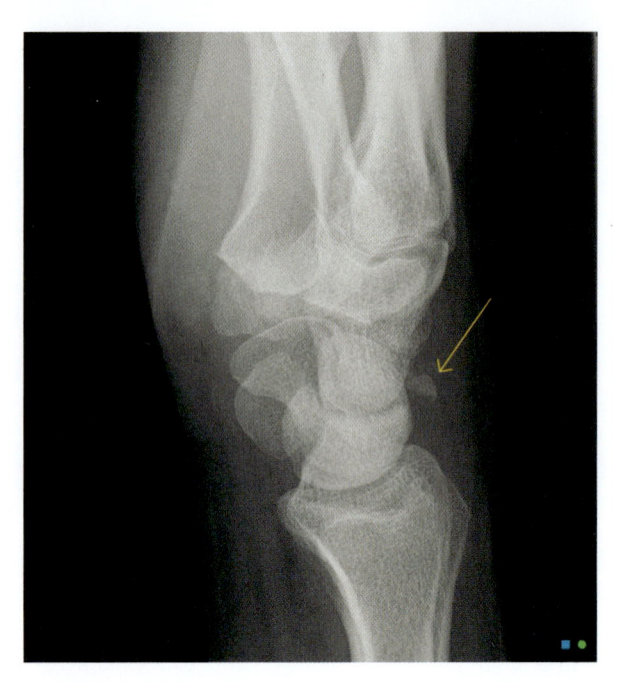

Figure 26.17 Lateral radiograph of triquetral flake fracture (arrow)

practice is excision of the fractured hook followed by three weeks wrist immobilisation (in preference to open reduction and internal fixation).[8,60] The pain only dissipates slowly, but the patient can usually resume sport six weeks after surgery. The long-term outcome of this approach is not known.

Triquetral fracture

Fractures of the triquetrum are the second most common carpal fracture. The two primary injury patterns are a fracture of the triquetral body, or the cortical, dorsal flake fracture which accounts for 93% of all triquetral fractures.

One mechanism of injury for the flake fracture is the ulna chiselling an avulsion fragment following a fall into forced ulnar deviation and dorsiflexion. A less common cause is a high-velocity dorsal blow forcing radial deviation and palmar flexion.[61]

The athlete will present with point tenderness over the dorsum and a painful wrist with flexion. Precise palpation of the fracture is difficult due to its ulnar position. Diagnosis is then dependent upon anteroposterior, lateral and oblique pronated view radiographic scans (Fig. 26.17). CT is a useful tool for occult fractures.

With respect to the flake fractures, the athlete must understand that it is not the bone that is the problem, but rather the soft tissue injury and potential loss of stability. Cast immobilisation is essential for three to four weeks to ward off instability. Graded range of motion can begin then with a removable splint for protection, with full function usually restored by eight weeks.[62]

The less common triquetral fracture is through the body of the bone following a high-energy collision. Any diagnosis of a fracture must be investigated thoroughly with 12–25% of these associated with perilunate fracture dislocation. Surgery using pins or a compression screw will depend on the degree of displacement and the diagnosed presence of concomitant injury.

Lunotriquetral dissociation

Lunotriquetral dissociation is an injury that is frequently missed on initial presentation, yet is the second most common form of carpal instability. The injury is often the result of a backwards fall onto an externally rotated, dorsiflexed, supinated and radially deviated hand. Physical examination is unlikely to reveal significant bruising or swelling. There will be pain at end range of pronation and supination and with pronated grip. Ballottement of the joint may be uncomfortable, and relief may be experienced with posterior displacement of the pisiform.[63]

Conservative management can be successful in managing this condition and is preferable to surgery at least in acute settings. The wrist should be splinted or casted for six weeks, at which time a weaning and ulnar-sided strengthening program can begin. The use of a pisiform boost type of splint may be beneficial in chronic cases. Athletes should be aware that the process of recovery from either conservative or surgical management can take up to six months.[63, 64] Biomechanical studies indicate that training of extensor carpi ulnaris (ECU) may be beneficial; however, this is yet to be demonstrated clinically.[65]

Triangular fibrocartilage complex tear

The triangular fibrocartilage complex (TFCC) lies between the ulna and the carpus. It is the major stabiliser of the distal radioulnar joint. The 'complex' consists of the triangular fibrocartilage, ulnar meniscus homologue, ulnar collateral ligament, numerous carpal ligaments and the ECU tendon sheath (Fig. 26.18a). Only the periphery of the TFCC is vascular and able to heal if damaged. The central avascular portion cannot heal and usually requires debridement once injured.

The TFCC is commonly injured in racquet or stick sports and those that create repetitive ulnar and compressive loading like gymnastics, weightlifting, boxing and surfing. In water skiers it is considered a traction injury.[1] It should be investigated following distal radius fracture and wherever DRUJ instability exists. The patient complains of ulnar-sided pain that worsens with grip, rotation and weight-bearing.[66]

Examination reveals tenderness and swelling over the dorsal ulnar aspect of the wrist, pain on resisted wrist dorsiflexion and ulnar deviation (Fig. 26.2k), a clicking sensation on wrist movement and reduced grip strength. Sharp pain with deep palpation is known as a positive foveal sign and indicates an ulnatriquetral ligament injury and/or a disruption of the TFCC at the base of the ulna styloid (fovea), which is associated with DRUJ instability (Fig. 26.2l).[13, 66] The 'press test' may also be helpful in diagnosing TFCC tears and differentiating from other conditions like ECU tendinopathy (Fig. 26.2m). The patient creates an axial ulnar load by attempting to lift his or her weight up off a chair using the affected wrist. A positive test replicates the presenting symptom.[14]

High-quality MRI (Fig. 26.18b) can image the TFCC and this is an increasingly popular investigation for ulnar-sided wrist pain.[67] Estimates of sensitivity and specificity are about 60% and 90%, respectively,[68] which suggests that a negative MRI should not be used to rule out the condition if it is clinically suspected. Interestingly, ultrasonography shows promise for matching MRI in the detection of TFCC lesions; however, arthroscopy remains the gold standard and should be considered as early as possible for the athlete wanting a rapid return to play.[69, 70]

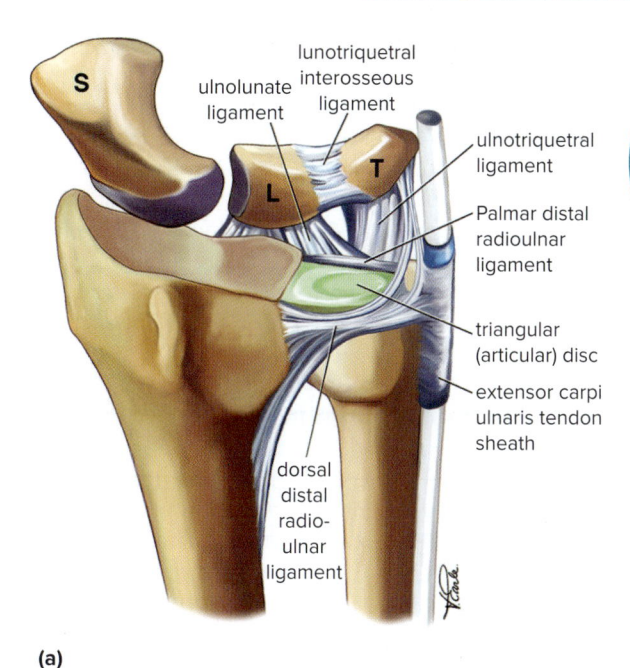

Figure 26.18 Triangular fibrocartilage complex (TFCC) (a) TFCC and surrounding ligaments (b) Coronal MRI of foveal tear of TFCC off ulna

Arthroscopy permits accurate diagnosis and excision of any torn cartilage if required. If the ulna is longer than the radius (positive ulnar variance), it impinges on the triangular fibrocartilage and predisposes it to tearing.

PART B Regional problems

It may be necessary to shorten the ulna as well as excising the torn fibrocartilage.[71]

Treatment after surgery will likely involve a period of immobilisation, followed by a carefully graded return to full motion and grip strength.[66] Conservative management involves a short period of splinting followed by specific strapping to offload the TFCC, coupled with stabilisation exercises involving ECU and pronator quadratus, and likely technical adjustment. It is rarely as successful for treatment of central and foveal tears as it is for smaller, peripheral tears.

Distal radio-ulnar joint instability

The thickened dorsal and volar aspects of the triangular fibrocartilage act as the dorsal and volar ligaments of the distal radio-ulnar joint. Subluxation of the ulnar head occurs because of avulsion of these ligaments. It may be either volar or dorsal. Dorsal subluxation of the ulnar head associated with a tear of the volar radio-ulnar ligament is more common and may be due to repetitive or forceful pronation in contact sports, tennis or gymnastics. Dorsal displacement of the ulnar styloid process during pronation may be detected on true lateral radiograph. Treatment requires repair of the TFCC.[72]

Extensor carpi ulnaris tendon injuries

The ECU resides in the sixth dorsal wrist compartment and helps stabilise the DRUJ.[65, 73] It has its own subsheath just distal to the ulnar styloid, which prevents subluxation from the distal ulnar groove. Its angular path from its origin on the lateral epicondyle to the tendon insertion at the base of the fifth metacarpal is exaggerated with ulnar deviation and supination (Fig. 26.19a).

The subsheath is designed in such a way that it stretches and deforms in response to forces. It can fail abruptly with hypersupination and flexion, but more usually fails as fibrous tearing occurs over a period of time due to repetitive forearm supination, wrist flexion and ulnar deviation.

The tendon can either sublux (a partial loss of excursion beyond the volar lip of the notch, which occurs in up to 45% of asymptomatic persons) or it can dislocate with a complete loss of continuity. Presentation will be ulnar-sided wrist pain that intensifies with active contraction or stretching of the tendon. Instability will be obvious as the tendon subluxes volarly, often with an audible flick, and ultrasound imaging is useful.[74, 75] Weight-bearing through the palm should not be painful unless other structures like the TFCC are involved.

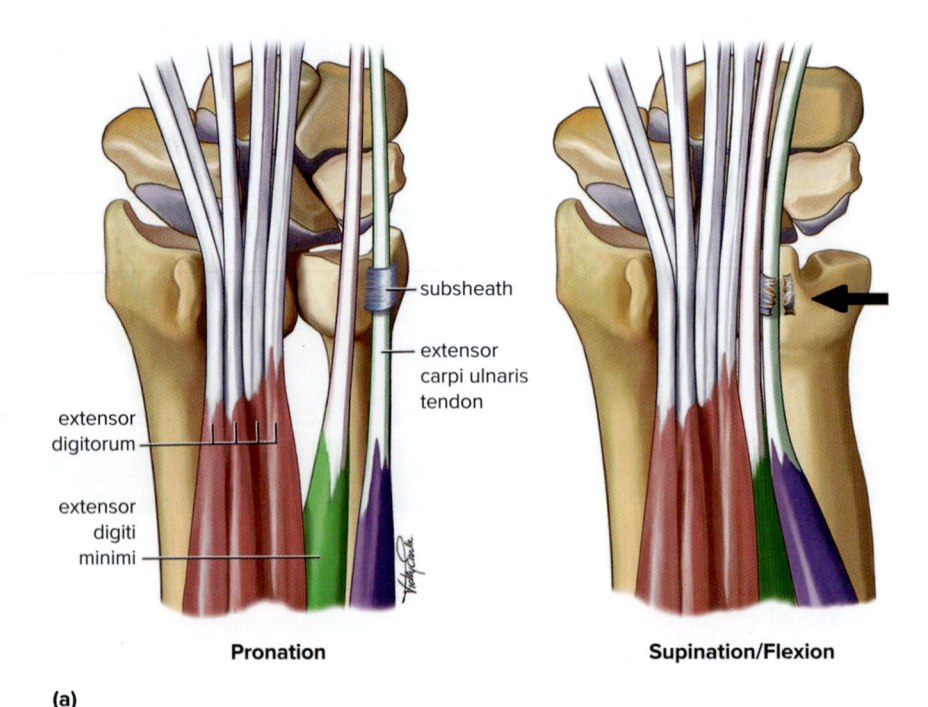

Figure 26.19 Extensor carpi ulnaris (ECU) tendon (a) Tendons at the wrist showing supination position where the ECU tendon is most likely to sublux and tear subsheath

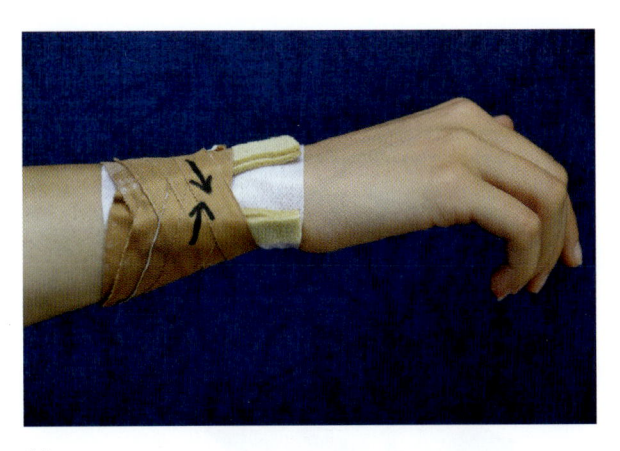

(b)

Figure 26.19 (cont.) (b) Tennis-specific taping method that unloads and blocks the wrist with TFCC and/or ECU injury. Readers are directed to Stroia et al.[78] for a complete description of the method

Athletes at risk are those who require grip and extremes of wrist motion in supination, for example golfers, cricketers, weightlifters and rodeo riders.[76] Tennis players with double-handed backhands are at particular risk as the hand closest to the racquet head moves rapidly into a supinated, flexed and radially deviated posture.[77]

If there is no tendon rupture, initial treatment can be conservative. The arm is splinted in radial deviation, extension and neutral to pronation. If stability remains a problem, the cast should extend to include the elbow at 90°.[75] The splint is worn for 1–4 weeks, depending on the severity of the symptoms. A strengthening and control program is then initiated with taping to stabilise the ECU within the ulnar groove (Fig. 26.19b).[78] Failure of conservative management is an indication for surgical reconstruction of the sheath with or without recontouring of the sulcus. Anticipated return to play is at three months following surgery.[79]

Other tendinopathies around the wrist

Any of the flexor and extensor tendons around the wrist may become painful with excessive activity. On examination, there is tenderness and occasionally swelling and crepitus. The principles of treating tendinopathies apply—management should include attention to biomechanics (ergonomics), progressive strengthening and functional rehabilitation.[25]

CAUSES OF WRIST NUMBNESS AND HAND PAIN

Patients may present with wrist numbness or paraesthesia. This suggests a neurological pathology, most likely carpal tunnel syndrome or ulnar nerve compression.

Carpal tunnel syndrome

The median nerve may be compressed as it passes through the carpal tunnel along with the flexor digitorum profundus, flexor digitorum superficialis and flexor pollicis longus tendons (Fig. 26.20). This condition is characterised by burning volar wrist pain with numbness or paraesthesia in the distribution of the median nerve (thumb, index finger, middle finger and radial side of the ring finger). Nocturnal paraesthesia is characteristic. The pain can radiate to the forearm, elbow and shoulder. Tinel's sign may be elicited by tapping over the volar aspect of the wrist (Fig. 26.20). A positive Phalen's test will reproduce symptoms in up to 60 seconds when the patient rests both elbows on a table with forearms vertical and their wrists flexed by gravity.

The most important aspects in diagnosis are the history and physical examination, but nerve conduction studies can help confirm the diagnosis and may predict how the patient will respond to surgery.[80] Patients with carpal tunnel syndrome should be checked for diabetes mellitus, as it is a known risk factor.

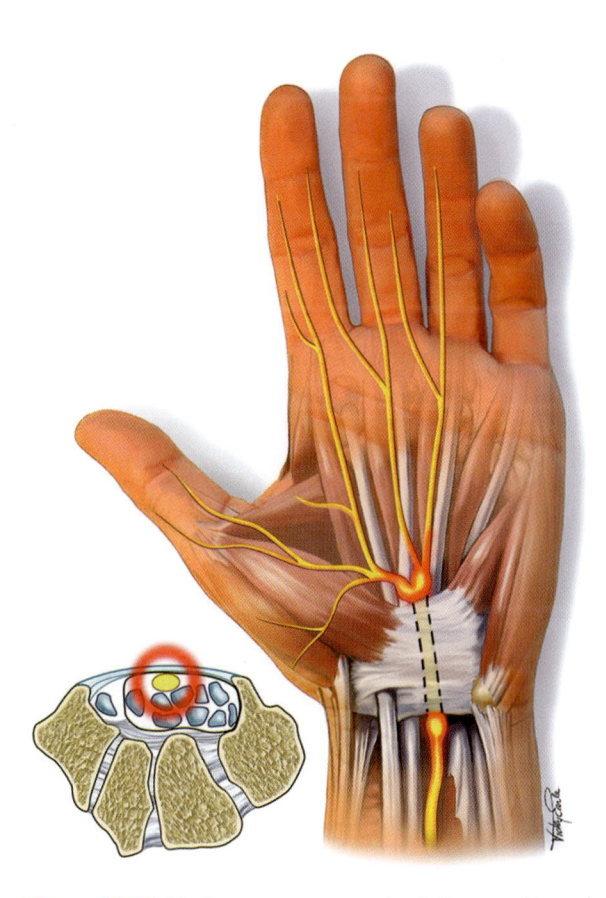

Figure 26.20 Median nerve compression in the carpal tunnel

PART B Regional problems

(a)

(b)

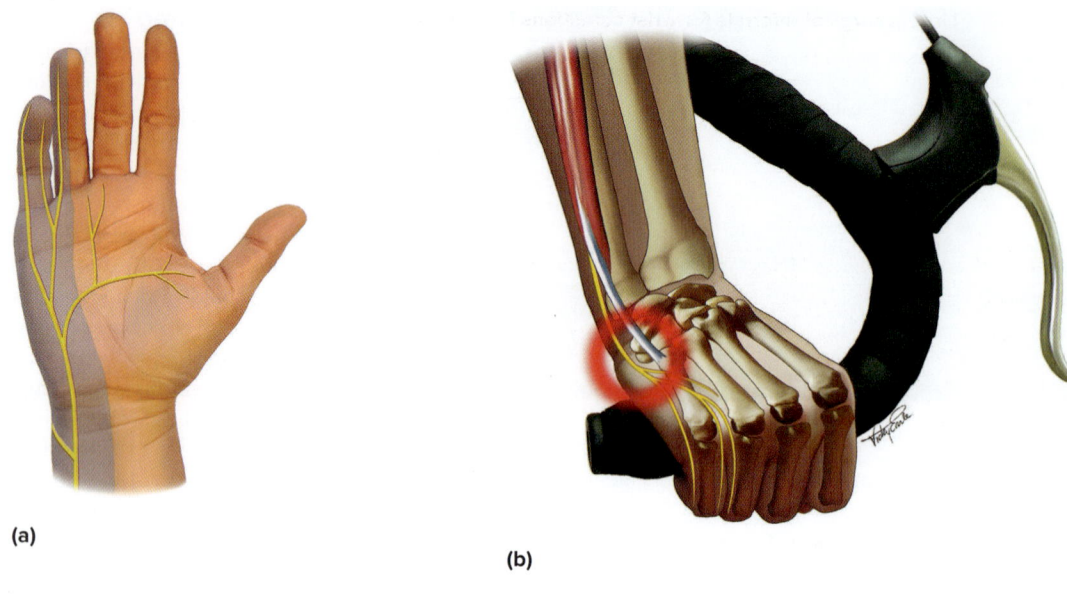

Figure 26.21 Ulnar nerve compression (a) Ulnar nerve (b) Mechanism of nerve compression in cycling

Mild cases may be treated conservatively with non-steroidal anti-inflammatory drugs (NSAIDs) and splinting.[81,82] A single corticosteroid injection may provide temporary relief,[82,83] but persistent cases require surgical treatment.[84] Surgery may be either open or endoscopic, and systematic reviews to date show no difference between the two techniques for symptom relief.[85]

Ulnar nerve compression

The ulnar nerve may be compressed at the wrist as it passes through Guyon's canal, sometimes with ulnar artery thrombosis. It is called hypothenar hammer syndrome, and it is most commonly seen in cyclists due to supporting body weight over a long duration when cycling,[86] because of poor bike fit or a failure to use several relaxed handlebar grip positions (Fig. 26.21). It also occurs in karate practitioners, and one study highlighted the risk of hand neurovascular changes in baseball players, especially catchers, from repeated trauma associated with catching a ball.[87] Within Guyon's canal, the nerve lies with the ulnar artery between the pisiform bone on the ulnar side and the hamate radially.

Symptoms include pain and paraesthesia to the little finger and ulnar side of the fourth finger. Weakness usually develops later. For cyclists, non-surgical treatment involves splinting, NSAIDs and changes to bicycle set up. In particular, the grip position should be assessed, and moving the saddle backwards may reduce the amount of weight going through the cyclist's upper limbs. Surgical exploration of Guyon's canal may be required.

SURGERY FOR WRIST CONDITIONS

Traditional indications for surgery are a failure of conservative treatment together with an applicable surgical procedure that has proven outcome results. In many weekend athletes this holds true. However, in professional athletes with a limited career time span, the career goals impact heavily on both the indication and the timing of surgery.

In the management of intersection syndrome, aggressive use of early surgery with immediate return to elite rowing means less loss of condition and changes to technique that may impact on the sports results and hence the career of the rower. The use of more sturdy fixation than normal for a wrist fracture allows return to sport earlier and with more confidence. The risks of surgery must be discussed with the individual athlete to measure the risk–benefit ratio and to discuss the subsequent rehabilitation. (See Chapter 2–shared decision making). Table 26.4 indicates conditions where an early surgical opinion and liaison with the athlete support team are warranted.

Wrist pain CHAPTER 26

Table 26.4 Urgent surgical referrals for wrist conditions in sports

Injury	Common sports	Management
Fractured radius	All high-impact sports	Immediate assessment of need for surgery (X-ray/specialist)
Fractured scaphoid	Contact sports/riding sports	Early diagnosis by X-ray or CT scan and early surgery best option
Extensor carpi ulnaris (ECU) dislocation or subluxation	Wrist rotation sports (especially tennis)	Early splinting but often requires surgery
Perilunate dislocation	Contact sports	Emergency joint reduction and pinning (median nerve at great risk)
Kienböck's disease (avascular necrosis of lunate)	All sports but especially golf and tennis	Splint very early but most require specialist reconstruction
Acute carpal tunnel syndrome	Any sports	Numbness must be treated urgently to avoid long-term disability
Forearm compartment syndrome (acute)	Crush injuries (high impact)	Decompression urgently

WRIST REHABILITATION

The key factor in wrist rehabilitation is the balance between the need to immobilise or restrict movement and the requirement to restore full range of movement.

Wrist splinting

Correct positioning of a wrist within a cast or splint is crucial to its potential to heal. Commercially available splints rarely fit well enough, and so custom fabrication is recommended for most conditions. If immobilisation of the fingers is not required, then the cast should end at the distal palmar crease to allow full finger flexion. Casting of non-displaced scaphoid fractures does not always require the thumb to be included, but it is preferred to do so.[88]

The material used will depend on the injury, with plaster or fibreglass best for fractures, and thermoplastic more suited to tendinopathies, strains, postoperative splinting and protection during activity. The rules governing the use of splints in sport vary widely between competitions and levels, making it the treating clinician's responsibility to know what is permissible.

Post-immobilisation wrist rehabilitation

A wrist that has been casted or splinted for an extended period of time will be stiff and weakened when the cast is removed. Management of the expectations of the athlete is paramount. There is no point in restoring full wrist motion at the expense of stability and control. Oedema must be minimised and compression bandages and wraps are useful. Ongoing use of a splint may be required overnight or in between exercise sessions to minimise pain and inflammatory responses. Its presence can also be a reminder to the patient not to do too much in the initial stages.

Joint mobilisation, stretching, active movement in all planes and graduated strengthening should begin as soon as healing permits, as well as the incorporation of functional activities such as bouncing a ball. The dart thrower's motion (mid-range radial extension to ulnar flexion) is a stable movement that can be used for early mobilisation in situations where ligamentous injury has not been ruled out.[89]

Functional wrist strengthening and neuromuscular training exercises may include:

- bouncing a ball
- ball/towel stretch on a table or wall
- holding a racquet, rolling a ball on strings
- light catching (alter the ball size)
- throwing a ball at a mini-trampoline
- slosh pipe (an unstable weight created by putting water inside a plastic pipe)
- gyro-ball
- tossing ball, underhand/overhand
- TheraBand™
- wrist weights
- weight-bearing progression through putty, ball, wobble board
- putting
- curling a cricket bat
- rotation with a hammer.

PART B — Regional problems

REFERENCES

References for this chapter can be found at www.mhhe.com/au/CSM5e

Chapter 27

Hand and finger injuries

with HAMISH ANDERSON and GREGORY HOY

> *Star midfielder Daniel Kerr says he's willing to risk permanent damage to his injured finger if it means helping the Eagles reach and win another Grand Final. West Coast's bid for a third straight grand final, and back-to-back premierships, was dealt a shattering blow last week when Kerr had to undergo surgery on a ruptured tendon in the ring finger of his left hand.*
> Superfooty AFL, 29 August 2007

Sports-related injuries account for up to 15% of all hand injuries seen in accident and emergency departments.[1] Some hand injuries are potentially serious and require immobilisation, precise splinting and/or surgery. Finger injuries are often neglected by athletes in the expectation that they will resolve spontaneously. Athletes often present too late for effective treatment, especially with ligamentous injuries and joint instability.

The importance of early assessment and management must be stressed so that long-term deformity and functional impairment can be avoided. Many hand and finger injuries require specific rehabilitation and appropriate protection upon resumption of sports. Joints in this region do not respond well to immobilisation, which often exacerbates oedema and stiffness. Hence, surgical stabilisation and protected stabilisation with active motion splints are becoming commonplace for sports-related hand injuries.

As in all injury management, return to occupation is important, and if the occupation is sport, then more aggressive management options are often employed.

The sport-specific causes of pain in the hand are shown in Table 27.1. The anatomy of this area is demonstrated in Figure 27.1.

CLINICAL APPROACH
History
The mechanism of injury is the most important component of the history of acute hand injuries. A direct, severe blow to the fingers may result in a fracture, whereas a blow to the point of the finger may produce an interphalangeal dislocation, joint sprain, or long flexor or extensor tendon avulsion.

A punching injury often results in a fracture at the base of the first metacarpal or to the neck of one of the other metacarpals (usually the fifth), or carpo-metacarpal (CMC) joint instability. An avulsion of the flexor digitorum profundus tendon, most commonly to the fourth finger, is suggested by a history of a patient grabbing an opponent's clothing while attempting a tackle.

Lack of active motion is an important warning sign of significant injury. Associated features such as an audible crack, degree of pain, swelling, bruising and loss of function should also be noted.

Patient outcome measures are also useful, particularly in determining levels of function in chronic cases. The Michigan Hand Outcomes Questionnaire and the Disabilities of the Arm, Shoulder and Hand are widely used evaluations[3-5] (Table 27.2).

Physical examination
At the outset of examination, examine the posture of the hand, the protection of movement and the deformities compared to the other (hopefully) uninjured hand. Ask the athlete to make a fist and open, and to oppose the thumb to each finger on each side.

Carefully palpate the bones and soft tissues of the hand and fingers, looking for tenderness. The examiner should always be conscious of what structure is being palpated at any particular time. The joints should be examined to determine active and passive range of movement

PART B Regional problems

Table 27.1 Sport-specific hand conditions

Injury	Common name	Common sports	Management
Flexor digitorum profundis avulsion	Jersey finger	Tackling sports: rugby, all football codes	Early: Surgical repair Late: (>6 weeks) two-stage reconstruction
Flexor tendon pulley rupture (especially A2 and A4)	Climber's finger	Rock climbing and mountaineering	Taping (preventative) Splints (acute) or surgical pulley reconstruction
Sagittal band rupture MCPs 2,3,4	Boxer's knuckle	Boxing	Sagittal band reconstruction
Ulnar digital nerve neuroma	Bowler's thumb	10-pin bowling	Padding to thumb hole Surgical neurolysis
Ulnar collateral ligament rupture MCP thumb	Skier's thumb (gamekeeper's thumb)	Skiing, football ('thumb plant')	Splint if incomplete Surgical reconstruction if Stener lesion
Radial collateral ligament tear MCP thumb	AFL thumb	Australian rules football	Tape +/− splint to finish season Surgical reconstruction
CMC index/middle subluxation and carpal bossing	Boxer's hand	Boxing, martial arts	Splints (for competition without surgery) Resect bossing (short term) CMC fusion
Hook of hamate fracture		Batting and clubbing sports	Early: Protect Late: Excision of hook of hamate
Stress fracture scaphoid		High board diving	Splint or cast for 6 weeks
Stress reaction lunate (differential diagnosis: Stage 0 Kienböcks disease)		Golf, tennis	Splint or cast for 6 weeks Change technique

and stability. Stability should be tested both in an anteroposterior direction and with ulnar and radial deviation to assess the collateral ligaments. Do not forget that a depressed fragment of bone in a joint may produce a false positive test when stretching the redundant collateral ligament. The cause of any loss of active range of movement should be carefully assessed and not presumed to be due to swelling. Normal range of motion for the second to fifth digits is approximately 80° of flexion at the distal interphalangeal, 100° of flexion at the proximal interphalangeal and 90° of flexion at the metacarpophalangeal (MCP) joint. A common injury site that can be overlooked is the volar plate, a thick fibrocartilagenous tissue that reinforces the phalangeal joints on the palmar or volar surface.

The extensor tendons of the hand are often divided into six compartments. At the wrist on the dorsal side of the hand, the tendons are encased in synovial sheaths as they pass under the extensor retinaculum (Fig. 26.1). When palpating in the most radial compartment, also known as compartment one, the examiner identifies abductor pollicis longus and extensor pollicis brevis, the tissues involved in de Quervain's tenosynovitis. Lister's tubercle is located on the dorsal surface of the distal end of the radius. The extensor pollicis longus angles sharply around this bony prominence and it can damage or even rupture the tendon after a serious wrist fracture.

The anatomical snuffbox is composed of the extensor pollicis longus and brevis and the abductor pollicis longus. The floor of the snuffbox is the scaphoid and scaphotrapezial joint. Clinically this is a significant region for several reasons. Tenderness may suggest scaphoid fracture. The deep branch of the radial arterial passes through, as well as the superficial branch of the radial nerve. Consequently, if a cast or splint is applied too tightly, it can lead to numbness in the thumb.

Examination of the fingers and hand involves:

1. Observation and sensation testing as per the wrist (Chapter 26). Special note should be made of the hand arches and any deformities at the proximal or distal interphalangeal joints.
   a. hand at rest
   b. hand with clenched fist (Fig. 27.2a)

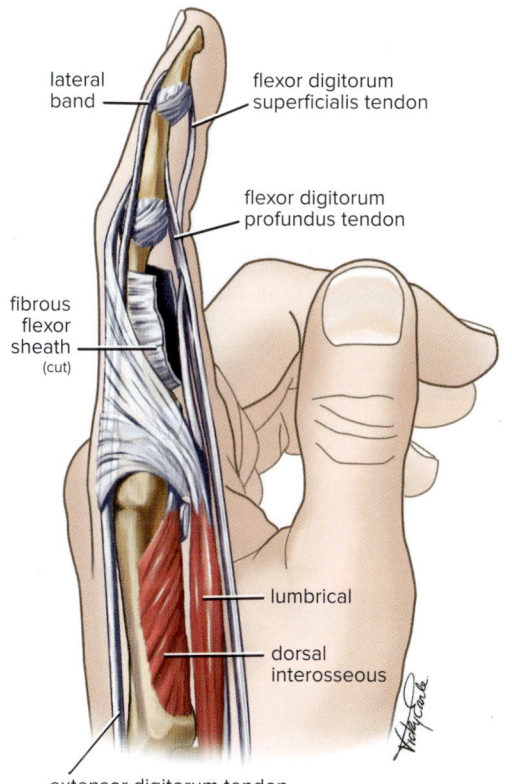

Hand and finger injuries   **CHAPTER 27**

3. Active movements–thumb
   a. flexion
   b. extension
   c. opposition (Fig. 27.2b)
4. Resisted movements (to test tendon integrity)
   a. flexor digitorum profundus (Fig. 27.2c)
   b. flexor digitorum superficialis (Fig. 27.2d)
   c. extensor tendon (Fig. 27.2e)
5. Special test
   a. ulnar collateral ligament of the first MCP joint (Fig. 27.2f)
   b. IP joint collateral ligaments

Sensitivity and specificity of testing the stability of the ulna collateral ligament of the first MCP joint has been demonstrated to improve significantly to 100% and 87.5% post injection of local anaesthetic to the joint. The accessory collateral ligament at the proximal interphalangeal (PIP) joint is tested for lateral laxity in extension, whereas the cord collateral ligament is stress tested with the PIP joint flexed to 45°.[2]

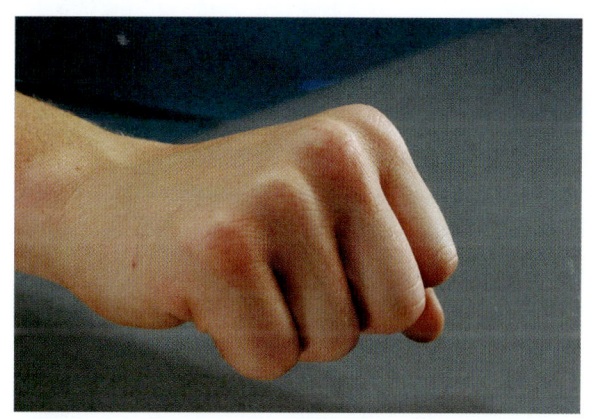

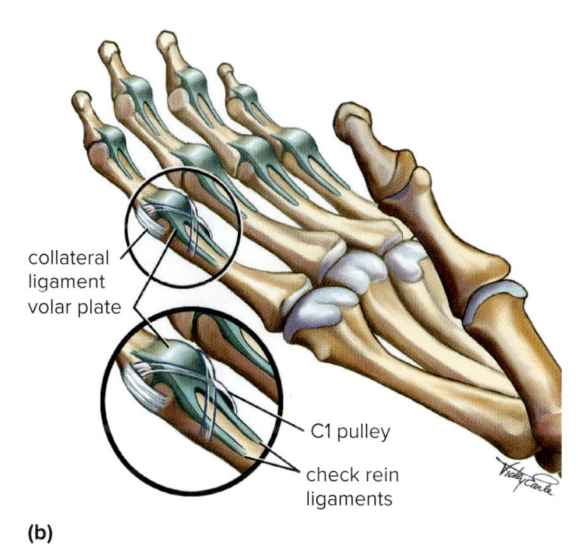

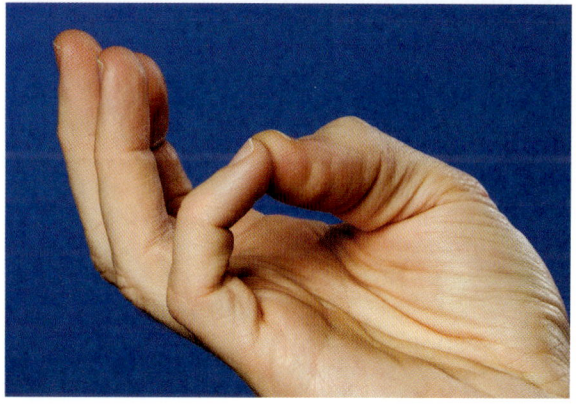

Figure 27.1 Anatomy of the metacarpals and fingers (a) Muscles and tendons (b) The volar plate

2. Active movements–fingers (all joints)
   a. flexion
   b. extension
   c. abduction
   d. adduction

Figure 27.2 (a) Attitude of hand with clenched fist (b) Thumb movement—opposition

(c)

(e)

(d)

(f)

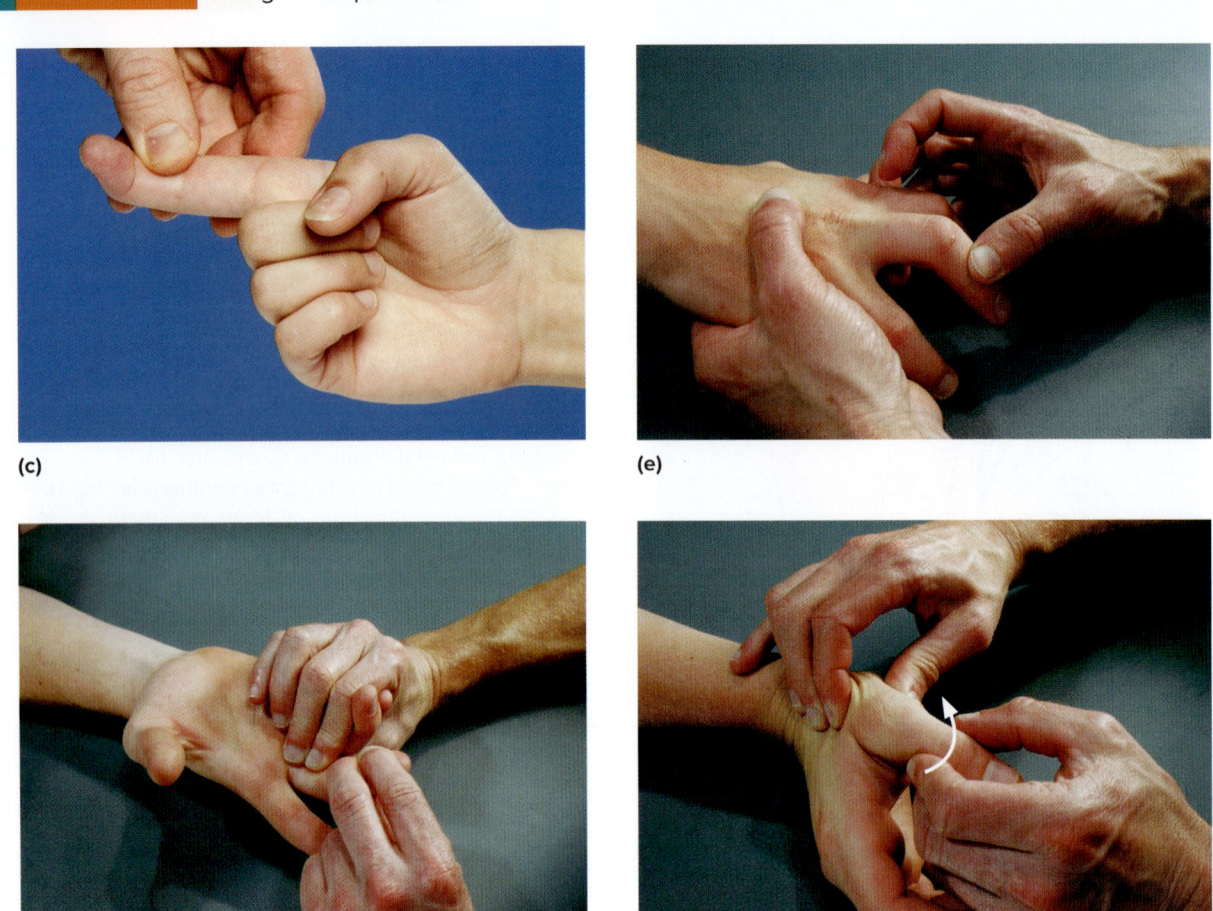

Figure 27.2 (cont.) (c) Tendon integrity—flexor digitorum profundus. The patient flexes the DIP joint with the PIP joint held in extension (d) Tendon integrity—flexor digitorum superficialis. The patient flexes the PIP joint with the other DIP joint held in extension (e) Tendon integrity—extensor tendon. The patient extends the PIP joint with the MCP joint in extension (f) Special test—the ulnar collateral ligament of the thumb is tested with 10° of flexion at the first MCP joint

Key outcome measures
Refer to Table 27.2 (Refer also to Chapter 16 Patient reported outcome measures in sports medicine).

> **PRACTICE PEARL**
>
> All traumatic finger injuries should be X-rayed.

Investigations
Routine radiographs of the hand include the PA, oblique and lateral views. Ideally, 'dislocations' need to be radiographed before reduction to exclude fracture and after reduction to confirm relocation. Even when pre-reduction radiographs are not performed because reduction has occurred on the field, post reduction films should be obtained after the game. Care should be taken with lateral views to isolate the affected finger to avoid bony overlap.

The use of more sophisticated investigation techniques is now more routine. CT scans show subtle avulsions and 3D CT scans are useful for understanding fracture patterns and methods of reduction. Single-photon emission computed tomography (SPECT) imaging combined with CT scans can show hot spots and stress reactions in bone as well as excluding bone lesions in some circumstances. MRI scanning is now very common for ligament and tendon injuries to grade and assist surgical decision making. Ultrasound is still widely indicated in dynamic imaging such as with subluxing tendons, the Stener lesion in the thumb, and siting tendon-ends in ruptures and lacerations.

PRINCIPLES OF TREATMENT
The functional hand requires mobility, stability, sensitivity and freedom from pain. It may be necessary to obtain

Hand and finger injuries — CHAPTER 27

Table 27.2 Patient-reported outcome measures (PROMs) for hand and finger injuries and pain

Michigan Hand Outcomes questionnaire
1. Hand-specific assessment covering function, ADLs, pain, work performance, aesthetics and satisfaction
2. x items: 37
3. Score range x–y
4. Test–retest reliability: >0.81[3]
5. Validity: High validity demonstrated
6. MDC95%: Varies according to diagnosis
7. MCID: Varies according to diagnosis
8. Available online: Yes
Disability of the Arm, Shoulder and Hand questionnaire (DASH and Quick DASH)
1. Measures physical function, symptoms and quality of life in people with musculoskeletal disorders of the upper limb
2. x items: DASH 30; Quick DASH 11
3. Score range x–y: 0 (no impairment)—100 (poor)
4. Test–retest reliability: DASH >0.96;[4] QuickDASH >0.91[5]
5. Validity: DASH >0.70;[4] QuickDASH > 0.70[6]
6. MDC95%: DASH 12.75%;[4] QuickDASH 11.2%[5]
7. MCID: 10.83%;[4] 8%[5]
8. Available online: DASH and QuickDASH

stability by surgical methods. However, conservative rehabilitation is essential to regain mobility and long-term freedom from pain. Treatment and rehabilitation of hand injuries is complex. As the hand is unforgiving of mismanagement, practitioners who do not see hand injuries regularly should ideally refer patients to an experienced hand therapist, or at least obtain advice while managing the patient.[7]

Inflammation and swelling are obvious in the hand and fingers. During the inflammatory phase, the therapist must aim to reduce oedema and monitor progress by signs of redness, heat and increased pain. During the regenerative phase (characterised by proliferation of scar tissue), the therapist can use supportive splints and active exercises to maintain range of motion. During remodelling, it is appropriate to use dynamic and serial splints, and active and active assisted exercises, in addition to heat, stretching and electrotherapeutic modalities.[8]

Oedema control

Oedema can be controlled through splinting, compression, ice, elevation and electrotherapeutic modalities (Chapter 17). Splinting needs to be in the intrinsic plus position, with the wrist in 30° of dorsiflexion, the MCP joints flexed to 70° and the PIP joint extended to 0° with the thumb abducted (Fig. 27.3). Splints are periodically removed to allow exercise. Fist-making exercises are used to maintain joint movement and to help remove oedema. During exercise, the hand should be elevated. Short, frequent exercise periods are optimal.

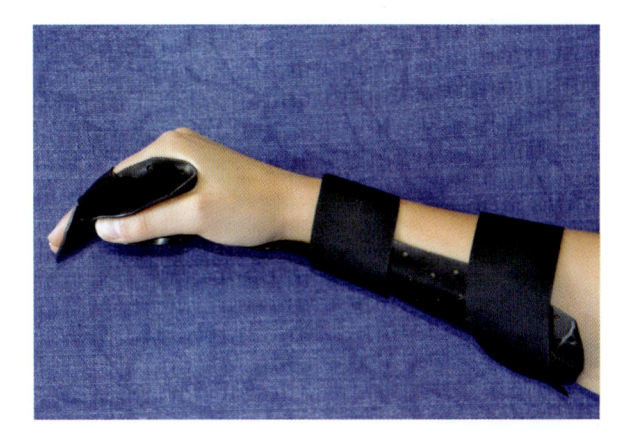

Figure 27.3 The 'intrinsic plus' position for splinting of hand injuries: 30° of wrist dorsiflexion, 70° of MCP flexion and minimal PIP flexion

PART B   Regional problems

Compression in the hand can be achieved with a compression glove and by using a Coban™ elastic bandage: a 2.5 cm size is appropriate for fingers. If applicable, active tendon gliding and range of motion exercises in combination with elevation can assist in the reduction of swelling. Electrotherapeutic modalities can be useful in the control of oedema.

Exercises

Exercises may be active, active assisted or resisted. Tendon lacerations or ruptures are generally treated by protocols determined by the surgical technique and preferences of the treating surgeon.

Exercise prescription for other injuries includes:

- blocking exercises, which isolate an injured joint or muscle by immobilising neighbouring joints with the other hand
- composite flexion exercises (e.g. tendon gliding exercises)
- extension exercises
- active assisted exercises in which the patient takes a joint through the available range of motion and then the therapist assists in gaining slightly greater range with overpressure.

Taping and splinting

The most commonly used method of taping is 'buddy taping' (Fig. 27.4). Its role is to provide a vehicle for active assisted exercise. The uninjured digit provides additional stability and encourages full range of motion.

An injury to the finger can often be managed successfully with a conservative approach using the protection of some form of splint. Thin thermoplastic–1.6 mm or less is ideal–can be remoulded to accommodate changes in swelling or protocol. Finger sleeves (Fig. 27.5a) can be made of neoprene or Lycra® to manage oedema, pain or chronic flexion deformity, and both can be reinforced with thin thermoplastic if extra stability is required.[9]

Splints can have padding added and be taped on for protection during sporting activity. The goal is to provide stability, but not at the expense of limiting movement and impeding performance.[10] The use of splints during a game is entirely dependent upon the athlete, his or her sport and the rules governing the sport at that level.

> **PRACTICE PEARL**
>
> 1.6 mm thermoplastic can be softened sufficiently in a hot cup of water to make a splint on the sidelines.

In the acute phase of injury, static splints are used to reduce oedema. Dynamic splints can also be used in the repair phase of injury to provide some force along joints and encourage increased range of motion (Fig. 27.5b and c). With dynamic splinting, the splint should be worn with less tension for a longer period.[9, 10]

METACARPAL FRACTURES
Fracture of the base of the first metacarpal

Fractures of the base of the first metacarpal commonly occur as a result of a punch connecting with a hard object, such as an opponent's head, or a fall on the abducted thumb. There are two main types of fracture: (1) the extra-articular transverse fracture of the base of the first metacarpal about 1 cm distal to the joint (Fig. 27.6a) and (2) a Bennett's fracture/dislocation (or Rolando comminuted fracture/dislocation) of the first carpo-metacarpal joint (Fig. 27.6b).

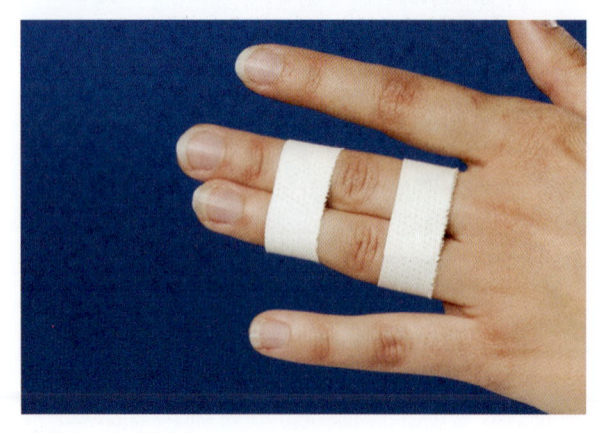

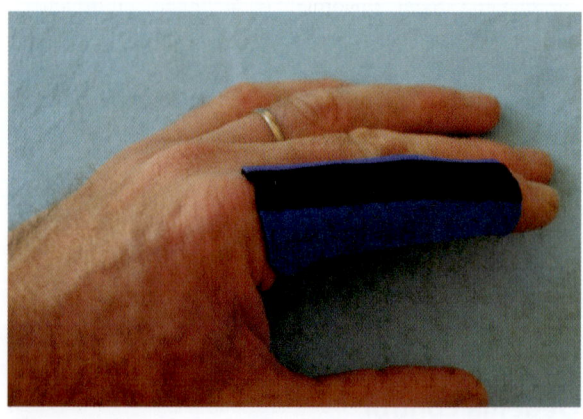

Figure 27.4 Buddy taping of fingers

(a)

Figure 27.5 Splints used to treat fixed flexion deformity (a) Neoprene finger sleeve provides gentle extension also addresses chronic oedema

Hand and finger injuries   CHAPTER 27

(b)

(c)

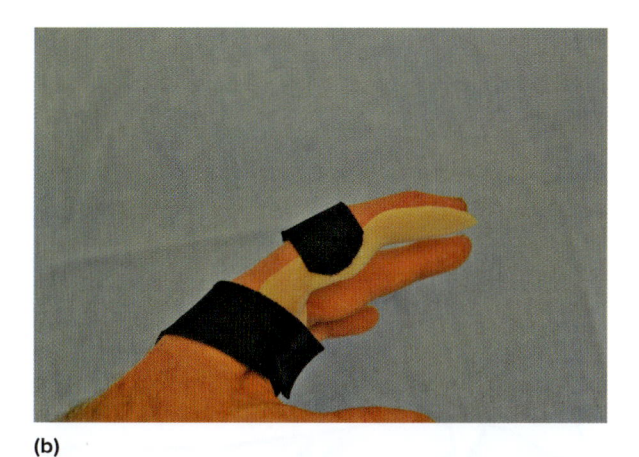

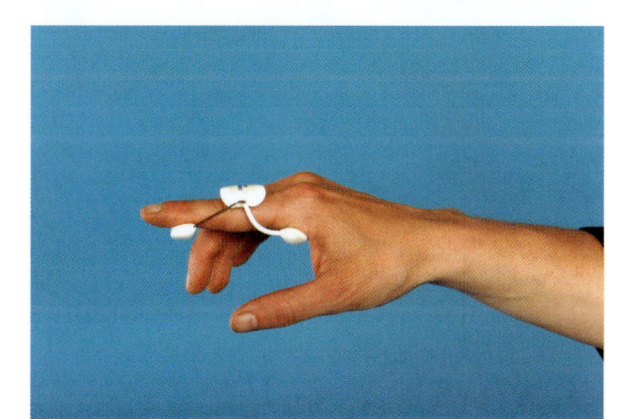

Figure 27.5 (cont.) (b) Static progressive (also known as a 'belly gutter') splint. This simple finger gutter splint has a 'belly' underneath the PIP joint. It is usually put on half an hour before bed with a gentle tension on the central strap. This provides a progressive and controlled end-range stretch into extension overnight (c) A commercial dynamic (spring) finger-based PIP extension splint. This splint is only suitable for contractures of less than 40° and does permit active flexion

The transverse fracture near the base of the first metacarpal results in the thumb lying flexed across the palm. Reduction of this fracture involves extension of the distal segment of the metacarpal. This fracture can be immobilised in a short arm spica cast, but now more commonly internal fixation allows both anatomical reduction and early active movement. This produces prompt return to activity, and less delay in recovery from loss of position. The often-quoted 'surgery only as a last resort' is less relevant today with better surgical training, better imaging and modern surgical implants.

A Bennett's fracture dislocation of the first carpo-metacarpal joint occurs as a result of axial compression

(a)

(b)

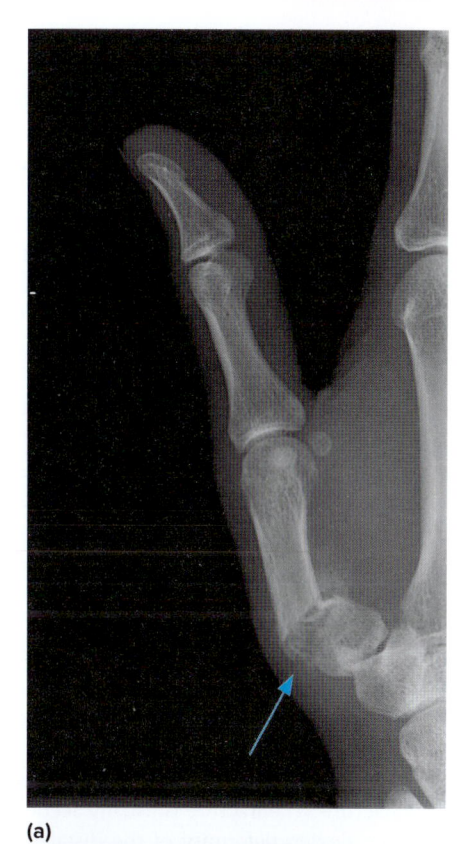

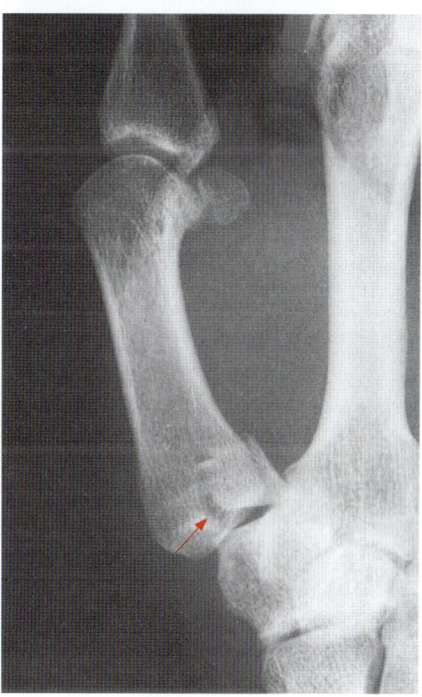

Figure 27.6 Fractures of the base of the first metacarpal (arrows) (a) Healing transverse fracture (b) Bennett's fracture

495

PART B Regional problems

when the first metacarpal is driven proximally, shearing off its base. A small medial fragment of the metacarpal remains attached to the strong volar ligament and the main shaft of the metacarpal is pulled proximally by the unopposed pull of the abductor pollicis longus muscle. This injury should be referred to a hand surgeon.

Treatment in recreational athletes requires closed reduction and percutaneous Kirschner wire fixation together with cast immobilisation for 4–6 weeks. Upon removal of the cast, mobilisation of the surrounding joints is required and, if early return to sport is required, a protective device should be worn.

Professional athletes will have anatomical reduction, plate fixation and early active movement. Patients not engaging in contact sport find soft neoprene braces (Fig. 27.7) supportive and comfortable after a Bennett's fracture and other common hand injuries. These are not replacements for firmer splints and braces that might be needed when trauma can be anticipated.

Fractures of the other metacarpals

Fractures of the second to fifth metacarpals may also occur as the result of a punch, contact with ball and ground, and direct hits at hockey, cricket, baseball, etc. When seen in the fourth and fifth metacarpals, it is referred to as a 'boxer's fracture'. The fracture is usually accompanied by considerable flexion deformity of the distal fragment which is countered by the extra dorsiflexion available at the MCP joint to make up for this deformity. This results in surprisingly little functional disability (Figs 27.8 and 27.9).

The acceptable angulation for fractures of the neck of the fourth and fifth metacarpals is up to 30°, as long as there is little rotational deformity. Up to 10° angulation is acceptable in the second and third metacarpals. However, prominence of the metacarpal head in the palm of the hand may be a problem for tennis players and athletes who require a firm grip.

Treatment involves splinting or casting in a position of 70° of flexion of the MCP joints to prevent shortening of the collateral ligament and subsequent stiffness (Fig. 27.10a). Check that this position does not displace the fracture. The splint may be removed after 2–3 weeks and non-contact sport resumed immediately with

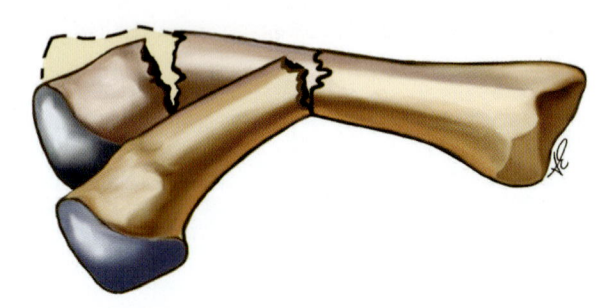

Figure 27.8 In metacarpal fractures, the more proximal the fracture, the more the knuckle will drop

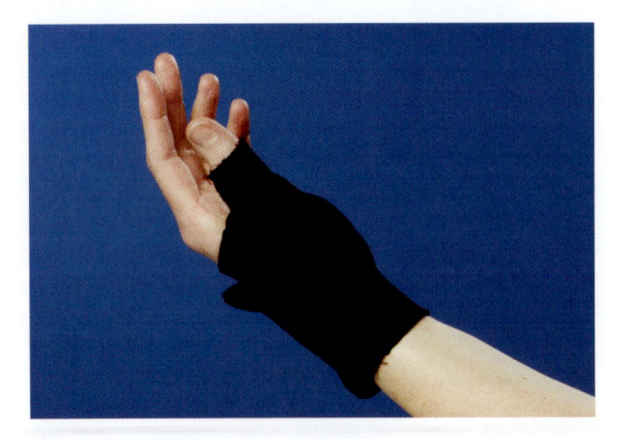

Figure 27.7 Soft neoprene splints can provide support during rehabilitation after a hand injury

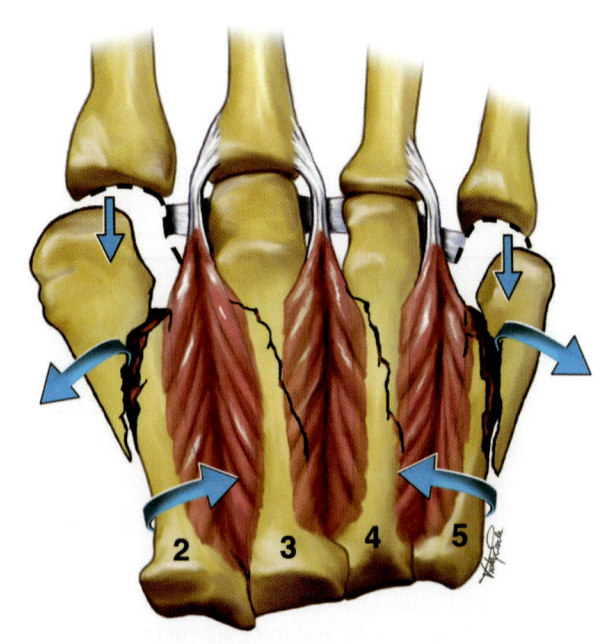

Figure 27.9 Spiral fractures of the second and fifth metacarpals (border digits) are more unstable than those of the third and fourth metacarpals as only one side of the border metacarpals is supported by the strong, deep transverse intercarpal ligaments

Hand and finger injuries   CHAPTER 27

protection (Fig. 27.10b). Unprotected return to contact sport is more controversial, and recently suggestions of aggressive return to play 1–2 weeks after strong plating in professional sports have been put forward.

Shortened, rotated and intra-articular fractures of the metacarpals require anatomical reduction and fixation. In displaced fractures, this usually involves plating from the dorsal or lateral aspect to correct angulation and rotation. Check for rotation of finger fractures clinically (as subtle rotation causes 'crossing' of metacarpals and affects grip) and not by using radiographs. Un-displaced fractures can be immobilised in a gutter splint with flexion of the MCP joint.[11]

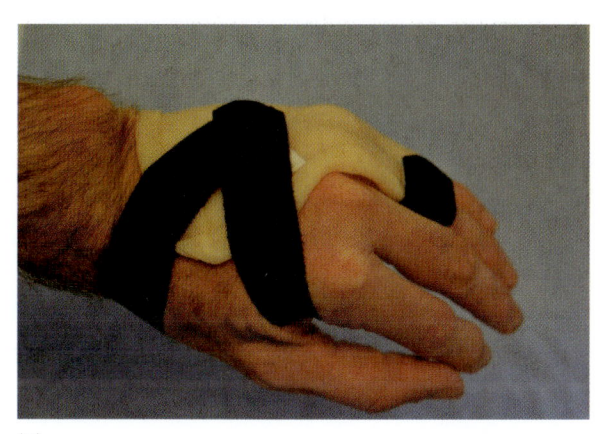

FRACTURES OF PHALANGES
Proximal phalanx fractures
Fractures of the proximal phalanx may lead to functional impairment due to the extensor and flexor tendons coming into contact with callus and exposed bone, and due to imbalance of the extensor expansion with flexors creating 'Z' deformities through the PIP and distal interphalangeal (DIP) joints in hypermobile individuals.

Un-displaced fractures require weekly radiographs to ensure movement has not occurred. If further stability is needed, the adjacent finger can be buddy taped, but it is more common now to pin, wire or plate these fractures to regain stability and allow hand therapy to achieve better early results. Splints are removed after a maximum 3–4 weeks but ideally earlier to improve function. Unstable fractures require urgent surgical referral.

Rotational deformity of phalangeal fractures may not be obvious in extension so the fingers should be examined end on with PIP and DIP flexion to reveal any deformity present. All rotated fractures need open reduction and possibly internal fixation.

Middle phalanx fractures
Fractures of the middle phalanx involve hard cortical bone. Generally oblique or transverse, these fractures heal slowly. The central slip of the extensor tendon attaches dorsally to the base of the bone and the flexor digitorum inserts on the volar surface more distally. Thus, fractures distal to the flexor tendon attachment show flexion of the proximal fragment and extension of the distal fragment.

Stable fractures are immobilised in a splint for 3 weeks (70° of MCP joint flexion and 0° of PIP joint flexion). When the splint is removed, range of motion exercises are begun.

Unstable fractures, or intra-articular fractures involving more than 25% of the PIP joint surface, require open reduction and internal fixation. Small-calibre Kirschner wires or screws are used and range of motion exercises are begun as soon as fixation is considered to be stable in order to avoid stiffness.

Volar plate avulsion fractures can occur at the PIP joint following a hyperextension injury (and often a joint subluxation or dislocation). This injury is very common,

(a)

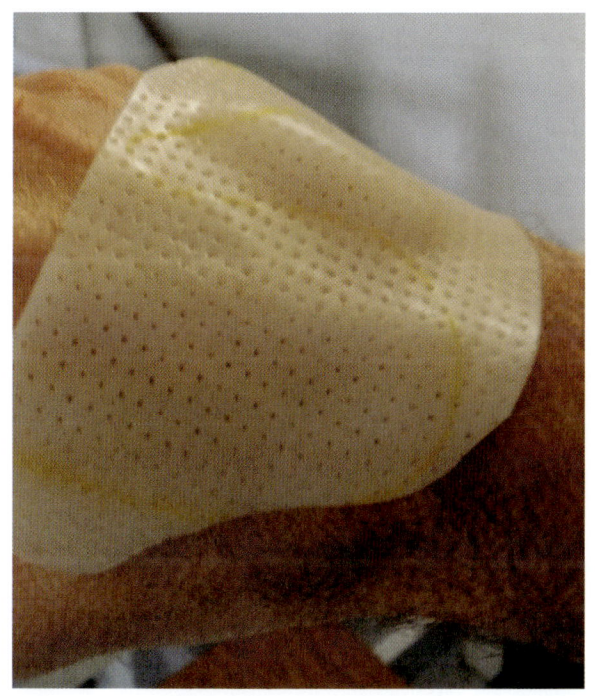

(b)

Figure 27.10 Splints used in the management of fracture of the fifth metacarpal (a) The treatment splint should position the MCP joints of the 4th and 5th fingers in 70° of flexion, leaving the IP joints free to move (b) Protective splint used for early return to sport when appropriate. Note the bubble over the fracture site to accommodate swelling

497

PART B Regional problems

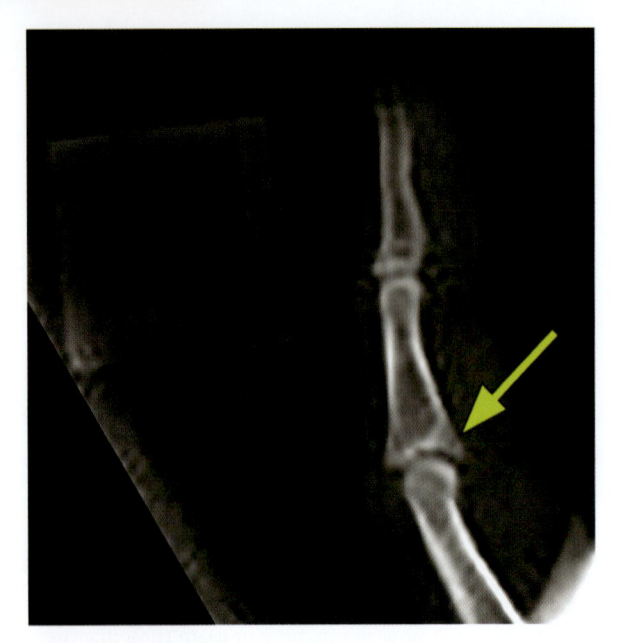

Figure 27.11 Radiograph confirms the subtle nature of a volar plate avulsion

converts a closed fracture to a compound fracture and requires careful prevention or prophylaxis of infection. A percutaneous K-wire from the tip down across fracture and DIP joint allows early function but not contact sport.

> **PRACTICE PEARL**
>
> Most distal phalangeal fractures heal in 4–6 weeks.

DISLOCATIONS OF THE CARPO-METACARPAL JOINTS

Most carpo-metacarpal (CMC) subluxations (with or without fractures of the carpal bones) occur with hitting, such as martial arts, or impact with the ground. Plain radiograph demonstrates the incongruence and the subluxation (Fig. 27.12). While splints can protect temporarily, the best treatment of this injury is reduction and pinning (acutely) or fusion of the CMC joints involved (usually index and middle finger metacarpals to trapezoid and capitate) if chronic.[13]

Dorsal dislocation of the MCP joints of the fingers is uncommon and usually occurs in the index finger or thumb. It has been called the 'irreducible dislocation' because the metacarpal head is pushed through the volar plate of the MCP joint and caught between the lumbrical and long flexor tendons with a buttonholing effect. Suspect this injury when examination reveals hyperextension of the involved MCP joint with ulnar deviation of the finger overlapping the adjacent finger.

An attempt to reduce the dislocation may be made by increasing the deformity and pushing the proximal phalanx through the tear in the volar plate. However, open reduction is sometimes required. The MCP joint is

and usually ignored owing to an unawareness of the potential consequences. The typical anatomy is shown above in Figure 27.1b and the radiographic appearance is shown in Figure 27.11.

Non-randomised controlled trials have compared early mobilisation with splinting and found that mobilisation has led to good functional outcomes,[12] although extension blocking helps prevent hyperextension and recurrent dislocations. Often flexion deficits occur when the volar fragment and scarred volar plate are too thick and interfere with tight grip. Excision of the fragment and volar plate arthroplasty (VPA) helps eliminate this problem.

Distal phalanx fractures

Fractures of the distal phalanx are usually caused by crushing injuries, such as fingers being jammed between a fast-moving ball and a stick or bat. They are usually non-displaced.

Often a splint and compression dressing will provide adequate treatment for non-displaced fractures. Much of the pain associated with these fractures can be due to subungual haematoma. Significant subungual haematoma requires nail bed exploration and excision as the nail bed is often disrupted. In this case surgical repair may be required to prevent future nail deformity. This represents a compound fracture and should be treated as such.

Perforation of the nail to drain a subungual haematoma is a relative contraindication in this instance as it

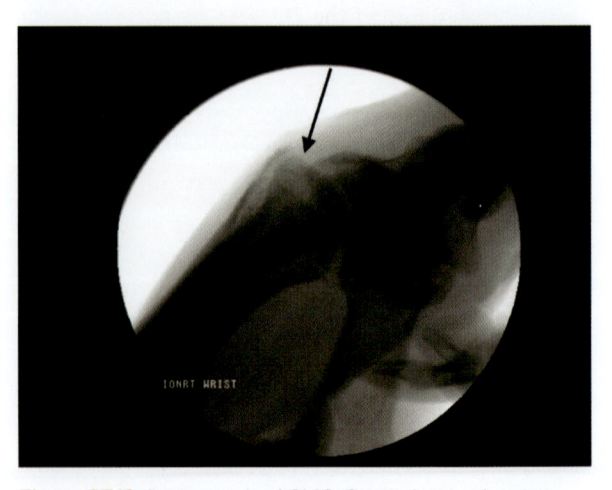

Figure 27.12 Radiograph of CMC. Sagittal view showing dorsal subluxation of metacarpal (arrow)

usually stable after reduction in 30° of MCP flexion and early movement can be commenced in a dorsal splint allowing full flexion but preventing the last 30° of MCP joint extension. The immobilisation is maintained for 5-6 weeks. Associated osteochondral fractures require open reduction and internal fixation, and the collateral ligaments should be checked (even by MRI if required) to ensure accurate reduction.

DISLOCATIONS OF THE FINGER JOINTS
Dislocations of the PIP joint

Dorsal PIP joint dislocations are the most common hand dislocation. They usually result from a hyperextension stress with some degree of longitudinal compression such as may occur in ball sports. This may produce disruption of both the volar plate and at least one collateral ligament. Ideally, radiographs should precede reduction to confirm the diagnosis and exclude an associated fracture. In practice, reduction often occurs on or beside the playing area so it is vital that radiography be performed afterwards. If a fracture is present, the stability of the joint must be tested.

If the joint is stable post-reduction, a splint is not necessary and buddy taping to prevent hyperextension with active movement is recommended. If the joint is unstable, then the joint should be splinted in flexion beyond the point of instability and gradually extended to neutral over a period of 3-4 weeks[14] (Fig. 27.13).

Fixed flexion deformities are common following this injury in spite of treatment; however, if left untreated, a hyperextension deformity and instability may develop. Swelling around the joint can last for several months and should be managed using an elastic pressure bandage or neoprene sleeve, soft tissue treatment and electrotherapeutic modalities.

Volar dislocations of the PIP joint are uncommon and are often resistant to closed reduction. There is almost always an associated rupture of one or more collateral ligaments along with disruption of the extensor central

> **PRACTICE PEARL**
>
> If radiographs reveal an associated fracture of the volar lip of the middle phalanx involving more than one-third of the joint surface, open reduction and internal fixation are usually required to restore stability.

slip insertion. This injury predisposes to the development of a boutonnière (buttonhole) deformity and should be treated aggressively with either surgery or a splint, holding the PIP joint of the affected finger in extension for 6 weeks while encouraging DIP movement. Surgery requires

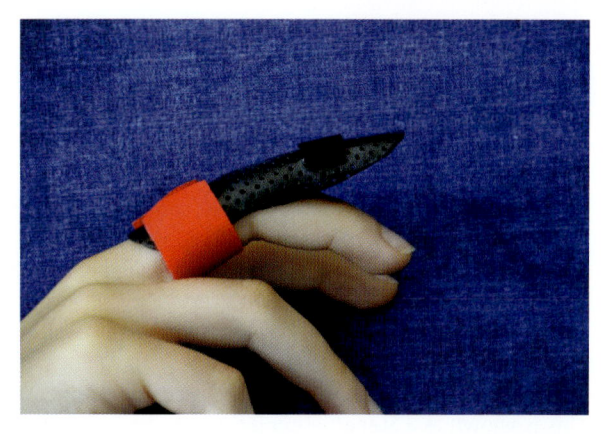

Figure 27.13 Splinting following a PIP joint dislocation. This dorsal block splint allows flexion but stops full extension at the PIP joint

prevention of flexion for 6 weeks and so significant loss of game time occurs in mid-season injuries. Waiting until the end of the season risks a fixed boutonnière deformity which often heals poorly with or without surgery.

Dislocations of the DIP joint

Dislocations of the DIP joint are most often due to a ball hitting the tip of the finger forcing hyperextension. They are commonly associated with a volar skin laceration. Reduction is achieved by traction and flexion. The joint is usually stable post reduction, but should still be splinted for 3 weeks in 10° of flexion.[15] Controlled active flexion is permitted during this time if the joint is stable, and can be progressed gradually from that point. Collateral ligament injuries are rare. Failure to achieve reduction of the joint should be investigated, and flexor tendon function must be assessed as avulsion can occur with this injury.[16]

The less common volar dislocation occurs in association with a fracture and usually involves damage to the extensor tendon. This presents with the mallet finger deformity. Thus, all mallet fingers must be radiographed to exclude fracture. If volar dislocation has occurred, open repair may be indicated depending on the size and position of the fracture fragment.[17]

LIGAMENT AND TENDON INJURIES
Sprain of the ulnar collateral ligament of the first MCP joint

Initially known as 'gamekeeper's thumb', and more recently 'skier's thumb', this injury is one of the most common injuries to the hand and is found in all sports, especially those requiring stick holding or ball handling. Damage to the collateral ligaments of the thumb has an adverse effect

499

on the hand's strength and precision.[18] This is particularly appreciated in pinching tasks such as holding a key (Fig. 27.14a).

Diagnosis is typically made clinically, with stress testing of the metacarpal joint of the thumb done in neutral and at 30° of flexion (Fig. 27.2f). Laxity in a radial direction of greater than 15° with soft end feel compared to the contralateral thumb is an indication of a complete rupture. Less than 15° indicates an incomplete tear. Radiographs are required to rule out an avulsion fracture.[18, 19]

Surgical repair is required for complete tears because the anatomy of the ulnar aspect of the metacarpal joint can preclude opposition of the ends of the ruptured ligament. This is known as a Stener lesion for which surgical repair is mandatory (Fig. 27.15). In general, surgical management using suture anchors with pinning of the MCP joint is preferred for full tears, with inconsistent results reported for conservative treatment.[18, 20] However although results are better if repaired acutely, delayed repair is still successful, making the timing of surgery dependent upon factors specific to the athlete such as the sport and the time of season.[21]

Incomplete tears are splinted in a hand-based thumb spica with the thumb MCP joint placed in slight radial deviation and return to play dependent upon the athlete. The splint is worn full-time for 6 weeks, at which time a weaning and active motion protocol is initiated with strengthening at 8–10 weeks, and return to play with taping and/or a protective dorsal gutter splint for another 2–3 months (Fig. 27.14b). Postoperative rehabilitation is similar, with return to protected play as early as 2 weeks after surgery.[19, 22]

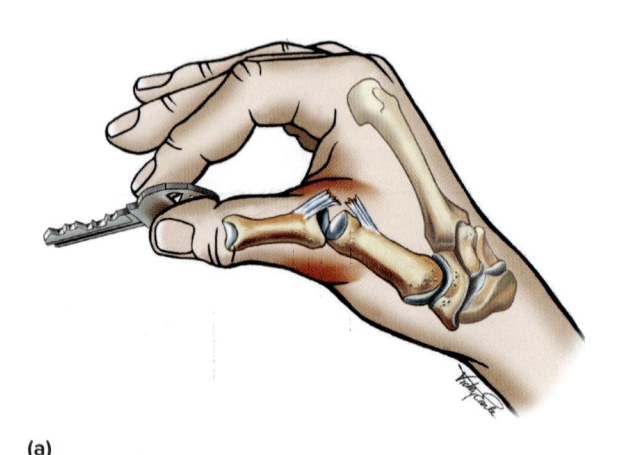

Sprain of the radial collateral ligament of the first MCP joint

Tears of the radio-collateral ligament at the MCP joint of the thumb are not as common as ulnar-sided injury and the management is mostly conservative. The major difference is that Stener-type lesions are extremely rare due to differences in anatomy. The injury occurs as a result of an ulnar directed force, be it from a punch or from a ball. Stability is usually not the chief presenting problem, with pain on grip and stiffness being the chief complaints, making delayed surgery more acceptable. Stress testing is positive with greater than 15° of laxity compared to the contralateral side and confirmation made radiologically.[18]

Management is usually conservative, with hand-based spica splinting in a position that minimises the pull of the adductor pollicis for 6 weeks, followed by an extended period of protected taping and splinting in play. Surgery is required for large tears with volar subluxation and chronic cases, with presentation often more delayed than for UCL injuries.[21, 23] Immobilisation is required for 4–6 weeks afterwards, and protection in play for 2–3 months, with good long-term results reported.[24] Surgery is often indicated between seasons for contact sport athletes due to chronic instability.

Capsular sprain of the first MCP joint

Capsular sprains of the first MCP joint are an extremely common injury in ball-handling sports. They result from a hyperextension injury and are prone to recurrence. Treatment involves active rehabilitation and protection of the joint from hyperextension. This is achieved with the use of a thermoplastic brace over the dorsal aspect of the MCP joint.

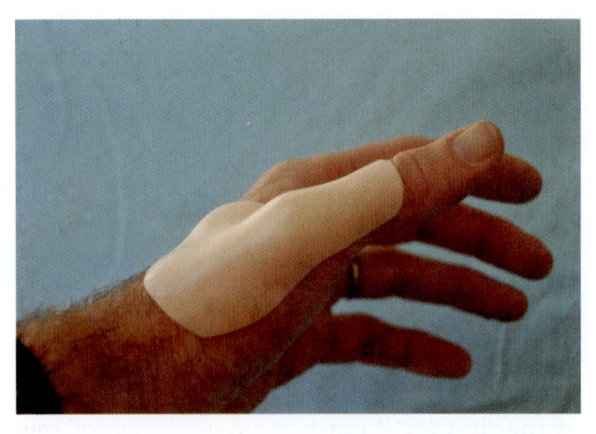

Figure 27.14 Complete ligament tear of the first MCP joint (a) Pinching is affected (b) Protective splint worn under tape during return to sport. A hole can be created over the MCP joint to permit some flexion but still restrict deviation

Hand and finger injuries

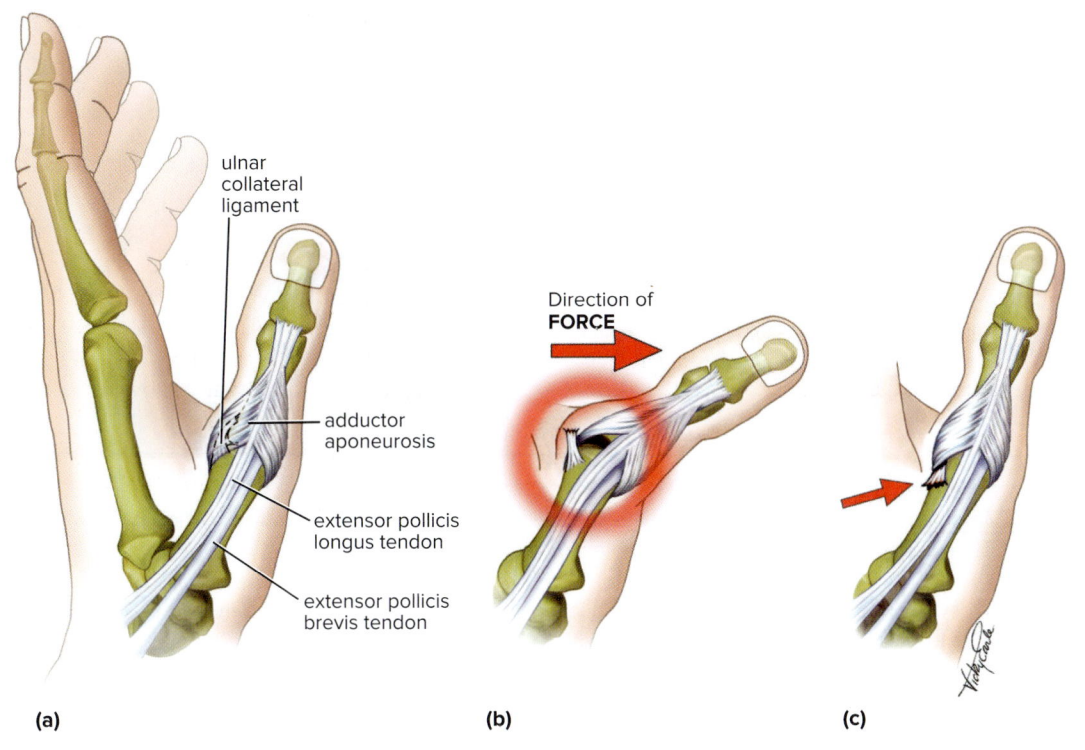

CHAPTER 27

Figure 27.15 Mechanism of formation of a Stener lesion of the thumb (a) Anatomy (b) Valgus stress opens up the joint and the adductor aponeurosis slips past the distal end of the proximal portion of the ruptured ulnar collateral ligament (c) As alignment returns to normal, the adductor aponeurosis catches the proximal portion of the ulnar collateral ligament and flips it back proximally to form the Stener lesion

PIP joint sprains

The collateral ligaments of the PIP joints are commonly injured as a result of a sideways force. Partial tears of the collateral ligament are painful, but remain stable on lateral stress. Complete tears show marked instability with lateral stress. This injury also includes hyperextension stress to the volar plate, which may avulse its insertion from the base of the metacarpal.

Stable tears should be treated by 10 days of finger-based splinting with the PIP in neutral, followed by buddy taping (Fig. 27.4), swelling management and active exercises. If the joint is unstable the splint should be fashioned in 10° of flexion greater than the point of instability (Fig. 27.13). This splint should then be gradually extended towards neutral, adjusting weekly over a period of 3 weeks. Active flexion within this controlled arc is permitted and encouraged.[25] Complete tears of the collateral ligament should ideally be treated with surgical repair, although in most cases conservative management provides an adequate result.[26]

Volar plate injuries without dislocation may heal normally, but also may produce a painful PIP joint or a lax volar plate with repeated sprains and arthritis. Cortisone injected into the joint helps with chronic pain, but sometimes a volar plate arthroplasty is indicated to prevent further complications.

Combined tears of the volar plate and either collateral ligament may lead to a 'windscreen wiper' effect on the condyles of the proximal phalanx and eventual deformity. Repair is a better option.

Mallet finger

Mallet finger is a flexion deformity resulting from either avulsion of the extensor tendon from the distal phalanx or following rupture of the tendon proximal to its insertion into the distal phalanx (Fig 27.16a). As a result, it can be classified as bony or soft (Table 27.3). It affects the ulnar three digits 90% of the time and commonly results from a ball striking the extended fingertip, forcing the DIP joint into flexion while the extensor mechanism is actively contracting. This produces disruption or stretching of the extensor mechanism over the DIP joint and is often seen in baseball catchers, fielders, football receivers, cricketers and basketball players.[27]

PART B   Regional problems

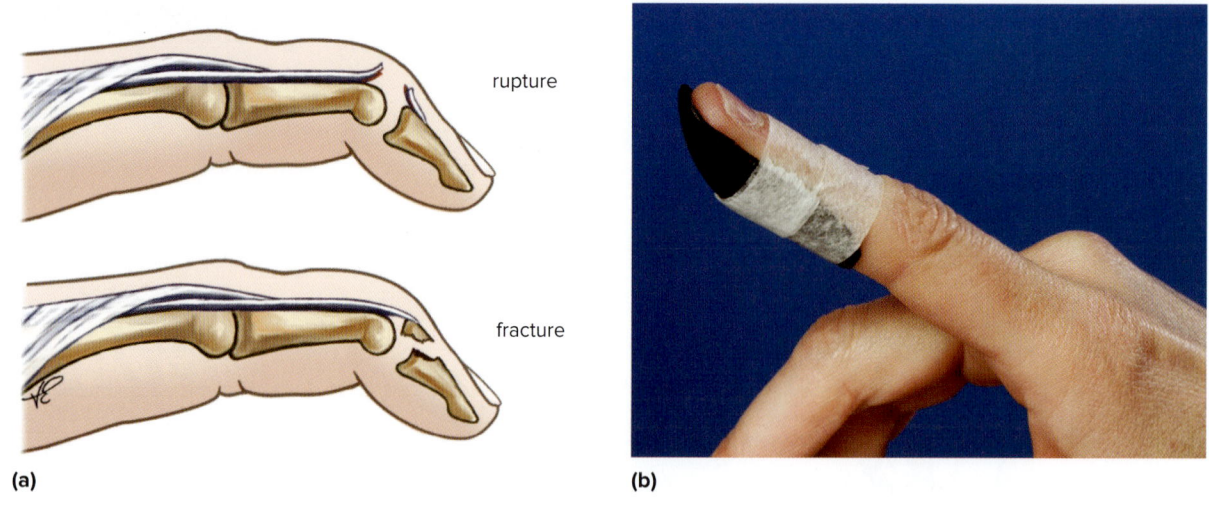

Figure 27.16 Mallet finger (a) Mechanism of deformity—rupture or avulsion (b) Stack splint. A dorsal splint is preferred for early return to sport because it will permit some tip protection and allow palmar sensation

Examination reveals tenderness over the dorsal aspect of the distal phalanx and an inability to actively extend the DIP joint from its resting flexed position. If left untreated, a chronic mallet finger type deformity develops. This flexion deformity is caused by the unopposed action of the flexor digitorum profundus tendon.

Radiography must be performed to exclude an avulsion fracture of the distal phalanx or injury and subluxation to the DIP joint. The avulsion fracture is only considered significant if greater than one-third of the joint surface is involved. Any volar subluxation requires open reduction and internal fixation to correct the joint position (the subluxation).[27] A fracture dislocation of the epiphyseal plate may occur in children. Most of these injuries are type II epiphyseal injuries and closed management is preferred.

Treatment of uncomplicated mallet finger involves splinting the DIP joint in slight hyperextension for a period of 6 weeks for a bony mallet and up to 8 weeks for a soft mallet injury, with regular monitoring. The splint is then worn for an additional 4 weeks while engaging in sporting activity and at night (Table 27.3). Treatment is reinstituted at any sign of recurrence of a lag. The splint may be made of metal or plastic and applied to either the volar (Fig. 27.16b) or the dorsal surface. Patients with dorsal splints maintain pulp sensation, which may

Table 27.3 Mallet finger treatment protocol

	Type of injury	
	Bony mallet	**Soft mallet**
Continuous splinting	Thermoplastic palmar splint for 6 weeks (2/52 more if lag)	Thermoplastic palmar splint for 8 weeks (2/52 more if lag)
Weaning protocol		
Week 1 after continuous splinting period over	Off for 1 hour am, 1 hour pm On all other times	As for bony
Week 2	Off for 2 hours am, 2 hours pm On all other times	As for bony
Week 3	Off for 4 hours am, 4 hours pm On all other times	As for bony
Week 4	Off during day, on during sleep and sport	As for bony
Weeks 5 and 6	Tape for sport. Initiate exercises to increase DIP flexion if required	Tape for sport

Hand and finger injuries CHAPTER 27

be more suitable should the athlete insist on returning to sports before the injury has healed. The finger should be kept dry and examined regularly for skin slough and maceration.[28]

When treating mallet finger, emphasise to the patient that the joint must be kept in hyperextension at all times during the first 6–8 weeks, even when the splint is removed for cleaning. If a patient is not prepared to do this, then surgery should be considered. The consequences of not splinting are a chronic mallet finger type flexion deformity with osteophyte formation and degeneration of the DIP surface, and hyperextension at the PIP joint.

Chronic swan neck deformity

There is commonly confusion between the presentation of swan neck and boutonnière deformities (Fig. 27.17). Hyperextension of the PIP with DIP joint flexion is characterised as a swan neck deformity. It can be a sequela to mallet finger injury or volar plate disruption.[28] Chronic cases will demonstrate instability of the PIP joint with visible snapping and discomfort. Fine motor activities become difficult and the finger can lock. Given that palliative treatment can be provided with dorsal blocking, game-day taping or functional figure-eight splints (Fig. 27.18),[29] many athletes opt to delay surgical reconstruction to the end of their season or career.

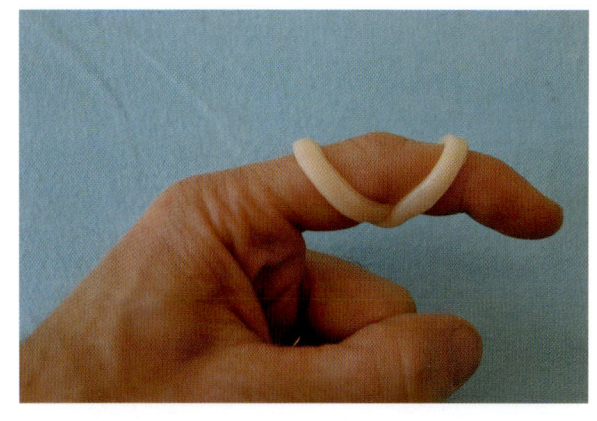

Figure 27.18 Functional figure-eight splint for swan neck deformity preventing hyperextension but permitting PIP flexion

Boutonnière deformity

Injury to the extensor tendon of the finger just proximal to its insertion on the middle phalanx can result in a boutonnière deformity, characterised by PIP joint flexion and DIP joint hyperextension. It is a common injury in ball handling sports like basketball, football and volleyball.[30, 31] With the central slip damaged, the lateral bands of the extensor mechanism migrate volarly and proximally, flexing the PIP joint and extending the DIP joint. This is then exacerbated by the now unopposed flexor digitorum superficialis. Without correction, ligaments will contract and the position become entrenched (Fig. 27.19).[32]

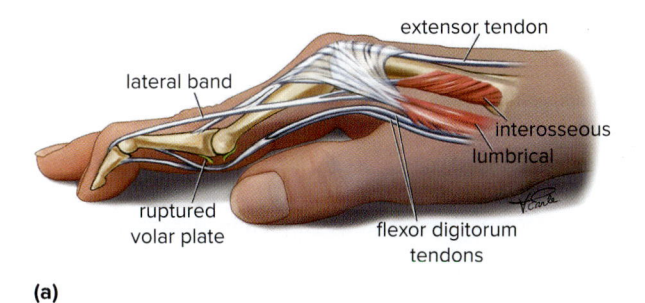

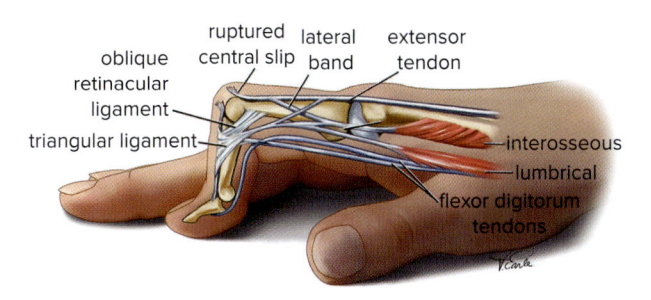

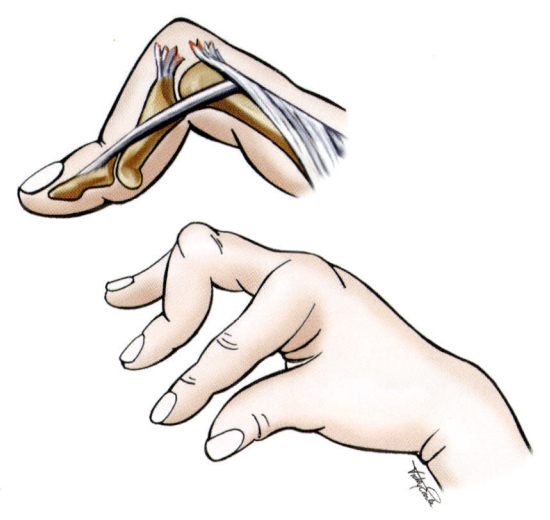

Figure 27.17 There is commonly confusion between the presentation of (a) swan neck and (b) boutonnière deformities

Figure 27.19 Boutonnière deformity

503

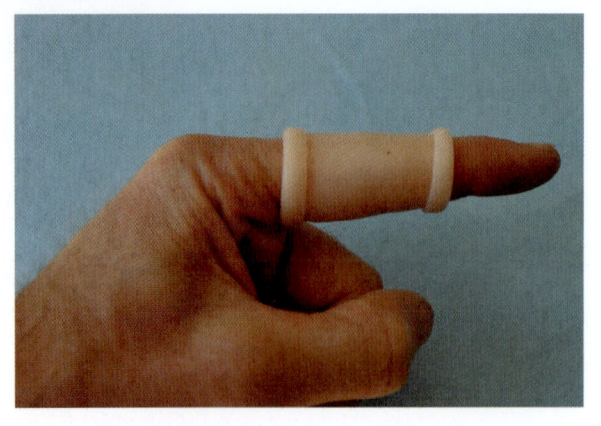

Figure 27.20 Barrel splint holding the PIP in extension but permitting DIP flexion

The deformity may not be immediately obvious and can take several weeks to develop, making an early accurate assessment important, but also highlighting the need for ongoing evaluation where injury is suspected.[32, 33] Typically there will have been blunt trauma to the dorsum of the PIP or an instance of PIP joint hyperflexion. Open laceration requires immediate surgical consult and intervention. There will usually be significant swelling, and radiographs may show an avulsion fracture. The central slip can be tested by hyperextending the MCP joint and then asking the athlete to actively extend the PIP joint. If this can be done fully, the central slip is intact.[32]

Management of the closed injury involves extension splinting of the PIP joint continuously for 6–8 weeks, encouraging regular active DIP joint flexion (Fig. 27.20). Ongoing night splinting may be required. Controlled active PIP joint flexion protocols introduced after 3 weeks of PIP joint extension have been shown to have fewer complications but require consistent monitoring, and are best instituted by a skilled hand therapist.[33, 34]

Surgical repair of open or chronic injuries often requires reconstruction and/or pinning of the PIP joint, which can preclude a return to sport for 6 weeks until the pin is removed. Reconstruction of a chronic injury is more successful if a flexion contracture has been reduced to a more neutral position with a splint.[32] For the athlete with a closed boutonnière, if they can play with a splint that maintains PIP extension, then immediate return is possible.[30, 31]

Avulsion of the flexor digitorum profundus tendon ('jersey finger')

This injury is most commonly seen in the ring finger and may be caused by the player grabbing an opponent's clothing, resulting in the distal phalanx being forcibly extended while the athlete is actively flexing. The patient often feels a 'snap'. The condition is often referred to as 'jersey finger'.

Examination may reveal the finger assuming a position of extension relative to the other fingers. There is an inability to actively flex the DIP joint of the affected finger. Radiography should be performed to exclude an associated avulsion fracture of the distal phalanx. A bone fragment may be seen volar to the middle phalanx or PIP joint. A lump may be palpated more proximally in the finger corresponding to the avulsed tendon.

> **PRACTICE PEARL**
>
> Treatment is urgent surgical repair with reattachment of the profundus tendon to the distal phalanx. This must take place within 10 days of the injury.

Late treatment requires the use of a two-stage operation, with a silicon rod being placed for some months in the finger to create the tendon sheath gap for the tendon graft to slide in. This is sometimes considered too big an operative insult, and fusing the DIP joint without grafting the tendon gives a nearly acceptable result.

Lacerations and infections of the hand

Lacerations to the fingers and hand occur frequently in sport as a result of contact with equipment such as the undersurface of a football boot. All lacerations have the potential to become infected and should, therefore, be thoroughly cleaned with an antiseptic solution and observed closely for signs of infection. Tetanus toxoid should also be administered where appropriate.

A particular concern is a laceration of the hand, often over the MCP/PIP joint, caused by teeth, usually from a punch to the mouth. These injuries should always be assumed to be contaminated and an immediate course of a broad-spectrum antibiotic should be commenced. The wound should not be closed.

Lacerations over volar DIP or PIP joints may represent compound dislocations. If this has occurred, the joint has been contaminated and the patient requires hospital admission for surgical debridement and repair. Otherwise septic arthritis may follow.

OVERUSE CONDITIONS OF THE HAND AND FINGERS

Important but sometimes overlooked are the overuse problems associated with the hand. These include trigger finger, flexor pulley injuries and other small joint injuries that are commonly seen in rock climbers.[35-37] Trigger finger is caused by a tenosynovitis in the flexor tendon that is large enough to be impeded by the proximal A1 (annular) pulley located at the base of the finger. Diagnosis is made clinically, with the patient presenting with often painful clicking and locking of the finger as it actively flexes. Ultrasound is used for confirmation. Conservative treatment involves splinting to prevent metacarpal flexion only, and local treatment to reduce the enlarged tendon. Corticosteroid injection is often advocated first, and then surgical release of the impeded A1 pulley.[38,39]

Rock climbers put chronic severe stresses on the flexor tendons and can damage or tear the important A2 and/or A4 pulleys, producing bowstringing. This often appears to be simple swelling initially, but can become quite severe. Most serious climbers wear tape or circular splints to control the tension, but surgical reconstruction may be required.

SURGICAL REFERRALS FOLLOWING HAND AND FINGER INJURY

There are a number of conditions that require urgent referral to a hand surgeon. These are shown in Table 27.4.

Exercises for the hand

Exercises following hand injury should be prescribed so as to include both intrinsic and extrinsic hand musculature. The tendon gliding sequence of exercises does this well, and passive stretches that push into these positions should also be encouraged when appropriate in the case of hand and finger stiffness (Fig. 27.21). Strengthening exercises utilising Theraputty®, grippers and stress balls are useful once the injured finger is stable but should not be introduced before joint or fracture stability is achieved. Building up the handles on a barbell or chin-up bar will increase grip strength demands, weight plate pinches will isolate intrinsic muscles, and finger extensors and the interossei can be worked using rubber bands.

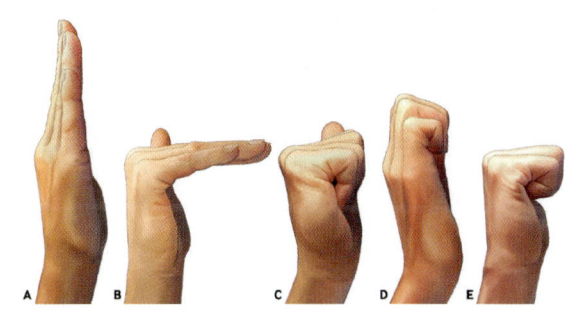

Figure 27.21 Tendon gliding sequence of exercises

Table 27.4 Urgent surgical referrals for sports hand conditions

Injury	Common sports	Management notes
Flexor digitorum profundus avulsion	Tackling sports, including rugby and all football codes	Early: acute surgical repair Late (>6 weeks): two-stage reconstruction
All compound lacerations	Contact sports and/or motor sports and/or cycling i.e. high velocity sports	Surgical washout (local or general) Explore to exclude foreign bodies (especially teeth, soil) and debride
Sagittal band rupture MCPs 2,3,4	Boxing	Sagittal band reconstruction (not as urgent)
Mallet fracture/dislocation	Ball sports	Joint reduction and pinning
Ulnar collateral ligament rupture, MCP thumb	Skiing, football ('thumb plant')	Splint if incomplete Surgical reconstruction if Stener lesion
Bennett's/Rolando fracture base of 1st MC	Contact sports	Must reduce joint surface for good result
Rotated fracture, middle phalanx	Contact sports	Does not tolerate shortening or rotation
Rotated fracture, proximal phalanx	Contact sports	Often leaves stiff PIP if left unreduced
Rotated metacarpal fracture	Contact sports	Causes crossover of fingers; quicker return in professional sports
CMC subluxation and dislocation	Boxing, martial arts	Must be reduced to maintain strength and power; if late needs CMC fusion

PART B Regional problems

REFERENCES

References for this chapter can be found at www.mhhe.com/au/CSM5e

Chapter 28

Thoracic and chest pain

with KEVIN SINGER and JEFF BOYLE

*I want to apologise to my fans. I broke my rib and again I am out of the fight.
I really wanted to come back, I'm not sure if I will ever come back.*

Khabib Nurmagomedov, UFC, October 2015

THORACIC PAIN

As with neck pain (Chapter 23) and low back pain (Chapter 29), it is frequently difficult for the clinician to make a precise diagnosis in patients with pain in the region of the thoracic spine given the interplay between the thorax, upper limb, neck, low back, and the cardiorespiratory and visceral systems. The most common musculoskeletal problems are disorders of the thoracic intervertebral joints and the numerous rib articulations as this region of the spine contributes stability to the axial skeleton. The thorax never sleeps as, even at rest, this complex interplay of joints, ligaments and muscles moves with respiration.

Injury to the intervertebral disc, the facet joints (also named zygapophyseal joints) or other nociceptive structures (Chapters 5 and 6) of the thoracic spine may lead to local or referred pain. Clinical presentation of these often articular problems is varied. Pain and altered motion are the dominant features when one or more intervertebral segments or rib joints are involved. There may be associated abnormalities of the paraspinal and periscapular muscles as well as increased neural mechanosensitivity (Chapter 6). Thoracic intervertebral joint problems frequently refer pain to the lateral or anterior chest wall. Prolapse of a thoracic intervertebral disc is rare in athletes; however, it may be under-reported given the often diffuse symptoms that arise.[1, 2] Appropriate imaging studies are often necessary to rule out this diagnosis. The astute clinician keeps all diagnostic options open when considering the thoracic region.

In adolescents, the most common cause of thoracic region pain is Scheuermann's disease (Chapter 44), a disorder of the growth plates of the thoracic vertebral endplates associated with an accentuated lower thoracic kyphosis. A list of the causes of pain in the region of the thoracic spine is shown in Table 28.1. The surface,

Table 28.1 Causes of thoracic pain

Common	Less common	Not to be missed
Intervertebral joint sprain	Rib stress reaction/fracture	Cardiac causes
• Disc	Fracture of the rib posteriorly	Peptic ulcer
• Zygapophyseal joints	Thoracic disc prolapse	Tumour (e.g. carcinoma of the breast with bony metastasis)
Paraspinal muscle strain	T4 syndrome	
Costotransverse joint sprain		Herpes zoster
Costovertebral joint sprain		
Scheuermann's disease (adolescents)		
Postural imbalance of neck and shoulder and upper thoracic spine		

PART B Regional problems

muscle and cross-sectional anatomy of this area are shown in Figure 28.1.

Vague symptoms must alert the astute clinician to consider the possibility of visceral origins as convergence of pain pathways may mimic somatic disorders (Chapters 5 and 6). The literature reporting occult pain presentations of thoracic-like pain encourages caution when assessing an individual with unresolved, at times over-investigated, symptoms.[3,4] Consider 'red flags' (see Chapter 7).

Assessment

History

The patient often complains of pain between or around the scapulae. The pain may be central, unilateral or bilateral, and have commenced suddenly as a result of a specific movement or have been of gradual onset without discernible precipitating incident. Symptoms may be elicited by any active movement–particularly rotation (Fig. 28.2) or lateral flexion.[5] The T4–8 segments show greater ranges of axial motion compared with the stiffer upper and lower segments. Note any associated sensory symptoms such as paraesthesia or numbness. Although dermatomal patterns are more predictable in the thoracic region, symptoms may depart from such conventions. Vague pain noted in the region of the shoulder may relate to disturbance of the cervicothoracic junction[6] and, similarly, buttock, hip or inguinal region symptoms may have a low thoracic origin.[5] The behaviour of symptoms relative to activity or diurnal variation will assist in classification of the condition (Fig. 28.3).

If you have established a musculoskeletal cause of symptoms, consider aspects of the clinical presentation relative to SINS (Severity, Irritability, Nature and Stage) to inform clinical reasoning and management. The Severity of the condition helps to determine the vigour of any prescribed activity or physical treatment; Irritability, or ease of aggravation, relates to the volume of prescribed activity or physical treatment; Nature refers to the type of condition (e.g. fracture, instability, neurological (radicular?, somatic?; see Chapter 6); and Stage means being relative to an acute, subacute or chronic classification.

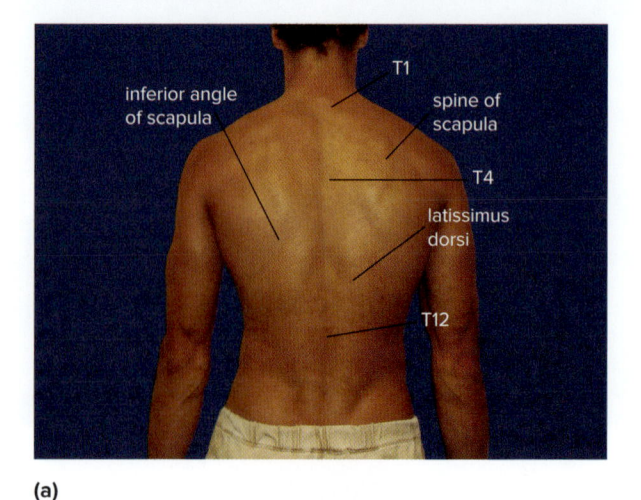

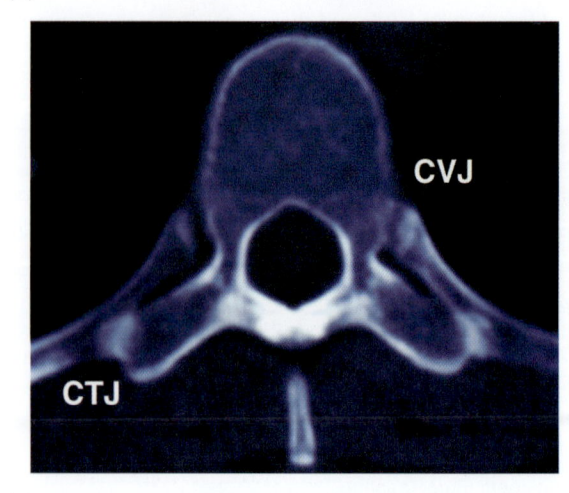

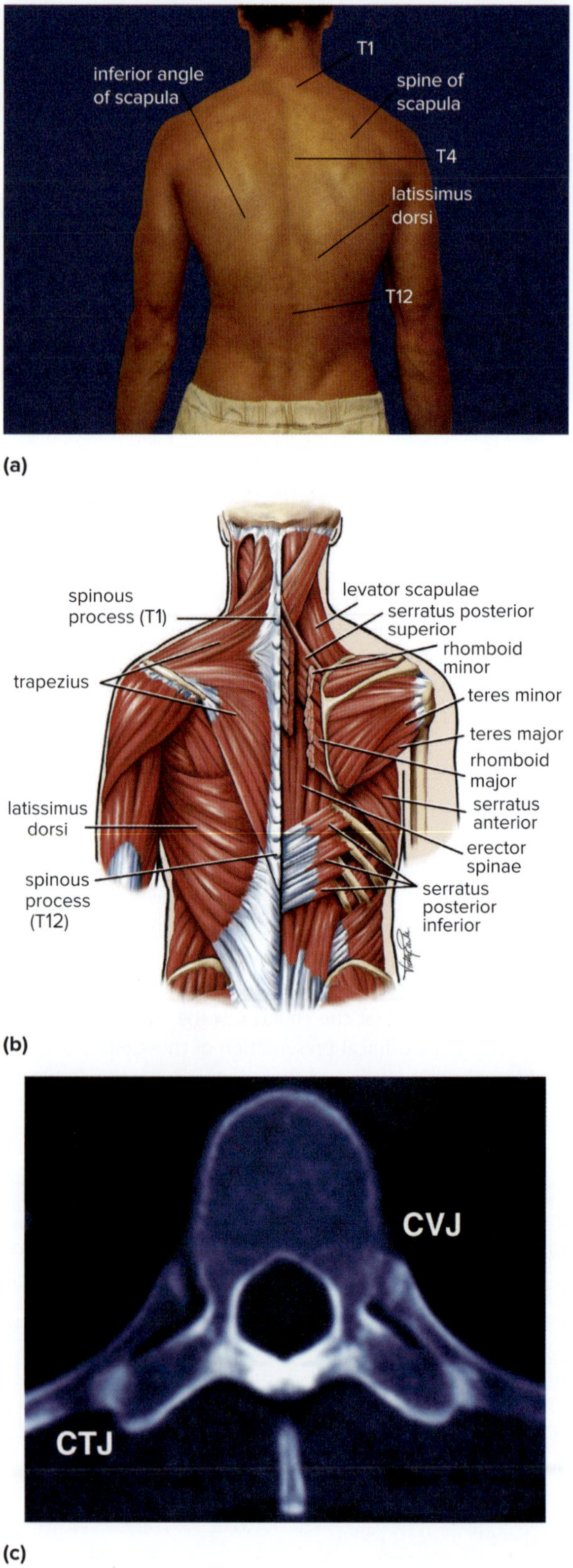

Figure 28.1 Anatomy of the thoracic spine region (a) Surface anatomy (b) Muscles of the thoracic spine region (c) Axial computed tomography (CT) image of the typical motion segment from the lower thoracic region. The most accessible rib articulation for palpation and mobilisation is the costotransverse joint (CTJ), with the costovertebral joint (CVJ) attached firmly to the lateral margin of the vertebral body, invertebral disc and base of the pedicles

Thoracic and chest pain CHAPTER 28

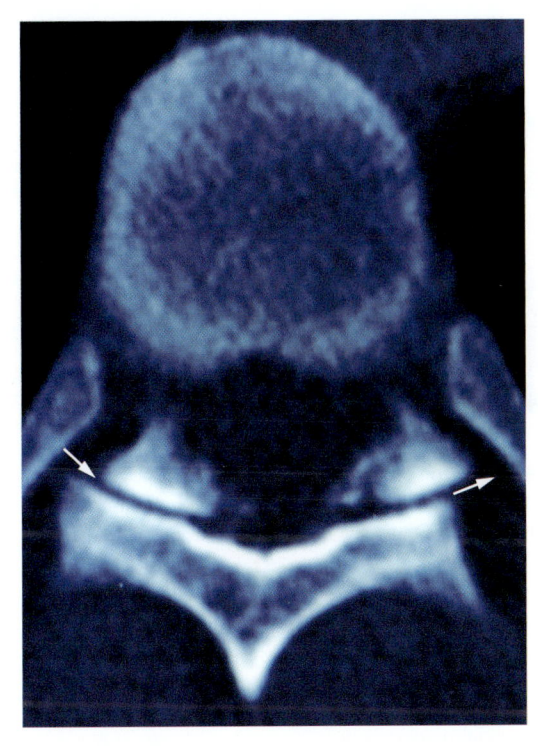

Figure 28.2 Axial CT depicting the nature of thoracic zygapophyseal joint translation in response to induced segmental rotation

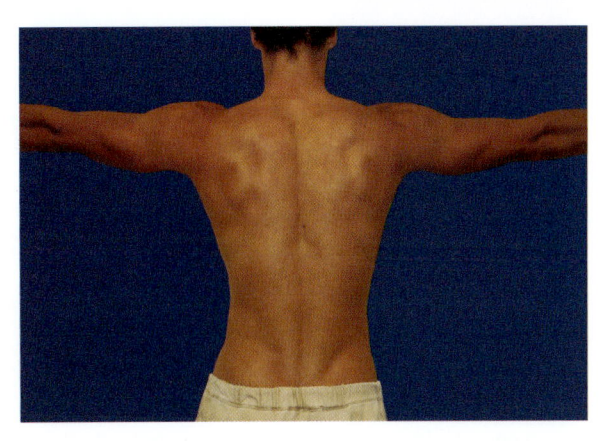

Figure 28.4 Examination of the patient with thoracic pain begins with observation and testing active movements

Physical examination

In the thoracic spine region, assess range of motion and mobility of each intervertebral segment and carefully palpate the paraspinal and periscapular soft tissue. Examine the lower cervical and upper lumbar spine and perform a neurological examination for altered mechanosensitivity.

1. Observation (Fig. 28.4)
   a. any asymmetry, scoliosis or kyphosis should be noted
   b. muscle spasm
   c. skin changes (sweating or erythema may suggest an autonomic response)
2. Active movements
   a. flexion
   b. extension
   c. rotation.

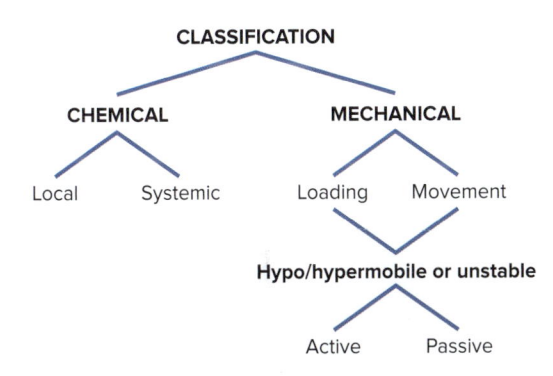

Figure 28.3 Flowchart of thoracic region disorders. Classification facilitates the differential diagnosis and better outcomes through prescription of condition-specific treatment.

In the thoracic region, carefully consider the potential for non-musculoskeletal causes. Red flags may include systemic illness, malignancy, unexplained weight loss, fever or night pain. As Professor Gwen Jull was fond of saying, 'If the voice in the back of your head tells you something is not right, listen to that voice' (and refer/investigate appropriately).

Active movements are assessed in the cardinal planes for range of motion, symptom reproduction, and aberrant patterns of movement that may be antalgic or indicate dysfunction. Combinations of these movements in two planes may help guide treatment (Fig. 28.5).[7] A consistent pattern in which a movement that stretches the symptomatic area produces symptoms which are increased by the addition of movement in another plane that also has a stretch effect may suggest an extra-articular source of symptoms (myofascial, nerve, joint capsule), while a pattern consistent with symptoms primarily on compressive movements may indicate an intra-articular source. Mixed patterns may suggest multiple tissue involvement.

PART B   Regional problems

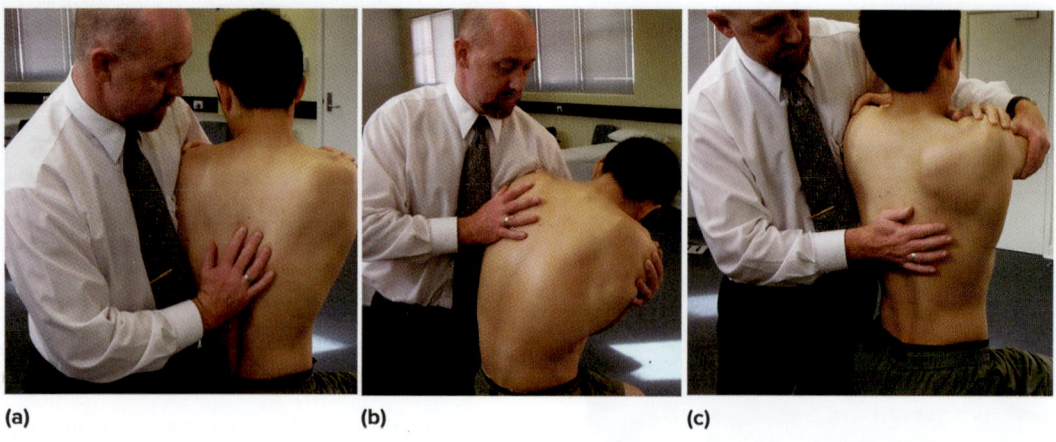

Figure 28.5 Combined movement assessment is performed by determining the most symptomatic primary movement; this movement is then repeated in the two extremes of another plane. For example, the primary symptomatic movement of axial plane left rotation (a) is subsequently performed in two positions in the sagittal plane—flexion (b) and extension (c)

3. Palpation
   a. soft tissue
   b. assess segmental unilateral mobility by posterior to anterior directional pressure over the transverse process (Fig. 28.6a)
   c. assess rib mobility by posterior to anterior directional pressure over the angle of the rib with the scapular protracted (Fig. 28.6b)
   d. zygapophyseal
   e. costotransverse joints and, indirectly, the costovertebral joints
   f. paraspinal muscles
   g. anterior palpation of sternal, chondral and clavicular joints.

Soft tissue is palpated for tenderness, swelling, spasm, and trigger points while bony and chondral structures are assessed for tenderness and deformity and for motion anomalies.

4. Special tests
   a. springing of the ribs and costochondral junctions
   b. maximal inspiration
   c. cough/sneeze
   d. neural tissue sensitivity tests (slump test–Chapter 15)
   e. cervical spine examination (Chapter 23)
   f. lumbar spine examination (Chapter 29)
   g. muscle strength testing.

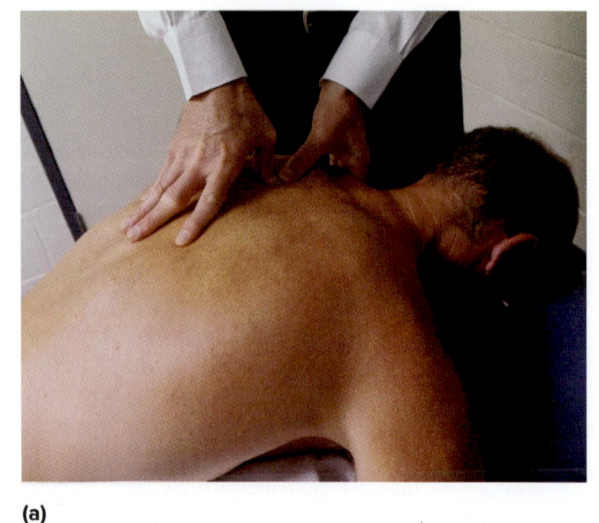

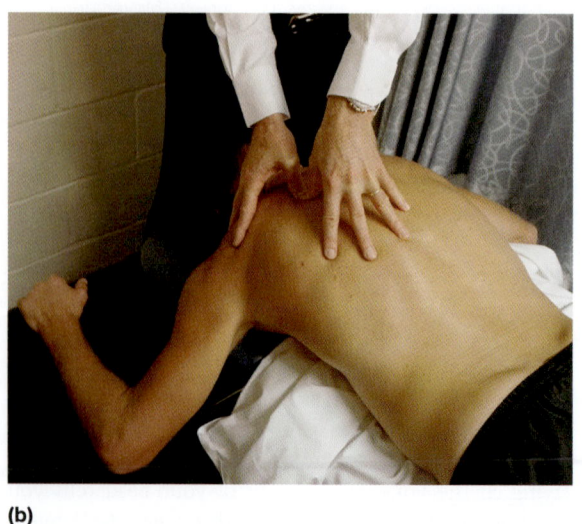

Figure 28.6 (a) Assess segmental unilateral mobility by posterior to anterior directional pressure over the transverse process (b) Assess rib mobility by posterior to anterior directional pressure over the angle of the rib with the scapular protracted

Investigations

Plain radiograph of the thoracic spine region is not routinely indicated as it usually adds little to the clinical picture. It may, however, demonstrate the presence of intervertebral growth plate abnormalities, indicate Scheuermann's disease, or show the presence of a secondary neoplastic disorder affecting the thoracic spine or ribs. Computed tomography (CT) and magnetic resonance imaging (MRI) scans may be indicated to exclude serious pathology in the presence of red flags such as unexplained weight loss or nocturnal pain. These imaging modalities may confirm a thoracic intervertebral disc prolapse or help stage neoplastic disease. Atypical pain patterns unresponsive to routine management should also signal the need for investigation, even in the young athlete (see also Chapters 5 and 6).

Thoracic intervertebral joint disorders

Intervertebral joint injuries involving the intervertebral discs, rib articulations and zygapophyseal joints are the most common cause of pain in this region. They may be of sudden or gradual onset. Examination may reveal hypomobility of one or more intervertebral segments associated with local tenderness over the spinous processes, the zygapophyseal joints, the costotransverse joints or the surrounding paravertebral muscles. However on occasion, pain rather than stiffness may be the main presenting feature.

Treatment aims to restore full mobility by mobilisation or manipulation techniques. Passive overpressure (Fig 28.7) can be used to assess treatment response (feel for resistance and assess pain response). Soft tissue therapy and graded specific exercise may be required to restore normal function in the paravertebral and periscapular muscles. Passive techniques include digital ischaemic pressure and sustained myofascial tension. Trigger points in the paraspinal muscles are common and may be treated with appropriate soft tissue techniques. Use of dry needling techniques for trigger points may be used with caution; avoid complications such as pneumothorax.

Note that there is considerable variation in joint anatomy at the transitional junctions of the spine, particularly at the thoracolumbar junction.[8] These variations may contribute to subtle differences in segmental mechanics and injury patterns. While some zygapophyseal joints are remarkably asymmetrical, others may show a morphology that acts to constrain motion which should not be perceived as unusual hypomobility (Fig. 28.8). However, the transitional segments between the thoracic and lumbar regions are disposed to severe strain or injury during overload and these segments account for the highest incidence of spine-related trauma, particularly from high-energy sports (e.g. skiing, equestrian events, jet ski, motorcross).[9]

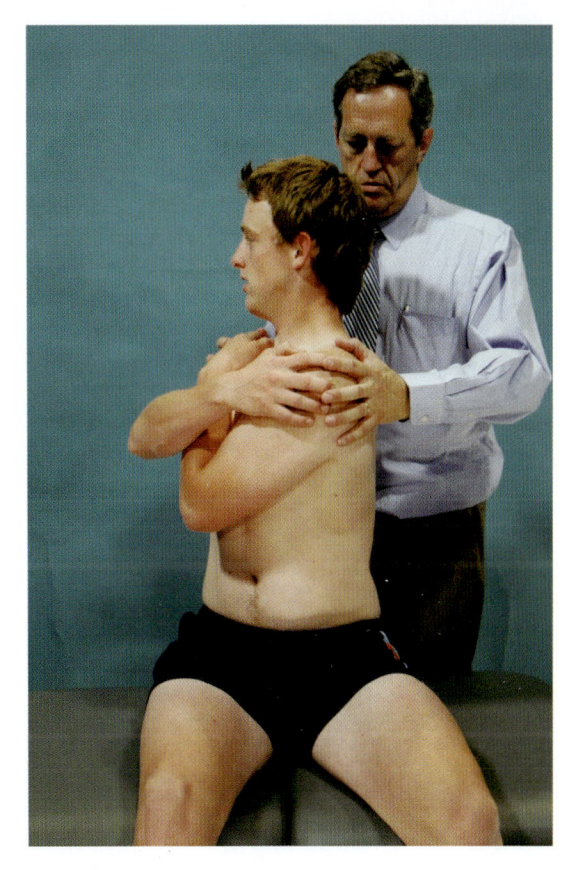

Figure 28.7 Thoracic rotation overpressure applied passively at the end of active range to assess for resistance and pain response

Costovertebral and costotransverse joint disorders

Disorders of the rib articulations include inflammatory spondyloarthropathies (such as ankylosing spondylitis), degenerative change (such as osteoarthritis) and mechanical joint sprains. Costotransverse joint problems are associated with localised tenderness and restricted mobility of the joints. This is often evident on deep inspiration and active movement as the ribs rotate in a predictable pattern relative to thoracic motion. Treatment may include mobilisation of the costotransverse joints, which will also have a modest influence on the deeper costovertebral articulations. There is no quality evidence to support image-guided corticosteroid injection as treatment when the condition remains unresponsive to standard management. A common problem of these small synovial joints may be derangement of intra-articular synovial fold inclusions which occupy the periphery of the internal joint cavity (Fig. 28.9). These conditions are usually amenable to mobilisations or manipulation.[10]

PART B Regional problems

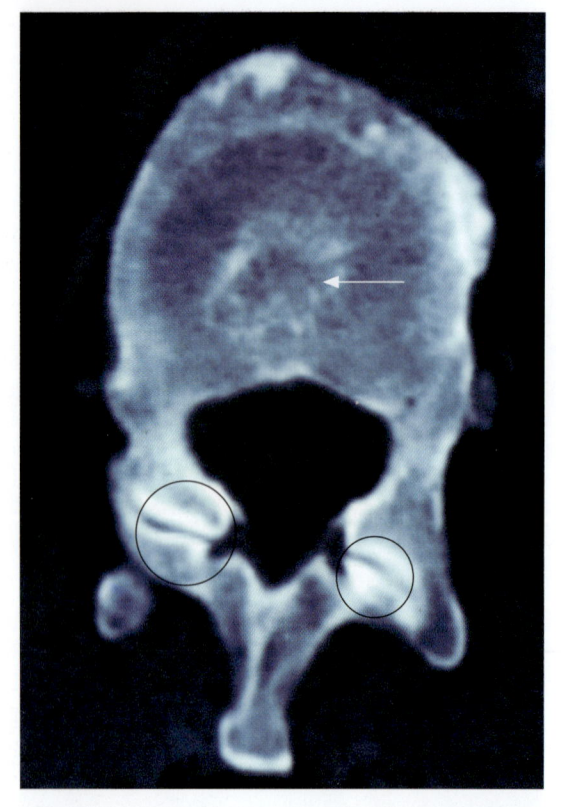

(a)

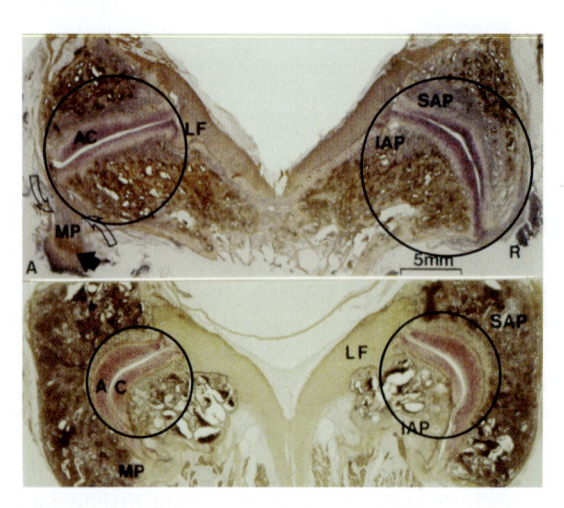

(b)

Figure 28.8 Zygapophyseal joint abnormalities (a) Axial CT scan highlighting marked zygapophyseal joint tropism (rotation in response to load) (circled); a central Schmorl's node is noted within the endplate (arrow) (b) Horizontal histological section (100 μm) through the zygapophyseal joints of the thoracolumbar junction to demonstrate variations in articular morphology from asymmetric (top image) to an enclosing morphology which constrains motion (lower image)

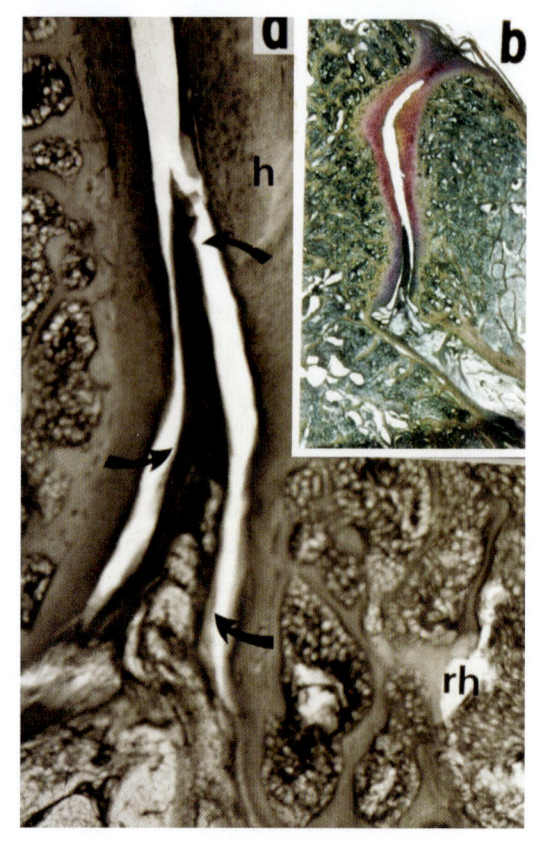

Figure 28.9 Painful costovertebral joint synovial inclusions (black arrows). Horizontal histological section through the dorsal region of a costovertebral joint demonstrates a long fibro-fatty synovial inclusion within the joint cavity. Entrapped innervated inclusions may contribute to localised thoracic pain which can often be relieved through manipulation

Scheuermann's disease

Scheuermann's disease is the most common cause of pain in the thoracic spine region in adolescents and is characterised by an accentuated low thoracic kyphosis arising from multiple vertebral endplate irregularities involving four or more vertebral bodies (Fig. 28.10). This condition is described in Chapter 44. Accentuated kyphosis may also arise from habitual training postures which involve loading into flexion.[11, 3] Extended training periods in one posture (e.g. cycling) tend to be associated with adaptive changes, and modification to training postures may need to be considered when recommending long-term management.

Thoracic intervertebral disc prolapse

Prolapse of a thoracic intervertebral disc is a relatively rare condition that may be under-reported in the athletic

Thoracic and chest pain CHAPTER 28

community.[1, 12] The segments that tend to be most commonly involved are the larger discs of the lower thoracic segments. MR images are shown for a T12–L1 disc prolapse (Fig. 28.11). The pathology of thoracic disc prolapse is shown in Figure 28.12. The clinical

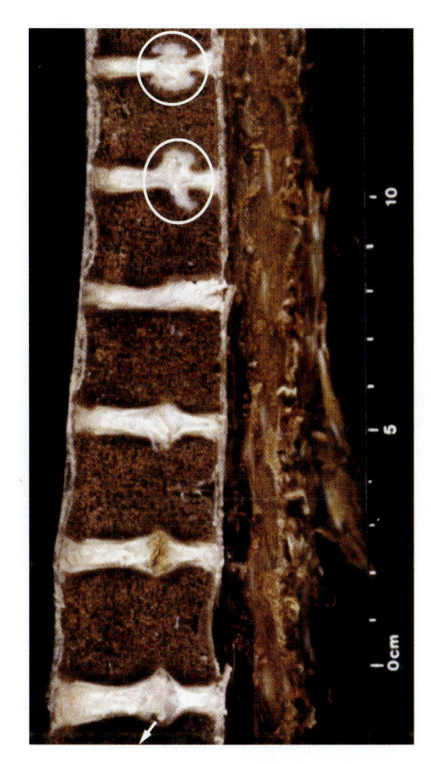

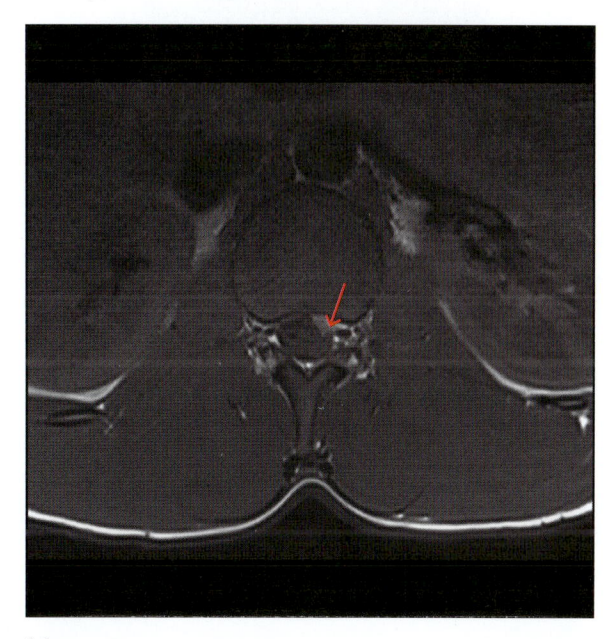

Figure 28.10 Multiple endplate lesions (Schmorl's nodes) evident within the lower thoracic vertebral bodies (circles) typical of Scheuermann's disease

(a)

(b)

(c)

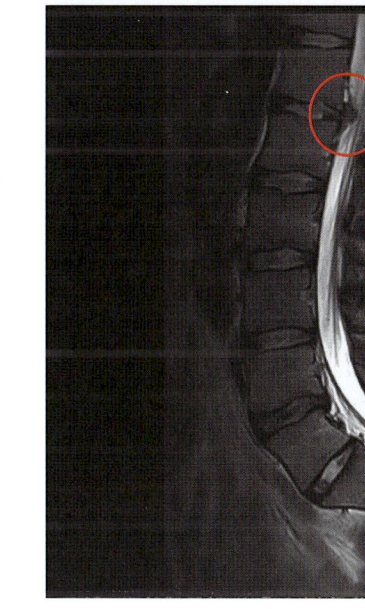

Figure 28.11 MRI of T12–L1 disc prolapse in a 26-year-old Australian rules footballer (a) T1-weighted axial MRI demonstrating left para-central displaced disc fragment (arrow) (b) T2-weighted axial MRI highlighting internal disc derangement (arrowheads) and disc herniation (arrow) (c) T2-weighted saggital image showing disc fragment (circled) at T12-L1. It impinges on the spinal cord

513

PART B Regional problems

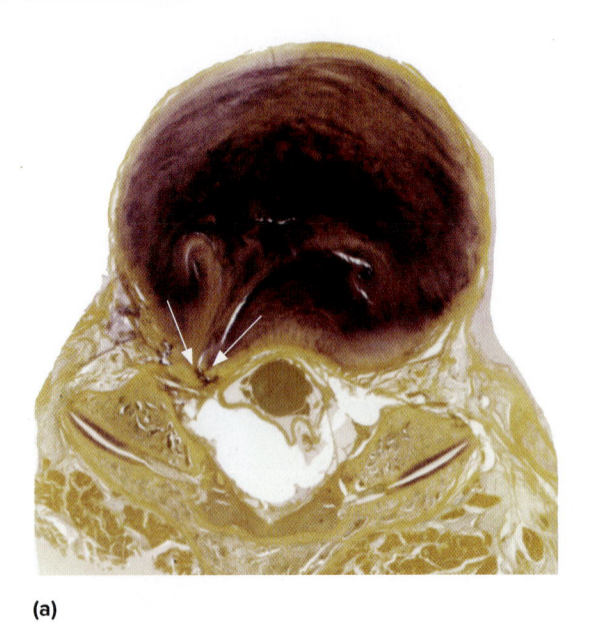

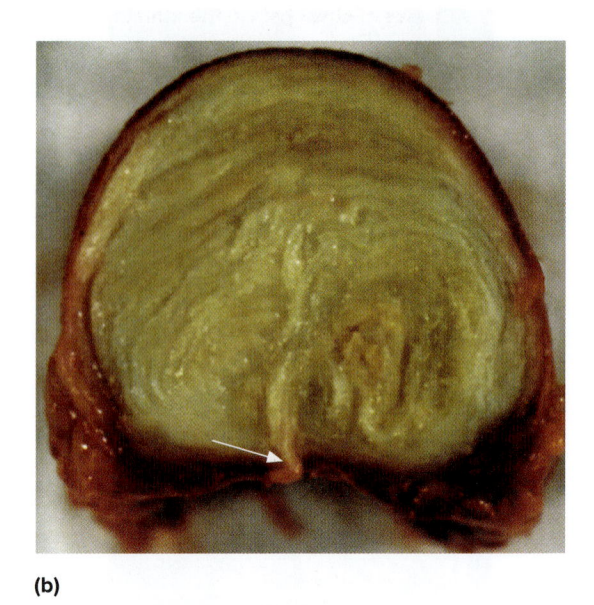

Figure 28.12 Thoracic disc prolapse (a) Haemotoxylin and eosin (H&E) stained horizontal section at T10–11 depicting a posterolateral prolapse of the intervertebral disc (arrows). Such prolapses are most common in the lower thoracic segments given the greater volume and height of these discs and loading patterns involving flexion and rotation (b) Macroscopic horizontal section of a T11–12 disc to demonstrate a midline annular fissure and small central prolapse (arrow), which is a common presentation for thoracic disc lesions

presentation involves local back pain with radicular pain radiating in the distribution of the affected thoracic spinal nerve/s. However, pain from a thoracic disc prolapse often does not follow a characteristic radicular pattern so this may confuse the diagnosis (see also Chapters 5 and 6).[2, 13] Consider this potential diagnosis and refer for axial imaging and relevant pain intervention if you suspect the diagnosis.

T4 syndrome
Occasionally, patients present with diffuse arm pain and sensory symptoms such as bilateral paraesthesias in the hands, generalised headache and interscapular tightness which is attributed to intervertebral joint problems around the upper thoracic region. This vague constellation of symptoms has been labelled the T4 syndrome.[14] Although not verified clinically, it speculates that the sympathetic nervous system contributes to symptoms. Examination often reveals hypomobility of the upper to middle thoracic segments together with a forward head position and shoulder protraction. Restoration of sagittal postural alignment of the head in relation to the thorax, shoulder retraction, improved neck and scapular muscle endurance, and mobilisation or manipulation of affected joints may relieve symptoms.

Postural imbalance of the neck, shoulder and upper thoracic spine
Common muscle imbalances relative to shoulder dysfunction include weakness of the scapula retractors, particularly inferior and middle trapezius, and serratus anterior. Stronger muscles will often exhibit increased tone and decreased length, and commonly include scalenus posterior, pectoralis minor and both rhomboid major and minor.[15] These muscle imbalances may adversely influence segmental thoracic and rib articulation accessory motion.[16]

CHEST PAIN
Chest pain occurs not infrequently in athletes, usually due to musculoskeletal causes. In mature athletes, the possibility that pain is of cardiac origin must be considered. This possibility is increased in the presence of associated symptoms, such as palpitations or shortness of breath, or when there is a family history of cardiac disease. Male endurance athletes who perform high-intensity training are susceptible to atrial fibrillation, either as paroxysmal episodes or as a persistent form.[17] Other causes of chest pain include peptic ulceration, gastroesophageal reflux, chest infection and malignancy.

The most common cause of chest pain in the athlete under 35 years is referred pain from the cervical or

Thoracic and chest pain CHAPTER 28

Table 28.2 Causes of chest pain in the athlete

Common	Less common	Not to be missed
Rib trauma	Costochondritis	Cardiac causes
• Fracture	Sternocostal joint sprain	Peptic ulceration
• Contusion	Intercostal muscle strain	Gastroesophageal reflux
Referred pain from the thoracic spine	Rib stress fracture	Pneumothorax
Sternoclavicular joint disorders	Fractured sternum	Herpes zoster
Side strain		Pulmonary embolism

thoracic spine. Thus, patients presenting with anterior or lateral chest wall pain require a thorough examination of the cervicothoracic spine and thorax.

A list of possible causes of chest pain in athletes is presented in Table 28.2. The surface anatomy of this region is shown in Figure 28.13.

It may be difficult to distinguish between chest pain of cardiac origin and pain referred from the thoracic spine. They may both be unilateral and related to exercise. The clinical features of these two causes of chest pain in the athlete are considered in Table 28.3.

Major trauma to the chest wall is a medical emergency. Injuries sustained in contact sport commonly affect the ribs, resulting in either bruised or fractured ribs. These may lead to secondary dysfunction of the thoracic zygapophyseal joints, which can cause persistence of pain. Sternoclavicular and costochondral joint injuries

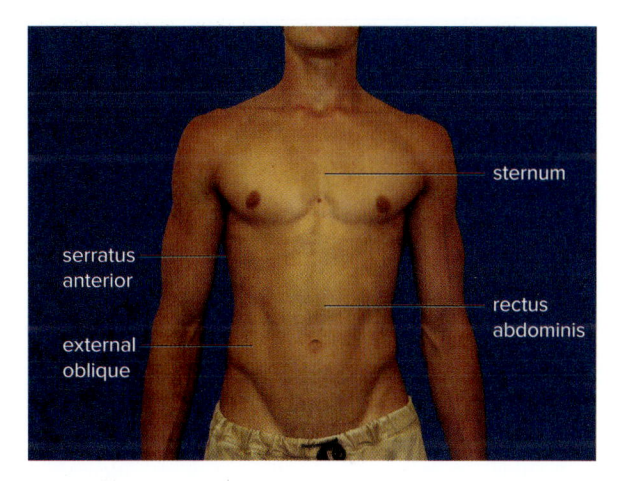

Figure 28.13 Surface anatomy of the anterior chest to assess for symmetry

Table 28.3 Comparison of clinical features of chest pain of cardiac origin and chest pain referred from the thoracic spine

Feature	Referred pain from thoracic spine	Myocardial ischaemia
Age	Any age, especially 20–40 years	Older (>35 years), greater likelihood with greater age
History of injury	Sometimes	No
Site and radiation	Spinal and paraspinal, arms, lateral chest, anterior chest, substernal, iliac crest	Retrosternal, parasternal, jaw, neck, inner arms, epigastrium, interscapular
Type of pain	Dull, aching, occasionally sharp, sudden onset and offset, severity related to activity, site and posture	Constricting, vice-like ('clenched-fist' sign), may be burning, gradual onset and offset
Aggravation	Deep inspiration, postural movement of thorax, certain activities (e.g. slumping or bending, walking upstairs, lifting, sleeping or sitting for long periods)	Exercise, activity, heavy meals, cold, stress, emotion
Relief	Maintaining erect spine, lying down, firm pressure on back (e.g. leaning against wall)	Rest Glyceryl trinitrate (GTN)
Associations	Chronic poor posture, employment requiring constant posture such as at a keyboard or computer	Cardiac risk factors such as family history, obesity, smoking, dyspnea, nausea, tiredness, pallor, sweating, vomiting

are not uncommon. Intercostal muscle strains have been considered a cause of chest wall pain but, on close clinical examination, many patients with this presentation are actually suffering referred pain from the thoracic spine. Stress fractures of the ribs occur in sports such as rowing, tennis, golf, gymnastics and baseball pitching where rapid torsion loads are common. The aetiology of chest wall muscle injury from violent overload is exemplified by cricket fast bowlers who induce a rapid alternation between muscle lengthening followed by rapid eccentric contraction during delivery. This action can result in a strain injury at the rib or costal cartilage insertion of the internal oblique muscle over the lower four ribs.

Clinical assessment
History
A history of trauma to the chest wall will lead the clinician to suspect a rib injury. In the absence of trauma, the history should distinguish between musculoskeletal conditions and other cardiac, gastrointestinal and respiratory causes. It is important to elicit the type of pain and the location of the pain. Associated symptoms such as palpitations, shortness of breath and sweating may indicate that the pain is cardiac in nature. A history of productive cough may suggest pain is of respiratory origin, while symptoms of food-related pain or a burning, boring pain behind the sternum should alert the clinician to include gastroesophageal reflux or peptic ulceration in the differential diagnosis.

Pain aggravated by deep inspiration or coughing may be musculoskeletal in nature or indicative of a respiratory problem. Associated thoracic and, to a lesser extent, cervical or lumbar pain may suggest the thoracic spine or rib joints as possible sources of the patient's chest pain. An increase in pain with trunk rotation might add to this suspicion.

Examination
Examination of the patient with chest wall pain should include palpation of the painful area and of possible sites of referral, especially the thoracic spine. Examination of the thoracic spine has been described earlier in this chapter. The cardiovascular and respiratory systems must always be examined. The abdomen should be examined for sources of referred pain.

Investigations
If there has been significant rib trauma, a chest radiograph should be performed to exclude the presence of a pneumothorax. Specific rib views may be necessary to detect rib fractures. Chest radiography will indicate cardiac size and may reveal evidence of respiratory infection.

MRI (nuclear imaging/CT where MRI not available) may be required to detect stress fractures or other reactive bony conditions.

Electrocardiography and other cardiac investigations, including a stress ECG and an echocardiograph, may be performed if there is clinical suspicion of cardiac dysfunction. A Holter monitor may be indicated to help detect occult cardiac pacing irregularities. Gastroscopy may be indicated if peptic ulceration or reflux is suspected.

Rib trauma
A direct blow to the chest may result in trauma to the ribs. This may range from bruising to an undisplaced or displaced rib fracture or to costal cartilage displacement (Fig. 28.14). Typically, the patient complains of pain aggravated by deep inspiration or coughing. Examination reveals local tenderness over one or more ribs.

A pneumothorax or rarely, a haemopneumothorax, may occur as a result of a rib fracture. Any athlete with rib trauma must undergo a respiratory examination to exclude these conditions. It is also important to consider trauma to underlying structures such as the liver, spleen and kidneys.

Radiographs may confirm the presence of a rib fracture, although it is not essential as treatment is symptomatic. Injury to the upper four ribs is unusual as they are somewhat protected. The lower two ribs are likewise rarely fractured as they are not attached to the sternum.

Treatment consists of analgesia and encouragement of deep breathing to prevent localised lung collapse. A fractured rib can be extremely painful. It will continue to be painful and tender to palpation for at least 3 weeks. Bruised ribs may also be painful and tender for up to 3 weeks.

Return to sport for athletes with an undisplaced rib fracture is appropriate when pain settles. Protective padding or splints may be used in contact sports after a rib

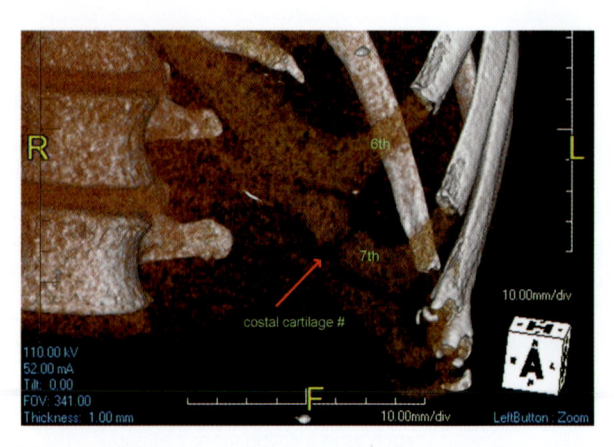

Figure 28.14 Fracture of the costal cartilage in a 30-year-old footballer

Thoracic and chest pain **CHAPTER 28**

injury. Local anaesthesia may be used for short-term pain management where indicated and with due care to avoid causing a pneumothorax. Contusion of the costochondral joints can be painful. Local treatment consists of cold therapy and strapping to splint the region.

Referred pain from the thoracic spine

Referred pain to the chest may or may not be associated with a history of thoracic spine pain. On examination, there will usually be marked tenderness and stiffness, either centrally over the spinous processes of the thoracic vertebrae or, more commonly, on the same side as the chest pain over the thoracic zygapophyseal or costovertebral joints. There is also often associated tenderness in the soft tissues surrounding the thoracic spine, especially the paravertebral muscles. Active trigger points may develop and contribute to the referred pain. Referred pain, however, may not follow predictable patterns, which requires the clinician to explore symptoms and to rule out visceral disorders.[5, 13]

Local treatment aims to restore full range of motion of the involved thoracic intervertebral segments by mobilisation or manipulation. Soft tissue therapy to surrounding areas may be helpful. This includes digital ischaemic pressure to painful sites, and sustained myofascial tension and other massage techniques where chronic muscle and soft tissue tightness is established. Dry needling of involved trigger points may also be considered.

> **PRACTICE PEARL**
>
> Referred pain from the thoracic spine is probably the most common cause of chest wall pain in the young athlete.

Sternoclavicular joint problems

The sternoclavicular (SC) joint is the sole articulation between the upper extremity and the axial skeleton. The joint itself is diarthrodial, with an articular disc interposed between the two bones (Fig. 28.15). The articular surface of the medial clavicle is much greater than the sternal articulation. Only about 25% of the medial clavicle's surface articulates with the sternum at any one time, making the SC joint the joint with the least bony stability in the body.

The integrity of the joint comes from the strong surrounding ligaments, including the anterior, posterior, superior and inferior SC ligaments and the interclavicular, costoclavicular and intra-articular disc ligaments. The epiphysis of the medial clavicle is the last to ossify and fuse, at around 18 and 25 years of age, respectively. Another feature of this joint is the number of vital structures located directly posterior to the joint. These include the subclavian veins and artery, the trachea, the oesophagus and the mediastinum.

The SC joint can be injured by a direct blow or, more commonly, indirectly from a blow to the shoulder and is

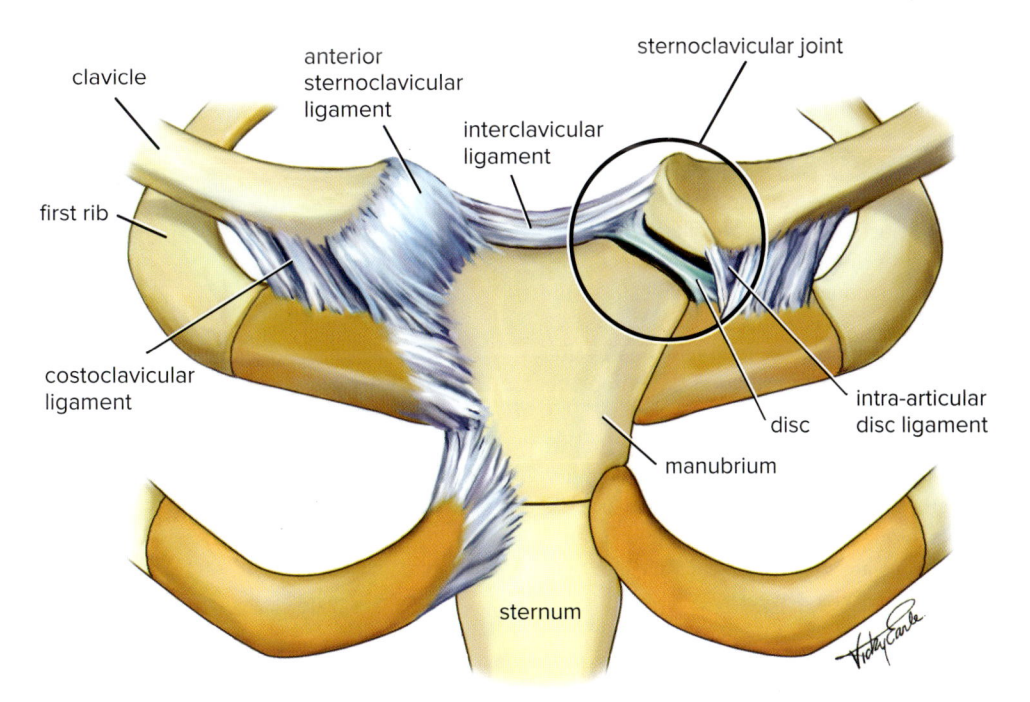

Figure 28.15 Anatomy of the sternoclavicular joint

PART B   Regional problems

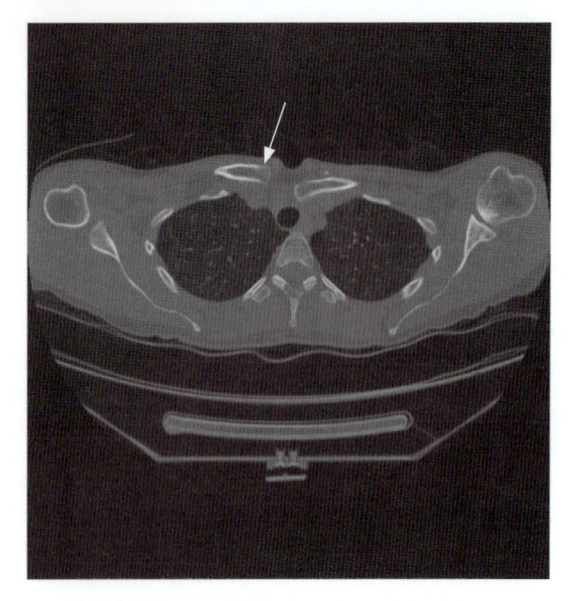

Figure 28.16 CT scan of anterior sternoclavicular joint dislocation showing clear asymmetry between the dislocated side (arrow) and the normal articulation

seen in upper limb weight-bearing sports (e.g. gymnastics). Simultaneous injuries of the acromioclavicular (AC) and SC joints are reasonably common.[18-20]

Traumatic injuries of the SC joint can be divided into first and second-degree sprains involving the joint capsule, subluxations, and dislocations involving rupture of the SC and/or costoclavicular ligaments and fractures of the medial clavicle. Subluxations and dislocations are further divided into anterior (more common; Fig. 28.16) and posterior (more dangerous given the adjacent neurovascular structures).[21-23]

Patients present with local pain and swelling depending on the severity of the injury. Anterior subluxations can be treated symptomatically by a figure-of-eight bandage for 1-2 weeks. Anterior dislocations can be reduced with lateral traction on the abducted arm and direct pressure over the medial clavicle. Dislocations are immobilised for 3-4 weeks in a clavicular strap. If the joint redislocates after closed reduction, a period of observation is appropriate. Many patients remain asymptomatic.

Posterior dislocations should be reduced closed under general anaesthesia as soon as possible after the injury. Traction is applied to the patient's abducted arm and the medial clavicle is brought forward manually or with a towel clip. Reductions are generally stable and are held with a figure-of-eight strap for 4 weeks.

Costochondritis

Costochondritis occurs at the plane joints between the sternum and ribs. It is characterised by activity-related pain and tenderness localised to the costochondral junction, usually over the T2-5 segments. Tietze's syndrome describes a painful inflammation of usually a single costochondral joint, although the sternoclavicular joint may be involved.[24]

Treatment consists of nonsteroidal anti-inflammatory drugs (NSAIDs), local physiotherapy and gentle mobilisation of the costochondral joints. This can prove an extremely difficult condition to treat. Corticosteroid injection to the costochondral junction may be of some assistance in refractory cases.

Stress fracture of the ribs

Stress fracture of the ribs has been reported with a number of sports and is due to excessive muscle traction at the attachments to the ribs.[25-28] Stress fracture of the first rib is seen in baseball pitchers and appears to occur at the site of maximal distraction between the upward and downward muscular forces on the rib. This stress fracture tends to heal poorly. The injury has also been reported in golfers, generally on the leading side (i.e. left ribs in a right-handed player).

Anterolateral stress fractures of the ribs (Fig. 28.17), mainly the fourth and fifth ribs, are commonly seen in rowers. This stress fracture is thought to be due to excessive action of the serratus anterior muscle. The biomechanics of the rowing action (Chapter 9) should be assessed and discussed with the coach and athlete to determine the possible cause/s and changes to technique where indicated. The concept of excess rib cage

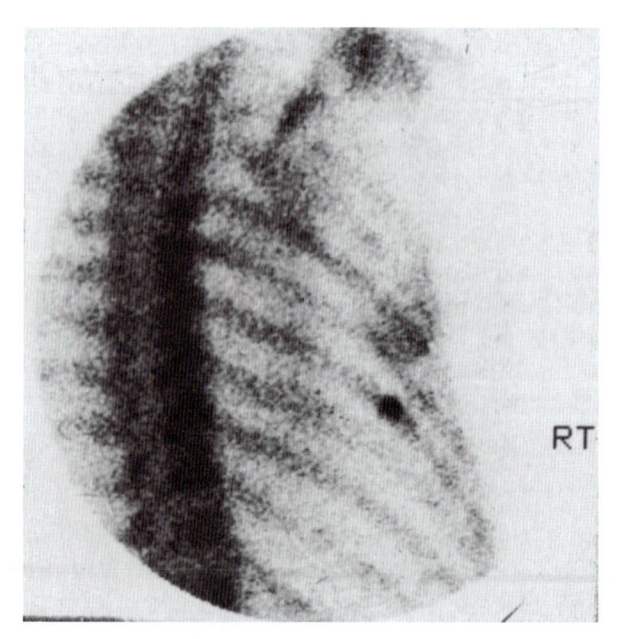

Figure 28.17 Isotopic bone scan of a stress fracture of the ribs

compression coupled with excessive isometric thoracic muscle contraction in the beginning of the drive phase in rowing has been proposed as the mechanism.[28-30]

Side strain

with ANDREW NEALON

'Side strain' is an injury sustained by athletes that is characterised by pain and focal tenderness of the lateral trunk over the inferior rib cage.[31, 32] It has most commonly been reported in cricket fast bowlers[31, 33-35] and baseball players,[32, 36, 37] and has also been reported in case studies in a golfer, javelin thrower, rower,[31] rugby player[35] and professional tennis player.[38] The injury typically occurs on the side contralateral to the bowling arm in fast bowlers.[31] In major league baseball the majority of injuries occur to the side contralateral to the throwing arm in pitchers, and the side facing the pitcher in batters.[32] It is evident that side strain is most commonly reported in sports that require highly repetitive, unilateral, asymmetrical and explosive actions that place great demand on the trunk.[39]

Clinical features

The athlete typically presents with sudden pain and focal tenderness over the lateral aspect of the lower costal margins,[31-32, 35-38] and may initially have considerable pain to breathe deeply,[31, 36, 38] cough and roll over in bed.[39] Palpation is typically reported to reproduce pain. Diagnosis is primarily clinical, although imaging with MRI or ultrasound is common practice in elite sport.[39]

Pain is commonly reproduced by movements associated with the initial mechanism of injury.[31] Trunk lateral flexion range of motion is a common clinical test and is typically reduced and limited by pain when moving both towards and away from the injury side.[39] Isometric resisted shoulder adduction on the injury side may also reproduce symptoms.[39]

Pathology and epidemiology

The pathology of side strain has been described in MRI[31] and ultrasound[35] studies as a tear of the internal oblique muscle from its rib or costal cartilage attachment with acute oedema and haemorrhage (Fig 28.18). Rib oedema and stripping of the rib periosteum have also been reported in a significant proportion of cases.[31] This suggests that some side strain injuries involve both soft tissue and bony pathology though the effect of this on recovery time is yet to be determined.[39] Injury from the undersurface of the eleventh rib is most common, followed by the tenth and then ninth ribs.[31] The relationship between imaging findings and recovery time is yet to be determined and is the subject of current research.

> **PRACTICE PEARL**
>
> Cricket fast bowlers are particularly vulnerable to side strain injury, with over half of the fast bowlers playing regularly at first class level in Australia and England reporting at least one episode during their career.

The injury tends to occur most commonly in the early twenties and often during the early stages of a player's career at first class level. Side and abdominal strain contributed the second highest incidence of all body areas over the past two decades in the most recent Australian first class cricket injury report, causing the third highest total player unavailability behind only lumbar stress fractures and thigh and hamstring strains.[40] It also comprised 5% of all injuries in major league baseball.[32] Injury surveillance studies in both cricket and baseball suggest that the incidence of side strain injury has increased in recent years.[32, 40]

The mechanism of side strain injury is difficult to establish, although it is typically incurred in a single specific activity, such as bowling or throwing, and prevents further play.[39] It has been postulated to occur due to sudden eccentric contraction of the internal oblique muscle after the lengthening that occurs during the wind-up phase of bowling or throwing.[31] However, trunk lateral flexion range of motion during the fast bowling action exceeds the range demonstrated in standing by a mean of 29%[41]

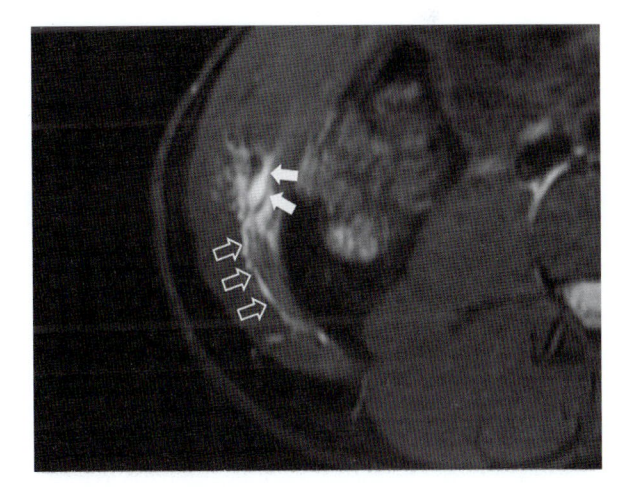

Figure 28.18 MRI (axial proton density image with fat saturation) of a side strain injury of the right internal oblique muscle. Focal grade II tearing of the internal oblique muscle is shown (solid arrows) just below the muscle attachment to the periosteum of the undersurface of the tenth rib. Intermuscular haemorrhage (open arrows) tracks between the internal and external oblique muscles

and compression of the lower ribcage versus the iliac crest may also be a factor. Side strain is most commonly sustained during the early stages of the competitive playing season.[32, 42] This suggests that adjusting to the demands of competition intensity may be a risk factor for this injury.[39]

Management

Treatment includes resting until pain has resolved during respiration followed by the restoration of strength and lateral flexion mobility of the trunk with graduated return to sports-specific activity. The repetitive nature of the sports commonly associated with side strain mean that high volumes of strengthening exercise need to be performed in the rehabilitation phase so that the athlete can cope with the demands of sport upon returning to play.[39]

Recovery time can be prolonged. Case series of cricket and baseball players report times of 4-10 weeks to return to play.[39] Currently ongoing research in first class cricket in Australia and England indicates that while about 20% of first class cricket fast bowlers return to pre-injury level of competition within 3 weeks, almost 50% require more than 5 weeks. In excess of 7 weeks was required for over 20% of fast bowlers. Major league baseball surveillance reports that baseball players spent a mean time of 4-5 weeks on the disability list over the 20 years to 2010.[32]

> **PRACTICE PEARL**
>
> Recurrence is common—30% of cricket first class bowlers suffered a further injury.

This is most common in the first 12 months, with 20% of all cases recurring in this time. In the only published case series of first class cricket fast bowlers to date, six out of ten cases were recurrences.[33] Baseball data reports a lower recurrence rate of 12%.[32]

Costoiliac impingement symptoms following side strain injury are also common, experienced by over a third of fast bowlers upon their return to bowling during rehabilitation and persistent in 20% of cases at time of return to competition. Currently it is unknown if such symptoms are associated with risk of recurrence. Non-remitting pain has led to surgery in cricket fast bowlers, with excision of the involved rib resolving symptoms.[34]

Despite its high prevalence in sports such as cricket and baseball, knowledge on side strain remains limited. The relationship between clinical assessment measures, MRI findings and time to return to play in first class cricket fast bowlers is the subject of current research.

Conclusion

Disorders of the thoracic region in athletes can be complex given the interactions between musculoskeletal, cardiorespiratory and visceral systems, and their convergence in innervation patterns. Athletic training and competition impose unique strains on the thorax and thoracic spine, particularly during the important skeletal development years, which may give rise to a variety of stress or overuse responses.

In considering a differential diagnosis, the clinician needs to consider the biomechanics of the activity and common soft tissue and joint disorders of the thoracic region, and to be alert to the potential for occult symptoms masquerading as musculoskeletal problems. Similarly, symptoms suggestive of a musculoskeletal presentation may indeed arise from cardiac or visceral systems which can require timely referral and intervention.

REFERENCES

References for this chapter can be found at www.mhhe.com/au/CSM5e

Chapter 29

Low back pain

by PETER O'SULLIVAN and ALEX KOUNTOURIS, with JOEL PRESS and MARIA REESE

> *My MRI shows I have a damaged disc at L5/S1. I am disappointed that I can never play basketball, golf and go for a run ever again. A neurosurgeon says he can perform a fusion. Is there anything else I can do?*
>
> 24-year-old athlete with disabling low back pain

Low back pain (LBP) is the leading cause of disability in the world affecting both the general population and athletes alike. In this chapter we outline a contemporary, multidimensional understanding of LBP and detail a clinical perspective of assessing and managing the disorder.

The anatomy of the low back is shown in Figure 29.1.

EPIDEMIOLOGY

Back pain affects up to 85% of the population at some time in their lives. LBP is rarely reported before the age of 10; however, during adolescence there is a rapid increase in the reporting of LBP reaching near-adult rates (lifetime prevalence of 70%) at the age of 17 years. While the majority (70-80%) improve from an *acute* episode over a 3-month period irrespective of treatment, between 50-80% will have at least one *recurrent* episode. However, for up to 20-30%, LBP can become *persistent* and disabling, limiting sporting activity, physical functioning and impacting on a person's quality of life.[1]

LBP is the most common cause of disability in those under the age of 45, and the most expensive healthcare problem in those between the ages of 20 and 50. Back problems account for a significant percentage (25% in the United States) of workers' compensation claims. LBP is also a common cause of lost time from sport. Of great concern is that in spite of enormous financial resources being spent on radiological imaging, treatments and medicating for LBP, the chronicity and disability rates are increasing.[2] The estimated annual cost of LBP in the United States, for example, is over US$40 billion.

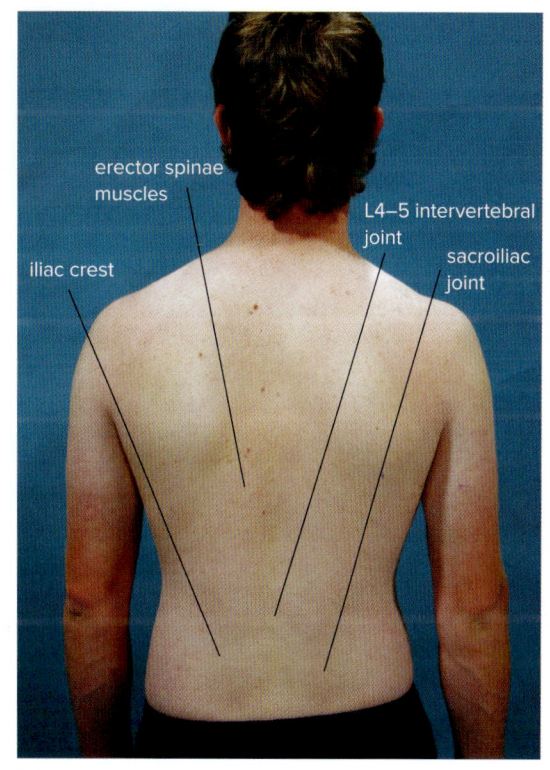

Figure 29.1 Anatomy of the low back (a) Surface anatomy

PART B   Regional problems

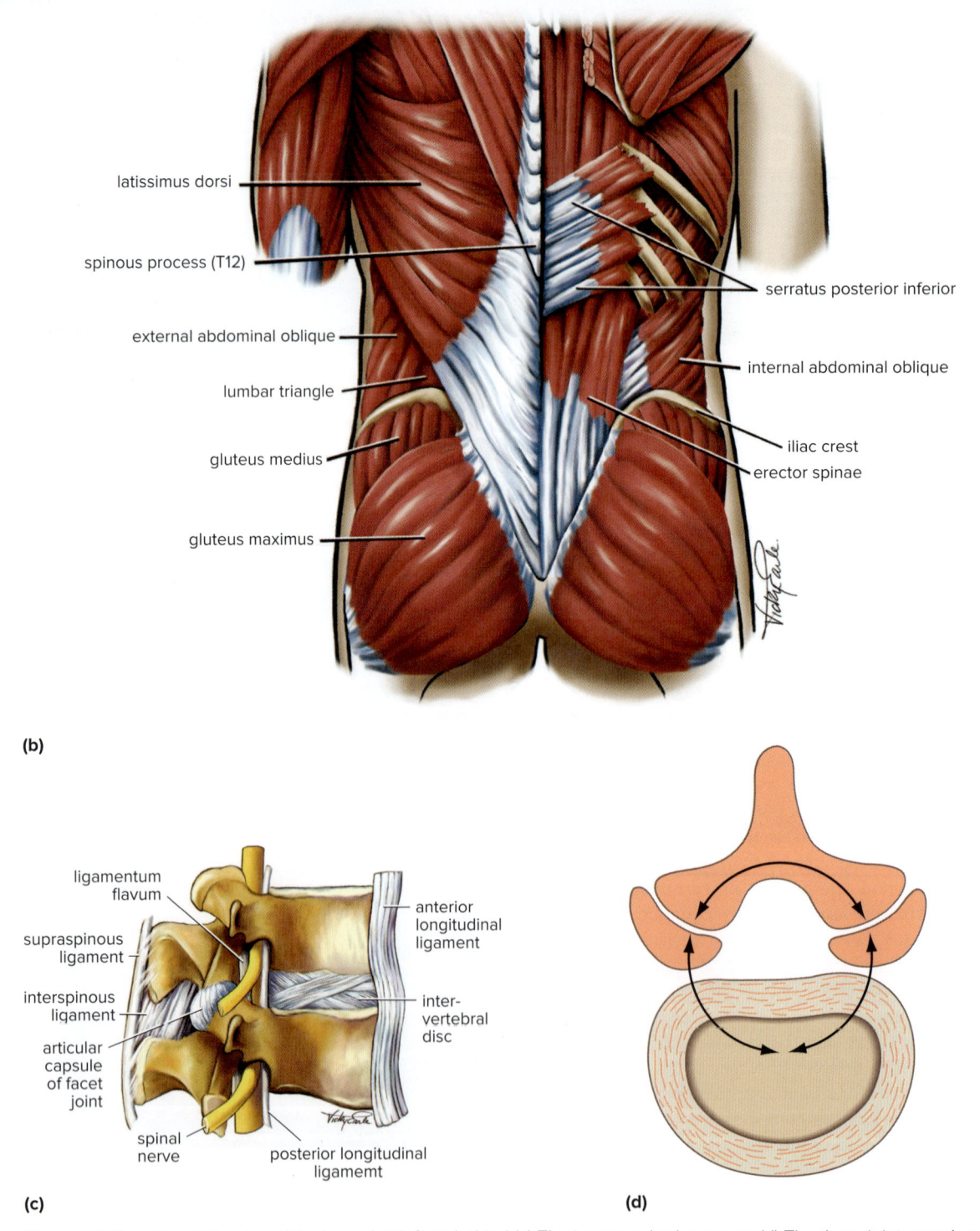

Figure 29.1 (cont.) (b) Muscles of the lower back from behind (c) The intervertebral segment (d) The three-joint complex consisting of the intervertebral disc and the two zygapophyseal (facet) joints

522

Low back pain   CHAPTER 29

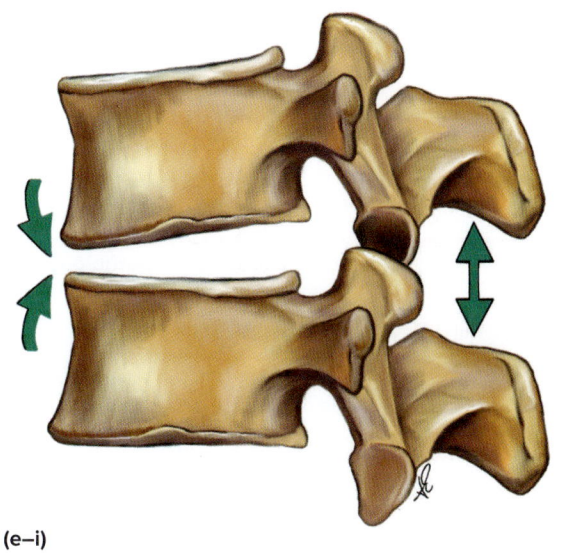

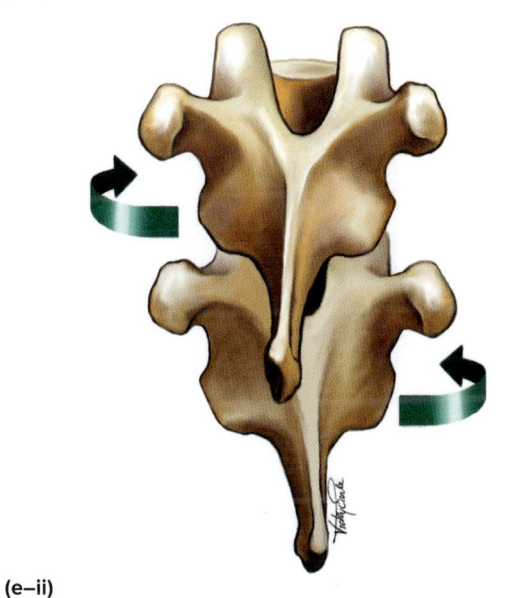

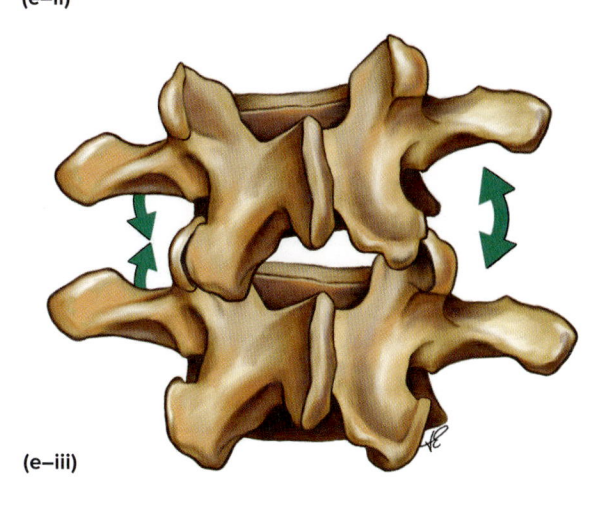

The multidimensional nature of low back pain

Once serious and specific pathology has been excluded, LBP in an athlete is frequently considered to be caused by an injury to the spine's structures. This is in spite of the fact that a clear mechanism of injury or even biomechanical strain often cannot be identified. Consequently, clinicians often reinforce the belief to the athlete that LBP is due to tissue damage, with treatments being directed at treating spinal structures.

In contrast, contemporary evidence supports the concept that LBP disorders in both sporting and non-sporting populations are associated with a complex combination of factors which may include pathoanatomical, physical, lifestyle, psychological, social, neurophysiological and genetic, all of which can predispose to LBP as well as maintain a vicious cycle of pain, distress and disability.[1, 3] This may present as LBP associated with an acute injury, repeated strain or in the absence of any tissue strain. The combination of contextual risk factors for the individual will determine levels of pain experienced, disability behaviours and coping strategies, as well as the risk for pain recurrence and chronicity. A detailed understanding of the various risk factors for LBP is required in order to provide a clear framework for clinicians to both examine and direct effective treatment and management.

TRIAGE

When a person presents with LBP, the clinician must first triage him or her to rule our serious and specific pathology (Fig. 29.2, right column and left column).

Serious pathology

For 1-2% of patients, LBP may be associated with serious pathology such as malignancy, infection or inflammatory disorder. The strongest factor suggestive of malignancy is a previous history of malignancy; for infection, a previous history of intravenous drug use coupled with fever; and for inflammatory disorder, an insidious onset of non-mechanical pain linked to night pain and morning stiffness.[4]

Specific pathoanatomical diagnoses

For another 5-10% of patients with LBP, a definitive diagnosis can be made based on spinal imaging linked to careful clinical examination.

- In sporting populations, fractures related to direct trauma, such as a transverse process fracture (e.g. from a knee in the back) or compression fracture of the vertebra

Figure 29.1 (cont.) (e) Segmental motion: (i) flexion/extension (sagittal plane motion); (ii) torsion (transverse plane motion); (iii) side bending (frontal plane motion) showing compressive and torsional forces

PART B Regional problems

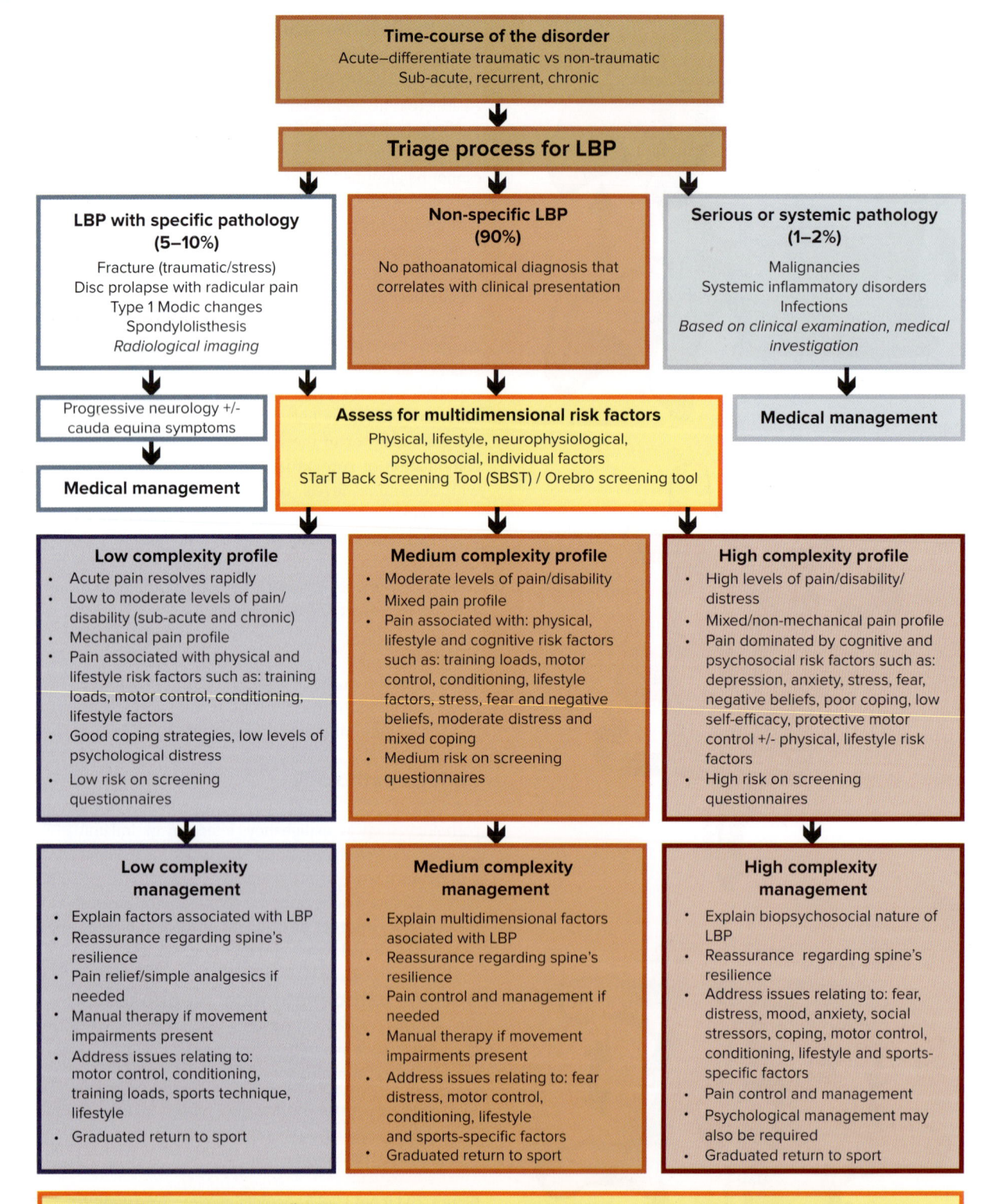

```
┌─────────────────────────────────────┐
│     Time-course of the disorder     │
│ Acute–differentiate traumatic vs    │
│ non-traumatic                       │
│ Sub-acute, recurrent, chronic       │
└─────────────────────────────────────┘
                  ↓
┌─────────────────────────────────────┐
│       Triage process for LBP        │
└─────────────────────────────────────┘
```

LBP with specific pathology (5–10%)
- Fracture (traumatic/stress)
- Disc prolapse with radicular pain
- Type 1 Modic changes
- Spondylolisthesis
- *Radiological imaging*

Non-specific LBP (90%)
- No pathoanatomical diagnosis that correlates with clinical presentation

Serious or systemic pathology (1–2%)
- Malignancies
- Systemic inflammatory disorders
- Infections
- *Based on clinical examination, medical investigation*

Progressive neurology +/− cauda equina symptoms → **Medical management**

Assess for multidimensional risk factors
Physical, lifestyle, neurophysiological, psychosocial, individual factors
STarT Back Screening Tool (SBST) / Örebro screening tool

Medical management

Low complexity profile
- Acute pain resolves rapidly
- Low to moderate levels of pain/disability (sub-acute and chronic)
- Mechanical pain profile
- Pain associated with physical and lifestyle risk factors such as: training loads, motor control, conditioning, lifestyle factors
- Good coping strategies, low levels of psychological distress
- Low risk on screening questionnaires

Medium complexity profile
- Moderate levels of pain/disability
- Mixed pain profile
- Pain associated with: physical, lifestyle and cognitive risk factors such as: training loads, motor control, conditioning, lifestyle factors, stress, fear and negative beliefs, moderate distress and mixed coping
- Medium risk on screening questionnaires

High complexity profile
- High levels of pain/disability/distress
- Mixed/non-mechanical pain profile
- Pain dominated by cognitive and psychosocial risk factors such as: depression, anxiety, stress, fear, negative beliefs, poor coping, low self-efficacy, protective motor control +/− physical, lifestyle risk factors
- High risk on screening questionnaires

Low complexity management
- Explain factors associated with LBP
- Reassurance regarding spine's resilience
- Pain relief/simple analgesics if needed
- Manual therapy if movement impairments present
- Address issues relating to: motor control, conditioning, training loads, sports technique, lifestyle
- Graduated return to sport

Medium complexity management
- Explain multidimensional factors asociated with LBP
- Reassurance regarding spine's resilience
- Pain control and management if needed
- Manual therapy if movement impairments present
- Address issues relating to: fear distress, motor control, conditioning, lifestyle and sports-specific factors
- Graduated return to sport

High complexity management
- Explain biopsychosocial nature of LBP
- Reassurance regarding spine's resilience
- Address issues relating to: fear, distress, mood, anxiety, social stressors, coping, motor control, conditioning, lifestyle and sports-specific factors
- Pain control and management
- Psychological management may also be required
- Graduated return to sport

Underpinned by a strong therapeutic relationship which emphasises person centred care, active management planning and consideration of the patient's 'life' context goals and expectations

Figure 29.2 Clinical framework for the profiling and targeted management of LBP

(loading injury), can occur in the lumbar spine. Stress fractures of the pars interarticularis may also present, usually during the adolescent growth phase, in association with increased training exposures to sports that involve cyclical spinal loading such as cricket fast bowling, tennis, weightlifting, throwing sports and gymnastics. The natural history for these injuries is favourable, with conservative management involving a period of relative rest from pain-aggravating activities with a graduated return to full function.

- Spondylolysis or spondylolisthesis are present in 5% of the pain-free population and have genetic predisposition. They correlate poorly with pain and disability, but may become symptomatic in sporting populations that involve repeated spinal bending and loading. Their natural history is positive with good conservative care, unless the listhesis is high grade (>3) and/or when it is associated with neural compromise.
- While disc protrusions are present in pain-free populations, LBP associated with acute radicular pain +/− neurological deficits that correlates with imaging findings of disc prolapse, is considered a specific cause of LBP and associated leg pain. This may be linked to a history of a sudden increase in exposures to repeated spinal loading with flexion and rotation, and is considered to result in radial fissuring in people genetically vulnerable to disc prolapse. Although very painful in the acute phase, the natural history for disc prolapse is favourable and, for the majority, the prolapse resolves over time. Only in the case of progressive neurological deficit and/or cauda equina symptoms is imaging and surgical review required.
- Vertebral endplate oedema (Modic type 1 changes) is also associated with LBP and can be observed on magnetic resonance imaging (MRI) scan (T1-weighted view). It reflects an active inflammatory process of the subchondral bone of the vertebral endplate. This may be linked to repeated biomechanical loading of an underlying degenerate disc and tends to be more prevalent in middle-aged populations. When symptomatic, this may present as disabling pain associated with loading, movement and night pain. However, the natural history for these presentations is good with appropriate conservative management.
- Spinal canal stenosis is rare in young and middle-aged athletes as the condition is related to advanced degenerative changes, but may occasionally be seen in older athletes. It is typically characterised by diffuse pain in the buttocks or legs, aggravated by standing and walking, and relieved by sitting, lying and lumbar flexion. This may be managed conservatively with exercises that reduce the lumbar lordosis and enhance hip extension mobility to reduce extension loading. Where this approach fails, surgical review may be indicated.

It must be understood that in pain-free populations, there is a high prevalence of abnormal findings on MRI scans (Table 29.1).[5] These findings are poor predictors of future back pain and do not correlate well with levels of pain and disability.[6] This makes a true pathoanatomical diagnosis difficult to achieve, reinforcing the need for careful clinical examination. Early MRI imaging for minor back strains results in poorer prognosis, increased instances of sick leave and a higher possibility of surgery.[7]

This highlights the potential iatrogenic influence that imaging plays in LBP and confirms that clinicians need to take great care in communicating radiology findings in a manner that is evidence based and does not create fear and anxiety, causing the patient to catastrophise their

Table 29.1 Age-specific prevalence estimates of degenerative spine imaging findings in asymptomatic patients

Imaging finding	Age						
	20	30	40	50	60	70	80
Disc degeneration	37%	52%	68%	80%	88%	93%	96%
Disc signal loss	17%	33%	54%	73%	86%	94%	97%
Disc height loss	24%	34%	45%	56%	67%	76%	84%
Disc bulge	30%	40%	50%	60%	69%	77%	84%
Disc protrusion	29%	31%	33%	36%	38%	40%	43%
Annular fissure	19%	20%	22%	23%	25%	27%	29%
Facet degeneration	4%	9%	18%	32%	50%	69%	83%
Spondylolisthesis	3%	5%	8%	14%	23%	35%	50%

Reproduced with permission from Brinjikji et al. 2015[5]

PART B Regional problems

condition. Even when a specific diagnosis can be made, consideration of the multidimensional factors that can influence pain and disability (listed in the next section) is important and may need to be addressed for optimal management of the disorder.

Low back pain without a pathoanatomical diagnosis

> **PRACTICE PEARL**
>
> For the majority of patients who present with LBP (85–90% of patients), no definitive structural diagnosis can be made, leaving a management vacuum and a diagnosis of 'non-specific low back pain'. However, the experienced clinician can usually identify a clear pattern of tissue sensitisation linked to specific spinal structures.

FACTORS CONTRIBUTING TO LOW BACK PAIN

A major recent paradigm shift has been the recognition that non-specific back pain can be strongly associated with a variety of different modifiable physical, lifestyle, psychosocial and neurophysiological risk factors that provide the clinician with the opportunity to target management.[1, 5] We explore those in turn.

Physical factors
Extrinsic factors

Each sport carries a different risk for LBP. An increased risk of LBP is linked to specific sports associated with high volumes of sustained and cyclical loading of the spine especially when coupled with rotation and side bending. For example, sports such as cycling, field hockey and rowing are associated with increased flexion loading +/− rotation strain, whereas sports such as dance, gymnastics, tennis and fast bowling in cricket are associated with increased extension strain coupled with side bending and rotation. These sport-specific factors interplay closely with training loads, volumes and technical aspects of the sport, which are closely related to the reporting of LBP.[8] Considering these extrinsic factors in conjunction with the coach and sport demands, and in line with the intrinsic factors of the individual, is important for targeted management.

Intrinsic factors

There is evidence that non-neutral spinal postures in standing (sway, hyperlordotic and flat back) are associated with an increased risk of LBP.[9] These postures are linked to changes in spinal loading as well as altered motor control patterns of the trunk and the hip region.[10] There is also evidence that these habitual postures influence movement patterns and may represent a 'signature' upon which more complex motor patterns develop.[11] These postural patterns, when interacting with sport-specific related extrinsic factors, may result in end-range tissue strain sensitising the spinal structures. This can result in directional patterns of pain sensitisation (flexion/extension/lateral [side bending] or multidimensional) in the presence or absence of tissue injury.[12]

In the acute phase of an LBP disorder following a traumatic injury and/or when associated with pathology, muscle guarding and movement impairments may be protective and adaptive. However, in the absence of tissue injury or when pain persists past tissue healing time, 'protective muscle guarding' may become unhelpful, provocative and maladaptive. This may reflect a response to a person's perception of underlying sense of threat, fear or vulnerability in the absence of ongoing pathology or tissue injury.[12, 13]

In this case, increased protective trunk muscle co-contraction may increase spinal stiffness and compressive loading, which may provoke pain-sensitive structures. This is similar to the 'limp' that occurs when a person sprains their ankle and that then persists beyond the natural tissue healing time, predisposing the person to recurrent and/or persistent pain.

Persistent motor control deficits (as described below) can also potentially leave a person vulnerable to increased tissue loading. These patterns are not stereotypical and are commonly associated with directional patterns of sensitisation with spinal movement and loading.[12, 13]

There is also evidence that people with LBP present with proprioceptive deficits specific to these patterns,[14] as well as changes in the cortical mapping of the motor cortex,[13] which may act to reinforce the maintenance of provocative patterns of movement. This highlights the need for an individualised mind–body approach to rehabilitation.

Deconditioning and muscle weakness in one body region, secondary to habitual postures and movement patterns, avoidance or sedentary behaviours, can also alter patterns of motor control in a proximal region. For example, weakness of the gluteal or lower limb muscles has been shown to increase lateral trunk shift and increased levels of trunk muscle co-contraction with single-leg loading resulting in increased spinal loading.[15] This may be linked to pain associated with sports involving limb loading. On the other hand, deficits in back muscle strength and endurance may render a person vulnerable to flexion loading strain in a sport such as rowing or hockey.[14, 16]

Lifestyle factors

Sedentary behaviour, sudden increases in activity levels, abdominal obesity, sleep deficits and disruption, excessive alcohol and smoking are all known to be risk factors that can act both peripherally and centrally to sensitise spinal structures.[17-19] These may be important targets for management.

Psychosocial factors
Cognitive factors
Negative beliefs, as well as fear of pain, movement and activity, are strong predictors of disability levels.[20] Healthcare professionals provide a critical role in transferring beliefs with regard to back pain to their patients. Language such as 'your back is unstable' may be interpreted as 'my back is damaged and it's dangerous to move'. A comment that states a 'lack of core stability' may lead the patient to believe that 'my back is weak and vulnerable and I need to be vigilant to protect when I move'. Words such as 'disc degeneration' and 'wear and tear' may also have long-lasting negative effects.[21, 22]

These may contribute to: fear of pain, movement and sporting activity; pain hypervigilance; and catastrophising linked to the belief that pain equals harm. Low levels of confidence and self-efficacy are also related to higher disability levels and this is often related to poorer coping strategies.[23] In some athletes, this may manifest as 'avoidance' of movement and/or sporting activity and dependence on passive treatments, while for other athletes 'endurance' coping strategies may present where they overexert themselves with pain-provoking activities in spite of significant pain exacerbation.[24] This can lead to an activity 'boom' (i.e. overactivity), followed by 'bust' (i.e. inactivity) pattern.

The responsibility of the clinician is to use language and management strategies that build confidence and empower the patient to develop effective self-management strategies while reducing reliance on passive therapies.[21] It is known that negative back pain beliefs and fear are also associated with avoidance behaviours and protective muscle guarding highlighting the close body-mind relationship with LBP.[25] Inquiring and screening for an athlete's pain beliefs, levels of fear and thoughts about pain are essential for effective management.[21, 26]

Emotional factors
Emotional factors such as stress, anxiety, depression, anger and frustration can act to reinforce maladaptive behaviours, further enhancing the pain experience and disability levels.[3] They can also influence pain processing, both centrally and peripherally, through dysregulation of the hypothalamic-pituitary-adrenal axis, altered immune and neuro-endocrine function, and cortical changes. They are commonly associated with LBP in sporting populations[27] and require screening and enquiry.[26] Screening for comorbid mental health disorders (anxiety disorder, obsessive compulsive disorder, panic disorder and depression) is important, especially when an athlete is disabled and distressed.

Social stressors
Work- and sports-related stress, expectations of the coach, media, family stress and cultural factors can all have an influence on pain beliefs, coping and vulnerability and need to be considered in the context of the athlete.[3] Significant life stress events are predictive of LBP disorders and should be screened for when the pain experience is disproportionate to the pain history (i.e. disproportionate pain responses to mechanical loading) and when pain develops in the absence of a clear history of tissue loading.

Neurophysiological factors
LBP is associated with complex changes in both the peripheral and central nervous system. There is growing evidence that persistent LBP is also associated with changes in the neuro-immune and neuro-endocrine systems, sensorimotor cortex, and associated with a loss of endogenous pain inhibition related to genetic/environmental interactions.[3] These factors are thought to contribute to the various sensorimotor changes observed by clinicians in a clinical setting, ranging from anatomically specific to more widespread pain disorders.[28]

Proportionate pain responses to mechanical loading
In sporting populations, LBP disorders are often localised to an anatomical region and present with proportionate pain responses relative to specific patterns of biomechanical loading (i.e. pain is clearly linked to directional patterns of spinal loading and movement).[28] There is growing evidence that cyclical spinal loading that involves either end-range or combined spinal movements (sagittal with side bending and/or rotation) with compressive loading can result in pain sensitisation of spinal structures without demonstrable 'tissue damage'.

In these cases, any of the nociceptive structures of the lumbopelvic region may be associated with LBP. These structures may include the vertebral endplate, annulus fibrosis of the intervertebral disc which are the main load-bearing structures, the laminae, zygapophyseal joints and surrounding ligamentous structures which provide resistance to end-range loading and torsion, the dura mater and nerve structures, as well as muscles and their fascia. All of these structures are richly innervated and may become sensitised by different combinations of the multidimensional risk factors reported earlier.

In the case of referred or 'neurogenic' pain where leg pain presents with signs of neural tissue sensitivity (positive single-leg raise [SLR] and slump tests), this may be associated with sensitisation of the nerve root epineurium in the absence of nerve root compression.[29] The potential lumbar spine nociception generators are listed in Table 29.2. By using skillful palpation, the clinician may be able to localise pain to discrete spinal levels associated

PART B Regional problems

Table 29.2 Lumbar spine pain generators

- Nucleus pulposus
- Annulus fibrosus
- Facet joints
- Ligaments
- Muscles
- Nerve
- Synovium

with localised muscle tension and tenderness (trigger points); however, the ability to identify the sensitised structure/s with confidence (i.e. disc versus facet joint) based on clinical examination is limited.

Disproportionate pain responses to mechanical loading

Inflammatory pain is usually a sequel to tissue injury or trauma. It is characterised by constant pain at rest that may be provoked with movement or loading. This pain should settle with expected healing time and may respond to non-steroidal anti-inflammatory drugs (NSAIDs). Inflammatory pain may also be associated with a repetitive tissue strain mechanism (i.e. after an hour on a rowing ergometer or bowling 10 overs in cricket).

For others with LBP, their symptoms may be more widespread, variable and demonstrate disproportionate pain responses relative to biomechanical loading (i.e. pain that is provoked with minimal biomechanical stress or aggravated by levels of stress, anxiety, low mood, disrupted sleep and/or fatigue rather than biomechanical factors). In these cases, pain is often more bothersome, distressing and disabling; and the underlying pain mechanisms are commonly linked to central pain processes (central sensitisation) and widespread tissue hypersensitivity rather than clear nociceptive processes.

This may present clinically as pain provoked by minor mechanical provocation in all directions of spinal movement and/or loading, and associated with widespread tissue hyperalgesia and multiple trigger points in surrounding muscles. On the other hand, it may present as a person who is distressed, anxious and hypervigilant, but with an absence of clear clinical signs.

The identification of widespread tissue sensitivity to palpation, cold and/or movement may be clinical indicators of central sensitisation. Localisation of pain to discrete spinal levels is usually difficult in these cases. These presentations are also more likely to present with comorbid anxiety, depression, heightened levels of distress as well as non-specific health complaints (i.e. fatigue, nausea, headaches, stomach pain, sleep disturbance and so on).

Treating the sensitised tissue structures (with injections or manual techniques) may result in short-term relief, be unsuccessful or indeed exacerbate the pain disorder, resulting in more distress. In contrast, care that targets the underlying mechanisms of the disorder (i.e. sleep, mood and stress-related factors) is required and likely to be more effective.

Many with LBP may present with a mixed pain picture where consideration of all multidimensional factors is required.

Individual considerations

There is growing evidence to support the idea that genetic variations have a powerful influence on pain processing as well as tissue structure (i.e. what you see on an MRI scan).[3] These factors interact with biopsychosocial factors in the presentation of LBP. This can explain how two people with similar MRI findings can have very different pain experience and disability levels.

The presence of health (irritable bowel, fatigue, restlessness) and pain (headaches, migraines) comorbidities are important as they may reflect the level of the allostatic load on the athlete (physiologic consequences of adapting to repeated or chronic stress).[30] It has been identified that these factors are predictive of episodes of LBP which may be mediated via neuro-immune processes.

The athlete's goals, expectations and readiness for change are also known to be important considerations in the assessment, management and prognosis of people with LBP and need to be considered.[31, 32]

CLINICAL APPROACH

A clinical reasoning process, based on the patient's 'story', screening questionnaires[26] and clinical examination, determines the relative weighting, dominance and relevance of the variety of factors with regard to the individual's disorder (Fig. 29.2). This allows the clinician to prioritise and target treatment and management.

History

The aim of the interview is to hear the story of LBP from the patient's own perspective. This involves the pain history, gaining a clear understanding of the mechanism of injury or biomechanical aggravation if present. Where LBP is of insidious onset, it is essential to understand changes in training load, contextual stressors and lifestyle factors.

Determination of the location of the pain, any radiation to the buttocks or legs, the aggravating and relieving factors (postures, movements and activities), and the presence of any associated features including sensory and motor symptoms is important. Any previous history of back pain and response to treatment in the past is noted. Understanding directional patterns of pain provocation and relief (such as flexion, extension or combinations of movement and/or loading) and how easily the pain is aggravated is important in gaining an insight into patterns of tissue sensitivity, and for directing the physical examination as well as the type and intensity of treatment.

Where LBP is distressing and/or disabling, screening for psychosocial factors including levels of stress, anxiety, fear, focus on pain and mood are critical as well as levels and patterns of sleep. Understanding the person's beliefs about their pain, fear of pain and/or movement, coping strategies, as well as any patterns of avoidance or persistence provides insight into their levels of self-efficacy.

Understanding personally relevant goals and expectations for treatment as well as their current levels of training, activities of daily living and future sporting commitments is also important. Screening for general health, levels of energy/fatigue, comorbid pain and health complaints is necessary.

Review of radiology, where present, allows for consideration of imaging relative to the clinical presentation, as well as an opportunity to reassure the patient regarding their spine's structural integrity if no specific pathology is present.

Screening for potentially serious symptoms include:

- cauda equina symptoms (e.g. bladder or bowel dysfunction)
- spinal cord symptoms (e.g. difficulty walking, tripping over objects)
- sensory symptoms (e.g. pins and needles, paraesthesia)
- motor symptoms (e.g. muscle weakness)
- systemic symptoms (e.g. weight loss, malaise)
- severe night pain.

The use of standardised self-reporting measures for pain (Numeric Pain Rating Scale (NPRS), body chart), disability (patient-specific functional scale, Oswestry Disability Index or Roland Morris Disability Questionnaire), psychosocial distress (STarT Back Screening Tool, Orebro multidimensional screening tool) are also recommended as screening tools to identify the complexity profile of the athlete and as a way of quantifying the effects of treatment (Table 29.3). Having the

Table 29.3 Patient-reported outcome measures (PROMs) for LBP

Roland Morris Disability Questionnaire
- Self-administered questionnaire that evaluates pain and function in LBP[33]
- 24 items
- Score range: 0–24
- Test-retest reliability: 0.91[34] (same day), 0.93[35] (1–14 days) and 0.86[36] (3–6 weeks)
- Construct validity: SF-36 physical functioning 0.85;[37] SF-36 role – physical 0.70;[37] SF-12 physical component summary scale 0.80[37]
- Minimal detectable change (MDC)95%: 8.6–9.5[38]
- Minimal clinically important difference (MCID): 4[33]
- Available online: www.rmdq.org

Orebro Musculoskeletal Disability Questionnaire
- Self-administered questionnaire to assist in early identification of yellow flags and if an individual is at risk of developing work disability due to pain[39–41]
- 25 items
- Score range: 0–210
- Test-retest reliability: 0.80[39]
- MDC95%: NA
- MCID: NA
- Available online: www.worksafe.vic.gov.au/health-professionals

STarT Back Screening Tool
- Self-administered questionnaire to distinguish subgroups of patients with LBP based on the presence of physical and modifiable psychosocial prognostic variables[42]
- 9 items (4 regarding physical symptoms and 5 regarding psychosocial contributors)[42]
- Score range: 0–9
- Test-retest reliability: overall score 0.73–0.79[43]/psychosocial subscale 0.69–0.76[43]
- MDC95%: NA
- MCID: NA
- Available online: www.keele.ac.uk/sbst/startbacktool

continued

PART B   Regional problems

Table 29.3 *Cont.*

Disability Anxiety Stress Scale (DASS)

- Self-administered questionnaire evaluating anxiety, depression and tension/stress
- 42 items (14 depression, 14 anxiety and 14 tension/stress)
- Score range: 0–126
- Test-retest reliability: depression 0.71, anxiety 0.79 and stress 0.81[44]
- MDC95%: NA
- MCID: NA
- Available online: www2.psy.unsw.edu.au/dass/down.htm

Tampa Scale for Kinesiophobia

- Self-administered questionnaire evaluating fear of movement and re-injury[45]
- 17 items
- Score range: 17–68
- Test-retest reliability: 0.93 (CLBP),[45] 0.78 (acute LBP)[46]
- Construct validity: pain catastrophising scale 0.51/FABQ physical activity 0.53
- MDC95%: 9.2[47]
- MCID: NA
- Available online: www.worksafe.vic.gov.au/health-professionals

painDETECT Questionnaire

- Self-administered questionnaire to determine the presence of neuropathic pain in adults with LBP[48]
- 9 items (7 symptoms, 1 pain course pattern and 1 pain radiation)[48]
- Score range: 0–38
- Test-retest reliability: 0.93[49]
- Predictive validity: Sn 0.85[48]/Sp 0.80[48]
- MDC95%: NA
- MCID: NA
- Available online: www.pfizerpatientreportedoutcomes.com/order-measures

NA = Not available

patient fill in at least the body chart, as well as a disability and a psychosocial screening questionnaire prior to examination is considered best practice.

Physical examination

Examination of the patient with LBP may include the following test elements.

- Assessment of functional postures, movements and sports-specific activities nominated during the interview as pain provoking and relieving. This is first carried out to observe for patterns of pain provocation, motor control strategies, guarded movement, protective behaviours, patterns of avoidance and levels of confidence.
- Assessment of the pattern, timing and range of spinal movement in relation to the whole kinetic chain. This is important in order to identify the adopted movement strategies.
- Repeated and/or sustained movements can be tested to determine patterns of pain provocation and easing (in the case of central back pain), as well as pain centralisation (where symptoms move peripheral to central, seen as a positive clinical finding) and peripheralisation (where symptoms move peripherally, seen as a negative clinical finding) in the case of leg pain. Finding a patient's directional preference or centralising the patient's pain during the physical examination can help guide management.[50]
- Combined movement testing can be useful to establish patterns of pain provocation related to combined spinal movement and loading. For example, in a tennis player with LBP related to the serve, combined movement testing of backward bending combined with side bending and rotation may reproduce symptoms.
- Palpation of the back and trunk muscles is to determine levels of muscle tension during spinal movements. For example, where the back muscles are activated during

backward bending or the abdominal wall activates during forward bending, this is seen as an abnormal muscle bracing motor control strategy.
- Functional tests can be applied during these provocative functional tasks to determine whether altering the spinal posture, the movement pattern or level of muscle tension increases or reduces the pain experience during functional tasks. For example, where pain is related to lumbar spine flexion during lifting/loading tasks, enhancing the anterior pelvic tilt with relaxation of the thoracic spine can be tested during lifting to determine whether this reduces the pain experience. In contrast, where pain is related to lumbar spine extension during lifting/loading/ backward bending tasks, then enhancing posterior pelvic tilt to reduce lordosis can be tested. Where pain is related to loading in neutral spine positions, relaxation of the abdominal wall with diaphragm breathing in conjunction with a relaxed thoracic posture can be used. Where pain is provoked by frontal or rotation plane activities then modify these activities by addressing control within these planes. These functional tests can provide an insight as to whether the identified motor control strategies (i.e. protective muscle guarding) protective (adaptive) or provocative (maladaptive).
- Assessment of spine 'stiffness' and patterns of tissue sensitivity in muscles and joints with palpation examination.
- Screening for lower limb (squat and lunge) strength and endurance is conducted where pain is associated with sustained and/or repeated spinal loading (i.e. running, jumping, limb loading).
- Screening for back muscle strength and endurance (squat hold or Sorensen test) is conducted where there is a pain associated with a clear loss of control into lumbar flexion.
- Testing for neurological deficits in the presence of radicular pain and signs of nerve compression.

These examination goals can be met by following this clinical routine.

1. Observation movement patterns in sitting, lying, standing, bending
2. Active movements
   a. flexion (Fig. 29.3a)
   b. extension (Fig. 29.3b)
   c. lateral flexion (Fig. 29.3c)
   d. combined movements–quadrant position (Fig. 29.3d)
   e. single-leg extension (Fig. 29.3e)
3. Passive movements
   a. overpressure may be applied at the end of range of active movements
   b. muscle length (e.g. psoas, hamstring, gluteals)
   c. hip quadrant
4. Palpation
   a. spinous processes (Fig. 29.3f)
   b. over the zygapophyseal joints
   c. inferior sulcus sacroiliac joint (Fig. 29.3g)
   d. over the iliolumbar ligament
   e. paraspinal muscles (Fig. 29.3h)
   f. quadratus lumborum (Fig. 29.3i)
   g. gluteal muscles
5. Assessment of strength
   a. lower limb (e.g. double leg squat, single-leg squat; Fig. 29.3j, lunge)
   b. Sorensen (or Biering-Sorensen) test (Fig. 29.3k)
6. Special tests
   a. straight leg raise/slump test (Chapter 15)
   b. prone knee bend/femoral slump
   c. sacroiliac joint stress tests and active straight leg raise (Chapter 30)
   d. neurological examination

The clinical utility of various clinical assessment findings are outlined in Table 29.4.

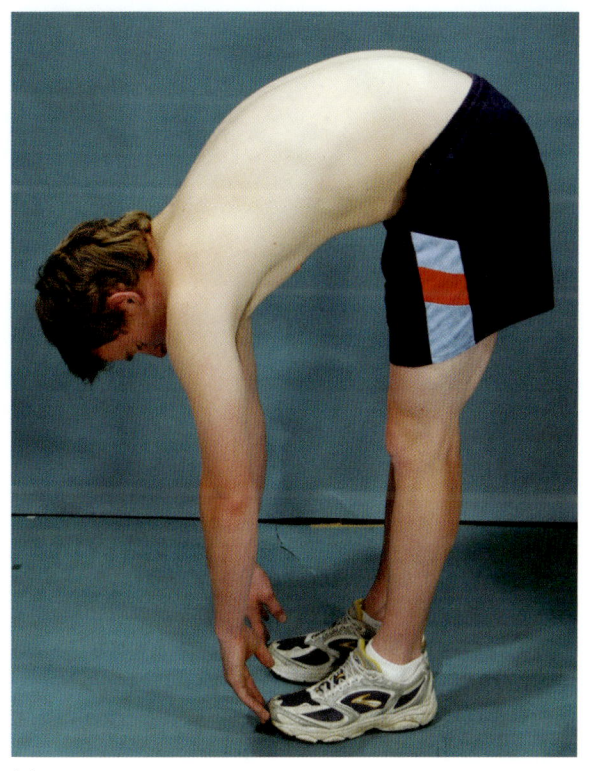

(a)

Figure 29.3 (a) Active movement—flexion. Look at symmetry of movement on both sides of the back, range of movement and, if restricted, whether it is due to pain or stiffness

531

PART B   Regional problems

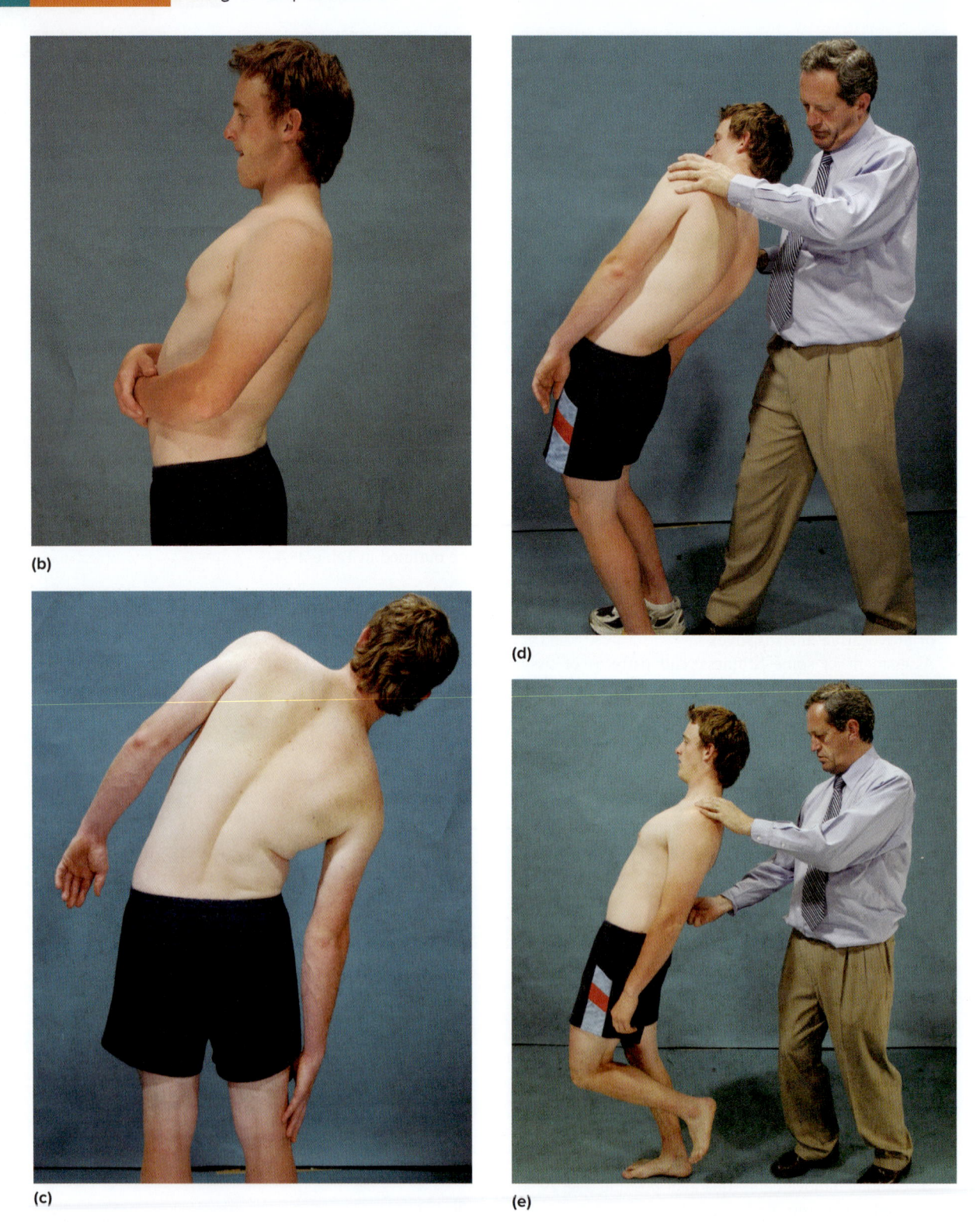

Figure 29.3 (cont.) (b) Active movement—extension. Assess degree of lumbar extension and any symptoms provoked. Patient should maintain pelvis in neutral position (c) Active movement—lateral flexion (d) Active movement—combined movement (quadrant position—extension, lateral flexion, rotation) (e) Single-leg extension

Low back pain   CHAPTER 29

(f)

(h)

(g)

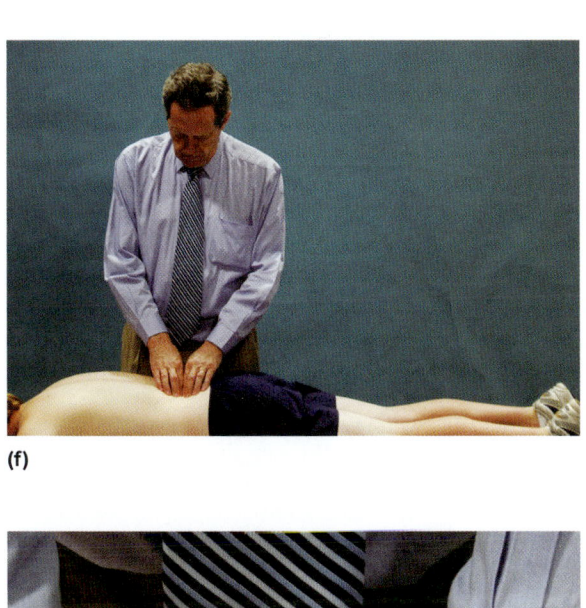

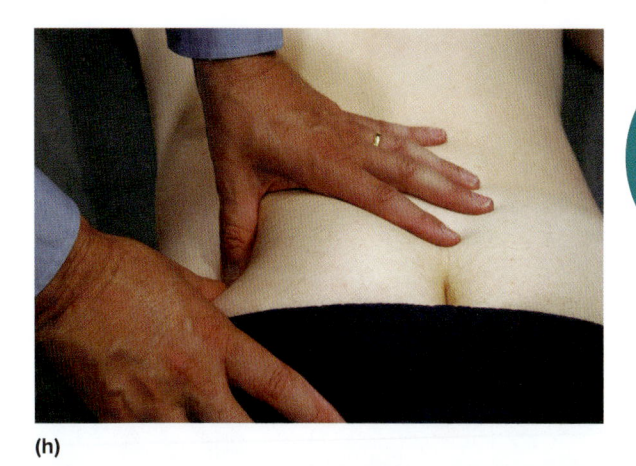

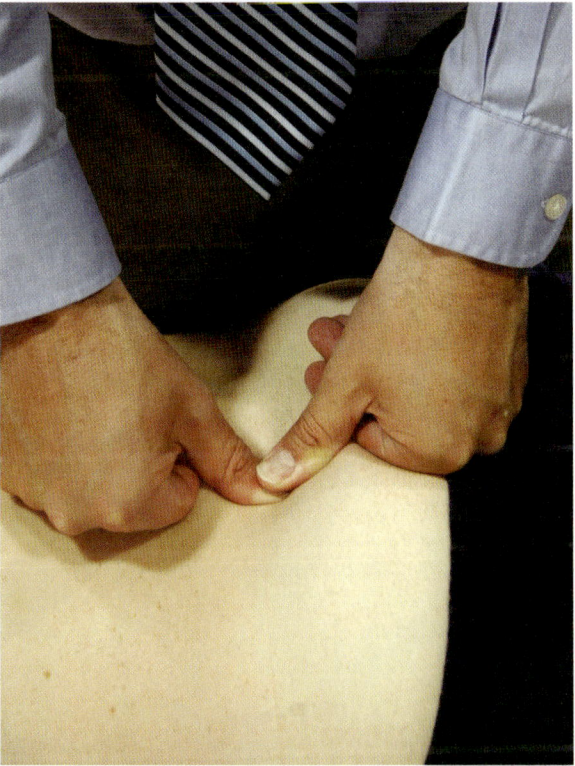

(i)

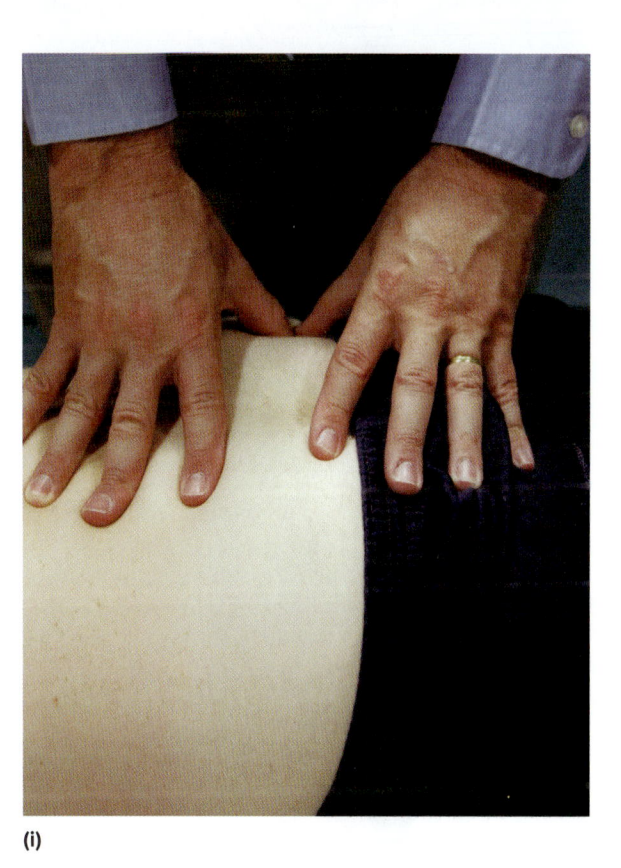

Figure 29.3 (cont.) (f) Palpation—intervertebral joints. Palpate over spinous processes, apophyseal joints and transverse processes. Assess degree of tenderness and amount of muscle guarding (g) Palpation—sacroiliac region. Palpate over the sacroiliac joints and iliolumbar ligaments (h) Palpation—muscles and fascia. Palpate paraspinal and gluteal muscles for generalised increase in muscle tone and focal areas of tissue tension, including active trigger points (i) Palpation—quadratus lumborum between the iliac crest and the rib cage

PART B   Regional problems

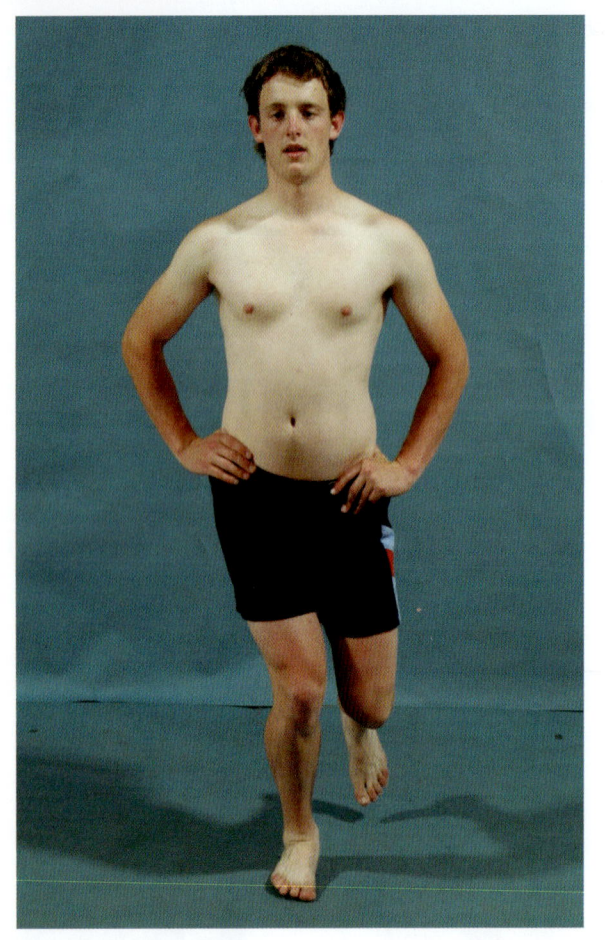

Investigations

In the management of most cases of LBP, investigations are not required. However, there are certain clinical indications for further investigation. Radiography should be performed if traumatic fracture or spondylolisthesis is suspected. Radioisotopic bone scan may be helpful in cases of suspected stress fracture of the pars interarticularis.

When specific pathology is suspected or LBP is distressing, disabling and progressive, and further diagnostic imaging is needed, MRI is often the imaging modality of choice. MRI can evaluate for a variety of possible sources of nociception including lumbar disc herniation, nerve root compression, spinal stenosis and bony stress reactions. MRI can also be used to image the internal structure of the discs. Degenerated discs that have lost fluid have a characteristic appearance on MRI (Fig. 29.4). MRI may confirm the presence of bone oedema of the vertebral endplate. The clinician must be wary, however, of placing too much emphasis on this investigation, as abnormalities shown on MRI may not necessarily be responsible for all or any of the patient's pain–they commonly reflect normal age-related changes.[57] MRI studies with and without contrast can be beneficial in patients with prior history of lumbar spine surgery and to help identify malignancy or metastatic disease.[58, 59]

Unlike MRI, computed tomography (CT) scanning is unable to provide further information on the internal structure of the intervertebral disc, yet it can be used in cases of suspected nerve root compression where MRI is either contraindicated or unavailable. The presence and

(j)

Figure 29.3 (cont.) (j) Single-leg squat functional test—double-/single-leg squat. If the patient's pain has not already been reproduced, functional tests such as squat, lunge, hop, step-up, step-down or eccentric drop squat should be performed (k) Sorensen test—patent maintains the horizontal position for as long as possible or for a set time (e.g. 240 seconds)

(k)

Low back pain CHAPTER 29

Table 29.4 Diagnostic accuracy of clinical tests (history, physical exam) in patients with low back pain

Test	What is a positive finding?	Sensitivity	Specificity	LR+	LR−
Lumbar disc herniation with radiculopathy					
Sensory deficits[51]	Altered or reduced sensation on side of suspected radiculopathy	40	59	1.1	0.93
Motor paresis[51]	Altered or reduced strength on side of suspected radiculopathy	22	79	1.1	0.96
Reflex deficits[51]	Altered or reduced reflexes on side of suspected radiculopathy	29	78	1.3	0.87
Passive straight leg raise[52]	Pain below the knee at any angle	92	28	1.3*	0.28*
Crossed straight leg raise[52]	Pain below the knee at any angle	28	90	2.8*	0.8*
Slump test[53]	Reproduction of radicular pain	84	83	4.9	0.19
Ankylosing spondylitis					
Measurement of chest expansion[54]	<2.5 cm change from maximum expiration to maximum inspiration	91	99	91	0.09
Spondylolysis					
Single-leg hyperextension test[55]	Pain in lumbar spine	50–73	17–46	0.7–1	1.0–1.5
Spondylolisthesis					
Lumbar spinous process palpation[55]	Presence of a lumbar spinous process step deformity	60	87	4.7	0.5
Zygapophyseal joint pain					
Extension rotation test[56]	Pain with either active motion or passive overpressure of movement	100	22	1.3	0.00

LR+ = Positive likelihood ratio; LR− = Negative likelihood ratio; NA = not available; * = estimated from available research data
See Chapter 14 for a guide to interpreting test sensitivity, specificity and likelihood ratios

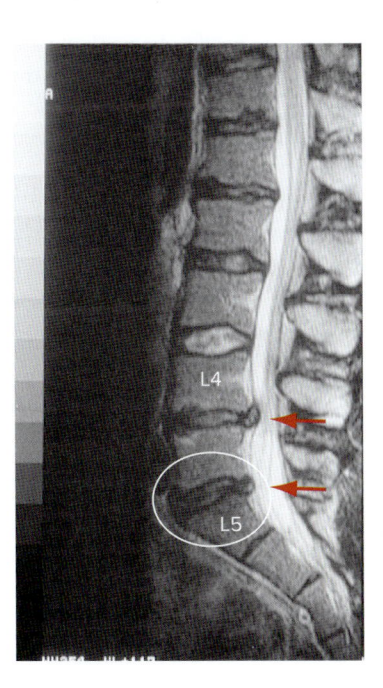

acuity of a pars interarticularis defect can be determined with reverse gantry CT scanning.

MANAGEMENT OF SPECIFIC LBP DISORDERS

Stress fracture of the pars interarticularis/lumbar spondylolysis

Lumbar spondylolysis is a term used to describe radiologically confirmed lesions in the posterior vertebral arch, in the region of the pars interarticularis.[60-64] The term includes a spectrum of bone stress injuries (stress reactions and stress fractures) and defects (non-united fractures). Traditionally spondylolysis was considered

Figure 29.4 Sagittal T2-weighted image of the lumbar spine showing decreased fluid (dark signal) in the L4/5 and L5/S1 intervertebral discs. Also noted are small disc herniations (arrows) at both levels. The clinical significance of these findings is debated (see below)

an injury of the pars interarticularis, but with the advancement of imaging techniques it is apparent that it commonly involves the adjoining pedicle and lamina.[65, 66]

The incidence of spondylolysis in the general population is 4–9% and varies with race and sex.[60, 67-70] In the athletic population, the incidence of spondylolysis is much higher, affecting predominantly adolescents involved in sporting activities that require repetitive spinal loading.[71, 72] It is particularly common in tennis players, platform or springboard divers, gymnasts, soccer players, volleyball players, track and field athletes and ballet dancers.[73-79] Cricket fast bowling, which involves a combination of repetitive trunk rotation, extension and lateral flexion during the delivery stride, has one of the highest incidence of spondylolysis of any sport.[80-84] The biomechanics of cricket fast bowling are described in Chapter 9.

The reports of spondylolysis in the athletic populations can sometimes be misleading because they often include symptomatic and asymptomatic spondylolysis together, and there is typically no differentiation between active bone stress injuries (stress reactions and stress fractures) and symptomatic chronic non-united fractures or defects.

> **PRACTICE PEARL**
>
> When considering spondylolysis it is important to have a clear understanding of the terminology, pathology, clinical presentation and radiology because the management of spondylolysis will vary depending on the morphology of the spinal abnormality.[62]

Terminology

The terminology used to subcategorise spondylolysis is not universal, but there are basically two main types of lesions that are distinctly different in regards to pathology, clinical presentation and radiological features.[60, 62]

1. Active bone stress lesions. These can be subcategorised to reflect the progression along the bone stress continuum:
   a. pre-spondylolytic bone stress
   b. stress reaction
   c. stress fracture.
2. Non-united stress fractures. These are often referred to as chronic defects.

The broad spectrum of spondylolytic pathology is reflected in vastly different clinical features ranging from asymptomatic to debilitating pain.[85, 86] The clinical presentation is also typically varied and complex; and best appreciated by the radiological characteristics that traverse the bone stress continuum (Table 29.5).

The earliest stage in the bone stress continuum is *pre-spondylolytic bone stress* that is characterised by the absence of symptoms, but a radiological appearance of bone stress on imaging such as MRI or nuclear medicine but with no fracture line (Table 29.5). The absence of symptoms means that it is a condition typically identified in radiology-based screening programs or incidentally when imaging for another injury.[87]

Stress reactions have similar radiological characteristics to pre-bone stress lesions but are symptomatic, highlighting a progression of bone stress continuum, such as more advanced microfractures (Table 29.6). It is possible that the intensity and extent of the signal on MRI may be greater in stress reactions than in pre-bone stress conditions; however, this has not been scientifically validated. At the final stage of the bone stress continuum are *stress fractures*, which are the most advanced bone stress injuries and identified radiologically by the presence of active bone stress (similar to stress reactions) but with a visible fracture line (partial or complete).

Spondylolytic stress fractures are prone to non-union and should therefore be considered as high-risk stress fractures like the navicular and fifth metatarsal stress fractures (Chapter 4). This explains the high rate of non-united spondylolytic fractures (also known as defects) reported in the published literature. A clear distinction between active stress fractures and non-united defects is essential as the management strategies need to be vastly different.

It is therefore important to understand the difference in pathology, clinical presentation and radiological features between active spondylolytic bone pathology and chronic defects.

Clinical presentation

There is no scientific research that outlines the clinical features of spondylolysis. The few papers published highlight a clinical picture that is similar to many other lumbar spine conditions.[61] Kobayashi et al. reported

Table 29.5 Radiological and clinical definition of athletic spondylolytic lesions

Diagnosis	Bone stress (MRI and scintigraphy)	Cortical breach (X-ray, CT, MRI)	Symptoms
Pre-symptomatic bone stress	Yes	No	No
Stress reaction	Yes	No	Yes
Stress fracture	Yes	Yes	Yes
Chronic non-united defect	No	Yes	Yes or no

Low back pain CHAPTER 29

that key clinical tests were unable to differentiate pain from spondylolytic injury or other back pain.[61] There are also no scientifically validated tests that differentiate spondylolysis between active bone stress injury (stress reaction or fracture) and chronic non-united defects. It is understandable that some clinical features would be similar because the source pain is from the same anatomical location of the posterior vertebral arch.

In active spondylolytic bone stress injuries, pain is typically of gradual onset and often related to changes in training volume and/or repeated cyclical loading of the spine. Pain is localised to the lumbar region, with occasional radiating pain to the buttock and posterior thigh.[61, 62, 88, 89] Pain often begins as low grade or 'stiffness', but typically progresses (in severity) quickly with continued activity (loading). The pain is typically mechanical in nature, particularly reproduced by spinal side flexion, rotation and hyperextension.[68, 88-90] Clinical tests that load the ipsilateral posterior vertebral arch and facet joints, such as active and passive lumbar extension and ipsilateral side flexion (or a combination of these movements), reproduce symptoms.[61, 91, 92] The single-leg extension test or stork test (Fig. 29.3e) had been advocated as a possible clinical test that can specifically differentiate spondylolytic pain from other sources of pain; however, studies have demonstrated that this is not a valid test for spondylolysis.[93, 94] Localised palpation tenderness and muscle spasm are also common features of spondylolytic injury and may be useful in identifying the specific vertebral level involved.[94]

Imaging

The lack of scientifically validated clinical tests means that radiological imaging has an important role in establishing the diagnosis when spondylolysis is suspected. It is important to use imaging tests that:

1. differentiate spondylolysis from other sources of back pain
2. confirm the presence of active bone stress pathology
3. establish the stage of the bone stress continuum (Table 29.6 and Fig. 29.5).

What the various imaging modalities provide

Traditionally, spondylolysis was identified on the oblique radiograph with the classic 'Scotty dog' appearance confirming the presence of a spondylolytic lesion (Fig. 29.5a and b).[64] However, with advancements in other imaging modalities, plain radiography has a very limited role in detecting spondylolytic lesions because it does not allow differentiation of early active bone stress and does not provide the same level of detail of spondylolytic lesions as other imaging techniques.[61, 68, 99]

CT (Fig. 29.5c and d), MRI (Fig. 29.5e and f) and scintigraphy (Fig. 29.5g) are therefore the most commonly used imaging modalities when spondylolysis is suspected, with each modality having its advantages and disadvantages in evaluating spondylolytic injury. Sometimes a combination of modalities is required for accurate diagnosis and to differentiate clinically suspected spondylolysis from other sources of back pain.

Bone oedema (high signal on T2 fat saturated sequence) on MRI or increased tracer uptake on scintigraphy (particularly single-photon emission computed tomography [SPECT]) indicates active bone stress injury.[99, 100] Early comparisons between SPECT and MRI in detecting clinically relevant bone stress had favoured SPECT at detecting early stage bone stress spondylolysis.[93] However, with advances

Table 29.6 Imaging appearances along bone stress continuum

	Pre-spondylolytic bone stress	Stress reaction	Stress fracture	Non-united defect
Plain radiograph[61, 68]	Unreliable	Unreliable	Unreliable	Scotty dog appearance (oblique view), particularly larger defects (Fig. 29.5a and b)
CT[61, 68]	Unreliable—possible bone sclerosis	Unreliable—possible bone sclerosis	Cortical or trabecular fracture (partial or complete) with irregular/sharp edges (Fig. 29.5c)	Well-defined defect with smooth edges, incomplete ring sign or lysis (Fig. 29.5d)
MRI[61, 95, 96]	High-signal bone oedema evident (Fig. 29.5e)	High-signal bone oedema evident (Fig. 29.5e)	Fracture line—complete or incomplete (Fig. 29.5f)	Defect evident
Scintigraphy[68, 97, 98]	Increased uptake (Fig. 29.5g)	Increased uptake (Fig. 29.5g)	Increased uptake (Fig. 29.5g)	No increase in uptake

PART B   Regional problems

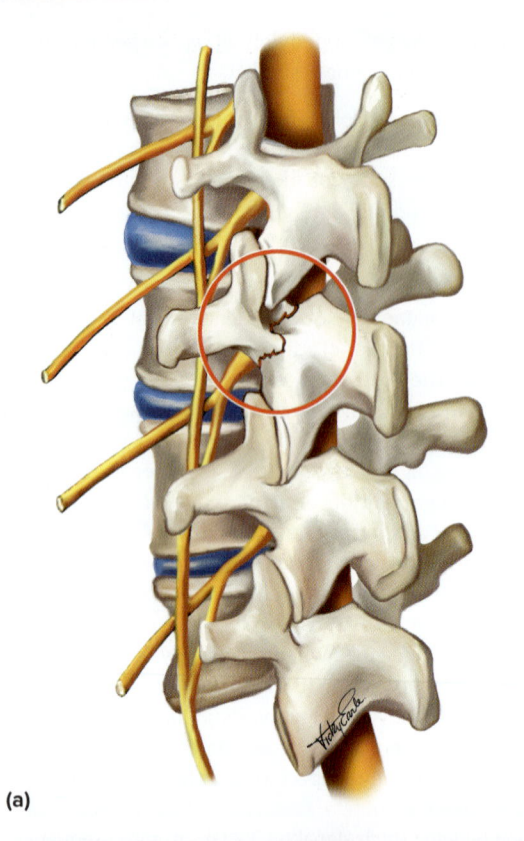

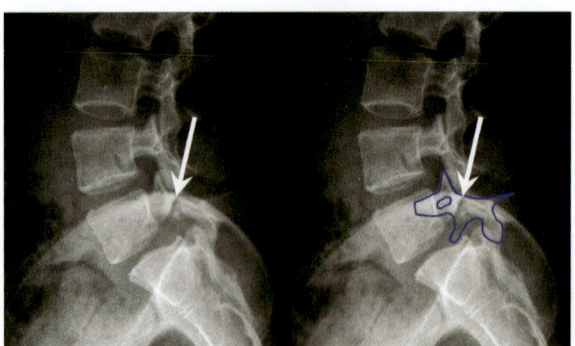

Figure 29.5 (a) Stress fracture of the pars interarticularis (b) Plain radiograph (arrow) demonstrating the 'Scotty dog' appearance of lumbar pars interarticularis stress fracture (c) Sagittal CT scan of pars interarticularis stress fracture (arrow). Note the possible impingement between the inferior articular facet of the vertebra below and the pars interarticularis of the vertebra above (d) CT scan demonstrating chronic defects (arrows) at the pars interarticularis (e) MRI demonstrating bone oedema (high signal between arrows) at the posterior vertebral arch

(b) IMAGING IN SPORTS-SPECIFIC MUSCULOSKELETAL INJURIES 2016, P. 551, ALI GUERMAZI, FRANK W ROEMER, MICHEL D CREMA. © SPRINGER INTERNATIONAL PUBLISHING SWITZERLAND 2016. WITH PERMISSION OF SPRINGER

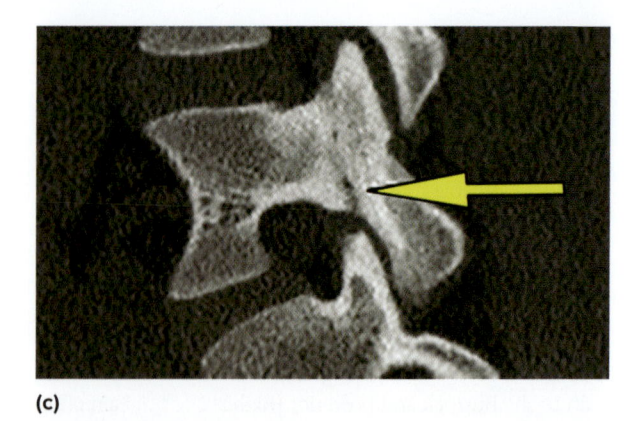

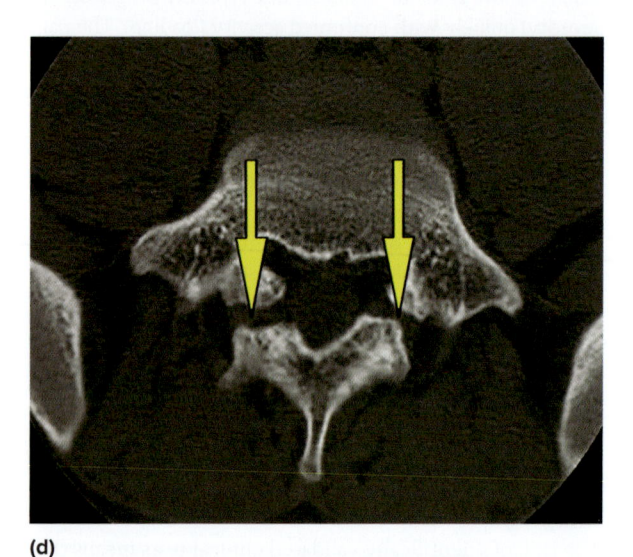

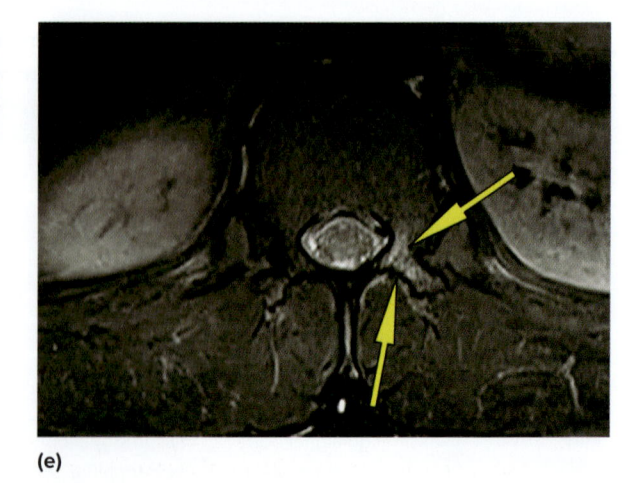

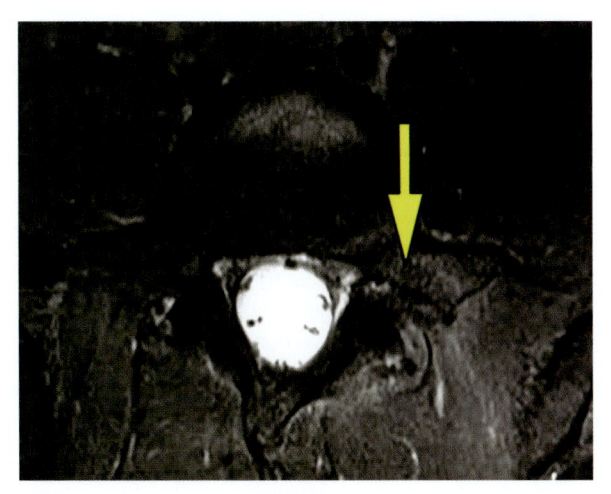

Low back pain　CHAPTER 29

(f)

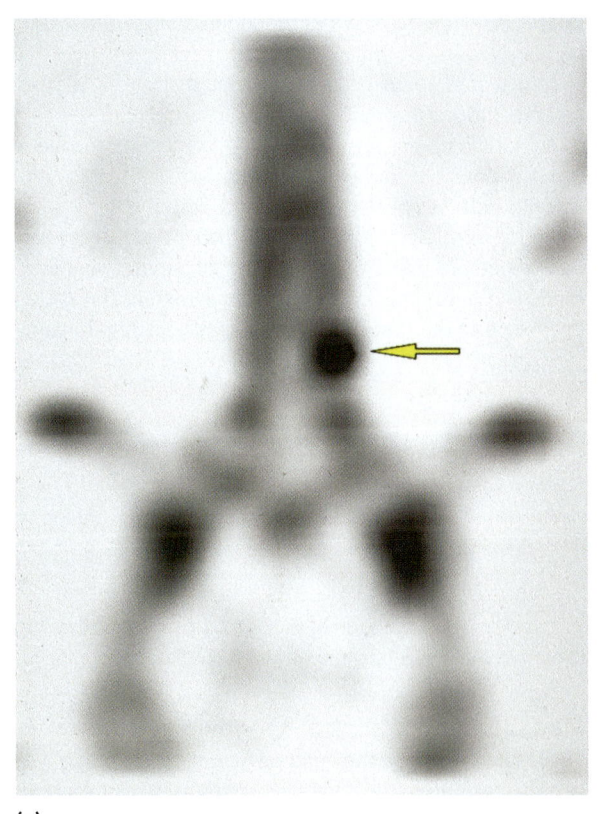

(g)

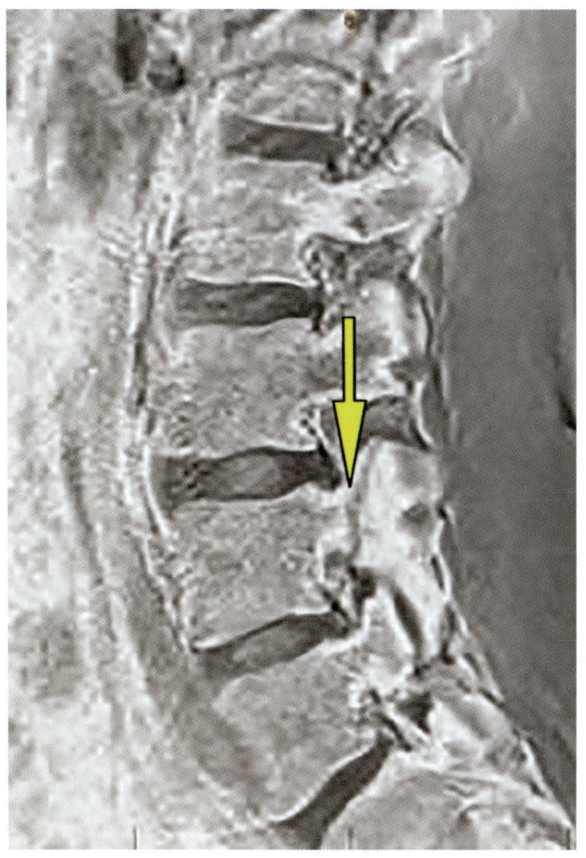

(h)

Figure 29.5 (cont.) (f) T2-weighted fat-suppressed axial MRI of L5 vertebral body, showing left-sided pars inter-articularis defect (arrow). There is mild bone marrow oedema (bright signal) surrounding the defect, most noteworthy in the left transverse process (g) Scintigraphy (SPECT) demonstrating increased uptake at the posterior vertebral arch (arrow) (h) MRI 3D T1 fat-suppressed image that allows better visualisation of the fracture (arrow)

in MRI imaging technology (higher powered magnets and image sequences) and the associated improvements in radiologists' ability to interpret abnormal signal, MRI is the first choice of imaging modality for detecting bone stress particularly as it does not involve ionising radiation.

Apart from detecting bone stress, MRI can be used to identify the presence of spondylolytic stress fractures, although thin-slice reverse gantry CT imaging remains the gold standard for imaging these fractures.[68]

CT provides the most detail of a fracture and allows for the grading of spondylolytic lesions as early stage (hairline fractures), progressive stage (wider fractures) or terminal (chronic sclerotic pseudoarthrosis).[95, 101] The staging of stress fractures is important because early stage lesions have a much better chance of bone healing, compared to progressive lesions, while terminal defects have no ability to heal.[100-102] With advances in MRI, reconstructed fat suppressed T1 MRI images (Fig. 29.5h) can image fractures and non-united defects that would usually require CT imaging.[95, 96, 98]

PART B   Regional problems

The usefulness of MRI extends beyond making the initial diagnosis, with the presence or absence of MRI bone oedema an important determinant of whether bone healing is possible in spondylolytic stress fractures.[102] Sequential MRI imaging following spondylolytic stress fractures has also been used in the management of spondylolysis, with the gradual resolution of bone oedema on monthly scans correlating with bone healing and the resolution of pain.[100]

As discussed earlier, non-union is a common outcome following spondylolytic stress fractures in athletic populations.[85, 103] Unlike some other stress fractures such as the navicular and fifth metatarsal, athletes with non-united spondylolytic stress fractures can remain asymptomatic and return to playing, even at the elite level.[85, 103] MRI, plain radiograph and CT imaging can detect chronic defects as sclerotic scar-filled clefts. These fibrous defects are prone to becoming symptomatic with mechanical loading, but the pain is similar to that from other nociceptive structures such as the intervertebral discs or facet joints. To determine if the defect is the source of pain, the gold standard is radiologically guided local anaesthetic injection into the defect and re-assessing key clinical tests.[90]

Pathogenesis

As with other bone stress injuries, the pathogenesis for athletic spondylolysis involves localised repetitive bone loading that consistently exceeds the normal bone strain threshold.[60, 104, 105] The posterior vertebral arch is loaded during trunk extension, rotation and side flexion movements.[106] It is possible that these movements either lead to shear forces or bony impingement that result in microfractures (early bone stress) and eventually lead to symptomatic stress (macro) fractures.[106-108]

High ground reaction forces contribute to athletes exceeding the bone strain threshold. For example, cricket fast bowlers can have weekly bowling loads of 150 to 300 deliveries or 5000 to 7000 deliveries per year, with ground reaction forces of 7-10 times body weight per delivery.[109]

The magnitude and frequency of load required to fracture the posterior vertebral arch is unknown, but individual variations (intrinsic factors) may predispose some athletes to lower fracture thresholds than others. Age influences the fracture threshold for spondylitic bone stress, with younger and skeletally immature athletes at greatest risk.[72] Bone geometry is also important as a lower proportion of cortical to trabecular bone at the pars region increases risk of fracture.[110] Other intrinsic factors such as shorter interfacet distances,[105, 111] increased coronal facet joint orientation,[112] excessive lumbar lordosis[105, 111, 113] and increased pedicle length[114] are associated with spondylolytic injury.

As discussed previously, spondylolytic stress fractures are prone to non-union, which results in a scar-filled defect and eventually a pseudoarthrosis.[60, 95, 100-102, 115] The reason for the high rates of non-union are unknown, but likely to be related to either an inadequate period of unloading to allow healing, or because of a delay in confirming the diagnosis (continue playing sport) that may disrupt the bone's attempt at healing. The non-united defect eventually fills with scar tissue to form a pseudoarthrosis.

The histological appearance of the scar tissue is that of a fibrocartilaginous mass that has similar properties to ligamentous tissue combined with a small amount of osseous particles, and has been described as enthesis-like, resembling a ligament–bone junction.[115] The enthesis-like nature of the spondylolytic mass allows it to stabilise the vertebral arch and absorb tensile forces.[115] This enthesis-like material suggests that pain from spondylolytic defects can be analogous to a joint or tendon pathology and should be managed in the same manner once symptomatic.

When non-union occurs and enough time is allowed for the fibrocartilaginous mass to mature and stabilise, some athletes can return to an elite level of athletic participation.[85] It is not clear why some athletes with chronic defects cope and others do not, and why some defects remain asymptomatic and others painful. It is likely that repetitive mechanical loading or single high-force trauma (e.g. landing in a lumbar hyperextension) causes disruption of the fibrocartilaginous tissue, leading to pain.

> **PRACTICE PEARL**
>
> The pseudoarthrosis and nature of the enthesis-like mass suggest that symptomatic defects should be managed as chronic (or acute on chronic) joint or tendon injuries.

In rare cases, herniation of the fibrocartilaginous mass can cause nerve root impingement and radicular symptoms.[115]

Management of lumbar spondylolysis

The difference in the pathogenesis of spondylolysis between symptomatic bone stress injuries (stress reactions and fractures) and non-united defects highlights the importance of accurate diagnosis and that management strategies need to be appropriate for the pathology.

> **PRACTICE PEARL**
>
> Management of spondylolysis needs to be considered as two separate entities: active bone stress injury and symptomatic non-united defects.

Active spondylolytic bone stress injury

The key management goals for active spondylolytic bone stress injury (stress reactions and stress fractures) are the resolution of symptoms, bone healing, return to pre-injury function and avoidance of recurrence. All four goals are interrelated and bone healing is key to the process.[86, 89, 116, 117]

Conservative management can produce excellent clinical and radiological outcomes, particularly in young athletic populations.[86, 88, 118-123] However, return-to-sport times range from 3–6 months and complex cases take up to 12 months.[86, 89, 101, 102, 121, 123, 124] This reflects the physiology of bone healing and correlates with imaging resolution of bone oedema on MRI and bone union on CT.[100] It reflects the need to invest time in a well-planned rehabilitation program that addresses musculoskeletal and biomechanical deficiencies.

The type of exercise and loading activities should be guided by clinical symptoms, bone healing times, imaging and clinical assessment. To simplify this, the rehabilitation program can be divided into three distinct periods that have specific focus.

Weeks 0–8: fracture healing phase

The aim is to protect the stress fracture and create an environment to enhance bone healing. For stress reactions, the aim is to prevent the progression to a stress fracture, and for stress fractures it is to attain bone healing and avoid non-union.

The most important aspect of the early management is to cease sporting activities that load and stress the posterior vertebral arch, such as running, jumping and landing. It also includes ceasing other training activities such as resistance-based strength training that involves axial loading[125] and avoiding repeated or end-range trunk positions, particularly extension, rotation and side flexion that may load the posterior elements of the vertebrae.[101]

It is not clear whether any specific exercises can improve fracture healing, reduce recurrence rates or enhance return-to-sport times, but when planning rehabilitation, prescribe exercises that can minimise muscle atrophy, address lumbopelvic deficiencies and improve the lower limb kinetic chain deficiencies that are often present in the young athletes with spondylolysis.[71] In particular, prescribe exercises that focus on strength, control and flexibility of the lumbopelvic region, such as abdominal strengthening and 'core stabilising'.[123] Lumbar extensor muscle endurance has been linked with the development of lumbar bone stress injury in cricket fast bowlers and should be considered in those identified to have insufficient strength and endurance.[126]

> **PRACTICE PEARL**
>
> A good starting point with the rehabilitation program is lower limb body weight exercises such as squatting, bridging and lunging to address strength and control deficits, while minimising excessive lordosis and developing a base for strength training later in the rehabilitation program.

Exercises to improve lumbopelvic control are also appropriate to minimise the effects of deconditioning of the trunk postural muscles, particularly in athletes with ongoing pain. It is important to closely monitor clinical signs during this part of the rehabilitation program, as any reproduction of symptoms during or after the exercise could be a sign of disruption of the fracture site. General exercise such as walking and cycling is safe and can be used to maintain cardiovascular fitness.

The use of thoracolumbar bracing can be considered during this stage to restrict spinal movements during daily activities and protect the fracture. There are some published reports that demonstrate good clinical and radiological (bone healing) outcomes with the use of strict protocols for bracing following lumbar bone stress injuries.[71, 100, 123] The brace needs to be worn almost all day and for months to enhance the potential for healing. A practical approach to brace treatment might be to use it in athletes who have pain at rest or with daily activities during the early period post-injury, in those with excessive lumbar lordosis, if there is radiological evidence of delayed bone healing, or with bilateral stress fractures.[71, 123]

Weeks 9–16: protected reloading phase

During this stage, there should be total resolution of key clinical signs, while daily activities and rehabilitation exercises should also remain pain-free. The introduction of low-impact activities that specifically load the lumbar spine can commence and theoretically stimulate bone healing through the process of mechano-transduction.[127]

Typically, the bone oedema will be less apparent on MRI during this stage, indicating resolution of bone stress, and in most cases should have totally resolved by 12 weeks post injury.[100] It is unknown how MRI bone oedema correlates with physiological bone healing, but Sakai et al. demonstrated that the resolution of bone oedema in active spondylolytic injury occurred between 3–4 months post injury and correlated well with bone healing observed on CT imaging and resolution of symptoms.[100]

The progression from body weight to loaded strength exercises such as dumbbell leg squats and lunges is an appropriate transition, while lumbopelvic control exercises can also be progressed to more functional trunk positions. Body weight exercises involving trunk rotation and extension can commence to gradually load the spine and stimulate healing.

Jogging can commence during this period with a gradual transition to higher intensity running by (approximately) week 12 onwards if symptoms and imaging suggest that healing is progressing without complication. In the latter part of this stage, functional submaximal dynamic exercises (e.g. plyometric) or sports-specific drills can commence at lower intensity and volume. For example, hopping or jumping activities for athletes involved in sports such as basketball and volleyball, kicking drills for sports such as football (soccer) and Australian football, or drills that mimic specific activities such as cricket fast bowling can commence.

The commencement and progression of exercises and activities should be guided by consistent absence of localised LBP and no change in clinical symptoms on key tests. If there is any deterioration in clinical presentation, the progression of exercises should be reviewed until symptoms resolve. Additionally, if imaging demonstrates that bone healing is delayed, these milestones should be held back until satisfactory progress is evident.

Week 17 onwards: transition to return to full function and sport

This is an important and often neglected part of the rehabilitation process that should involve careful monitoring of symptoms, reassessment of key physical competencies, addressing biomechanical changes and gradually introducing unrestricted load until there is a full return to pre-injury function. All daily activities, training exercises and key clinical tests should remain pain-free during this stage.

Radiologically, evidence of advanced bone healing would be expected during this stage. In particular, resolution of MRI bone oedema has been demonstrated by 16 weeks post injury and coincides with bone healing on CT imaging.[100] Repeating an MRI (fracture views shown in Fig. 29.6) and/or limited (only the appropriate vertebral segment) CT scan at approximately 16 weeks post injury is useful to determine the bone healing response.

> **PRACTICE PEARL**
>
> Although radiological healing is an encouraging sign in the recovery process, it is unknown how this correlates with physiological bone healing.

The key rehabilitation principle for this stage is the gradual increase in rehabilitation and training loads to allow a safe transition to return to play. As part of the process, unrestricted strength training can be progressed to ballistic exercise. Running and other conditioning methods can become sports specific, but it is important to monitor both workload intensity and volume during this stage, so the transition from the training ground to playing arena is graduated appropriately avoiding 'spikes' in workloads, that have been shown to be linked with athletic injuries.[128, 129] Sport-specific exercise and training is gradually progressed so that intensity and workload are at a level required to return to competition. Once again, an exacerbation of LBP in the region of the previous injury and reproduction of pain with key clinical tests should be seen as a sign to slow down or to cease the activity.

Symptomatic non-united fractures or chronic defects

When spondylolytic stress fractures fail to heal, the remaining defect fills with scar tissue that offers enough

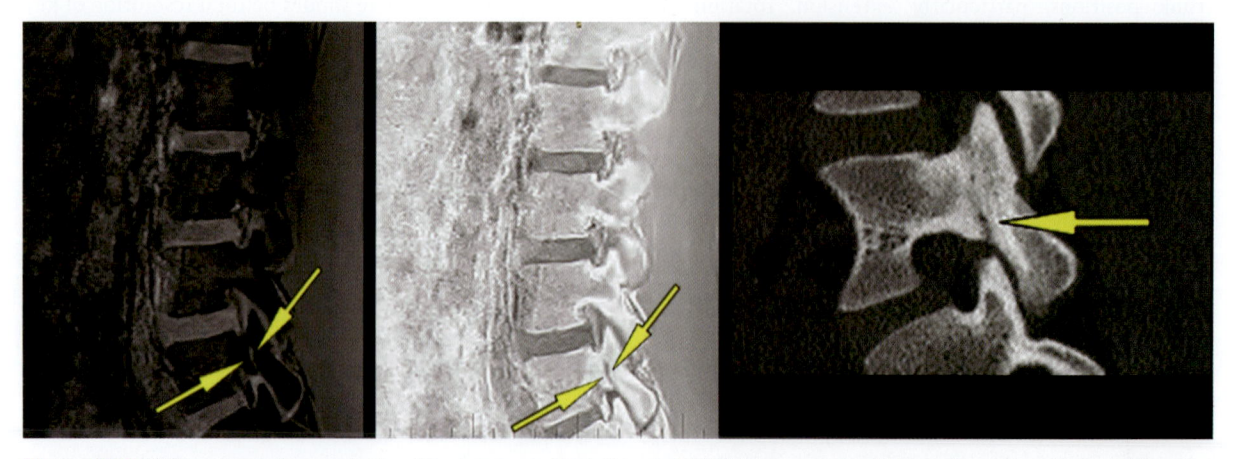

Figure 29.6 Different imaging modalities. The image on the left is an MRI T1 fat-suppressed three-dimensional image. The second is the same MRI image inverted (black becomes white) to make it look similar to CT. The third is the CT image of the same patient on the same day. Note the similarity between the CT and MRI images

stability to the segment to allow some athletes to return to unrestricted pre-injury function, even at the elite level. It is unknown how many athletes with non-united spondylolytic stress fractures fail to return to pre-injury level of activity, but there are numerous reports of athletes competing at the elite level with (often asymptomatic) chronic lumbar defects.[80] If an athlete does return to sporting activities with a non-united defect, episodic or ongoing pain is common if the fibrous scar tissue is disrupted and irritated with mechanical loading.

An exacerbation of pain from a non-united spondylolytic defect needs to be managed as an acute or chronic injury. The acute component is likely to be inflammatory in nature due to mechanical disruption of the fibrous scar and can respond to appropriate anti-inflammatory management strategies. The chronic nature of the defect does mean that there is virtually no possibility of bone healing, so this should not be considered as a viable management goal.[101, 102, 121]

Symptom management
With little prospect of bone healing, the main aim of treatment is to reduce pain and restore function. While the exact source of pain is unknown, disruption and inflammation of the fibrous scar is a likely mechanism so the use of these anti-inflammatory methods should be considered as well as analgesic medication and possibly oral corticosteroids.

Radiologically guided corticosteroid and local anaesthetic injection within the defect (Figure 29.7) has considerable merit. The short-acting local anaesthetic is useful in determining if the defect is the source of pain, while the corticosteroid can provide the localised anti-inflammatory response thereby reducing pain and allowing a faster transition through the rehabilitation program and return to function.[90]

Unloading phase
The nature of the fibrous tissue within the bony defect, particularly that it is histologically similar to ligament and tendon, suggests that the management of non-union should be similar to the management of those tissues. Importantly, a brief period of unloading to allow irritability of the fibrocartilaginous scar to resolve may be required, with rest from aggravating (sporting) activities required if pain does not settle. The length of the unloading period needs to be guided by the nature of the pain and typically involves initially reducing exposure to provocative activities that involve repetitive trunk extension, rotation and side flexion or any other aggravating activity.

The length of the unloading phase and the transition to reloading should depend on the reduction of symptoms and improvement in painful clinical tests.

> **PRACTICE PEARL**
>
> Unlike acute bone stress injuries, total resolution of pain of non-union is not necessary, but careful monitoring of response to reloading is important.

It may be possible that athletes can return to sport with some low-grade pain as long as the pain characteristics remain manageable with increase in load and during the transition to sporting function. In this sense, the unloading phase for chronic symptomatic pars defects is similar to tendinopathy, where the unloading phase serves to reduce but not always eliminate pain.[130]

Summary
Lumbar spondylolysis is a complex condition with little scientific evidence underpinning the clinical tests to differentiate it from other causes of lower back pain. Even more complex is understanding the stage in the bone stress continuum as this is important in the management of spondylolysis. Advances in imaging have improved the understanding of this condition, particularly the stage in the bone stress continuum and differentiating active bone stress injury from symptomatic non-united defects. The management of spondylolysis needs to consider the clinical features and the imaging. The management of active spondylolysis needs to focus on bone healing that takes months, while symptomatic non-united fractures can be treated symptomatically, reducing the recovery period.

Spondylolisthesis
Spondylolisthesis (Fig. 29.8a) refers to the anterior displacement of part or all of one vertebra forwards on another. It is often associated with bilateral pars defects that usually develop in early childhood and have a definite family predisposition. Pars defects that develop due to athletic activity (stress fractures) rarely result in spondylolisthesis.

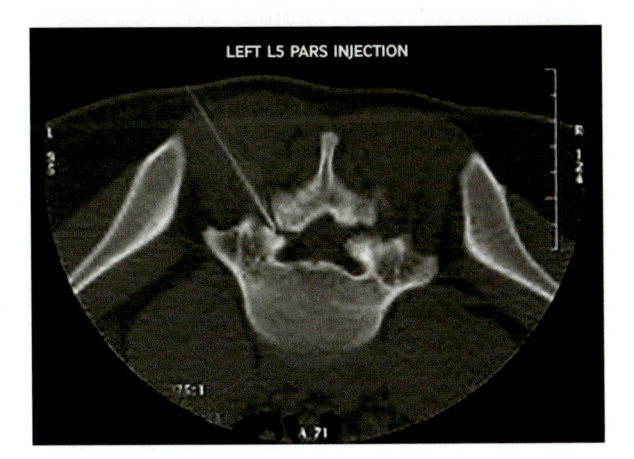

Figure 29.7 Guided injection into the chronic pars defect

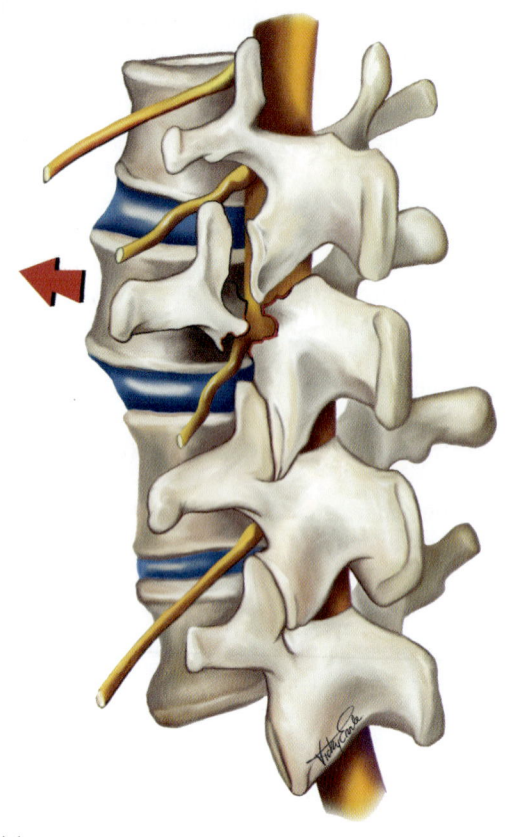

PART B   Regional problems

(a)

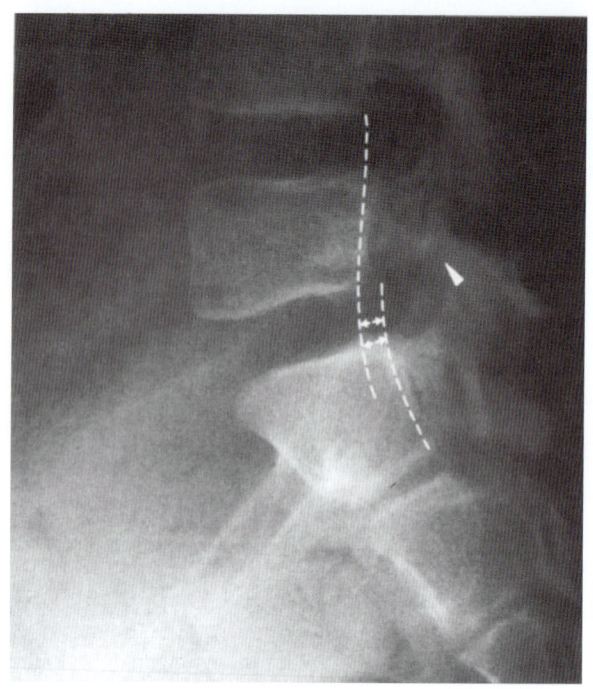

(b)

Figure 29.8 Grade I spondylolisthesis and pars defect (a) Anterior slip (arrow) (b) Plain radiograph (single arrow shows the defect; dotted lines show the method of measuring slippage)

Spondylolisthesis is most commonly seen in children between the ages of 9 and 14. In the vast majority of cases, it is the L5 vertebra that slips forwards on the S1. The spondylolisthesis is graded according to the degree of slip of the vertebra. A grade I slip denotes that a vertebra has slipped up to 25% over the body of the vertebra underlying it; in a grade II slip the displacement is greater than 25%; in a grade III slip, greater than 50%; and in a grade IV slip, greater than 75%. It is rare for a slip to progress once the athlete has reached maturation. Lateral X-rays best demonstrate the extent and possible progression of vertebral slippage (Fig. 29.8b). A recent systematic review suggests that spondylolisthesis is not predictive of LBP in the general population.[131] However, in an athletic population it may become symptomatic.

Clinical features
Spondylolisthesis is often asymptomatic and the patients may be unaware of the defect. However, LBP, with or without leg pain associated with the spondylolisthesis, may develop in response to various biopsychosocial factors and is frequently aggravated by extension activities and postures. On examination, there may be a palpable step off corresponding to the slip.

Treatment
In considering the treatment of this condition, it is important to remember that the patient's LBP is not necessarily being caused by the spondylolisthesis. First, it is important to reassure the athlete that spondylolisthesis is common in the pain-free population and the natural history for these disorders is usually very good. Addressing the various biopsychosocial features of the disorder described above is central to management.

Treatment of athletes with grade I or grade II symptomatic spondylolisthesis is usually non-surgical, and rehabilitation exercise approaches are shown to be effective.[132] Athletes with grade I or grade II spondylolisthesis may return to sport after their rehabilitation program, when they have minimal pain on extension and have good spinal control during functional and sports-specific activity. If the symptoms recur and are distressing, activity should be modified.

Athletes with grade III or grade IV spondylolisthesis should avoid high-speed or contact sports. Treatment is initially conservative, yet if a patient continues to experience symptoms after a 6-month non-surgical treatment period, he/she may be considered for surgical fixation. Other indications for surgery include growing children with a

Low back pain   CHAPTER 29

slip >50%, progressively worsening neurological signs and radiological evidence of further displacement.[133]

Acute radiculopathy +/− nerve root compression

Acute radiculopathy is usually the result of an acute disc prolapse when the contents of the nucleus pulposus of the intervertebral disc are extruded through the annulus fibrosis into the spinal canal, irritating the nerve root (Fig. 29.9). The irritation of the nerve root may be due to direct mechanical compression by the nuclear material and/or as a result of the chemical irritation caused by the prolapse, and is usually very painful and distressing.

Prolapse usually occurs in discs that have been previously weakened by one of the processes mentioned already. Disc prolapse usually occurs between the ages of 20 and 50 years and is more common in males than females. The L5–S1 disc is the most commonly prolapsed disc and L4–5 the next most common.

Clinical features

Typically, a patient with a disc prolapse presents with acute LBP and radicular leg pain following a relatively trivial movement, usually involving forward bending. This is frequently preceded by a period of rapid increase in repeated flexion loading (such as a sudden increase in rowing training volumes). On occasion, the presentation may be painless, with weakness or sensory symptoms only (in the case of nerve compression).

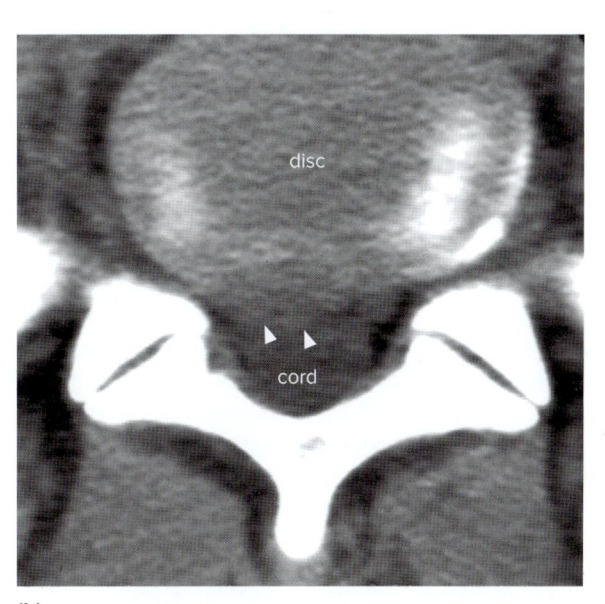

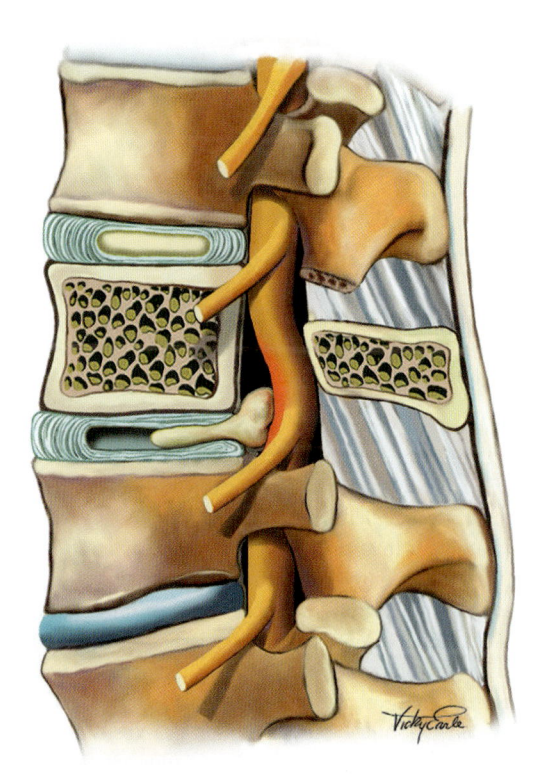

Figure 29.9 Disc extrusion compressing nerve root (a) Spinal cord compression from severe disc prolapse (b) Axial CT scan. Arrowheads point to the border between the bulging disc (anterior) and the compressed cord (posterior) (c) Sagittal MRI showing prominent posterior L3–4 disc bulging (arrow) and cauda equina compression. The L4–5 disc (arrowhead) is also abnormal (compressed) but not protruding

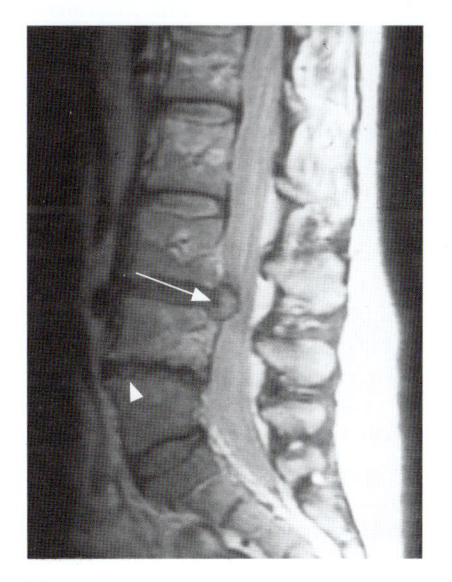

545

PART B   Regional problems

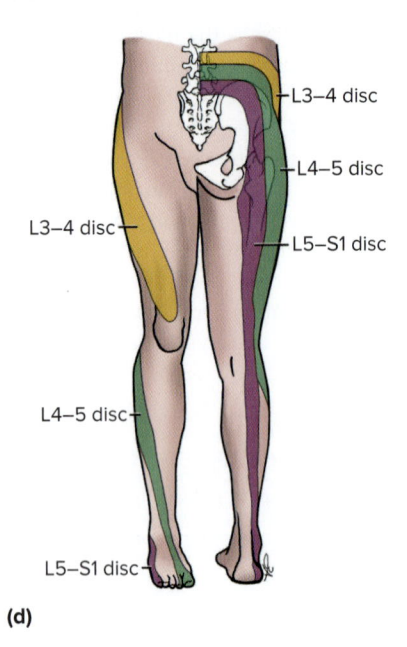

Figure 29.9 (cont.) (d) Common areas of pain radiation with disc prolapse at the L3–4, L4–5 and L5–S1 levels

The symptoms depend on the direction of the prolapse. Posterior herniations are more likely to cause LBP with later development of leg pain, whereas posterolateral herniations may cause radicular symptoms without LBP. Sharp, lancinating pain in a narrow band down the leg is common with radicular pain and is associated with nerve root irritation and positive SLR, accompanied by pins and needles, numbness and weakness. Pain is often aggravated by sitting, bending, lifting, coughing or sneezing. Pain is usually eased by lying down, particularly on the asymptomatic side, and is often less after a night's rest.

On examination, the patient often demonstrates a list to one side that is usually, although not always, away from the side of pain (Fig. 29.10). This is a protective scoliosis and reflects an adaptive motor response. Examination may be difficult if there is severe pain and irritability. Straight leg raise is usually limited (less than 30° in severe cases) and all active movements of the lumbar spine, particularly flexion, are usually restricted by muscle guarding. Palpation usually reveals muscle spasm with marked tenderness but occasionally it may be unremarkable. A neurological examination should always be performed when pain extends past the buttock fold or there are subjective sensory and/or motor changes.

Treatment

It is important to educate the patient that the natural history for disc prolapse is excellent for the majority, with resolution of symptoms and reabsorption of the prolapse occurring

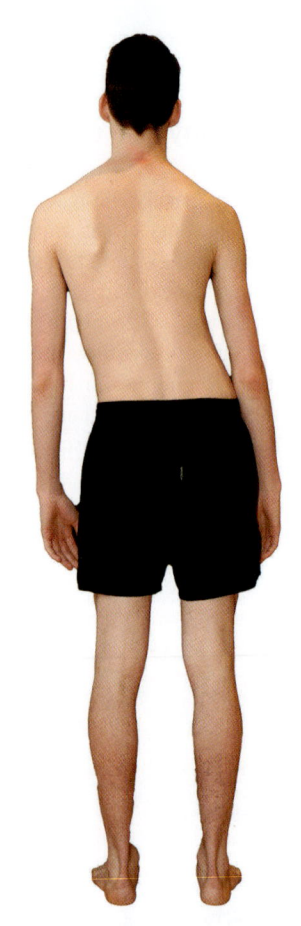

Figure 29.10 List to the left, commonly associated with pain on the right

over a 3–6 month period of time. The 2-year outcomes for surgical compared to non-surgical interventions are the same.[134] However, any deterioration in bladder function or neurological deficits must be monitored and reported immediately for investigation and surgical review.

In the acute phase (1–5 days), if pain is severe, adopting positions of maximum comfort with administration of analgesics and NSAIDs is indicated. The patient should minimise sitting and keep active with gentle walking. In the absence of nerve compression (neurological signs), gentle spine mobility exercises such as extension and/or rotation exercises (Fig 29.11) may provide pain relief and if so should be commenced as soon as possible. However, if exercises cause an increase in peripheral (i.e. lower extremity) symptoms and/or neurological signs, they should be ceased immediately.

Mobilisation techniques should be performed with care. Rotational positioning (Fig. 29.11) may be effective in providing pain relief. Manipulation is contraindicated in conditions with severe pain, muscle guarding and acute neurological signs and symptoms.

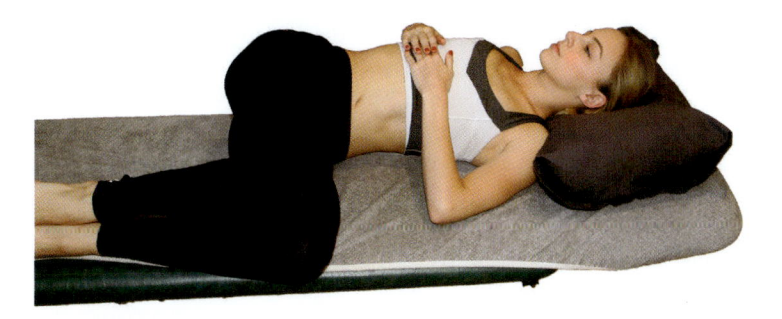

Figure 29.11 Rotation exercise for acute LBP

A transforaminal epidural injection of corticosteroid may help if there is no significant improvement in symptoms and signs with rest, and pain levels are distressing. Selective nerve root blocks using only local anaesthetic can be helpful to confirm a particular nerve root as a source for radicular leg pain. A transforaminal epidural steroid injection can be performed to provide pain relief from the implicated irritated nerve root. These injections are more specific and concentrate the medication around the nerve root as compared to interlaminar or caudal epidural steroid injections that cover a larger area yet place a more dilute injectate at each level.[135]

Epidural injections with a long-acting local anaesthetic +/− a corticosteroid are a treatment for radicular leg pain and not a treatment for LBP.[136] However, there is little research evidence for the efficacy of these procedures in chronic radicular pain.

As the acute episode settles, restoration of normal pain-free movement to the area can be assisted with localised mobilisation and gentle stretching. Following restoration of range of movement, optimising patterns of spinal control, conditioning and adjustment of sporting technique is important in order to optimise stress on spinal structures and prevent recurrence. This is discussed later in this chapter.

Spinal surgery should only be considered when nerve root compression results in persistent: bladder or bowel symptoms, progressive sensory or motor abnormalities, or where radicular pain is intractable despite adequate conservative management. Various surgical options exist including microsurgical decompression, open laminectomy or percutaneous discectomy using a needle aspiration technique.

While complications are rare, it is important for the clinician to advise the patient of the potential risks for each of the interventions just discussed, which include infection, bleeding, worsening pain, allergic reaction, vascular and neural injury, as well as intravascular injection.[135]

Vertebral endplate oedema (Modic type 1 changes)

A patient with vertebral endplate oedema typically presents with persistent, severe and disabling localised LBP. Pain is usually constant (at rest and at night) and exacerbated with loading and movement. Diagnosis is based on MRI with finding of oedema of the vertebral endplate proximal to a degenerate disc (Fig. 29.12).

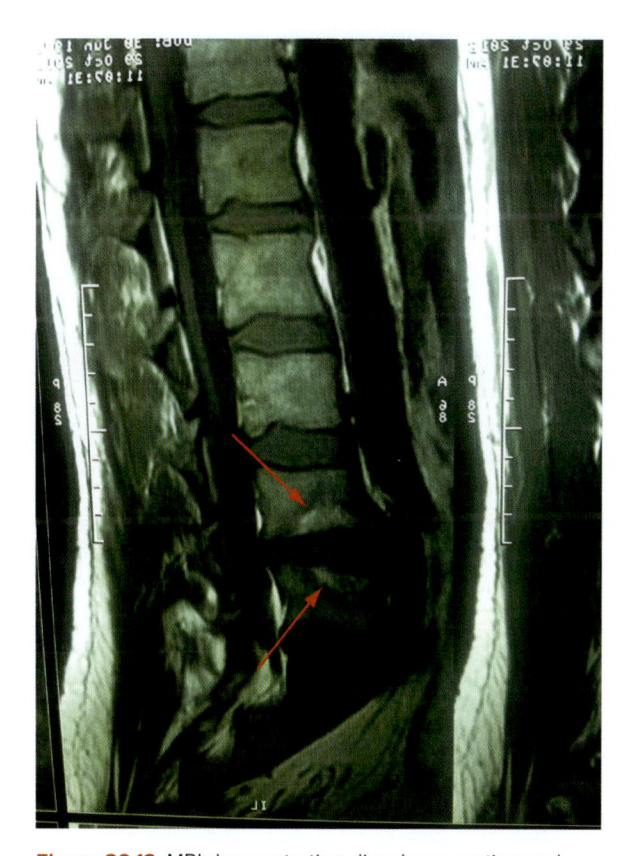

Figure 29.12 MRI demonstrating disc degeneration and moderate intensity signal Modic type 1 changes (arrows)

547

Treatment

Management is consistent with other LBP disorders (outlined in the next section) and involves addressing the relevant extrinsic and intrinsic risk physical factors, as well as lifestyle and psychosocial factors in conjunction with medical management (anti-inflammatory medication). A period of relative unloading from sport, combined with regular unloaded cardiovascular exercise (water- based/ exercise bike), is usually required to allow the inflammatory process to settle, followed by a gradual return to sport. The natural history is good.

There is some preliminary evidence to suggest that these MRI findings, when presenting secondary to a disc prolapse, may represent an underlying low-grade infection. One randomised controlled trial (RCT) reported benefit with treating this using broad-spectrum antibiotics, although replication trials are required to confirm this.[137]

MANAGEMENT OF NON-SPECIFIC LBP DISORDERS

Once the patient has been triaged to exclude serious and specific pathology (Fig. 29.2), treating the symptom of pain when it is acute, severe and distressing is very important. However, there is growing evidence to support that targeting the modifiable beliefs and behaviours that drive pain and disability may be more effective than simply treating the symptom of pain in order to achieve long-term changes and especially where LBP is persistent and/or recurrent.[16, 138]

An integrated person-centred, goal-orientated management approach for LBP is adapted to the time course and complexity of the patient's profile. The focus of this process is directed by the findings taken from the examination with regard to the primary contributing factors, across the different domains, linked to the patient's disorder.

> **PRACTICE PEARL**
>
> Developing a strong clinical alliance underpins the therapeutic process. Effective communication encompassing therapist empathy, active listening, responsiveness, validation of the patient, confidence, warmth and friendliness are central to clinical outcomes.

Any management approach in the athlete must be applied in discussion with the coach and in consideration of managing training loads.

Clinical approach
Effective patient education

As LBP can often be distressing and associated with increased fear, catastrophising, vigilance, anxiety and worry, providing the athlete with a clear understanding of the underlying mechanisms linked to the disorder and directions for treatment and management is central to any intervention. This may involve:

- providing effective patient-centred education regarding the multidimensional mechanisms that drive their pain and disability, as well as clear expectations for prognosis and management
- education regarding the influence of beliefs, fear, vigilance, levels of mood, anxiety, stress, worry, sleep deficits and levels of fatigue on pain physiology
- addressing negative beliefs and fear regarding pain with positive information regarding the spine's resilience and providing epidemiological advice regarding MRI findings if relevant[21]
- education regarding the importance of optimal motor control, body relaxation and conditioning, and the interplay this has with sports-specific biomechanical demands and training loads to influence tissue strain and sensitivity
- promoting active coping strategies for pain and installing confidence
- facilitating goal-orientated behavioural change regarding stress management, sleep, physical activity, pacing and diet
- feedback, which is critical and involves:
  mindfulness of the body's responses to pain and
  visual feedback with the use of mirrors, video and written instruction.

> **PRACTICE PEARL**
>
> Effective, evidence-based patient education and targeted reassurance is a treatment in its own right. (See also Chapter 5 which underscores that explaining pain is a treatment in its own right.)

Pain relief

There is strong evidence that symptomatic treatments for LBP (such as manual therapy, soft tissue therapy, needling, spinal injections and pharmacology), while providing a window of short-term pain relief, have little impact on the long-term trajectories of LBP. Therefore, these treatments need to be closely integrated with active management strategies that address the relevant biopsychosocial factors identified in the examination. They should be seen as creating a window of opportunity to enhance functional capacity, but should not be relied on as a treatment in itself. Furthermore, creating a reliance on passive therapies may be unhelpful in the long term as it likely reduces the patient's levels of self-efficacy and internal locus of control.

Functional restoration

Restoration of full range of relaxed spinal movement is the first priority. Once this has been achieved, then pain-provocative postural and movement patterns and protective behaviours are identified (specific to the individual), broken down into component parts and retrained in a mindful and relaxed manner in order to provide strategies that enable the athlete to actively control their pain during functional tasks (see later section).

These 'new' postural and movement patterns are gradually targeted towards the activities and movements that provoke pain and/or are avoided by the patient in order to reduce the threat value of the task and normalise it. These 'new' patterns are then integrated into the patient's daily life and sporting activities in a graduated manner. Targeted strengthening and conditioning is incorporated as required by the functional goals of the patient and the specific demands of the sport.

Addressing lifestyle aspects

Addressing lifestyle factors such as sleep hygiene, body–mind relaxation (using meditation techniques), activity pacing, healthy diet, reducing sedentary behaviours, alcohol consumption and drug taking where relevant is also important.[17]

Multidisciplinary care

In situations where pain is severe and a barrier to rehabilitation, integrating care with medical management may be indicated. Where psychological comorbidities dominate, combined psychological management may be required.

Acute severe low back pain

Acute severe LBP associated with a clear history of a significant sudden or repeated high-level biomechanical loading of the lumbar spine, where there is no sign of disc prolapse and radiculopathy or risk of fracture, should be considered an acute tissue strain. The pain response may involve local sensitisation and an inflammatory sequel related to affected spinal structures, which may involve the vertebral endplate, intervertebral disc, zygapophyseal joints and/or associated ligamentous structures.

> **PRACTICE PEARL**
>
> As clinical examination cannot accurately determine the specific source of pain, a 'structure specific' diagnosis cannot be made with any confidence. Reassuring the athlete that these 'tissue strains', while very painful, have an excellent natural history if managed well, is important.

However, it must also be noted that severity of symptoms and levels of distress for acute LBP are often a poor indicator of levels of tissue damage, and acute pain may also reflect the level of underlying tissue sensitisation

and contextual distress of the individual. This may be characterised by an athlete who presents with acute pain and distress linked to a minor mechanical loading event or an insidious onset of pain. Careful questioning commonly identifies high levels of contextual stress, anxiety or mood fluctuations coupled with lifestyle factors (such as sleep deficits and fatigue) as precipitating factors in these presentations.

These disorders should not be treated as an 'injury', with care being directed to reassure the person that they aren't 'damaged', but that their spinal structures are sensitised by contextual factors in their life. These disorders usually settle quickly with confident management that targets reassurance, body relaxation and functional restoration while addressing contextual stress and lifestyle-related factors. Careful correlation between the history of pain (i.e. injury mechanism/s), lifestyle factors, contextual stresses, psychosocial screening and disability levels can help differentiate these groups.

Clinical features

The patient presents with high ratings of pain and disability of sudden onset. The pain is usually in the lower lumbar area, but it may radiate to the buttocks, hamstrings or lower leg, and is somatic in nature, with the patient complaining of a deep-seated ache. The patient with acute, sudden onset of LBP often adopts a fixed, guarded position and movements are severely restricted. Palpation of the lumbar spine reveals areas of marked tenderness with associated muscle spasm.

Management

Successful management of acute severe low back pain requires education, pain control and progressive rehabilitation to permit the patient to regain function.

Education

Once triage has been completed to rule our serious and specific pathology, educate the patient that pain is associated with acute sensitisation of spinal structures. Reinforce that levels of pain do not equate well to degree of damage and that a severe pain experience can be related to sensitisation of spinal structures, amplified by sleep deficits, contextual stress, lower mood, heightened anxiety, fear and muscle guarding, and so on. Keeping the athlete calm, relaxed and positive is central to effective management. Reassure the patient that these disorders are very painful, but self-limiting and with an excellent natural history.[21]

Pain control and functional restoration

Initially, encourage the patient to adopt the position of most comfort and relax using diaphragm breathing. This position is often supine crook lying depending on the

PART B Regional problems

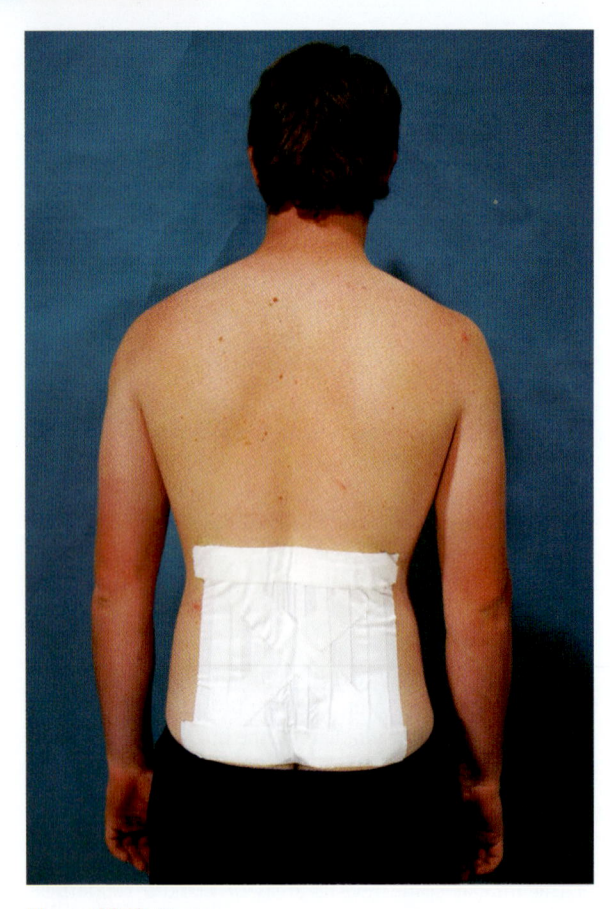

Figure 29.13 Taping

patient's pattern of sensitisation. Following this, these management strategies may be helpful:

- Movements that aggravate pain should initially be limited, whereas movements that reduce or minimise pain should be encouraged.
- Relative rest in the position of most comfort may be continued for up to 48 hours if pain is severe and disabling and related to biomechanical loading. Bed rest longer than 48 hours has been shown to be detrimental.[139]
- Taping of the low back (Fig. 29.13) for the first 48 hours can reduce acute back pain, provide reassurance, allow trunk muscle relaxation and allow quicker functional restoration.
- Analgesics may control the pain and reflex muscle spasm. NSAIDs may help reduce inflammation if a clear pattern of tissue injury is present.
- Exercise in a direction away from the movement that initially provoked the patient's symptoms should be commenced as early as possible.

For example, for those patients in whom lumbar flexion aggravates their symptoms (linked to flexion strain), extension exercises can be performed. The degree of extension should be determined by the level of pain sensitivity and pattern of pain provocation. Initially, lying prone may be sufficient. Later, extension of the lumbar spine by pushing up onto the elbows may be possible. Eventually, further extension with straight arms can be achieved.

In patients for whom extension movements aggravate their pain (usually linked to an extension pattern of strain), flexion exercises can be performed (Fig. 29.14). For these patients, prolonged posture involving extension, such as standing with excessive lumbar lordosis, should be minimised in the acute phase (48 hours).

If a side bending or rotational strain has occurred, then rotation and side bending away from the direction of tissue strain and pain provocation can be performed.

PRACTICE PEARL

Exercises should be discontinued if peripheralisation or exacerbation of symptoms occurs (i.e. increasing pain in the lower extremity).

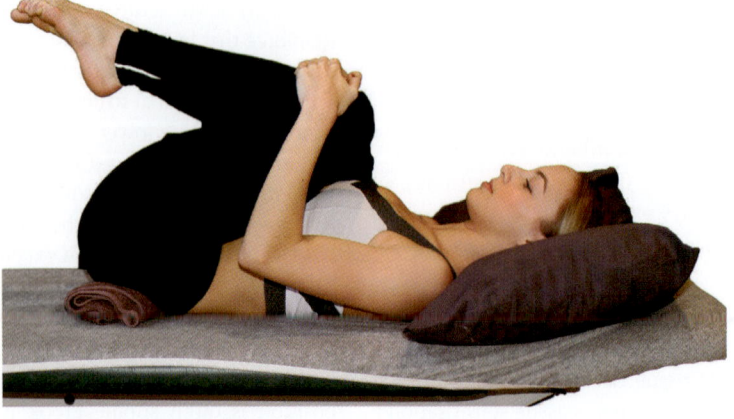

Figure 29.14 Flexion exercise

Manual therapy has a limited role in treating severe LBP where there has been a clear history of tissue trauma. Gentle mobilisation techniques, such as non-provocative physiological movements of the spine, may assist the patient to relax and move; however, the patient's response must be monitored. If there is deterioration of symptoms, mobilisation should be ceased. The mobilisation should be performed in the position of comfort adopted by the patient and in the direction of pain 'easing'.

Similarly, gentle soft tissue therapy may be helpful in relieving pain and muscle spasm. Traction has not been found to be helpful in patients with acute LBP. Manipulation should not be attempted in the presence of marked muscle spasm.

In the absence of a clear history of tissue strain, manual therapy can be very helpful to relax the person and facilitate functional restoration in a graded manner and with respect to pain.

Subacute low back pain

Once the acute phase (up to 48 hours) of severe LBP has passed with reduction in pain and muscle spasm, graduated exercise therapy can be commenced. The aim of this stage of therapy is to first restore normal relaxed spinal movement. This can be facilitated with the use of pain-relieving manual and soft tissue treatments (outlined below) in conjunction with exercise therapy.

Once normal spinal movement has been restored, this is gradually integrated into functional postures and movements of daily living with attention to confident relaxed body control and other multidimensional factors associated with the onset of the pain disorder based on their complexity profile (see below). Once the person's symptoms settle and spinal movement is normalised (usually within 1-3 weeks), then a graduated return-to-sport program is developed.

The over-arching aims are to provide a clear understanding to the patient of their disorder, enhance pain controllability and return the athlete to their desired level of activity with confidence. An exacerbation prevention and management plan is also important where recurrent back pain is a feature of the disorder. To monitor the effectiveness of the treatment, regular screening questionnaires are helpful in order to monitor levels of pain, disability and distress.

Passive treatments for low back pain

Passive treatments for LBP (where the patient is the recipient of the treatment rather than being actively involved) may be helpful where pain acts as a barrier to functional activation. These treatments can be used as a window of opportunity in the acute or subacute phase to provide pain relief, to activate the athlete. It is important for the clinician to recognise that passive therapies only provide short-term pain relief and they do not change the natural history of the disorder on their own.

Where active pain control strategies can be integrated with these treatments, such as mindfulness and relaxation techniques as well as exercise, functional activation and lifestyle modifications, they should be actively encouraged. Passive treatments should not be used in isolation and they have a limited role in recurrent and persistent LBP disorders (see below). Passive therapies include the following.

Pharmacological treatment

There is some evidence that NSAIDs are effective for short-term symptomatic relief in patients with LBP.[140] There is no evidence that one type of NSAID is more effective than another. There is no evidence to support the long-term use of NSAIDs, both in relation to their lack of effectiveness and their significant incidence of side effects. Other medications with good evidence of short-term effectiveness for pain control include skeletal muscle relaxants for acute LBP and tricyclic antidepressants for chronic LBP.[141] Gabapentin has fair evidence for effective pain relief for radicular type pain.[141]

Mobilisation and manipulation

Mobilisation and manipulation techniques may be helpful for short-term pain relief (Chapter 17) and to restore spinal movement impairments detected on examination. These techniques affect multiple structures and can be adapted to the pattern of movement impairment that presents. Mobilisation techniques used in the treatment of LBP include:

- posteroanterior (PA) central pressure (Fig. 29.15a)
- posteroanterior unilateral pressure (Fig. 29.15b)
- rotational mobilisation (Fig. 29.15c).

Posteroanterior central mobilisation and rotations are used in patients with central or bilateral pain with movement impairments into extension. Posteroanterior unilateral mobilisation and rotation mobilisation techniques may be

continued

PART B Regional problems

used for unilateral pain with sagittal and/or frontal plane movement impairments. The strength of the mobilisation technique used will depend on the level of tissue sensitivity and response to treatment. Mobilisation techniques can also be used to reassure the patient that movement is beneficial and not to be feared.

Soft tissue treatments

Tension and hypersensitivity of the myofascial structures is common with LBP and are related to pain-related muscle guarding and associated tissue hyperalgesia. This commonly involves the back muscles (lumbar multifidus and erector spinae), quadratus lumborum, abdominal wall and hip muscles (flexors, abductors and extensors). Tender focal areas of tension/'thickening' in the myofascial structures may be palpated.

Treatment of these areas with the use of soft tissue techniques and dry needling can result in short-term pain reduction and relaxation of guarded muscles. Soft tissue techniques may consist of transverse gliding, sustained longitudinal pressure on the tense bands emanating away from the most sensitive point and sustained firm pressure on the painful point (Fig. 29.16). Treatment is aimed at reducing tissue tension and sensitivity.

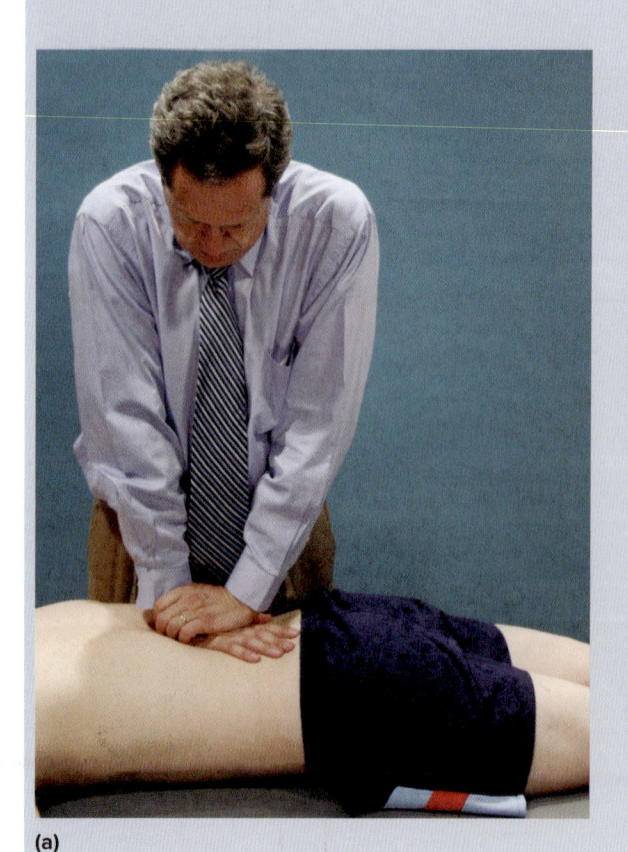

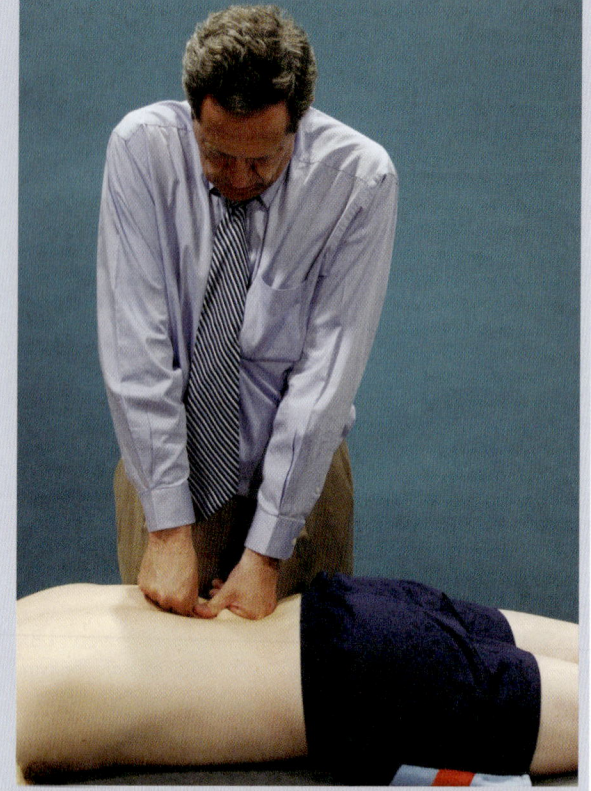

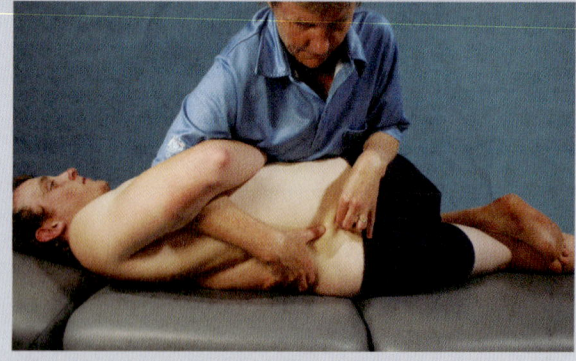

Figure 29.15 Mobilisation techniques (a) Posteroanterior central—The therapist performs an oscillating movement over the spinous processes using thumbs or heels of the hands. Elbows are extended and pressure is exerted through the shoulders and arms (b) Posteroanterior unilateral—Thumbs are placed over the apophyseal joints (c) Manipulation—rotation. With the patient positioned as shown, the therapist exerts a short sudden forward thrust on the ilium while maintaining strong counterpressure on the shoulder. This position can be used for manipulation or mobilisation

Low back pain CHAPTER 29

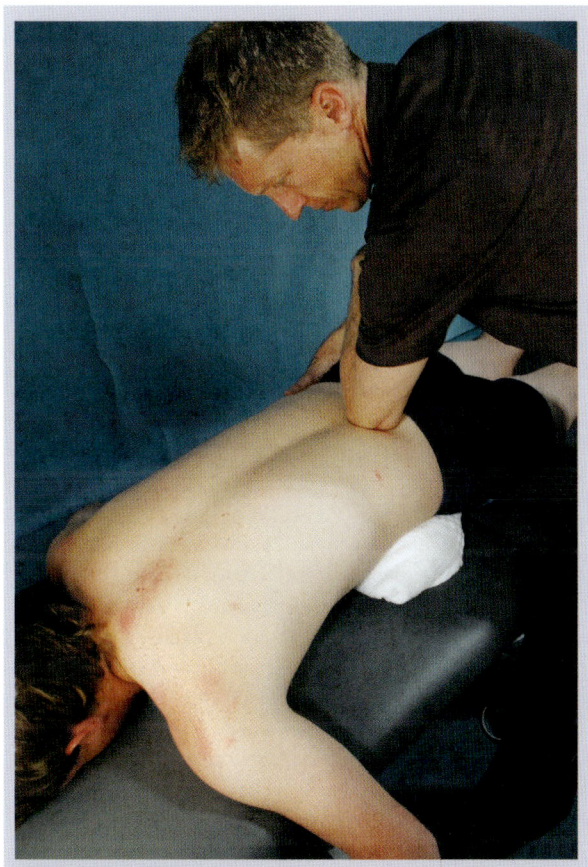

Figure 29.16 Soft tissue techniques (a) Sustained ischaemic pressure at each segmental level (b) Sustained ischaemic pressure using the knuckles to the quadratus lumborum in the position of sustained stretch

Dry needling to sensitised myofascial structures (Fig. 29.17) may also reduce pain and muscle tension in the short term, thus providing a window to facilitate the restoration of movement and function.

After treatment directed to either the articular and/or myofascial structures, the patient should be provided mobility exercises to maintain and restore the functional capacity.

Neurodynamic treatments
Neural tissue sensitisation may be linked to an LBP disorder when it is associated with peripheral referral of pain into the leg. If neural provocation tests such as the slump test and straight leg raise are limited (reflecting protective motor responses to a sensitised nerve), aggravate the patient's peripheral symptoms, and nerve palpation is associated with hyperalgesic responses, this may indicate peripheral sensitisation of the epineurial structures. Management of these pain states may respond to mobilisation of the articular and myofascial structures proximal to the nerve tissue (see above). Gentle mobilisation of the neural tissue (Fig. 29.18), if the structures are not highly sensitised, may also be

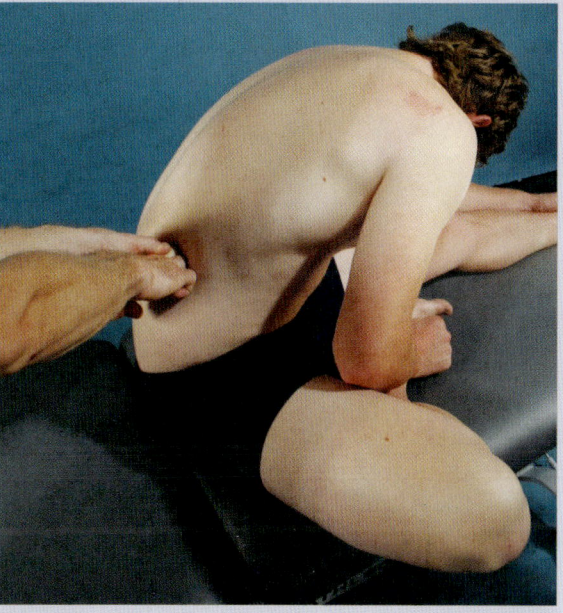

beneficial. However, 'stretching' of the nerve is **not** advisable as it may result in provocation of the disorder

Spinal injections: What is the evidence?
Where localised mechanically provoked pain persists, acting as a barrier for functional restoration, spinal injections may create a window of relief to enhance functional capacity. It must be noted that these techniques are usually short acting and so must be integrated with cognitive functional restoration programs. Some clinicians argue that this should occur once the pain has become chronic (i.e. 3-month duration) while others argue that interventional techniques may aid in the identification of the pain generator and may help expedite the athlete's recovery.[135]

When compared to target-specific diagnoses achieved through accurate local anaesthetic injections done under image intensifier, our ability to make a specific diagnosis using clinical skill or imaging is very limited.

Structures that may become sensitised with LBP are:

- zygapophyseal joints
- intervertebral discs

continued

553

PART B Regional problems

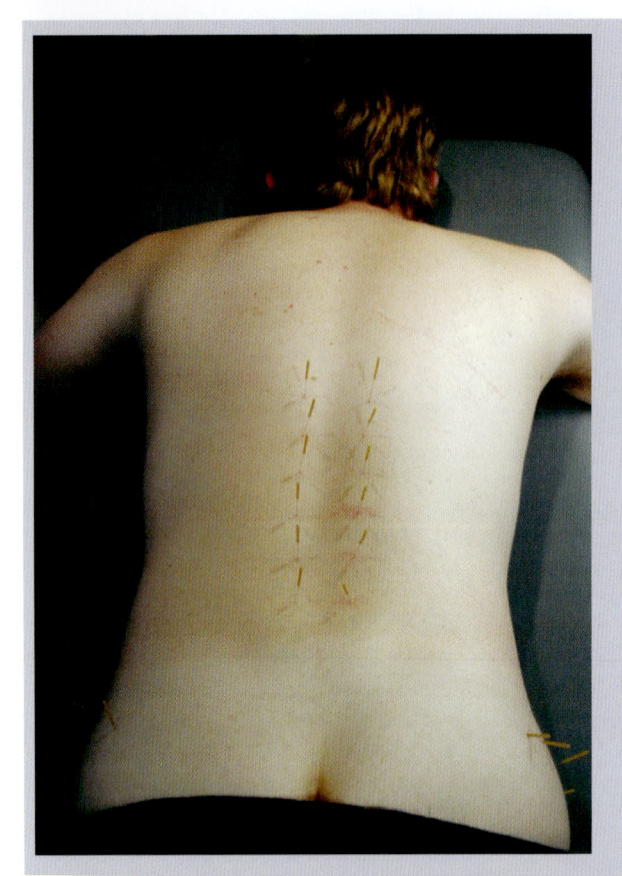

Figure 29.17 Dry needling of trigger points in the paraspinal and gluteal muscles

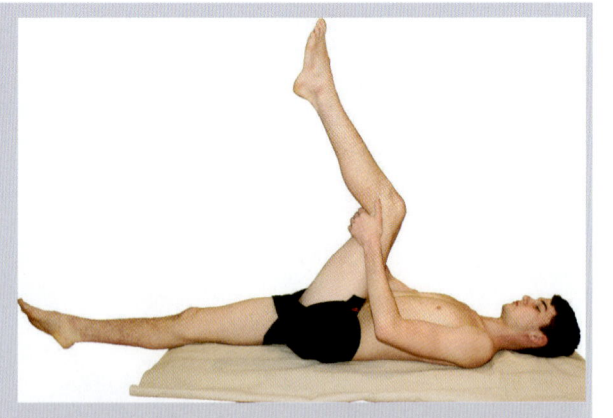

Figure 29.18 Gentle mobilisation of the neural tissue

- sacroiliac joints
- nerve root sensitisation (i.e. pain radiating into the lower extremity without neurological signs).

These areas may be diagnosed and at times treated by the use of specific interventions outlined below.

Zygapophyseal joint pain can be diagnosed with medial branch blocks as the medial branches of the dorsal rami of the spinal nerves above and below the joint innervate each lumbar zygapophyseal joint. These procedures involve using an image intensifier to place a needle onto the appropriate medial branches that supply a zygapophyseal joint and injecting local anaesthetic onto the nerve. To block one joint, two nerves must be blocked; to block two adjacent joints, three nerves must be blocked. The patient then completes a pain chart and if the pain goes away for the duration of the anaesthetic, the clinician can be approximately 60% sure of the diagnosis. A second block with a different local anaesthetic is then done. If there is concordant pain relief, then the diagnostic confidence is approaching 90%.[142]

If the two medial branch blocks confirm the pain generator is the zygapophyseal joint, a radiofrequency neurotomy procedure can be performed. Radiofrequency neurotomy utilises an electrical current to ablate the medial branches to provide long-term symptom relief from zygapophyseal joint mediated pain.[135] This technique has a 90% chance of 60% pain relief and a 60% chance of 90% pain relief for lumbar zygapophyseal pain.[143] Note that zygapophyseal joint injections lack diagnostic and therapeutic validity.

Diagnostic criteria for *discogenic pain* are not clearly defined.[135] While discography is available and often used to aid in the diagnosis of discogenic pain, it lacks diagnostic validity and reliability.[144] Additionally, clinicians should be aware that discography can lead to accelerated progression of degenerative changes and carries a significant risk of infection.[145, 146] Several interventional options have been proposed to treat discogenic pain including nucleoplasty, corticosteroid injection, anaesthetic injection and intradiscal electrothermal therapy (IDET). However, there is little quality evidence to support these interventions.[135]

Sacroiliac joint pain can be diagnosed with a sacroiliac joint injection of anaesthetic performed with image guidance. With a control block, diagnostic confidence can approach 90%. An injection of anaesthetic and corticosteroid into the sacroiliac joint can provide symptomatic relief. Additionally, radiofrequency neurotomy can be performed for sacroiliac joint mediated pain with evidence for a 60% chance of more than 50% pain relief and with a 30% chance of 90% pain relief.[147] While some people advocate prolotherapy for sacroiliac joint problems, evidence for this is currently inconclusive.

Selective *nerve root blocks* using only local anaesthetic can be helpful to confirm a particular nerve root as a source for radicular leg pain as well as provide pain relief as stated earlier (radicular pain with nerve compression section).

Recurrent/persistent low back pain: a clinical sub-grouping approach

For a significant group of people (10–15%), LBP may persist beyond natural healing time following a tissue injury. For others, LBP develops insidiously and becomes persistent. This group of people together consume the majority of the healthcare resources.

> **PRACTICE PEARL**
>
> Genetic, physical (maladaptive movement patterns), neurophysiological (tissue sensitisation), psychosocial (fear, catastrophising, low self-efficacy, poor coping responses, stress, anxiety and depression) and lifestyle (sleep deficits and disruption, fatigue) are all risk factors for LBP persistence.

A combination of a person's negative thoughts and emotional and behavioural responses to pain (such as protective muscle guarding and/or avoidance) can set up a vicious cycle of pain sensitivity and disability.

Screening and identification of these factors early in the presentation of an LBP disorder is important to target treatment and prevent chronicity. Passive therapies for symptom palliation in this group should be avoided.

> **PRACTICE PEARL**
>
> Persistent LBP disorders can be broadly sub-grouped into low-, medium- and high-complexity categories (Fig. 29.2).[21, 148]

In the rest of this chapter we outline the approach to this common group of patients according to the clinical subgroupings shown in Figure 29.2.

Low-complexity profile

A large group of athletes will present with low-complexity profiles. This profile is characterised by low to moderate levels of pain and disability, and with minimum distress. They predominantly have localised LBP with proportionate pain responses linked to specific movements, postures and activities (i.e. pain is provoked with spinal movements and loading but relieved when movements are ceased). They are commonly able to continue to participate with sport and have high levels of self-efficacy and active pain coping strategies. They present as low risk on psychosocial screening questionnaires.

Factors underlying this disorder may be ongoing sensitisation of spinal structures due to sport demands and training loads coupled with intrinsic physical factors (provocative motor control patterns +/− deconditioning). This may also be coupled with other sensitising factors such as sleep disturbance or deficits and fatigue. Identification of the underlying modifiable drivers of the disorder is important for management.

Clinical presentation

Athletes with LBP complain of pain that is usually intermittent (provoked and relieved with specific postures, movements and activities), or constant only when following sustained provocative activities. Pain is relieved quickly when the provocative movement or activity ceases. The pain may be central or unilateral and is often described by the patient as a 'band across the lower back' +/− somatic pain in the buttock and/or hamstring.

On examination, impairments in spinal movement are uncommon; however, motor control impairments (patterns of movement linked to end-range strain of the lumbar spine) are usually observed. These clinical presentations are characterised by clear directional patterns of pain provocation.[12, 149] They can be identified by trained therapists and present an opportunity for targeted rehabilitation.[150, 151]

The following patterns are to illustrate the heterogeneous nature of lumbar spine motor control. While they are common clinical patterns, the clinician should not rigidly adhere to these presentations, but rather use them as a broad framework to guide management.

Active extension pain pattern

Some people with LBP present with a pattern of pain sensitivity-associated extension loading and movement activities associated with maintaining lumbar hyperlordosis with co-contraction of the back extensors and abdominal wall muscles. This is called an 'active extension pattern' where a person actively holds their back in lordosis during functional tasks (such as sitting, forward and backward bending and lifting), resulting in extension loading of sensitised spinal structures (Fig. 29.19). This is also often associated with an inability to relax the back muscles during forward bending in standing and sitting.[13]

These pain disorders may be exacerbated with loaded squat exercises in the gym, and sports that involve spine extension coupled with side bending and extension such as tennis, fast bowling in cricket, throwing sports, swimming, running, dance and gymnastics. These patterns may be associated with conditioning deficits of the posterior hip muscles (gluteal and hamstrings) as well as tension of the hip flexors, resulting in anterior pelvic rotation. Spinal repositioning deficits in these cases demonstrate a tendency to reposition into lumbar extension from neutral.

On palpation, these presentations are commonly associated with increased muscle tension of the back muscles and quadratus lumborum and a lack of flexibility of the hip flexors. They report relief with lumbar flexion postures and movements.

PART B   Regional problems

(a) Active extension pattern-pain provoked with lumbar extension movements and loading

(b) Active extension pattern-corrected

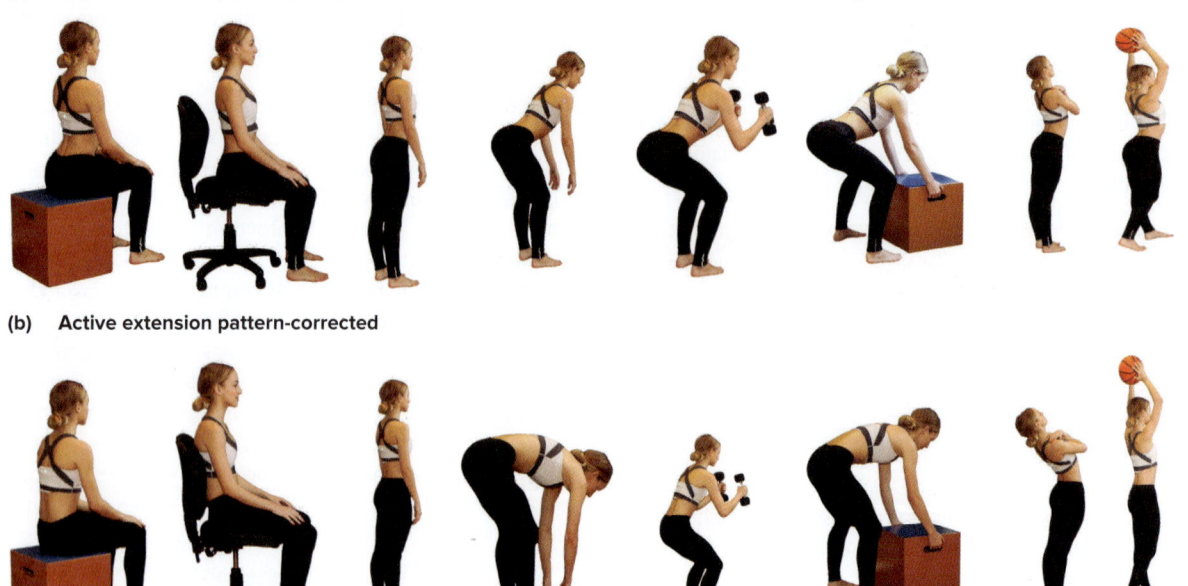

Figure 29.19 Active extension pattern (a) An 'active extension pattern' where a person actively holds their back in lordosis during functional tasks (such as sitting, forward and backward bending and lifting), resulting in extension loading of sensitised spinal structures (b) Correcting the active extension pattern with focus on posterior rotation of the pelvis and relaxation of the back extensor muscles, in order to reduce extension loading

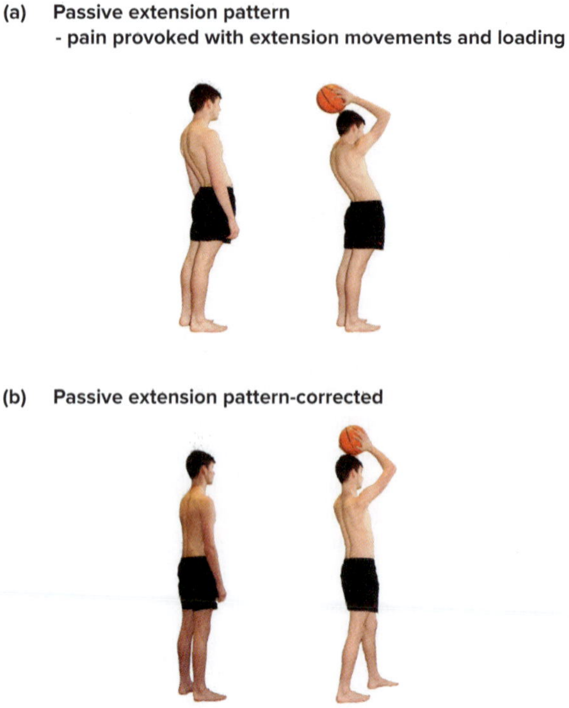

(a) Passive extension pattern
    - pain provoked with extension movements and loading

(b) Passive extension pattern-corrected

Passive extension pain pattern

The other presentation related to extension pain sensitivity is associated with a sway posture in standing and a tendency to hinge through the lower lumbar spine, while maintaining the thoracic spine in flexion, during backward bending (Fig. 29.20). This results in focal stress to the lower lumbar spine and is commonly associated with the sports that involve backward bending, especially throwing sports, ballet and gymnastics and/or sports that involve overhead arm activities (such as tennis and throwing sports).

These cases often present with conditioning deficits of the iliopsoas and thoracic erector spinae muscles, and poor eccentric control of the upper abdominal wall muscles (tendency to maintain thoracic flexion). Spinal repositioning deficits in these cases demonstrate a tendency to reposition into thoracic flexion.

On palpation, these presentations are commonly associated with increased muscle tension of the upper

Figure 29.20 Passive extension pattern (a) Sway posture in standing and a tendency to hinge through the lower lumbar spine, while maintaining the thoracic spine in flexion, during backward bending (b) Correcting their sway posture with thoracic extension and upper abdominal wall relaxation, during standing and backward bending

abdominal wall muscles. They report relief with lumbar flexion and when correcting their sway posture with thoracic extension and upper abdominal wall relaxation, during standing and backward bending (i.e. to reduce lower lumbar extension) (Fig. 29.20).

Flexion pain pattern

In other cases, where LBP has a flexion pattern of pain sensitivity, this is associated with a tendency to initiate forward bending and lifting from the lower back while fixing the pelvis into posterior rotation. This may either be associated with thoracolumbar flexion or lower lumbar flexion with thoracolumbar extension and upper abdominal wall activation (Fig. 29.21).[12, 13, 152] This results in flexion loading stress to the lumbar spine and is associated with activities such as loaded squats in the gym and sports such as cycling, rowing and field hockey.

These cases often present with conditioning deficits of the hip flexors and lumbar back extensors and over-activation of the trunk flexors during bending activities. Spinal repositioning deficits in these cases demonstrate a tendency to reposition into lumbar flexion from neutral. On palpation, these presentations are commonly associated with increased tension, loss of eccentric relaxation and/or loss of flexibility of the gluteal and hamstring muscles.

Lateral pain pattern

In other cases, LBP is associated with pain sensitivity related to lateral loading and spinal movements in the frontal plane. These presentations are associated with frontal plane motor control deficits of the hip (Trendelenburg) and/or thoracolumbar (lateral shift), which results in lateral loading strain to the low back (Fig. 29.22). These cases often present with conditioning deficits of the hip abductor (gluteal) muscles on the side of pain. Spinal repositioning deficits in these cases demonstrate a tendency to reposition into a lateral shifted position.

On palpation, these presentations are commonly associated with increased tension of the quadratus and lateral abdominal wall muscles on the side of pain. These presentations are common in sports related to limb loading such as running and jumping, landing sports.

Rotational plane pain pattern

In other cases, LBP is associated with pain sensitivity related to rotational movement and activities. This may be seen in sports such as tennis, golf and hockey. In many cases, these pain disorders are linked to control deficits in other planes (i.e. active extension, flexion, frontal plane). Lumbar spine rotation is more limited when the spine is at the end range of flexion, extension or side bending, and therefore the addition of rotation to end-range sagittal postures may increase spinal loading to the lumbar spine (Fig. 29.23).

In other cases, rotational strain may be placed on the spine due to a dynamic impairment of hip or thoracic spine rotation, resulting in increased rotational strain being placed on the lumbar spine. Assessment of the relative flexibility and control through the whole kinetic chain is important when assessing these disorders.

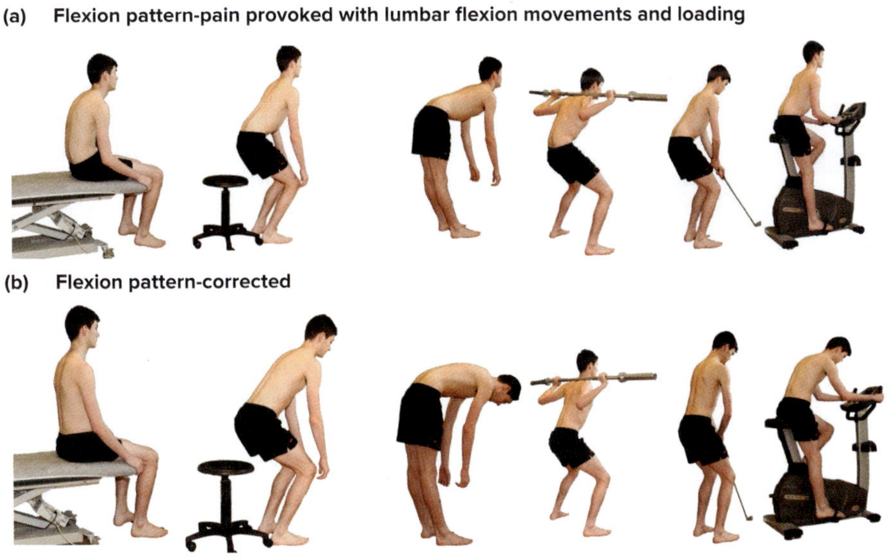

Figure 29.21 Flexion pattern (a) Lower lumbar flexion with thoracolumbar extension and upper abdominal wall activation resulting in flexion loading (b) Correction of the flexion pattern via anterior pelvic tilt and relaxation of the thoracic spine into more flexed posture

PART B   Regional problems

(a)   Lateral control pattern-pain provoked with lateral lumbar movements and loading

(b)   Lateral control pattern-corrected

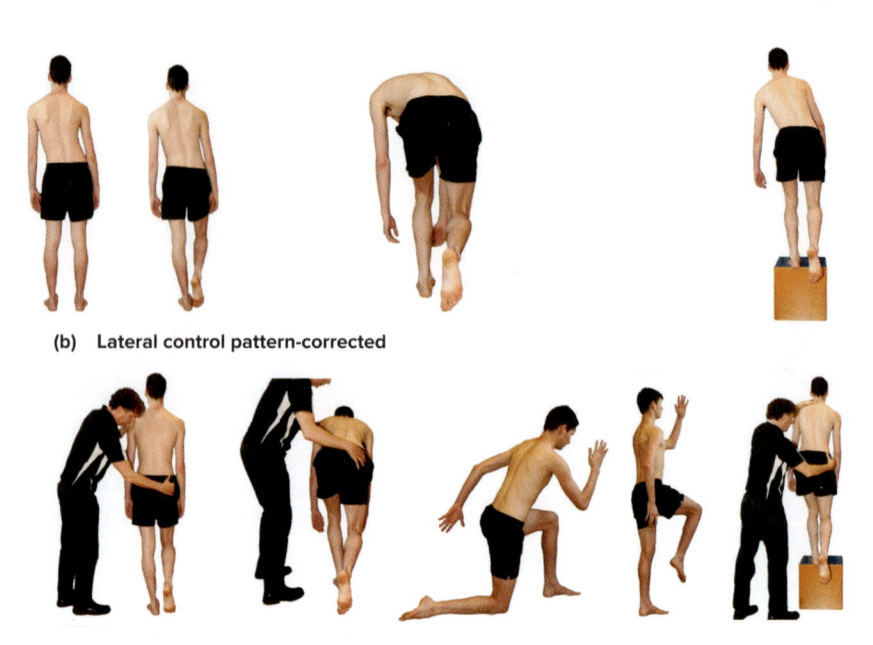

Figure 29.22 Lateral control pattern (a) Lateral pain pattern associated with frontal plane motor control deficits of the hip (Trendelenburg) and/or thoracolumbar (lateral shift), which results in lateral loading strain to the low back (b) Correction of the frontal plane control focuses on gluteal activation and correction of the Trendelenburg and/or lateral shift

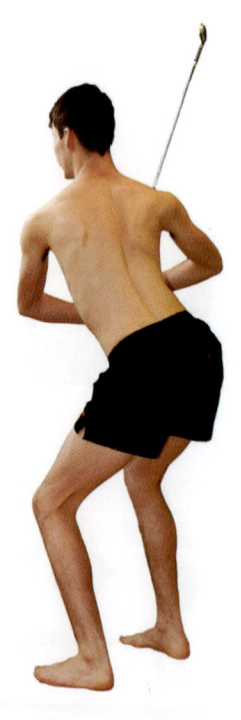

Figure 29.23 The addition of rotation to end-range sagittal postures (e.g. extension) may increase lumbar spine loading (image exaggerated for illustrative purposes)

Multidirectional pain pattern
In other cases, LBP may present where the spine is sensitive to movement in more than one plane (i.e. flexion, extension, rotational or lateral). This may be associated with high levels of underlying tissue sensitivity and related to a combination of various motor control strategies as described previously (i.e. passive extension and flexion pattern). These people may have difficulty finding a pain-relieving movement direction (Fig. 29.24). Neutral spine positions with trunk muscle relaxation may provide some relief. Spinal repositioning deficits in these cases demonstrate a tendency to overshoot in different directions and these are often associated with high levels of thoracic muscle co-contraction (abdominal wall and back muscles).

Management
Management of these disorders involves targeting the cognitive, physical and lifestyle factors underlying the disorder.[16, 138] The cognitive aspects of the intervention involve educating the athlete regarding the factors associated with LBP and providing reassurance regarding the spine's resilience. Manual therapy is only used if movement impairments are present and provide a barrier to functional activation.

Functional rehabilitation strategies are directed by the clinical presentation of the athlete as outlined below. Motor control training is integrated with the use of

Low back pain CHAPTER 29

(a) **Multi-directional pattern (passive extension and flexion)**
- pain provoked with lumbar flexion and extension movements and loading

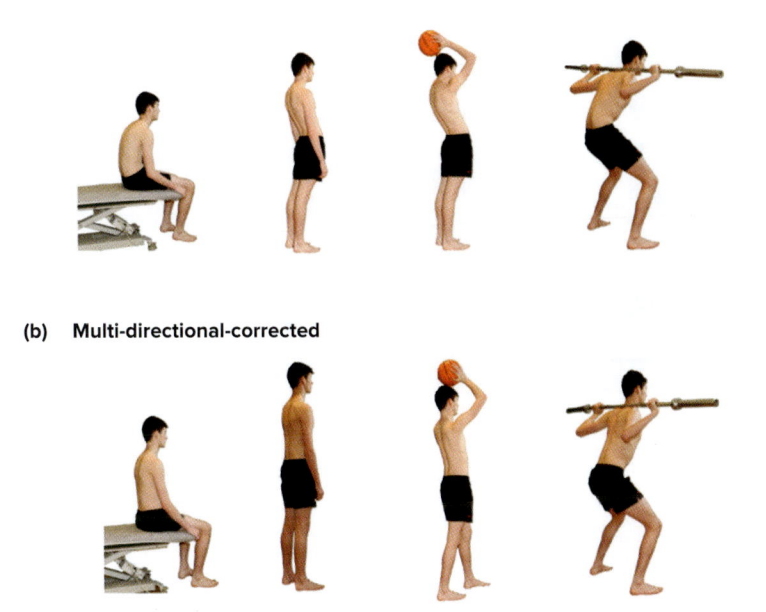

(b) **Multi-directional-corrected**

Figure 29.24 Multidirectional pattern (a) Pattern associated with pain provoked in more than one direction. In this case, a combination of both passive extension and flexion control patterns is observed (b) Correction of these patterns

mirrors and video so the athlete has a clear understanding of how they move. Postural correction should always reduce their LBP during provocative tasks.

The training is then integrated back into conditioning and sports-specific programs. Modifying training volume and technical aspects of the sport may be important to integrate with this. Lifestyle factors are also addressed when present.

Active extension pain pattern

The athlete is provided strategies to reduce their lumbar lordosis with posterior pelvic rotation exercises (initiated via the posterior hip muscles and not the abdominal wall). This may first be taught in supine crook lying and progressed to sitting to reduce anterior tilt and relax their back muscles. This is then progressed into sit-to-stand and squat positions (Fig. 29.19). In standing, posterior pelvic tilt is instructed in order to reduce the lumbar lordosis. If the athlete is unable to relax their back and/or hip muscles, then soft tissue work (Fig. 29.25a) and muscle stretching can be carried out (Fig. 29.25b).

These patterns are then integrated into conditioning-based exercises (squat and single-leg squat exercise) with weights that target the gluteal muscles, as well as sports-specific exercises (training forward and backward bending) (Fig. 29.19).

Passive extension pain pattern

The athlete is provided strategies to correct their postural sway in standing by increasing their thoracic and upper lumbar lordosis with control of the pelvis augmented with the posterior hip muscles. If the athlete is unable to relax their upper abdominal wall and extend their thoracic spine, then soft tissue work directed to the upper abdominal wall can be used, and lateral costal diaphragm breathing exercise integrated with thoracic spine extension mobilisation techniques (Fig. 29.20).

Squatting is trained with thoracic extension and neutral lordosis. Backward bending is trained by facilitating upper lumbar and thoracic extension with hip extension in order to reduce focal extension stress. These movement patterns are then integrated with conditioning exercises that target postural control in a sport-specific exercise, with mirror feedback as appropriate.

Flexion pain pattern

The athlete is provided strategies to reduce lumbar flexion with anterior pelvic rotation exercises. This may first be taught in supine crook lying and progressed to sitting in order to facilitate anterior tilt without over-activation of the thoracic erector spinae and abdominal wall. This is then progressed into sit-to-stand and squat positions facilitating the movement with anterior pelvic rotation and a relaxed thoracic spine (Fig. 29.21).

These movement patterns are then integrated into conditioning-based exercises that reinforce these motor patterns (Fig. 29.21), as well as sports-specific exercises.

559

PART B   Regional problems

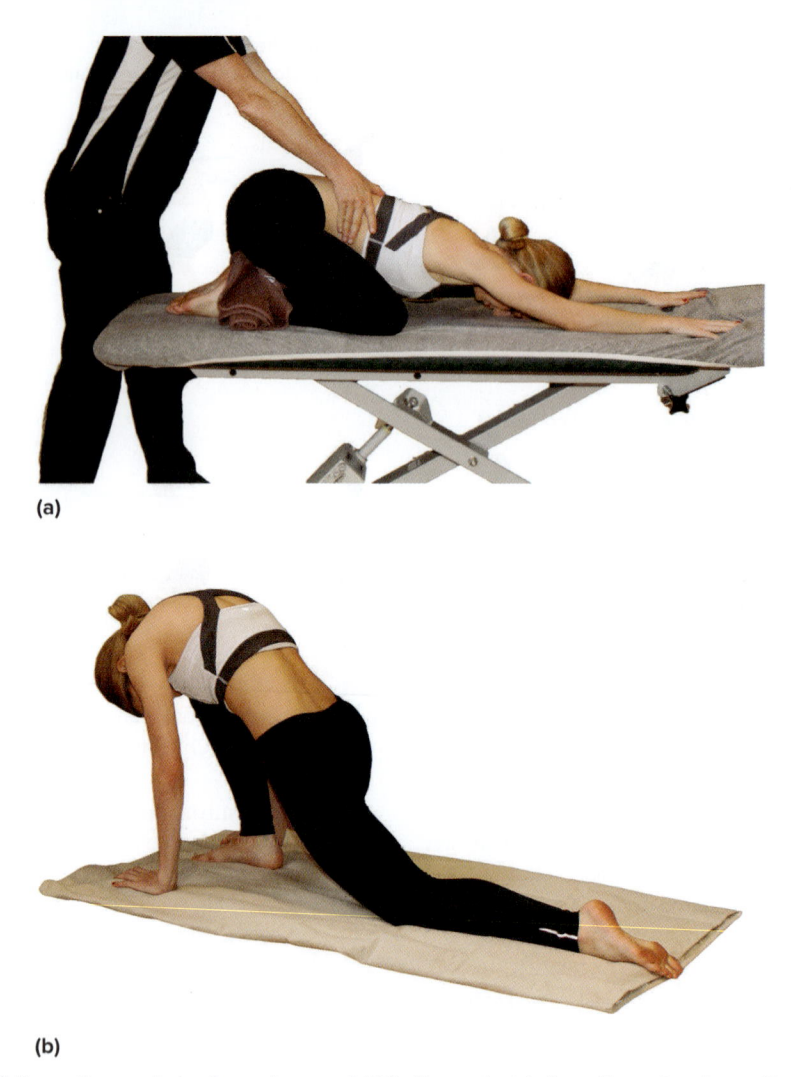

Figure 29.25 (a) Soft tissue therapy to lumbar extensors (b) Hip flexor stretch for active extension pattern

Utilising this cognitive functional approach has been found to be effective in rowers with flexion-related LBP.[16]

Lateral pain pattern
The athlete is provided strategies to control their frontal plane postural control in sitting, sit to stand and standing by centring their head position in relation to the pelvis. This is progressed to single-leg standing (with or without support), single-leg squatting with careful attention to control of the hip/pelvis (preventing Trendelenburg pattern) as well as the thoracolumbar spine alignment relative to the pelvis (nose in line with navel). Training can be integrated with conditioning exercises that target single-leg loading and load transfer, progressing towards dynamic loading and sports-specific exercises (Fig. 29.22).

Rotational plane pain pattern
The athlete is provided strategies to control their spine during provocative rotational movements. In some cases, this may involve adjustments to spinal posture as outlined earlier (Fig. 29.23). In other cases, this involves addressing impairments of movement of thoracic rotation (usually linked to co-contraction of the oblique abdominal wall muscles). This involves teaching relaxed thoracic spine rotation with breathing control (lateral costal breathing) during rolling, sitting, standing and functional rotational tasks. Where there is an impairment of hip rotation, addressing this with soft tissue work stretching and then active functional integration is trained. This can then be integrated into conditioning-based exercises with the use of pulleys.

Multidirectional pain pattern

The nature of the training is an integration of any of the previously mentioned motor control strategies dependent on the athlete's presentation (Fig. 29.24). For example, this may involve training the control of both the forward and backward bending movement and single-leg loading (see Fig. 29.2, central pillar). This is integrated into functional and conditioning programs as required.

Medium-complexity profile

A moderate number of athletes will present with medium-complexity profiles. (See Fig. 29.2, central pillar.)

Clinical presentation

This sub-group profile is characterised by moderate levels of pain, disability and distress. These athletes often avoid sporting activities due to pain. They may have a mixed pain picture with both pain at rest and with mechanical loading of the spine. Negative cognitive factors are dominant in these disorders such as negative beliefs (i.e. 'my discs are crumbling'), high levels of fear (i.e. 'I am too frightened to dance'), catastrophising (i.e. 'I think my back will collapse', 'it will never get better'), hypervigilance (i.e. 'I can't stop thinking about my back pain'), low levels of self-efficacy (i.e. 'I don't have any way to control the pain', 'I can't play sport with the pain'). They may also report high levels of contextual stress (i.e. 'my current stress levels are 7–8/10').

These cognitive factors are related to pain amplification,[153] and in some may be linked to high levels of protective muscle guarding, slow cautious movement patterns and protective movement behaviours (i.e. bracing of the hands on the thigh with bending, breath holding, avoidance of limb loading). These movement behaviours are usually superimposed upon the movement patterns described under the low-complexity profile. With high levels of fear, it is common to see movement impairments (loss of functional range of movement), reflected in high levels of trunk muscle guarding associated with feared movement direction (Fig. 29.26).

In other cases, the level of distress may be disproportionate to the clinical presentation (i.e. high levels of pain and distress, but with pain-free movement and functional activity, no tissue hyperalgesia but pain with attention and at rest).[154] Lifestyle factors such as high levels of contextual stress, activity avoidance and poor sleep hygiene are common. These athletes present as medium risk on screening questionnaires.

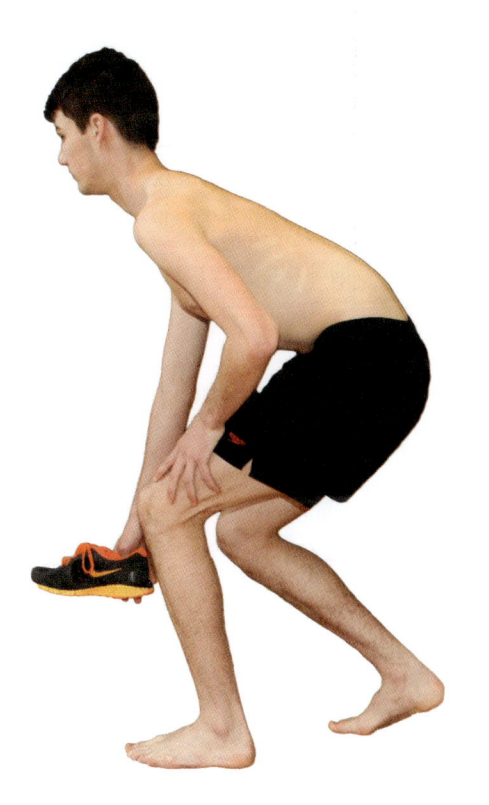

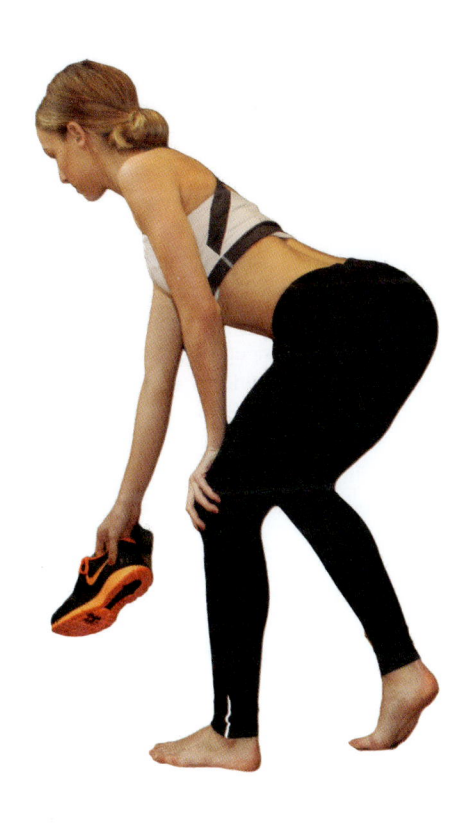

Figure 29.26 Protective patterns (a) Protective pattern with thoracic extension and bracing of the hand (b) Protective pattern with lumbar extension and bracing of the hand

Management

Education regarding the multidimensional factors associated with LBP is essential for the person to understand that their LBP is not related to 'damage', but due to sensitised spinal structures related to negative thoughts, fears and pain-related behavioural responses. Reassurance regarding the spine's resilience is essential.

> **PRACTICE PEARL**
>
> High levels of fear and catastrophising are addressed through education as well as providing the athlete with pain-control strategies such as relaxation, mindfulness techniques and graded movement training in a relaxed manner back towards fear activities where this is a barrier.

This is directed by their pain-related movement profile as outlined in the low-complexity group. (See also Fig. 29.2.)

Where movement impairments prevent functional activation, manual therapy and soft tissue techniques can be used to relax guarded muscles, so as to reinforce that spinal movement can be trusted. The athlete is gradually exposed to the feared movement pattern (i.e. fear of lumbar flexion is initially trained in supine with posterior pelvic tilt, hip flexion, lumbar flexion in stand and then progressed to standing). Once motor control patterns have been normalised, these are gradually integrated back into conditioning programs and then into the person's sport.

Where there is an absence of clinical signs linked to the patient's LBP, it is critical to reassure the athlete to reduce their focus on the back and trust the resilience of the spine. Manual therapies and specific exercises that direct attention to the back in these cases may be unhelpful.

Addressing lifestyle factors such as stress management (meditation techniques), sleep hygiene, alcohol intake and minimising sedentary behaviours is also important where indicated. Graduated physical activation is also central to this process where this has been avoided, and ideally this should be linked to their sport. This may require a graduated, paced process to recovery to avoid a boom–bust activity pattern.

High-complexity profile

A small group of athletes present with high-complexity profiles. (See Fig. 29.2, right column.)

Clinical presentation

This profile is characterised by moderate to high levels of pain, disability and distress. They will almost certainly be avoiding sporting and social activities due to their pain, or be exercising obsessively with pain. They usually have a mixed pain picture and may present as widespread and constant pain that is exacerbated with minimal movement provocation. Consequently, they may easily flare up with minimal physical examination.

The other presentation as outlined earlier is the complaint that pain is distressing, but with an absence of clinical findings. In this profile pain is often worse at rest and when focused on, and better when moving and distracted. This profile is often linked to underlying anxiety and hypervigilance. These athletes also commonly report comorbid pains (headaches, migraine, stomach pain) as well as nonspecific health complaints (i.e. fatigue, lack of energy).

These athletes present with similar negative cognitive factors as outlined in the medium-complexity profile, (i.e. negative beliefs, high levels of fear, stress, hypervigilance, low self-efficacy and poor coping). They commonly have catastrophic beliefs about their pain (i.e. 'my pelvis is out', 'my disc is stuffed') coupled with high levels of perceptual body distortion. In addition, these athletes present with high levels of emotional distress, heightened anxiety levels and depressed mood. It is important to screen as to whether the athlete has a diagnosed comorbid anxiety and/or depressive disorder and if so whether this is being actively managed. These presentations usually present with maladaptive functional behaviours, muscle guarding and avoidance as outlined in the medium-complexity profile. This may also be coupled with hyperarousal (apical rapid breathing, agitation, sweating, fidgeting).

The athlete may also present with pain behaviours such as constant touching of the back, habitual self-manipulation and rubbing of the area, grimacing and an inability to relax. This may also be coupled with negative lifestyle factors (sleep disturbance, inactivity, alcohol intake and social isolation). These athletes may also tend to become reliant on passive therapies. They present as high risk on screening questionnaires.

Management

A cognitive functional approach that provides a biopsychosocial understanding of pain, pain control strategies through body relaxation, mindfulness, movement retraining and functional activation is central to this process.[155] Education regarding the multidimensional factors associated with LBP is essential so that the person understands that their thoughts, emotions and behaviours can influence their pain responses and behaviours. Reassurance regarding the spine's resilience is central to the therapeutic process. Before movement training can be initiated, the athlete may need to be trained to relax using slow relaxed-diaphragm breathing, body relaxation and mindfulness techniques.

The approach to movement training is then guided by their movement profile (outlined in low-complexity profile). Focus is placed on discouraging protective movement behaviours (propping of the hands, breath holding and tensing with movement). Pain behaviours (i.e. self-manipulation, repeated stretching and touching of the spine) are also actively discouraged.

> **PRACTICE PEARL**
>
> Graduated physical activation and addressing maladaptive behaviours is usually more difficult in this group due to the dominance of central nervous system pain features. (See also Chapter 5.)

Consequently, minimal movement may result in pain flares and over-zealous clinicians may find the athlete distressed with a pain flare. Slow graduated physical activation with a clear paced program to return to sporting activity is usually required. Addressing lifestyle factors such as sleep disturbance, contextual life stress and activity avoidance is central to this process. The use of exercise and sleep diaries may assist this process.

The presence of uncontrolled comorbid anxiety, panic disorder, depression and/or high levels of contextual stresses in the athlete's social life may necessitate psychological referral. Central nervous system pain features and sleep disturbances may require medical referral for targeted pharmacological treatments to provide a window of opportunity for functional restoration.

Reliance on passive therapies and interventional medicine is usually unhelpful and provocative and should be avoided in these cases.

REHABILITATION FOLLOWING LOW BACK PAIN

Developing an ongoing plan based on the risk profile of the athlete is important in order to minimise the future risks. This includes managing *physical risk factors* such as training loads, technical skills, optimising body posture and control, conditioning and fitness specific to the sport's requirements. The nature of this training is specific to the individual presentation of the athlete. Integrating this into gym-based conditioning programs is crucial.

It also involves managing *psychosocial* and *lifestyle* risks such as energy levels, emotional and psychological health, stress resilience, incorporating relaxation strategies, sleep hygiene, healthy diet and minimising sedentary behaviours. There are many online resources to support both the clinician and the athlete in this process.

Sporting technique

Poor technique in sporting activities may increase stress on the structures of the lumbar spine. The technique should be assessed with the aid of a coach and in some cases with high-speed film and biomechanical analysis. Any necessary corrections should be made under supervision and with the guidance of the coach. Examples of sport-specific technique factors linked to lower back pain are covered in Chapter 9.

Optimal motor control

There is a lot of controversy regarding core stability exercises in LBP. Systematic reviews support the idea that 'stabilisation' exercises are not more effective than general exercise for LBP.[156] Furthermore, studies investigating muscle changes suggest that changes in the stabilising muscles are not prognostic of superior outcomes. While trunk muscle strength and conditioning is critical for many sports, as previously reported, recurrent and chronic LBP is often associated with higher levels of co-contraction of the trunk muscles. Hence, rehabilitation programs need to be sports specific and attend to the individual impairments of the athlete rather than be prescriptive.

Control of the lumbar spine is influenced greatly by both the thoracic spine and the hip pelvic region. Hence, optimising control of the lower back involves attending to control of these proximal and distal regions. Adequate strength of the lower limbs is essential in sports involving limb loading to adequately dampen ground reaction forces and ensure trunk control. The double- and single-leg squat is an excellent rehabilitation exercise combining motor control and strengthening. Similarly, a lack of upper body (upper limb and thoracic) strength and control can compromise lumbar spine mechanics in sports demanding use of the upper limbs (e.g. tennis, cricket, throwing and swimming). In these cases, maintaining a balanced exercise program that ensures optimal control of these regions is important.

Flexibility

Depending on the sport and the individual, addressing the relative flexibility of the hip muscles and/or the thoracic/shoulder girdle regions, as well as the lumbar spine, is important. Commonly, tense or 'shortened' muscles (i.e. erector spinae, hip flexors, gluteals, hamstrings, rectus abdominis, quadratus lumborum, pectorals and latissimus dorsi) may influence the biomechanics and motor control strategies of the lumbar spine. For example, tightness of the hamstrings may result in greater flexion strain of the lower back in a rower. Conversely, tight hip flexors may result in increased lumbar spine extension in a dancer or runner. On the other hand, tightness of the latissimus dorsi may result in excessive side bending of the lumbar spine in a fast bowler in cricket. The tension in these muscles should be addressed as part of the rehabilitation program. The various techniques are shown in Figure 29.27.

CONCLUSION

The clinical approach to the athlete with LBP requires a multidimensional perspective. The first is to triage the athlete in order to rule out serious and specific

PART B Regional problems

pathoanatomical disorders. The second is to identify the dominance and presence of potential physical, psychosocial and lifestyle risk factors that may be influencing pain and disability profiles both in the presence and absence of specific pathology. The integration of screening questionnaires is critical in this process.

> **PRACTICE PEARL**
>
> Considering non-specific LBP as a feature of sensitisation of the spine structures, rather than 'damage to the spine', is critical to change the clinician's and the athlete's mindset to their problem.

In the acute phase of a disorder, providing pain control, restoration of function and then targeting the intervention based on the individual's biopsychosocial profile allows for targeting of care. When LBP is persistent, identification of underlying modifiable drivers of pain sensitisation and disability is critical. This is tailored to the complexity profile of the athlete. In high-complexity cases, multidisciplinary care may be required.

There is growing evidence that an individualised approach is more effective than traditional structural, biomechanical approaches to LBP. Encouraging the athlete to develop a positive view of the spine's resilience, enhancing optimal motor control and confidence in their spine, as well as guiding the patient to make healthy lifestyle choices, are goals of this process.

Muscle	Self-exercise	Assisted exercise	Myofascial release
Erector spinae	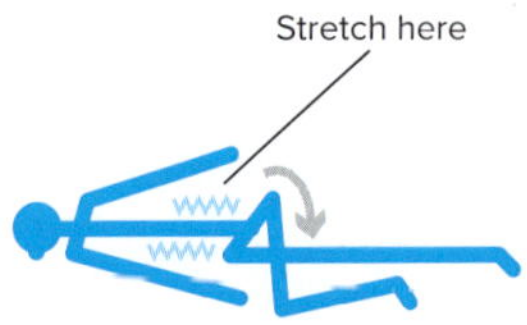 Stretch here	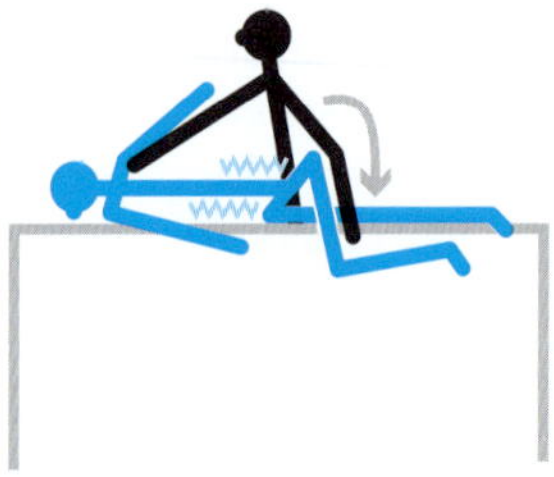	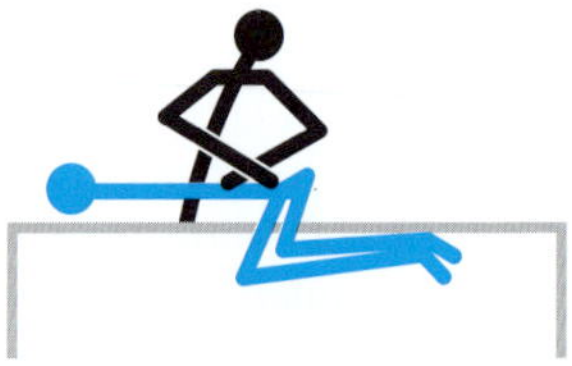 Patient is side-lying. Therapist's wrists are crossed over each other to provide traction.
Psoas	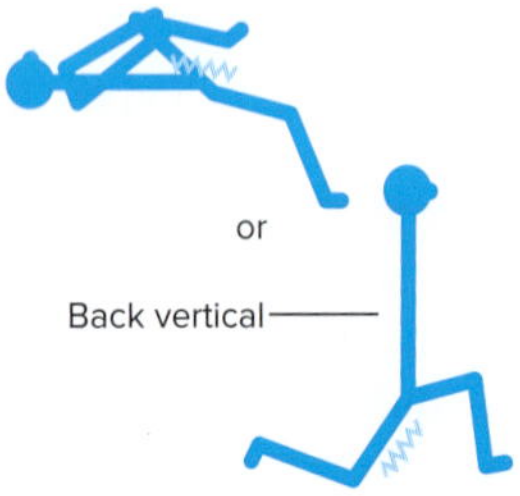 or Back vertical	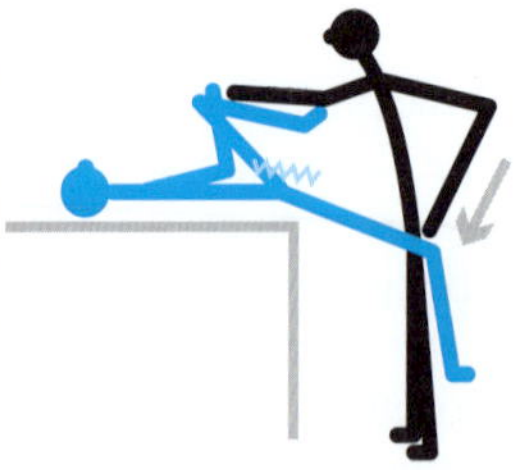	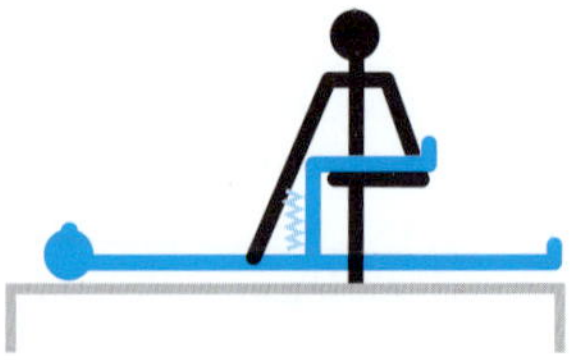 Therapist's hand is over the psoas. Hip is extended from the flexed position.
Iliotibial band	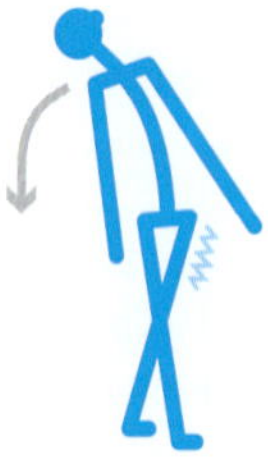	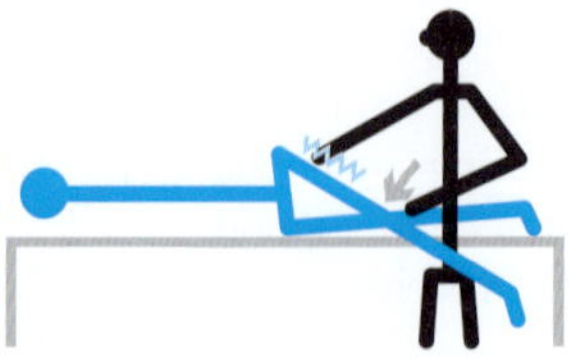 Patient is side-lying and facing away. Hip is extended and adducted.	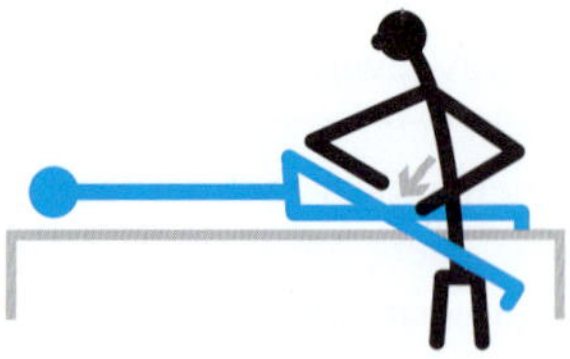 Patient is side-lying and facing away. Therapist uses elbow/forearm to perform release.

Figure 29.27 Techniques used to treat tightness of individual muscles

564

Low back pain　　CHAPTER 29

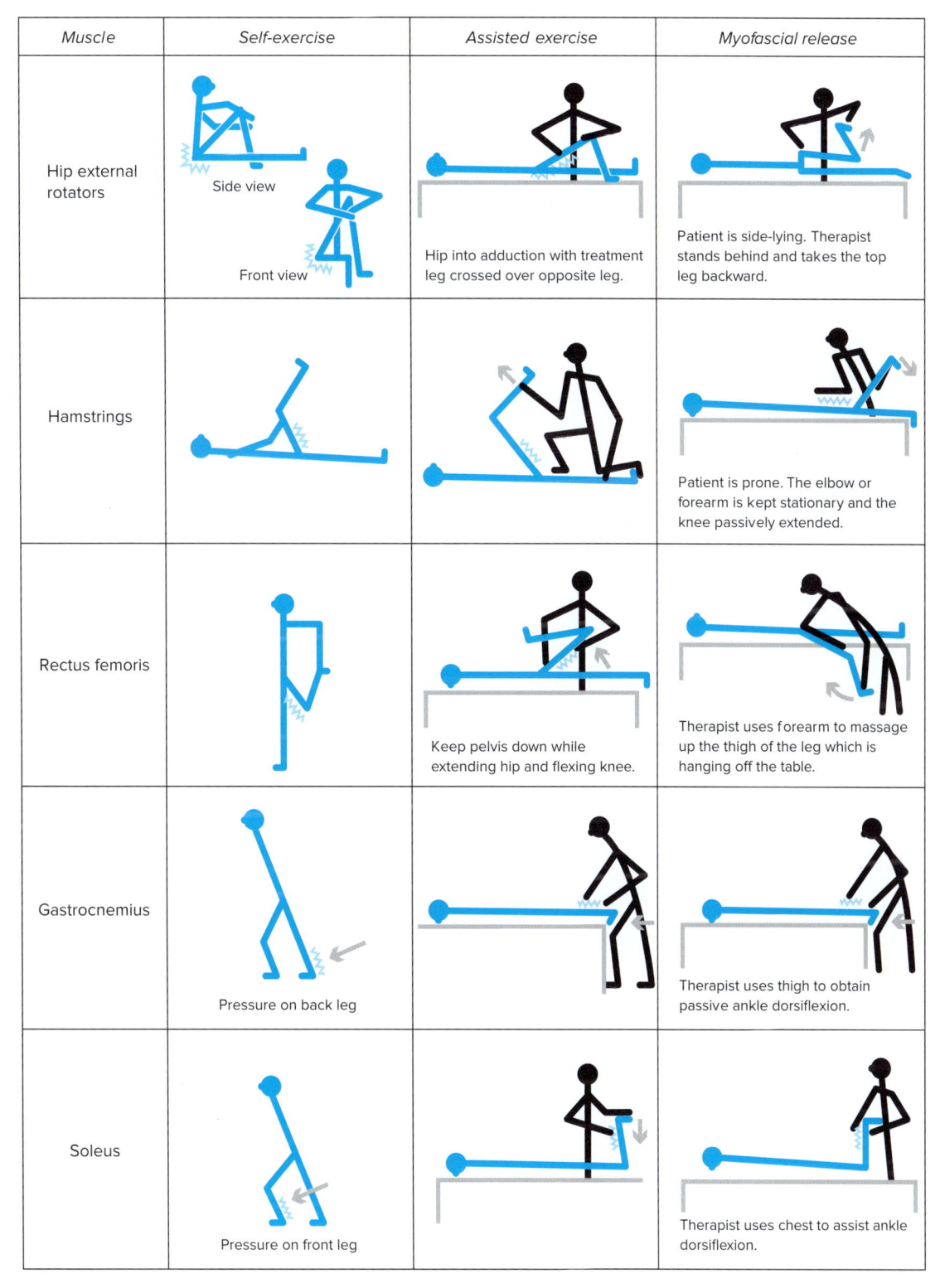

Muscle	Self-exercise	Assisted exercise	Myofascial release
Hip external rotators	Side view / Front view	Hip into adduction with treatment leg crossed over opposite leg.	Patient is side-lying. Therapist stands behind and takes the top leg backward.
Hamstrings			Patient is prone. The elbow or forearm is kept stationary and the knee passively extended.
Rectus femoris		Keep pelvis down while extending hip and flexing knee.	Therapist uses forearm to massage up the thigh of the leg which is hanging off the table.
Gastrocnemius	Pressure on back leg		Therapist uses thigh to obtain passive ankle dorsiflexion.
Soleus	Pressure on front leg		Therapist uses chest to assist ankle dorsiflexion.

Figure 29.27 (cont.) Techniques used to treat tightness of individual muscles

565

PART B Regional problems

REFERENCES

References for this chapter can be found at www.mhhe.com/au/CSM5e

Chapter 30

Buttock pain

with ADAM MEAKINS

Running has substantially shaped human evolution, it is one of the most transforming events in human history. We have literally evolved to run and our big incredible butts are evidence of this.

Professor Dan Lieberman, evolutionary biologist, Harvard University

The assessment and diagnosis of an athlete with buttock pain can be a challenge for the clinician due to the complex anatomy as well as the many different structures that can refer pain into this area. Buttock pain can be experienced by a wide variety of athletes, but higher incidence is often seen in those who are involved in running, sprinting and kicking sports. Buttock pain can be either sudden or gradual in onset, it can occur in isolation or with low back, posterior thigh and even groin pain, and it can also be due to direct trauma from falls or collisions. A list of causes of buttock pain can be found in Table 30.1. Anatomy of the buttock region can be found in Figure 30.1.

CLINICAL APPROACH

Assessment of any reported buttock pain should always first try to ascertain if there is any involvement from the lumbar spine. This can be challenging due to the complex nature of low back pain especially in chronic states. For more on low back pain and lumbar spine assessment and treatment see Chapter 29.

Detailed, comprehensive and careful questioning around the onset, duration and nature of the buttock pain, together with identifying the aggravating and easing factors will help guide the clinician to probable causes and help plan the physical examination.

However when taking a history it is important for the clinician to focus not only on the painful area, but to recognise the many other factors that can contribute to injury and pain in athletes. Time should be taken to explore and obtain a detailed history of an athlete's lifestyle and other psychosocial factors. For example, lack of sleep, chronic levels of stress and fatigue have been found to contribute to injuries and recovery in athletes.[1-4] It is also important for a clinician to assess an athlete's psychological status. High levels of fear of re-injury, anxiety and catastrophisation have been shown to affect assessment and treatment outcomes.[5, 6]

Table 30.1 A list of causes of buttock pain

Common	Less common	Not to be missed
Myofascial pain	Piriformis syndrome	Spondyloarthropathies
Referred from lumbar spine	Ischiofemoral impingement	Ankylosing spondylitis
Proximal hamstring tendinopathy	Posterior thigh compartment syndrome	Psoriatic arthritis
Sacroiliac joint dysfunction	Ischial tuberosity injury	Reactive arthritis (Reiters)
	Proximal hamstring tendon rupture	Stress fracture sacrum
	Avulsion fracture (children)	Stress fracture pubic ramus
	Gluteus medius tendinopathy (see Chapter 31)	Malignancy
		Bone/joint infections

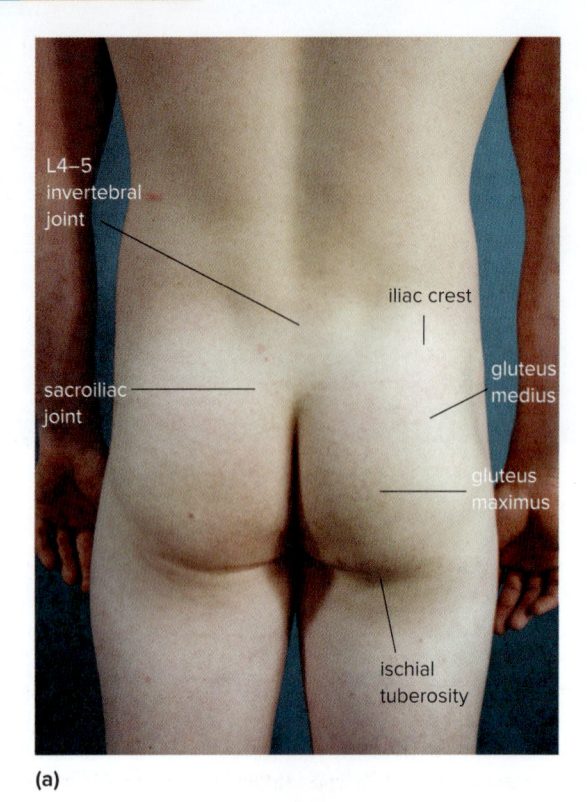

PART B Regional problems

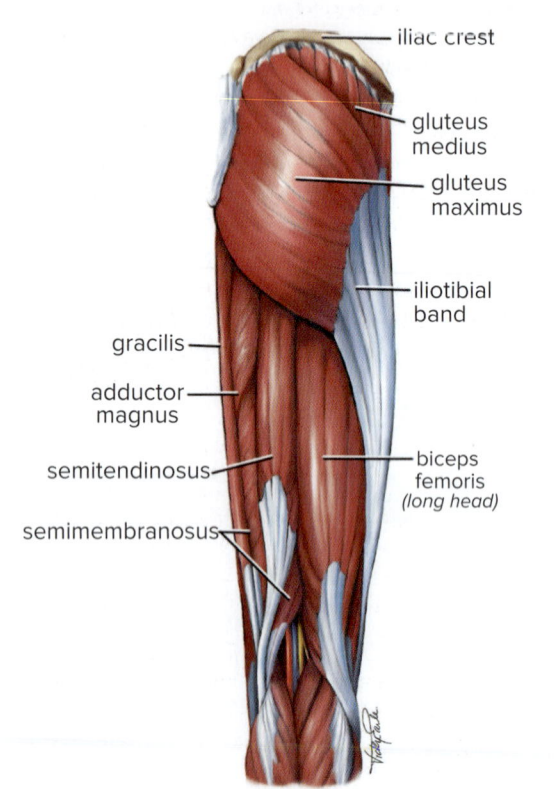

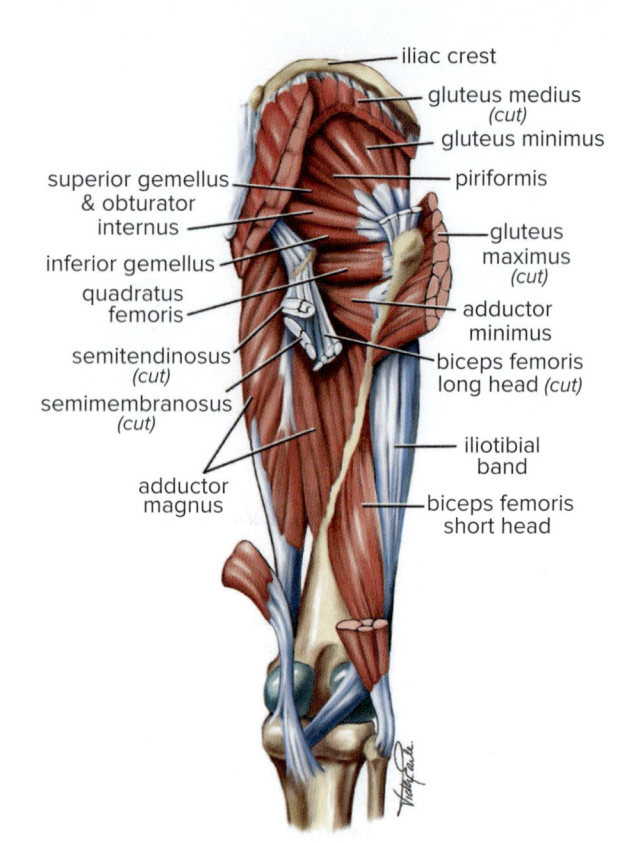

Figure 30.1 Anatomy of the buttocks (a) Surface anatomy (b) Superficial muscles (c) Deep muscles

There are many physical examination tests described in the literature to diagnose specific structures or pathologies of buttock pain. However, the clinician should exercise caution when a positive or negative test is found in isolation, as the specificity and sensitivity (see below) of most of these tests are poor. A combination of objective tests combined with a good thorough subjective history will give the clinician much more confidence in his or her diagnosis.

History

The onset of buttock pain can be reported either as sudden during a sporting activity or as a gradual insidious onset afterwards. Buttock pain that is deep, diffuse and hard to localise, accompanied with low back pain may suggest some lumbar spine involvement. However, it must be remembered that buttock pain without low back pain does not mean the lumbar spine is not involved.

Buttock pain combined with posterior thigh pain, with or without low back or neural symptoms, can be suggestive of a lumbar radiculopathy. However, consideration must also be given to facet joint and hamstring pathology.

Buttock pain felt around the ischial tuberosity (Fig. 30.1) or Tuber area (Fig. 30.2) may be suggestive of proximal hamstring pathology and/or ischiogluteal bursitis. Buttock pain felt more axially or directly over the sacroiliac joint, sometimes referred to as the Fortin area (Fig. 30.2), may suggest a sacroiliac joint or ligament dysfunction.[7] However, location of pain alone should never be used in isolation to make a diagnosis.

Buttock pain reproduced with movements and activities is also not diagnostic in isolation as many structures can be aggravated concurrently. However, it may give clues to possible structures as a source of pain. Suspicion of lumbar spine involvement is increased if low back, buttock or posterior thigh pain is either increased or decreased on repeated lumbar spine movements.[8, 9]

Diurnal variation of buttock pain can be useful to establish a diagnosis. Morning pain and stiffness that lasts more than 30 minutes and eases with light activity is highly suggestive of inflammatory conditions such as sacroiliitis and ankylosing spondylitis, although further tests are needed to confirm.

Physical examination

A visual inspection of the buttock and pelvic area with the lumbar spine and upper thigh is essential. Observation of bruising around the ischial tuberosity and down the posterior thigh may indicate a proximal hamstring avulsion in those with a history of severe sudden traumatic onset of buttock pain when sprinting or running.

Observation of muscle atrophy and gross asymmetry should be noted. However, there are questions about the clinical usefulness of many of the commonly used observational tests to assess spinal curves and pelvic positions and postures. It is known that there are wide normal variations in skeletal morphology, posture and positions in the population.[10-12] Despite popular belief there is no evidence that any spinal or pelvic position or posture is more associated with pain or a risk of increased incidence of injury.[13-17]

Palpation of the lumbar spine, pelvis and buttocks for pain provocation may assist in the identification of a pathological structure, but again it cannot be used in isolation to make a diagnosis. Palpation tests to determine hypermobility or hypomobility of the spine and pelvic joints are commonly used, but are of questionable clinical utility. The very small movements that do occur around the sacroiliac joint make the ability to detect these with palpation highly unlikely.[18]

The reliability of all pelvic palpation tests used to assess sacroiliac joint movement is poor.[19, 20] Palpation tests used to detect joint stiffness or laxity have been shown to have wide variation in forces applied by therapists.[21] When combined with wide variations in individual stiffness, it makes any interpretation of joint hyper- or hypomobility completely unreliable and down to individual clinician perception.[22] Finally it has been shown there is no correlation between spinal joint stiffness and pain.[23]

Neurodynamic examination tests (Chapter 15) may be included if there is a suspicion of lumbar radiculopathy as a cause of buttock pain. However, there are issues with false positives and the diagnostic accuracy of these tests, meaning again they cannot be used in isolation.[24]

Physical examination of the buttock can be divided into observation, movement and resistance tests, both isolated and dynamic.

1. Observation static
   a. stance
      i. alignment (shifted, inability to stand straight)
      ii. atrophy (glutes/hamstrings)
      iii. bruising (ischial tuberosity/posterior thigh)
   b. single-leg stance
      i. pain
      ii. balance
      iii. Trendelenburg sign
2. Observation dynamic (checking for pain/control/alignment)
   a. gait
      i. antalgic/Trendelenburg
   b. squat
   c. single-leg squat
      i. valgus knee
      ii. hip internal rotation
      iii. trunk compensation

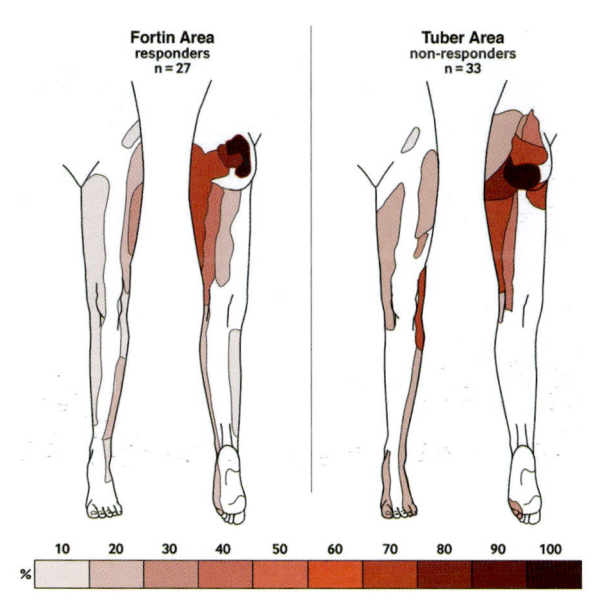

Figure 30.2 Fortin and Tuber pain areas

PART B Regional problems

   d. Lunge
      i. forward
      ii. backward
      iii. lateral
3. Active movements–lumbar spine
   a. standing flexion
   b. standing extension
   c. standing single-leg extension (pars interarticularis test)
   d. standing lateral flexion
   e. standing and seated rotation
   f. combined/functional movements
4. Active movements–hip, standing
   a. flexion
   b. extension
   c. abduction
   d. adduction
5. Active movements–hip, supine
   a. flexion (Fig. 30.3a)
   b. abduction
   c. adduction
   d. FABER
6. Passive movements–hip, supine
   a. log roll
   b. hip quadrant
   c. FABER
   d. FADIR
7. Passive movements–hip, prone
   a. extension (Fig. 30.3b)
   b. external rotation
   c. internal rotation
8. Resisted movements–supine
   a. hip flexion (psoas)
   b. straight leg raise (rectus femoris)
   c. external rotation (in 90° flexion)
   d. internal rotation (in 90° flexion)
   e. double-leg bridge (Fig. 30.3c)
   f. single-leg bridge
9. Resisted movements–side-lying
   a. hip abduction in neutral (TFL/glute med) (Fig. 30.3d)
   b. hip abduction in 30° flexion (glute med)
10. Resisted movements–prone
    a. hip extension (glute max/hamstrings)
    b. knee flexion (hamstrings)
11. Palpation
    a. sacroiliac joint (Fortin area)
    b. ischial tuberosity (Tuber area) (Fig. 30.3e)
    c. gluteal muscles
    d. lumbar spine vertebral segments
    e. lumbar spine paraspinal muscles

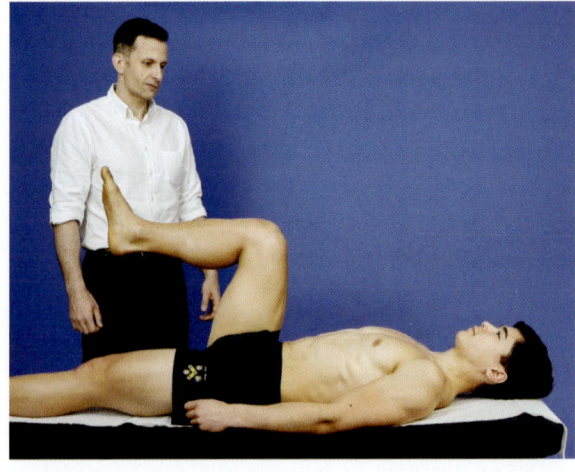

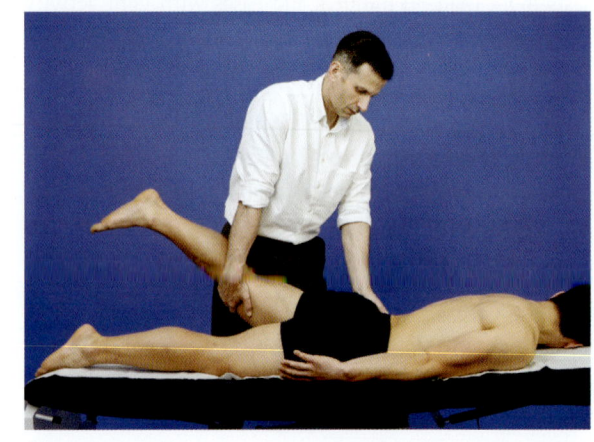

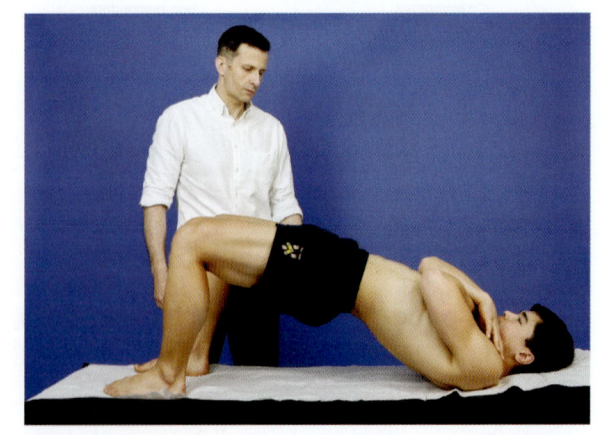

Figure 30.3 Examination (a) Active hip flexion with knee at 90° (b) Passive hip extension (c) Double-leg bridge

Buttock pain CHAPTER 30

(d)

(e)

(f)

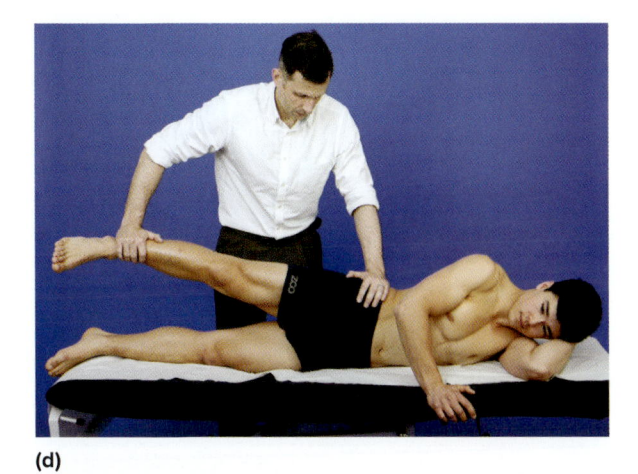

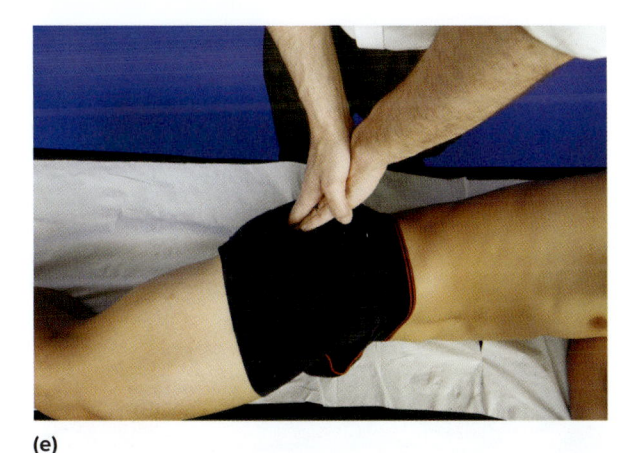

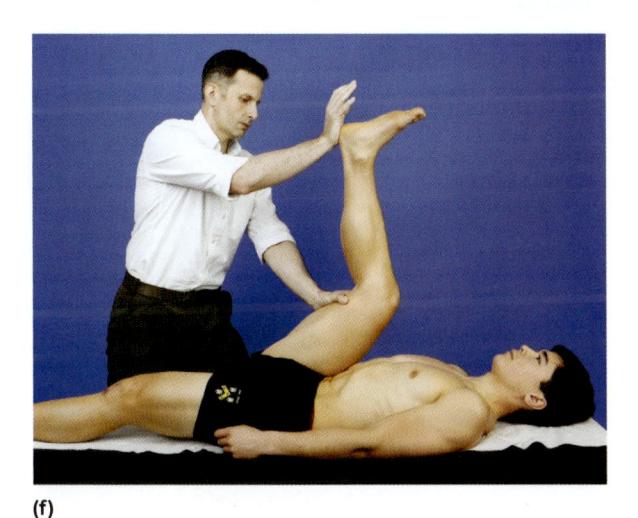

Figure 30.3 (cont.) (d) Resisted hip abduction in side-lying, hip in neutral (e) Palpation of the ischial tuberosity (f) Modified bent knee stretch

(g)

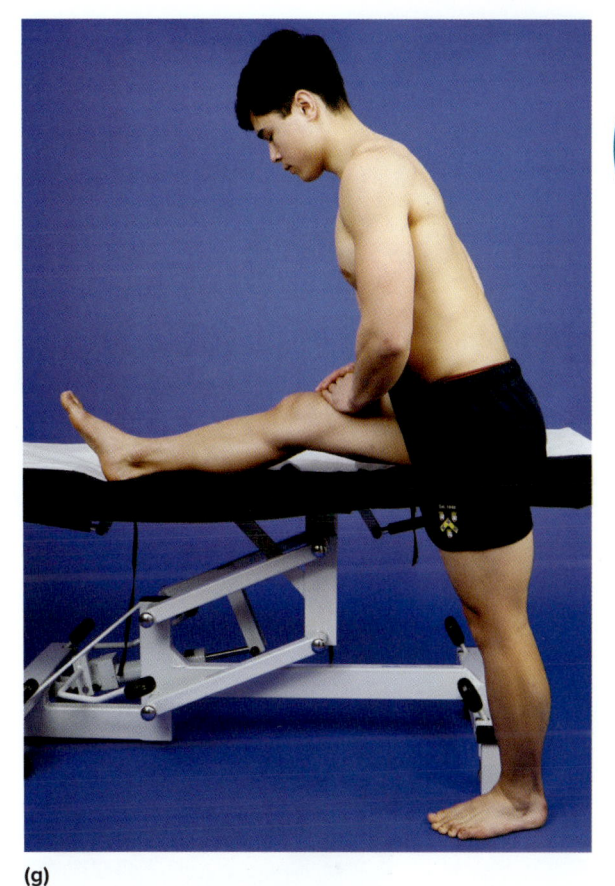

Figure 30.3 (cont.) (g) Puranen–Ovara stretch test

12. Neurodynamic tests (Chapter 15)
    a. slump
    b. straight leg raise
    c. special tests–proximal hamstring tendinopathy
    d. bent knee stretch test
    e. modified bent knee stretch test (Fig. 30.3f)
    f. Puranen–Ovara stretch test (Fig. 30.3g)
    g. supine plank test (Fig. 30.3h)
13. Special tests–sacroiliac joint
    a. Gaenslen's torque test (Fig. 30.3i)
    b. Patrick's test (FABER) (Fig. 30.3j)
    c. femoral shear/thigh thrust test (Fig. 30.3k)
    d. distraction test (Fig. 30.3l)
    e. compression test (Fig. 30.3m)
    f. sacral thrust test (Fig. 30.3n)
    g. active straight leg raise test (Fig. 30.3o)
14. Special tests–piriformis
    a. active side-lying piriformis test (Fig. 30.3p)
    b. passive seated piriformis test (Fig. 30.3q)
    c. FAIR test (Fig. 30.3r)

PART B   Regional problems

(h)

(i)

(j)

(k)

(l)

(m)

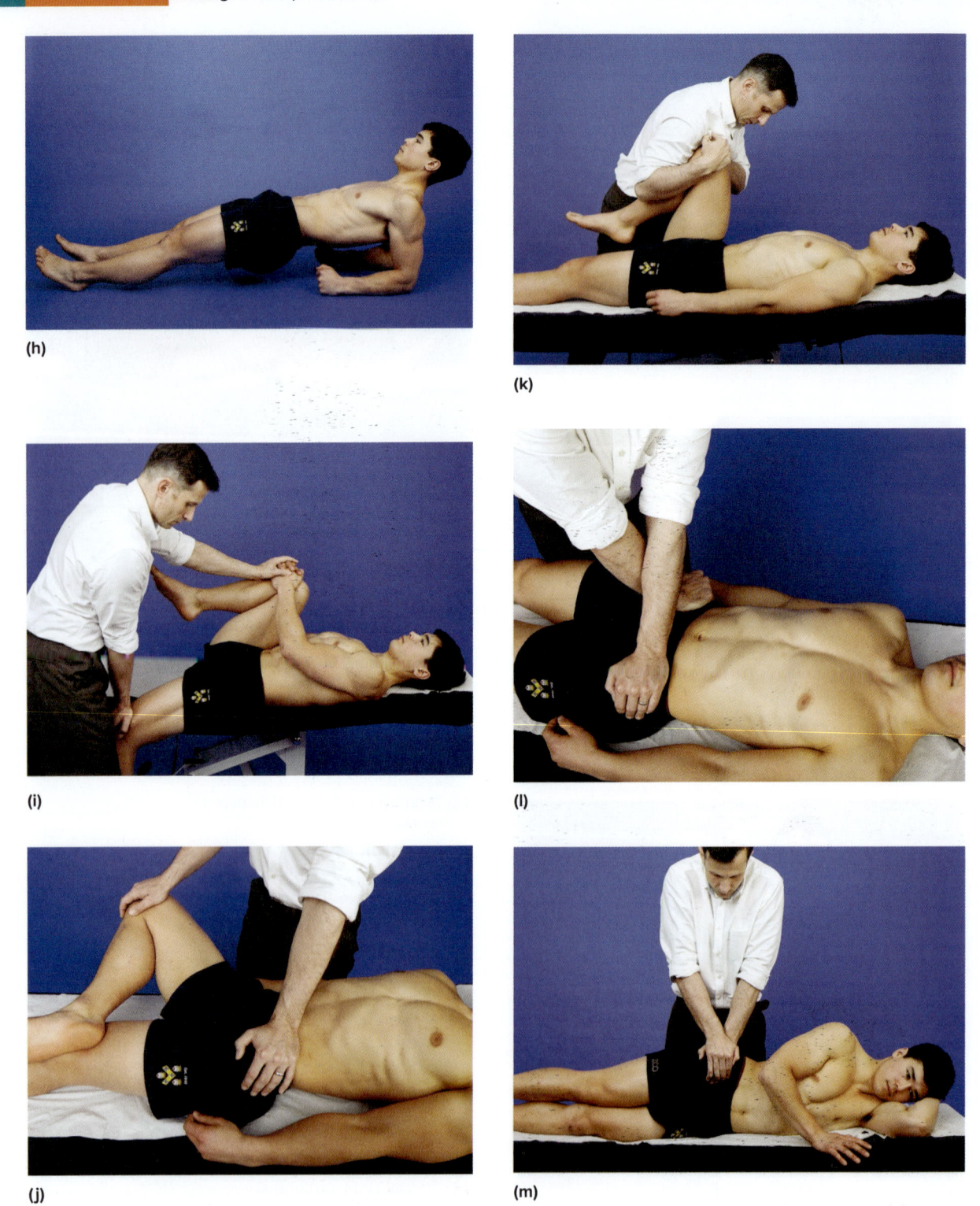

Figure 30.3 (cont.) (h) Supine plank test (i) Gaenslen's torque test (j) Patrick's test (FABER) (k) Femoral shear/thigh thrust test (l) Distraction test (m) Compression test

572

Buttock pain CHAPTER 30

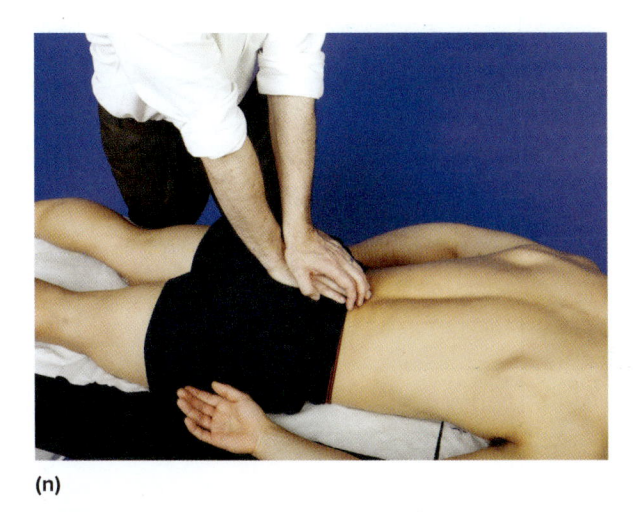

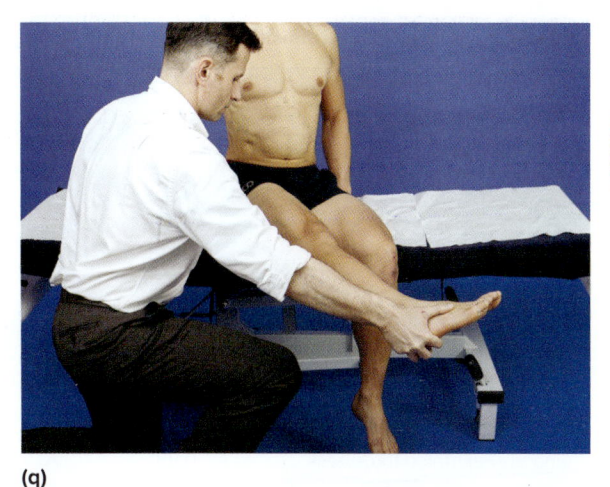

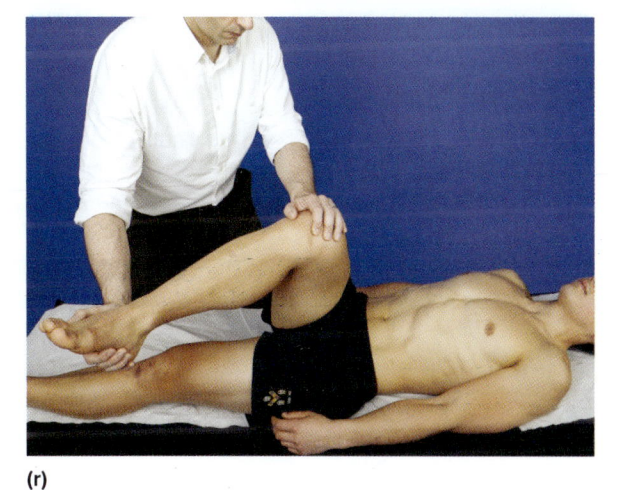

Figure 30.3 (cont.) (q) Passive seated piriformis or PACE test (active resisted abduction with patient seated with hip flexed 90°) (r) FAIR (passive flexion, adduction and internal rotation of the hip, with patient in supine)

Sensitivity and specificity of tests for buttock pain
Refer to Table 30.2.

Key outcome measures
There is no validated outcome measure for general buttock pain. However, the VISA-H is a validated outcome measure that can be used for monitoring progress for those with proximal hamstring tendinopathy.[25] It consists of eight questions to assess severity of symptoms, function and sporting activity.

Investigations
Pelvic radiographs can be used if there is suspicion of bony trauma as the cause of buttock pain such as a pubic ramus

Figure 30.3 (cont.) (n) Sacral thrust test (o) Active straight leg test (p) Active side-lying piriformis test or Beatty test (active resisted abduction with patient side-lying with the hip flexed 90°)

PART B Regional problems

Table 30.2 Specificity and sensitivity of tests for buttock pain

	Sensitivity	Specificity	Positive likelihood ratio	Negative likelihood ratio
Proximal hamstring tendinopathy special tests				
Bent knee stretch test	0.84	0.87	6.5	0.18
Modified bent knee stretch test	0.89	0.91	10.2	0.12
Puranen-Ovara stretch test	0.76	0.82	4.2	0.29
Supine plank test	NA	NA	NA	NA
Sacroiliac joint special tests				
Gaenslen's torque test	0.50	0.77	2.21	0.65
Patrick's test (FABER)	0.40	0.99	NA	NA
Femoral shear/thigh thrust test	0.88	0.69	2.80	0.18
Distraction test	0.60	0.81	3.20	0.49
Compression test	0.69	0.69	2.20	0.46
Sacral thrust test	0.63	0.75	2.50	0.50
Active straight leg raise test	0.58	0.97	NA	NA
Van der Wurff cluster (3 or more +ve from tests 1, 2, 3, 4, 5)	0.85	0.79	4.02	0.19
Laslett's cluster (2 or more +ve from tests 3, 4, 5, 6)	0.88	0.78	4.00	0.16
Gluteal sciatic nerve entrapment/piriformis syndrome special tests				
Straight leg raise	0.15	0.95	3.20	0.90
Active side-lying piriformis test	0.78	0.80	3.90	0.27
Passive seated piriformis test	0.52	0.90	5.22	0.53
FAIR test	0.88	0.83	5.20	0.14

fracture or ischial tuberosity avulsion in the younger athlete. Loss of sacroiliac joint definition on a pelvic X-ray strongly suggests a spondyloarthopathy, but needs to be confirmed with blood tests and MRIs.

Lumbar X-rays can be used if a pars interarticularis fracture is suspected; however, these can be difficult to see and oblique views are best when looking for the 'Scotty dog' collar sign (see Chapter 29).

If there is a suspicion of a stress fracture or reaction of the pars interarticularis, ishium, scarum or pubic rami, then magnetic resonance imaging (MRI) should be considered. Isotopic bone or CT scans may also be an option but careful consideration should be given to exposure to radiation, especially in the younger athlete. Caution must also be used when interpreting imaging, because joint problems such as spondylosis or spondylolistheses can be very common in asymptomatic athletes.[26]

MRI can be used to confirm other soft tissue structures as a cause of buttock pain such as ischiogluteal bursitis, proximal hamstring tendinopathy and prolapsed intervertebral disc. Again, caution is advised when interpreting imaging of the lumbar spine, as many so-called pathological findings are often seen in asymptomatic patients.[27]

Diagnostic ultrasound scanning can be used to assess tendons and bursa around the buttock area. However, they are highly user dependent and the reliability of the findings is based on the clinician's skill and interpretation.[28]

MYOFASCIAL BUTTOCK PAIN

Strains to the lumbar, buttock and posterior thigh muscles, sacroiliac ligaments and other soft tissues are arguably the most common cause of back and buttock pain in athletes. It is estimated that up to 97% of all sporting injuries are soft tissue in nature.[29] A soft tissue injury is often reported as a fairly localised pain that is aggravated by continued activity or resistance.

The buttocks provide locomotion and power, but also have important stabilising roles. The buttock muscles can often become overloaded, strained and painful during

Buttock pain — CHAPTER 30

sports, and this may be due to poor training program design, training error, or a biomechanical deficit or muscle weakness. Palpation of the soft tissue is used to locate areas of myofascial pain, feeling for localised areas of tightness, muscle knots or taut bands. These are commonly referred to as 'trigger points' (see Chapter 4) and may be adverse areas of sustained muscle fibre contractions.[30]

Examination

A lack of gluteal muscle strength can be a common cause for buttock pain in an athlete. A common sign of gluteal muscle weakness is the Trendelenburg sign.[31] This is a drop of the contralateral pelvis, or a compensated hitch or lateral lean of the trunk when standing on one leg. This can be difficult to notice in fit and strong individuals, and can sometimes only be identified when the athlete is fatigued or asked to stand on one leg for extended periods.[32]

To assess the strength of the gluteal muscles in athletes, isometric manual muscle testing can be used. For more accurate objective assessment and monitoring, hand-held dynamometry has been shown to have good reliability.[33] However, there are limitations on hand-held dynamometry testing due to individual examiner strength differences.[34]

There is debate around the best positions to assess and strengthen the gluteal muscles.[35, 36] However, resisted side-lying hip abduction (Fig. 30.3d) is seen to produce high levels of activation in the gluteus medius and resisted prone hip extension produces high levels in the gluteus maximus.[37] These clinical tests are simple, quick and easy to perform.

Treatment of myofascial buttock pain

If weakness is found in the gluteal muscles, a well-rounded, progressive strength and conditioning program needs to be adopted to address it that incorporates both isolated and functional multi-joint compound exercises in weight-bearing positions. For more on exercise prescription see Chapter 10. The levels of EMG activity of various exercises involving the gluteal muscles are shown in Figure 30.4.[38]

Treatment for tender tight muscle bands or 'trigger points' is often performed with soft tissue techniques such as ischaemic pressure with thumb or elbow, or via invasive techniques such as dry needling or injections.[39]

Gluteus maximus activation

Exercise	%MVIC
Prone plank	9
Lunge - backward trunk lean	19
Bridging on Swiss ball	20
Side-lying hip abduction	21
Lunge - forward trunk lean	22
Bridging on stable surface	25
Clam - 30° hip flexion	34
Lunge - neutral trunk	36
Clam - 60° hip flexion	39
Single-leg bridge	40
Sideways lunge	41
Lateral step-up	41
Transverse lunge	49
4 point kneel with opposite arm/ leg lift	56
Single-leg mini squat	57
Retro step-up	59
Wall squat	59
Single-leg squat	59
Single-leg deadlift	59
Forward step-up	74

% Maximal Voluntary Isometric Contraction (MVIC)

(a)

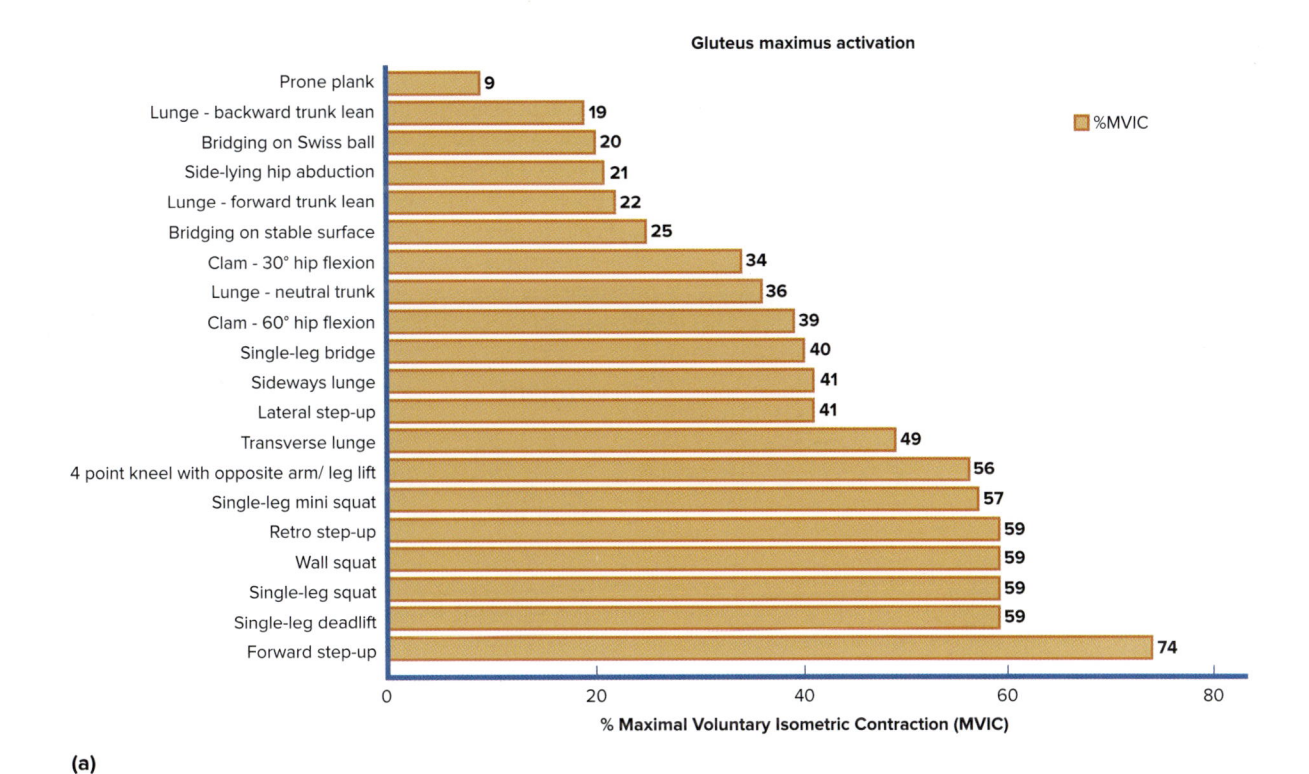

Figure 30.4 Exercises and the levels of electromyographic activity of (a) Gluteus maximus

PART B Regional problems

Gluteus medius activation

Exercise	%MVIC
Prone plank	27
Bridging on unstable surface	28
Lunge - neutral trunk position	34
Single-leg mini-squat	36
Retro step-up	37
Clam - 60° hip flexion	38
Sideways lunge	39
Clam - 30° hip flexion	40
Lateral step-up	41
4-point kneel with opposite arm/leg lift	42
Forward step-up	44
Single-leg bridge	47
Transverse lunge	48
Wall squat	52
Side-lying hip abduction	56
Pelvic drop	57
Single-leg deadlift	58
Single-leg squat	64
Side-bridge to neutral spine position	74

% Maximal Voluntary Isometric Contraction (MVIC)

(b)

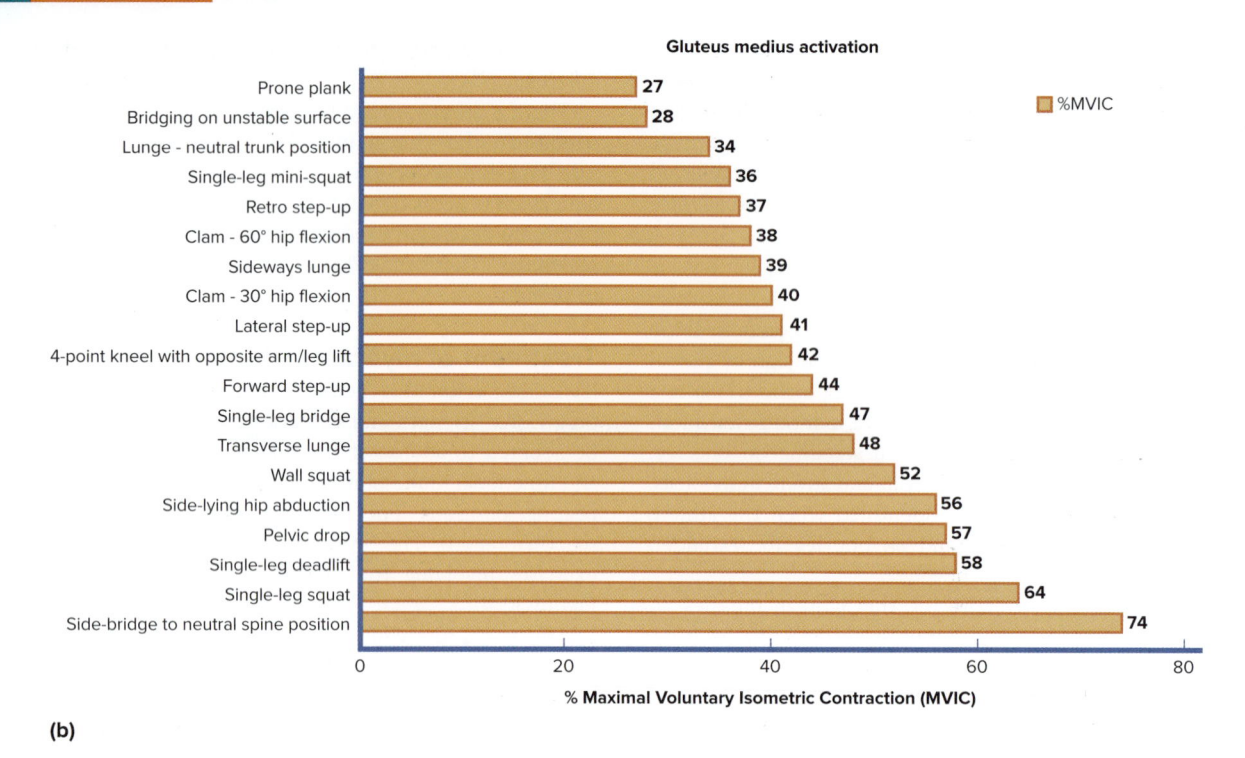

Figure 30.4 (cont.) Exercises and the levels of electromyographic activity of (b) Gluteus medius[38]

REFERRED PAIN FROM THE LUMBAR SPINE

Buttock pain can often be referred from the lumbar spine and be associated with or without concurrent low back pain. For more on the assessment and treatment of the lumbar spine see Chapter 29.

The most common lumbar spine structures that can cause buttock pain are the zygapophyseal (facet) joints or intervertebral discs. An athlete with either of these may describe a dull, deep diffuse pain in the buttock that can vary in intensity and location.

Pain may be aggravated with repeated lumbar spine movements as well as prolonged static postures, such as sitting or standing. Palpation of the vertebral segments and paraspinal muscles may provoke local and referred pain.

Examination

Repeated movements of the lumbar spine in one direction can cause low back and buttock pain to centralise, and when repeated in the other direction can cause the pain to peripheralise. This is highly suggestive of a discogenic lumbar radiculopathy.[9] Lumbar facet joint pathology can be almost conclusively ruled out if seated lumbar extension and combined rotation testing is negative.[40, 41]

Lumbar radiculopathy can also present with neural symptoms, such as pain and paraesthesia into the posterior thigh or further distally. Buttock pain caused by nerve root compression or irritation can be aggravated with neurodynamic testing, such as the slump and straight leg raise tests (Chapter 15).[42]

However, it has been shown that pain that is not specific to lumbar radiculopathy, such as that associated with hamstring issues, may lead to false positives for the straight leg raise test and can inflate the sensitivity of these tests.[24]

Treatment

Treatment of lumbar spine disorders requires an integrated multimodal approach to reflect the complex nature of low back pain. This can include passive treatment, such as manual therapy, but the primary focus should always be on active rehabilitation looking to restore mobility, movement and strength, with consideration given to any psychological factors, such as fear or apprehension that can contribute to increased central sensitisation. An individualised progressive strength and conditioning program should incorporate clear patient-centred goals and objectives based on a realistic schedule for increasing exposure, duration and intensity to activity, with the ultimate goal being to return the athlete to play and competition. See Chapter 29 for more on treatment of low back pain.

Buttock pain | CHAPTER 30

PROXIMAL HAMSTRING TENDINOPATHY

The hamstrings are a commonly strained and injured muscle group during sporting activity. Although not as common as acute hamstring muscle tears (Chapter 34), proximal hamstring tendinopathy is a commonly encountered problem in sports that involve long distance running, jumping or repeated hip flexion. Tendinopathy has an unclear pathogenesis and there is even a lack of consensus over terminology; however, it is usually characterised as an activity overload-related condition culminating in pain, impaired performance and extended periods of rehabilitation.[43]

Functional anatomy

The attachment of the three hamstrings onto the pelvis and the ischiogluteal bursa is complex (Fig. 30.5). All three hamstring tendons blend into a common tendon before they insert onto the ischial tuberosity. The hamstrings cross both the hip and knee joint, which means they are exposed to large eccentric tensile forces during activities that involve both hip flexion and knee extension, such as when decelerating the leg and foot to place it on the ground in the late swing phase of running.

The proximal hamstring tendon is also subject to high compressive loads when the hip is flexed (Fig. 30.6). This compression of the proximal hamstring tendon against the ischial tuberosity is absorbed and attenuated by the ischiogluteal bursa that is positioned between them.

The actions of the hamstrings are classically described as knee flexion and hip extension. However, as they also attach onto the tibia, their role in lower limb function and biomechanics, including the foot and ankle, cannot be overlooked.[44]

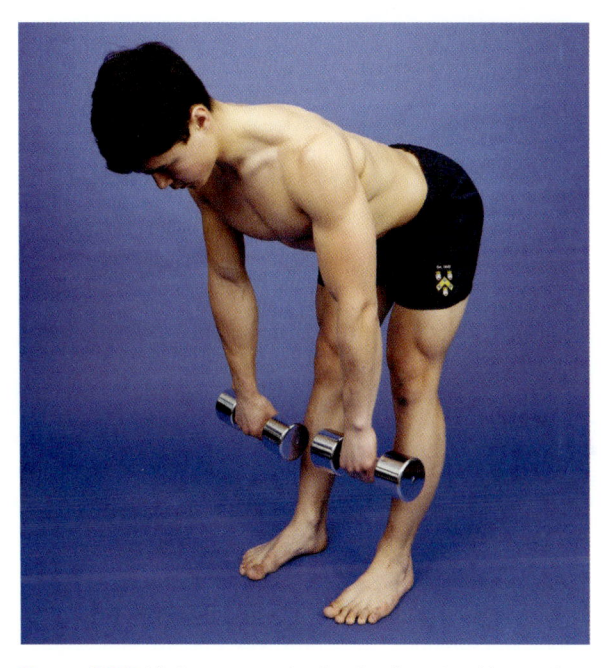

Figure 30.6 High compressive loads of proximal hamstring with the hip in flexion. Ensure spine is straight

Proximal hamstring tendinopathy (PHT) was first described in 1988 as 'high hamstring syndrome',[45] with the common features of pain felt around the lower gluteal region and down the posterior thigh. PHT occurs frequently in association with ischiogluteal bursitis, but no clinical test can differentiate between these two conditions, except for MRI or ultrasound imaging. However, as the mechanisms and subsequent management are similar for both of these conditions, apart from the use of injection therapy for recalcitrant ischiogluteal bursitis, there is no need to separate them clinically.

PHT is experienced by athletes across a wide variety of sports, but it is often seen in middle and long distance runners, and occasionally sprinters.[46] Initially, PHT pain is mild during the sport or activity, but it soon progresses and completely stops the athlete from performing. PHT pain can then progress to be felt in normal daily activities, such as walking and climbing stairs, sitting for prolonged periods or when stretching the hamstrings or gluteal muscles.

PHT is often misdiagnosed in the early stages as a pulled hamstring muscle or mild sciatica. Early identification of PHT is critical, however, as it often progresses rapidly and recovery times can extend significantly if it is not managed appropriately in the early stages.

The primary cause of PHT is mechanical overload of the tendon, and the most common factor in its aetiology is a sudden change or increase in training duration, intensity or method. Therefore, a thorough and detailed subjective history of the athlete's training history is essential.

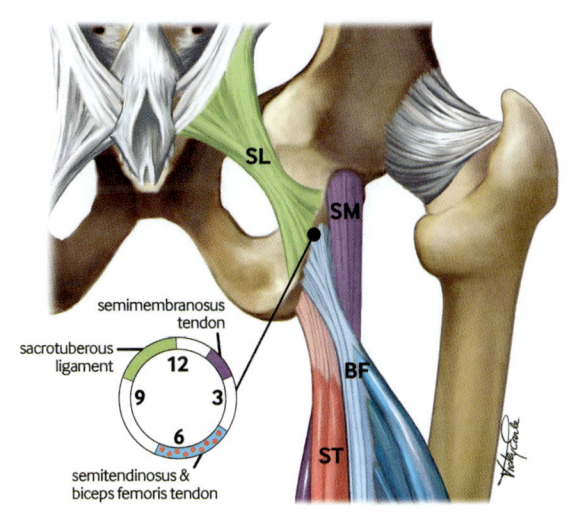

Figure 30.5 Proximal hamstring anatomy

577

Attention should be given to any sudden increase in amount or intensity, or to activities that involve greater hip flexion movements, such as hill sprints, weighted deadlifts, lunges or squats. These activities create high levels of proximal hamstring tendon compression against the ischial tuberosity which, if not progressed steadily or given enough time for adaptation, can be a primary factor for development of tendinopathy.[47, 48]

Examination

Physical assessment of an athlete with suspected PHT must first exclude the lumbar spine of any involvement. Lumbar flexion can aggravate the pain of PHT by compressing the proximal hamstring tendon against the ischial tuberosity and reproducing pain.

Neurodynamic testing can also be highly provocative for PHT simply due to the action of stretching the hamstring tendon insertion, but also by compressing the tendon onto the ischial tuberosity. In addition, the close proximity of the proximal hamstring tendon to the sciatic nerve can produce false positives due to biochemical irritation or even in some chronic cases due to fibrous adhesions developing around the sciatic nerve.[49]

PHT pain is usually well reproduced on passive stretch tests such as the bent knee stretch, modified bent knee stretch (Fig. 30.3f) and Puranen-Ovara tests (Fig. 30.3g). These tests have been shown to have high inter-examiner reliability (range 0.82–0.88) and very high intra-examiner reliability (range 0.87–0.93). Sensitivity and specificity together with predictive values and likelihood ratios of these tests are shown in Table 30.2.[50]

Pain is also well reproduced on strong isometric contraction of the hamstrings, such as in the supine plank position (Fig. 30.3h) and on direct palpation of the ischial tuberosity, which is usually best performed in side-lying to avoid the bulk of the gluteals.[46]

Imaging of the suspected PHT and the ischiogluteal bursa can be used to confirm diagnosis. MRI (Fig. 30.7) and ultrasound scans can often show a thickened tendon, intra-substance heterogeneity and increased signal intensity.[51]

Treatment

Research into the conservative treatment of PHT is limited to just a few case studies.[52, 53] However, using the principles and research into other tendinopathies (Chapter 4) can help guide the management of PHT.

Initial treatment

Treatment for PHT should be focused to reduce pain and minimise compression of the tendon against the ischial tuberosity. Advise the athlete against stretching the hamstrings or gluteal muscles and to avoid positions of sustained hip flexion, such as prolonged sitting, as much as possible.

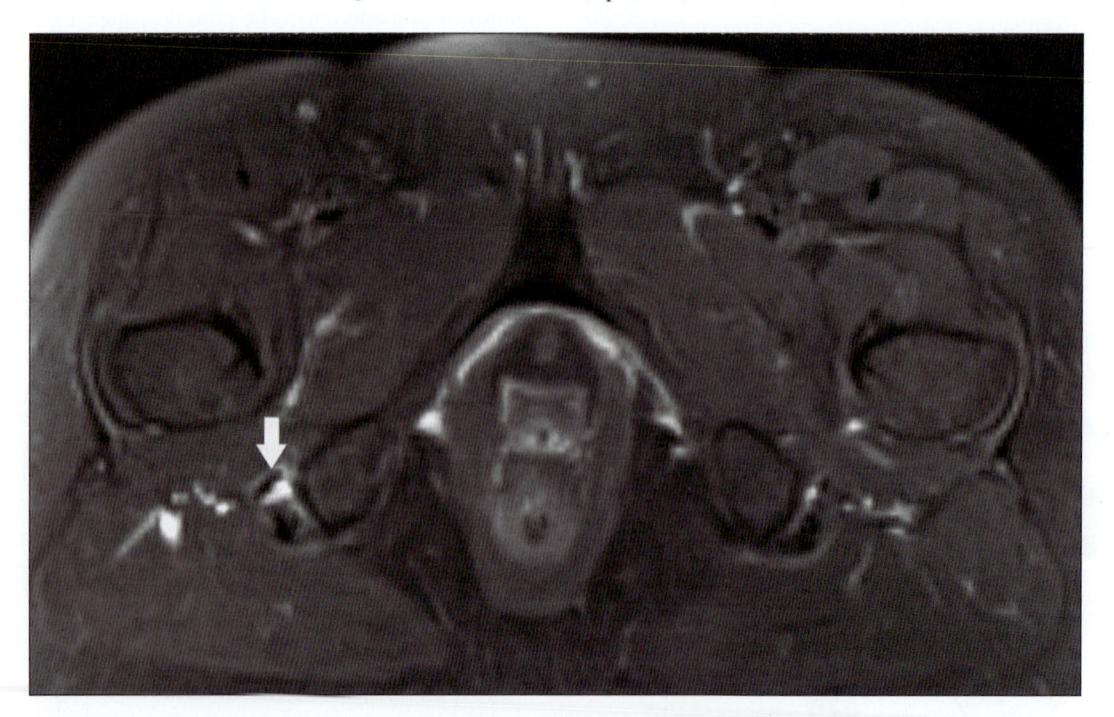

Figure 30.7 T2 fat-suppressed axial MR image showing high T2 signal (arrow) equal to that of fluid involving right common hamstring origin at ischial tuberosity, consistent with partial tear

IMAGING IN SPORTS-SPECIFIC MUSCULOSKELETAL INJURIES, 2016, P.520, ALI GUERMAZI, FRANK W ROEMER, MICHEL D CREMA. © SPRINGER INTERNATIONAL PUBLISHING SWITZERLAND 2016. WITH PERMISSION OF SPRINGER

Buttock pain CHAPTER 30

Treatment can also be directed towards relieving symptoms, using soft tissue techniques on the posterior thigh and gluteals, applying ice and prescribing analgesic medication if needed. Manual therapy techniques, such as deep transverse frictions across the ischial tuberosity and proximal hamstring tendon, are not advocated due to their potential to increase adverse compressive forces. Although they may provide a transient analgesic effect, the forces applied do not break adhesions or increase blood flow significantly.[54]

> **PRACTICE PEARL**
>
> Primary treatment for any tendinopathy must always be staged, progressive loading.[55]

This is no different in PHT and it should begin immediately. Initially in the acute, irritable and painful stages the musculotendinous unit loading should be done well within pain tolerance and in positions that do not compress the tendon.

Isometric contractions can also be very beneficial in the early stages of tendinopathy, producing an analgesic effect as well as maintaining load through the musculotendinous unit. Although the pain reducing effects of isometric contractions are not completely understood, they are believed to be via both peripheral and central nervous system mechanisms.[56] The most effective 'dosage' of isometric contractions is not fully known, but long duration, 45–60 seconds, at as near as pain tolerance allows to maximal force, seems to have the greatest effect. This should be done regularly and intermittently throughout the day in groups of 3–5 repetitions at a time.[57] Good examples are the prone hamstring curl (Fig. 30.8) and the supine bridge position (Fig. 30.9a).

Hydrotherapy can also be useful in the early reactive stages to allow loading and movement, while reducing weight-bearing forces and so pain. As pain and irritability reduces, loading of the hamstrings is progressed steadily, aiming to create the mechanical forces needed to stimulate cellular activity to promote healing as well as restore strength, endurance and capacity to the tendon.[58]

Clear instructions should be given to the athlete that pain during and after tendinopathy loading is normal and to be expected, but it has to be monitored and managed sensibly every 24 hours to ensure daily loading can be completed. Using the visual analogue scale as a guide can be useful. Keeping pain under 4–5/10 when performing rehabilitation exercises seems best to prevent flare ups and allows daily progression.[59]

As the tendon continues to settle, heavier, slower, eccentric resistance training should be used for the hamstring muscles.[60] Eccentric phases of exercise allow for greater forces over greater durations of time to be tolerated within the musculotendinous unit compared to concentric phases. However, the loading should not focus solely on eccentric contraction. Concentric muscle action is also important, and a mixed and varied program of exercises incorporating both has been shown to achieve good results with tendinopathy.[61]

Intermediate stage treatment

Intermediate PHT rehabilitation exercises should incorporate eccentric action as well as increased load and resistance while minimising positions of high tendon compression. Prone hamstring curls (Fig. 30.8) are a simple, effective method to load hamstrings without any adverse compression, and can be easily adapted, depending on symptoms, with either increased or decreased load, intensity, speed of contraction and range of movement.

Body weight exercises, such as bridges, can be simply and easily progressed into more challenging variations. For example, simply doing them in single leg positions (Fig. 30.9a) or elevating the feet (Fig. 30.9b) or varying the amount

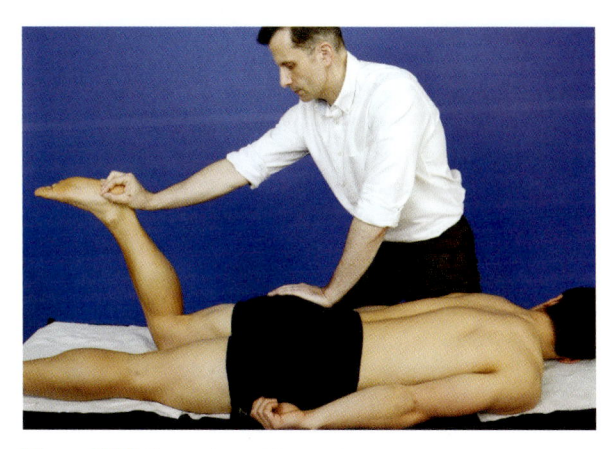

Figure 30.8 Prone hamstring curl

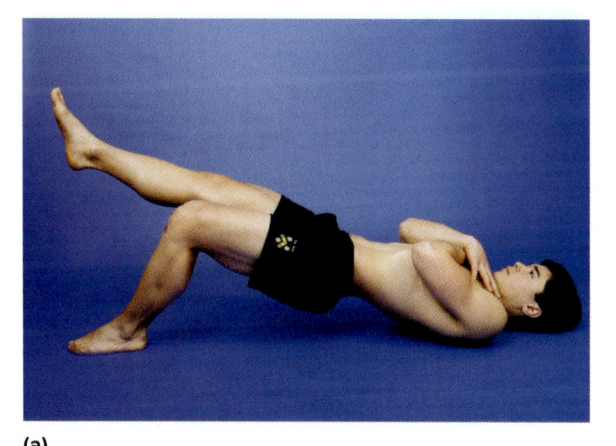

(a)
Figure 30.9 (a) Single-leg hamstring bridge

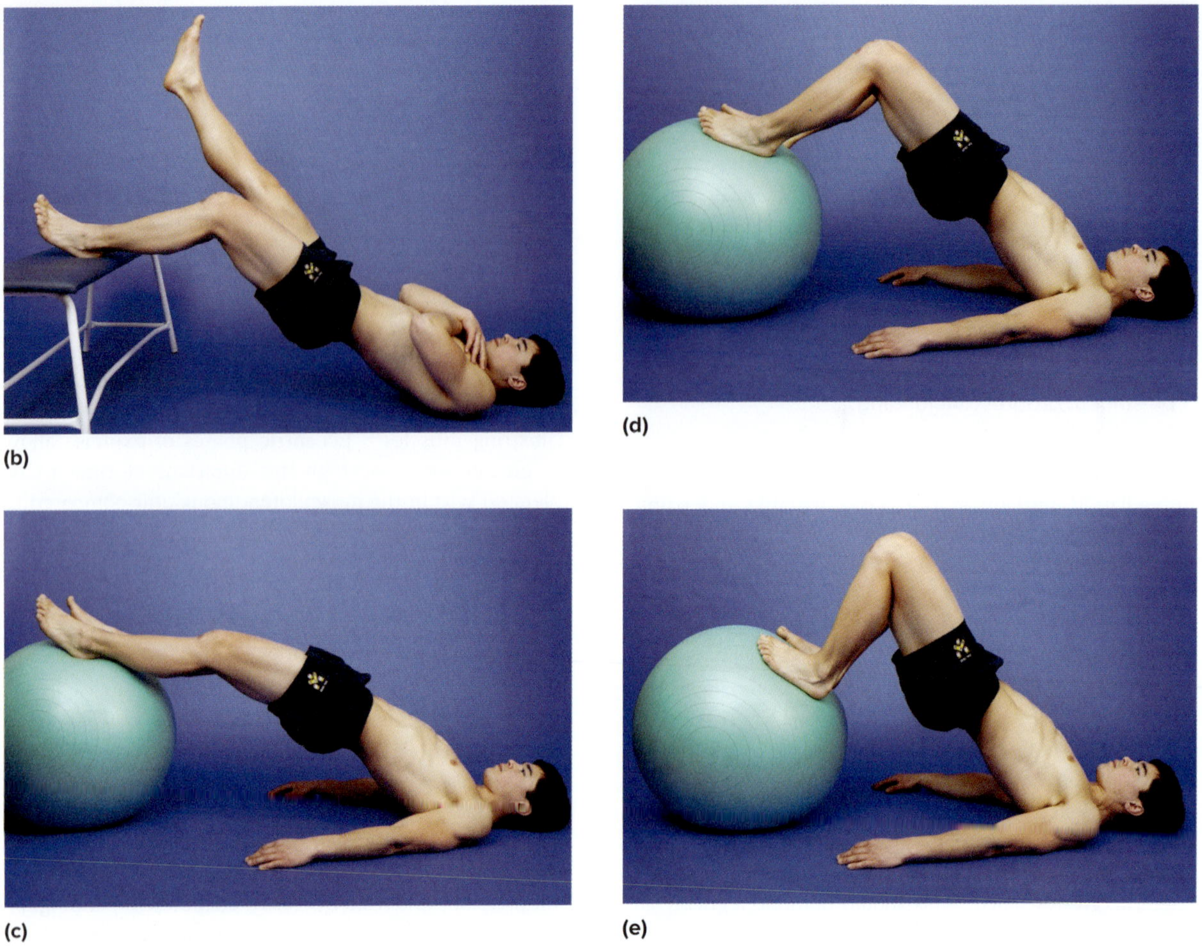

PART B   Regional problems

(b)

(d)

(c)

(e)

Figure 30.9 (cont.) (b) Elevated single-leg hamstring bridge (c) to (e) Gym ball hamstring curls

of knee flexion or extension allows for greater or less force in the hamstrings to be felt. Bridging on a gym ball is a good progression for the intermediate stage of rehabilitation. It adds a dynamic component to the exercise as well as involving and element of proprioceptive training (Fig. 30.9 c,d,e).

As symptoms continue to reduce, exercises in weight-bearing upright positions can be included. These exercises can also progressively introduce compressive forces by increasing the amount of hip flexion to allow the proximal hamstring tendon to start to adapt to them. Exercises such as 'good mornings' (Fig. 30.10a), deadlifts (Fig. 30.10b) and squats (Fig. 30.10c) are good examples, and can be easily and simply progressed by increasing the amount of hip flexion or increasing external loads carried or performing them on the single leg.

During the tendon loading phase, consideration should be given to identifying and addressing any weaknesses found in the kinetic chain or any biomechanical deficits seen around the lumbopelvic area. Static alignment tests, such as planks and their different variations which ask an athlete's lumbopelvic area to resist external forces over a period of time, can give clues to potential weak areas that need addressing.

Dynamic tests, such as single-leg squats and lunges as well as functional tests that mimic an athlete's activity as closely as possible, can give a therapist clues to any possible biomechanical imbalances and lack of proprioceptive ability that may also be a causative factor, while also continuing the appropriate loading for the PHT.

There is no one best or more validated method to assess lumbopelvic strength or biomechanics. Each assessment will be based on, and guided by, the athlete's level of ability and sport, as well as the therapist's own clinical reasoning, experience and preference. Information taken from these tests is to be used with caution and is not to be used in isolation. There is scant evidence and little consensus on the role that biomechanics does or does not have in tendinopathy incidence.

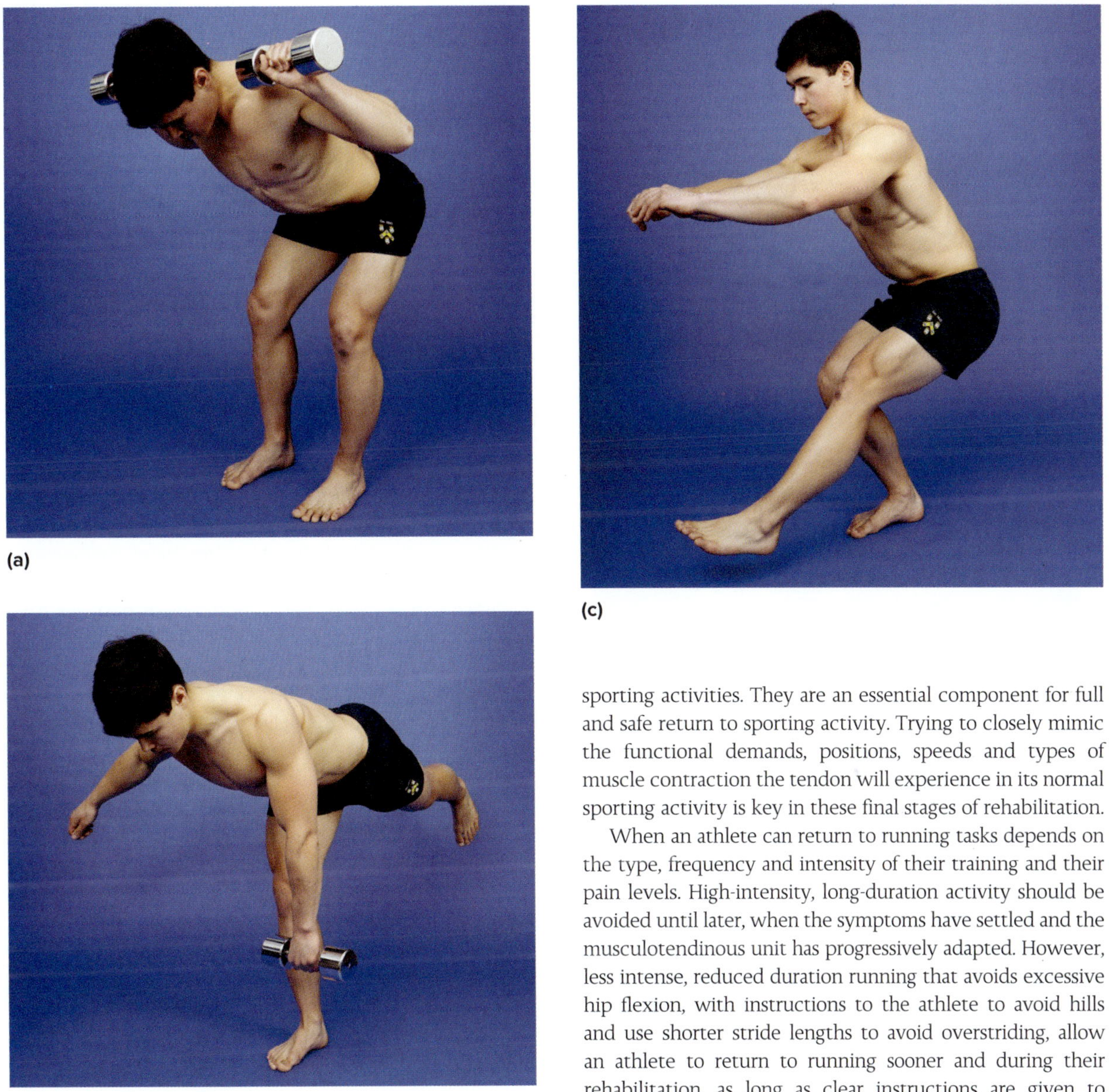

Buttock pain **CHAPTER 30**

Figure 30.10 (a) Loaded double-leg good mornings (b) Single-leg RDL (Romanian dead lift)/toe touches (c) Single-leg squat

Final stage of treatment

The final stages of rehabilitation should include progressive higher speed, plyometric and ballistic movements, such as bounding, hopping and jumping, heel flicks and high knee drives (Fig. 30.11). These types of activities expose the musculotendinous unit to sudden changes in eccentric and concentric action, and allow it to adapt to the normal stretch shortening cycle required in most sporting activities. They are an essential component for full and safe return to sporting activity. Trying to closely mimic the functional demands, positions, speeds and types of muscle contraction the tendon will experience in its normal sporting activity is key in these final stages of rehabilitation.

When an athlete can return to running tasks depends on the type, frequency and intensity of their training and their pain levels. High-intensity, long-duration activity should be avoided until later, when the symptoms have settled and the musculotendinous unit has progressively adapted. However, less intense, reduced duration running that avoids excessive hip flexion, with instructions to the athlete to avoid hills and use shorter stride lengths to avoid overstriding, allow an athlete to return to running sooner and during their rehabilitation, as long as clear instructions are given to monitor pain levels both during and after activity.

SACROILIAC JOINT DYSFUNCTION

The sacroiliac joint (SIJ) is a highly debated and controversial source of low back and buttock pain in sports, with it often being accused of moving too little, too much or even subluxating or popping out of position.

> **PRACTICE PEARL**
>
> SIJ dysfunction is a broad term and is often used as a scapegoat for low back and buttock pain that has no clear diagnosis.

581

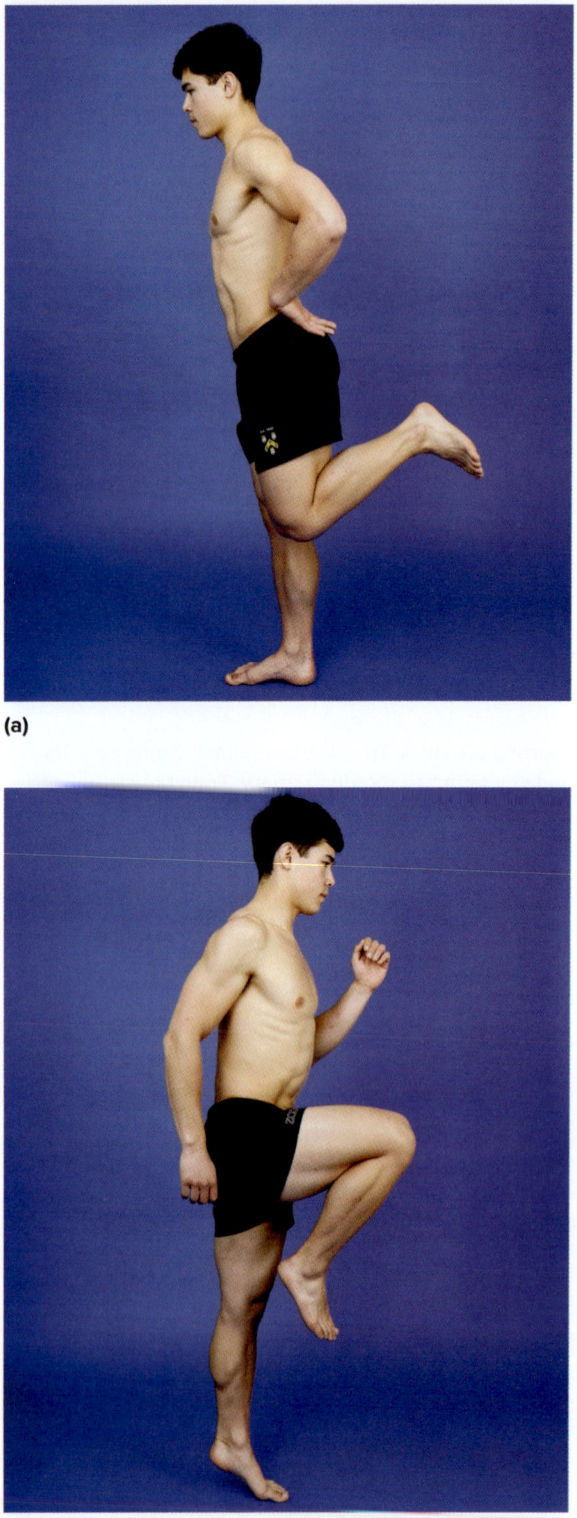

PART B Regional problems

Figure 30.11 (a) Heel flicks (b) High knee drives

The prevalence of SIJ dysfunction varies greatly in the literature, with estimates ranging between 15–30%[62] and even as high as 50% in certain sporting populations.[63]

The true prevalence of SIJ dysfunction is extremely difficult to establish, not only due to the complex anatomy of the SIJ with its many ligaments and myofascial structures that can be a source of pain, but also due to the multifactorial nature of low back and buttock pain.

To confuse matters further, many of the gold standard tests, such as imaging and diagnostic local anaesthetic, cannot be relied upon for the SIJ. Imaging alone cannot differentiate symptomatic from non-symptomatic SIJs;[64] local anaesthetic injections leak out of the joint and affect other tissues and nerve roots around the pelvis.[65]

There is also controversy and disagreement on how and why the SIJ can cause pain. It is commonly believed that poor spinal or pelvic positions or poor posture may be factors in SIJ dysfunction, with excessive anterior or posterior tilt of the pelvis adversely stressing and sensitising either the joint itself, its many ligaments or the myofascial tissue across it.[66] However, there is no evidence that spinal or pelvic positions or postures have any association with pain or incidence of injury.

Poor strength of the pelvic floor, abdominal or lumbar spine muscles is also often proposed as a causative factor for SIJ dysfunction, in the belief that it allows for excessive SIJ movement and shear forces.[67, 68]

However, there are doubts around this commonly held theory. There is no correlation between excessive movement of the SIJ and pelvic pain post-partum.[69] It is even questionable if excessive movement actually occurs at the SIJ, even in those with diagnosed widespread hypermobility joint syndromes and chronic pelvic pain.[18]

Finally, despite claims for the need to improve trunk and pelvic strength to increase the stability of the SIJ, we have no idea what amount of trunk and pelvic muscle activity is needed to provide sufficient stability to the SIJ during different tasks, or if it is even a causative factor in developing SIJ pain.

All this uncertainty around the pelvis often leaves the clinician confused and frustrated when trying to determine whether the SIJ is or is not, dysfunctional or a source of pain, let alone how best to manage it.

Functional anatomy

The sacroiliac joints are highly specialised joints that permit a stable, yet slightly flexible platform for the transmission of forces between the lower limb and the rest of the body. The SIJs are large, flat, part synovial, part fibrotic joints that have a highly congruent surface that provides a large friction coefficient, which together with its many strong ligaments, allows for effective and

Buttock pain CHAPTER 30

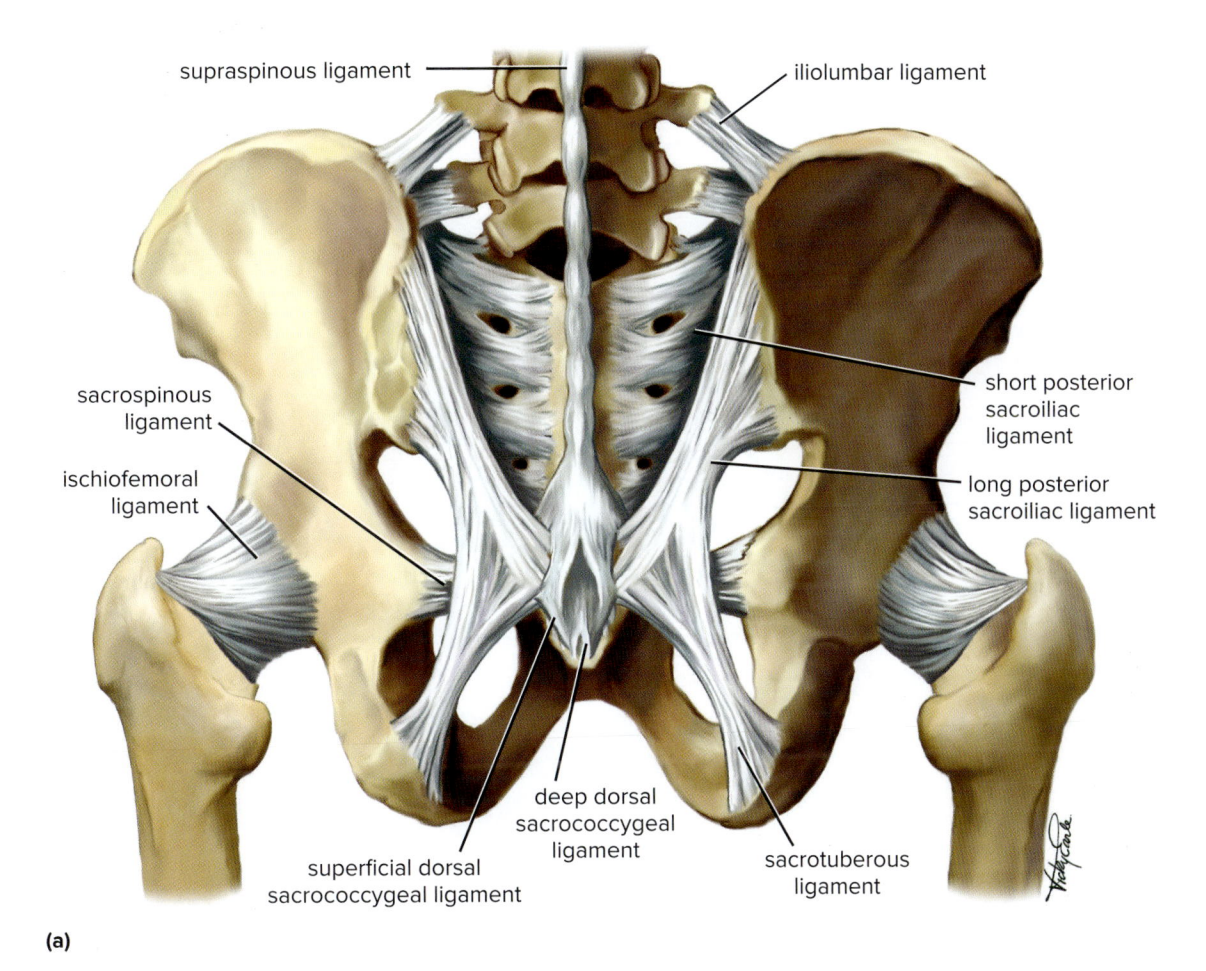

Figure 30.12 Sacroiliac joint anatomy (a) Posterior view

efficient transfer of force with minimal movement.[70] The anatomy of the SIJ ligaments can be seen in Figure 30.12.

There is wide variation described in the literature as to how much normal movement occurs at the SIJ. Some describe up to 8 mm of translation,[71] while others describe much less, between 1.4 and 3.1 mm.[72] However, it is agreed that although there is movement at the SIJ, it is minimal.

During movement, SIJ kinematics are highly complex due to the interaction of the many forces from the upper and lower limbs as well as the spine. Rotational movements at the pubic symphysis are an essential component for the pelvis to function as a unit allowing for simultaneous opposite direction movements of the SIJ to occur during gait. During lumbar flexion the sacrum is tilted anteriorly and produces a force on the innominate bones that creates an external rotation and outflaring movement, this is often described as 'nutation'. The opposite occurs during lumbar extension and is usually called 'counter-nutation'.[73]

The role of the trunk musculature in providing movement, stability and control around the SIJ is also complex. The abdominals, gluteals, hamstrings, latissimus dorsi, spinal extensors and the extensive thoracolumbar fasica are all reported to work together in cross-like slings, assisting in the locking of the SIJ during movement. The term 'force closure' is often used to describe this effect of these muscles on the SIJ.[74]

Clinical features

An athlete with SIJ dysfunction can report a deep, diffuse, usually unilateral buttock pain that may be triggered after a change in activity level. A full and detailed history of an athlete's training record must be thoroughly explored to locate any potential trigger. The onset, location and sensations of SIJ pain can closely mimic that of a lumbar spine issue. However, SIJ pain is more likely to be reported below the level of L5 and possibly more directly over the SIJ, but rarely over the ischial tuberosity. Pain can also

PART B Regional problems

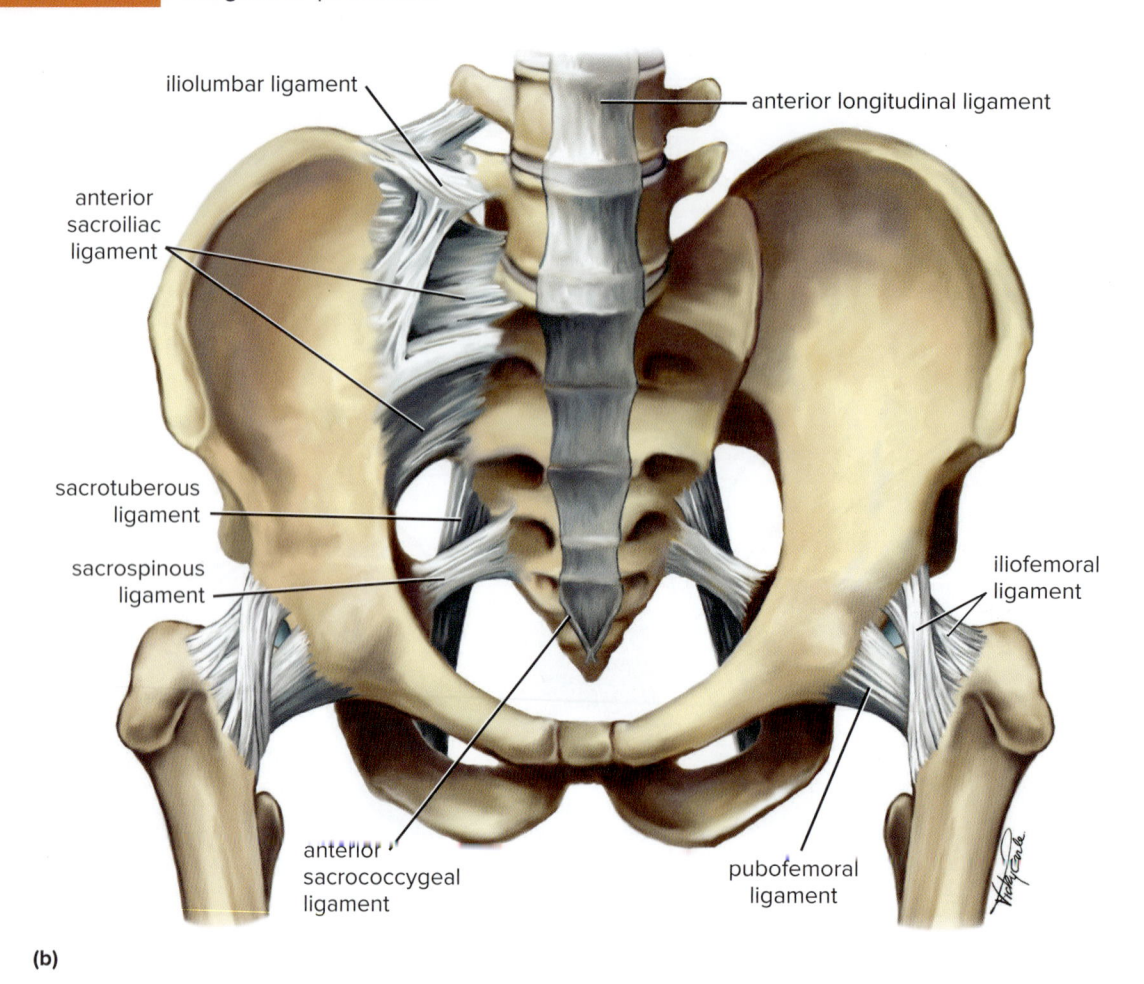

Figure 30.12 (cont.) Sacroiliac joint anatomy (b) Anterior view

occasionally be felt bilaterally and sometimes refer distally down the posterior and lateral thigh.[75]

Aggravating factors tend to be activities that increase forces or loads through the SIJ, such as sitting, walking, lumbar spine movements, and sporting tasks. Easing factors can be resting in supine positions, but side-lying can be uncomfortable.

Examination of the athlete with suspected SIJ pain should look globally at the quality of movement of the gait, hip and lumbar spine movements and check to see if any directional preference is produced with repeated movements which may indicate discogenic or lumbar radiculopathy symptoms rather than SIJ dysfunction.[8] The use of identifying the bony landmarks of the ASIS and PSIS to ascertain if the pelvis is symmetrical or in good alignment has little clinical utility and will not help in the diagnosis or treatment planning.

Other common tests used to assess the SIJ position, alignment or its hypermobility or hypomobility have also been shown to have poor specificity or sensitivity and again have no place in an evidence-based clinical assessment.[19, 20, 76] In fact it has been demonstrated that using palpation tests that feel for movement of the SIJ exaggerate the small SIJ movements by up to five times.[71]

The best way to determine if the SIJ is a source of buttock pain is with a cluster of pain provocation tests.[7, 9] These tests can be seen in Figure 30.3 and the sensitivity and specificity of the combinations are shown in Table 30.2.

The active straight leg raise test (ASLR) has also been proposed as a valid test to assess the ability of the SIJ to withstand load (Fig 30.3o).[9] When it produces a sensation of heaviness or pain, it is thought to highlight trunk or pelvic muscle weakness or altered motor control that reduces SIJ force closure.[77, 78] However, when a positive ASLR test is measured, the increased movement is found at the symphysis pubis joint not the SIJ.[79] It is also not known if a positive ASLR test is a cause or an effect of SIJ dysfunction, as experimentally induced SIJ pain in normal pain-free subjects has been shown to produce a positive test.[80]

Treatment

The management of a patient with suspected SIJ dysfunction must be multimodal to reflect the psychosocial nature of pain, as well as the complex anatomy, biomechanics and relationships that this area has with surrounding structures.

Manual therapy techniques in and around the pelvis, lumbar spine and buttocks, such as soft tissue massage, joint mobilisations and manipulations have been advocated.[81] It must be remembered, however, that the SIJ is highly congruent and well supported by immensely strong ligaments and muscles, therefore these techniques do not and cannot change or alter an SIJ's physical position or affect its biomechanical properties in any way.[82]

The effects achieved with manual therapy around the SIJ are not fully understood, but it appears they are due more to central and peripheral neuromodulation of the soft tissue and joint mechano- and nociceptors that reduce sensations of stiffness and pain rather than biomechanical or structural mechanisms (see Chapters 6 and 7).[83]

Other passive treatment modalities such as taping, pelvic belts and braces have also been suggested to offer relief from SIJ pain. They are often thought to help assist weak trunk muscles in the force closure of the pelvis.[84,85] However, the exact mechanism of action of SIJ belts is still unknown.[86]

Corticosteroid injections in and around the SIJ can help alleviate pain in the short term, but, as previously mentioned, the injected material often leaks out from the joint and can affect other surrounding tissues, which needs to be considered.

The use of sclerosing prolotherapy injections has been advocated in the management of SIJ pain.[87] There is a belief that these injections act as a trigger for fibrosis of the sacroiliac ligaments and help restore stability around the joint.[88] Good quality robust trials using control groups and placebo treatments are lacking with prolotherapy injections, and their use is usually based on anecdotal information.

Although initial treatments for an athlete with SIJ dysfunction can focus on pain relief and symptom modification, ultimately the primary treatment is to restore the capacity of the SIJ and its surrounding tissues to withstand load, stress, shear and strain with a progressive strengthening and functional exercise rehabilitation program.

In the initial stages this may begin with non weight-bearing exercises that focus on the muscles of the posterior chain, the erector spinae, gluteals and hamstrings. Exercises already mentioned in the proximal hamstring tendinopathy section can be used to good effect here.

Exercises such as bridges and their progressions can be combined with exercises that also strengthen the abdominals. Progression of exercises should include moving into weight-bearing positions, focusing on a single plane of movement, such as squats and deadlifts, progressing the resistance and load as symptoms improve. More complex movements involving different and multiple planes of movement, and variable loads and speeds, can be incorporated as the athlete improves, ultimately looking to return the athlete back to full participation in his or her sport.

LESS COMMON CAUSES OF BUTTOCK PAIN

Piriformis syndrome

Another highly debated diagnosis of buttock pain is piriformis syndrome or impingement. This diagnosis was first described in 1947 as an enlarged or inflamed piriformis muscle mechanically compressing the sciatic nerve causing buttock and posterior thigh pain.[89] The anatomy of the piriformis muscle and its relation to the sciatic nerve can be seen in Figure 30.13. Variation in the path of the sciatic nerve around or even through the piriformis has been described as a potential cause for this condition.[90]

It has been proposed that up to 5% of all buttock pain is related to piriformis syndrome.[91] However, there is disagreement over the true prevalence, with some authors arguing that piriformis syndrome is a neurological condition and therefore can only be diagnosed with electro-diagnostic evidence of a neurological deficit.[92] Others think that piriformis syndrome is a myalgia that occurs secondary to insufficiency or weakness of the larger hip and buttock muscles, such as the gluteals.[93]

Piriformis syndrome may be more common in sports that involve frequent hip flexion, internal rotation and adduction, such as cycling, skiing, dance and gymnastics. It can occur with a gradual insidious onset as well as through a traumatic event. Pain is usually reported in the mid buttock area and described as deep and diffuse. It tends to increase with seated positions more than standing and pain may be felt when stretching the buttocks.

Clinical examination of an athlete with suspected piriformis syndrome should try to exclude the more common causes of pain such as the lumbar spine, sciatic neuropathy, hamstring tendinopathy, and the SIJ and its ligaments.

The straight leg raise (SLR), the active side-lying piriformis test (Fig. 30.3p) and passive seated piriformis test (Fig. 30.3q) have been investigated to check their sensitivity and specificity to diagnose sciatic nerve

PART B   Regional problems

(a)

(b)

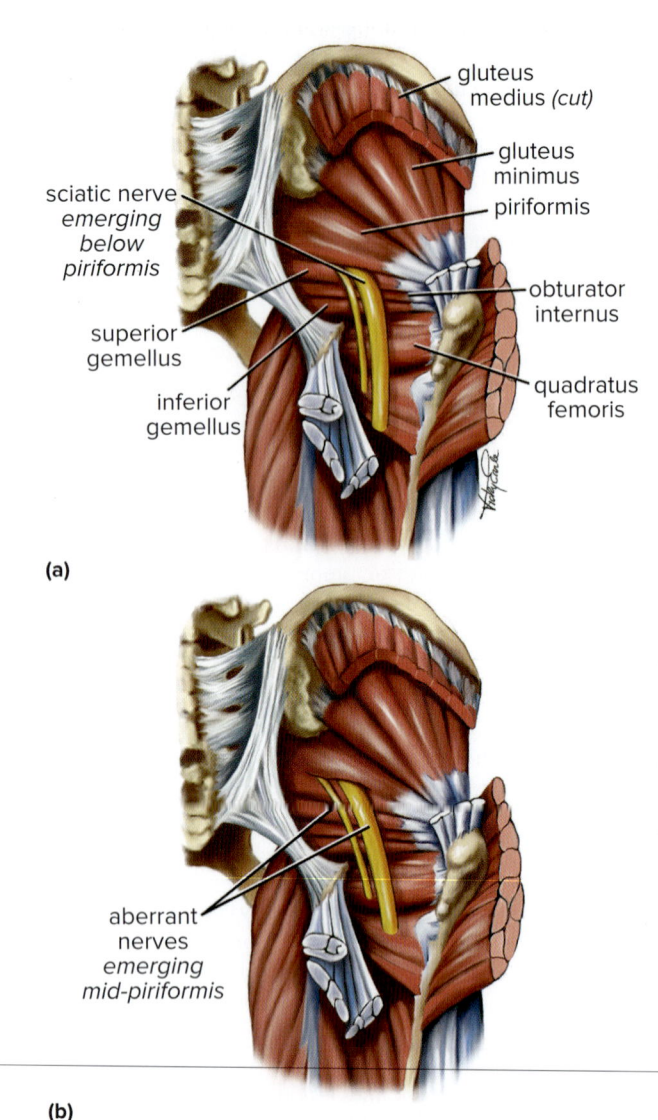

Figure 30.13 Course of the sciatic nerve in the buttock (a) Normal (b) Aberrant

(a)

(b)

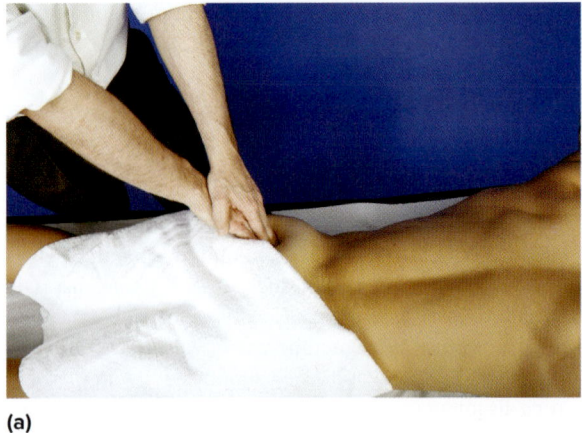

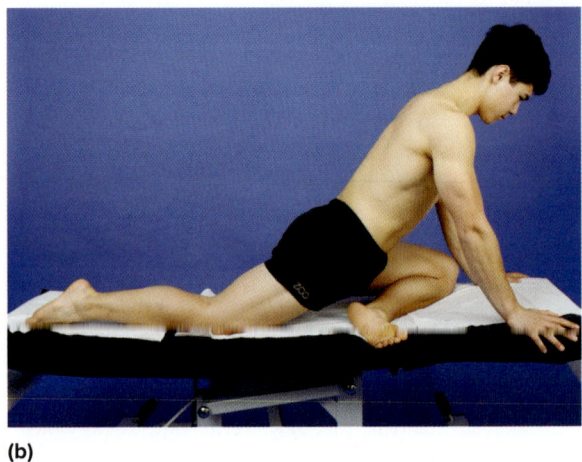

Figure 30.14 Treatment of tight piriformis muscle (a) Soft tissue therapy—piriformis. Sustained longitudinal pressure to the belly of the piriformis muscle, initially in passive external rotation and then moving into internal rotation (b) Stretching of hip external rotators

entrapment in the deep gluteal region and can be seen in Table 30.2.[94]

Special tests used to confirm piriformis syndrome are active resistance tests for the piriformis challenging its actions of hip extension from flexion and external rotation, and are often called the PACE and Beatty tests. Other special tests for piriformis syndrome are passive stretch tests of the muscle in positions of hip flexion and internal rotation, often called the FAIR and Freiberg tests. However, these tests have not shown reproducible validity and so must be used with caution as they also stress other structures. These tests can be seen in Figure 30.3.

As with other causes of buttock pain, treatment should first be prioritised to help reduce pain and modify symptoms. This may be achieved with manual therapy techniques, such as soft tissue massage (Fig. 30.14a) and stretching of the piriformis (Fig. 30.14b). Self-applied methods using tennis and golf balls can be taught.[95] Although the evidence is limited, there can be a role for local anaesthetic injections in the management of piriformis syndrome; however, there seems no advantage in adding corticosteroid to these.[96]

Once symptoms have reduced, the focus should be directed towards strengthening the buttock muscles and their actions of hip extension and abduction. These have already been described in the myofascial pain section in this chapter.

586

Surgical treatment by open or arthroscopic release has been described in a few cases, but these are uncontrolled case studies and should only be considered as a last resort in chronic, refractory cases.[97, 98]

Ischiofemoral impingement

The skeletal morphology of the hip joint is well known as a source of impingement in athletes. A rarer type of hip impingement between the lesser trochanter of the femur and the ischium exists, called ischiofemoral impingement (IFI), and this can manifest as atypical groin or buttock pain.

IFI is believed to be due to abnormal or repeated contact between the lesser trochanter of the femur and the ischium, usually when in positions of hip extension, adduction and external rotation, for example when ballet dancers perform their poses and positions.[99] It could also hypothetically be caused by weakness or fatigue of the hip and pelvic abductors allowing for a Trendelenburg position of excessive pelvic adduction during sports or tasks. This abnormal pelvic and leg position could cause adverse contact, compression and then injury to the quadratus femoris (QF) muscle, a strong adductor and external rotator of the femur and hip stabiliser.

True prevalence of IFI is not fully known, but estimates are around 4% with it predominantly seen in females (84%) and around 40% of cases being bilateral.[100]

An athlete with IFI can present with a similar presentation as an adductor or proximal hamstring tendinopathy, with pain felt in the deep buttock and/or groin when they perform sport or activity, that progressively worsens until it is felt in normal daily activity.[101] Painful popping and clicking sensations can be reported with IFI and can be misdiagnosed as a snapping iliopsoas or labral injury. IFI can also cause neural symptoms due to the close proximity of the QF muscle to the sciatic nerve.[102]

There are no clinical diagnostic special tests for IFI. IFI should be suspected when movements that compress the QF muscle, such as combined hip extension, adduction and external rotation, reproduce pain; however, these should not be used in isolation and should not be relied upon to diagnose IFI.

To diagnose IFI, an MRI is needed that shows QF muscle oedema and/or a reduced space between the ischial tuberosity and lesser trochanter of the femur (Fig. 30.15).[103]

Treatment

Conservative management options for IFI are initially to provide advice and education regarding activity modification to reduce symptoms and allow for soft tissue recovery. Manual therapy can help reduce soft tissue pain, if needed. Once pain has settled, a progressive strengthening program should be started to address any weakness found around the hip, trunk or lower limb that may have predisposed the QF to adverse compression. Consideration should also be given to biomechanical effects, for example, ensuring there is no adverse or unnecessary crossing of the feet over the mid line when running, as well as to good lumbopelvic control during sporting activities.

The surgical management of IFI is highly controversial as it involves resection of the lesser tuberosity. This has risks to the blood supply to the femoral head as well as risks to the sciatic nerve and so should only be considered in the most extreme cases.[104]

Posterior thigh compartment syndrome

Compartment syndrome develops due to increased soft tissue oedema or bleeding that increases tissue pressures within myofascial compartments, compressing

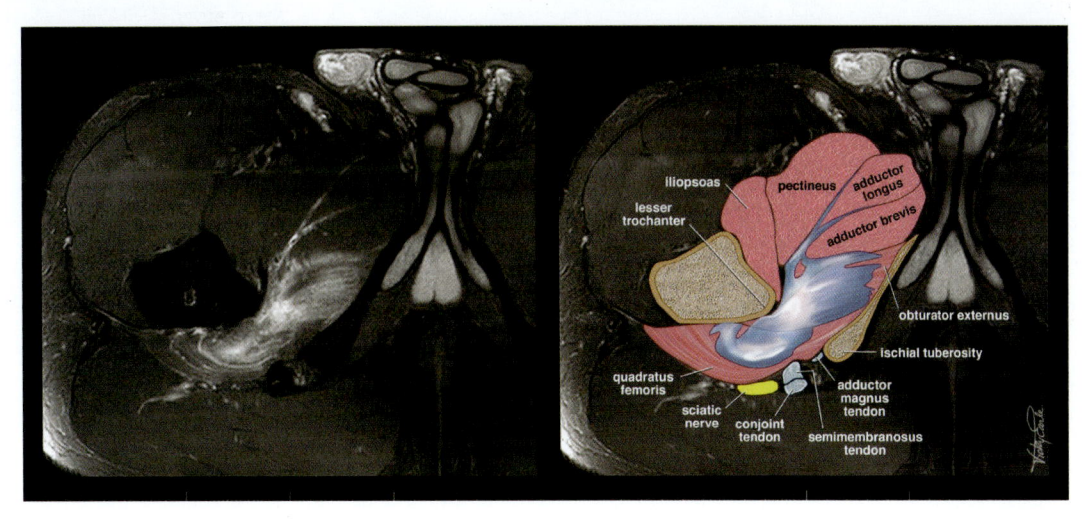

Figure 30.15 MRI showing muscle oedema of the quadratus femoris muscle secondary to ischiofemoral impingement

and compromising the soft tissues, vascular and neural structures.[105] Posterior thigh compartment syndrome is a rare type of compartment syndrome, which causes buttock and posterior thigh pain.

Posterior thigh compartment syndrome can be associated with a traumatic event, such as a blow or a fall onto the buttocks or posterior thigh. It has been reported with acute traumatic hamstring muscle tears or tendon avulsions.[106, 107] It can also be atraumatic and caused by long periods of immobilisation and inactivity.[108]

Posterior thigh compartment syndrome pain is usually diffuse and progressive. It can be accompanied with distal neural and vascular occlusion type symptoms of weakness and paraesthesia. Examination reveals distended, tense and difficult to manipulate soft tissues, possibly with visible bruising if traumatic.

To confirm a diagnosis of compartment syndrome, elevated internal tissue pressures need to be recorded (Chapter 38), with levels between 30-50 mmHg being found to cause muscle necrosis if left more than 4-8 hours.[109] Early diagnosis and careful monitoring of this condition is essential to ensure symptoms do not deteriorate and to avoid any serious complications or adverse effects, such as tissue ischaemia or permanent neural injury.

Conservative management should be directed to help reduce compartment pressures with gentle active and passive movements, and elevation of the limb. Gentle soft tissue massage may help alleviate symptoms. In cases that do not respond with conservative management, or if compartmental pressures worsen, partial surgical fasciotomy is recommended.[110]

Proximal hamstring tendon rupture

Complete disruption of the proximal hamstring tendon at its attachment onto the ischial tuberosity is rare compared to the more commonly encountered hamstring muscle tears or strains in sport. However, complete proximal hamstring tendon ruptures are seen in sports that have a risk of traumatic sudden hip flexion with the knee remaining in near full extension, such as water skiing, gymnastics and motorcross.[111]

These traumatic mechanisms cause the athlete to experience sudden, severe pain, frequently with a sensation of tearing or popping around the upper posterior thigh and usually the patient will not be able to bear weight.[112]

Over the next few hours to days, significant bruising and swelling will emerge extending down the posterior thigh. An observable and palpable deformity may be seen and felt in the posterior thigh on active knee extension when prone. Knee extension will be grossly weak and walking will be difficult due to pain. Confirmation of the extent of the avulsion is best done with MRI (Fig. 30.16) or ultrasound scanning.

Treatment

The decision between conservative and surgical management for proximal hamstring rupture injury is not clear. Some advocate conservative treatment if there is less than 2 cm of retraction seen on imaging.[113] Others suggest all are surgically repaired to ensure complete return of normal muscle strength and power and to maximise chances for return to sport.[114]

Conservative management of complete hamstring ruptures is often challenging due to the large slow resolving haematoma that can complicate the healing

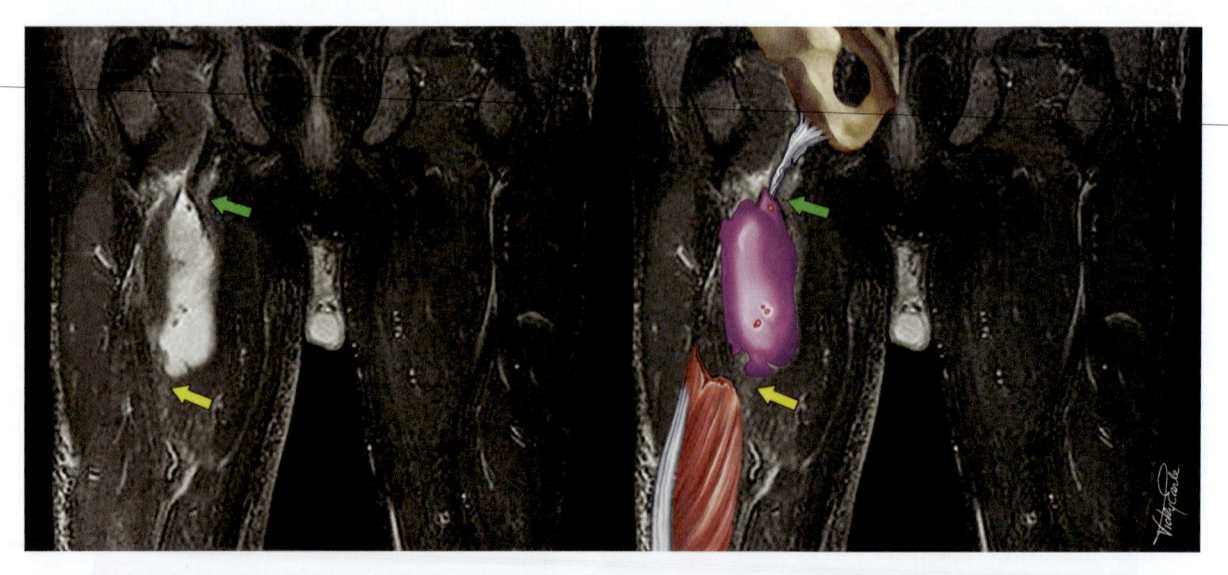

Figure 30.16 MRI showing proximal hamstring rupture. The proximal (green arrow) and distal (yellow arrow) ends of the ruptured tendon are shown with the intervening region of haemorrhage which is the bright signal (white) in the left panel and overdrawn in purple proximal to the retracted muscle in the right panel

process and encourage excessive scarring. This can lead to complications such as adhesions to the sciatic nerve, sometimes called 'hamstring syndrome' and that might even need surgical release.[49]

Conservative treatment for hamstring avulsions should first recognise and ensure that the athlete's expectations are realistic and he or she is fully aware of the extended time this injury will take to recover. Treatment should focus on pain relief and offloading the hamstrings with crutches until weight-bearing can be tolerated. Gentle active and passive movement should be encouraged to prevent joint stiffness and encourage organised scar tissue formation; pool work is a good option here. Manual therapy needs to be used with caution so as not to interfere with normal healing processes. Once weight-bearing is comfortable then a progressive strengthening and conditioning program can begin. However long-term deficits in strength, power and endurance can persist.[115]

Surgical repair for hamstring avulsions is becoming an increasingly popular management option for both acute and chronic hamstring avulsions, with higher levels of patient satisfaction and return to play, greater strength and endurance, and less pain.[116] These injuries are discussed further in Chapter 34.

Avulsion fracture of ischial tuberosity

Avulsion fractures of the ischial tuberosity are similar to complete proximal hamstring tendon ruptures, but are usually seen only in adolescents. They occur when the hamstring tendon fractures the ischial tuberosity, pulling it away from the pelvis.[117] They are most commonly seen in adolescent football and gymnastics.[118]

The age range for these injuries is between 11–17 years old (mean 13.8 years) with the mechanism of presentation usually being exactly the same as a proximal hamstring tendon rupture, a sudden acute pain being felt with a sensation of popping or tearing during a rapid hip flexion movement and an inability to weight-bear.[118]

Examination is the same as with a proximal hamstring tendon rupture, with bruising and swelling developing over the following few hours and days, weakness and pain on prone knee extension, and possibly a visible and palpable deformity of the hamstrings. Confirmation of an avulsion fracture can be made with an ultrasound or MR scan but it can also be seen on a plain radiograph showing a displaced bony fragment away from the ischium (Fig. 30.17).

Management is usually conservative and should be treated the same as a proximal hamstring tendon rupture, by offloading the hamstrings with crutches and with gentle active and passive movements to avoid joint stiffness. Once able to weight-bear, a progressive strengthening and return to play program can commence. However, if the bony fragment is seen to be displaced more than 2.5 cm,

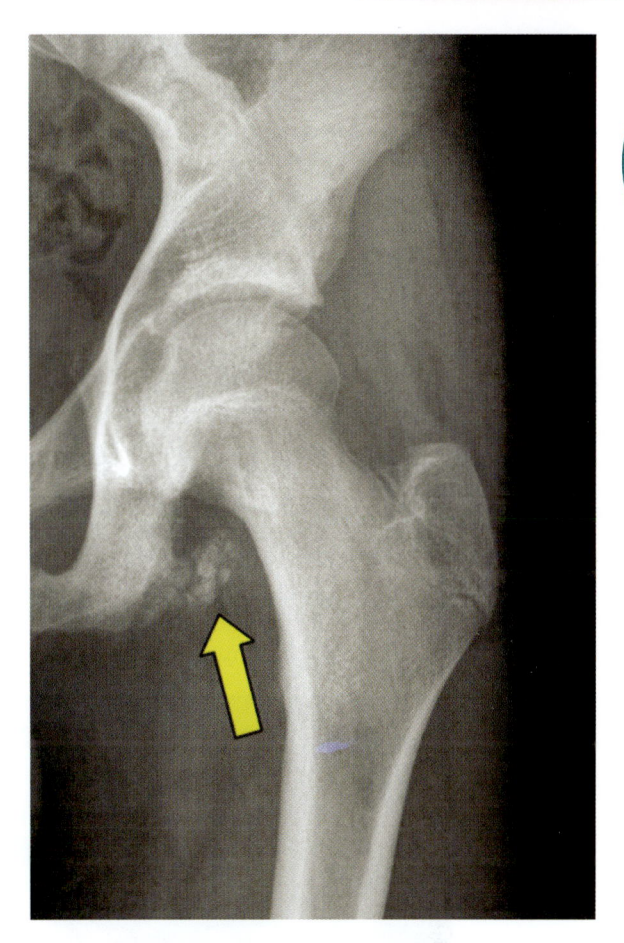

Figure 30.17 Radiograph of an avulsion fracture of the hamstring tendon from the ischial tuberosity
COURTESY OF KYLE NAGLE

surgery may be recommended to restore congruity of the tendon and ensure return to sport.[119]

CONDITIONS NOT TO BE MISSED

Spondyloarthropathies

Buttock pain can be one of the first symptoms associated with a group of systemic inflammatory disorders, such as ankylosing spondylitis. There will usually be no history of trauma, rather a non-specific, insidious onset of buttock pain that is resistant to usual conservative treatments lasting for more than 3 months.

Ankylosing spondylitis is more prevalent in Caucasian races and has a mean age of onset around 23 years. It is rarely seen after the age of 40. It has a male-to-female ratio of 3:1. Buttock and spinal pain and stiffness is commonly reported, lasting more than 30 minutes first thing in the morning, and movement and exercise reduces the pain.[120] These conditions also tend to be associated with multiple joint pains and other enthesopathies in athletes, such as plantar fasciopathy or tendinopathies, and may have extra articular symptoms as well, usually affecting the eyes.[121]

Diagnosis follows observation of a combination of subjective symptoms, imaging and genetic testing for the HLA B27 gene. However, in early manifestations imaging can appear normal. The New York criteria has been suggested as an aid to diagnosis.[122]

Treatment consists of patient advice and education regarding activity modification, with the emphasis on physical exercise and mobility. Nonsteroidal anti-inflammatory medications, corticosteroid injections and the use of disease-modifying anti-rheumatic drugs (DMARDs) have also been found to help.[123]

Stress fracture of the sacrum

Sacral stress fractures are a rare and uncommon cause of buttock pain in the athlete, however the diagnosis is often missed or delayed due to a lack of awareness. There is little epidemiological data, but they are most frequently seen in osteopenic female runners, possibly secondary to menstrual and/or eating disorders (Chapter 4).[124]

The clinical presentation can be variable and very similar to a SIJ dysfunction. The main complaint is usually acute low back or pelvic pain, associated with a severe reduction in mobility and a possible radiation to the leg, groin, buttocks and thighs.

Symptoms are increased with weight-bearing activity, and improve with rest and lying supine. Tenderness over the sacral area is common. There can often be associated tenderness over the symphysis pubis, due to the high incidence of pubic rami fractures in association with sacral stress fractures.[125] Neurological defects are usually absent.

Physical examination may reveal many positive tests for SIJ dysfunction including sacral tenderness on lateral compression; the flexion-abduction-external rotation (FABER) test, Gaenslen's test and the squish test are often positive.[126] Diagnosis of a sacral or pubic ramus fracture is done with imaging. Radiographs can be inconsistent as they will only show complete fractures and even then abdominal and bowel contents can shadow fracture lines.[127] MRI (Fig. 30.18) and CT scans are the best options.

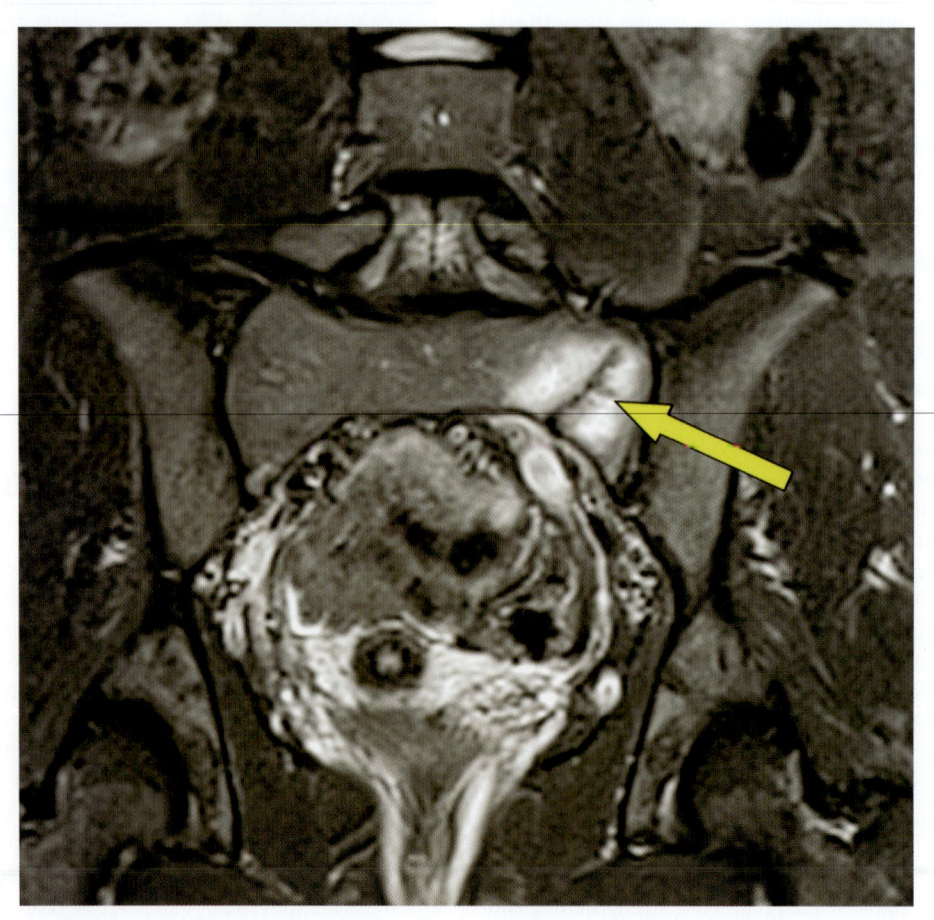

Figure 30.18 Coronal MRI of a sacral stress fracture (arrow)
IMAGING IN SPORTS-SPECIFIC MUSCULOSKELETAL INJURIES, 2016, P.646, ALI GUERMAZI, FRANK W ROEMER, MICHEL D CREMA. © SPRINGER INTERNATIONAL PUBLISHING SWITZERLAND 2016. WITH PERMISSION OF SPRINGER

There are no guidelines for best practice in the management of sacral stress fractures, with some advocating 3-6 months non weight-bearing, and others just a week or two.[128]

The use of non-steroidal anti-inflammatory medications is not recommended in the presence of fractures due to the potential detrimental effects they can have on bone healing (Chapter 4).[127, 129]

The principle treatment is a short period of rest to reduce pain and then progressive early mobilisation to encourage weight-bearing stimulation of osteoblastic activity as well as maintaining bone density, muscle tone and tension, and limiting atrophy and stiffness.

Hydrotherapy is a good early option as body weight can be loaded or offloaded depending on symptoms. As pain continues to settle, a progressive strengthening and conditioning program can be designed and implemented. It has been suggested that return to running activity can be as soon as 2 months after diagnosis, despite pain remaining for around 6 months.[130]

REFERENCES

References for this chapter can be found at www.mhhe.com/au/CSM5e

Chapter 31

Hip pain

with JOANNE KEMP, KAY CROSSLEY, RINTJE AGRICOLA, ANTHONY SCHACHE and MICHAEL PRITCHARD

> ...Lionel Messi returned to Barcelona early from international break due to an inflammation in his hip, pain that has also plagued other players such as Raul, Xabi Alonso, Aduriz, Busquets and a host of Athletic Club's current squad. There are different options in terms of treatment, and each player has undergone their own decision towards recovery to get back onto the pitch as quickly as possible.
>
> www.Marca.com, 4 September 2016

Recently, the hip joint has been recognised as a possible cause of problems in the athletic population. This is reflected in the published literature describing hip pathology and its treatment. The advent of magnetic resonance imaging (MRI) and then hip arthroscopy increased the awareness of hip labral pathology and anatomical variants that can lead to femoroacetabular impingement (FAI) syndrome as a potential underlying cause of hip and groin pain in young and middle-aged people. Lateral hip pain is also increasingly recognised as a substantial clinical problem.

EPIDEMIOLOGY

Pain reported by patients as being in the hip region ('hip pain' for convenience in this chapter) is a common cause of activity restriction in athletes. Hip and groin pain is the third most common injury reported in the Australian Football League (AFL),[1] accounting for between 5-15% of all AFL-related injuries,[2] and is commonly seen in many other sports, including tennis, football of all codes and hockey. People with 'cam'-type FAI are four times more likely to develop hip pain over 4 years than those without this morphological variant.[3] Burnett et al. demonstrated that 92% of patients with arthroscopically confirmed labral tears complained of moderate to severe groin pain.[4] Philippon et al. described labral tears and FAI in 100% of professional National Hockey League ice hockey players presenting for hip arthroscopy for the treatment of longstanding hip and groin pain.[5] However, cam-type morphology is also associated with labral and cartilage hip damage in asymptomatic males where adjusted odds ratios range from 2.45 to 2.77.[6] Therefore the relationship between activity, pain, morphology and pathology is complex and not fully understood.

The likelihood of an athlete sustaining an injury to the hip joint can be increased by the demands of the sport, in particular sports that require repetitive hip flexion, adduction and rotation,[7] but may also be caused by inherent or acquired individual anatomical variations within the joint, such as FAI or developmental dysplasia of the hip.[5, 8-13]

Intra-articular hip pathologies, including chondral and labral pathology contribute to a reduced ability to participate in sporting or physical activities as well as pain and reduced function during activities of daily living.[14] In addition, people with pathology such as FAI, labral tears and chondral pathology have impairments in hip range of motion, hip muscle strength, balance and functional task performance.[14, 15] These physical impairments are themselves associated with further pain, limitations in daily activities, sporting participation and quality of life in affected individuals.[16] Given the increased recognition of hip pathology as a source of hip and groin pain in active individuals, it is important that clinicians have a thorough understanding of likely diagnoses and appropriate treatment options in these patients.

FUNCTIONAL ANATOMY AND BIOMECHANICS

The hip has three functions, which are to allow mobility of the lower limb, to transmit loads between the upper body, trunk and lower limb, and to provide a stable base in weight-bearing activities. The anatomy of the hip allows it to perform these functions.

PART B Regional problems

The hip joint is supported by a number of dynamic and passive supports, which include its bony morphology, passive restraints such as capsule and ligaments, and a complex system of interplaying muscle groups. The biomechanics of the hip joint are generally under-reported in the literature and as such are poorly understood. An appreciation of the functional anatomy of the hip and the role of the various structures surrounding the hip will assist in this understanding (Fig. 31.1).

Morphology

The hip joint (femoroacetabular joint) is a tri-planar synovial joint, formed by the head of femur inferiorly and the acetabulum superiorly. The acetabulum sits within the bony pelvis and is normally anteverted (forward facing) by approximately 23° (Fig. 31.2a).[17] The acetabulum also faces inferiorly and laterally.

The head of femur is also anteverted, which refers to the angle between the axis of the femoral neck and the transcondylar axis of the knee (Fig. 31.2b). This angle is normally between 10-15° in adults. The head of femur also faces superiorly and medially.

Any orientational or morphological deviation from this normal anatomy can result in unnecessary stresses within the hip joint. An undercoverage of the femoral head by the acetabulum as seen in acetabular dysplasia can place high static loads on the anterosuperior acetabular cartilage due to a decreased contact area. In contrast, an overcoverage of the femoral head by the acetabulum can lead to 'pincer'-type FAI. A cam deformity can lead to a biomechanically imperfect hip joint, as it may cause cam-type FAI. The anteversion of the proximal femur and acetabulum and the neck-shaft angle can in turn influence the susceptibility of the hip joint to FAI. The concept of FAI will be discussed in more detail below.

This morphological structure allows the hip to achieve its 3° of movement, flexion and extension, adduction and abduction, and external and internal rotation. It also allows the athlete to move freely in three planes of movement.

Acetabular labrum

The acetabulum forms the socket of the hip joint and is lined with articular cartilage. The acetabular labrum (Fig. 31.3) is a ring of fibrocartilage and dense connective tissue which is attached to the bony acetabular rim. The acetabular labrum is thinnest in its anterior aspect.

The blood supply of the labrum enters through the adjacent joint capsule. Only the outer third of the labrum is vascularised.[19] The labrum is innervated by a branch of the nerve to quadratus femoris and also by the obturator nerve.[20] Nocioceptive free nerve endings are distributed throughout the acetabular labrum, while labral cells are capable of releasing cytokines when damaged, suggesting a pain and inflammation-producing capacity.[21-23] In addition, the labrum contains nerve end organs which suggest that, as well as a capacity to mediate pain, it can also assist in proprioception and generate neurosecretion that may assist in connective tissue repair.[20]

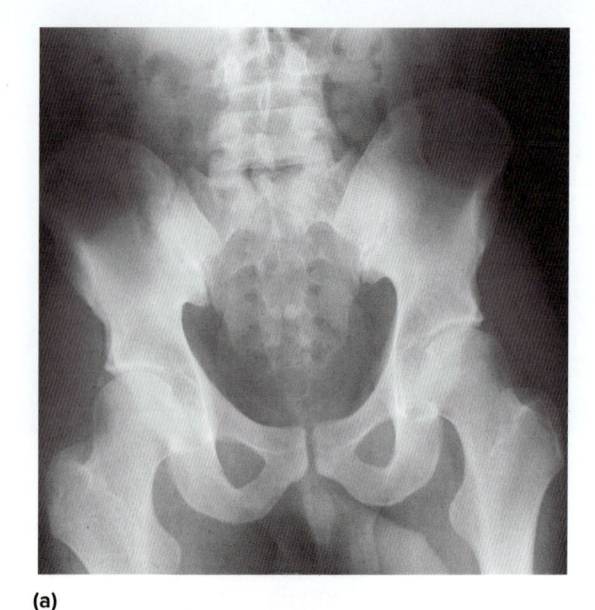

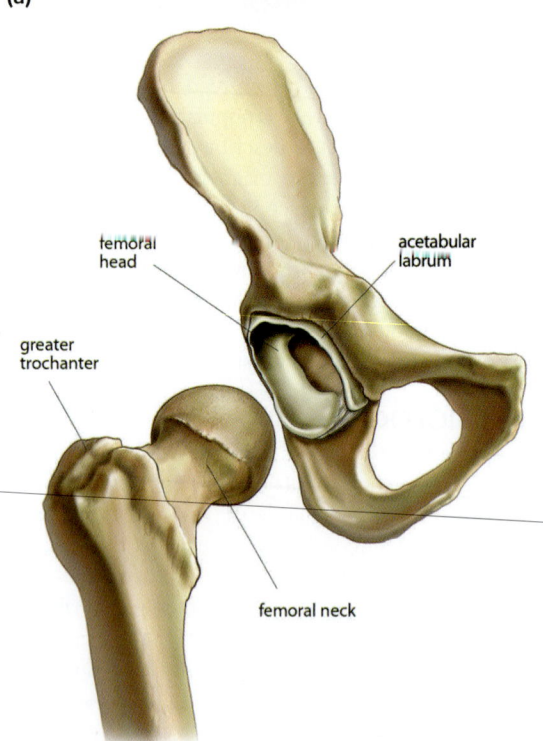

Figure 31.1 Anatomy of the hip and groin area (a) Plain radiograph of the pelvis (b) The hip joint

Hip pain   CHAPTER 31

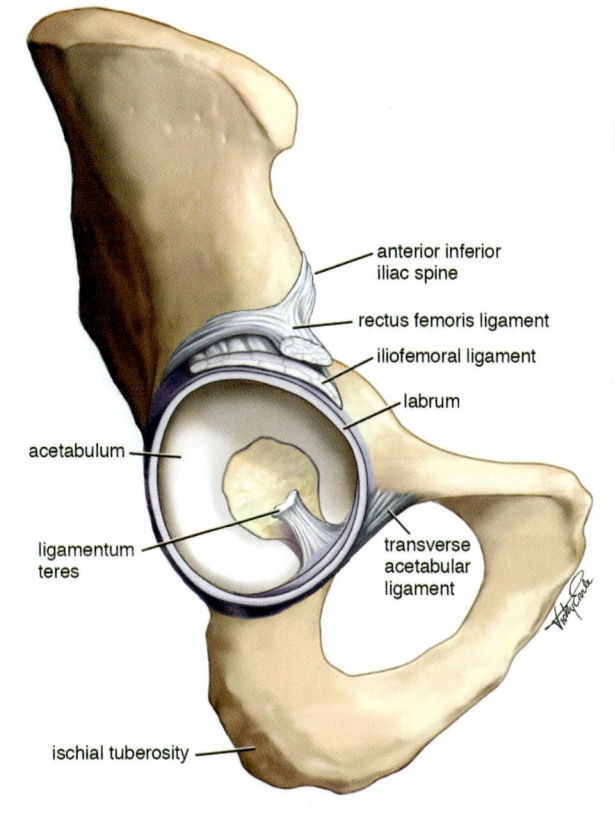

Figure 31.3 Transverse acetabular ligament, acetabular labrum and ligamentum teres (resected)

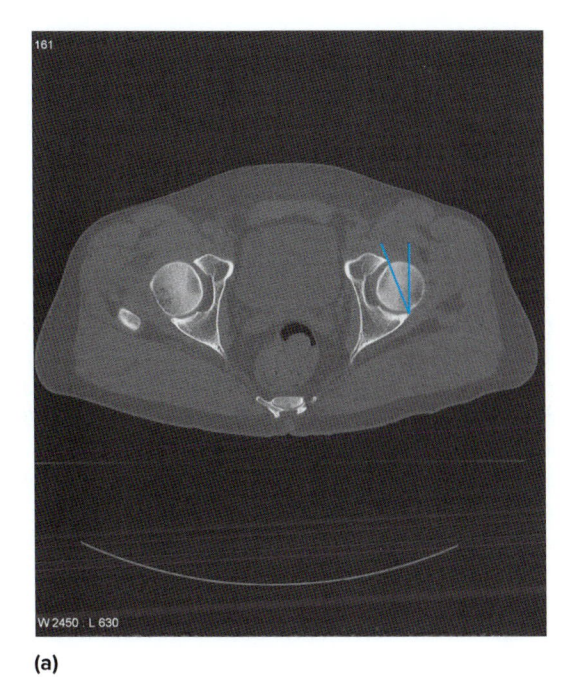

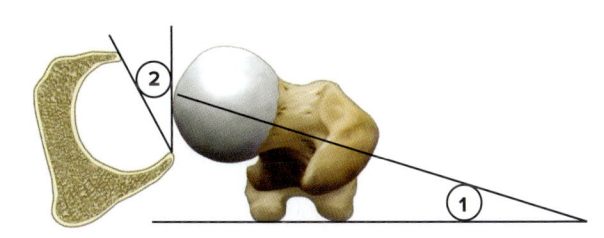

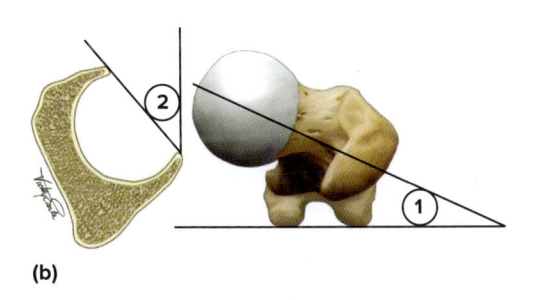

Figure 31.2 (a) Computed tomography showing acetabular anteversion[17] (b) Transverse views of a normal hip (upper figure) and a dysplastic hip (lower figure)[18] (1) Angle of torsion—rotation of the femoral neck relative to the shaft (transcondylar axis), normally 10–15° of anteversion. Dysplastic hips usually have increased angle (2) Acetabular anteversion angle—the anterior direction of the acetabulum is normally 20–40° of anteversion. Dysplastic hips usually have increased angle but it may be decreased

The acetabular labrum has several functions. These are primarily to deepen the acetabulum, to distribute the contact stress of the acetabulum over a wider area (increasing contact area by 28%)[24], and to assist in synovial fluid containment and distribution by virtue of the fluid seal mechanism.[22, 24, 25] The acetabular labrum is continuous with the acetabular rim and adjacent acetabular articular cartilage, providing nutrition to, and assisting in, modulating loads within the acetabulum of the hip.

Normally, the fluid seal of the labrum and synovial fluid pressure is greatest in activity involving external rotation of the femur, while activity involving flexion and internal rotation (impingement) reduce the fluid seal and synovial fluid pressure.[26] Also people with cam-type FAI do not achieve maximal fluid seal and synovial fluid pressure during external rotation.[27] Given that adequate labral seal and synovial fluid pressure are essential for labral and cartilage nutrition, this has the potential to cause problems. These findings may help explain why hip impingement is associated with hip pain and pathology such as labral and chondral lesions, and why people with cam-type FAI are more susceptible to these associated pathologies.

595

Ligaments of the hip

The transverse acetabular ligament (Fig. 31.3) traverses the acetabular notch, connecting the anterior and posterior edges of the labrum. The deepest layer of labral tissue blends into this ligament. The transverse acetabular ligament is under greatest load in weight-bearing, when the head of femur relocates in the acetabulum, widening the acetabular notch and placing the transverse acetabular ligament under a tensile load.[25]

Originally thought to be a histological vestige that becomes redundant early in childhood, it is now assumed that the ligamentum teres (Fig. 31.3) plays an important proprioceptive role, especially in weight-bearing activities.[28]

The hip capsule contains ligaments that act together to restrain excessive motion of the hip joint. These are the iliofemoral ligament, the pubofemoral ligament and the ischiofemoral ligament (Fig. 31.4). The iliofemoral ligament ('Y ligament of Bigelow') reinforces the anterior capsule and originates from the anterior iliac spine, fanning into an inverted Y shape to insert into the intertrochanteric line. It is taut in hyperextension and also provides stability in relaxed standing. The pubofemoral ligament arises from the anterior surface of the pubic ramus and inserts into the intertrochanteric fossa. It is taut in abduction and extension and also reinforces the anterior capsule. The ischiofemoral ligament arises from the posterior surface of the acetabular rim and labrum and extends into the femoral neck just proximal to the greater trochanter. Its fibres run in a spiral pattern and are also taut in hyperextension. These three ligaments act to restrain hyperextension, which is of particular relevance in relaxed standing.

Chondral surfaces

Both articular surfaces of the hip are lined with articular cartilage. These chondral surfaces rely upon adequate function of the synovium and movement of synovial fluid within the joint to provide nutrition, as articular cartilage is avascular. As detailed above, the degree of synovial fluid distribution is affected by the functional position of the hip, as well as by the presence of cam-type FAI, indicating that both the position of the hip and cam-type FAI may impact on cartilage nutrition. Both acetabular labrum and ligamentum teres have been reported to attach to synovium, and thus both may also play a role in the nutrition and normal function of articular cartilage within the hip joint.

In a normal, healthy hip joint, the articular cartilage assists in smooth movement as well as absorbing loads, protecting the subchondral bone and adjacent intra- and extra-articular structures. Glycosaminoglycans (GAGs) are molecules contained within the extracellular matrix of cartilage. They provide the strength and shock-absorbency characteristics typical of healthy cartilage. When reduced, the strength of cartilage and its ability to absorb forces are greatly inhibited. Lower levels of GAGs are reported in the early stages of osteoarthritis (OA) and also in people with cam deformity, pain on impingement testing and painful FAI.[29] There is an increased risk of chondral injury when coexisting labral pathology and cam-type FAI are present,[14] while it has been suggested that chondral injury may represent hip OA in its earlier stages.[30]

It appears that the interrelated nature of cam-type FAI, labral pathology and chondral injury all contribute to the breakdown of normal hip function and that abnormal hip mechanics may also contribute to these pathologies. Strategies that are focused on optimising the mechanics of the hip joint may be important targets when improving function, reducing pain and slowing hip-joint disease progression.

Muscle function

Dynamic hip stability is provided by a complex interplay between various muscles surrounding the hip joint. In particular, the primary hip stabilisers provide a posterior, medial and inferior force on the femur to control the

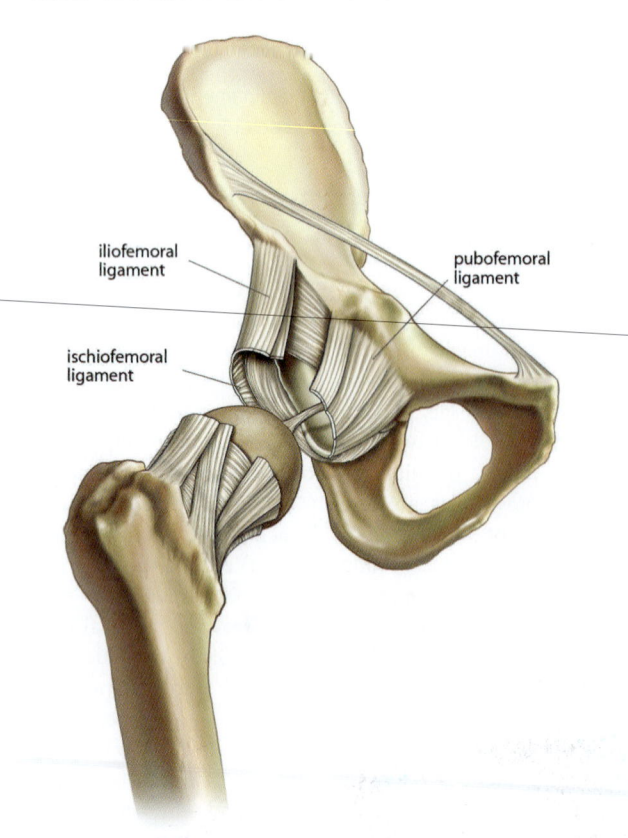

Figure 31.4 Capsular ligaments of the hip

Hip pain   CHAPTER 31

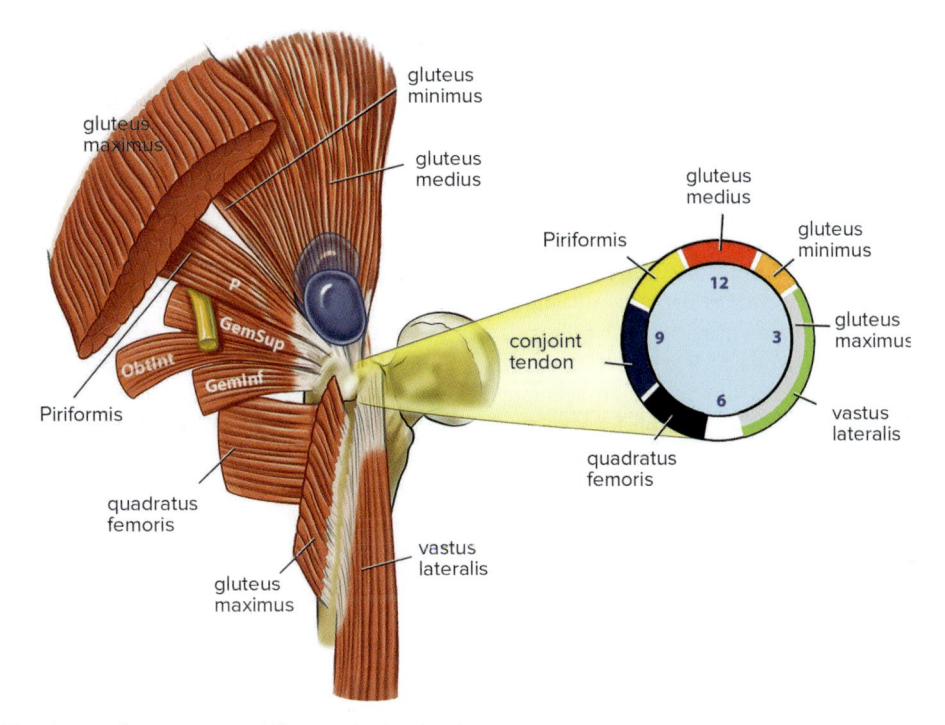

Figure 31.5 Muscle attachments around the greater trochanter

> **PRACTICE PEARL**
>
> The concept of deep hip stabilisers as the hip 'rotator cuff'[31] has grown in popularity in recent years.

position of the head of femur within the acetabulum.[32] Ultimately, the dynamic control provided by the deep hip stabilisers has potential to minimise stress on vulnerable structures, such as the anterosuperior acetabular labrum and the anterosuperior acetabular rim (Fig. 31.5).

Reports detail the role of hip muscles with respect to muscle morphology, primary action of joint movement and lines of action in relation to the axes of joint movement.[31, 33, 34] Some muscles have greater capacity to generate torque over larger ranges of motion (prime movers), while other muscles are better placed to act as dynamic hip joint stabilisers.

Short hip stabilising muscles

The six short hip external rotators (obturator internus and externus, the superior and inferior gemellus, quadratus femoris and piriformis), also known as short hip stabilising (SHS) muscles, provide hip joint compression and hence dynamic stability during most weight-bearing and nonweight-bearing activities.[33] The gluteus medius is the dominant hip abductor and is the primary lateral stabiliser of the hip during one-leg stance activities.[34]

Clinical biomechanics

For the patient with hip pain and/or pathology, the clinician should also consider the lines of actions for each of the deep hip stabilisers.[33] For example, although all of the SHS muscles provide dynamic hip stability in the anatomic position, the quadratus femoris also has a line of action that is inferomedial. Therefore, it has a greater capacity to resist superior translation of the hip. Similarly, the gluteus maximus and four SHS muscles (piriformis, gemellus inferior and superior, obturator internus) have a line of action that is posteromedial and may be able to resist anterior force of the hip.[35]

In contrast, although the gluteus medius is an important lateral stabiliser of the hip, its line of action is both medial and superior[33] and it is the greatest contributor to both medial and superior hip contact force during walking.[35] Furthermore, the anterior fibres of gluteus medius and minimus become hip internal rotators when the hip is flexed. The relevance of these factors to the rehabilitation of the patient with hip pain and pathology will be described below.

In healthy people without hip pain, men are generally stronger than women in most hip muscle groups, while there is no difference between the dominant and non-dominant leg.[36] Hip muscle strength can be measured reliably in the clinic using hand-held dynamometry.[36, 37] In certain populations, the relationships between agonist and antagonist muscle groups have been reported,

597

providing further evidence of how hip muscles function together in healthy groups[37, 38] and how this function might be impaired in people with hip pain and pathology.

CLINICAL APPROACH

Hip region pain can be multifactorial and therefore difficult to diagnose. Hip pain also commonly coexists with groin-related pathology, such as the adductor, iliopsoas, inguinal and pubic-related entities (Chapter 32). These entities can present as hip pain. This makes definitive diagnosis and provision of appropriate management programs difficult and often multifactorial.[39] Therefore, the key to the effective management of hip pain is an accurate diagnosis of the likely source of and reason for the pain and understanding important differential diagnoses. The causes of hip pain are shown in Table 31.1.

> **PRACTICE PEARL**
>
> One major issue facing clinicians when encountering a patient with pain in the hip and groin region is the poor specificity of the majority of clinical tests,[40] making accurate diagnosis of the source of pain difficult (see also Chapter 14).

Fortunately, a number of clinical tests have good or excellent sensitivity, meaning clinicians can have a reasonable degree of certainty that a patient with a negative test finding does not have pain whose source is the hip joint.

A second issue is the potential for intra- and extra-articular sources of hip pain, as well as remote factors to contribute to the patient's symptoms. Finally, imaging modalities are useful, but are not equal or superior to arthroscopy when diagnosing hip pain. Therefore, clinicians need to consider a range of possible sources of pain when making the diagnosis from a combination of subjective and objective findings and imaging results.

Hip region pain and associated pathologies have not been well managed in the athletic population until recently. A large cohort study of patients with FAI in the USA indicated that most patients had hip pain for 12–36 months.[41] Weir and colleagues reported a mean duration of hip and groin pain in athletes of 22 weeks,[42] with the maximum duration 250 weeks (5 years), while many other studies report symptom duration of greater than 2 years.[18] Byrd and Jones reported an average of 7 months from initial assessment and multiple other diagnoses being made before a definitive diagnosis of hip pathology was made.[43]

In the fourth edition of *Clinical Sports Medicine*, we mentioned the debate regarding the efficacy of hip arthroscopy as an appropriate intervention for athletes with hip pain. The efficacy of both surgical and non-surgical interventions for hip pain remains unknown. The danger of both surgical and non-surgical procedures being perceived as being fashionable is that practitioners can become polarised in their opinions and not assess each case and therefore the most appropriate intervention on its merits. Future studies determining the efficacy of both surgical and non-surgical management of hip pain are essential.

When assessing the hip, the reliability and clinical utility of assessment findings should be considered. These are contained in Table 31.2. A comprehensive discussion of the key components of a clinical history, physical examination and appropriate referral for investigations is outlined below.

History

The only feature from a clinical history with known validity is painful clicking; it has a low likelihood ratio (Table 31.2). This indicates that a patient without painful clicking is unlikely to have a labral tear. Nonetheless, it is important to obtain a full history from a patient prior to undertaking a physical examination or obtaining any investigations. This history should include:

- age, general health, past medical history (including presence or absence of childhood conditions such as 'clicky hips', slipped upper femoral epiphysis or infantile dysplasia), past family history of hip pain and hip OA (there is a greater risk of FAI if it is present in other family members[50]) and medications
- weight and height (BMI >25 can increase severity of symptoms of OA and tendinopathy, as well as increase joint loads; also, patients with FAI and related pathology tend to have a BMI >25[14, 41])
- exact mechanism of injury (if known), was onset sudden or insidious?
- time since onset of symptoms (patients with FAI often have had symptoms for 1–3 years[41])
- pattern of symptoms since onset (worsening, improving or not changing)
- presence of mechanical symptoms such as locking, clicking or giving way (suspect labral or possibly ligamentum teres pathology)
- location of pain (hip pathology may present as groin, lower back, lateral hip, buttock or thigh pain[51] and secondary sources of pain such as muscle spasm, which complicate the assessment)
- Note that lateral hip pain is usually *not caused* by hip joint pathologies

Table 31.1 Causes of hip pain

Common	Less common	Not to be missed
Anterior pain		
Labral tear Chondropathy Osteoarthritis Synovitis Ligament teres tear Hip joint instability (hypermobility or developmental dysplasia of the hip) Groin-related pain (see Chapter 32)	Stress fracture of the neck of femur (see Chapter 32) Traction apophysitis (anterior inferior iliac spine–rectus femoris; anterior superior iliac spine–sartorius; lesser trochanter–iliopsoas)	Avascular necrosis of the head of femur Synovial chondromatosis Slipped capital/upper femoral epiphysis Perthes' disease (see Chapter 44) Tumour
Lateral pain		
Gluteus medius tears and tendinopathy	Referred pain lumbar spine Pain from the trochanteric bursa	Fracture of neck of femur Nerve root compression Tumour
Posterior pain		
Posterior labral tear Posterior chondral lesion Ligamentum teres tear Posterior micro-instability secondary to anterior impingement	Referred pain lumbar spine and pelvic joints Proximal hamstring-related pain (see Chapter 34) Sciatic nerve entrapment in short posterior rotators (see Chapter 30)	Nerve root compression Tumour

- nature of pain (intensity, severity, constancy, time of day, latency will provide clues as to presence of inflammation, synovitis, bursitis or tendinopathy in addition to intra-articular pathology)
- neurological signs and low back pain (the lumbar spine can refer pain to the hip and should be eliminated as a potential primary source of pain)
- aggravating factors (be specific regarding position of hip and potential for impingement during these activities, how long it takes for these activities to provoke pain and latent pain)
- current level of activity (frequency and intensity, differentiate between upper and lower limb workouts. Tendon pain tends to be load dependent over a period of 3 days, thus aggravating factors related to gluteal tendinopathy may be difficult to determine if the person has very limited 'unloaded leg days')
- factors easing pain (be specific regarding positions of ease as well as time required for pain to ease)
- current sporting history (including level of sport, such as community, state, national; and position played within the team as certain positions will place the hip under more load
- previous sporting history (certain sports played may increase the likelihood of a hip injury such as dancing, gymnastics, martial arts, tennis and hockey)
- desired level of future sporting activity (this is important to establish in order to determine level of intervention as well as future risk of injury)
- activities of daily living, including occupation, length of time spent sitting, amount of hip flexion and rotation, and degree of manual labour within occupation, family situation including the presence of young children
- any past treatment, including investigations, conservative treatment or surgical intervention.

During the history, appropriate patient reported outcome measures (PROMs) should be given to the patient to complete to establish a baseline score for severity of the condition, to explore specific areas of concern and to allow accurate monitoring of the patient's progress over time (see below).

PART B Regional problems

Table 31.2 Diagnostic accuracy of clinical tests (history, physical exam) in patients with hip pain

Assessment finding	What is a positive finding?	Sn	Sp	LR−	LR+
History					
Labral tear					
Painful clicking in hip[44]	Clicking	100	85	0.00	6.7
Physical examination tests					
Intra-articular pathology (not specific)					
Flexion, abduction and external rotation (FABER)[40]	Pain	42–81	18–75	0.72–0.73	1.1–2.2
Scour test[45]	Pain	50	29	0.70	1.72
Thomas test[46]	Pain and reduced range	89	92	0.12	11.1
Labral tear					
Flexion, adduction and internal rotation (FADIR) (vs magnetic resonance arthrogram)[40]	Pain	94	9	0.48	1.02
FADIR (vs arthroscopy)[40]	Pain	99	5	0.15	1.06
Flexion internal rotation[40]	Pain	96	25	0.27	1.12
Femoral fracture					
Patellar-pubic percussion[40]	Reduced percussion on side of pain	95	86	0.07	6.11
Gluteal tendinopathy					
Trendelenburg[40]	Drop in NWB pelvis	61	92	0.25	6.83
Resisted hip abduction[40]	Weakness and pain	71	84	0.37	5.50
Resisted internal rotation[47]	Weakness and pain	55	69	0.66	1.77
Resisted external de-rotation test[48]	Pain	88	97.3	0.12	32.6
Single-leg stance hold for 30 seconds[48]	Pain during single-leg stance	100	97.3	0.0	37
Combination of findings	Number of variables present	Sn	Sp	LR−	LR+
Hip OA (vs X-ray)[49]					
Squatting aggravates symptoms	5/5	14	98	0.87	7.3
Lateral pain on active hip flexion	≥4/5	48	98	0.53	24.3
Scour test positive	≥3/5	71	86	0.33	5.2
Pain with active hip extension	≥2/5	81	61	0.31	2.1
Passive internal rotation ≤25°	≥1/5	95	18	0.27	1.2

Sn = sensitivity; Sp = specificity; LR− = negative likelihood ratio; LR+ = positive likelihood ratio. High sensitivity indicates a test is useful for ruling out a condition (good screening tool), while high specificity indicates a test is useful for ruling in a condition (good diagnostic tool).

Blue = large change in likelihood (LR− <0.1, LR+ >10). This indicates that a positive test is likely to indicate a 'true-positive' finding, while a negative test is likely to indicate a 'true-negative' finding, meaning the test has high clinical utility.

Red = rarely important change in likelihood (LR− >0.5, LR+ <2.0). This indicates that a positive test is unlikely to indicate a 'true-positive' finding, while a negative test is unlikely to indicate a 'true-negative' finding, meaning the test has poor clinical utility.

Hip pain   CHAPTER 31

Physical examination

In this section, the clinical tests that are valid are identified with a double asterisk (**). Other tests that have not had their validity reported but are likely to be useful are also listed.

Examination involves:

1. Observation
   a. standing:
      i. general lower limb alignment
      ii. femoral alignment
      iii. muscle tone and symmetry
   b. walking
      i. pain
      ii. limp
      iii. lateral pelvic stability 'Trendelenburg sign'
2. Active movements
   a. hip flexion/extension
   b. hip abduction/adduction
   c. hip internal**/external rotation at 90° flexion
3. Passive movements
   a. flexion (Fig. 31.6a)
   b. anterior impingement test**–flexion, adduction and internal rotation (FADIR) (Fig. 31.6b)
   c. internal rotation at 90° flexion**
   d. flexion, abduction and external rotation** (FABER or Patrick's test) (Fig. 31.6c)
   e. quadriceps muscle stretch
   f. psoas muscle stretch/impingement (Thomas position) (Fig. 31.6d)
4. Tests of muscle function
   a. adductor squeeze test** (Fig. 31.6e)
   b. hand-held dynamometry of hip muscle strength bilaterally
      i. flexion/extension
      ii. adduction/abduction
      iii. internal/external rotation

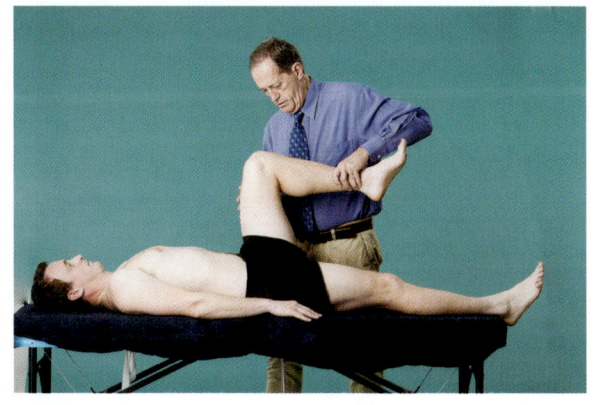

Figure 31.6 (a) Measurement of hip flexion range of motion

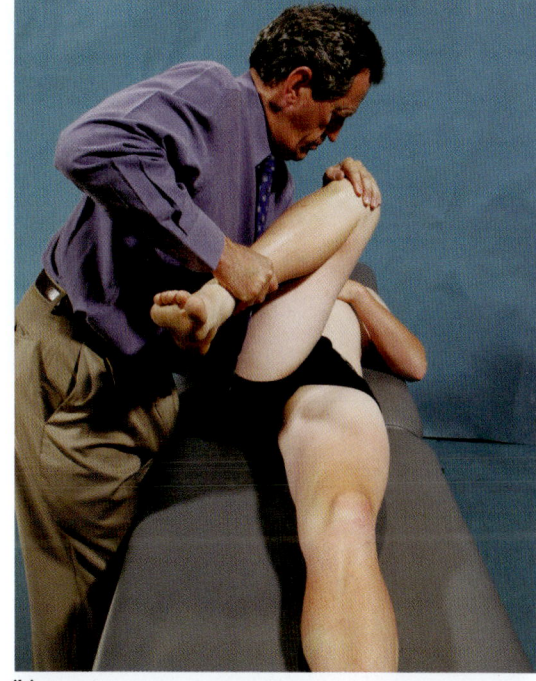

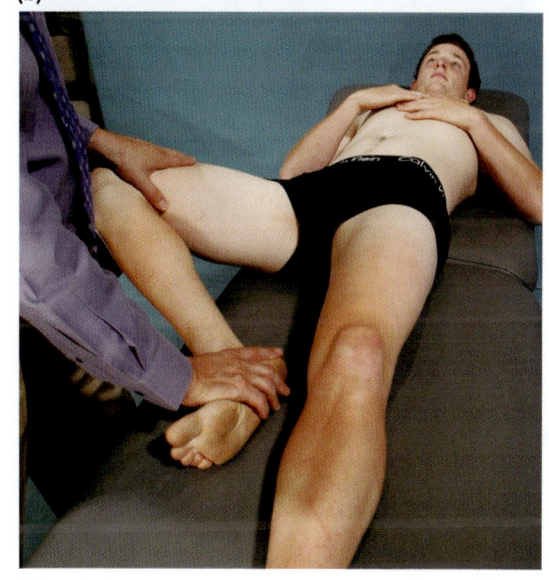

Figure 31.6 (cont.) (b) Passive movement—anterior impingement (hip quadrant: flexion, adduction and internal rotation—FADIR) (c) Passive movement—flexion, abduction and external rotation (FABER or Patrick's test). Range of motion, apart from extreme stiffness/laxity, is not that relevant. Some caution needs to be exercised, as it is possible to sublux an unstable hip in this position. Pain felt in the groin is very non-specific. Pain in the buttock is more likely to be due to sacroiliac joint problems. However, pain felt over the greater trochanter suggests hip joint pathology

601

PART B   Regional problems

(d)

(e)

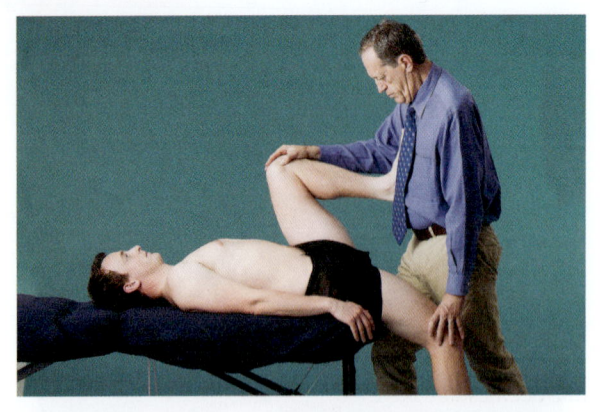

(f)

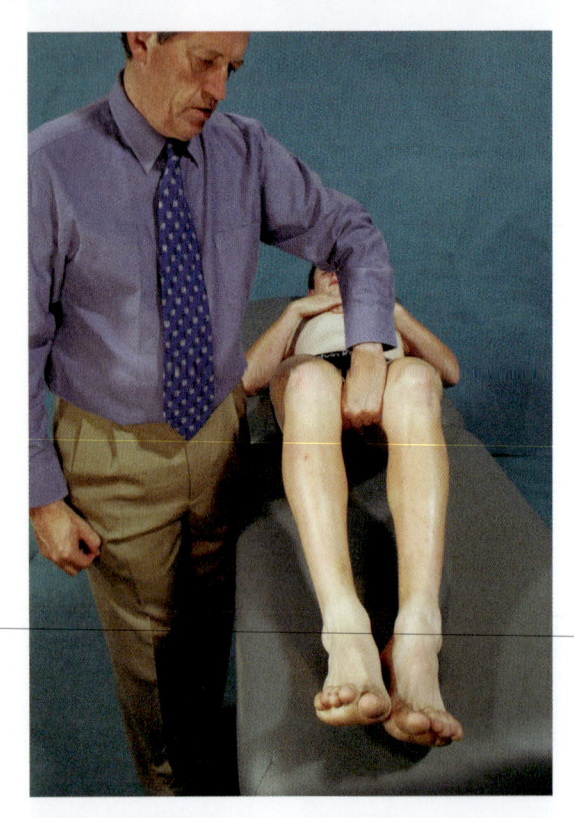

(g)

Figure 31.6 (cont.) (d) Passive movement—psoas stretch (Thomas position). Pain in the hip being stretched suggests psoas abnormality. Pain in the hip being compressed can be significant for anterior impingement of the hip joint (e) Resisted movement—squeeze test. Examiner places fist between knees as shown. Patient then adducts bilaterally against the fist (f) De-rotation test—in 90° flexion, the hip is taken into external rotation and the patient asked to return the leg to the axis of the table against resistance. The test result is positive when the usual pain is reproduced (g) Palpation of iliopsoas in muscle belly and at anterior hip joint

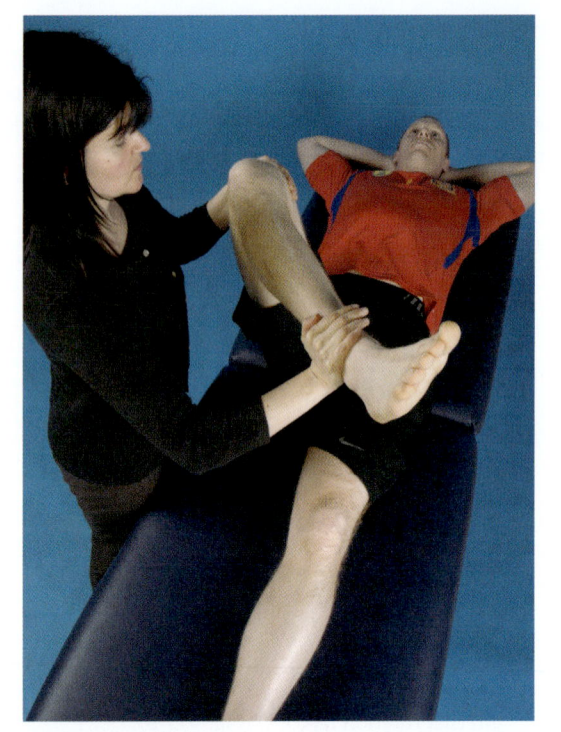

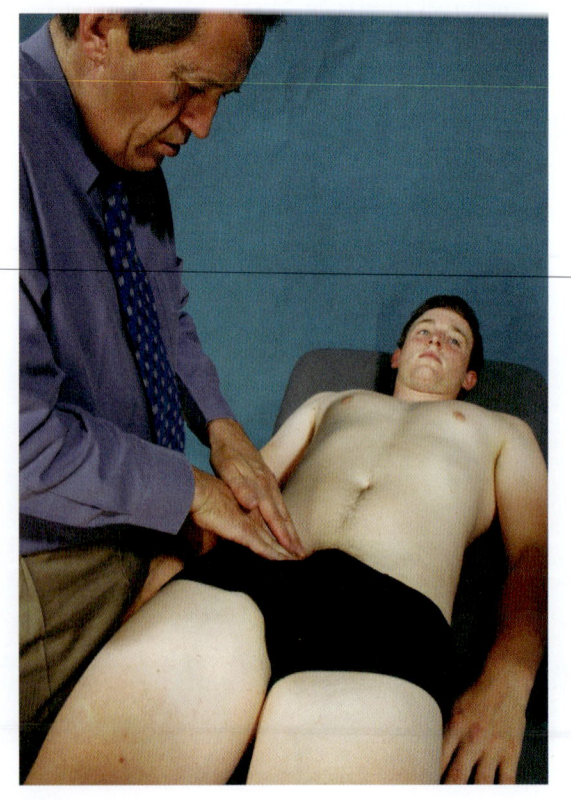

Hip pain   CHAPTER 31

   iv. de-rotation test**[48] (Fig. 31.6f). In 90° flexion, the hip is taken into external rotation and the patient asked to return the leg to the axis of the table against resistance. The test result is positive when the usual pain is reproduced.
5. Palpation
   a. anterior hip joint line
   b. adductor muscles/tendons/entheses
   c. pelvis including pubis symphysis, ischial tuberosities and proximal hamstring attachment
   d. iliopsoas in muscle belly and at anterior hip joint (Fig. 31.6g)
   e. superficial hip abductors including tensor fasciae latae, gluteus medius and superior gluteus maximus
   f. greater trochanter and tendons of gluteus medius and minimus
6. Functional movements
   a. double-leg and single-leg squat, looking at range of motion, femoral alignment and balance
   b. hopping (to reproduce pain)
   c. forward hop
   d. step up and down forwards on the affected leg (observe stability, pain level and pain location)
   e. side step up and down on the affected leg
   f. hip hitch (in neutral, internal rotation), keeping the knee extended. Identify the pain location and severity. Reproduction of sacroiliac joint or low back pain probably indicates a low back or sacroiliac joint problem rather than a hip problem
   g. kicking (if appropriate)
   h. balance and proprioception in dynamic tasks
   i. trunk strength and control (for example, side bridge test).

Key outcome measures

A patient-reported outcome measure (PROM) is the gold standard when evaluating an outcome in a clinical population (Chapter 16). When choosing a PROM, the psychometric properties of all possible PROMs should be considered, specific to the patient. Other questionnaires such as the Hip Outcome Score (HOS)[55] and the Modified Harris Hip Score[55] are not recommended as their validity and responsiveness have not been established.

> **PRACTICE PEARL**
>
> We recommend the Copenhagen Hip and Groin Outcome Score (HAGOS),[52] the Hip Dysfunction and Osteoarthritis Outcome Score (HOOS)[53] or the international Hip Outcome Tool-33 (iHOT-33)[54] (Table 31.3).

Investigations

Plain radiography, MRI and ultrasonography are the mainstay of imaging for diagnosis of hip pathology. Plain radiographs are often overlooked by clinicians, but usually should be the first investigation ordered as they can provide valuable information. FAI can often be seen on an anteroposterior view or a lateral view of the pelvis, such as a Dunn view (Fig. 31.7), cross-table view or frog-leg view

Table 31.3 PROMs for hip pain

Copenhagen Hip and Groin Outcome Score
• Self-administered questionnaire evaluating symptoms and function in patients with hip and groin pain
• Six subscales scored separately: symptoms, pain, activities of daily living, sport and recreation, physical activities and quality of life
• Raw scores converted to score from 0 to 100 (100 = best possible score)
• Test–retest reliability: ICC 0.82–0.91
• MDC95%: 8–19 points
• MCID: 6–10 points
• Available online: www.koos.nu
Hip Dysfunction and Osteoarthritis Outcome Score
• Self-administered questionnaire evaluating symptoms and function in patients with hip arthroscopy, hip osteoarthritis and intra-articular causes of hip pain
• Five subscales scored separately: pain, other symptoms, daily living, sport and recreation, and quality of life
• Raw scores converted to score from 0 to 100 (100 = best possible score)
• Test–retest reliability: ICC 0.93–0.96
• MDC95%: 9–17 points
• MCID: 6–11 points
• Available online: www.koos.nu

continued

PART B Regional problems

Table 31.3 • Cont.

The international Hip Outcome Tool-33
• Self-administered questionnaire evaluating symptoms and function in younger, active patients with a variety of hip pathologies • Thirty-three items • Each of the 33 items scored out of 100. Points summed and divided by number of items to get an overall score out of 100 (100 = best possible score) • Test–retest reliability: ICC 0.78 • MDC95%: 16 points • MCID: 6 points • Available as appendix to Mohtadi et al. 2012[54]

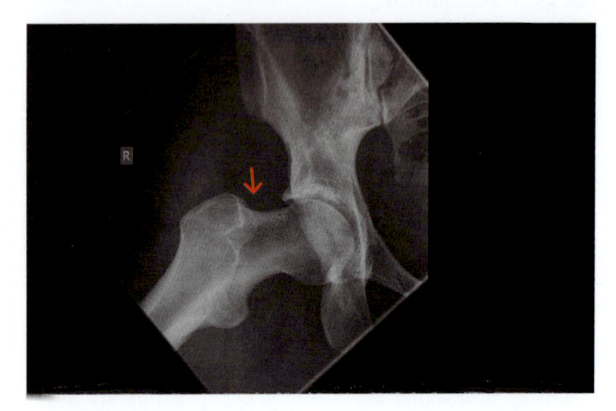

Figure 31.7 Dunn 45° flexion view indicating sclerotic cam lesion at femoral head–neck junction (arrow), pincer impingement at acetabulum and bony cyst at femoral head–neck junction

of the hip. Similarly, these plain radiographs can also guide the clinician to the presence of OA and abnormalities in morphology such as acetabular dysplasia, acetabular retroversion or anteversion, the presence of os acetabulare, and not-to- be missed pathologies such as a slipped upper femoral epiphysis, Perthes' disease, tumours, fractures of the neck of femur and avascular necrosis. Unfortunately, a plain radiograph does not provide information about soft tissue injuries such as labral, chondral, ligamentum teres or tendon pathology.

MRI is commonly used in the diagnosis of soft tissue injuries of the hip. Pathologies such as labral tears, ligamentum teres tears, tendon and bursae pathology, and occasionally chondral defects may be seen on an MRI scan. In recent years, the sensitivity and specificity of MRI to these injuries has improved (see Table 31.4), although false-negative results are often noted. Therefore, imaging findings should be taken in combination with the patient's history and physical examination in order to obtain a correct diagnosis.

Due to the depth of the joint, diagnostic ultrasound is not especially useful for the diagnosis of intra-articular hip pathology; however it can be useful in determining the presence of bursae of the greater trochanter or iliopsoas tendon, and tendinopathy of these regions. Real-time ultrasound can be used to assess the function of the deep lumbar and hip stabilising muscles.

Diagnostic injections of local anaesthetic are used frequently in the hip to determine the presence of intra-articular pathology of the hip. These are generally performed under imaging guidance. A reduction in symptoms following an injection generally confirms the presence of intra-articular pathology, although a negative response does not necessarily indicate that no pathology is present, and further investigation and management may still be warranted.

Surgeons may obtain specific computed tomography (CT) scans pre-operatively to assist them in planning surgery for the treatment of FAI, but these are not routinely used in clinical practice for diagnosis of the source of hip pain.

PREDISPOSING FACTORS FOR HIP PAIN

A number of intrinsic and extrinsic factors can contribute to hip region pain (Fig. 31.8). Such factors may be modifiable or non-modifiable. Modifiable factors should be targeted for treatment as they can alter the loads on the hip joint.

Extrinsic factors may include the type of sport played, particularly those involving repeated combined hip flexion, abduction and adduction, and loaded rotational or twisting movements. These factors may also include the volume of sport and activity undertaken, footwear worn or type of surface played upon. Of these extrinsic factors, the type of sport and volume of load undertaken are probably the most important when evaluating the athlete with hip pain. Sport and activity involving repeated hip flexion, abduction and adduction; and rotation and twisting are reported throughout the literature as influencing the likelihood of the development of hip pathology. The clinician must examine these loads in

Hip pain — CHAPTER 31

Table 31.4 Diagnostic accuracy of imaging tests in patients with hip pain

	Sn	Sp	LR−	LR+
Gluteal tendinopathy				
Ultrasound	79–100	100		
MRI[56]	33–100	92–100		
Labral tear				
Ultrasound[57, 58]	82–94	0–60	0.30	2.05
CT[59, 60]	92–97	87–100		
Multidetector CT (MDCT)[61–64]	88–100	87–100		
MRI[65]	66	79		
MRI + contrast (magnetic resonance arthrography—MRA)[65, 66]	87	64		
Cartilage				
CT[59, 67, 68]	66–88	40–94		
MRI	59	94	0.44	9.83
MRA[66 59, 68–71]	49–97	33–100		
FAI				
MRI[65]	66	79	0.43	3.14
MRA[72]	91	80	0.11	4.55
CT	92–97	87–100		

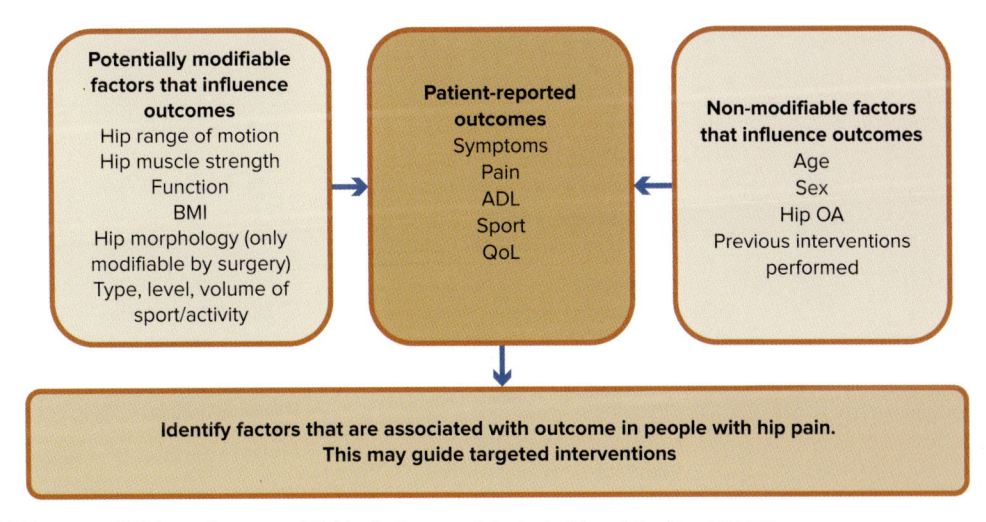

Figure 31.8 How modifiable and non-modifiable factors contribute to hip-related symptoms

Potentially modifiable factors that influence outcomes
- Hip range of motion
- Hip muscle strength
- Function
- BMI
- Hip morphology (only modifiable by surgery)
- Type, level, volume of sport/activity

Patient-reported outcomes
- Symptoms
- Pain
- ADL
- Sport
- QoL

Non-modifiable factors that influence outcomes
- Age
- Sex
- Hip OA
- Previous interventions performed

Identify factors that are associated with outcome in people with hip pain. This may guide targeted interventions

detail and modify accordingly for those athletes that are experiencing hip pain.

Intrinsic factors can also influence the development of hip pain and pathology. These factors may also alter loads within the joint, predisposing the hip to injury. Intrinsic factors are either 'local', 'remote' or 'systemic', and must be considered for comprehensive assessment of the athlete with hip pain. Identifying these factors via a thorough assessment is essential if the clinician is to successfully modify the loads within the joint to protect potentially

PART B   Regional problems

vulnerable structures. An understanding of all possible contributing factors to hip pain will assist the clinician in devising a targeted treatment plan.

Local factors
A number of modifiable local factors can contribute to hip pain and are potential targets for treatment, as shown in Table 31.5.

Remote factors
Proximal and distal remote factors may contribute to the development of hip pain. Those factors that are modifiable should be targeted when planning treatment programs for patients with hip-related pain.

Proximal factors
Increased pelvic tilt and/or lumbar hyperextension may increase the load on the anterior margins of the hip, due to the more distal placement of the anterior acetabular rim. Patients with increased pelvic tilt and reduced trunk strength can have increased acetabular retroversion and reduced femoral internal rotation range.[73] This increased load may be a source of increased hip pain and eventually anterior hip pathology. The clinical assessment of pelvic symmetry and lumbar spine is outlined in Chapter 29.

Inadequate control of the lumbopelvic segments may result in a number of asymmetries, which alter the loads on the hip joint. In particular, lateral pelvic tilt may increase the load on both the lateral and medial structures of the hip joint, due to the increased adductor and internal rotation moment seen on the stance leg.

Hip and lumbopelvic control can be assessed using the single-leg squat (Chapter 8), other single-leg activities, gait or sport-specific activities. In some cases, the athlete should also be videoed whilst running, particularly when fatigued, as altered control may become more pronounced. The demands on the lumbopelvic region for the individual's sport must be considered, as this may predispose certain athletic groups to fatigue and subsequently altered load on the hip joint.

Table 31.5 Local factors that can contribute to hip-related pain and their possible mechanisms

Factor	Possible mechanisms	Confirmatory assessments
Reduced hip flexion range of motion	Structural • Cam and/or pincer impingement • Chondrolabral pathology	Plain radiograph • Anteroposterior pelvis • Dunn view 45°/90° Positive FADIR (Fig. 31.6b) MRI
Reduced hip internal rotation range of motion	Structural • Acetabular retroversion • Cam and/or pincer impingement • Femoral retroversion • Osteoarthritis changes (osteophytes)	Plain radiograph • Anteroposterior pelvis • Dunn view 45°/90°
	Functional • Reduced strength hip internal rotators • Tight gluteals and piriformis • Muscle spasm	Hand-held dynamometry Muscle-length tests
Increased hip rotation range (external rotation and/or internal rotation)	Structural • Acetabular anteversion • Acetabular dysplasia • Capsular laxity	Plain radiograph
Altered movement patterns	Reduced muscle strength • Reduced hip abductor, adductor, extensor strength, external rotator strength Muscle inhibition, disuse atrophy Reduced performance in single-leg squat, neuro-motor control and balance tasks	Hand-held dynamometry Palpation, observation, real-time ultrasound Functional and balance tests

Hip pain — CHAPTER 31

Distal factors

Increased subtalar pronation may lead to an increase in tibial internal rotation. This in turn may lead to an overload on the iliotibial band (ITB) and the lateral structures of the hip. Increased ITB tension results in increased compression over the greater trochanter and the development of gluteus medius and minimus tendinopathy and trochanteric bursitis. Increased tibial internal rotation may also create increased internal rotation of the femur, thus heightening load on the hip, particularly in athletes with an increased risk of impingement. The clinical assessment of the subtalar joint is outlined in Chapter 41.

Adequate range of ankle dorsiflexion during the stance phase of gait is essential in order to minimise excessive loads further up the kinetic chain. In addition, reduced ankle dorsiflexion range can increase the amount of adduction at the knee in single-leg squatting tasks, therefore potentially increasing hip impingement. If this movement is limited, the gait pattern may be altered to achieve onward forward propulsion of the athlete. One adaptation commonly seen is an increase in hip adduction and rotation at the middle of the stance phase of gait. This may increase load on the hip joint in similar ways outlined above. The clinical assessment of ankle dorsiflexion range of motion is outlined in Chapter 41.

Systemic factors

Common 'systemic' factors contributing to hip joint loads include patient age, sex, BMI and family/genetic predisposition. Of these, BMI is the only factor that is potentially modifiable. Patients with a BMI >25 should be advised to seek appropriate guidance to reduce BMI to a healthy level. Other non-modifiable factors should be considered when considering a patient's likely outcomes, prognosis and expectations, as well as appropriate surgical versus non-surgical treatment options.

FEMOROACETABULAR IMPINGEMENT

Femoroacetabular impingement (FAI) is defined as a pathological mechanical process by which morphological abnormalities of the acetabulum and/or femur combined with vigorous hip motion can damage the soft tissue structures within the hip joint itself.[74] For the clinical diagnosis of FAI, the hip should be symptomatic. There are two types of FAI which differ in both the anatomical site of the morphological abnormality and the mechanism by which it causes intra-articular damage.[75]

Types of FAI—cam and pincer impingement

The first FAI type is 'cam impingement', in which the morphological abnormality is located on the femoral side of the hip joint. The cam deformity is extra bone formation at the anterolateral head–neck junction, causing a non-spherical femoral head.[11] During hip motion, particularly flexion and internal rotation, the cam deformity can be forced into the acetabulum, causing shear forces at the chondrolabral junction (Fig. 31.9b).[8]

The second type of FAI is referred to as 'pincer impingement' (Fig. 31.9c). This refers to a morphological or orientational abnormality of the acetabulum leading to an over-coverage of the femoral head. This can either manifest as a deep acetabulum or as a retroverted acetabulum, which are most commonly seen anteriorly. Particularly during hip flexion, the femoral neck can impinge against the over-covered acetabulum, causing an impaction on the labrum. This type of impingement might lead to labral and also cartilage damage throughout the acetabulum in a small thin strip around the labrum.[8]

A cam deformity and a pincer deformity may exist together and when this leads to symptoms it is referred to as a mixed type of FAI. It is very important to recognise that a cam deformity or a pincer deformity will not always cause FAI. Susceptibility is highly dependent on many co-factors including other anatomical characteristics of the hip such as femoral and acetabular version, on the type and intensity of hip movement, and on the vulnerability of the labrum and cartilage itself.[76]

Prevalence of FAI

As the mechanical impingement seen in FAI is difficult to quantify, most studies on the prevalence of FAI have

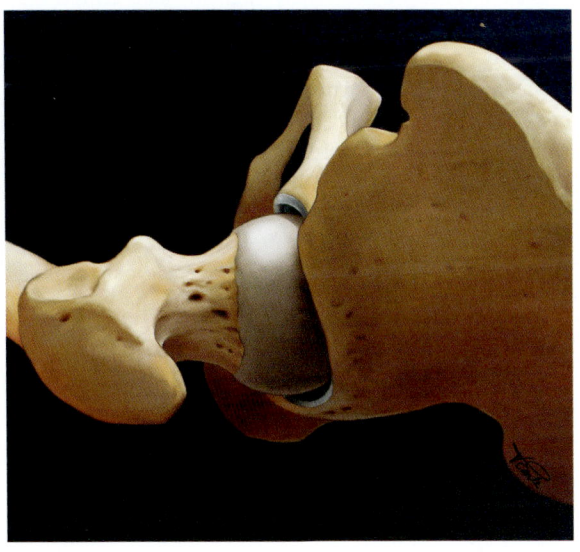

(a)

Figure 31.9 Hip joints with and without FAI
(a) Hip joint without FAI

607

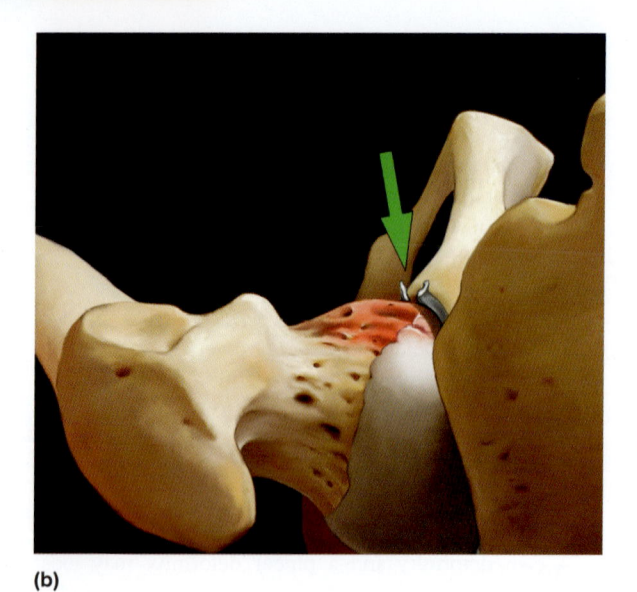

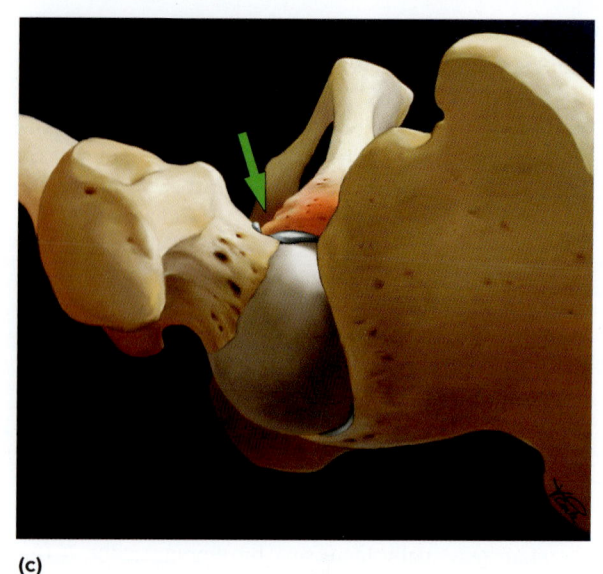

Figure 31.9 (cont.) (b) Cam lesion—additional bone arises as a 'bump' on the femoral surface (c) Pincer lesion—bone spur extends from the acetabular surface

focused on the morphology, that is, the presence of a cam or pincer deformity. It is important that the clinician understands that the morphology that can lead to FAI is highly prevalent and is in itself not a pathology.

The prevalence of cam deformity in the general asymptomatic population has been estimated at around 10–25%.[6, 77] Cam deformity is more prevalent in males (25–50%) than in females (0–10%).[6] Interestingly, the prevalence can be extremely high in male athletes—up to 89%—compared to only 9% in non-athletic controls.[78]

Pincer deformities are generally more prevalent in women, but the prevalence varies widely between studies because of the heterogeneity in what is considered a pincer deformity. General over-coverage is a condition in which the femoral head is positioned deep in the acetabulum or when there is an overgrowth of the acetabular rim. This type of pincer deformity is present in about 20% of the population.[79, 80] When focal over-coverage or acetabular retroversion is also taken into account, the prevalence can be as high as 60%.[81] Whether the latter should be regarded as a pincer deformity is still under debate.[82] It is unknown if pincer deformity is more prevalent among athletes.

Aetiology

Hip loading during adolescence is emerging as a key factor in the aetiology of a cam deformity. Cam deformity was first recognised by Murray et al. in 1971,[83] and more recently,[78] hip loading during skeletal maturation has appeared to be related to development of a cam deformity (Fig. 31.10a and b). Since 2011, two cohort studies described the development of a cam deformity during adolescence.[78, 84] The prevalence was higher in both football players and basketball players than in non-athletic controls.[78, 84] In these young athletes, the extra bone formation in the anterolateral head-neck junction becomes radiographically visible from around the age of 13 years and the cam deformity develops gradually until the growth plate closes.[85] After growth plate closure, the morphology of the proximal femur appears to change minimally.[85] This is supported by the high prevalence of cam deformity in adult athletes participating in high-impact sports ranging from 60% to 89%.[78, 81, 86] Therefore, a cam deformity is most likely a bone adaptation in response to vigorous hip loading when the growth plate is still open. During the time of skeletal maturation, there might be a dose-response relationship between the intensity of sports practice and the development of a cam deformity. Genetics might also play a role, as a cam deformity might have a familial pattern, with siblings being three times more likely to have a cam deformity than controls.[50] The aetiology of a pincer deformity is unknown and there are no studies available that investigate how a pincer deformity develops.

Association with pain and pathology

A prerequisite of the FAI definition is the presence of hip pain and symptoms. Without hip pain, the diagnosis of FAI cannot be made. The presence of a cam or a pincer deformity in isolation have been associated with hip pain

Hip pain   CHAPTER 31

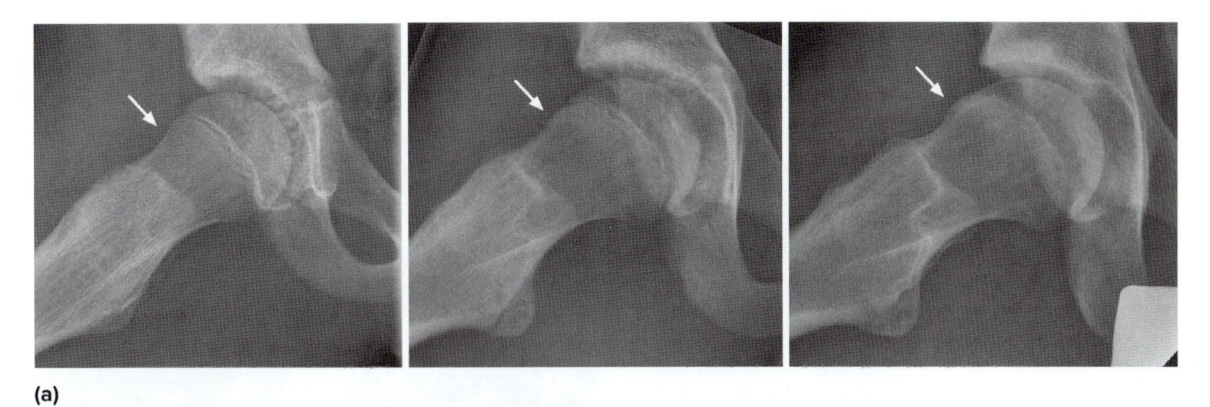

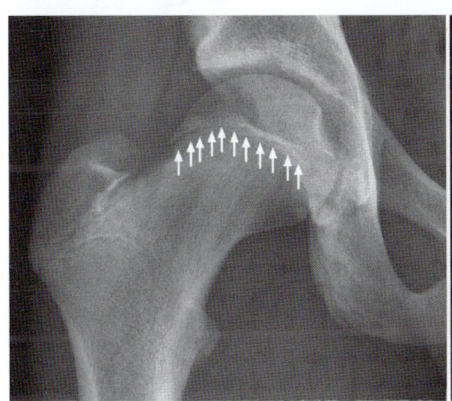

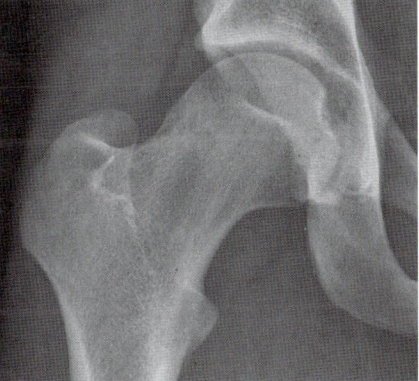

Figure 31.10 (a) Development of a cam deformity over time during skeletal maturation (b) Extension of the growth plate towards the femoral neck during the development of a cam deformity

in young adults,[87] but only 26% of people with a cam deformity complain of hip pain.[88] Asymptomatic young adults with a cam deformity have a 4.5 times higher risk of developing hip pain within 4 years than those without a cam deformity. This was shown in a cohort of 170 subjects, in which 16% of asymptomatic hips with a cam deformity at baseline had at least one episode of hip pain lasting longer than 6 weeks within the next 4 years.[3]

However, athletes might have a higher risk of developing hip pain resulting from a cam deformity, particularly when they experience repetitive movements of flexion and internal rotation of the hip. In American football (gridiron) players, the presence of a cam deformity is associated with greater hip and groin symptom prevalence, whereas a pincer deformity is not.[89] In ice hockey players, hip pain together with symptoms of FAI is associated with a cam deformity at a mean age of 19 years.[90] The association between a cam deformity and hip pain is likely also true for other sports requiring movements of deep flexion, rotation and pivoting.

Following the anterolateral location of a cam deformity, the anterosuperior region of the acetabulum is mostly affected corresponding to the site where the cam deformity is forced into the acetabulum with flexion and internal rotation.[8] This results locally in high shear forces at the acetabular chondrolabral junction. Resultant damage to the labrum can progress to its detachment from the acetabular rim and involvement of the acetabular cartilage. This can range from slight softening and swelling of the cartilage in the early stage, to delamination of the cartilage from the subchondral bone in later stages, a so-called carpet lesion. The size of the cam deformity is positively correlated with more severe cartilage damage.[91]

> **PRACTICE PEARL**
>
> Cam impingement is associated with intra-articular pathology, whereas the association between pincer impingement and intra-articular pathology is less clear.

Severe intra-articular hip damage is already seen in athletes around their twenties. Even in asymptomatic males with a mean age of 20 years, those with a cam deformity are 2.8 times more likely to have labral lesions and a decreased combined femoral and acetabular cartilage thickness of 0.19 mm.[6] In the presence of a pincer deformity, labral lesions and a more circumferential pattern of acetabular cartilage damage have been described based on intra-operative findings, but epidemiological data on intra-articular hip pathology in those with asymptomatic pincer deformities is lacking.[8]

Osteoarthritis

A cam deformity is associated with hip OA, whereas the association between a pincer deformity and OA is conflicting. Since a cam deformity is present immediately after skeletal maturity, prospective studies to evaluate the risk for developing OA would require a long-term follow-up of decades. Therefore, current cohort studies consist mostly of individuals aged over 40 years. In this population, there is strong evidence that a cam deformity is a risk factor for development of OA.[76, 92] A prospective study found that a cam deformity conferred a four times higher risk of developing OA within 5 years and up to 10 times higher risk with a greater cam deformity.[93] Individuals with a cam deformity and decreased internal rotation ≤20° had a 53% chance of developing OA compared to only 2% in people without these features. Most other case-control, cross-sectional and retrospective cohort studies also show an increased risk for OA.[79, 94, 95] Regarding the higher prevalence of cam deformity in athletes and the higher chance to experience FAI in the presence of a cam deformity because of the repetitive movements they undertake, athletes might even be more likely to develop OA due to cam-type FAI.

The relationship between pincer deformity and OA is less clear. Some studies show a moderately increased risk for having OA in the presence of a pincer deformity,[79] while others, including higher-quality studies, showed no association or even a protective effect of a pincer deformity on development of OA.[94, 96]

> **PRACTICE PEARL**
>
> This association between FAI and increased incidence of other hip pathology has resulted in considerable debate regarding the benefit of prophylactic surgery to correct deformity associated with FAI in athletes who do not have hip or groin pain. As there is no conclusive evidence at this stage which indicates that all athletes with FAI will develop other hip pathology, prophylactic surgery to correct deformities in athletes who do not have signs of hip pathology is not recommended.

The early identification of FAI in athletes with hip and groin pain is essential. Unfortunately there is no gold standard for clinical diagnosis of FAI. Clinical signs that are often reported to indicate the presence of FAI include

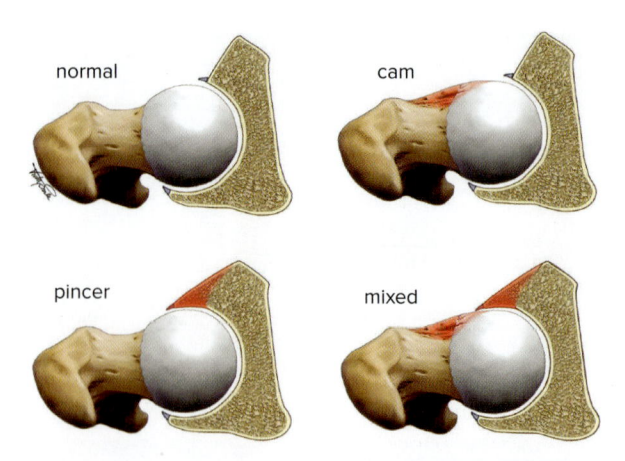

Figure 31.11 Appearances of the different types of FAI

reduced range of hip internal rotation, particularly when the hip is flexed, and a positive FADIR test. Unfortunately these tests are not specific to detect FAI and may result in a high number of false-positive results. Therefore, radiological examination is required.[42] Plain radiographs can be useful and generally a plain anteroposterior view of the pelvis will indicate the presence of FAI when read by an experienced radiologist (Fig. 31.11).

Athletes who present with FAI should be encouraged to avoid the position of impingement as much as possible. This position of impingement is usually flexion, internal rotation and adduction or any combination of these (Fig. 31.12). This may involve activity modification on a day-to-day basis, as well as during athletic pursuits. For example, in ball sports this may involve playing in a different position which requires less time changing direction and getting down low to the ball. It may also involve reducing the time spent on the field. Maximising dynamic neuromotor control around the hip will also assist in achieving this goal.

LABRAL TEARS

Acetabular labral tears (Fig. 31.13) are seen frequently in the athletic population, with 22% of athletes with groin pain having labral tears, and 55% of patients with mechanical symptoms and hip pain having labral tears.[18, 22, 44, 97] The aetiology of labral tears is well described in the literature. However, studies have also shown that there is a high prevalence of labral tears in the asymptomatic population, especially as people age, and as with many other parts of the musculoskeletal system, pain does not always match pathology.

Pathology

The presence of both cam-type FAI [5, 8, 11, 98, 99] and developmental dysplasia of the hip (DDH)[100, 101] can increase the risk of a labral tear. Mechanisms include impingement

Hip pain   CHAPTER 31

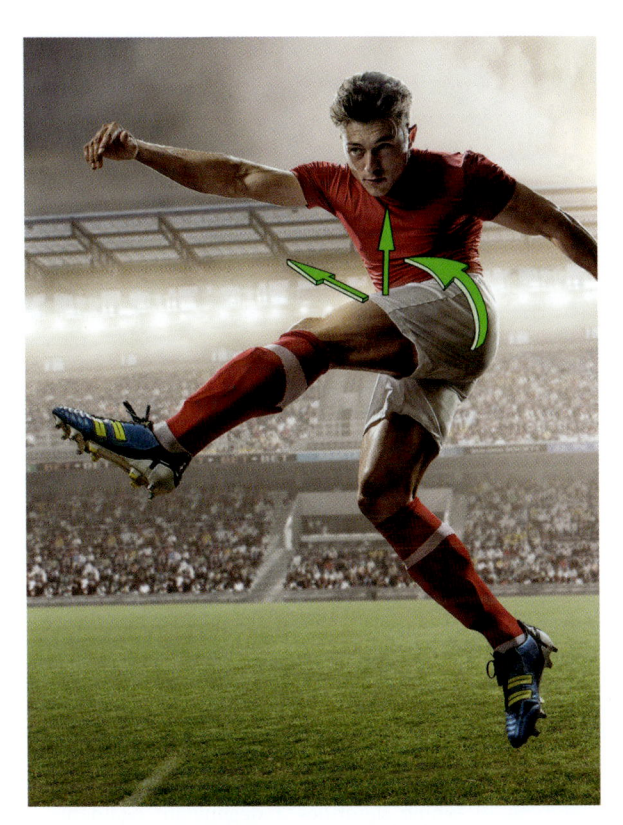

Figure 31.12 Hip impingement during kicking motion—flexion, internal rotation and adduction
ISTOCK/VICKY EARLE

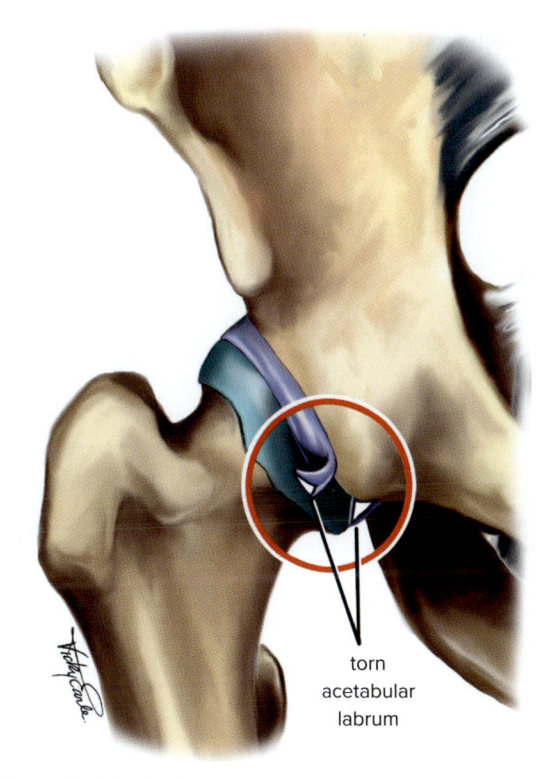

Figure 31.13 Labral tear

of the labrum in the presence of FAI and increased shear forces on the outer joint margins, including the labrum, in the presence of DDH. In addition, patients with labral tears are 40% more likely to have coexisting chondropathy.[14] The inability of a damaged labrum to adequately sustain chondral nutrition via the synovial fluid, as well as the reduced load-bearing capacity of a damaged labrum, may provide an explanation for these findings.

The prevalence of labral tears in the USA and Europe is greatest anteriorly.[18, 22, 97, 102] Various causes for the high number of anterior labral tears have been postulated, including reduced thickness of the labrum anteriorly, the prevalence of FAI lesions seen anteriorly resulting in anterior impingement, and common functional activities, especially those with repetitive twisting and pivoting of the hip.[5] The reduced bony support seen anteriorly in the hip due to the anteverted position of the acetabulum, which results in higher shear forces on anterior soft tissue structures, is also a likely cause of labral pathology. It has been shown that in the last 20–30% of the stance phase of gait and in more than 5° of hip extension, increased forces are placed on anterior soft tissue structures by the head of femur.[18, 103]

Tears of the acetabular labrum are usually classified as type I or type II tears.[22, 104] Type I is described as a detachment of the labrum from the articular hyaline cartilage at the acetabular rim. Type II is described as cleavage tears within the substance of the labrum. The location of these tears relative to the vascularisation of the labrum influences the potential for healing of the tear and the most appropriate type of intervention. Recently it has been suggested that the innervation of the labrum may allow for the capacity for regeneration and repair.[20]

Clinically, the identification of labral tears in patients remains difficult. The patient often complains of mechanical symptoms such as locking, clicking, catching and giving way. The location of pain is usually reported to be within the anterior hip or in the anterior groin region, although some patients report pain in the posterior buttock.

Clinical examination is also difficult. While clinical tests such as FADIR (Fig. 31.6b) and FABER (Fig. 31.6c) have high sensitivity, meaning a negative test will rule out intra-articular hip pathology, they have low specificity, meaning they are not good at determining which intra-articular hip structure is the cause of pain (Table 31.2). The Thomas test (Fig. 31.6d) has a high likelihood ratio, where a positive test (pain on testing) is likely to indicate the presence of intra-articular hip pathology (Table 31.2). This may also reflect the common situation of multiple intra-articular

611

PART B   Regional problems

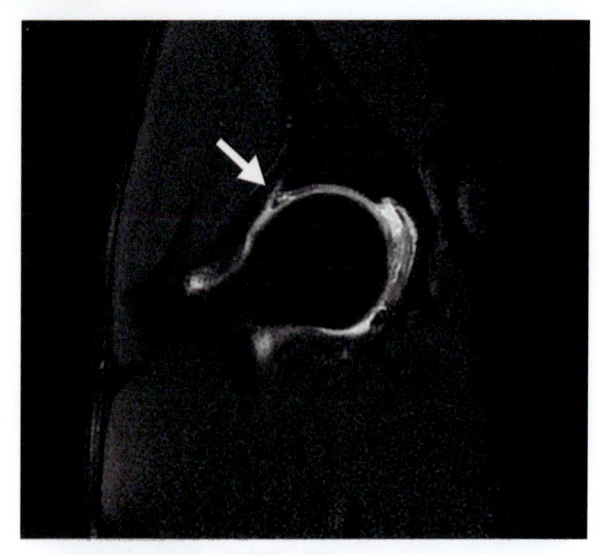

Figure 31.14 T1 fat suppressed coronal MR image showing an anterior-superior labral tear (arrow)

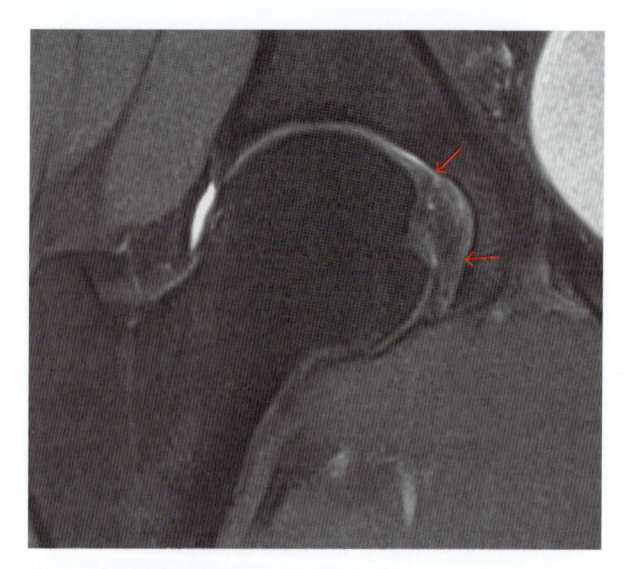

Figure 31.15 Coronal T2-weighted MR arthrogram of a hypertrophied, irregularly thickened, partially torn ligamentum teres that carries greater signal than a normal dark ligament (between arrows)

hip pathologies coexisting. The diagnostic accuracy of radiological investigations for labral tears has improved in recent years, with MRI and MRA (magnetic resonance arthrography) (Fig. 31.14) both having a reasonable degree of sensitivity and specificity (Table 31.4).[40, 66] However, labral tears may be suspected but not confirmed until patients present for hip arthroscopy, which remains the gold standard to diagnose labral pathology.[18, 22]

Athletes with labral pathology may respond to conservative management and this should always be trialled prior to undergoing surgery. Management should be directed to unloading the damaged labrum which is almost always anterior and/or superior. Repetitive hip flexion, adduction or abduction and rotation at the end of range should be avoided through activity modification. Improving hip joint neuromotor control via activation of the deep stabilising muscles, initially in an unloaded then a progressively loaded manner, appears to assist in the unloading of the labrum.

Gait retraining may also be undertaken to minimise excessive hip extension at the end of stance phase of gait, as increased hip extension has been demonstrated to increase the loads on anterior hip joint structures.[105] Neuromotor control of the hip should be maximised as outlined above, and any remote factors influencing the mechanics of the hip should be addressed.

LIGAMENTUM TERES TEARS

Ligamentum teres tears (Fig. 31.15) are commonly reported in athletes undergoing hip arthroscopy and are being reported more frequently in the literature. Studies have found up to 70% of athletes undergoing hip arthroscopy for FAI and labral tears also have tears of the ligamentum teres.[5] Tears of the ligamentum teres are classified as type I which is a partial tear, type II which is a complete rupture and type III which describes a degenerate ligament.[106] Ligamentum teres tears can occur in isolation, but often coexist with FAI, dysplasia and synovitis, probably due to the altered joint loads seen in these conditions.

The mechanism of injury for ligamentum teres most commonly involves forced flexion and adduction, and often internal or external rotation.[106] Twisting motions and hyperabduction injuries have also been reported to cause a tear to this ligament. With the likelihood of the ligamentum teres playing a large proprioceptive and stabilisation role of the hip becoming increasingly recognised, the prompt diagnosis and management of these injuries in the athlete is essential. Likewise, any surgical procedure that sacrifices the ligamentum teres through open dislocation should be carefully considered.

If suspected, the principles of management are similar to those of labral pathology, with a particular emphasis on regaining neuromotor control, excellent proprioception and avoiding positions that place the ligament under most stress using activity modification.

SYNOVITIS

Synovitis (Fig. 31.16) is often seen in athletes with other intra-articular hip pathology, whether it is FAI, labral tears, ligamentum teres tears or chondropathy. It is rarely seen as a primary entity. Synovitis can cause considerable pain in the hip joint, with night pain and pain at rest being common presentations.

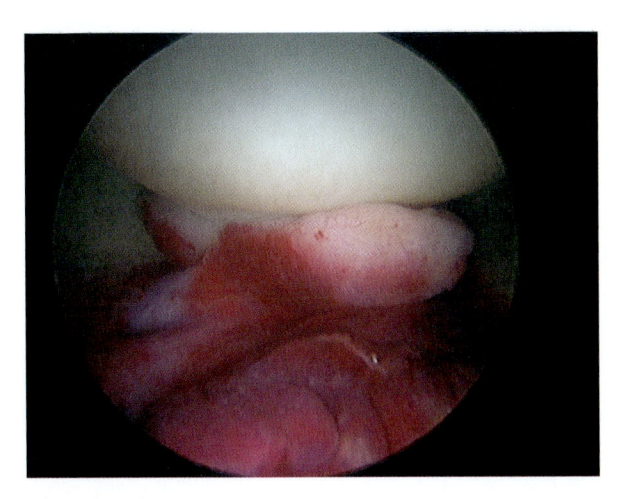

Hip pain   CHAPTER 31

Figure 31.16 Synovitis

Synovitis is a concern to the clinician due to the pain and associated changes in muscle activation that are seen around the hip in the presence of pain. In addition, the implications of synovial dysfunction on cytokine production, nutrition and hydration of articular cartilage, which may already show signs of chondropathy, is significant for the long-term health of the hip joint.

Management should aim to address the other coexisting pathology, restore normal neuromotor control around the hip, modify loads as well as introduce anti-inflammatory measures such as oral non-steroidal anti-inflammatory drugs (NSAIDs) or intra-articular injections. Peak synovial fluid pressure is reduced in positions of hip flexion and internal rotation, already reducing potential nutrition to chondral surfaces.[26] When synovitis is present, these positions should be avoided to try and optimise movement of synovial fluid through the joint.

CHONDROPATHY

Changes to the chondral surfaces of the hip are often seen in conjunction with other hip pathologies (Fig. 31.17). It is well reported that the presence of FAI,[8, 9, 13, 14, 107] decreased acetabular anteversion,[10] labral pathology[14, 18, 101] and DDH[9, 10, 101] can increase the risk of chondropathy and ultimately OA of the hip. In patients with significant labral pathology, chondral loss is often up to 70% of the full thickness or Outerbridge grade III or IV.[108] It is also proposed that the presence of longstanding synovitis may also affect the nutrition of chondral surfaces, possibly exacerbating chondral damage.

The presence of chondropathy at arthroscopy is associated with worse patient-reported outcomes, up to 3 years post-operatively, especially compared to healthy controls. In addition, outcomes are unlikely to improve over time.[14] Patients with severe chondral

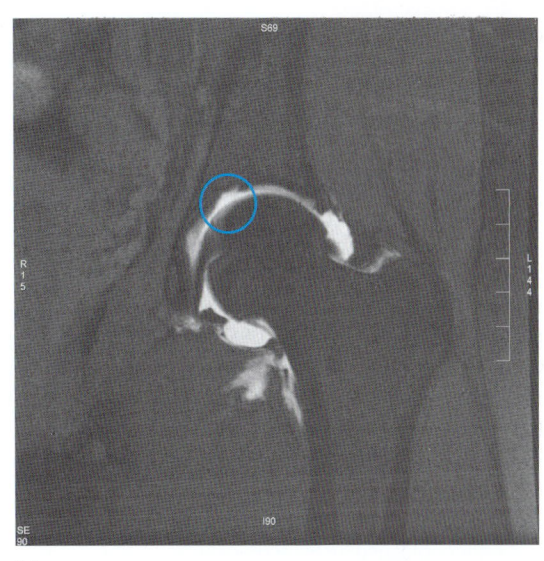

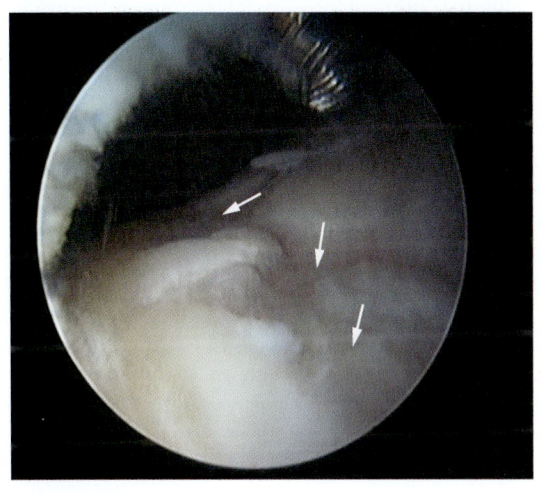

(a)

(b)

Figure 31.17 (a) Coronal MR arthrogram showing full thickness chondral defect in the central acetabulum (b) Arthroscopic view of severe chondral damage secondary to FAI

lesions are more likely to have worse outcomes than those with mild lesions[14] and have a much higher risk of progressing to total hip replacement within 2 years of an arthroscopic procedure.[109] Outcomes for people with severe chondral lesions look similar to those reported for people with advanced hip OA,[14] and it is now thought that chondropathy may represent hip OA in its early stages.

The majority of chondral lesions are seen on the anterior or superior aspect of the acetabular rim, at the chondrolabral junction. This is not surprising considering that this is also the location for the majority of cam and pincer lesions and the majority of labral tears (see above). DDH also involves a reduction in the bony coverage of the femoral head by the acetabulum, thus the anteriorly directed forces of the femoral head will be concentrated on a smaller surface area on the anterior aspect of the joint.

The clinical diagnosis of chondropathy is unlikely to be confirmed with plain radiographs because early chondral changes will not be visible, unless the disease is well advanced. MRI may identify earlier chondral lesions, although the extent of chondropathy is often only evident on hip arthroscopy.[14] The presence of FAI, labral tears and DDH should also increase the suspicion of chondropathy as these often coexist. Clinical tests such as FADIR, which have high sensitivity for intra-articular pathology, may increase suspicion of a chondral lesion; however, this is often only confirmed arthroscopically.

Chondropathy is difficult to manage and may be difficult to confirm in the early stages without arthroscopic confirmation. If suspected, the management again is similar to that of labral pathology, as the majority of chondral lesions of the hip occur in the anterior aspect of the acetabular rim at the chondrolabral junction. As such, this region should be unloaded in the same fashion as labral pathology, with an emphasis on regaining normal neuromotor control of the hip. Recent evidence has shown atrophy in the inferior gluteus maximus and hypertrophy in gluteus medius in early OA, with atrophy also occurring in gluteus medius in severe OA.[110, 111] As chondropathy is likely to represent hip OA in its early stages, aspects of treatment that have been described as being effective for hip OA should be introduced. This may include weight reduction where appropriate, lifestyle factors, general fitness programs, aquatic exercise programs and specific strengthening exercises for hip muscles.

Attempts to minimise synovitis should also be made as the synovium and synovial fluid plays an important role in articular cartilage nutrition. As outcomes of hip arthroscopy for individuals with significant chondral loss are generally worse than for those with no chondral loss and the risk of hip replacement is high,[5, 109, 112-114] conservative measures should be attempted first and in some cases the athlete counselled to modify the amount of weight-bearing activities they undertake.

HIP INSTABILITY

Hip instability is increasingly being recognised as an important potential source of hip pain. Gross instability of the hip is seen in DDH and generalised hypermobility, while localised directional instability may be present in cam-type FAI (as a contra-coup lesion), ligamentum teres tears (due to reduced proprioception), hips with large amounts of anteversion (as capsular insufficiency anteriorly) and in 'normal' hips that are subjected to extremes of range of motion, such as dancers and gymnasts. There is no good clinical or radiographic test for instability and diagnosis is usually one of clinical suspicion when extremes of range of motion, poor balance, poor control in functional tasks, observable excessive translation of the femoral head, and clicking and clunking are present. Treatment for hip instability involves restoring hip muscle strength, improving balance and functional control, modification of functional tasks to avoid extremes of range, and education regarding the risks of repeated activity in unsafe and extremes of range. Some surgeons have reported treating hip instability by arthroscopic shortening of the hip capsule, but outcomes for this procedure are unknown. In extreme cases of DDH and abnormal acetabular version, patients may consider major orthopaedic procedures such as peri-acetabular osteotomy.

TREATMENT OF HIP IMPAIRMENTS

This section will describe the impairments associated with hip pathology and explain how to treat them. The subsequent section will then outline the application of those same principles of management to patients post hip arthroscopy.

Principles of rehabilitation of the injured hip

Rehabilitation of the injured hip requires careful consideration of the interplay between pain and loading (including progression of exercises and activities). Importantly, due to its role in all activities of daily living, including simple activities such as sit-stand, standing and walking, it is hard to 'rest' the hip. Given this, it appears the most provocative loading for the hip occurs when rotational loads, loading at extremes of range and overload in the impingement position occur, rather than excessive amounts of walking, running or other weight-bearing activities that do not involve extremes of rotation, impingement and other end-range positions. It is vital that the patient and the clinician have a good understanding around monitoring joint loads and the loading response.

Unfortunately, there is no level I or II evidence that supports the ideal rehabilitation program or evaluates the effectiveness of particular principles of rehabilitation of the hip. However, the general principles of management of hip pathology are straightforward and are consistently reported in clinical commentaries available concerning rehabilitation of the hip.[5, 18, 115-118] In addition, several recent studies have detailed the physical impairments that exist in people with hip pain and pathology, around which an impairment-based rehabilitation guideline can be based.

Hip pain CHAPTER 31

The most commonly reported physical impairments seen in hip pain and pathology:

1. reduced hip joint range, especially flexion and internal rotation[15, 119, 120]
2. reduced hip muscle strength in all hip muscles, especially abductors and adductors (men and women), extensors (mostly women) and external rotators (mostly women)[15, 119, 121, 122]
3. reduced balance in single-leg dynamic tasks[123]
4. increased femoral adduction in single-leg squats
5. reduced trunk muscle strength
6. alterations in gait biomechanics (primarily reduced range of hip motion in gait)[124, 125]
7. reduced functional performance, especially in hopping and squatting tasks[15]
8. probably adverse loading within the hip due to morphology, changes in range of motion, hip muscle weakness and poor functional performance
9. abnormalities of the kinetic chain.

Nine principles of rehabilitation for hip pain patients

1. Restore hip range of motion

Hip range of motion may impact on load within the hip. Hip flexion[35, 127] and hip extension[127] may increase load on the anterior[103, 127] and superior[35] regions of the hip. As most FAI lesions and associated hip pathology occur in the anterior and superior regions of the hip,[41, 88] loads associated with these regions of the hip require consideration. Range of motion may be limited in this group if movement at the end of range loads damaged tissue in a manner that provokes pain. Often a patient's range of motion is limited to protect damaged regions of the hip and, as such, gaining greater range of motion may also worsen symptoms. Manual techniques such as soft tissue release and needling, stretching and muscle activation may improve range, but should be done with respect to the athlete's pain during and after treatment.

Table 31.6 Best available evidence reports of impairments seen in patients with hip pain

Impairment	Deficit observed	Level of evidence**	References
Range of motion			
	↓ Flexion range of motion†	3b	15
	↓ Abduction range of motion†	3b	15
	↓ Internal rotation range of motion in 90°‡	4	119
	↓ External rotation range of motion in 90°†‡	3b, 4	15, 119 (Two only in females)
	↑ Extension range of motion‡	4	119
Strength			
	↓ Flexion strength†Ω	3b, 4	15, 126
	↓ Extension strength‡	4	119
	↓ Abduction strength†‡¥	3b, 4	15, 119, 122
	↓ Adduction strength†‡	3b, 4	15, 119
	↓ Internal rotation in 0° strength¥	4	122
	↓ External rotation in 0° strength ¥	4	122
	↓ Internal rotation in 90° strength‡¥	4	119, 122
	↓ External rotation in 90° strength†‡¥	3b, 4	15, 119, 122
Neuromuscular activity			
	↓ Tensor fasciae latae activity in hip flexion maximal voluntary contraction	3b	15
Gait			
	↓ Frontal plane hip range of motion (abduction/adduction) †	3b	15
	↓ Sagital plane hip range of motion (flexion/extension) †	3b	15
	↓ Internal rotation range of motion †	3b	15

continued

PART B Regional problems

Table 31.6 Cont.

Impairment	Deficit observed	Level of evidence**	References
Activity limitations			
	↓ Squatting depth	3b	15
	↓ Sagittal plane range of motion when ascending stairs	3b	15
	↓ Maximum hip extension range of motion when ascending stairs	3b	15
	↓ Internal rotation range of motion when ascending stairs	3b	15
Balance			
	↑ Medial lateral range in single-leg squats‡	4	123
Patient reported outcomes			
	↑ Pain§	4	38
	↑ Stiffness§	4	38
	↓ Sports participation§	4	38
	↓ Quality of life§	4	38
	↓ Activities of daily living§	4	38

‡ chondrolabral pathology; ¥ chronic hip joint pain; † symptomatic femoroacetabular impingement; § severe chondropathy; Ω labral pathology; ** NHMRC levels of evidence

Blue = supported by meta-analyses (systematic reviews) or randomised controlled trials
Orange = supported by nonrandomised studies and case series
Black = supported by expert opinion, clinical guideline
Red = current evidence does not support

2. Restore hip muscle strength

Restoration of hip muscle strength should follow these principles.

Phase 1: Deep hip stabiliser retraining

The SHS muscles are those with the greatest capacity to provide dynamic stabilisation of the hip (see above). Retraining of these deep hip stabilisers may be undertaken in the early stages of rehabilitation. As with other pain conditions,[128] clinical observation indicates that pain appears to inhibit effective activation of the SHS muscles. Therefore, pain must be well controlled.

The initial step involves educating the patient in the role of the SHS muscles to provide dynamic hip stability, and the location and actions of these muscles. The second step involves facilitating independent contraction of these muscles. This is often best commenced in 4-point kneeling (Fig. 31.18a), where the patient is taught to activate the SHS muscles and then perform an isometric external rotation or adduction contraction against minimal resistance. The aim is to produce a low-level tonic hold of these muscles. In this position (90° hip flexion), the contribution from the larger external rotator (gluteus maximus) is reduced (see section on joint structure

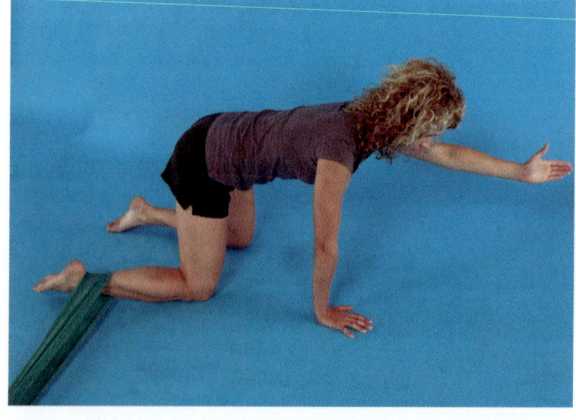

(a)

Figure 31.18 Deep hip stabiliser strengthening exercises (a) Activation of the SHS muscles in 4-point kneel with TheraBand™ resistance. The degree of difficulty can be progressed by decreasing or increasing the level of resistance, changing the speed of activation and increasing the number of repetitions. The challenge to the core can also be increased by lifting one hand off the floor in this position, and the degree of hip flexion or extension and abduction or adduction can be altered based on the needs of the athlete

Hip pain CHAPTER 31

(b)

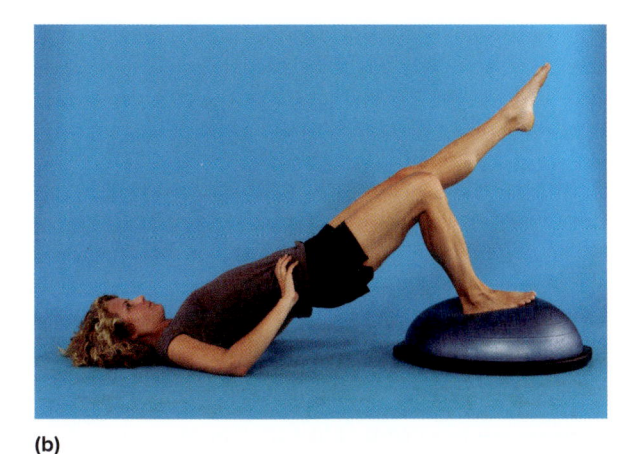

Figure 31.18 (cont.) (b) Progression of activation of deep hip stabilisers into a closed chain position, ensuring adequate deep hip external rotators, gluteus maximus, lateral pelvic and core stability

and muscle function), thus enabling more specificity of activation for the SHS muscles.

Both the patient and the clinician must be confident that the deep hip stabilisers are activated and a real-time ultrasound (RTUS) machine may assist with providing feedback. Progression of the retraining includes providing different levels of resistance, number of repetitions and speed of movements. Other progressions include increasing the amount of hip flexion and decreasing the support (i.e. lifting one hand) to increase the balance demands and challenge to lumbopelvic stability.

Further progressions include activation of the deep hip stabilisers (Fig. 31.18b) in a variety of degrees of hip range of motion and in various functional positions as the activity of the athlete demands, and these can be assessed using an RTUS in these varying positions. For example, an athlete that performs regularly in positions of hip flexion such as a deep squat should ultimately perform muscle activation in this position.

Phase 2: Gluteus maximus retraining

Gluteus maximus plays an important role in generating extension, adduction and external rotation torque, and has the potential to provide hip stabilisation by resisting anterior hip force.[33, 35] Facilitation of independent gluteus maximus contraction may be best commenced in prone (Fig. 31.19a and b), where the patient is taught to perform an isometric external rotation contraction against minimal resistance (low-level tonic hold of these muscles). As with the SHS muscles, feedback may assist in ensuring that the muscle is activated. Since the gluteus maximus is more superficial, feedback may be provided by palpation, surface electromyography biofeedback or RTUS machine.

(a)

(b)

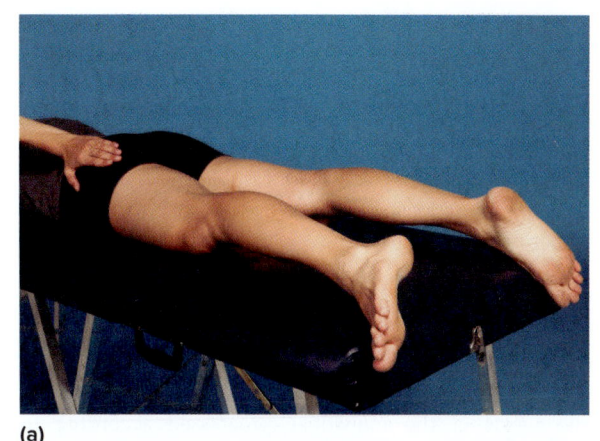

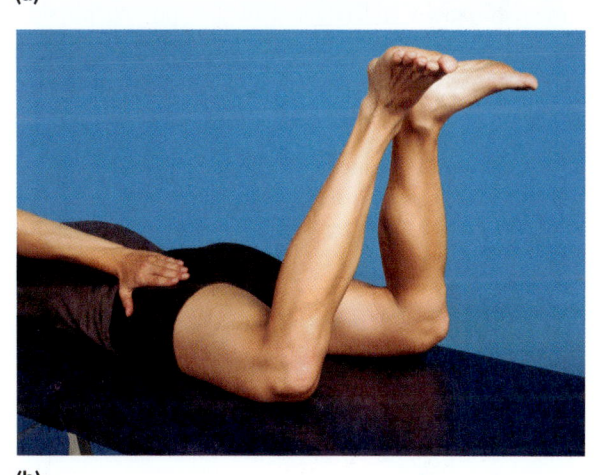

Figure 31.19 Gluteus maximus retraining exercises. Two examples of activation of gluteus maximus, in combination with short hip external rotator (SHER) muscles in prone. RTUS assessment can also be undertaken in this position (a) Prone—knee extension (b) Knee flexion

The activation of the gluteus maximus should be undertaken in a variety of degrees of hip range of motion as the functional demands of the athlete's activity require and can be assessed using an RTUS in these varying positions. For example, hip abduction and external rotation or hip adduction and internal rotation for an athlete who performs cutting manoeuvres, or in hip flexion for an athlete that is required to perform in a deep squatting position. It should be then progressed from open chain to closed chain and then functional positions.

Phase 3: Generalised strengthening exercises

Generalised hip strengthening exercises should only be commenced when the patient and clinician are confident that the key stabilising muscles can be activated and the activation maintained. During this phase, the aim

PART B Regional problems

is to restore muscle function (strength, endurance) and proprioception. This phase remains low impact (Fig. 31.20a). Exercises should initially be undertaken with specific activation of the deep stabilisers prior to completing the exercises. This ensures that the athlete has adequate control of the hip prior to placing it under load, which will assist in protecting vulnerable or damaged structures within the hip.

Generalised hip strengthening exercises should be undertaken, based on clinical assessment, for example targeting hip abductors (predominantly gluteus medius), for those with reduced hip abduction strength.

Strengthening exercises need to be targeted to the needs of the individual, progressed according to patient responses and targeted to the sporting/physical requirements. For example, an athlete who regularly jumps and lands such as a netballer or gymnast should incorporate these actions into their rehabilitation program (Fig. 31.20b).

Exercises are frequently commenced in prone (to ensure specificity and isolation of muscle activations) or in 4-point kneeling and then progressed into functional/weight-bearing positions, bilaterally and then unilaterally (Fig. 31.20c-e). Such exercises also address the rehabilitation goals of balance and functional task performance.

3. Improve balance and proprioception
Retraining of balance can commence immediately in low-impact dynamic functional tasks and be progressed as symptoms and performance allow. It is important that during balance tasks, the athlete is reminded of correct alignment of the pelvis and femur, and to maintain activation of the SHS muscles to facilitate control.

4. Improve hip control in functional task performance
Reducing load on the anterior aspect of the hip joint may require assessment and treatment of movement patterns during functional tasks. Patients with chondrolabral pathology demonstrate reduced balance and increased femoral adduction during a single-leg squat.[123] This potentially places the hip into a position of impingement and loads vulnerable anterior structures.

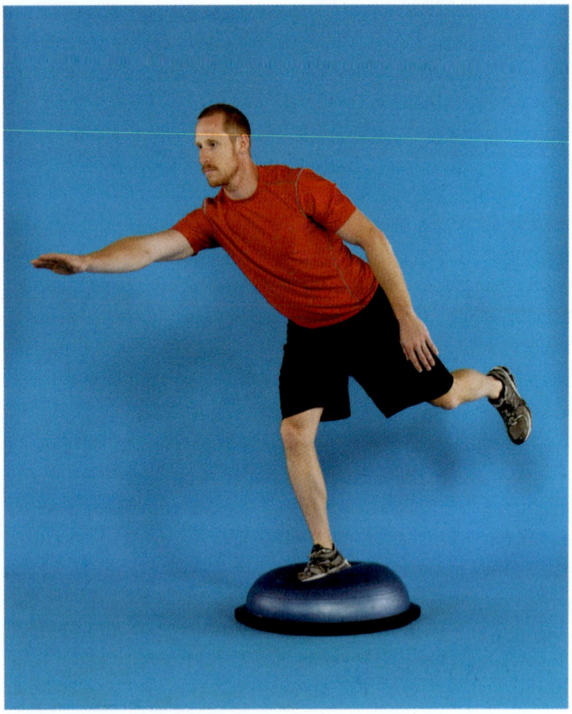

(a)

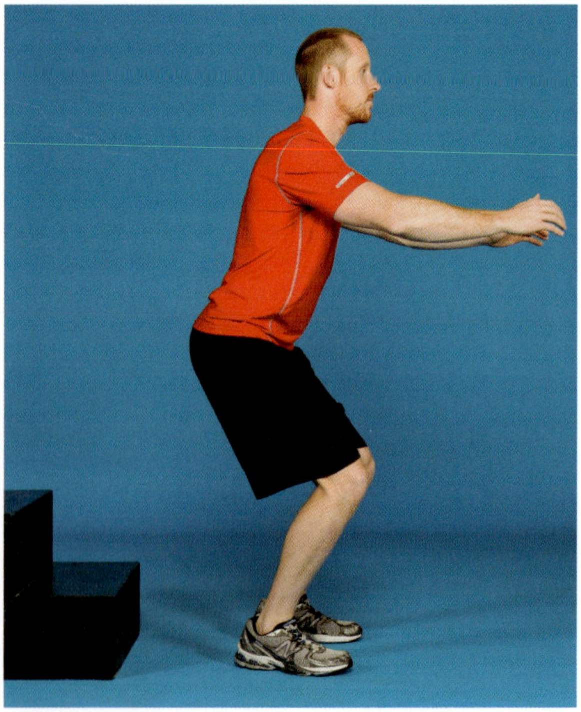

(b)

Figure 31.20 Generalised hip strengthening exercises (a) An example of low-impact functional retraining of deep hip stabilisers, ensuring adequate activation of these muscle groups in a challenging situation without excessive impact or load through vulnerable hip structures (b) A jumping and landing task ensuring adequate activation of deep hip, lateral pelvic and core stabilisers at take-off and landing

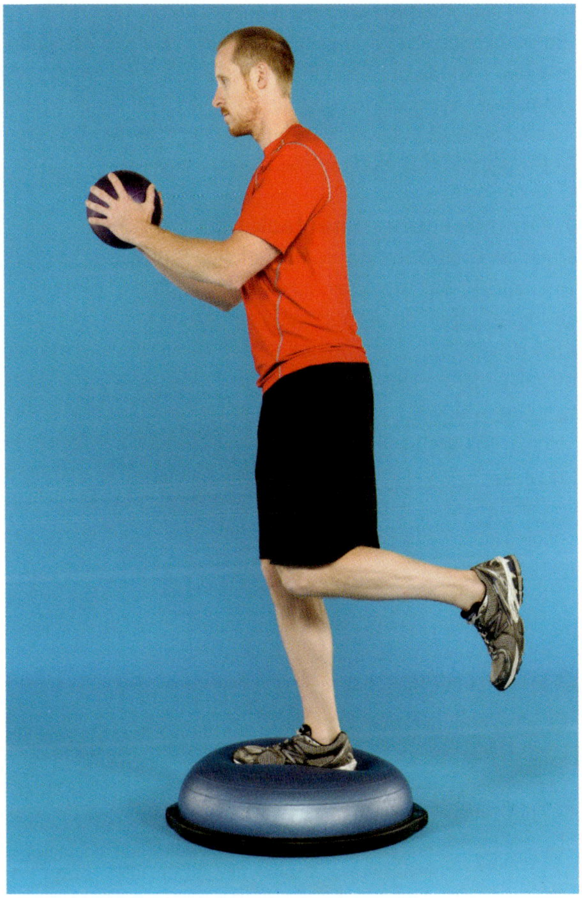

Hip pain CHAPTER 31

(c)

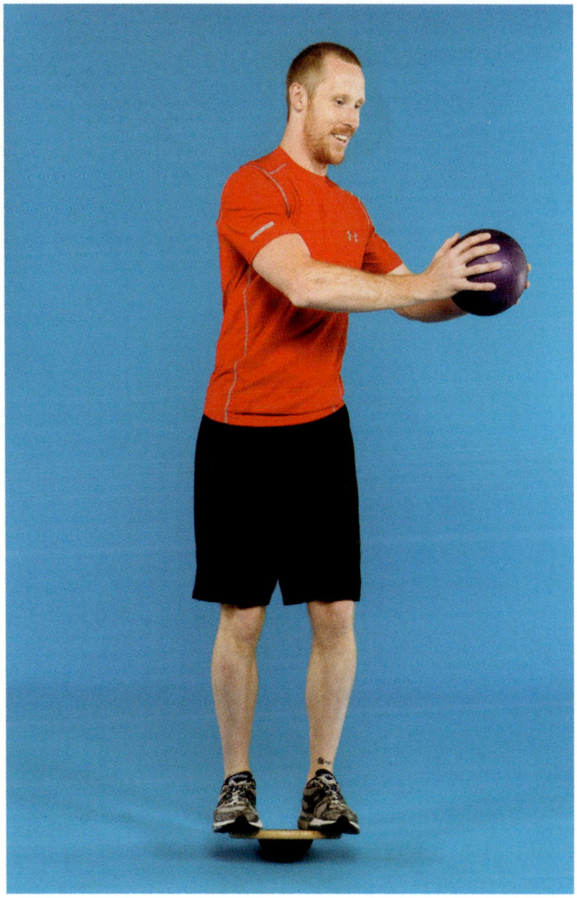

(d)

Figure 31.20 (cont.) (c) and (d) Two examples of later-stage functional activities with concurrent SHER muscle activation, core activation, and functional balance and proprioceptive challenges

Improving the motions of the hip (i.e. reducing hip internal rotation and adduction) and trunk lateral lean may reduce load on the anterior hip. This may be addressed through hip abductor, adductor and rotator strengthening; balance, trunk strength and movement retraining programs described previously. Increased femoral adduction during single-leg tasks will result in increased impingement and may prolong the athlete's symptoms. Adequate femoral control without excessive adduction must be gained in all balance and functional tasks.

Athletes with specific strength deficits of the trunk, hip abductors and hip adductors should address these in targeted strength programs as well as in functional and balance retraining. Adequate control of the femur during single-leg tasks is essential before an athlete can return to sport (see box), especially when fatigued. This can be achieved using specific motor-control training of functional tasks as well as training to address strength-endurance to prevent fatigue-related loss of control.

5. Improve trunk muscle strength

Trunk muscle strength is an important target for athletes with hip pain, given that it is impaired in people with hip pathology, and when reduced, increases acetabular retroversion and impingement. Principles of exercise prescription to optimise spinal stiffness and mobility are given in Chapter 11. When the patient performs trunk exercises, the clinician should ensure the exercises are pain free and the hip is not placed in positions of impingement. The patient should avoid over-using secondary trunk muscles such as iliopsoas, as this may increase impingement and hip pain. Exercises such as sit-ups, where the hip flexors are commonly used, may exacerbate these symptoms and should be avoided.

PART B Regional problems

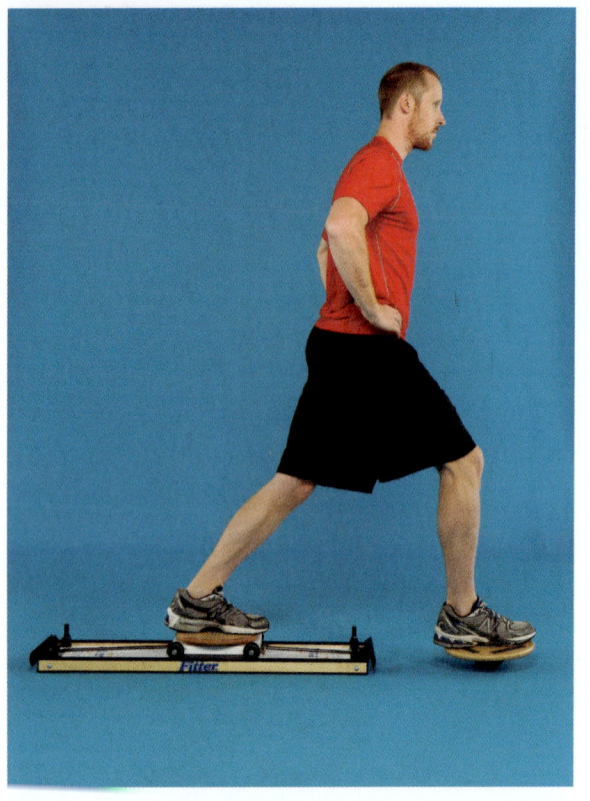

change and cutting manoeuvres specific to the athlete's functional demands. If required, it should also include stairs and hill training (up and down). Generally, patients with hip pain have a reduced step length to avoid increased joint loading seen at end-range hip extension. Any modification to gait should not increase the athlete's hip pain.

7. Optimise functional task performance

Once good neuromotor control of the deep hip stabilisers and global hip muscles has been regained, functional and sports-specific activities should be assessed and then undertaken, both to retrain these movement patterns, but also ensure the athlete can cope with these activities without failing.

Any retraining of functional activities should focus on pre-activation of the deep hip stabilisers, adequate control of the lumbar spine and pelvis during the activity, and correct alignment of the femur during weight-bearing tasks (Fig. 31.21).

Retraining of hip stabilisers should be performed in the positions that place the hip at greatest risk of overload, such as direction change and pivoting, deep squatting and kicking. They should also be undertaken in a repeated fashion, again to ensure the athlete does not fail in a controlled environment.

8. Address adverse loading

The most effective way to unload and protect specific structures of the hip varies slightly for different pathologies, based on our understanding of the functional anatomy and biomechanics of the hip. When addressing the loads on structures outlined below, the principles of management of neuromotor control and remote factors should also be applied. Managing the load on the hip can be particularly difficult as the athlete may need to increase provocative loads on the hip in daily tasks. Thus it is vital that the ability to climb stairs, squat, put on shoes and perform

(e)

Figure 31.20 (cont.) (e) Example of a later-stage functional exercise incorporating deep hip and core stability with proprioceptive and neuromotor control retraining

6. Optimise gait biomechanics

Specific activities to normalise gait biomechanics and improve gait performance and endurance are outlined in Chapter 8 and should be progressed in a structured, graduated fashion. It should also include running, direction

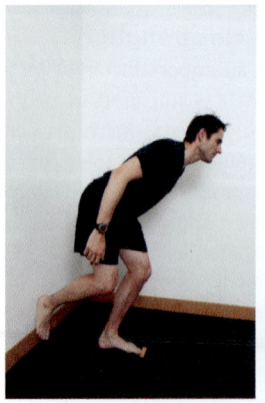

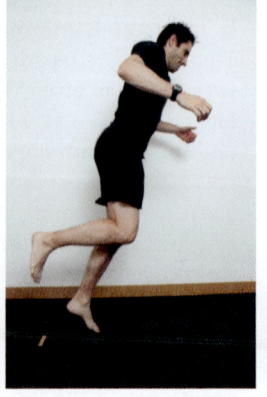

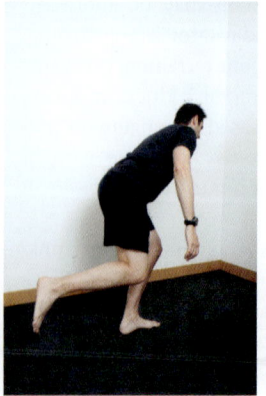

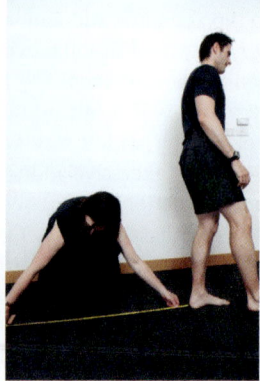

Figure 31.21 Retraining of functional activities—single-leg hop for distance

Hip pain CHAPTER 31

Criteria for returning to sport as the final stage of hip rehabilitation

The decision regarding a patient's readiness to return to sport is made using clinical judgment of the individual's functional capacity. In the absence of robust scientific evidence, the following criteria are suggested:

- performance on the one-leg hop test (or other single-leg functional tests) at least 90% of the uninjured side (if unilateral symptoms)
- performance on strength tests at least 90% of the uninjured side (if unilateral symptoms)
- performance of functional tasks and sporting activity that does not reproduce hip pain, and that the athlete has adequate control of the hip to avoid impingement, even under conditions of fatigue.

---

everyday activities such as getting in and out of a chair is undertaken in such a way that these activities do not aggravate the underlying pathology.

9. Address other remote factors that may be altering the function of the kinetic chain

As outlined previously, a number of remote factors (e.g. lumbopelvic control, ankle dorsi-flexion range) are likely to influence the rehabilitation of hip pain and pathology. Therefore, all potential contributing factors should be addressed and treated appropriately.

Surgical management of the injured hip

Hip arthroscopy is now commonly performed to manage intra-articular hip pathologies, including FAI, labral tears, chondropathy and ligamentum teres tears.[129] Hip arthroscopy has revolutionised hip surgery, since this minimally invasive procedure is associated with considerably less morbidity than open procedures. Internationally, the number of hip arthroscopy procedures now performed is growing rapidly. In the USA, the number of hip arthroscopies has increased 18-fold in the past decade[41] and in Australia it has doubled in recent years. Hip arthroscopy is a technically challenging orthopaedic procedure and should only be undertaken by high-volume, fellowship-trained surgeons.

Clinically, patients presenting for hip arthroscopy surgery tend to be grouped into two categories–those diagnosed with morphological variations, with or without soft tissue injuries, requiring surgical intervention, and those not requiring bony intervention but presenting with soft tissue injuries requiring intervention.

The first group includes patients with FAI, which may be cam, pincer or mixed impingement. This group may also have coexisting labral pathology, ligamentum teres pathology or chondral lesions.

The second group includes those with soft tissue pathologies, but without morphological change requiring surgical intervention. This group may include labral pathology, ligamentum teres pathology, chondral lesions or any combination of these. They may have coexisting issues such as dysplasia or hypermobility, which predispose them to such injuries, but do not themselves require surgical intervention. This group may also include patients with essentially normal morphology, but who undergo a massive single episode of excessive range (usually rotation), which causes trauma to the associated soft tissues.

The body of evidence examining outcomes following hip arthroscopy is growing rapidly. Systematic review evidence shows that patients without chondropathy have favourable outcomes for up to 10 years (no osteoplasty) and 3 years (with osteoplasty).[129] Patients with chondropathy have worse outcomes than those without, especially when chondral damage is severe, and risk progressing to total hip replacement within 2 years.[109] Prior to surgery, it is important that patients trial the conservative treatments outlined above. There are still no known published randomised controlled trials examining the effectiveness of hip arthroscopy, although these studies are underway internationally and will provide definitive evidence of the efficacy of hip arthroscopy for subgroups of patients with intra-articular hip pathology in the coming years. The majority of the literature focuses on outcomes following surgery for FAI, labral pathology, chondropathy or combined pathology, and is level III and IV evidence.

Rehabilitation following hip arthroscopy

Rehabilitation following hip arthroscopy has been described in the literature in a number of clinical commentaries and a systematic review.[115, 117, 130, 131] Rehabilitation programs essentially follow the same conservative principles of management outlined above. The individual pathology treated during hip arthroscopy should influence the post-operative rehabilitation program to ensure it is adequately unloaded and protected whilst healing. This generally involves a period of partial weight-bearing as tolerated on crutches until a pain-free normal gait pattern is achieved.

Generally osteoplasties performed for the correction of FAI must be protected for at least 6 weeks, while microfracture surgery performed for chondral defects may be protected through non and partial weight-bearing for at least 3 months.

Labral debridement and repairs should be protected for at least 6 weeks, ensuring the athlete avoids potential positions of impingement through activity modification and normalisation of neuromuscular control around the hip.

Injuries to the ligamentum teres should be protected for at least 6 weeks by avoiding end-range positions that place the ligament under stress, and ensuring excellent neuromotor and proprioceptive control around the hip.

During this initial protective phase, the athlete should commence active rehabilitation of the deep hip stabilisers, initially in an isolated fashion and then progressing into functional activity in a safe manner. The therapist should also address any overactivity of the secondary stabilisers such as the long adductors, the proximal gluteals, the tensor fasciae latae and the hip flexors in this period.

Once this protective phase is complete, the athlete should undertake a dynamic rehabilitation program ensuring full strength of all muscle groups around the hip, and normal function of the whole kinetic chain and sports-specific activity. A full assessment of the muscle strength and function around the hip using RTUS and hand-held dynamometry at this time can also assist in providing targeted exercise programs to address any ongoing residual deficits in strength or muscle activation. Generally, most athletes return to full sport between 3 and 5 months postoperatively following hip arthroscopy, although this will vary depending on the level and type of sport played, as well as the specific pathology and surgery performed.

LATERAL HIP PAIN

with ALISON GRIMALDI

Lateral hip pain signals very different pathologies to the medial or anterior hip region pain the chapter has focused on so far. It is a common presentation particularly among distance runners and women over the age of 40. Local soft tissue pathology may mimic or coexist with hip joint and lumbar spine pathologies so a full differential diagnosis as described earlier in this chapter will be required. Hallmarks of a local pathology include specific areas of pain and tenderness either at the greater trochanter or iliac crest.

Greater trochanteric pain

Patients with trochanteric pain complain of pain and significant tenderness over the greater trochanter, particularly lying on their side at night. The pain may radiate from the greater trochanter, most commonly down the lateral aspect of the thigh to the knee, and occasionally extending into the upper lateral leg along the line of the ITB. Tasks that involve a single-leg weight-bearing phase such as standing on one leg to dress, ascending stairs or hills and particularly those involving higher eccentric loads or a stretch-shortening cycle, such as running, bounding or hopping, are usually reported as provocative.

Traditionally the primary local source of trochanteric pain was thought to be the trochanteric bursa; however, there are a number of soft tissue structures at the greater trochanter that have nociceptive capacity. Less common findings include thickening of one or more of the three associated bursae and the region of the ITB crossing the greater trochanter.[132-134]

> **PRACTICE PEARL**
>
> Imaging studies have demonstrated that soft tissue pathology in this patient population most commonly presents in the gluteus medius and/or minimus tendons.

The same pathological mechanism is likely to underlie all of these local soft tissue changes, and therefore the relative local contributions to nociception may be less pertinent in early conservative management than attending to the underlying issues. While medical comorbidities may compromise tendon function and load-bearing status,[135-137] mechanical loading is a potent driver of biological processes responsible for soft tissue structure and health.[138, 139]

Relevant anatomy

Mechanical load within the local soft tissues will be influenced by the relative anatomical relationship between these tissues and the underlying bony greater trochanter in different postures and dynamic function. As the gluteus medius and minimus tendons wrap around the greater trochanter on their course to their insertion sites, they are separated from the underlying bone by their relevant bursae (subgluteus medius and subgluteus minimus bursae) (see Fig. 31.5 for general anatomy of this region).

The trochanteric bursa, often now referred to as the subgluteus maximus bursa, sits superficial to these tendons and beneath the thick, fibrous ITB. This relationship is illustrated in Figure 31.22. Mechanical load may be applied longitudinally (tensile load) or transversely (compressive load) across the tissues. Excessive compressive load is an important aetiological factor in the development of insertional tendinopathies,[140, 141] engendering changes within the soft tissues that may ameliorate compression but subsequently reduce tensile loading capacity.

Role of compression in pathology

The gluteal tendons and bursae may become compressed between the underlying greater trochanter and overlying ITB, while the ITB itself may also be exposed to compression against the greater trochanter. Compression increases tenocyte production of larger

Hip pain   CHAPTER 31

> **PRACTICE PEARL**
>
> Compressive loading of the trochanteric soft tissues may be accumulated during static postures such as standing 'hanging on one hip' in adduction, sitting with knees crossed or together, or during dynamic functional tasks completed with excessive lateral pelvic tilt or shift.

proteoglycan molecules (aggrecan and versican)[142] that bind water within the tendon resulting in a thicker tendon more resistant to compression. There may also be a shift within a compressed tendon to cartilage-like cells, which are particularly robust for compressive loading. Thickening of the associated bursae and the ITB are also likely to represent a response to excessive compression. Unfortunately this seemingly successful adaptation to compression results in reduced tensile loading capacity of a tendon due to concurrent disorganisation and enzymatic resorption of large type 1 collagen fibres.[143]

Tendons that have adapted to compression may then fail at lower tensile strain rates.[141] Consistent with this scenario, gluteal tendons in those with lateral hip pain have been shown to be either thicker than normal (likely in the earlier adaptive stage), or attenuated and thinner with partial or full thickness tearing (later stage when the compromised collagen fibres yield under tensile loads).[132, 72]

Compressive loading of the lateral soft tissues is strongly influenced by hip joint position and particularly by hip adduction. Birnbaum and colleagues determined that, as the hip moves from neutral adduction, where the ITB exerts 4 N of compressive load on the greater trochanter and intervening tissues, loads rise nine-fold by 10° of adduction and over 25-fold by end-range, 40° adduction.[144] Running with a midline or cross-midline striking pattern, on the camber of a road or the same direction around a track, may increase the risk of developing lateral hip pain,[145, 146] perhaps due to the cumulative loading stimulus.

Iliac crest pain
Lateral hip pain may also emanate from soft tissue sources at the iliac crest, with local pain and tenderness over the region of origin of the TFL and ITB and adjacent fascia, with pain radiating most commonly over the anterolateral hip towards the greater trochanter. In such patients, thickening, increased water content and partial tearing have been noted on MRI in the TFL tendon of origin, the proximal ITB and the gluteal aponeurotic fascia that covers the gluteus medius, all of which anchor along the iliac crest.[134, 147, 148] While an in vivo study such as Birnbaum et al.'s[144] has not been replicated at the iliac crest, it is reasonable to conceive that, as the hip moves into adduction, the ITB and the gluteal aponeurotic fascia will also wind firmly around the iliac crest, with the iliac tubercle providing the most prominent bony cam region. In running athletes, this condition is an overuse injury with reports of gradual onset worsening with activity over a number of months.[134, 148] The clinican should be aware of the same issues as for greater trochanteric pain–assessing and controlling exposure to hip adduction during static postures and functional loading.

Examination of the patient with lateral hip pain
Distinct tenderness on direct palpation over the greater trochanter or iliac tubercle is a key finding that determines

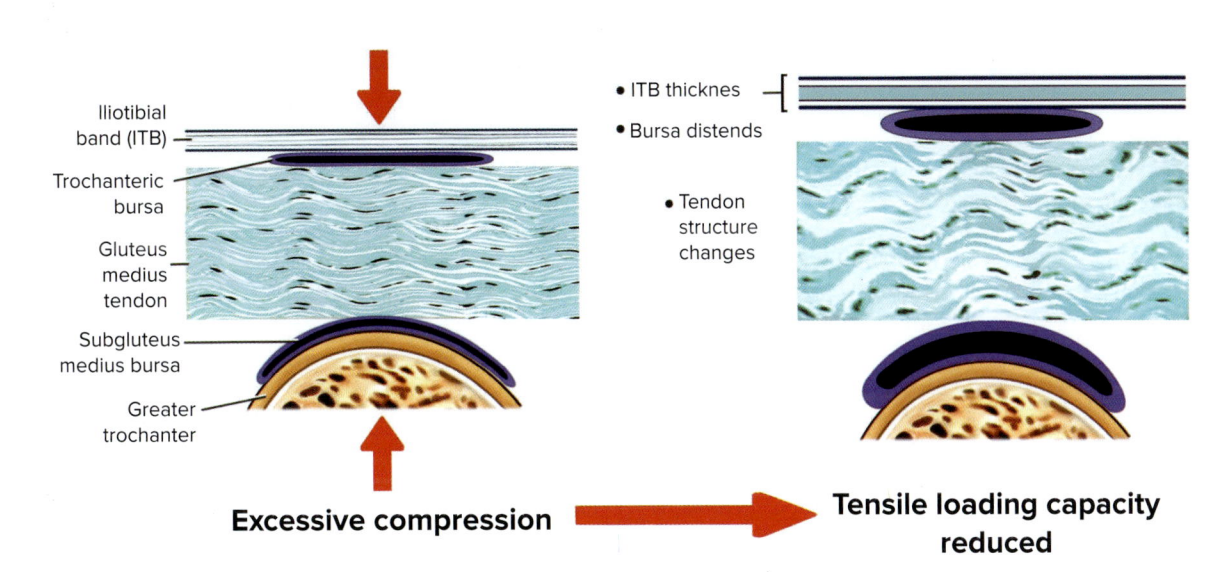

Figure 31.22 Adaptation of soft tissue of the greater trochanter to compressive loading. Structural changes include production of larger proteoglycans, a hydrophilic gel matrix, increased water content and a shift to cartilage-like cells

whether lateral hip pain is originating from a local soft tissue source. A lack of local tenderness would strongly indicate that other more remote conditions should be considered. However, tenderness alone is not sufficient for a firm diagnosis. Lumbar screening and a full hip joint assessment, as described in the preceding physical examination section, should be undertaken. Range of motion tests are usually unremarkable, helping to differentiate from primary hip joint pathology. Similarly, the FABER test is usually not significantly limited in range, but reproduction of lateral hip pain on this test, in the absence of difficulty manipulating shoes and socks (which is usually associated with limited FABER), has been shown to be useful in differentiating local greater trochanteric pain from hip OA.[149]

Despite the anecdotal assumption that those with lateral hip pain have tightness in the lateral soft tissues of the hip and thigh, particularly the ITB, the adduction range on the Ober's or Modified Ober's test is not correlated with the presence of gluteal tendon pathology.[150] About 25% of participants were positive for local pain at the greater trochanter during the Ober's test.[150] This may reflect the potentially provocative action of compressing the soft tissues between the greater trochanter and the ITB. This adducted position will also wrap the proximal ITB and TFL tendon around the iliac tubercle and therefore may be clinically useful as part of a test battery. Diagnostic utility of the Ober's test for proximal ITB/TFL pathology is currently unknown, as no clinical tests apart from palpation have been described or analysed for such conditions.

Passive compressive tests may become more valuable with the addition of an active tensile load. Isometric abduction tests have, however, only been described to date from a hip-neutral or abducted position. While abductor muscle weakness is common in those with lateral hip pain and is important to assess, the diagnostic usefulness of such tests is limited by the fact that patients with no lateral hip pain or other conditions also commonly present with hip abductor muscle weakness.[150] Pain reproduction on resisted hip abduction showed some weak diagnostic properties.[150] Further research is required to assess whether isometric abduction performed in an adducted hip posture may be more useful in differential diagnosis of lateral hip pain.

In a meta-analysis of diagnostic accuracy of clinical hip tests, the only test to show a strong ability to influence the likelihood of a positive diagnosis of gluteal tendinopathy was the resisted external rotation de-rotation test (Fig 31.6f).[40] The test winds the ITB and fasciae latae over the greater trochanter in hip flexion and external rotation, and then superimposes an active contraction of the gluteus medius and minimus via resisted internal rotation, combining compressive and tensile loads across the greater trochanter. Adding hip adduction will further increase compressive load and therefore may be useful as a test variation.

(a)

(b)

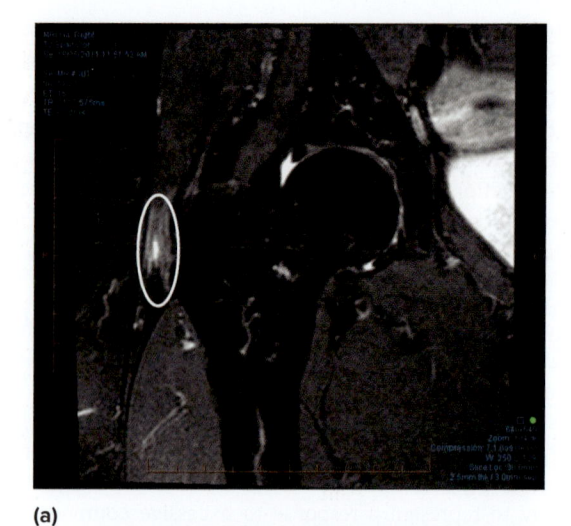

Figure 31.23 MRI appearances of gluteus medius abnormalities (a) Coronal fat-suppressed T2 image showing tendinopathy of the gluteus medius tendon near its greater trochanteric insertion (b) Fat-suppressed T1 image showing partial tear of the gluteus medius tendon (arrows)

Functional movement tests are employed to highlight functional deficits and may provide helpful treatment direction. These tests generally do not perform well as diagnostic tests as dysfunction around the hip and pelvis is common to many lower quadrant disorders. One exception may be the 30-second sustained single-leg stance test as described by Lequesne et al.[48] When performed as a pain provocation test, rather than a traditional Trendelenburg test, reproduction of pain over the greater trochanter within 30 seconds of standing on one leg was shown to have good sensitivity and specificity for the detection of gluteal tendinopathy.

Diagnostic ultrasound can be performed to determine if thickening is present in the bursae or ITB or to look for thickening, thinning or hypoechoic changes that are consistent with tendinopathy and tears.[72, 132, 133] MRI is the gold standard for assessing tendinosis and tears of the gluteus medius and minimus tendons (Fig. 31.23).[151, 152] While imaging studies are useful as an adjunct to clinical assessment where the diagnosis is unclear or the patient is failing to respond to treatment, they should not be used as a stand-alone medium for determining the source of lateral hip pain. This is due to the high prevalence of soft tissue abnormalities in this region that may occur in the absence of lateral hip pain.[152]

Treatment of the patient with lateral hip pain

The principles of treating lateral hip pain are consistent with other insertional tendinopathies. First, manage the pain by controlling soft tissue loads at the greater trochanter or iliac crest. Introduce graduated strengthening of the involved musculotendinous complex, aiming to improve load tolerance and optimise abnormal movement patterns. Return to sport is closely monitored to ensure volume of tendon load is controlled, time for adaptation is allowed and recurrence is avoided.

Managing pain

Managing pain will primarily involve removing or minimising potentially provocative loads and instituting pain-relieving loading techniques. Reduction of compressive loading will require minimisation of sustained, repetitive or loaded end-range adduction. Positional habits such as sitting with knees crossed or together or standing 'hanging on one hip' in adduction should be discouraged. Sleeping postures should also be addressed, educating the patient to sleep in supine, quarter from prone or, if side-lying is unavoidable, to use pillows between the legs to reduce adduction of the uppermost side. An eggshell overlay for the lowermost side is recommended.

ITB and gluteal stretches involving hip adduction should be avoided. Provocative physical activities should be suspended or modified, such as long-distance, high-speed and hill running or, for the more severe presentation, all running may need to be temporarily suspended. Runners should stay on the flat or run in straight lines rather than on a camber or around a track; plyometric drills such as jumping, bounding and hopping particularly using stairs or boxes should be avoided.

While corticosteroid injection may reduce pain in the short term via interactions with local neuropeptides and neurotransmitters,[153, 154] the effect is not long lasting. It fails to address the underlying pathoaetiological issues and may even hinder a tendon's capacity to respond appropriately to loading (see Chapter 17) via the downregulation of fibroblastic production of collagen.[155, 156]

Shock wave therapy reduces lateral hip pain.[154, 157] However, it is recommended that shock wave therapy is reserved for those who fail a load management and exercise approach.[158, 159]

Managing load: First line treatment

Exercise for the hip abductor musculature begins with isometric abduction in neutral or slight hip abduction to minimise compression. This may be completed in side-lying (affected side up with pillows between legs) (Fig. 31.24a), supine with a belt around the lower thighs or standing (Fig. 31.24b). The patient should *slowly* ramp up the contraction to a 25% maximum voluntary isometric contraction level initially, which allows time for a good gluteus minimus and medius recruitment, and avoids dominance of the TFL. The level of force development may be increased if well tolerated and early and dominant gluteal contraction is achieved. The primary aim at this point is pain relief, provided by isometric exercise via activation of segmental and/or extra-segmental descending pain inhibitory mechanisms,[160, 161] and now recommended in the early management of lower limb tendon pain.[162, 163]

The strengthening phase includes exercises that directly target the hip abductors and functional loading tasks with a focus on strict control of hip adduction through graduated levels of difficulty (Fig. 31.25). Spring-resisted sliding platforms such as Pilates reformers provide frontal plane weight-bearing resistance with applied load easily titrated and progressed.

> **PRACTICE PEARL**
>
> Side-lying 'clams' (hip abduction/external rotation–hip adduction/internal rotation) are generally provocative, possibly due to the compression and friction that the ITB imparts on the soft tissues as it passes over the greater trochanter; they should therefore be avoided.

Bridging (Fig. 31.26) and functional strengthening progressions (Fig. 31.27) begin with bilateral loading, progressing to offset and then single-leg tasks, allowing hand support where necessary to optimise pelvic control and minimise hip adduction and therefore compression, which is the first priority.

Athletes can then progress to more complex sports-specific tasks, as described in the management of hip joint

PART B   Regional problems

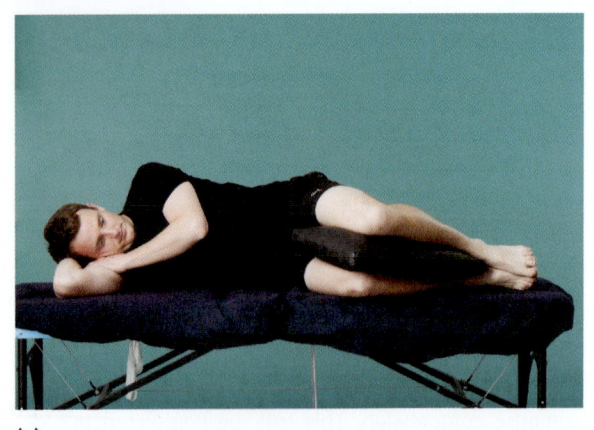

(a)

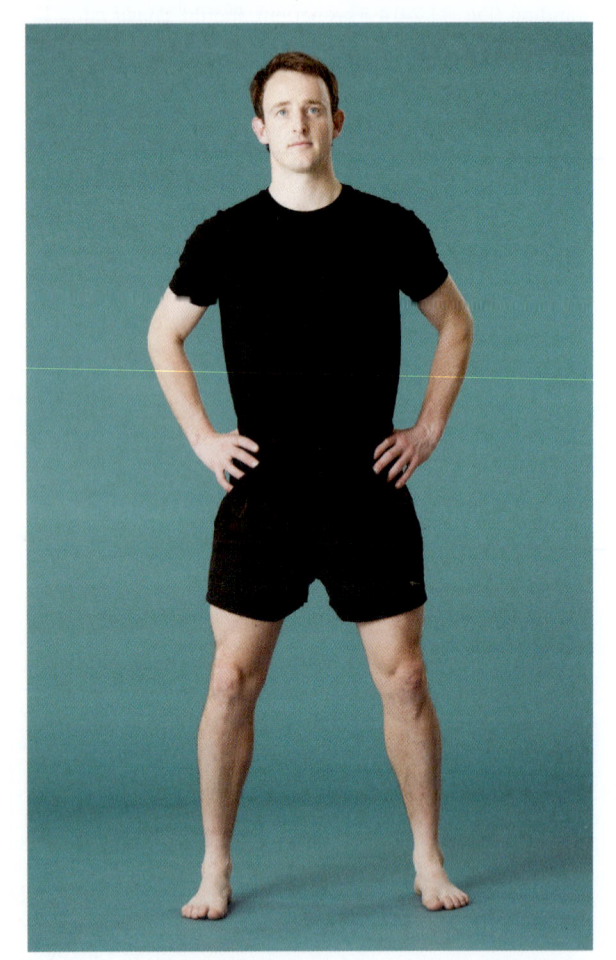

(b)

Figure 31.24 Examples of positions for pain-relieving isometric abduction exercises for lateral hip pain (a) Side-lying 'preparation for lifting' (b) Standing in slight abduction

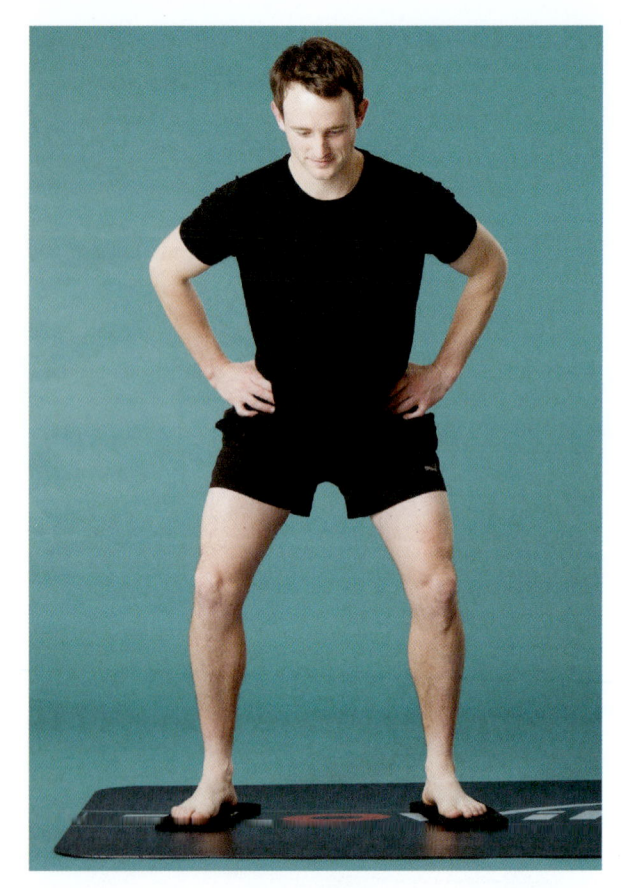

Figure 31.25 Resisted hip abduction exercise (sliding) in weight-bearing

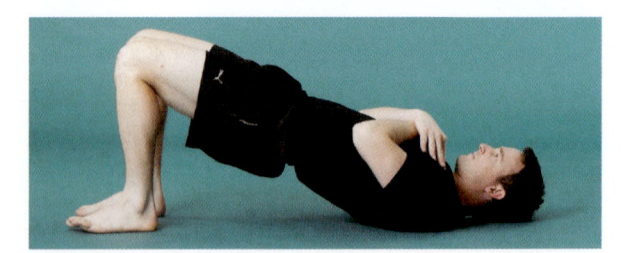

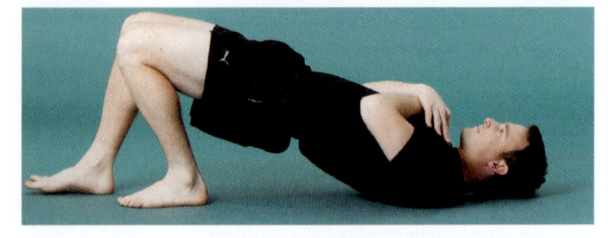

(a)

(b)

Figure 31.26 Examples of basic bridge progressions (a) Double-leg bridge—equal weight-bearing (b) Offset bridge—gluteals of 'close side' foot do most of the work

626

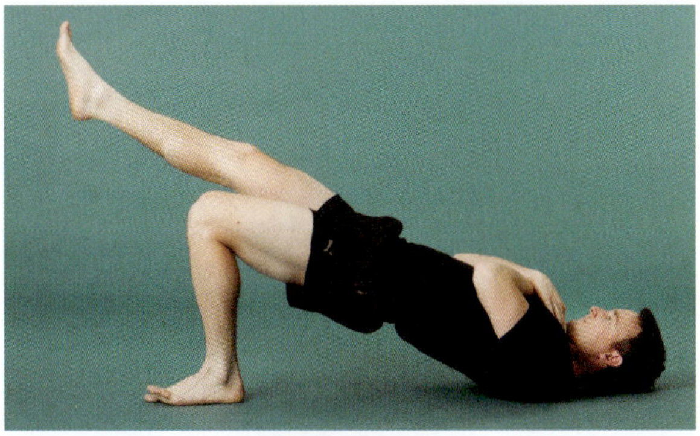

Hip pain   CHAPTER 31

(c)

Figure 31.26 (cont.) (c) Single-leg bridge—pelvis controlled in a level position by the gluteals of the weight-bearing side throughout the hip flexion/extension movement

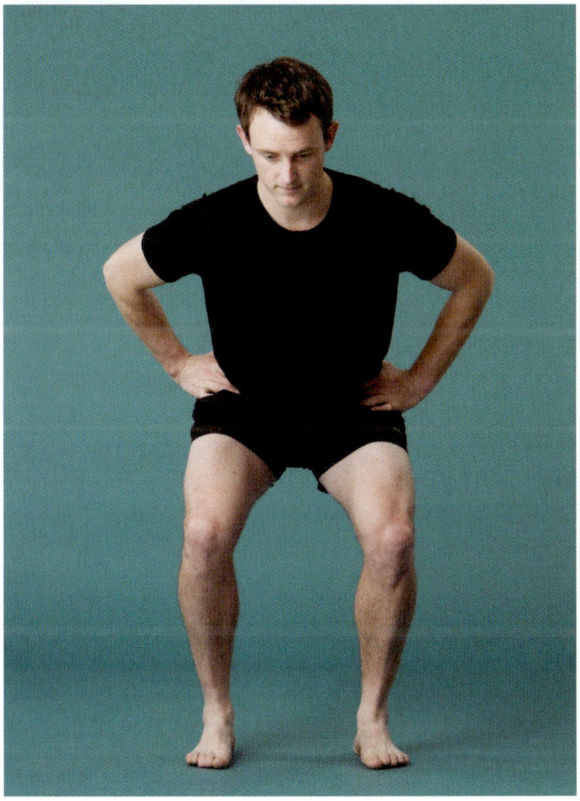

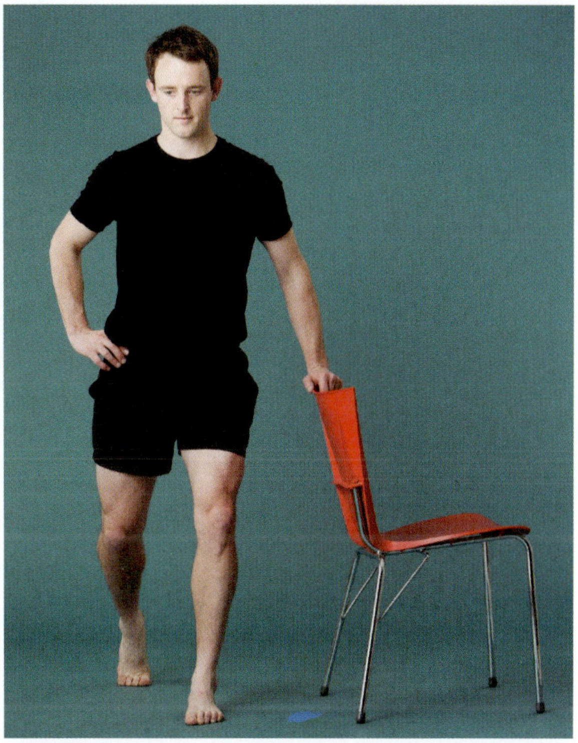

(b)

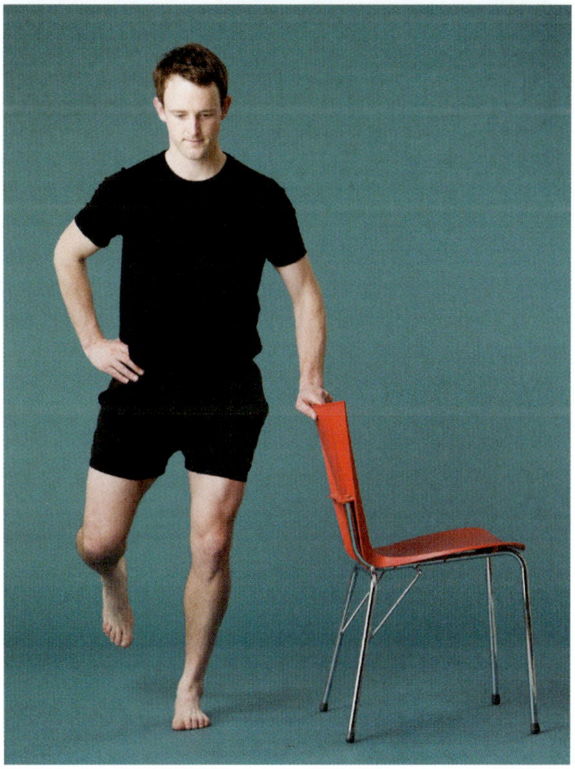

(a)

Figure 31.27 Examples of functional strengthening progressions (a) Double-leg squat—equal weight-bearing (b) Offset squat—gluteals of front side do most of the work (c) Single-leg squat—pelvis controlled in a level position by the gluteals of the weight-bearing side throughout the hip flexion/extension movement

(c)

627

PART B Regional problems

(d)

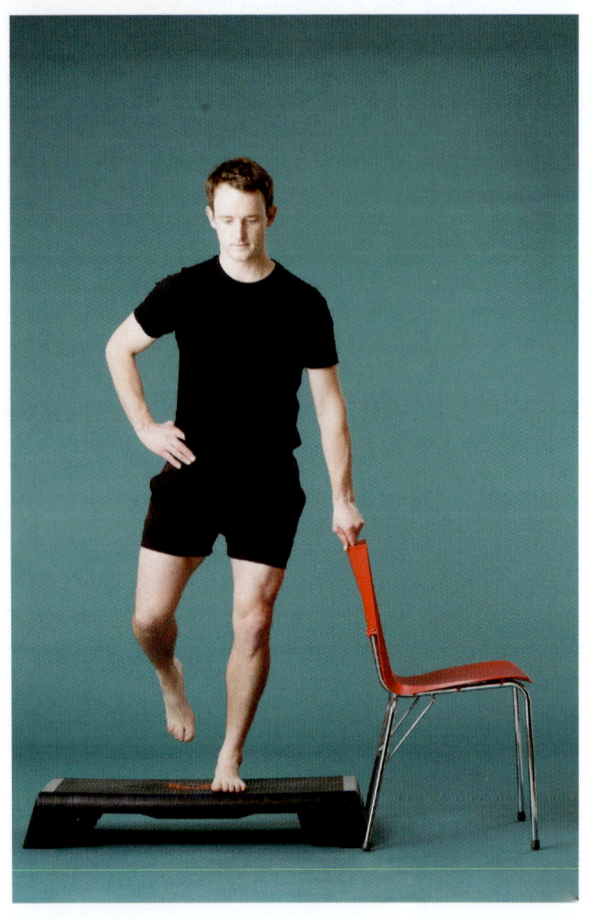

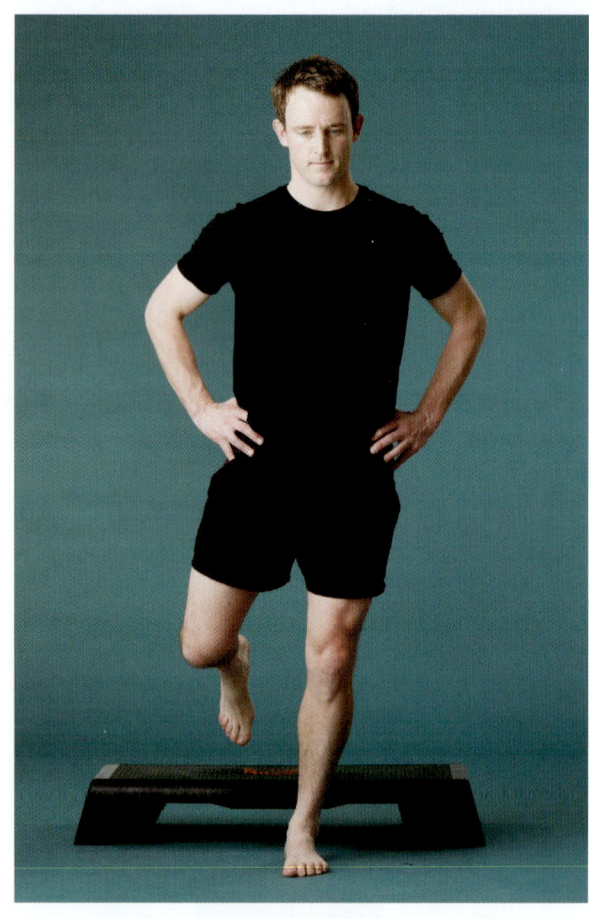

(e)

Figure 31.27 (cont.) (d) Step up (e) Landing training—requires control of pelvic and femoral alignment during a dynamic landing task

pathologies earlier in this chapter. For running athletes, visual biofeedback and increases in cadence have been shown to be effective in reducing peak hip adduction.[164] Increasing cadence by 10% enhanced pre-activation of gluteus medius prior to stance phase and improves in lateral pelvic control during the subsequent stance phase.[165] As stretching into adduction is to be avoided, athletes may require massage, needling or home use of a trigger ball or vibratory hand-held massager to control muscle soreness or tightness arising secondary to the loading program.

For those who fail conservative management, usually older non-athletic individuals, there are surgical options that include ITB release around the greater trochanter ± bursectomy and tendon repair as required.[166-169] While outcomes are generally reported as good to excellent, athletes are much less likely to progress to a surgical intervention.

REFERENCES

References for this chapter can be found at www.mhhe.com/au/CSM5e

Chapter 32

Groin pain

with ADAM WEIR, PER HÖLMICH and KRISTIAN THORBORG

Soccer was my first love, and I enjoyed playing on the left wing until a groin injury forced me out of the game in 2008.
Chad le Clos, South African swimming gold medallist

This chapter discusses both acute and longstanding groin injuries in athletes. It covers the anatomy where the complexity and degree of interconnections is highlighted. Epidemiology and risk factors have been updated using systematic reviews. The 2015 Doha agreement meeting on terminology and definitions in groin pain in athletes is included and the chapter follows the terminology agreed upon during this expert meeting. Clinical examination and assessment is covered including a practical guideline for systematic assessment of an injured athlete. There is a new section on imaging highlighting the lack of evidence in this area. Treatment with specific sections on adductor, iliopsoas, inguinal and pubic-related groin pain as well as acute groin injuries is covered with suggestions for rehabilitation.

ANATOMY

The word groin most likely originates from the ancient English word *grynde* which meant abyss or void. Confusion surrounding the groin region has made clinicians refer to this region as the 'Bermuda triangle' of the body.[1] In this section, we explain and simplify the complex anatomy of the groin. The groin region, where the abdomen meets the lower limbs via the pelvis, contains not only musculoskeletal structures, but also important internal organs and urogenital structures. In this section we focus on the musculoskeletal anatomy of the groin. The anatomy of the hip joint is described in Chapter 31.

We will focus on the pubic symphysis, hip adductors, hip flexors, abdominals and the inguinal region. An overview of the anatomy is depicted in Figure 32.1a.

Pubic symphysis

The pubic symphysis is a secondary cartilaginous joint connecting the two pubic rami. It is supported superiorly by ligaments and inferiorly by the superior pubic ligament and the inferior or arcuate pubic ligament respectively.[2] The joint is lined with hyaline cartilage. A fibrocartilaginous disc separates the two pubic bones. The pubic symphysis is the site of numerous musculotendinous attachments, which act to dynamically stabilise the anterior pelvis and the transference of large

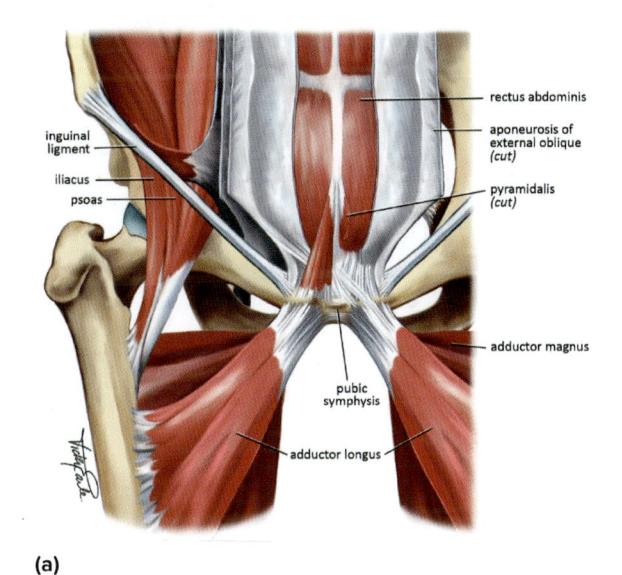

Figure 32.1 (a) Overview of the anatomy of the groin

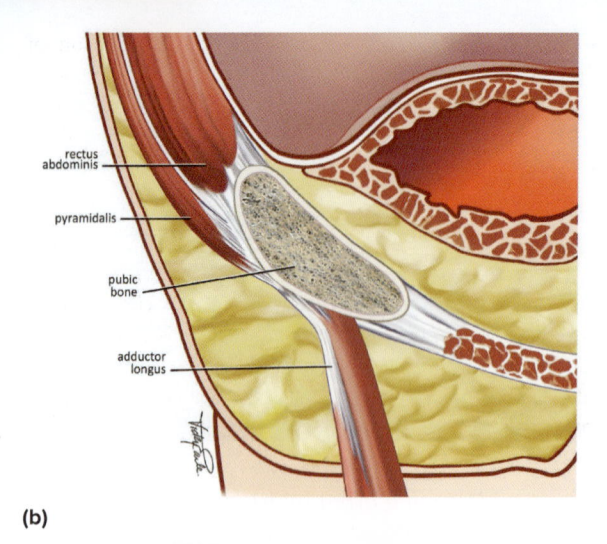

PART B   Regional problems

(b)

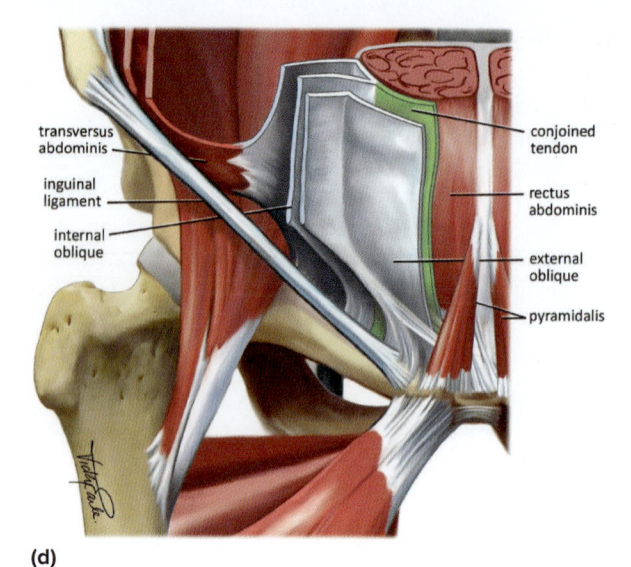

(d)

Figure 32.1 (cont.) (d) Anatomy of the muscles in the inguinal region

the most commonly injured groin muscle in soccer[3, 4] and the adductor longus is the most commonly injured adductor muscle.[5] It inserts at the middle one-third of the linea aspera of the femur and has an interesting proximal origin. The origin is predominantly muscular (around 60%). The anterior tendinous portion continues across the front of the symphysis to fuse with the distal rectus and external oblique forming an aponeurosis.[6] This aponeurosis has fibres that insert from the adductors and rectus directly into the pubic symphysis joint capsule and disc.[2] The adductor longus not only acts as an adductor but also as an important hip flexor when the hip is in an extended position, and therefore is also highly involved in kicking.[7]

The anatomy of the aponeurosis on the anterior side of the pubic symphysis in shown in Figure 32.1b.

Hip flexors

The iliopsoas is the primary hip flexor but rectus femoris, sartorius, tensor fascia lata and a number of hip adductors also contribute to hip flexion. The iliopsoas is made up of the iliacus, which originates from the iliac fossa in the pelvis and the psoas muscle.[8] The psoas arises from the vertebral bodies of T12 and L1–5 and the intervertebral discs. The two muscles converge distally to form the iliopsoas. Although the tendon is often depicted as a common tendon, the lateral portion of the iliacus extends distally to insert directly onto the femur and at the level of the hip joint there are distinct tendons.[8]

The distal iliopsoas tendon anatomy is shown in Figure 32.1c.

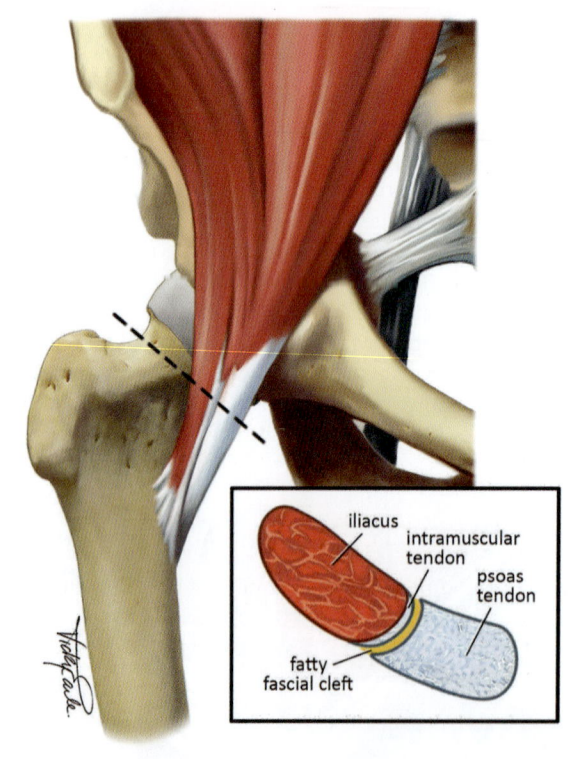

(c)

Figure 32.1 (cont.) (b) Anatomy of the aponeurosis on the anterior side of the pubic symphysis (c) Anatomy of distal iliopsoas tendon

forces acting across this joint, especially during specific sporting activities such as kicking and cutting.

Hip adductors

The hip adductors include pectineus, gracilis and adductor longus, brevis and magnus. The adductors are

Inguinal region
The anatomy of the inguinal canal is complex and extensively described in detail in classic anatomical texts. The abdominal muscles–transversus abdominis, internal and external obliques and the rectus abdominis–are all intimately related in this region. The inguinal ligament is formed by a distal shelving of the external oblique and the conjoined tendon from a convergence of transversus abdominis and the internal oblique at the medial ends. The conjoined tendon also inserts into the lateral rectus sheath.[9]

The anatomy of the muscles in the inguinal region is shown in Figure 32.1d.

Summary of anatomy
The anatomy of the groin has clinical implications as it demonstrates a high degree of confluence of the muscle, tendon, bone and joint structures. This connectivity means that pain provocation or stress tests do not load a single anatomical structure in isolation. This may explain why patients who present with groin pain often have diffuse, poorly localised pain and multiple clinical findings.

EPIDEMIOLOGY
Groin pain and injury is common with sports that involve kicking, rapid acceleration and deceleration, and sudden change of direction.[10, 11] Until recently, there was no agreement on terminology, definitions or classification of groin pain in athletes.[12] This makes comparing epidemiological studies difficult for two main reasons. Firstly, multiple injury definitions and classifications systems have been used; some combined hip and groin, some classify groin separately, and almost all use different terminology for various groin injuries, which are often not specifically described.[13] Additionally, the nature of injury onset is often poorly reported (e.g. acute versus chronic; traumatic versus overuse).

The second difficulty is that groin injury is often only recorded when an athlete misses a training session or match. Therefore, the prevalence of groin injury may be underestimated as those athletes who continue to train and play through injury often are not recorded.

Incidence—soccer
A recent systematic review on the incidence of groin pain in soccer included 34 articles.[14] In general, there was risk of bias in the studies due to participant selection (18 studies), exposure (17 studies) and precision of the estimates given (18 studies).

The main findings of the review were:

- groin injuries in male club soccer accounted for 4–19% of all injuries
- groin injuries in female club soccer accounted for 2–14% of all injuries

- analysis of 29 studies found a higher proportion of groin injuries in men (12.8%) than women (6.9% with an absolute difference of 5.9%, 95% with a confidence interval of 4.6–7.1%)
- groin injury rates in males were 0.2–2.1/1000 hours and 0.1–0.6/1000 hours in women (rate ratio 2.4, 95% with a confidence interval of 2.0–2.9).

In adductor-related injuries in elite male soccer the re-injury rate has been reported to be 15%.[3] The recovery period for a re-injury in elite soccer players is almost twice as long compared to the original injury emphasising the importance of avoiding re-injury by finishing treatment properly the first time.[3]

Incidence—elite sports other than soccer
A recent review identified 31 papers where more than 10 team seasons of groin or groin region injury incidence were reported.[11] These studies used varying injury definitions and also considered varying injury categories from general to specific (all groin/hip region injuries, groin injuries, adductor muscle strains, intra-articular hip injuries). The main findings were as follows.

- When playing the same sport, males had greater injury incidence of groin injury than females (RR 2.45, 95% with a confidence interval of 2.06–2.92).
- The sports with a high rate of groin injury were ice hockey and the football codes where field kicking is common (Australian rules football, Gaelic football).
- Within the football codes, player positions involving more kicking had a higher incidence.
- Uniform injury classification and definitions would improve comparison of results across studies.

Prevalence
As mentioned previously, using only time loss or medical attention definitions to count athletes as being injured probably misses many less-severe injuries. The injuries leading to time loss are thought to represent the tip of the iceberg. A study on football players showed that 49% had experienced groin pain in the previous season and that this had lasted longer than 6 weeks in 31%.[15]

Distribution of acute injuries
Few studies have closely examined which proportion of groin injuries has an acute onset. In a Danish study of 998 soccer players it was found that on the 58 injuries registered, 20 had acute onset, 31 were classified as overuse and 7 could not be classified.[4] This would suggest that acute onset injuries represent a significant proportion of the total injuries in soccer players. Defined terminology using specific classification systems for

injury distribution have not been used in many studies. The study of 998 soccer players used a terminology and classification system almost identical to the one we use in this chapter (see section below) to classify the 58 injuries.[4] Of the 58 injuries, 16 (27%) could not be classified and 24% had multiple entities. Adductor-related groin pain was the most frequent injury (51%) with iliopsoas (30%) and abdominal (19%) also being diagnosed frequently.

A recent study examined acute onset groin injuries in 110 athletes presenting to a sports medicine hospital within 7 days of injury.[5] The majority (76%) were football code players with 10% basketball and 8% handball players. In the football codes 40% of the injuries occurred during kicking, where change of direction was the most frequent activity (31%) during onset in other sports. Clinical examination and imaging (MRI or ultrasound) were performed in all 110 athletes. The majority of injuries affected the adductors (66%), with iliopsoas (17–25%) and rectus femoris (15–23%) injuries also being frequent.

Other case series have examined the distribution of groin pain in those presenting to different clinicians in multiple countries. These series found adductor-related groin pain,[16] inguinal-related groin pain[17] and hip-related groin pain[18] to be the most common problems. As these studies all suffer from referral bias, they are less helpful than studies where a single cohort is followed over time. They do, however, all report multiple problems occurring in a significant number of those who present.

> **PRACTICE PEARL**
>
> Adductor-related groin pain is the most common groin injury in the football codes and ice hockey.

RISK FACTORS

A lack of agreement on definitions and terminology of groin pain and the various definitions of when injury is present make the literature on risk factors challenging to understand. A previous comprehensive review[19] was updated in 2015.[20] This systematic review covered 29 studies and summarised literature with a levels-of-evidence approach. The majority of studies were prospective cohort studies. The review found that there was level 1 and 2 evidence that the following are associated with an increased risk of groin injury in athletes:

- previous groin injury (level 1)
- higher level of play (level 1)
- reduced hip adduction (absolute and relative to abduction) strength (level 2)
- lower levels of sport-specific training (level 2).

Whittaker et al. also highlighted that to date there has been virtually no investigation of the relationship between exposure/athletic load and risk. Future studies should be large enough to ensure around 50 injury cases to examine for moderate to strong associations and include clear injury definitions.[20]

Where risk factor studies should ideally be prospective in design, cross-sectional and case control studies allow multiple factors to be examined in smaller populations. While no prospective relationship can be determined, these factors can be considered in future studies on risk factors, investigations and treatment. A systematic review with a meta-analysis examining these cross-sectional factors differentiating athletes with and without groin pain was carried out in 2015.[21] Seventeen cross-sectional studies were included, of which 10 were high quality. In total, 62 different measures were investigated. Eight studies were suitable for meta-analysis. Meta-analysis showed that athletes with hip and groin pain had:

- pain and lower strength on adductor squeeze test
- reduced hip internal rotation and bent knee fall out, but that hip external rotation was the same as controls.

For other factors, a levels-of-evidence synthesis was performed. There was strong evidence that athletes with hip and groin pain have an association with:

- lower patient-reported outcome (PROM) scores
- altered trunk muscle function.

TERMINOLOGY AND DEFINITIONS

A systematic review on the treatment of groin pain in athletes included 72 studies, in which 33 different diagnostic terms were used.[13] The 'Doha agreement meeting on terminology and definitions in groin pain in athletes' was convened to attempt to resolve this problem.[22] The aim was to agree on a standard terminology, along with accompanying definitions. A Delphi process was used to inform agreement. Unanimous agreement on the following terms and definitions was reached. Some considerations are presented here as a preamble to the terms.

> **PRACTICE PEARL**
>
> The preferred umbrella term was 'groin pain in athletes'. This was favoured over others (e.g. athletic pubalgia, athletic groin pain, sports groin pain, athletes' groin) because it is clearly descriptive and cannot be misunderstood to be a diagnostic term.

A number of previously popular terms were considered and rejected during the meeting. The terms that the group chose not to recommend were: adductor and iliopsoas tendinitis or tendinopathy, athletic groin pain, athletic pubalgia, biomechanical groin overload, Gilmore's groin, groin disruption, hockey-goalie syndrome, hockey groin, osteitis pubis, sports groin, sportsman's groin, sports hernia and sportsman's hernia. The term 'entity' was chosen to reflect the recognisable pattern of symptoms and signs exhibited by the athlete.

To ensure generalisability and straightforward use in everyday practice, a clinically based classification system is recommended. This means that a thorough history and physical examination are essential. In the history, in all cases the athlete should report pain in the affected region that worsens on exercise. Palpation is important to identify the painful structures and must be precise, as numerous structures in the groin region are in close proximity and can refer pain to overlapping areas. The term 'tenderness' is defined in this system as discomfort or pain when the area is touched and that the athlete recognises this to be their specific injury pain.

Pain on resistance testing should also be felt in the affected structure. For example, in adductor-related groin pain, the pain on resisted adduction testing should reproduce the athlete's recognisable pain in the adductors. Pain felt in a different location (e.g. the inguinal region on resisted adduction testing) would not signify adductor-related groin pain. The techniques of physical examination are covered in the 'Clinical overview' section.

Classification
Acute groin injuries
Acute injuries refer to the manner in which the athlete first felt the pain (i.e. sudden onset). In general, the system proposed in this section could potentially be used to classify the majority of acute groin injuries into entities. There is far less literature on acute groin injuries when compared to longstanding groin pain.

Consequently, a careful history–along with examination comprising palpation, resistance testing and stretching–is critical. In cases with severe pain, it may be hard to perform a thorough physical examination. It should be recognised that some acute groin injuries such as proximal rectus femoris injuries do not readily fit into the current Doha classification system. Further work will be needed to refine this system to fully encompass the entire spectrum of acute groin injuries.

Longstanding groin pain
The exact duration considered to be longstanding is not further defined. Longstanding groin pain can start either gradually or suddenly and does not refer to the mechanism of onset, but only to the duration of symptoms.

The classification system has three major subheadings of groin pain in athletes.

1. *Defined clinical entities for groin pain:*
   - adductor related
   - iliopsoas related
   - inguinal related
   - pubic related.

   The locations of the four entities for groin pain are shown in Figure 32.2.

2. *Hip-related groin pain.* Pain from the hip joint (Chapter 31) should always be considered as a possible cause of groin pain.

3. *Other conditions causing groin pain in athletes.* Besides the defined clinical entities and the hip, there are many other possible causes for groin pain in athletes. A high index of clinical suspicion is needed to identify these and clinicians need to be alert to the possibilities, especially when the complaints cannot easily be classified into one of the common defined

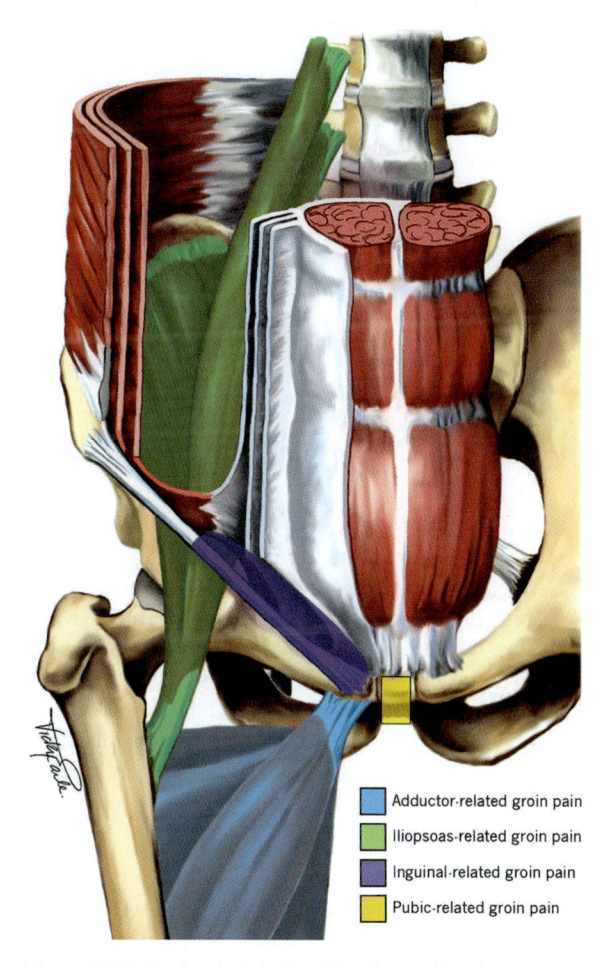

Figure 32.2 Defined clinical entities for groin pain
REPRODUCED WITH PERMISSION OF BRITISH JOURNAL OF SPORTS MEDICINE

PART B Regional problems

Table 32.1 Overview of some possible causes of groin pain in athletes

Entities defined during Doha agreement meeting	Other musculoskeletal causes	Not to be missed
Adductor-related groin pain Iliopsoas-related groin pain Inguinal-related groin pain Pubic-related groin pain Hip-related groin pain	Inguinal or femoral hernia Post-hernioplasty pain Nerve entrapment: – obturator – ilioinguinal – genitofemoral – iliohypogastric Referred pain – lumbar spine – sacroiliac joint Apophysitis or avulsion fracture – anterior superior iliac spine – anterior inferior iliac spine – pubic bone	Stress fracture – neck of femur – pubic ramus – acetabulum Hip joint – slipped capital femoral epiphysis (adolescents) – Perthes' disease (children and adolescents) – avascular necrosis /transient osteoporosis of the head of the femur – arthritis of the hip joint (reactive or infectious) Inguinal lymphadenopathy Intra-abdominal abnormality – prostatitis – urinary tract infections – kidney stone – appendicitis – diverticulitis Gynaecological conditions Spondyloarthropathies – ankylosing spondylitis Tumours – testicular tumours – bone tumours – prostate cancer – urinary tract cancer – digestive tract cancer – soft tissue tumours

clinical entities. An unclear relationship between the pain and loading during sport, nocturnal or extremely severe pain or a lack of response to treatment should trigger more suspicion. There are numerous possible causes, a number of which are listed in Table 32.1. The main categories are orthopaedic, neurological, rheumatological, urological, gastrointestinal, dermatological, oncological and surgical; however, this list is not exhaustive as many rare conditions could possibly cause pain in the groin region.

A careful history and physical examination covering more than only the musculoskeletal system, and appropriate additional investigations or referrals are critical for identifying other possible causes. Some of these conditions are discussed in more detail at the end of this chapter.

CLINICAL OVERVIEW

As previously alluded to, it is important to appreciate the anatomy of the hip and groin, and undertake a careful history and examination. The clinical approach can be difficult as the anatomy around this region is complex and often multiple pathologies coexist. Pain may be difficult to localise and be accompanied by vague symptoms. An insidious onset with varying locations of the pain may also cloud the clinical presentation.

History

The athlete experiences groin pain, which is usually located in the medial upper thigh around the proximal adductors and pubic rami. The pain can also be more central in the upper thigh inferior to the inguinal ligament around the hip joint/distal iliopsoas region. The pain frequently starts in one region and is unilateral, but it can gradually spread to other regions and become bilateral. Pain superior to the inguinal ligament can be felt in the region of the inguinal canal. Groin pain in athletes is aggravated by exercise, with running, twisting/turning and kicking being the most challenging activities. The athlete and coach usually notice a decrease in sports performance, especially related to performing explosive sporting actions such as kicking, accelerating/decelerating, turning and so on.

Pain pattern

The onset of groin pain in athletes can be acute or gradual, but with both types of onset, groin pain can become longstanding. In the early stages, the longstanding groin pain patient typically presents late during the physical activity or after activity, with pain and stiffness next morning. The pain and stiffness then gradually lessen with daily activities and warming-up for the next training session or match. When the condition worsens, pain is present immediately upon exercise. Non-steroidal anti-inflammatory drugs (NSAIDs) tend to decrease pain, but will usually not result in a lasting cure. Short periods of rest reduce the severity of the symptoms, but on resumption of sporting activities the pain often returns to its original intensity and severity. The natural history is one of progressive deterioration with continued activity until symptoms prevent participation in the sporting activity.

Where is the pain located?

The localisation of the pain is important in determining which structure may be causing the pain. Adductor-related groin pain is often located at the attachment of the adductor longus tendon to the pubic bone. Iliopsoas-related groin pain is located more centrally in the groin and proximal thigh. The type of activity that aggravates the pain gives a clue to the primary site of the problem. Side-to-side movements, kicking, twisting and turning activities which aggravate the pain suggest adductor-related groin pain. Straight-line running or jogging suggests iliopsoas-related groin pain. Pain with sit-ups and/or coughing, may suggest an inguinal-related groin pain. Note that these clinical observations are guidelines rather than hard and fast rules, as many of the symptoms overlap.

Pain that becomes progressively worse with exercise may suggest a stress fracture or an apophysitis in young athletes. A history of associated pain such as low back or buttock pain indicates that the groin pain may be referred from another site (such as the hip, the sacroiliac joint or the spine). A full training history should be taken to determine if any recent changes in training (e.g. a generalised increase in volume or intensity, the introduction of a new exercise or an increase in a particular component of training) may have led to the development of the groin pain.

Clinical examination

Clinical examination includes the adductor muscles, the pelvic bones, the hip joint, the hip flexors (including tensor fascia lata and sartorius) and the lower abdominal muscles. The lumbar spine and sacroiliac joints should also be examined. Pelvic alignment must be assessed and large leg length discrepancies (>2 cm) noted.

Examination involves the following.

1. Observation
    a. standing
    b. walking Fig. 32.3a
    c. squatting, running, jumping
2. Active movements
    a. hip flexion/extension (Chapter 31)
    b. hip abduction/adduction
    c. hip internal/external rotation
    d. lumbar spine movements (Chapter 29)
3. Passive movements
    a. passive movement–adductor muscle stretch (Fig. 32.3b)
    b. modified Thomas Test (Fig. 32.3c)
4. Resisted movements
    a. resisted movement–single leg (Fig. 32.3d)
    b. resisted movement–squeeze test
        i. with hips in 45° flexion (Fig. 32.3e-i)
        ii. with hips in neutral (Fig. 32.3e-ii)
    c. hip flexion (Fig. 32.3f)
    d. abdominal muscles (Fig. 32.3g)
5. Palpation
    a. adductor (Fig. 32.3h)
    b. psoas above inguinal ligament (Fig. 32.3i)
    c. psoas below inguinal ligament (Fig. 32.3j)
    d. inguinal region–external inguinal ring (Fig. 32.3k)
    e. inguinal region–scrotal invagination (Fig. 32.3l)
    f. pubic symphysis (Fig. 32.3m)
6. Hip-related groin pain
    a. examination of the hip joint (Chapter 31)
7. Screening for other pathology
    a. stress fractures–neck of femur and pubic ramus
    b. thoracic spine (Chapter 28) and lumbar (Chapter 29)
    c. sacroiliac joint (Chapter 30).

Assessment of severity

While clinical examination is essential for diagnosing and classifying groin pain in athletes, it gives little objective information on the severity of the condition. The severity, insights into the impairments, activity limitations and accompanying participation restrictions can be measured with strength, range of motion and patient-reported outcome tools.

Strength

The assessment of muscle strength provides better understanding of the degree of impairment in athletes

PART B Regional problems

(a)

(b)

(c)

(d)

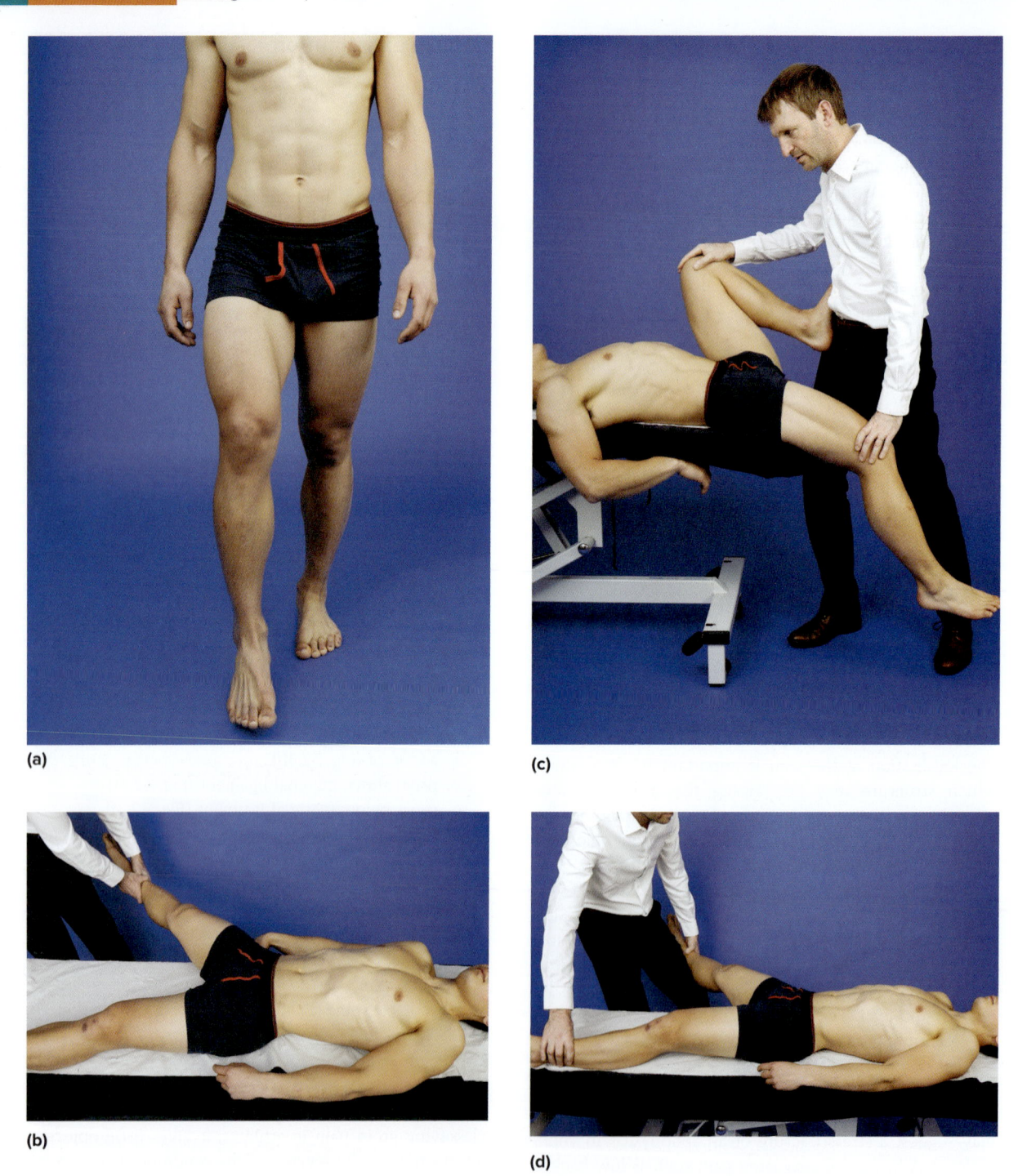

Figure 32.3 Examination of the patient with longstanding groin pain (a) Walking—assess lower limb alignment from in front, particularly for evidence of excessive internal or external hip rotation and muscle wasting (b) Adductor muscle stretch—tightness or the presence of pain (c) Passive stretching of the hip flexors for tightness or the presence of pain. Following stretching, the athlete can push upwards with the leg to assess hip flexor strength in outer range and for the presence of pain during strength testing (d) Resisted movement—adductors in outer range—for strength and the presence of pain

Groin pain CHAPTER 32

(e)-(i)

(f)

(e)-(ii)

(g)

(h)

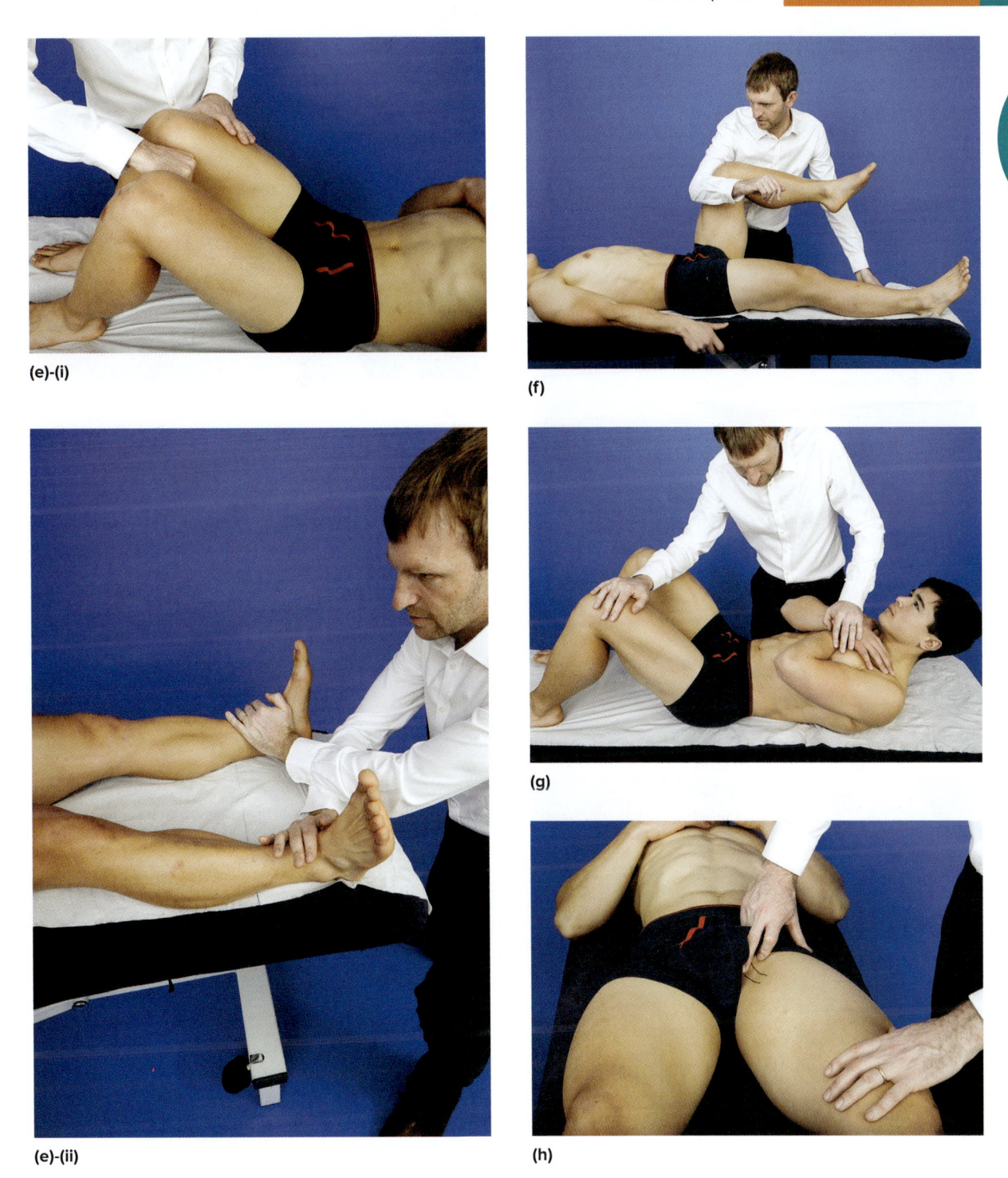

Figure 32.3 (cont.) (e) (i) Squeeze test—resistance testing of the adductors with the hip in 45° flexion (ii) Squeeze test—resistance testing of the adductors with the hip in neutral and long lever for strength and the presence of pain (f) Hip flexors with the hip in 90° flexion—for strength and the presence of pain (g) Resistance testing of the abdominals for strength and the presence of pain (h) Palpation of the proximal adductors for tenderness

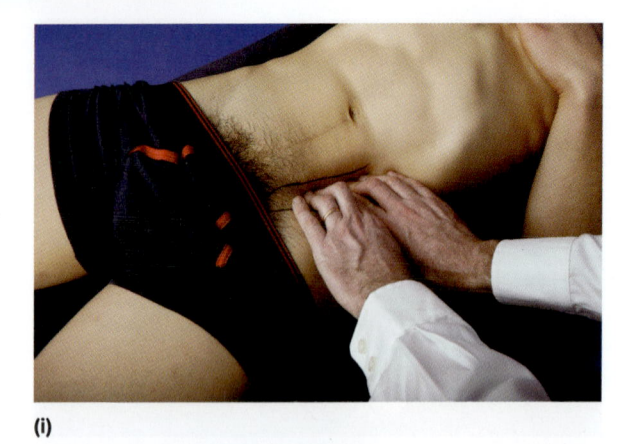

PART B Regional problems

(i)

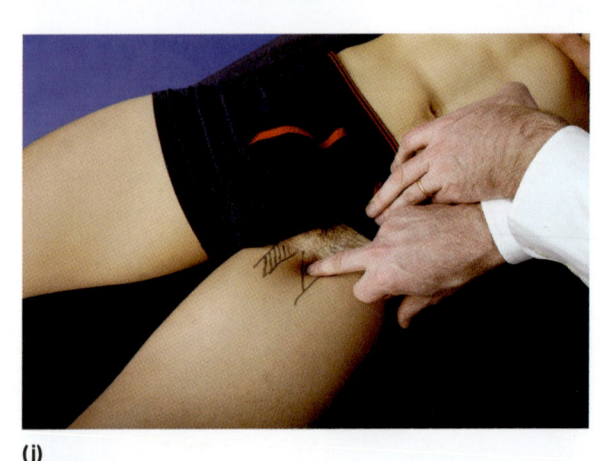

(j)

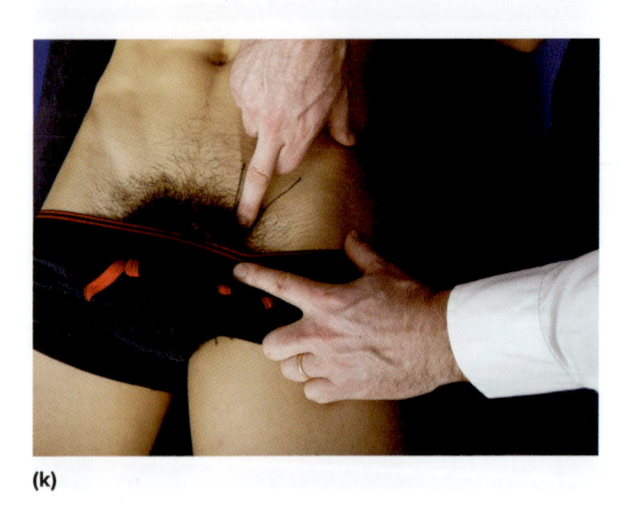

(k)

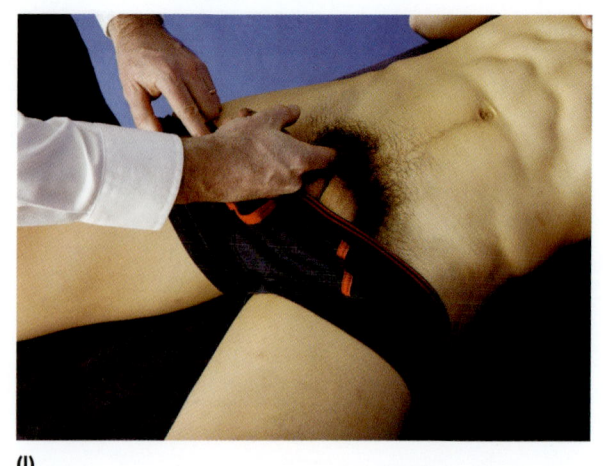

(l)

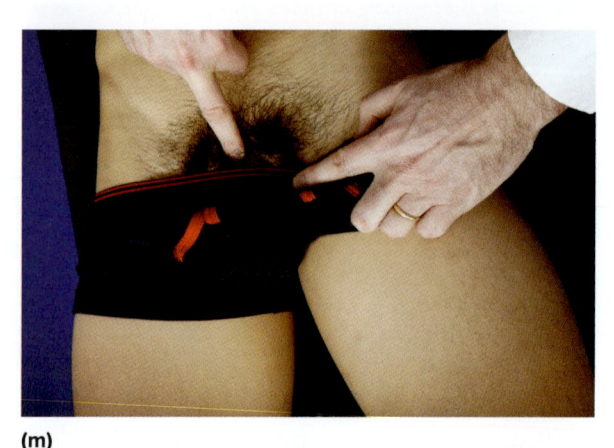

(m)

Figure 32.3 (cont.) (i) Abdominal portion of the psoas for tenderness (j) Palpation of the distal iliopsoas for tenderness (k) Transabdominal palpation of the external inguinal ring for tenderness (l) Scrotal invagination for palpation of the inguinal ring and canal for tenderness and/or hernia (m) Palpation of the pubic symphysis for tenderness

with groin pain. It can be quantified objectively, and is a great help in monitoring clinical progress or deterioration. Adductor strength can be reliably assessed using hand-held dynamometry and quantified either unilaterally (Fig. 32.4a) or as a squeeze test (Fig. 32.4b and c) and is especially relevant in athletes with adductor-related or pubic-related groin pain. It may also be relevant to include abductor strength (Fig. 32.4d) before return to sport in athletes with adductor-related groin pain or acute injury, as an eccentric hip adductor/abductor ratio of <0.8 appears to increase the risk of future adductor injuries.

For isometric and eccentric measures, the minimal detectable change when using the same tester is around 10–15%, while being around 20% for the isometric adduction/abduction (ADD/ABD) ratio.[23] While eccentric ratios for ice hockey players[24] and isometric ratios for soccer players seem to be around 1.0,[25] these ratios may be sport-specific. Clinically, this means that reductions in strength of 15% can be measured at the individual level. This may indicate that athletes either have, or are

(a)

(c)

(b)

(d)

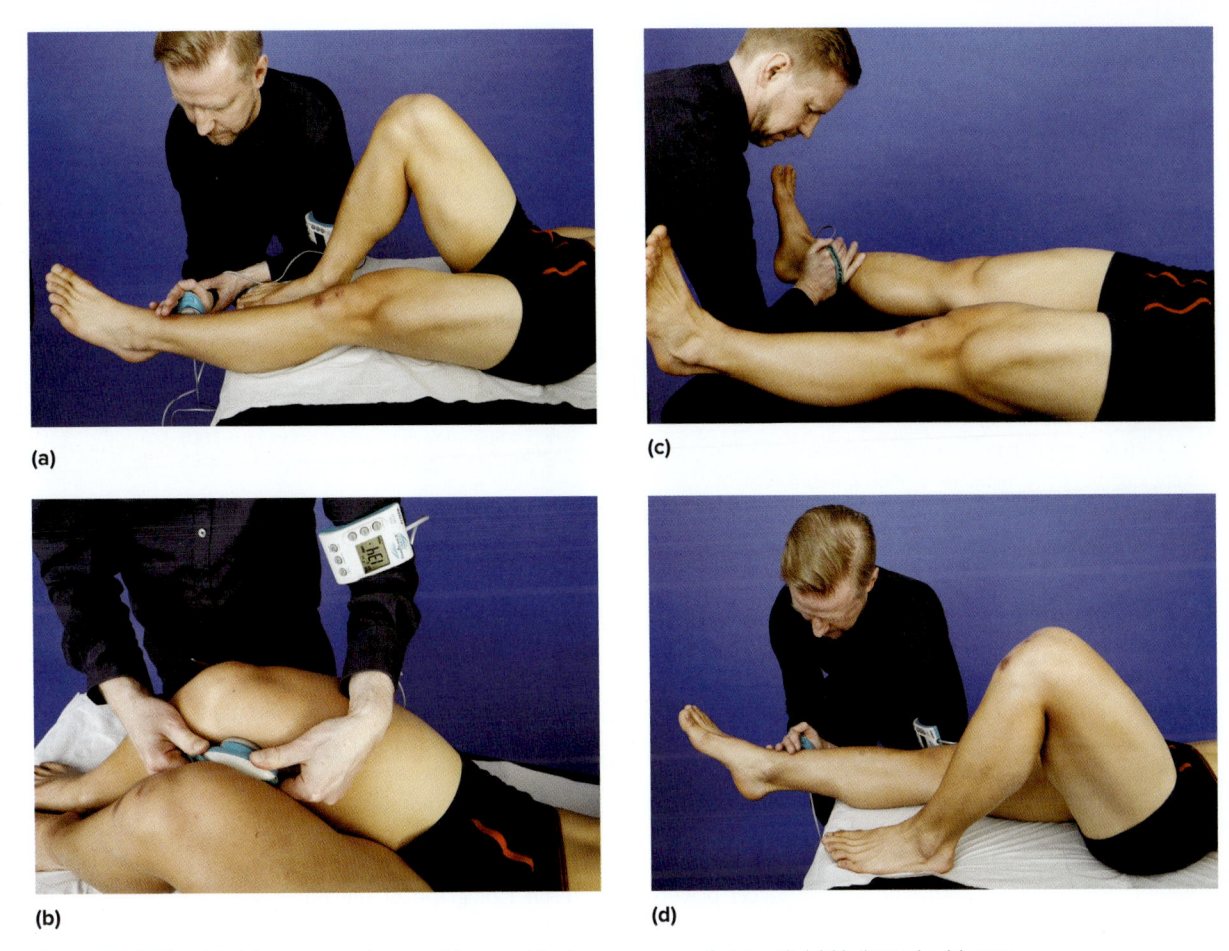

Figure 32.4 Hand-held dynamometry provides an objective measure of strength (a) Unilateral adductor (b) Bilateral (squeeze) in hip and knee flexion (c) Squeeze in hip abduction (d) Abductor

at increased risk, of developing groin pain. Studies in European and Australian soccer players and Gaelic football players with groin pain have shown that strength deficits of around 20% or more seem to exist in eccentric strength and during the squeeze test.[26–29]

Range of motion
Passive hip joint internal rotation range of motion in degrees can also be reliably assessed using a goniometer or inclinometer, although severe restrictions in passive range of motion are more closely related to hip intra-articular conditions, and less often to groin pain related to tendon attachments and the pubic bone. Assessment of the hip joint is demonstrated in Chapter 31.

Patient-reported outcome measures (PROMs)
The use of validated outcome measures should also be encouraged. In a systematic review from 2015 on the clinimetric properties of PROMs for young physically active individuals with hip and/or groin pain, the Copenhagen Hip and Groin Outcome Score (HAGOS) was recommended.[30] HAGOS is reliable, valid and responsive in athletes with hip and/or groin pain, and therefore not restricted to any specific pathology or entity. Reference values for soccer players have been provided.[31] It measures six relevant subsets related to groin pain in athletes, including pain, symptoms, activities of daily living, participation in physical activity, sports function and quality of life. Reference values have been given for soccer players without groin pain, and while their average and upper boundary is 100 points, the lower boundary goes down to 70 points in the sporting function and participation scores.[32] On average, Gaelic footballers and soccer players with adductor-related groin pain display scores in the area of 50 points and below when having had pain for at least 4 weeks.[26, 27]

Imaging
The current evidence for the use of radiographs, MRI and ultrasonography in groin pain is based on relatively

PART B Regional problems

Outcome measures

Physical assessments should include some of the following valid and reliable measures according to relevance to the clinical findings. The following measures are of relevance.

Strength (hand-held dynamometer (HHD) or sphygmomanometer)
- hip adduction strength—squeeze, isometric, eccentric (Fig. 32.4(a)–(c))
- hip abduction strength—isometric, eccentric, eccentric ADD/ABD ratio (Fig. 32.4(d))
- hip flexion strength—isometric, eccentric

Range of motion (goniometer or inclinometer)
- hip internal rotation
- hip external rotation
- hip abduction
- hip extension (Thomas test position)

Patient-reported outcome measures (PROM)
- Copenhagen Hip and Groin Outcome Score, six subscales
  1. Pain (0–100)
  2. Symptoms (0–100)
  3. Activities of daily living (0–100)
  4. Sport and recreation (0–100)
  5. Participation in physical activity (0–100)
  6. Quality of life (0–100).

few heterogeneous studies which are of varying methodological quality.[33] The correlation between clinical findings, athletes' symptoms and the identified radiological abnormalities is quite weak.

Two recent studies have illustrated this.[34,35] Branci et al. compared the standardised MRI findings of three groups of male adult athletes matched for level of sports activity.[34] Positive MRI findings were significantly more frequent in soccer players compared with non-soccer players irrespective of whether or not the soccer players had symptoms, suggesting that these MRI changes may be associated with soccer play itself rather than clinical symptoms. In a 4-year prospective cohort study of young soccer academy players using serial clinical and imaging assessments, Robinson et al. found a high prevalence of positive imaging findings, including pubic bone marrow oedema (BMO), in asymptomatic soccer players as well as in those with injury.[35] These two studies show that imaging should not be used in isolation when diagnosing groin pain in athletes.

Radiography

Plain radiographs of the pelvis are commonly recommended in many cases to evaluate the hip joints and the pubic bones. If the patient history and the clinical examination suggest that the groin pain could be hip-related, an anteroposterior pelvic radiograph and a true lateral radiograph should be obtained. The α angle, the centre-edge (CE) angle and other relevant measurements can be examined, looking for any bony morphology that can result in femoroacetabular impingement (FAI).

FAI morphology has been found to coexist with longstanding adductor-related groin pain and the presence of FAI morphology is not necessarily a sign of hip joint pathology (Chapter 31).[36] In this study of athletes with longstanding adductor-related groin pain, 94% had at least one radiographic sign of FAI on the X-ray. In a different cohort of athletes with longstanding adductor-related groin pain who also had plain radiographs performed, follow-up was done after 8-12 years. The study found no evidence that bony hip morphology related to FAI or dysplasia prevented successful outcome of an exercise treatment for this musculotendinous injury.[37]

Plain radiograph of the pubic symphysis often shows osteolytic changes, irregular widening and sclerosis along the rami of the os pubis in soccer players. Historically these changes were interpreted as a diagnosis using the term 'osteitis pubis' (Fig.32.5a). These changes can also be seen before radiographic changes are present as pubic BMO on MRI. As described earlier, this is not that specific for injury, but probably reflects the considerable strain that the pelvic girdle is exposed to in the kicking sports in particular.[34]

It is likely that there is a continuum of bone stress and that there is not a strong relationship between the degree of stress and the pain felt by an athlete. This was alluded to by Harris et al. in 1974,[38] and the case control study of Branci et al.[34] found that higher grades of pubic BMO, along with protrusion of the disc in the symphyseal joint, were associated, but not strongly, with pain compared to soccer-playing controls. A bone biopsy study of athletes with pubic-related groin pain found evidence of new woven bone formation but a lack of inflammation, and so using the term 'osteitis pubis' cannot be recommended.[39]

In the skeletally immature adolescent athlete, plain radiographs are used to detect osseous avulsions in musculotendinous distraction injuries and epiphysiolysis of the growth plate of the femoral neck. The plain radiograph is also a good primary examination for

Groin pain CHAPTER 32

neoplasms of the bone. Even in seemingly healthy athletes, this should be considered as a possible cause of unexplained groin pain or when there is an unusual response to treatment. Radiographs are often used as a first-line investigation if a pelvic stress fracture is suspected; if a stress fracture is visible, radiographs can confirm the clinical suspicion. Clinicians should note that radiographs are frequently negative when stress fractures are present and cannot be used to rule out stress fractures.

Magnetic resonance imaging

Magnetic resonance imaging (MRI) is a very sensitive, but not always equally specific, imaging technique. It is used widely, but the results should be interpreted with caution.[33] The high sensitivity means that when imaging athletes with MRI many 'abnormalities' will be seen, but that the clinical relevance of these findings is doubtful in terms of making a diagnosis or estimating prognosis. Ongoing studies are examining the value of MRI in the diagnosis of acute groin injuries and the results are promising. Some common MRI findings are pubic BMO, adductor tendon changes and findings around the aponeurosis anterior to the symphysis.

Pubic BMO is a common finding. Studies have shown that the percentage of athletes without groin pain found to have BMO on MRI is high (31–61%).[34, 40, 41] To date, no studies have examined the effect of the presence/absence or grade of BMO on the time to recovery.

Changes in MRI signal of the adductor tendon around the proximal insertion have been referred to as 'enthesopathy',[42] 'tendinopathy'[34] and 'pubic aponeurosis defect'.[43] This demonstrates the confusion with regard to describing these virtually identical radiological findings of increased signal intensity in the proximal adductor tendon. Some have found the reliability of determining if adductor tendon signal changes are present to be poor,[44] while others found it to be good.[35]

The differing terminology may explain why some studies found changes in the tendon to be present in more than 70% of asymptomatic players,[34] while others in only 11%.[41] As with pubic BMO, there have been no studies to date examining whether athletes who have adductor tendon signal changes take longer to recover than those without. In other tendons, only weak associations have been found between structure and symptoms, and a normalisation of tendon structure after treatment was not associated with better outcome.[45]

The secondary cleft sign (Fig. 32.5c) was first described as being present when contrast medium injected into the pubic symphysis extended beyond the midline or inferior to the joint.[46] Other groups used a high signal intensity line extending laterally and inferiorly from the

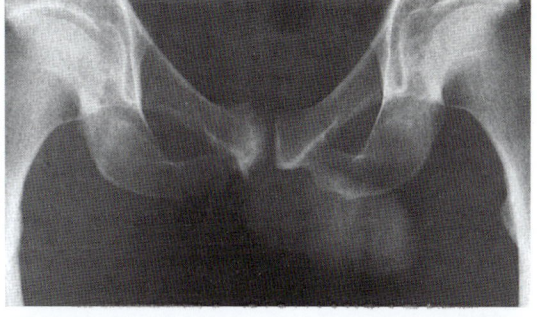

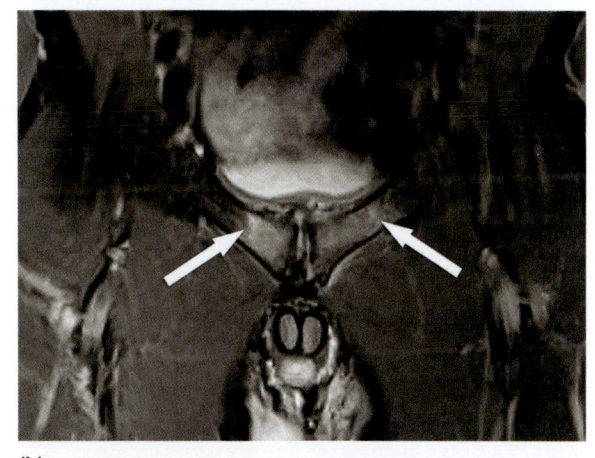

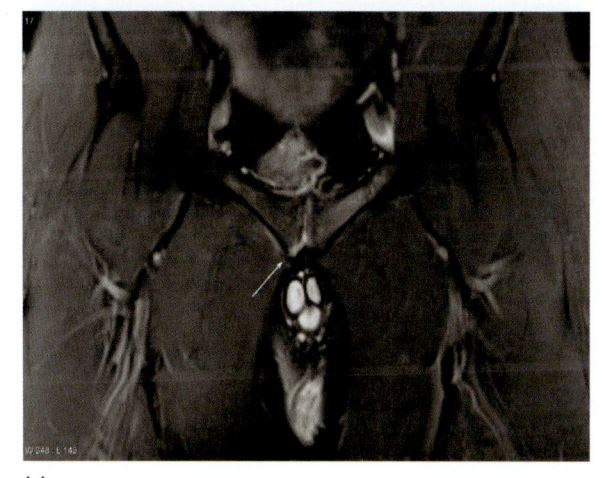

Figure 32.5 (a) X-ray showing characteristic moth-eaten appearance consistent with longstanding pubic bone stress (b) MRI BMO. Arrows point to BMO in pubic bones on both sides of symphyseal joint (seen as diffuse increased signal intensity on fluid sensitive sequences) (c) MRI secondary cleft. Hyperintense cleft (arrow) on fluid-sensitive sequences, extending inferiorly and laterally to the symphyseal joint

641

PART B   Regional problems

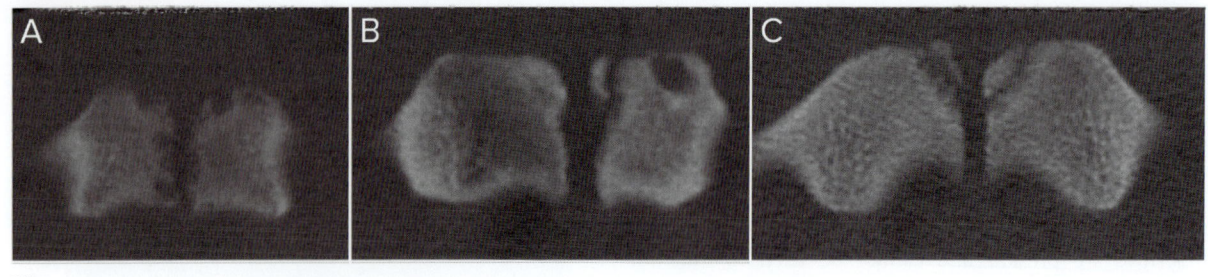

Figure 32.5 (cont.) (d) CT scans demonstrating stress-related changes at the pubis: (A) Cystic changes; (B) Asymmetrical irregularities and cystic changes; and (C) Unilateral widening of the pubic apophysis

inferior part of the symphysis of fluid sensitive sequences, without the use of contrast, to define the secondary cleft.[34] The secondary cleft was initially found to be present in two-thirds of athletes with groin pain and absent in 70 control subjects who were rowers.[46] Later studies found it to be present at similar prevalences in soccer players with and without groin pain,[34] and in a prospective study of young asymptomatic soccer players it did not predict the onset of groin pain.[35] Again there is a lack of data on how the presence of a secondary cleft on MRI may affect the prognosis.

> **PRACTICE PEARL**
>
> In summary, the common MRI findings of pubic BMO, adductor tendon changes and secondary cleft are found frequently in healthy players, and in general do not discriminate well between those with and those without pain.

There is a lack of data on how these findings should influence treatment decisions and their meaning for helping make a more accurate prognostic prediction.

Stress fractures, neoplasms and other occult bony injuries are rare and when suspected, but not visible on radiography, MRI is the best investigation. Even in seemingly healthy athletes, these should be considered as a possible cause of unexplained groin pain.

Ultrasonography
Ultrasonography (US) has gained increasing popularity in recent years (Chapter 15). Scientific evidence for its use in groin injuries is very limited.[33] It has shown promise with other muscle and tendon injuries.[47, 48] There is a significant discrepancy between the widespread clinical use and experience gained in many countries, and the amount of data available in the literature to help clinicians improve interpretation of findings.

Computed tomography scan
Computed tomography (CT) scan offers excellent visualisation of the pubic symphysis joint, but requires high doses of radiation. Its general use in the young athletic population cannot be advised due to the significant radiation risk and a lack of data on normal findings in the athletic population. An interesting recent paper which examined CT scans of young males who had undergone CT scans for reasons other than groin pain showed that the pubic apophysis closes in the late teens and early twenties (Fig. 32.5d).[49] While the apophysis can be visualised well on CT, it can also be clearly seen on MRI, which is safer and therefore the preferable modality.

Radioisotopic bone scan
Given the high radiation dose of bone scans, and the fact that MRI allows good visualisation of both bony and soft tissue structures in the pelvis, the use of bone scan as a routine investigation for groin pain in athletes cannot be recommended.

ACUTE GROIN INJURIES
An acute groin injury usually involves one or more musculotendinous structures.[5] The lesion can be in the musculotendinous junction, but in some cases the tendon itself or the entheses where the tendon inserts into the bone is the site of the injury. These injuries usually happen during explosive actions such as kicking, reaching with the leg, sudden change of direction or other movements where the muscle is being stretched during forceful contraction.[5]

Diagnosis
The most common acute injury in the groin is to the adductors, especially the adductor longus, which has been verified both clinically and with diagnostic imaging.[5] Good agreement between clinical diagnosis and diagnostic imaging seems to exist for acute adductor longus injuries.[5]

However, acute injuries to other musculotendinous structures such as the iliopsoas, proximal rectus femoris or the inguinal canal/conjoined tendon are more difficult to localise clinically in the acute stage. Acute injuries to iliopsoas and rectus femoris are not infrequent and should be considered relevant differential diagnoses that may need imaging to be correctly identified.

In the acute stage, ultrasound has shown clinical promise as a simple method for localising specific structures in the groin, due to the visualisation of oedema or structural derangement. MRI has advantages when considering the underlying symphysis joint and adjacent bone, thus allowing for more complete assessment, and may be less operator dependant. Diagnostic imaging may therefore play an important differential diagnostic role when examining acute groin injuries, but may also have a role in guiding treatment choices from a very early stage in relation to which structures and what kind of tissue should be targeted in the rehabilitation of the particular injury. At the present time, however, there is no evidence that the use of imaging does lead to better clinical outcomes or more accurate prediction of the duration of injury.

If the initial injury is not treated appropriately in the first place or if a player is returned to sport too quickly, it may develop into a more longstanding injury. If the athlete does not get appropriate treatment and continues to participate, the injury pattern may start to resemble the more overuse type where more and more sport-specific activities become problematic. This type of injury can then take months to recover from and what started out as minor acute injury can develop into a longstanding problem.

The actual percentage of acute groin injuries that progress to longstanding groin pain in athletes is unknown. There is currently limited data on the recovery times for acute groin injuries.

LONGSTANDING GROIN PAIN

The Doha agreement confirms our approach to the classification of longstanding groin pain into the four clinical entities: adductor-related groin pain, iliopsoas-related groin pain, inguinal-related groin pain and pubic-related groin pain.[22] As demonstrated in the 'Epidemiology' section an athlete can have more than one entity, in which case multiple entities can be diagnosed. The criteria for the diagnosis of each clinical entity are highlighted in each of the following sections in italics.[22]

Adductor-related groin pain

Adductor-related groin pain is the most common acute and longstanding groin injury.[3-5] Acute groin injuries are described elsewhere in this chapter and this section focuses on longstanding groin pain.

The patient with longstanding adductor-related groin pain usually complains of pain medially in the groin, most pronounced around the insertion of the adductor longus tendon at the pubic bone. The pain may radiate distally along the medial thigh. Pain during sprinting, cutting changes of direction and kicking the ball are common complaints.

Diagnostic criteria

The diagnostic criteria for adductor-related groin pain are *adductor tenderness* (Fig. 32.3h) AND *pain on resisted adduction testing* (Fig. 32.3d).[22]

Evidence for treatment of groin pain in athletes

A systematic review from 2015 on the treatment of groin pain in athletes identified 72 studies.[13] All studies were assessed for their methodological quality with a scoring system. The majority of studies (90%) were case series, of which 80% were retrospective. Only four studies were high quality. Twenty-five per cent reported on conservative treatment and 75% on surgical treatment for groin pain. A significant association was found with methodologically weaker studies reporting higher treatment success percentages. There has been no significant improvement in the quality of studies published over the last 30 years. A level-of-evidence approach was used to synthesise the results.

There is moderate evidence that for longstanding adductor-related groin pain:

- supervised active physical training results in a higher success and percentage of athletes returning to play than passive physical therapy modalities
- multi-modal treatment including manual adductor manipulation can result in a faster return to play, but not a higher treatment success, than a partially supervised active physical training program
- partial release of the adductor longus tendon seems effective for return to sport over time.

Additionally, there is moderate evidence that, for athletes with inguinal-related groin pain, laparoscopic hernia repair results in lower pain and a higher percentage returning to play than conservative treatment.

Treatment

The treatment of both acute and longstanding adductor-related groin pain will be considered together. The basis of the treatment of these conditions is exercise therapy and is based on Professor Per Hölmich's seminal paper published in *The Lancet* in 1999 which was the first randomised controlled trial (RCT) to examine treatment regimes in adductor-related groin pain.[50] The original exercise program is shown in full in the box below.

The exercise program comprises two modules. The first module consists of specific isometric and dynamic exercises to reactivate the adductor muscles and probably also modulates the pain.[51] The athlete can have difficulties activating these muscles, probably as a result of negative feedback caused by the pain. The second module includes heavier resistance training as well as challenging balance and coordination exercises. The exercise program is performed three times a week, alternating with the exercises from module 1 on the days in between.[50]

The total length of the exercise training period is between 8 and 12 weeks. Absence from training is necessary as the functionality and strength of the adductor muscle group has to be re-established and pain brought under control without provocation by sport. Stationary cycling and general fitness training not involving the adductors can be allowed if pain-free.

Jogging is allowed after 6 weeks as long as it does not provoke any groin pain. When the patient is able to jog and undergo his or her regular treatment without pain, the treatment program is completed and the athlete is allowed to gradually progress to demanding sports-specific training followed by sports participation. No stretching of the adductor muscles should be done during this 2–3 month exercise training period.[50]

Injection of corticosteroids at the adductor enthesis is not recommended, as there is no documented long-term beneficial effect and it might make it more difficult to monitor the training program needed to cure the groin pain. It is the experience of the authors that adductor tenotomy is extremely rarely indicated.

Many rehabilitation programs for adductor-related groin pain have used the Hölmich exercises as their basis.

Professor Per Hölmich's 1999 exercise program: an evidence-based foundation for contemporary rehabilitation programs

This program consists of static and dynamic exercises aimed at improving the muscles stabilising the pelvis and the hip joints, in particular the adductor muscles. The program consists of two parts.

- Module 1: Two-week familiarisation program—adductor activation.
- Module 2: More demanding exercises with heavier resistance training and balance and coordination. The training program is performed three times a week and the exercises from module 1 are performed on the days in between the treatment days. The total length of the training period is 8–12 weeks. Sport activities are not allowed in the treatment period. Pain-free bike riding is allowed. After 6 weeks, pain-free jogging is allowed. Return to sport is allowed when neither treatment nor jogging causes any pain.

Stretching of the adductor muscles is not advised, but stretching of the other lower extremity muscles, particularly the iliopsoas, is recommended.

Module 1: Static and dynamic exercises (2-week base training program)

Static

1. a. Adduction for 30 seconds against a soccer ball placed between the feet when lying in the supine position with the knees fully extended and the first toe pointing straight upwards.
1. b. Adduction for 30 seconds against a soccer ball placed between the knees when lying in the supine position with the knees and the hips flexed at 45° and the feet flat on the floor pointing straight ahead (Fig. 32.6a).

Exercises 1a and b should be repeated 10 times with 15-second recovery periods between each contraction. The force of the adduction should be just sufficient to reach the point where pain begins.

Dynamic

1. c. Sit-ups from the supine position with the hip and knee joints flexed at 45° and the feet against the floor. The sit-ups are performed as a straight abdominal curl and also with a quarter twist towards the opposite knee: five sets of 10 with 15-second recovery periods.
1. d. In the same starting position as for the sit-ups but clamping a soccer ball between the knees, the player does a combination of a sit-up while pulling the ball towards the head (Fig. 32.6b and c). The exercise is performed rhythmically and with accuracy to gain balance and coordination: five sets of 10 with 15-second recovery periods.
1. e. Wobble board training for 5 minutes.
1. f. Adductor lateral slide. Using a sliding board with an extremely smooth surface (or a very smooth floor) and wearing a low-friction sock on the sliding foot, one foot is positioned next to the sliding board and the other foot on

Groin pain CHAPTER 32

the board parallel to the first one. The foot on the board slides out laterally and is then pulled back to the starting position. The foot should be pressed against the surface through the whole exercise with as much force as can be tolerated within the patient's threshold of pain (Fig. 32.6d).

1. g. Forward slide. The same procedure is also done with the foot on the board placed in a 90° angle to the foot outside the board. Both exercises 1f and g are performed continuously for 1 minute with each leg in turn.

All the above exercises should be commenced carefully and the number of sets and range of motion gradually increased respecting pain and exhaustion.

Module 2: Dynamic exercises

This entire module is done twice at each training session for three training sessions per week with a day in between. *Note:* Module 1 is done on alternate days, so players are training a total of 6 days per week. Exercises 2a to e are done as five sets of 10 repetitions.

2. a. Lying on one side with the lower leg stretched and the upper leg bent and placed in front of the lower leg, the lower leg is moved up and down, pointing the heel upwards.
2. b. Lying on one side with the lower leg bent and the upper leg stretched, the upper leg is moved up and down, pointing the heel upwards.
2. c. Begin by standing at the end of a high couch and then lie prone so that the torso is supported by the couch. The hips are at the edge of the couch at 90° of flexion and the feet are on the floor. From this position, both hips are slowly extended so both legs are lifted to the greatest possible extension of hips and spine; legs are then lowered together.
2. d. Standing abduction/adduction using ankle pulleys/elastic bands. Begin with a low weight and gradually increase the weight but keep it submaximal (Fig. 32.7).
2. e. Standing on one leg, the knee of the supporting leg is flexed and extended rhythmically and in the same rhythm swinging both arms back and forth independently ('cross-country skiing on one leg') (Fig. 32.8). The non weight-bearing leg is not moved.

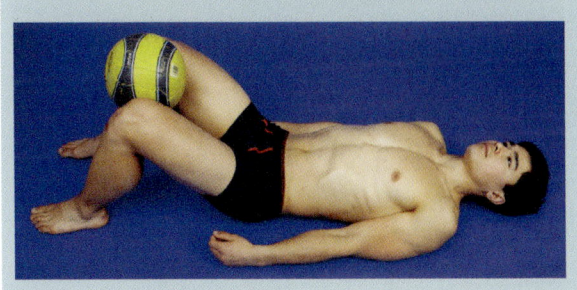

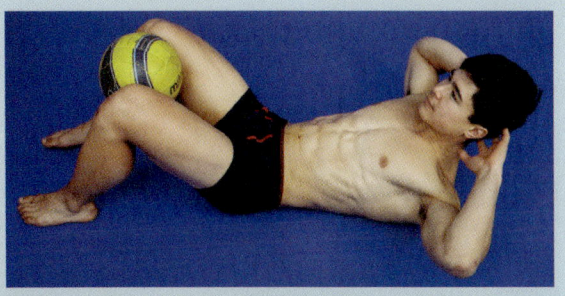

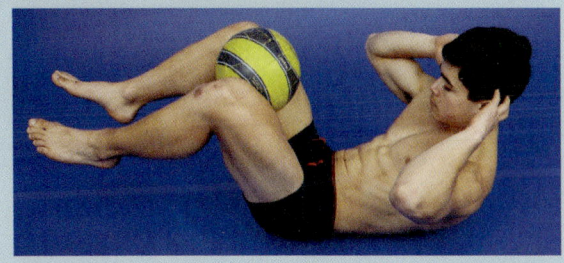

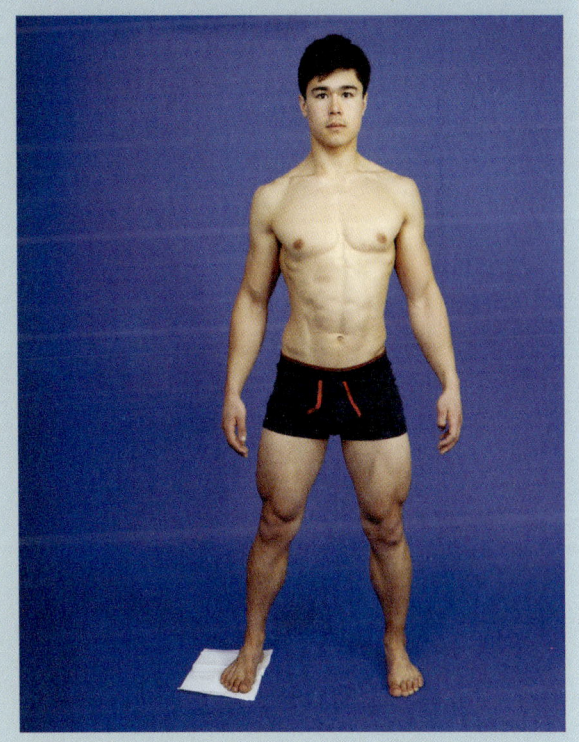

Figure 32.6 (a) Isometric exercise—adduction (b) and (c) Dynamic sit-ups for abdominals (d) Adductor lateral slide

continued

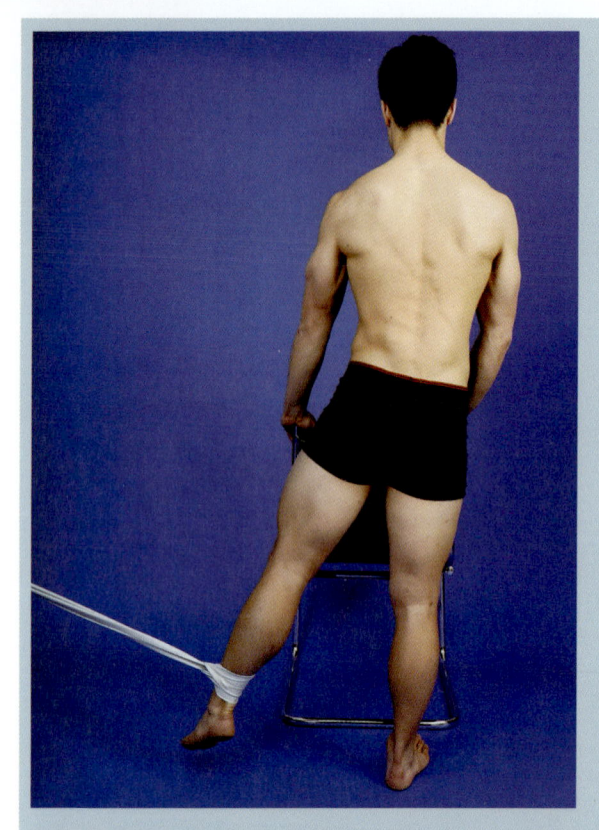

PART B Regional problems

Figure 32.7 Standing hip adductor strengthening with elastic band. Dynamic strength and coordination exercise with emphasis on maximal concentric, isometric and eccentric strength of adductor muscles, with co-activation from contralateral

   The balance and position is kept accurately and the exercise is stopped when this is no longer possible. Progression of the exercise is obtained by holding a 1 kg weight in each hand.
2. f. 'Fitter' training for 5 minutes.
2. g. Standing on the sliding board, side-to-side skating movements on the sliding board are done as five sets of 1-minute training periods with 15-second recovery.

Practical tips

- Supervision is important—the patient should be instructed by a physiotherapist, a clinician, an athletic trainer or another qualified person who has been trained in the details of the program.
- Exercises such as 1d and 2e are very important, especially at the end of the training period, but they are technically difficult.
- The athletes can do the program at home or at the gym or fitness club, but we recommend physiotherapist supervision for three to four times within the first 2 weeks

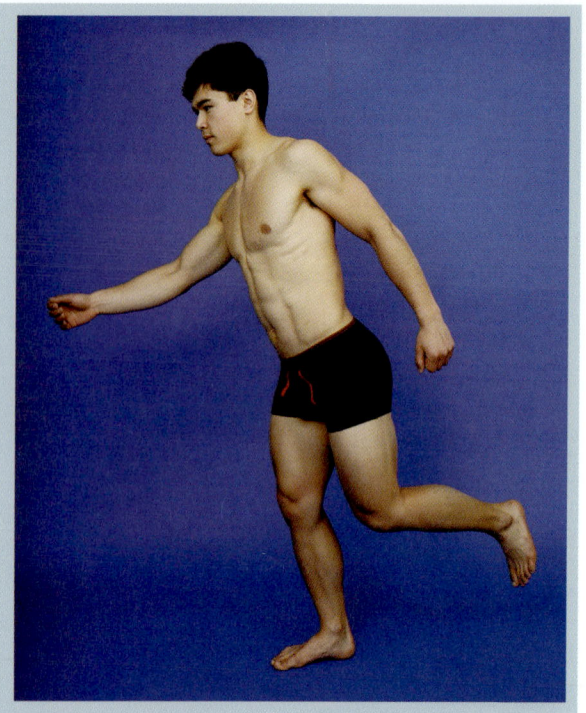

(a)

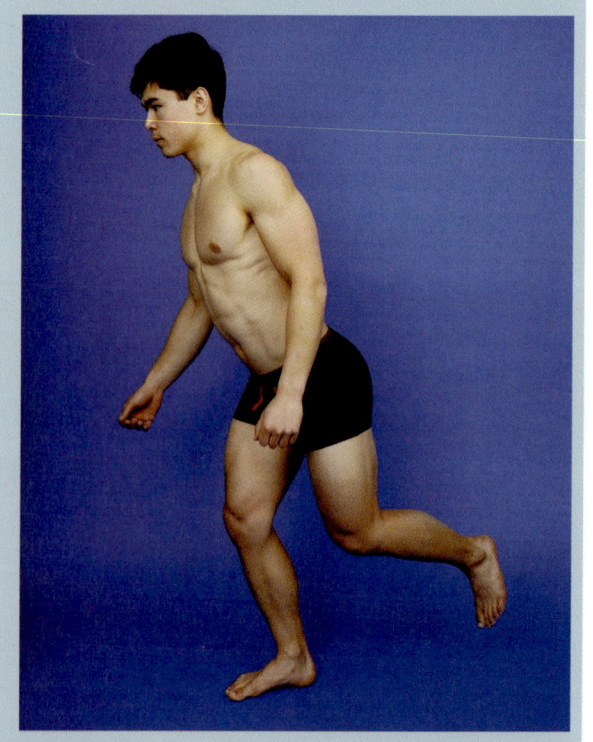

(b)

Figure 32.8 (a-c) Cross-country skiing. Dynamic hip flexion on one leg with coordinated arm swing

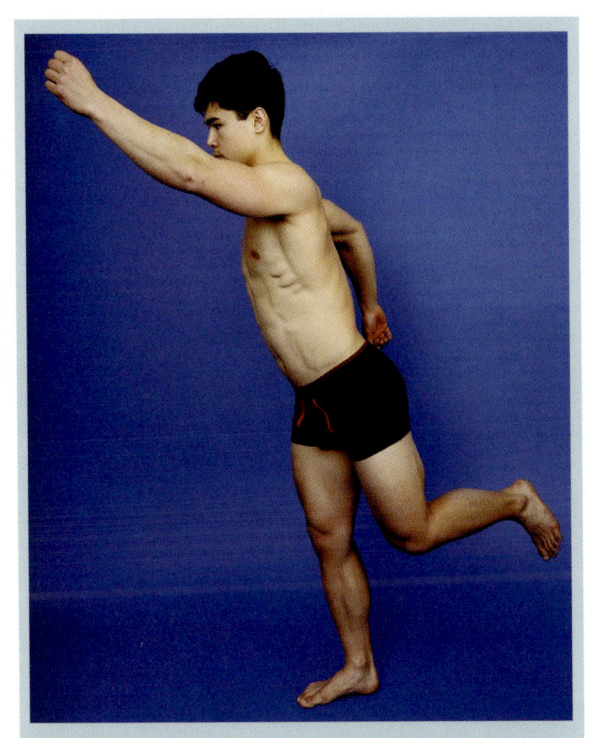

Groin pain CHAPTER 32

Reflecting this more contemporary approach, the following rehabilitation program is divided into four phases, each with a different rehabilitation focus. In general, the rehabilitation program works from focus and isolation on the specific injured tissues towards integration of the specific structures into sports-specific function and return to sport based on individual and continuous assessment of:

- injury (structural) status
- functional status
- performance status; and finally
- sports participation status, at specific time points during the rehabilitation period.

PRACTICE PEARL

The rehabilitation of acute groin injuries can be divided into four main phases prior to pre-injury competitive level:

1. acute/subacute phase
2. conditioning phase
3. sports-specific phase
4. return-to-sport phase.

1. Acute/subacute phase

The acute and subacute phase is characterised by musculotendinous pain and/or inflammation at the musculotendinous junction (MTJ), in the tendon or at the insertional enthesis. This phase focuses on the initiation of tissue repair and/or regeneration, but also includes effects of possible disuse as a result of injury. The primary goals to be addressed during this phase are protection of the injured structure, control of pain and inflammation, normalisation of flexibility within restrictions and preventing excessive muscular inhibition using isometric contractions with no or minimal pain provocation.

Criteria for progression to conditioning phase
The criteria for progression to the conditioning phase are:

- no or minimal pain with all exercises and clear muscle activation during isometric contractions
- active hip abduction range of movement (ROM) of at least 50% of the non-injured side.

2. Conditioning phase

This phase focuses on tissue repair and/or regeneration. In this phase gradual and progressive loading of adductor, hip flexor and abdominal muscles is commenced while still respecting the structural injury and underlying healing processes depending on the location of the injury (MTJ, tendon, aponeurosis or insertion) at this early stage.

(c)

Figure 32.8 (cont.)

and after that a visit every 10–14 days to check the technique and ensure progression.
- Patience is the key to success.
- Patients often make good progress in the first few weeks, but symptoms can plateau from that period until the 6–9 week period, when there is a positive 'breakthrough'.
- It is important to use pain as a guide to how much to do. Muscle soreness similar to that after a regular practice in the sports field is not a problem, but if the patient experiences pain from the injury, the intensity of the exercises should be adjusted.
- Pain medication including NSAIDs should be avoided.
- Athletes should continue with some of the exercises on a regular basis (1–2 times a week) for at least a year after total recovery and return to sport.
- The athlete must appreciate that successful rehabilitation of longstanding groin pain takes a minimum of 8–12 weeks.

PRACTICE PEARL

An advance in recent years has been that rehabilitation programs have evolved from time-based protocols such as that used by Hölmich, to criteria-based protocols (see Chapter 18).

Gentle dynamic muscle exercises are commenced starting off with a low load from 20–30 repetitions maximum (RM). Strength training machines, side-lying using the weight of the leg and standing exercises with elastic bands (Fig. 32.7b) can be used for targeting the adductor longus muscle and at least two different exercise types should be used with 3 × 20 repetitions of each.

The musculotendinous conditioning should focus on concentric, isometric and eccentric contractions during these exercises of the specific injured tissues structure. For the abdominals, abdominal crunches in supine, frontal rolling exercises with Swiss ball, modified planks or training in a machine should also be performed using the same principles as applied for the adductors. For the hip flexors, isometric hip flexion in various degrees of range of motion, hip flexor training with elastic bands, and hip flexion work in a machine or with free weights should also be performed using the same principles as applied for the adductors and the abdominals. All these exercises should be performed 3 times a week with at least one day of rest in between sessions.

Pain during exercises must not be neglected, but some discomfort and pulling may be felt during early initiation of these exercises. A general rule of thumb is that pain and discomfort should be less than 3/on a numerical rating scale (NRS) during exercise and that initial pain levels before exercise are reached shortly after exercises are finished. Increasing morning pain and stiffness, compared to the initial state, is also a good indicator that the exercises have been progressed too quickly. Once the patient is pain-free, pain-free walking can begin and be gradually increased in speed and distance.

The criteria for when the patient may return to running are when:

- brisk walking is pain-free
- resisted hip adduction testing and squeeze testing is pain-free
- there is minimal adductor guarding.

Criteria for progression to sports-specific phase

The criteria for progression to the sports-specific phase are:

- no or minimal pain with all phase 2 exercises and normal execution (no compensation strategies to avoid loading injured structures) of dynamic exercises of adductor, hip flexor and abdominal muscles
- active ROM at least 80% of the non-injured side and adductor strength of at least 60% of the non-injured side; which means that the athlete will be able to do (i) 20 repetitions maximum using the same resistance based on 20 repetitions maximum from the uninjured side, and/or able to do 20 repetitions of exercises for adductors (side-lying adductor lifts), (ii) 20 repetitions for abdominals (abdominal crunches lying supine) and (iii) 20 repetitions for hip flexors (hip flexions against your own hand lying supine) on the floor with proper form, and with no or minimal pain.

3. Sport-specific phase

The primary goals to be addressed during this phase are restoration of musculotendinous endurance and strength, aerobic and anaerobic capacity, and neuromuscular control/balance/coordination. Dynamic muscle strengthening exercises for the adductor and hip flexor muscles in standing, using elastic band resistance, are continued starting off with a load of 20 RM progressing towards 10 RM. The same principle is applied for abdominal exercises where a Swiss ball is used.

The musculotendinous conditioning should focus on slow heavy concentric, isometric and eccentric contractions during these exercises. Exercises on a sliding board (Fig. 32.6d) are commenced by introducing 5 to 10 sets of 1 minute of skating from side to side. All these exercises should be performed three times a week with at least one day of rest in between. Pain during exercises must not be neglected and the same guidelines accepting pain 0–2 on an NRS as stated earlier apply.

Various progressive running and kicking regimens can be used. An example is described below.

- The regime starts with 50–100 m run-throughs with 5–10 m acceleration and deceleration phases with walk recovery, depending on running demands of the specific sport. Patient should commence with 6–8 repetitions on alternate days. Key criteria (adductor guarding, squeeze test) should be assessed immediately after each session and again the next morning. The running program can be progressed further by replacing walk recovery with jog recovery. The aim should be to build up to 20 run-throughs and jog back.
- Lateral running (gradual change of direction such as figure of eight) can be commenced when the above running program is completed pain-free, the hip flexion test is still pain-free with no crossover sign, there is no adductor guarding and, in addition, the squeeze test is pain-free. Figure-of-eight running should commence slowly with very gradual change of direction, then gradually increase both speed and sharpness of changes of direction.
- Finally, Copenhagen hip adductor exercises (Fig. 32.9) should be incorporated starting at level 1 with 3–5 repetitions on each side (change top leg). Then progress to intermediate level 2 with 7–10 repetitions on each side and then level 3 with 12–15 repetitions on each side. All exercises above should be performed 2–3 times a week, with a day of rest from these exercises in between.

Initial agility drills should be performed with proper form, with no clear and visible compensation strategies

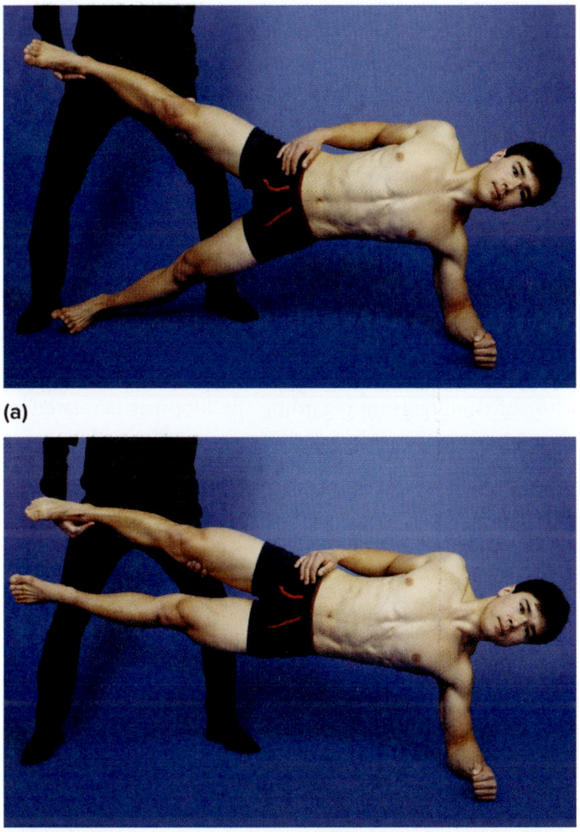

Groin pain　CHAPTER 32

injured structures) of dynamic exercises of adductor, hip flexor and abdominal muscles
- active ROM of nearly 100% of the non-injured side and adductor strength of at least 80% of the non-injured side, able to do 3 × 10 RM, by using the same resistance based on 10 RM from the uninjured side for hip adductors or flexors, or able to do 3 × 10 side-lying adductor lifts with external load of at least 5 kg, and able to do 3 × 10 hip flexor exercises lying supine using the weight of the leg as the external weight and 3 × 10 abdominal crunches lying over Swiss ball with proper form, and with no or minimal pain.

4. Return-to-sport phase

The return-to-sport phase is characterised by activities that focus on returning the athlete to full sporting function and participation, with successful return to previous functional and sporting level and the prevention of re-injury. The primary goals during this phase are maintenance of musculotendinous endurance and strength, aerobic and anaerobic capacity, and improving neuromuscular control/balance/coordination.

Dynamic muscle exercises using the elastic bands are continued with a load of 8-10 repetitions maximum, with focus on different and increasing speeds of eccentric contractions. Copenhagen adductors are continued at level 3 and exercises on a sliding board are continued by introducing 10-20 times 1 minute of skating from side to side. All these exercises should be performed 2-3 times a week with at least one day of rest from strength training in between.

Criteria for return to pre-injury competitive level

Participation in the specific sport, on an individual level or with the rest of the team, progressing from 30 minutes to 90 minutes of training and participating in 1-3 weeks of full training before full return to sport (match/competition activity) can be commenced, depending on the severity of the initial injury (the more severe the longer participation period before full return).

Key clinical signs suggestive of 'excessive loading' during rehabilitation

As the therapist must continually guard against the player 'overdoing' rehabilitation, we share the following signs that appear to suggest excessive loading and deterioration during rehabilitation:

- pain on passive hip abduction
- adductor muscle 'guarding' with increased muscle tone on passive combined hip external rotation and abduction
- pain and weakness with resisted adduction and squeeze testing.

Figure 32.9 (a) Copenhagen adductor exercise (b) A partner exercise where the player is lying on the side of the non-dominant leg with one forearm as support on the floor and the other arm placed along the body. The dominant leg is held at approximately the height of the hip of the partner, who is holding the leg with one hand supporting the ankle and the other supporting the knee. (Fig. 32.9a) The player then raises the body from the floor and the non-dominant leg is adducted so that the feet touch each other and the body is in a straight line (Fig.32.9b)

during maximal and forceful actions such as accelerating, decelerating, twisting turning and kicking.

In kicking sports, short stationary kicking can be commenced when adduction and squeeze tests are pain-free without crossover. The player may gradually increase the kicking distance and then start shorter kicking on the run. The last stage in the kicking program is long kicks at full pace and kicking around the body.

Criteria for progression to return-to-sport phase

The criteria for progression to the return-to-sport phase are:
- no or minimal pain with all exercises and normal execution (no compensation strategies to avoid loading

PART B Regional problems

Other non-surgical treatments for adductor-related groin pain

Compression shorts

Compression shorts can be used in cases where athletes continue to train and play despite ongoing symptoms. This can be either in cases where therapy does not result in a complete resolution of symptoms or where, for whatever reasons, athletes return to the field without having completed rehabilitation. They can also be useful when athletes are not fully confident after longstanding injuries.

Compression shorts reduce pain during athletic activities without a significant effect on performance. A study of 29 healthy athletes wearing two types of shorts used surface electromyography (EMG) of the adductor muscles during a 45° cutting movement. When wearing compression shorts with directional reinforcement properties, athletes had reduced adductor muscle activity during cutting.[52] The reduced muscle activity may be one mechanism by which compression shorts reduce pain. The reductions in pain are only small and to what extent this may postpone recovery has not been studied.

Manual therapy

A case series followed by an RCT have studied the effects of a multimodal treatment program, including an adductor muscle manipulation, stretching and a graded running program, in longstanding adductor-related groin pain.[53, 54] The RCT was evaluated as being high quality in a recent systematic review which concluded that multimodal treatment including manual adductor manipulation can result in a faster return to play, but not a higher treatment success, than a partially supervised active physical training program.[13]

There are a number of clinical scenarios in which manual therapy including adductor manipulation (Fig. 32.10a and b) or soft tissue therapy (Fig. 32.10c) can be considered. It can be offered as a standalone treatment, but should be considered more as an adjunct to active exercises in cases where:

- exercise therapy has not given a satisfactory result.
- 'weekend warriors' are not motivated or able to perform exercise therapy for the required intensity and duration manual therapy might be of help.

Iliopsoas-related groin pain

Iliopsoas-related groin pain is the second most common injury in the groin region.[3-5] It is characterised by pain in the anterior part of the proximal thigh, more laterally than adductor-related groin pain. Iliopsoas-related groin pain can present in isolation, but may also be part of the disturbed muscle balance in the region when other structures are injured. It is an important differential diagnosis for hip-related groin pain; not only because of the pain location, but also since the iliopsoas with its close relation to the hip joint as an anterior stabiliser tends to get involved whenever there is a hip or groin problem. It seems to be a muscle that frequently gets involved in compensating for the overload.

Diagnostic criteria

The diagnostic criteria for iliopsoas-related groin pain are *iliopsoas tenderness* (Fig. 32.3i and j) and *iliopsoas-related groin pain is more likely if there is pain on resisted hip flexion AND/OR pain on stretching the hip flexors* (Fig. 32.3f).[22]

Treatment

Most of the literature regarding the iliopsoas is related to the snapping hip and in recent years to hip arthroscopy. The painful iliopsoas muscle and/or tendon in athletes have not been the focus of any evidence-based research. The authors' preferred treatment of iliopsoas-related groin pain aims to strengthen the hip flexor muscles (Fig. 32.11) using isometric, concentric and eccentric contractions,[55] and combining this with a series of pelvic stabilisation and balance exercises.

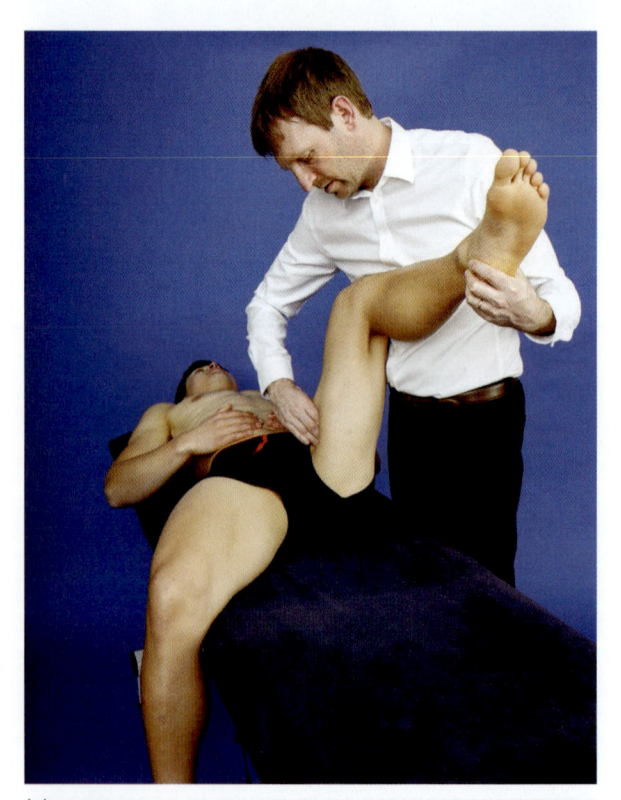

(a)

Figure 32.10 Manipulation of the adductors (a) Using the left hand to hold the heel, the right hand takes a hold of the muscle belly of the adductors

Groin pain CHAPTER 32

B

(c)

(b)

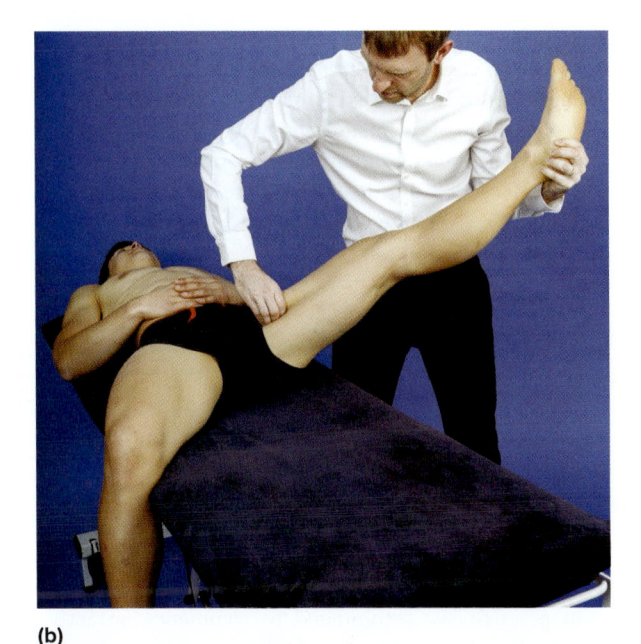

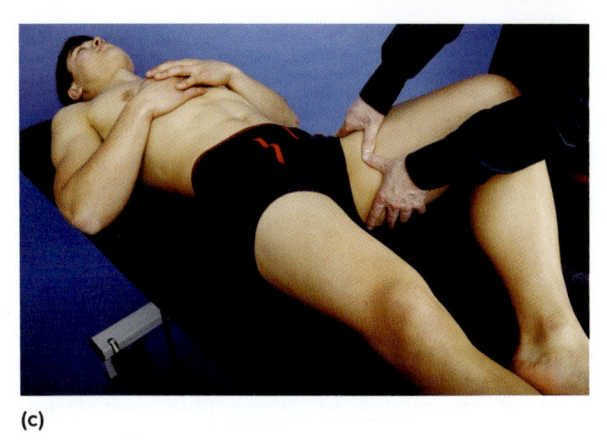

Figure 32.10 (cont.) (b) The left hand brings the hip into forced abduction and external rotation to apply the maximal tolerable stretch to the adductor group, while the right hand controls the tension; the motion is circular and flowing (c) Soft tissue therapy to the adductors

(a) (b)

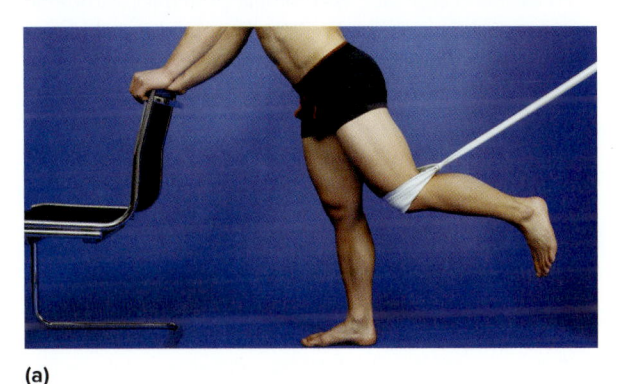

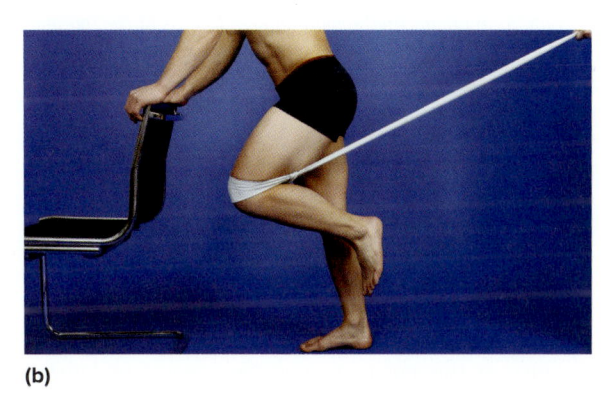

Figure 32.11 Hip strengthening exercises. Standing hip flexor strengthening with elastic band from start position (a) to finish position (b). Dynamic strength and coordination exercise with emphasis on maximal concentric, isometric and eccentric strength of hip flexor muscles. With elastic band fixated from above (here) the emphasis will be on rectus femoris and adductor longus in relevant kicking position, whereas if elastic band is fixated from below then the emphasis will be on strengthening the iliopsoas by focusing on optimal resistance towards full hip flexion

Additional physiotherapy, including stretching, soft tissue therapy and trigger point stimulation for symptomatic relief, might also be helpful. In most cases, players can return to play in 4–6 weeks. If the strength training is not progressing satisfactorily because it is too painful to perform the exercises, it is often possible to decrease the pain with an ultrasound guided local corticosteroid injection along the iliopsoas tendon.

Causes for groin pain can be seen in isolation or alongside each other in the same patient and the treatment needs to be directed at all entities that are diagnosed. The general exercises aiming at the coordination and synergies of the muscles and joints related to the hip and pelvis are along the same lines in most programs. However, it is very important that the individual entities are addressed individually with specific strengthening and endurance exercises.

In the internal coxa saltans (snapping psoas) the patient feels a snap happening during activity in the groin region when the hip is extended from the flexed position. The snap can sometimes be audible. If the snapping is very uncomfortable or painful it can, in our experience, be treated with a strengthening and stretching program in the majority of cases. On rare occasions, a partial release of the tendon at or close to the insertion may be performed with good results. The surgery can be performed as an open or arthroscopic/endoscopic procedure.[56]

651

Inguinal-related groin pain

Inguinal-related groin pain is probably one of the areas surrounded by the most confusion when dealing with groin pain in athletes. This entity has been defined in multiple ways, been given numerous differing nomenclatures and been the subject of much debate. Differing terminology has emerged from different geographical regions and the terms 'sports hernia', 'sportsman's hernia', 'sportsman's groin', 'posterior wall weakness', 'incipient hernia', 'Gilmore's groin' and 'hockey groin' have all been used in the past.[22] A consensus statement from the British Hernia Society proposed the term 'inguinal disruption', which can be used when three out of five possible findings are present.[57] This statement was the subject of some debate as it introduced yet another term into the fray and was not part of a wider classification system.[58]

Diagnostic criteria

The diagnostic criteria for inguinal-related groin pain are:

- *pain in inguinal canal region and tenderness of the inguinal canal* (Fig. 32.3k–l); *no palpable inguinal hernia is present*
- *more likely if aggravated with abdominal resistance* (Fig.32.3g) or *Valsalva/cough/sneeze.*[22]

There is no attempt made to describe any possible underlying pathology, as the exact substrate is still unknown. Bulging of the posterior wall, bulging causing entrapment neuropathy, tendinopathy of the inguinal ligament, tears of the external oblique aponeurosis and tearing of the conjoined tendon have all be proposed as being 'the pathology' underlying the problem. The authors feel that at this point in time, the issue of underlying pathology has yet to be resolved.

The confusion surrounding inguinal-related groin pain probably explains some of the difficulties when diagnosing and treating this condition. The actual prevalence remains unknown and this is clearly illustrated by the variety in reporting this in the literature.

A 1995 Australian case series from a sports physician on 189 cases of groin pain in athletes defined 'incipient inguinal hernia' as chronic pain above the pubic tubercle, increased by activities such as running or kicking,[17] local tenderness over the conjoined tendon area and posterior inguinal wall laxity at surgical exploration. In this series, 50% of the athletes were found to have incipient inguinal hernia. This is in stark contrast to a series of 207 athletes from Hölmich in 2007, who defined 'sports hernia' to be the presence of tenderness of the external inguinal ring and conjoined tendon and close to its insertion on the pubic tubercle in the absence of a visible or palpable inguinal hernia.[59] In this series, 4 of the 207 athletes (2%) were classified as having 'sports hernia'.

A prospective study examining new cases of groin pain in soccer players over the course of a season in Denmark defined 'abdominal-related groin pain' as the presence of pain on palpation of the abdominal muscle insertion together with pain on abdominal flexion against resistance. Eleven of the 58 entities (19%) were abdominal-related and in 9 of the 11 cases this coexisted with the presence of adductor-related groin pain.[15]

Treatment

When considering treatment options for inguinal-related groin pain, it is important to consider the available evidence. The systematic review discussed earlier in the section 'Evidence for treatment' noted that there 'were no studies focused on the conservative treatment of sport's hernia with a well-described treatment protocol'.[13] It should be noted that only case series with more than 10 subjects were included so some smaller previous series which report success were not included.[60, 61]

In practice, we recommend to commence an active exercise-based approach with similar principles as those in the program earlier described for longstanding adductor-related groin pain. This approach aims to strengthen the abdominal muscles, including isometric, concentric and eccentric contractions, in combination with a series of adductor and abductor-strengthening exercises, pelvic stabilisation and balance exercises. The abdominal exercises used in the adductor program (Fig. 32.6b and c) can be used as a starting point,[50] progressing into more strenuous exercises for the abdominal wall through plank exercises (Fig. 32.12a) and then into modified plank exercises with high muscle activation of both internal and external obliques.[62] A Swiss ball can also be used in the late stage conditioning phase before return to sport to mimic some of the external loads and forceful eccentric/concentric contractions that the abdominals go through, especially in kicking, throwing or shooting (ice hockey) (Fig. 32.12b and c).[63]

As with the adductor program, the total length of the exercise training period is dependent on criteria-based progression, but is generally between 8–12 weeks. Absence from training is again necessary as the functionality and strength of the abdominal muscle group has to be re-established, and pain brought under control without continued provocation by the sport that first precipitated the injury. Stationary cycling and general fitness training not involving the abdominals can be allowed if they can be done without pain. Jogging is again allowed after 6 weeks as long as it does not provoke any groin pain.

When the patient is able to jog and undergo his or her regular treatment without pain, the treatment program is completed. The athlete is allowed to gradually progress to demanding sports-specific training followed by sports

Groin pain CHAPTER 32

participation. No excessive stretching of the abdominal or the adductor muscles during this 2–3 month exercise training period is recommended as it can put unnecessary strain on the adductor and abdominal complex.

Surgery

In cases where conservative treatment is not successful or surgery is considered for other reasons, it should be noted that there have been no comparative studies on the superiority of different techniques. A study comparing laparoscopic to open hernia repair is currently ongoing.[64]

A review identified 12 surgical studies on open hernia repair, 10 studies on laparoscopic hernia repair and 16 studies in which combined procedures (including adductor tenotomy) were performed.[13] Additional neurectomy was performed in 12 studies. There was only one high-quality study identified in the review.[65] The studies with the weakest methodological score reported the highest treatment success. This is important to take into consideration when using these published results to help inform patient decisions in clinical practice.

The one high-quality RCT compared laparoscopic hernia repair to conservative treatment in cases of 'sportsman's hernia (athletic pubalgia)'.[65] This was defined as athletes having more than 3 months history of pain above the inguinal ligament. There was pain on palpation of the deep inguinal ring and in cases where there was also pain on the pubic bone, pubic tubercle or adductors, or bone marrow oedema seen on the MRI, the athletes were also included.

The study randomised 60 athletes to treatment with either a bilateral totally extraperitoneal (TEP) laparoscopic hernia repair or conservative treatment. Unfortunately, the conservative treatment protocol is only described briefly as being total rest from their sports, active physiotherapy, steroid injections into the painful area and oral anti-inflammatory analgesics. This treatment was given 3 times a week for 90 minutes for 8 weeks and was supervised by the club physiotherapist.

This study found that 97% of those treated with surgery had returned to sport at 1 year compared to 50% of the conservative group. Until now this is the only high-quality study comparing surgery with conservative treatment. The poor description of the conservative treatment makes interpretation for clinical practice challenging, but it seems that some patients may benefit from conservative treatment and will be able to return to sport without having surgery. As complications from surgery are not uncommon in this region, non-surgical treatment should be considered and exhausted first.

Figure 32.12 (cont.) (c) Dynamic abdominal strengthening with eccentric emphasis.

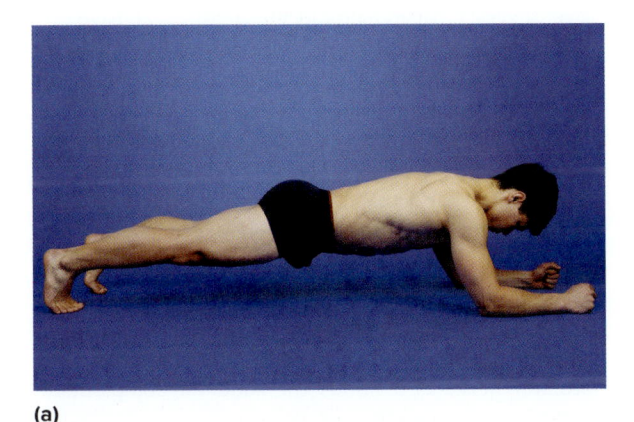

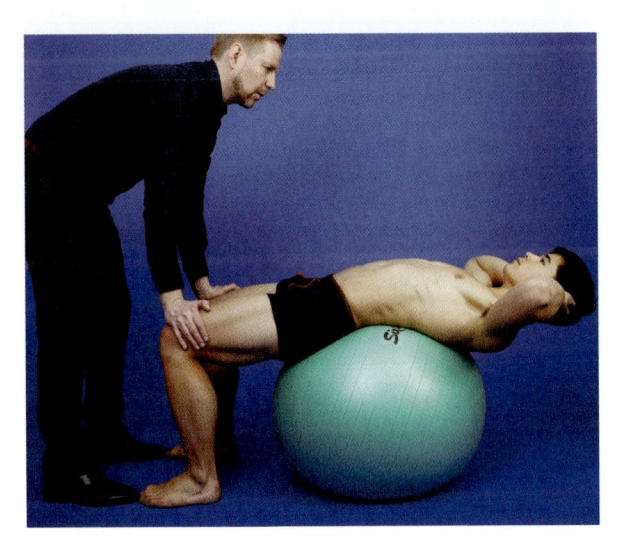

Figure 32.12 (a) Long lever planks with static maximal trunk muscle activation (b) Swiss ball curls

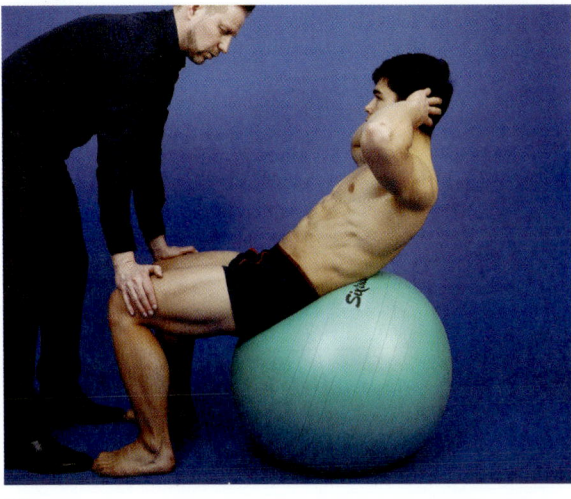

653

The consensus agreement from the British Hernia Society noted that there was no proven best surgical technique.[57] This means that local availability along with the experience and preference of the surgeon are likely to be important when decisions are made as to which type of surgery to perform.

Inguinal hernia

Inguinal hernias occur in athletes as in the general population. They can be either direct or indirect. Small hernias may become painful as a result of exertion. Symptoms may include a characteristic dragging sensation to one side of the lower abdomen aggravated by increased intra-abdominal pressure, such as coughing. On examination, there is occasionally an obvious swelling and the hernia can be palpated. In cases of a symptomatic inguinal hernia, the treatment consists of surgical correction of the defect.[66]

Pubic-related groin pain

No epidemiological data are available in the literature regarding how common pubic-related groin pain is.

Diagnostic criteria

The diagnostic criteria for pubic-related groin pain are:

- local tenderness of the pubic symphysis and the immediately adjacent bone (Fig. 32.3m)
- no particular resistance tests to test specifically for pubic-related groin pain could be identified.[22]

Verrall et al. described clinical signs including pubic symphysis and superior pubic ramus tenderness as part of a bone stress-related problem.[67] The presence of BMO on MRI in the pubic bone was also a part of the diagnosis. The clinical criteria included the presence of at least 6 weeks of groin pain, located in the adductor and/or pubic bone region and present during and/or after sporting activity. No particular resistance tests to test specifically for pubic-related groin pain have been identified, but squeeze testing seems to be the most relevant.[68]

In a study of 10 Australian rules football players with longstanding groin pain, using the criteria mentioned, biopsy was taken from the area in the superior pubic rami where MRI showed BMO. Histologically new woven bone was found and this was considered to represent a repair process that was the pathological stress reaction that was causing the groin pain. No controls with BMO but without symptoms were included and as such it is not known if the woven bone is a normal reaction to the stress the bone is receiving playing football or it is a sign of pathology.[39]

Treatment

The treatment for this condition as described by Verrall et al. consists of mainly unloading the lower extremities and gradually increasing load again over a period of 3–4 months moving from rest from all weight-bearing running activities for 12 weeks over a period with stationary cycling, a stepping device and a gradual return to running activity.[69] The athletes were allowed to return to football training when 30 minutes of pain-free interval running was tolerated. There is no evidence-based treatment available.

COMPLETE ADDUCTOR AVULSIONS

Complete proximal adductor avulsions (Fig. 32.13) are not common, but in American football (National Football League) the mean time for return to play in players treated conservatively for an acute adductor longus rupture was reported to be 6 +/− 3 weeks (range, 3–12 weeks).[70] A recent study of two different adductor ruptures in a soccer player suggests that adductor longus ruptures can have very different recovery times. In this study, normal hip adductor strength was obtained after 52 weeks for the first injury, but after 10 weeks for the second injury.[71] This highlights the importance of measuring hip adductor strength by using a hand-held dynamometer, as this gives important information on the actual recovery process of the adductors, which cannot be obtained from diagnostic imaging.

LESS COMMON INJURIES
Obturator neuropathy

Obturator neuropathy is a fascial entrapment of the obturator nerve as it enters the adductor compartment

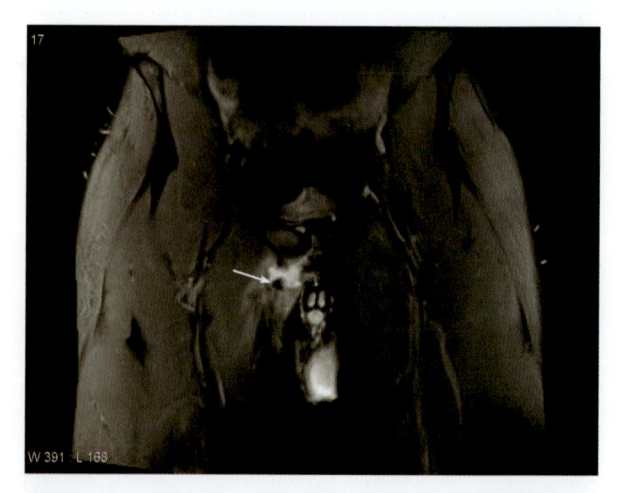

Figure 32.13 MRI coronal short tau inversion recovery (STIR) view of adductor avulsion. Images display acute rupture and retraction of adductor longus tendon on right side (arrow), with acute oedema (high intensity) and haemorrhage in surrounding muscle tissues

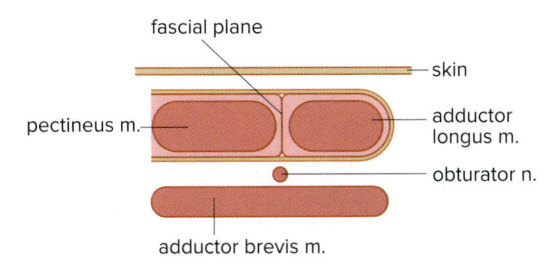

Figure 32.14 Obturator neuropathy—fascial arrangement

(Fig. 32.14). Obturator neuropathies have been reported to occur in Australian rules football and rugby. It has distinct clinical features that separate it from other causes of groin pain.[72, 73]

Obturator neuropathy presents as exercise-related groin pain, which initially is located in the proximal groin but with increasing exercise radiates towards the distal medial thigh. There may be associated weakness or a feeling of a lack of propulsion of the limb during running but numbness is very rarely reported. At rest, examination findings can be non-specific, with pain on passive abduction of the hip, and pain and weakness on resisted hip adduction. The ipsilateral pubic tubercle is often tender. The essential component of the physical examination is to exercise the patient to a level that reproduces the symptoms followed by immediate examination of the patient. This examination will reveal weakness of resisted adduction and numbness over the distal medial thigh. The diagnosis is confirmed by needle EMG, which shows chronic denervation patterns of the adductor muscle group.

Conservative treatment of this condition, including sustained myofascial tension over the adductor compartment, neural stretches, spinal mobilisation and iliopsoas soft tissue techniques, is generally unsuccessful.

The definitive treatment of this condition is surgical. An oblique incision is made in the proximal groin. The plane between the adductor longus and pectineus is identified and dissected, revealing the obturator nerve under the fascia over the adductor brevis. This fascia is divided and the nerve is freed up to the level of the obturator foramen. The fascial anatomy here is important, with the fascia of the adductor longus curving around the muscle medially and passing back deep to the muscle to become the fascia over the adductor brevis, which is thought to be responsible for the fascial entrapment of the obturator nerve. Post-surgical management includes wound management, soft tissue techniques and a graduated return to full activity over a period of 4–6 weeks.

Other nerve entrapments

A number of superficial nerves in the groin may become entrapped and should be considered as possible causes of groin pain. The ilioinguinal nerve supplies the skin around the genitalia and the inside of the thigh and may produce pain as a result of entrapment. The genitofemoral nerve innervates an area of skin just above the groin fold. The lateral cutaneous nerve of the thigh is the most common nerve affected. This nerve supplies the outside of the thigh. This condition is known as 'meralgia paraesthetica' and is described in Chapter 33.

Pudendal nerve entrapment requires the presence of the following criteria: pain in the territory of the pudendal nerve (from the anus to the penis or clitoris); pain that is predominantly experienced while sitting; pain that does not wake the patient at night; pain with no objective sensory impairment; and pain relieved by diagnostic pudendal nerve block.[74]

Treatment of these conditions is usually not necessary as they often spontaneously resolve. Meralgia paraesthetica is sometimes treated with a corticosteroid injection at the site where the nerve exits the pelvis, 1 cm medial to the anterior superior iliac spine. Occasionally, the nerve needs to be explored surgically and the area of entrapment released.

Stress fractures of the neck of the femur

Stress fracture of the neck of the femur is another cause of groin pain. The usual history is one of gradual onset of groin pain, poorly localised and aggravated by activity. Examination may show some localised tenderness but often there is relatively little to find other than pain at the extremes of hip joint movement, especially internal rotation. Plain radiograph may demonstrate the fracture if it has been present for a number of weeks but this investigation should not be relied on to rule out the condition; isotopic bone scan and MRI (Fig. 32.15) are the most sensitive tests.

Stress fractures of the neck of the femur occur on either the superior or tension side of the bone or on the inferior or compression side (Fig. 32.16). Stress fractures of the superior aspect of the femoral neck should be regarded as a surgical emergency and treated with either urgent internal fixation or strict rest. The concern is that such stress fractures have a tendency to go on to full fracture, which compromises the blood supply to the femoral head.

Stress fractures of the inferior surface of the femoral neck are more benign and can be treated with an initial period of non weight-bearing rest followed by a period of weight-bearing without running. They require at least 6 weeks of rest and usually considerably longer. Following the period of rest, a further 6 weeks of progressive loading will take the patient back to full training. Biomechanical (Chapter 8), nutritional and endocrine risk factors (Chapter 4) should be assessed and treated as appropriate.

PART B   Regional problems

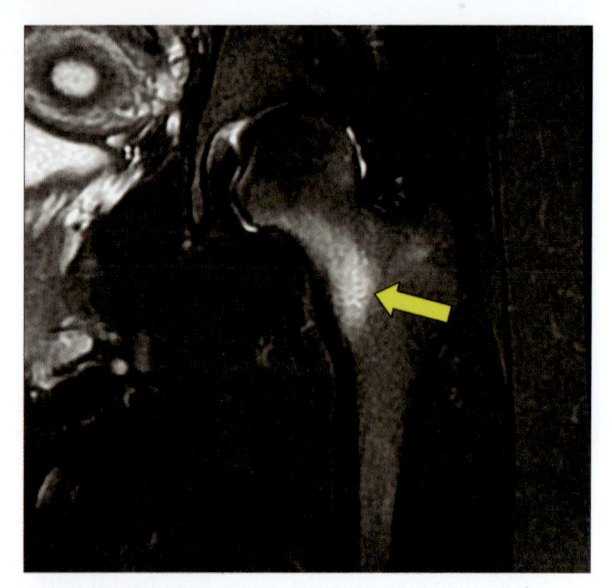

Figure 32.15 MRI showing stress fracture neck of femur
IMAGING IN SPORTS-SPECIFIC MUSCULOSKELETAL INJURIES, 2016, P.741, ALI GUERMAZI, FRANK W ROEMER, MICHEL D CREMA. © SPRINGER INTERNATIONAL PUBLISHING SWITZERLAND 2016. WITH PERMISSION OF SPRINGER

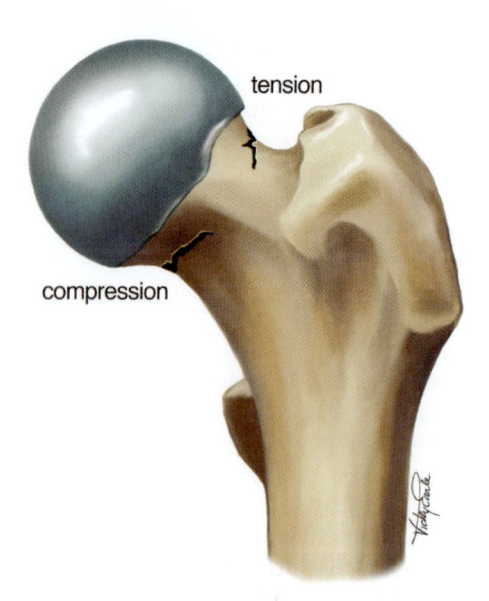

Figure 32.16 Stress fractures of the neck of femur—superior or tension fracture on the superior aspect of the femoral neck, and inferior or compression fracture on the inferior side

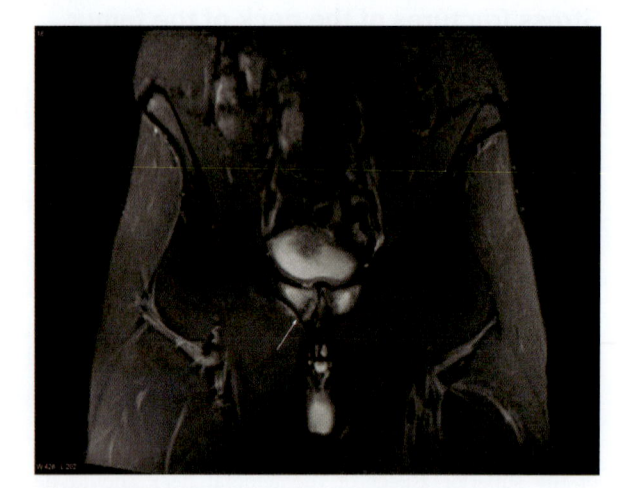

Figure 32.17 MRI stress fracture of the inferior pubic ramus. Images show subcortical hypointense line (arrow) representing bony stress fracture parallel to the symphyseal joint surface in the inferior pubic ramus

Stress fracture of the inferior pubic ramus

Stress fracture of the inferior pubic ramus, especially in distance runners, is an important differential diagnosis of adductor tendinopathy. There is usually a history of overuse and localised tenderness, which is not aggravated by passive abduction or resisted adduction. In this condition, pain is often referred to the buttock.

A stress fracture may not be visible on plain radiograph for several weeks, whereas a radionuclide bone scan will demonstrate a focal area of increased activity within hours and an MRI (Fig. 32.17) will show a focal area of bone oedema. As with any stress fracture, aetiological factors must be considered. Stress fractures of the inferior pubic ramus in females may be associated with reduced bone density, low initial aerobic fitness and nutritional insufficiency. Prolonged amenorrhoea is also linked with this stress fracture (Chapter 4).

Treatment consists of relative rest from aggravating activities such as running until there is no longer any local tenderness. Fitness should be maintained with swimming or cycling with gradual return to weight-bearing over a number of weeks. Predisposing factors such as a negative energy intake, muscular imbalance or biomechanical abnormality also require assessment and intervention.

Preventative strategies can be incorporated, especially in the female military/elite athlete population. Strategies may include pre-training interventions focusing on improving aerobic fitness to reduce fatigue fractures, and calcium and vitamin D supplementation.[75, 76] Female recruits who report no menses during the year previous to recruitment should also be observed closely.[76]

Referred pain to the groin

The possibility of referred pain to the groin should always be considered, especially when there is little to find on local examination. A common site of referral to the groin is the sacroiliac joint (SIJ) and this should always be assessed in any examination of a patient with groin pain. The SIJ may also refer pain to the scrotum in males and labia in females. The assessment and treatment of sacroiliac problems are discussed in Chapter 30.

The lumbar spine may refer pain to the groin. The lumbar spine and thoracolumbar junction should always be examined in a patient with groin pain. Neurodynamic tests, such as the slump and neural Thomas tests, should be performed as part of the assessment (Chapter 15). Variations such as the addition of adduction or hip rotation may reproduce the patient's pain.

A positive neurodynamic test result requires further evaluation to determine the site of the abnormality. The position of reproduction of pain can be used to correct neural tightness by stretching. Active trigger points may also refer to the groin and should be treated with soft tissue therapy.

As mentioned in the section 'Terminology and definitions' there are many other conditions that can give rise to groin pain. When athletes present with groin pain that is not typical in nature, has no clear relationship with loading, nocturnal pain or pain associated with other non-musculoskeletal symptoms, one must think broadly in terms of possible differential diagnosis.

PREVENTION OF GROIN INJURIES

By late 2016, seven RCTs had investigated prevention of sports injuries where data on groin injuries had been included. These seven studies were evaluated and analysed in a systematic review and the data was pooled in a meta-analysis.[77]

The studies examined the effect of different prevention interventions, predominantly looking at strengthening, coordination and balance exercises, and there were more than 2000 subjects in control and intervention groups, respectively. In total 157 injuries occurred, 68 in the intervention group and 89 in the controls. While the reduction is around 20%, this was not statistically significant. This means that at present, despite the number of trials examining groin injury prevention, there is no proven effective intervention. Due to the use of time loss definitions in the majority of studies, many overuse injuries will not have been registered, which is a limitation in the existing literature. Furthermore, compliance was not recorded in three studies and in the other four, compliance was less than intended.

Despite these limitations, including an active exercise strategy for strengthening and improving muscle function, load transfer and tolerance in the pelvic region may induce a relevant reduction of groin injuries. No reports of adverse events in relation to such a strategy have been documented. Clinicians and athletes should weigh up the time and effort that needs to be invested against the possible reduction to decide whether to implement in their setting.

Possible prevention strategies

A number of measures can be considered in clinical practice. Given the fact that previous injury is a risk factor, athletes with a history of groin pain should be given extra attention. Research on soccer players during the start of a new season has shown that those who had groin pain in the previous season still had reduced function and residual symptoms after the summer break.[78] In this light. it would seem prudent for athletes with groin pain in season to use the off-season to concentrate on treatment and recovery rather than simply resting.

A careful examination should be done at the end of the season, as described in the 'Clinical overview' section. Any deficits found can be used to target improvements in the off-season and should be combined with sports-specific training. A study from elite ice hockey showed that those players who performed the least sports-specific training in the off-season had triple the risk for a groin injury in the next season.[79]

Little is known about the specific relationship between training load and groin pain. Recent literature from other fields has highlighted that athletes who have a rapid rise in training load, without sufficiently accumulating training to have ensured readiness are prone to injury. As such, careful consideration of training load can be part of groin injury prevention, but is likely to be part of a more general prevention strategy than only aimed at the hip or groin.

Monitoring players for changes in hip muscle strength in an attempt to predict the onset of groin pain was performed in a study on Australian rules football players.[80] Elite junior players (n = 86, 16-18 years old), were measured using squeeze tests on a weekly basis. They were also monitored for the presence of groin pain in the previous week. When they reported having groin pain 2 weeks in a row, this was considered to be the start of a groin injury.

The variation of the squeeze strength scores across the season was 2-3%. Twelve players developed groin pain and their strength in the week before the onset of the pain was reduced by 12+/−3% from their own baseline. As such, monitoring of strength and the onset of groin pain can be used to allow early detection and hopefully aid prevention. Furthermore, in those footballers where groin pain is encountered through continuous screening and examination, early detection and management seem to be highly relevant as a groin pain duration of only 1-2 weeks is associated with a much better HAGOS score at the beginning of the pre-season/new season, compared to individuals with longer durations of groin pain in the previous season.[78]

REFERENCES

References for this chapter can be found at www.mhhe.com/au/CSM5e

Chapter 33

Anterior thigh pain

with ZUZANA MACHOTKA

It was the quad in my right leg, the tendon just kept tearing. I couldn't get back to the point of playing and obviously after having a really good start last season, and not playing again, it was frustrating.

Joel Paris, promising Australian cricket fast bowler

The anterior thigh region (Fig. 33.1) is a common site of sporting injuries. Quadriceps muscle strains and contusions constitute the majority of these injuries; however, referred pain from the hip, sacroiliac joint (SIJ) or lumbar spine may also cause anterior thigh pain.[1] Stress fracture of the shaft of the femur is a less common but important diagnosis. A summary of the causes of anterior thigh pain is shown in Table 33.1.

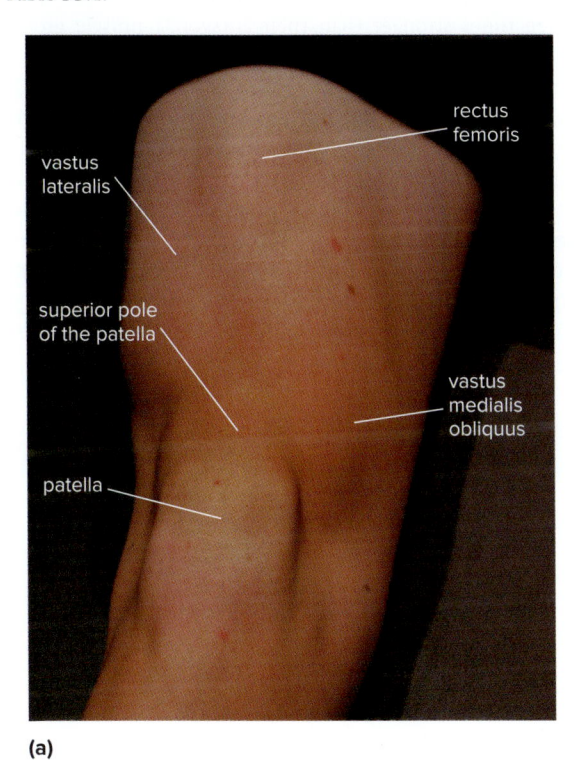

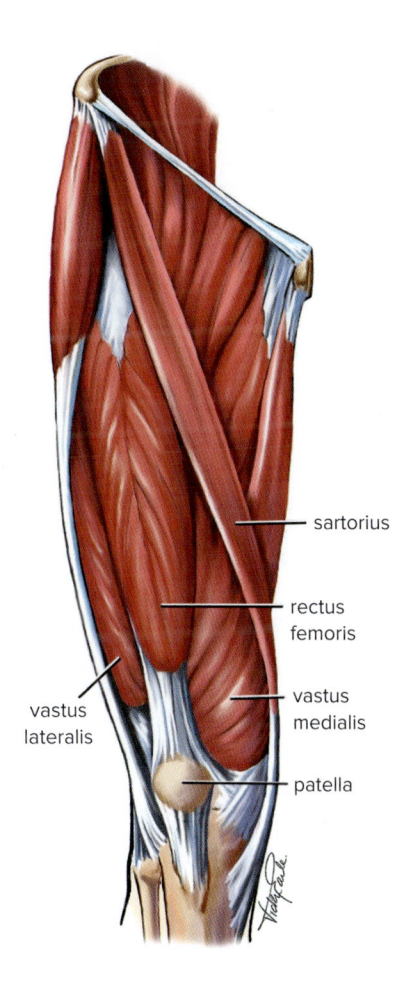

Figure 33.1 Anatomy of the anterior thigh (a) Surface anatomy (b) Muscles of the anterior thigh

659

PART B   Regional problems

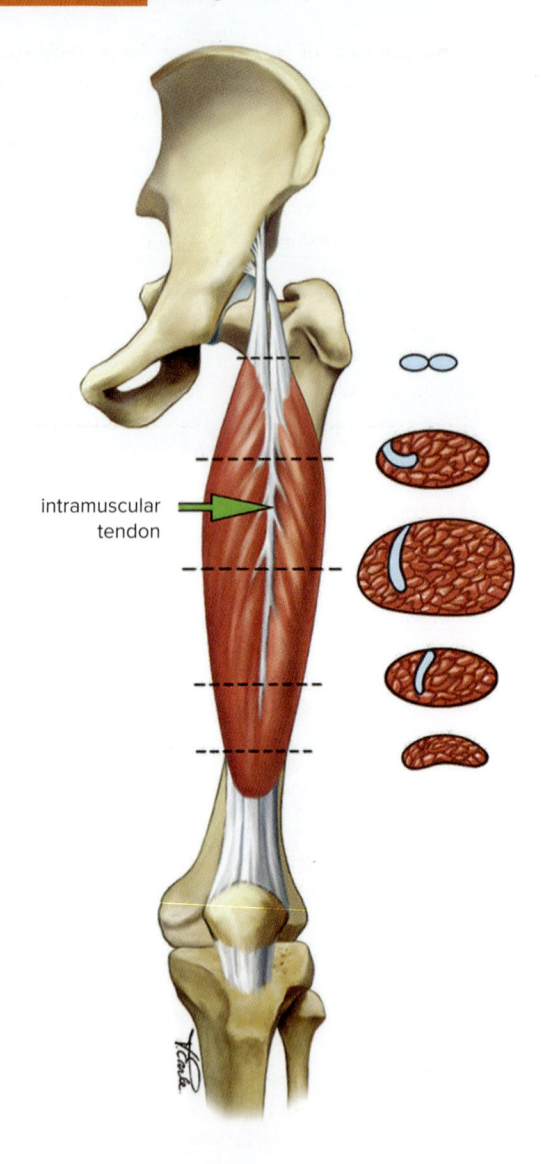

EPIDEMIOLOGY

Lower limb injuries, particularly thigh muscle injuries, are common in sport. In athletics, thigh muscle strains account for up to 13.5% of all injuries.[1] In professional soccer, up to a third of injuries involve lower limb muscles and 19% of all muscle injuries involve the quadriceps.[2, 3] Recurrent quadriceps muscle injuries are associated with a significantly longer period of rehabilitation and time to return to sport. Therefore, an accurate initial diagnosis and a structured rehabilitation program are essential to ensure a safe return to sport.

FUNCTIONAL ANATOMY AND BIOMECHANICS

The thigh musculature is divided into anterior, medial and posterior compartments by intermuscular septa. The anterior compartment is the largest of the three, and includes the femur, quadriceps femoris and sartorius muscles. The quadriceps include the rectus femoris, vastus lateralis, vastus medialis and vastus intermedius muscles (Fig. 33.1b). Concentric contraction of the quadriceps muscles extends the knee against gravity, which is important in such activities as rising from sitting and climbing up stairs. Eccentrically, the quadriceps muscles have an important role in lowering body weight, for example during walking/running down hills and down stairs. The quadriceps muscles contribute enormously to acceleration and power during jumping and running. As a consequence, the quadriceps can be up to three times stronger than their antagonist muscle group, the hamstrings.[4]

The rectus femoris is the only quadriceps muscle to cross the hip joint and has two heads at its origin (Fig. 33.1c). Proximally, the direct head of the rectus femoris originates from the anterior inferior iliac spine and the indirect head originates from above the acetabulum. The two heads form a conjoint tendon just beneath their origin. The direct head is more superficial and has connections with the deep fascia of the thigh (fascia lata). The indirect head contributes to a deep

Figure 33.1 (cont.) (c) Central tendon of the rectus femoris

Table 33.1 Causes of anterior thigh pain

Common	Less common	Not to be missed
Quadriceps muscle contusion ('cork thigh', 'charley horse') Quadriceps muscle strain • distal rectus femoris • proximal rectus femoris Myositis ossificans	Referred pain • upper lumbar spine • sacroiliac joint • hip joint Stress fracture of the femur Sartorius muscle strain Avulsion of the apophysis of rectus femoris Nerve entrapment • lateral cutaneous nerve • femoral cutaneous nerve	Slipped capital femoral epiphysis Perthes' disease (Chapter 44) Tumour (e.g. osteosarcoma of the femur) Acute compartment syndrome of the thigh

musculotendinous junction or 'central tendon', which can travel up to two-thirds of the muscle belly (Fig. 33.1c).[5-7] This complex anatomy and its biarthrodial (i.e. two joint) nature, may be why the rectus femoris is the most commonly strained quadriceps muscle.[8]

Distally, all four quadriceps muscles insert into the superior pole of the patella and continue to form the patellar tendon which, in turn, attaches to the tibial tuberosity. Overlying the quadriceps muscles is the sartorius muscle. The sartorius muscle passes medially from the anterior superior iliac spine to the superior/medial surface of the tibia in an arrangement called the pes anserinus (Chapter 37). The sartorius flexes, abducts, and laterally rotates the hip joint, flexes the knee joint and provides restraint to knee valgus forces. Despite its functional importance, the sartorius is less prone to strain injury because it works synergistically with other hip and thigh muscles.

The adductor canal is located deep to the sartorius muscle and extends from the apex of the femoral triangle (Chapter 32) to the adductor hiatus–the gateway to the popliteal fossa. The femoral artery and vein, saphenous nerve, and the nerve to vastus medialis are bundled together within the adductor canal. This site is commonly used to administer anaesthesia (femoral nerve block). Quadriceps weakness can occur following a femoral nerve block and should be monitored postoperatively because the quadriceps can atrophy rapidly following periods of immobilisation or decreased activation.[9, 10]

CLINICAL APPROACH

In the anterior thigh, primary diagnoses frequently include contusions and strains. However, it is important that clinicians consider important factors that may influence the diagnosis and subsequent rehabilitation. These can include:

- details of previous injuries, including rehabilitation methods, time frames and outcomes
- the magnitude of any impairments in quadriceps strength, control and activation
- any hypermobility or hypomobility, particularly of the hip, knee and ankle joints
- psychological factors such as motivation, pain tolerance and readiness to return to sport.

History

The two most important aspects of the history of a patient with anterior thigh pain are the exact site of the pain and the mechanism of injury. The site of the pain is usually well localised in cases of contusion or muscle strain. Contusions can occur anywhere in the quadriceps muscle but they are most common anterolaterally or in the vastus medialis obliquus. Muscle strains generally occur in the midline of the thigh anteriorly.

The mechanism of injury may help differentiate between muscle strains and contusions. A contusion is likely to be the result of a direct blow, whereas a muscle strain usually occurs when an athlete is striving for extra speed when running or extra distance when kicking. In contact sports, however, the athlete may have difficulty recalling the exact mechanism of injury.

Whether or not the athlete was able to continue activity, the present level of function and range of motion, night pain and the degree of swelling are all guides to the severity of the condition. Determine whether the POLICE regimen was implemented initially (see Chapter 17) and whether there were any aggravating factors (such as continued activity).

Gradual onset of poorly localised anterior thigh pain in a distance runner worsening with activity may indicate a stress fracture of the femur. Burning pain and associated paraesthesia suggest nerve involvement, and poor location of pain can suggest a referred pain from other areas such as the SIJ, hip joint and upper lumbar spine. Bilateral pain suggests the pain is referred from the lumbar spine.

Physical examination

In anterior thigh pain of acute onset, the diagnosis is usually straightforward and examination can focus on local structures. In anterior thigh pain of insidious onset, diagnosis is more difficult and examination should include sites that refer pain to the thigh–the lumbar spine, SIJ and hip.

Muscle tightness and altered muscle activation around the pelvis and thigh can lead to asymmetries further down the kinetic chain. These asymmetries can alter how ground reaction forces are absorbed, particularly during high impact activities such as jumping and sprinting, thus predisposing athletes to further injury. In the patient with anterior thigh pain, assessing and treating muscle imbalances is often necessary to optimise movement patterns and address risk factors for further injury.

The aim of the examination is to determine the exact site of the abnormality and to assess range of motion and muscle strength. Functional testing may be necessary to reproduce the symptoms.

1. Observation (look for muscle bulk, wasting, swelling and position of patella. During activity, observe muscle activation, pelvic control, patella tracking and any signs of a limp)
    a. standing
    b. walking
    c. supine
2. Active movements (are there any asymmetries?)
    a. hip flexion
    b. knee flexion
    c. knee extension
    d. active straight leg raise[11]

PART B   Regional problems

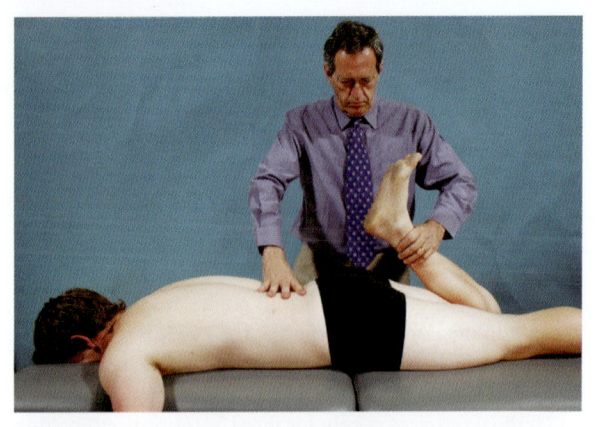

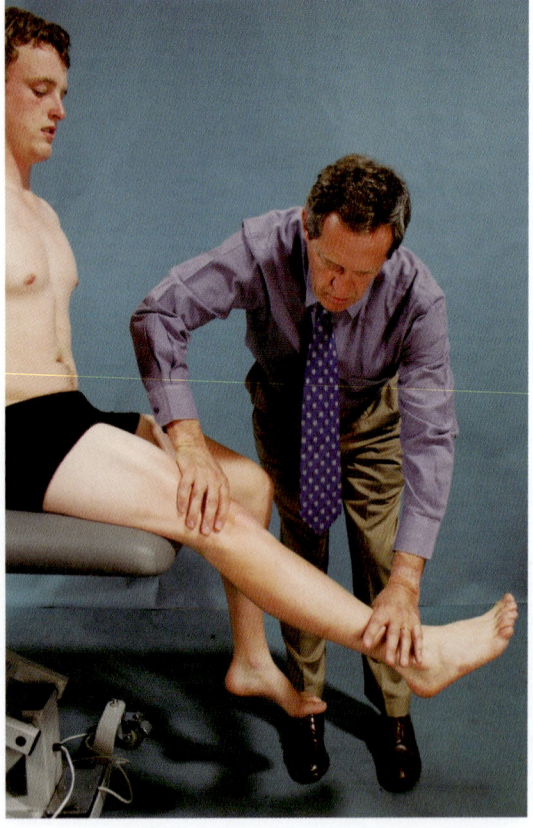

(a)

(b)

(c)

Figure 33.2 Examination of the patient with anterior thigh pain (a) Passive movement—quadriceps stretch. A passive stretch of the quadriceps muscles is performed to end of range. Passive hip extension may be added to increase the stretch on the rectus femoris, which may reproduce the patient's pain (b) Resisted movement—knee extension. With the hip and knee flexed to 90°, the knee is extended against resistance (c) Resisted movement—hip flexion

3. Passive movements (consider what determines the end feel e.g. muscle spasm)
   a. hip and knee (e.g. hip quadrant, knee hyper-extension)
   b. muscle stretch (e.g. quadriceps) (Fig. 33.2a)
   c. patella glides (Chapter 36)
   d. Thomas test (Chapter 32)

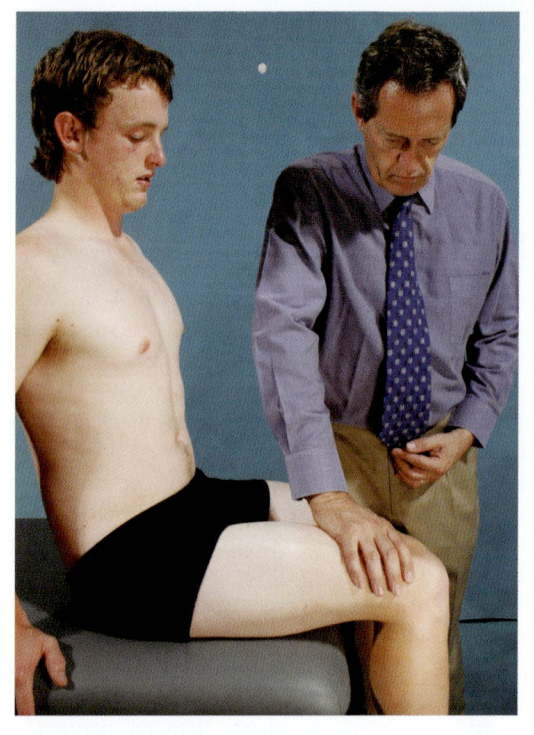

4. Resisted movements (isometric or concentric. Graded using a 0–5 scale or with a hand-held dynamometer)
   a. knee extension (Fig. 33.2b)
   b. straight-leg raise
   c. hip flexion (Fig. 33.2c)
5. Functional tests
   a. squat (Fig. 33.2d) (single leg, ¼ squat vs full)
   b. jump (vertical jumps, box jumps)
   c. hop (on the spot, hop for distance)[12, 13]
   d. kick (short vs long distance)
   e. lunge (forward vs reverse eccentric lunges)
6. Palpation (consider firmness and if able, map out area of tenderness)
   a. sartorius and quadriceps muscles (Fig. 33.2e)
   b. femoral artery (the proximal two-thirds of a line drawn from the mid-inguinal ligament point to the adductor tubercle with the thigh flexed, abducted, and laterally rotated represents the course of the femoral artery and nerve)

Anterior thigh pain CHAPTER 33

(d)

(e)

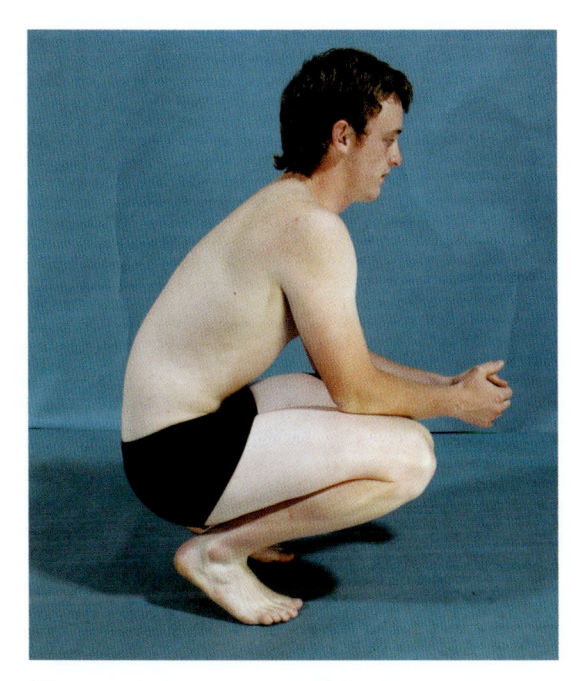

(f)

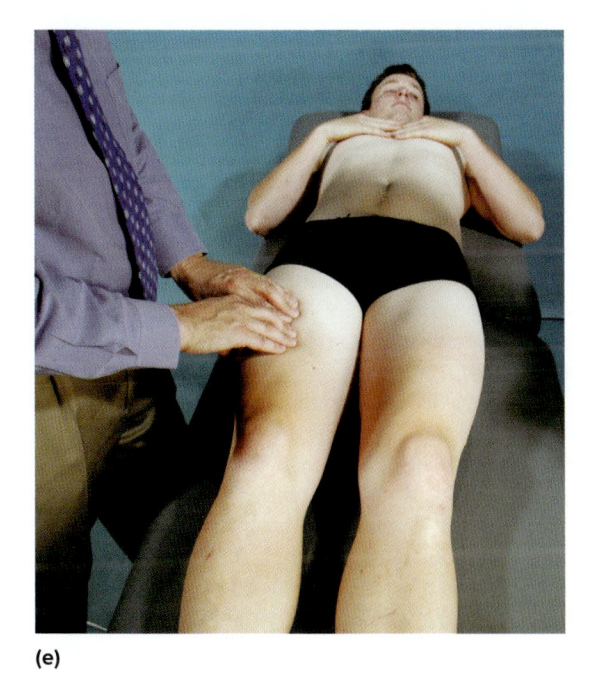

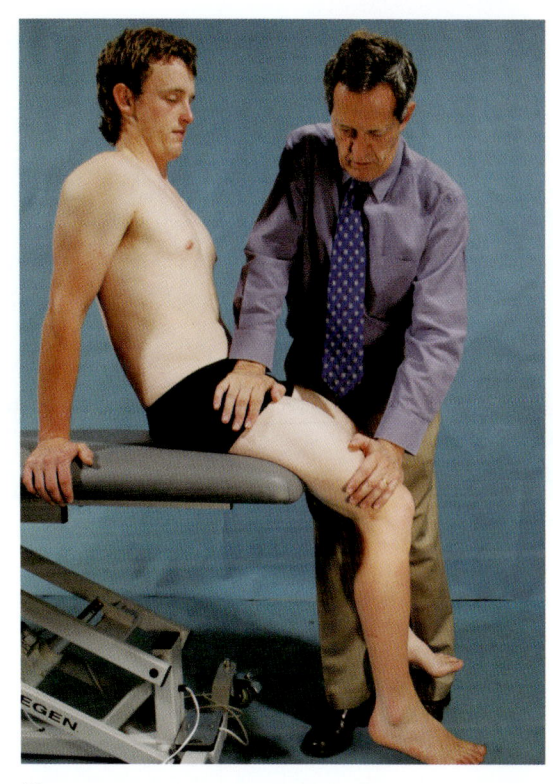

(g)

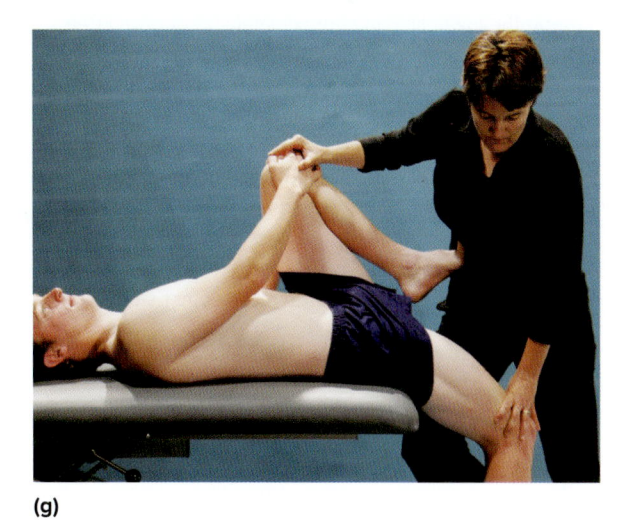

Figure 33.2 (cont.) (d) Functional movements—squat. If the previous activities have failed to reproduce the patient's pain, functional movements should be used to reproduce the pain. These may include squat, hop or jump (e) Palpation—the anterior thigh is palpated for tenderness, swelling and areas of focal muscle thickening. A focal defect in the muscle belly may be palpated, especially with active muscle contraction (f) Special tests—the fulcrum test for the presence of a femoral stress fracture. This is performed with pressure over the distal end of the femur. Reproduction of the patient's pain may be indicative of a femoral stress fracture (g) Special tests—neurodynamic test (modified Thomas test). The patient is placed in the psoas stretch position. Cervical and upper thoracic flexion is added and then the clinician passively bends the patient's knee (using his or her own leg). Reproduction of the patient's symptoms indicates a neural contribution

PART B   Regional problems

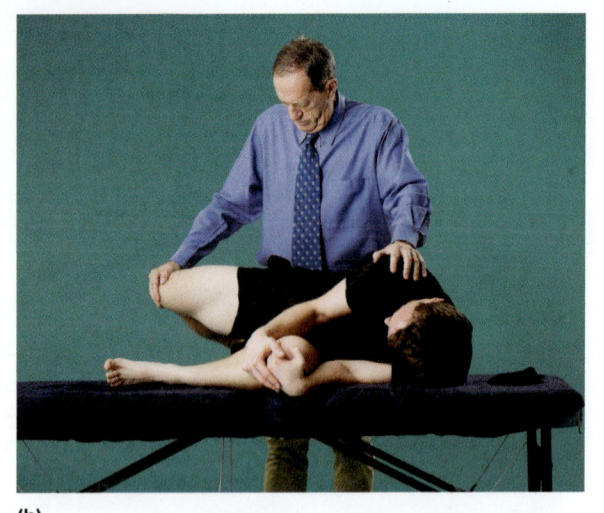

Figure 33.2 (cont.) (h) The side-lying slump test—an extension of the standard prone knee bend test and focuses on the neural-sensitive structures of the anterior thigh (e.g. femoral nerve). Test starts with the subject in a side-lying position. Subject holds lower leg for stability in a comfortable, not fully flexed, position with head in cervical flexion. The assessor/therapist stands behind subject supporting the upper leg in a neutral hip position, maintaining neutral hip abduction/adduction throughout the test. With one hand over hip, the other hand is used to support the lower limb in approximately 90 degree knee flexion. Resting symptoms should be recorded (e.g. stretch through anterior thigh). The subject's hip is then extended, noting any changes in resting symptoms and/or position of thigh with onset of symptoms. If no symptoms are evoked, the leg is extended to the point of firm hip resistance. The subject is then asked to extended their neck and report any change in symptoms. The assessor should monitor for any changes in hip resistance before returning to starting position. Test should be repeated on the other side

7. Special tests
   a. fulcrum test (Fig. 33.2f) (this test is reported to have excellent sensitivity and specificity for mid-shaft femoral stress fractures)[14, 15]
   b. neurodynamic testing (modified Thomas test Fig. 33.2g, femoral nerve test,[16] prone knee bend[17], side-lying slump Fig. 33.2h)
   c. lumbar spine (Chapter 29)
   d. SIJ (Chapter 30)
   e. knee jerk reflex (present, strong, endurance)

Key outcome measures
There are currently no patient-reported outcome measures that are specific to anterior thigh pain that can be used to monitor treatment progression. However, the lower extremity functional scale (LEFS) is a reliable (ICC=0.92) and valid questionnaire that can be used to evaluate function for a variety of musculoskeletal conditions, including anterior thigh pain.[18, 19] The LEFS involves rating the difficulty of performing 20 functional activities from 0 (extremely difficult) to 4 (no difficulty). The highest possible score of 80 indicates a high level of function. The LEFS has a minimum detectable change of ±9 points, a standard error of measurement of 4 points and a minimal clinically important difference of ±9 points.[18, 19]

It is important to achieve symmetrical quadriceps strength following an anterior thigh injury. The gold standard measure of quadriceps strength is isokinetic dynamometry; however, few clinicians have access to this equipment. Hand-held dynamometers offer a clinically feasible alternative. Isometric quadriceps strength testing with a hand-held dynamometer has been found to be reliable (ICC=0.96) and to correlate moderately with isokinetic testing (r=0.62).[20] However, due to variability in quadriceps strength between individuals, the minimum detectable change and minimal clinically important difference in quadriceps strength for patients with anterior thigh pain is not known.

Investigations
Investigations are usually not required in athletes with anterior thigh pain, although magnetic resonance imaging (MRI) may have a role in the evaluation of the severity of rectus femoris strains, especially where injuries to the central tendon are suspected.[5, 6]

If a quadriceps contusion fails to respond to treatment, plain radiographs may demonstrate myositis ossificans. This is usually not evident until at least 3 weeks after the injury. Ultrasound examination or MRI will confirm the presence of a haematoma and may demonstrate early evidence of calcification.

If a stress fracture of the femur is suspected, plain radiograph is indicated. If this is normal, an isotopic bone scan or MRI can be ordered to further rule out the condition.

Although hip pathology most often refers to the groin (Chapter 32), it can refer to the anterior and occasionally lateral, thigh. In adults, hip impingement or osteoarthritis are likely diagnoses; in adolescents, consider a slipped capital femoral epiphysis (Chapter 44) or avulsion fracture, particularly when coupled clinically with an abnormal gait pattern. When thigh pain is associated with restricted or painful hip motion, imaging may be indicated.

QUADRICEPS CONTUSION
Quadriceps contusion, known colloquially as 'charley horse' or 'cork thigh', is an extremely common injury caused by blunt trauma to the thigh. The injury affects both the connective tissue and muscle fibres. As the fibres are disrupted during blunt trauma, the intervening space fills up with blood, which later forms clots.

Anterior thigh pain   CHAPTER 33

Table 33.2 Distinguishing features of minor quadriceps contusion and grade I quadriceps muscle strain

Diagnostic features	Quadriceps contusion	Grade I rectus femoris muscle strain
Mechanism	Contact injury	Non-contact
Pain onset	Immediate or soon after	After cool down (next day)
Behaviour of pain (24 hours post-trauma)	Improves with gentle activity	Painful with use
Location	Usually lateral or distal	Rectus femoris muscle belly (proximal or middle-third)
Bruising/swelling	May be obvious early	May be absent or delayed
Palpation findings	Tenderness more obvious, lump may feel ovoid or spherical, becomes progressively harder	May be difficult to find or may be a small area of focal tenderness with a characteristic ring of inflammation surrounding it Muscle spasm in adjacent fibres proximally and distally
Effect of gentle stretch	May initially aggravate pain	Not associated with pain
Strength testing	No loss of strength except pain inhibition	Loss of strength (may need eccentric or functional testing to reproduce pain)

It can sometimes be difficult to distinguish clinically between a contusion and a muscle strain (Table 33.2).

Quadriceps contusion is common in contact sports such as soccer and basketball. In sports such as hockey, lacrosse, and cricket, sporting equipment, such as a hockey stick, ball or puck travelling at high speed may cause a contusion.

Examination confirms an area of tenderness and swelling with worsening pain on active contraction and passive stretch. In severe cases with extensive swelling, pain may be severe enough to interfere with sleep. Assessing the severity of the contusion during the initial assessment is important when planning rehabilitation and return to sport.

Severity can be divided into mild, moderate and severe[21] and an appropriate time to return to sport can vary from several days to a number of weeks.[21-23] The degree of passive knee flexion after 24 hours can be used as a clinical indicator of the severity of the haematoma (Table 33.3).[22]

In severe cases it is important to identify the exact muscle(s) involved. MRI together with ultrasound are the most appropriate investigations.[24] Ultrasonography is useful in determining the precise location of the haematoma.[25, 26] MRI can provide greater insight into the extent and location of the haematoma and may provide greater prognostic value than ultrasound. An example of an MRI of a severe haematoma is shown in Figure 33.3.

Table 33.3 Grading of quadriceps contusion

Severity	Clinical features	Active knee flexion (°)
Mild	May or may not remember incident Usually can continue activity Sore after cooling down or next morning Normal gait, tender on palpation Minimal loss of strength	>90°
Moderate	Usually remembers incident but can continue activity, although may stiffen up with rest (e.g. half-time or full-time) Some pain on contraction Antalgic gait, tender on palpation May have associated knee effusion	45–90°
Severe	Usually remembers incident May not be able to control rapid onset of swelling/bleeding Difficulty with full weight-bearing Tender over large area (tracking) Obvious bleeding Loss of strength and function	<45°

PART B   Regional problems

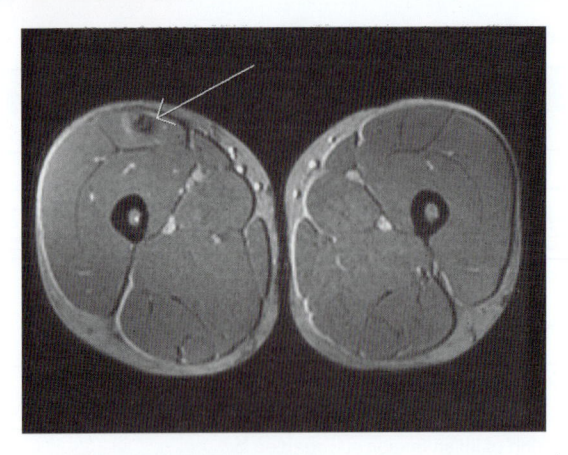

Figure 33.3 MRI appearance of severe haematoma (arrow) of the vastus intermedius muscle

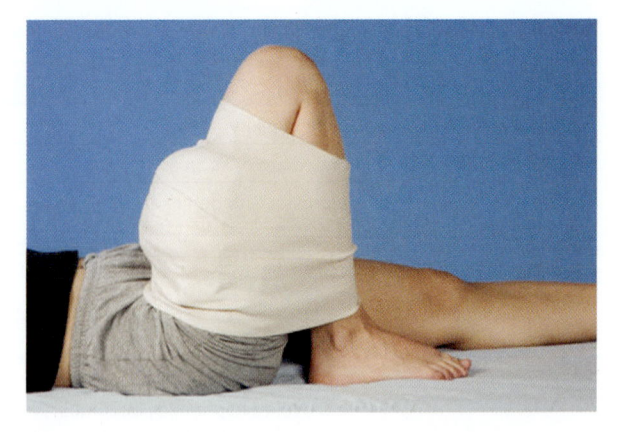

Figure 33.4 Ice and compression treatment of an acute thigh contusion in a position of maximal pain-free stretch

It is important to appreciate that blood from contusions of the lower third of the thigh may track down to the knee joint and irritate the patellofemoral joint. This has been demonstrated in a study of quadriceps contusion in rugby players.[27] Quadriceps circumference and the knee brush/swipe test, used to detect swelling around the knee, were associated with greater recovery time, more missed games and a greater number of treatments sought.

Treatment of quadriceps contusion

The most important period in the treatment of a thigh contusion is the first 24 hours following the injury. A player who suffers a thigh contusion should be removed from the field of play and receive the POLICE regimen (Chapter 17). If full weight-bearing is painful, crutches can help unload the muscle and can emphasise the serious nature of the condition to the athlete, team mates and coaches.[22] Generally the treatment of a thigh contusion can be divided into four stages:

- stage 1–control of haemorrhage
- stage 2–restoration of pain-free range of motion
- stage 3–functional rehabilitation
- stage 4–graduated return to activity.

A summary of the types of treatment appropriate for each stage is shown in Table 33.4. Progression within each stage, and from one stage to the next, depends on the severity of the contusion and the rate of recovery. For severe contusions, regular ice and compression over 2–3 days should be commenced straightaway. Massage, electrotherapy and stretching should be avoided in the first 3 days. After the initial period, electrotherapy with non-thermal effects (e.g. pulsed ultrasound) may be considered; however, evidence of the effectiveness of such interventions continues to be limited.[28, 29]

> **PRACTICE PEARL**
>
> In the acute management of a thigh contusion, ice should be applied in a position of maximal pain-free quadriceps stretch (Fig. 33.4). Immobilising the knee in 120° of flexion immediately after injury and for the first 24 hours may be beneficial.[30] This is done by bandaging the entire lower limb. The patient then mobilises with crutches.

In the first 7–10 days after a moderate-to-severe contusion there is a considerable risk of re-bleed. The athlete must be careful not to aggravate the bleeding by excessive activity, alcohol ingestion or the application of heat. Care should also be taken with stretching and it should be pain-free in the initial stages. The aim of soft tissue therapy in the first few days after a thigh contusion is to promote lymphatic drainage. Excessively painful soft tissue therapy will cause bleeding to recur and is contraindicated for 48 hours following contusion.

Loss of range of motion is the most significant finding after thigh contusion and range of movement must be regained in a gradual, pain-free progression before return to athletic activity is considered. In a study of military cadets, Ryan et al. found average disability times of 13 days for mild contusions, 19 days for moderate contusions and 21 days for severe contusions.[22]

Protective padding, such as thigh pads and athletic pants with removable pads, may help attenuate direct contact forces to the anterior thigh. It has been suggested that athletes in high-risk sports should consider wearing thigh-protective padding routinely.[31] Players such as ruckmen in Australian rules football, forwards in

Anterior thigh pain CHAPTER 33

Table 33.4 Treatment of moderate quadriceps contusion or grade II muscle strain

Stage	Weight-bearing	Acute management	Soft tissue therapy	Stretching	Strengthening
1. Control haemorrhage	Crutches if FWB	POLICE, compression to include knee joint if lower-third of thigh (Fig. 33.4)	Contraindicated	Gentle active stretch to onset of pain (no hold of stretch) (Fig. 33.5a)	Static muscle contraction if pain-free
2. Restore pain-free range of motion	Progress to WB and FWB as tolerated	Maintain compression bandage when limb is dependent. Ice after exercise	Grade I–II longitudinal gliding away from site of injury. Grade II transverse gliding away from site of injury	Increase active stretches to passive stretches to regain ROM	Static muscle contraction, inner-range to through-range (Fig. 33.6a). Stationary exercise: bike. Pool: pain-free (walk/swim/kick). Concentric and eccentric exercises (Fig. 33.6b), reverse Nordics (Fig. 33.6c)
3. Functional rehabilitation	FWB	NA	Longitudinal gliding. Transverse gliding	Maintain stretch (Fig. 33.5b)	All stage 2 exercises gradually increasing repetitions, speed and resistance. Include pulleys, rebounder, profitter, wall squats, step-downs (Fig. 33.6d). Hopping/jumping, running. Increase eccentric exercises
4. Graduated return to sport	FWB	NA	Myofascial release techniques in knee flexion (Fig. 33.7)		Kicking action with pulleys. Multidirectional activities. Figure of eight. Jumping. Plyometrics. Graduated specific sporting activities. Must complete full training before return to sport. Heat-retaining brace may be helpful

ROM = range of motion; PWB = partial weight-bearing; FWB = full weight-bearing

667

PART B   Regional problems

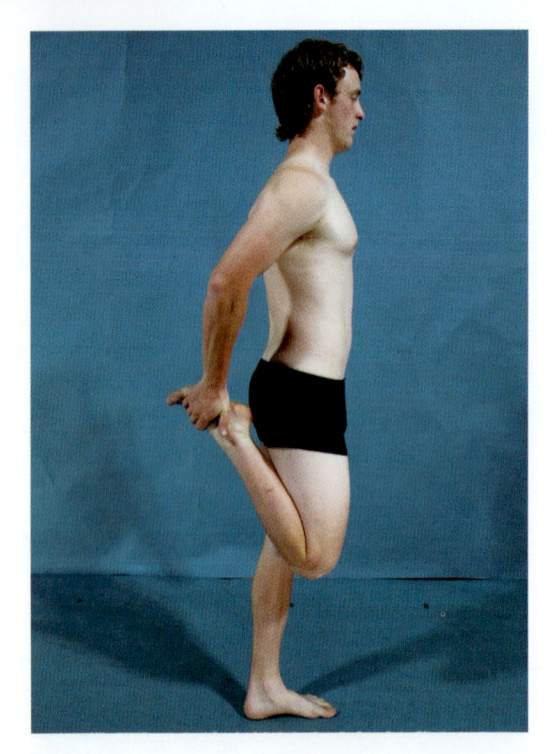

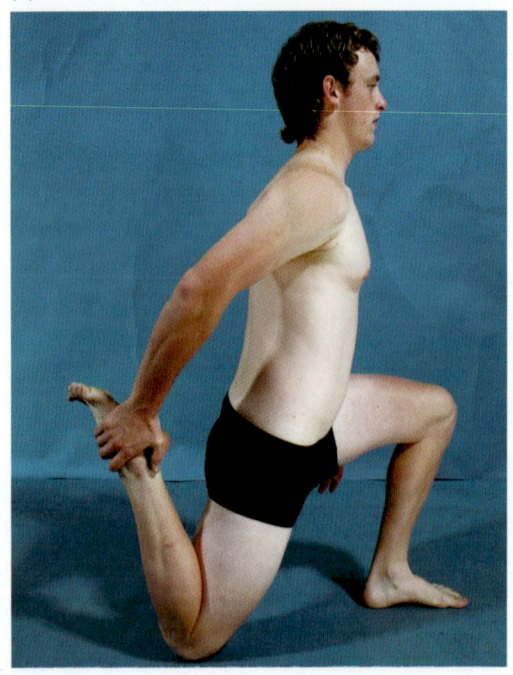

Figure 33.5 Quadriceps stretching exercises (a) Standard quadriceps stretch while standing. It is important to have good pelvic control and not to lean forward while performing the stretch (b) Passive stretch. The tension of the stretch can be altered by adding hip extension

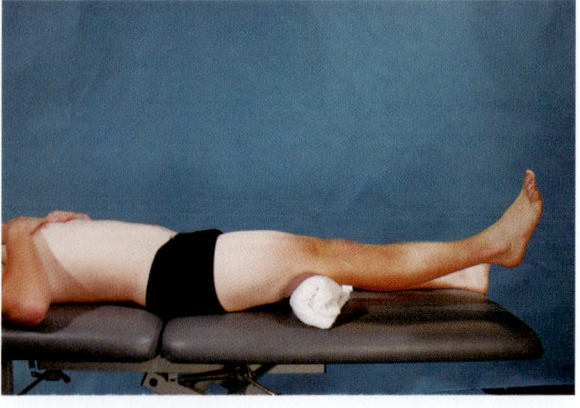

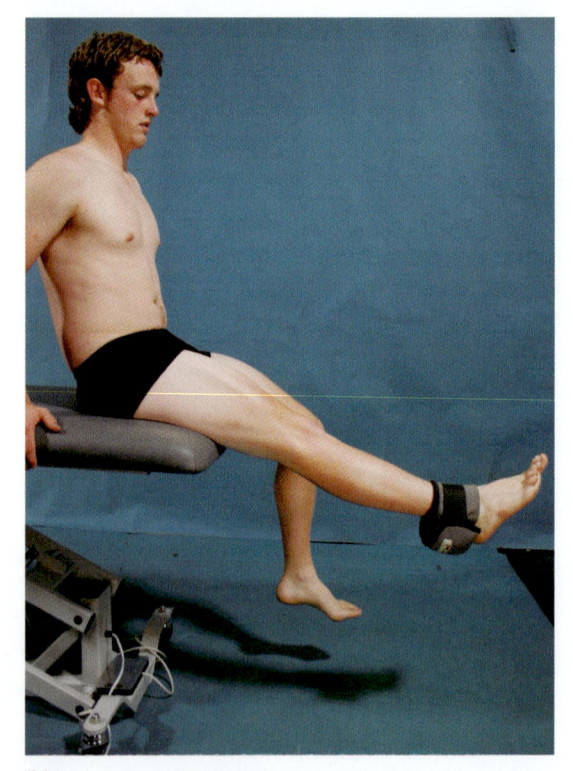

Figure 33.6 Quadriceps strengthening exercises (a) Active quadriceps exercises. Initially inner-range quadriceps strengthening is performed with a rolled towel under the knee as shown. The range is slowly increased, depending on symptoms, until through-range quadriceps contraction can be performed without pain (b) Resisted quadriceps. Concentric and eccentric exercises are performed against gradually increased resistance. Knee extension involves concentric contraction of the quadriceps muscle, while lowering the foot from extension involves eccentric quadriceps contraction

Anterior thigh pain　　CHAPTER 33

(c-i)

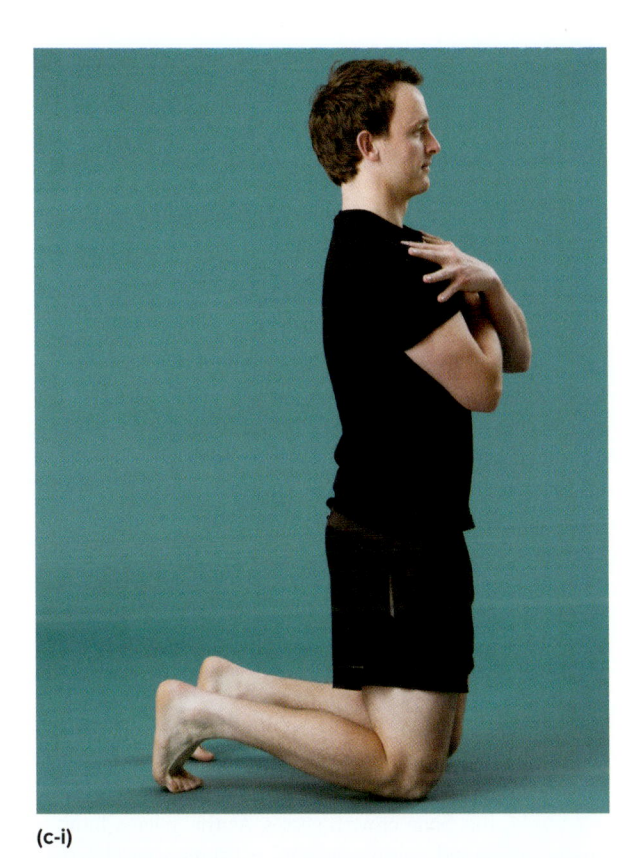

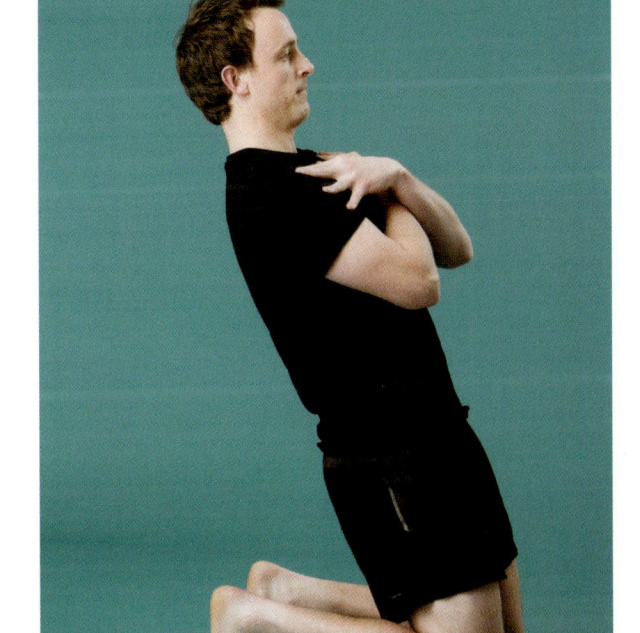

(c-ii)

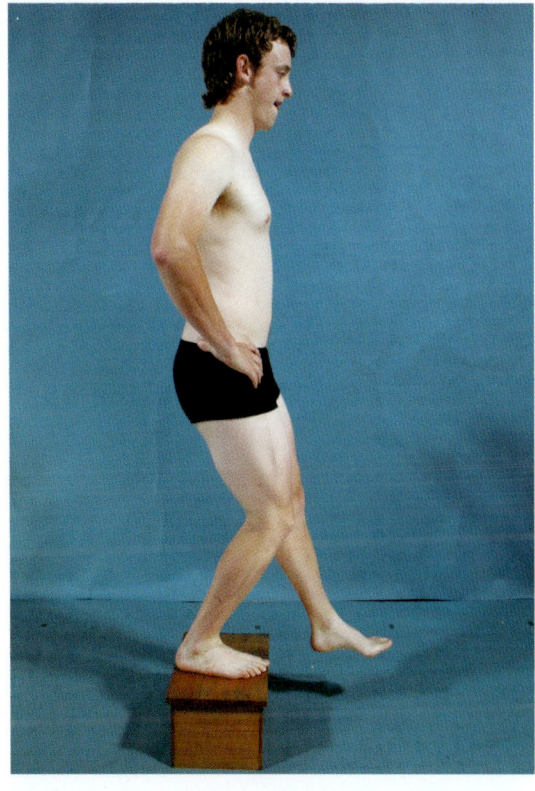

(d)

Figure 33.6 (cont.) (c) (i) and (ii) Reverse Nordics. Similar to the hamstring Nordic curl exercise but in the opposite direction. Subject/athlete starts in a kneeling upright position (i). The subject/athlete goes as far as they can (ii) until feeling a stretch in anterior thigh or until they cannot maintain neutral trunk position. Focus is placed on the knee being the pivot point while maintaining neutral trunk position throughout exercise (i.e. not breaking at the hips or increasing lumbar lordosis). Exercise can be performed either with ankles in full plantar flexion or on toes. Progressions include arms outstretched with hand weights or arms over head with a medicine ball (d) Functional exercises. A variety of functional exercises can be performed in the late stage of rehabilitation: squats, wall squats, stepdowns (shown), shuttle. Most of these involve both eccentric and concentric contraction of the quadriceps

basketball, and running backs in American football may sustain a series of minor contusions during the course of a game, which may have a cumulative effect and impair performance. Protective padding may help to reduce the severity of contusions; however, evidence for its effectiveness is currently limited.

PART B   Regional problems

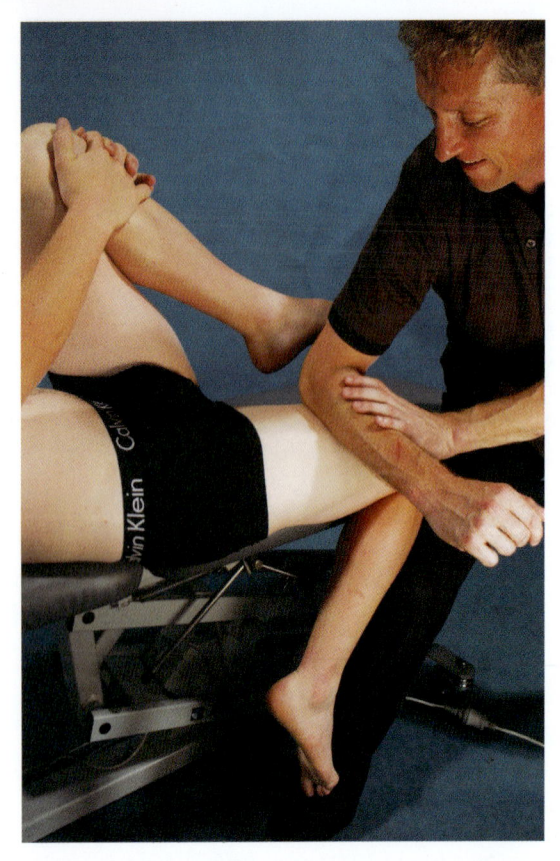

Figure 33.7 Soft tissue therapy—sustained myofascial tension in the position of maximal hip extension and knee flexion

Complications related to contusion

Compartment syndrome of the thigh

Intramuscular haematoma of the thigh after a blunt contusion may result in high intra-compartmental pressures and a diagnosis of compartment syndrome of the thigh. Symptoms often include pain and paraesthesia, and occur with intra-compartmental pressures greater than approximately 20 mmHg.[32] Pressures of greater than 30 mmHg over a duration of more than 6 hours can lead to irreversible damage.[32, 33] Unlike other compartment syndromes, there is no evidence that this condition needs to be treated by surgical decompression unless it occurs in conjunction with other significant injuries or medical conditions, for example fractured femur, coagulation defects.[33] A number of cases of surgery have been reported, but none described necrotic muscle or subsequent clinical evidence of muscle fibrosis, restriction of knee motion or loss of function.[34]

A case study detailing conservative management of an amateur soccer player who sustained a high-impact injury from an opposing player has been published.[32] Conservative treatment included rest from any lower limb activity for the first 48 hours followed by gentle range of motion exercises of the hip and knee. This routine was slowly progressed over the following months and the athlete returned to soccer after 6 months. Success with conservative treatment can be achievable, but often requires a prolonged rehabilitation period.[32]

Myositis ossificans

Occasionally, after a thigh contusion, the haematoma calcifies; that is, osteoblasts replace some of the fibroblasts in the healing haematoma and bone tissue is deposited within the muscle. This condition is known as myositis ossificans. The estimated incidence of myositis ossificans following a thigh contusion ranges from 9% to 20%.[35] It is unclear why some contusions develop calcification and others do not; however, the more severe the contusion, the more likely that an athlete will develop myositis ossificans.[35] Intramuscular contusions appear to be more susceptible to the development of myositis ossificans than intermuscular contusions.

In the acute phase, that is, the first week following the injury, there is a proliferation of fibroblasts into the area of injury.[36] The following 10 days, the sub-acute phase, are characterised by the infiltration of osteoblasts. In the final stage, bone is deposited within the muscle. By approximately 6–7 weeks, this bone growth ceases. At this stage a lump is often palpable and a plain radiograph (Chapter 3, Fig. 3.7a) can help to confirm the diagnosis. Ultrasound can demonstrate the myositis ossificans (Fig. 33.8a) however, MRI (Fig. 33.8b) is more sensitive in detecting the inflammatory oedema that precedes myositis ossificans and therefore may be more useful in the early stages.[36]

Symptoms of myositis ossificans include ongoing pain in the injured area, morning or night pain, decreased range of motion, local tenderness, stiffness and a palpable mass.[37] On palpation, the developing myositis ossificans has a characteristic 'woody' feel. If there is no convincing history of recent trauma, the practitioner must rule out differential diagnoses such as tumours (Chapter 7).[38]

The risk of myositis ossificans is especially high if the contusion results in prone knee flexion of less than 45° 2–3 days after the injury. Thus, particular care should be taken when managing a severe thigh contusion, as a significant re-bleed may result in the development of myositis ossificans. Inappropriate treatment after muscle injury, such as heat, massage and forced stretching, may increase the risk of developing myositis ossificans.[39] The incidence of myositis ossificans appears to be increased when a knee effusion is present.

Once myositis ossificans is established, there is very little that can be done to accelerate the resorption process. Treatment may include local electrotherapy to

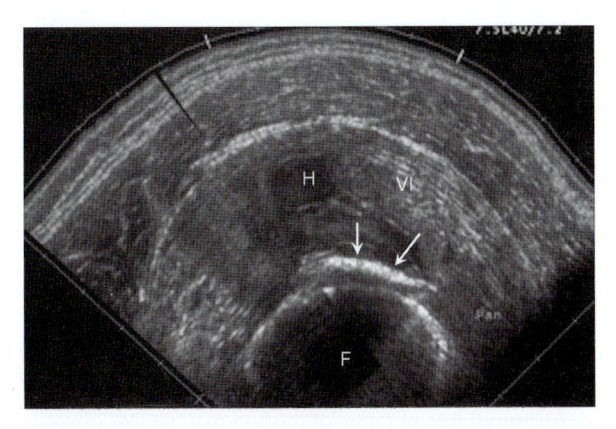

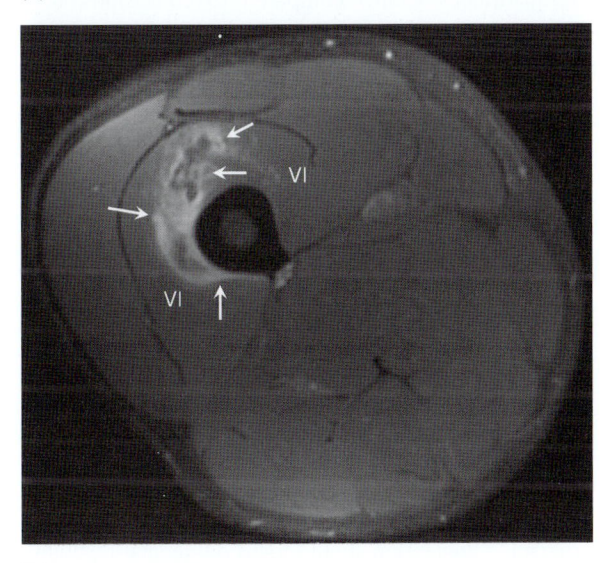

Anterior thigh pain   CHAPTER 33

high-risk presentations such as severe contusions or those close to bone.[35] A corticosteroid injection is absolutely contraindicated in this condition. Surgery is contraindicated in the early stages and only considered when the margins of the ectopic bone are smooth on investigation, suggesting bone maturity. It must be noted that surgery can lead to recurrence post-surgery.[35]

QUADRICEPS STRAIN

Strains of the quadriceps muscles are common and usually occur during sprinting, jumping or kicking. Fatigue, weakness, muscle imbalance and sprinting/kicking sports are proposed risk factors for quadriceps strains.

In soccer, quadriceps strains are often associated with over-striding when decelerating during running or under-striding during the deceleration phase of the kicking leg when kicking a ball on the run.[45] Among professional soccer players, quadriceps muscle injuries cause more missed games than hamstring and groin muscle injuries, and re-injury rates are high.[3] Strains are most common in the rectus femoris muscle, which is more vulnerable to strain than the other quadriceps muscles, because it passes over two joints–the hip and the knee.

Figure 33.8 Myositis ossificans (a) Ultrasound appearance 6 weeks after injury showing resolving haemorrhage (H) in the vastus intermedius (VI) with development of ossification (arrows). F = femur (b) MRI appearance with fluid and oedema (arrows) in the vastus intermedius

(A) AND (B) IMAGING IN SPORTS-SPECIFIC MUSCULOSKELETAL INJURIES, 2016, P.81, ALI GUERMAZI, FRANK W ROEMER, MICHEL D CREMA. © SPRINGER INTERNATIONAL PUBLISHING SWITZERLAND 2016. WITH PERMISSION OF SPRINGER

> **PRACTICE PEARL**
>
> The most common site of strain is the distal musculo-tendinous junction of the rectus femoris (see below). Management of this type of rectus femoris strain and of strains of the vasti muscles is relatively straightforward; rehabilitation time is short. Strains of the proximal rectus femoris are not as straightforward and are considered in a separate section later in the chapter.

reduce muscle spasm and gentle, painless range of motion exercises. Shock wave therapy has been suggested to improve function for patients with myositis ossificans; however, evidence for its effectiveness is limited.[40, 41] Acetic acid iontophoresis has been shown to be helpful in two case studies,[42, 43] while one case study described the intravenous use of bisphosphonate pamidronate.[44] However, neither method is widely used.

Indomethacin, which reduces new bone formation, has been prescribed as a preventative measure in

Distal quadriceps muscle strain

The grading of muscle strains such as distal quadriceps strains (Fig. 33.9a) has recently been reviewed and is discussed in Chapter 3. The athlete feels the injury as a sudden pain in the anterior thigh during an activity requiring explosive muscle contraction. There is local pain and tenderness, pain on stretching and resisted knee extension, and, if the strain is severe, swelling and bruising. If the athlete reports burning or paraesthesia, assessment should rule out femoral nerve injury and neural mechanosensitivity.

Pain on resisted active contraction and on passive stretching are typical signs in quadriceps strains. An area of local spasm is palpable at the site of pain.

Complete tears of the rectus femoris occur with sudden onset of pain and disability during intense

671

PART B Regional problems

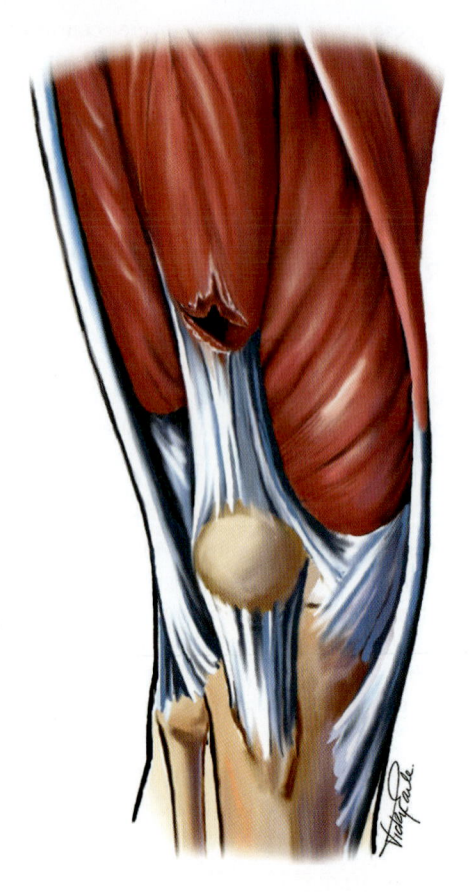

activity. A muscle fibre defect is usually palpable when the muscle is contracted. In the long term, they resolve with conservative management, often with surprisingly little disability.[46]

Treatment

The principles of treatment of a quadriceps muscle strain are similar to those of a thigh contusion. The various treatment techniques shown in Table 33.4 are appropriate for the treatment of quadriceps strain; however, progression through the various stages may be slower for more severe injuries.

Although loss of range of motion may be less obvious for quadriceps strains compared to contusions, it is important that the athlete regains pain-free range of movement as soon as possible. Loss of strength may be more marked than with a thigh contusion and strength retraining should be emphasised in the rehabilitation program, with respect to the stage of healing. As with the general principles of muscle rehabilitation, the program should commence with low-resistance, high-repetition concentric strengthening exercises, and progress to higher resistance and eccentric strengthening exercises.

General fitness can be maintained by activities such as swimming (initially with a pool buoy) and upper body training. Functional retraining such as running and kicking should be incorporated as soon as it is safe to do so. Full training must be completed prior to return to sport. Unfortunately, quadriceps strains often recur; therefore, it is important to maintain an ongoing preventative program.[47] Prevention should focus on general flexibility of muscles of the thigh and leg, adequate balance of concentric and eccentric strength of the hip flexors and knee extensors and adequate core stability. Exercises based on deceleration under specific sport situations should be included in prevention programs for rectus femoris muscle injuries.

Proximal rectus femoris strain

Strains of the proximal rectus femoris (Fig. 33.9b) can occur either at the conjoint tendon or at the deep musculotendinous junction of the indirect head.[5, 7, 48] A strain occurring at this musculotendinous junction has a worse prognosis than one occurring peripherally in the muscle belly.

Diagnosis of these deeper injuries is difficult because the physical assessment findings are often inconclusive. MRI can help diagnosis in this instance and demonstrates what is termed a 'bull's eye lesion'[49] (Fig. 33.10). A bull's eye lesion is present when a disruption is seen around the deep part of the proximal tendon.

Figure 33.9 Two types of quadriceps strains (a) The more common occurs at the distal musculotendinous junction of rectus femoris and has a better prognosis (b) The less common occurs in the proximal rectus femoris and takes longer to repair
ADAPTED FROM HASSELMAN ET AL. P.495

Management of proximal rectus femoris strains is influenced by the location and severity of the injury, and the age and athletic demands of the individual. Most proximal rectus femoris strains are managed conservatively and surgical intervention is typically reserved for injuries that involve significant damage to the central tendon (Fig. 33.9). Conservative management aimed at symptom relief and avoidance of re-injury is recommended for most strains.

A study involving 10 professional soccer players reported that players took an average of 3.8 months to return to full training and playing after surgery.[50] Another study reported that professional Australian rules footballers took an average of 27 days to return to full training following central tendon lesions compared to 9 days for peripheral rectus femoris strains and 4.5 days for strains of the vasti muscles.[51]

The use of platelet-rich plasma (PRP) injections has been suggested for these recalcitrant injuries. This treatment is discussed more fully in Chapter 17. There is little evidence for its efficacy in the treatment of muscle injuries.

Complete rectus femoris tear

Complete tears of the rectus femoris muscle are uncommon due to the length of the musculotendinous junction (approximately two-thirds of the muscle belly).[5] In three case studies of complete rectus femoris tears the time from injury to when the athlete sought treatment ranged from 5–7 months.[51]

The initial injury may be described as a deep tearing sensation. Patients complain of a tender anterior thigh mass, and weakness and/or pain with activities such as running and kicking. The anterior thigh mass may be associated with muscle retraction.[5] These signs and symptoms are likely due to the indirect (central tendon) and direct heads of the proximal tendon acting independently, creating a shearing phenomenon in contrast to what occurs in the normal rectus femoris.[8] Unlike typical strains, which present as focal lesions on MRI, rectus femoris proximal musculotendinous junction injuries have a longitudinal distribution of increased signal along the tendon (Fig. 33.10).[5]

Avulsion injury

Adolescent athletes participating in sports that involve sprinting may sustain an avulsion injury of the anterior inferior iliac spine (AIIS)–the proximal attachment of the direct head of the rectus femoris muscle. These injuries are uncommon in skeletally mature athletes. Patients with greater than 2 cm displacement of the fragment from the AIIS, as determined by X-ray, may require surgery. However, most patients do not require surgery and return to sport after 10–12 weeks.[52]

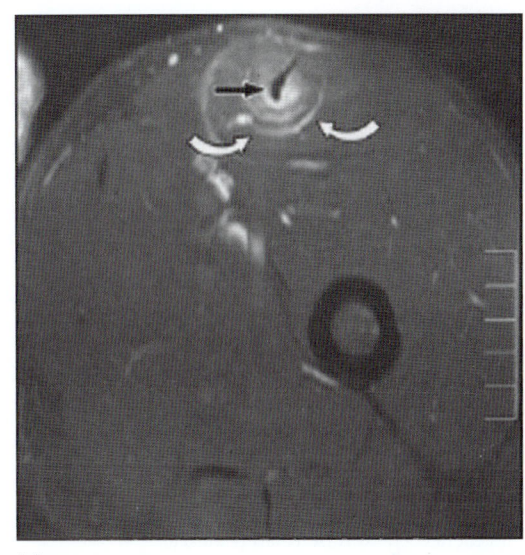

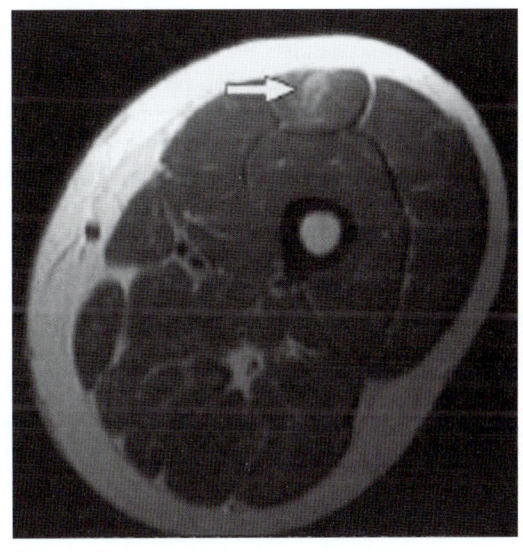

Figure 33.10 MRI of the proximal rectus femoris musculotendinous junction (a) MRI of a proximal rectus femoris tear in a 19-year-old man shows the characteristic 'bull's-eye' sign; this is made up of a halo of increased signal (white signal highlighted by white arrows) around the deep tendon (black tendon highlighted with a black arrow) (b) A comparable MRI of a similar injury, which differs only in the tendon having a low-signal intensity inside the bright halo (arrow). This is consistent with fatty atrophy in the tendon—the results of the injury having occurred a reasonable time in the past (chronic)

Injury to the indirect head of rectus femoris may be associated with concomitant injury to the hip joint labrum; or a HALTAR lesion (Hip Anterosuperior Labral Tear with Avulsion of Rectus femoris).[52] This injury has been described in both skeletally mature and skeletally immature athletes and is analogous with the SLAP lesion of the shoulder (Chapter 24). Athletes with rectus femoris injuries who do not progress as expected through rehabilitation may have sustained a concomitant hip labral injury and may require further investigation.

Prevention

Warming up to reduce the risk of injury is common practice in sport. Stretching is commonly performed as part of the warm-up by athletes; however, recent evidence suggests that static stretching does *not* reduce the incidence of exercise-related injury.[53-56]

Furthermore, static stretching has been associated with impairments in muscular performance, particularly in the quadriceps and hamstring muscle groups.[54, 57, 58] On the other hand, studies have shown that dynamic stretching can enhance muscular performance, but as yet, no consensus exists on the most appropriate exercise parameters (e.g. duration and frequency).[57, 59-61] Dynamic stretches for the anterior thigh muscles can include walking quadriceps stretches, high knee pulls, forward leg swings, walking lunges and various running drills.

In addition to integrating dynamic stretching into the athlete's warm up, stretching and mobility exercises may also need to be addressed after and between training sessions and games. Prevention strategies for rectus femoris injuries include improving general flexibility of muscles of the thigh and leg, and a focus on both concentric and eccentric strength of the hip flexors and knee extensors.

The iliopsoas muscle has a mechanical relationship with the femoral nerve. If the iliopsoas muscle becomes restricted, the mobility of the femoral nerve may also be affected, in the same way that hamstring muscle restrictions can affect the mobility of the sciatic nerve (Chapter 34). Similarly, because the iliopsoas muscle functions synergistically with the rectus femoris in sprinting and kicking, iliopsoas weakness may increase the demand placed on the rectus femoris muscle.[7]

> **PRACTICE PEARL**
>
> Flexibility and strengthening programs should address both the rectus femoris and the iliopsoas muscles, rather than considering these muscles in isolation.[7]

In sprinting, the risk for rectus femoris injuries may be highest during the acceleration (eccentric muscle actions in the early swing phase) and deceleration phases. Exercises that simulate this eccentric loading should therefore be included in prevention programs for rectus femoris muscle injuries. Exercises such as the reverse Nordic curl (Fig. 33.6c), forward deceleration and reverse lunge (with/without overhead medicine ball, Fig. 33.11) may improve the capacity of the rectus femoris to tolerate eccentric loads during sport.[7]

Adequate core strength and activation is necessary to counteract torsional forces of the spine, pelvis, and lower limb, particularly during kicking and changing direction. Preventative programs should therefore emphasise strength and activation of the trunk and gluteal muscles, using both isolated and functional tasks.

LESS COMMON CAUSES

Stress fracture of the femur

Stress fractures are common in the athletic population and are categorised as overuse injuries (Chapter 4). Femoral stress fractures can occur around the femoral neck, intertrochanteric and subtrochanteric regions (Chapter 32), and the femoral shaft.[62] Stress fractures in the distal femur can occur following anterior cruciate ligament (ACL) reconstruction surgery using transfemoral fixation and may be more common in athletes using accelerated rehabilitation programs.[63, 64] Stress fracture of the shaft of the femur should be suspected in an athlete, especially a long distance runner, who complains of a dull and poorly localised ache in the anterior thigh.[14]

Risk factors for developing femoral stress fractures include training errors, hard training surfaces (e.g. concrete), and poor footwear (ill-fitting, worn and inflexible such as military boots).[62, 65] Intrinsic risk factors include leg length discrepancies and excessive foot pronation or supination.[65]

Pain may be referred to the groin or knee and the athlete may present with an antalgic gait (especially in the case of femoral neck stress fractures).[66] Clinical assessment should include an assessment of lower limb alignment, particularly leg length and foot posture. Local tenderness, warmth and swelling may be present. The fulcrum test is a pain-provocation test that can be used to confirm the diagnosis (Fig. 33.2f).

Plain radiography may not be sensitive enough to detect changes in bone structure in the initial stages of a femoral stress fracture; however, MRI (Fig. 33.12) has excellent specificity (100%) and sensitivity (86–100%) for identifying femoral stress fractures.[65] Isotopic bone scans have excellent sensitivity (74–84%) but poor specificity (33%).[65, 67]

Anterior thigh pain CHAPTER 33

(a) (b)

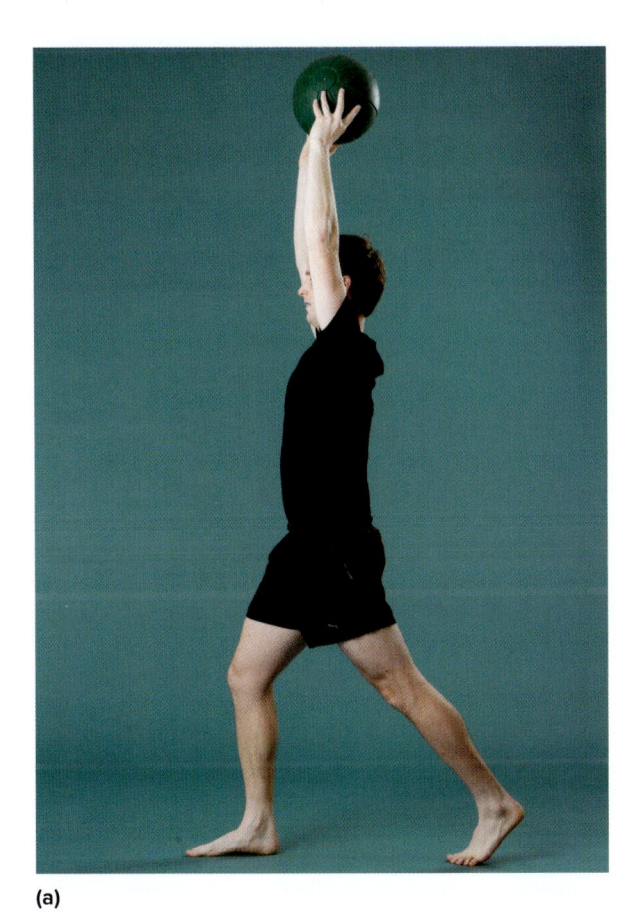

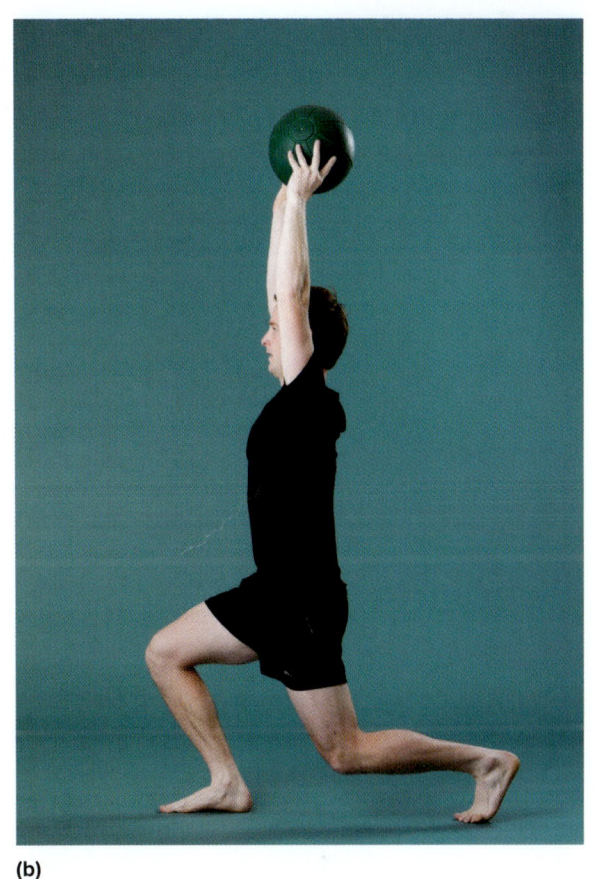

Figure 33.11 Reverse lunge with overhead medicine ball: Subject starts in a comfortable split lunge position (a), medicine ball over head. Subject then performs a backwards lunge (b), focusing on placing weight through the behind leg until thigh is vertical. The knee should remain behind the toes of the forward leg

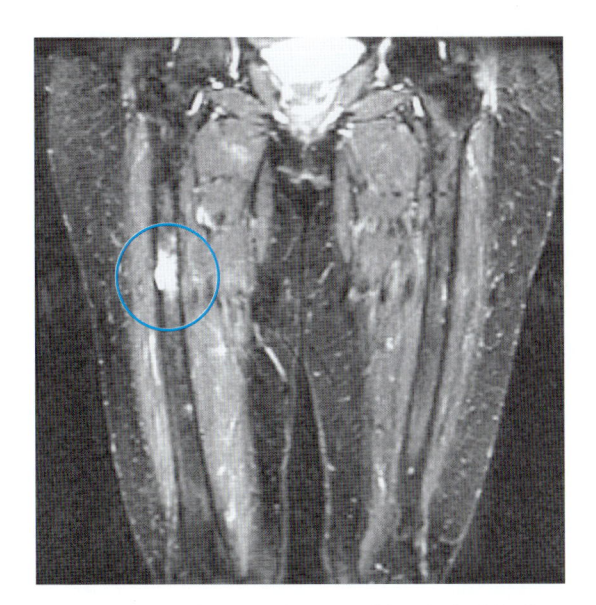

Figure 33.12 MRI of a stress fracture of the shaft of the femur

False positives associated with bone scans include bone infections and tumours. Differentiating between a bone stress reaction and a stress fracture on a bone scan can be challenging because the size of the uptake on the scan may not correlate with the magnitude of the pathology.

Stress fractures are more prevalent among female athletes. The 'female athlete triad', discussed in Chapter 4, is a specific risk factor of stress fractures in females (low energy availability with or without disordered eating, menstrual dysfunction and low bone mineral density).[68, 69]

> **PRACTICE PEARL**
>
> There may be tenderness over the shaft of the femur that can be aggravated if the patient sits with the leg hanging over the edge of a bench, particularly if there is downward pressure placed on the distal femur, the so-called 'hang test' or 'fulcrum test' (Fig. 33.2f).

Treatment of femoral stress fractures depends on the location and type of fracture, but all treatment should initially involve rest from painful activities and maintenance of aerobic fitness with cycling, deep water running or swimming. Weight-bearing as tolerated is often permitted; however, cam boots and crutches may be considered for athletes who are unable to weight bear without pain. Underwater and anti-gravity treadmills may be beneficial for these athletes.[70] Surgery is indicated where a fracture has become displaced.

When the fulcrum test is completely negative, on average after 7 weeks, it is thought to be safe to initiate return-to-sport progressions in rehabilitation.[15] To avoid associated complications, such as a complete fracture, bone healing must be confirmed before the athlete returns to play.[9]

In females with stress fractures, menstrual disturbance information should be sought and corrected where possible through the aid of bone mineral density tests and endocrine function tests. Nutritional input may be considered for those identified with eating disorders.

Lateral femoral cutaneous nerve injury ('meralgia paraesthetica')

Lateral cutaneous nerve of thigh (LFCN) injury, also known as 'meralgia paraesthetica', can be a cause of anterolateral thigh pain.

Anatomy

The LFCN is a sensory nerve that originates from the lumbar plexus (L2, L3 spinal nerves) and runs along the lateral border of the psoas major muscle, across the iliacus muscle, and exits the abdomen under the inguinal ligament close to the anterior superior iliac spine (ASIS). From here it crosses the sartorius muscle and divides into anterior and posterior branches.

The posterior branch pierces the fascia lata and runs distally supplying the skin of the lateral thigh from the greater trochanter to mid-thigh region. The anterior branch supplies the skin approximately 10 cm below the inguinal ligament and distally to the proximal knee. It should be noted that the anatomical course can have many variations between individuals and is susceptible to compression injury where it exits the pelvis.[71]

Clinical biomechanics

Repeated hip flexion and extension during sporting activity (e.g. gymnastics) can irritate the nerve, and entrapment can occur around the ASIS between the ilium and the inguinal ligament.[72] Obesity and pregnancy increase intra-abdominal pressure and can compress the nerve via the distended abdomen where the nerve leaves the pelvis.[73] Tight-fitting garments and athletic compression garments can lead to symptoms. Entrapment as a result of wearing weight belts in scuba divers has also been reported.[74]

The LFCN is susceptible to injury via blunt trauma around the ASIS and the anterior thigh, especially in contact sports such as rugby.[72] Repeated falls from a balance beam in gymnastics may also cause injury.[74] Surgical procedures are a risk factor for LFCN injury, irritation and entrapment.[32, 75, 76] Injury to the LFCN has been reported following hip arthroscopy because this nerve lies approximately 3 mm from the anterior portal.

Clinical features

Symptoms include pain, burning, numbness, and paraesthesia of the anterolateral thigh without loss of reflex or motor control.[74, 75] Sporting activity can aggravate symptoms, while sitting may alleviate symptoms by altering the length and tension within the nerve and associated tissues.[71, 72, 77] Differential diagnoses include femoral nerve injury and referred pain (discussed below). Sensory changes and symptoms exacerbated by hip extension can help to confirm the diagnosis.[71]

Management

Treatment is often conservative, with a period of rest and manual therapy until symptoms have resolved. One case series has suggested that Kinesio taping is beneficial, but evidence continues to be limited.[78] Anti-inflammatory medications can be beneficial in the early phases.[75] If symptoms do not settle quickly, other interventions such as a local injection of corticosteroid and surgical interventions (either nerve decompression or neurectomy) can be considered, but these interventions currently have limited evidence.[73] Thigh and hip pads can be used as preventative strategy in high-contact sports.[72]

Femoral nerve injury

The femoral nerve passes between the psoas major and the iliacus muscles and exits the abdomen deep to the inguinal ligament through the femoral canal. In the upper thigh, the nerve gives off motor branches to the quadriceps, sartorius and pectineus muscles. The sensory branches supply the skin of the anterior thigh. The femoral nerve then continues distally as the saphenous nerve.

Injury to the nerve can occur secondary to hyperextension of the hip, such as seen in gymnasts, dancers, soccer players, basketball players and long jumpers.[72, 74] Gymnasts and dancers performing manoeuvres that involve extreme hip extension coupled with knee flexion are susceptible to femoral nerve injury.[74]

Previously, injury was thought to be due to traction placed on the nerve. However, it is now thought to be secondary to muscle strain of the iliopsoas muscle, where

Anterior thigh pain CHAPTER 33

the local haematoma causes compression of the nerve.[72, 74] Psoas bursitis can also lead to compression and irritation.[74]

Pain is often located around the inguinal region. Reduced power of the knee extensors and/or reduced knee jerk may also be present.[72, 74] Sometimes, despite motor changes, sensation can be normal.[74]

Conservative treatment is normally trialled first until symptoms settle. Return to sport is possible when strength in the lower limb is regained.

Referred pain

Referred pain may arise from the hip joint, SIJ, lumbar spine (especially upper lumbar) and neural structures. Patients with referred pain may not have a history of injury and may have few signs suggesting local abnormalities. An increase in neural mechanosensitivity may suggest that referred pain is contributing to thigh pain. The modified Thomas' test (Fig. 33.2g) is the most specific neurodynamic tension test for a patient with anterior thigh pain.

If the modified Thomas' test reproduces anterior thigh pain and altering the neural mechanosensitivity (e.g. passive knee flexion/extension) affects the pain, the lumbar spine and psoas muscle should be examined carefully. Any areas of abnormality should be treated and both the local signs (e.g. reproduction of pain with functional testing) and neurodynamic tests should be repeated to assess any changes. The slump knee bend test (side-lying slump) (Fig. 33.2h) has good reliability, excellent sensitivity and specificity, and can be used in patients with suspected lumbosacral radicular pain.[16, 79] The test is considered positive if the symptoms can be reproduced and if the intensity of the symptoms can be influenced by changing the nerve tension.[16]

As with any soft tissue injury, local and referred factors may contribute to the patient's symptoms. Commonly there is hypomobility of the upper lumbar intervertebral segments on the affected side associated with a tight psoas muscle. Mobilisation of the hypomobile segments and/or deep soft tissue treatment to the psoas muscle will often reduce symptoms (Fig. 33.13).

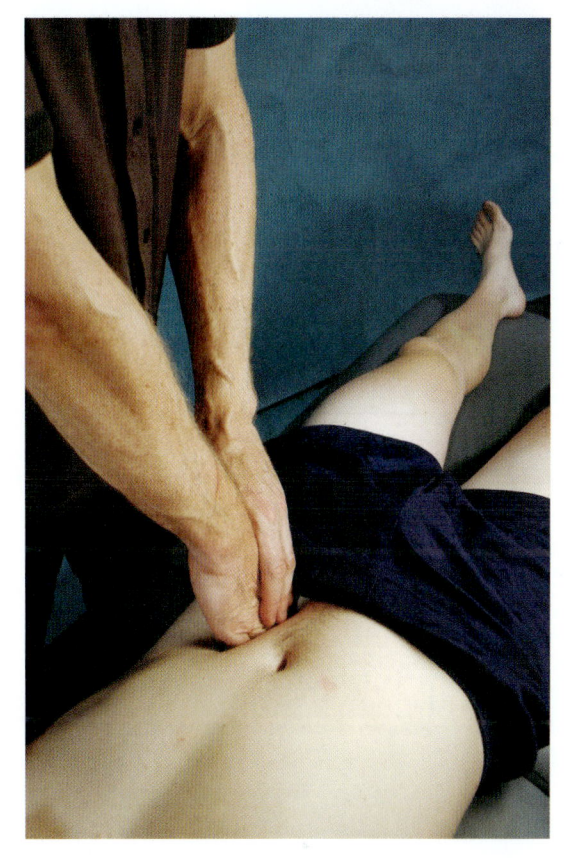

Figure 33.13 Deep soft tissue treatment to the psoas muscle

REFERENCES

References for this chapter can be found at www.mhhe.com/au/CSM5e

Chapter 34

Posterior thigh pain

with CARL ASKLING and ANTHONY SCHACHE

You know, this is a different hamstring–I did my left hamstring, I've done the right side of my back, I've just done my right hammy . . . obviously I've got injury concerns at the moment, now I have to go back and do what the experts tell me to give myself the best chance of being fully fit.

Michael Clarke, Australian cricket captain, December 2014

Pain in the 'hamstring region' can prove very frustrating for recreational and amateur athletes and may be career threatening for professional athletes. Hamstring muscle strains are the most common cause of posterior thigh pain, but referred pain to this area is also common. The average number of days until return to play (RTP) for hamstring injuries depends on the severity of the injury, but has been found to range between 18-60 days in elite level soccer players.[1]

The incidence of recurrence is high. Up to one-third of hamstring injuries will recur, with the greatest risk being during the initial 2 weeks following return to sport.[2]

In this chapter, we focus on:

- relevant anatomy which is critical to diagnosis, prognosis and management
- clinical distinction between the major pathologies in the patient with posterior thigh pain
- the role of diagnostic imaging for this injury
- treatment approaches for the two types of acute hamstring injuries and for referred pain
- the indications for considering early or late surgical treatment
- how to make the often difficult return-to-play decision
- preventing the rightfully feared setback–hamstring strain recurrence.

FUNCTIONAL ANATOMY

The hamstring muscle group (Fig. 34.1) consists of three main muscles: biceps femoris, semimembranosus and semitendinosus. Biceps femoris has two heads: a long head and a short head. The long head is innervated by the tibial portion of the sciatic nerve (L5, S1-3), whereas the short head is innervated by the common peroneal portion (L5, S1-2).

The proximal hamstring complex (Fig. 34.1c) is a common site for pathology and has a complex anatomical arrangement.[3]

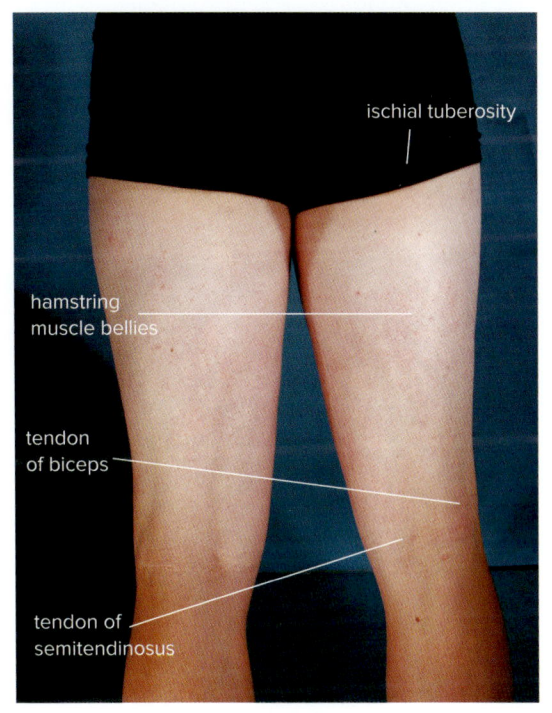

Figure 34.1 Anatomy of the posterior thigh (a) Surface anatomy

PART B Regional problems

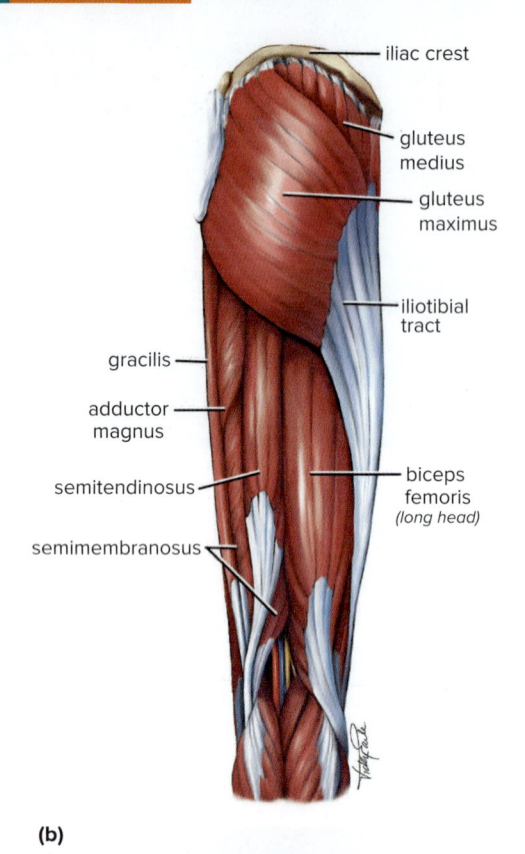

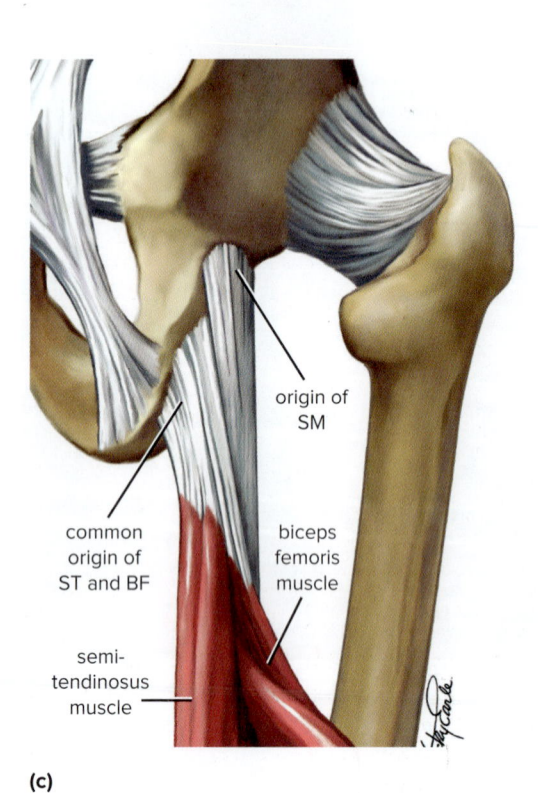

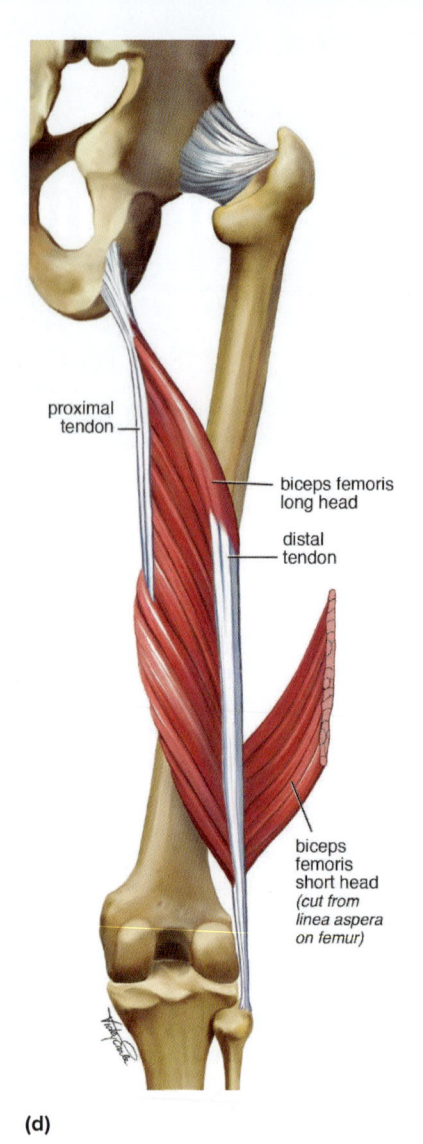

Figure 34.1 (cont.) (b) Muscles of the posterior thigh (c) Proximal hamstring origin (d) Anatomical arrangement of the long and short heads of biceps femoris

The long head of biceps femoris and semitendinosus share a common proximal tendon that arises from the medial facet of the ischial tuberosity. Semitendinosus muscle fibres originate from the ischial tuberosity and the medial aspect of the common tendon; the biceps femoris long head muscle fibres originate from the lateral aspect of the common tendon approximately 6 cm below the ischial tuberosity (Fig. 34.1d). The proximal free tendon of semimembranosus arises from the lateral facet of the ischial tuberosity and has a length of more than 10 cm. Moving distally, it extends medially passing ventral (deep) to the semitendinosus/biceps femoris long head common proximal tendon.

The short head of biceps femoris arises from the linea aspera and thus only acts about the knee joint. Semitendinosus inserts onto the anteromedial surface of the proximal tibia (as part of the pes anserine muscle group), whereas semimembranosus inserts onto the medial tibial condyle. Biceps femoris long head and short head form a common distal tendon that has several insertions, including the lateral femoral condyle, fibula head, popliteus tendon and arcuate popliteal ligament.[4]

Both the proximal and distal tendons of the biceps femoris extend approximately 60% of the length of the muscle (Fig. 34.1d).[5] As such, the biceps femoris muscle-tendon junction (a common site of injury) has a relatively unique arrangement that comprises two parts: the proximal muscle-tendon junction extending along the medial border and the distal muscle-tendon junction extending along the lateral border, with an area of overlap in the mid-zone of the muscle belly.

The ischiocondylar portion of the adductor magnus functions as if it was a 'hamstring' due to its anatomical alignment and innervation. Adductor magnus is a strong hip extensor muscle, especially when the hip is flexed. The ischiocondylar portion is innervated by the tibial portion of the sciatic nerve, like the majority of the hamstring group.

CLINICAL APPROACH

The key to effective management of posterior thigh pain is correct diagnosis. The clinician must determine whether the injury to the posterior thigh is an acute muscle injury (e.g. strain or contusion) or pain referred from elsewhere (e.g. lumbar spine). This differentiation can sometimes be challenging.

In healthy individuals, a strain to a large muscle group such as the hamstrings is the result of substantial force. The athlete will typically recall a particular point in time that the incident occurred and whether a significant force was applied to the muscle. The incident may be related to an eccentric contraction (e.g. sprinting) or it may be associated with an excessive stretch (e.g. ballet dancing).

Tethering of neural structures or fascial strains in the posterior thigh can also occur as an incident; however, appropriate examination will reveal whether the injury has a neuromechanical or fascial component. Although the clinical examination may not present differently to a low-grade strain, the absence of evidence of muscle injury on magnetic resonance imaging (MRI) (10–20% of posterior thigh pain presentations) should make the clinician highly suspicious of a referred cause of pain.[6–9]

The causes of posterior thigh pain are shown in Table 34.1.

History

Because there are different causes of posterior thigh pain, the clinician should use the history to develop a differential diagnosis that can then be refined further with a physical examination that is then appropriately structured.

Clinicians consider a wide range of factors in the history of the patient with posterior thigh pain. Some of these include the following.

1. Level of activity
   a. Has a change in training coincided with injury?
   b. Is there an adequate base of training?
2. Occupation/lifestyle
   a. What factors outside of sport could be aggravating the condition (e.g. prolonged sitting at work, repetitive bending over with young children)?
3. Incident
   a. Yes: consider strain, fascial/neural trauma.
      If there was an incident, then what was the mechanism of injury? This information will help determine optimal rehabilitation exercises. Also, what was the severity of the pain experienced at the time of the injury? This information is important because a greater maximum pain score (visual analogue scale [VAS] 0–10) is associated with a longer time to RTP. For example, a VAS pain score of greater than 6 out of 10 has been shown to be significantly associated with an RTP time of >40 days.[8, 10, 11]
   b. No: consider overuse, referred pain, alternative abnormality.
4. Immediate impact on function
   a. Being forced to stop participating in sport within 5 minutes of the initial incident is associated with an increased time to RTP.[11]
5. Progress following injury
   a. Slow: indicates a more severe injury
   b. Erratic: strain is being aggravated by activity or injury is not a strain.
6. Ability to walk pain-free within one day following injury. A study involving Australian rules football players found that those who could not walk pain-free within 1 day

> **PRACTICE PEARL**
>
> Clinicians should be reticent to diagnose an acute muscle strain in the absence of a convincing history of injury. Without a strong history of injury, consider referred pain.

PART B Regional problems

Table 34.1 Causes of posterior thigh pain

Common	Less common	Not to be missed
Hamstring muscle strains • Type I • Type II • Recurrent Hamstring muscle contusion Referred pain • Lumbar spine • Neural structures • Gluteal trigger points	Referred pain • Sacroiliac joint Tendinopathy • Biceps femoris • Semimembranosus/semitendinosus Bursitis • Semimembranosus • Ischiogluteal Fibrous adhesions 'Hamstring syndrome' (Chapter 30) Chronic compartment syndrome of the posterior thigh Apophysitis/avulsion fracture of the ischial tuberosity (in adolescents) Nerve entrapments • Posterior cutaneous thigh • Sciatic Adductor magnus strains Myositis ossificans, hamstring muscle	Tumours • Bone tumours Vascular • Iliac artery endofibrosis

were four times more likely to require >3 weeks to RTP compared to those who could.[12] Note, however, that a more recent study involving athletes from a variety of sports did not confirm this relationship.[13]

7. Aggravating factors
   a. Incident related: useful for specificity of rehabilitation (e.g. acceleration injuries require acceleration in the rehabilitation program)
   b. Non-incident related: eradication or modification for recovery and prevention (e.g. sitting at a computer causing back/hamstring pain requires ergonomic modification).
8. Behaviour with sport
   a. Warms up with activity, worse after: inflammatory pathology
   b. Starts with minimal or no pain, builds up with activity but not as severe after: claudicant, either neurological or vascular
   c. Sudden onset: mechanical (e.g. strain).
9. Night pain
   a. Sinister pathology
   b. Inflammatory condition.
10. Site of pain
    a. Posterior thigh and/or lower back: lumbar referral or neuromotor/biomechanical mediator
    b. Buttock, sacroiliac joint (SIJ) without lower back symptoms: gluteal trigger points
    c. Ischial: tendinopathy/bursitis/apophysitis/avulsion.
11. Presence of neurological symptoms
    a. Nerve involvement
12. Recurrent problem
    a. Extensive examination and rehabilitation required
    b. History of hamstring injury in the previous season is a strong predictor of risk of recurrence. For example, Australian Football players with a recent history of hamstring injury are 20 times more likely to suffer a recurrence within 3 weeks of RTP than those without a history.[12]

> **PRACTICE PEARL**
>
> Two items in the above list are particularly important:
> • 3-the severity of the pain at the time of injury
> • 12-whether it is a recurrent problem.

Physical examination

The examination further refines the distinction between local injury (i.e. acute muscle strain), referred pain or other unusual causes. A practical approach to assess various factors that commonly cause posterior thigh pain is outlined below.

1. Observation
   a. standing (Fig. 34.2a)
   b. walking
   c. lying prone
2. Active movements
   a. lumbar movements
   b. hip extension
   c. standing leg swing
   d. supine active knee extension (Fig. 34.2b)

Posterior thigh pain CHAPTER 34

3. Passive movements
   a. hamstring muscle stretch (Fig.34.2c)
4. Resisted movements
   a. knee flexion in isolation
   b. hip extension in isolation
   c. combined contraction–single leg bridge (Fig.34.2d)
5. Functional tests
   a. running
   b. kicking
   c. sprint starts
6. Palpation
   a. hamstring muscles (Fig.34.2e)
   b. ischial tuberosity
   c. gluteal muscles (Fig.34.2f)

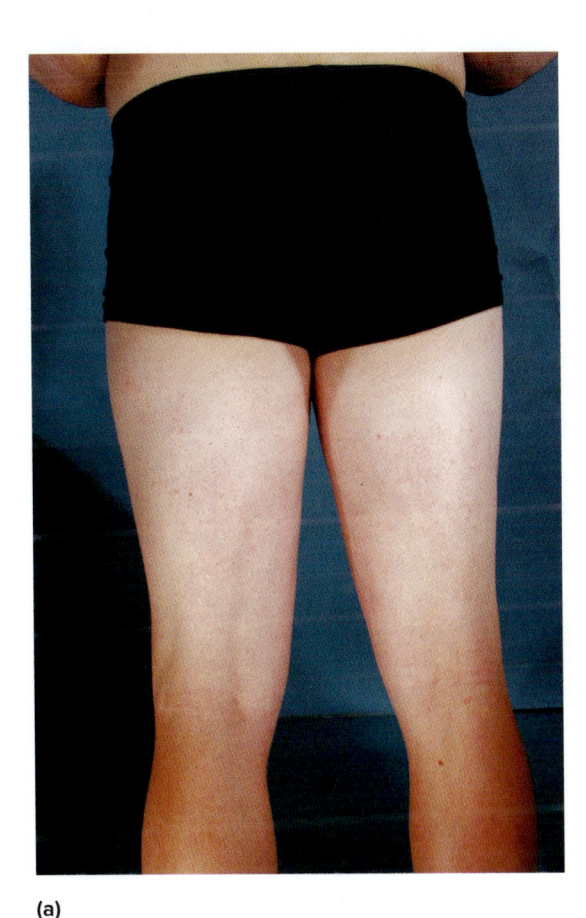

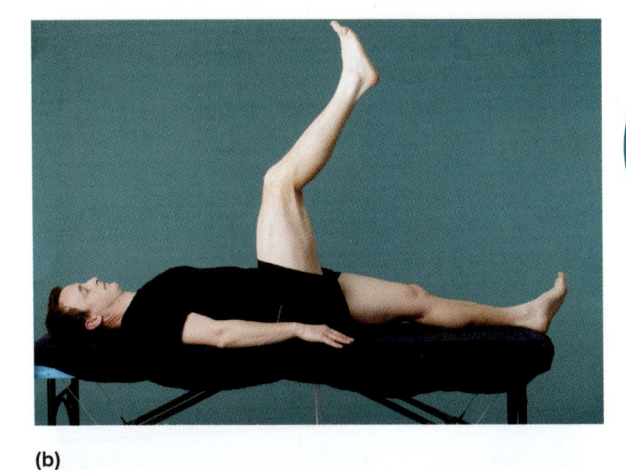

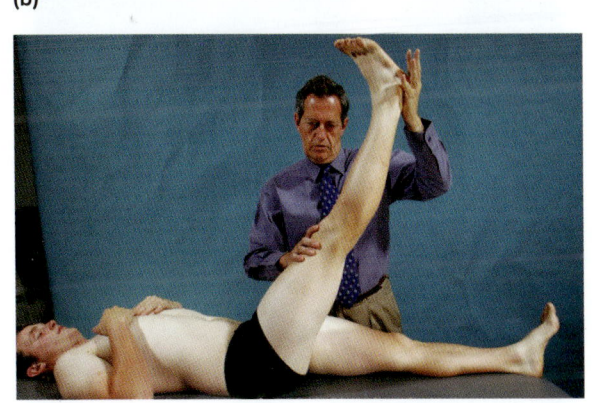

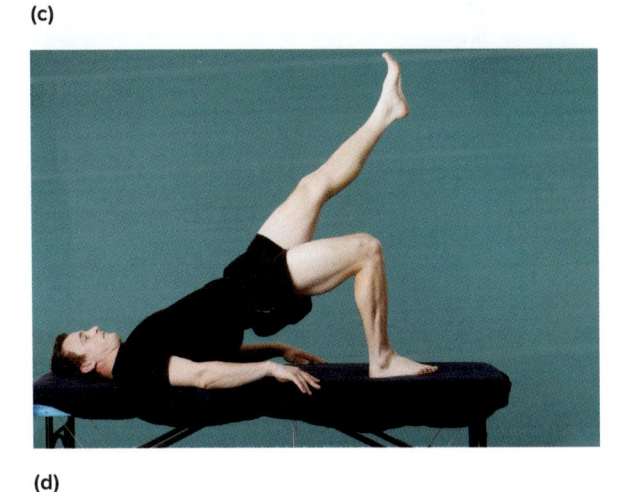

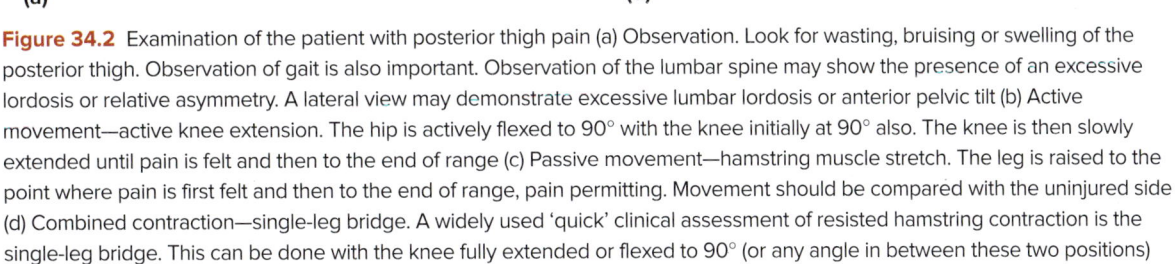

(a)

(b)

(c)

(d)

Figure 34.2 Examination of the patient with posterior thigh pain (a) Observation. Look for wasting, bruising or swelling of the posterior thigh. Observation of gait is also important. Observation of the lumbar spine may show the presence of an excessive lordosis or relative asymmetry. A lateral view may demonstrate excessive lumbar lordosis or anterior pelvic tilt (b) Active movement—active knee extension. The hip is actively flexed to 90° with the knee initially at 90° also. The knee is then slowly extended until pain is felt and then to the end of range (c) Passive movement—hamstring muscle stretch. The leg is raised to the point where pain is first felt and then to the end of range, pain permitting. Movement should be compared with the uninjured side (d) Combined contraction—single-leg bridge. A widely used 'quick' clinical assessment of resisted hamstring contraction is the single-leg bridge. This can be done with the knee fully extended or flexed to 90° (or any angle in between these two positions)

683

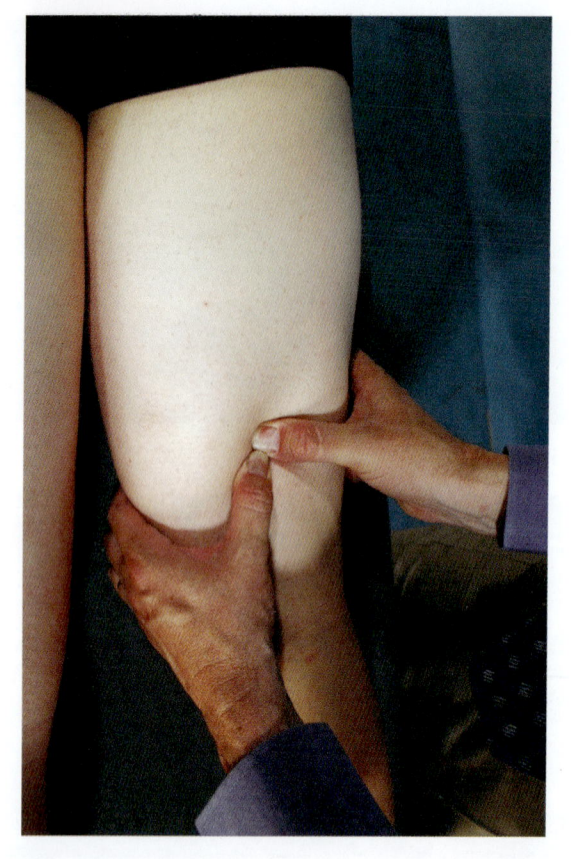

PART B   Regional problems

(e)

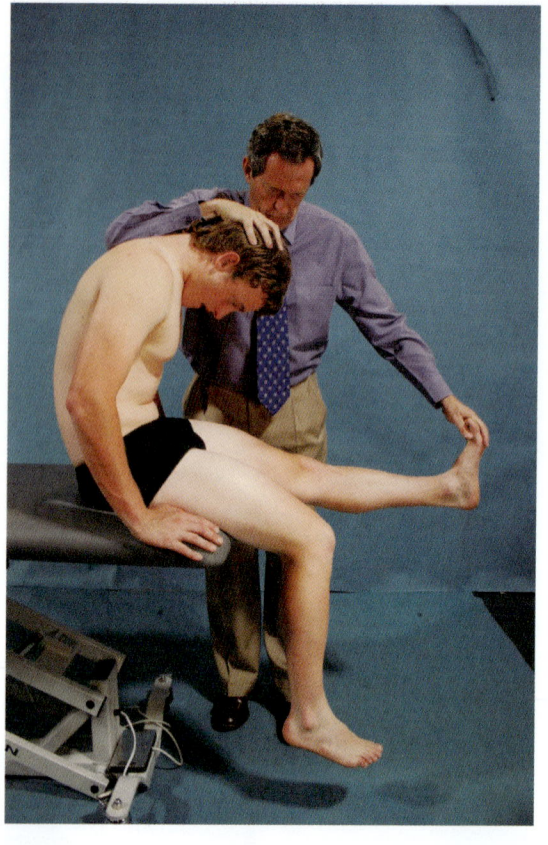

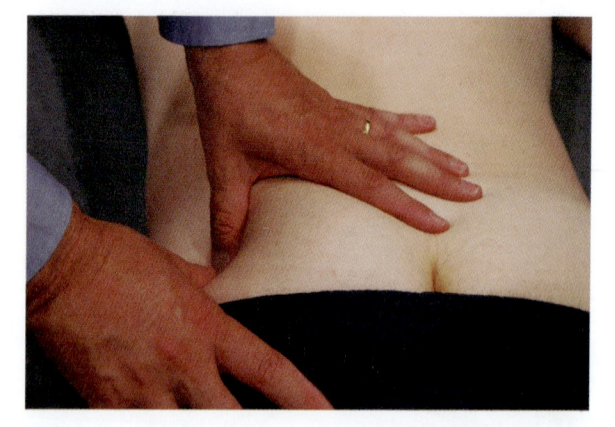

(f)

(g)

Figure 34.2 (cont.) (e) Palpation. Palpate carefully bearing the underlying anatomy in mind to determine the location of an acute muscle strain (e.g. medial versus lateral hamstring, proximal versus distal etc.) (f) Palpation—gluteal muscles. Palpate the gluteal muscles for trigger points that are taut bands, which are usually exquisitely tender locally and may refer pain into the hamstring muscle (g) Special tests—slump test. The slump test (Chapter 15) is an essential part of the examination of the patient with posterior thigh pain. It helps the clinician differentiate between hamstring muscle injuries and referred pain to the hamstring region from the lumbar spine

7. Special tests
   a. neuromechanical tests: slump test (Fig.34.2g)
   b. lumbar spine examination (Chapter 29)
   c. sacroiliac joint (Chapter 30)
   d. assessment of lumbopelvic stability (Chapter 11)
   e. biomechanical analysis (Chapter 8).

Investigations

Investigations of posterior thigh pain can be very useful but clinicians must interpret these findings together with the rest of the examination. Appropriate imaging may include ultrasound (Fig. 34.3a), MRI (Fig. 34.3b) and at times, computed tomography (CT). MRI is the most

Posterior thigh pain CHAPTER 34

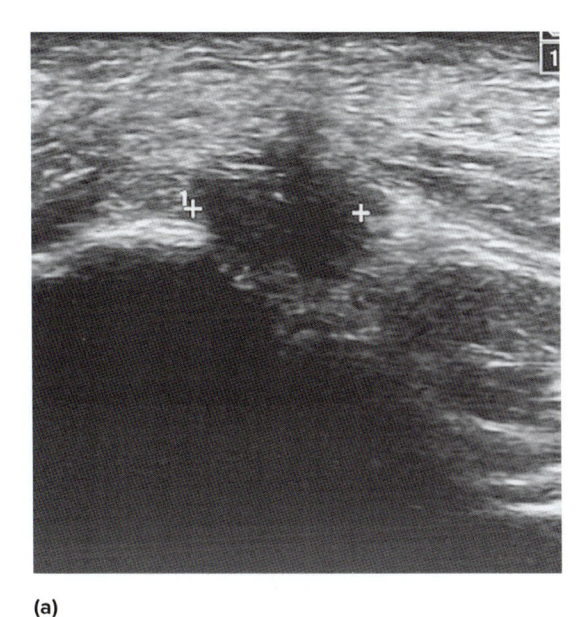

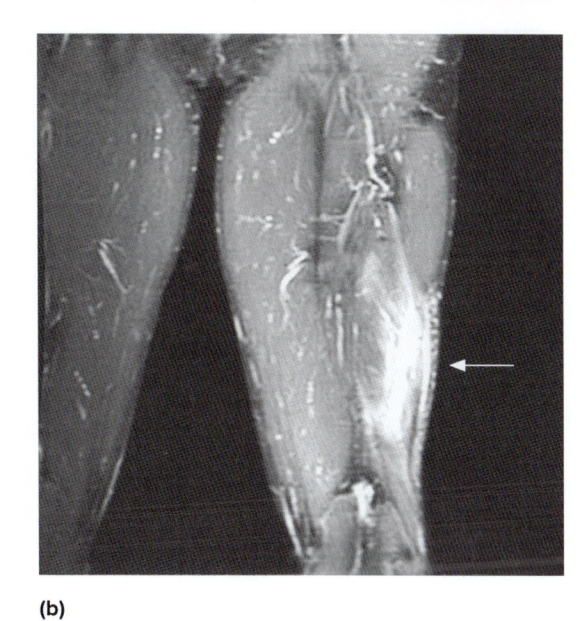

Figure 34.3 Imaging of hamstring injuries (a) Ultrasound showing hypoechoic area (between electronic callipers, +) (b) MRI demonstrating area of oedema in hamstring consistent with biceps femoris muscle tear

popular option (especially for the elite-level athlete) because it is non-invasive and capable of providing high-resolution images.[13–16]

> **PRACTICE PEARL**
>
> MRI can help identify the presence and location of pathology, contribute to determining the likely prognosis in certain instances, and monitor healing over time.

Integrating the clinical assessment and investigation to make a diagnosis

Table 34.2 summarises elements of the history, physical examination and investigations that point to whether the diagnosis is likely to be an acute hamstring muscle injury or referred pain to the posterior thigh.

ACUTE HAMSTRING MUSCLE STRAINS

Before outlining type I and type II hamstring injuries, we briefly outline the epidemiology of these injuries

Table 34.2 Clinical features of hamstring muscle tear and referred hamstring pain

Acute hamstring strain (type I or II)	Referred pain to posterior thigh
Sudden onset	May be sudden onset or gradual feeling of tightness
Moderate to severe pain	Usually less severe, may be cramping or 'twinge'
Disabling—difficulty walking, unable to run	Often able to walk/jog pain-free
Markedly reduced stretch	Minimal reduction in stretch
Markedly reduced contraction with pain against resistance	Full or near to full muscle strength against resistance
Local haematoma, bruising	No local signs
Marked focal tenderness	Variable tenderness, usually non-specific
Slump test negative	Slump test frequently positive
May have gluteal trigger points	Gluteal trigger points that reproduce hamstring pain on palpation or needling
May have abnormal lumbar spine/SIJ signs	Frequently have abnormal lumbar spine/SIJ signs

together. As the differentiation of acute hamstring injuries into two types has only recently been recommended, it is not possible to confidently separate epidemiological data.

> **PRACTICE PEARL**
>
> In the large majority of hamstring strains, the injured muscle is biceps femoris (83% of all hamstring injuries). Semimembranosus injuries are uncommon (12%) and semitendinosus injuries are rare (5%).[1]

Epidemiology

Acute hamstring strains are common in many popular sports, including the various football codes, field hockey, cricket and athletics. For example, hamstring strains are the most common injury in Australian rules football, constituting 15% of all injuries, with an incidence rate of six injuries per club (approximately 40 players) per season and a cost of 21 missed matches per club per season.[17] Similarly, in English soccer, hamstring strains make up 12% of all injuries, with an incidence rate averaging five injuries per club per season, resulting in 15 matches and 90 days missed.[18, 19]

Approximately 180 hamstring injuries occur in the 30 teams in the American National Football League (NFL) each year, so the incidence of approximately six injuries per team per season is similar to the AFL. Mean days lost per injury has been found to be 13.2.[20] Twelve per cent of all injuries in European elite-level soccer are hamstring injuries. A typical 25-player squad experiences 4-6 hamstring injuries during a season with a mean of 14.3 days lost per injury (standard deviation 14.9).[21] A study of American collegiate soccer players noted that men were 64% more likely than women to sustain a hamstring strain.[22]

The average injury severity has been reported to be between three to four missed matches per injury.[17, 23] Hamstring injuries in ballet have not been captured as well as in football codes but estimates of lifetime prevalence of hamstring injury are as high as 51% (34% acute, 17% overuse).[24]

With respect to epidemiology of recurrence, acute hamstring strains have the highest recurrence rate of any injury, with a rate of 20% in AFL,[25] 16.5% in American NFL[20] and 16% in European soccer.[21] It has also been shown in collegiate soccer that recurrence is more common for men than women.[22]

Type I and type II acute hamstring strains—not all acute hamstring injuries are the same!

There are at least two distinctly different types of acute hamstring strains (types I and II), distinguished by different injury situations. The more common, type I, hamstring strains occur during high-speed running (Fig. 34.4a).[26–32] Type II hamstring strains occur during movements leading to extensive lengthening of the hamstrings in hip flexion combined with knee extension, such as high kicking, sliding tackle and forward split (Fig. 34.4b), and may occur at slow speeds.[26–29, 31]

Type I strains (the high-speed running type) usually involve the long head of biceps femoris, most commonly at

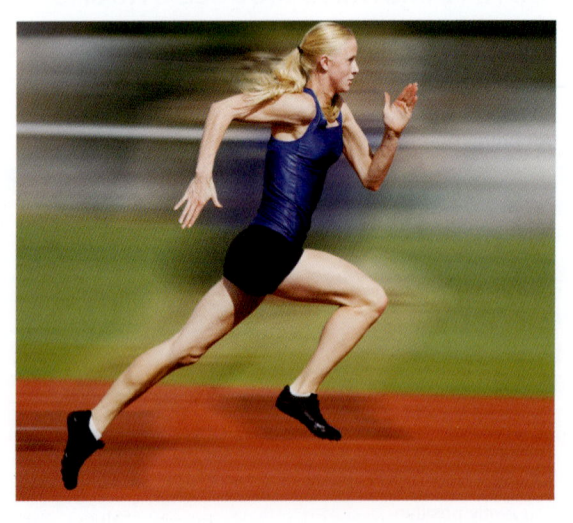

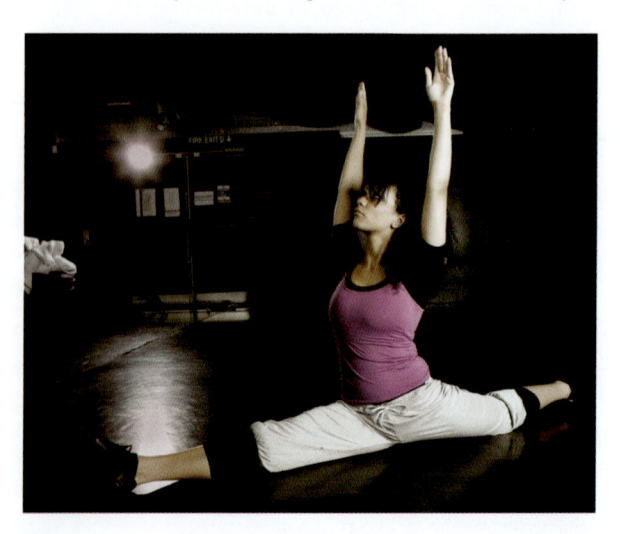

(a)   (b)

Figure 34.4 (a) Sprinting is the classic activity that causes type I hamstring strains (b) Type II hamstring strains occur with maximal stretching (e.g. dancer's forward split shown with right hamstring under tension)
(A AND B) ISTOCKPHOTO

Posterior thigh pain CHAPTER 34

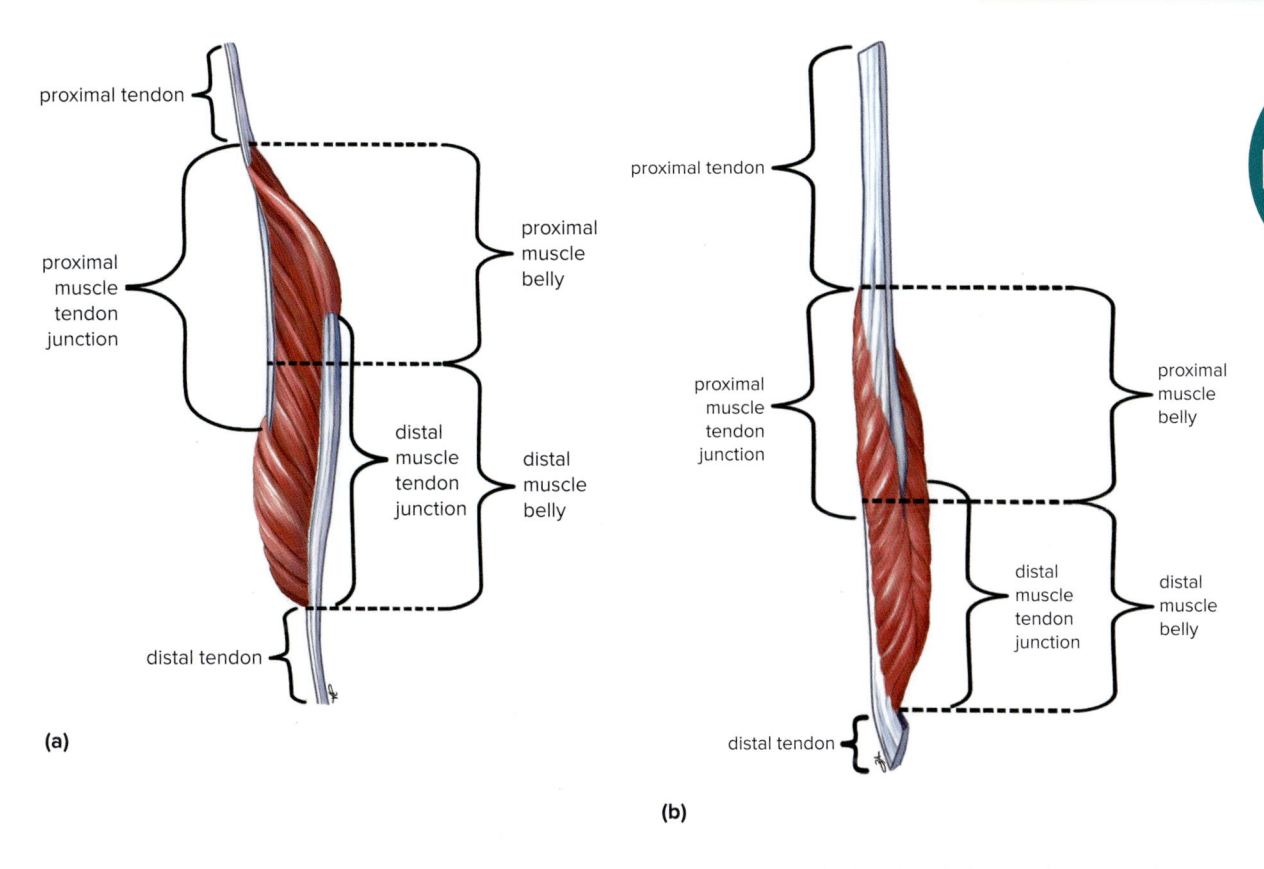

Figure 34.5 (a) Type I strains (the high-speed running type) are mainly located to the long head of biceps femoris and typically involve the proximal muscle–tendon junction (b) Type II injuries (the stretching type) are typically located close to the ischial tuberosity and involve the proximal free tendon of semimembranosus[31]

the proximal muscle-tendon junction (Fig. 34.5a).[26, 27, 30–32] In contrast, type II injuries (the stretching type) are typically located close to the ischial tuberosity and involve the proximal free tendon of semimembranosus (Fig. 34.5b)[27, 31] thus the stretching type of hamstring strain can in fact be considered a primary tendon injury.[33]

Type I strains (e.g. high-speed running) generally cause a more marked acute decline in function, but typically require a shorter rehabilitation period than type II stretching-type hamstring strains (Fig. 34.6).[34] The injury mechanism and location can give us important information about the prognosis of the injury.[26–28, 30, 34] The injury location can be determined both by maximal pain palpation and by MRI during the first 2 weeks after injury occurrence. The closer the site of maximum pain palpation to the ischial tuberosity, the longer the rehabilitation period. An injury site closer to the ischial tuberosity has been reported to be associated with a longer rehabilitation period;[26, 27, 31, 32, 35] however, a recent study by Moen did not confirm this relationship.[13] MRI should always be performed when a total rupture is suspected.

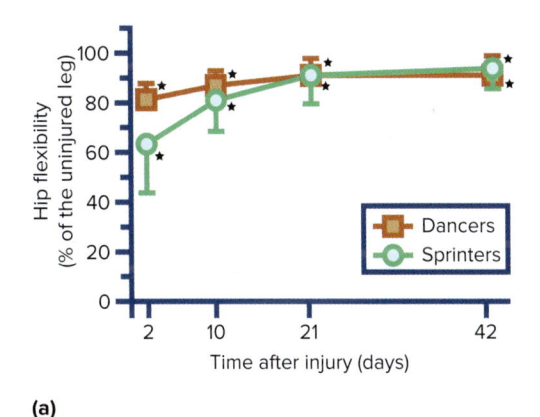

Figure 34.6 Comparison of hamstring injuries in sprinters (type I) and dancers (type II) (a) Hip flexibility (range of motion) of the injured leg expressed as a percentage of the uninjured leg in the sprinters (n=18) and dancers (n=15). The sprinters' injuries (type I) resulted in more reduction in flexibility, but similar times to return to near pre-injury flexibility levels[34]
REPRODUCED WITH PERMISSION OF BRITISH JOURNAL OF SPORTS MEDICINE

PART B   Regional problems

(b)

(c)

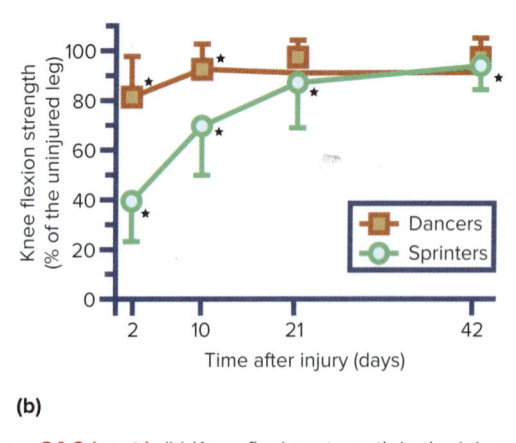

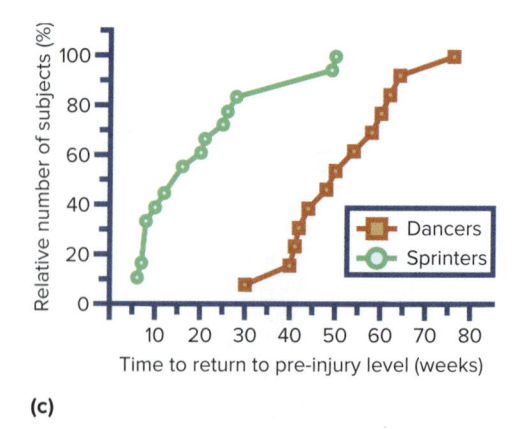

Figure 34.6 (cont.) (b) Knee flexion strength in the injured leg expressed as a percentage of the uninjured leg in the sprinters (n=18) and dancers (n=15) showing markedly increased reduction in strength in the sprinters' injuries (type I) (c) Relative number of subjects in each group plotted against the corresponding time, in weeks, to return to pre-injury level of performance (n=18 for the sprinters type I and n=13 for the dancers type II) demonstrating the prolonged rehabilitation time for type II injuries[34]
REPRODUCED WITH PERMISSION OF BRITISH JOURNAL OF SPORTS MEDICINE

Type I acute hamstring strain: sprinting-related

Although there are a variety of sports skills that can potentially heavily load the hamstrings (e.g. kicking, twisting, jumping, hurdling), sprinting is the most commonly reported mechanism of type I acute hamstring muscle strain.[8, 23, 36, 37]

Why do hamstrings fail during sprinting? Biomechanical studies suggest that hamstrings are most vulnerable to injury during the terminal swing phase of sprinting,[38, 39] a time in the stride cycle where they are highly activated as they work eccentrically to decelerate the swinging tibia and control knee extension in preparation for foot strike.[40]

Patients who present with type I acute hamstring strain typically complain of sudden onset pain in the hamstring region that usually stops them. On examination, careful palpation and testing will usually locate the injury in the long head of biceps femoris, often the proximal muscle-tendon junction.[26, 27, 31, 32] Type I strains are generally associated with a more marked acute decline in function than type II strains.

If imaging is deemed necessary (e.g. if presence of type I acute hamstring strain is unclear on clinical grounds), then MRI (Fig. 34.7) would be the current recommended imaging modality because it is non-invasive and of high resolution. The only disadvantage is cost (rarely an issue for the elite athlete). MRI can be helpful in accurately identifying the location of the injury (semimembranosus versus biceps femoris long head versus semitendinosus; distal versus proximal; tendon versus muscle-tendon junction versus epimysium).

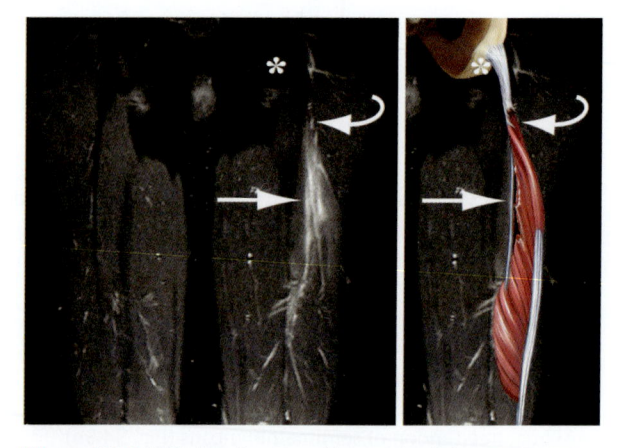

Figure 34.7 MRI showing type I hamstring injury

For two reasons, the role of MRI in predicting prognosis following type I acute hamstring muscle strains is currently uncertain. First, simple clinical parameters (Table 34.2) are just as good if not better predictors of prognosis than MRI-based parameters.[11, 13] Second, most of the studies investigating the prognostic value of MRI-based parameters are considered to have a high risk of bias and thus findings must be interpreted cautiously,[15] although a recent high-quality study has found increased cranio-caudal length of lesion on MRI to be positively correlated with longer time to RTP.[41] If there is a clinical suspicion of total tendon rupture, then MRI should always be performed.

Type II acute hamstring strain: stretch-related (dancers)

Type II acute hamstring strains more commonly occur in sports that necessitate large amplitude movements and ballistic limb actions, such as ballet dancing and gymnastics. The common mechanism of injury in these instances is an excessive stretch into hip flexion.

In contrast to type I injuries, the stretching-type injuries typically are located close to the ischial tuberosity and involve the proximal free tendon of semimembranosus.[26, 27, 35, 42] MRI shows the site of the type II injury close to the ischial tuberosity (Fig. 34.8).

Although type II hamstring strains can cause a less dramatic acute limitation than type I strains, their rehabilitation period is often longer than that of type I strains.[26, 27, 34] It is important to directly inform the athlete that the rehabilitation is likely to be prolonged. Unrealistically optimistic information will only reinforce the disappointment and frustration of the injured athlete. The athlete can often do quite demanding rehabilitation training early on, as long as pain-provoking exercises are avoided. Passive stretching and heavy load exercises seem to aggravate the stretch-type of hamstring injuries by increasing pain.

Prognosis of hamstring injuries

The following factors have been shown to be associated with increased length of time to RTP, although in some instances the evidence is conflicting.

- Time (days) to walk normal pace pain-free has been shown to be significantly associated with RTP time (>1 day = 4 times more likely to take >3 weeks). Combining this with a past history of hamstring injury within 12 months resulted in a 93% chance of taking longer than 3 weeks to return in elite AFL players.[12] However, note that a more recent study involving athletes from a variety of sports has failed to confirm this relationship.[13]
- Days to jog pain-free has been found to be a strong predictor of time to RTP.[8]

  - 1–2 days ≤ 2 weeks to RTP
  - 3–5 days ≥ 2 weeks to RTP
  - >5 days ≥ 4 weeks to RTP

- MRI-negative 'hamstring strains' are associated with relatively rapid time to RTP and are relatively common (10–20%).[6, 8, 9, 43]
- Several studies have found the more proximal the site of injury, the more prolonged the time to RTP,[26, 27, 31] although this relationship was not confirmed in a recent study.[13]
- Injury to the intramuscular ('conjoint' or 'central') tendon of biceps femoris long head is associated with a long time to RTP (e.g. around 3–4 months), much longer than an injury only involving the muscle-tendon junction or epimysium.[35, 44–46] (See below.)
- A 'kicking' or 'slow-stretching' mechanism of injury is associated with a longer rehabilitation period than a high-speed running mechanism, even though initial signs and symptoms may actually present as far less severe.[26, 27, 34]
- Greater self-predicted time to RTP.[13]
- Forced to stop training/playing within 5 minutes following onset of pain.[11]
- Greater maximum pain intensity experienced at the time of injury.[10, 11]
- Longer length of hamstring tenderness with palpation (cm).[11]
- Passive range of motion deficit (injured versus uninjured side) recorded within a few days of injury occurrence using the passive straight leg raise test[13] or the active knee extension test.[47]
- Longer craniocaudal length of lesion on MRI.[6, 41]

> **PRACTICE PEARL**
>
> Clinicians need to watch out for the type I acute hamstring muscle strain of the proximal biceps femoris long head that is associated with a longitudinal split or partial rupture of the proximal conjoint tendon (as visualised on MRI). These particular injuries require a prolonged rehabilitation period.

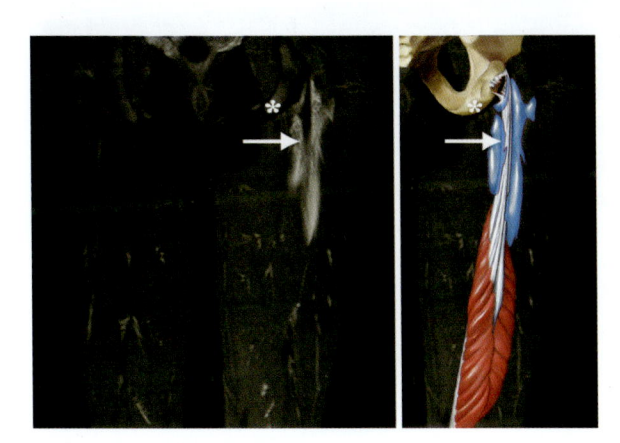

Figure 34.8 MRI shows the site of the type II injury close to the ischial tuberosity

PART B   Regional problems

INTRAMUSCULAR TENDON INJURIES

Injuries to the musculotendinous junction of the proximal or distal intramuscular tendons (Fig.34.1d) are common. Occasionally the tendon itself is injured. On MRI scanning, the disrupted intramuscular tendon has a wavy retracted appearance as opposed to its normal taut cord-like appearance (Fig. 34.9a). Sometimes the tendon failure occurs like a piece of string, with disrupted tendon strands overlapping each other and offering some scaffold for healing to occur (Fig. 34.9b). In some cases, there is longitudinal delamination and splitting of the intramuscular tendon (Fig. 34.9c), which otherwise appears continuous. In other cases, the tendon may retract and create a gap (Fig. 34.9d).

These injuries have particular clinical significance due to prolonged healing rates and possible increased risk of recurrence.[44, 46] It is increasingly thought that surgical intervention for this latter pathology offers a predictable and steadfast pathway for healing. An example of a spilt proximal intramuscular tendon is shown on MRI (Fig. 34.9e) and surgical appearance (Fig. 34.9f). Regardless, of whether conservative or surgical treatment is employed, studies have shown that the RTP time frame is typically 8-10 weeks. High resolution MR scans can help in making the distinction as to whether strands of the disrupted intramuscular tendon rachis remain in broad continuity or are separated and retracted.

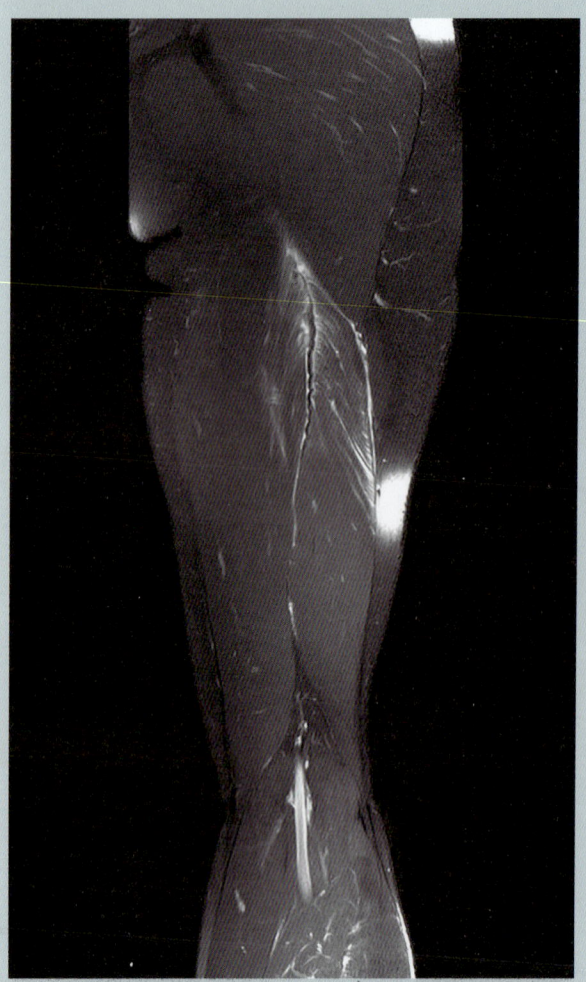

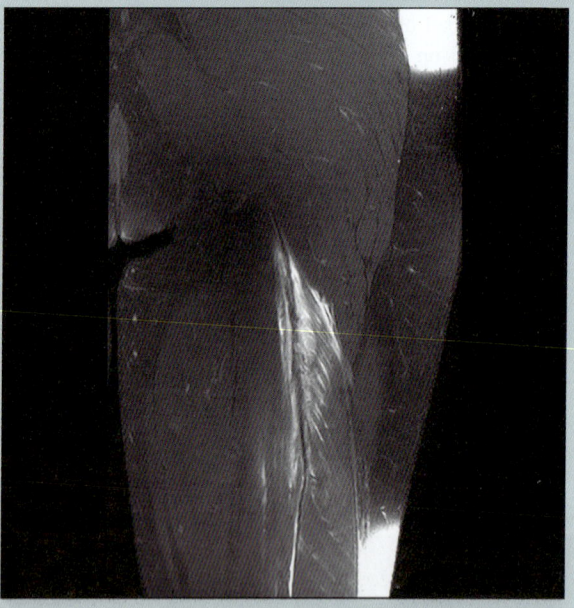

Figure 34.9 Appearances of injury to the intramuscular biceps femoris tendon (a) A wavy retracted appearance as opposed to its normal taut cord-like appearance (b) Disrupted tendon strands overlapping each other and offering some scaffold for healing to occur
COURTESY OF DR TOM ENTWISTLE

Posterior thigh pain CHAPTER 34

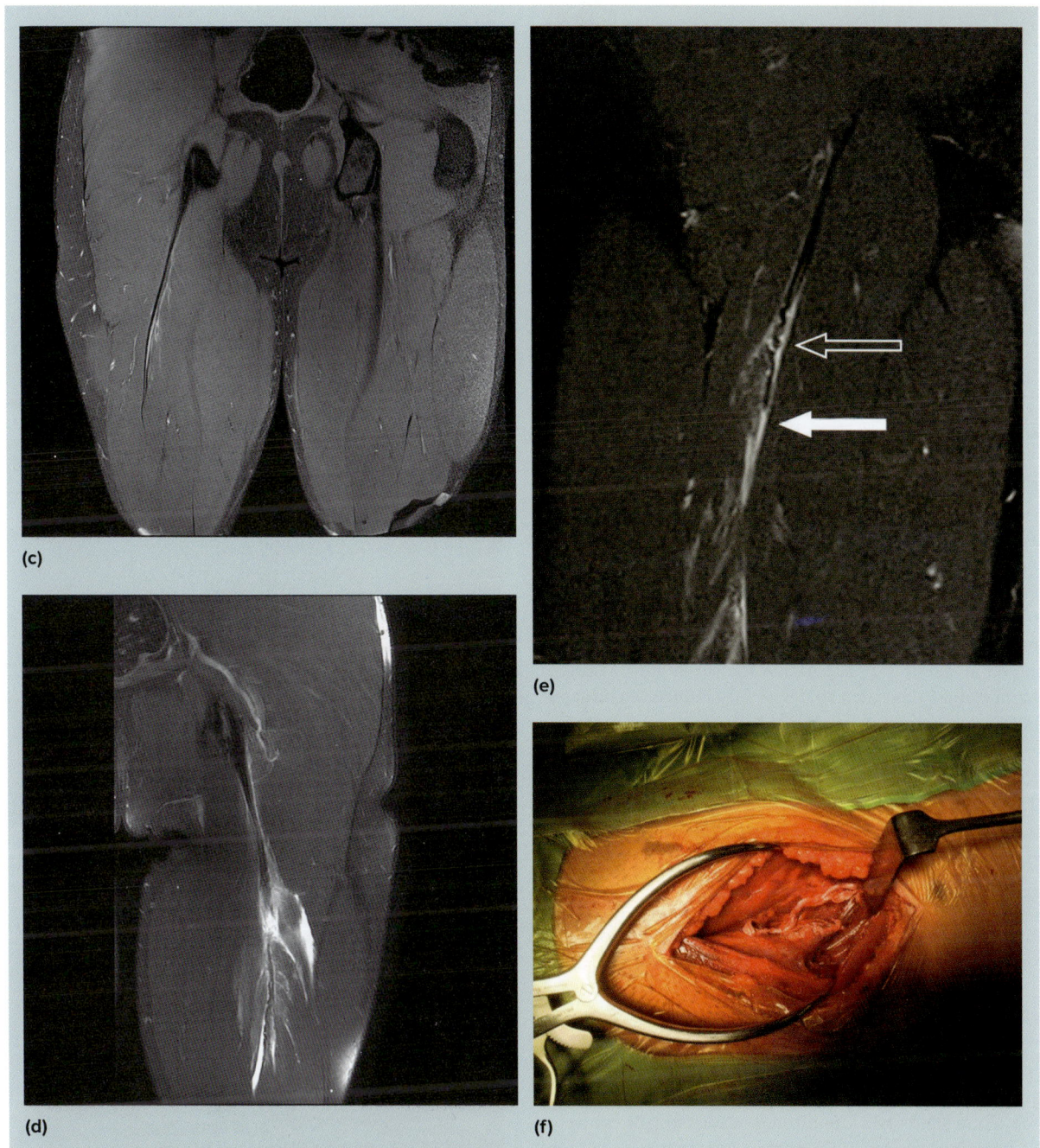

Figure 34.9 (cont.) (c) Longitudinal delamination and splitting of the intramuscular tendon (d) The tendon retracts and creates a gap (e) Disruption of the intramuscular tendon. Compare (e) The MRI appearance of a disrupted intramuscular tendon, showing wavy line indicative of tendon disruption (open arrow) and area of tendon retraction (closed arrow) with (f) The surgical appearance of the same injury. After surgery to repair the defect, the athlete made a successful RTP at 9 weeks
(a-d) COURTESY OF DR TOM ENTWHISTLE (f) COURTESY OF JULIAN FELLER

Management of hamstring injuries

Six RCTs evaluated the efficacy of a particular intervention for the rehabilitation of acute hamstring strains.[26, 27, 41, 48–50] While these studies have provided clinicians with some important information, more research is required to fully elucidate the best treatment

691

PART B Regional problems

> **PRACTICE PEARL**
>
> Progression through phases of rehab program must NOT be time-dependent. Sometimes what initially appears to be a rather minor injury can take an extended period to fully recover and vice versa. Progression must be based on successfully achieving key functional and/or clinical criteria (see Table 34.3).

options, particularly with regards to avoiding recurrence following RTP. Hence, the approach below remains largely based on clinical experience. Management of acute hamstring strains is summarised in Table 34.3.

Rehabiltation programs require a basic structure, but should never be a 'recipe'. Treat each case on its merits. The following is a suggested structure, which is similar to that recommended by other experienced clinicians.[43, 51]

Acute management phase

Acute injuries should always be assessed thoroughly before any treatment is administered. The fundamental objective of the acute management phase is to facilitate myofibre regeneration and minimise fibrosis. If strategies aimed at minimising scar tissue formation are instituted immediately, then such strategies may reduce the chances of injury recurrence.

Rest, ice, compression, elevation

Traditionally, the most common treatment in the first few days or thereabouts following type I acute hamstring strain is the rest, ice, compression, elevation (RICE) program. For example, applying ice for 10–15 minutes using a cold pack, every 3–4 hours, for the first few days until acute symptoms settle. Compression can be achieved in-between times via an elastic bandage or Tubigrip™ stocking.

Muscle activation

Although RICE would still be the recommended initial approach, recent research in cell therapy and tissue engineering is indicating an additional role for controlled and monitored exercise (or muscle contraction) regimens. Muscle contraction promotes angiogenesis (i.e. the formation of new blood vessels and the expansion of existing vascular trees) and in doing so increases the likelihood of delivering muscle-derived stem cells to the injured region. These cells are likely derived from the vascular endothelium and offer great potential for providing long-term myofibre regeneration.[52] Another aim of early pain-free muscle contractions is to prevent neuromuscular inhibition around the injured area. Note that this recommended approach to muscle healing is consistent with the concept of 'mechanotherapy'.[53]

The commencement of frequent (e.g. 3–4 times per day), low-grade, pain-free muscle contractions (e.g. simple isometric hamstring contractions or active prone knee bends) immediately following injury would appear advantageous (Fig. 34.10). Such exercises should be biased as much as possible towards selective activation of the injured muscle.

Medical therapies

A number of different medical therapies have been used in the management of acute hamstring muscle injuries. There is little evidence to support their use.[54]

Despite the widespread use of nonsteroidal anti-inflammatory drugs (NSAIDs) in the treatment of hamstring injuries, the two randomised controlled studies

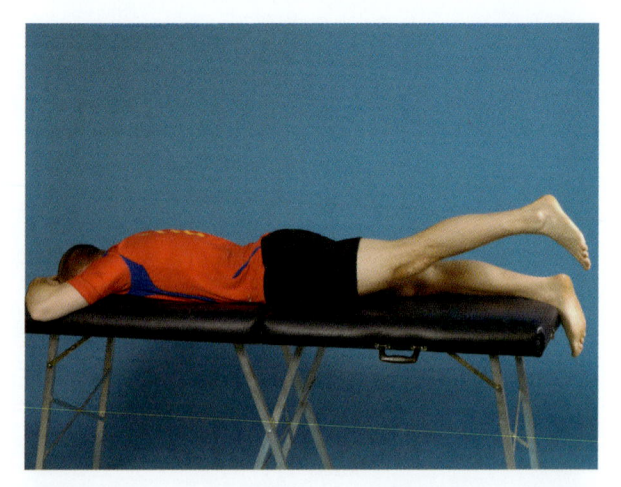

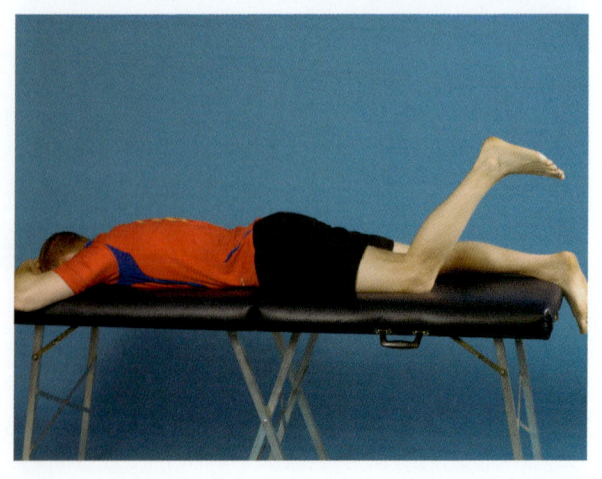

Figure 34.10 Early pain-free muscle contraction (a) Single-leg hip extension exercise with whole leg a few centimetres off the plinth (b) Active prone knee bends

failed to show beneficial or superior effects of NSAIDs compared to analgesics or placebo on acute muscle strain injuries.[12, 55] It is likely that simple analgesics are just as effective without the long-term risks on skeletal muscle and the gastrointestinal system associated with NSAIDs.

One study showed favourable results with intramuscular corticosteroid injection in American football players with acute hamstring injuries.[56] Previously, the use of corticosteroids in acute muscle strains had been clearly contraindicated because they were thought to delay elimination of haematoma and necrotic tissue, as well as retard muscle regeneration. There are concerns regarding the retrospective nature of the NFL study and lack of control group, so we caution against the use of corticosteroids in this situation in light of the fact that there have been no further studies confirming these results.

The pros and cons of delivering growth factors via autologous blood or platelet-rich plasma (PRP) injections are discussed in Chapter 17. A number of studies have investigated the effect of PRP administration specifically in hamstring muscle injuries.

One study suggested that a single autologous PRP injection combined with a rehabilitation program was significantly more effective in treating hamstring injuries than a rehabilitation program alone;[57] however, a number of subsequent studies of higher quality have shown no significant benefit.[58–60] At this stage, there is insufficient evidence to recommend the use of PRP in acute hamstring muscle injuries.

The combined injection of Traumeel® S and Actovegin®, a deproteinised calf-blood haemodialysate, immediately after a hamstring muscle injury and again at days 2 and 4 post-injury to the area of the muscle strain and the lumbar spine is common practice in sports medicine in Germany, and has been used elsewhere in some instances, despite the lack of any controlled trials supporting its use.[61, 62] A pilot study with limited subjects and a poor methodology reported a significant difference in subjective recovery and the RTP time in athletes following the intramuscular administration of Actovegin into grade I muscle tears, but there is no further evidence available.[63]

In summary, there is currently no good scientific evidence to support the use of any medication in the management of hamstring muscle injuries.

Criteria for progression to subacute phase

Once the athlete is pain-free with walking and adequate/sufficient force can be generated without pain on resisted hamstrings contraction, then jogging can commence and gradually increased.

In some instances, the athlete can experience considerable improvement in clinical signs and symptoms within 4–6 days post-injury. However, the clinician must remember that the healing process is still in its initial stages and the risk for re-injury is high, as the injured tissue is unlikely to be able to tolerate maximal loads. The criteria for progression to the subacute phase are shown in Table 34.3.

Table 34.3 Criterion-related rehabilitation of hamstring muscle strains

Phase	Key criteria
1. Begin running/active rehabilitation (i.e. begin subacute phase)	Pain-free walking Adequate force with resisted muscle contraction
2. Return to full training (i.e. begin functional phase)	Complete resolution of **any** symptoms with maximal resisted muscle contraction Equivalent tenderness upon palpation (left = right) Full and symptom free range of movement/flexibility (left = right) Successful completion of a structured running program (i.e. maximum sprinting speed achieved at the end of the running program is comparable to the athlete's previously recorded benchmark when uninjured Successful completion of appropriate rehabilitation exercises Successful completion of controlled functional (sports-specific) tasks simulating the original injury mechanism
3. Return to play (RTP)	Successful completion of **at least one** full week of normal training load with no adverse reaction in any clinical and/or functional signs and symptoms Additional quantitative tests of hamstring function (e.g. hand-held dynamometry, isokinetic dynamometry, Askling H-test (below), the single-leg bridge capacity test, performance on Nordic eccentric hamstring exercise); compare data for injured limb to uninjured limb or to data collected prior to injury No adverse psychological characteristics, such as apprehension regarding RTP or fear of re-injury

PART B Regional problems

Subacute/conditioning phase

Stretching

The role of targeted hamstring stretching in the rehabilitation of hamstring strain injury should be considered on an individual basis (Fig. 34.11). There is some limited evidence to suggest that rate of recovery can be increased with an increased daily frequency of hamstring-stretching exercises.[49] Consequently, to prevent long-term loss of range of motion (e.g. perhaps from significant scar tissue), a controlled stretching program can be instituted. However, in our clinical experience, most athletes regain their normal range of motion without the need for excessive or aggressive hamstring-stretching regimens.

It may be more important to focus on stretching of other structures. For example, tight hip flexor muscles, if present, may place the athlete at greater risk of hamstring strain.[64, 65]

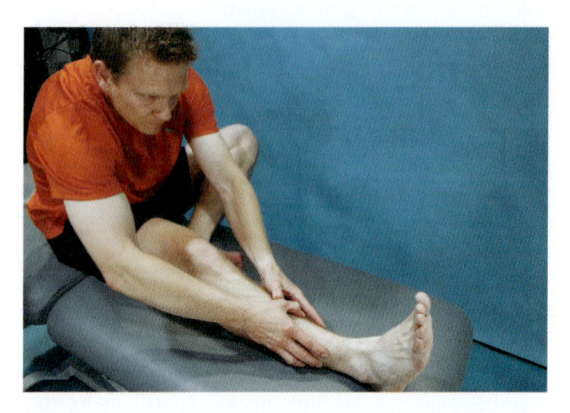

Manual therapy

A comprehensive clinical examination of the lumbar spine, sacroiliac and buttock regions should be instituted at an early stage to assess whether or not these regions have any contribution to the presenting injury. For example, Cibulka et al. reported that mobilisation of the sacroiliac joint was of some benefit in the treatment of acute hamstring strains.[48]

Neural mobility restriction is frequently present in hamstring injuries secondary to bleeding around the sciatic nerve. Neural mobilising exercises should be performed to reduce adhesions. Neural mobilising can be performed in the hamstring stretch position (Fig. 34.11) by adding gentle cervical flexion.

Soft tissue techniques can be used in the treatment of hamstring strains. Sustained compression (Fig. 34.12a) and sustained myofascial tension (Fig. 34.12b) are used, gently at

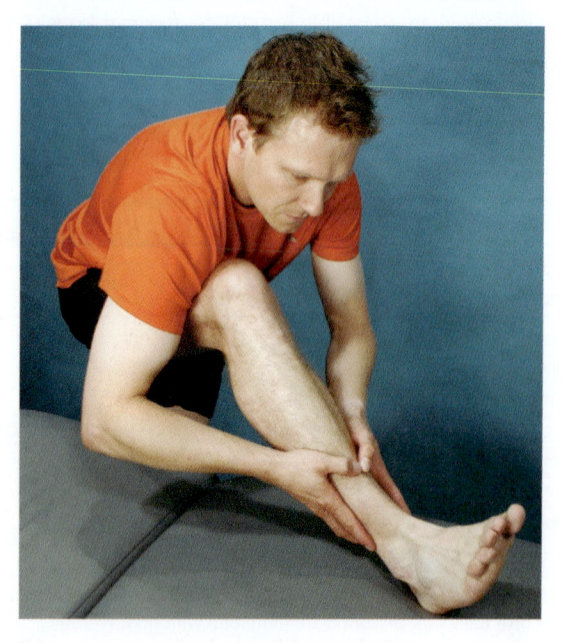

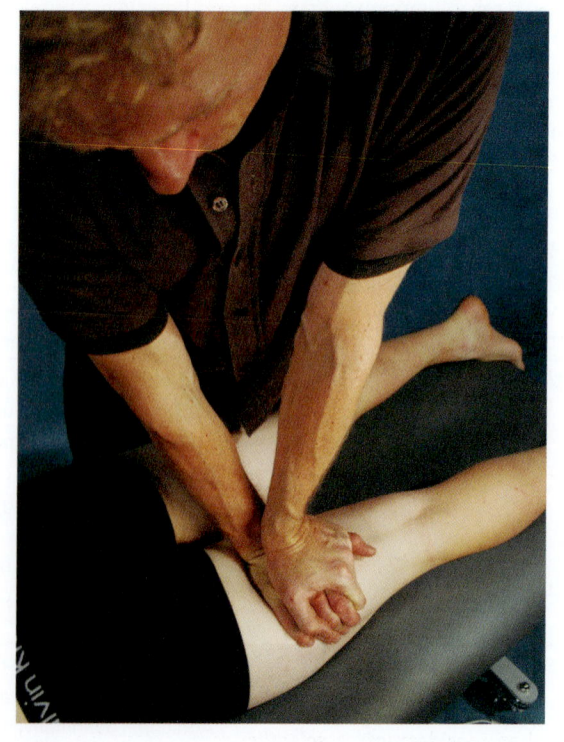

Figure 34.11 Hamstring stretches (a) Hamstring stretch with contralateral knee flexion. The lower leg can be placed in different degrees of external and internal rotation to maximise the effectiveness of the stretch (b) Hamstring stretch with bent knee results in maximal stretch to the upper hamstrings

Figure 34.12 Soft tissue techniques in the treatment of hamstring injuries (a) Sustained compression force to hamstring

Posterior thigh pain   CHAPTER 34

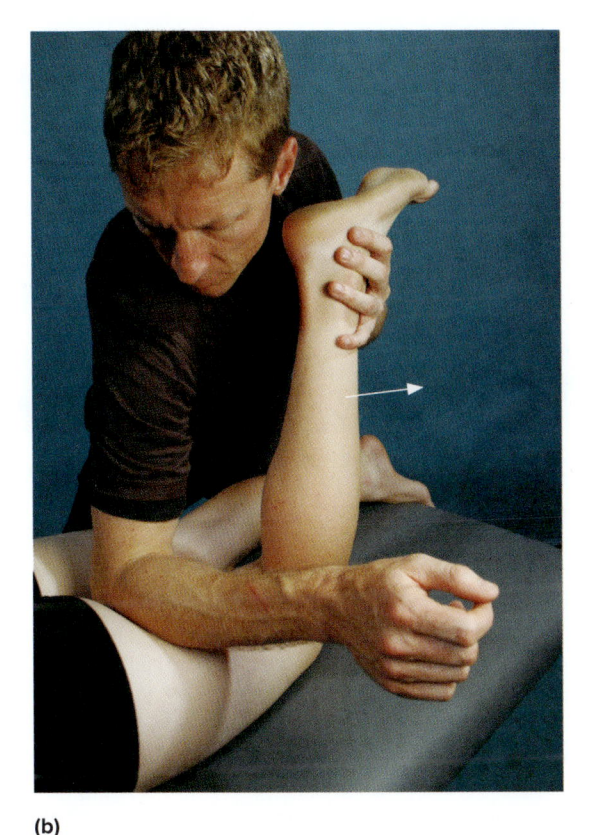

Figure 34.12 (cont.) (b) Sustained myofascial tension combined with passive knee extension. The hand or the elbow (illustrated) is kept stationary and the release is performed by passively extending the knee (arrow)

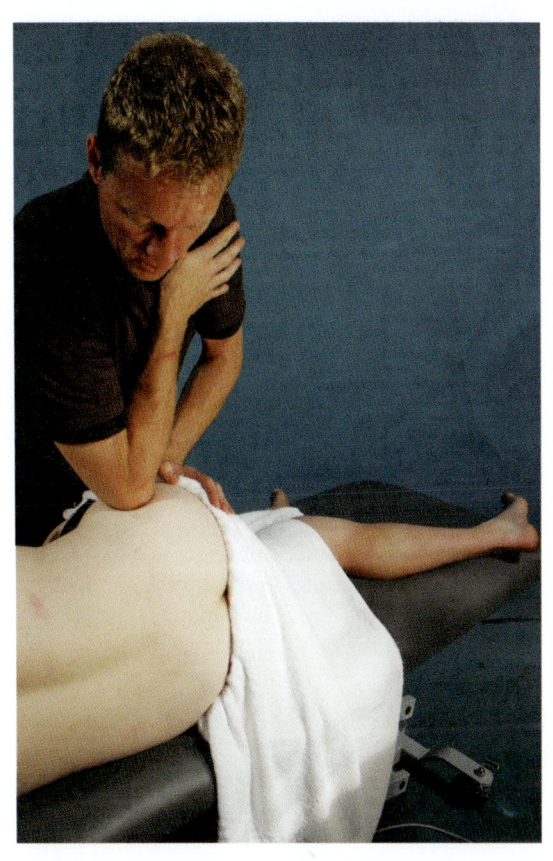

Figure 34.13 Treatment of the gluteal region in a side-lying position using elbow ischaemic pressure

first and then more vigorously. Longitudinal massage along the muscle may assist in optimising scar reorganisation. Abnormalities of the gluteal muscles may be associated with hamstring strains. These regions may be treated in a side-lying position using elbow ischaemic pressure with the tissue on stretch (Fig. 34.13).

Strengthening for hamstring muscles

Strengthening is an essential component of the rehabilitation and prevention of hamstring injuries. When designing a strengthening program, the clinician needs to consider the following parameters: the type of contraction (i.e. eccentric/isometric/concentric), the length of the muscle-tendon unit (i.e. lengthened/optimal/shortened) and the speed of contraction (i.e. slow/fast rate of force development). A further consideration is selective recruitment (i.e. medial versus lateral), as different exercises tend to preferentially activate different parts of the hamstring muscle group.[66-68] A comprehensive strengthening program will therefore require a variety of exercises.

Most hamstring strain researchers probably agree that the strains occur when the hamstring muscle group is extensively lengthened, especially in the stretching-type[35, 42] injury, but also in the sprinting type of injury.[40, 69]

It is also generally accepted that retraining needs to be specific to muscle function and as much as possible to the specific hamstring muscle injured (i.e. most commonly biceps femoris long head).[70-73]

Based on this concept, training programs for the rehabilitation of hamstring injuries should include exercises emphasising eccentric muscle contractions and extensive lengthening. It is also recommended to use exercises that load the hamstrings about the hip and the knee simultaneously, since three of the four hamstring muscles are bi-articular.

Recent clinical trials have shown that a rehabilitation program emphasising lengthening-type exercises (L-protocol) is more effective after acute hamstring injuries in elite footballers/sprinters/jumpers than a program

PART B Regional problems

containing inner range exercises such as supine single leg bridging and standing hip extension against a pulley.[26, 27]

The L-protocol (lengthening) consists of three exercises (the extender, the diver and the glider) specifically aimed at loading the hamstrings during extensive lengthening, shown and explained in detail in Figures 34.14. The extender is aimed mainly at increasing flexibility, the diver is a combined exercise for hamstring strength and trunk/pelvis stabilisation, and the glider is more of a specific eccentric hamstring exercise. The L-protocol could be started 3–5 days after injury occurrence and no pain should be provoked.[26, 27]

Another recent clinical trial[41] compared a rehabilitation program containing progressive running and eccentric strengthening to a program containing progressive agility and trunk stabilisation exercises. The time taken to RTP was similar for both programs.

There are a wide variety of strengthening exercises that load the hamstrings eccentrically and involve simultaneous hip and knee joint motions. Figure 34.15 illustrates some of the more popular exercises:

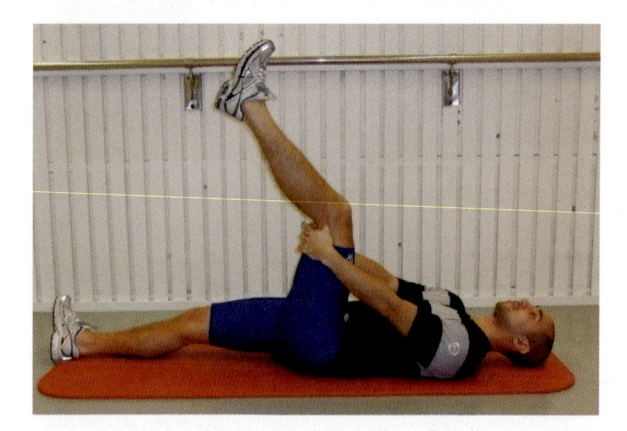

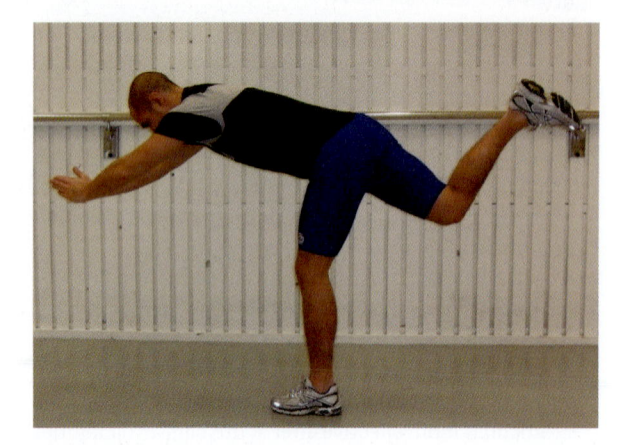

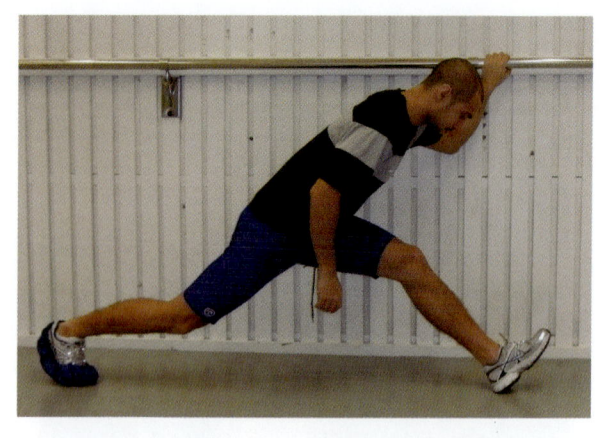

(a)

(b)

(c)

Figure 34.14 The L-lengthening protocol recommended by Askling (a) The Extender (aimed mainly at increasing flexibility) The subject should hold and stabilise the thigh of the injured leg with the hip flexed approximately 90° and then perform slow knee extensions to a point just before pain is felt. Perform twice every day, 3 sets with 12 repetitions (b) The Diver (combined exercise for hamstring strength and trunk/pelvis stabilisation) The exercise should be performed as a simulated dive, that is, as a hip flexion (from an upright trunk position) of the injured, standing leg and simultaneous stretching of the arms forwards and attempting maximal hip extension of the lifted leg while keeping the pelvis horizontal; angles at the knee should be maintained at 10–20° in the standing leg and at 90° in the lifted leg. Due to its complexity, this exercise should be performed very slowly in the beginning. Perform once every other day, 3 sets with 6 repetitions (c) The Glider (a specific eccentric strength exercise). The exercise is started from a position with upright trunk, one hand holding onto a support and legs slightly split. All the body weight should be on the heel of the injured (here left) leg with approximately 10–20° flexion in the knee. The motion is started by gliding backwards on the other leg (note low-friction sock) and stopped before pain is reached. The movement back to the starting position should be performed with the help of both arms, not using the injured leg. Progression is achieved by increasing the gliding distance and performing the exercise faster. Perform once every third day, 3 sets with 4 repetitions
REPRODUCED WITH PERMISSION OF BRITISH JOURNAL OF SPORTS MEDICINE

- standing single leg hamstring catches with TheraBand™ (Fig. 34.15a)
- single-leg bridge catch (Fig. 34.15b)
- single-leg ball roll-outs (Fig. 34.15c)
- single-leg slide-outs (Fig. 34.15d)
- Nordic drops (Fig. 34.15e)
- single-leg reverse deadlift with kettle bell (Fig. 34.15f)
- Yo-Yo (Fig. 34.15g)
- L-protocol: extender, glider, diver (Fig. 34.14).

Posterior thigh pain CHAPTER 34

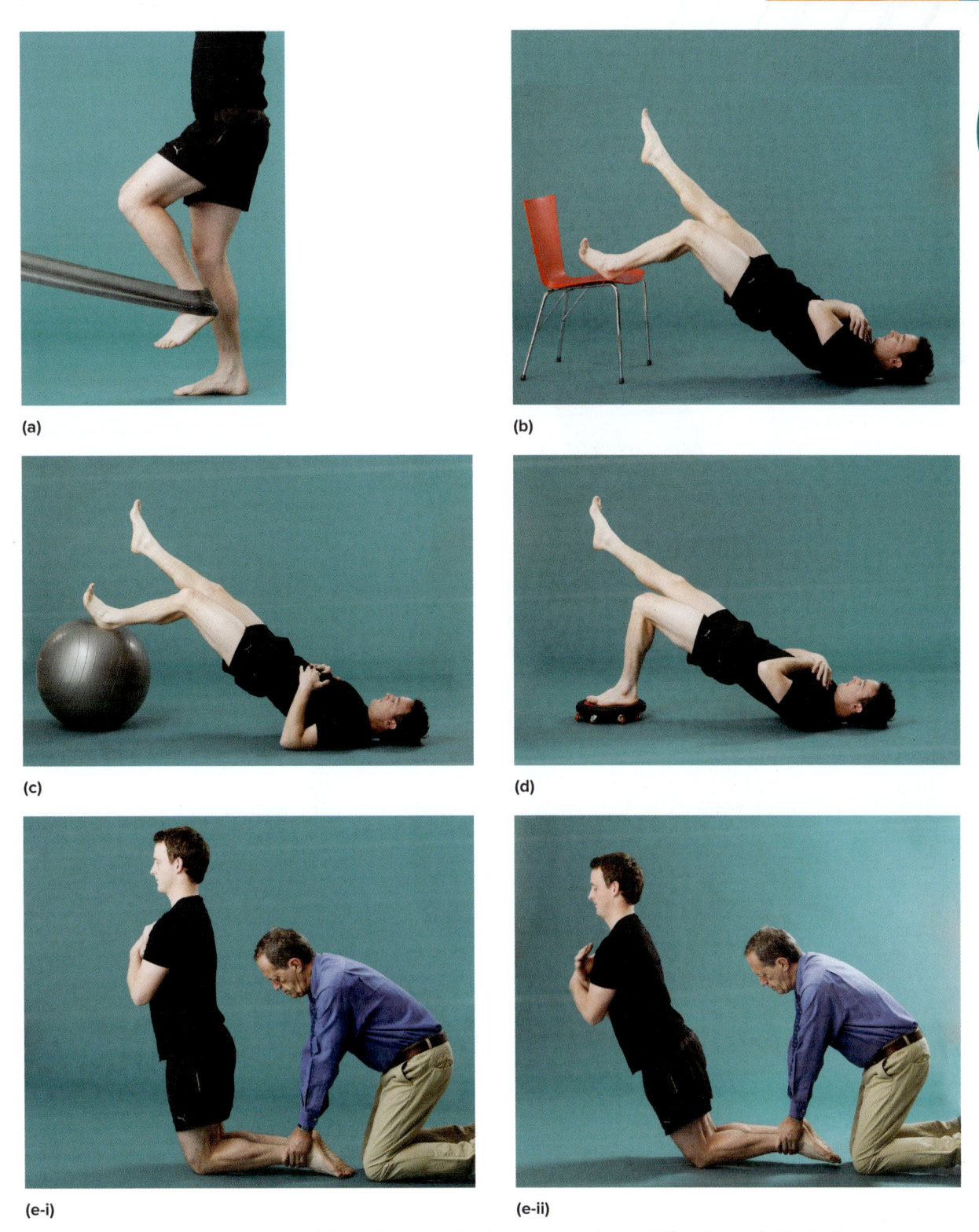

Figure 34.15 Strengthening exercises (a) Standing single-leg hamstring catches with TheraBand™ (b) Single-leg bridge catch (c) Single-leg ball roll-outs (d) Single-leg slide-outs (e) Nordic eccentric hamstring exercise (drops): patients allow themselves to fall forwards and then resist the fall for as long as possible using their hamstrings

PART B   Regional problems

(f)

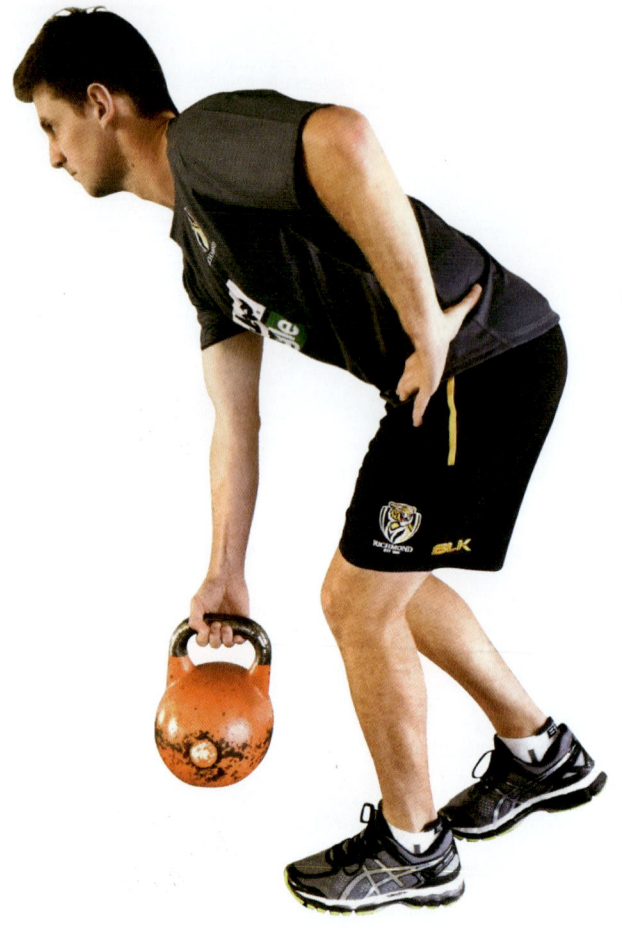

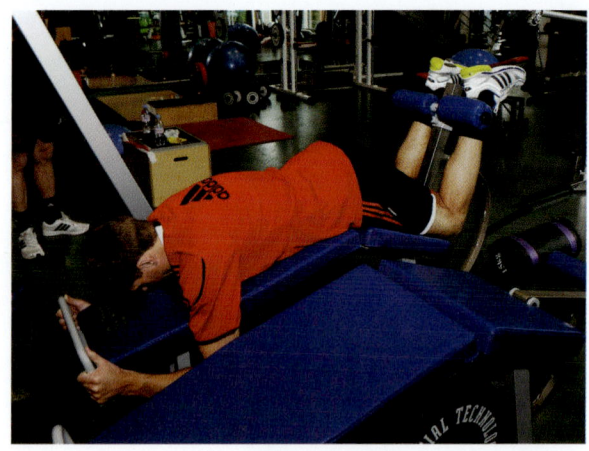

(g)

Figure 34.15 (cont.) (f) The single-leg reverse dead lift. The athlete holds a kettle bell in one hand and flexes forward at the hip while maintaining the lumbar spine in a neutral position. Note that in this instance the non weight-bearing limb is NOT used as a counter lever to specifically increase the load on the hamstrings of the weight-bearing limb. The exercise can be progressed by increasing the weight of the kettle bell, the depth of movement (i.e. the amount of hip flexion) and the speed of movement (i.e. drop/catch) (g) Yo-Yo machine

One study has confirmed the efficacy of the Nordic drops in developing hamstring strength.[74] Other studies have shown that Nordic exercises are effective in preventing both new and recurrent hamstring injuries (see below).[75–77]

The Nordic strengthening program shown in Table 34.4 is based on the Mjolsnes and Arnason studies.[74, 75] It is designed for a 5–10 week pre-season training program. Because of the eccentric load, it is important to ensure that there is at least one day between sessions and that the loads are adjusted if excessive delayed onset muscle soreness (DOMS) results, as this may affect compliance. If the program is continued in-season, then one session per week is adequate.

Generally, low grade/minor hamstring injuries or first-time injuries will progress quickly; therefore, functional strength may be adequate to allow return to sport. In this situation, an exercise such as the single-leg bridge catch (Fig. 34.15b) is probably sufficient.

More severe or recurrent injuries require more advanced strength exercises and high-level eccentric loading (e.g. Nordic eccentric hamstring exercise, single-leg reverse dead lift, L-protocol). Eccentric muscle training results in muscle damage and DOMS in those unaccustomed to it. Therefore, any eccentric strengthening program should allow adequate time for recovery, especially in the first few weeks.

Strengthening for hamstring synergists
Rehabilitation must not be restricted to the hamstring muscles alone–it must also include exercises to target muscles that assist the hip extensor function of the hamstrings, such as the gluteus maximus and adductor magnus muscles. Thus, if gluteal and adductor magnus strength is inadequate in a sprinting athlete, it is possible that the hamstrings will be overloaded.

The gluteus maximus acts during running to control trunk flexion of the stance leg, decelerate the swing

Posterior thigh pain   CHAPTER 34

Table 34.4 Pre-season training protocol for Nordic hamstring exercises

Week	Sessions per week	Sets and repetitions	Load
1	1	2 × 5	Load is increased as subject can withstand the forward fall longer. When managing to withstand the whole range of motion for 12 repetitions, increase load by adding speed to the starting phase of the motion. The partner can also increase loading further by pushing at the back of the shoulders
2	2	2 × 6	
3	3	3 × 6–8	
4	3	3 × 8–10	
5–10	3	3 × 12/10/8	

leg and extend the hip.[78] Therefore, any alteration in gluteus maximus activation, strength or endurance may place greater demand on the hamstrings to control hip extension of the stance leg and decelerate the leg during the swing phase. Overall, the gluteus maximus provides powerful hip extension when sprinting.[79]

The hip extensor moment arm of the gluteus maximus is largest when the hip is in extended, whereas the hip extensor moment arm of the adductor magnus is largest when the hip is flexed.[80] Thus, the gluteus maximus is a strong hip extensor of the extended hip, whereas the adductor magnus is a strong hip extensor of the flexed hip.

To improve gluteus maximus activation, strength and endurance, initially teach good motor patterns and isolate the gluteus maximus from hamstrings, commencing bridges with both legs then progressing to one leg, and finally progress to high load hip extension exercises such as the barbell hip thrust (Fig. 34.16a).[81] Other hip extensor strength exercises that load both the gluteus maximus and adductor magnus in addition to the proximal hamstrings include squats (Fig. 34.16b) and deep lunges (Fig. 34.16c).[66, 79, 82]

Neuromuscular control exercises

Neuromuscular control of the lumbopelvic region, including anterior and posterior pelvic tilt, may be required to promote optimal function of the hamstrings in sprinting and high-speed skilled movement. For example, a rehabilitation program focusing on progressive agility, neuromuscular control and lumbopelvic stability exercises has been shown to be more effective in preventing injury recurrence than a more traditional stretching and simple strengthening exercise program.[50] Furthermore, the time taken to RTP appears to be similar for progressive agility and trunk stabilisation exercises compared to progressive running and eccentric strengthening.[41] Progressive agility and trunk stabilisation exercises include fast feet drills, side-stepping, karaoke side-stepping, single-leg balance

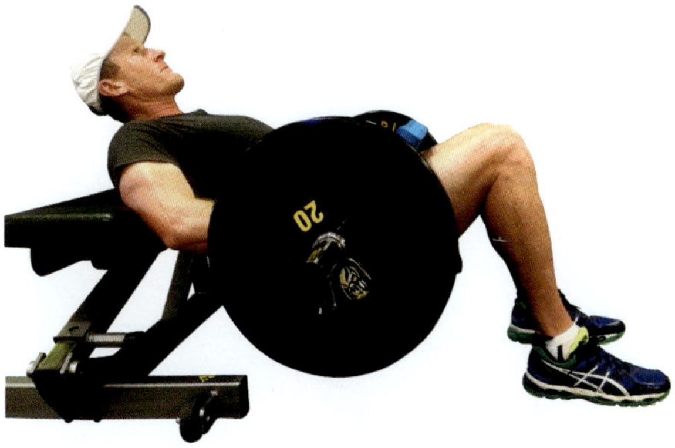

Figure 34.16 Gluteus maximus and adductor magnus strengthening exercises: barbell hip thrust (a) starting with hips flexed and (b) moving hips into extension

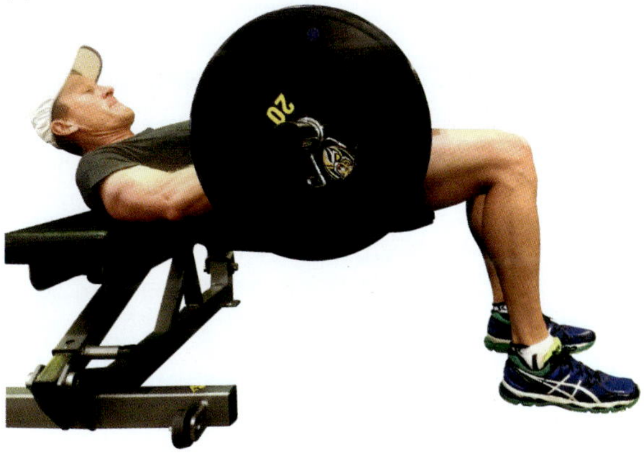

699

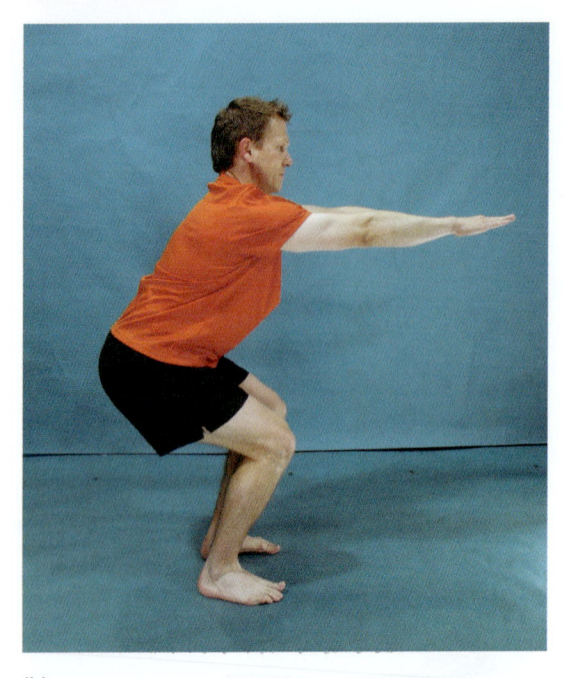

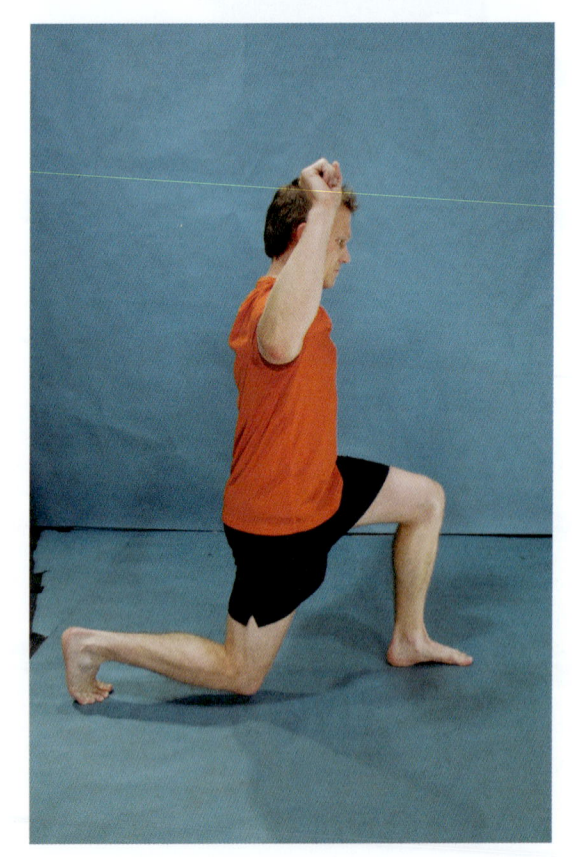

(Fig. 34.17), single-leg stand windmill touches (moving in and out of a body weight arabesque position) and supine single-leg bridging.[41, 50]

It may also be important to consider motor control exercises for the deep lumbar spine stabilisers (e.g. multifidus). Such exercises can involve isolated activations in prone lying, and then progress to functional postural control exercises against gravity (e.g. sit-to-stand action, inclining the trunk forwards by flexing at the hip while maintaining an extended posture at the lower lumbar spine, performed against resistance). Recent studies have found motor control training to be effective in reducing lower-limb injuries in Australian rules football players.[83, 84]

Other examples of advanced neuromuscular control exercises for the lumbopelvic region and entire lower extremity are discussed in Chapter 11.

Functional progression

Early commencement of a structured running program is an important part of the rehabilitation

Figure 34.16 (cont.) (b) Squat (c) Deep lunge

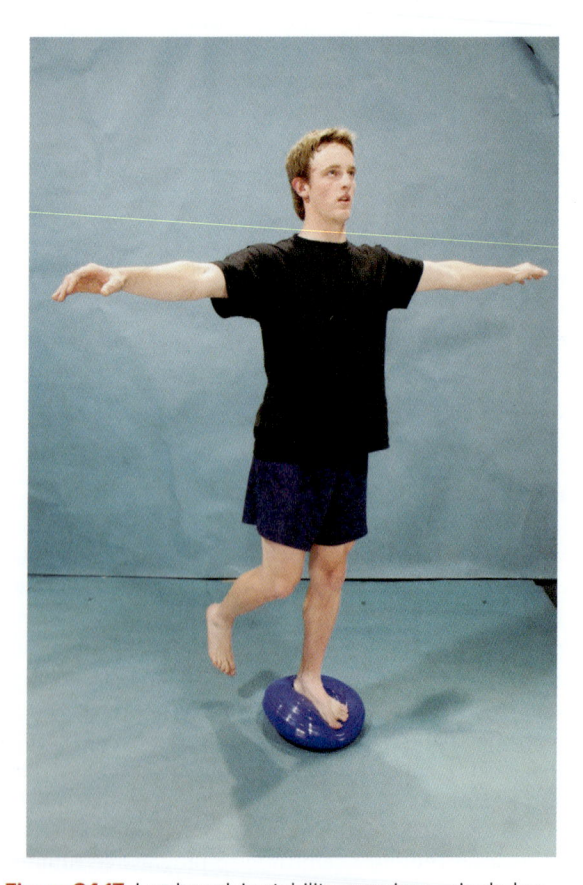

Figure 34.17 Lumbopelvic stability exercises—single-leg balance. A quarter squat can be added

Posterior thigh pain CHAPTER 34

Key principles to consider when designing a running program following hamstring muscle strains

1. Running sessions may be completed 5–6 times per week in the initial stages of the rehabilitation process when volume and intensity is low (if so desired). However, once the sessions become more advanced, a day on/day off approach is recommended (i.e. 3 times per week). Running on a day on/day off basis allows the athlete sufficient time to recover and adapt between sessions. The clinician can assess key clinical signs the following day and make a judgment as to whether or not the athlete has tolerated or reacted adversely to the load. The structure of the next running session can then be planned accordingly.
2. Running can commence once the athlete is capable of producing adequate force with resisted muscle contraction and has no pain with walking or other everyday activities. Begin with slow jogging intervals and then progress to fartlek-type running as tolerated (e.g. 15–20 repetitions of a 10-second walk followed by a 20-second jog followed by a 30-second run).
3. Once the athlete is capable of achieving approximately 50% pace without symptoms or apprehension, then running may be progressed to a structured running program that involves repeated strides over a distance of 60–90 m at a prescribed intensity. In order to increase the dose of high-speed running in the latter stages of the rehabilitation process, extra interval running at a safe intensity can be completed in addition to the structured running program (e.g. 150 m or 200 m repetitions).
4. Load on the hamstrings increases with faster running.[40] Therefore, running speed both within a session and from one session to the next should always be progressed in a graduated manner. Rapid increments in running intensity must be avoided, especially during the early stages of the rehabilitation process.
5. The warm-up prior to running should consist of jogging as well as footwork and agility drills.[41, 50]
6. Sprinting technique drills should also be integrated into the running program (e.g. as part of the warm-up). Sprinting technique drills have been shown to be effective in improving an athlete's lower-limb joint position sense (or proprioception).[85] Furthermore, poor lower-limb joint position sense has been linked with greater risk of hamstring strains in Australian rules football players.[86]
7. Sport-specific training drills should be included in the final stages of the rehabilitation process.[87] Ideally, these drills should simulate as closely as possible the original mechanism of injury.

process following a hamstring muscle strain. The basic principles of the running program are outlined in the box above. Once the athlete has successfully completed all running progressions as well as relevant sport-specific activities, and all strength and neuromuscular control exercises have been advanced to a sufficient level, then the athlete can progress to the next stage— the RTP phase.

> **PRACTICE PEARL**
>
> Progression of hamstring strain rehabilitation is NOT time dependent, but rather progressed on the basis of clinical signs (key outcome measures).

RTP phase

It is extremely difficult to decide when the athlete is ready to RTP after a hamstring strain.[2, 43, 50, 88] These difficulties may be reflected in a conspicuously high injury recurrence rate, particularly within a few weeks after the return.[36, 89] This vulnerability to strain persists, though gradually reduces, for many weeks following RTP.[17]

RTP rehabilitation programs that rely solely on subjective measures such as 'pain-free movements' may result in deficits in neuromuscular control, strength, flexibility, ground reaction force attenuation and production, and lead to asymmetries between legs during normal athletic movements.[79] These deficits and deficiencies could persist into sport practice and competition, and ultimately increase the risk of re-injury and limit athletic performance.

A criteria-based approach to rehabilitation that includes objective and quantitative tests has the potential to identify deficits and address them in a systematic progression (i.e. algorithm) during the stages of returning to sport. While validated criteria to assess whether an athlete can safely RTP are still lacking, criteria that should be considered by the clinician when making this assessment include:

- no difference in tenderness with palpation for the injured versus uninjured hamstring[14]
- full range of movement (equal to uninjured leg) measured via:
    - active/passive straight leg raise test[90, 91]
    - active knee extension test[14]
- pain-free maximal isometric contraction

PART B   Regional problems

- objective strength assessments measured via:
    - hand-held dynamometer[92] or isokinetic dynamometer[93, 94]
    - performance with the Nordic eccentric hamstring exercise (e.g. using the NordBord[88] to measure the force from each lower limb independently during the exercise–see below)
    - performance with the single-leg bridge capacity test[95]
- Askling's H-test[96] (see box below)
- completion of structured running program:
    - maximum sprinting speed achieved at the end of the running program is comparable to the athlete's previously recorded benchmark when uninjured
- functional tests:
    - repeat maximum accelerations from a standing start over a variety of distances (e.g. 5 m, 10 m, 15 m, 20 m)
    - high-intensity weaving/cutting and random (unanticipated) agility activities
    - successful execution of sport-specific activities (e.g. bending over to gather a ground ball while running at speed for Australian rules football players)
- successful completion of a sufficient amount of standard training sessions (e.g. 1 to 2 weeks)
- evaluation of an athlete's psychological status regarding readiness for RTP and fear of re-injury.

While it is recommended that athletes do not RTP following hamstring strains until all clinical signs and

Askling's H-test

Askling's H-test is a complement to the clinical examination before return to sport.[96] Notably, this active test must not be performed before all clinical tests, including those of passive flexibility, indicate complete recovery. During the test, the subject should be positioned on a bench in a supine position with the contralateral leg and the upper body stabilised with straps (Fig. 34.18). A knee brace ensures full knee extension of the tested leg and the foot of the tested leg should be kept in a slightly plantar-flexed position. No warm-up exercises are to be performed before the test. The uninjured leg is tested before the injured leg. The instruction to the subject is to perform a straight leg raise as fast as possible to the highest point without taking any risk of injury. A set of three consecutive trials are performed, preceded by one practice trial with submaximal effort. After the three active test trials, the subject is to estimate experience of insecurity and pain on a VAS scale, from 0 to 100. In the study by Askling, Nilsson and Thorstensson, the athletes noted an average insecurity estimation of 52 for the injured leg and 0 for the uninjured leg, respectively.[96]

The active test seems to be sensitive enough to detect differences both in active flexibility and in insecurity after acute hamstring strains at a point in time when the commonly used clinical examination fails to reveal injury signs. If insecurity persists, the test should be repeated until no insecurity is reported. The athlete is then allowed to return to sport.

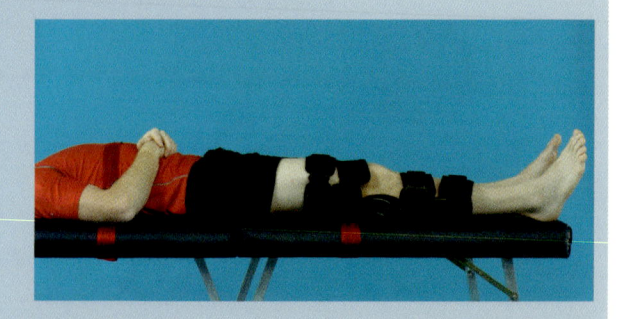

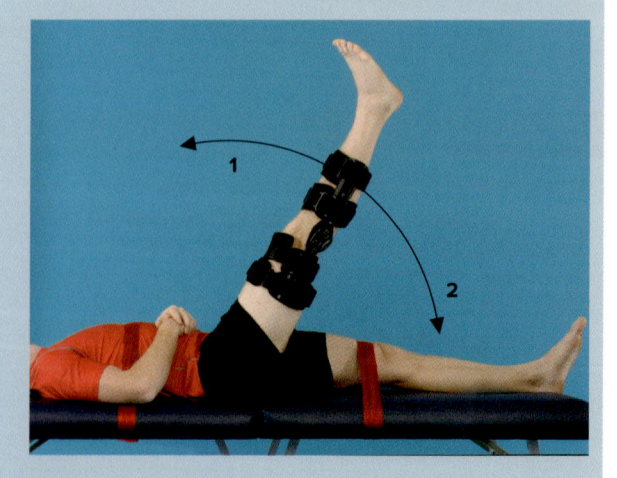

Figure 34.18 Askling's hamstring apprehension test
(a) Starting position (b) Maximal hip flexion

symptoms have fully resolved,[14] clinicians should recognise that many athletes are capable of coping with advanced functional progressions and making a successful RTP despite in some instances having residual strength deficits of 10% of more[94, 97] and persisting increased signal intensity on MRI.[6, 97, 98] These characteristics may take up to 6 months to fully resolve.[97] Hence, MRI appearance does not seem to be a valid indicator of readiness to RTP.

MRI can monitor tissue healing, but the extent of healing on MRI that is sufficient for an athlete to RTP with minimal risk for recurrence is presently not known. It is therefore evident that RTP following hamstring muscle strains rarely coincides with complete healing from the injury, making the timing of RTP a very challenging management decision for the clinician. The issue of RTP has been suggested to be one of risk minimisation (not risk elimination), as there appears to be trade-off between quick RTP and likelihood for recurrence.[99] This trade-off must be acknowledged and carefully considered by the clinician on a case-by-case basis.

The length of time until RTP depends on the severity of the injury. In most cases, an athlete with a mild hamstring strain who is optimally managed will be able to successfully RTP within approximately 18 days.[1]

A practical tip to reduce the incidence of recurrence is to restrict game time when first returning from hamstring injury to minimise fatigue and reduce overall exposure to high-risk activities. In this way, RTP can be gradually progressed over several weeks.

> **PRACTICE PEARL**
>
> It is important to persist with a well-structured strength and neuromuscular control exercise program after RTP to lessen the likelihood of recurrence. All elements of the program should be continued until all impairments have been resolved. These strength sessions must be carefully scheduled to allow recovery time before exposing the athlete to high-risk activities again.

RISK FACTORS FOR ACUTE HAMSTRING STRAIN

We discuss risk factors here because patients rarely present for 'primary prevention'—to avoid hamstring injuries before they have one. We review risk factors for acute hamstring strain to identify those which may be mitigated. As with all injuries (Chapters 3 and 4), risk factors for acute hamstring strains may be intrinsic (person-related) or extrinsic (environment-related) factors. Two systematic reviews were published on this topic in 2013.[100, 101]

Factors that appear to predict risk of hamstring strain are discussed in the following section. Other factors have been evaluated, but do not appear to be risk factors. Such factors include:

- body mass index[36, 102, 103]
- height[36, 37, 102, 103, 105]
- weight[36, 102, 103, 105]
- functional performance tests (e.g. countermovement jump, 40 m sprint tests, gross performance with the Nordic eccentric hamstring exercise, hamstring length measurement).[103]

Intrinsic risk factors

Age

A number of studies have shown that athletes of an older age are at increased risk of acute hamstring strain, even when the confounding factor of previous injury is removed.[37, 102–105] Australian rules football players aged 23 years or more were almost four times as likely to sustain an acute hamstring strain before their younger counterparts during the season.[37]

Older athletes may be at heightened risk due to increased body weight and reduced hip flexor flexibility.[65] It has also been speculated that the high risk of older athletes to acute hamstring strain is related to degenerative changes at the lumbosacral junction.[106]

Past history of injury—a critical factor

Past history of injury is a critical factor for the development of another hamstring injury. It has been well demonstrated that a prior history of acute hamstring strain is a strong risk factor for future injury.[100, 101] In comparison to athletes without a history of hamstring strain, recent studies have found that those with a history do not appear to display appreciable differences in running mechanics;[107–109] however, they do display evidence of neuromuscular inhibition,[110–112] specific strength deficits,[110, 112] as well as altered muscle-tendon morphology (muscle atrophy, reduced muscle fascicle length, presence of scar tissue)[97, 113, 114] and contraction mechanics.[115]

It may be that future risk of re-injury in athletes who have suffered a hamstring strain is explained by the presence of one or more of these characteristics. Clinical interventions (e.g. exercise, manual therapy) aimed at addressing or minimising the impact of such characteristics are therefore of great importance.

Athletes with a history of injury to other areas of the lower limb also have an increased likelihood of acute hamstring strain. These include:

- knee–major knee injury (anterior cruciate reconstruction, patellar dislocation)[105, 116]
- groin–history of groin pain (bone oedema MRI)[105]
- calf muscle strain[104]
- lumbar spine–major injury (i.e. episode which required radiological investigation with a specific recorded clinical diagnosis).[105]

Strength

Numerous studies have evaluated whether strength quantified via an isokinetic dynamometer is a risk factor for hamstring strain. While intuitively reduced muscle strength would appear to predispose to hamstring strain, the evidence is mixed. Such conflicting findings may relate to the difficulty in quantifying muscle strength in a systematic manner; that is, what type of contraction (isometric, concentric, eccentric), what strength parameter or index to measure (peak torque, knee angle at which peak torque occurs, hamstring/quadriceps ratio, hamstring to hip flexor ratio, strength asymmetry), as well as the level of motivation of the athletes.

A recent systematic review and meta-analysis evaluating the existing evidence regarding risk factors for hamstring strain reported a somewhat counterintuitive outcome concerning strength; specifically, that increased quadriceps strength is a risk factor for hamstring strain but reduced hamstring strength is not.[100] This result might be a consequence of some of the previously outlined issues with measuring strength, but it might also be a consequence of previous risk factor studies not taking the multifactorial nature of hamstring injuries into account.[117] Clinicians aiming to design evidence-based hamstring injury prevention programs for athletes are therefore advised to be cautious about how findings from risk factor studies are interpreted.

To further understand the role that hamstring strength has in creating injury risk, a prospective study has recently been completed investigating whether or not eccentric hamstring strength, measured during the Nordic hamstring exercise, is a risk factor for hamstring strain in elite Australian rules football players.[118]

In this study, a novel field-testing device, the NordBord (Fig. 34.19), was used to record eccentric strength while players performed the Nordic hamstring exercise. Force was recorded by connecting uniaxial load cells between the braces holding the ankles and the base of the testing device, allowing the force output for each lower limb to be recorded independently. Peak force during the exercise from a single lower limb averaged 330 N for uninjured football players. Players with a peak force of less than 279 N at the end of the pre-season were found to have a 4.3 fold greater risk of sustaining a hamstring strain during the season. Similar results have also recently been reported in elite soccer players.[119] Taken together, these findings suggest that athletes with low levels of eccentric hamstring strength are at greater risk of injury.

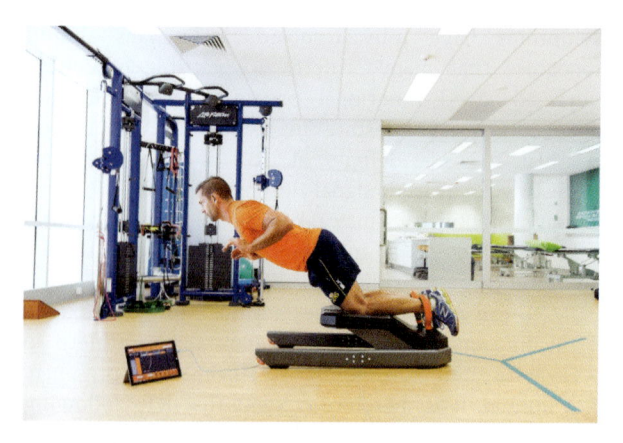

Figure 34.19 The NordBord test

Musculotendon morphology

While the available evidence is somewhat limited at this stage, intrinsic musculotendon morphological properties may have a role in determining an individual's risk for hamstring strain. For example, the width of the proximal biceps femoris long head tendon exhibits high variability among healthy athletes,[120] and tissue strains in the muscle fibres immediately adjacent to the proximal musculotendinous junction have been found to be higher in individuals with a narrow proximal tendon width.[121, 122] Thus, it is possible that athletes with a narrow proximal tendon have an increased risk for proximal biceps femoris long head strains.

Smaller muscle fascicle length might be another morphological property associated with greater risk for injury, as it has been recently reported that athletes with a history of unilateral hamstring strain have reduced muscle fascicle length in the biceps femoris long head on the injured side compared to the contralateral uninjured side and compared to people without a history of injury.[114] Furthermore, a recent prospective study has found that risk of hamstring injury is significantly greater for soccer players with biceps femoris long head fascicle lengths shorter than 10.56 cm.[119]

Other factors

Other intrinsic risk factors for acute hamstring strain which have only limited supporting evidence include (but are not limited to): ethnicity,[23, 105] reduced ankle dorsiflexion lunge range of motion,[123] reduced quadriceps flexibility[91, 123] and poor lower-limb joint position sense.[86]

There is conflicting evidence regarding whether or not reduced hamstring flexibility (e.g. assessed via the active and/or passive knee extension test) is a risk factor for hamstring strain. Most studies indicate that reduced hamstring flexibility is not a risk factor;[37, 102, 103, 123] however, two studies have reported the contrary.[91, 124]

Extrinsic risk factors

Fatigue
It has long been speculated that fatigue is a risk factor for an acute hamstring strain, but there is very little evidence to support or refute this claim. Verrall et al. found that 85% of acute hamstring strains occurred after the first quarter of a competitive match or after the first 15 minutes of a training session.[8] Furthermore, Woods et al. found that 47% of their acute hamstring strains occurred towards the end (during the final third) of the first and second halves of the match.[23] Such observations suggest fatigue may be a factor, but further research is required.

Player position
There is limited evidence that different playing positions are associated with a higher risk of hamstring strain. Goalkeepers have a significantly lower risk for hamstring strain than outfield players in soccer[23] and rugby forwards have a reduced risk of hamstring strains compared to backs.[36] In American football, the speed position players, such as the wide receivers and defensive secondary, as well as players on the special teams units, are most commonly injured.[20]

PREVENTION OF HAMSTRING STRAINS
A systematic review published in 2010 concluded that there is insufficient evidence from randomised controlled trials to draw conclusions on the effectiveness of interventions used to prevent hamstring injuries in people participating in football or other high-risk activities for these injuries.[125] However, recent studies have provided strong evidence indicating that eccentric hamstring strength training with good compliance is an effective intervention for preventing hamstring strains.[126]

Eccentric hamstring strength training
High-quality studies have demonstrated that eccentric strength training for the hamstring muscles can prevent hamstring strains in athletes.[75–77, 127]

In Petersen's study,[76] there was a significant reduction (approximately 3-fold) in the 'total' number of hamstring injuries (i.e. new plus recurrent injuries) and a significant reduction (approximately 7-fold) in the number of recurrent injuries for the intervention group, which undertook a 10-week progressive pre-season eccentric training program of Nordic exercises (Table 34.4) followed by a weekly seasonal program. There was also an approximate 2.5-fold reduction in the number of new hamstring injuries in the intervention group, but this effect did not reach statistical significance.

Arnason's study also showed a reduction in hamstring injuries with a Nordic exercise program,[75] while a positive effect on prevention of hamstring injuries in soccer players was also found for an eccentric/concentric strengthening program using a Yo-Yo flywheel ergometer.[126] Most recently, van der Horst et al. investigated the preventive effect of the Nordic hamstring exercise in amateur soccer players and found a significant reduction in the incidence of hamstring strains but not the severity.[77]

In contrast to the aforementioned studies, two other studies have investigated the effectiveness of the Nordic hamstring exercise. Gabbe et al.[128] reported a minimal effect only, while Engebretsen et al.[129] reported no effect. However, both of these studies suffered from poor compliance, which most likely explains the less favourable results.[125]

Balance exercises/proprioception training
Proprioceptive exercises or balance training may be an effective strategy for preventing hamstring injuries.[130–132] A positive effect was found in one study,[130] while two other studies failed to show any effect.[131, 132]

In the German study, 24 elite female soccer players of a premier league soccer team included an additional soccer-specific proprioceptive multistation training program over 3 years.[130] Progression in level of difficulty from easy to complex was a main feature of the exercises. The duration of each exercise was between 15 and 30 seconds.

The following exercises were implemented:

1. single-leg stand on right and left foot
2. jump forwards in single-leg stand with flexed knee at landing and balancing
3. jump backwards in single-leg stand and balancing
4. row jumping single foot
5. row jumping bipedal
6. obstacle course forwards and backwards
7. obstacle course sideways
8. bipedal jumping on forefoot
9. sideways jumping in single-leg stand
10. sitting on a wobble board with balancing torso
11. jumping forwards over a line, landing with flexed knees and balancing
12. standing on both hands and feet with diagonal balancing.

PART B   Regional problems

All exercises were performed with no additional weight; that is, players had to bear only their own body weight on one or two legs or all extremities depending on the exercise. In addition, balance training was implemented in soccer-specific match play training on balance boards.

At the end of the 3-year proprioceptive balance training intervention, non-contact hamstring injury rates were reduced from 22.4 to 8.2/1000 hours. Furthermore, the more minutes of balance training performed, the lower the rate of hamstring injuries.

Sport-specific training

In seasonal sports such as Australian rules football and soccer, hamstring strains occur far more frequently during official matches/games than training sessions. Hence, sport-specific training during the pre-season is considered to be an important strategy for preventing hamstring strains during the competitive season.[133]

The aim of sport-specific training during the pre-season is to gradually expose the hamstring muscles to the sorts of high-risk activities that are regularly encountered during the competitive season (e.g. repetitive sprinting, maximum accelerations, kicking, running with trunk flexion), thereby improving the ability of the hamstrings to withstand these activities. For instance, Verrall et al. demonstrated a significant reduction in the incidence of hamstring strains in one Australian rules football club following the introduction of sprint training, stretching once fatigued and sport-specific training drills during the pre-season.[87]

A promising clinical approach for the high-risk athlete

Another potential strategy for preventing hamstring strains, especially for the athlete with a past history of injury, is to try to identify (via clinical examination) those who have reacted adversely to a high-intensity activity (e.g. match/game or training session). In some instances, high-intensity activities may result in aberrant levels of muscle damage and/or fatigue. Athletes can be assessed 1–2 days following a match/game throughout the competitive season and high-risk activities can be modified accordingly for those who display positive clinical signs (e.g. pain and inhibition with resisted muscle contraction and overt tenderness with palpation).

Isometric maximum voluntary contractions may be most suitable for this purpose because they are quick and easy to perform for the clinician, no expensive equipment is necessarily required and they are relatively safe for the athlete. Recent research has demonstrated the potential capability of isometric maximum voluntary contractions of the hamstrings to detect the presence of neuromuscular inhibition for up to 72 hours following a soccer match.[134, 135]

A simple, clinically applicable approach for measuring isometric maximum voluntary contractions has been described by Schache et al.[136] A digital sphygmomanometer can be used as an inexpensive way to quantify the athlete's hamstring strength. Alternatively, a portable force plate can be used to obtain data in newtons (N).[135] Data can be collected in different positions that change the way load is distributed on the hamstrings; for example, with the athlete positioned with their knee flexed to 90° and heel resting on a firm surface (Fig. 34.20a) or with the athlete positioned in supine with their knee extended and heel resting on a small step performing a single-leg bridge (Fig. 34.20b). Both of these positions mimic commonly used pain provocation tests for the hamstrings. Other clinically applicable and reliable methods for recording isometric maximum voluntary contractions of the hamstrings involve the use of a hand-held dynamometer or load cell and are performed in various prone or seated positions against either therapist resistance or external belt fixation.[92, 137, 138]

The overall objective is to identify those athletes who have painful and/or inhibited hamstring muscles. It is then up to the clinician to use these findings together with the athlete's history and other clinical examination findings to decide whether or not an intervention is required, and if so, what type of intervention (e.g. manual therapy, specific exercise therapy, activity modification). Clinically applicable tests of hamstring strength are also very useful outcome measures for monitoring healing following acute hamstring strains.[34]

(a)

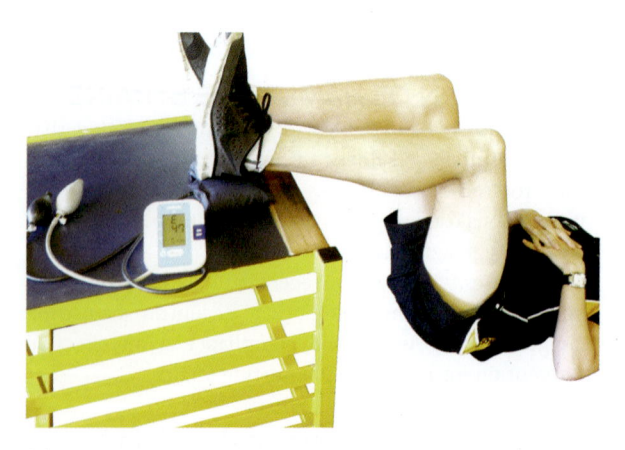

Figure 34.20 Schache's hamstring maximum voluntary contraction (MVC) test.[136] The set-up used to measure an isometric MVC of the hamstrings with the digital sphygmomanometer (a) The athlete is positioned with his or her knee flexed to 90° and heel resting on a firm surface

Posterior thigh pain   CHAPTER 34

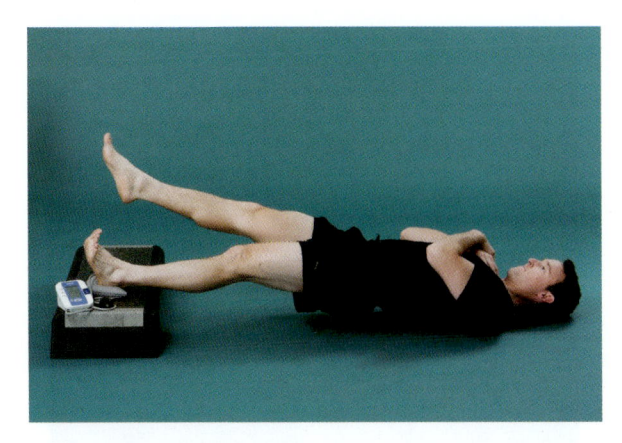

(b)

Figure 34.20 (cont.) (b) The athlete positioned in supine with their knee extended and heel resting on a small step performing a single-leg bridge

REFERRED PAIN TO POSTERIOR THIGH

The possibility of referred pain should always be considered in the athlete presenting with posterior thigh pain. Hamstring pain may be referred from the lumbar spine, the SIJ or from soft tissues; for example, the proximal fibres of the gluteus maximus, and especially the gluteus medius and the piriformis muscle. Often, there is a history of previous or current low back pain.

The slump test (Fig. 34.2g) should be used to detect neural tightness. The test is positive when the patient's hamstring pain is reproduced and subsequently relieved with reduction of the neural tension by neck extension. Examination may reveal reduced range of movement of the lumbar spine, tenderness and/or stiffness of lumbar intervertebral joint(s) or tenderness over the area of the SIJ.

A positive slump test is strongly suggestive of a referred component to the patient's pain. The slump test has been advocated as a method of treatment of hamstring pain in Australian rules football players.[139] Nevertheless, a negative slump test does not exclude the possibility of referred pain and the lumbar spine should be carefully examined to detect any intervertebral segment hypomobility. Careful palpation of the hip musculature, especially the extensors, abductors and external rotators, should also be performed.

Trigger points

Trigger points are common sources of referred pain to both the buttock (Chapter 30) and posterior thigh. The most common trigger points that refer pain to the

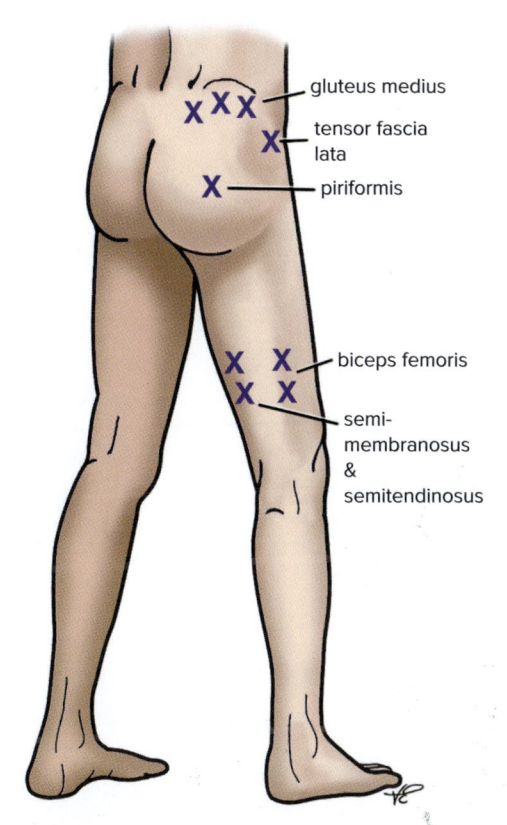

Figure 34.21 Pattern of referred pain to the hamstrings from trigger points

mid-hamstring are in the gluteus minimus, gluteus medius and piriformis muscles (Fig. 34.21).

The clinical syndrome associated with posterior thigh pain without evidence of hamstring muscle injury on MRI and reproduction of the patient's pain on palpation of gluteal trigger points is now well recognised and extremely common.[140]

The clinical features are described earlier in Table 34.2. The patient will often complain of a feeling of tightness, cramping, 'twinge' or a feeling that the hamstring is 'about to tear'. On examination there may be some localised tenderness in the hamstring, although it is usually not focal and there is restriction in hamstring and gluteal stretch. Firm palpation of the gluteal muscles will detect tight bands that contain active trigger points, which when firmly palpated are extremely tender, refer pain into the hamstring and may elicit a 'twitch response'.

Treatment involves deactivating the trigger point either with soft tissue massage techniques (Fig. 32.22a) or dry needling (Fig. 32.22b). Following the local treatment, the tight muscle groups (the gluteals and hamstrings) should be stretched.

PART B   Regional problems

(a)   (b)

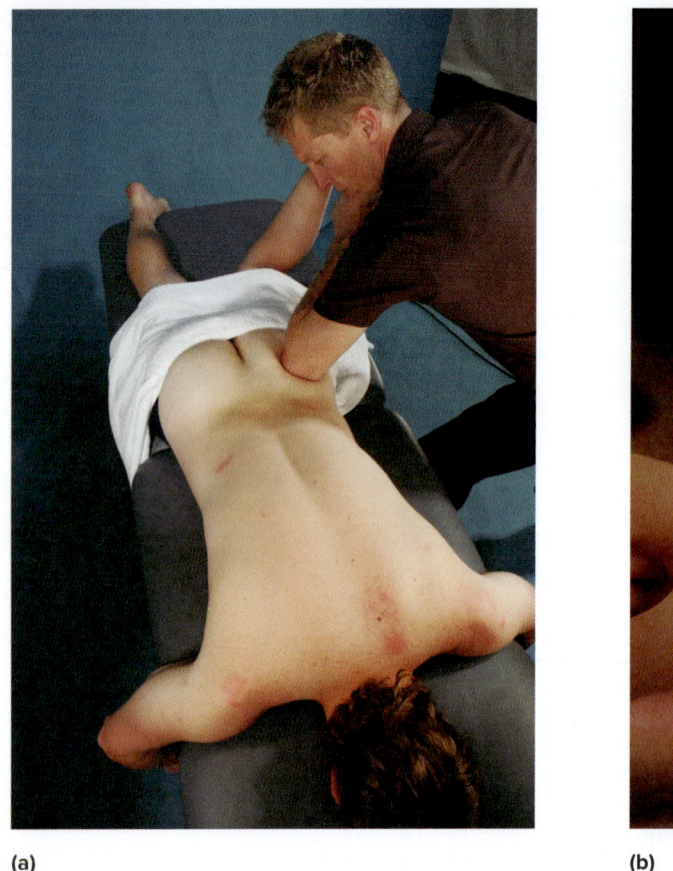

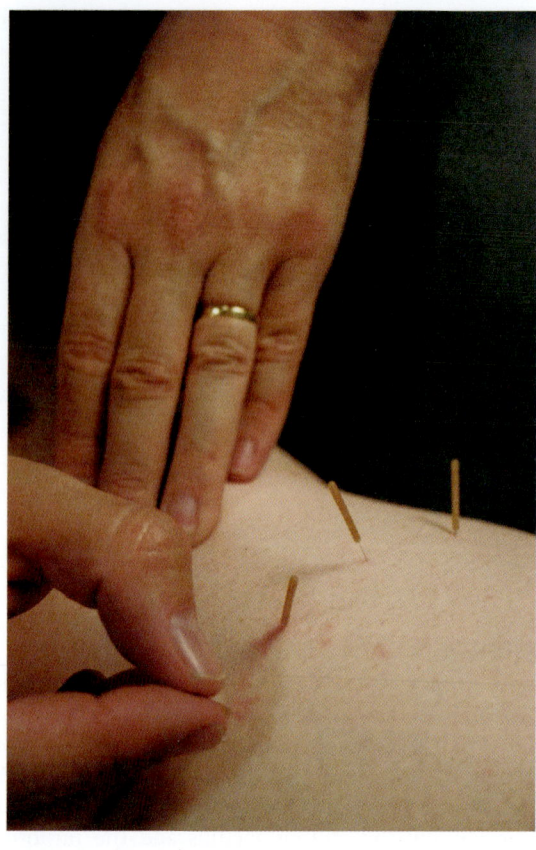

Figure 34.22 Treatment of gluteal trigger points (a) Elbow pressure (b) Dry needling

Lumbar spine

The lumbar spine is a source of pain referral to the posterior thigh. Unfortunately, it is difficult to distinguish between sources based on the behaviour and distribution of the pain. Pain may be referred from the disc, zygapophyseal joints, muscles, ligaments or any structure that can produce pain locally in the lumbar spine.[141]

Nerve root compression may also be a cause of hamstring pain. Diagnostic blocks and provocation injections have been advocated to isolate sources of pain in the lumbar spine. However, in the clinical setting, this is often not possible. It is important to examine the lumbar spine carefully (Chapter 29). This will assist in the identification of the lumbar spine as a source of hamstring pain. It is also important to remember that the lumbar spine may be a cause of lumbar pain indirectly. For example, the lumbar spine may cause a biomechanical block to hip extension, resulting in overload of the SIJ and referred pain to the hamstring group.

True nerve root compression is usually more definitive in its presentation. The patient may have associated neurological symptoms, such as numbness and loss of foot eversion. The management of these injuries usually involves an extended period of rest and, in certain cases, an epidural injection. In extreme cases, surgical decompression of the nerve root may be warranted.

Spondylolisthesis and spondylolysis (Chapter 29) have both been associated with hamstring pain and tightness.[142] Examination findings of positive lumbar quadrant tests or single-leg standing lumbar extension suggests either of these conditions and these spinal pathologies can be confirmed on MRI or CT scan.

Stabilisation programs are the treatment of choice as the deep abdominal muscles are deficient in people with back pain as a result of spondylolisthesis and spondylolysis.[143] In severe cases, clinicians have resorted to corticosteroid injection (+/− neuroablation using pulsed radiofrequency) under X-ray control into the deficient pars interarticularis.[144] This procedure is only supported by low-level evidence, but it may reduce pain from spondylolysis.

Not all hamstring pain associated with the lumbar spine is due to sport-related loading of the lumbar spine. The lumbar spine can cause pain as a result of prolonged sitting

Posterior thigh pain — CHAPTER 34

or bending forwards. Athletes in sedentary occupations should be aware that poor sitting posture can aggravate lumbar-mediated posterior thigh pain.

Travel involving prolonged sitting prior to training and competition may cause injury. Prolonged sitting results in sustained lumbar flexion whereas running requires good lumbar extension. When the lumbar spine is required to suddenly 'switch' from one activity to the other, this may cause problems. Care should be taken to limit prolonged sitting and to provide adequate lumbar support.

Sacroiliac complex

SIJ abnormalities can refer pain into the hamstring or cause indirect pain in the hamstring similar to the lumbar spine. Problems of the SIJ are discussed in Chapter 30.

OTHER HAMSTRING INJURIES

Avulsion of the hamstring from the ischial tuberosity

with RAJ SUBBU and FARES HADDAD

The proximal hamstring complex is frequently injured in athletes, with 12% of hamstring injuries being in the proximal complex and 9% being complete ruptures.[145] Traditionally, these occur in waterskiing, sprinting and hurdling; however, they are increasingly being recognised in a variety of different sports, commonly soccer and rugby.[146] The injuries are typically associated with a very forceful eccentric contraction of the hamstrings where the hip is rapidly flexed with the knee in full extension.

Patients present with a history of hearing a pop or snap at time of injury, complaining of acute pain at the buttock crease, an antalgic gait, and loss of hip and knee function with reduced hamstring power. Physical examination may reveal swelling and massive ecchymosis in the posterior aspect of the thigh, which may even track distally. There may also be a positive bowstring sign when the patient is assessed in the prone position with a palpable lack of tension on passive flexion of the knee to 90°. Palpation at the gluteal crease evokes pain and there is decreased power in both flexion of the knee and extension of the hip. Tenderness proximally with symptoms and signs of sciatic nerve irritation should alert the clinician to the possibility of an avulsion injury.

Once clinically assessed, radiological imaging is required to confirm the diagnosis. MRI and ultrasonography remain the imaging modalities of choice (Fig 34.23).[145] With greater severity of injury there is a greater amount of haemorrhage, oedema and fluid involving a larger longitudinal and cross-sectional area.[145] Studies have compared MRI and ultrasonography, and MRI has been shown to consistently demonstrate large areas of oedema and greater sensitivity in picking up subtle fluid changes and exact anatomical area of injury.[147] A specific MRI classification for proximal avulsion injuries has been described based on the anatomical location and amount of retraction of the proximal complex (Table 34.5).[147] Typically, type 5 injuries are delayed presentations, indicating that the tendons may retract with time (Fig 34.23b).

Treatment has previously been based on the amount of retraction from the ischial tuberosity with less than 2 cm being treated conservatively, which may lead to decreased hamstring strength, function and prolonged rehabilitation.[148] A recent study of 112 proximal avulsion injuries has shown that surgical repair is indicated in all proximal avulsion injuries despite the amount of retraction.[146]

The timing of surgery is important regarding RTP. Subbu et al. reported that the average time to RTP for those with surgical repair within 6 weeks of initial injury was 16 weeks (range 12–32), 25 weeks (range 18–40) within 6 months and 29 weeks (24–41) after 6 months of initial injury.[146] Return to full pre-injury level of sport was on average 9 weeks faster for those with surgical repair within 6 weeks of injury compared with those within 6 months, and 13 weeks faster compared with those with surgical repair performed more than 6 months after injury.[146]

(a)

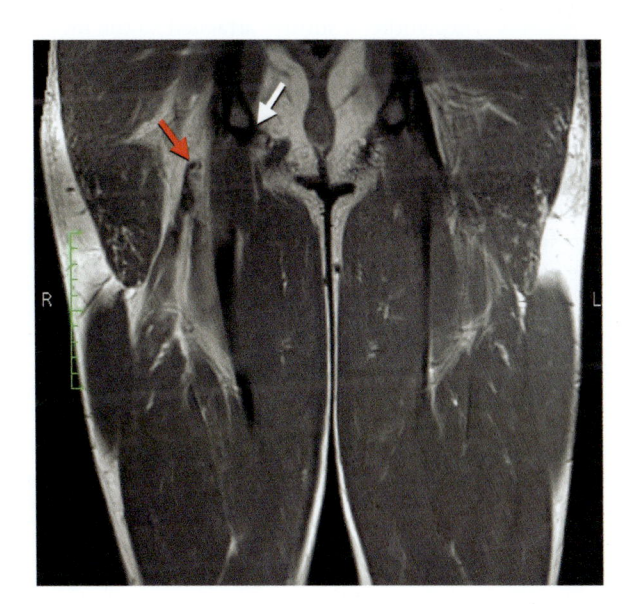

Figure 34.23 (a) MRI showing acute complete avulsion of the conjoint tendon of semitendinosus and biceps femoris with retraction (red arrow). Semimembranosus intact (white arrow)

PART B   Regional problems

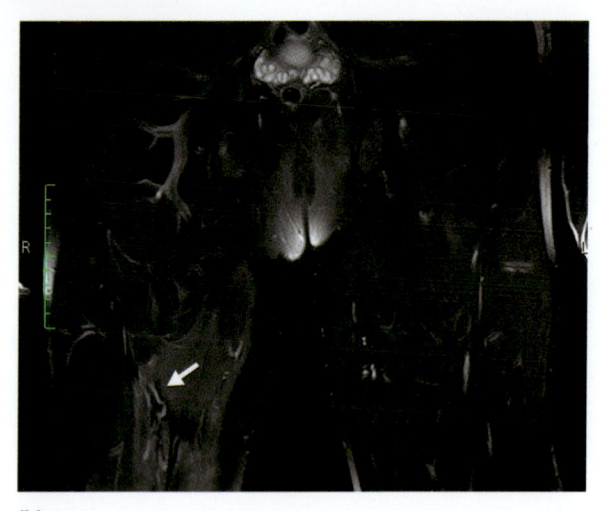

Figure 34.23 (cont.) (b) MRI showing chronic complete avulsion of the entire proximal hamstring complex with diffuse increased signal and early muscle atrophy. Ischial tuberosity fragment identified (arrow). Consistent with type 5b injury

A structured rehabilitation program should be centred on using the first 4 weeks as healing time while protecting the surgical repair. The next 4 weeks are used to regain range of motion and function and then a graduated return to sport-specific activity.[149] Each patient should be given an individualised rehabilitation program depending on the complexity of surgery and the level of activity to be achieved. A rehabilitation guide is outlined in Table 34.6.

Early diagnosis and surgical interventions are associated with less complex surgery, fewer postoperative complications, more efficient rehabilitation and a faster return to pre-injury levels of activity.

Upper hamstring tendinopathy

Tendinopathy of the proximal hamstring tendon or 'high hamstring tendinopathy' is increasingly being recognised as an important cause for chronic pain in the active population (Chapter 30). Patients usually present with subacute onset of deep buttock or posterior thigh pain/stiffness that is exacerbated by repetitive activity (such as long-distance running) and is often aggravated by sitting, stretching and aggressive strengthening. MRI is more sensitive than ultrasound in detecting pathological abnormalities involving the proximal hamstring tendons, but note that many typical findings such as intratendinous and peritendinous signal as well as ischial tuberosity oedema can also be seen in asymptomatic individuals.

Initial treatment in clinical practice should include a graduated strengthening program, largely comprising isometric and slow isotonic exercises under high load. However, patients sometimes fail to respond to this conservative regimen. The use of ultrasound-guided injections of corticosteroid and local anaesthetic has been shown to be safe and effective in reducing pain in the short term, but is associated with a high recurrence rate when used in isolation.[150] This procedure should be performed in conjunction with a progressive strengthening program to achieve optimal results and avoid recurrent injury.

The surgical procedure involves retrieving the retracted complex with suture anchors that have a metal peg, which are fastened into the ischial tuberosity. The synthetic sutures attached to the metal peg can then be passed through the mobilised tendon to fashion a well-tensioned bone–tendon approximation. When surgery is delayed, the procedure becomes more complex with greater retraction of the proximal complex; a larger, vertical incision is required for greater exposure and there is an increased risk of damage to the sciatic nerve, with it becoming embedded within the retracted complex. When surgery is delayed until after 6 weeks, patients inevitably require postoperative bracing which consequently delays the rehabilitation process.

Table 34.5 MRI classification of proximal avulsion injuries[147]

Type	Level of injury
Type 1	Osseous avulsions (generally seen in paediatric patients)
Type 2	Avulsions at the musculotendinous junction
Type 3	Incomplete tendon avulsions
Type 4	Complete avulsions with no/minimal retraction
Type 5a	Complete avulsions with retraction but NO sciatic nerve involvement
Type 5b	Complete avulsions with retraction AND sciatic nerve involvement

Table 34.6 Rehabilitation protocol for proximal avulsion injuries

Weeks	Rehabilitation guide
1–2	Avoid hip flexion beyond 60°
	Wound care
	Avoid sitting on affected ischial tuberosity
	Calf pumps
	Non weight-bearing
3–4	Start passive knee flexion and hip extension
5–6	Bear toe weight if possible
7–10	Encourage to bear full weight
	Hydrotherapy
	Passive and active range of motion—avoid extremes
	Begin core work
	Begin closed chain exercises
11–14	Expect normal gait
	Encourage strength work
	Progress to fast walk/jog
15–16	Consider isokinetic testing
	Heavy weight training
	Potentially running

A rehabilitation program utilising eccentric training, lumbopelvic stabilisation and trigger point dry needling has been suggested.[151] Shock wave treatment has also been shown to be effective in relieving symptoms associated with high hamstring tendinopathy.[152]

In order to document the severity of the tendinopathy, the VISA-H questionnaire has recently been developed.[153]

LESS COMMON CAUSES
Nerve entrapments
The hamstring group is supplied by the tibial branch of the sciatic nerve except for the short head of the biceps femoris, which is supplied by the peroneal branch of the sciatic nerve. These nerves arise from the lumbosacral plexus, specifically from the roots of L5, S1 and S2.

Nerve damage can occur at a variety of sites, resulting in pain in the posterior thigh. Compression of the nerve roots of the sacral plexus will often result in pain into the hamstring group. Usually this is distinguished from other conditions by the identification of associated neurological symptoms such as alteration in sensation, loss of the Achilles reflex or weakness in muscles not in the hamstring group, such as the ankle evertors.

The sciatic nerve may be damaged or compressed at any point along its pathway as a result of direct impact or pelvic trauma. Compression of the nerve at the level of the piriformis has been described as an alternative cause of sciatica.[154] However, work by McCrory et al. suggests that it is not only the piriformis, but also the other hip external rotators that may cause compression of the sciatic nerve.[155]

The peripheral nerves may also be a source of posterior thigh pain. The posterior cutaneous nerve of the thigh (PCNT) and the inferior cluneal nerve supply the skin over the posterior thigh. The PCNT has been described as the source of pain in piriformis syndrome as an alternative to the sciatic nerve.[155] If symptoms do not extend below the knee and there is no associated loss of neurological function in the structures supplied by the sciatic nerve, then the PCNT should be considered.

Ischial bursitis
It is often difficult to distinguish between high hamstring tendinopathy and ischial bursitis. Both conditions present as pain at the origin of the hamstring muscle. An inflamed bursa is not readily palpated; however, athletes tend to complain of pain when sitting on hard surfaces where the ischium is under pressure. Ultrasound or MRI can confirm the presence of a fluid-filled bursa.

Anti-inflammatory medications combined with ice and rest are of limited benefit. Corticosteroid injections can be performed under radiographic control but the results are not always satisfactory.

Adductor magnus strains
Adductor magnus strains are rare, but when they do occur, behave similarly to a hamstring strain. The mechanism tends to be more of a rotatory action of eccentric internal rotation on one hip or landing with sudden deep hip flexion. Prognosis tends to be far better than hamstring strains; therefore, it is important to differentiate it from strains in the hamstring. The key to differentiating this condition is careful palpation to elicit the precise location of the tissue damage. Side-lying on the affected leg allows that hamstring group to fall laterally so that ready access can be made to the adductor magnus.

Compartment syndrome of the posterior thigh
Although nowhere near as common as lower leg compartment syndromes, the posterior thigh can be affected by a compartment syndrome. Patients present with dull pain, stiffness, cramps and weakness of the posterior thigh during and after training.[156] Two groups of patients with this syndrome are seen–endurance athletes without a history of trauma and those with a history of hamstring injury. Conservative management has not been successful and posterior fasciotomy of the thigh appears to be an effective treatment.[156]

PART B Regional problems

Vascular

Endofibrosis of the external iliac artery usually produces pain in the lateral and anterior thigh or calf (Chapter 39). However, in some cases pain may be experienced in the posterior thigh. This condition is associated with cycling and has been observed in triathletes.[157] The pain is claudicant in nature. Pain may arise after 15–20 minutes of exercise but usually stops immediately with the cessation of exercise.

On examination, a bruit is heard during the exercise that causes the pain. Diagnosis may be confirmed with echography or arteriography. If the condition is affecting performance, then surgical treatment is indicated.

REFERENCES

References for this chapter can be found at www.mhhe.com/au/CSM5e

Chapter 35

Acute knee injuries

with RICHARD FROBELL, RANDALL COOPER, HAYDEN MORRIS, and MARK HUTCHINSON

The thing is I have no ACL. So unless I get surgery, there's nothing really magical that I can do that's going to make it better. I just can get my leg stronger, my muscle stronger and try and support it a little more. But that has a small impact. My knee is loose and it's not stable and that's the way it's going to be from here on out.

Lindsey Vonn, Olympic gold medal skier

For many athletes, the most fearful injury is that of the acute knee–it can spell the end of a professional career. Even for recreational athletes, an acute knee injury may be the catalyst for early arthritis. Acute knee injuries are common in all sports that require twisting movements and sudden changes of direction, especially the various types of football, basketball, netball and alpine skiing.

FUNCTIONAL ANATOMY

The knee joint can be divided into two parts: the tibio-femoral joint with its associated collateral ligaments, cruciate ligaments and menisci; and the patellofemoral joint, which obtains stability from the medial and lateral retinaculum and the large extensor mechanism tendons (quadriceps and patella tendons) which encase the patella distally before its insertion on the proximal tibia. Most commonly we refer to the tibiofemoral joint as the knee joint. The anatomy of the knee joint is shown in Figure 35.1.

The two cruciate ('cross') ligaments, anterior and posterior, are often referred to as the 'crucial' ligaments, because of their importance in providing knee stability. They are named anterior and posterior in relation to their

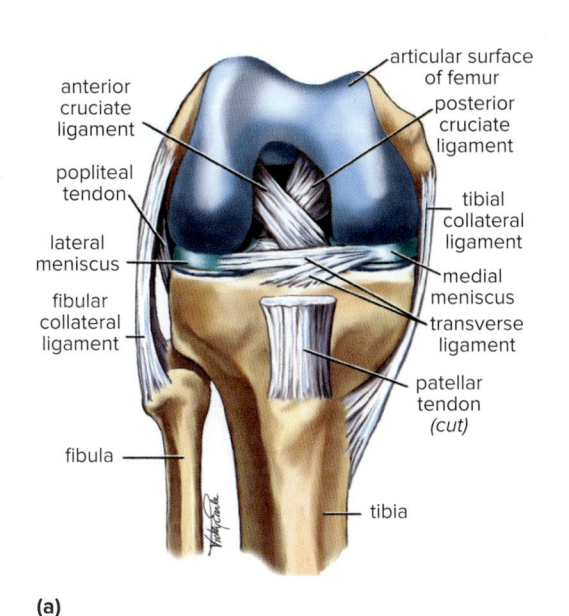

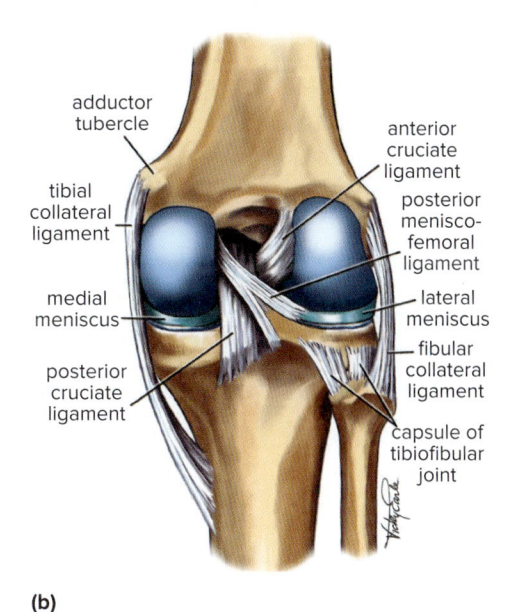

Figure 35.1 Anatomy of the knee joint (a) The knee joint (anterior view) (b) The knee joint (posterior view)

attachment to the tibia. The anterior cruciate ligament (ACL) prevents forward movement of the tibia in relation to the femur and controls rotational movement of the tibia under the femur. The posterior cruciate ligament (PCL) prevents the femur from sliding forwards off the tibial plateau.

The ACL is essential for control in pivoting movements. If the ACL is not functional, the tibia may rotate under the femur in an anterior–lateral direction such as when an athlete attempts to land from a jump, pivot or stop suddenly. The PCL stabilises the body (femur) above the tibia. In its absence, the femur wants to shift forwards on the tibia. This shift forwards is accentuated when one tries to run down an incline plane or down stairs.

The two collateral ligaments, the medial and lateral, provide medial and lateral stability to the knee joint. The superficial medial (or tibial) collateral ligament (MCL) is extracapsular. The deep layer, or coronal ligaments, attaches to the joint margins and has an attachment from its deep layer to the medial meniscus. The MCL prevents excessive medial opening (i.e. valgus) of the tibial–femoral joint.

The lateral (or fibular) collateral ligament (LCL) is a narrow strong cord with no attachment to the lateral meniscus. It prevents lateral opening of the tibia on the femur during varus stress; it also stabilises the upright knee in single-leg stance phase of gait.

The medial and lateral menisci are intra-articular and attach to the capsule layer at the level of the joint line. The menisci buffer some of the forces placed through the knee joint and protect the otherwise exposed articular surfaces from damage. By increasing the concavity of the tibia, they contribute to stabilising the knee. As the menisci contribute to joint lubrication and nutrition, it is important to preserve as much of them as possible after injury.

CLINICAL APPROACH

The acute knee injury of greatest concern to the athlete is the tear of the ACL. Meniscal injuries are common among athletes, either in isolation or combined with a ligament injury (e.g. of the MCL or ACL). Importantly, the articular cartilage of the knee is often damaged in association with ligament or meniscal injuries. Cartilage damage, depending on the size and/or location, can accelerate the development of arthritis.[1]

A list of acute knee injuries occurring in sport is shown in Table 35.1.

'Does this patient have a significant knee injury?'

To answer this critical question, consider the following elements of the patient's story:

- the mechanism of injury (low-energy force versus high-energy force)
- the amount of pain and disability at the time of injury
- the presence and timing of onset of swelling which may be a clue to haemarthrosis (joint bleeding)
- the degree of disability on presentation to the clinician
- patient-specific vulnerabilities (previous injury, medical comorbidities that can affect bone and/or tendon health).

In the majority of cases, an acute knee injury can be diagnosed with an appropriate history and examination. The main goals of assessment are:

1. to determine which structures have been damaged
2. to determine the extent of damage to each structure
3. to determine the degree of joint/limb disability to provide safe and timely initial management.

History

It is absolutely critical to invite the patient to tell his or her own story of the injury. Once the patient has explained what happened, the clinician may elicit additional aspects of the history.

Table 35.1 Causes of acute knee pain

Common	Less common	Not to be missed
Medial meniscus tear	Patellar tendon rupture	Fracture of the tibial plateau
MCL sprain	Quadriceps tendon rupture	Avulsion fracture of tibial spine
ACL sprain (rupture)	Acute patellofemoral contusion	Osteochondritis dissecans (in adolescents)
Lateral meniscus tear	LCL sprain	
Articular cartilage injury	Bursal haematoma/bursitis	Complex regional pain syndrome type 1 (post injury)
PCL sprain	Acute fat pad impingement	
Patellar dislocation	Avulsion of biceps femoris tendon	Quadriceps muscle rupture
	Superior tibiofibular joint injury	

Note: all these conditions may occur in isolation or, commonly, in association with other conditions

Important components include:

- a description of the precise mechanism of injury and the subsequent symptoms (e.g. pain and giving way)
- demonstration by the patient if possible, on the uninjured knee, of the stress applied at the time of injury
- the location of pain – pain associated with cruciate ligament injuries is often poorly localised (or emanates from the lateral tibial plateau); pain from injuries to the collateral ligaments is usually fairly well localised
- severity of pain – this does not always correlate with the severity of the injury, although most ACL injuries are usually painful immediately.

> **PRACTICE PEARL**
>
> The degree and time of onset of swelling can reflect either intra-articular or extra-articular injury and thus, provides an important clue to the injured structure (Table 35.2). Intra-articular swelling (i.e. haemarthrosis) is usually voluminous (obvious) and develops within 1 or 2 hours following injury.

The causes of haemarthrosis are:

- major ligament rupture
   - ACL
   - PCL
- patellar dislocation
- osteochondral fracture
- peripheral tear of the meniscus, more common medially
- Hoffa's syndrome (acute fat pad impingement)
- bleeding diathesis (rare).

Note: Lipohaemarthrosis (fat and blood in the knee) is caused by intra-articular fractures. Lipohaemarthrosis will present in a similar manner to haemarthrosis.

> **PRACTICE PEARL**
>
> An effusion that develops after a few hours or, more commonly, the following day represents reactive synovitis and is a feature of meniscal and chondral injuries. There is usually little effusion with collateral ligament injuries.

> **PRACTICE PEARL**
>
> If the patient volunteers having heard a 'pop', a 'snap' or felt a 'tear', the injury should be considered as an ACL tear until proven otherwise.

Patients presenting with a sensation of something having 'moved' or 'popped out' in the knee may be thought to have a patellar dislocation. However, this symptom is more commonly associated with an ACL rupture. There may be associated 'clicking' or 'locking' and this is often seen with meniscal injuries. Locking is classically associated with a loose body or displaced meniscal tear. Locking does not mean locked in one knee position, but is used when significant loss of passive range of motion is present, especially loss of full extension. It is helpful to ask the patient in what 'position' the knee locks. If the patient reports that the knee locks when it is straight and does not bend, this usually is a manifestation of patellofemoral pain and injury–the kneecap is unable to engage in the groove secondary to pain.

The symptom of 'giving way' can occur with instability, such as in ACL deficiency. Instability may also occur with meniscal tears, articular cartilage damage, patellofemoral pain (Chapter 36) or severe knee pain. In the latter cases of knee *pain* instability, a careful history will reveal more of a 'jackknife' (collapsing) phenomenon in flexion rather than a true 'give way' in extension. Patients with recurrent patellar dislocation and those with loose bodies in the knee can describe similar sensations. If a patient reports feeling unstable on steps, this is most often a reflection of quadriceps weakness and/or pain and rarely represents true kneecap instability.

The comprehensive history will also include:

- the initial management of the injury
- the degree of disability
- a history of previous injury to either knee or any previous surgery
- the patient's age, occupation, type of sport and leisure activities and the level of sport played.

If the patient is a good historian, the diagnosis will be obvious in most cases.

Table 35.2 Time relationship of swelling to diagnosis

Intermediate (0–2 hours) – haemarthrosis	Delayed (6–24 hours) – effusion	No swelling
ACL rupture Patellar dislocation Major chondral lesion MCL sprain (deep)	Meniscus Smaller chondral lesion	MCL sprain (superficial)

PART B Regional problems

Physical examination

Examination includes:

1. Observation
   a. standing
   b. walking
   c. supine (Fig. 35.2a)
2. Active movements
   a. flexion
   b. extension
   c. straight leg raise
3. Passive movements
   a. flexion (Fig. 35.2b)
   b. extension (Fig. 35.2c)
4. Palpation
   a. patellofemoral joint (including patellar and quadriceps tendons, medial and lateral retinaculum)
   b. MCL
   c. LCL
   d. medial joint line (Fig. 35.2d)
   e. lateral joint line
   f. posterior structures (e.g. hamstring tendons, Baker's cyst, gastrocnemius origins, best done in the prone position)
5. Special tests
   a. presence of effusion (Fig. 35.2e)
   b. stability tests
      i. MCL (Fig. 35.2f)
      ii. LCL (Fig. 35.2g)
      iii. ACL
         1. Lachman's test (Figs 35.2h–k)
         2. anterior drawer test (Fig. 35.2l)
         3. pivot shift test (Fig. 35.2m)
      iv. PCL
         1. posterior sag (Fig. 35.2n)
         2. reverse Lachman's test
         3. posterior drawer test (Fig. 35.2o)
         4. external rotation test–active and passive
      v. patella
         1. medial and lateral patella translation (or mobility)
   c. flexion/rotation
      i. McMurray's test (Fig. 35.2p)
      ii. Apley's grind test
   d. patellar apprehension test (Fig. 35.2q)

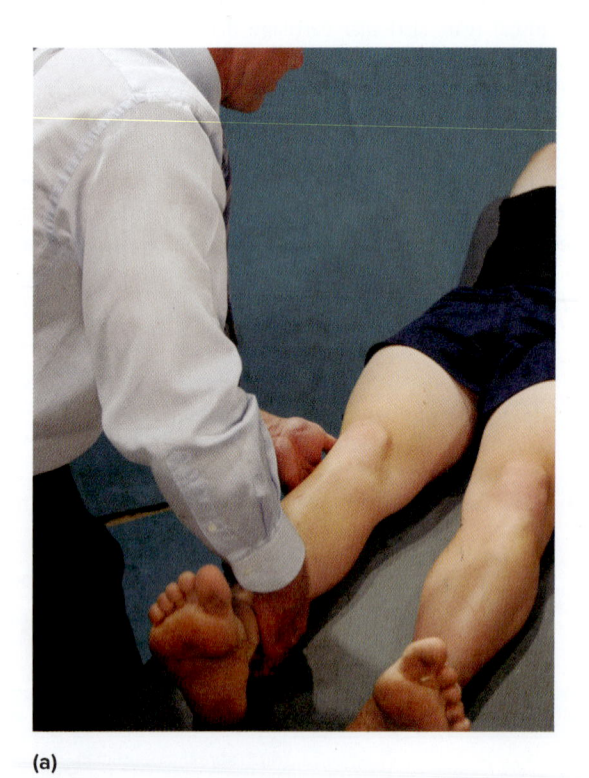

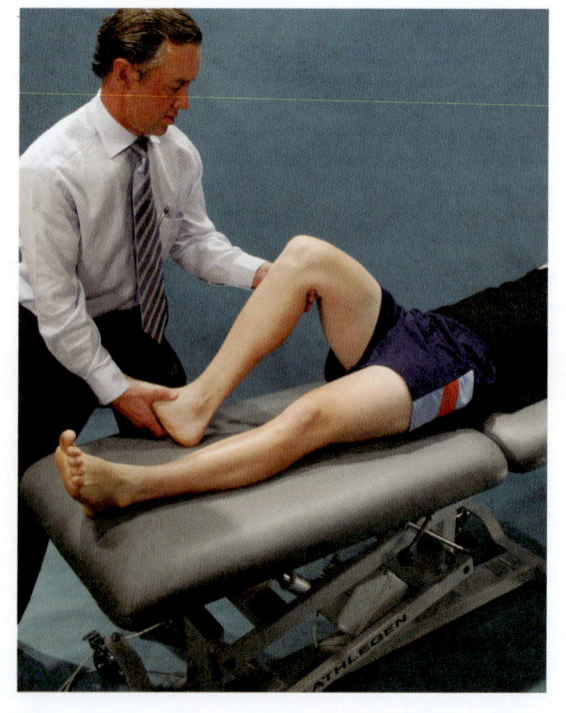

(a)

(b)

Figure 35.2 Examination of the patient with an acute knee injury (a) Observation—supine. Look for swelling, deformity and bruising (b) Passive movement—flexion. Assess range of motion, end feel and presence of pain

Acute knee injuries CHAPTER 35

  e. patellofemoral joint (Chapter 36)
  f. functional tests
     i. squat test (helps to assess functional valgus collapse of knee)
     ii. hopping on the spot
     iii. pelvic bridge/plank arrow (helps assess core strength)

The clinical utility of the various special tests for diagnosing acute knee injuries is shown in Table 35.3.

Key outcome measures

Patient-reported outcome measures (PROMs) for acute knee injuries are shown in Table 35.4.

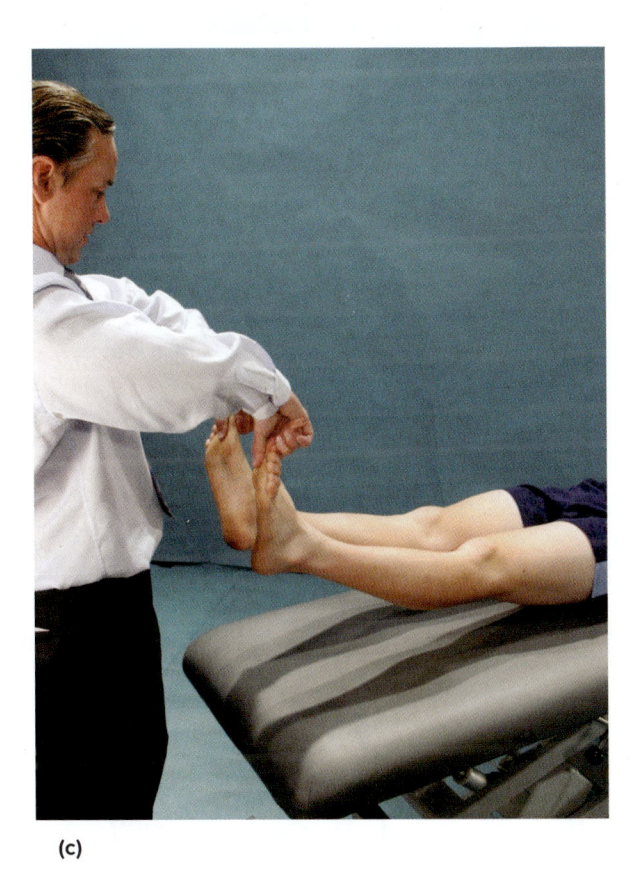

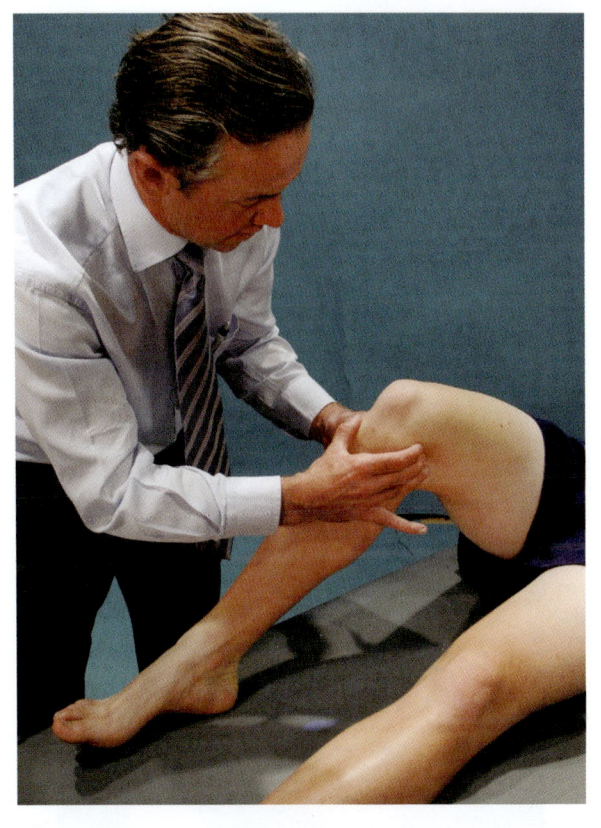

(c)

(d)

(e)

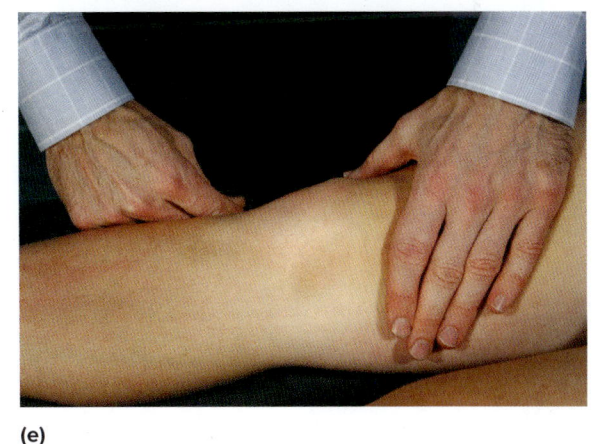

Figure 35.2 (cont.) (c) Passive movement—extension. Hold both legs by the toes, looking for fixed flexion deformity or hyperextension in ACL or PCL rupture. Overpressure may be applied to assess end range. This procedure may provoke pain in meniscal injuries (d) Palpation—medial joint line. The knee should be palpated in 45–90° of flexion (e) Special tests—presence of effusion. Manually drain the medial subpatellar pouch by stroking the fluid in a superior direction. Then 'milk' the fluid back into the knee from above on the lateral side while observing the pouch for evidence that fluid is re-accumulating. This test is more sensitive than the 'patellar tap'. It is important to differentiate between an intra-articular effusion and an extra-articular haemorrhagic bursitis

PART B Regional problems

(f)

(g)

(h)

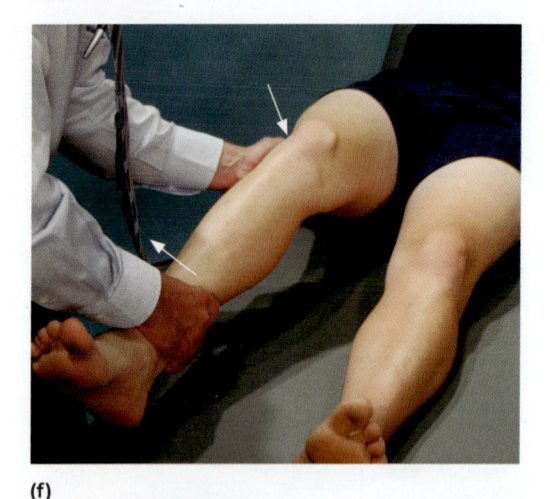

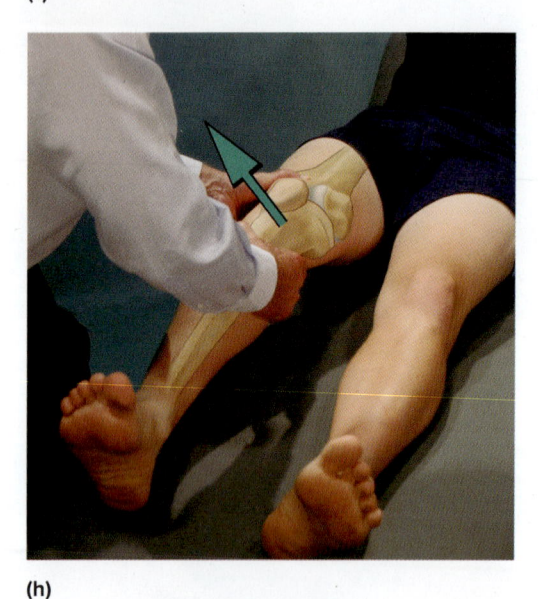

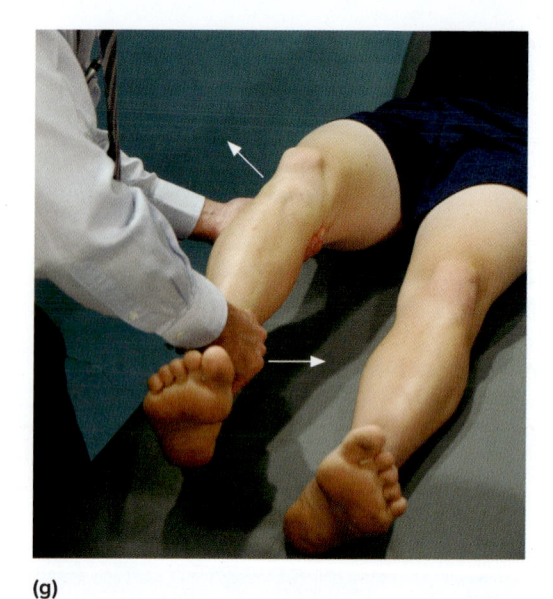

Figure 35.2 (cont.) (f) Stability test—MCL. This is tested first with the knee in full extension and then also at 30° of flexion (illustrated). The examiner applies a valgus force, being careful to eliminate any femoral rotation. Assess for onset of any pain, extent of valgus movement and feel for end point. If the knee 'gaps' at full extension, there must be associated posterior cruciate injury (g) Stability test—LCL. The LCL is tested in a similar manner to the MCL except with varus stress applied (h) Stability test—Lachman's test. Lachman's test is performed with the knee in 15° of flexion, ensuring the hamstrings are relaxed. The examiner draws the tibia forwards, feeling for laxity and assessing the quality of the end point. Compare with the uninjured side (i) The ACL is slightly slack in the start position (j) When the ACL is intact, the ligament snaps tight and the examiner senses a 'firm'/'sudden' end feel (k) When the ACL is ruptured, the Lachman's test results in a 'softer'/'gradual' end feel

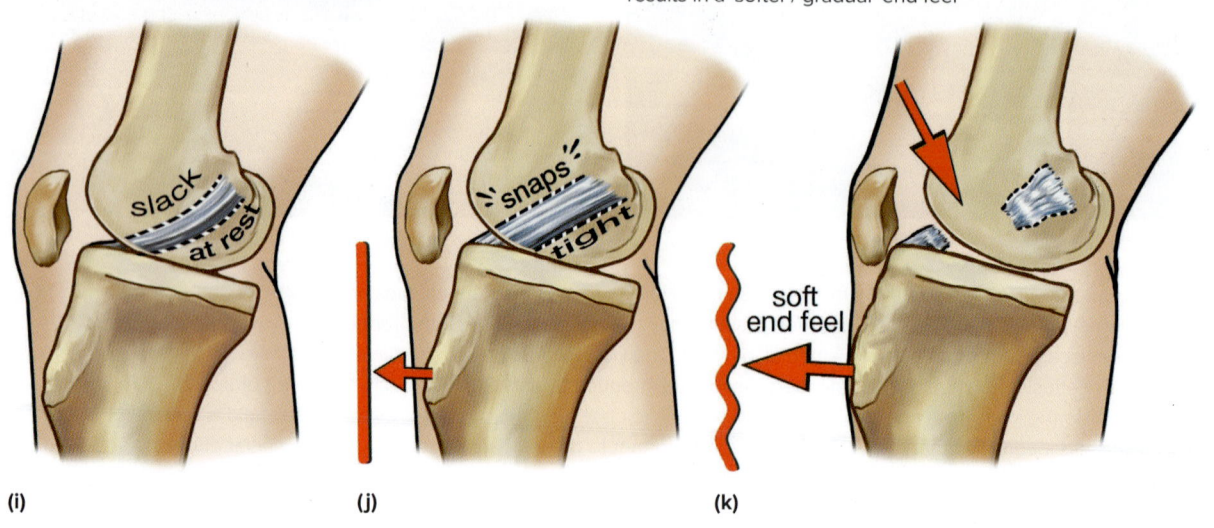

(i)   (j)   (k)

Acute knee injuries CHAPTER 35

(l)

(m)

(n)

(o)

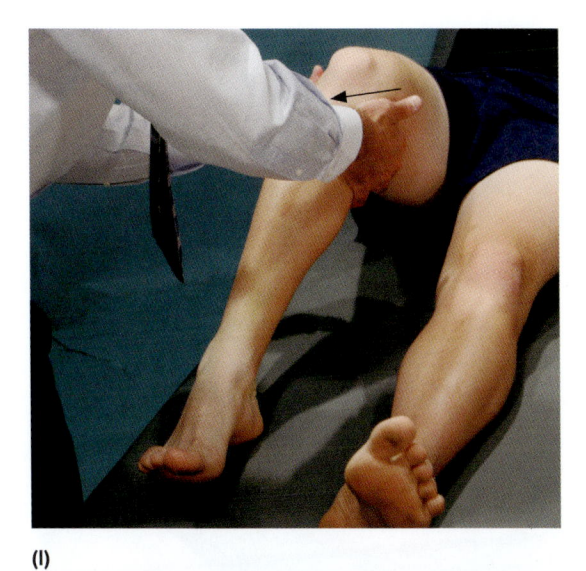

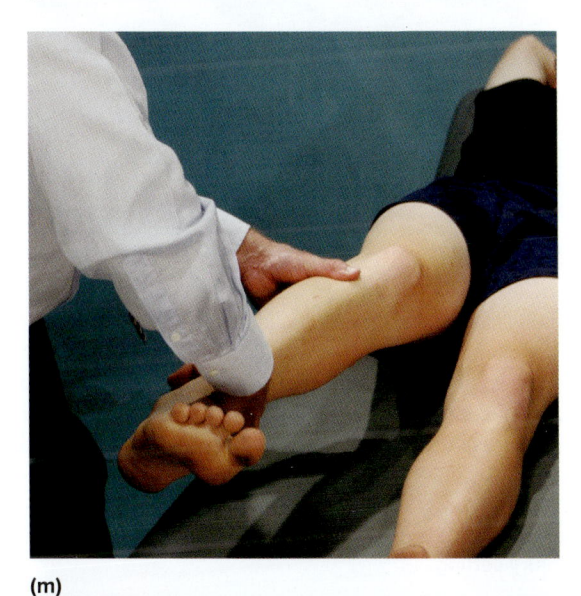

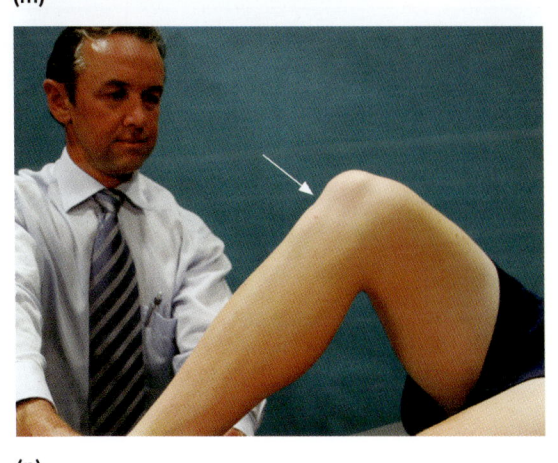

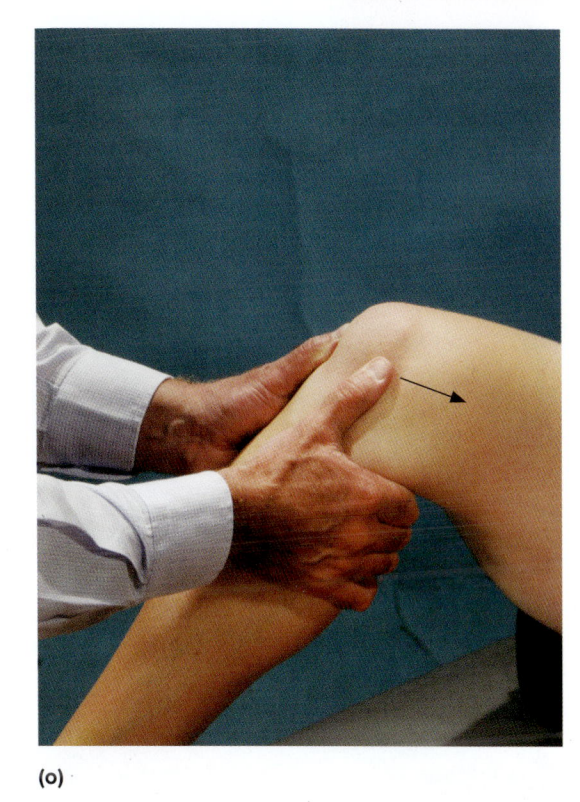

Figure 35.2 (cont.) (l) Stability test—anterior drawer test. This is performed with the knee in 90° of flexion and the patient's foot kept stable. Ensure the hamstrings are relaxed with the index finger on the femoral condyles. The tibia is drawn anteriorly and assessed for degree of movement and quality of end point. The test can be performed with the tibia in internal and external rotation to assess anterolateral and anteromedial instability respectively (m) Special test—pivot shift test. With the tibia internally rotated and the knee in full extension, a valgus force is applied to the knee. In a knee with ACL deficiency, the condyles will be subluxated. The knee is then flexed, looking for a 'clunk' of reduction, which renders the pivot shift test positive. Maintaining this position, the knee is extended, looking for a click into subluxation, which is called a 'positive jerk test' (n) Stability test—posterior sag. With both knees flexed at 90° and the patient relaxed, the position of the tibia relative to the femur is observed. This will be relatively posterior in the knee with PCL deficiency (o) Stability test—posterior drawer test. With the knee as for the anterior drawer test, the examiner grips the tibia firmly as shown and pushes it posteriorly. Feel for the extent of the posterior movement and quality of end point. The test can be repeated with the tibia in external rotation to assess posterolateral capsular integrity

PART B   Regional problems

(p)

(q)

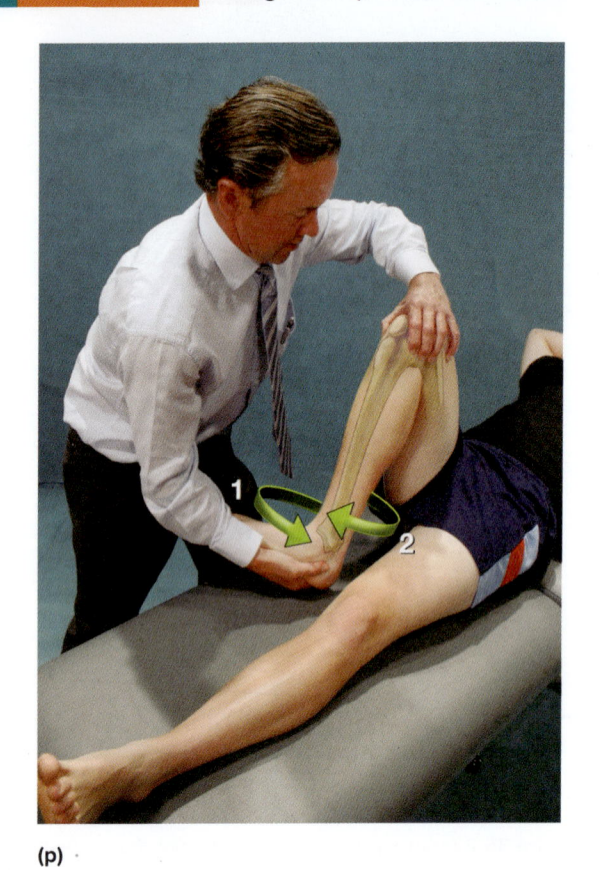

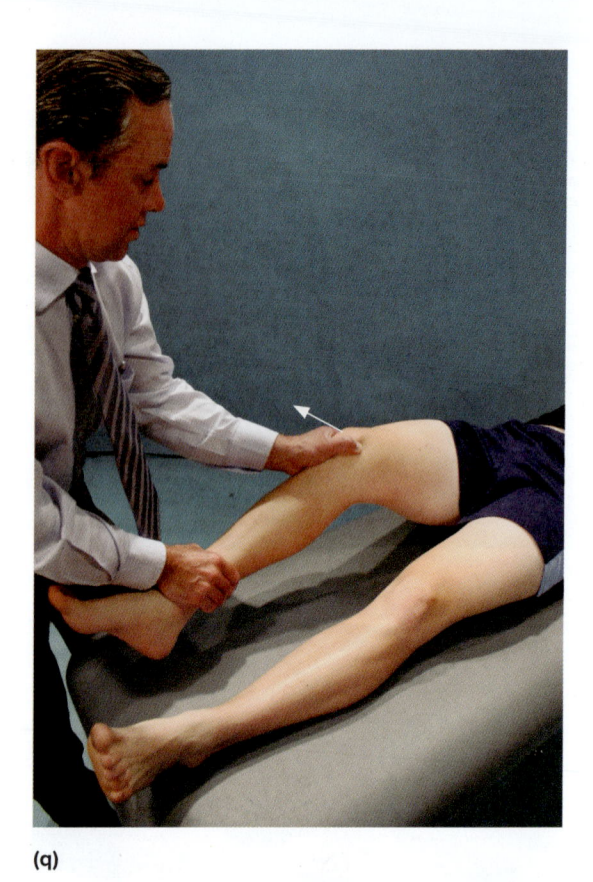

Figure 35.2 (cont.) (p) Flexion/rotation test—McMurray's test. The knee is flexed and, at various stages of flexion, internal and external rotation of the tibia are performed. The presence of pain and a palpable 'clunk' is a positive McMurray's test and is consistent with meniscal injury. If there is no clunk but the patient's pain is reproduced, then the meniscus may be damaged or there may be a patellofemoral joint abnormality (q) Special test—patellar apprehension test. The knee may be placed on a pillow to maintain 20–30° of flexion. Gently push the patella laterally. The test is positive if the patient develops apprehension with a sensation of impending dislocation

Table 35.3 Diagnostic accuracy of tests used in the acute knee injury setting

	What is a positive finding?	Sensitivity	Specificity	LR+	LR−
Knee fracture					
Ottawa knee decision rule[2]	One of the following: • age ≥ 55 years • tenderness head of fibula • isolated tenderness of patella • inability to flex beyond 90° • inability to weight-bear more than 4 steps	98.5	49	1.9*	0.05
ACL injury					
Lachman's test[3]	Soft end feel for tibial translation	81	81	4.5	0.22
Anterior drawer[3]	>5 mm anterior tibial translation	38	81	4.5	0.67
Pivot shift[3]	Anterior subluxation of tibia	28	81	5.4	0.84

720

Table 35.3 Cont.

	What is a positive finding?	Sensitivity	Specificity	LR+	LR−
PCL injury					
Posterior drawer[4]	>5 mm posterior tibial translation	22–100	98	50.1	0.11
Posterior sag sign[4]	Posterior sagging of tibia	46–100	100	88.4	0.28
Reverse Lachman's[4]	Soft end feel for tibial translation	63	89	5.9	0.41
Meniscal tear					
McMurray's test[5]	Palpable or audible click or pain	61	84	3.2	0.52
Joint line tenderness[5]	Reproduction of patient's pain	83	83	4.0	0.52
Apley's test[6]	Pain	61	70	2.0	0.56
MCL injury					
Valgus stress test at 30°[7]	Pain	78	67	2.3	0.30
	Laxity	91	49	1.8	0.20
LCL injury					
Varus stress test at 30°	Pain/laxity	NA	NA	NA	NA

LR+ = positive likelihood ratio; LR− = negative likelihood ratio; NA = not available; see Chapter 16 for a guide to interpreting test sensitivity, specificity and likelihood ratios
* estimated from available research data

Table 35.4 Patient-reported outcome measures for acute knee injuries

International Knee Documentation Committee (IKDC) Subjective Knee Evaluation Form

- Self-administered questionnaire evaluating symptoms, function and sports activities due to knee impairment
- Eighteen items (7 items for symptoms, 10 items for sport activities and 1 item for current knee function)
- Score range 0–100
- Test-retest reliability: 0.845–0.93[8–10] (ACL injuries) 0.95[11] (meniscal injuries)
- Construct validity: Lysholm score 0.62–0.89,[10, 12–15] SF-36 physical function 0.71,[16] Cincinnati Knee Rating System 0.87–0.946[17]
- MDC 95%: 8.8–15.6[11, 18]
- MCID: (Sn) 11.5,[19] (Sp) 20.5[19]
- Available online in a range of languages: American Orthopaedic Society for Sports Medicine, www.sportsmed.org/aossmimis

Knee Injury and Osteoarthritis Outcome Score (KOOS)

- Self-administered questionnaire evaluating a patient's opinion about their knee and associated problems[20]
- Five domains: Symptoms and stiffness (7 items), Pain (9 items), ADL function (17 items), Sport and recreational activity function (5 items) and Quality of life (4 items)
- Score range 0–100 (0 = extreme symptoms and 100 = no symptoms)
- Test-retest reliability: Symptoms and stiffness (cartilage lesions 0.9/ACL 0.89), Pain (cartilage lesions 0.91/ACL 0.87), ADL function (cartilage lesions 0.93/ACL 0.87), Sport and recreational activity function (cartilage lesions 0.92/ACL 0.84) and Quality of life (cartilage lesions 0.95/ACL 0.88)[21]
- Construct validity: SF-36-bodily pain (cartilage lesions 0.72/ACL 0.66), SF-36 physical function (cartilage lesions 0.63/ACL 0.65)[21]
- MDC 95%: Symptoms and stiffness (cartilage lesions 30.8/ACL 15.6), Pain (cartilage lesions 26.3/ACL 12.7), ADL function (cartilage lesions 29.7/ACL 12.9), Sport and recreational activity function (cartilage lesions 29.9/19.2) and Quality of life (cartilage lesions 20.5/ACL 16.3)[21]
- MCID: NA
- Available online in a range of languages: Professor Ewa Roos, Institute of Sports Science and Clinical Biomechanics, www.koos.nu/

continued

Table 35.4 Cont.

Lysholm Knee Scoring Scale

- An eight-item knee-specific scale initially designed for the purpose of assessing knee ligament function that can be self-administered or clinician administered
- Eight items related to knee function
- Score range 0–100 (100 = no symptoms or disability)
- Test–retest reliability: 0.88–0.97[15, 22–25]
- Construct validity: Fulkerson Knee Instability Scale 0.93,[25] Kujala Anterior Knee Pain Scale 0.86,[26] SF-12 physical function 0.54[24] and SF-12 role physical 0.48[24]
- MDC95%: 8.9–10.1[15, 22–25]
- MCID: Has not been established[20]
- Available online in a range of languages; original scale is freely available from the paper:[22] www.ncbi.nlm.nih.gov/pubmed/4028566

Tegner Activity Scale

- A standardised method to grade work and sporting activity level; the questionnaire can be self-administered or clinician administered and was developed initially to be used in combination with the Lysholm knee score
- One item
- Score range 0–16 (16 = increased frequency of participation in athletic activity)
- Test–retest reliability 0.82–0.92[15, 23, 25]
- Construct validity: SF-12 physical function 0.46,[23] Lysholm Knee Scoring Scale 0.35[24]
- MDC95%: 1[23]
- MCID: Has not been established[20]
- Original scale is freely available from the original paper:[22] www.ncbi.nlm.nih.gov/pubmed/4028566

Activity Rating Scale

- Self-administered, knee-specific questionnaire that evaluates activity level of various knee disorders[20]
- Four items related to frequency of athletic activity[20]
- Score range 0–16 (16 = more frequent participation in athletic activities)[20]
- Test–retest reliability 0.97 (mixed knee pathologies)[27]
- Construct validity: Tegner Activity Scale 0.66,[27] Cincinnati Knee Rating System 0.67[27]
- MDC95%: Has not been established[20]
- MCID: Has not been established[20]
- Available online: www.aaos.org/uploadedFiles/PreProduction/Quality/Measures/pdf-MARX%20SCALE-%20english.pdf

SF = Short Form Health Survey; MDC = minimal detectable change; MCID = minimal clinically important difference; Sn = sensitivity; Sp = specificity; ADL = activities of daily living

Investigations

Plain radiography (AP)

Should you perform a plain radiograph in cases of an acute knee injury? More than 90% of radiographs ordered to evaluate knee injuries are normal. The Ottawa knee X-ray decision rules may be helpful (Table 35.5).[28]

The main aim of performing an a plain radiograph in cases of moderate and severe acute knee injuries is to detect a fracture:

- tibial avulsion fracture associated with an ACL or PCL injury
- a tibial plateau fracture following a high-speed injury or knee loading injury
- an osteochondral fracture after patellar dislocation.

The classic radiograph series should include an anterior-posterior (AP) view, a lateral view and a patellar tangential view (skyline or sunrise view). Additional oblique views can assist in identifying subtle loose bodies. A notch view can image cruciate avulsions and assess notch width as a factor for ACL injury. Weight-bearing views are ideal to assess for associated arthrosis. For children, comparative images of the contralateral side may be helpful in identifying subtle physeal injuries. Finally, stress radiographs can assist in defining the severity of ligamentous injuries.

If surgery is considered, preoperative films are justified.

Magnetic resonance imaging

Magnetic resonance imaging (MRI) is reliable, safe and accurate in the diagnostic work-up of acute knee injuries.

Acute knee injuries CHAPTER 35

Table 35.5 Criteria for knee X-ray based on Ottawa knee rule[*]

A knee radiograph is indicated after trauma only when at least one of the following is present:
- patient age more than 55
- tenderness at the fibular head
- tenderness over the patella
- inability to flex the knee to 90° (this captures most haemarthrosis, fractures)
- inability to weight-bear for four steps at the time of the injury and when examined.

To these, we suggest adding a high index of suspicion for:
- high-speed injuries
- children or adolescents (who may avulse a bony fragment instead of tearing a cruciate ligament)
- if there is clinical suspicion of loose bodies.

[*] The Ottawa knee rule was designed for use in the emergency department setting

Even when a ligament disruption is diagnosed by physical exam, MRI can add value by demonstrating the extent of associated injury to cartilage and meniscus. Patellar and quadriceps tendon injury can also be assessed.

> **PRACTICE PEARL**
>
> MRI does not substitute for a good physical examination.

MRI should never be ordered in the absence of a thorough history and physical examination and MRI findings should be interpreted in the light of the clinical findings. For example, a relatively high proportion of asymptomatic knees, especially in athletes >35-40 years, have meniscus tears.[29] Thus, evidence of a meniscal tear on MRI, but not associated with pain, local tenderness and positive examination findings, might be a 'red herring' (irrelevant) not in need of treatment.

MRI can be very useful when a primary patellar dislocation is suspected clinically and can help to detect osteochondral avulsion fractures that require surgical assessment. As the avulsed fragment swells (and deteriorates), there is limited window of time for surgical fixation. Usually it needs to be identified and treated within 10–14 days of the injury.

Significant knee injuries are associated with MRI findings of oedema in the subchondral region–a bone bruise or bone marrow lesion (BML). Clinically, a BML is associated with pain, tenderness, swelling and delayed recovery. The presence of a BML indicates articular cartilage damage,[30, 31] but its clinical relevance is discussed later in this chapter.

The role for diagnostic arthroscopy

The concept of 'diagnostic arthroscopy' predates knee MRI. Today, it remains a diagnostic option in settings where MRI is not available. In the developed world, arthroscopy may be performed to seek pertinent intra-articular pathology in those rare cases when the patient has persistent pain and swelling not responding to treatment and MRI is normal.

Ultrasound examination

As outlined in Chapter 15, ultrasound examination can detect complete and partial patellar or quadriceps tendon tears, the size and location of bursal swelling and identify intra-versus extra-articular swelling if necessary. Ultrasound is not as efficacious for intra-articular injuries such as cruciate ligament or osteochondral injury. When radiography and MRI are available, ultrasound in a clinic/hospital setting adds little value to the assessment of the acute knee. As a sideline instrument, it can help confirm the diagnosis of a complete patellar or quadriceps tendon rupture and facilitate definite transfer, referral and treatment of that patient.

MENISCAL INJURIES

Acute meniscal tears occur when the shear stress generated within the knee in flexion and compression combined with femoral rotation exceeds the meniscal collagen's ability to resist these forces.[32] The medial meniscal attachment to the medial joint capsule decreases its mobility, thereby increasing its risk for injury compared with the more mobile lateral meniscus.[33]

Experienced clinicians consider patients with meniscal injury to be on a continuum where the two anchors of the continuum can be considered as being:

1. the young patient with the morphologically pristine articular surfaces in whom substantial forces damage the previously pristine meniscus, and
2. the older (>40 years) patient in whom an 'acute' presentation of knee pain arises from a knee that already has features of (asymptomatic) articular cartilage damage and has menisci that already had (asymptomatic) degenerative features.

PART B   Regional problems

Patients will fall along this continuum–and where they fall should influence management (see the section on treatment). Degenerative meniscal tears occur in the older population frequently without an inciting event and also without symptoms.[29] (See box below.)

The different types of meniscal tear are shown in Figure 35.3.

Clinical features

The history can provide a mechanism and a sense of the severity of meniscal tears. The clinical features can include the following.

- The most common mechanism of meniscal injury is a twisting injury with the foot anchored on the ground; this rotational force is often caused by another player's body.
- The twisting component may be of comparatively slow speed. This type of injury is commonly seen in football and basketball players.
- The degree of pain associated with an acute meniscal injury varies considerably. Some patients may describe a tearing sensation at the time of injury.
- A small meniscal tear may cause no immediate symptoms; it may become painful and cause knee swelling over 24 hours.
- Small tears may also occur with minimal trauma in the older athlete as a result of degenerative change of the meniscus.
- Patients with more severe meniscal injuries, such as a longitudinal ('bucket handle') tear, present with more

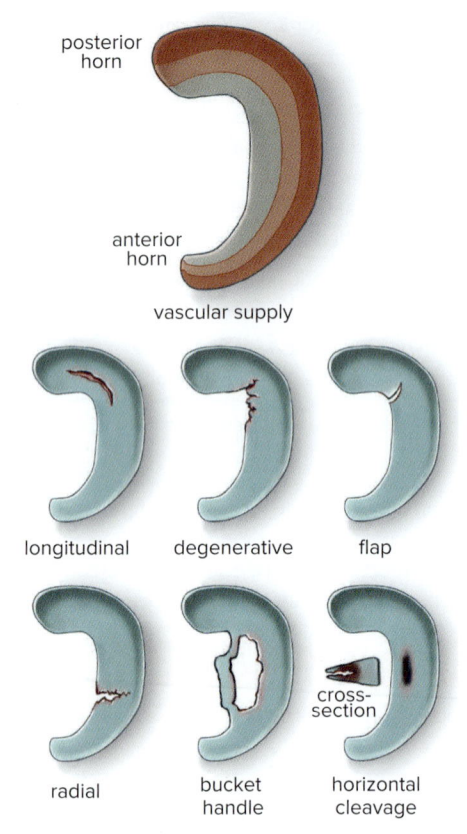

Figure 35.3 Meniscus tear orientation and zones of vascularity; these drawings are of a medial meniscal tear

Degenerative meniscus lesions

Adapted from the ESSKA Meniscus Consensus project (www.esska.org)

A degenerative meniscus lesion is a slowly developing lesion, typically involving a horizontal cleavage of the meniscus, generally in a middle-aged or older person. Such meniscus lesions are frequent in the general population and often incidental findings on knee MRI. There is often no clear history of an acute knee injury.

The prevalence of meniscus lesions in the general population:

- age 50–59 years ≈ 25%
- 60–69 years ≈ 35%
- 70–79 years ≈ 45%
- patients with knee osteoarthritis ≈ 75–95%.

There is very limited evidence that pain in the degenerative knee is directly attributable to a degenerative meniscus lesion, even if the lesion is considered to be unstable. Great caution must be taken before arriving at the conclusion that the degenerative meniscus lesion is the direct cause of the patient's knee symptoms.

Knee radiographs should be used as a first-line imaging tool to support a diagnosis of osteoarthritis or to detect certain more rare pathologies of the knee. Therefore, at least anteroposterior weight-bearing semi-flexed knee radiographs including a lateral view should be included in the work-up of the middle-aged or older patient with knee pain.

Knee MRI is typically not indicated in the first-line work-up of middle-aged or older patients with knee joint symptoms. However, knee MRI may be indicated in selected patients with refractory symptoms or in the presence of 'warning flags' or localised symptoms indicating more rare disease. If a surgical indication is considered, based on history, symptoms, clinical

Acute knee injuries CHAPTER 35

exam and knee radiographs, knee MRI may be useful to identify structural knee pathologies that may (or may not) be relevant for the symptoms.

When should arthroscopic partial meniscectomy (APM) be proposed?

- Surgery should not be proposed as a first line of treatment of degenerative meniscus lesions.
- After 3 months with persistent pain/mechanical symptoms despite appropriate rehabilitation: for a degenerative meniscus with normal X-rays/abnormal MRI (grade III meniscus lesion), APM may be proposed.
- Surgery can be proposed earlier for patients presenting with considerable mechanical symptoms.
- No arthroscopic surgery should be proposed for a degenerative meniscus lesion with advanced osteoarthritis on weight-bearing radiographs.

Most of the published randomised control trials (RCTs) found no difference in terms of clinical outcomes after surgery compared to non-operative treatment.

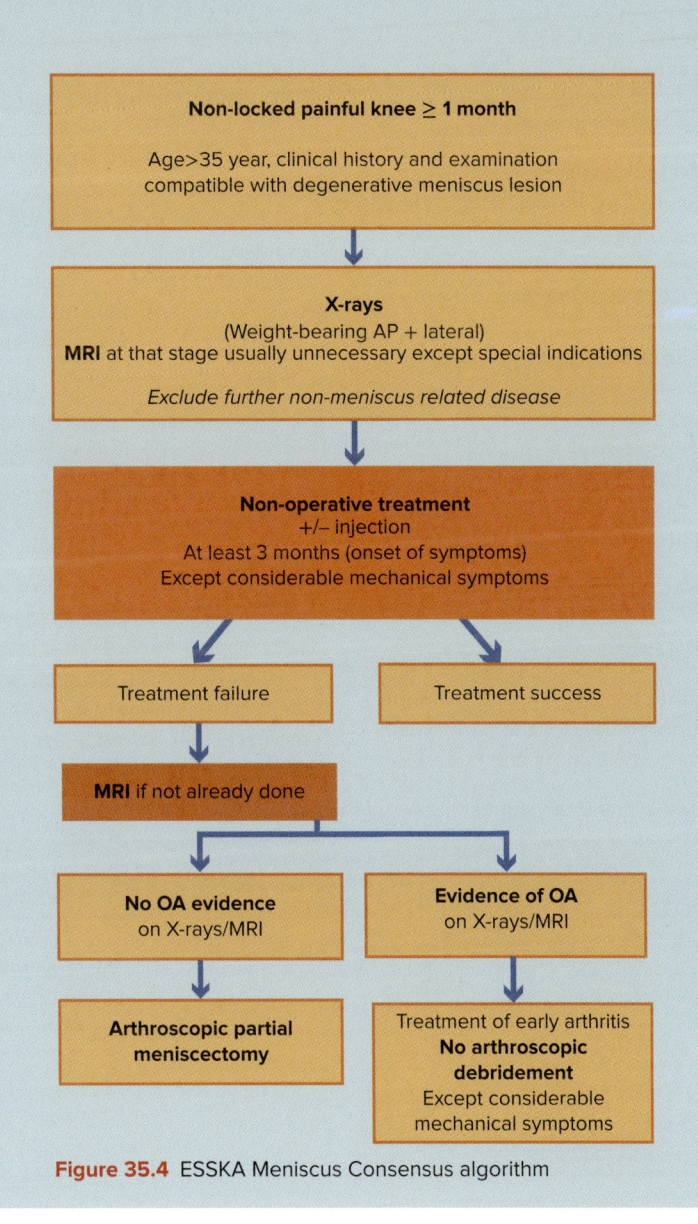

Figure 35.4 ESSKA Meniscus Consensus algorithm

severe symptoms. Pain and restriction of range of motion occur soon after injury. Intermittent locking may occur as a result of the torn flap, the 'bucket handle', impinging between the articular surfaces. This may unlock spontaneously with a clicking sensation. This often occurs in association with ACL tears. In these patients, a history of locking may be due to either the ACL or the meniscal injury.

On examination, the signs of a meniscal tear include:

- joint line tenderness (palpated with the knee flexed at 45-90°)
- joint effusion–this is usually present, although absence of an effusion does not necessarily rule out meniscal damage
- pain–usually present with knee hyperflexion, such as squatting, especially with posterior horn tears
- restricted range of motion of the knee joint–this may be due to the torn meniscal flap or the effusion.

The flexion/rotation (McMurray's) test (Fig. 35.2p) is positive when pain is produced by the test and a clunk is heard or felt that corresponds to the torn flap being impinged in the joint. However, it is not necessary to have a positive McMurray's test (i.e. a clunk) to make a diagnosis of a torn meniscus. The hyperflexion portion of the McMurray's test provokes pain in most meniscal injuries. Pain produced by flexion and external rotation suggests medial meniscal damage, whereas pain on internal rotation indicates lateral meniscal pain. Asking patients where they feel pain during hyperflexion manoeuvres gives a suggestion of the location of the tear, medial or lateral. MRI is the investigation of choice. This can aid management if the MRI shows either a complex tear versus minimal damage or, more rarely, a peripheral meniscus tear.

Treatment

The management of meniscal tears varies depending on the severity of the condition, the age of the patient and the presence of mechanical pathology. At one end of the spectrum, a small tear or a degenerative meniscus tear, presenting with pain but not with mechanical symptoms such as locking or range of motion (ROM) restriction, should initially be treated conservatively.[34]

In a highly publicised paper published in the *New England Journal of Medicine* in 2013, the outcomes after arthroscopic partial meniscectomy in patients without knee osteoarthritis but with symptoms of a degenerative medial meniscus tear, were no better than those after a sham surgical procedure.[35] A recent trial compared exercise therapy with arthroscopic partial meniscectomy in middle-aged patients with degenerative meniscal tears and found no clinically relevant difference between the two groups in Knee injury and Osteoarthritis Outcome Score (KOOS) at 2 years. At 3 months, muscle strength had improved in the exercise group.[36]

An algorithm for the management of degenerative meniscal lesions is shown in the box above.

On the other hand, a large painful 'bucket handle' tear, causing a locked knee, requires urgent arthroscopic surgery. The majority of meniscal injuries fall somewhere between these two extremes and the decision on whether to proceed immediately to arthroscopy must be made on the basis of the severity of the symptoms and signs, as well as the demands of the athlete. Table 35.6 provides some clinical guidance for choosing either conservative or surgical treatment.

> **PRACTICE PEARL**
>
> Physical examination features and MRI can predict those patients with early osteoarthritis and a meniscus tear who might benefit from arthroscopic surgery.[37] The highest likelihood of benefit from arthroscopic partial meniscectomy came in patients with clinical findings of increasing pain (as distinct from stable pain) as well as locking when these were complemented by MRI findings of a displaced meniscal tear but no marrow lesions.[37]

Table 35.6 Clinical features of meniscal injuries that may affect prognosis

Factors that may indicate non-surgical treatment is likely to be successful	Factors that may indicate surgery will be required
Symptoms develop over 24–48 hours following the injury	Severe twisting injury, athlete is unable to continue playing
Minimal injury or no recall of specific injury	Locked knee or severely restricted ROM
Able to weight-bear	Positive McMurray's test (palpable clunk)
Minimal swelling	Pain on McMurray's test with minimal knee flexion
Full range of movement with pain only at end of ROM	Presence of associated ACL tear
Pain on McMurray's test only in inner range of flexion	Little improvement of clinical features after 3–6 weeks of non-surgical treatment
Previous history of rapid recovery from similar injury	
Early degenerative changes on plain radiographs	

ROM = range of motion

Non-surgical management of meniscal injuries

Non-surgical management of relatively minor meniscal injuries will often be successful, particularly in the athlete whose sporting activity does not involve twisting activities. The principles of non-surgical management are the same as those following partial meniscectomy (Table 35.7), although the rate of progress may vary depending on the clinical features.

The criteria for return to sport following meniscal injury, treated surgically or non-surgically, are shown below. If appropriate rehabilitation principles have been followed, then the criteria will usually all be satisfied:

- no effusion
- full range of movement
- normal quadriceps and hamstring function
- normal hip external rotator function
- good proprioception
- functional exercises performed without difficulty
- training performed without subsequent knee symptoms
- simulated match situations undertaken without subsequent knee symptoms.

Surgical management of meniscal injuries

The aim of surgery is to preserve as much of the meniscus as possible. Some meniscal lesions are suitable for repair by arthroscopic meniscal suture. The decision as to whether or not to attempt meniscal repair is based on several factors, including acuity of the tear, age of the patient, stability of the knee, and tear location and orientation. The outer one-third of the meniscus rim has a blood supply and tears in this region can heal.

The tear with the best chance of a successful repair is an acute longitudinal tear in the peripheral one-third of the meniscus in a young patient.[38] Degenerative, flap, horizontal cleavages and complex meniscal tears are poor candidates for repair.[33] Young patients have a higher success rate of healing the meniscus. Peripheral meniscus tears in otherwise stable knees without concomitant ligament damage have a reduced success rate.[39]

Partial tears may require removal of the damaged flap of the meniscus. Patients with degenerative tears with no or minimal cartilage wear will be less symptomatic than those patients with concomitant cartilage damage.

Rehabilitation after meniscal surgery

Rehabilitation should always commence prior to surgery and in some cases surgery can be avoided because 'prehabilitation' leads to full recovery. For patients scheduled for surgery it is important to:

- reduce pain and swelling with the use of electrotherapeutic modalities and gentle ROM exercises
- maintain strength of the quadriceps, hamstrings, and hip abductor and extensor muscles
- protect against further damage to the joint (patient may use crutches if necessary)
- explain the surgical procedure and the postoperative rehabilitation program to the patient.

The precise nature of the rehabilitation process will depend on the extent of the injury and the surgery performed (Table 35.7). Arthroscopic partial meniscectomy is usually a straightforward procedure followed by a fairly rapid return to activity. Some athletes with a small isolated medial meniscal tear are ready to return to sport after 4 weeks of rehabilitation.

> **PRACTICE PEARL**
>
> The rehabilitation process usually takes longer if there has been a more complicated tear of the meniscus, especially if the lateral meniscus is injured.

The presence of associated abnormalities, such as articular cartilage damage or ligament (MCL, ACL) tears, will necessarily slow down the rehabilitation process.

The time to return to pre-injury level of competition is significantly longer after lateral than medial meniscectomy in elite professional soccer athletes. Lateral meniscectomy has a higher incidence of adverse events in the early recovery period, including pain/swelling and the need for further arthroscopy. It is also associated with a significantly lower rate of return to play (RTP).[40]

If the athlete returns to play before the knee is properly rehabilitated, he or she may not experience difficulty during the first competition, but may be prone to develop recurrent effusions and persistent pain.

> **PRACTICE PEARL**
>
> A successful return to sport after meniscal knee surgery should not be measured by the time to play the first match. Clinicians must consider the player's longer term performance (season, multiple seasons). Is there acceleration of osteoarthritis?

Close monitoring is essential during post-meniscectomy rehabilitation as the remaining meniscus and underlying articular cartilage slowly increase their tolerance to load-bearing activities. Constant reassessment after progressively more difficult activities should be performed by the therapist monitoring the rehabilitation program. The development of increased pain or swelling should result in the program being slowed or revised accordingly.

PART B Regional problems

Table 35.7 Rehabilitation program for both non-surgical management of meniscal injury and following arthroscopic partial meniscectomy

Phase	Goal of phase	Time post-injury	Physiotherapy	Exercise program	Functional/sport-related activity
Phase 1	Control swelling Maintain knee extension Knee flexion to 100°+ 4/5 quadriceps strength 4+/5 hamstring strength	0–1 week	Cryotherapy Electrotherapy Compression Manual therapy Gait re-education Patient education	Gentle ROM (extension and flexion) Quadriceps/VMO setting Supported (bilateral) calf raises Hip abduction and extension Hamstring pulleys/rubbers Gait re-education drills Light exercise bike	Progress to FWB and normal gait pattern
Phase 2	Eliminate swelling Full ROM 4+/5 quadriceps strength 5/5 hamstring strength	1–2 weeks	Cryotherapy Electrotherapy Compression Manual therapy Gait re-education Exercise modification and supervision	ROM drills Quadriceps/VMO setting Mini-squats and lunges Leg press (double, then single-leg) Step-ups Bridges (double, then single-leg) Hip abduction and extension with rubber tubing Single-leg calf raises Gait re-education drills Balance and proprioceptive drills (single-leg)	Swimming (light kick) Exercise bike Walking
Phase 3	Full ROM Full strength Full squat Dynamic proprioceptive training Return to running and restricted sport-specific drills	2–3 weeks	Manual therapy Exercise/activity modification and supervision	As above—increase difficulty, repetitions and weight where appropriate Jump and land drills Agility drills	Running Swimming Road bike Sport-specific exercises (progressively sequenced) (e.g. running forwards, sideways, backwards, sprinting, jumping, hopping, changing direction, kicking)
Phase 4	Full strength, ROM, and endurance of affected limb Return to sport-specific drills and restricted training and match play	3–5 weeks	As above	High-level sport-specific strengthening as required	Return to sport-specific drills, restricted training and match play

FWB = full weight-bearing; ROM = range of motion; VMO = vastus medialis obliquus

Acute knee injuries   CHAPTER 35

MEDIAL (TIBIAL) COLLATERAL LIGAMENT INJURY

Injury to the MCL usually occurs as a result of a valgus stress to the partially flexed knee. This can occur in a non-contact mechanism such as downhill skiing or in contact sports when an opponent falls across the knee from lateral to medial. MCL tears are classified on the basis of their severity into grade I (mild, first degree), grade II (moderate partial ruptures, second degree) or grade III (complete tears, third degree).

In patients with a grade I MCL sprain, there is local tenderness over the MCL on the medial femoral condyle or medial tibial plateau but usually no swelling. When a valgus stress is applied at 30° of flexion, there is pain but no increased laxity. Ligament integrity is intact.

A grade II MCL sprain is produced by a more severe valgus stress. Examination shows marked tenderness, sometimes with localised swelling. A valgus stress applied at 30° of knee flexion causes pain. Some laxity (typically <5 mm) is present but there is a distinct end point. The knee is stable at full extension; ligament integrity is compromised but intact throughout its length.

A grade III tear of the MCL results from a severe valgus stress that causes a complete tear of the ligament fibres. The patient often complains of a feeling of instability and a 'wobbly knee'. The amount of pain is variable and frequently not as severe as one would expect given the nature of the injury. On examination, there is tenderness over the ligament and valgus stress applied at 30° of flexion reveals gross laxity without a distinct end point. A minor valgus instability is usually also found at full extension. This test may not provoke as much pain as incomplete tears of the ligament due to complete disruption of the nociceptive fibres of the ligament.

Grade III MCL injuries are frequently associated with a torn ACL. The presentation of medial joint line tenderness and lack of full extension is more a reflection of MCL injury than meniscal pathology. The lateral meniscus is more at risk because the mechanism of injury typically opens the medial side and compresses the lateral side.

While swelling is uncommon in grade 1 sprains, it may occasionally be seen with grade 2 injuries. In grade 3 sprains, there is associated capsular tearing (deep fibres and superficial) and fluid escapes; some degree of swelling is common although a tense effusion is not present.

Distal MCL injuries have a tendency to recover more slowly than proximal lesions.[41]

Treatment

A hinged knee brace (Fig.35.5a) provides support and protection to the injured MCL for a period of 4–6 weeks, during which time the athlete undertakes a

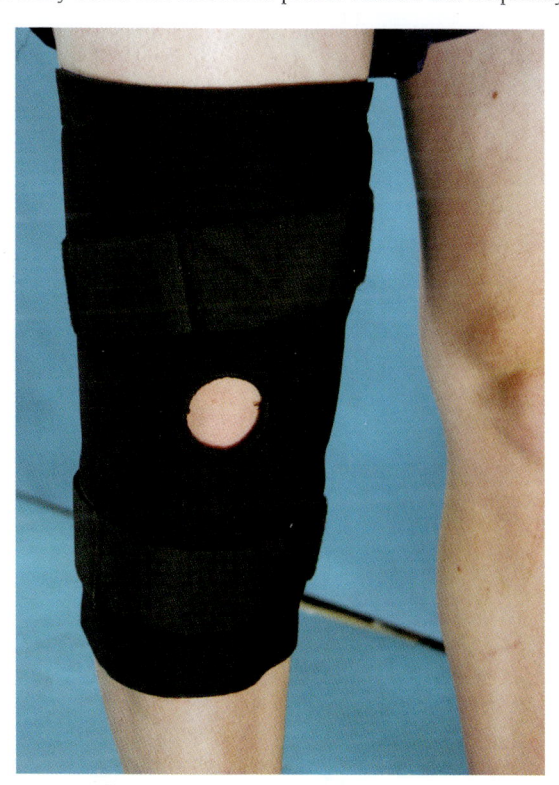

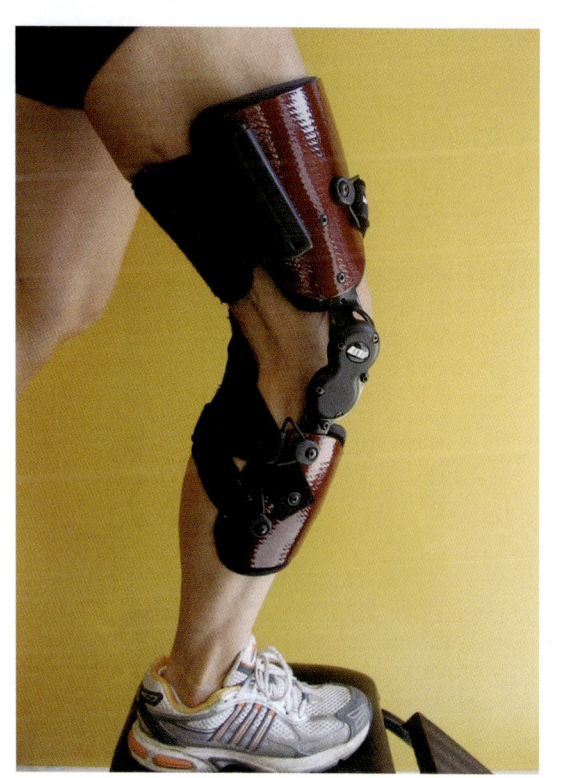

(a)

(b)

Figure 35.5 Splints (a) Hinged knee brace (b) Limited-motion knee brace

comprehensive rehabilitation program. The brace and the exercise promote early healing of the ligament and any associated capsular injury.

In one study, there were no differences between patients with grade III MCL injuries that were treated non-surgically (i.e. bracing) or surgically, thus non-surgical treatment is recommended.[42] A typical rehabilitation program for milder MCL injuries (grade I and mild grade II) is shown in Table 35.8.

The more severe MCL injury (the severe grade II or grade III tear) could be treated with a limited-motion knee brace (Fig.35.4b) and requires a longer period of rehabilitation and a rehabilitation program as shown in Table 35.9.

Table 35.8 Rehabilitation of a mild MCL injury (see Figs 35.5 and 35.6)

Phase	Goal of phase	Time post-injury	Physiotherapy treatment	Exercise program	Functional/sport-related activity
Phase 1	Control swelling Knee flexion to 100°+ Allow +20° extension 4/5 quadriceps strength 4+/5 hamstring strength	0–1 week	Cryotherapy Electrotherapy Compression Manual therapy Gait re-education Patient education	Gentle ROM (flexion mainly) Quadriceps/VMO setting Supported (bilateral) calf raises Hip abduction and extension Hamstring pulleys/rubbers Gait re-education drills	Progress to FWB and normal gait pattern
Phase 2	Eliminate swelling Full flexion ROM Allow +10° extension 4+/5 quadriceps strength 5/5 hamstring strength Return to light jogging	1–2 weeks	Cryotherapy Electrotherapy Compression Manual therapy Gait re-education Exercise modification and supervision	ROM drills Quadriceps/VMO setting Mini-squats and lunges Leg press (double, then single-leg) Step-ups Bridges (double, then single-leg) Hip abduction and extension with rubber tubing Single-leg calf raises Gait re-education drills Balance and proprioceptive drills (single-leg)	With hinged knee brace Straight-line jogging Swimming (light kick) Road bike
Phase 3	Full ROM Full strength Full squat Dynamic proprioceptive training Return to running and restricted sport-specific drills	2–4 weeks	Manual therapy Exercise/activity modification and supervision	As above—increase difficulty, repetitions and weight where appropriate Jump and land drills Agility drills	Progressive running Swimming Road bike Sport-specific exercises (progressively sequenced) (e.g. running forwards, sideways, backwards, sprinting, jumping, hopping, changing direction, kicking)
Phase 4	Full strength, ROM, and endurance of affected limb Return to sport-specific drills and restricted training and match play	3–6 weeks	As above	High-level sport-specific strengthening as required	With hinged knee brace Return to sport-specific drills, restricted training and match play

FWB = full weight-bearing; ROM = range of motion; VMO = vastus medialis obliquus

Acute knee injuries CHAPTER 35

Table 35.9 Rehabilitation of a moderate-to-severe MCL injury (see Figs 35.6 and 35.7)

Phase	Goal of phase	Time post-injury	Physiotherapy treatment	Exercise program	Functional/sport-related activity
Phase 1	Control swelling Knee flexion to 90°+ Allow +30° extension 4/5 quadriceps strength 4+/5 hamstring strength	0–4 weeks	Limited-motion knee brace (limited 0–30°) Cryotherapy Electrotherapy Compression Manual therapy Gait re-education Patient education	Exercises done in brace Gentle flexion ROM Extension ROM to 30° only Quadriceps/VMO setting Supported (bilateral) calf raises Hip abduction and extension Hamstring pulleys/rubbers Gait drills	Initially NWB/PWB Progress to FWB Walking (normal gait pattern)
Phase 2	FWB Eliminate swelling Full ROM 4+/5 quadriceps strength 5/5 hamstring strength	4–6 weeks	Removal of brace 4–6 weeks Cryotherapy Electrotherapy Compression Manual therapy Gait re-education Exercise modification and supervision	ROM drills Quadriceps/VMO setting Mini-squats and lunges Leg press (double, then single-leg) Step-ups Bridges (double, then single-leg) Hip abduction and extension with rubber tubing Single-leg calf raises Gait re-education drills Balance and proprioceptive drills (single-leg)	Swimming (light kick) Road bike Walking
Phase 3	Full ROM Full strength Full squat Dynamic proprioceptive training Return to light jogging Return to running and restricted sport-specific drills	6–10 weeks	Manual therapy Exercise/activity modification and supervision	As above—increase difficulty, repetitions and weight where appropriate Jump and land drills Agility drills	Straight-line jogging with hinged knee brace (no earlier than 6 weeks) Running Swimming Road bike Sport-specific exercises (progressively sequenced) (e.g. running forwards, sideways, backwards, sprinting, jumping, hopping, changing direction, kicking)
Phase 4	Full strength, ROM and endurance of affected limb Return to sport-specific drills and restricted training and match play	8–10/12 weeks	As above	High level of sport-specific strengthening as required	Return to sport-specific drills, restricted training and match play

FWB = full weight-bearing; NWB = non weight-bearing; PWB = partial weight-bearing; ROM = range of motion; VMO = vastus medialis obliquus

PART B   Regional problems

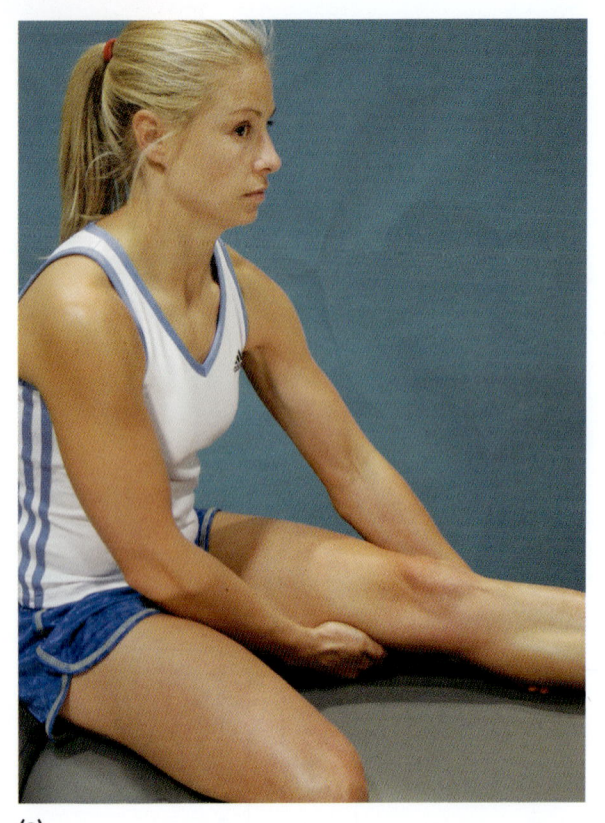

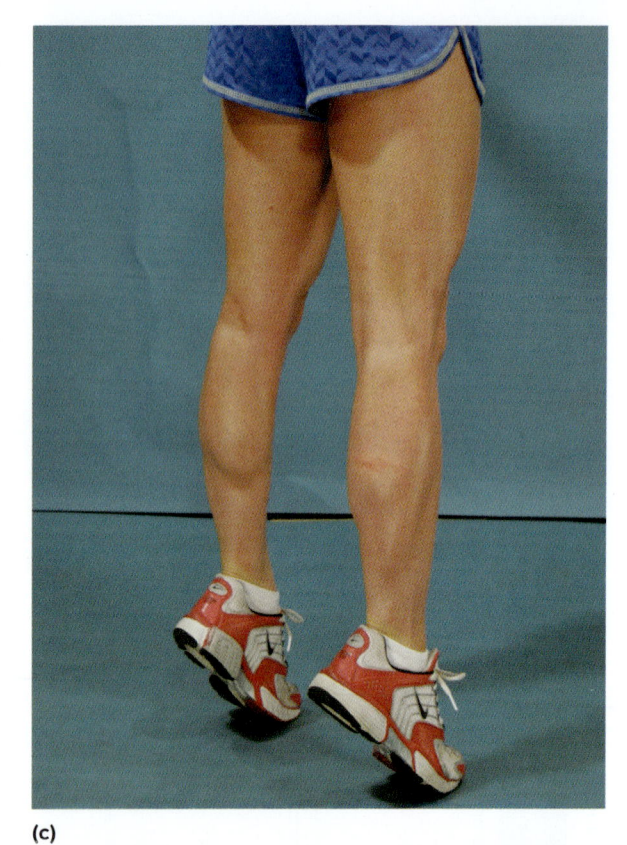

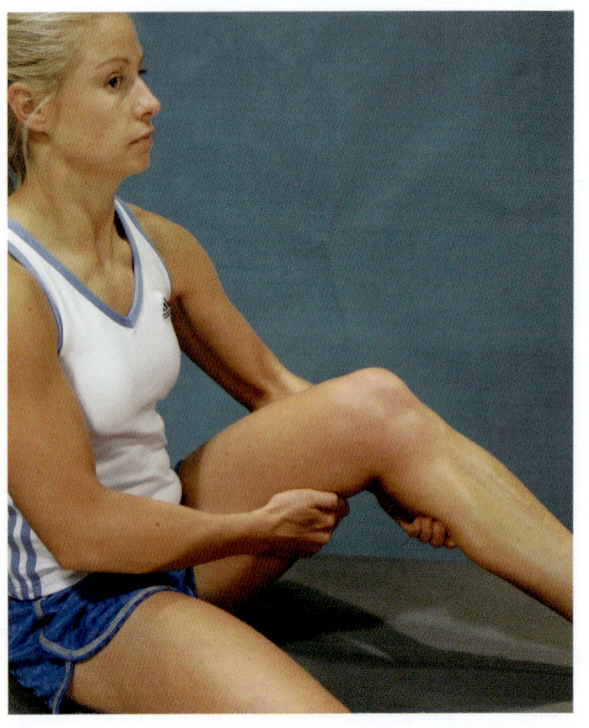

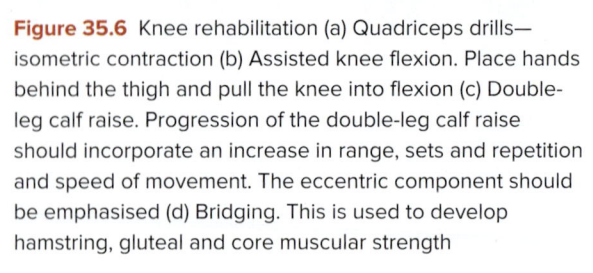

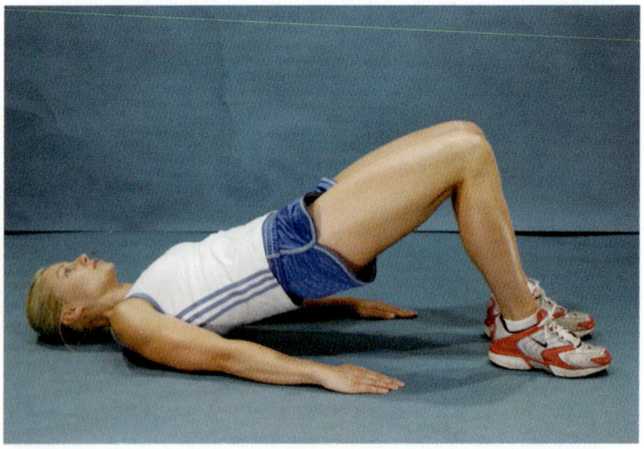

(a)

(b)

(c)

(d)

Figure 35.6 Knee rehabilitation (a) Quadriceps drills—isometric contraction (b) Assisted knee flexion. Place hands behind the thigh and pull the knee into flexion (c) Double-leg calf raise. Progression of the double-leg calf raise should incorporate an increase in range, sets and repetition and speed of movement. The eccentric component should be emphasised (d) Bridging. This is used to develop hamstring, gluteal and core muscular strength

Acute knee injuries CHAPTER 35

(e)

(f)

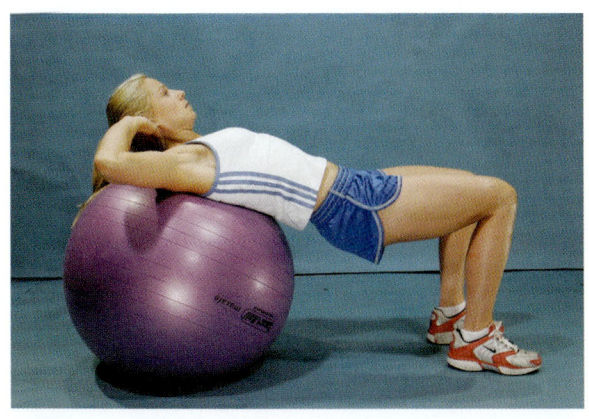

(g)

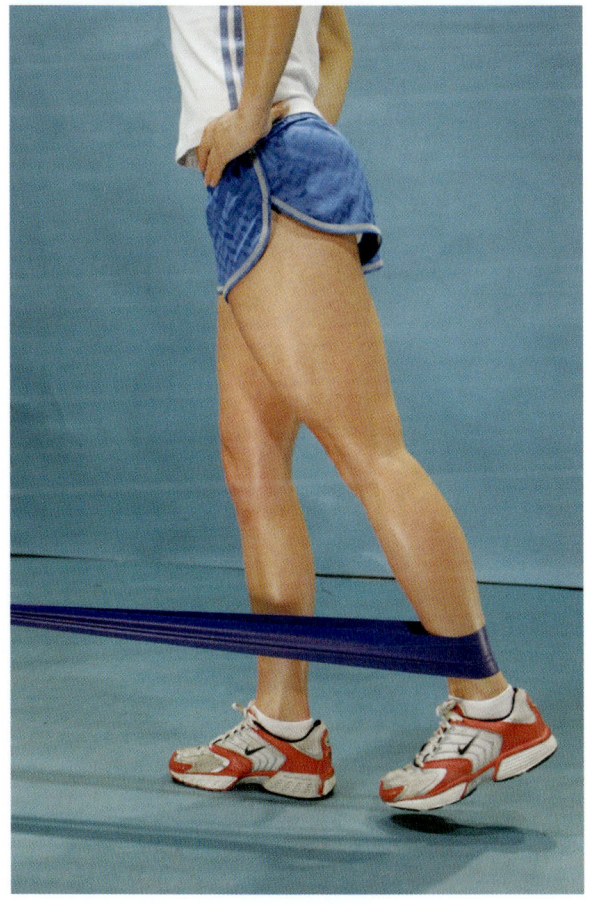

(h)

Figure 35.6 (cont.) (e) Bridging with Swiss ball. A Swiss ball may be used to progress the exercise (f) Hip extension— with rubber tubing (g) Hip abduction with rubber tubing (h) Rubber tubing eccentric stride catch—standing

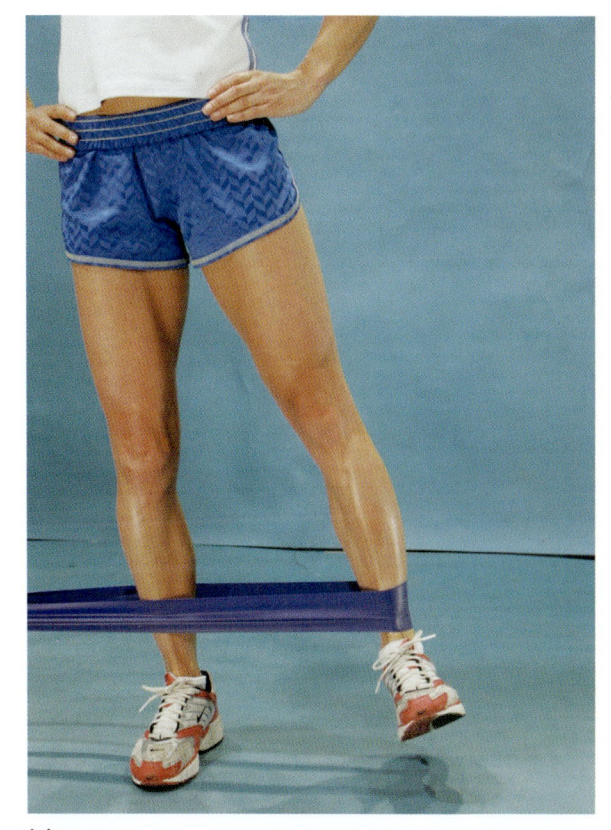

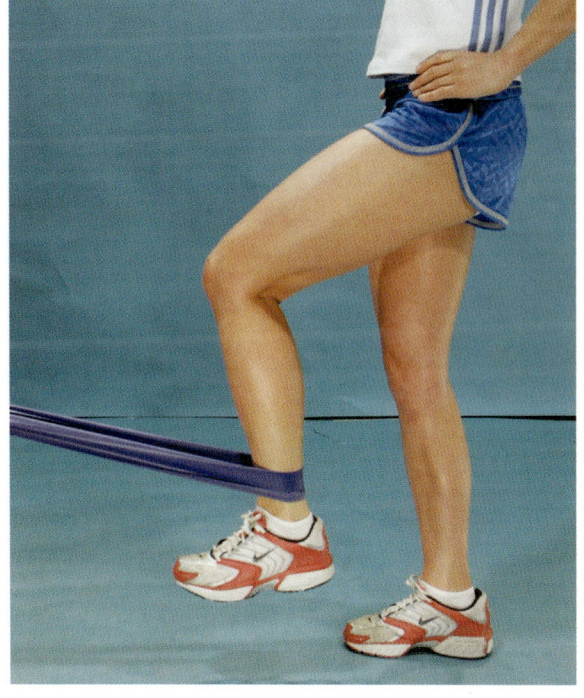

PART B   Regional problems

(i)

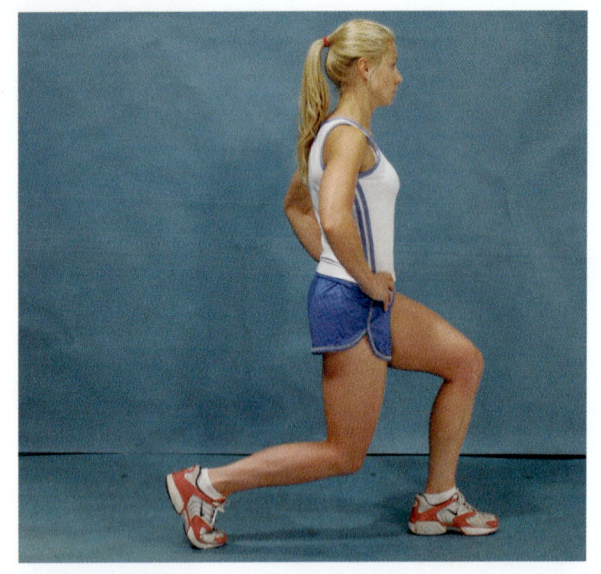

(j)

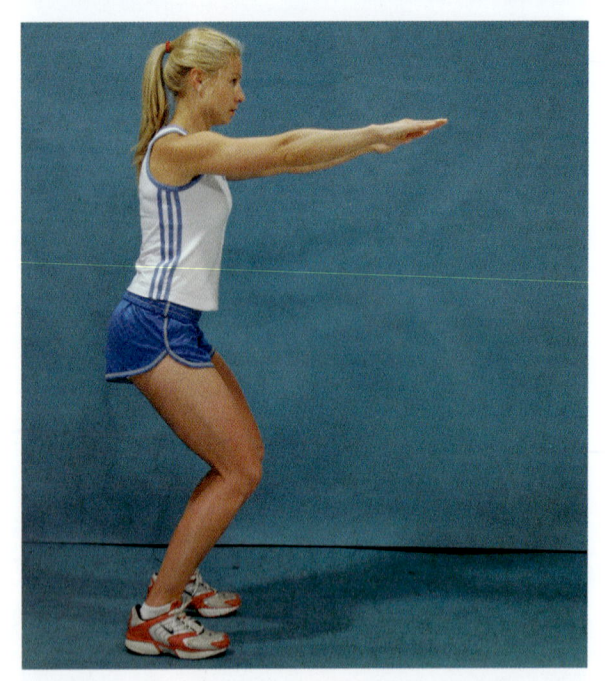

(k)

(l)

Figure 35.6 (cont.) (i) Lunge—performed as shown. Progression involves a combination of increasing the number of sets and repetitions, increasing the depth of the lunge and finally by holding additional weight (j) Double-leg quarter squat (k) Single-leg half squat. All squat exercises should be pain-free. The squat may be aided by the use of a Swiss ball. Particular attention must be given to technique and control of the pelvis, hip and knee. Progression of the squat is similar to that of progression of the leg press exercise (l) Arabesque single-leg squat

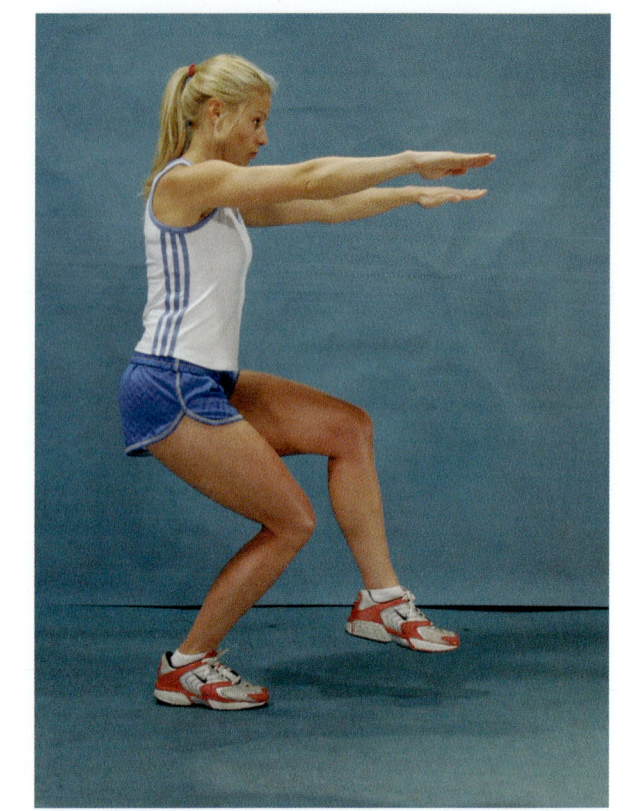

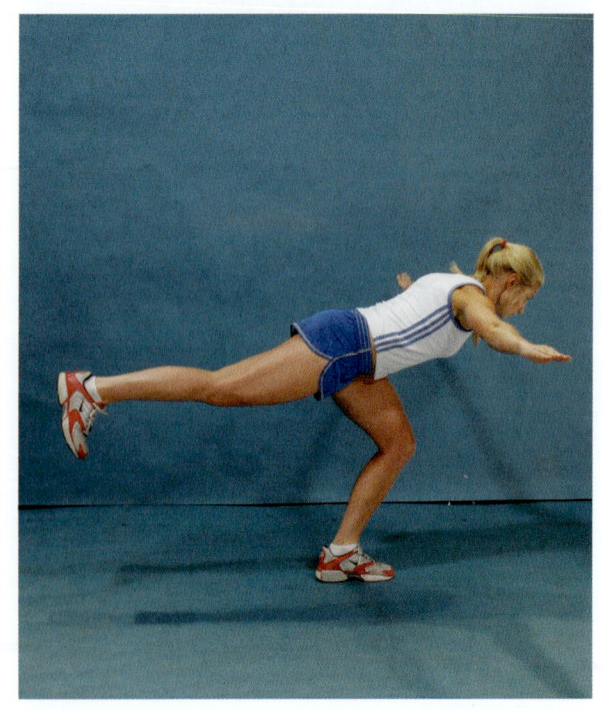

Acute knee injuries   CHAPTER 35

(m)

(n)

(o)

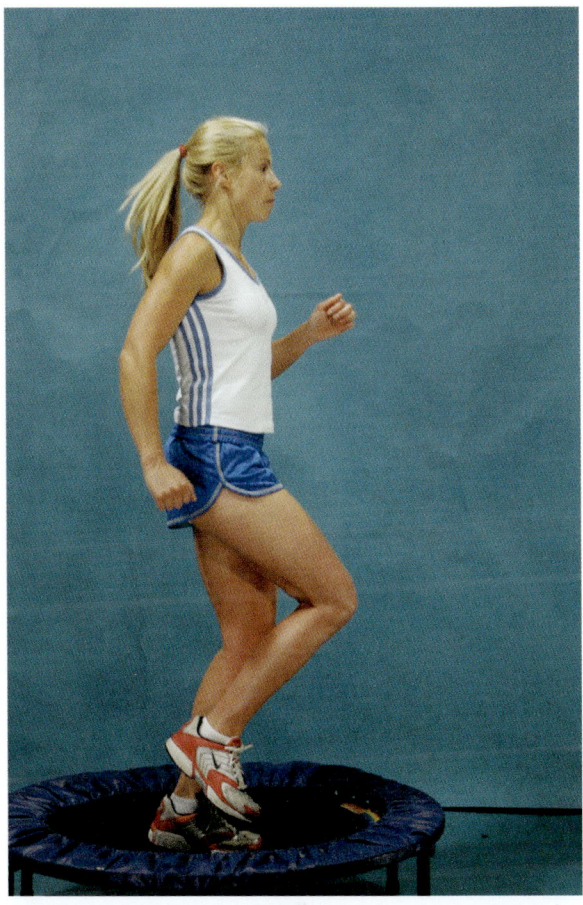

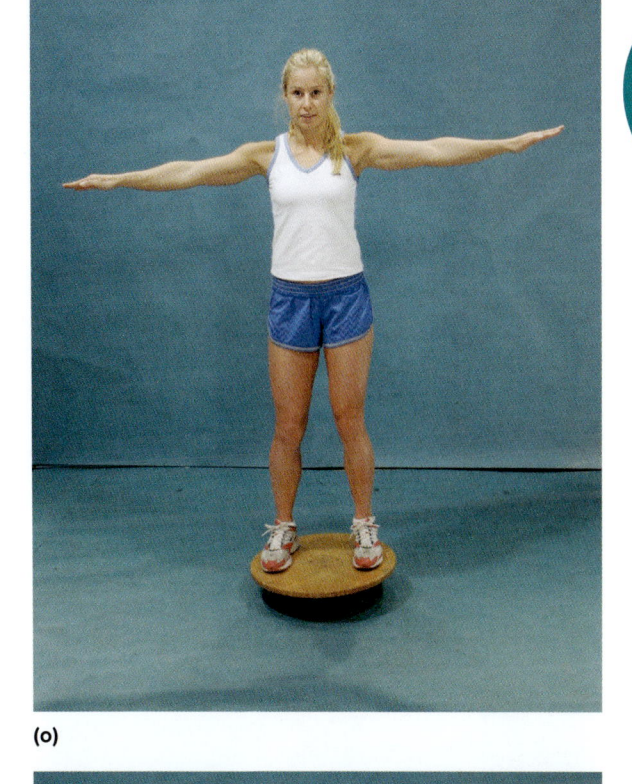

(p)

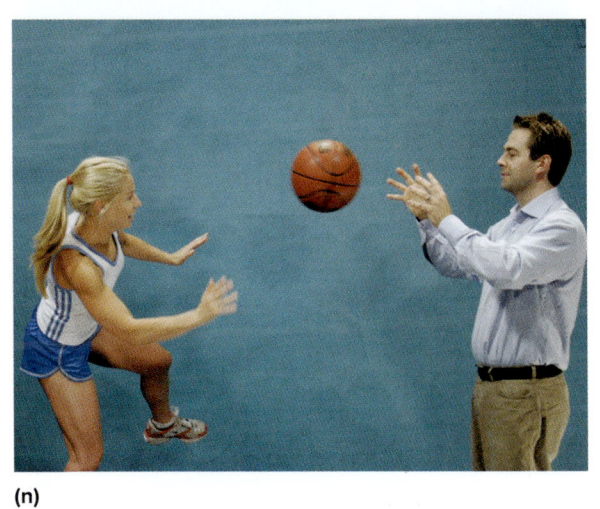

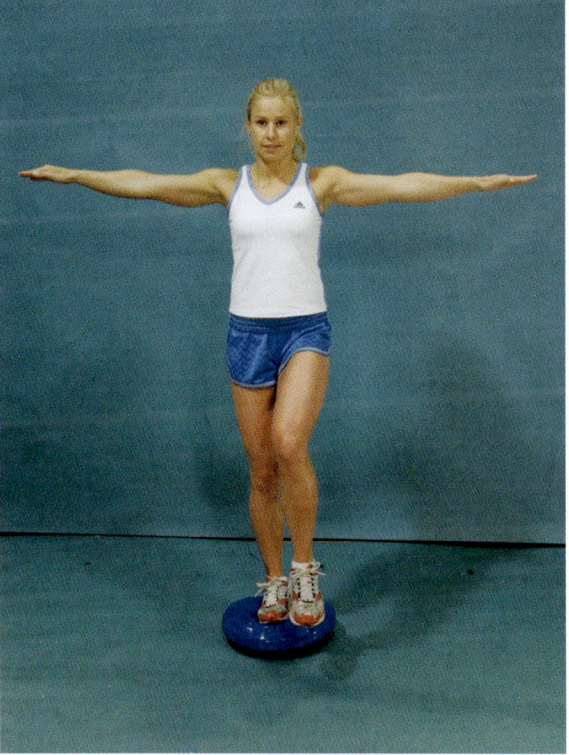

Figure 35.6 (cont.) (m) Rebounder—jogging. A good way to introduce higher impact activity. (n) Static proprioceptive hold/throwing ball. Ball throwing or 'eyes-closed' exercises can provide an excellent functional challenge (o) Wobble board (p) Dura disc balance

PART B   Regional problems

(a)

(b)

(c)

(d)

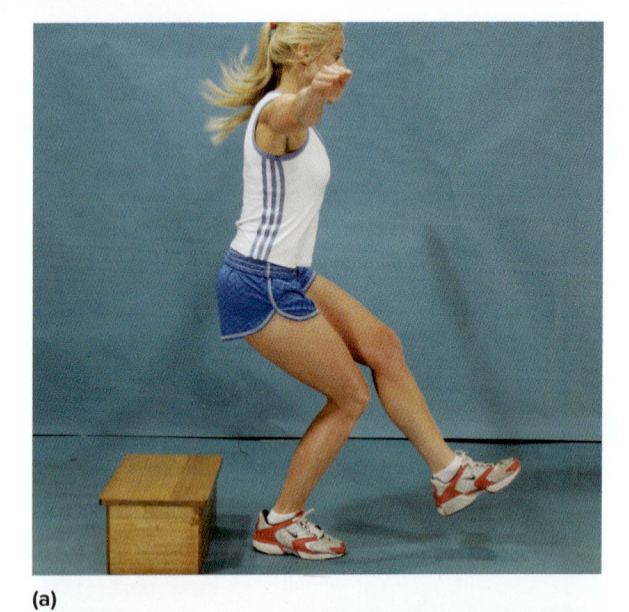

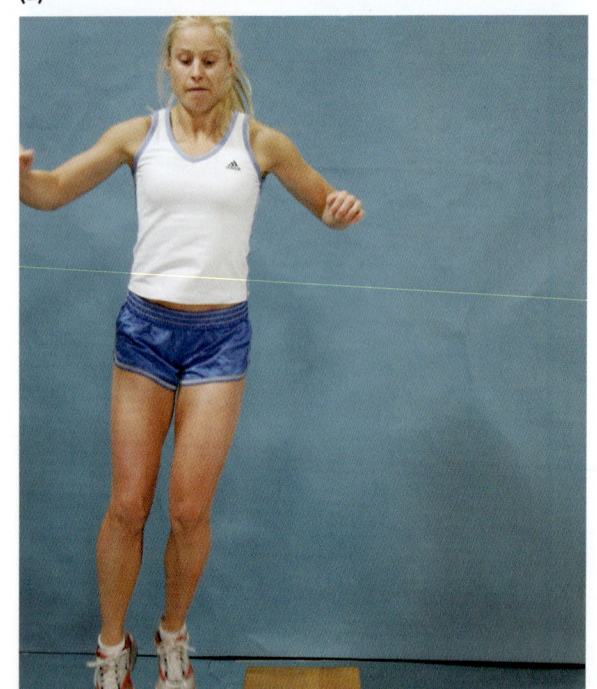

Figure 35.7 Functional activities (a) Jump and land from block. This exercise may be used to replicate functional movements in many sports. Begin the exercise from a small height and jump without rotation. This exercise can be progressed by increasing the height of the jump and rotating 90° during the jump (b) Plyometric jumps over block—lateral plyometric exercises should only be included in the later stages of rehabilitation. Each plyometric exercise should be sport-specific

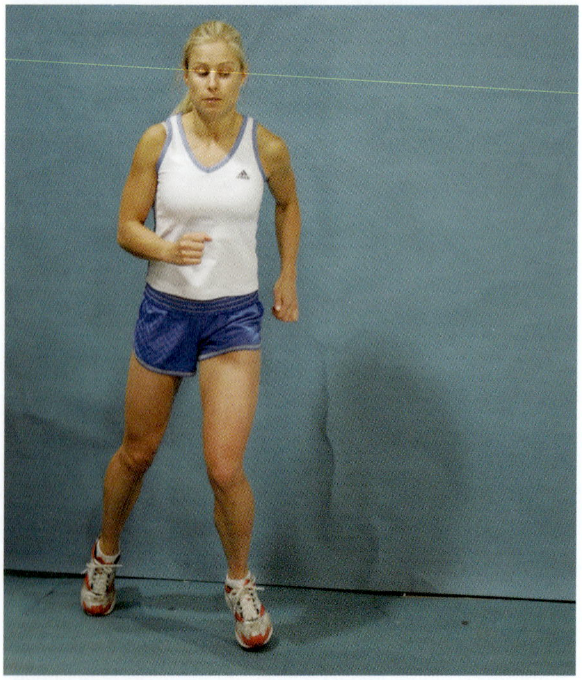

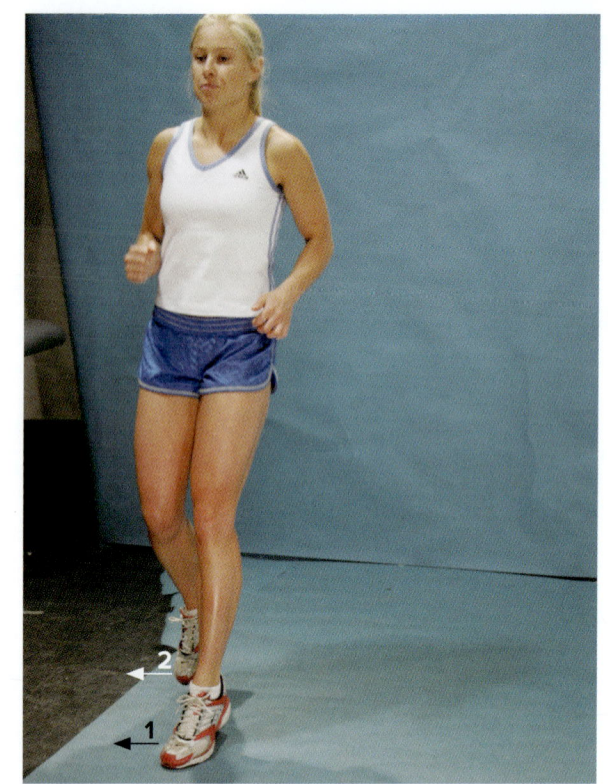

Figure 35.7 (cont.) (c) Carioca exercises—crossover stepping exercise (d) Figure-of-eight running

ANTERIOR CRUCIATE LIGAMENT INJURIES

The annual incidence of ACL tears is 81 per 100 000 inhabitants aged 10-64 years in Europe.[43] In the United States more than 200 000 ACL reconstructions are performed annually at a cost of over US$2 billion.[44, 45]

ACL injuries occur most frequently in sports involving pivoting and sudden deceleration (e.g. football, basketball, netball, soccer, European team handball, gymnastics, downhill skiing). The incidence rate of ACL tears is between 2.4 and 9.7 times higher in female athletes competing in similar activities.[46-51]

A genetic predisposition to ACL tear has been proposed; nonetheless, although specific gene polymorphisms and haplotypes have been identified, it is difficult to come to a conclusion on the basis of the existing literature. More studies are needed in larger populations of different ethnicities. Gene-gene interactions and gene expression studies in the future may delineate the exact role of these gene polymorphisms in ACL tears.[52]

Although ACL tears can occur in isolation, this is relatively uncommon. More frequent are those occurring in combination with associated injuries, such as meniscal tears, articular cartilage injuries or MCL injuries.[53] Principally, all ACL injuries have associated BMLs that are visible on MRI and form a footprint of the injury mechanism.[30]

> **PRACTICE PEARL**
>
> As the torn ACL is only one part of a more complex problem in most ACL injured knees, the diagnosis 'ACL injury' may underplay the severity of an acute knee injury.

Anatomy of the ACL

The ACL is one of four main ligaments that stabilise the knee joint and provides nearly 90% of the stability to anterior translation. The femoral insertion site of the ACL is located on the lateral intercondylar wall 43% of the distance from the proximal to distal femoral articular margin and, in the anterior to posterior dimension, 2.5 mm plus the radius of the ACL footprint anterior to the posterior articular margin.[54] The ACL's insertion on the tibial plateau is 15 mm anterior to the PCL insertion and two-fifths of the width from the medial to lateral tibial spine.[54]

The two bundles that make up the ACL are named according to their tibial insertion. The anteromedial (AM) bundle inserts anteriorly and medially on the tibia, near the medial intercondylar tubercle, while the posterolateral (PL) bundle inserts posteriorly and laterally on the tibia. The fibres of the AM bundle are isometric overall, while the PL bundle fibres are anti-isometric. This means that

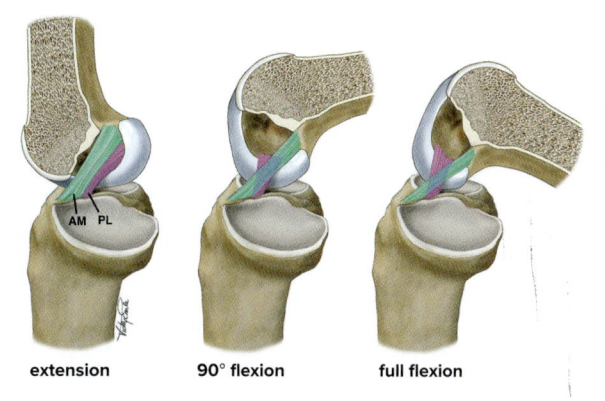

Figure 35.8 ACL bundles during knee flexion. From extension to full flexion, the posterolateral (PL) bundle femoral insertion moves in an arcuate path around the anteromedial (AM) bundle femoral insertion

the length of one portion of the ACL fibres varies during flexion-extension movements.[55]

During flexion, the PL bundle wraps around the AM bundle at the femur; the femoral insertion of the PL bundle forms an arc around the AM bundle's femoral insertion (Fig. 35.8) The anterior fibres of the AM bundle are more isometric, but nevertheless they are less taut between 0° and 30° flexion, which allows them to deform (deformation with superior concavity) as they make contact with the anterior side of the intercondylar notch, thereby allowing full knee extension. Conversely, they are continuously under tension between 30° and 130° flexion.

The posterior fibres of the PL bundle are the least isometric fibres; they are all parallel and completely taut in extension. Between 0° and 90° flexion, they gradually relax and then become taut again beyond 90° flexion. The PL bundle seems to have the most control over tibial rotation due to its more lateral position.[55]

An intact ACL stabilises the femur on the tibia and prevents anterior tibial translation and rotation during agility exercises, jumping, deceleration and pivoting with sudden changes of direction.

Mechanism of ACL injury

In ball sports, two common mechanisms cause ACL tears:

1. a cutting manoeuvre[56-58]
2. single-leg landing.

Cutting or sidestep manoeuvres are associated with dramatic increases in the varus–valgus and internal rotation moments, as well as deceleration. The typical ACL injury occurs with the knee externally rotated and in 10° to 30° of flexion when the knee is placed in a valgus position as the athlete takes off from the planted foot and internally rotates their upper body with the aim of suddenly changing direction (Fig. 35.9a).[59, 60] The ground reaction force falls medial to the knee joint during a cutting manoeuvre and this added force may tax an already tensioned ACL and lead to failure. Similarly, in the landing injuries, the knee is close to full extension.

High-speed activities such as cutting or landing manoeuvres require eccentric muscle action of the quadriceps to resist further flexion. It is hypothesised that vigorous eccentric quadriceps muscle action may play a role in disruption of the ACL. Although this normally may be insufficient to tear the ACL, it may be that the addition of a valgus knee position and/or rotation could trigger an ACL rupture.

One question that is often asked is why the ACL tears in situations and manoeuvres that the athlete has performed many times in the past. Frequently, there is some external factor that renders the athlete susceptible. The athlete could be off balance, be pushed or held by an opponent, be trying to avoid collision with an opponent or have adopted an unusually wide foot position. These perturbations may contribute to the injury by causing the athlete to plant the foot so as to promote unfavourable lower extremity alignment; this may be compounded by inadequate muscle protection and poor neuromuscular control.[60] Fatigue and loss of concentration may also be relevant factors.

What has become recognised is that unfavourable body movements in landing and pivoting can occur, leading to what has become known as the 'functional valgus' or 'dynamic valgus' knee, a pattern of knee collapse where the knee falls medial to the hip and foot. This has been called by Ireland the 'position of no return' or perhaps it should be termed the 'injury-prone position' since there is no proof that one cannot recover from this position (Fig. 35.9b).[61] Intervention programs aimed to reduce the risk of ACL injury are based on training safer neuromuscular patterns in simple manoeuvres such as cutting and jump-landing activities.

The mechanism of ACL injury in skiing is different from that in jumping, running and cutting sports such as football and basketball. In skiing, most ACL injuries result from internal rotation of the tibia with the knee flexed greater than 90°, a position that occurs when a skier who is falling backwards catches the inside edge of the tail of the ski.[62] Intervention programs in skiing are aimed at increasing the skier's awareness of patterns that are injurious to the knee and giving alternative strategies in the hope of avoiding these patterns altogether.

Clinical features

The typical features of the history include the following.

- The patient often describes an audible 'pop', 'crack' or feeling of 'something going out and then going back'.
- Most complete tears of the ACL are extremely painful, especially in the first few minutes after injury.
- Athletes are often initially unable to continue their activity. Occasionally pain will limit further activity and this is usually associated with a large tense effusion. This is the clinical feature of a haemarthrosis. Occasionally, swelling is minimal or delayed.
- At times the athlete tries to recommence the sporting activity and feels instability or a lack of confidence in the knee. Occasionally the athlete may resume playing and suffer an acute episode of instability.

Most athletes with an ACL tear present to a sports medicine practitioner between 24 and 48 hours following the injury. At this stage, it may be difficult to examine the knee. The best time to examine a patient with this condition is in the first hour following the injury before the development of a tense haemarthrosis, which limits the examination. After a few days, when the swelling has started to settle and the pain is less intense, the examination becomes easier to perform in most cases.

After ACL rupture, the examination findings are typical:

- athletes have restricted movement
- they may have widespread mild tenderness
- lateral joint tenderness is often present (this is likely due to the impact pain from the collision of tibia and

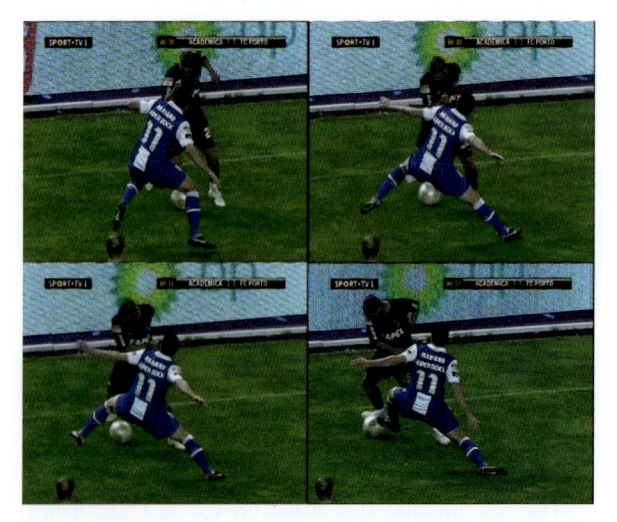

(a)

Figure 35.9 Abnormal positions that may lead to ACL injury
(a) The typical position during the cutting manoeuvre which leads to ACL injury
REPRODUCED WITH PERMISSION OF BRITISH JOURNAL OF SPORTS MEDICINE

Acute knee injuries CHAPTER 35

	muscles involved	Position of safety	body position	body position	Point of 'no return'	muscles involved
back			normal lordosis	forward flexed, rotated opposite side		
hips	extensors abductors gluteals		flexed neutral abduction adduction, neutral rotation	adduction internal rotation		flexors adductors iliopsoas
knee	flexors hamstring		flexed	less flexed, valgus		extensors quadriceps
tibial rotation	plantar flexors		neutral	internal or external		dorsiflexors
landing pattern	gastrocnemius posterior tibialis		both feet in control balanced	one foot out of control unbalanced		peroneals tibialis anterior

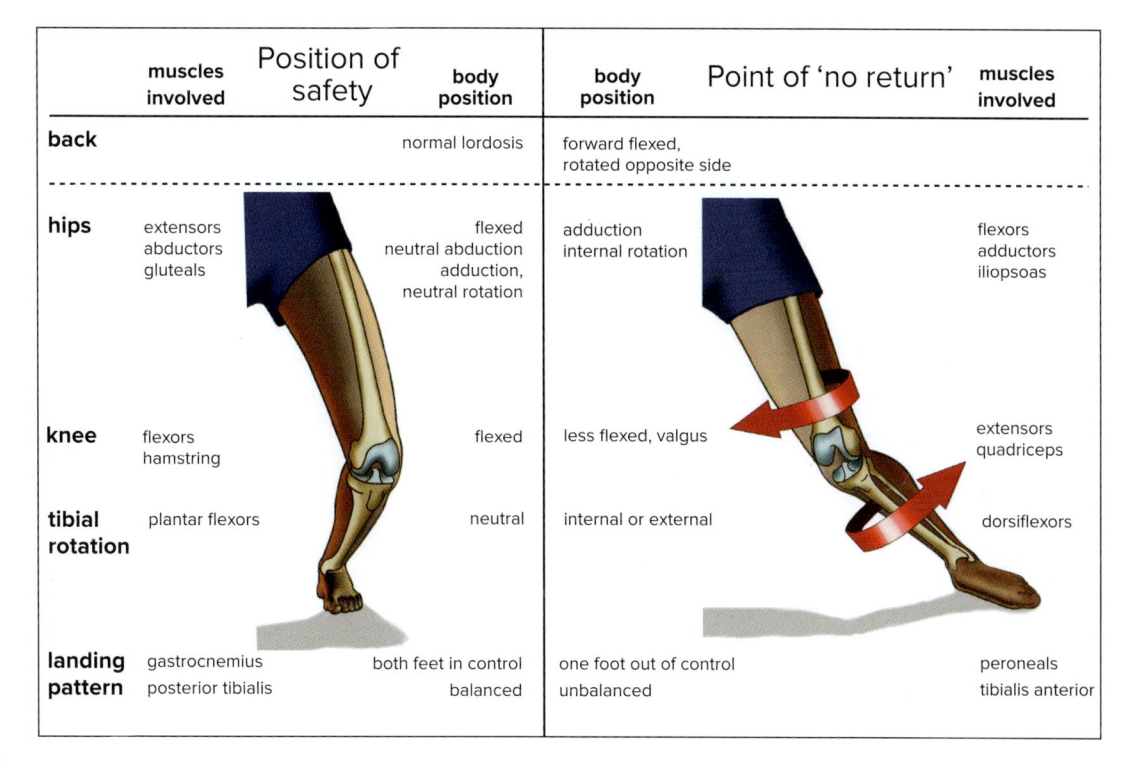

(b)

Figure 35.9 (cont.) (b) The positions of safety and of 'no return'

femur at the time of injury occurring in the valgus position) resulting in a bone marrow lesion (BML)
- medial joint line tenderness may be present if there is an associated medial meniscus injury.

> **PRACTICE PEARL**
>
> The Lachman's test is positive in ACL disruption and is the most useful test for this condition.

The Lachman's test (Figs 35.2h–k) is a core competency for clinicians who see patients with knee injuries. It is judged on both the degree of anterior translation and the quality of the endpoint.[3, 63] With an effusion, maximum anterior tibial excursion may be restricted, but the quality of the endpoint is indistinct.

A positive pivot shift (or jerk) test (Fig. 35.2m) is diagnostic of ACL deficiency, but it requires the patient to have an intact MCL and iliotibial band, as well as the ability to extend the knee almost to full extension.[3] In cases of acute injuries, especially with associated injury (e.g. meniscal tear), the pivot shift test is difficult to perform as the patient is unable to relax sufficiently. The anterior drawer test (Fig. 35.2l) is usually positive in cases of ACL tears but is the least specific test.[3] It should always be compared with the other side as often there is a degree of anterior tibial translation with this test which is quite variable within the population.

A plain radiograph of the knee should be performed when an ACL tear is suspected. Although radiographs are often normal, it may reveal an avulsion of the ligament from the tibia or a 'Segond' fracture at the lateral margin of the tibial plateau (Fig. 35.10); this has always been regarded as pathognomonic of an ACL rupture.[64] More recent studies have suggested that the Segond fragment is actually an avulsion of the anterior lateral ligament of the knee (the mid third capsular ligament) and represents a more severe injury than an isolated ACL tear.[65] Experienced clinicians and radiologists may also detect signs of increased joint fluid on plain radiographs.

MRI may be useful in demonstrating an ACL injury (Fig. 35.11) when the diagnosis is uncertain clinically, and will also demonstrate the typical bone bruise associated with ACL tears (see box below and Fig. 35.11). However, MRI should be used mainly to detect associated meniscal

PART B   Regional problems

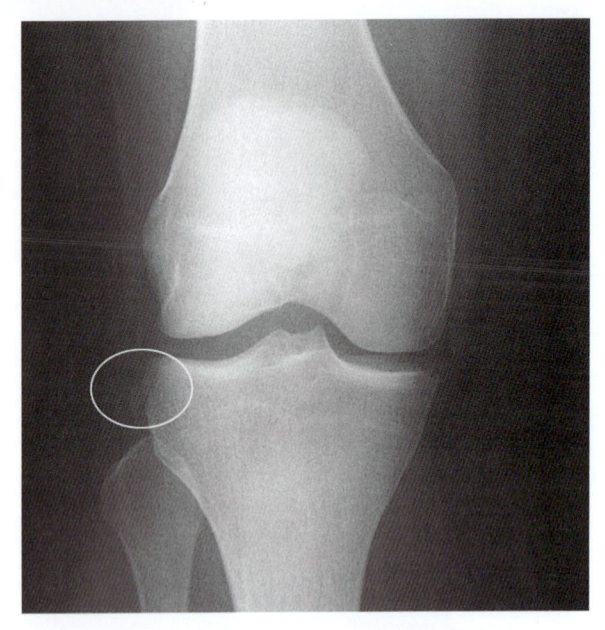

Figure 35.10 X-ray showing a Segond fracture

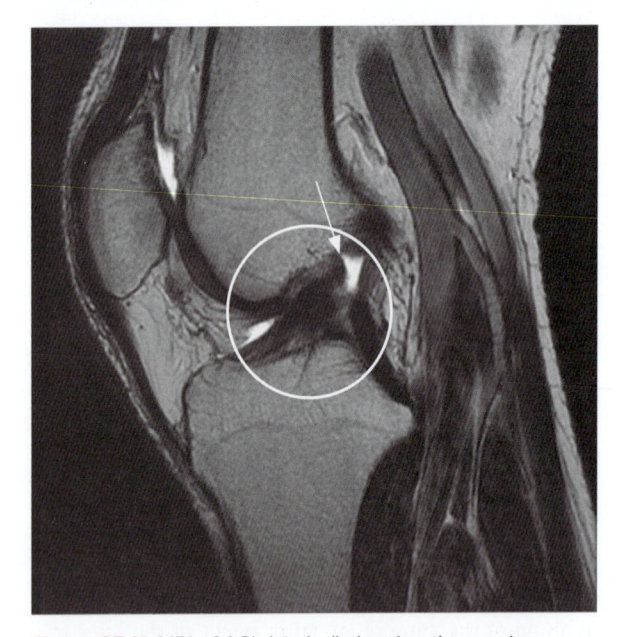

Figure 35.11 MRI of ACL (circled) showing the precise location of the tear (arrow)

tears and cartilage injuries when these injuries are suspected clinically.

Surgical or conservative treatment of the torn ACL?

The optimal treatment of the torn ACL is not known, and there are several areas of controversy regarding the

What is a bone bruise?

A post-traumatic bone marrow lesion (BML) (commonly referred to as a 'bone bruise') is only visible on MRI and accompanies an ACL injury in 80–98% of cases.[30, 50] The most common site is the lateral femoral condyle (Fig. 35.12a–c) and the lateral tibial condyle (Fig.35.12d). The BML is most likely caused by impaction between the posterior aspect of the lateral tibial plateau and the lateral femoral condyle during displacement of the joint at the time of the injury. The presence of a BML indicates impaction trauma to the articular cartilage.[31]

The degree to which BMLs result in permanent injury to the cartilage continues to be investigated. At present it is not clear whether the presence of a BML is significant in the long term. Whether patients with a BML are more prone to osteoarthritis is a hot topic; one report indicated there was no difference in the longer term outcome between those with and without a post-traumatic BML.[66] Whether the presence of a BML should slow the rehabilitation process is also not clear but most clinicians favour a conservative course of treatment in this regard and limit pounding activities for 3 months post bone bruise.

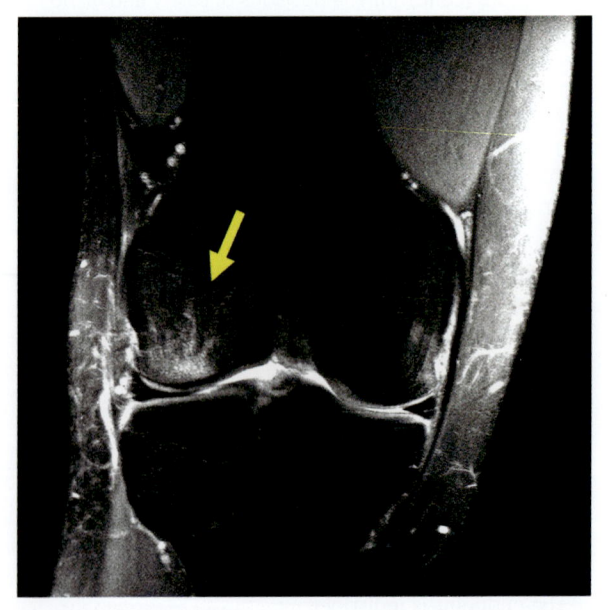

(a)

Figure 35.12 Bone bruising, evident on MRI, is an important diagnostic and prognostic feature often associated with ACL injury (a) Anteroposterior coronal MRI of a lateral femoral condyle bone marrow oedema in association with an ACL rupture. In radiology exams, this is considered pathognomonic of an ACL rupture until proven otherwise

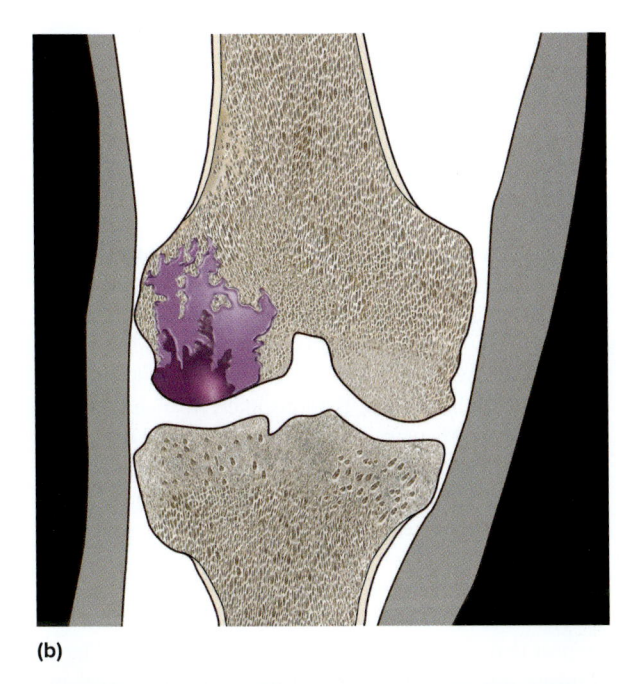

Acute knee injuries CHAPTER 35

(b)

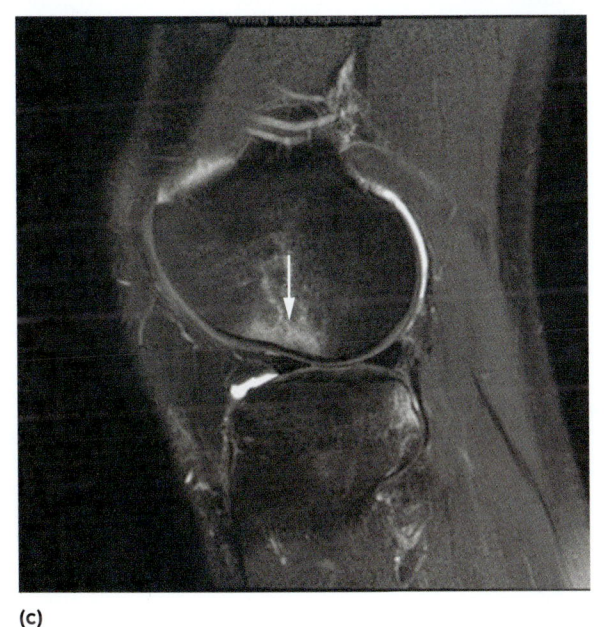

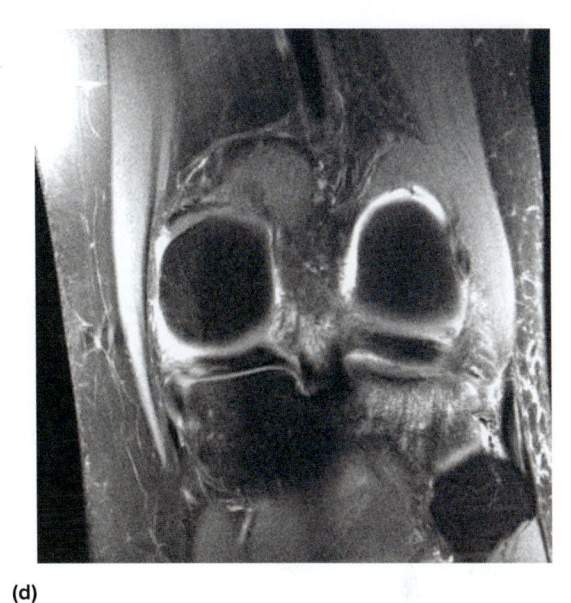

(d)

Figure 35.12 (cont.) (b) The pathological appearance of a lateral femoral condyle bone marrow oedema in association with an ACL tear (c) Sagittal MRI appearance of the femoral condyle BML (d) The tibial plateau often also suffers bone marrow oedema; posterolateral tibial bruising (arrowheads in this coronal MRI) is also pathognomonic of ACL injury

(c)

management of ACL injuries. These include: the relative merits of non-surgical versus surgical management; the use of braces to prevent ACL injury or control the ACL-deficient knee; whether surgery should be performed immediately after the injury or should be delayed; whether a delayed reconstruction is to be performed weeks, months or even years after injury; the relative merits of the various surgical techniques; and the benefit of different rehabilitation programs.

There is only one RCT that has compared the results of a surgical and a non-surgical treatment strategy.[67, 68] In this study, 121 patients aged 18–35 with acute ACL injuries were randomly divided into two treatment groups: rehabilitation plus early ACL reconstruction; or rehabilitation alone with the possibility of a later ACL reconstruction if this was deemed necessary. Professional athletes and those who did not regularly practice sport were excluded from the study whereas competitive athletes on a subprofessional level and recreational athletes were included in the trial. After both 2 and 5 years, there were no differences in terms of knee function reported by the patient, return to sports or surgical treatment of meniscus injury between the groups. However, after 2 years 39% and after 5 years 51% of the group treated with initial rehabilitation needed to have an ACL reconstruction.

This study is used by the proponents of non-surgical rehabilitation treatment with an option of later reconstruction stating that the results at 2 years and 5 years were the same as the group who underwent early surgical reconstruction.[67, 68] The proponents of early surgical reconstruction use the 51% of the non-surgical group who required later reconstruction by 5 years as support for their claim as well as arguing that the delay in reconstruction may lead to an increased risk of associated injuries of the meniscus and/or articular cartilage.[69]

Well-structured and extensive rehabilitation seems to be crucial for patients with ACL injury. Still, rehabilitation only is not sufficient for some 50% who are likely to need surgery in order to cope with their injury. Little is known about individual factors related to a good treatment outcome and thus the decision on selecting patients for surgery or rehabilitation is difficult.

Early phase instability at rest (i.e. within the first 3 months after injury) was not a good predictor for the need for later surgical treatment, whereas instability after 3 months was a relatively good prospective predictor.[70] The following factors should be considered when deciding whether or not to take the surgical option:

- the age of the patient
- the degree of instability in function
- a repairable meniscus tear
- associated knee injuries (e.g. MCL tear, meniscal tear)
- the patient's desire to return to jumping and pivoting sports
- the patient's occupation (e.g. firefighter, police).

The use of functional tests to help 'predict' those that may need operative ACL treatment is currently being investigated. Early reports suggest performing screening examination after 10 sessions of progressive exercise therapy was of value in helping to inform decision making for ACL reconstruction. Those who had surgery were also younger and had a higher activity level.[71]

A systematic review of the factors related to the need for surgical reconstruction after ACL rupture reviewed seven studies, three of which were of high quality.[72] Based on these studies, neither sex (strong evidence) nor the severity of knee joint laxity (moderate evidence) can predict soon after ACL injury whether a patient will need ACL reconstruction following non-operative treatment. All other factors identified in this review either had conflicting or only minimal evidence as to their level of association with the need for surgical reconstruction.

Still, it is important to note that there is limited evidence in determining who will benefit from what treatment. Most decisions are made in consensus between the treating clinician and the patient and are based on empiric knowledge rather than scientific evidence.

The degree of instability may be assessed by a number of parameters. It is important to note that instability at rest (i.e. at clinical examination of the knee) is not a reliable indication of the functional instability experienced by the patient. However, as recurrent episodes of giving way indicate functional instability, this is likely to be a reliable indication of disability and an increased likelihood of needing surgery.

> **PRACTICE PEARL**
>
> For patients presenting with a history of 'giving way' or a history of instability in function despite adequate strength, an ACL reconstruction is recommended.

Many surgeons would advocate ACL reconstruction in patients with concomitant meniscal injuries (50% prevalence) that could be repaired. The decision is also influenced by the demands placed on the knee. A young athlete who wishes to return to a pivoting sport, such as football or basketball, is more likely to need an ACL reconstruction than an athlete who is prepared to confine activity to those sports that do not involve a large amount of twisting, turning and pivoting. However, some of the patients in this category do perform well after 2 years, also after rehabilitation alone.[67] It is likely that repeated episodes of giving way increase the risk of developing knee osteoarthritis but there is no scientific evidence to support that an ACL reconstruction reduces the incidence of future osteoarthritis. A recent report did not reveal any differences in the frequency of osteoarthritis between surgically reconstructed and non-surgically treated patients 10 years after ACL injury.[73]

Another important factor to assess is the likelihood of the patient adhering to a comprehensive, time-consuming rehabilitation program. If the patient indicates a lack of willingness to undertake appropriate rehabilitation, treatment may not be successful. It is important to also note that the results of an ACL reconstruction are dependent on a successful postoperative rehabilitation. Other factors to consider are the cost of surgery, rehabilitation and the amount of time off work.

In summary, surgery is generally recommended for athletes wishing to participate in a high-speed sport with constant change of direction and pivoting. Rehabilitation without surgery, however, has been shown to be an alternative for this patient category.[67] A trial of non-surgical management does not rule out the possibility of eventual later surgery when indicated.

Surgical treatment

There are numerous surgical techniques used to treat ACL injuries. As ACL tears are usually in-substance tears and therefore not suitable for primary repair, reconstruction of the ACL (ACLR) is the surgical treatment of choice. ACLRs are performed 'arthroscopically aided' through small arthroscopic incisions (see box below). Arthroscopic surgery utilises small incisions to help visualise the inside of the joint and facilitates tunnel placement of the ACL graft. Depending on the type of graft, incisions to harvest the graft and secure tunnel access for graft fixation will be made as well.

Acute knee injuries CHAPTER 35

What happens during ACL reconstruction surgery?

The surgical reconstruction technique involves harvesting the tendon (patellar or hamstring, Fig. 35.13a) through a small incision and threading the tendon through tunnels drilled in the bones. The most crucial parts of the operation are locating the points of entry of the tibial and femoral tunnels and then the fixation of the graft.

The tibial attachment should be in the centre of the previous anterior cruciate attachment (at the level of the inner margin of the anterior portion of the lateral meniscus). The femoral attachment is to the position of optimal or maximised isometry. This is a position in the intercondylar notch on the femur at which the graft is at a fixed tension throughout the range of knee movement.

Once the graft attachment areas have been delineated and prepared, the graft is fixed by one of a variety of different methods. These methods include interference screw fixation (Fig. 35.13b), staples or the tying of sutures around fixation posts. The better the quality of graft fixation, the more comfortable one is in advancing rehabilitation in the first weeks after surgery.

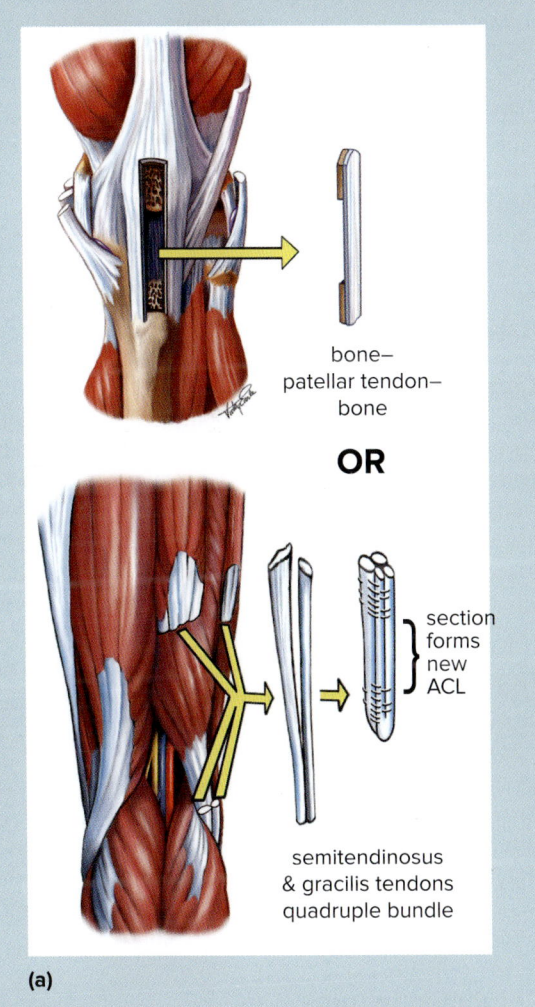

Figure 35.13 The key steps in the process of ACL reconstruction (a) Harvesting graft tissue for the patellar tendon (top panel) or semitendinosus and gracilis tendon ('hamstring graft') ACL reconstruction (b) Replacing the ruptured ACL with the graft tendon tissue; interference screw shown (c) After surgery—the knee with the new graft or 'neoligament' in place

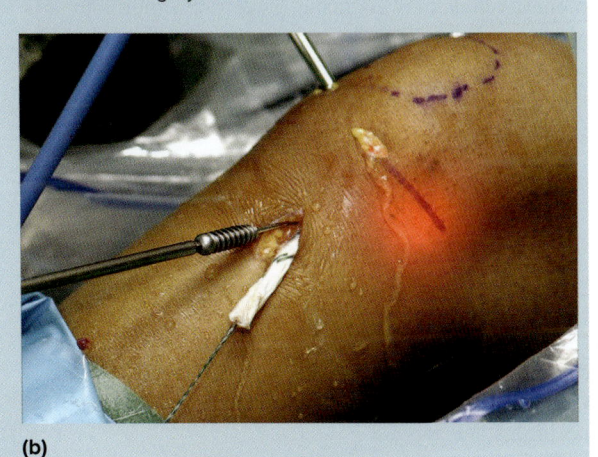

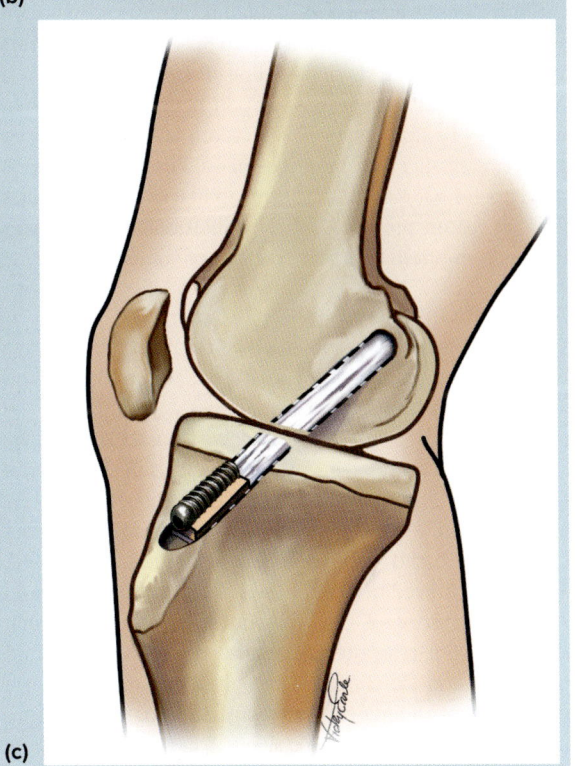

743

Type of graft

The aim of an ACLR is to replace the torn ACL with a graft that reproduces the normal kinetic functions of the ligament. In most cases, an autogenous graft, taken from around the knee joint, is used. The most common grafts used are the bone–patellar tendon–bone (BTB) autograft involving the central third of the patellar tendon or a multi-stranded hamstring (semitendinosus +/− gracilis tendons) graft using the ipsilateral limb. Other autograft choices include the quadriceps tendon and autografts from the contralateral limb. Allografts (donated tissue from cadaveric specimens) have also been used with the potential benefit of reducing harvest site morbidity but introducing questions of graft incorporation or disease transmission (e.g. HIV, hepatitis, bacterial). Graft choice is dependent on a number of factors including surgeon competency and familiarity with the various techniques.

Patellar tendon versus hamstring tendon graft

There is debate on graft choice, in particular patellar tendon versus hamstring tendon. Reviews of the numerous research papers comparing the two techniques have shown very little difference in outcome measures and there is no universal agreement on which technique is superior.[74,75] Each case should be considered on its merit, taking into account some of the differences in potential postoperative issues.

For example, after patellar tendon reconstruction, pain with kneeling is common and up to 50% of patients report anterior knee pain with kneeling. Patients who have a hamstring graft ACL reconstruction have decreased end-range knee flexion power. The incisions used for hamstring grafts are smaller and more cosmetic. Potential problems need to be addressed in the rehabilitation program and for that reason we advocate rehabilitation regimens with different emphasis for the two types of surgery.

Autograft versus allograft

There has been considerable debate regarding the relative merits of autograft (using the patient's own tissue) and allograft (using another person's tissue). A summary of the nine RCTs and 10 systematic reviews showed statistically significant differences in favour of autograft for clinical failure, the Lachman test, the instrumented laxity test and the Tegner score.[76] When subgroup analyses were conducted based on whether irradiation was used, autograft achieved better clinical outcomes than irradiated allograft in terms of the Lysholm score, clinical failure, the pivot shift test, the Lachman test, the instrumented laxity test and the Tegner score. In addition, there were no significant differences between the autograft and non-irradiated allograft groups for all eight indices. The authors concluded that autograft had greater advantages than irradiated allograft with respect to function and stability, whereas there were no significant differences between autograft and non-irradiated allograft.

Single bundle versus double bundle

The ACL has two distinct bundles: the anteromedial (AM) bundle and the posterolateral (PL) bundle. It is possible to reconstruct the bundles individually (anatomic double-bundle ACL reconstruction) particularly in large knees. Double-bundle ACL reconstruction (DBACLR) restores the native footprint of the ligament and is definitely superior to isometric ACLR. Whether or not double-bundle anatomic is better than single-bundle anatomic is as yet undecided.

Meta-analyses have suggested that double bundle may result in superiority in rotational stability, the degree of osteoarthritis (OA) changes, and subjective function score postoperatively compared with the single-bundle procedure[77] and less anterior laxity.[78] However, there was no difference on functional outcomes between the treatment procedures at long-term follow-up. Given the lack of conclusive evidence of superiority and the doubling of implant costs involved with double-bundle ACLR, single bundle is probably the procedure of choice at this point in time.

Timing of surgery—early or late

The timing of ACL reconstruction after an acute injury has come under review. Traditionally and with very little evidence in support, ACLRs were performed as soon as practical after the injury. However, there is some evidence that delaying the surgery may decrease the postoperative risk of arthrofibrosis (see 'Soft tissue stiffness').[79] Initial reports suggested 3 weeks as the appropriate delay in surgery but now focus is more on the condition of the knee rather than the actual time. The injured knee should have little or no swelling and have near full ROM; the patient should have a normal gait.

A systematic review examined 22 articles (3583 patients).[80] Eight articles promoted early reconstruction, whereas the majority of articles found no difference in outcome between early and delayed surgery. Two articles were inconclusive. The authors concluded that there were few or no differences in subjective and objective outcomes related to timing of ACL reconstruction.

Combined injuries

Injuries of the ACL rarely occur in isolation and thus most of all ACL injuries occur in combination with other injuries. The presence and extent of associated injuries may affect the way in which the ACL injury is managed. Associated injury to the MCL (grades II–III) poses a particular problem due to the tendency to develop stiffness after this injury. Most orthopaedic surgeons would initially treat the MCL injury in a knee brace for a period of 4–6 weeks, during which time the athlete would undertake a comprehensive rehabilitation program (see below). This allows for early healing of the ligament injury and any potential capsular injury, reducing the risk of chronic valgus instability.

ACL injuries are frequently associated with chondral damage. The majority of the literature supports the clinical relevance of cartilage lesions which are correlated with a poorer outcome after ACL reconstruction.[81]

Injuries to the posterolateral corner which may occur in conjunction with an ACL injury are considered later in the chapter.

Rehabilitation after ACL injury

Traditionally, most rehabilitation principles have been evaluated as postoperative rehabilitation protocols due to the frequent use of ACL reconstruction as the treatment of choice. However, rehabilitation alone, performed according to a protocol similar to that used postoperatively, was recently shown to provide similar 2-year outcomes as the combination of ACL reconstruction plus rehabilitation.[67] Thus, rehabilitation may be performed in a similar setting regardless of whether or not additional reconstructive surgery is performed.

Rehabilitation after ACL injury has changed dramatically over time, resulting in greatly accelerated rehabilitation programs.[82] The speed at which an ACL injury is rehabilitated must take into account the time it takes for soft tissues to heal and remodel as well as the neuromotor control and coordination of the athlete. The most important aims are: reduction of pain, swelling and inflammation; and regaining ROM, strength and neuromuscular control.[83] The major change over the past few years is the incorporation of a core stability program along with increased emphasis on proprioceptive and balance exercises. These exercises have been used in successful ACL prevention programs (see Chapter 12). Despite the widespread acceptance of these elements into rehabilitation programs, the two RCTs have not shown convincing evidence of their efficacy.[84, 85]

The rehabilitation program is shown in Table 35.10. The time frames in the table are a guideline only and must be adjusted depending on the progress of the individual patient. It is essential to rehabilitate each patient individually, taking into consideration the extent of damage to the knee (e.g. articular cartilage damage), the patient's adherence to the exercise program, the amount of knee stiffness, which varies considerably between patients, and the eventual functional aims of the patient (e.g. daily activities, high-level sport). The patient must be taught to monitor the signs and symptoms around the knee following each work-out. Ice may need to be applied if pain, inflammation or swelling is present.

The timing of return to sport (see next section) is dependent on several different factors, including knee stability, neuromotor function, the nature of the sport, the therapist's and coach's opinion, and the confidence of the patient.

Neuromotor function and muscle strength should be regularly assessed during rehabilitation and prior to return to play. An excellent functional test that can be easily conducted in the clinical setting during the later stages of rehabilitation is the single-leg hop test. The patient performs the single-leg hop by hopping as far as possible using the injured leg, with distance being measured. Athletes with good function are able to land confidently, and 'stick it'. Those with functional disability step further or take another small hop. Comparison should be made with the uninjured leg. Another way of testing function is by incorporating sport-specific drills. Isokinetic testing may be used to evaluate muscle strength. Quadriceps and hamstring strength should approximate that of the uninjured leg. In the light of all these factors and the varying progress of different athletes and the sport to which they are returning, the time for return to sport after ACL injury may vary from 4–12 months.

The use of a brace on return to sport is not necessary but may help the athlete's confidence. Several systematic reviews and RCTs on the topic do not recommend the use of postoperative brace after ACLR. Bracing does not seem to help with pain, function, rehabilitation and stability.[74]

The research into the effectiveness of various rehabilitation techniques has generally been of poor quality and thus limited conclusions can be drawn. The Orthopaedic Section of the American Physical Therapy Association publishes clinical practice guidelines, including the level of supporting evidence, for treatment of knee sprains based on an international classification of functional disability.[86] The MOON Group (a collection of orthopaedic surgeons) has developed, in conjunction with their physiotherapists, rehabilitation guidelines based on a systematic review of the available evidence.[87]

Considerations in rehabilitation after ACLR

When performed after ACLR, management principles have changed as surgical techniques have changed. There is a better understanding of the initial graft strength and the strength of various graft fixation techniques. There is no difference in joint laxity or clinical outcome between those who underwent accelerated rehabilitation compared to those with a non-accelerated program at 2 years post-surgery.[88]

Without an open arthrotomy, the extensor mechanism has been better preserved with reduced joint adhesions. The principle of complete immobilisation has been replaced with protected mobilisation, with a resultant dramatic decrease in stiffness and increase in ROM of the knee joint. This has allowed earlier commencement of a strengthening program and rapid progression to functional

PART B Regional problems

Table 35.10 Rehabilitation following ACL reconstruction (see Figs 35.5 and 35.6)

Phase	Goal of phase	Time post-surgery	Physiotherapy treatment	Exercise program	Functional/sport-related activity
Prehabilitation (preoperative rehabilitation)	No/minimal swelling Restore full ROM, particularly extension General 4+/5 lower limb strength or better Patient education—anatomy, surgical procedure, rehabilitation commitment, and goal setting	NA	Cryotherapy Electrotherapy Compression Manual therapy Gait re-education Exercise modification and supervision	Dependent on ability of patient In early stages, follow the exercise program from phase 1 and progress to phase 2 If patient has high level of function, start with exercise program from phase 2 and progress weights and repetitions as appropriate	Walking Bike riding Swimming (light kick and no breaststroke)
Phase 1	PWB–FWB Eliminate swelling 0–100° ROM 4+/5 quadriceps strength 5/5 hamstring strength	0–2 weeks	Cryotherapy Electrotherapy Compression Manual therapy Gait re-education Patient education	Gentle flexion ROM Extension ROM to 0° Quadriceps/VMO setting Supported (bilateral) calf raises Hip abduction and extension Hamstring pulleys/rubbers Gait drills	Nil
Phase 2	No swelling Full knee hyperextension Knee flexion to 130°+ Full squat Good balance and control Unrestricted walking	2–12 weeks	Cryotherapy Electrotherapy Compression Manual therapy Gait re-education Exercise modification	ROM drills Quadriceps/VMO setting Mini squats and lunges Leg press (double-leg, then single-leg) Step-ups Bridges (double-leg, then single-leg) Hip abduction and extension with rubber tubing Single-leg calf raises Gait re-education drills Balance and proprioceptive drills (single-leg)	Walking Exercise bike

Table 35.10 (cont.)

Phase	Goal of phase	Time post-surgery	Physiotherapy treatment	Exercise program	Functional/sport-related activity
Phase 3	Full ROM Full strength and power Return to jogging, running, and agility Return to restricted sport-specific drills	3–6 months	Manual therapy Exercise/activity modification and supervision	As above—increase difficulty, repetitions, and weight, where appropriate Jump and land drills Agility drills	Straight-line jogging Swimming (light kick) Road bike Straight-line running at 3 months Progressing to sport-specific running and agility (progressively sequenced) (e.g. running forwards, sideways, backwards, sprinting, jumping, hopping, changing directions, kicking)
Phase 4	Return to sport	6–12 months	As above	High-level sport-specific strengthening as required	Progressive return to sport (e.g. restricted training, unrestricted training, match play, competitive match play)

FWB = full weight-bearing; PWB = partial weight-bearing; ROM = range of motion; VMO = vastus medialis obliquus

exercises. The average time for rehabilitation after ACLR to return to sport has been reduced from around 12 months to 6-9 months before the injured individual could regain sporting activity. The importance of early return to sports in relation to later osteoarthritis development needs to be determined.

Rehabilitation must commence from the time of injury, not from the time of surgery, which may be days, weeks or months later if needed at all.[89] The initial management aims to reduce pain, swelling and inflammation, thus reducing the amount of intra-articular fibrosis and resultant loss of ROM, strength and function. Treatment should commence immediately after injury, including interferential stimulation, ultrasound and transcutaneous electrical nerve stimulation (TENS), as well as strengthening exercises for the quadriceps, hamstring, hip extensor, hip abductor and calf muscles. Pain-free ROM exercises should also be performed.

Additional muscle strengthening and neuromuscular rehabilitation prior to surgery can improve outcomes.[90, 91] This is often referred to as 'pre-habilitation' or 'pre-hab'. This period is also an opportunity for the clinician to explain the hospital protocol and the progression and goals of the rehabilitation program. The therapist should set a realistic goal, taking into consideration the individual patient. It is helpful to provide a written explanation as well. If necessary, the postoperative knee brace should be fitted and the use of crutches taught.

Immediately following surgery, weight-bearing status is largely determined by concomitant injuries (e.g. meniscal repair, intra-articular fracture or function of other ligaments). Isolated ACLRs are typically treated as weight-bearing as tolerated, using a brace and/or crutches until adequate quadriceps muscle strength is restored. Instructions should be given regarding the use of crutches as the patient will progress from limited weight-bearing to full weight-bearing for the first 2 weeks.

The rehabilitation programs for patellar tendon and hamstring tendon graft ACLRs are slightly different due to the need to prevent the particular complications associated with each type of reconstruction. Potential problems with the patellar tendon graft are kneeling pain, patellar tendinopathy and/or reduced patellar mobility (see the next section). Therefore, attention must be paid to this area during the rehabilitation program with the use of soft tissue therapy to the patellar tendon, accompanied by a strengthening program for the tendon and patellar taping (Chapter 35) to prevent patellofemoral and fat pad problems. The hamstring graft should be treated as though the patient has had a hamstring tear (Chapter 34), with an appropriately paced rehabilitation program to restore full ROM and strength.

Problems encountered during ACL rehabilitation
Problems that are not treatment dependent
Low back pain
Low back pain is not uncommon in the early stages of the rehabilitation program possibly due to the use of crutches, altered gait patterns or altered sleep patterns. It usually occurs in patients who have a prior history of low back pain.

Problems in non-surgically treated patients
Instability
The main problem that may occur in the rehabilitation of non-surgically treated patients is remaining functional instability. All non-surgically treated patients should have a scheduled appointment with the treating clinician within the first 3 months after injury. When having complaints on symptomatic instability or lack of trust in their knee due to instability despite a successful rehabilitation, an ACLR could be recommended. This is especially true for patients still wishing to resume sporting activities.

Symptomatic meniscus tears
Another problem that may increasingly occur among this group is a symptomatic meniscus tear. Unlike those undergoing ACLR, the non-surgically treated patient does not routinely undergo surgery for meniscus tears associated with their initial injury. Some of these meniscus tears remain asymptomatic, some might heal but some will develop to be symptomatic. Here it is important to differentiate between symptoms adhering to the injured meniscus and symptoms related to the ACL injury and to treat that symptomatic injury. When such problems are encountered, the best option is to let an experienced orthopaedic surgeon assess the injury and discuss treatment alternatives with the patient.

Problems in surgically treated patients
Apart from surgical complications (e.g. infection, deep venous thrombosis, graft harvest site morbidity), a number of secondary problems may occur during the postoperative rehabilitation process.

Patellar region pain
Patellofemoral pain may occur on the injured or the uninjured side. Patients may present with typical symptoms of patellofemoral pain (Chapter 36) but often will not comment on the presence of anterior knee pain as they assume that it is part of the normal process following surgery. The patient should always be asked about symptoms at the front of the knee and the patellofemoral joint should be examined at each visit.

Such factors may be the same as those that predispose a person without ACLR to having patellofemoral pain (Chapter 36), such as altered patellofemoral alignment, altered lower limb mechanics (including internal hip rotation and adduction, apparent knee valgus), quadriceps and hip muscle insufficiencies; or may have developed as part of the ACL injury and reconstruction process. For example, following ACLR, some people have fat pad thickening and oedema, often associated with patella baja or alta, insufficient restoration of quadriceps and hip muscle strength and control, altered tibial rotation (relative to the femur), or persistent loss of knee extension or flexion range. Some of these factors may be aggravated by persistent swelling and/or pain. Such factors should be evaluated and treated as appropriate.

Closed chain activities such as squats and lunges are preferred to open chain activities, as open chain loaded knee extension results in larger patellofemoral forces in the functional knee flexion range of 0° to 60°.[92] To minimise patellofemoral force, open chain exercises should be performed between 60° and 90° of knee flexion, while closed chain exercises should be maintained to <60° flexion. However, loaded knee extension at knee flexion angles <60° is thought to strain the ACL graft; clinicians need to exercise caution during early strengthening interventions in this knee range.[93] Notably, patellofemoral problems occur not only with patellar tendon graft reconstructions but also with hamstring tendon graft reconstructions with considerable morbidity.[94]

The infrapatellar fat pad may be damaged by the arthroscope and can be the source of considerable discomfort after ACL reconstruction. Taping techniques (Chapter 36) can be used to unload the fat pad.

Another complication seen after patellar tendon ACL reconstruction is inferior displacement of the patella (patella baja) due to traction on the patella by tight infrapatellar soft tissue structures. Patellar tendinopathy (Chapter 36) is also seen following ACL reconstruction, especially with patellar tendon grafts.

A common and as yet unexplained finding in cases of chronic ACL insufficiency and following reconstruction is trochlea chondral damage. Factors related to the development and persistence of chondral damage in the tibiofemoral and patellofemoral compartments are currently being studied.[95,96]

Lower limb stiffness
Stiffness in the foot and ankle commonly occurs as a result of a period of non weight-bearing and the wearing of a brace. Tightness of the Achilles tendon is common. These problems may not be recognised until the patient returns to running. Full ROM of these joints should be maintained early in the rehabilitation program with mobilisation and stretching in addition to active plantarflexion/dorsiflexion exercises.

Soft tissue stiffness (arthrofibrosis following surgery)
The rehabilitation program and its rate of progression will be influenced by the intrinsic tissue stiffness or laxity of the patient. This depends on the nature of the patient's collagen and appears to correlate with generalised ligamentous stiffness or laxity throughout the body. Patients with stiff soft tissues may develop a large bulky scar with adhesions after ACLR. These patients are usually slow to regain full flexion and extension and the knee may require passive mobilisation by the therapist. Patients tend to have tight lateral structures around a stiff patellofemoral joint. This is known as arthrofibrosis or stiff knee syndrome.[97]

Treatment involves encouraging active movement, early passive mobilisation, soft tissue therapy and encouraging early activity. Efforts to control swelling are critical. It may be helpful to remove the brace earlier than usual in these patients. Severe cases may require arthroscopic scar resection as well as a vigorous rehabilitation program.

As mentioned previously, delaying the surgery until all signs of the haemarthrosis have resolved and full ROM has been regained in particular full extension, reduces the incidence of arthrofibrosis in ACL reconstructions.

Soft tissue laxity
The group of patients classified as having 'loose' soft tissue are characterised by generalised increased ligamentous laxity. These patients tend to rapidly gain good ROM in extension and flexion. They are treated by prolonging the time in the brace to prevent hyperextension and restricting the range available. ROM exercises are discouraged, mobilisation contraindicated and full extension work reduced to avoid stretching the graft. The rehabilitation program is slowed in these patients to allow time for the graft to develop as much scar tissue as possible.

Muscle weakness
Muscle weakness occurs following ACL reconstruction despite significant regeneration of the tendon used for the graft (hamstring or patellar).[98,99] A systematic review found that the majority of studies could demonstrate specific muscular imbalances in the ACL-reconstructed leg with control or the contralateral leg with the knee flexors and extensors involved.[100] In addition, some recent studies have also shown deficits of the hip muscles after ACLR.

Muscular deficits are pronounced within the first 6 months after surgery, but they can persist up to 2 years and longer. The muscular deficits after ACLR are graft related. Extensor deficits are associated with patellar tendon grafts; flexion deficits are associated with hamstring grafts. There is limited evidence with inconsistent study results that there is a difference in postoperative flexor strength between patients with semitendinosus tendon autograft and semitendinosus/gracilis tendon autograft.

The authors of the systematic review recommended that isokinetic examination of flexor and extensor strength should be used as one criterion to decide if an athlete can be allowed to return to unrestricted sporting activities and that the rehabilitation protocol after ACLR should focus on the used graft and aim on negotiation of graft-related muscle weakness. Training to improve hip muscle strength may help to prevent a dynamic valgus during landing positions.[100]

Proprioception

Postural control is impaired following ACLR. A systematic review included 10 studies evaluating 644 participants at a mean 29 months follow-up.[101] In static balance tasks, there was a trend towards improved postural control in the control group for eyes-open but not eyes-closed conditions. Only four studies evaluated dynamic balance and the results from these were somewhat mixed. They concluded that there appeared to be a trend towards impaired static and dynamic postural control in patients following ACLR surgery, although the limited number of studies and differing methodologies made conclusions tentative.

Patients with ACL injury have poorer proprioception than people without such injuries when measured using joint position sense and threshold to detect passive motion techniques respectively. Patients had poorer proprioception in the injured than uninjured leg and the proprioception of people whose ACL was repaired was better than those whose ligament was left unrepaired.[102]

A review of 22 studies covering a total of 479 patients with a mean age of 27.3 showed that patients after ACLR have altered gait patterns that can persist for up to 5 years after surgery.[103]

Psychological problems

Psychological responses are important factors in RTP after ACLR.[104] In one study, 56 out of 187 athletes (31%) had returned to their pre-injury level of sports participation at 12 months. Significant independent contributions to returning to the pre-injury level by 12 months after surgery were made by psychological readiness to return to sport, fear of re-injury, sport locus of control and the athlete's estimate of the number of months it would take to return to sport, as measured preoperatively and at 4 months postoperatively.

Another study looked at fear of injury and found that athletes participating in sport 2–7 years following their ACL reconstruction generally appear to do so without fear of re-injury.[105] However, they commented that gender, the timing of surgery following injury and the level of sport the athletes returned to may be associated with fear of re-injury following surgery.

Patient psychological factors are predictive of ACLR outcomes.[106] Self-confidence, optimism and self-motivation are predictive of outcomes, which is consistent with the theory of self-efficacy. Stress, social support and athletic self-identity are predictive of outcomes, which is consistent with the global relationship between stress, health and the buffering hypothesis of social support.

In a review of psychosocial factors influencing the recovery of athletes with ACL injury a high internal health locus of control and a high self-efficacy were useful cognitive factors to facilitate the recovery.[107] Athletes with a low level of fear of re-injury had the best knee outcome after the injury followed by a reconstruction. In addition, athletes who returned to sport had less fear of re-injury, and were more experienced and established athletes compared with athletes who did not return to sport. Furthermore, researchers showed that there was a positive relation between goal setting and adherence, which in turn yielded a positive relation with the outcome of the rehabilitation of an ACL injury. There were several psychosocial interventions that appeared to be facilitating the rehabilitation process.

Outcomes after ACL treatment

While the general consensus among the surgical and sporting communities is that those sustaining an ACL injury can and often do make a full recovery after ACLR surgery, research findings suggest otherwise. Four main outcome measures are used to determine the success or failure of ACL treatment:

1. the patient's own perspective of (self-reported) knee function
2. return to pre-injury sporting activities
3. re-injury rate
4. prevalence of osteoarthritis.

Self-reported knee function

The recommended assessment of outcome after ACL injury has changed over the last 15 years. Traditionally, outcome was obtained by an observer, often using a scoring scale such as the Lysholm Knee Scoring Scale,[22] the Cincinnati Knee Ligament Rating Scale[108] or the International Knee Documentation Committee (IKDC).[109] It is well known that treating surgeons underestimate symptoms and overestimate function when compared to the patient's own opinion. This was also confirmed after ACL reconstruction in a study from 2001.[110] Thus, the patients' own perspective of knee function has been in focus over the last two decades and the use of validated self-administered questionnaires has been promoted. Patient-reported outcomes are generally good at a minimum of 10 years following ACL reconstruction.[111]

After ACLR, data from large samples could be obtained from registries, mainly from Sweden, Norway and Denmark. Here, a large improvement could be seen over the first 2 years after surgery, suggesting that the self-reported knee function is greatly improved by treatment. However, a report from the Swedish ACL registry with data from more than 2000 individuals reported that self-reported knee-related quality of life, knee pain and knee symptoms were much worse after ACL reconstruction[112] as compared to an age-matched community-based sample.[113]

Little is known about self-reported knee function after non-surgical treatment. In an RCT comparing surgical and non-surgical treatment strategies, no differences were found between the two treatment arms after 2 and 5 years.[67, 68] The results were comparable to those previously reported after ACLR.

Eleven studies reported quality of life (QoL) in 473 ACL-deficient individuals, at a mean of 10 (range 5–23) years following ACL rupture.[114] Eight studies reported knee-related QoL using the Knee injury and Osteoarthritis Outcome Score QoL subscale (KOOS-QoL); scores were impaired compared to population norms. Health-related QoL, measured with the SF-36 domain scores in five studies, was similar to population norms, but impaired compared to physically active populations. Meta-analysis revealed no significant differences in KOOS-QoL and SF-36 scores between ACL-deficient and ACL-reconstructed groups.

In summary, both surgical and non-surgical treatment has been shown to improve self-reported knee function after ACL injury. There exists no scientific evidence to support superiority of one treatment over the other. Two years after injury, ACL-injured patients report a worse outcome than an age-matched community-based sample, which indicates that none of the current treatment options are successful in restoring knee function from the patients' own point of view.

Return to sport

One of the major aims of treatment of ACL injury is to restore the knee and to return the athlete to pre-injury activity levels. This is also the main argument for surgical treatment. Reports of return to sports following ACL injury do not use a consistent definition and thus results should be interpreted with some caution. One frequent source of misinterpretation is that the definition of return to pre-injury activity is vague and includes one, and sometimes two, levels below the actual pre-injury activity level on a 10-graded scale.

Following ACLR, there is a large variation in reports of return to sport, with rates from 65–88% being able to return to sport within the first year.[115-118] In a meta-analyses of 392 patients, 72% (n = 281) had returned to their pre-injury activity level 2 years after ACLR.[119]

A report on elite soccer players showed a return to sports rate of 94% after ACLR.[120] The authors speculate that one of the main contributing facts might be the extraordinary care and rehabilitation provided by the team physiotherapist in these professional soccer clubs. In contrast, another publication showed that only 63% of NFL athletes returned to NFL game play at an average of 10.8 months after ACL surgery.[121] A success rate around 70% is not excellent for a surgical treatment option but it should be noted that some of these athletes do not return to sports for reasons other than knee problems. However, the proportion of such individuals is not well described.

A systematic review examined 69 articles, reporting on 7556 participants.[122] On average, 81% of people returned to any sport, 65% returned to their pre-injury level of sport and 55% returned to competitive-level sport after surgery. Symmetrical hopping performance and the contextual factors of younger-age males playing elite sport and having a positive psychological response favoured returning to the pre-injury level sport. Another systematic review found weak evidence in 16 articles suggesting that variables associated with return to sport included higher quadriceps strength, less effusion, less pain, greater tibial rotation, higher Marx Activity score, higher athletic confidence, higher preoperative knee self-efficacy, lower kinesiophobia and higher preoperative self-motivation.[123]

In a recent review, Nagelli and Hewett advocate waiting 2 years before RTP after ACL reconstruction.[124] They presented evidence showing that at 2 years after ACLR, biological healing (absence of bone bruises, ACL graft maturation and sensory restoration) has occurred and functional recovery (biomechanical and neuromuscular control and quadriceps strength) of the knee has normalised or is not significantly different from baseline.[124] Therefore, delaying a return to high-level activity for high-risk athletes until 2 years after ACLR will restore knee joint homeostasis and significantly reduce the risk of subsequent injury. They do, however, acknowledge the potential deleterious impact on an athlete's career if he or she misses 2 years of their sport.

Among patients treated non-operatively, the return to sports rates vary even more than among those treated surgically. Scientific reports suggest a range from 19% to 82% for return to pre-injury activity.[67, 125-127] While there is no firm evidence to support that return to pre-injury sports is more likely after ACL reconstruction than after non-surgical treatment, individuals active on a professional or subprofessional level often lack the possibility to wait and see and thus undergo surgery in most cases. Athletes who successfully return to sport after non-operative treatment could represent a group gaining functionally stable knees without fully restored stability at rest. Factors associated with success after non-surgical treatment need to be better explored.

There is some evidence that those returning to pre-injury sports after ACL injury may stop playing earlier than their non-injured counterparts.[127-129] In the only study in which the reduction in sport participation can be related to a control group, Roos et al.[126] found that only 30% of those who had ACL injury were active after 3 years compared with 80% of controls and that after 7 years none of the elite injured players were active regardless of the type of treatment. In addition, previously injured athletes retire at a higher rate than athletes without previous ACL injury.[130] The reason for this may be that many of the athletes who return to sport experience significant knee problems such as instability, reduced ROM and/or pain.[125]

Criteria for RTP after ACL reconstruction

As previously mentioned, strength deficits persist following ACLR.[100] Various authors have recommended the use of isokinetic testing as a possible objective marker for RTP. In a review of the various protocols used in isokinetic testing involving 39 studies, the variables that were most commonly used were concentric/concentric mode of contraction (31 studies), angular velocity of 60°/s (29 studies), three to five repetitions (24/39 studies), ROM of 0-90° (6 studies) and using gravity correction (9 studies).[131] Eight studies reported strength limb symmetry index scores as part of their RTP criteria. The authors concluded that there was no standardised isokinetic protocol following ACLR and that isokinetic strength measures have not been validated as useful predictors of successful RTP.[131]

In the only prospective study that addressed neuromuscular control and coordination, poor neuromuscular control was a risk factor for ACL graft rupture.[132] In this study of 56 athletes, transverse plane net moment impulse at the hip, dynamic frontal plane knee ROM, side-to-side differences in sagittal plane, knee moment at initial contact and deficits in postural stability were associated with a three times greater risk of ACL graft rupture.[132]

A review of guidelines used for RTP identified three objective criteria used to allow release to sports activities.[133] The most common was lower extremity muscle strength, followed by lower limb symmetry, and knee examination parameters of range of knee motion and effusion. Twelve studies listed one criterion for release to sports, eight studies listed two criteria and one study recommended three criteria.

A recent study followed 158 male professional athletes who underwent an ACLR and returned to their previous professional level of sport.[134] Before players returned to sport they underwent a battery of discharge tests (isokinetic strength testing at 60°, 180° and 300°/s, a running T-test,[135] single-hop, triple-hop and triple crossover-hop tests). The criteria for each test was as follows:

- isokinetic test at 60, 180 and 300°/s: quadriceps deficit <10% at 60°/s
- single-hop: limb symmetry index >90%
- triple-hop: limb symmetry index >90%
- triple crossover-hop: limb symmetry index >90%
- on-field sports-specific rehabilitation: fully completed
- running T-test <11 s.[135]

The athletes returned to their previous competitive level a mean of 229 days after surgery (range 116-513 days). Of these, 26 (16.5%) sustained an ACL graft rupture and 11 (7.0% of 158) sustained a contralateral rupture of their native ACL. Athletes who did not meet the specific discharge criteria before return to sport and were not fully discharged from ACLR rehabilitation by the surgeon had a four times greater risk of sustaining an ACL graft rupture (73%) compared with those who returned to their sport after passing the necessary criteria (27%). The study also looked at hamstring to quadriceps ratio and found that those who had a lower ratio at 60°/s had a greater risk of ACL graft rupture (HR 10.6 per 10% difference, 95% confidence interval of 10.2 to 11, $p = 0.005$). The authors concluded that two factors were associated with increased risk of ACL graft rupture: 1. not meeting all six of the discharge criteria before returning to team training; and 2. decreased hamstring to quadriceps ratio of the involved leg at 60°/s.[134]

Re-injury rate

The rate of graft re-rupture after 10 years is approximately 6%. It appears that the risk of re-rupture or a graft failure is highest within the first 12 months after an ACL injury.[136] After the first 12 months, the overall increase in risk is divided fairly evenly between the reconstructed knee and the contralateral knee.[137]

The aetiology of ACL graft failure is varied and often more than one cause exists. In general, the aetiology of ACL graft failure can be dividing into five categories: 1. surgical technique; 2. trauma; 3. poor graft incorporation and healing (failure of ACL graft to undergo the ligamentisation process); 4. arthrofibrosis; 5. inadequate rehabilitation. The most common reasons for failure due to surgical technique are non-anatomic tunnel placement, failure to address associated ligamentous laxity or secondary restraints at the time of the primary reconstruction, graft impingement, inadequate strength of the primary ACL graft and abnormal graft tension (under or overtensioning).

Early failures (<3 months) are usually related to loss of fixation and infection. Midterm failures (3-12 months) are most frequently due to errors in surgical technique, aggressive physical therapy, premature return to full activity or unrecognised loss of secondary restraints. Late failures (>12 months) are usually related to trauma.

The risk of a contralateral ACL injury is similar to that of a rupture of the graft (i.e. about 6%).[137, 138] When reviewing the literature, it appears to be clear that the risk of contralateral ACL injuries is greater than the risk of first-time ACL injuries.[137] The most prominent risk factor for a contralateral ACL injury is the return to a high level of activity. There are some indications that young age at the initial ACL injury and at the subsequent ACLR,[139] ACLR with patellar tendon autograft (compared to hamstring tendon autograft) and a narrow intercondylar notch can increase the risk for a contralateral ACL injury. Female gender does not seem to be a risk factor for a contralateral ACL injury. Altered biomechanics and altered neuromuscular function as a result of the initial ACL injury, affecting both the injured and the uninjured leg, most likely, further increase the risk for a contralateral ACL injury.

Data from non-surgically treated individuals are lacking. One prospective investigation of consecutively recruited ACL injured patients, initially treated conservatively without ACLR with later surgical intervention only when deemed necessary, where the patients were advised to avoid contact sports, found an annual incidence of contralateral ACL injuries of 0.4% over 15 years.[127]

Revision surgery

If failure of the original ACL graft occurs, a revision procedure can be performed. Outcomes of revision surgery are predictably not as good as in primary reconstruction. In a meta-analysis including studies with 300 revision ACLRs and 413 primary ACLRs, patients who had had revision surgery reported inferior Lysholm Knee Scoring Scale scores, had inferior clinician-reported knee function as assessed with the objective IKDC classification and pivot shift test and more radiographic evidence of tibiofemoral osteoarthritis (50% versus 25%) compared with patients who had had primary surgery.[140]

A previous review included 31 articles which documented rate of return to sport and showed that whereas 73% had good objective and satisfactory subjective results, 57% of patients did not return to the same level of sport activity, significantly inferior to that of a primary procedure.[141]

Osteoarthritis

A frequent consequence of ACL rupture is the increased risk of knee osteoarthritis (OA).[142] Following ACL injury, rates of radiographic knee OA are typically reported to be approximately 50% at 10–20 years post-injury.[142, 143] As ACL injury frequently occurs in adolescents and young adults, these individuals typically develop OA before they reach 40 years, which would not be expected in the absence of joint trauma. An ACL injury is therefore said to be responsible for *early-onset* knee OA.

Current evidence does not indicate that ACLR reduces the rate of OA development.[144, 145] Indeed, higher rates of OA may be evident following surgical compared to non-surgical management of the ACL-deficient knee, which may be related to the return to high-impact cutting and pivoting sports activity, which non-operative treatment algorithms often advise against.[146, 147]

An ACL rupture causes a significant disruption to the homeostasis of the knee. The considerable force required to rupture a healthy ACL is consistent with the frequent presence of subchondral BMLs,[148] articular cartilage damage[149] and meniscal tears.[148, 150] The considerable mechanical impact to the articular cartilage and subchondral bone can disrupt the cartilage matrix and alter cell metabolism,[151, 152] which can predispose to OA development even in the absence of altered mechanical loading.[151] However, the altered mechanical environment following an ACL injury is thought to be a fundamental driver for post-traumatic OA development.[153, 154]

The instability and altered kinematics following ACL injury are theorised to shift load bearing to areas of cartilage unaccustomed to such load, potentially contributing to the early onset of OA.[153] Perhaps altered kinematics in the setting of already damaged cartilage is most deleterious following ACL injury, as cartilage response to load is dependent on the health of the cartilage.[153] Abnormal knee kinematics persist despite ACLR, which might explain why rates of OA are not reduced with surgical stabilisation.[155] Dynamic knee joint loading and OA development may also be affected by prolonged muscle weakness, in particular quadriceps weakness, which can persist for years after ACL injury.[156]

Inherent biomechanical characteristics preceding ACL injury may also be implicated in the development of post-traumatic OA. Specifically, high external knee abduction loads during a jump-landing task can predict ACL injury in young female athletes,[157] while increased external knee abduction moments during gait have been associated with lateral tibiofemoral OA following ACLR.[158]

The unique biomechanical characteristics following ACL injury, including high knee abduction loads, may contribute to the distinct patterns of post-traumatic disease typically observed.[159] Pre-injury kinematic and kinetic patterns are likely to persist following ACL injury, irrespective of surgical reconstruction, although targeted neuromuscular training may help to decrease knee abduction loads.[160]

Importantly, post-traumatic knee OA displays distinct patterns of disease compared to a typical non-traumatic OA presentation. Post-traumatic OA affects the medial and lateral tibiofemoral compartment equally, likely reflecting the local factors unique to ACL injury and reconstruction.[158, 159]

Patellofemoral OA is also particularly prevalent at all time points following ACLR regardless of autograft type[161, 162] and early signs of patellofemoral deterioration are evidence as early as 1 year post-surgery.[163] Altered biomechanics, including tibial rotations and knee flexion, may play a role in patellofemoral OA following ACLR[164, 165] and lower limb function or the presence of patellofemoral cartilage lesions can predict the presence of poorer prognosis following ACLR.[166] Post-traumatic OA should therefore be considered a distinct entity and clinicians should pay particular attention to the status of the patellofemoral joint following ACLR.

The increased risk of OA development following ACL injury and reconstruction appears to be driven by factors such as concomitant trauma to other knee structures, altered kinematics and loading environment, and muscle weakness. However, systemic factors that increase the risk of incident non-traumatic OA, such as older age, female sex and higher body mass index (BMI), also appear to accentuate the development of post-traumatic OA. The interaction of local and systemic risk factors likely creates an imbalance of biochemical markers, leading to cartilage degradation and ultimately OA. This is summarised in Figure 35.14.

Sex difference

In light of the increased prevalence of ACL injuries in female athletes discussed previously, attention has been paid to possible differences in outcome after ACLR between males and females. The majority of studies show increased post-surgical laxity in females, but no difference in graft failure, activity level, or subjective or functional assessment.[115, 167-171]

The most recent review included 13 studies.[172] Meta-analysis revealed no difference in graft failure risk (eight studies), contralateral ACL rupture risk (three studies) or postoperative knee laxity on physical examination (six studies). There was no evidence of a clinically important difference in patient-reported outcomes according to sex.

However, one study of several thousand patients treated with ACLR from the Swedish ACL registry showed

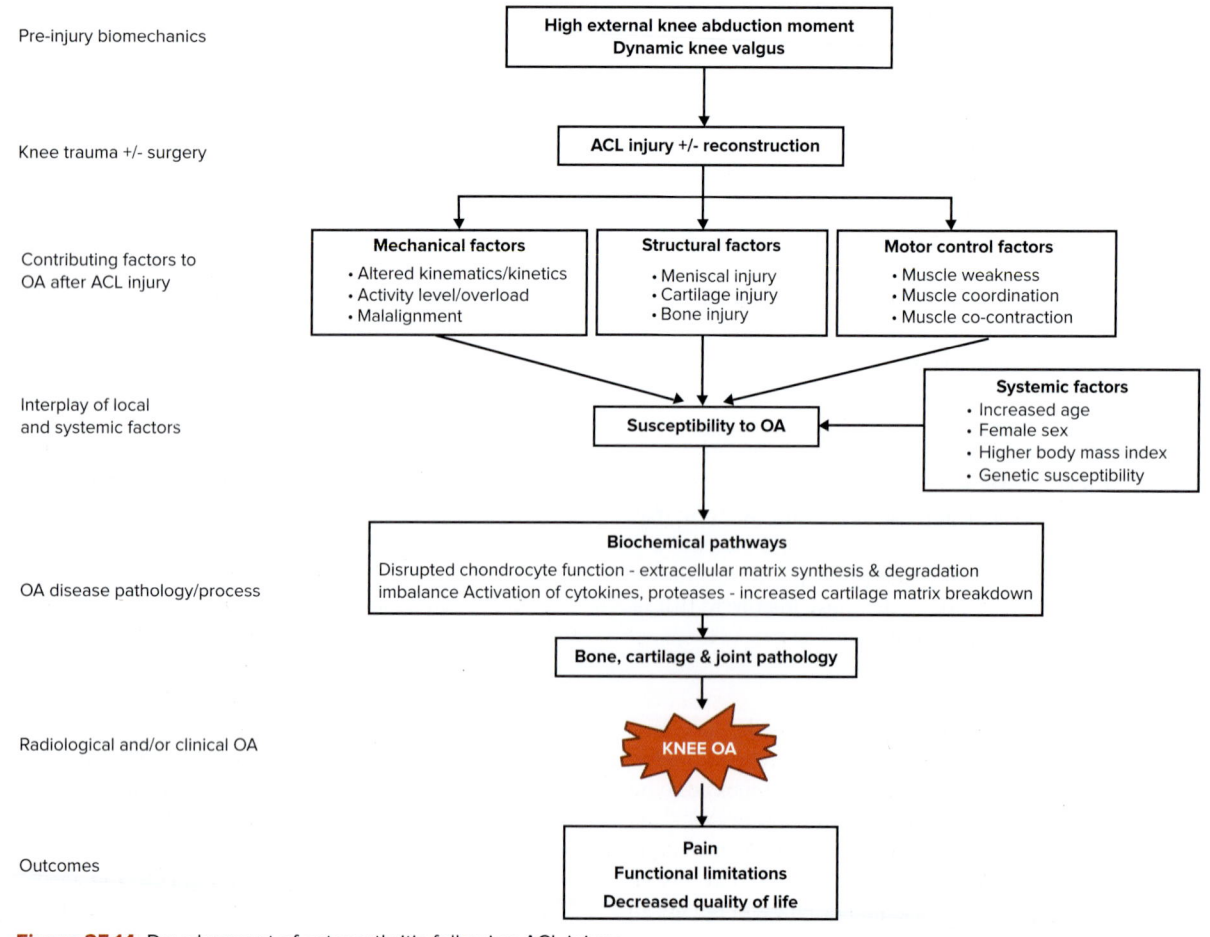

Figure 35.14 Development of osteoarthritis following ACL injury
COURTESY DR ADAM CULVENOR

Acute knee injuries — CHAPTER 35

significant gender differences in the self-reported outcome 1 and 2 years after surgery.[112] The authors reported that female patients showed worse outcomes than male patients before surgery and at 1 and 2 years after ACLR, and suggested that possible sex differences should be analysed in future studies on evaluation after ACL injury/reconstruction.

Age

Younger athletes have been shown to have a higher chance of graft rupture than older athletes.[173] A 10-year difference in age was associated with a 2.6 times greater chance of ACL graft rupture. Among 1820 patients after primary ACLR, younger athletes had a higher activity level and a higher incidence of ACL re-injury.[174] Based on data from the Swedish National Knee Ligament Register, the combination of being young and playing soccer is a substantial risk factor for revision surgery.[175]

Results after ACL reconstruction in patients older than 40 years and comparison with younger populations were recently the subject of a systematic review.[176] Twelve studies with a total of 452 patients were included. The mean patient age was 47.8 years (range, 40–66 years) with a mean follow-up of 53.3 months (minimum, 24 months). Lysholm scores improved from 53.9 to 90.5 in the 11 operative studies. IKDC scores of A or B were found in 81%. Tegner activity scores averaged 4.7 pre-injury, fell to 2.9 preoperatively and returned to 4.7 postoperatively. The reported failure rate was 2.3%. There were few complications and failure rate was similar in younger patients. The data confirm that ACLR can be recommended to patients older than 40 years who wish to maintain an active lifestyle or have symptomatic instability with daily activities.

Partial ACL tear

Approximately 5–15% of ACL injuries are thought to be partial tears.[177] There is no consensus on the definition of a partial ACL tear. The presence of an intra-substance incomplete tear of the ACL on MRI (Fig. 35.15) or at arthroscopy is generally regarded as being the gold standard diagnosis. Rather than an anatomical diagnosis, a functional assessment of stability is more practical from a treatment viewpoint.

If clinical instability is present and the pivot shift is positive, then ACL instability is diagnosed. Most would consider a 'partial' tear to be associated with a negative pivot shift test. Controversy centres around whether a complete tear of one of the two bundles (anteromedial and posterolateral) should be considered under the definition of a partial tear and whether some asymmetrical laxity on Lachman's test albeit with a definite end point should be included.[178] The partial tear is often described on MRI reports as a percentage of ACL remaining.

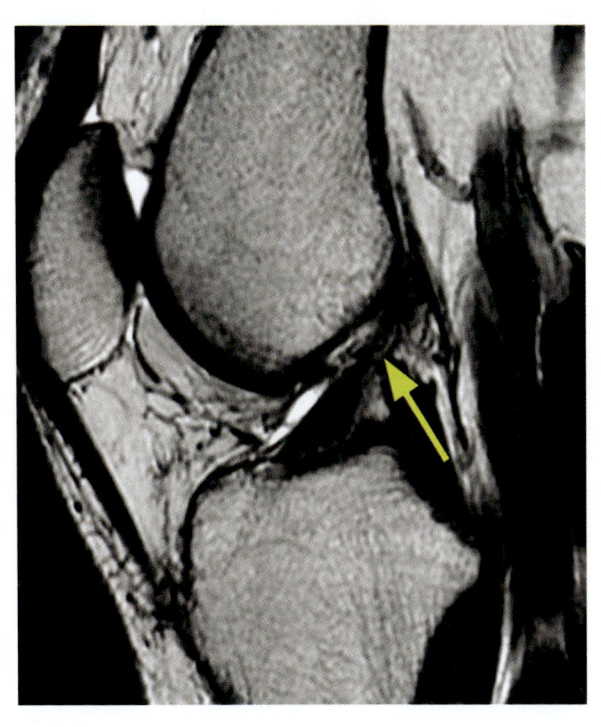

Figure 35.15 Sagittal T2 image showing partial ACL rupture characterised by increased T2 signal (yellow arrow) and some fibre disruption within its proximal aspect. The normal angle and some continuous fibres distinguish this partial tear from a full-thickness rupture

The management of partial ACL tears depends on the degree of instability. A clinically and functionally stable partial tear can be treated non-surgically with the option of later surgery if needed. Unstable lesions especially in those who wish to play high-intensity sports can be treated surgically either with a full knee reconstruction or augmentation of the remaining ligament. Degenerative changes were present in 15% of patients 8 years after partial ACL tear managed conservatively.[179]

Prevention of ACL injuries

Prevention of ACL injuries is thoroughly discussed in Chapter 12. Risk factors and prevention programs including the FIFA-11 are described in detail.

ACL rupture in children with open physes

Rupture of the ACL in children with open physes presents an additional challenge to the treating practitioner. This topic is covered extensively in Chapter 44.

POSTERIOR CRUCIATE LIGAMENT INJURIES

The PCL is composed of two bundles, the larger anterolateral (AL) bundle and the smaller posteromedial (PM) bundle, which are most readily identified at their femoral locations.

However, at their tibial attachment to the PCL facet, the bundles are more compact and difficult to separate. Historically, the two bundles of the PCL were believed to function independently, with the ALB primarily functioning in flexion and the PMB in extension. However, in light of recent biomechanical investigations, a more synergistic and co-dominant relationship between the two bundles has been validated. Ahmad et al. investigated the spatial orientation of the PCL bundles and reported that changes in the orientation of each bundle during knee flexion and extension prevented either bundle from exercising complete dominance in the restraint of posterior tibial motion.[180]

The PCL has historically been considered a primary restraint to posterior tibial translation and more recent studies have also identified it as a secondary restraint to rotation, particularly between 90° and 120° of flexion.[181] Complete sectioning of the PCL has reportedly led to a significant increase in posterior tibial translation at 0° to 120° of flexion and an increase in internal rotation at 90° to 120° of flexion. The magnitude of abnormal translation and rotation appears to depend on whether one or both of the bundles are injured. An isolated tear of either PCL bundle results in a minimal clinically important increase in posterior tibial translation. Generally, the literature supports that the PCL has a more expansive role in providing rotational stability than previously thought, and it is important to assess internal and external rotation stability when considering PCL injury.[181]

PCL injury typically presents concurrently with other knee injuries, including ACL, MCL or posterolateral corner (PLC) injury or, less commonly, in isolation. Recent studies have helped to clarify and elucidate the prevalence of concurrent ligament injuries with a complete (grade III) PCL tear.[181] A majority of grade III PCL tears are associated with multi-ligament knee injuries, with one study reporting that 79% of multi-ligament knee injuries involved the PCL in a trauma setting.[182] Furthermore, 46%, 31% and 62% of PCL injuries have been reported to be concomitant with ACL, MCL and PLC knee injury in a trauma setting, respectively.[183]

PCL injuries are often associated with meniscal and chondral injury. The incidence of associated meniscal tears varies from 16% to 28%. Longitudinal tears of the anterior horn of the lateral meniscus are the most common location. There is also a high incidence of radial tears in the middle or posterior lateral meniscus.[184] The incidence of significant chondral damage with isolated PCL injury was not thought to be as high as with ACL injury, but one study showed chondral damage in 52% of those with PCL tears, with lesions of grade III or more found in 16%.[184]

Clinical features

The mechanism of PCL injury is usually a direct blow to the anterior tibia with the knee in a flexed position (i.e. dash-board injury). This can be from contact with an opponent, equipment or falling onto the hyperflexed knee. Hyperextension may also result in an injury to the PCL and posterior capsule.

> **PRACTICE PEARL**
>
> Whereas a patient with an ACL or MCL injury often describes the feel of a distinct 'pop' or 'tear', PCL tears typically have vague symptoms such as unsteadiness or discomfort.

A patient with an acute isolated PCL injury may have a mild-to-moderate effusion, pain in the posterior aspect of the knee or pain with kneeling. In a case of subacute or chronic PCL injury, the patient may describe vague anterior knee pain, pain with deceleration and descending inclines or stairs, or pain with running at full stride.

On examination, there is usually minimal swelling as the PCL is an extrasynovial structure. The posterior drawer test (Fig. 35.2o) is the most sensitive test for PCL deficiency. This is performed in neutral, internal and external rotation. A posterior sag of the tibia (Fig.35.2n), and pain and laxity on a reverse Lachman's test, may be present. PCL rupture is particularly disabling for downhill skiers, who rely on this ligament for stability in the tucked up position adopted in racing.

PCL tears are graded I, II and III on the position of the medial tibial plateau relative to the medial femoral condyle at 90° of knee flexion (the posterior drawer position). The tibia normally lies approximately 1 cm anterior to the femoral condyles in the resting position. In grade I injuries, the tibia continues to lie anteriorly to the femoral condyles but is slightly diminished (0-5 mm laxity). In grade II injuries, the tibia is flush with the condyles (5-10 mm laxity). When the tibia no longer has a medial step and can be pushed beyond the medial femoral condyle (>10 mm laxity), it is classified as a grade III injury.

It is important to distinguish between isolated PCL injury and a combined PCL and posterolateral corner injury. In isolated PCL tears, there is a decrease in tibial translation in internal rotation due primarily to the influence of the MCL.[185]

Plain radiographs are advocated when one is examining the presence of avulsion fracture fragments, Segond fractures, fibular head avulsions and lateral joint space widening. Any perceptible degree of posterior tibial sag should be documented. Stress radiographs provide reproducible objective assessment of the degree of posterior tibial translation between the injured and normal contralateral knee.[186] It has been reported that partial PCL tears result in <8 mm of increased posterior tibial translation, isolated complete PCL tears in 8-12 mm and combined complete PCL tears (usually with a PLC injury) in >12 mm.[187]

MRI has a high predictive accuracy in the diagnosis of the acute PCL injury,[188, 189] but a lesser accuracy in chronic injuries.[190] The normal appearance of a PCL is a well-defined continuous band of low signal intensity in all pulse sequences with a maximum anteroposterior diameter of 6 mm when measured on sagittal T2-weighted images. Conversely, a torn PCL (Fig 35.15) has been reported to have an abnormally large (>7 mm) anteroposterior diameter.[191]

Bone bruises are seen in over 80 % of acute grade II and III PCL injuries on MRI. In contrast to the bone bruises associated with ACL tears, which commonly occur on the posterior tibia and lateral femoral condyle, the location of bone bruises observed with PCL injuries is less predictable. Bone bruises in the medial compartment were significantly more often associated with a PCL-PLC combined injury, while lateral compartment bone bruises were significantly more often associated with a concomitant PCL-MCL injury.[192]

Treatment

Grade I, II and most grade III PCL injuries can generally be managed non-surgically with a comprehensive rehabilitation program. A suggested program emphasising intensive quadriceps exercises is shown in Table 35.11. More severe injuries (grade III) should be immobilised in extension for the first 2 weeks.

The PCL has been reported to have an intrinsic healing ability after injury, although this healing may occur in a lax or attenuated position. Therefore, in cases of acute isolated PCL injury, non-operative management has been recommended. However, acute multi-ligament knee injuries with a concomitant or chronic PCL tear are believed to be best treated by surgery.[180] The use of a brace (e.g. the Jack or Rebound PCL brace) that applies a constant or dynamic anterior force to counteract the posterior sag of the tibia, may help to increase healing after PCL injury by reducing the ligament to a more physiological position.[193]

Patients with isolated PCL tears have a good functional result despite ongoing laxity after an appropriate rehabilitation program. Regardless of the amount of laxity, half of the patients in one large study returned to sport at the same or higher level, one-third at a lower level and one-sixth did not return to the same sport.[194] Other studies have shown that knee instability did not correlate with return to sport or knee satisfaction.[195-197]

Although favourable non-operative results have been observed, the long-term consequences of isolated PCL deficiency remain unknown.[198] Boynton and Tietjens have observed deterioration at extended follow-up of non-operative treatment despite good early results.[199] In 38 patients with isolated tears with a mean follow-up of 13.4 years, eight patients had subsequent meniscal injuries and surgery. Of the remaining 30 patients with normal menisci, over 80% had occasional pain and over 50% had occasional swelling. With time, an increase in articular cartilage degeneration was seen on plain radiographs. Investigators who evaluated isolated PCL tears that were treated with non-operative rehabilitation programs reported radiographic evidence of arthritic changes in 23% of patients at 7-year follow-up[200] and 41% at 14-year follow-up.[201] However, only a small percentage of the patients in the long-term follow-up had moderate or severe osteoarthritis (11%), and the majority of patients had good strength and subjective outcome scores, although stress radiographs were not reported.[180]

Indications for surgical repair

Operative management is reserved for acute or chronic isolated grade III PCL injuries with symptoms of pain or instability which have failed an adequate rehabilitation program treatment, or PCL insufficiency in the setting of a multi-ligamentous knee injury.[198] Complete PCL tears, as indicated by PCL stress radiographs with an increased anteroposterior laxity measurement of >8 mm, combined with repairable meniscal body or root tears are a possible indication for PCL reconstruction.[180]

Similar to ACL reconstruction, grafts can be either autograft (hamstring tendon or bone–patellar tendon–bone) or allograft, single or double bundle. Single-bundle PCL reconstruction is typically indicated for symptomatic chronic PCL injuries, either in isolation or combined with other knee ligamentous injury, and for acute, multi-ligament PCL injuries. Recent efforts have focused on an anatomic single-bundle reconstruction using arthroscopic and radiographic reference points instead of the historical non-anatomic 'isometric' reconstruction that has been reported to result in initial joint overconstraint and increased laxity over time.

Controversy exists regarding the use of transtibial versus tibial inlay techniques of PCL reconstruction. In the transtibial

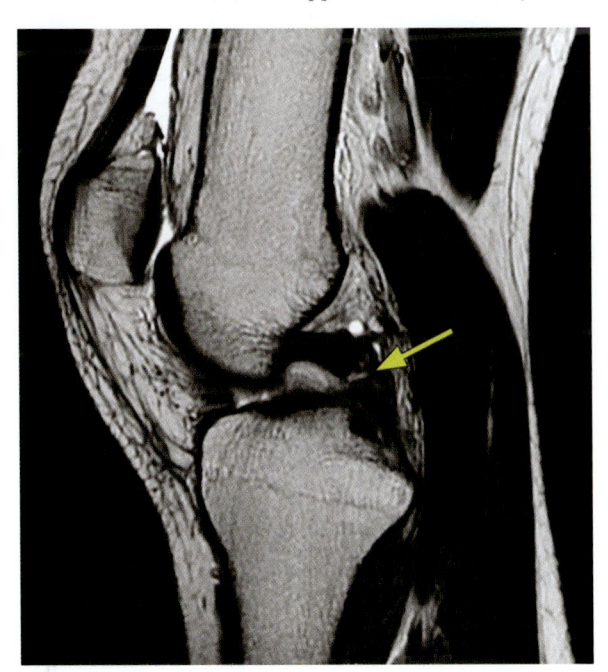

Figure 35.16 Sagittal T2 MRI showing a defect with associated oedema (arrow) in the midsubstance of the PCL

PART B Regional problems

Table 35.11 Rehabilitation of a PCL tear (see Figs 35.6 and 35.7)

Phase	Goal of phase	Time post-injury	Physiotherapy treatment	Exercise program	Functional/sport-related activity
Phase 1	PWB–FWB Eliminate swelling 0–100° ROM 4+/5 quadriceps strength 5/5 hamstring strength	0–2 weeks	Jack or Rebound PCL brace Cryotherapy Electrotherapy Compression Manual therapy Gait re-education Patient education	Gentle flexion ROM Extension ROM to 0° Quadriceps/VMO setting Supported (bilateral) calf raises Hip abduction and extension Hamstring pulleys/rubbers Gait drills	Nil
Phase 2	No swelling Full ROM 4+/5 quadriceps strength 5/5 hamstring strength	2–4 weeks	Cryotherapy Electrotherapy Compression Manual therapy Gait re-education Exercise modification	ROM drills Quadriceps/VMO setting Mini-squats and lunges Leg press (double, then single-leg) Step-ups Bridges (double, then single-leg) Hip abduction and extension with rubber tubing Single-leg calf raises Gait re-education drills Balance and proprioceptive drills (single-leg)	Walking Exercise bike
Phase 3	Full ROM Full strength and power Return to jogging, running and agility Return to restricted sport-specific drills	4–6 weeks	Manual therapy Exercise/activity modification and supervision	As above—increase difficulty, repetitions and weight where appropriate Jump and land drills Agility drills	Straight-line jogging Swimming (light kick) Road bike Straight-line running Progressing to sport-specific running and agility (progressively sequenced) (e.g. running forwards, sideways, backwards, sprinting, jumping, hopping, changing directions, kicking)
Phase 4	Return to sport	6–10 weeks	As above	High-level sport-specific strengthening as required	Progressive return to sport (e.g. restricted training, unrestricted training, match play, competitive match play)

FWB = full weight-bearing; PWB = partial weight-bearing; ROM = range of motion; VMO = vastus medialis obliquus

technique, the tibial and femoral tunnels are drilled and the graft must make an acute turn as it surfaces from the tibial tunnel and changes direction before entering the knee joint. Subsequent graft abrasion and attenuation may result in graft rupture or laxity.[202] This sharp turn has been implicated in the residual posterior knee laxity observed clinically after transtibial PCL reconstruction. The tibial inlay was developed as an alternative to the transtibial technique to avoid this problem. In tibial inlay reconstruction, the graft is fixed directly to the PCL's native insertion site on the tibia.[198]

Double-bundle PCL reconstructions have evolved as an alternative to single-bundle reconstructions with the same indications for surgery. As reported by biomechanical studies, the AL and PM bundles perform in a co-dominant manner and these roles theoretically would not be restored by a single-bundle PCL reconstruction.[203] Therefore, an anatomic double-bundle PCL reconstruction may be able to more closely restore native kinematics than the single-bundle technique.

Results of surgical reconstruction are generally good,[204, 205] but one review[206] suggested that the rate of graft failure was 11.6%. In the isolated PCL studies, 50–82% of patients were able to return to pre-injury activity level. The most commonly reported complications after PCL reconstructions are residual posterior laxity, usually defined as more than 4 mm of increased posterior translation on PCL stress radiographs, and flexion loss due to prolonged immobilisation of the knee in extension.

Since PCL graft healing times have been reported to be almost double the time of ACL graft healing, it has been suggested that PCL reconstruction patients should be kept non weight-bearing for 6 weeks. Patients are placed in an immobiliser brace in extension after surgery for 3 days before transitioning to a dynamic or static anterior drawer knee brace. The Jack Brace and the Rebound® PCL brace which apply increasing force as a function of flexion angle, are the only currently available dynamic braces and it has been recommended that the brace of choice should be worn at all times for up to a minimum of 24 weeks postoperatively.[207]

LATERAL COLLATERAL LIGAMENT TEARS

Lateral (or fibular) collateral ligament (LCL) tears are much less common than MCL tears. In contrast to the common pattern of isolated MCL injury, an injury to the lateral side of the knee usually requires higher magnitude of force and thereby affects additional structures in the area. Isolated injuries to the LCL involve forces of lower magnitude, resulting in lower-grade damage to the ligament. Isolated high-grade injuries to the LCL are therefore fairly rare.[208]

Posterolateral corner injuries

Posterolateral corner injuries are being increasingly recognised. In a consecutive series of 187 patients with an acute knee injury and a complete ligament tear found on MRI, the incidence of grade III PLC injuries was 16%.[209]

The posterolateral corner (PLC) of the knee was once referred to as 'the dark side of the knee' due to the limited understanding of the structures, biomechanics and possible treatment options.[210] A number of studies in recent years have led to a heightened understanding of the PLC and biomechanically validated reconstruction techniques. Posterolateral corner injuries are commonly associated with ACL or PCL tears. The LCL, popliteofibular ligament, arcuate ligament, oblique popliteal ligament, fabellofibular ligament, posterolateral capsule, popliteus tendon, biceps femoris tendon, lateral head of the gastrocnemius, lateral meniscus and the iliotibial band may all be involved in the injury pattern to some degree.

The three major static stabilisers of the PLC are the LCL, the popliteus tendon (PLT) and the popliteofibular ligament (PFL).[211] The PLC structures provide the primary restraint to varus forces of the knee as well as posterolateral rotation of the tibia relative to the femur in cases of cruciate deficient knees. These structures are also important secondary stabilisers to anterior and posterior tibial translation.

Mechanisms of injury usually cause force at multiple vectors of varying magnitude–with varus, extension, rotation and translation all playing a role. A common mechanism of injury to the PLC is a direct blow to the anteromedial knee. However, hyperextension and non-contact varus stress injuries can also damage the PLC. Most often, PLC tears are associated with ACL and/or PCL injuries, justifying close examination for a PLC injury for every cruciate ligament tear.[210]

Frequently reported symptoms include pain, perceived side-to-side instability near extension, increased difficulty walking on uneven ground or up and down stairs, bruising and swelling. This instability and difficulty walking can present as a varus thrust gait seen during the initiation of the stance phase.[212] It is not uncommon for the patient to complain of paraesthesia of the common peroneal nerve distribution or foot drop. Common peroneal nerve injury has been reported to occur in up to one-third of PLC injuries.[213]

The varus stress (Fig. 35.2g) test should be performed in both full extension and at 20–30° of flexion. Lateral compartment gapping in comparison to the contralateral side with the knee flexed to 30° indicates an injury to the LCL and potentially to the secondary stabilisers of the PLC. If stability is restored when tested in full extension, an isolated injury to the LCL is presumed. However, if the varus instability persists in full extension, a combined LCL, PLC and cruciate ligament injury is assumed.[210]

A routine radiographic work-up with standing anteroposterior (AP), lateral and axial views should be performed to rule out the presence of fractures. A standing long-leg AP view should be obtained in chronic cases because the limb alignment should be corrected using an osteotomy prior to or at the same time as a reconstruction procedure. Additionally, varus and PCL stress radiographs can be used to obtain objective quantification of the amount of lateral compartment varus gapping and a combined PLC and PCL injury, respectively.[214]

MRI allows identification of concurrent lesions such as meniscus tears, cartilage lesions and occult fractures. It has been shown to have 90% sensitivity and specificity for IT band, biceps tendon, LCL and PLT injury. The only PLC structure with lower diagnostic accuracy values was the popliteofibular ligament, with 68.8% sensitivity and 66.7% specificity.[209] For optimal MRI diagnostic accuracy for PLC injuries, an imaging sequence using 2 mm slices in a coronal oblique plane following the obliquity of the PLT should be employed. Bone bruise patterns are found in 81% of all PLC injuries, usually on the anteromedial femoral condyle. Together, these imaging techniques are excellent tools to augment the diagnosis of PLC injury.[214]

Non-surgical management

Good results have been reported for non-surgical treatment for grade I and II injuries with minimal radiographic changes at 8 year follow-up following the use of an early mobilisation protocol.[215] However, poor functional outcomes for non-operatively treated grade III PLC injuries with persistent instability and degenerative changes have been reported.[216] Increased forces on the PCL and ACL reconstruction grafts have been reported if concurrent PLC injuries are not addressed.[217]

Surgical management

Surgical treatment of PLC injuries is the treatment of choice for patients with isolated grade III PLC injuries, combined PLC injuries and failed non-operative treatment.[214] Acute surgical treatment (<3 weeks) results in improved outcomes and can avoid the need for an additional procedure for limb alignment correction that may be necessary in chronic cases. Patients treated acutely may undergo repair or reconstruction procedures. Primary repairs of LCL and PLTs avulsions, without midsubstance injury, may be performed within 2-3 weeks after the injury. After that point, the tissue becomes retracted and scars down, making it nearly impossible to reattach the injured structures to their native anatomic locations. Improved outcomes have been demonstrated with primary repair of avulsed ligament structures and augmentation of midsubstance ligament injuries.

Several reconstruction techniques have been described and can be broadly categorised as biceps tendon transfer, fibular-based sling or anatomic-based reconstruction of the LCL, PLT and popliteofibular ligament.[218] Outcomes following reconstruction have been shown to be significantly better than those following repair.[219, 220] A recent systematic review found the repair of acute grade III PLC injuries with staged cruciate reconstruction was associated with a 38% failure rate, whereas a more robust reconstruction-focused approach for PLC injuries with concurrent reconstruction of cruciate injuries resulted in an overall mean 9% failure rate.[218]

Surgical reconstruction of a chronic LCL tear is difficult. Surgical techniques include variations of fibular slings, capsular shifts and anatomic-based techniques (fibular tunnel and tibial tunnel). A recent systematic review included 15 studies with a total of 456 patients of which 59% had combined PCL injuries, 23% had combined ACL injuries, 6% had combined ACL and PCL injuries and 12% had isolated PLC injuries.[221] Cruciate ligament tears were treated simultaneously with PLC reconstruction in the majority of the 15 studies. Surgical management of these chronic PLC injuries had a 90% success rate and a 10% failure rate according to the authors' objective assessment of outcomes.[221]

In chronic injuries (greater than 6 weeks from injury), lower extremity alignment should be evaluated and corrected with an osteotomy prior to ligament reconstruction because failure to address malalignment can lead to increased stress and stretching of the reconstruction grafts and failure.[222] A varus knee with lateral and/or posterolateral instability is associated with worse results.

ARTICULAR CARTILAGE DAMAGE

Chondral defects are seen in 3.4-62% of knee arthroscopies, while full-thickness focal lesions with an area of at least 1-2 cm^2 are seen in 4.2-6.2% of all arthroscopies in patients younger than 40 years of age.[223] The incidence is higher in athletes.

Epidemiology

A systematic review included 11 studies containing 931 athletes of which 40% were professionals (US National Basketball Association and National Football League).[223] The overall prevalence of full-thickness focal chondral defects in athletes was 36%. Fourteen per cent of athletes were asymptomatic at the time of diagnosis. Patellofemoral defects (37%) were more common than femoral condyle (35%) and tibial plateau defects (25%). Medial condyle defects were more common than lateral (68% versus 32%) and patella defects were more common than trochlea (64% versus 36%). Meniscal tear (47%) was the most common concomitant knee pathological finding, followed by ACL tear (30%) and then medial collateral ligament or lateral collateral ligament tear (14%).

Articular cartilage damage may occur as an isolated condition in which chondral or subchondral damage is the primary pathology or in association with other injuries, such as ligamentous instability resulting from MCL, ACL or PCL injuries or patellar dislocations.

Table 35.12 Outerbridge classification of chondral defects

1. Softening
2. <1 cm (<0.4 in.) partial thickness lesion
3. >1 cm (>0.4 in.) defect, deeper
4. Subchondral bone exposed

Table 35.13 International Cartilage Repair Society (ICRS) classification of chondral defects

1. Superficial lesions
   A. Soft indentation
   B. Superficial fissures or cracks
2. Lesions <50% cartilage depth
3. A. Lesions >50% depth
   B. Down to calcified layer
   C. Down to but not through subchondral bone
   D. Blisters
4. Full thickness into subchondral bone

Articular cartilage damage may also be seen in association with meniscal injury and patellar dislocation.

Quantifying chondral injury

Chondral injury is graded according to the Outerbridge classification and more recently the International Cartilage Repair Society (ICRS) grading system (Tables 35.12 and 35.13). Articular cartilage damage varies from gross, macroscopically evident defects in which the underlying bone is exposed (grade IV), to microscopic damage that appears normal on arthroscopy but is soft when probed (grade I).

Articular cartilage damage in the knee has both short-term and long-term effects. In the short term, it causes recurrent pain and swelling. In the longer term, it accelerates the development of osteoarthritis. Various methods have been used to encourage healing of articular cartilage defects. These include microfracture (piercing the subchondral bone with an 'ice pick' to recruit pluripotential stem cells from the marrow), mosaic plasty such as Osteoarticular Transfer System Surgery or OATS (osteochondral plugs are taken from the trochlea margin and implanted within the injured area) and autologous chondrocyte implantation (ACI), where cultured chondrocytes (harvested from the patient and cultured in the laboratory) are re-implanted to the chondral defect. Gene therapy and bone morphogenetic proteins are currently in the experimental stage.

Management

There is currently considerable debate as to the efficacy of the various treatments and as yet no consensus on optimal treatment has been reached. Although short-term reduction of symptoms has been shown with these treatments, long-term reduction of arthritic disability has not been shown. Successful results also vary according to size and location of the articular lesion and between treatments. As yet, no method of treatment has been able to reproduce true hyaline cartilage with its complex layered structure.

A systematic review to determine which surgical technique/s have improved outcomes and enabled athletes to return to their pre-injury level of sports, and which patient and defect factors significantly affect outcomes after cartilage repair or restoration identified 11 studies for inclusion (658 subjects).[224] Only one RCT was identified. All other studies were prospective cohorts, case-control studies, or case series reporting results after microfracture, ACI or OATS. Better clinical outcomes were observed after ACI and OATS versus microfracture. Results after microfracture tended to deteriorate with time. The overall rate of return to pre-injury level of sports was 66%. The timing of return to the pre-injury level of sports was fastest after OATS and slowest after ACI. Defect size of less than 2 cm^2, preoperative duration of symptoms of less than 18 months, no prior surgical treatment, younger patient age and higher pre-injury and post-surgical level of sports all correlated with improved outcomes after cartilage repair, especially ACI. Results after microfracture were worse with larger defects. The rate of return to sports was generally lower after microfracture versus ACI or OATS and if a patient was able to return to sports, performance was diminished as well.

Another review surveyed the literature regarding factors used in determining a course of surgical treatment for symptomatic cartilage lesions of the knee to determine which factors affect treatment outcomes and should be incorporated in the treatment algorithm.[225] Twenty-seven studies examining 1450 human (1416 in vivo; 34 cadaveric) and 90 animal subjects met inclusion criteria. Female sex and higher BMI significantly predicted cartilage loss rates and recovery after microfracture and autologous matrix-induced chondrogenesis. Defect size and location significantly predicted treatment outcomes. Sizes >2-4 cm demonstrated worse outcomes after microfracture treatment. Defect size did not consistently affect autologous chondrocyte implantation or osteochondral autograft transplantation outcomes. Intra-articular lesion location was related to intralesional subchondral bone contact and microfracture outcome. Corrected patellofemoral and tibiofemoral alignment improved clinical outcome when realignment procedures were done concurrently with cartilage repair.

The authors concluded that the choice of the appropriate repair technique for focal knee cartilage defects is multifactorial and suggested a treatment algorithm which should consider frequently used factors such as defect size, location, knee alignment and patient demand. However, patient sex and BMI could also be considered. Patient age was not significantly associated with clinical outcome.

An effective method of promoting scar tissue formation in damaged articular cartilage is by continuous passive motion. Continuous passive motion has been shown to stimulate formation of hyaline-like fibrocartilage in the chondral defect, especially in the immediate postoperative period. This should be supplemented by low load, non weight-bearing exercise such as swimming and cycling. Following articular cartilage injury, the athlete may have to modify his or her training to reduce the amount of weight-bearing activity and substitute activities such as swimming and cycling.

When an injury (e.g. patellar dislocation, ACL or MCL tear) requires a lengthy period of partial or non weight-bearing, particular attention must be paid to preserving the integrity of the articular cartilage. This is done with continuous passive motion, a hydrotherapy program, swimming or cycling.

Other methods of reducing stress on the damaged articular cartilage include correction of biomechanical abnormalities, attention to ensure symmetry of gait and the use of a brace to control any instability. Pool running, mini-trampoline and the AlterG® Anti-Gravity Treadmill® may be used in the early stages of running and agility work to reduce load bearing. Proprioceptive exercises and strength exercises are also important.

ACUTE PATELLAR TRAUMA

Acute trauma to the patella (e.g. from a hockey stick or from a fall onto the kneecap) can cause a range of injuries from fracture of the patella to osteochondral damage of the patellofemoral joint with persisting patellofemoral joint pain. In some athletes, the pain settles without any long-term sequelae.

If there is suspicion of fracture, a plain radiograph should be obtained. It is important to be able to differentiate between a fracture of the patella and a bipartite patella which is a benign finding present in 1–2% of the population. A skyline view of the patella should be performed in addition to normal views.

If there is no evidence of fracture, the patient can be assumed to be suffering acute patellofemoral pain. This can be a difficult condition to treat. Treatment consists of nonsteroidal anti-inflammatory drugs (NSAIDs), local electrotherapy (e.g. interferential stimulation, TENS) and avoidance of aggravating activities such as squatting or walking down stairs. Taping of the patella may alter the mechanics of patellar tracking and therefore reduce the irritation and pain (Chapter 36). If taping provides symptom relief, rehabilitation and altered loading by strengthened quadriceps could be beneficial.

Fracture of the patella

Patellar fractures can occur either by direct trauma, in which case the surrounding retinaculum can be intact, or by indirect injury from quadriceps contraction, in which case the retinaculum and the vastus muscles are usually torn.

Fractures should be described by fracture orientation and position (e.g. transverse, inferior pole), degree of comminution and displacement (especially affecting the articular surface). Vertical fractures are possible but rare. A well-corticated fragment in the superolateral quadrant is more than likely part of a bipartite patella and not an acute fracture. Avulsion fractures are most commonly located at the inferior pole of the patella and often encountered in the paediatric population as patellar sleeve fractures. In the adult population, avulsion fractures occur at the origin of the patellar tendon and often cause disruption of the extensor mechanism.

The goals of treatment are a functional extensor mechanism, articular congruity and full, painless motion of the knee. Undisplaced fractures of the patella with normal function of the extensor mechanism can be managed non-surgically, initially with an extension splint. Over the next weeks as the fracture unites, the range of flexion can be gradually increased and the quadriceps strengthened in the inner range.

Transverse fractures are best treated with a tension-band technique (traditionally two axial Kirschner wires with a figure-of-eight wire anteriorly) which neutralises tension forces anteriorly and converts them into stabilising compressive forces at the articular surface. This technique is stronger than a simple cerclage wire in transverse fractures and can be combined with screw fixation in simple and in more comminuted fractures to increase stability.[226]

Small fragments may be excised or repaired with suture or screw fixation if possible. Every effort should be made to preserve and stabilise as much of the patella as possible to maintain the moment arm and avoid loss or poor outcomes which can occur when greater than 40% of the patella is removed. Removal of the entire patella may be contemplated for patients with massively comminuted fractures. Excision addresses the pain related to the fracture but decreases the mechanical advantage the patella provides to the extensor mechanism. The loss of quadriceps strength after total patellectomy can be as great as 49% and enough loss to preclude climbing stairs or getting out of a chair. Therefore, total patellectomy should be considered only after all techniques for salvage have been exhausted.[226]

Patella dislocation

Mean annual incidence of patellar dislocation varies with age group: it is between 5.8 and 7.0 per 100 000 person-years in the general population, but 29 per 100 000 in 10–17 year olds. Women are at greater risk than men, as are young subjects; the risk decreases with age. Patellar dislocation may have long-term consequences: instability of patellar origin, pain, recurrent dislocation and patellofemoral osteoarthritis.

Anatomy

Normally, the two patellar joint surfaces, medial and lateral, are symmetric and congruent with the femoral trochlea. Trochlear morphology remains relatively constant but, with growth, the thick trochlear cartilage thins in the middle, creating an illusion of a trochlear 'hollow'. The peripatellar soft tissue and particularly the medial patellofemoral ligament (MPFL) and vastus medialis obliquus (VMO) muscle contribute significantly to joint stability. The MPFL inserts to the femur between the medial epicondyle and the adductor tubercle and to the superomedial edge of the patella (Fig. 35.17).[227]

The MPFL provides 50-80% of the mechanisms counteracting lateral patellar glide.[228] Lateral patellar dislocation renders it incompetent, promoting recurrence of dislocation.[229] Neighbouring structures, such as the patellomeniscal or patellotibial ligaments and the superficial medial retinaculum, make lesser contributions to patellar stability. The VMO muscle is very important, acting as a dynamic stabiliser, and is intimately related to the MPFL.[227]

Patella dislocation occurs when the patella is displaced laterally (Fig. 35.18a), leaving its confines within the trochlea groove of the femoral condyle. Acute patellar dislocation may be either traumatic with a history of a traumatic force, followed by development of a haemarthrosis or atraumatic, which usually occurs in young girls with associated ligamentous laxity. Often the latter do not have a history of significant trauma and the dislocation is accompanied by mild-to-moderate swelling.

The typical mechanism underlying patellar dislocation is a movement of the knee in flexion and valgus without direct contact, accounting for 93% of traumatic patellar dislocations.[230] Most patients report a sensation of slippage, intense pain and secondary effusion, often suggestive of knee sprain. True traumatic dislocation, caused by direct tangential force dislocating the patella laterally, also occurs. Almost all patients with traumatic patellar dislocation show haemarthrosis, MPFL lesion and medial patellar wing fracture. Osteochondral fracture occurs in 25% of traumatic patellar dislocations. The recurrence risk is increased 6-fold in the case of history of ipsi- or contralateral patellar dislocation.[227]

Predisposing factors

Predisposing factors for patellar dislocation are either primary or secondary.[227] Primary disposing factors are:

- trochlear dysplasia
- elevated distance between the tibial tubercle (TT) and the trochlear groove (TG)
- patella alta (high patella)
- patellar tilt.

Secondary predisposing factors are:

- elevated Q angle with TT lateralisation and genu valgum
- elevated femoral anteversion with compensatory lateral tibial torsion
- vastus medialis hypoplasia
- ligament hyperlaxity with genu recurvatum
- patella dysplasia.

Clinical features

Patients with traumatic patellar dislocation usually complain that, on twisting or jumping, the knee suddenly gave way with the development of severe pain. Often the patient will describe a feeling of something 'moving' or 'popping out'. Swelling develops almost immediately. The dislocation usually reduces spontaneously with knee

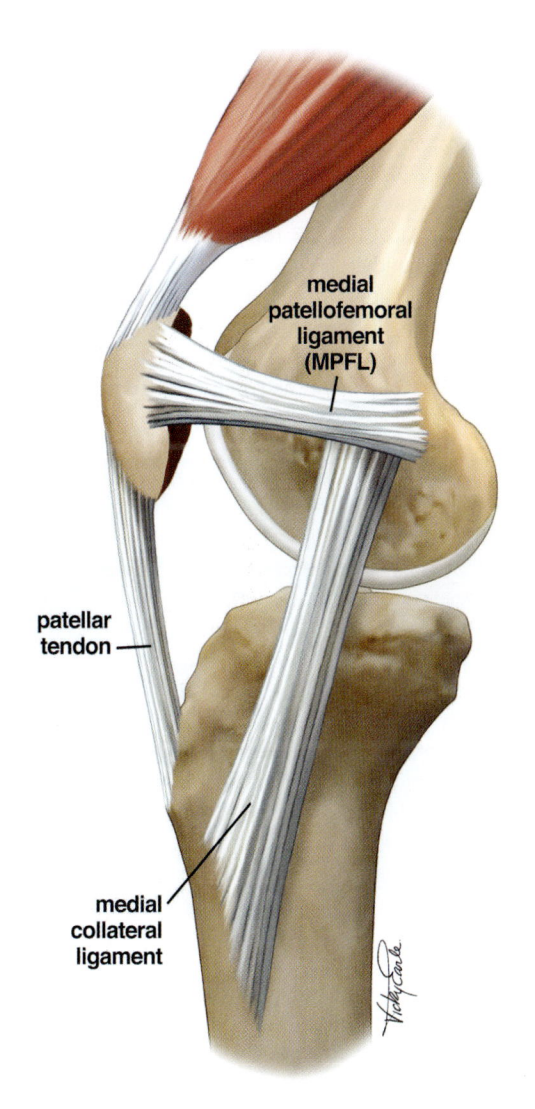

Figure 35.17 Anatomy showing the MPFL

PART B Regional problems

extension; however, in some cases this may require some assistance or regional anaesthesia (e.g. femoral nerve block).

The main differential diagnosis of an acute patella dislocation is an ACL rupture. Both conditions have similar histories of twisting, an audible 'pop', a feeling of something 'going out' and subsequent development of haemarthrosis.

On examination, there is usually a gross effusion, marked tenderness over the medial border of the patella and a positive lateral apprehension test (Fig. 35.2q) when attempts are made to push the patella in a lateral direction. Any attempt to contract the quadriceps muscle aggravates the pain and the patient often finds a painless rest in full extension.

Radiographs, including anteroposterior, lateral, skyline and intercondylar views, should be performed to rule out osteochondral fracture or a loose body.

The Merchant view may reveal bone avulsion of the medial facet of the patella and enables analysis of patellofemoral centring. The avulsion involves either the patellar insertion of the MPFL or the more distal patellomeniscal ligament insertion. Osteochondral fractures of the inferomedial pole of the patella are highly suggestive of traumatic patellar dislocation, but are overlooked on 30-40% of initial radiographs.

Computed tomography (CT) scan can assess osseous risk factors such as patellofemoral malalignment, osteochondral defects, patellar tilt and lateral subluxation, elevated TT-TG distance and trochlear dysplasia.

MRI is more specific in precisely determining involved structures and thus guiding treatment decision making. It assesses the patellofemoral joint cartilage surfaces and also the medial patellar stabilising structures (medial retinaculum, MPFL and VMO).[231] In patellar dislocation, MRI reveals: haemarthrosis; osteochondral lesions and bone oedema of the medial patellar facet (Fig. 35.18b); and bone oedema of the lateral femoral condyle (Fig. 35.18c). Concave deformity of the inferomedial patella, due to impaction, is a specific sign of lateral patellar dislocation Figure 35.18d) illustrates the three components of the injury: rupture of the MPFL; injury to the inferomedial pole of the patella; and bone bruising to the femoral lateral condyle.

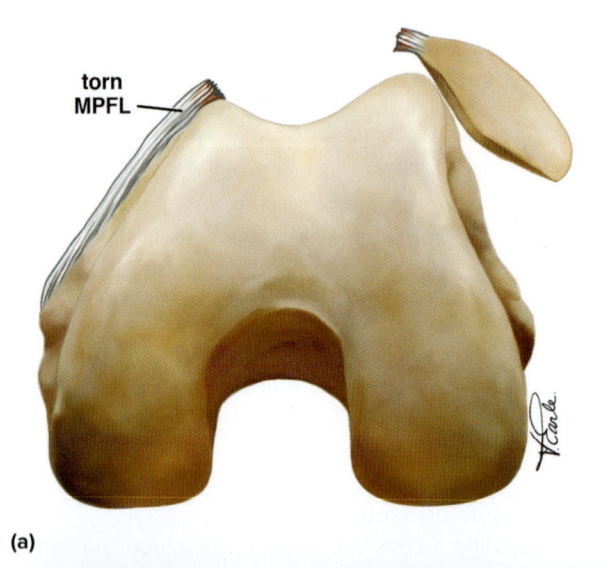

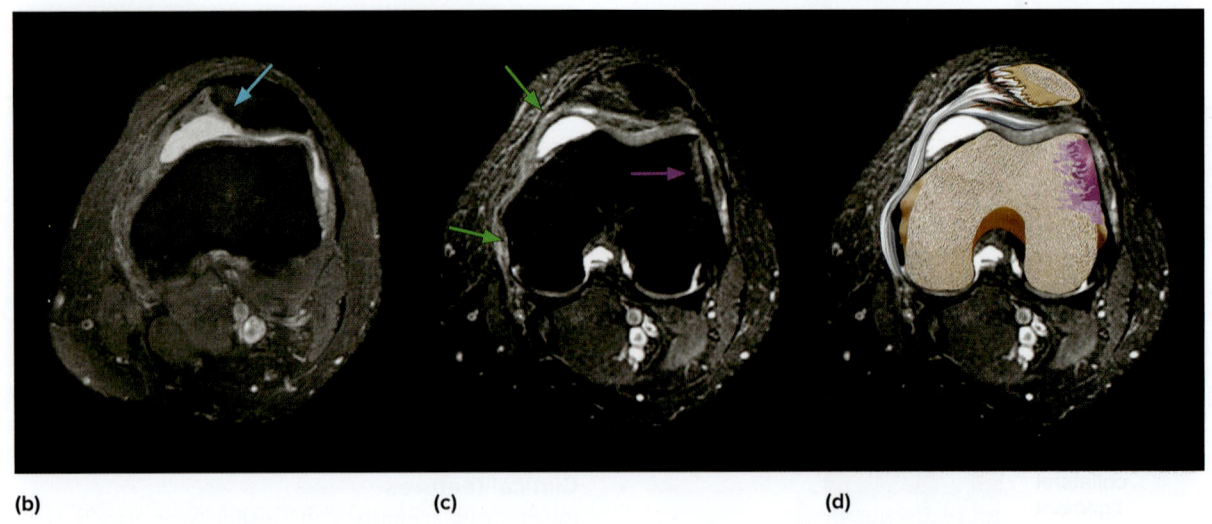

Figure 35.18 (a) The patella dislocates laterally tearing the MPFL (b) Axial fat-suppressed T2 MRI of the left knee. Blue arrow shows patellar chondral injury. (c) The torn MPFL is highlighted with the green arrow. Abnormal high signal represents oedema at the site of MPFL tear. Purple arrow at right of image shows bone marrow oedema at the lateral femoral condyle, the impact zone when the patella dislocates (d) Diagram demonstrating the three components of the injury—the torn MPFL, the articular damage at the inferomedial corner of the patella and the bone oedema at the lateral condyle

Treatment

The initial management of a first-time traumatic patellar dislocation is controversial, with no evidence-based consensus to guide decision making. Most first-time traumatic patellar dislocations have been traditionally treated non-operatively; however, there has been a recent trend towards initial surgical management.

Following a systematic review of 70 level I–IV studies looking at study design, mean follow-up, subjective and validated outcome measures, re-dislocation rates and long-term symptoms, the authors recommended initial non-operative management of a traumatic dislocation except in several specific circumstances.[232] These include:

- the presence of an osteochondral fracture
- substantial disruption of the medial patellar stabilisers
- a laterally subluxated patella with normal alignment of the contralateral knee
- a second dislocation
- in patients not improving with appropriate rehabilitation.

Arthroscopy should be performed in case of an intra-articular loose body secondary to a chondral lesion or osteochondral fracture. When an osteochondral fracture involves more than 10% of the patellar joint surface or involves the weight-bearing surface of the lateral femoral condyle, the osteochondral fragment should so far as possible be fixed by open surgery, for instance using resorbable pins; if this is not possible, micro-fracturing may stimulate cartilage regrowth. As the MPFL and medial retinaculum tend to be torn in acute traumatic patellar dislocation, stabilisation surgery may be required.

According to Duthon, surgery for patellar dislocation patients can be classified under three categories according to whether there are predisposing factors and whether the dislocation is inaugural or recurrent.[227]

1. Inaugural dislocation without predisposing factors. Immediate surgical repair of the patellar stabilising structures (VMO, MPFL, medial retinaculum) is recommended in athletic patients. Bone avulsion at the patellar insertion of the MPFL is known not to show consolidation even with proper immobilisation; functional results of non-operative treatment are unsatisfactory and fixation is recommended.
2. Inaugural dislocation with predisposing factors. Surgical repair of the patellar stabilising structures (VMO, MPFL, medial retinaculum) is recommended when risk factors for recurrence such as trochlear dysplasia, patella alta, elevated TT-TG distance, are present.
3. Recurrent dislocation. In recurrent patellar dislocation, surgery is recommended due to severe apprehension constituting a disability in everyday life, and to prevent chondral lesions which, in the long term, would cause patellofemoral osteoarthritis. The type of surgery is determined by the presence of one or more risk factors and therefore may involve:

- lowering the tibial tubercle
- patellar tenodesis
- tibial tubercle medialisation
- sulcus-deepening trochleoplasty
- vastus medialis plasty.

While patellar dislocations are increasingly being managed with surgery, there is no good evidence of a benefit over conservative management. Hing et al. performed a literature review of five studies for the Cochrane Database.[233] No significant difference emerged for risk of recurrent dislocation, Kujala patellofemoral score or need for surgical revision.

The most important aim of rehabilitation after patellofemoral dislocation is to reduce the chances of a recurrence of the injury. The therapist should aim to restore normal range of knee motion (full flexion and extension) and to reinforce the quadriceps to restore dynamic patellar balance.

As a result, the rehabilitation program is lengthy and emphasises core stability, pelvic positioning, vastus medialis obliquus strength and stretching of the lateral structures when tight. Similar to ACL intervention exercises, rotational control of the limb under the pelvis is critical to knee and kneecap stability. A suggested rehabilitation program is shown in Table 35.14.

Bracing could be helpful for these patients in combination with extensive rehabilitation. The patella brace usually has a hole for the patella and a lateral rim to prevent lateral dislocation. Bracing does not prevent recurrent instability but may be helpful for those with symptomatic instability.

LESS COMMON CAUSES
Patellar tendon rupture

The patellar tendon occasionally ruptures spontaneously. This is usually in association with a sudden severe eccentric contraction of the quadriceps muscle, which may occur when an athlete stumbles or when attempting a powerful take off manoeuvre (e.g. long jump event in track and field competition). There may have been a history of previous corticosteroid injection into the tendon. A previous history of patellar tendinopathy is uncommon.

Patients complain of a sudden acute onset of pain over the patellar tendon accompanied by a tearing sensation and are unable to stand. On examination, there is a visible loss of fullness at the front of the knee as the patella is retracted proximally. The knee extensor mechanism is no longer intact and knee extension with a straight leg cannot be initiated.

Table 35.14 Rehabilitation program following patellar dislocation (see Figs 35.6 and 35.7)

Phase	Goal of phase	Time post-injury	Physiotherapy treatment	Exercise program	Functional/sport-related activity
Phase 1	Control swelling Maintain knee extension Isometric quadriceps strength	0–2 weeks	Extension splint (removal dependent on surgeon/physician) Cryotherapy Electrotherapy PFJ taping Manual therapy	Quadriceps drills (supine) Bilateral calf raises Foot and ankle Hip abduction	Progress to FWB
Phase 2	No swelling Full extension Flexion to 100° 4+/5 quadriceps strength 5/5 hamstring strength	2–6 weeks	Cryotherapy Electrotherapy Compression Manual therapy Gait re-education Exercise modification	ROM drills Quadriceps/VMO setting Mini-squats and lunges Bridges (double, then single-leg) Hip abduction and extension with rubber tubing Single-leg calf raises Gait re-education drills Balance and proprioceptive drills (single-leg)	Walking Exercise bike
Phase 3	Full ROM Full strength and power Return to jogging, running, and agility Return to restricted sport-specific drills	6–8 weeks	Manual therapy Exercise/activity modification and supervision	As above—increase difficulty, repetitions and weight, where appropriate Single-leg squats Single-leg press Jump and land drills Agility drills	Straight-line jogging Swimming (light kick) Road bike Straight-line running Progressing to sport-specific running and agility (progressively sequenced) (e.g. running forwards, sideways, backwards, sprinting, jumping, hopping, changing directions, kicking)
Phase 4	Return to sport	8–12 weeks	As above	High-level sport-specific strengthening as required	Progressive return to sport (e.g. restricted training, unrestricted training, match play, competitive match play)

FWB = full weight-bearing; PFJ = patellofemoral joint; ROM = range of motion; VMO = vastus medialis obliquus

Surgical repair of the tendon is needed and must be followed by intensive rehabilitation. Full recovery takes 6-9 months and there is often some residual disability.

Bursal haematoma
Occasionally, an acute bursal haematoma or acute pre-patellar bursitis occurs as a result of a fall onto the knee. This causes bleeding into the pre-patellar bursa and subsequent inflammation. This usually settles spontaneously with firm compression bandaging. If not, the haematoma should be aspirated and the bloodstained fluid removed. Anti-inflammatory medication may also be appropriate. This injury is often associated with a skin wound (e.g. abrasion) and therefore may become infected. Adequate skin care is essential. If the bursa recurs, then aspiration followed by injection of a corticosteroid agent may be required. If conservative treatment fails, arthroscopic excision of the bursa is indicated.

Fat pad impingement
Acute fat pad impingement (often incorrectly referred to as 'Hoffa's syndrome') usually occurs as a result of a hyperextension injury. As the fat pad is the most sensitive part of the knee, this condition may be extremely painful.[234] There may be an inferiorly tilted lower pole of the patella predisposing to injury. On examination, tenderness is distal to the patella but beyond the margin of the patellar tendon. A haemarthrosis may be present.

This can be an extremely difficult condition to treat. The basic principles of treatment are a reduction of aggravating activities, electrotherapeutic modalities to settle inflammation and resumption of range of movement exercises as soon as possible. Taping of the patella may help in reducing the amount of tilt and impingement (Chapter 36). If conservative management is not successful, arthroscopic joint lavage and resection of the fat pad can be helpful.

Fracture of the tibial plateau
Tibial plateau fracture is seen in high-speed injuries such as falls while skiing, wave-jumping or horseriding. This condition needs to be excluded when diagnosing collateral ligament damage with instability. The patient complains of severe pain and inability to weight-bear. Fractures are associated with a lipohaemarthrosis, which can be detected on a horizontal lateral X-ray by the presence of a fat fluid level. CT scan is helpful in defining the fracture.

Minimally displaced fractures should be treated by 6 weeks of non weight-bearing in a hinged knee brace (Fig. 35.5a). Displaced fractures (Fig 35.19) or fractures with unstable fragment/s require internal surgical fixation. Displaced vertical split fractures may be fixed percutaneously during arthroscopy.

Tibial plateau fractures are commonly associated with meniscal or ACL injuries. In these cases, arthroscopic assessment is required. Following recovery from a tibial plateau fracture, weight-bearing activity may need to be reduced as the irregular joint surface predisposes to the development of osteoarthritis.

Superior tibiofibular joint injury
Acute dislocation of the superior tibiofibular joint occurs occasionally as a result of a direct blow. The patient complains of pain in the area of the joint and may be aware of obvious deformity. The common peroneal nerve may be damaged with this injury.

Sprain of the tibiofibular joint is more common. The patient complains of local pain aggravated by movement and, on examination, there is local tenderness and some anteroposterior instability. Treatment consists of rest and local electrotherapeutic modalities. Rarely, a chronic instability of the superior tibiofibular joint develops, but these cases may need surgical stabilisation.

Ruptured hamstring tendon
Spontaneous rupture of one of the distal hamstring tendons at the knee occurs occasionally during sprinting. Sudden onset of pain is localised to either the biceps femoris tendon or the semitendinosus tendon. Pain and weakness is present with resisted hamstring contraction. When these injuries involve the tendon portion of the hamstring unit, it may be amenable to surgical exploration and repair, followed by protection in a limited-motion brace.

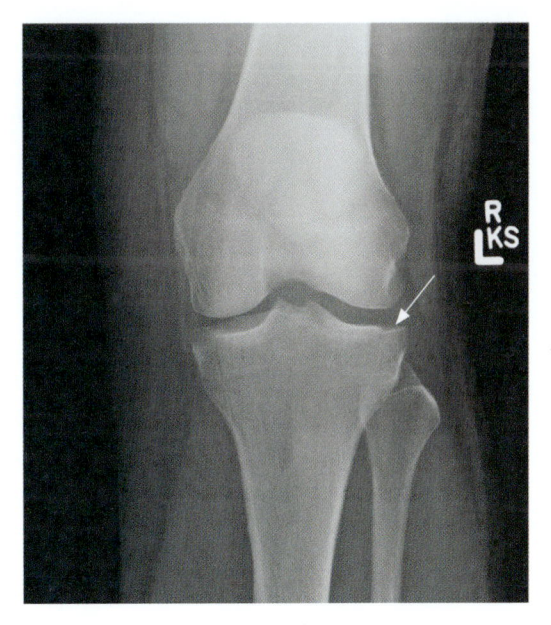

Figure 35.19 X-ray of a tibial plateau fracture

PART B   Regional problems

REFERENCES

References for this chapter can be found at www.mhhe.com/au/CSM5e

Chapter 36

Anterior knee pain

by KAY CROSSLEY and JILL COOK with SALLIE COWAN, ADAM CULVENOR, SEAN DOCKING, MICHAEL RATHLEFF and EBONIE RIO

> *The New York Knicks announced today that Carmelo Anthony will have season-ending left knee surgery. The procedure, which will be performed by Team Orthopedist Dr. Answorth Allen, includes a left knee patella tendon debridement and repair.*
> www.NBA.com, 18 February 2015

Anterior knee pain is the most common presenting symptom in many physiotherapy and sports physician practices.[1, 2] It contributes substantially to the 20-40% of family practice consultations that relate to the musculoskeletal system.[3] Anterior knee anatomy is shown in Figure 36.1.

In this chapter, we:

- outline the clinical approach to assessing the patient with anterior knee pain, particularly with a view to distinguishing the common conditions–patellofemoral pain (PFP) and patellar tendinopathy
- detail contemporary management integrating high level evidence (Chapter 2) with the best of clinical experience
- discuss less common causes of anterior knee pain such as fat pad impingement, which may mimic features of both PFP and patellar tendinopathy
- highlight new research investigating PFP in adolescents, patellar tendinopathy and patellofemoral osteoarthritis (OA).

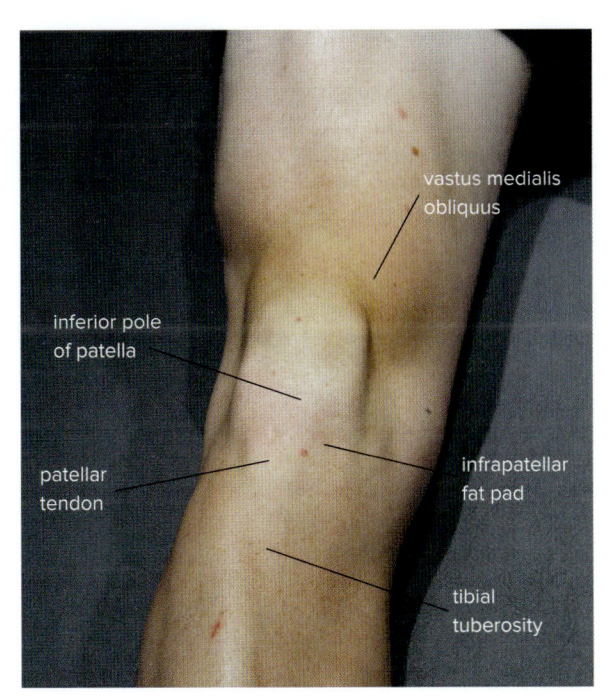

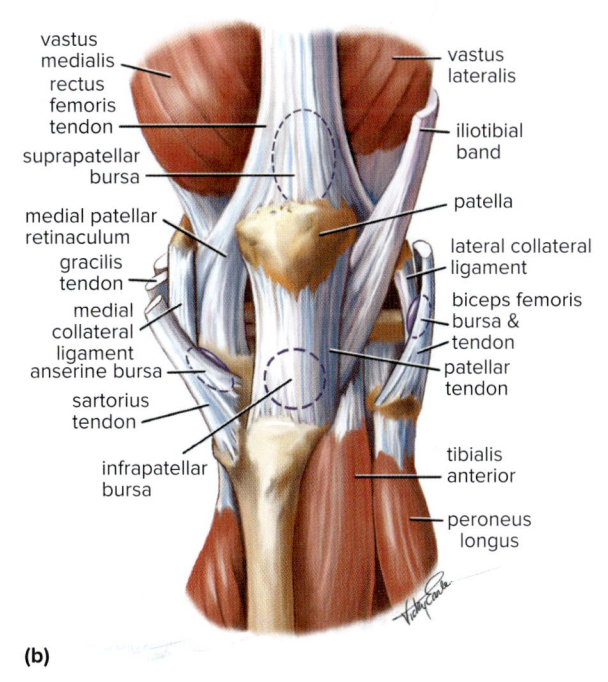

Figure 36.1 Anterior knee (a) Surface anatomy (b) Anatomy

PART B Regional problems

CLINICAL APPROACH

Distinguishing between PFP and patellar tendinopathy as a cause of anterior knee pain can be difficult. Rarely, both conditions may be present. Causes of anterior knee pain are listed in Table 36.1.

History

A number of important factors can be elicited from the history of a athlete presenting with anterior knee pain. These include the specific location of the pain, the nature of aggravating activities, the history of the onset and behaviour of the pain, as well as any associated clicking, giving way or swelling.

Although it may be difficult for the patient with anterior knee pain to be specific about the location of pain, this symptom provides an important clue as to the likely diagnosis. For example, retropatellar or peripatellar pain suggests that the patellofemoral joint (PFJ) is a likely culprit, lateral pain localised to the lateral femoral epicondyle increases the likelihood of iliotibial band syndrome as the diagnosis (Chapter 37). Patellar tendon pain will be localised to the inferior pole of the patella and the patient can point to it with a single finger. The pain remains localised both at rest and on loading with the decline squat. The location of pain (and source) appear to be associated with different changes to motor drive, indicating that the rehabilitation approaches are likely to be different.[4]

The onset of PFP is typically insidious and unrelated to an acute injury. However, it may present secondary to an acute traumatic episode (e.g. falling on the knee) or consequent to another knee injury (e.g. meniscal, anterior cruciate ligament) or knee surgery. The patient presents with a diffuse ache, which is usually exacerbated by PFJ-loaded activities, such as ascending/descending stairs or running. Sometimes PFP is aggravated by prolonged sitting ('movie-goer's knee'), but sitting also tends to aggravate patellar tendinopathy symptoms and therefore is not diagnostic of PFP. Pain during running that gradually worsens is more likely to be of patellofemoral origin, whereas pain that occurs at the start of activity, settles after warm-up and returns after activity is more likely to be patellar tendinopathy. While the pathologies of patellar tendinopathy and PFP may co-exist, in practice they rarely present as co-existing clinical entities. Table 36.2 is an aid to differentiate PFP and patellar tendinopathy based on clinical history and presentation.

The type of activity that aggravates the anterior knee pain also aids diagnosis. Consider two contrasting scenarios that a patient may report as causing pain at the infrapatellar region. In one case, precipitating activities, such as basketball, volleyball, high, long or triple jumps, that involve repetitive loading (specifically energy storage and release) of the patellar tendon suggest the diagnosis of patellar tendinopathy. On the other hand, if a freestyle swimmer reported pain following tumble turning or vigorous kicking in the pool, where there had been no energy storage and release load on the tendon but a forceful extension of the knee, the practitioner should suspect an irritated fat pad. The mechanism of injury and the aggravating features are critical to an accurate diagnosis.

A history of crepitus may suggest PFP. A feeling that the patella moves laterally at certain times suggests patellofemoral instability. An imminent feeling of giving way may be associated with patellar subluxation, PFP or meniscal abnormality. Although frank, dramatic giving way is usually associated with anterior cruciate ligament

Table 36.1 Causes of anterior knee pain

Common	Less common	Not to be missed
Patellofemoral pain	Synovial plica	Referred pain from the hip
Patellar tendinopathy	Pre-patellar bursitis	Osteochondritis dessicans
	Quadriceps tendinopathy	Slipped capital femoral epiphysis
	Infrapatellar bursitis	Perthes' disease
	Patellofemoral instability	Tumour (especially in the young)
	Fat pad impingement	
	Sinding–Larsen–Johansson lesion in adolescents (Chapter 44)	
	Tenoperiostitis of upper tibia	
	Stress fracture of the patella	
	Osgood–Schlatter lesion in adolescents (Chapter 44)	

Anterior knee pain — CHAPTER 36

Table 36.2 Comparison of the clinical features of patellofemoral pain and patellar tendinopathy

Signs	Patellofemoral pain	Patellar tendinopathy
Onset	Running, steps/stairs, hills, any weight-bearing activities involving knee flexion	Activities involving jumping and/or changing direction
Pain	Non-specific or vague; may be medial, lateral or infrapatellar; aggravated by activities that load the PFJ	At the inferior pole of patella, aggravated by energy storage loads such as jumping
Tenderness	Usually medial or lateral facets of patella but may be tender in infrapatellar region; may have no pain on palpation due to areas of patella being inaccessible	Localised to inferior pole of patella; this tenderness can exist in jumping athletes without patellar tendinopathy
Swelling	May have small effusion, swelling, suprapatellar or infrapatellar	Tendon may be increased in thickness; no joint swelling
Clicks/clunks	Occasional	No
Crepitus	Occasionally under patella	No
Giving way	Rarely, due to quadriceps weakness/inhibition or subluxation	Rarely, due to quadriceps weakness/inhibition
Knee range of motion	May be decreased in severe cases but usually normal	Normal
Quadriceps contraction in extension	Can be painful, often normal	Often painful
PFJ movement	May be restricted in any direction. Commonly restricted medial glide due to tight lateral structures	Normal PFJ biomechanics
Functional testing	Squats, stairs may aggravate. PFJ taping should decrease pain	Decline squats aggravate pain; PFJ taping has less effect

(ACL) instability (Chapter 35), giving way resulting from pain-induced muscle inhibition is not uncommon in people with various types of anterior knee pain.

A history of previous knee injury or surgery may be important; PFP is a well-recognised complication of posterior cruciate ligament injury and following anterior cruciate ligament reconstruction (Chapter 35). Patellar tendinopathy may be present after ACL reconstruction using bone-patellar tendon-bone grafts.

Knee pain and/or effusion may result in inhibition of the quadriceps (reduced magnitude and delayed timing of electromyography (EMG) onset) commonly termed 'pain-induced muscle inhibition'. This inhibition appears to be more profound in the vastus medialis obliquus (VMO), especially at smaller knee effusion volumes.[5, 6] Preferential inhibition of the VMO has potential to set up an imbalance in the medial and lateral forces on the patella, predisposing to PFP.[7] Significant knee swelling is rare in atraumatic anterior knee pain and generally suggests additional intra-articular abnormality. However, a small effusion may be present with PFP.

Previous treatment and the patient's response to it should be noted. If treatment was unsuccessful, it is essential to determine whether the failure was due to incorrect diagnosis, inappropriate treatment or poor patient adherence.

Physical examination

The primary aim of the clinical assessment is to determine the most likely cause of the patient's pain. It is critical to reproduce the patient's anterior knee pain as location of tenderness and aggravating factors are key to the differential diagnosis. This is usually done with either a double or single leg squat (Fig. 36.2c). A squat done on a decline board (Fig. 36.2d).[8] is very painful in people with patellar tendinopathy. It is essential to palpate the anterior knee carefully to determine the site of maximal tenderness, although palpation soreness by itself is not diagnostic; for example, the patellar tendon can be tender on palpation in asymptomatic athletes.[9]

Many clinical tests outlined below have not been evaluated for their clinical utility. Those that have been evaluated for PFP and patellar tendinopathy are outlined in Tables 36.3 and 36.4. The best tests to identify people with PFP are pain during activities (squatting, stairs, prolonged sitting) and pain during an isometric quadriceps contraction, although these tests fall well below the recommended cut offs for a diagnostic test (LR + >10).[10] A combination of these tests may provide greater diagnostic accuracy.[10]

PART B Regional problems

Examination includes the following.

1. Observation
   a. standing (Fig. 36.2a)
   b. walking
   c. supine (Fig. 36.2b)
2. Functional tests
   a. double then single-leg squat (Fig. 36.2c)
   b. step-up/step-down
   c. jump/hop
   d. lunge
   e. single-leg decline squat (Fig. 36.2d)

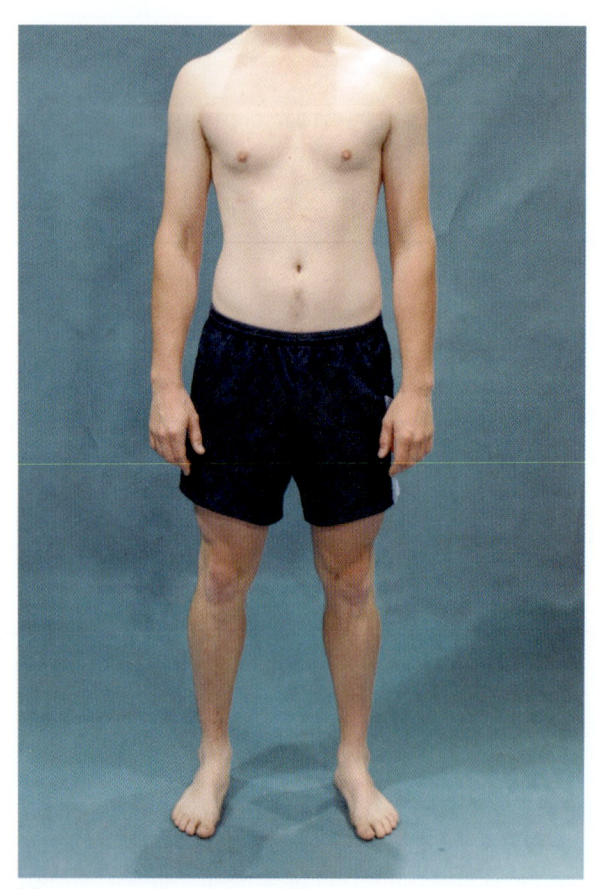

Figure 36.2 Examination of the anterior knee
(a) Observation—standing. Observe the patient from the front to examine lower limb alignment including femoral torsion, patellar alignment and any signs of muscle wasting (b) Observation—supine. Observe for lower limb alignment, effusion, position of the patella, and any evidence of patella tilt or rotation (c) Functional test—double/single-leg squat If the patient's pain has not already been reproduced, functional tests such as squat, lunge, hop, step-up, step-down or eccentric drop squat should be performed

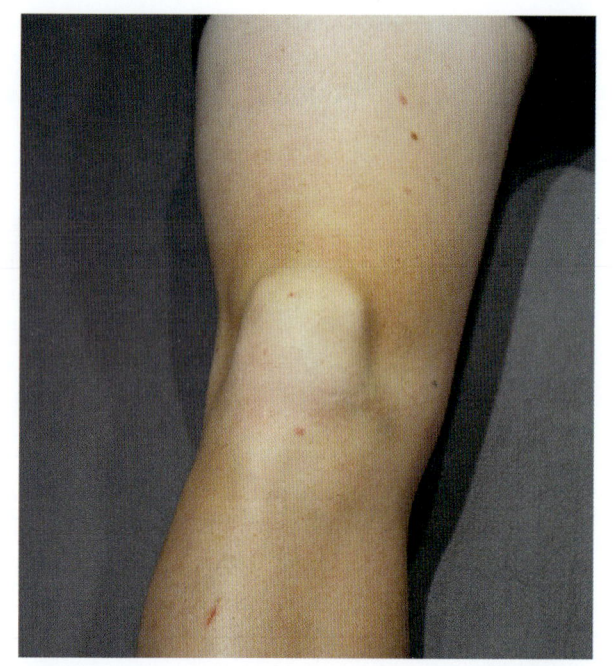

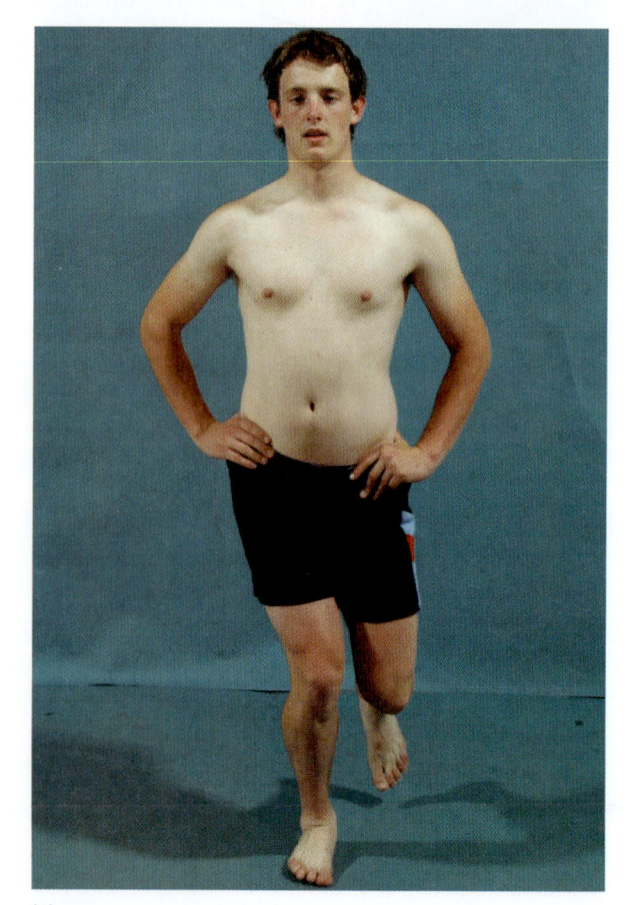

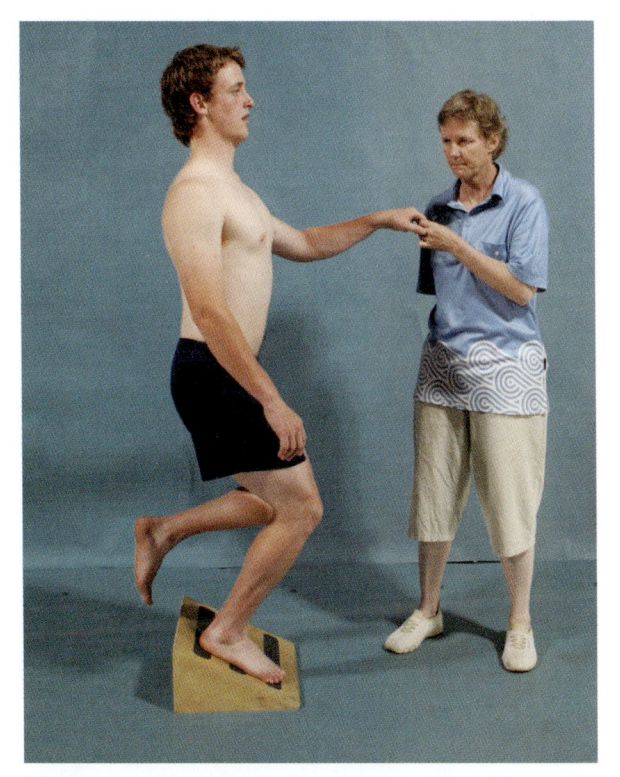

Anterior knee pain   CHAPTER 36

(d)

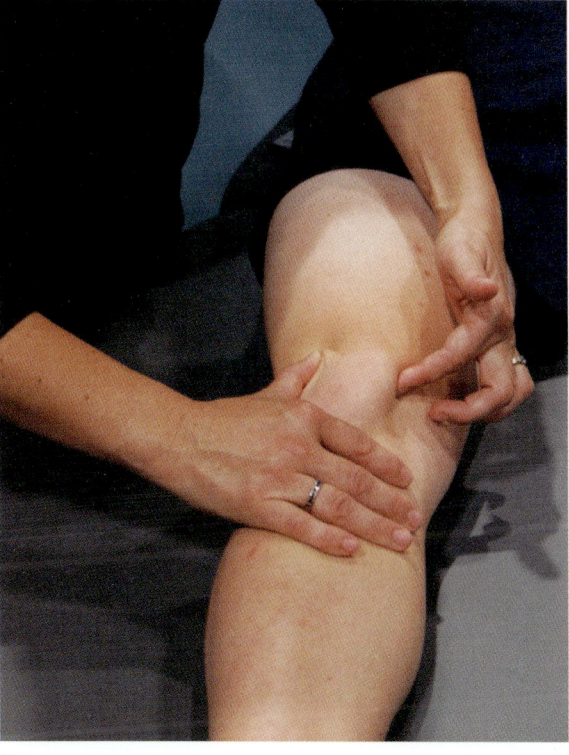

(f)

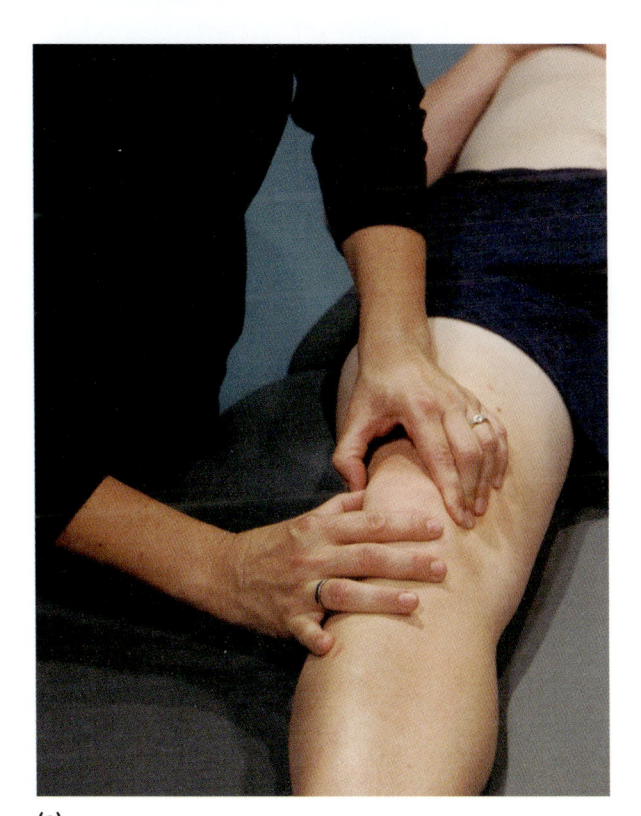

Figure 36.2 (cont.) (d) Functional test—single-leg squat on decline board (e) Palpation—patella, and medial and lateral facets are palpated for tenderness (f) Patellofemoral joint assessment—mobility of the patella—medial glide

3. Palpation
    a. patella–medial and lateral facets (Fig. 36.2e)
    b. medial/lateral retinaculum
    c. patellar tendon
    d. tibial tubercle
    e. effusion–swipe test, ballotment test
4. PFJ assessment
    a. quadriceps function
    b. mobility of patella
        i. superior glide
        ii. inferior glide
        iii. medial glide (Fig. 36.2f)
        iv. lateral glide–look for apprehension
    c. tracking of patella in passive knee flexion/extension
5. Flexibility and range of motion
    a. lateral soft tissue structures
    b. quadriceps
    c. hamstring
    d. iliotibial band
    e. gastrocnemius
    f. soleus

(e)

PART B Regional problems

Table 36.3 Diagnostic accuracy of examination tests for patellofemoral pain

Test	What is a positive finding?	Sensitivity	Specificity	LR+	LR−
Pain during functional tests (history or examination)					
Squatting[10]	Pain	91	50	1.8	0.2
Stair climbing[10]	Pain	72	43	1.3	0.6
Kneeling[10]	Pain	84	50	1.7	0.3
Prolonged sitting[10]	Pain	72	57	1.7	0.5
Patellar palpation					
Medial tenderness[11]	Pain	48	71	1.6	0.7
Lateral tenderness[11]	Pain	41	71	1.4	0.8
Palpation of patellar borders[10]	Pain	47	68	1.5	0.8
Passive mobility tests					
Passive gliding patella[11]	Pain	48	47	0.9	1.1
Patella translation superior to inferior[12]	Reduced ROM	63	56	1.4	0.7
Patella translation medial to lateral[12]	Reduced ROM	54	69	1.8	0.7
Patellar tendon mobility[12]	Reduced ROM	49	83	2.8	0.6
Patella inferior pole tilt[12]	Reduced ROM	19	83	1.1	0.9
Special tests					
Patella apprehension test[13]	Pain or apprehension	15	89	1.3	1.0
Resisted isometric quads[10]	Pain	39	82	2.2	0.8

LR+ = positive likelihood ratio; LR− = negative likelihood ratio
See Chapter 14 for a guide to interpreting test sensitivity, specificity and likelihood ratios

Table 36.4 Diagnostic accuracy of examination tests for patellar tendinopathy

Test	What is a positive finding?	Sensitivity	Specificity	LR+	LR−
Palpation					
Palpation of the patellar tendon attachment[9]	Pain	68	9	0.5	0.2

LR+ = positive likelihood ratio; LR− = negative likelihood ratio; NA = not available
See Chapter 14 for a guide to interpreting test sensitivity, specificity and likelihood ratios

   g. knee flexion/extension
   h. tibial rotation
   i. hip and lumbar spine range of motion–all planes
6. Special tests (to exclude other pathology)
   a. examination of knee joint with respect to acute injury (Chapter 35)
   b. examination of hip joint (Chapter 31)
   c. examination of lumbar spine (Chapter 29)
   d. neurodynamic tests (neural Thomas test, slump test, prone bent knee test-Chapter 9)

Patient-reported outcome measures

Patient reported outcome measures (PROMs) are considered gold standard to evaluate outcomes in a clinical population. When choosing a PROM, the psychometric properties of all possible PROMs should be considered, specific to the patient. For PFP, three scales (the anterior knee pain scale, and visual analogue scales for usual and worst pain) have adequate psychometric properties for use (Table 36.5). The patient specific functional scale[14] is also a useful clinical PROM, but has not been

Anterior knee pain — CHAPTER 36

Table 36.5 Patient-reported outcome measures for patellofemoral pain

Anterior knee pain scale (AKPS), also known as Kujala scale
- Self-administered questionnaire that evaluates pain and function in anterior knee pain[15]
- 13 items
- Score range 0–100 (100 is best score)
- Test-retest reliability: 0.81–0.90[16]
- MDC95%: 19.7[16]–9.7[17]
- MCID: 8–10[17]

Visual analogue pain scale when usual pain (VAS-U)
- Self-administered questionnaire to evaluate pain on a 100 mm visual analogue scale during usual activities in the past week[17]
- Score range 0–100 (100 is worst imaginable pain)
- Test-retest reliability: 0.56–0.77[16]
- MDC95%: 33[16]–17[17]
- MCID: 15–20[17]

Visual analogue pain scale when worst pain (VAS-W)
- Self-administered questionnaire to evaluate pain on a 100 mm visual analogue scale during worst (most aggravating) activities in the past week[17]
- Score range 0–100 (100 is worst imaginable pain)
- Test-retest reliability: 0.56–0.79[16]
- MDC95%: 30[16]–17[17]
- MCID: 20[17]

specifically validated for PFP. For each scale, the patient needs to improve by more than the Minimal Detectable Change (MDC), to be greater than the error associated with the measurement and greater than the Minimal Clinically Important Difference (MCID), to have a clinically meaningful change. See Chapter 16 for more details on PROMS and how to use them in clinical practice.

Investigations

Imaging may be used to confirm a clinical impression obtained from the history and examination. Structural imaging includes plain radiography, ultrasound, CT, and MRI. Occasionally, radionuclide bone scan is indicated to evaluate the 'metabolic' status of the knee (e.g. after trauma, or in suspected stress fracture).

Most patients with PFP will require either no imaging or plain radiography consisting of a standard AP view, a true lateral view with the knee in 30° of flexion and an axial view through the knee in 30–40° of flexion. Plain radiography can detect bipartite patella, apophyseal changes at the patellar tendon attachments and osteoarthritis, as well as rule out potentially serious complications such as tumour or infection. Although CT and three-dimensional CT can assess the PFJ morphology, MRI is gaining increasing popularity as an investigation of PFP and the unstable patella.[18] These imaging techniques can identify features including bone lesions, chondral lesions, tendinopathy and synovitis. However, the importance of such features to symptoms or progression of disease remains unknown.[19]

MRI displays high signal abnormality in patellar tendinopathy. Ultrasound hypoechogenicity and excessive vascularity also indicate a potential diagnosis of patellar tendinopathy.[20] However, in asymptomatic athletes or those with symptoms from another source in the anterior knee, the patellar tendon can be abnormal on imaging,[21,22,23] and the clinician should be wary of using imaging findings diagnostically.

PATELLOFEMORAL PAIN

In this section we:
- define the condition and underscore its significance
- review clinically relevant functional anatomy
- alert the clinician to predisposing factors and how to identify them–this may prove critical for effective long-term treatment
- summarise the results of RCTs that have added high-quality evidence (Chapter 2) to guide clinical treatment.

PART B   Regional problems

What is patellofemoral pain?

> **PRACTICE PEARL**
>
> Patellofemoral pain is the preferred term used to describe pain in and around the patella.

Synonyms include patellofemoral pain syndrome, anterior knee pain and chondromalacia patellae. Patellofemoral pain (PFP) is an 'umbrella' term used to embrace all peripatellar or retropatellar pain in the absence of other pathologies.[24] Since the cause of the pain may differ between patients, it is appropriate to review the potential sources of PFP.[25]

Numerous structures in the PFJ are susceptible to overload. A number of extra- and intra-articular components of the knee can generate neurosensory signals that ultimately result in the patient feeling pain (see box below). Patellofemoral articular cartilage is avascular and aneural. However, a cartilage lesion may lead to chemical or mechanical synovial irritation, bone oedema or erosion, all of which can result in pain.[26, 27]

Peripatellar synovitis, in the absence of obvious cartilage damage, must be considered as a primary cause of PFP.[28] Soft tissues such as the lateral retinaculum are also implicated as a potent source of PFP.[29, 30-32] Other important sources of pain are the synovium and infrapatellar fat pad.[33-36]

So how does an increase in PFJ load result in PFP? Dye and Vaupel[37] described a concept whereby injury to the PFJ musculoskeletal tissues results from supraphysiological loads–either a single maximal load or lower magnitude repetitive load. Injury to these tissues initiates a cascade of events encompassing inflammation of the peripatellar synovium through to bone stress. Thus, a number of different pain-sensitive structures can give rise to the conscious sensation of PFP (Chapters 5 and 6).[37]

The 'pain' in patellofemoral pain

Local and central contributors to PFP
Pain is a complex protective mechanism (Chapters 5 and 6). Although nociception is an input to the brain that may result in the output of pain, the brain considers many other inputs before deciding to create pain, some of which may be far more decisive than the level of nociception. The experience of knee pain is modulated at different sites in the body, both locally and centrally within the brain and spinal cord. This means that both local peripheral nociceptors and facilitated central pain pathways, may influence the pain that is experienced by the patient. Current thinking in the field of pain science teaches us that pain reflects the perception of threat more so than the state of injury to tissues. Pain, such as perceived in the PFJ, is considered a driver of behaviour to protect tissues.

Do people with PFP have hyperalgesia?
The pathways involved in PFP are starting to be evaluated. Compared with pain-free controls, female adolescents presenting with longstanding PFP have hypersensitivity highlighted by reduced pressure pain thresholds (PPTs) around the knee and more distally around the tibialis anterior muscle.[38] The distal hyperalgesia may reflect segmental spreading of hyperalgesia.[39] Identification of pressure pain hyperalgesia (decreased PPT) may be clinically important and associated with poorer recovery as previously shown in adult patients with acute whiplash injury and after total knee replacement. However, early reports indicate that low PPTs around the knee or tibialis anterior are not associated with a worse prognosis and PPTs tend to increase when patients recover.[40] This implies a nociceptive contribution to PFP.

How does facilitated central pain mechanism affect the pain experience in PFP?
Conditioned pain modulation (CPM) (primarily a descending inhibitory mechanism) is also impaired in young female adults with longstanding PFP.[40] Less efficient CPM mechanisms are evident in patients with musculoskeletal pain conditions, such as myofascial temporomandibular disorders, chronic low back pain and fibromyalgia. A reduced potency of the descending control can make the entire neuroaxis more vulnerable to pain. However, in the study of female adolescents with PFP, the CPM mechanisms were highly variable, ranging from an efficient CPM system to severely impaired CPM. This suggests that central pain mechanisms may be a factor we need to consider in some, but not all, patients with PFP. Furthermore, there is emerging evidence that some people may be more vulnerable to pain due to genetic and other factors.

Clinical signs that may suggest facilitated central pain mechanisms
In a clinical setting the following signs may suggest facilitated central pain mechanisms:
- disproportionate pain, implying that the severity of pain and related reported or perceived disability are disproportionate to the nature and extent of the injury
- presence of diffuse pain distribution, allodynia and hyperalgesia.

If this fits with your patient with longstanding PFP and he or she does not respond to your normal exercise protocol, you might want to consider the following items.

Guidelines for clinical management of longstanding PFP in respect to a heightened/hypersensitive central pain presentation
(adapted from Nijs et al[41])
- Be conservative when estimating the initial training load; prefer a lower baseline and then progress from there depending on symptom flaring.
- Monitor symptom flares after exercise and progress exercises depending on response.
- Let the patient know that minor symptom flares are natural during the initial stages of exercise therapy, but should cease once an exercise routine is established.
- Allow increased pain during and shortly following exercise but avoid continuously increasing pain intensity over time.
- Use aerobic exercise as well as motor control training.
- Include exercise of non-painful parts of the body (including cross-education and strength training of the other limb).
- Use multiple and long recovery breaks in between exercises.

What is patellofemoral osteoarthritis?

Patellofemoral osteoarthritis (OA) can be a considerable source of anterior knee symptoms and functional limitations,[42] with a growing body of evidence indicating that patellofemoral OA occurs before tibiofemoral disease[43] and can affect young to middle-aged adults.[44] Specific risk factors for early-onset patellofemoral OA development include a history of patellofemoral dysfunction (i.e. pain, dislocation, cartilage lesions), ACL rupture, and meniscal tears. Evidence updates, to highlight the importance of patellofemoral OA, are outlined in the box below.

Patellofemoral osteoarthritis as a source of anterior knee pain in active young adults

Is patellofemoral OA related to PFP?
The best available evidence suggests that PFP and patellofemoral OA may exist on a continuum;[45] retrospective recall of PFP is associated with radiographic[46] and MRI[47] features of patellofemoral OA. While not all patients with PFP will develop patellofemoral OA, PFP should be considered to be more than simply a benign, self-limiting condition and therefore be managed with appropriate evidence-based interventions.

Is patellofemoral OA a consequence of acute knee injuries?
Anterior cruciate ligament injury increases the risk of tibiofemoral and patellofemoral OA.[48] Five years after ACL injury, radiographic patellofemoral OA is evident in 19% of knees, regardless of conservative or surgical management or graft type used,[49] while MRI evidence of patellofemoral OA is observed in 17% of individuals at 1 year following ACL reconstruction.[50] By 10 years after ACL reconstruction, almost 50% of people will demonstrate radiographic patellofemoral OA.[51] Meniscal tears requiring partial meniscectomy, either in association with ACLR[52] or in isolation,[53] are associated with 2–5 times greater odds of patellofemoral OA development than knees without meniscal pathology over the following 8–20 years.

The mechanisms driving the development of post-traumatic patellofemoral OA following ACL and meniscal injury are not well understood, but may relate to concomitant damage to the PFJ at the time of initial trauma, or inherent biomechanics that are risk factors for both PFP and ACL injury (e.g. high knee abduction moments).[54]

Patellofemoral trauma, such as patellar dislocation, doubles the risk of patellofemoral OA at 13 years post-injury (22% vs 11%), irrespective of non-operative or surgical management.[55] The onset of post-traumatic patellofemoral OA may be mediated by the presence of a patellofemoral articular cartilage lesion—a particularly common finding in the unstable PFJ (97%),[56] which predicts future cartilage loss[57] and the development of radiographic patellofemoral OA.[51]

Can we identify people with or at high risk for patellofemoral OA?
The presence of knee crepitus and history of patellar pain are associated with patellofemoral joint OA (but not tibiofemoral joint OA) in women.[58] However, clinical examination findings and knee pain location have limited ability to discriminate those with patellofemoral OA from those with tibiofemoral OA.[24] Future studies may shed some light on diagnostic tests to recognise or predict patellofemoral OA in people with PFP.

Where to now for research and clinical practice?
The sensitivity of MRI to detect joint changes in the earliest stages of disease and recently proposed MRI-OA criteria[59] offer promise for early OA diagnosis, enabling studies of risk factors for early onset patellofemoral OA and evaluating interventions to be tested early in the disease process.

PART B Regional problems

Functional anatomy
At full extension, the patella sits lateral to the trochlea. During flexion, the patella moves medially and comes to lie within the intercondylar notch until 130° of flexion, when it starts to move laterally again.[35] With increasing knee flexion, a greater area of patellar articular surface comes into contact with the femur, thus offsetting the increased contact load that occurs with flexion. Loaded knee flexion activities subject the PFJ to loads ranging from 0.5 times body weight for level walking to seven to eight times body weight for stair climbing.[36]

Factors that may contribute to patellofemoral pain
Patellofemoral pain is likely to be initiated by increased or unaccustomed PFJ loads. Factors that influence PFJ load can be considered in two categories: extrinsic and intrinsic. During physical activities the extrinsic load is created by the body's contact with the ground (ground reaction force) and is therefore moderated by body mass, speed of gait, surfaces and footwear. The number of loading cycles and frequency of loading are also important. During weight-bearing activities, any increase in the amount of knee flexion will increase the PFJ load. Therefore, when an individual experiences an increase in the magnitude of the PFJ load (e.g. higher training volume, increased speed of running), this may overload the PFJ structures sufficiently to initiate pain. Note that activities with a high eccentric component, such as bounding, will overload the PFJ structures but are more likely to lead to patellar tendon pain.

Intrinsic factors can influence both the magnitude and the distribution of the PFJ load. Distribution of load is influenced by the alignment of the patella within the femoral trochlea, also known as patella tracking. Intrinsic factors that can influence patella tracking may be considered as 'remote' or 'local'. Considering the patient as a whole, 'remote' factors that affect patella tracking include femoral and tibial rotations. These factors can in turn be influenced by hip muscle strength, trunk kinematics, subtalar pronation and muscle flexibility (discussed below).[60] Local factors that influence patella movement include bony shape of the patella and trochlea, soft tissue tension and neuromuscular control of the medial and lateral components of the vasti.[61]

Therefore, when the initial subjective and objective examinations are completed and the diagnosis of PFP is confirmed, the clinician should assess the contribution of various extrinsic and intrinsic factors to the development of PFP.

> **PRACTICE PEARL**
>
> Although the history provides valuable information pertaining to extrinsic factors, clinical examination is usually required to evaluate the key intrinsic contributing factors ('remote' and 'local'). This comprehensive assessment is crucial in the planning treatment.

'Remote' intrinsic factors
The following 'remote' intrinsic factors may contribute to PFP developing (see also Chapter 8):

- increased hip/femoral internal rotation
- Increased hip adduction
- increased apparent knee valgus/external tibial rotation
- poor trunk and pelvic control
- pronated foot type
- sagittal plane motions.

It is important to assess the patient in static postures and during functional activities. Some factors may become more obvious during specific functional tasks, such as the step-down or single-leg squat and hopping or landing from a jump, where the postural demands are high. Once a potential contributing factor has been identified, the clinician must investigate the mechanisms that may require intervention (Table 36.6a–d).

Increased femoral/hip internal rotation
Increased femoral/hip internal rotation motions are associated with PFP[62-65] and may contribute to its development.[66] Clinical observation of the patient in standing reveals internally rotated femurs, often manifesting as 'squinting patellae'–the patellae both face medially. During tasks of increasing load, further internal rotation of the thigh can often be observed and may be visualised as an apparent knee valgus.

Increased hip adduction motions
Increased hip adduction motion may increase valgus load on the knee during dynamic tasks[62] and has been associated with PFP.[63-68] Clinical observation of the patient in standing may not reveal any abnormality. During functional tasks such as a single-leg squat, adduction of the thigh can often be observed and is usually associated with a pelvic drop towards the non weight-bearing leg.

Increased apparent knee valgus and/or increased tibial external rotation
Genu valgum (knee valgus or abduction) may be associated with PFP and observed in standing. This

Anterior knee pain CHAPTER 36

Table 36.6a Remote factors that can contribute to patellofemoral pain syndrome and their possible mechanisms—increased femoral internal rotation

Increased femoral/hip rotation	Possible contributing factors	Confirmatory assessments
	Structural: • femoral anteversion	Imaging—MRI, radiography
	Inadequate strength/control: • hip external rotators • hip abductors • hip extensors • lumbopelvic muscles	Clinical assessment: • manual muscle test (Figs 28.3a, b) • hand-held dynamometer • biofeedback
	Range of motion deficits: • inadequate ankle dorsiflexion range • inadequate hip external rotation range	Range of motion tests: • clinical inclinometer (Chapter 8) • figure '4' or FABER test (Fig. 31.6c)
	Altered movement patterns	Biomechanical/gait assessment (Chapter 8): • can the patient correct the movement pattern when asked to focus on it?

Table 36.6b Remote factors that can contribute to patellofemoral pain syndrome and their possible mechanisms—increased hip adduction

Increased hip adduction	Possible contributing factors	Confirmatory assessments
	Inadequate strength/control: • hip external rotators • hip abductors • hip extensors • lumbopelvic muscles • trunk muscles	Clinical assessment: • manual muscle test • hand-held dynamometer • side-bridge tests • biofeedback
	Altered movement patterns	Biomechanical/gait assessment (Chapter 8): • can the patient correct the movement pattern when asked to focus on it?

may be exaggerated during gait, possibly associated with a midstance valgus thrust. Additionally, increased hip adduction/internal rotation or a lateral pelvic drop during the step-down and single-leg squats (potentially owing to weakness of the gluteus medius) may be observed as an increase in apparent knee valgus posture. Knee abduction is associated with PFP.[63,-65, 67, 69, 70] Increased structural or functional tibial rotations can affect PFJ loads directly and also through transferred rotations to the femur. Importantly, tibial rotations are strongly coupled with the motion of the subtalar joint. Although there is little data on the assessment or treatment of structural tibial rotation in isolation, experienced clinicians often address functional rotation in association with femoral or subtalar rotations (see treatment outline later).

PART B Regional problems

Table 36.6c Remote factors that can contribute to patellofemoral pain syndrome and their possible mechanisms—increased knee valgus/tibial external rotation

Increased apparent knee valgus/tibial external rotation	Possible contributing factors	Confirmatory assessments
	Structural: • genu varum • tibial varum • coxa varum	Radiographic: • long leg X-ray Clinical assessment: • goniometer/inclinometer
	Inadequate strength/control: • hip external rotators • hip extensors • hip abductors • quadriceps • hamstrings • lumbopelvic muscles	Clinical assessment: • manual muscle test • hand-held dynamometer • biofeedback
	Altered movement patterns	Biomechanical/gait assessment (Chapter 8): • can the patient correct the movement pattern when asked to focus on it?

Table 36.6d Remote factors that can contribute to patellofemoral pain syndrome and their possible mechanisms—increased trunk lean

Increased trunk lean	Possible contributing factors	Confirmatory assessments
	Inadequate strength/control: • trunk extensors/flexors/rotators • hip abductors/adductors • hip extensors/flexors • lumbopelvic muscles	Clinical assessment: • manual muscle test • hand-held dynamometer • biofeedback
	Inadequate strength/control: • hip external rotators • hip extensors • hip abductors • quadriceps • hamstrings • lumbopelvic muscles	Clinical assessment: • manual muscle test • hand-held dynamometer • biofeedback
	Altered movement patterns	Biomechanical/gait assessment (Chapter 8): • can the patient correct the movement pattern when asked to focus on it?

Trunk and pelvic motions

The trunk represents the largest proportion of body mass and hence any alterations to trunk and pelvic motions can influence lower limb loads, including those of the PFJ. Although not studied as frequently as other segments, recent studies have focused on trunk and pelvic motions and their influence on PFJ loads.[71] Increased trunk flexion is associated with lower PFJ stress.[71] Furthermore, people with PFP exhibited greater anterior (forward) and ipsilateral trunk lean and contralateral trunk drop, compared to controls.[63, 65, 72, 73] Clinical observation of the patient in standing may not reveal any abnormality. During functional activities such as a single leg squat, ipsilateral trunk lean may be observed, often in association

Anterior knee pain CHAPTER 36

with contralateral pelvic drop. Observing the patient from the side may reveal inadequacies in sagittal plane motion (i.e. too much or too little forward trunk lean or anterior pelvic tilt).

Dynamic foot function
Dynamic foot function (e.g plantar loading) and static foot posture (e.g. increased pronation, navicular drop, arch height mobility) are associated with PFP and may contribute to its development.[63, 65, 66, 74-78] Static foot posture can be observed clinically in standing and during gait (Chapter 8).

Sagittal plane
Recently, studies have focused on frontal plane and transverse plane motions when evaluating people with PFP. Sagittal plane impairments should also be considered. In particular, loss of knee flexion[79-81] and greater trunk flexion[72, 73, 82] are features of people with PFP. While some of these adaptations may serve to reduce PFJ reaction force and hence joint stress, over time they may be associated with atrophy of key muscle groups (especially quadriceps) or increased frontal plane knee loads[83] with potential for further damage to the PFJ.[84] Hence, all patients should be observed from the side, to check for loss of sagittal plane motions.

Local contributing factors
Local factors that can contribute to the development of PFP are in three main categories (Table 36.7):

- patella position
- soft tissue contributions
- quadriceps (vasti) dysfunction.

Patella position
Clinical examination provides valuable information on the structural and functional relationships of the PFJ

Table 36.7 Local factors that can contribute to patellofemoral pain

Factor	Structural observations	Functional observations (with quadriceps contraction)
Patella position		
Lateral displacement	• Patella displaced laterally, closer to the lateral than medial femoral condyle • Restricted medial glide (Fig. 36.2f)	• Patella moves laterally
Lateral tilt	• Difficult to palpate lateral border, high medial border • Lateral tilt increases with passive medial glide	• Patella tilts laterally
Posterior tilt	• Inferior patella pole displaced posteriorly, often difficult to palpate due to infrapatellar fat pad	• Inferior pole moves further posteriorly. A 'dimple' may appear in the infrapatellar fat pad
Patella alta	• High-riding patella	• NA
Soft tissue contributions		
Tight lateral structures	• Lateral patella displacement or tilt • Palpation of lateral structures (Fig. 36.3)	• Lateral patella displacement or tilt
Compliant medial structures	• Lateral patella displacement or tilt	• Lateral patella displacement or tilt
General hypermobility	• NA	• Increased patellar mobility in all directions
Quadriceps (vasti) dysfunction		
Reduced activity of quadriceps (general)	• Reduced muscle bulk of quadriceps	• Reduced muscle strength
Delayed onset or reduced magnitude of VMO relative to VL	• Reduced muscle bulk of VMO	• Poor quantity/quality of VMO • Assess in functional positions • Biofeedback can assist (Fig. 36.4)

(Table 36.7). The clinician should carefully assess passive and active movement of the patella in all directions: medial (Fig. 36.2f), lateral, superior, and inferior glides, as well as rotations. Although the tests for patella position are not functional and may not be repeatable,[85, 86] clinical examination of the patella position remains a useful tool for clinical decision making.

Soft tissue contributions

The contribution of the superficial and deep soft tissues to the PFJ mechanics can, in part, be obtained from the structural and functional assessments of patella position. Palpation around the thigh, knee and lower leg allows the clinician to ascertain the compliance of soft tissues which may be contributing to PFP (Fig. 36.3).

Quadriceps (vasti) dysfunction

Individuals with PFP produce less quadriceps torque[87-89] and have smaller quadriceps size[90] than those without pain, and quadriceps weakness increases the risk of PFP development.[91]

There is controversy in the literature regarding an imbalance in vasti activation in PFP.[92-101] Inadequate vasti motor control could increase lateral patellar shift[102] or patellofemoral pressure.[103] Balanced activation of VMO and VL has long been believed to be disrupted in people with PFP, but the literature is inconsistent regarding imbalances in vasti activation or size and PFP pain.[99-101, 104-107] These inconsistencies may in part be accounted for by a wide variation in methodology and also by inherent heterogeneity in the PFP population, meaning that some, but not all, may have delayed VMO onset. Furthermore, the role of delayed EMG onset on medial vasti force production remains unknown.

Clinical examination of the vasti (medial and lateral components) provides some insight into their role in a patient's presentation (Table 36.7, Fig. 36.4). Frank muscle wasting and weakness may be obvious, but seemingly normal muscle bulk does not ensure normal function. If VMO dysfunction is suspected, then its ability to contract synchronously with the rest of the quadriceps should be evaluated. The vasti function should be assessed in a number of positions or activities, including those that are functionally relevant to the patient.

Treatment of PFP

Effective treatments usually integrate several different treatment techniques that target the local PFJ factors, in addition to the more remote (distal and proximal) factors. Different techniques, including exercise, manual therapy, taping, bracing and foot orthoses can be used in isolation or in combination, depending on the patient's presentation, the clinician's expertise and the preferences of both patient and clinician.[108] An integrated approach to management of a patient with PFP generally includes the following components:

- exercise
- taping
- manual therapy
- foot orthoses
- bracing.

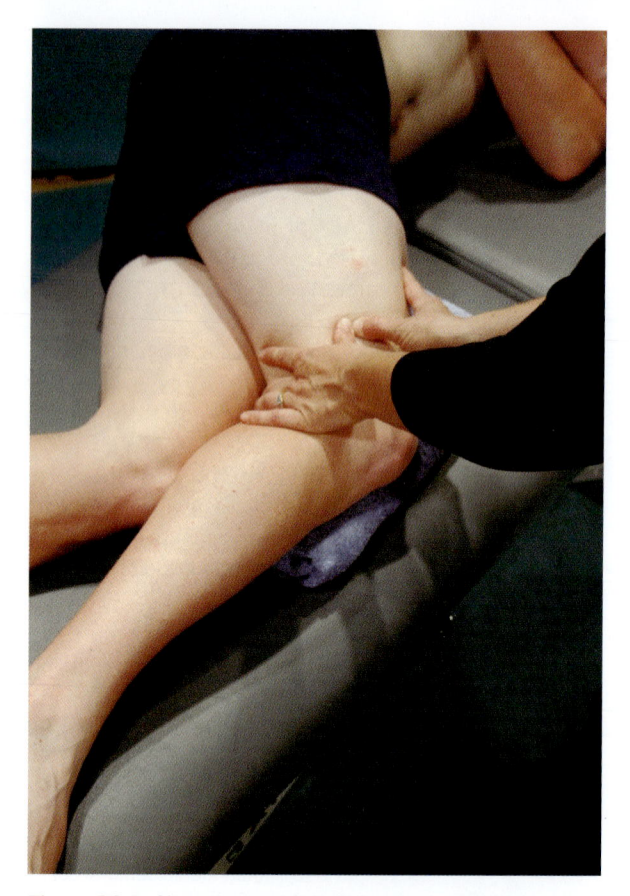

Figure 36.3 Clinical assessment of lateral soft tissue contribution. The iliotibial band and lateral retinacular structures are palpated for any reduced compliance

> **PRACTICE PEARL**
>
> The first priority of treatment is to reduce pain. Rest from aggravating activity usually suffices but it may require ice, a short course of oral analgesics (rarely) or techniques such as mobilisation (Fig. 36.7). Taping should have an immediate pain-relieving effect; when it does, this strongly suggests that the diagnosis is PFP (Fig. 36.6).

Anterior knee pain CHAPTER 36

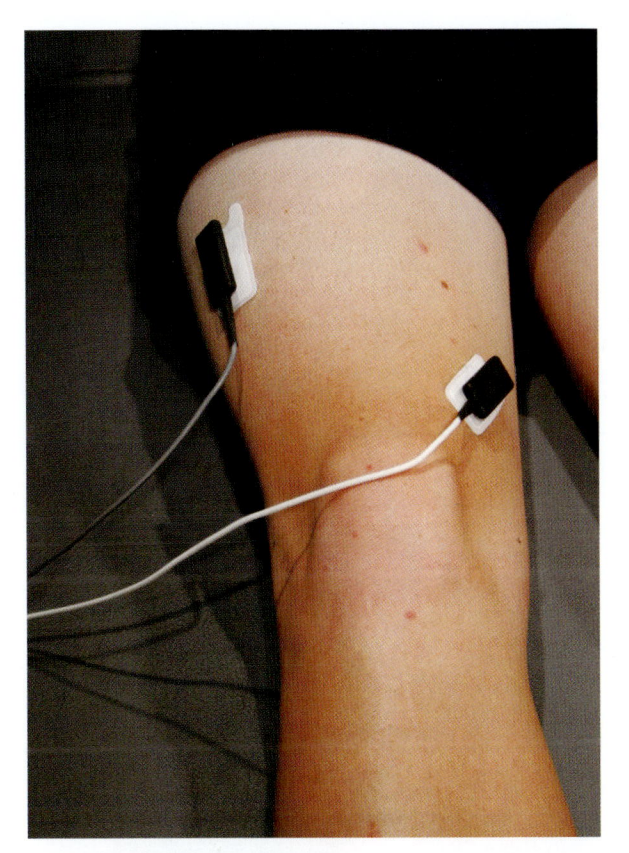

Figure 36.4 Clinical examination of neuromotor control of the vasti. The quality (amount and timing) of the vastus medialis obliquus and vastus lateralis component of the quadriceps can be assessed in a number of positions, including supine, sitting and standing. In these positions the patient is asked to contract the quadriceps. The clinician can either observe or palpate the quality of the contraction in these positions. A surface EMG biofeedback (illustrated) may be used to provide useful information to the clinician on the relative contribution of the vasti during quadriceps contractions across the various positions

Exercise

Exercise is a cornerstone of PFP management. Usual components include:

- quadriceps retraining
- hip muscle retraining
- strengthening/endurance building for lower limb and trunk muscles
- coordination and balance training
- retraining of functional activities (including sports- or work-related).

Not all patients will require all components. Using a pain monitoring system[109] (where pain levels scoring 0–3 on a 10 cm numerical pain scale are considered acceptable during exercise) may avoid pain-induced muscle inhibition and enhance adherence to an exercise program. Pain levels up to 5 (out of 10), momentarily during exercise or immediate following exercise are acceptable, but not extending to the following morning. Patellar taping may be required to ensure pain-free exercise.

Quadriceps retraining programs

Retraining the quadriceps can reduce PFP and symptoms,[108, 110-113] as well as enhance VMO activation relative to VL.[114] Patients cannot activate the VMO in isolation and no exercise appears to be preferential for activation of the VMO. Most people will not require a specific focus or emphasis on their VMO. However, for those who appear to have difficulty with VMO activation, it may be necessary to find and use training positions where the patient can attain a consistent VMO activation.

It may be necessary for the patient to learn to contract the VMO. By palpating the VMO while contracting their quadriceps in various degrees of knee flexion, hip abduction or knee rotation and/or in different activities the patient can receive feedback on the contraction. A dual-channel biofeedback machine may also be used (Fig. 36.4). The patient should attempt to recruit the VMO during all quadriceps contractions. Other strategies may assist VMO activation, including imagery or visual cues, facilitation techniques (e.g. palpation, dry needles/acupuncture), other forms of feedback (e.g. real-time ultrasound, tactile or visual) or inhibitory techniques to reduce over-activity in the VL or lateral hamstrings (e.g. inhibitory taping, feedback).

Initially, quadriceps exercises may commence in sitting with the knee at 90°, the foot on the floor and in this position, the patient may palpate the VMO to facilitate muscle activation (Fig. 36.5a). To ensure the quadriceps are trained in positions where they are required to function, the patient should begin training in a weight-bearing position and perform functional exercises with steadily increasing load and difficulty as soon as possible.

Progression is based on their ability to maintain control and the absence of significant pain (2–3 out of 10). Lower load exercises may include lunges, squats and step-ups. Further progressions can be made from minimal weight-bearing (using hand rails or other supports) to full weight-bearing (eventually including added loading) and through various knee flexion ranges.

The final aim of quadriceps training is to achieve a carry-over from functional exercises to functional activities. The patient should perform small numbers of exercises frequently throughout the day. A series of graded quadriceps exercises is demonstrated in Figure 36.5.

PART B   Regional problems

(a)

(b)

(c)

(d)

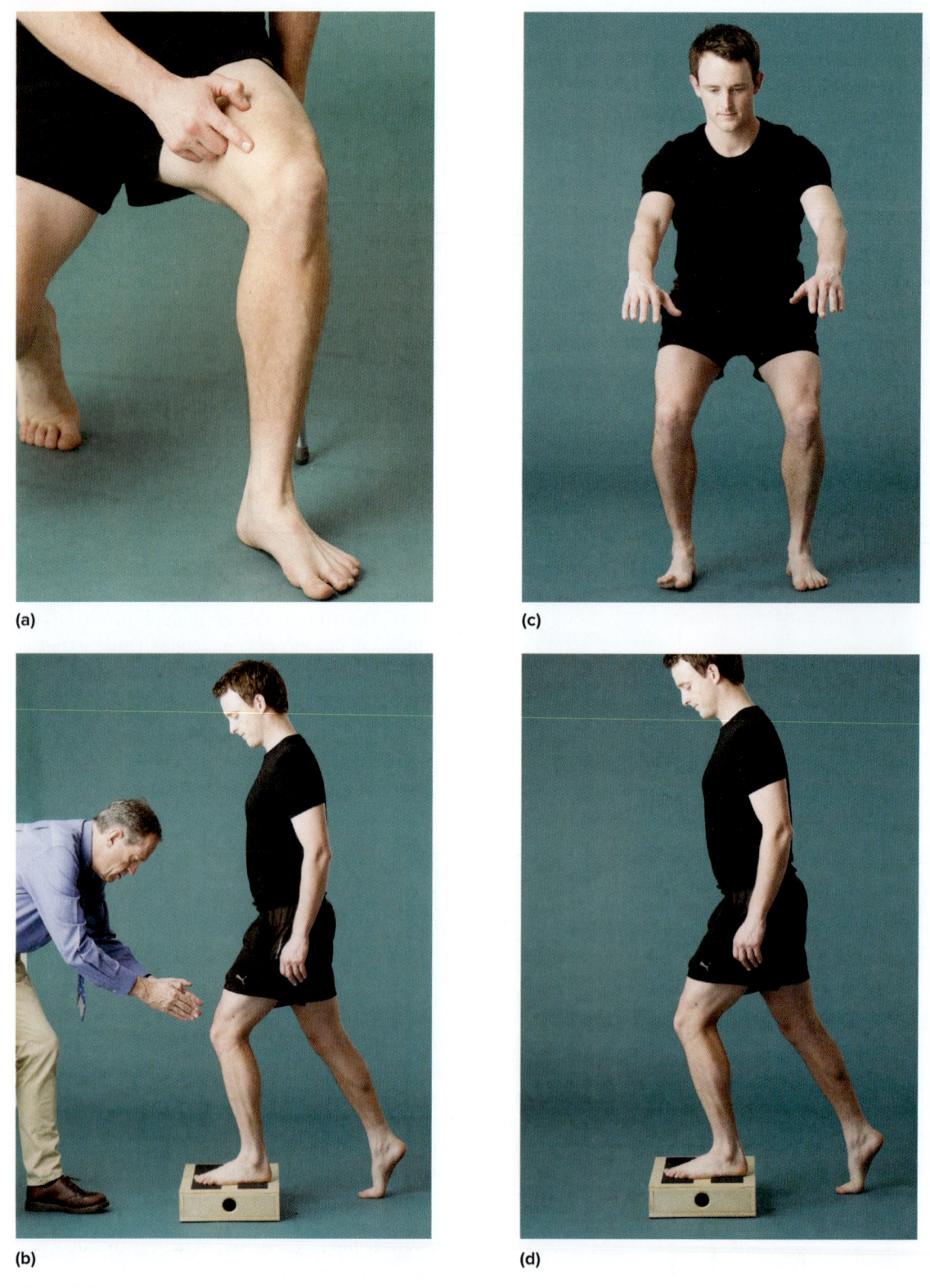

Figure 36.5 (a) Retraining focuses on increasing the patient's ability to activate their VMO, ideally with little VL activity or lateral hamstring co-contraction (b) Step-up with feedback on knee position (c) Double-leg squat (d) Step-up

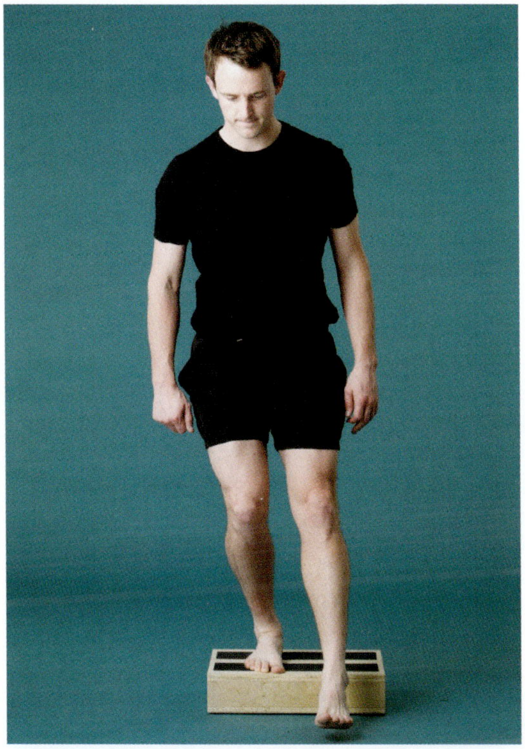

Anterior knee pain   CHAPTER 36

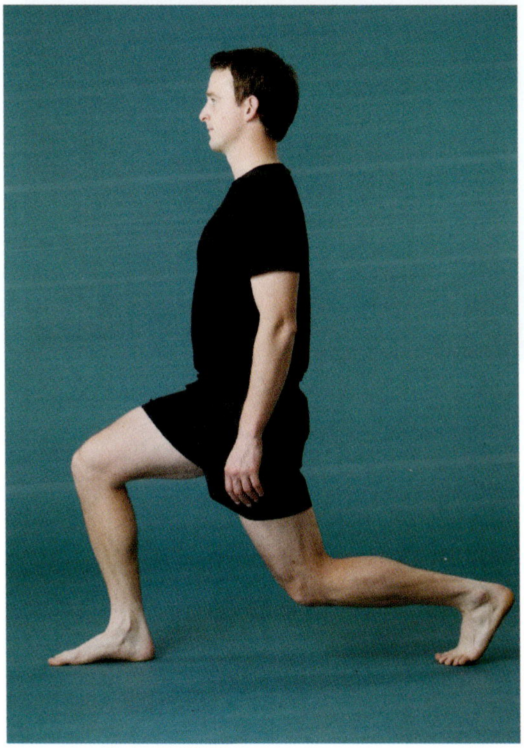

Figure 36.5 (cont.) (g) Standing on one leg, with single-leg squat catching a ball

Hip retraining programs

Retraining the hip abductors, external rotators and extensors is thought to stabilise the lateral pelvis and to control internal hip rotation and adduction. Such strengthening programs have been associated with pain reduction in patients with PFP.[115] Indeed, evidence suggests that hip retraining is an essential component to any PFP rehabilitation. The principles for retraining hip muscle function are the same as above, with exercises performed initially in non weight-bearing positions and then progressed to weight-bearing positions (Fig. 36.5). It is critical to ensure that the targeted muscles are being activated during the retraining program. For example, if your assessment reveals that hip external rotator retraining is required then the retraining programs must be activating the hip external rotators. More detail on hip retraining exercises is available in Chapter 31. The focus of all retraining exercises is on quality, then quantity.

As soon as it is possible and practical, the patient must be taught to activate the hip abductors, extensors and

Figure 36.5 (cont.) (e) Single-leg step-down (f) Lunge

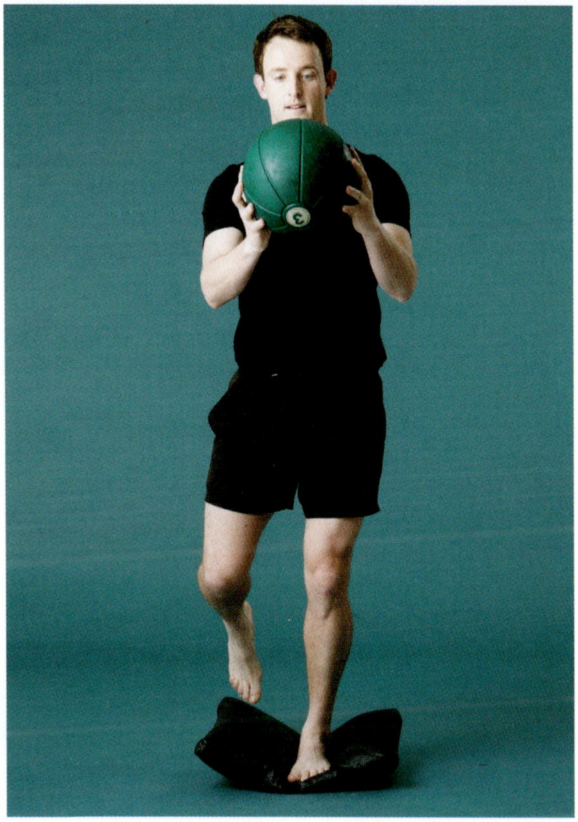

785

external rotators, in combination with other lower limb muscles during functional exercises. The emphasis of all retraining exercises will be on maintaining the activation of these muscles and correct alignment of the hip (i.e. neutral rotation) during weight-bearing flexion tasks (e.g. lunge, step up and step down. Some patients may require retraining of their movement patterns during functional or potentially aggravating activities.[116]

Lower limb strengthening/endurance-building exercises

Adequate strength and endurance, especially in the quadriceps, hip, trunk and calf muscles, is likely to be important for all patients. Strengthening programs can be commenced early (see above for maintaining control and monitoring pain) in the patient's treatment, and progressed according to patient response and American College of Sports Medicine guidelines.[117] A generalised quadriceps strengthening program can effectively relieve patellofemoral pain and improve function.[112] However, patients with poor vasti or hip coordination may first need to address their motor control deficits. The available evidence does not support the effectiveness of one exercise regimen over another.

Movement retraining

This is required in the final stage of the exercise-based interventions in order to return to high loaded activities involving knee flexion during full weight-bearing (e.g. stair descent, deep squats), or higher intensity activities such as running. Patients need additional training to facilitate progression to these high PFJ loading activities. Motor control, strength and endurance in the quadriceps and global muscles (e.g. calf, hip and trunk muscles), balance and coordination should be trained in these higher loading tasks. Exercise choice and progression decisions are based on the patient's needs, their ability to maintain control and the absence of significant pain. More detail on movement (and running) retraining is available in Chapter 8.

Patellar taping

The aim of taping is to correct the abnormal position of the patella in relation to the femur. Although patellar taping reduces PFP substantially and immediately,[118] the precise mechanism of the effect is still being investigated. It is possible that pain relief following patella taping could be due to subtle changes in patella position and PFJ contact area[119] and/or changes in motor control or proprioceptive input.[120] Regardless of the mechanism, patella taping is an effective interim measure to relieve PFP and can increase adherence to an exercise program and/or enable pain-free activities of daily living.

A commonly used technique involves taping the patella with a medial glide (Fig. 36.6a). It may also require correction of abnormal lateral tilt (Fig. 36.6b), rotation (Fig. 36.6c) or inferior tilt (Fig. 36.6d). The taping is performed with rigid strapping tape. It is important that the clinician recognises a posteriorly displaced inferior pole of the patella, as taping the patella too low will increase the patient's symptoms. Taping to 'unload' the fat pad (effectively to 'lift' the patella away from

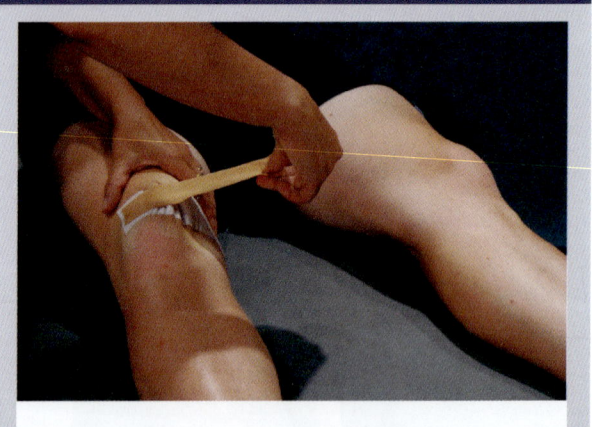

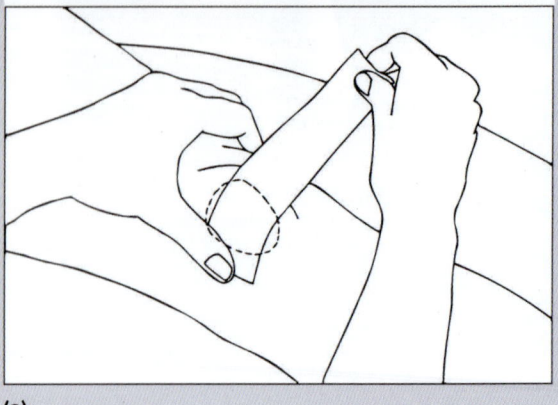

Figure 36.6 Patellar taping techniques (a) Patellar taping (medial glide). Tape is applied to the lateral aspect of the patella. The patella is glided medially and the tape is anchored to the skin over the medial aspect of the knee. When taping is completed, skin creases should be evident on the inside of the knee, indicating adequate tension on the patella

(a)

Anterior knee pain   CHAPTER 36

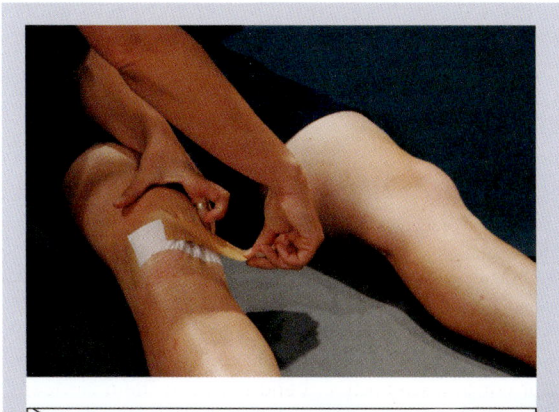

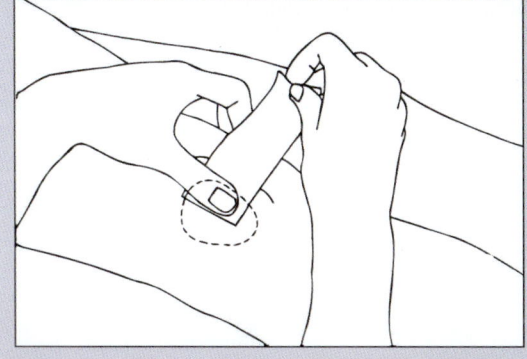

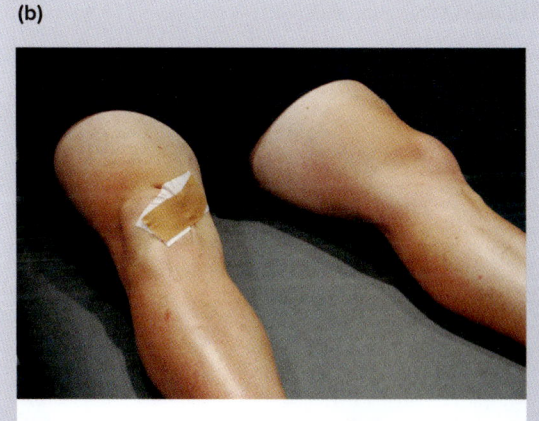

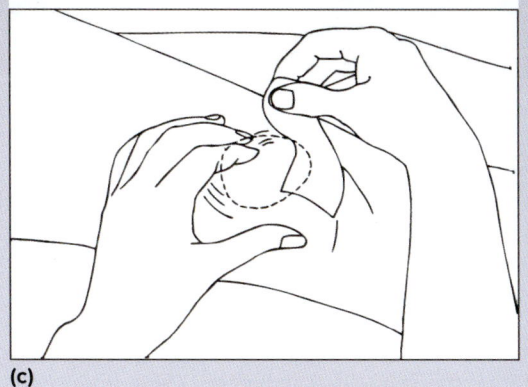

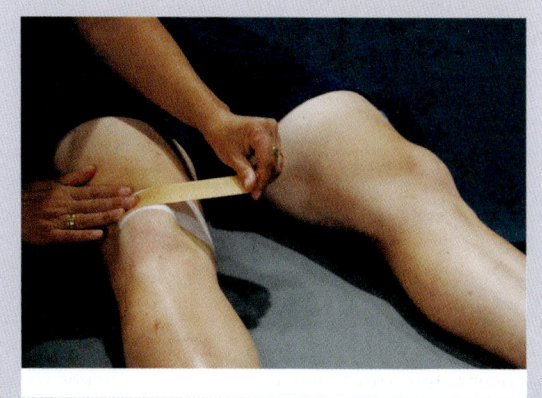

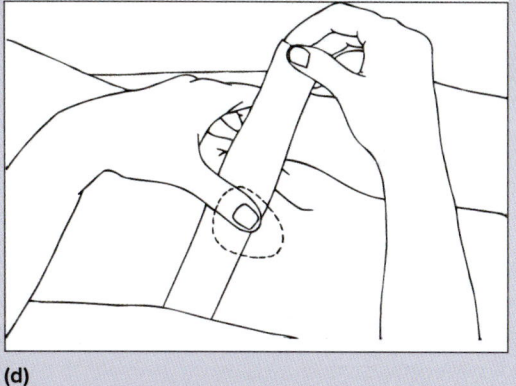

Figure 36.6 (cont.) (b) Patellar taping (correction of lateral tilt). Tape is applied to the medial aspect of the patella and secured to the soft tissue on the inner aspect of the knee (c) Patellar taping (correction of rotation). Tape is applied to the inferior pole of the patella and taken medially and superiorly to rotate the patella (d) Patellar taping (correction of inferior tilt). Tape is applied across the superior pole of the patella with sufficient firmness to elevate the inferior pole

the fat pad) can also be used, either alone or in conjunction with the above techniques (see below, 'Fat pad irritation/impingement' for more details; Fig. 36.15).

Patella taping effects should be assessed immediately using a pain-provoking activity such as a single- or double-leg squat. If the tape has been applied correctly and is going to be a useful treatment option, the post-taping squat will be less painful. If all or some pain persists, the tape should be altered, possibly including a component for tilt or rotation or both. Note that if patella tape does not make a substantial (at least 50%) reduction in the patient's pain, the initial diagnosis should be revisited.

If patients are able to perform strengthening exercises pain-free without tape, then exercises should be performed

continued

tape free. Some people, however, require tape to perform the exercises and, initially, to continue their sporting activities. Acute cases of PFP may initially need tape applied 24 hours a day until the condition settles. The tape time is then gradually reduced.

Adverse skin reactions can occur beneath the rigid tape. Therefore, the area to be taped should be shaved and a protective barrier applied beneath the rigid strapping tape to reduce both the reaction to the zinc oxide in the tape adhesive and the reaction to shearing stresses on the skin. This can be achieved with adhesive gauze tape (Hypafix® or Fixomull®) applied to the area to be taped. A protective barrier or plastic skin can also be used in patients with extremely sensitive skin. If skin irritation still occurs, the patient must be advised to remove the tape. Treatment with a hydrocortisone cream may be necessary. Patients with fair skin seem to have particularly sensitive skin and need to be monitored closely.

Manual therapies

Manual therapies, such as joint and soft tissue mobilisation, manipulation and massage may relieve symptoms associated with PFP. Joint mobilisations can include patellofemoral or tibiofemoral joint glides, whereas soft tissue therapies might involve massage of tight lateral retinacular structures or the fascia/muscles of the thigh (predominantly anterolateral). Applied passively by either the patient or clinician, these techniques are designed to optimise movement and facilitate the exercise program. When applied by the clinician, the patient may be in a side-lying position with the knee flexed. The therapist glides the patella medially using the heel of the hand for a sustained stretch (Fig. 36.7). Other simple stretching techniques can be performed by the patient, usually in sitting, with the knee flexed approximately 30–90°. Studies evaluating efficacy of such techniques applied in isolation do not show benefit,[121] supporting the clinical practice to include manual therapy as part of a combined approach to management and not performed in isolation.

Attention must also be paid to improving the compliance of the hip flexors, quadriceps, hamstring and calf muscles as well as the iliotibial band if required, through stretches, soft tissue techniques (Fig. 36.8) or dry needling. Restoration of optimal muscle and fascial length is the goal. Further detail on soft tissue techniques including dry needling are available in Chapter 17.

In-shoe foot orthoses

Prefabricated in-shoe foot orthoses, combined with active retraining of the extrinsic muscles of the foot, improve pain and physical function in people with PFP.[111] Although the mechanisms underpinning the clinical effects are unclear, it appears both neuromuscular and mechanical factors need to be considered when prescribing in-shoe foot orthoses.[122] A clinical decision-making paradigm has been proposed to assist with orthosis prescription for people with PFP[123] (see also Chapter 8).

Pain reduction during aggravating activities with either anti-pronation taping or an orthosis, may indicate

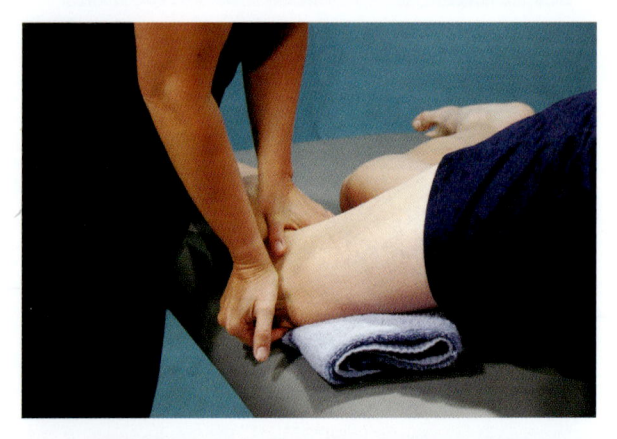

Figure 36.7 Mobilisation of the patella (supine or side-lying)

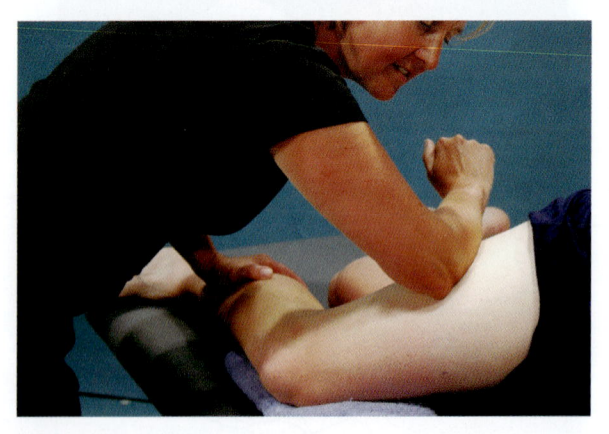

Figure 36.8 Soft tissue therapy—myofascial tension of the iliotibial band

which patients are more likely to have a favourable response to orthoses.[124, 125] Older people with less severe pain and a more mobile midfoot are more likely to experience success with orthosis intervention.[123] Additionally, the clinician might consider customised foot orthoses or changing footwear, although the efficacy of these interventions is unknown. These interventions are discussed in Chapter 8.

Anterior knee pain CHAPTER 36

Braces

Some braces (Fig. 36.9) are commercially available to maintain medial glide. Patella braces reduce patella displacement, increase patella contact area[126] and reduce PFJ stress[127] in individuals with PFP. However, an RCT of such a brace did not find any benefit of the brace over a 'sham' knee sleeve or a general quadriceps strengthening program.[128] Braces are less specific than taping and do not specifically address tilt or rotation; but they may have a role in those patients who are unable to wear tape or who suffer recurrent patella subluxation or dislocation.

Evidence base for physical and exercise interventions

A number of systematic reviews and meta-analyses of randomised clinical trials have assessed the efficacy of physical interventions for PFP (Table 36.8). Level I evidence supports the use of multimodal interventions (combination of retraining, strengthening, balance/coordination, functional retraining, taping and manual therapy)[112] and also for individual treatments in isolation.[112,129,130] Proximal (mostly hip) rehabilitation programs, when combined with a quadriceps program, decreases pain in the short and medium term, and emerging evidence suggests that proximal retraining, either combined with quadriceps retraining or in isolation, may be superior to quadriceps retraining alone.[115] While tailored patellar taping produces immediate pain reduction, other techniques result in only small (untailored medial patellar taping) or negligible (kinesiotape) pain reductions in the immediate term.

Limited evidence supports better short-term outcomes with foot orthoses versus flat inserts,[112,129] versus 'wait and see',[131] and beneficial effects for exercise (versus control), closed chain exercises (versus open chain exercises) and acupuncture (versus control).[112] However, there is moderate evidence for no additive effectiveness of knee braces to exercise therapy on pain and conflicting evidence on function.[132]

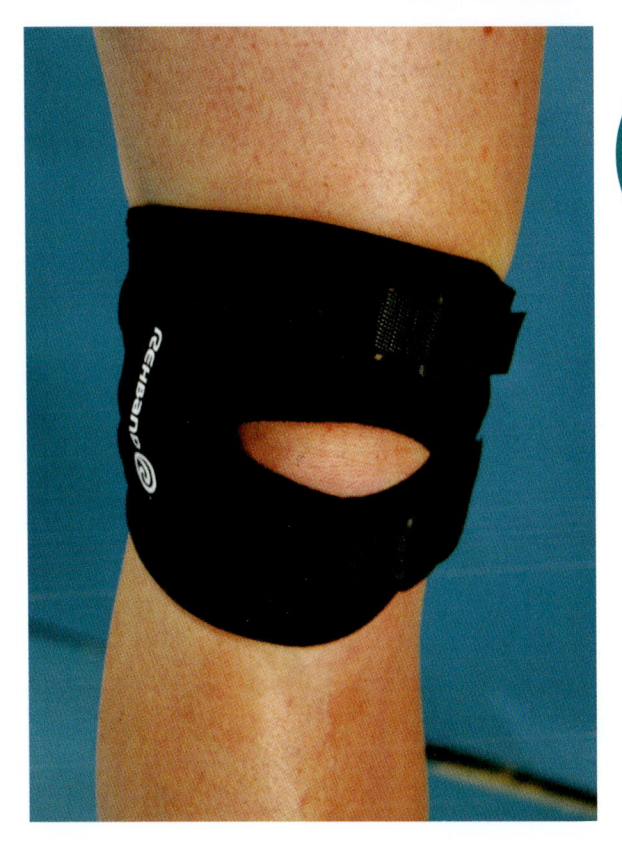

Figure 36.9 Patella stabilising brace

Table 36.8 Best available evidence for the physical and exercise interventions for patellofemoral pain (since 2010)

Intervention	Level of evidence	Reference	Supported by consensus statements[113] or Best Practice Guide[108]
Combined intervention (exercise, education, manual therapy, taping)	1	**Collins 2012**[133] **Bolgla 2011**[134]	Yes[113] Yes[108]
Exercise therapy	1	**van der Heijden 2015**[130] **Collins 2012**[133] **Lack 2015**[135] **Kooiker 2014**[136] **Clijsen 2014**[137]	Yes[113] Yes[108]
Hip muscle retraining	1	**van der Heijden 2015**[130] **Lack 2015**[135] **Bolgla 2011**[134] **Clijsen 2014**[137]	Yes[113] Yes[108]

continued

Table 36.8 Cont.

Intervention	Level of evidence	Reference	Supported by consensus statements[113] or Best Practice Guide[108]
Foot orthoses	1	**Barton 2010**[129] **Bolgla 2011**[134] **Collins 2012**[133] **Hossain 2010**[138]	Yes[113] Yes[108]
Patellar taping: immediate effects	1	**Barton 2014**[118] **Collins 2012**[133]	Uncertain[113] Yes[108]
Kinesiotaping	1	Kalron 2013[139]	Not included[113] Not included[113]
Patellar taping: medium/long-term effect	1	**Callaghan 2012**[140]	Uncertain[113] Yes[108]
Acupuncture	1	**Collins 2012**[133]	Uncertain[113] Yes[108]
Gait/movement retraining	5	Barton 2015[108]	Uncertain[113] Yes[108]
Mobilisation	1	**Collins 2012**[133]	No[113]
Bracing	1	**Swart 2012**[132]	Uncertain[113] No[108]
Electrotherapeutic agents	1	Lake 2011[141] **Collins 2012**[133]	No[113] No[108]

Blue = supported by meta-analyses (systematic reviews)
Black = expert opinion, clinical guidelines
Orange = insufficient evidence
Red = no evidence supporting its use
Bold text = reviews considered to be moderate or high quality

Although the interventions tested in clinical trials reflect some aspects of clinical practice, in many studies the interventions are not individualised to the patient's needs. Furthermore, some studies have evaluated one aspect of intervention in isolation. These studies have enabled the assessment of a single treatment strategy, but the study results may not be generalised to clinical scenarios. Therefore, while the evidence base for different combinations of physical or exercise therapies for PFP is increasing in quality and quantity, clinicians need to individualise their treatment approaches, thus targeting the treatment to their patient's presentations and requirements and clinician preferences and expertise.[108]

Addressing extrinsic contributing factors

Although the patient should reduce the load on the PFJ initially, it is essential that as rehabilitation progresses, any extrinsic factors that may have been placing excessive load on the PFJ (e.g. training, shoes, surfaces) be addressed.

Surgery: to be avoided

Experienced clinicians will have observed that surgery is now much less common for PFP than it was 30 years ago. This is likely to be due to the availability of evidence-based, exercise-based, physical interventions. To date, no surgical RCT has demonstrated the effectiveness of treatments such as chondroplasty or lateral release for PFP. Surgery should only be an option for athletes/patients whom have failed a number of attempts of conservative interventions. Poor surgical outcomes have been reported in the literature.[142]

> **PRACTICE PEARL**
>
> Patient education is an important element of effective treatment. A number of resources exist, including Barton and Rathleff www.patellofemoral.completesportscare.com.au/wp-content/uploads/2014/11/Managing-my-patellofemoral-pain_education_single-sheets.pdf.

Anterior knee pain CHAPTER 36

Patellofemoral osteoarthritis can be managed using an approach similar to patellofemoral pain

Can we prevent patellofemoral OA in people with patellofemoral pain or ACL injury?

Strategies targeting prevention of PFP and traumatic knee injuries are vital to prevent patellofemoral OA in active adults. Following knee injury or PFP, treatments to optimise patellofemoral biomechanics may reduce the risk of patellofemoral OA.

Until more research can determine which features of an individual makes them more likely to develop OA after PFP or knee injuries such as ACL or meniscal, interventions with potential to reduce PFJ stress (e.g. patellofemoral malalignment, low quadriceps strength, higher body mass, valgus knee malalignment) should be included as part of a treatment package. Furthermore, it is probably never too early to discuss the possibility of chronic knee pain, and the need for ongoing management of the knee.

How do we treat people with established radiographic patellofemoral OA?

Once patellofemoral OA has developed, non-surgical management is the preferred primary treatment. Although few clinical trials exist to inform best-practice management, multimodal physiotherapy treatment (i.e. exercise, education, manual therapy and taping)[143] and knee braces[144] may be efficacious. Patellar bracing may improve PFJ kinematics and knee pain, and shrink BMLs in those with patellofemoral OA.[145, 146] Although tibiofemoral and patellofemoral OA frequently coexist, it is inappropriate to assume that treatments designed for tibiofemoral OA are optimal for patellofemoral OA.

Can we optimise treatments for patellofemoral OA?

To improve treatments for those with patellofemoral OA, we need to recognise the clinical findings that identify and discriminate them from tibiofemoral OA.[24]

A number of factors associated with patellofemoral OA may alter the mechanics of the patellofemoral joint and increase joint stress, leading to OA. Identification of these impairments in patients with patellofemoral OA may lead to targeted and personalised interventions, with capacity to not only reduce the symptoms but have potential to slow disease progression. Such factors include:

- **Abnormal patellofemoral joint alignment and trochlear morphology** These are associated with patellofemoral OA (both radiographic and MRI features).
- **Muscle weakness** Quadriceps function, such as muscle size,[147] strength[148, 149] and muscle force,[150] is impaired in people with patellofemoral OA, and quadriceps weakness is a risk factor for patellofemoral OA.[151, 152] Impairment in proximal muscle function is also evident on patellofemoral OA.
- **Abnormal biomechanics** Abnormal movement patterns during functional activities may affect PFJ loading and stress,[153–155] which can lead to OA and pain[156–158] and are, therefore, potential targets for rehabilitation interventions. There is recent evidence that individuals with patellofemoral OA also demonstrate abnormal biomechanics during gait.[150, 152, 159–161] In the only longitudinal study to date, Teng et al. found that peak knee flexion moment and flexion moment impulse at baseline lead to progression of PFJ cartilage damage over 2 years.[162]

Note: Patellofemoral pain may predispose to the development of patellofemoral osteoarthritis and hence treatments should aim to not only reduce pain and symptoms but to address potential contributing factors.

How does our treatment need to change for adolescents with patellofemoral pain?

Patellofemoral pain is common in adolescents

Chances are that if you work in clinical setting you will see a lot of young patients with knee complaints. Up to 7% of the adolescent population may be affected (in varying severities) by PFP, making it one of the most common knee conditions among adolescents. Fifty percent of the adolescents with knee pain will, at some point, seek medical treatment, often through their general practitioner (in a Danish context).[163] This means that at some point, we are likely to meet them (and their parents) in the clinic. So how should we treat adolescents with PFP? Do they need to be treated differently to adults with PFP?

continued

PART B   Regional problems

Education and exercises
Combining exercise therapy and patient education is more effective than patient education alone in adolescents aged 15–19 with PFP.[164] Adding exercise therapy to patient education improves recovery rates in both the short term (3 months) and long term (24 months). However, not all adolescents respond favourably to the exercise therapy, and the overall recovery rate is lower than for adults. This suggests that exercise therapy is effective for some adolescents but not all. How can we improve the effect of exercise therapy among adolescents to ensure good outcomes?

Adherence and modifying the activity level are crucial
Two issues seem to be particular important when treating adolescents with PFP. One is adherence to exercise therapy, and the second is sports participation.[165] For highly active young adolescents, frequent sports participation is a risk factor for persistent knee pain and failure to modify sports participation may hinder recovery.[166, 167] This suggests that, in the group of highly active adolescents, PFP may result from excessive loading of the PFJ during sport and physical activity.[165] The clinical implication is that we need to educate both the adolescents and their parents to modify the adolescents' activity levels and make a gradual return to sport that is guided by symptoms.

The second important issue is adherence to exercise therapy. Adolescents with poor adherence (less than 1 exercise session per week) were 4 times less likely to be recovered after 12 months compared to those with good adherence (at least 3 exercise sessions per week)[164].

To improve adherence, it is essential that the adolescent and the parent are educated about the importance of adherence and understand why the exercises are important. If you suspect that the adolescent may not perform the prescribed home exercises, it might be relevant to focus on supervised exercises to improve outcomes.

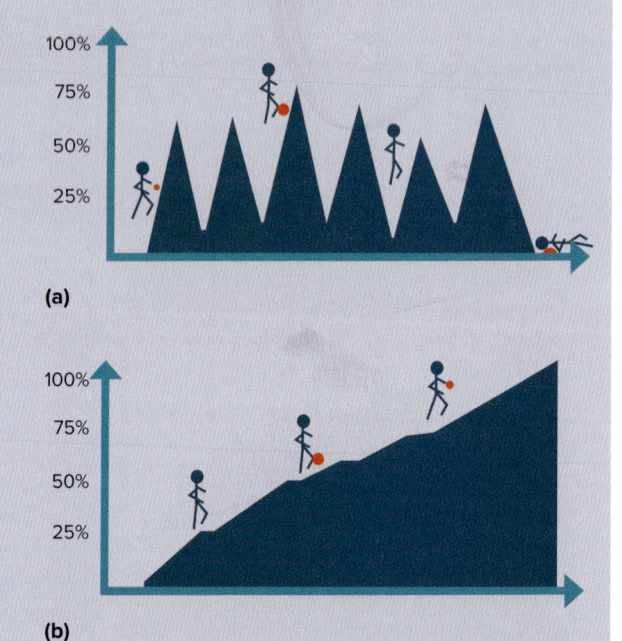

Figure 36.10 a and b Modifying the physical activity level may be key to successful treatment and to avoid recurrence of knee pain.

PATELLOFEMORAL INSTABILITY
Before discussing the causes of and treatments for, patellofemoral instability we need to clearly define the term. As is also the case at shoulder, 'instability', is not a synonym for 'dislocation'. Instability refers to excessive joint range of motion (and is often referred to as 'subluxation'). Patellofemoral instability may be primary (referred to as patellar subluxation) or secondary (meaning that the instability is due to previous acute patella dislocation) (see Chapter 35).

Primary patellofemoral instability
Factors that predispose to this condition include patella alta (a patella that is located more superiorly than normal), trochlear dysplasia and generalised ligamentous laxity. Patients usually describe sensations of instability (patella moving or slipping) and the pattern of tenderness around the patella may be similar to PFP or more generally distributed. Examination reveals patella hypermobility with apprehension and pain when the patella is pushed laterally by the clinician.

Treatment
Treatment of patellofemoral instability parallels that of PFP. The aim of acute management is to reduce pain and swelling. Patellar taping in combination with a knee extension brace may provide temporary immobilisation after an initial episode. The patient may use crutches for either partial or

> **PRACTICE PEARL**
>
> Rehabilitation to improve active support for the PFJ is paramount as dominant predisposing factors cannot be addressed easily (bony morphology and ligamentous laxity).

non weight-bearing in that instance. Rehabilitation requires a comprehensive multimodal approach, as outlined earlier for PFP to be commenced as soon as possible.

In acute situations, biofeedback and/or electrical stimulation may be required as an adjunct to vasti retraining. Taping (and/or bracing) may be part of long-term management. It is also vital to address any proximal and distal contributing factors (see above), maximise trunk and lower limb muscle strength and/or endurance and provide advice regarding avoiding aggravating activities.

Surgery is rarely indicated. Surgical approaches aim to correct the structural/anatomical predisposing factors, and techniques used include arthroscopic medial plication. Bony realignment procedures including 'trochleaplasties' have largely lost popularity in Scandinavia and Australia, but are performed in a limited number of countries including the United States. These interventions often do not have favourable outcomes, thus they should only be considered if a properly managed non-surgical program fails. An intensive rehabilitation program should be trialled prior to the athlete considering surgical options.

Secondary patellofemoral instability

Secondary instability results from a primary dislocation episode (see Chapter 35 for acute management) that is likely to have arisen because of rupture of the medial patellofemoral ligament. This ligament is the main static restraint to lateral patella translation (Fig. 35.17). It acts like a guy rope on a tent. Individuals with persistent patellofemoral instability after an acute dislocation may require additional investigations. Imaging (Fig. 35.18) may reveal evidence of osteochondral damage to the articular surface of the patella and femur as well as predisposing anatomical abnormalities.

Arthroscopy may be required to remove a loose osteochondral fragment, and, if appropriate, the medial patellofemoral ligament may need reconstruction.[168] As with surgery for primary instability, surgery for secondary instability also requires aggressive rehabilitation. Rehabilitation for secondary patellofemoral instability follows the same guidelines as primary patellofemoral instability. At the current time, there is limited evidence to suggest that surgical management of primary patella dislocation decreases the risk of recurrent dislocation.[169]

PATELLAR TENDINOPATHY

There have been substantial advances in understanding the management of this condition in the past decade. Successful management of the athlete with patellar tendinopathy requires thorough clinical and functional assessment and then appropriate load management.

Nomenclature

Patellar tendinopathy is otherwise known as 'jumper's knee' due to its frequency in jumping sports (e.g. basketball, volleyball and high, long and triple jumps).[170] However, the condition also occurs in athletes who change direction, as well as those who put large energy storage loads on their tendon, such as running downhill. The term 'patellar tendinitis' is a misnomer as the pathology underlying this condition is degenerative tendinosis rather than a purely inflammatory condition (see Chapter 4).[171] On balance, patellar tendinopathy is probably the most appropriate general label for this condition as it describes the clinical condition of pain and loss of function, independent of the underlying pathology.[172]

Clinical features

The clinical features of patellar tendinopathy are outlined in Table 36.2. The key to making an accurate clinical diagnosis is that the patient complains of well-localised (focal) pain at the attachment of the patellar tendon to the patella (Fig. 36.11). The tendon is frequently thickened. The pain is aggravated by jumping, changing direction and decelerating. Distal lesions are less common and midsubstance lesions are rarely reported.[173]

Clinicians should assess factors such as weakness of the lower limb musculature, including calf, quadriceps and gluteal muscles. This loss in muscle strength often results in dysfunction of the kinetic chain, especially in its ability to function as a spring. These deficits may predispose or be a consequence of pain, but either way are important to assess so that they may addressed in rehabilitation.

> **PRACTICE PEARL**
>
> Pain on palpation (i.e. tenderness) is not a useful test to diagnose tendinopathy in general (Chapter 14); it is not a helpful diagnostic test in patellar tendinopathy as pain at this site is common and does not indicate the pain is from the tendon. Most importantly, it is not a reliable outcome measure to assess response to rehabilitation.

Note that the proximal patellar tendon is often tender in jumping athletes with normal tendons therefore palpation has poor specificity for patellar tendinopathy. Also, some athletes with patellar tendon pathology are not tender at the junction of patellar tendon and the patella–hence the test does not have perfect sensitivity. Note that palpation is also not a useful test of recovery (outcome measure)–this is discussed later.

To make the diagnosis of patellar tendinopathy, the clinician must be able to reproduce the patient's focal

PART B   Regional problems

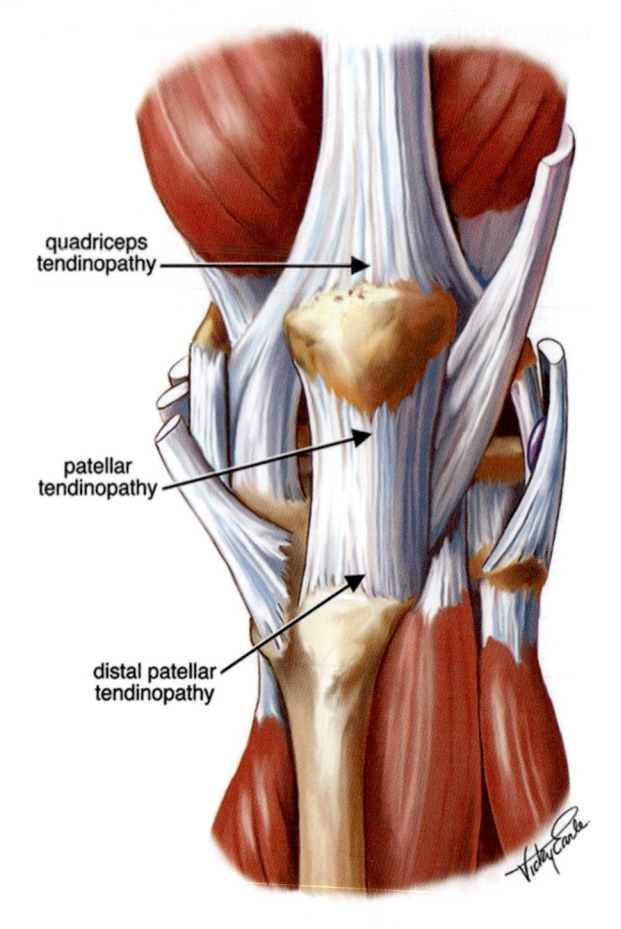

Figure 36.11 Sites of tendon pathology in the knee extensor mechanism. The most common presentation is patellar tendinopathy. Quadriceps tendinopathy is discussed later. Pain at the distal tendon (tibial tuberosity) can be associated with Osgood–Schlatter disease (Chapter 44)

pain when placing high loads on the tendon. The clinician should progressively increase the tendon load with functional activities, such as a squat, then progressing to a hop, to test the patient's ability to complete the task well and to reproduce the pain. In patellar tendinopathy the pain remains localised. If the pain becomes diffuse with loading, consider other diagnoses.

> **PRACTICE PEARL**
>
> Knee pain that is described as being diffuse with loading does not represent a clinical diagnosis of patellar tendinopathy (or tendon pain). Patients can perceive pain from the PFJ in the region of the patellar tendon.

In patellar tendinopathy, a useful outcome measure (Chapter 16) is pain on the decline squat (Fig. 36.2d). Document the amount of pain and the range when it occurs. An additional method to monitor the clinical progress of patellar tendinopathy is the VISA-P questionnaire (Table 36.9).[174, 175] This simple patient-completed questionnaire takes less than 5 minutes to complete.

Investigations

Ultrasound and MRI can image patellar tendon pathology. These imaging modalities have low sensitivity with better specificity for patellar tendinopathy (Fig. 36.12). Imaging findings need to be placed within the context of the clinical presentation and the loading history of the patient. Up to 50% of asymptomatic players in patellar tendon loading sports (e.g. volleyball, basketball) have imaging abnormalities.[22] These changes are best described as load-appropriate changes and do not contribute to making a clinical diagnosis.

Management: is the athlete still competing?

After making the diagnosis of patellar tendinopathy, the approach to management will vary if the player can keep competing or if the tendinopathy is at a level where the player needs to withdraw from competition and complete rehabilitation.

Factors that determine whether a player should keep playing or withdraw from competition are: the levels of (i) pain, (ii) function and (iii) effect on performance (Table 36.10). Players always want to keep playing and the clinician will support this where appropriate, but there are also times when the quality shared decision is for the player to withdraw from training and competition and undergo comprehensive rehabilitation.

As the player will want to keep competing in most cases, we address that scenario first. We discuss out-of-competition rehabilitation below.

The approach to 'in-season' treatment of the player with patellar tendinopathy

When the player presents with pain in-season, the clinician should discuss the key elements of treatment and explain that there is unlikely to be complete relief of pain during the season.

In-season management of patellar tendinopathy requires maintenance (or improvement) of strength in the affected muscle–tendon unit and the rest of the kinetic chain. Load reduction, correcting biomechanical factors and adjunct therapies such as soft tissue therapy to the affected muscle (not the tendon) are also appropriate in this scenario (detailed below).

Anterior knee pain — CHAPTER 36

Table 36.9 Victorian Institute of Sport Assessment (VISA-P) questionnaire (English version, this is available in numerous languages)[150]

1. For how many minutes can you sit pain-free? — POINTS
   0 min ─ 0 1 2 3 4 5 6 7 8 9 10 ─ 100 min

2. Do you have pain walking downstairs with a normal gait cycle? — POINTS
   Strong severe pain ─ 0 1 2 3 4 5 6 7 8 9 10 ─ No pain

3. Do you have pain at the knee with full active non-weight-bearing knee extension? — POINTS
   Strong severe pain ─ 0 1 2 3 4 5 6 7 8 9 10 ─ No pain

4. Do you have pain when doing a full weight-bearing lunge? — POINTS
   Strong severe pain ─ 0 1 2 3 4 5 6 7 8 9 10 ─ No pain

5. Do you have problems squatting? — POINTS
   Unable ─ 0 1 2 3 4 5 6 7 8 9 10 ─ No problems

6. Do you have pain during or immediately after doing 10 single-leg hops? — POINTS
   Strong severe pain ─ 0 1 2 3 4 5 6 7 8 9 10 ─ No pain

7. Are you currently undertaking sport or other physical activity? — POINTS
   - 0 ☐ Not at all
   - 4 ☐ Modified training ± modified competition
   - 7 ☐ Full training ± competition but not at same level as when symptoms began
   - 10 ☐ Competing at the same or higher level as when symptoms began

8. Please complete EITHER A, B, or C in this question.
   - If you have no pain while undertaking sport please complete Q8A only.
   - If you have pain while undertaking sport but it does not stop you from completing the activity, complete Q8B only.
   - If you have pain that stops you from completing sporting activities, please complete Q8C only.

   A. If you have no pain while undertaking sport, for how long can you train/practice? — POINTS
   | Nil | 1–5 min | 6–10 min | 11–15 min | >15 min |
   | 0 | 7 | 14 | 21 | 30 |

   OR

   B. If you have some pain while undertaking sport, but it does not stop you from completing your training/practice, for how long can you train/practice? — POINTS
   | Nil | 1–5 min | 6–10 min | 11–15 min | >15 min |
   | 0 | 4 | 10 | 14 | 20 |

   OR

   C. If you have pain that stops you from completing your training/practice, for how long can you train/practice? — POINTS
   | Nil | 1–5 min | 6–10 min | 11–15 min | >15 min |
   | 0 | 2 | 5 | 7 | 10 |

TOTAL SCORE ___ /100

REPRODUCED WITH PERMISSION OF ELSEVIER

PART B   Regional problems

(a)

(b)

(c)

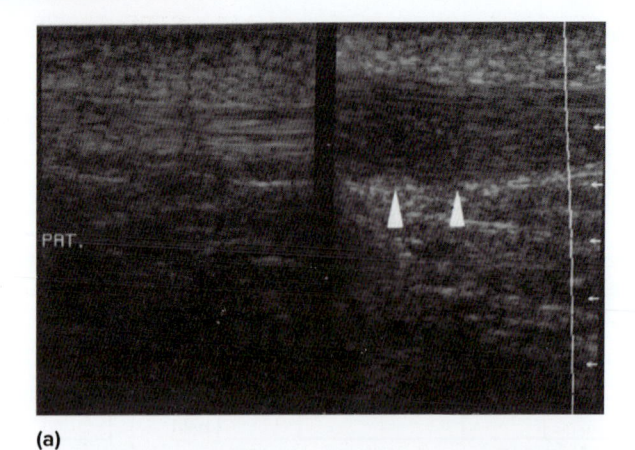

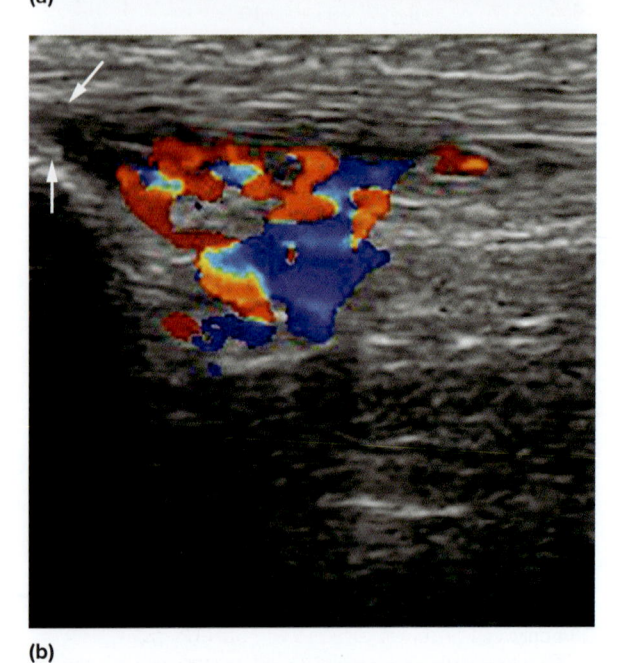

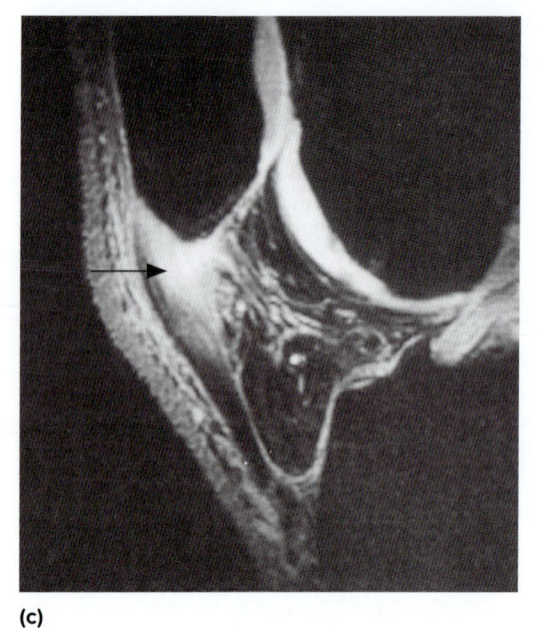

Figure 36.12 Ultrasound and MRI images of patellar tendinopathy in athletes (a) Ultrasound image (normal [left] and thickened [right] tendon). Arrowheads point to the posterior/deep edge of the patellar tendon (b) Ultrasound image with colour Doppler showing abnormal vascularity (blue and red signal) near the junction of the patellar tendon and the patella (arrows). (c) Sagittal slice MRI appearance of patellar tendinopathy

In-season treatment *does not include* heavy eccentric loading, power, and energy storage and release exercises, as the tendon is subjected to these frequently during training and competition. Injection therapies are contraindicated in-season because they require around 2–3 weeks out of sport after injection.

Table 36.10 Factors to take into account when making the decision about whether a player should keep competing or stop playing because of patellar tendinopathy. The decision should be shared between player and clinician

	Pain?	How limited is function?	Player's performance level	Likely clinical decision	Management strategy
Scenario 1 (often long-term)	Severe	Severely limited	Poor	Unable to compete—player understands he/she cannot play	Begin comprehensive out-of-competition rehabilitation program
Scenario 2 (often medium-term)	Tolerable	Moderate to severely limited	Adequate	Continue to compete but player is at risk of aggravating the tendon or suffering other injury	Maintain or improve function (see below)
Scenario 3 (more recent onset of symptoms)	Severe	Moderately limited	Adequate	Continue to compete but modify training/games to lower load	Use pain-relieving strategies (isometric exercise, medication)

Anterior knee pain   CHAPTER 36

This section outlines the physiotherapy approach to in-season management.

Relative load reduction: modified activity and biomechanical correction

There are numerous ways of reducing the load on the patellar tendon. The player must modify his or her training and perhaps game time, with reduction in the amount of jumping or sprinting in a session, the number of high load days each week or the total weekly training hours. Absolute rest is contraindicated and some continued lower limb load that does not include excessive energy storage loads (i.e. jumping, changes of direction, deceleration) on the tendon is critical to maintain tendon integrity, kinetic chain function and cardiovascular fitness.

Optimising biomechanics to improve the energy-absorbing capacity of the limb should be directed at both the affected musculotendinous unit and the hip and ankle. The ankle and calf are critical in absorbing the initial landing load and reduces the load transmitted to the knee.[176] Biomechanical studies reveal that only about 40% of landing energy is transmitted proximally.[177] Thus, the calf complex, and especially the soleus, must function well to prevent more load than necessary being placed on the patellar tendon.

Biomechanical correction should include assessment of both anatomy and function. Better landing techniques can decrease patellar tendon load. Compared with flat-foot landing, forefoot landing generates lower ground reaction forces and, if this technique is combined with a large range of hip or knee flexion, vertical ground reaction forces can be reduced by a further 25%.[177] Landing with weight further forward that uses all available dorsiflexion may also decrease patellar tendon load.[178, 179] Anatomical variants that may contribute to persistent patellar tendinopathy include limited ankle dorsiflexion and hallux rigidus. Tight hamstrings, quadriceps and calf muscles may increase the load on the patellar tendon. However, solely focusing on biomechanical correction without addressing kinetic chain strength and capacity will ultimately deliver an undesired outcome.

Isometrics for pain relief

Isometric exercises reduce pain and improve motor drive by reducing cortical inhibition.[4] (See also Chapter 4, Fig. 4.14) These exercises are best performed on weighted machines (Fig. 36.13) with single-leg isolated knee joint movement. Isometric exercise also is as effective as isotonic exercise in reducing pain in-season.[180, 181]

The specific parameters for isometric exercise are 45-second holds at 70% maximal voluntary isometric quadriceps contraction (MVC) with 2 minutes between each of the 5 repetitions. Long holds at mid-range with heavy weights are essential to the protocol but individual variations may be required.

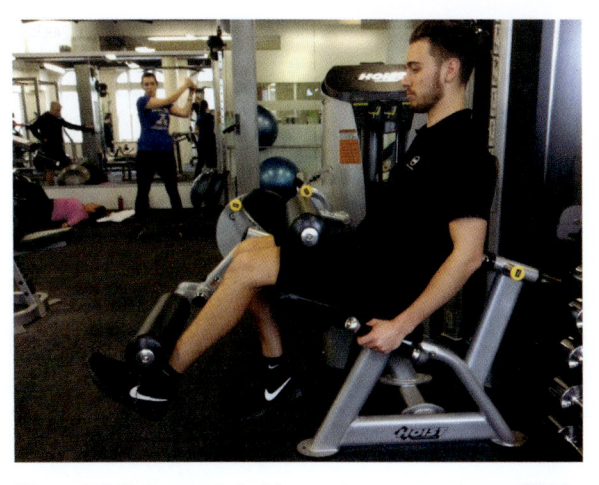

Figure 36.13 Isometric holds on a knee extension machine. Hold the highest weight possible for up to 45 seconds with good control

Strengthening

Strategies that maintain or improve strength of the entire kinetic chain are critical when managing a player during the season. Slow heavy-resistance training to maximise muscle strength prevents unloading weakness and atrophy, but may not improve performance or pain when competing.[182, 183]

Particular attention can be paid to the calf and gluteal muscles as these attenuate landing forces as well as improving quadriceps strength on the unaffected side. Cross-education means that quadriceps strength on the unaffected side can improve the strength of affected quadriceps by up to 20%.

The effect on cortical inhibition suggests that isometric exercises should also be used prior to quadriceps strength training throughout the four-stage program (Table 36.11) to improve the motor drive to the quadriceps.

Decline squat exercises (Fig. 36.14a) have traditionally been widely used, but are painful and can be detrimental when used during the season.[184, 185]

Soft tissue therapy

The use of friction to treat patellar tendinopathy remains a popular treatment, but lacks a logical theoretical construct and can further irritate the tendon. Studies that compared soft tissue therapy/transverse friction to other treatments demonstrated little benefit in reducing pain.[186, 187] Digital ischaemic pressure and sustained myofascial tension to tight muscles or trigger points in the quadriceps, hamstrings and calf muscles can be performed.

Pain reduction

Several strategies exist for reducing pain aside from the isometrics discussed earlier, all have to be considered against their potential to further irritate the tendon.

PART B Regional problems

Table 36.11 Four-stage strengthening program for treatment of patellar tendinopathy

Stage	Type of overload	Timing	Purpose	Activity	Maintain/kinetic chain exercise
1	Heavy load isometric exercise	0–1 months	Reduce pain	Weight-machine-based isolated quadriceps exercise	Begin isotonic exercise for calf and gluteals as well as quadriceps exercise for the other leg
2	Heavy load isotonic exercise	1–3 months	Improve strength, regain muscle bulk	Weight-machine-based heavy isotonic exercise	Isometrics before strength to reduce cortical inhibition Kinetic chain exercises
3	Energy storage exercises	3–4 months	Progressive high tendon load	Fast, body-weight-only knee flexion exercise to load the patellar tendon spring	Maintain isotonic exercise
4	Energy storage and release exercises	4–6 months	Sport-specific high tendon load	Jumping and change-of-direction exercises	Stop stage 3 exercise, maintain heavy load isotonic exercise
Return to training and competition	Sport-specific training	6+ months	Controlled-load return to sports activity	Sports drills with attention to frequency (2–3 times a week), volume and intensity	Maintain isotonic exercise

(a)

(b)

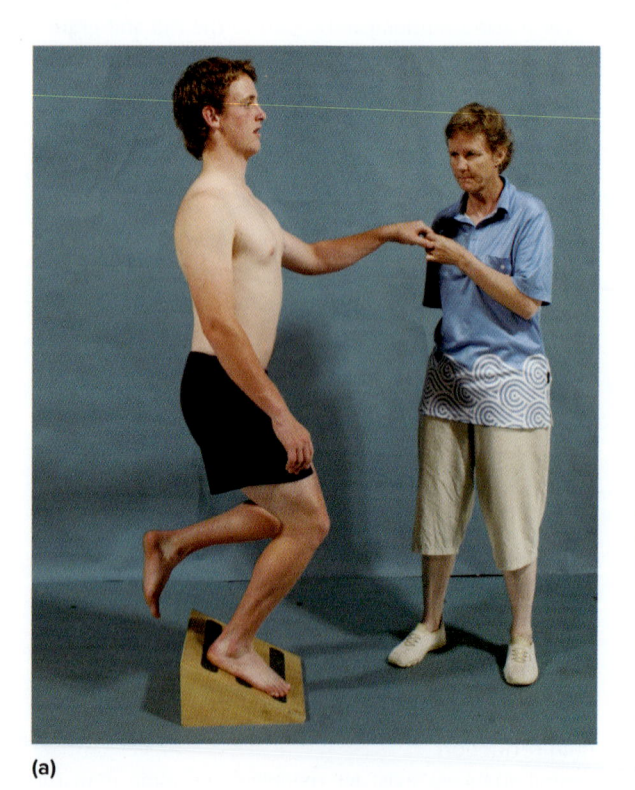

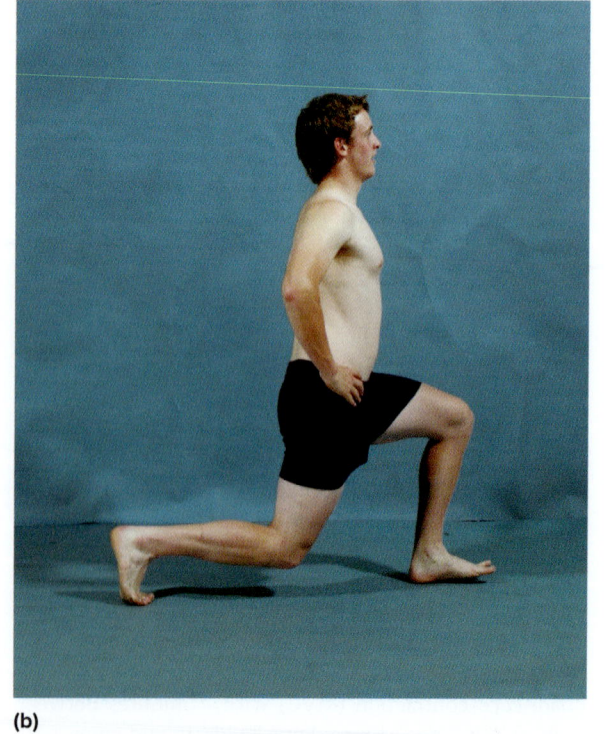

Figure 36.14 Patellar tendon eccentric strength training exercises (a) Single-leg squat on decline board (may aggravate pain and thus be detrimental in-season) (b) Lunge

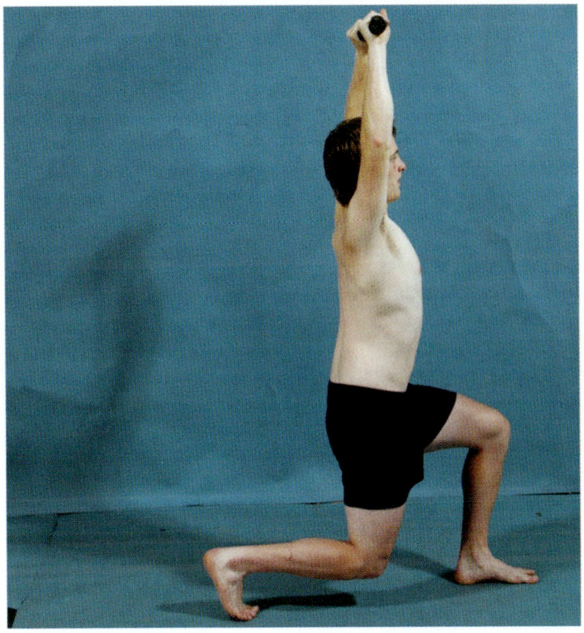

Figure 36.14 (cont.) (c) Lunge with weights

Cryotherapy
Cryotherapy (e.g. ice) is a popular adjunct to treatment but if the athlete finds no clinical benefit from this modality, there is no rationale for persisting.

Pharmacotherapy
Studies of pharmacotherapy in the treatment of patellar tendinopathy are limited to phoresis as few studies have investigated oral medications. The use of aprotinin in tendinopathy has some evidence, but is not recommended due to the risk of anaphylaxis after injection. Iontophoresis with corticosteroid improved outcome compared to phonophoresis, suggesting it may introduce corticosteroid into target tissue more effectively than phonophoresis.[188]

The model for tendinopathy proposed by Cook and Purdam suggests that early stage (reactive) tendinopathy could respond to medications that reduce cell activity and protein production.[189] Ibuprofen, doxycycline and green tea are hypothesised to improve pain and pathology in tendinopathy.[190]

Taping
Inferior patellar tendon taping reduced pain minimally and no more than placebo taping.[191]

Extracorporeal shock wave therapy
Extracorporeal shock wave therapy has been used to treat tendon pain. A systematic review including two RCTs showed variable results of randomised controlled studies; one RCT showed no benefit and the other showed better outcomes versus placebo in long-term tendon pain.[192]

Extracorporeal shock wave therapy may cause a neuropraxia to the nociceptive nerves resulting in decreased pain for several weeks. There is some animal evidence that it can have a negative effect on normal tendon structure within hours that remains for several weeks.[193]

The approach to out-of-competition treatment of the player with patellar tendinopathy
If the player needs to stop competing (see Table 36.10) an extensive out-of-competition exercise program is required to restore tendon, muscle and kinetic chain function. Resolution of the pathology is not required for recovery and good clinical outcomes can arise with limited changes in tendon structure.[194-196]

Another important concept that supports load-based rehabilitation is that a pathological tendon has adapted and has more aligned tendon structure than a structurally normal tendon.[197] This suggests that directing treatments at the area of pathology may be unnecessary and positive clinical outcomes may be due to improving the capacity of already present normal tendon structure.

The clinician will discuss the key elements of management and time frames for recovery/eventual return to play with the athlete, emphasising that there are no short cuts to recovery of function.

Conservative quadriceps rehabilitation of patellar tendinopathy requires appropriate strengthening, power, energy storage and release exercises, load reduction, and correction of biomechanical errors, along with adjunct therapies such as soft tissue therapy to the affected muscle (not the tendon). More invasive treatments, such as injection with substances that either affect the vessels (sclerotherapy with polidocanol), theoretically promote tendon repair (platelet rich plasma [PRP] injections) or augment matrix structure (prolotherapy), lack evidence.[198-200]

Relative load reduction
There are numerous ways of reducing the load on the patellar tendon without resorting to complete rest or immobilisation. Absolute rest is contraindicated; early rehabilitation with isometric and resistance training not only recovers muscle strength but reduces pain, so can be used immediately in the rehabilitation process. Variations on the isometric protocol outlined above may be required for individuals with high levels of pain. Although it is clear that long holds with heavy weights are required, it is unknown what is the most important (i.e. length of hold or external weight).

PART B   Regional problems

When and how should patellar tendon strengthening begin?

Therapists often have concerns as to when and how they should begin a strengthening program. Even athletes with the most severe cases of patellar tendinopathy should be able to begin some weight-based strength and other exercises (such as calf strength and isometric quadriceps work) in standing. However, the athlete who has not lost a lot of knee strength and bulk can progress quickly to the speed part of the program.

Both pain and the ability of the musculotendinous unit to do the work should guide the amount of strengthening to be done. If pain is a limiting factor, then the program must be modified so that the majority of the work occurs without aggravating symptoms within 24 hours of the exercise. A subjective clinical rating system, such as the VISA questionnaire (Table 36.9), administered at about monthly intervals, will help both the therapist and the patient measure progress.

If pain is under control, it is essential to monitor the ability of the limb to complete the exercises with control and quality. Exercises should only be progressed if the previous work load is easily managed, pain is controlled, and function is satisfactory.

Athletes with patellar tendinopathy tend to 'unload' the affected limb to avoid pain, so they commonly have not only weakness but also abnormal motor patterns that must be reversed. Strength training must graduate quickly to incorporate single-leg exercises (Fig. 36.14) as the athlete can continue to unload the affected tendon when exercising using both legs. Thus, exercises that target the quadriceps specifically (such as single-leg extensions) may have a place in the rehabilitation of patellar tendinopathy. Similarly, when the athlete is ready, increase the load on the quadriceps by having the patient stand on a 25° decline board to do squats. Compared with squatting on a flat surface, this reduces the calf contribution during the squat.

The therapist should progress the regimen by adding load and speed and then endurance to each of those levels of exercise. Combinations such as load and speed, or height and load, then follow. These end-stage exercises can provoke tendon pain, and are only recommended after a prolonged rehabilitation period, and when the sport demands intense loading. In several sports, it may not be necessary to add potentially aggravating activities such as jump training to the rehabilitation program, whereas in volleyball, for example, it is vital.

Finally, the overall exercise program must correct aberrant motor patterns such as stiff landing mechanics (discussed above) and pelvic instability. For example, weight-bearing exercises must be in a functionally required range, and the pelvis position must be monitored and controlled at all times. The common errors in rehabilitation strength programs are listed in Table 36.12.

Table 36.12 Why rehabilitation programs fail at various stages

Early failure	Late failure
Insufficient strength training	Failure to monitor the patient's symptoms
Progression of rehabilitation program too rapid	Rehabilitation and strength training end on return to training, instead of continuing throughout the return to sport
Inappropriate loads during rehabilitation (too little, too much)	No speed rehabilitation
	Plyometrics training performed inappropriately, not tolerated, or unnecessary

Restoring function

Strength, power and energy storage and release capacity are required for all the muscles, especially the anti-gravity muscles—the calf, quadriceps and gluteal muscles. An effective rehabilitation program embraces the principles outlined in Table 36.11. Commonly prescribed exercises are illustrated in Figure 36.14. When and how a strengthening program should begin is outlined in the box.

Several papers have documented the effectiveness of quadriceps strengthening exercises on patellar tendinopathy.[8, 201-205] These can be divided into two groups: those studies that investigated eccentric exercises on a decline board and those using other exercises.

The studies that have investigated the effectiveness of exercise on a 25° decline board–a method specifically loading the extensor mechanism of the knee by increasing the moment arm of the knee[203]–include two randomised trials which reported improvements in pain, function and return to sport with exercise, although time frames for improvement varied.[8, 204] In another study, compared to surgery, eccentric exercise on a decline board provided similar outcomes at 12 months.[205] Care with these exercises is required in the early painful stages as they can be provocative.

Other studies have investigated heavy load strengthening and report equally good results.[206] Three papers have suggested that exercise-based interventions such as squatting, isokinetics and weights reduced the pain of patellar tendinopathy.[186, 201, 202]

Soft tissue therapy, cryotherapy, pharmacotherapy, taping

Massage can be used for muscle soreness resulting from resistance training. Ice is of little benefit during rehabilitation, and medications and taping also have no place in this phase.

Biomechanical correction

Ongoing management of any range of movement deficits in the ankle and foot can be continued early in the rehabilitation program. Formal correction of running and jumping techniques, if required, are commenced once kinetic chain function has been mostly restored. However, solely focusing on biomechanical correction without addressing kinetic chain strength and capacity will ultimately deliver an undesired outcome.

Injection therapy

Neovascularisation is a cornerstone of degenerative tendon pathology and is the target of treatment by Alfredson and Ohberg's sclerosing injection.[207] In a high-quality RCT of elite athletes with patellar tendinopathy, investigators found that sclerosing injections with polidocanol resulted in a significant improvement in knee function and reduced pain in patients with patellar tendinopathy.[208] However, polidoconol has a neurotoxic effect that may underpin its effectiveness, rather than altering the vascularity.[209] This is supported by research that shows tendons that have substantial vascularity can remain pain-free.

Corticosteroid injections (CSI) have been compared to placebo and CSI improved symptoms so much so that all 12 athletes who had placebo injection subsequently had CSI. It is worthwhile noting that after initial improvement, 50% of athletes in the CSI group failed to return to sport and were referred to surgery.[210] Blood injection therapy (autologous blood, platelet rich plasma [PRP]) is being used clinically, but controlled trials show no additional benefit over placebo injection.[211] High volume injections and the addition of tendon cells are being used clinically with little or no quality research to show their efficacy.

Surgery

The only randomised trial to date that compared surgical treatment and conservative management of patellar tendinopathy was published in 2006.[212] There was no significant difference in outcome between groups; thus, surgical intervention provided no benefit over conservative management. Thus, the clinical implication is that surgery is not a 'quick fix' for patellar tendinopathy.[212]

A number of different surgical techniques have been proposed. There has been some enthusiasm for arthroscopic debridement of the anterior portion of the fat pad adjacent to the patellar tendon and results published to date appear similar to those of patients undergoing open surgery.[213, 214] Open surgery aims to remove the region of tendinosis from the proximal patellar tendon. A systematic review of 17 studies of surgery for patellar tendinopathy reported that outcomes were reasonable after both open and arthroscopic surgery, but that return to sport was faster with the arthroscopic surgery.[215]

We recommend surgery only after a thorough, high-quality rehabilitation program has failed. Surgeons must advise patients that while symptomatic benefit is very likely, return to sport at the previous level cannot be guaranteed (60–80% likelihood).[213, 216] Time to return to the previous level of sport, if achieved, is likely to take between 6 and 12 months.[213, 216]

Sudden, acute patellar tendon pain

The term 'partial tear' is often used when the player has a sudden painful episode, which may be associated with disability. A small partial tear of the patellar tendon is often diagnosed by ultrasonography following an event like this or as an incidental finding on ultrasound examination, and it is difficult to differentiate a tear from an area of tendinosis.[217, 218] Based on surgical specimens in the Achilles tendon, the ability of ultrasound to differentiate degenerative changes and partial tears are limited.

This type of partial tear occurs in degenerative tendinopathy and can be managed conservatively. There are few consequences in the patellar tendon as the tissue trauma is likely to be in an area of pathology of the patellar tendon and not in the normal, load-bearing tissue. If the pain and dysfunction after acute onset pain persists, further imaging and possible intervention may be justified to stimulate some healing response in the tendon.

LESS COMMON CAUSES OF ANTERIOR KNEE PAIN

Fat pad irritation/impingement

Fat pad syndrome was first described by Hoffa in 1903 to describe a condition where the infrapatellar fat pad was impinged between the patella and the femoral condyle due to a direct blow to the knee. More commonly, fat pad irritation occurs with repeated or uncontrolled hyperextension of the knee where it is impinged between the femur and tibia. The condition can be extremely painful and debilitating, as the fat pad is one of the most pain-sensitive structures in the knee.[25]

PART B Regional problems

Chronic fat pad irritation is relatively common and often goes unrecognised. The pain is often exacerbated by extension manoeuvres, such as straight leg raises and prolonged standing, so it needs to be recognised early so that appropriate management can be implemented.

Clinical findings include localised tenderness (at the inferior pole of the patella, deep to the tendon) and puffiness in the fat pad with the inferior pole of the patella appearing to be (or actually being) displaced posteriorly. Pain may be reproduced with active knee extension and passive overpressure in extension. Contracting the quadriceps with the knee extended may aggravate the pain during the acute phase. There may be quadriceps weakness. Patients often have hyperextension of the knees (genu recurvatum) associated with increased anterior pelvic tilt.

Thus, treatments should be directed to improve the control, strength and endurance of local (vasti), proximal and distal muscles as well as retraining to avoid uncontrolled and excessive terminal knee extension manoeuvres.

A popular clinical approach consists of treating the inferiorly tilted patella by taping across the superior surface of the patella to lever the inferior pole forward and relieve impingement of the fat pad (Fig. 36.6d). Unloading of the fat pad may be required to relieve the symptoms further.

To unload the fat pad, a 'V' tape is placed below the fat pad, with the point of the 'V' at the tibial tubercle coming wide to the medial and lateral joint lines. As the tape is being pulled towards the joint line, the skin is lifted towards the patella, thus shortening the fat pad (Fig. 36.15). Improving lower limb biomechanics is often helpful. Surgery should be avoided if possible. To date, there have been no RCTs of surgery for this condition.[219]

Osgood–Schlatter lesion

Osgood-Schlatter lesion is an osteochondrosis (Chapter 44) that occurs at the tibial tuberosity in children as they progress through puberty. It is much more common among boys of about 13–15 years (but these ages vary) than girls (age about 10–12) and results from excessive traction on the soft apophysis of the tibial tuberosity by the powerful patellar tendon. It occurs in association with high levels of activity during a period of rapid growth and is associated with a change in the tendon. Longitudinal imaging of the tendon in adolescents without pain shows that the attachment transitions to a normal attachment through a process that can be interpreted as osteochondritic.[220] As with all tendon-related pain, the clinician must be careful not to diagnose based on imaging findings.

Treatment consists of reassurance that the condition is self-limiting and muscle strength exercises. Whether or not to play sport depends on the severity of symptoms. Children with mild symptoms may wish to continue to play some or all sport; others may choose some modification of their programs. If the child prefers to cease sport because of pain, that decision should be supported. However, the amount of sport played does not seem to affect the time taken for the pain to disappear.

Sinding-Larsen–Johansson lesion

This rare lesion is one of the group of osteochondroses found in adolescents (Chapter 44). It is a clinically unimportant differential diagnosis in young patients with pain at the inferior pole of the patella, who can actually have patellar tendinopathy at a young age.

Quadriceps tendinopathy

Pain arising at the quadriceps tendon at its attachment to the patella occurs mainly in the older athlete and in weightlifters as the quadriceps tendon is loaded more in a deeper squat. It is characterised by tenderness at the superior margin of the patella and pain on resisted quadriceps contraction. Treatment follows the same principles as treatment of patellar tendinopathy. Differential diagnosis is suprapatellar pain of PFJ origin, plica and bipartite patella. Ruptures of the entire quadriceps attachment to the patella are not uncommon in middle-aged men and require surgery and extensive rehabilitation.

Bursitis

There are a number of bursae around the knee joint (Fig. 36.16). The most commonly affected bursa is the pre-patellar bursa. Pre-patellar bursitis ('housemaid's knee') presents as a superficial swelling on the anterior aspect of the knee. This must be differentiated from an effusion of the

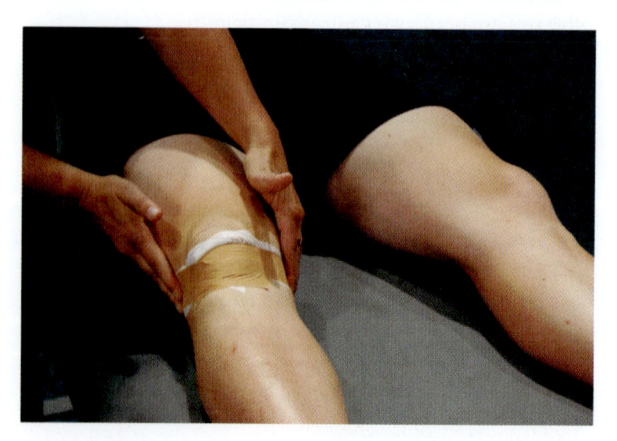

Figure 36.15 Fat pad unloading tape. Tape is applied in a 'V' from the tibial tuberosity to the joint lines. The fat pad region is pinched to unload the fat pad while applying the tape. This tape is often combined with taping of the superior pole of the patella (Fig. 36.6d) in the treatment of fat pad impingement

Anterior knee pain   CHAPTER 36

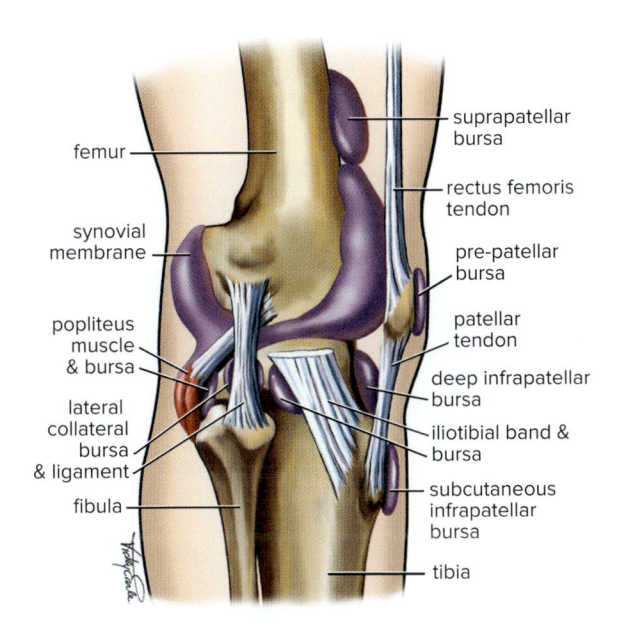

Figure 36.16 Bursae around the knee joint

knee joint. Acute infective pre-patellar bursitis, common in those who kneel a lot, should be identified and treated quickly. Infrapatellar bursitis can also cause anterior knee pain that may mimic patellar tendinopathy; this bursa forms part of an enthesis organ of the distal insertion and, thus, can be challenging to treat. Pes anserinus bursitis is often associated with an underlying rheumatological condition.

Treatment of mild cases of bursitis includes non-steroidal anti-inflammatory drugs (NSAIDs). More severe cases require aspiration and infiltration with a corticosteroid agent and local anaesthesia, followed by appropriate treatment of the enthesis if appropriate.

Synovial plica

The importance of the synovial plica, a synovial fold found along the supero-medial edge of the patella (see Fig. 36.17), has been a matter of considerable debate. An inflamed plica may cause variable sharp pain located anteriorly, medially or posteriorly. The patient may complain of sharp pain on squatting and it can mimic quadriceps tendinopathy. On examination, the plica is sometimes palpable as a thickened band under the medial border of the patella. It should only be considered as the primary cause of the patient's symptoms when the patient fails to respond to appropriate management of PFP. In this case and in the presence of a tender thickened band, arthroscopy should be performed and the synovial plica removed.

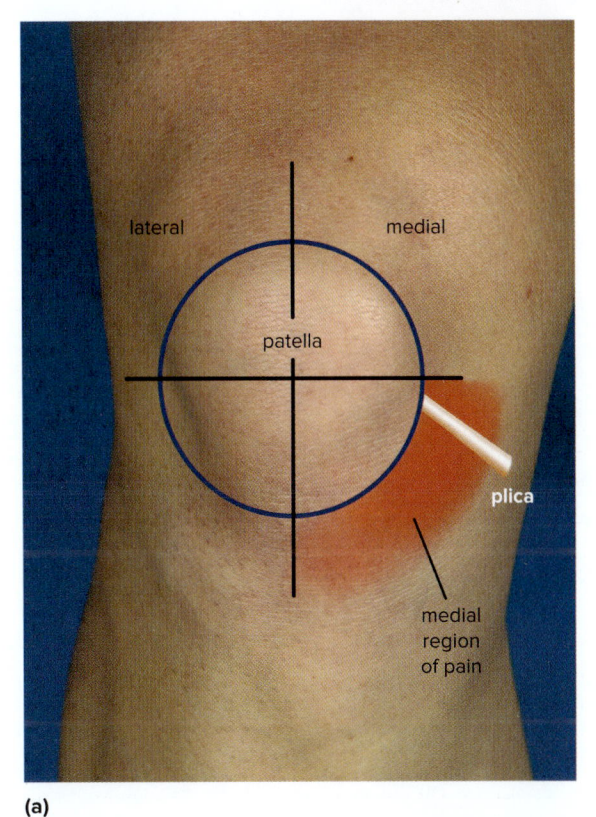

Figure 36.17 Synovial plica (a) Medial synovial plica presents with pain in the region highlighted (red). A band of tissue may be palpable (+/− tender) running from the medial patella to the epicondylar region (blue) (b) A frayed, thickened synovial plica photographed at arthroscopy. It catches between the patella above it and the femoral condyle

803

PART B: Regional problems

REFERENCES

References for this chapter can be found at www.mhhe.com/au/CSM5e

Chapter 37

Lateral, medial and posterior knee pain

with MARK HUTCHINSON

When I listened to other people—who seemed to have trouble even though their [knee replacements] went well—[I learned that] they didn't make the commitment to rehab . . . I can walk forever now—pain-free . . . I can hit a tennis ball again.

Billie Jean King, six years after her 2010 knee replacements

Although acute knee injuries and anterior knee pain are very common presentations in sports and exercise medicine practice, patients presenting with lateral, medial or posterior knee pain are not uncommon and can provide the clinician with both diagnosis and treatment challenges.

LATERAL KNEE PAIN

Athletes can present with the chief complaint of lateral knee pain for a number of underlying problems, including: lateral meniscus tears and cysts; bone bruises or cartilage injuries of the lateral compartment; patellofemoral syndrome or patellar instability; injuries of the posterolateral corner structures (popliteus, lateral collateral ligament, mid third capsular ligament anterolateral ligament); biceps insertional tendinopathy and injuries; tibiofibular joint instability; and iliotibial band syndrome at the knee.

Lateral knee pain (Fig. 37.1) is a particularly common problem among distance runners and cyclists, the most common cause of lateral knee pain being iliotibial band friction syndrome (ITBFS). Training errors as well as alignment and biomechanical abnormalities can precipitate ITBFS. Patellofemoral syndrome (Chapter 36) or instability may also present as lateral knee pain. In the older active person, lateral meniscus degeneration or lateral compartment osteoarthritis should be more strongly considered as part of the differential diagnosis. For sprinters and footballers, overuse injuries of the biceps femoris tendon and its insertion onto the fibula should be considered more highly in the differential diagnosis. The biceps femoris tendon may suffer compression and irritation as it passes posterolaterally to the knee and inserts into the head of the fibula, likely as a result of the repetitive flexion and rotation demands on the knee. Injuries of the superior tibiofibular joint may also cause lateral knee pain.

The astute clinician should always be conscious of the potential of associated injuries or referred pain involving the lateral aspect of the knee. Ligamentous injuries of the posterolateral corner are rarely isolated and frequently involve injury to the ACL or PCL. Lateral knee pain may also occur as a result of referred pain from the lumbar spine. The causes and differential diagnoses of lateral knee pain are shown in Table 37.1.

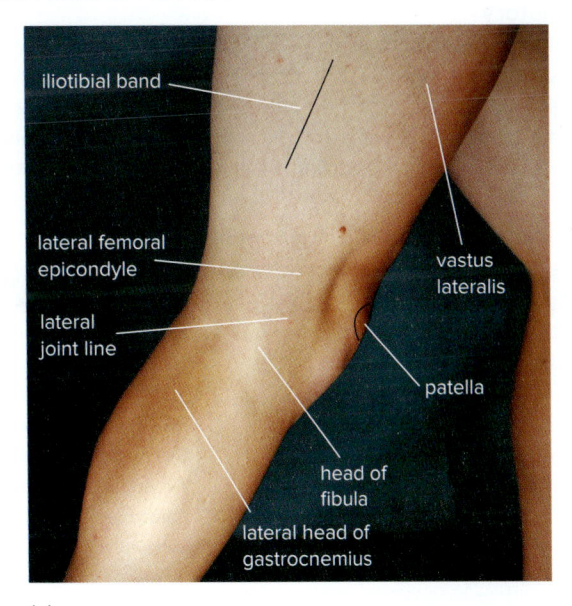

Figure 37.1 Lateral aspect of the knee (a) Surface anatomy

PART B Regional problems

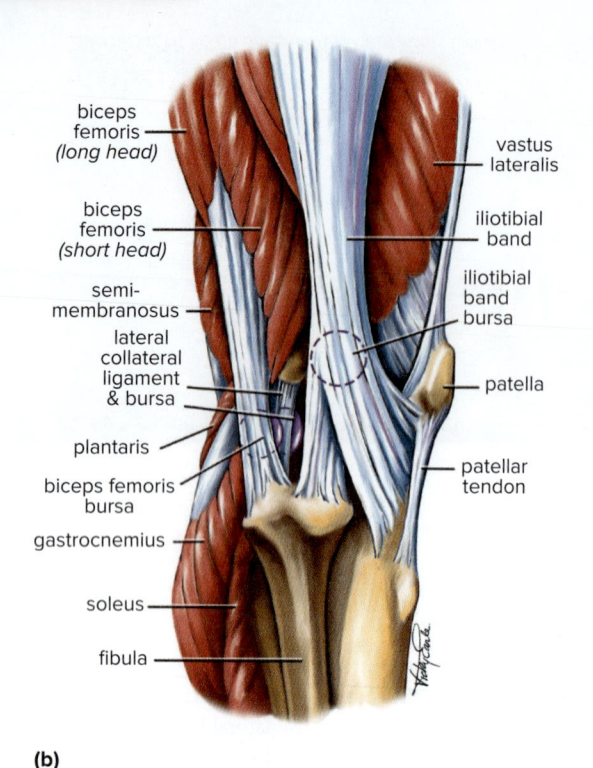

Figure 37.1 (cont.) (b) Anatomy of lateral aspect of the knee

Clinical approach
As with acute knee injuries (Chapter 35) and most musculoskeletal injuries, history and physical examination are key to an accurate diagnosis.

History
Most complaints involving the lateral aspect of the knee can be classified as either chronic, with no specific traumatic episode, or acute, where the athlete can recall a single event that initiated the complaint. A history of overuse or pain related to a change in training intensity suggests ITBFS or biceps femoris tendinopathy. ITBFS has been associated with acute ramping up of training period or distance, excessive downhill running and running on an uneven surface (particularly the downside leg on a canted/sloped road). Biceps femoris strains and tendinopathy have been correlated with sprinting or kicking activities.

The pain associated with biceps femoris tendinopathy flares up on initial activity and then starts to settle after warming up, usually recurring following cessation of activity or the next day. When left untreated, pain persists during exercise and the athlete may not be able to continue with sporting activity. ITB pain usually does not settle with ongoing activity and can be associated with a snapping sensation as well as swelling and pain localised proximal to the lateral joint line.

If the athlete can remember a single episode or event, then the clinician should consider such diagnoses as a bone bruise (bone marrow lesion [BML]) posterolateral corner ligament injury, proximal fibular subluxation, patellar instability or a lateral meniscus tear (Chapter 35). Lateral joint line pain associated with a sudden twisting event, accompanied by episodes of locking, is highly suggestive of a meniscus tear. The sensation of giving way may be secondary to intra-articular pathology such as a loose body, bucket-handle meniscus tear, or more commonly related to true ligamentous instability of the patella or posterolateral corner of the knee. As the population of active individuals who are over 50 years old increases, the diagnosis of lateral compartment osteoarthritis should be considered and it is possible for them to have an acute or chronic injury to a degenerative meniscus.

A complete history is necessary to avoid missing radicular or associated diagnoses. The presence of back pain may suggest referred pain from the lumbar spine. Associated neurological symptoms such as weakness and paraesthesia in the lower leg may indicate common peroneal nerve entrapment. Acute ankle injuries with

Table 37.1 Causes of lateral knee pain

Common	Less common	Not to be missed
Iliotibial band friction syndrome	Patellofemoral syndrome	Common peroneal nerve injury
Lateral meniscus abnormality	Osteoarthritis of the lateral compartment of the knee	Slipped capital femoral epiphysis
• Minor tear	Excessive lateral pressure syndrome	Perthes' disease
• Degenerative change	Biceps femoris tendinopathy	
• Cyst	Superior tibiofibular joint sprain	
	Posterolateral corner knee injury (Chapter 35)	
	Synovitis of the knee joint	
	Referred pain	
	• Lumbar spine	
	• Neuromechanical sensitivity	

Lateral, medial and posterior knee pain   CHAPTER 37

proximal fibular pain should raise suspicion of proximal tibiofibular joint instability or a *Maisonneuve* fracture (associated fracture of the proximal fibula).

Examination

Full assessment of the ligaments of the knee (Chapter 35) should be included in the examination. Biomechanical examination should also be performed.

1. Observation
   (a) standing
   (b) walking
   (c) supine
   (d) side-lying
2. Active movements
   (a) knee flexion
   (b) knee extension
   (c) repeated knee flexion (0–30°) (Fig. 37.2a)
   (d) tibial rotation
3. Passive movements
   (a) knee flexion/extension
   (b) tibial rotation (Fig. 37.2b)
   (c) superior tibiofibular joint
       (i) accessory glides (Fig. 37.2c)
   (d) muscle stretches
       (i) ITB (Ober's test) (Fig. 37.2d)
       (ii) quadriceps
       (iii) hamstring

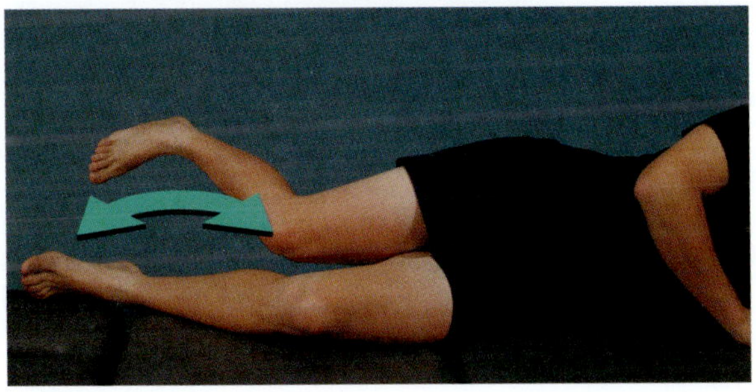

Figure 37.2 Examination of the patient with lateral knee pain (a) Active movements—repeated flexion from 0°–30°. This may reproduce the patient's pain if ITBFS is the case. It can be performed in a side-lying position (illustrated), standing or squatting (b) Passive movements—tibial rotation. This is performed in knee flexion to assess superior tibiofibular joint movement (c) Passive movements—accessory anteroposterior glide to superior tibiofibular joint (d) Passive movement—ITB stretch. This is performed in a side-lying position with the hip in neutral rotation and knee flexion. The hip is extended and then adducted. If the ITB is tight, knee extension will occur with adduction (Ober's test)

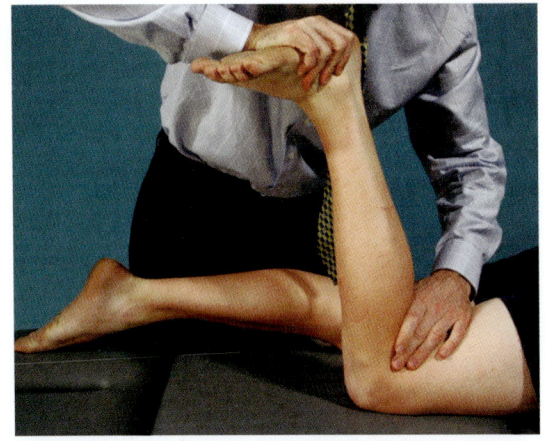

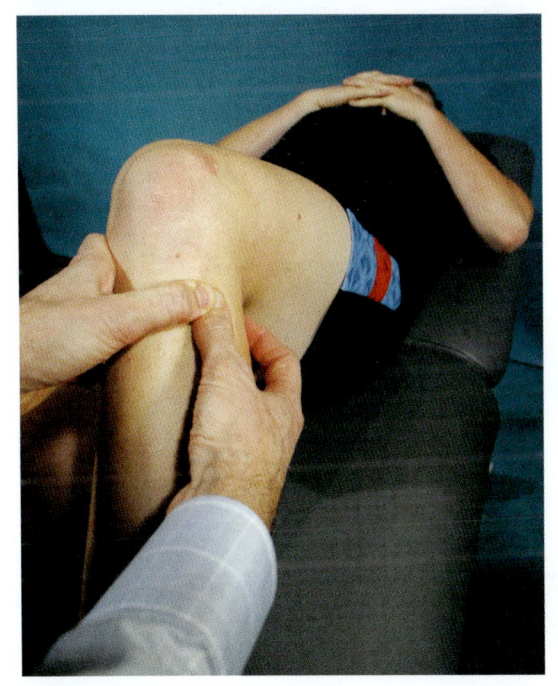

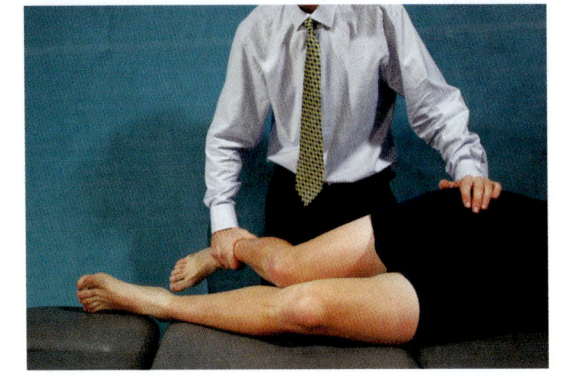

PART B   Regional problems

4. Resisted movements
   (a) knee flexion (Fig. 37.2e)
   (b) tibial rotation
5. Functional movements
   (a) hopping
   (b) squat/single-leg squat
   (c) jumping
6. Palpation
   (a) lateral femoral epicondyle (Fig. 37.2f)
   (b) lateral joint line
   (c) lateral retinaculum
   (d) lateral border of patella
   (e) superior tibiofibular joint
   (f) biceps femoris tendon
   (g) gluteus medius
7. Special tests
   (a) full knee examination (Chapter 35)
      (i) effusion (Fig. 37.2g)
      (ii) McMurray's test (Fig. 37.2h)
   (b) neural tension tests
      (i) prone knee bend
      (ii) slump (Fig. 37.2i)
   (c) lumbar spine (Chapter 29)
   (d) biomechanical assessment (Chapter 8) (Fig. 37.2j)

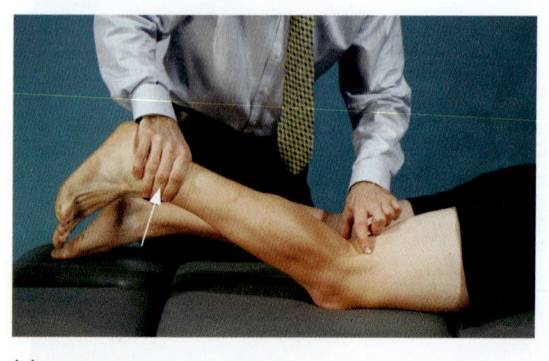

Figure 37.2 (cont.) (e) Resisted movement—knee flexion. Concentric or eccentric contractions may reproduce the pain of biceps femoris tendinopathy (f) Palpation—lateral femoral epicondyle (g) Special test—knee effusion. Manually drain the medial subpatellar pouch by stroking the fluid in a superior direction. (1) Then 'milk' the fluid back into the knee from above (2) while observing the pouch for reaccumulating fluid (h) Special tests—McMurray's test. The knee is flexed and, at various stages of flexion, internal and external rotation of the tibia are performed (arrow). The presence of pain and a palpable 'clunk' are a positive McMurray's test and are consistent with meniscal injury. If there is no 'clunk' but the patient's pain is reproduced, then the meniscus may be damaged or there may be patellofemoral joint abnormality

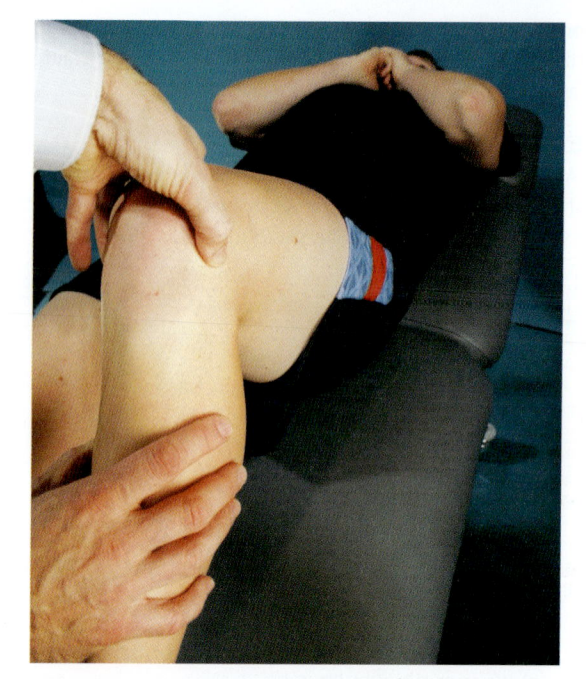

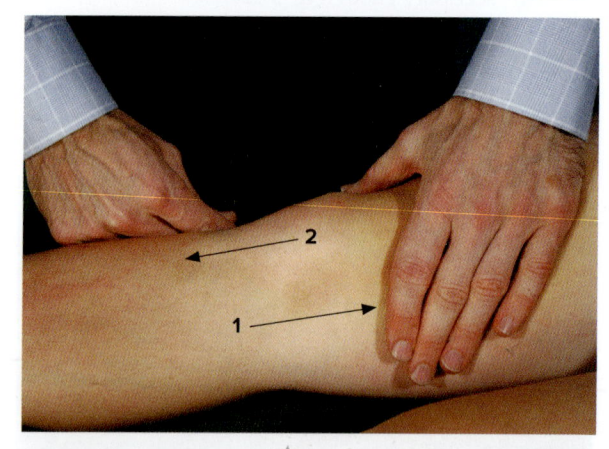

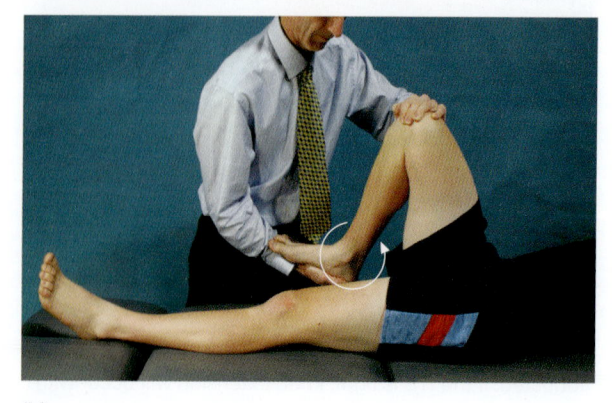

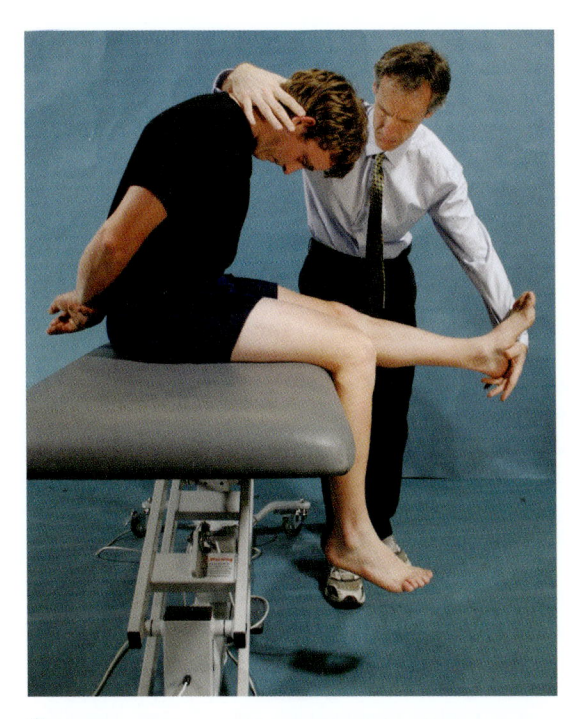

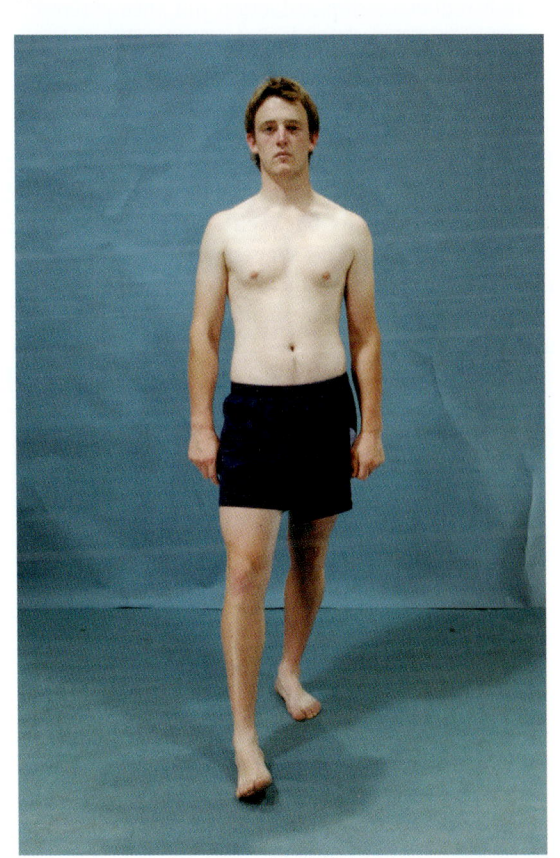

Lateral, medial and posterior knee pain CHAPTER 37

Investigations
Although the majority of patients with lateral knee pain do not require investigations, MR imaging can be useful in cases of persistent lateral knee pain when a degenerative lateral meniscus is suspected. Weight-bearing radiographs with the knee slightly flexed have an improved sensitivity for osteoarthritis when compared to standard radiographs obtained in a supine position. Full-length tibia/fibula films should be obtained when associated ankle injuries are present. When imaging is not readily available, a diagnostic local anaesthetic injection can be used to differentiate local soft tissue pain (e.g. ITBFS) from intra-articular or referred pain. If the clinician is concerned for the possibility of radiculopathy from the lumbar spine, electromyography or lumbar spine imaging may be indicated.

Iliotibial band friction syndrome
Iliotibial band friction syndrome (ITBFS) is an overuse injury presenting as lateral knee pain that is exacerbated by sporting activity. It is more commonly seen in runners, cyclists, defence force recruits and endurance athletes.[1-4] Incidence rates in running range from 1.6% to 12% and 1% to 5.5% in military populations.[3] In cycling ITBFS accounts for 15% to 24% of overuse injuries.[3]

Anatomy
Traditionally, ITBFS was considered to be the result of friction between the iliotibial band (ITB) and the underlying lateral epicondyle of the femur (Fig. 37.3) as the ITB switched from an extensor at 0–20° to a flexor at 20–90°. This friction was thought to contribute to local inflammation and irritation of an anatomical bursa lying between the tendon and the lateral femoral epicondyle (LFE).[5] However, anatomical studies have questioned or negated this theory.[2,4]

While both ultrasound and MRI can show thickening of the ITB over the lateral femoral condyle and often a fluid collection deep to the ITB at the same site,[6] studies do not support the presence of an anatomical bursa around the LFE.[2,4] Instead of a bursa, the authors claim that a richly innervated and vascularised layer of fat and connective tissue separates the ITB from the LFE and is the likely source of pain in ITBFS.[2,4]

It is important to note that the ITB is not a discrete band but a lateral thickening of the circumferential fascia lata that envelops the whole thigh like a stocking

Figure 37.2 (cont.) (i) Special tests—slump test
(j) Special tests—biomechanical assessment Full lower limb biomechanical assessment should be performed while standing, walking and lying. Abnormal pelvic movements (e.g. excessive lateral tilt) should be noted

PART B   Regional problems

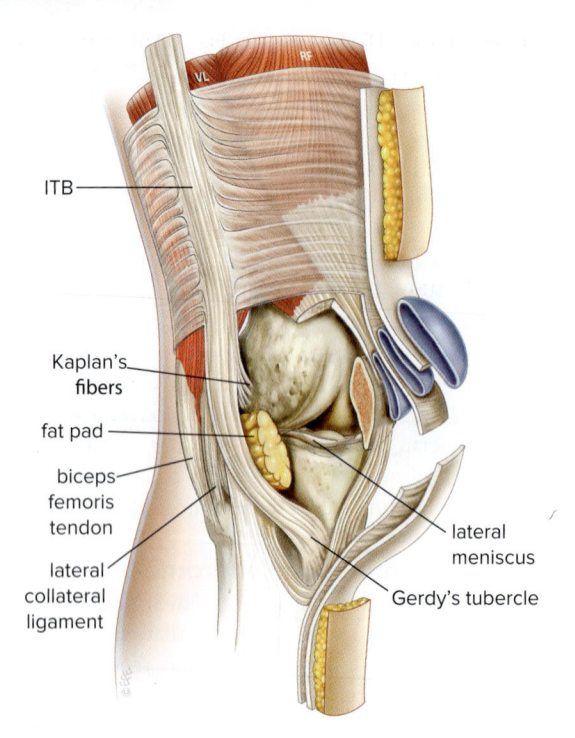

Figure 37.3 Anatomy of the iliotibial band insertion
FROM FRANKLYN-MILLER A. ET AL. *CLINICAL SPORTS ANATOMY*.
MELBOURNE: MCGRAW-HILL, 2010; P.269

(Fig. 37.3).[1,2,4] The ITB inserts along the length of the femur down the linea aspera via the lateral intermuscular septum.[1,2,4] Proximally, the tensor fascia lata muscle (TFL) inserts into the ITB, as does a substantial portion of the gluteus maximus muscle (GMax). The remaining portion inserts directly into the greater trochanter. Distally, the ITB crosses the LFE and is connected to the LFE by strong fibrous bands. The ITB continues, acting like a lateral ligament, from the LFE to insert onto the patella and Gerdy's tubercle on the tibia. The ITB can also project onto the fibula. This orientation demonstrates the close relationship between the ITB and the knee and hip complex and its role in lateral stability.

Clinical features

Typically, an athlete with ITBFS complains of an ache over the lateral aspect of the knee which is aggravated by running or cycling. The pain often develops at about the same distance/time during activity. Longer training sessions, downhill running or cambered courses are often aggravating factors.

On examination, tenderness is elicited over the LFE 2–3 cm above the lateral joint line (Fig. 37.2f). Crepitus and local swelling may also be felt. Repeated flexion/extension of the knee may reproduce the patient's symptoms. Ober's test (Fig. 37.2d) often reveals ITB tightness and may produce a burning sensation. Tightness may be secondary to shortening of the TFL and/or GMax muscles proximally or excessive development of the vastus lateralis, placing increased tensile load on the ITB. Imaging is not usually required to confirm the diagnosis of ITBFS.

Biomechanics

Understanding the anatomy and pathomechanics of the ITB should assist in better targeting therapeutic interventions. Movement of the ITB around the LFE is restricted by its strong fibrous band attachments. Traditional approaches involving the alteration of tension of the fascia lata and hip musculature may not achieve the intended outcomes and can result in an increase in compressive forces around the LFE,[2,4] leading to increased pain related to compression rather than a reduction in transverse frictional forces. The ITB clearly plays a role in stability around the hip through its tensioning effect. In hip adduction and flexion, an increase in pressure around the greater trochanter has been reported.[1] This pressure is further increased by knee flexion. The same pressure is reduced in hip abduction and knee extension. This is supported by surgical studies which have shown that ITB lengthening can lead to favourable outcomes in trochanteric bursitis presentations.[1]

It was originally thought that ITBFS was associated with repetitive knee flexion and extension movement. A biomechanical study found no significant difference in sagittal knee movements between an ITBFS population and matched controls.[5] This suggests that other planes of motion may be more relevant. For example, an increase in tibial internal rotation can augment compressive forces around the LFE by moving the ITB's distal attachment to the tibia more medially.[7]

> **PRACTICE PEARL**
>
> It is clear that the pathomechanics of ITBFS is complex and involves various segments along the kinetic chain. Tibial internal rotation may result from poor proximal control (increased hip adduction/internal rotation), a genu valgus strain and/or poor rearfoot mechanics.

An increase in hip adduction, especially during the loading phase of running, increases the eccentric demand on the hip abductors.[7]

Runners with ITBFS can have significant weakness of their hip abductors in the affected limb,[8] and decreased ability of the hip abductors to eccentrically control

Lateral, medial and posterior knee pain CHAPTER 37

adduction.[9] There is also often weakness in knee flexion and knee extension, with decreased braking forces.[10] Weakness and fatigue can result in increased compressive forces around the LFE and therefore lead to ITBFS.

Neural feedback from the richly innervated fat and connective tissue between the ITB and LFE may result in decreased tension in the hip abductors to reduce these compressive loads.[2] This can lead to hip muscle imbalances and altered biomechanics.

Treatment

Treatment of ITBFS should address not only local symptoms, but also each segment along the kinetic chain including foot alignment and hip biomechanics to assure more favourable long-term results. A guiding philosophy is that while the pathology is felt distally, treatment should be focused proximally.

Local treatment includes cryotherapy, topical non-steroidals and modalities such as shock wave therapy[11] applied to the area around the LFE. Oral NSAIDs may be helpful in the initial stages to reduce pain and allow therapy.[12] Corticosteroid injection (Fig. 37.4) has traditionally been used to inject the 'bursa'.[13] The inconsistent results from these injections can be attributed to a misunderstanding of the pathology. Whether there is a role for corticosteroid injections into the area of pain-sensitive tissue between the ITB and lateral femoral epicondyle is presently unclear. It is unlikely that they provide a cure; however, they may play a temporary role in relieving pain to allow rehabilitation. Caution should always be used when injecting steroids about ligaments for fear of weakening them.

Soft tissue treatment to the proximal ITB (Fig. 37.5a and b), dry needling (Fig. 37.5c) and self-massage with a foam roll (Fig. 37.5d) all help to reduce muscle tension and tone on the ITB. Stretching (Fig. 37.6) is routinely proposed as a treatment technique for ITBFS. However, because the ITB inserts into the entire length of the femur via the lateral intermuscular septum, stretching exercises may have a limited effect on the ITB itself. Stretching may have some effect on reducing the tension in the tensor fascia lata (TFL).[2,4] Stretching of the gluteus maximus muscle may prove more beneficial because of its close relationship to the ITB.

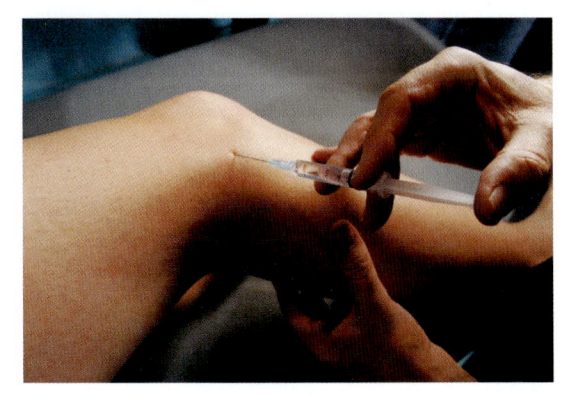

Figure 37.4 Corticosteroid injection, if used, is aimed deep to the ITB tendon—between it and the underlying LFE

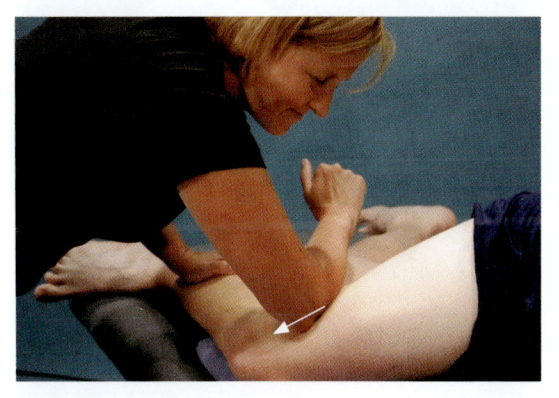

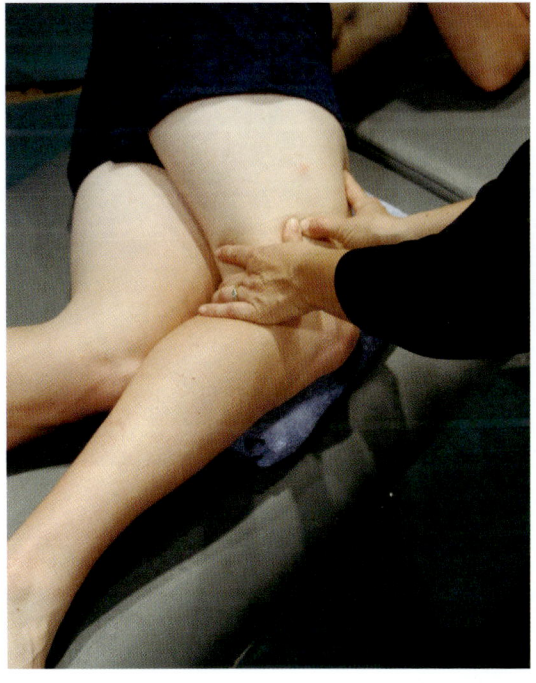

Figure 37.5 Treating tight myofascial structures
(a) Sustained myofascial tension to the proximal ITB
(b) Ischaemic pressure to the body of the ITB

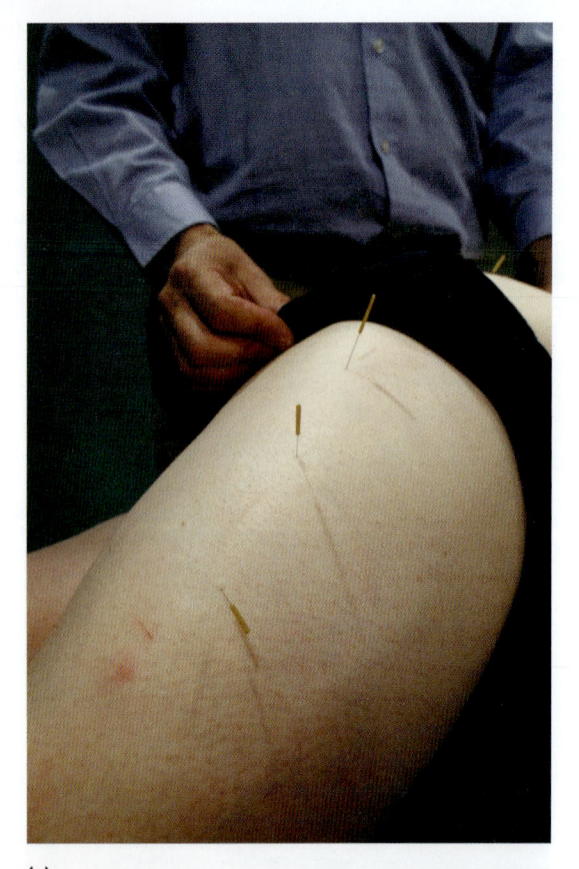

PART B   Regional problems

(c)

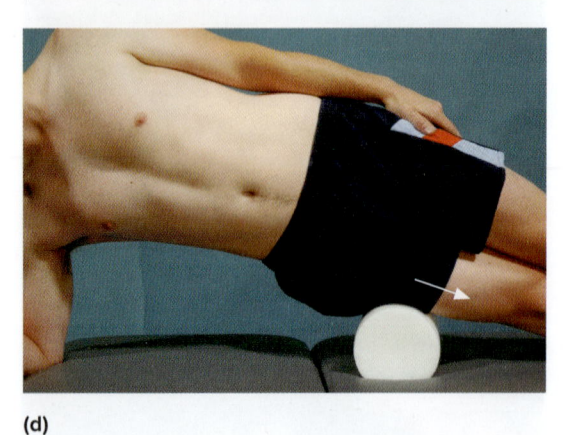

(d)

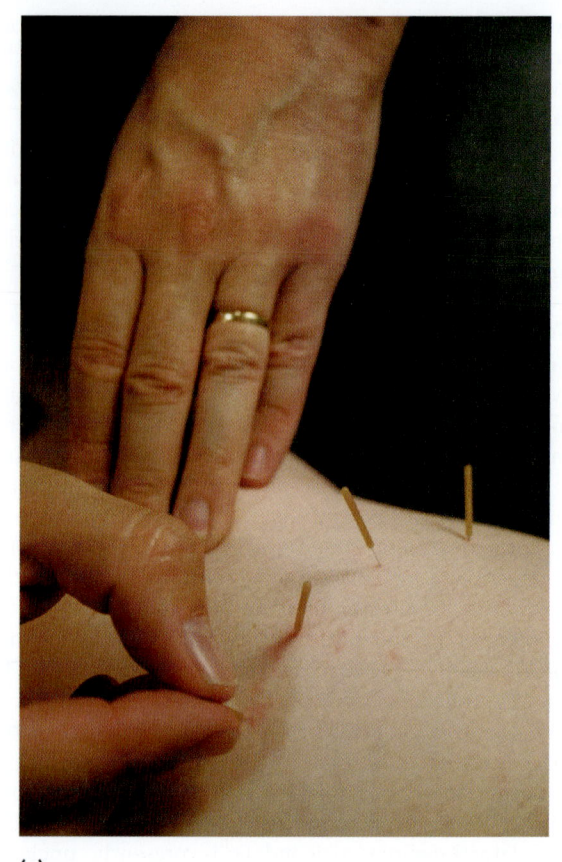

Figure 37.5 (cont.) (c) Dry needling to ITB trigger points (d) Foam roll self-massage to the ITB (e) Dry needling to gluteal trigger points

Tightness of the gluteal muscles and TFL are commonly associated with ITBFS. The presence of trigger points in the TFL, gluteus minimus and gluteus medius may contribute to ITBFS. Gluteal trigger point dry needling (Fig. 37.5e) and ischaemic pressure can reduce the tension and relieve local pressure around the LFE. Strengthening of the hip external rotators (Fig. 37.7a) and abductors (Fig. 37.7b) is an important component of the treatment of ITBFS in order to correct the underlying weakness and fatiguability of these muscles.

In rare and resistant cases, surgery may be considered. Surgery may be targeted proximally or distally. If the athlete has associated pain over both the greater trochanter and lateral aspect of the knee, then decompression/release of the ITB and excision of the 'bursa' or abnormal tissue can be done at either location or both. In patients with isolated distal pain over the lateral epicondyle, most surgeons will target the abnormal tissue by working arthroscopically beneath the ITB or via direct approach, splitting the ITB to address the abnormal tissue that lies beneath. It is essential to work aggressively with rehabilitation postoperatively as recurrence or residual pain is not uncommon.

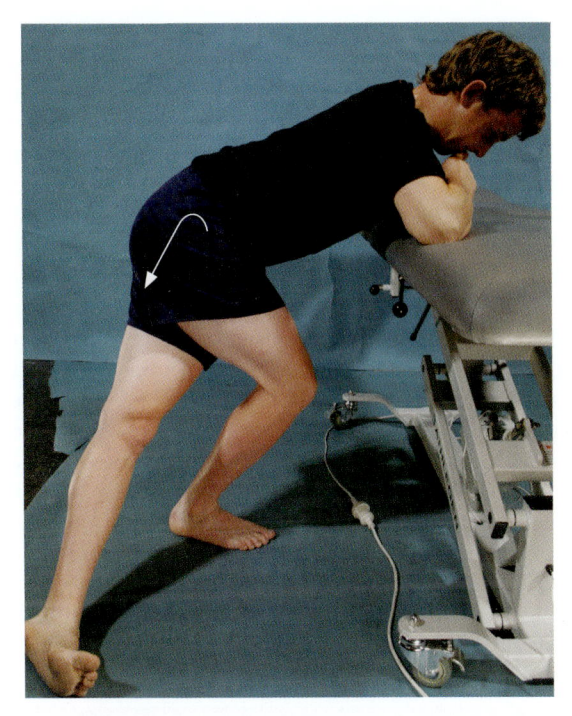

Lateral, medial and posterior knee pain CHAPTER 37

Figure 37.6 ITB stretch—the ITB on the left side is being stretched. The symptomatic leg is extended and adducted across the uninvolved leg. The patient exhales and slowly flexes the trunk laterally to the opposite side until a stretch is felt on the side of the hip

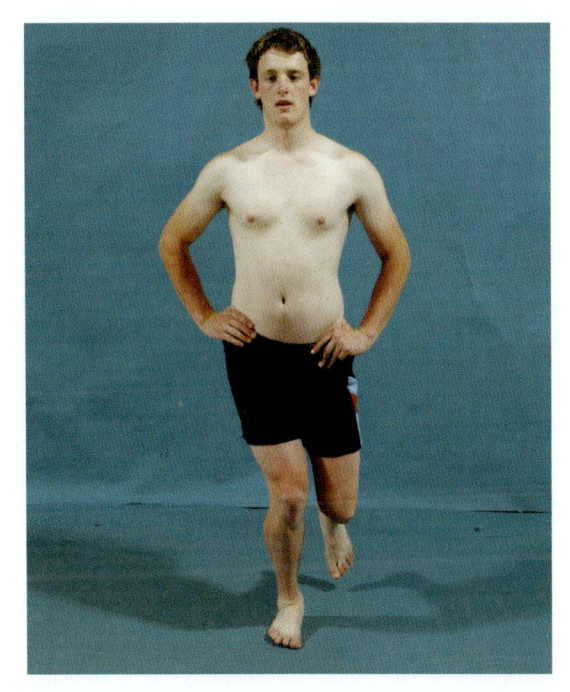

Lateral meniscus abnormality

When athletes present with lateral knee pain that is focused on the lateral joint line, lateral meniscus injury or pathology must be considered. The lateral meniscus is more circular than the C-shaped medial meniscus. It is loosely connected to the lateral joint capsule, has an unattached region through which the popliteus tendon passes and communicates with the PCL via the menisco-femoral ligaments. It is inherently more mobile than the medial meniscus. Acute meniscal injuries are discussed in Chapter 34.

> **PRACTICE PEARL**
>
> In children and early adolescents, diagnosing meniscal injury can be difficult due to vague subjective findings and difficulty in localising pain.[14] Meniscal injury in children is more common than previously thought and is underdiagnosed.[14]

A discoid (disc-shaped) lateral meniscus is an anatomical abnormality that has been reported in children. Most

(a)

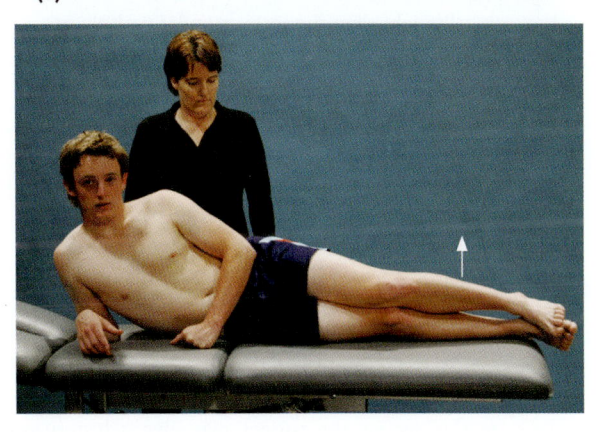

(b)

Figure 37.7 Strengthening exercises for the external hip rotators and abductors (a) Exercise involves the patient standing on one leg and slowly performing a squat, maintaining pelvic stability (b) Hip abduction is side-lying

commonly asymptomatic and presenting as an incidental finding on an MRI scan,[15] a discoid meniscus can also present as chronic 'snapping knee syndrome'. It is more common in the Asian population and may be bilateral. When symptomatic (i.e. painful, presence of joint effusion, symptoms of clicking and locking), it is either grossly unstable or associated with a degenerative meniscal tear, and treated arthroscopically with partial resection.[15]

813

PART B   Regional problems

Tenderness along the lateral joint line (2–3 cm below the lateral epicondyle and site of ITBFS) and a positive McMurray's test (pain with popping) is indicative of meniscal injury (Fig. 37.2h). Chronic degenerative meniscus tears can create a meniscus cyst which can be palpated as a soft, usually painful, bump over the lateral joint line. Radiographs can assist in ruling out other concerns, such as degenerative arthritis, osteochondritis dissecans, osteochondral loose bodies and tibial plateau fractures, within the differential diagnosis.[14, 15] MRI is over 90% accurate for intra-articular pathology but can be associated with false positives.[14]

Treatment of lateral meniscus pathology is based on the athlete's age, duration of symptoms, area of meniscal pathology (vascular areas compared with non vascular) and number of associated injuries such as cruciate ligament tear. Surgeons are more likely to repair meniscus injuries that appear in young athletes or that are large and in the peripheral vascular zone. Degenerative tears in older patients are usually less repairable. The outcomes of surgical repairs have a 90% success rate when performed with a concomitant cruciate reconstruction, compared with only 60–70% success rate when the meniscus tear is an isolated injury. Symptomatic meniscus cysts are usually treated by arthroscopically debriding the intra-articular pathology.

Less common causes of lateral knee pain
Osteoarthritis of the lateral compartment of the knee

Degenerative changes in the lateral compartment of the knee may also be the source of lateral knee pain, especially in older athletes. The pain can be caused by degeneration of the articular surface of lateral tibial plateau or femoral chondyle with or without degenerative changes of the meniscus. Contributing factors include functional demand, size and depth of the lesion, varus or valgus knee malalignment and obesity.[16, 17]

Early in the disease, the patient may give a history of increasing knee pain with activity, swelling, a grinding sensation and stiffness after a period of rest. As the disease progresses, the patient may start to experience more pain with activity, reduced function, morning stiffness or pain at night that may disturb sleep. In the early stages, examination may only reveal a small effusion or lateral joint line tenderness. McMurray's manoeuvre or varus and valgus stressing may exacerbate pain or create the sensation of grinding. A painful McMurray's is not specific for a meniscus tear unless associated popping or clicking occurs. In late stages, the grinding sensation becomes more obvious and the patient may have progressive alterations in their alignment.

The best imaging study is a weight-bearing plain radiograph in the plane of the tibial plateau with the knee slightly flexed. This has greater sensitivity than views taken with the patient supine. Other cartilage injuries that should be considered include osteochondritis dessicans in young patients, osteochondral injuries or loose bodies following acute trauma, and spontaneous osteonecrosis of the knee (SONK) in older patients.

Initial treatment of knee osteoarthritis targets symptom relief with cryotherapy, analgesia and NSAIDs. Modification of activity and exercise prescription are helpful, particularly when combined with weight loss in overweight patients. The efficacy of oral glucosamine and chondroitin sulphate and intra-articular hyaluronic acid injections (viscosupplementation) have been debated and in some reports have a similar efficacy to NSAIDs with very little risk of serious adverse effects (Chapter 17).[18, 19] Another alternative is the use of a deloader brace. Functional motor control assessment focusing on load distribution, such as single-leg squat, stair negotiation and gait, can identify biomechanical contributing factors.

Athletes may modify their activities to choose lower impact training (cycling and swimming rather than running) or reduced sporting challenges (doubles rather than singles tennis). Early identification of these factors may help delay further degeneration.

> **PRACTICE PEARL**
>
> Over the past decade, the efficacy of arthroscopic 'wash-outs' in the absence of mechanical pathology has shown no significant benefit over placebo.

Patients with severe clinical symptoms and joint space narrowing on radiographs may require unicompartmental[20] or, eventually, total knee replacement.

Excessive lateral pressure syndrome

Excessive lateral pressure syndrome (lateral patellar compression syndrome) occurs when there is excessive pressure on the lateral patellofemoral joint resulting from a tight lateral retinaculum. The lateral retinaculum is not one distinct anatomical structure but comprises several layers. A recent cadaveric study suggests there are three layers: a deep fascia layer (not attached to the patella), an intermediate layer (composed of the ITB and the quadriceps aponeurosis and their attachments to the patella) and the deepest layer consisting of the joint capsule.[21] Therefore, an increase in pressure around the lateral retinaculum will affect the joint capsule, the patellofemoral joint, the ITB and the quadriceps muscles. This can lead to bone strain on the lateral patella, inflammation of the lateral retinaculum and ITBFS.

Eventually the increased strain on the lateral patella may lead to chondral degeneration or the development of a vertical stress fracture. The stress fracture can be differentiated radiologically from a congenital bipartite patella by its sharper edges with no evidence of marginal sclerosis. MRI is useful to distinguish the two as a stress injury should have associated

Lateral, medial and posterior knee pain   CHAPTER 37

bone oedema.[22] Chronic changes and malalignment related to chronic cartilage degeneration of the lateral patellar facet are best seen on a tangential patellar view such as a sunrise view, which allows the clinician to assess patellar tracking, patellar tilt and patellar joint space narrowing.

Initial treatment consists of patellofemoral mobilisation and soft tissue therapy to the lateral retinaculum. Taping techniques rarely help. Surgical lateral retinacular release is reserved for patients with increased, uncorrectable, lateral patellar tilt with no patellar instability. If a lateral fragment is present, removal of fragment is occasionally required.[23]

Biceps femoris tendinopathy

Biceps femoris tendinopathy occurs with excessive acceleration and deceleration activities and is often associated with running and cycling. As with most tendinopathies it does not initially restrict sporting activity and therefore has a high risk of chronicity when not recognised early. Pain is described at the posterolateral corner knee, near and just proximal to the biceps insertion onto the fibular head. The pain usually settles after activity and post exercise; morning stiffness is common.

The pain is reproduced with resisted flexion, especially with eccentric contractions (Fig. 37.2e). The pain may be associated with tightness of the hamstring and gluteal muscles. Stiffness of the lumbar spine and poor core stability may also be contributing factors. The diagnosis is usually made clinically but ultrasound examination may reveal synovitis or tendinopathy.

Treatment is based on the general principles of the treatment of tendinopathy: a few days of relative rest and soft tissue therapy (Fig. 37.8) followed by progressive loading (Chapters 4 and 17). Strengthening of the hamstrings (Fig. 37.9) and the hip muscles, specifically the gluteus maximus, may also prove useful.[24] (See also Chapter 31 for the management of lateral hip pain.)

If prolonged pain and reduced function affect sporting activity despite quality conservative measures, surgical approaches may be considered. These include stripping of the paratenon, removal of degenerative tissue and other repair techniques for torn tendons.[25]

Superior tibiofibular joint injury

Injury to the superior tibiofibular joint (STFJ) is a rare but commonly missed cause of lateral knee pain. The STFJ is comprised of the articulation between the lateral condyle of the tibia and the fibular head. The joint capsule is strengthened by superior, anterior and posterior ligaments.[26, 27] The STFJ plays a role in tibiofemoral joint stability through its surrounding anatomical structures, which include the lateral collateral ligament, arcuate ligament, popliteofibular ligament, biceps femoris tendon and popliteus muscle.[27] The STFJ externally rotates

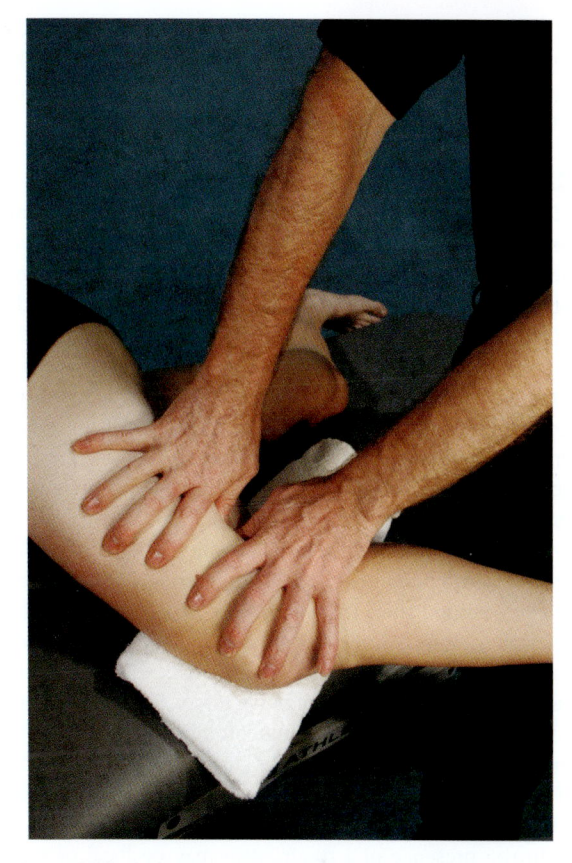

Figure 37.8 Soft tissue therapy in the treatment of biceps femoris tendinopathy. Ischaemic pressure at the musculotendinous junction (shown) and muscle belly can be effective

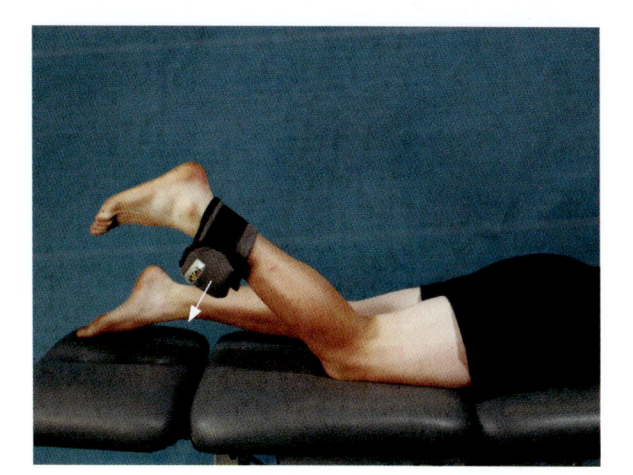

Figure 37.9 Eccentric strengthening exercises in the treatment of biceps femoris tendinopathy. Drop-and-catch is performed in prone positions. This may be progressed to include hip flexion (i.e. patient lying over the end of the bed)

during ankle dorsiflexion and is thought to dissipate torsional stresses from the ankle.[27] When injured, the STFJ can affect knee and ankle function and can be a source of lateral knee pain.

Clinical assessment

STFJ injury may result from twisting injuries or direct trauma resulting in capsuloligamentous sprains, subluxation or dislocation of the fibula. The mechanism of injury is often described as a combination of rotation and knee flexion (e.g. pivoting, cutting) and has been reported in sports such as rugby, soccer, skiing and the various forms of martial arts.[25] Additionally, STFJ injuries can be secondary to severe ankle injuries (a Maisonneuve variant) (Chapter 41). In the older athlete, osteoarthritis of the STFJ can accompany knee arthritis and can be confirmed by careful review of radiographic imaging.[26]

In the presence of an acute dislocation, the athlete may present with a prominent head of fibula, lateral knee pain and swelling around the STFJ. The athlete may report popping or clicking. Pain may be exacerbated by ankle movements and weight-bearing activities. It is important to immediately assess and rule out a peroneal nerve injury. STFJ injuries can be associated with popliteus tendon injury and injuries to the posterolateral corner of the knee.[26] Early recognition of posterolateral corner injuries is essential to optimising clinical and surgical outcomes for the patient (Chapter 35).[26]

In the presence of a sprain, pain may be local or may refer distally along the lateral calf. The STFJ is often tender, especially directly over the head of the fibula, and passive movement of the joint may be restricted by hamstring (biceps femoris) and peroneal muscle spasm. With these muscles relaxed, excessive movement may be detected on passive gliding (Fig. 37.2c).

Treatment

Acute and painful subluxations of the tibiofibular joint can be managed conservatively with immobilisation (approximately 2-3 weeks), followed by a progressive strengthening program of the hamstring and calf muscles.[25] Excessively mobile joints are more difficult to treat and can be associated with generalised hypermobility, especially in the female athlete. Predisposing factors, such as excessive pronation, which place greater torsional forces through the joint, should be assessed and may require correction. Dislocated joints require reduction with possible stabilising fixation.

Manual mobilisation can be an effective treatment for the stiff tibiofibular joint. Local electrotherapy may help relieve pain, but care must be taken as the peroneal nerve is quite close. Strengthening of the muscles around the knee, especially the tibial rotators (Fig. 37.15), may help stabilise the joint, reduce pain and improve function.

Occasionally a corticosteroid injection may be used. For patients with chronic pain or instability which impairs function, surgical options include arthrodesis and fibular head resection.[28] Proximal tibiofibular joint capsule reconstruction using a gracilis autograft can lead to subjective improvements and could aid return to sport.[25] However, strength may continue to be reduced.

Referred pain

Pain may refer from the lumbar spine to the lateral aspect of the knee. Referred pain is usually a dull ache and is poorly localised. The slump test may be positive. The lumbar spine should be examined in athletes presenting with atypical lateral knee pain.

MEDIAL KNEE PAIN

Like the lateral aspect of the knee, being able to evaluate and treat medial knee pain begins with an understanding of the basic anatomy and function of the structures on the medial aspect of the knee (Fig. 37.10). The medial collateral ligament (MCL) provides stability versus valgus stress of the knee and originates at the medial epicondyle and travels beneath the pes tendons to insert 10-15 cm distal to the medial joint line on the tibia. The sartorius, semitendinosus and gracilis tendons (pes anserine) serve to flex the knee and insert just anterior and proximal to the tibial insertion of the MCL. The medial patellofemoral ligament (MPFL)

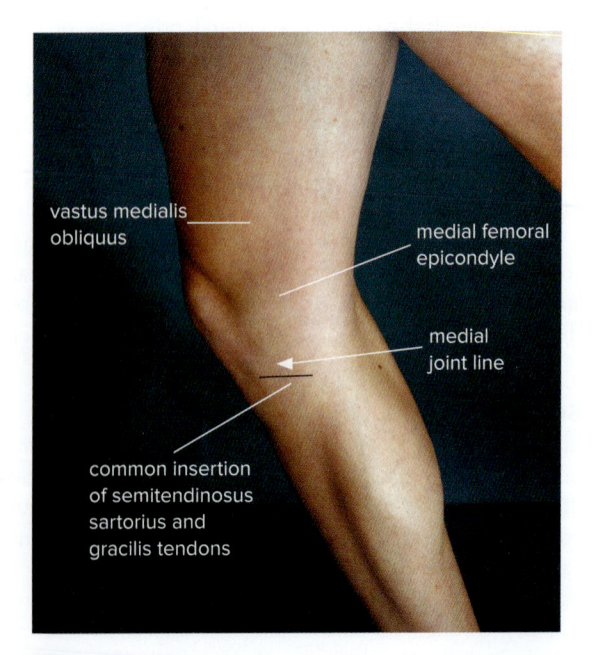

(a)

Figure 37.10 Medial aspect of the knee (a) Surface anatomy

Lateral, medial and posterior knee pain — CHAPTER 37

Patellofemoral syndrome

Anteromedial knee pain is common and is usually associated with patellofemoral syndrome or patellar mal-tracking. Patellofemoral syndrome is discussed in Chapter 36; however, some discussion is included here as it relates to the differential diagnosis of medial knee pain. Indeed, recent studies suggest that the MPFL may play a significant role in medial knee pain associated with patellofemoral syndrome.[29, 30]

When an athlete dislocates his or her patella, he or she will invariably injure the medial retinaculum and MPFL. Most of these will be injured in their mid-substance or off the femur; therefore, in addition to the sensation of apprehension and palpable effusion, the most common finding on examination is pain to palpation over the MPFL and medial retinaculum.

In chronic cases, pain over the MPFL and medial retinaculum may persist due to recurrent instability. Chronic inflammation of the medial retinaculum due to recurrent instability or repetitive irritation from knee flexion may present as a symptomatic plica (Chapter 36). Non-surgical treatments may include cryotherapy, taping, patellofemoral bracing and steroid injections. Surgical options can include arthroscopic resection of a resistant medial pica or medial patellofemoral ligament reconstruction targeting both pain and recurrent instability.[30]

Medial meniscus abnormality

Pain that is localised over the medial joint line is usually secondary to either meniscus tear or degeneration, or a cartilage injury in the medial compartment of the knee. In the young adult patient, a small tear of the medial meniscus may cause a synovial reaction and medial knee pain (Fig. 37.11). In the older patient, gradual degeneration of the medial meniscus can present as gradual-onset medial knee pain. The clinical scenario is similar to that described earlier for a lateral meniscal abnormality.

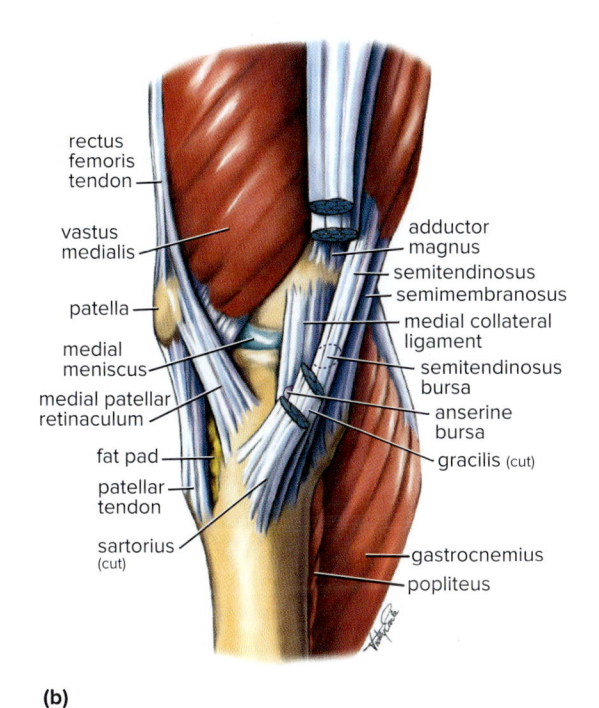

Figure 37.10 (cont.) (b) Anatomy
ADAPTED FROM THE CIBA COLLECTION OF MEDICAL ILLUSTRATIONS, REPRODUCED BY COURTESY OF CIBA-GEIGY LIMITED, BASEL, SWITZERLAND. ALL RIGHTS RESERVED

is a key stabilising structure for patellar stability and runs from the supero-medial border of the patella via the medial retinaculum to a point posterior to the femoral insertion of the MCL (Fig. 35.17). The medial meniscus is intimately attached to the MCL and may be injured with MCL injuries. Ultimately, injury to any of these structures can cause acute or chronic medial knee complaints in athletes. The causes of medial knee pain are shown in Table 37.2.

Table 37.2 Causes of medial knee pain

Common	Less common	Not to be missed
Patellofemoral syndrome	Synovial plica (Chapter 36)	Tumour (in the young)
Medial meniscus	Pes anserinus	Slipped capital femoral epiphysis
• Minor tear	• Tendinopathy	Referred pain from the hip
• Degenerative change	• Bursitis	Perthes' disease
• Cyst	Medial collateral ligament	
Osteoarthritis of the medial compartment of the knee	• Grade 1 sprain/bursitis	
	• Pellegrini-Stieda lesion	
	Referred pain	
	• Lumbar spine	
	• Hip joint	
	• Neural mechanosensitivity	

The athlete is generally aged over 35 years and complains of clicking and pain with certain twisting activities, such as getting out of a car, rolling over in bed, changing direction, and cutting and pivoting movements during sporting activity. Examination reveals joint line tenderness and a positive McMurray's test, that is, pain with a pop (Fig. 37.2h). MRI is the investigation of choice.

Like the lateral meniscus, treatment for medial meniscal injuries depends on the patient's age, chronicity, tear pattern, functional demands and associated ligamentous injuries (see Chapter 35). Conservative management is warranted for non-displaced or degenerative tears; however, if this fails, surgical intervention may be required. Complete meniscectomies are contraindicated as the remaining uninjured portion of the medial meniscus can continue to contribute to shock absorption.[31] Complete meniscectomies are associated with osteoarthritis. Assuming an appropriate tear pattern, meniscus repair is preferred, especially in younger athletes.

Osteoarthritis and chondral injuries of the medial compartment of the knee

Osteoarthritis (OA) of the knee generally affects older athletes (over the age of 50 years), but has been reported in adolescents and young adults.[32, 33] It is important to remember that OA affects not only articular cartilage, but also subchondral bone and synovium. Ligamentous, meniscal and chondral injury, as well as repetitive joint loading, can predispose the knee joint to OA.[32, 33]

Epidemiology

Risk factors for developing premature arthritis include obesity, sports participation, previous knee injury and genetic predisposition.[32, 33] Increasing obesity rates in children, specifically a body mass index (BMI) above the 95th percentile for height and weight ratios (for 2–19 year olds), has been linked to increased risk of musculoskeletal injury.[32, 33] Athletes participating in power sports, such as wrestling, boxing, weightlifting, and team sports, such as soccer, basketball and football, have a higher incidence of premature knee arthritis.[32, 33] However, some sports have a lower incidence of OA. These sports include cross-country skiing, walking and swimming.[32]

> **PRACTICE PEARL**
>
> In the early stages, it is very difficult to distinguish medial compartment OA clinically from medial meniscal injury.

A painful McMurray's manoeuvre may be present in either case. The sensation of grinding is consistent with arthritis while a palpable clunk during the McMurray's manoeuvre is more indicative of a meniscus tear. If weight-bearing radiographs are normal, MRI can distinguish the two conditions using specific articular cartilage sequences, including the technique of delayed gadolinium-enhanced MRI of cartilage (dGEMRIC), which estimates cartilage quality.[34]

Identifying and monitoring athletes at a high risk of OA can allow the opportunity for prevention and disease modifying interventions. Assessment of family history, previous knee injuries, muscle imbalances (specifically quadriceps weakness), lower limb biomechanics and body weight can be incorporated into a screening assessment. Preventive lower-limb-specific rehabilitation programs reduce the risk of lower limb injuries.[35-37]

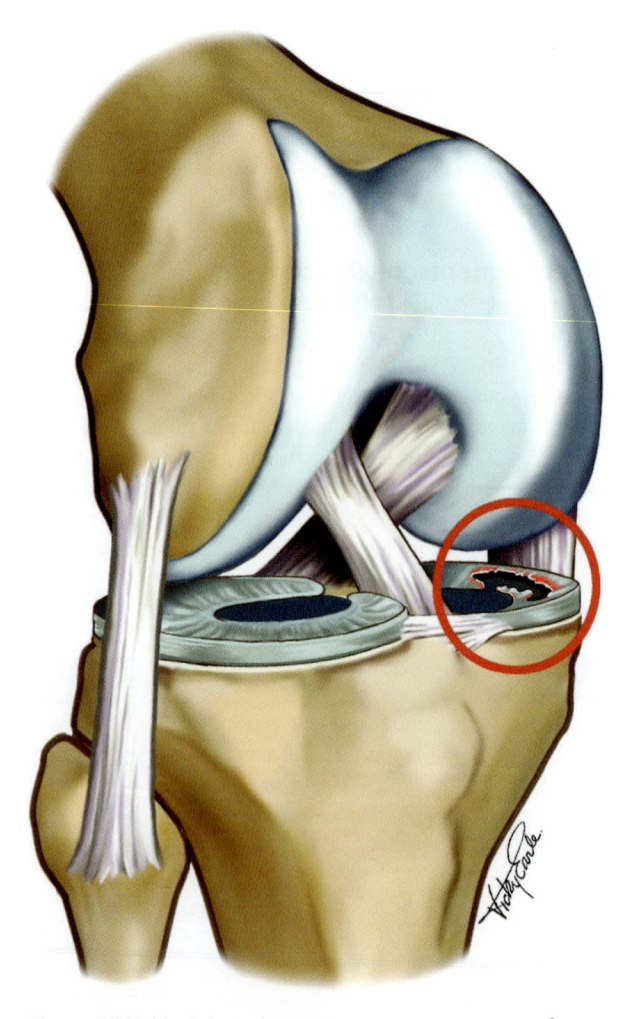

Figure 37.11 Medial meniscus tear—a common cause of medial knee pain

Treament

Initial management of osteoarthritis includes symptomatic relief with cryotherapy, analgesia and NSAIDs.[19] A randomised clinical trial found that a custom-made, valgus-producing functional knee (unloader) brace provided significant benefit in this population of patients aged in their 60s.[38] Biomechanical studies have shown that these braces maintain condylar separation.[39] The benefits of glucosamine and chondroitin sulfate supplementation and viscosupplementation injections have been debated but do not appear to have a deleterious effect other than cost (Chapter 17).[18, 40] Modification of activity and exercise prescription, together with weight loss, should be addressed early.

If clinical symptoms are persistent and severe, referral to an orthopaedic surgeon is warranted. Arthroscopic 'clean out' procedures for patients with arthritis but no mechanical pathology have fallen into disfavour but may be effective if mechanical symptoms are present. Surgical intervention may include high tibial osteotomy, unicompartmental replacement and total knee replacement. Interestingly, early surgical intervention to prevent OA has not been shown to be superior to non-surgical treatments;[32] indeed, some surgeries have been linked to the development of early degenerative changes in young adults, for example, ACL reconstruction.[41, 42]

Less common causes of medial knee pain
Pes anserinus tendinopathy/bursitis

Athletes who present with pain over the anteromedial aspect of the knee distal to the joint line should be evaluated for a stress fracture or pes anserine bursitis. A stress fracture would present with focal pain and pain with impact. Pes anserine bursitis is characterised by localised tenderness and swelling three fingerbreadths distal to the medial joint line but it can mimic medial meniscus pathology. Active contraction or stretching of the medial hamstring muscles can reproduce pain.

The pes anserinus ('goose's foot') is the combined tendinous insertion of the sartorius, gracilis and semitendinosus tendons at their attachment to the tibia (Fig. 37.10b). The area is richly innervated as each muscle (sartorius, gracilis, semitendinosus) is supplied by a different nerve (femoral, obturator and tibial respectively). The primary action of these muscles is to flex the knee; however, they play an important stability role by resisting valgus strain.[43, 44] The risk of injury to the pes anserinus is increased with excessive valgus stress. Excessive valgus stress can be the result of collateral ligament instability, meniscal pathology, muscle imbalances or valgus knee deformity.[44] The pes anserinus bursa lies between the pes anserinus insertion and the periosteum and may become inflamed as a result of overuse. The pes anserinus tendons themselves can also be compressed or irritated, resulting in a tendinopathy. Pes anserinus tendinopathy/bursitis is uncommon but may occur in swimmers (particularly breaststrokers), cyclists or runners.

Initial treatment follows the general principles of tendinopathy/bursitis management including cryotherapy, NSAIDS, electrotherapeutic modalities and eccentric stretching/strengthening. Ultrasound-guided corticosteroid injection into the bursa can be effective in reducing pain.[45] Advanced imaging such as MRI is rarely necessary, but may clarify the diagnosis or identify concomitant pathology in resistant cases.[45] For long-term results, biomechanical factors including the core, foot alignment and muscle imbalances, which can influence valgus forces, need to be addressed.

Chronic MCL injuries and Pellegrini–Stieda syndrome

Due to its excellent vascularity and multiple-layered anatomy, the medial aspect of the knee and in particular the MCL has an excellent healing potential with conservative treatment. Nonetheless, a few factors correlate with chronic medial knee pain due to resistant healing of the MCL.

Chronic repetitive valgus loading of the knee has been correlated with medial knee pain in breaststrokers. The repetitive whip kick can stress the MCL or nearby bursa. Treatment is usually symptomatic with rest, kick modifications, cryotherapy, NSAIDS followed by a gradual return when asymptomatic. Steroid injections are discouraged as they may weaken the MCL.

Pellegrini-Stieda syndrome is a disruption of the femoral origin of the MCL with calcification at the site of injury. It can be a difficult lesion to assess before radiological changes become evident. It may follow direct trauma or, less frequently, a grade 2 or 3 sprain of the MCL. Note that imaging abnormalities exist in asymptomatic individuals.[46]

> **PRACTICE PEARL**
>
> Pellegrini–Stieda syndrome is an important cause of knee stiffness. The patient complains of difficulty straightening the leg and twisting.

Examination reveals marked restriction in joint range of motion with a tender lump in the proximal portion of the MCL. Treatment consists of active mobilisation of the knee joint and infiltration of a corticosteroid agent to the tender MCL attachment if pain persists. Surgery may be indicated in the presence of significant bone formation and persistent symptoms (pain and stiffness).[47]

Injuries of the distal insertion of the MCL can be difficult to distinguish between the pes anserine insertion and a chronic MCL injury. In rare cases, the distal MCL is avulsed as a sleeve off its tibial insertion, leading to persistent pain and instability. Clinically, the patient

PART B Regional problems

will have pain 3–4 fingerbreadths distal to the joint line on the medial aspect of the knee. The key to clarifying the diagnosis with pes anserine bursitis is that a chronic injury of the MCL will be accompanied by valgus knee instability. If symptoms have been present for longer than 2 months, the potential for healing is poor and surgical repair is usually required.

Other causes of medial knee pain
Perhaps the most important thing to consider in an athlete with medial knee pain is not the knee at all. The most important thing is to consider the pathologies that can radiate to the knee and, if missed, lead to catastrophic outcomes.

For the skeletally immature athlete with medial knee pain, the clinician should always consider the possibility of a hip pathology such as slipped capital femoral epiphysis or Legg-Calvé-Perthes', disease (Chapter 44). For skeletally mature athletes, one must be aware that a femoral neck stress fracture (Chapter 32) can radiate pain to the medial knee. Since missing these diagnoses has potential catastrophic long-term implication on hip function, every athlete with medial knee pain should be screened with a simple hip examination assessing range of motion, looking for these associated pathologies. Radicular pain to the medial knee may also be caused by lumbar spine pathology such as a herniated disc but any potential catastrophic implication is usually more obvious, with associated paraesthesias or motor weakness.

POSTERIOR KNEE PAIN
The posterior knee is the most difficult and challenging region of the knee in which to make an accurate and specific diagnosis (Fig. 37.12). The anatomy is complex, there are multiple possible pathologies, structures are less superficial and the posterior knee pain is a common site of referred pain from the lumbar spine and from the patellofemoral joint. Reactive changes from other pathologies such as a knee effusion related to a meniscus tear may lead to pain and tightness of the back of the knee. The causes of posterior knee pain are shown in Table 37.3.

Clinical evaluation
Posterior knee pain precipitated by acceleration or deceleration (e.g. downhill running, kicking, sprinting) may trigger symptoms related to biceps femoris or popliteus tendinopathy.

History
Pain described as a poorly localised, dull ache that does not directly relate to activity is more suggestive of referred pain. The presence of low back pain, patellofemoral symptoms or other knee pathology may provide diagnostic clues.

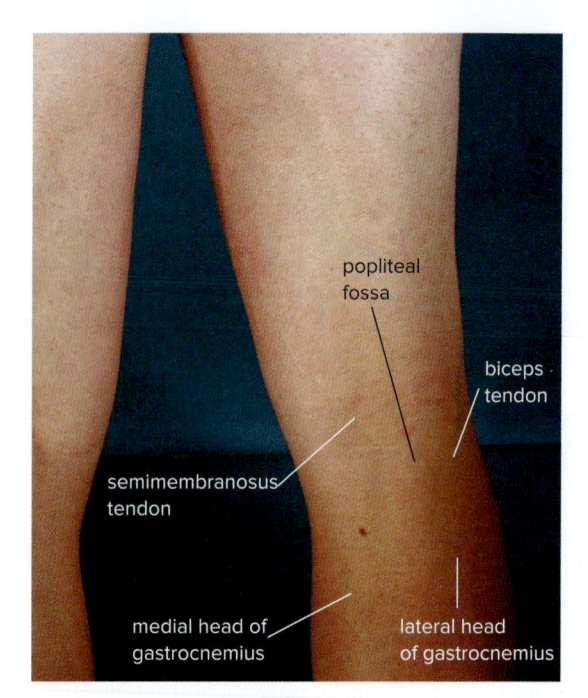

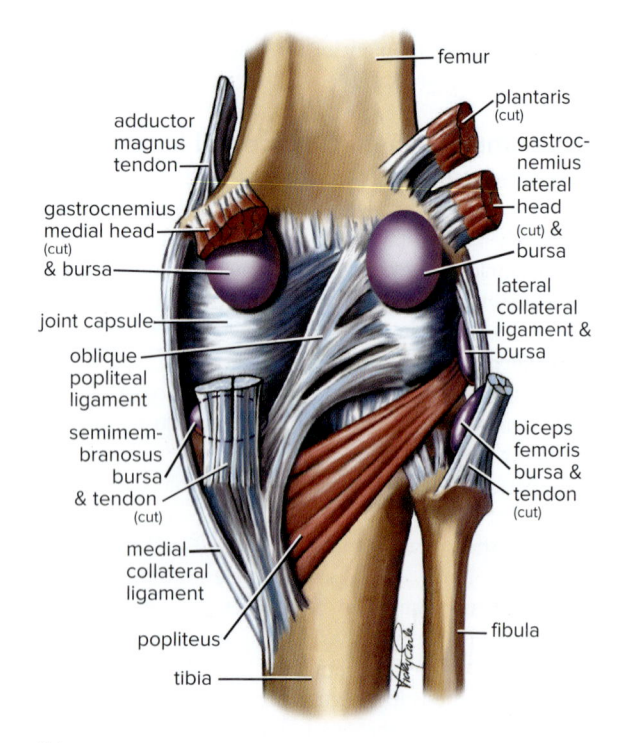

Figure 37.12 Posterior aspect of the knee (a) Surface anatomy (b) Anatomy
ADAPTED FROM THE CIBA COLLECTION OF MEDICAL ILLUSTRATIONS, REPRODUCED BY COURTESY OF CIBA-GEIGY LIMITED, BASEL, SWITZERLAND. ALL RIGHTS RESERVED

Lateral, medial and posterior knee pain — CHAPTER 37

Table 37.3 Causes of posterior knee pain

Common	Less common	Not to be missed
Knee joint effusion Baker's cyst Referred pain • Lumbar spine • Patellofemoral joint • Neural mechanosensitivity Biceps femoris tendinopathy	Popliteus tendinopathy Gastrocnemius tendinopathy	Deep venous thrombosis Claudication Posterior cruciate ligament sprain

Examination

In the examination of the posterior aspect of the knee, it is important to differentiate between local and referred causes of pain. The slump test may indicate whether the pain is referred from the lumbar spine or neural structures. It is also important to detect the presence of an effusion as this may be the cause of the posterior knee pain.

1. Observation
   (a) standing (Fig. 37.13a)
   (b) prone
2. Active movements
   (a) flexion
   (b) extension
   (c) tibial rotation
3. Passive movements
   (a) flexion
   (b) extension (with adduction and abduction)
   (c) tibial rotation
   (d) muscle stretch–hamstrings
4. Resisted movements
   (a) knee flexion
   (b) knee flexion in external tibial rotation (Fig. 37.13b)
   (c) external tibial rotation (Fig. 37.13c)
5. Palpation (Fig. 37.13d)
   (a) hamstring tendons
   (b) popliteus
   (c) joint line
   (d) gastrocnemius origin
6. Special tests
   (a) knee effusion
   (b) examination of knee joint (Chapter 35)
   (c) neural tension–slump test (Fig. 37.2i)
   (d) examination of lumbar spine (Chapter 29)
   (e) biomechanical examination (Chapter 8)
   (f) squat

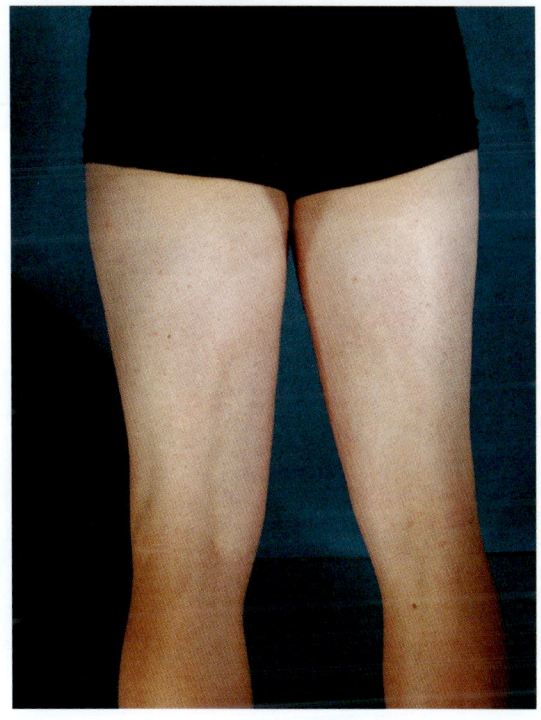

Figure 37.13 Examination of patient with posterior knee pain (a) Observation—standing. Obvious swelling or fullness of the posterior aspect of the knee joint suggests a Baker's cyst. Inspection may reveal a biomechanical abnormality (b) Resisted movements—knee flexion in external tibial rotation. Resisted contraction of the popliteus tendon

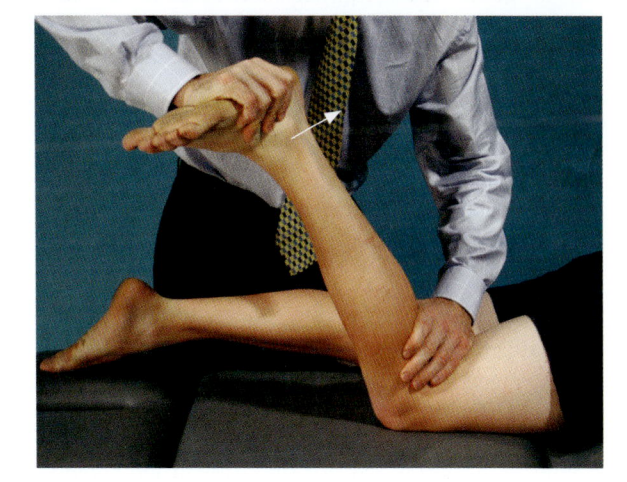

PART B Regional problems

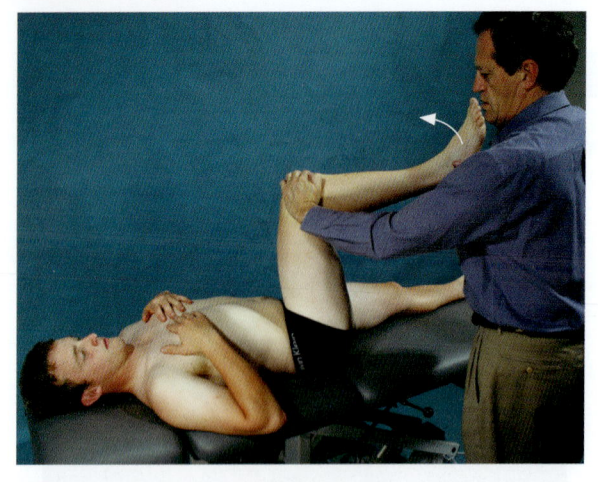

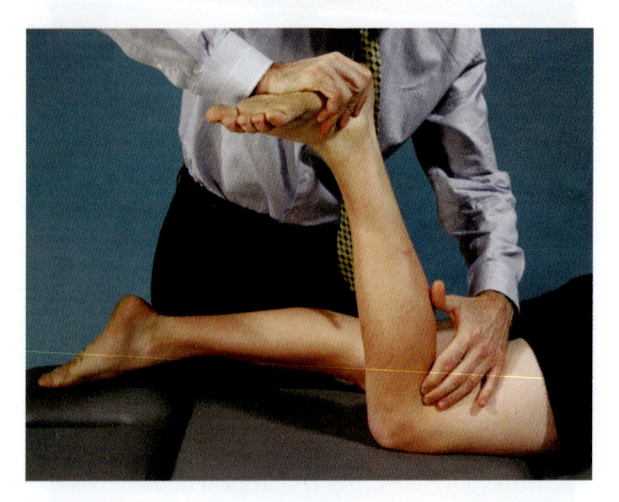

Figure 37.13 (cont.) (c) Resisted movement—popliteus. With the patient supine, hips and knees flexed to 90° and the leg internally rotated, the patient is asked to 'hold it there' while the examiner applies an external rotation force (d) Palpation. This should be performed with the knee in flexion. Tenderness can be elicited over the hamstring tendons (shown), gastrocnemius origin or popliteus. It is helpful for the patient to gently contract and relax individual muscles that are being palpated in order for the examiner to precisely pinpoint the site of pain

Investigations

Ideally, a good history and physical examination should lead to a confident diagnosis and obviate the need for additional investigations or advanced imaging. Nonetheless, it must be acknowledged that the anatomy and potential pathologies in the posterior aspect of the knee are complex and additional studies may be prudent to clarify the diagnosis. Since many patients with deep venous thrombosis are asymptomatic, the clinician should be readily willing to order venous Doppler studies if history and symptoms dictate. Radiographs may be reserved for resistant cases, but may reveal loose bodies in the posterior compartment of the knee. Diagnostic ultrasound may be used to confirm the presence of a Baker's cyst or identify a tendinopathy, and is a valid tool to guide targeted injections. In most cases, MRI is the investigation of choice if the initial diagnosis does not respond to treatment.

Baker's cyst

A Baker's cyst (popliteal cyst) is a synovial fluid filled mass located in the popliteal fossa.[48] The mass is often an enlarged bursa located beneath the medial gastrocnemius or semimembranosis muscles or both. It can be thought of as a chronic knee joint effusion (Fig. 37.14) that herniates between the two heads of the gastrocnemius.

In children the mass is often isolated and asymptomatic and resolves spontaneously. In adults the mass almost

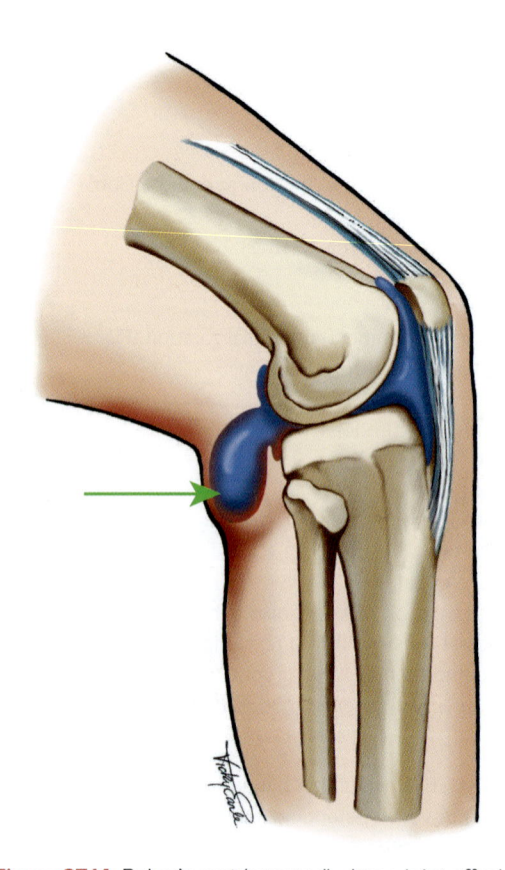

Figure 37.14 Baker's cyst (arrowed)—knee joint effusion herniating posteriorly; usually secondary to degenerative or meniscal pathology

always communicates with the knee joint and is secondary to intra-articular pathology.[48] Intra-articular pathology includes meniscal tears (most common), ACL deficiencies, cartilage degeneration and arthritis. The size of the mass may fluctuate.

Observation of an athlete's knee in standing often reveals a palpable, swollen, tender mass over the posteromedial joint line. End-of-range knee flexion can be restricted and painful. Deep squats and kneeling may also produce posterior knee pain. Due to its high association with intra-articular pathologies, a full assessment of the knee is warranted.

Radiographs may be of little use in the assessment of Baker's cyst, but may rule out other pathologies (e.g. calcification, loose bodies). Ultrasound can visualise the cyst but cannot assess intra-articular structures, which may be the underlying cause.[48] MRI will confirm the presence of the cyst and may identify the underlying intra- articular cause— it is considered the gold standard.[48, 49] Finally, aspiration can differentiate between inflammatory, infectious and mechanical aetiologies. Occasionally the cyst may rupture, leading to lower leg swelling that simulates venous thrombosis. A ruptured cyst usually displays a 'crescent sign'—an ecchymotic (bruised) area around the malleoli.

Initial treatment should involve addressing the underlying cause, (e.g. meniscal tear). Aspiration, together with steroid injection may be useful in the short term.[48, 50] Surgery may be indicated in symptomatic athletes presenting with a large, symptomatic mass. However, unless the underlying pathology is addressed, it is likely the mass will reform.

Biceps femoris tendinopathy

Biceps femoris tendinopathy has been described earlier under lateral knee pain.

Popliteus tendinopathy

The popliteus muscle arises from the posteromedial border of the proximal tibial metaphysis and travels proximally beneath the lateral head of the gastrocnemius to insert onto the lateral femoral condyle. It also has attachments to the fibula and the posterior horn of the lateral meniscus. A recent cadaveric study has confirmed the role of the popliteus tendon in limiting external and internal rotation, knee varus stresses and anterior translation of the femur (acts with the quadriceps and PCL).[51] Additionally, the popliteus has a role in unlocking the knee during initial flexion from an extended position and aids retraction of the posterior horn of the lateral meniscus to minimise compressive forces during knee flexion.

Clincal features

With its role in knee stability, the popliteal tendon could be thought of as the fifth ligament of the knee.[51] Therefore, assessment of tibial rotation during a routine knee stability assessment should be considered. Pain associated with the popliteus region may arise from the popliteus muscle, its tendon or the popliteus-arcuate ligament complex. Due to their close proximity, differentiation is difficult.

> **PRACTICE PEARL**
>
> Isolated popliteal muscle injuries are rare. Popliteal muscle injuries associated with lateral meniscus and PCL injuries are more common.[51, 52]

Posterior lateral instability is often associated with some degree of popliteal pathology.

Twisting activities can result in popliteal injuries, especially with associated posterior knee pain. Impingement of the popliteus tendon can occur with knee rotational instabilities (e.g. following posterior capsule–arcuate ligament strain) and overuse injuries are often associated with repetitive or prolonged acceleration/deceleration activities (e.g. downhill running).

Athletes typically present with posterior knee pain and may report some instability. The main clinical finding is tenderness on palpation along the proximal aspect of the tendon (Fig. 37.13d). With the athlete prone, palpation should begin near the posterolateral corner medial to the biceps tendon and then progress along the medial joint line. Resisted knee flexion in external tibial rotation may reproduce the athlete's pain (Fig. 37.13b).

Garrick and Webb[53] describe a test for the popliteus with the patient supine, hips and knees flexed to 90° and the leg internally rotated. The patient is asked to 'hold it there' while the examiner applies an external rotation force (Fig. 37.13c). It is important that the clinician assess both active and passive tibial rotation. Excessive rotation may be a result of repeated strain to the area. Knee flexion and extension range of motion at the end of range may be limited and also reproduce pain. Lower limb biomechanics should be assessed in terms of varus, valgus and rotational forces around the knee.

Soft tissue techniques and mobilisation may improve any restriction of tibial rotation or knee flexion/extension. Rehabilitation should focus on strengthening of the tibial rotators (Fig. 37.15) and hamstring muscles. Any weakness or fatigue in the quadriceps can add excessive strain on the popliteus and should be addressed, for example with a progressive strengthening program that includes tibial internal rotation.[54] Patients who fail to respond to initial treatment may benefit from corticosteroid injection posteriorly into the point of maximal tenderness or into the popliteus itself, guided by ultrasound.[55]

823

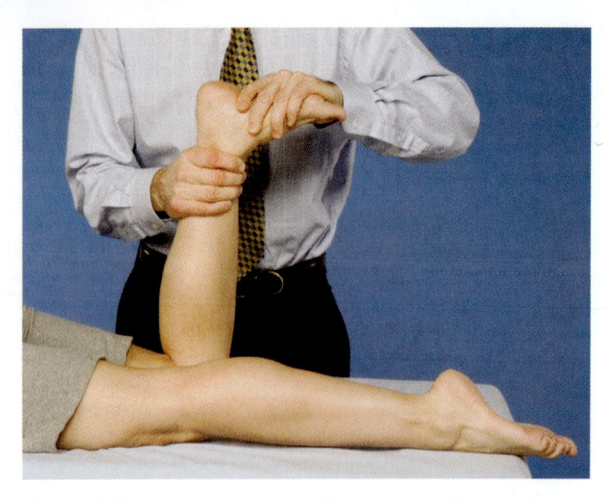

Figure 37.15 Strengthening the tibial rotators. This may be performed against manual resistance (illustrated), with pulleys, rubber tubing resistance or with an isokinetic machine

Pain may be reproduced on resisted knee flexion, calf raises with the knee in extension, jumping and hopping. Occasionally, stretching the gastrocnemius muscle can reproduce the athlete's pain. Possible biomechanical factors should be assessed, including muscle imbalances around the hip, knee and ankle. Knee stability, footwear and foot function should also be assessed.

Initial treatment may consist of activity modification, ice and local and generalised soft tissue therapy. A graduated/strengthening program is key to good long term results (Chapter 39).

Deep venous thrombosis

Deep venous thrombosis usually presents as calf pain (Chapter 39), but may occasionally present as posterior knee pain. It usually occurs after surgery or following a period of immobilisation. Due to the relative high incidence of asymptomatic deep venous thrombosis, it is important for the clinician to be liberal in the use of Doppler ultrasound or other vascular testing to rule it out, even with minimal suspicion. Distal swelling and some posterior knee pain or calf pain in an athlete who is on oral contraceptives, obese or post surgical, or who has a history of clotting problems, should be tested.

Claudication

Claudication can occasionally present as posterior knee pain. It can occur in young adults, not only in the older person. Popliteal artery entrapment syndrome usually presents as calf pain (Chapter 39).

Other causes of posterior knee pain
Gastrocnemius tendinopathy

The origin of the medial gastrocnemius at the posterior femoral condyle occasionally is susceptible to painful overuse injuries, especially in runners. This may result from excessive hill running or a rapid increase in mileage.

Examination may reveal local tenderness and associated trigger points in the medial gastrocnemius muscle belly.

REFERENCES

References for this chapter can be found at www.mhhe.com/au/CSM5e

Chapter 38

Leg pain

with MARK HUTCHINSON, WALTER KIM and MATT HISLOP

I saw it once like two years ago... And that was it, I didn't need to see any more after that.
Kevin Ware, commenting on his gruesome complete tibial fracture that occurred while contesting a loose ball in the NCAA in 2013.

The leg, defined as the anatomic region below the knee but above the ankle, is a common site of complaints among athletes, particularly distance runners. The term 'shin splints' is commonly used by runners as a non-specific reference to leg pain. The same term is also often used by health professionals to describe pain along the medial tibial border or to describe shin pain in general. Neither use of the term is pathologically precise. There are multiple causes with defined pathophysiology that should lead the clinician to a more specific diagnosis of leg pain in athletes. A more accurate and specific diagnosis allows for targeted treatment. Therefore, the term 'shin splints' should be abandoned in favour of a more specific, anatomic and diagnostic terminology.

This chapter focuses on four major pathologies that cause leg pain:

- medial tibial stress fracture
- anterior tibial cortical stress fracture
- medial tibial stress syndrome
- chronic exertional compartment syndromes.

CLINICAL APPROACH

Leg pain in athletes generally involves one or more of several pathological, anatomically specific processes.

1. Bone stress. A continuum of increased bone damage exists from bone strain to stress reaction and stress fracture.
2. Vascular insufficiency. This includes reduction in arterial inflow such as popliteal artery entrapment or vascular outflow due to venous insufficiency, thrombotic disease or vascular collapse due to elevated intracompartmental pressures.
3. Inflammation. This develops at the muscle insertions or along the tendons. Periosteal changes at the tibialis posterior and soleus, and fascia to the medial border of the tibia may be due to traction or a variation of the stress injury to bone.
4. Elevated intracompartmental pressure. The lower leg has a number of muscle compartments, each enveloped by a thick inelastic fascia. The muscle compartments of the lower leg are shown in Figure 38.1. As a result of overuse or inflammation, these muscle compartments may become swollen and painful, particularly if there is excessive fibrosis of the fascia.
5. Nerve entrapment.

The clarification between these processes and the narrowing of the differential diagnosis begins with the

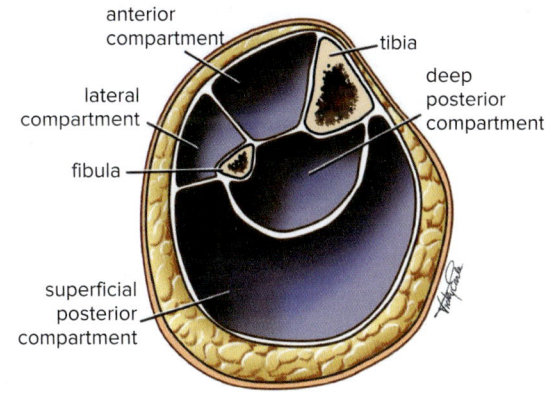

Figure 38.1 Cross-section of the lower leg (a) The various muscle compartments

PART B   Regional problems

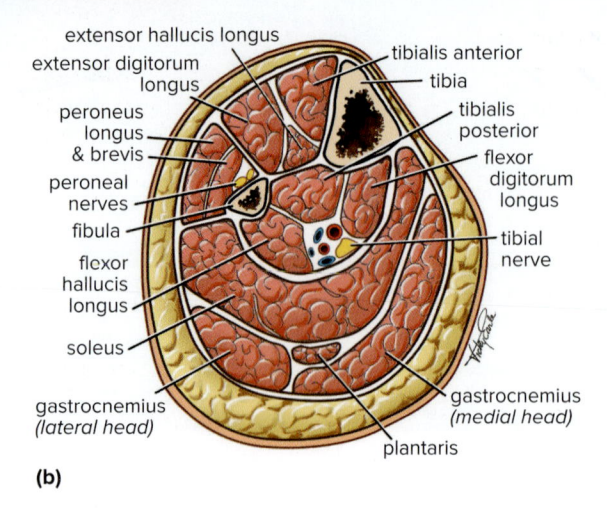

Figure 38.1 (cont.) (b) The individual muscles, nerves and vessels

history, narrowed by clinical examination findings, and confirmed with specific targeted imaging or clinical tests (Table 38.1). It is important to remember that two or three of these conditions may exist simultaneously. For instance, it is not uncommon to have a stress fracture develop in a patient with chronic periostitis. Periostitis or stress fracture may lead to intracompartmental swelling and tip a patient on the edge of symptomatic exertional compartment syndrome over the edge. This interrelationship is demonstrated in Figure 38.2. These co-existing conditions are usually managed differently and this explains why patients continue to have leg pain when only one condition has been addressed. The less common differential diagnoses for leg pain include tendinopathy, nerve entrapment, vascular claudication, neurogenic claudication, deep venous thrombosis (DVT), infection (osteomyelitis, cellulitis), metabolic bone disease, and tumours of bone and soft tissues, which may in rare cases affect prognosis and outcome of leg pain in athletes.

Role of biomechanics

Clinical experience suggests that abnormal biomechanics predisposes some individuals to pain on the anterior or medial border of the tibia (shin pain). Both extremes of foot type can contribute to the incidence of shin pain in athletes (Chapter 8). A rigid, cavus foot has limited shock absorption, thus increasing the impact pressure on the bone. In athletes with excessive pronation, the muscles of the superficial (soleus) and deep compartments (tibialis posterior, flexor hallucis longus [FHL], and flexor digitorum longus [FDL]) are placed at a relatively lengthened position and are required to contract eccentrically harder and longer to resist pronation after heel strike.

On toe off, these muscles must contract concentrically over a greater length to complete the transition to a supinated foot, creating a rigid lever for push off. With fatigue, these muscles fail to provide the normal degree of shock absorption. The chronic traction at the muscles' origins can lead to medial tibial stress syndrome. In chronic cases, this mechanism can contribute to the presentation of stress fractures or deep compartment syndromes.

The athlete with excessive pronation may also develop lateral shin pain or stress injuries of the fibula. Pronation of the fixed foot forces internal tibial rotation. With repetitive excessive pronation, the tibia and fibula are exposed to repetitive rotational (torque) stresses. These stresses are transferred across the fibula, tibia, and proximal and distal tibiofibular articulations. Based on these biomechanical stresses, overuse can lead to stress reactions or stress fracture, not only of the tibia but also of the fibula.

Motor imbalance can also lead to stress injuries in the lower extremity. Tight calf muscles, commonly the result of hard training, will restrict ankle dorsiflexion and increase the tendency for excessive pronation, leading to increased internal rotation of the tibia. Posterior tibial tendon weakness or deficiency can likewise contribute to foot pronation. Ankle instability secondary to chronic ankle sprains causes the athlete to overuse the peroneal tendons to compensate for ankle stability. This overuse can be just enough to send a athlete with borderline compartment syndrome over the brink to symptomatic complaints. To clearly understand biomechanics and have a foundation on which to create a differential diagnosis of leg pain, a complete knowledge of lower leg anatomy is essential (Figs. 38.1 and 38.3). When the presentation is atypical, one must expand the possibilities and consider a broad differential diagnosis for potential causes of leg pain in athletes (Table 38.2).

History

Taking a thorough history is essential for correct diagnosis of athletes with leg pain. Asking the right questions should narrow the diagnosis. Clarifying the pain complaints and assessing mechanism is key to the history. The history should be thorough and assess the presence of associated features with the pain such as paraesthesia or muscle hernia.[1] A complete history should include a broad review of systems to discover other facets such as metabolic issues, prior surgical procedures, developmental problems, contributing medical issues and social issues such as smoking. When the diagnosis does not classically fit the simple pain screen, a broader differential should be considered.

Leg pain CHAPTER 38

Table 38.1 The clinical characteristics and imaging features of common causes of shin pain in athletes

Condition	Pain	Effect of exercise	Associated features	Tenderness	Investigations
Bone stress reaction or stress fracture	Localised Acute or sharp Subcutaneous medial tibial surface or fibula	Constant or increasing Worse with impact	May be exacerbated by vibration with a tuning fork or therapeutic ultrasound (however, neither are a sensitive clinical test)	Subcutaneous medial tibial surface or fibula	Radiographs may be negative • Use magnified views • Look for callous or periosteal reaction MRI can stage severity and define prognosis but is also non-specific
Medial tibial stress syndrome	Diffuse pain on posteromedial border of tibia Variable intensity	Decreases as athlete warms up and stretches	Worse in the morning and after exercise Pes planus	Posteromedial edge of tibia at muscular insertions	Radiographs negative MRI shows diffuse oedema and periosteal thickening
Chronic exertional compartment syndrome	No pain at rest Ache, tightness, gradually building with exertion	Specific onset variable between athletes; usually 10–15 minutes into exercise Decreases with rest	Occasional muscle weakness or dysfunction with exercise Paraesthesia of nerve in affected compartment is possible	None at rest Anterior and lateral more common with exertion Occasionally related to palpable muscle herniation (superficial peroneal nerve)	Radiographs negative Bone scans negative Exertional compartment pressure testing is diagnostic Exertional MRI or infrared oxygen assessment may also be diagnostic
Popliteal artery entrapment	Pain in calf with exertion; not anterolateral 'Atypical compartment syndrome'	Worse with exertion especially active ankle plantar flexion	Pulses may be diminished with active plantar flexion (assessed by palpation or Doppler ultrasound)	Rarely in proximal calf	Radiographs negative MRI may reveal hypertrophic or abnormal insertion of medial gastrocnemius MR arteriography with provocative manoeuvres is diagnostic
Muscle-tendon injuries Strains Tendinopathy	Pain at pathologic site with resisted stretch	Pre-participation stretching usually helps	Short-term symptom relief with NSAIDs and ice	Pain can be at muscle belly, muscle–tendon junction, tendon or tendon insertion	Rarely required Radiographs usually negative MRI gives best view of soft tissue pathology

PART B   Regional problems

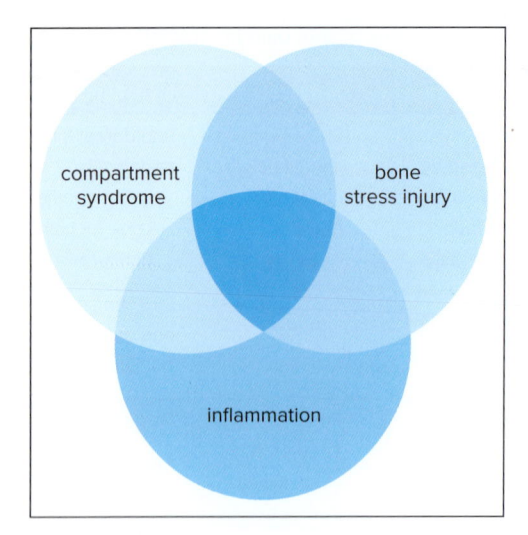

Figure 38.2 Possible interrelationship between the pathological sources of leg pain. These three entities need to be considered within a potentially critical factor—that of workload (represented by the surrounding box)

Physical examination

In the examination of the patient with leg pain, it is important to palpate the site of maximal tenderness and assess the consistency of soft tissue. At rest, the physical examination for certain diagnoses (specifically chronic exertional compartment syndrome) is often unrewarding and the patient may be completely asymptomatic. The astute clinician will ask the athlete to reproduce the pain or symptoms via exertion or impact. This can be done on the athlete's playing surface, on a treadmill, or in and about the clinician's office by having the athlete run stairs or run around the block. A complete examination should be sequential, repeated the same way with each patient, and include observation, analysis of muscle function and range of motion, anatomically directed palpation, functional testing and diagnosis-specific testing (Fig. 38.4)

1. Observation. Assess lower limb alignment (varus/valgus, tibial torsion, pes planus) swelling, bruising, asymmetry:
   a. standing (Fig. 38.4a)
   b. walking–assess gait mechanics (forwards, backwards, on toes, on heels)
   c. lying

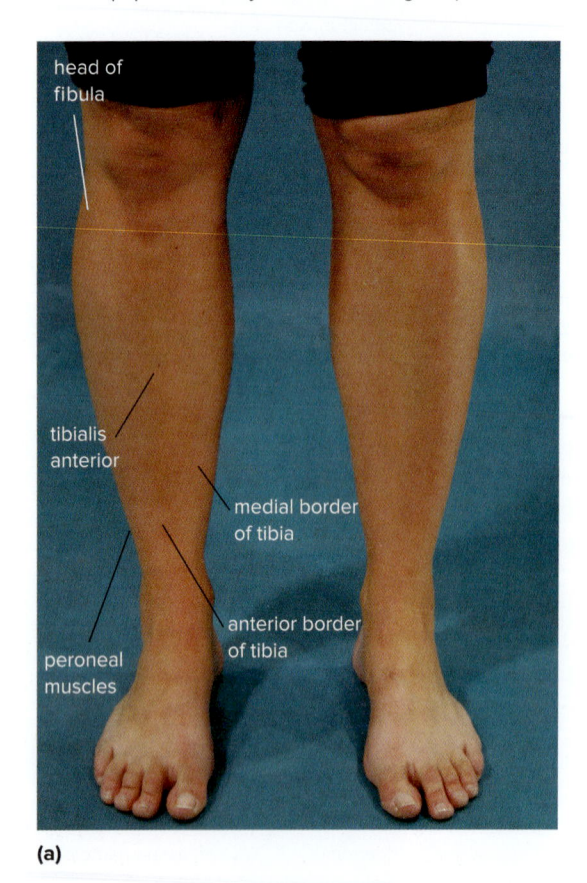

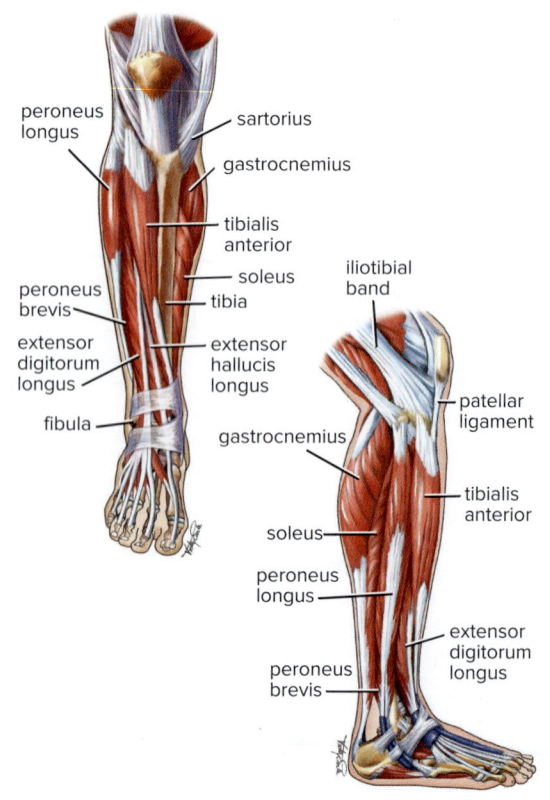

Figure 38.3 The leg (a) Surface anatomy (b) Anatomy of the lower leg from the front (left) and lateral aspect (right)

ADAPTED FROM THE CIBA COLLECTION OF MEDICAL ILLUSTRATIONS, REPRODUCED BY COURTESY OF CIBA-GEIGY LIMITED, BASEL, SWITZERLAND, ALL RIGHTS RESERVED

828

Leg pain — CHAPTER 38

Table 38.2 Causes of leg pain

Common	Less common	Not to be missed
Stress fracture • Medial tibia • Anterior tibia* **Acute fracture** **Medial tibial stress syndrome** **Periosteal contusion** **Chronic compartment syndrome** • Anterior • Lateral (peroneal) • Deep posterior	Stress fracture fibula Referred pain from spine Chronic compartment syndrome • Superficial posterior Vascular insufficiency/claudication DVT (Chapter 39) Popliteal artery entrapment Femoral endarteritis Atherosclerotic disease Superficial peroneal nerve entrapment Muscle herniations Baker's cysts or ganglion cysts Osgood–Schlatter's disease (Chapter 44) Pes anserine bursitis Proximal tibiofibular subluxation Electrolyte and metabolic dehydration cramping	Tumours • Osteosarcoma • Osteoid osteoma Infection (osteomyelitis, cellulitis) Acute compartment syndrome Chronic transition to acute compartment syndrome Chronic ankle injuries and Maisonneuve fracture ***Rare and unusual*** Syphilis Sickle cell anaemia Hyperparathyroidism Sarcoidosis Rickets Paget's disease Erythema nodosum

*Anterior tibial cortex stress fractures are less 'common' than medial tibial stress fractures but included here because of their clinical significance and because we discuss the two types of stress fractures in adjacent sections of this chapter.

---

2. Active movements. Assess motor function and range of motion:
   a. plantarflexion/dorsiflexion–check pulses in full plantar or dorsiflexion; if diminished, consider popliteal artery entrapment
   b. inversion/eversion
   c. flexion and extension of the knee will put the gastrocnemius/soleus complex in a contracted or relaxed position
3. Passive movements. Assess true joint range of motion. May exacerbate pain in compartment syndromes:
   a. plantarflexion (Fig. 38.4b)
   b. dorsiflexion (Fig. 38.4c)
   c. inversion/eversion
4. Resisted movements. Assess motor function. May exacerbate pain in muscle strains and tendinopathy:
   a. plantarflexion/dorsiflexion
   b. inversion/eversion
5. Functional tests:
   a. hopping (Fig. 38.4d)–requires motor strength and landing skills. Rigid landing on heels exacerbates the pain of stress fracture
   b. jumping
   c. running–may bring on pain of exertional compartment syndrome or popliteal artery entrapment symptoms. Athletes should always reproduce symptoms
   d. stair-climbing
6. Palpation. Evaluate pain distribution, warmth, swelling, pitting oedema, posterior cords or the presence of crepitus with motion:
   a. tibia (Fig. 38.4e)–focal pain indicates stress fracture, diffuse pain over posterior medial border of tibia indicates medial tibial stress syndrome
   b. fibula–the entire fibula should be palpated to identify focal pain related to a stress fracture. Severe eversion/external rotation ankle sprains may injure the syndesmotic connection between the tibia and fibula and be associated with a proximal fibula fracture (Maisonneuve fracture)
   c. gastrocnemius, plantaris and soleus muscles (Fig. 38.4f)–look for muscle strains and ruptures. Tennis leg is a partial rupture of the medial head of the gastrocnemius vs plantaris
   d. gastrocnemius-soleus aponeurosis (Fig. 38.4g)–assess for swelling and focal tenderness. May indicate tendinosis vs bursitis

829

PART B Regional problems

Key diagnostic questions

Question	Clinical significance of response
Was there an acute onset of pain?	Fractures and tendon ruptures are usually acute traumatic events. In athletes, the acute onset of pain may be preceded by low-grade chronic pain of a stress fracture or tendinopathy.
Is the pain chronic but stable?	Pain that is getting worse over time should raise concerns of a tumour.
Do you have a history of injury or prior leg pains?	Old fractures or injuries can lead to scar tissue, stiffness and pain.
Is the pain worse with impact?	Stress fractures are normally exacerbated with impact. Medial tibial stress syndrome and muscle strains may also be made worse with loading and resistance.
Is the pain worse with exertion?	Pain absent at rest, that presents with exertion is classic for exertional compartment syndrome. Nonetheless, popliteal artery entrapment can have a similar presentation with posterior rather than anterior/lateral pain.
Does the pain improve with warm-up and stretching?	Medial tibial stress syndrome and muscle strains will frequently improve with pre-participation stretching, while stress fractures and exertional compartment syndrome generally do not.
Does the pain get worse with stretching or resistance?	Providing resistance to the muscle–tendon units including their origins and insertions should exacerbate symptoms related to medial tibial stress syndrome and muscle–tendon strains and tendinopathy.
Where is the pain? Is the pain focal? Is the pain diffuse?	The anatomic site of pain is the best physical clue to diagnosis. Focal pain over bone should raise suspicion of a stress fracture; focal pain over the muscle–tendon is likely a muscle strain or tendinopathy; diffuse pain over the posteromedial border of the tibia is likely medial tibial stress syndrome.
Do you have swelling with the pain? Is it diffuse? Is it focal?	Localised swelling is possible with a contusion, a stress fracture or muscle herniation. Diffuse swelling may indicate more significant injury or vascular problems like a DVT. Medial tibial stress syndrome may have palpable swelling about muscle insertions on the posterior medial border of the tibia.
Do you feel electrical shooting pain? Do you have weakness with the pain? Do you get numbness with the pain?	Electrical shooting pain, dermatomal loss of sensation and sclerotomal loss of motor power usually indicate nerve injury, entrapment or radiculopathy. Always check the lumbar spine.
Does the pain get better with ice or non-steroidal anti-inflammatories (NSAIDs)?	Pathologies associated with inflammation should improve with cold therapy and anti-inflammatories. Osteoid osteomas (a benign bone tumour) are known to have significant response to aspirin.
Do you have pain at night?	Pain that wakes a patient up at night should raise concern about tumours.

   e. superficial and deep posterior compartment (Fig. 38.4h)
   f. anterior and lateral compartment–post-exertion palpation may reveal tenseness in exertional compartment syndrome or palpable localised mass due to muscle herniation

7. Special physical examination tests:
   a. stress fracture test (Fig. 38.4i)–vibration may exacerbate pain associated with a stress fracture. Applying a vibrating tuning fork along the subcutaneous border of the tibia is a convenient and inexpensive test easily applied in the training room

Leg pain CHAPTER 38

(a)

(b)

(c)

(d)

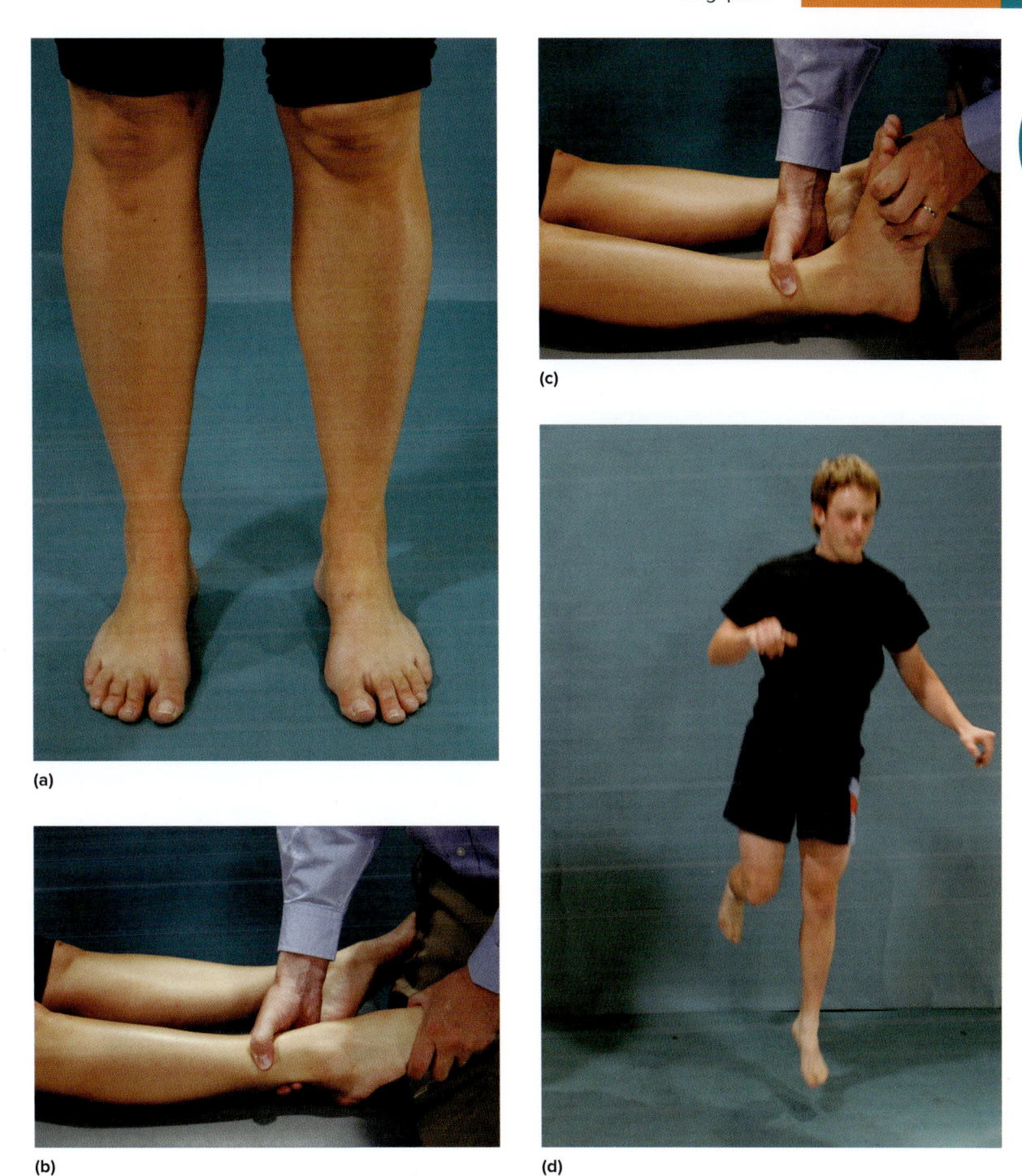

Figure 38.4 Examination of the patient with leg pain (a) Observation—standing. Assess lower limb alignment, swelling, bruising and any evidence of subperiosteal haematoma (b) Passive movement—plantarflexion. This may be restricted in anterior compartment syndrome (c) Passive movement—dorsiflexion. Measure the degree of passive dorsiflexion compared with the other side (d) Functional tests—hopping. If pain has not been reproduced, ask the patient to perform repeated movements, such as hopping, running or performing calf raises

PART B Regional problems

(e)

(f)

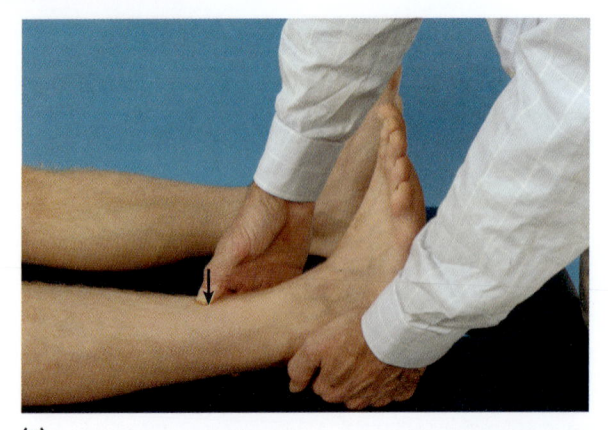

(g)

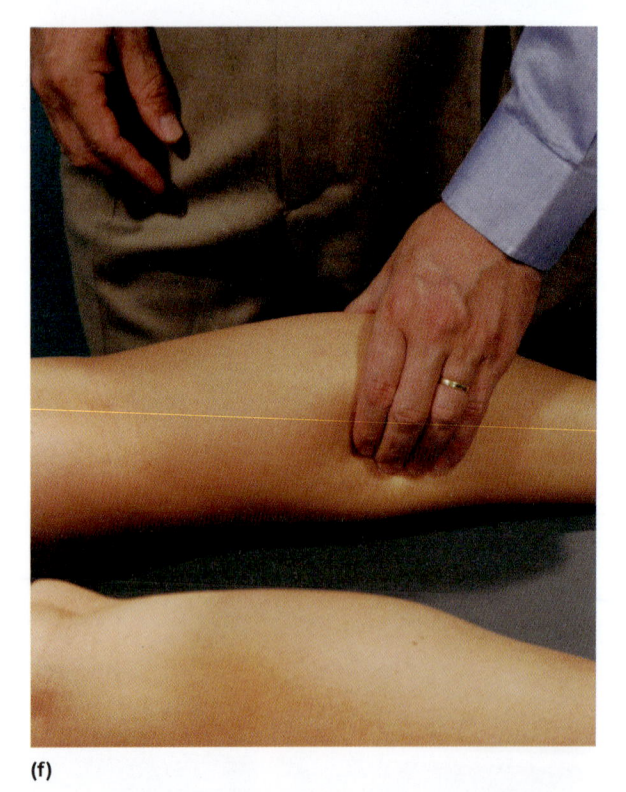

Figure 38.4 (cont.) (e) Palpation—tibia. Palpate for the exact site of focal tenderness. Determine if pain is diffuse, focal or multifocal. Bony irregularity or subtle swelling may occur along the medial tibial border with medial tibial stress syndrome or stress fractures (f) Palpation—soleus muscle belly. A pincer grip is used (g) Palpation—soleus aponeurosis. Palpate for sites of tenderness and associated taut bands that may be a precipitating factor in the development of inflammatory shin pain

or office; however, this test's sensitivity (35–92) and specificity (19–83) is not well established[2]

b. pain may also be exacerbated when therapeutic ultrasound is applied over a bone stress injury. However, this test has both poor sensitivity (64) and specificity (63),[2] and its use is not recommended.

c. biomechanical examination (Chapter 8).

Key outcome measures

The medial tibial stress syndrome score[3] is a valid and reliable outcome measure for medial tibial stress syndrome patients (Table 38.3). As there are few other tools to monitor leg pain, this questionnaire could also be used for patients with lower leg stress fractures. There are currently no questionnaires to monitor chronic exertional compartment syndrome.

Investigations

Following the history and physical examination, extended work-up should target the most likely diagnosis. Imaging options included radiographs, MRI, CT scan, angiography, ultrasound and nuclear medicine scans. Routine radiography is rarely obviously positive in the diagnosis of leg pain. Careful inspection may reveal a subtle radiolucent line

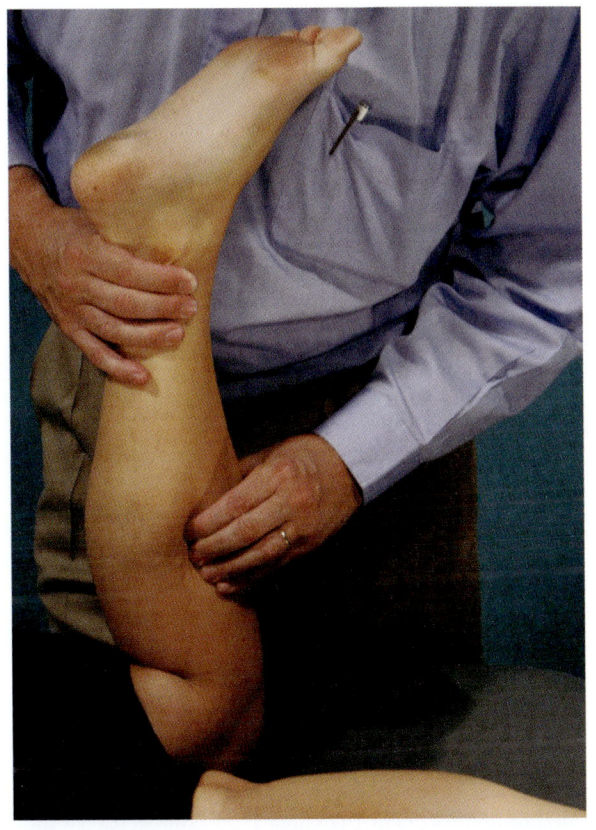

Leg pain CHAPTER 38

Table 38.3 Patient-reported outcome measures for leg pain

Medial tibial stress syndrome score
• Simple self-administered questionnaire that evaluates pain and function in patients with medial tibial stress syndrome • 4 items • Score range 0–10 • Test-retest reliability (1 week): 0.82 • Construct validity: moderate to strong correlation with items of RAND-36 and with changes in the volume and intensity of patients' sporting activities • MDC: 0.69 • MCID: 0.69 • Available online: www.sportsoutcomemeasures.com

indicating a stress fracture, but radiography has a very low sensitivity for stress fractures generally and that applies particularly at this site (tibia).

Historically, radioisotopic bone scan was the next test in line to confirm the presence of a stress fracture or medial tibial stress syndrome. For stress fractures, a discrete focal area of increased uptake is seen on either the tibia (Fig. 38.5a) or fibula. In chronic medial tibial stress syndrome, the bone scan may show patchy areas of increased uptake along the medial border of the tibia. The absence of uptake does not preclude the diagnosis of medial tibial stress syndrome. No identifiable changes on the bone scan are associated with compartment syndrome.[4]

> **PRACTICE PEARL**
>
> MRI is the investigation of choice in patients with leg pain on the basis of its sensitivity to evaluate bony lesions, marrow changes and soft tissue injuries and correlate these findings with clinical symptoms.[5]

Typically, a stress fracture will appear on MRI as an area of periosteal oedema (Fig. 38.5b). The severity of injury documented on MRI (bone oedema only, unicortical radiolucent line or bicortical radiolucent line) has been correlated with healing time.[6, 7] Medial tibial stress syndrome will appear with a broader area of oedema with thickening of the posterior medial periosteum or multiple small stress injuries of the bone. The MRI may also confirm the diagnosis of a muscle strain, muscle herniation, as well as benign (lipoma, cysts, osteoid osteoma) and malignant tumours. Magnetic resonance arteriography (MRA) with dynamic plantarflexion is the test of choice to confirm popliteal artery entrapment syndrome (Chapter 39).

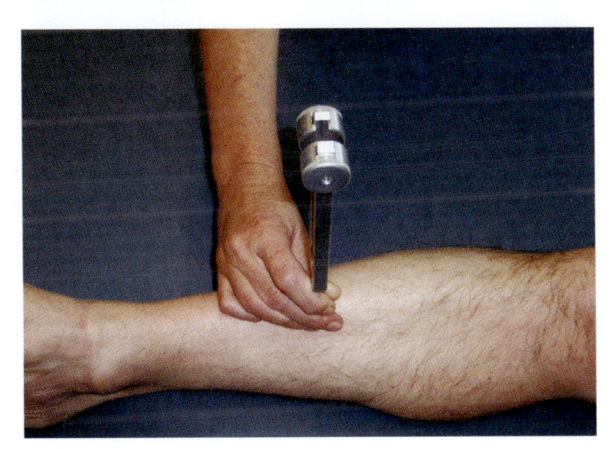

Figure 38.4 (cont.) (h) Palpation—deep posterior compartment. This is palpated through the relaxed overlying muscles. In compartment pressure syndrome, the entire compartment feels tight in contrast to the localised tissue tightness of chronic muscle strain. Muscle or fascial hernias are occasionally found. The superficial posterior compartment should also be palpated (i) Special test—stress fracture. Applying vibration using a tuning fork over the site of tenderness can provoke pain in the presence of a stress fracture

PART B   Regional problems

Investigation of chronic exertional compartment syndrome

For many years, it has been desirable to find a non-invasive method to confirm the diagnosis of chronic exertional compartment syndrome (CECS). Pre- and post-exertional MRI scans may reveal intracompartmental oedema confirming the diagnosis of an exertional compartment syndrome, but this is an expensive alternative. The role of MRI in the diagnosis of compartment syndromes is still unclear.[5, 8, 9] Recently, diffusion tensor magnetic resonance imaging (DTI) and ultrasound have emerged as potentially attractive non-invasive alternatives.

Ultrasound provides a non-invasive, cost-effective and readily available tool to diagnose CECS of the anterior compartment of the lower extremity.[10] Originally described by Gershuni et al.,[11] Martinson and Stokes[12] subsequently devised a technique using ultrasound to measure the thickness of the anterior compartment of the lower leg. Birtles et al.[13, 14] expanded upon this technique to measure anterior compartment thickness in patients with CECS versus control subjects when performing eccentric and isometric exercises. Rajasekaran et al. measured anterior compartment thickness in patients at pre- and post-exertion periods, defined as running for at least 5 minutes up to 7 mph on a 20% incline on a treadmill. Patients with CECS had a significant difference and percentage change in anterior compartment thickness at all post-exertional time points versus resting levels when compared to control subjects.[10]

The use of ultrasonography may also contribute to understanding the pathophysiology behind CECS. In CECS patients, a convexity in the anterior fascial layer was noted during the post-exertional period. The combined effect of fascial bowing with a significant increase in anterior compartment thickness among CECS patients appears to offer an alternative explanation to the fascial non-compliance theory secondary to repetitive overuse and inflammation in the causation of CECS. In addition, recent studies show no significant difference in fascial elasticity in patients with CECS versus control subjects in the anterior leg compartment, which lie in stark contrast to previous findings.[15]

DTI is a non-invasive MRI marker that can serve as a diagnostic probe for pathologic conditions involving skeletal muscles. Ischaemia, inflammation, and injury to the muscle all provoke degenerative changes in the myofibril and are able to be detected via DTI metrics such as mean diffusivity and fractional anisotropy. Patients with defined CECS via T2-weighted imaging (>20% change in signal intensity in each compartment) had significantly increased diffusion rates that were anisotropic in nature after exercise with the most affected compartments being the anterior and superficial posterior compartment.

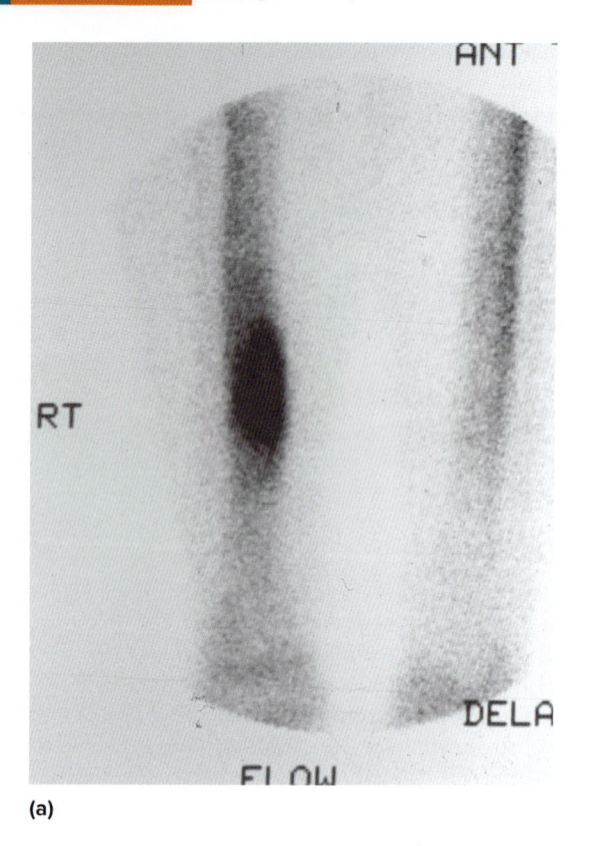

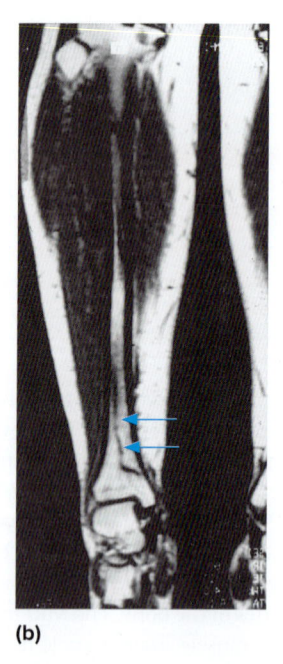

Figure 38.5 Characteristic appearances on imaging (a) Bone scan of tibial stress fracture (b) MRI of tibial stress fracture showing fracture line (arrows) in the presence of marrow oedema

This was postulated to be from elevated temperatures increasing water diffusion rates, structural dilation of the myofibrils or interfibre oedema with exercise. Further development of this technique may lead to its use in the diagnosis and evaluation of response to treatment in CECS patients.[16, 17]

> **PRACTICE PEARL**
>
> Intracompartment pressure measurement is the gold standard in confirming the diagnosis of chronic exertional compartment syndrome in the athlete.

Pre-exertion and immediate post-exertion measurements are essential to confirm the diagnosis. Devices used to measure the pressure have ranged from a wall blood pressure monitor with intravenous tubing and a three-way stopcock (Whiteside's technique), the transducer and pump used for an arterial line, laboratory systems and hand-held devices. In each case, the fascia is punctured percutaneously with a hollow bore needle, a needle with a side-port or by placement of a slit catheter.

A summary of the recommended techniques with appropriate exercises to produce pain is shown in Table 38.4.

The anterior compartment is relatively easy to find just lateral to the anterior border of the tibia with the lateral compartment being just lateral to the anterior compartment and anterior to the fibula. The deep posterior compartment or, if present, the tibialis posterior compartment may be more difficult to locate but is usually accessed posterior to the posteromedial edge of the tibia. Some experts recommend the use of ultrasound guidance to ensure correct catheter placement.[18]

> **PRACTICE PEARL**
>
> In clinical practice, the most widely used diagnostic criteria has been a basal intracompartmental pressure (ICP) of >15 mmHg, 1 minute post-exertion >30 mmHg and a 5 minute post-exertion >20 mmHg.[19]

There is currently no universally accepted method or ICP threshold for the diagnosis of CECS. Pressures between 10–20 mmHg or those that decrease with exercise are considered to be inconclusive. A systematic review showed the strength of evidence supporting these criteria to be weak, owing to the fact that there is high variability and inconsistency in pressure measurements, operator experience, catheter type used, volume of

Table 38.4 Compartment pressure testing

Compartment	Location of catheter	Exacerbating exercise	Compartment pressures (N=10 mmHg, post-exercise 5 min)
Deep posterior	Junction of lower and middle third of tibia Aim deep posteriorly just behind the posteromedial tibial border	Treadmill/running Stairs Run/jump Pulleys in PF/DF Repeated case raises Isokinetic PF with IV/EV Sports-specific challenges	>25 mmHg post exercise or an increase of >10 mmHg compared to resting baseline
Superficial posterior	Aim more posteriorly from deep posterior entry into medial gastrocnemius or soleus	Treadmill Stairs Repeated calf raises	Same as above
Anterior	Mid-belly of tibialis anterior Anterior to intermuscular septum (half-way between fibula and anterior border of tibia)	Repeated DF Treadmill/running Stairs Sports-specific challenges	Same as above
Lateral (Peroneal)	Mid-belly of peroneals Posterior to intermuscular septum	Repeated IV/EV Treadmill/running Stairs	Same as above

Ankle movements: PF = plantarflexion, DF = dorsiflexion, IV = inversion, EV = eversion

instilled fluid used and depth of catheter placement.[20] Admittedly, it is still the most common criteria used as there is no established technique that has been shown to be more effective.

Dynamic measurement of ICP has been introduced to address shortcomings associated with current static time driven methods of ICP measurement. This includes avoidance of multiple needle sticks and data collection that is reliable, extensive and not prone to artefact and technical issues associated with fluid-filled catheters/devices. Dynamic measurement allows changes in ICP to be matched to symptom development in real time during a standardised exercise challenge. This offers a more sensitive and specific method to diagnose CECS. Compared to the widely used Pedowitz criteria of ICP >30 mmHg 1 minute post exercise and ICP >20 mmHg 5 minutes post exercise, a threshold level of 105 mmHg achieved during active exercise was found to provide the greatest diagnostic validity in patients exhibiting symptoms of CECS. This indicates that continuous measurement of ICP throughout the duration of exercise improves its diagnostic utility in accurately diagnosing CECS.[21]

By increasing the diagnostic validity of methods used to diagnose CECS, we can potentially avoid poor outcomes after fasciotomy through better patient selection. By being able to differentiate between patients who exhibit symptoms of CECS but ultimately lack a pressure-related aetiology versus those that have a pressure-related condition, we can identify potential patients who stand to have a higher likelihood of a positive outcome after fasciotomy. Other authors have promoted the use of non-invasive methods such as near-infrared spectroscopy, and results are promising but require further validation.[9]

Additional work-up for more atypical causes of leg pain include:

- EMG/nerve conduction studies
  - peripheral nerve entrapments & metabolic neuropathy
- Ankle/brachial index
  - vascular claudication
- Venous Doppler
  - deep venous thrombosis
- Laboratory
  - CBC (complete blood count) with differential–infection or osteomyelits
  - ESR (erythrocyte sedimentary rate)–inflammation, rheumatologic conditions
  - sickle cell preparation–sickle cell anemia
  - urine analysis with uromyoglobin–rhabdomyolyis
  - CPK (creatine phosphokinase), myoglobin–rhabdomyolysis, myopathy
  - PT (prothrombin time), APTT (activated partial thromboplastin time)–deep venous thrombosis
  - D-dimer–deep venous thrombosis
  - metabolic panel–hypokalemia, hypocalcemia, hypomagnesium, etc
  - T_3 (triiodothyronine), T_4 (thyroxine), TSH (thyroid stimulating hormone)–thyroid myopathy.

MEDIAL STRESS FRACTURE OF THE TIBIA

Stress fractures are more commonly a cause of leg pain in athletes in impact, running and jumping sports. Overall limb and foot alignment as well as limb length discrepancy may also play a role. Runners with stress fractures have been shown to have a reduced cortical strength, a reduced cross-sectional area of cortical bone (thinner cortices) and reduced muscle cross-sectional area compared to athletes without a history of stress fractures.[22] The incidence of stress fractures increases on more rigid, unforgiving surfaces.

> **PRACTICE PEARL**
>
> Approximately 90% of tibial stress fractures will affect the posteromedial aspect of the tibia. The most common site is near the junction of the middle and distal thirds.

Proximal metaphyseal stress fractures may lead to more time loss from sport, as they do not respond as well to the functional bracing that allows earlier return to play. We discuss the dreaded 'anterior cortical tibial stress fracture' in a separate section.

Assessment

A typical posteromedial tibial stress fracture presents with the following clinical features:

- pain is gradual in its onset, aggravated by exercise, often with a recent history of an increase in training intensity
- pain may occur with walking, at rest or even at night.
- examination shows localised tenderness over the tibia.
- biomechanical examination may show a rigid, cavus foot incapable of absorbing load, an excessively pronating foot causing excessive muscle fatigue or a leg-length discrepancy
- tenderness to palpation along the medial border with obvious tenderness. Note that stress fractures of the posterior cortex occasionally produce symptoms of calf pain (Chapter 39) rather than leg pain
- bone scan and MRI appearances are of a stress fracture of the tibia, as shown in Figures 38.5a and 38.5b. MRI scans are particularly valuable, as the extent of oedema

Leg pain CHAPTER 38

and cortical involvement has been directly correlated with the expected return to sport[7]
- CT scan may also demonstrate a stress fracture (Fig. 38.6).

Treatment

Prior to initiating treatment or during the treatment plan, it is important to identify which factors precipitated the stress fracture. The most common cause is an acute or chronic change in training habits, such as rapidly increasing distance over a short period,[23] beginning double-practice days after a period of reduced training or changing to a more rigid playing surface. Footwear, abnormal biomechanics, and repetitive impact sports such as running and gymnastics have also been implicated. Systematic reviews have shown that the use of custom semi-rigid orthotics led to lower incidence of stress fractures in athletes and military recruits.[24] Coaches can play a key role in modifying training patterns to reduce the risk of these injuries.

In women, reduced bone density may increase risk of stress fracture.[25] All female athletes with a first time stress fracture should be screened for Relative Energy Deficiency in Sport (RED-S) (Chapter 4). Research has focused on reducing the vertical loading rate and ground reactive force by modifying stride length, gait retraining and running speed.[25-29] These studies suggest that a softer running style can prevent the development of stress fractures. This can be attained through:

1. a shorter stride length
2. slower running speeds
3. reduced mileage (reduces the number of impacts).

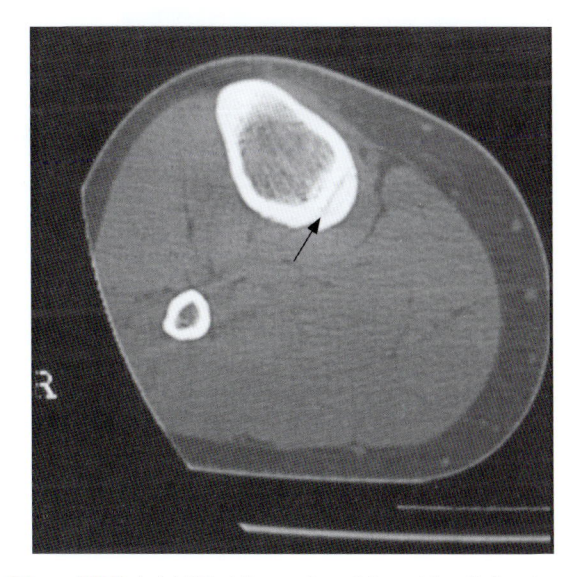

Figure 38.6 Axial CT at the region of the mid-calf showing the posteromedial aspect of the right tibia affected by a longitudinal stress fracture

The classic treatment plan is as follows:

- initial period of rest (sometimes requiring a period of non weight-bearing on crutches for pain relief) until the pain settles
- use of a pneumatic brace (Air-Stirrup® Leg Brace, Aircast®, New Jersey, USA), which has markedly reduced return to activity time compared with 'standard' recovery times in two of three studies [30, 31] and compared with a 'traditional treatment' group in the third.[32] In this latter study, the brace group returned to full, unrestricted activity in an average of 21 days compared with 77 days in the traditional group. The brace should extend to the knee as the mid-leg version may actually increase the stress across a midshaft stress fracture. Routine use of this treatment modality, implies rest and full-time use for 1-2 weeks. During that time, the athlete should notice excellent pain control while in the brace. If this positive response is achieved, then the athlete is allowed to gradually return to impact activities and play in the brace. If pain returns, the period of rest is extended. As long as the pain is well controlled, the athlete is allowed to return to full athletic participation in the brace. Most athletes will complete their competitive season using the brace as complete healing may not occur while the athlete is still loading the leg with or without the brace. Using this plan, there have been no reported cases of progression to complete catastrophic fracture of the tibia
- if pain persists, continue to rest from sporting activity until the bony tenderness disappears (4-8 weeks)
- once the patient is pain-free when walking and has no bony tenderness, gradually progress the quality and quantity of the exercise over the following month. Please note, the athlete is asked to continue to use a pneumatic brace to complete the current season until an appropriate period (4-8 weeks) of rest can occur
- cross-training with low-impact exercises including swimming, cycling, and water running maintains conditioning and reduces risk of recurrence
- pain associated with soft tissues distal to the fracture site can be treated using soft tissue techniques
- general principles of return to activity following overuse injury should be followed (Chapter 18).

Prevention of recurrence

- Determine whether excessive training and abnormal biomechanics precipitated the stress fracture.
- Inadequate calorie balance is a risk factor for stress fractures (Chapter 4).
- Alternative treatments including electrical stimulation and low-intensity pulsed ultrasound (LIPUS)[33, 34] have

837

been tried as a way to accelerate healing or prevent recurrence but have not proven effective (Chapter 17).
- Bisphosphonates have no place in the treatment or prevention of these stress fractures.[35]

STRESS FRACTURE OF THE ANTERIOR CORTEX OF THE TIBIA

> **PRACTICE PEARL**
>
> Stress fractures of the anterior cortex of the mid-shaft of the tibia need to be considered separately because they are prone to delayed union, non-union and complete fracture.

Stress fracture of the anterior cortex of the medial third of the tibia presents with diffuse dull pain aggravated by physical activity. The bone is tender to palpation at the site of the fracture and periosteal thickening as evidenced by a palpable lump may be present if the symptoms have been present for some months. Isotopic bone scan (Fig. 38.7a) shows a discrete focal area of increased activity in the anterior cortex. The radiographic appearance at this stage shows a defect in the anterior cortex, which is termed the 'dreaded black line' (Fig. 38.7b). This appearance is due to bony resorption and is indicative of non-union.

The mid-anterior cortex of the tibia is vulnerable to non-union for two reasons: it has a relatively poor blood supply and it is an area under tension due to the morphologic bowing of the tibia. Excessive anterior tibial bowing is often noted in association with this fracture. In general, the prognosis for these resistant stress injuries is guarded, with an elevated risk of delayed or non-union. One study presented some success with the use of pneumatic air braces in this population, avoiding the need for surgery.[36] The average return to unrestricted activities was 12 months with this form of treatment. Other options for treatment include pulsed electromagnetic stimulation, surgical excision and bone grafting and transverse drilling at the fracture site. Chang and Harris described five cases treated with intramedullary tibial nailing.[37] They had two excellent and three good results.

Treatment

Our current treatment protocol is as follows:

- immediate application of a pneumatic brace
- discontinuing anti-inflammatory medications and smoking
- thorough screening for associated nutritional, biomechanical and nutritional risk factors

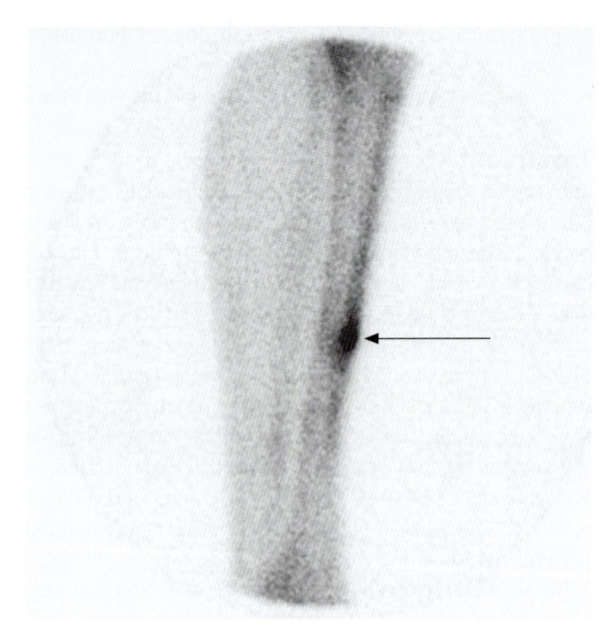

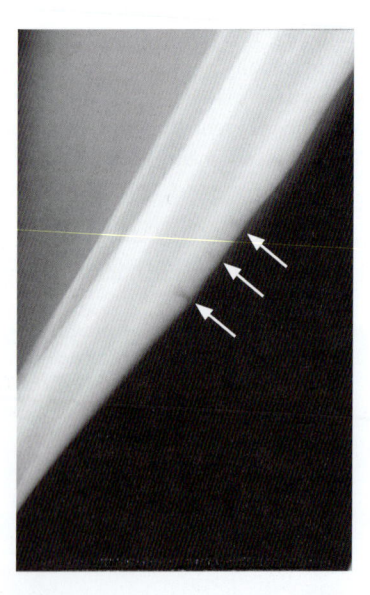

Figure 38.7 Stress fracture of the anterior tibial cortex (a) Bone scan appearance: lateral view highlights the anterior location of increased radioisotope uptake (b) Plain radiograph appearance of multiple 'dreaded black lines'

- for all elite-level athletes, application of electrical or ultrasonic bone stimulation
- if no progress by 4–6 months, intramedullary rodding (+/−) bone grafting, debridement or drilling is recommended.

MEDIAL TIBIAL STRESS SYNDROME

As noted previously, there has been a tendency in the past to categorise all shin pain, especially that which is not a stress fracture, under the term 'shin splints.'[38] Indeed, 'shin splints' is more of a vague symptom athletes describe for leg pain most commonly along the posterior medial border of their tibia. Imaging techniques such as CT and MRI allow us to make more precise anatomical and pathological diagnoses of patients with leg pain.

> **PRACTICE PEARL**
>
> The most descriptive term that accounts for the inflammatory, traction phenomena on the medial aspect of the leg more common in runners is medial tibial stress syndrome or medial tibial traction stress syndrome.

However, recent studies have argued that the process may be more similar to stress injury of the bone and argue that no inflammatory process is present.

The patient with medial tibial stress syndrome complains of diffuse pain along the medial border of the tibia (the junction of the lower third and upper two-thirds of the tibia), which usually decreases with warming up. The incidence has been reported between 4% and 35% in military personnel and athletes.[39, 40] More focal pain should alert the examiner to the possibility of a true stress fracture. The athlete can often complete the training session but pain gradually recurs after exercise and is worse the following morning. Historically, the tibialis posterior was thought to be the source of the pain, but more recently the soleus and flexor digitorum longus have been implicated.[39]

Risk factors

A number of factors may contribute to the increased stress and traction on the posterior medial aspect of the tibia. These include excessive pronation (Chapter 8), training errors, shoe design, surface type, muscle dysfunction, fatigue and decreased flexibility.[41] Other risk factors that have been reported include female sex, higher body mass index, greater internal and external rotation of the hip, increased calf girth, and a history of previous stress fractures or use of orthotics.[40, 42]

The biomechanics of medial tibial stress syndrome relates to the sequence of events that occurs with walking and running.[43] During midstance, foot pronation provides shock absorption and an accommodation to the varied terrain. The medial soleus is the strongest plantar flexor and invertor of the foot. The soleus muscle eccentrically contracts to resist pronation. Excessive pronation due to pes planus or overuse combined with repetitive impact loading leads to chronic traction over its insertion onto the periosteum on posterior medial border of the tibia leading directly to medial tibial traction stress syndrome and medial tibial stress syndrome.

Metabolic bone health may also contribute. Magnusson et al. found athletes with medial tibial stress syndrome had lower bone mineral density at the affected region compared with control and athletic control subjects.[44] Bone mineral density was also decreased on the unaffected side in subjects with unilateral symptoms.[44] These athletes regained normal bone mineral density after recovery from their symptoms.[45] Reduced bone density or bone load tolerance may contribute to the increased risk of medial tibial stress syndrome seen in female military recruits. A study examining possible risk factors for the development of medial shin pain in military recruits showed that females were three times as likely to develop the syndrome.[46] Beyond sex, no other risk factors of statistical significance were noted; however, increased hip range of motion (both internal and external rotation) and lower lean calf girth were associated with medial shin pain in the male recruits.[46]

Radiographs are normally negative with medial tibial stress syndrome. However, it is sometimes possible to see periosteal reactions or localised swelling. Isotopic bone scan may show patchy, diffuse areas of increased uptake along the medial border of the tibia. This is in contrast to stress fractures, which should show focal uptake. In the early stages of medial tibial stress syndrome, however, the bone scan appearance may also be normal. MRI was found to have similar sensitivity and specificity to isotope bone scan.[9] Interestingly, there were a number of abnormal bone scan and MRI appearances in the asymptomatic control group in that study.

Treatment

Most athletes will present with a long history of complaints, having tried a number of home remedies, stretches, medicines or cold treatment. Assessing previous treatments in terms of what provided relief and what exacerbated the problem is beneficial. While heat or whirlpool may improve flexibility and warm up muscles, it also increases the circulation to the region, which can increase symptoms.

The foundation of treatment is based on symptomatic relief, identification of risk factors and treating the underlying pathology. Symptomatic treatment begins

PART B　Regional problems

with rest, ice and analgesia as needed. Switching to pain-free cross-training activities such as swimming or cycling can keep the athlete active. Craig has suggested that no current method of treatment is better than rest alone; yet she still suggests the use of shock-absorptive insoles as promising.[39, 47]

In resistant cases, immobilisation and protected weight-bearing may be necessary to rest the chronic tension placed on the soleus insertion with repeated weight-bearing. Taping techniques are only effective if they control foot pronation.

A critical facet of treatment is based on a careful assessment of foot alignment and gait mechanics. Permanent relief can occasionally be achieved through appropriate footwear and the application of cushioned orthotics (for shock absorption assistance) with a semi-rigid medial arch support (to support the pronated foot). We have found positive results in our patients, at least in the initial phase, by treating them with the same knee-high pneumatic splint that we use for stress fractures (Air-Stirrup Leg Brace®, Aircast®, New Jersey, USA).

Alternative modalities can be effective in relieving pain and should be considered in patients with medial tibial stress syndrome. The entire calf muscle should be assessed for areas of tightness or focal thickening that can be treated with appropriate soft tissue techniques (Chapter 17). Digital ischaemic pressure may be applied to the thickened muscle fibres of the soleus, flexor digitorum longus and tibialis posterior adjacent to their bony attachment, avoiding the site of periosteal attachment, which may prove too painful (Fig. 38.8a). The effect may be enhanced by adding passive dorsiflexion and plantarflexion while digital ischaemic pressure is applied. Transverse frictions are commonly used in clinical practice to treat focal regions of muscle thickening in the soleus and flexor digitorum longus.

Abnormalities of the tibialis posterior may be treated through the relaxed overlying muscles. Sustained myofascial tension can be applied parallel to the tibial border, releasing the flexor digitorum longus and along the soleus aponeurosis in the direction of normal stress with combined active ankle dorsiflexion (Fig. 38.8b).

Physical therapy programs have focused on motor strengthening and flexibility, especially proprioceptive neuromuscular facilitation (PNF) stretching. In addition, electrical stimulation, iontophoresis and ultrasound have been attempted, with mixed results. Prolotherapy injection with agents intended to accelerate the healing process and platelet-rich plasma injections have also been performed, but very little quality research is available to validate their efficacy. In resistant cases, surgical release (with or without periosteal tissue resection or ablation)

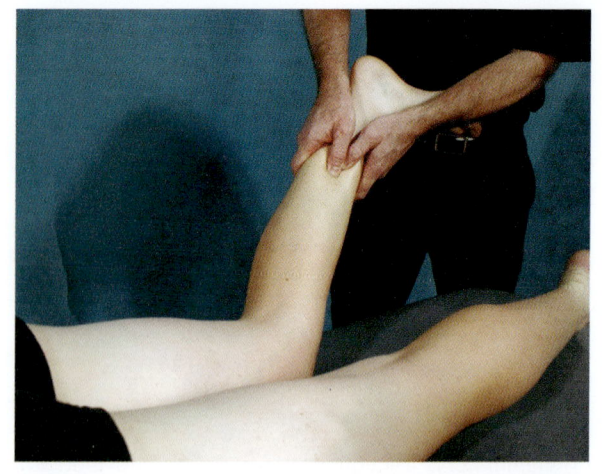

(a)

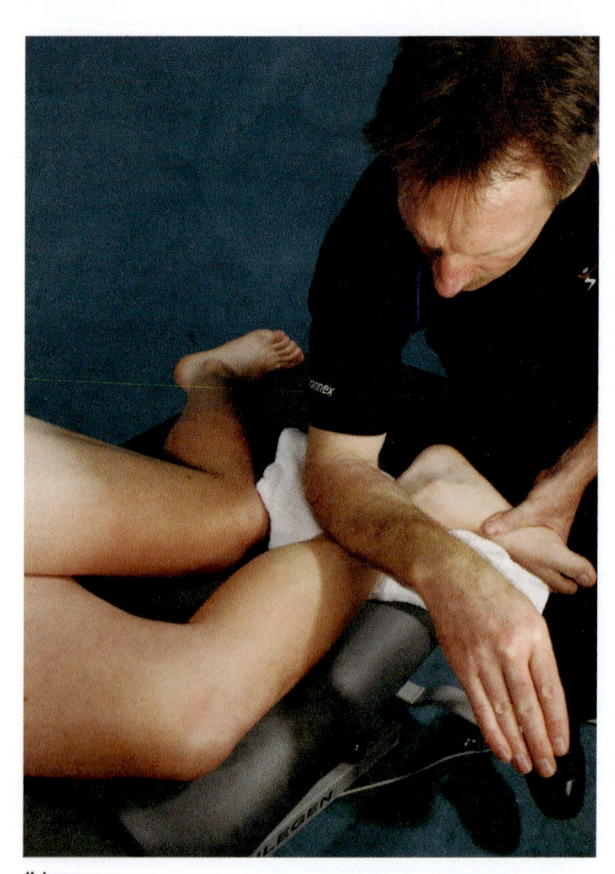

(b)

Figure 38.8 Soft tissue therapy in the treatment of shin pain (a) Digital ischaemic pressure to the medial soleus aponeurosis and flexor digitorum longus. This can be performed with passive and active dorsiflexion (b) Sustained myofascial tension along the soleus aponeurosis in the direction of normal stress combined with active ankle dorsiflexion

of the superficial and posterior compartments from its conjoined insertion onto the posteromedial border of the tibia can be performed with a projected success rate of 70% improvement in high-performance elite athletes.[38, 48]

CHRONIC EXERTIONAL COMPARTMENT SYNDROME

Compartment syndrome is defined as increased pressure within a closed fibro-osseous space causing reduced blood flow and reduced tissue perfusion subsequently leading to ischaemic pain and possible permanent damage to the tissues of the compartment.[49] This may be acute, chronic (exertional) or convert from chronic to acute. Together with stress fractures and medial tibial stress syndrome, CECS is a key differential diagnosis of leg pain in athletes, especially in distance runners and other endurance athletes. The syndrome is frequently bilateral. When the pain is in the calf, the clinician should also consider popliteal artery entrapment syndrome (Chapter 39).

Pathogenesis

While classically, exertional compartment syndrome was believed to be an ischaemic phenomenon like acute compartment syndrome, the exact aetiology of CECS is still unclear. Repetitive overuse followed by associated inflammation may lead to fibrosis and therefore reduced elasticity of the fascia surrounding the muscle compartments. As a result, when the patient exercises, the muscles attempt to expand but are unable to do so.

Biopsies have revealed abnormally thickened, non-compliant fascia. A series of biopsies at the fascial-periosteal interface revealed varying degrees of fibrocytic activity, chronic inflammatory cells, vascular proliferation and a decrease in collagen irregularity, which suggests attempted remodelling was taking place.[50] As a result of this stiffened, abnormal fascial compartment, when the patient exercises, the muscle attempts to expand, but is resisted by a less compliant fascia. This results in increased pressure and subsequent pain. As noted previously, ischaemia likely plays some role; however, this has not been well documented.

Within a tight fascial compartment, it is possible that normal metabolic activity during exercise leads to a sufficient increase in pressure to compromise tissue perfusion. Birtles et al. induced similar symptoms to those of compartment syndrome by restricting venous flow during exercise.[51] Edmundsson et al. noted that when patients with CECS had muscle biopsies at the time of their fascial release, laboratory analysis revealed lower capillary density, lower number of capillaries around muscle fibres and lower density of capillaries per muscle fibre area.[52-54] Thus, the reduced microcirculation likely contributed to the development or was secondary to the CECS.

Typical clinical features of CECS are the absence of pain at rest with increasing ache or pain and a sensation of tightness with exertion.

Symptoms usually resolve or significantly dissipate within several minutes of rest. Rarely, athletes will develop paraesthesia or motor weakness with exertion. At rest, physical examination is usually unremarkable. With exertion, the compartment may be tense on palpation, and it may be possible to see bulges or herniations in the leg.

The most common compartment involved is the anterior compartment, which presents as anterolateral pain with exertion. The other two common compartments are the lateral compartment, which may include paraesthesias in the distribution of the superficial peroneal nerve to the dorsum of the foot, and the deep posterior compartment, which is usually associated with posteromedial tibial pain. Symptoms arising from the superficial posterior compartment are rare.

Clinical features

Work-up and screening should always include an assessment of limb and foot alignment, evaluation of the biomechanical demands of the specific sport including training surface and shoe-wear, a history of previous injuries or trauma, and a screen for overlapping pathology such as stress fractures and medial tibial stress syndrome, as well as metabolic and nutritional factors. In one study, diabetes mellitus was implicated as a risk factor for developing CECS.[55] Radiographs are frequently obtained as an inexpensive screening tool for associated bone pathology.

The definitive diagnosis is made on the basis of intracompartmental pressure measurements (Table 38.4). The use of near-infrared spectroscopy has shown promise as a non-invasive alternative, but is expensive and has not yet become commonly used.[9] A study comparing near-infrared spectroscopy to MRI and intracompartmental pressure measurements found that the sensitivity of near-infrared spectroscopy (85%) was superior to either MRI or intracompartmental pressure measurements (both 77%).[9]

More recently, Williams and associates have suggested that non-painful neurosensory testing can be performed using a pressure-specified sensory device pre- and post-exertion, which may guide the clinician both in diagnosing CECS and in assessing the efficacy of treatment.[56] Other investigators have looked more deeply into advanced imaging techniques to assist with a non-invasive diagnosis of CECS, including ultrasound, Tc-99-tetrofosmin single-photon emission CT, a novel dual birdcage coil, in-scanner MRI protocols and DTI.[57, 58] Nonetheless, intracompartmental pressure measurements remains the gold standard.

PART B   Regional problems

Deep posterior compartment syndrome

Deep posterior compartment syndrome typically presents as an ache in the region of the medial border of the tibia or as chronic calf pain. Beware the multiple other causes of calf pain including popliteal artery entrapment syndrome (Chapter 39). The deep posterior compartment contains the flexor hallucis longus, flexor digitorum longus and tibialis posterior (Fig. 38.1). Occasionally, a separate fascial sheath surrounds the tibialis posterior muscle, forming an extra compartment that may provoke symptoms independent of the other compartments.

Active, passive or resisted motion of these muscles may exacerbate pain. The patient describes a feeling of tightness or a bursting sensation that increases with exercise. Distal symptoms such as weakness or pins and needles on the plantar aspect of the foot may indicate tibial nerve compression. Small muscle hernias occasionally occur along the medial or anterior borders of the tibia after exercise.

On examination, there may be tenderness along the medial aspect of the tibia, but this is often relatively mild. Due to the deep nature of the compartment, palpable fascial tightness is less obvious in comparison to anterior or lateral compartment syndromes. Nonetheless, the experienced clinician may be able to discern the difference between palpable tightness in the deep compartment and fascial thickening and induration found in association with medial tibial stress syndrome.

To measure deep posterior compartment pressures, the needle or catheter is inserted from the medial aspect through two layers of fascia aiming posterior to the tibia (Fig. 38.9). A range of exercises can be used to exacerbate complaints, such as running, jumping, stair climbing, repeated calf raises or resisted plantarflexion and dorsiflexion using elastics, pulleys or isokinetic resistance machines. Routinely, we ask patients to run 5 minutes into their pain to ensure a valid test. It is important to reproduce the patient's pain, otherwise the test is not considered valid.

Post-exertional measurements must be obtained immediately after ceasing exercise and may be repeated again after 10 minutes. Normal compartment pressures are regarded as being between 0 and 10 mmHg. Maximal pressure during exercise of > 25–30 mmHg, an elevation of pressures > 10 mmHg or a resting post-exercise pressure > 25 mmHg is necessary for the diagnosis of chronic compartment syndrome (Table 38.4). If the elevated pressure takes more than 5 minutes to return to normal, this may also be significant.

Treatment

Treatment of isolated deep posterior exertional compartment syndrome usually begins with a conservative regimen of reduced exercise and deep massage therapy.

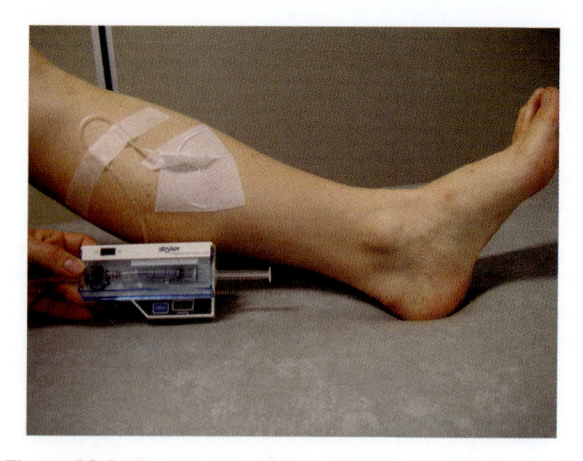

Figure 38.9 Compartment pressure testing—deep posterior compartment. The Stryker catheter is inserted into the deep posterior compartment

All contributing factors and overlapping diagnoses must be carefully considered. Effective soft tissue techniques include longitudinal release with passive and active dorsiflexion (Fig. 38.10) and transverse frictions. Dry needling of the deep muscles may also be helpful. Assessment and correction of any biomechanical abnormalities, especially excessive pronation, must be included.

Isolated deep posterior exertional compartment syndrome is uncommon and may be confused with medial tibial stress syndrome, popliteal artery entrapment syndrome, vascular claudication and stress fractures. Indeed, it is not surprising that initial treatment is the same as that for medial tibial stress syndrome. Unfortunately, if associated diagnoses or contributing factors cannot be identified and if pressures are elevated, symptoms are usually refractory to treatment. In this case, surgical release is necessary.

The surgical approach is along the posterior medial edge of the tibia and may be performed through a single or two small incisions. The saphenous vein lies directly along the path to the fascial insertion onto the posteromedial border of the tibia. Extreme care must be used to control all bleeding at the time of surgery as injury to one of the branches is common and increases the risk of postoperative haematoma or cellulitis.[59]

Some authors have suggested a benefit of fasciectomy (removal of a portion of fascial tissue) over fasciotomy (simple incision) due to concerns that the fascial insertion and sheath reforms.[18] They argue that this periosteal stripping serves an added role of treating any associated medial tibial stress syndrome and it assures release of any anatomic variations of tibialis posterior compartments. Due to the extensive nature of the procedure, which requires longer incisions and has increased risk of

Leg pain   CHAPTER 38

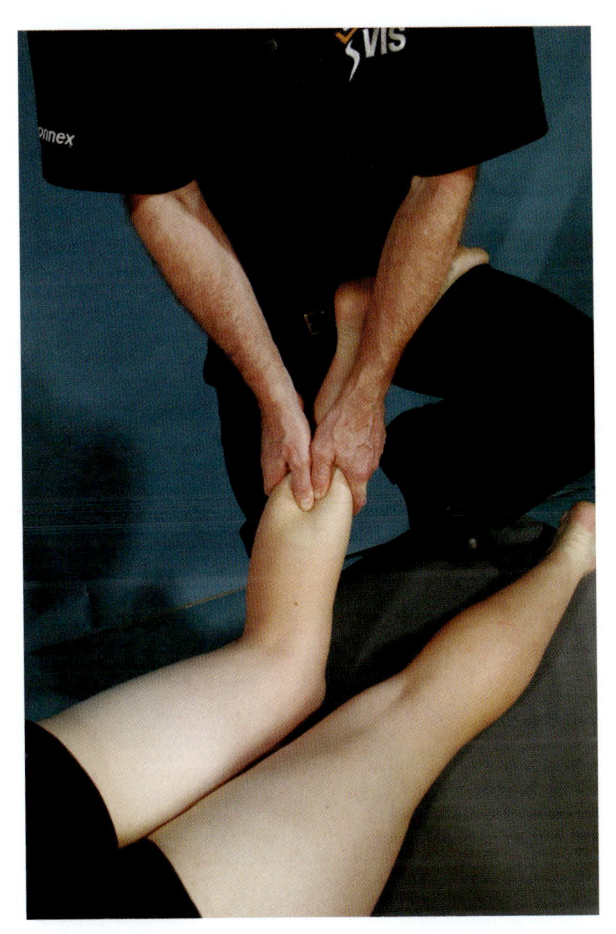

Figure 38.10 Soft tissue therapy in the treatment of posterior compartment syndrome—longitudinal release with active or passive dorsiflexion

compartment pathology, pain is felt just anterior to the fibula and paraesthesia may occur over the dorsum of the foot. The intermuscular septum (raphe) between the two compartments can be seen in thin individuals by looking for the indentation of skin when you squeeze the soft tissues between the anterior border of the tibia and fibula.

Clinical examination at rest will usually be normal or there may be palpable generalised tightness of the anterior or lateral compartment with focal regions of excessive muscle thickening. It is also important to assess the plantarflexors, especially the soleus and gastrocnemius. If these antagonists are tight, they may predispose to anterior compartment syndrome. Muscle herniation may be palpable with exertion most commonly occurring 5–7 cm proximally to the distal tip of the fibula where the superficial peroneal nerve penetrates through the lateral compartment fascia. Diagnosis of anterior and lateral exertional compartment syndrome is confirmed with pre- and post-exertional compartment testing (Table 38.4).

Treatment

Treatment is based on the same principles as for the deep posterior compartment. All contributing factors should be assessed and treated. Lowering the heel in the athlete's shoe or orthotics may reduce the load of the anterior muscles and alleviate pain. Soft issue techniques, such as sustained myofascial tension combined with passive and active plantarflexion (Fig. 38.11), transverse frictions and dry needling may alleviate symptoms.

Dr Andrew Franklyn-Miller has argued for much more attention to the biomechanics of running to treat CECS.[62, 63] To reduce load on tibialis anterior, he promotes midfoot landing rather than heel-strike and an increased cadence of 5–10%. Other gait adjustments are made according to individual assessment, such as reducing the vertical tibial angle at foot strike, promoting a smooth gait pattern, a more anterior centre of mass and a shortened stride length.[62]

A study conducted among military personnel studied the effect of using a forefoot strike pattern among individuals with CECS symptoms for at least 10 months who had an initial hindfoot strike gait pattern.[64] Six weeks after the implementation of forefoot strike technique, subjects had reduced post-running ICP, reduced pain during running and increased running distance. Improvements were maintained at the 1-year follow-up, where subjects also had an improved 2-mile time trial performance. Most importantly, surgical intervention was not required in any of the individuals.[64]

Another non-operative CECS management strategy is the use of botulinum toxin. It reduces muscle hypertrophy and provide analgesic properties in treating myofascial conditions involving contractures and hypertrophy.[65] In one case series, intramuscular injection of botulinum

complications, we recommend this extensive approach only in revision cases. In addition, we believe it is prudent to limit treatment to the most affected compartment in patients who have positive anterior or lateral compartment pressures, but only borderline pressures in the deep compartment. This may reduce the risk of postsurgical complications, which is elevated when releasing the posterior compartments.[59-61]

Anterior and lateral exertional compartment syndromes

The anterior compartment contains the tibialis anterior, extensor digitorum longus, extensor hallucis longus and peroneus tertius muscles, as well as the deep peroneal nerve. The lateral (peroneal) compartment contains the peroneus longus and brevis tendons as well as the superficial peroneal nerve. For anterior compartment pathology, exertional pain occurs just lateral to the anterior border of the shin. Paraesthesia may also occur in the first web space. For lateral

PART B Regional problems

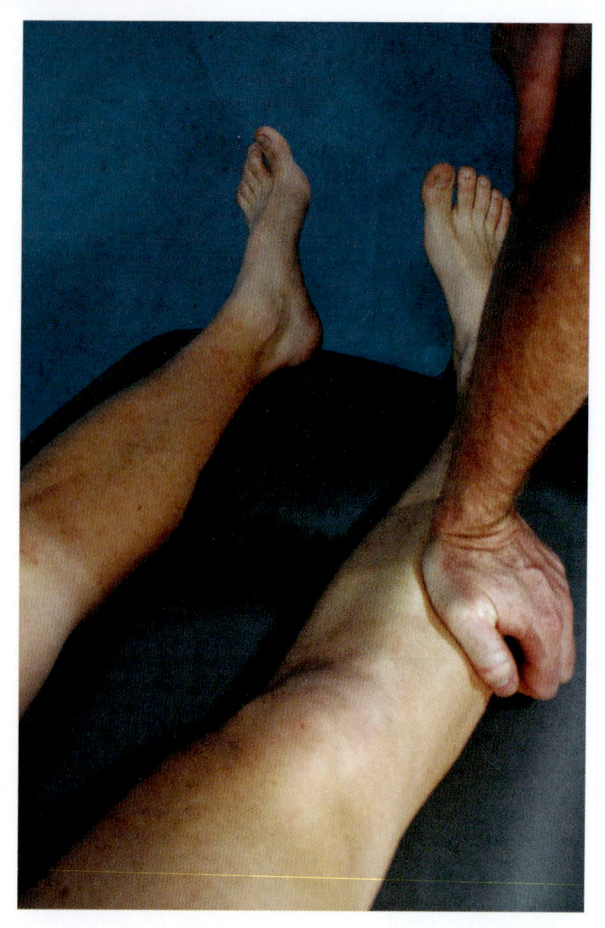

Figure 38.11 Soft tissue therapy in the treatment of anterior compartment syndrome. Sustained myofascial tension with active or passive plantarflexion

Acute compartment syndromes

Acute compartment syndromes are usually associated with trauma. Intracompartmental pressures are significantly elevated and do not subside with rest. Immediate surgical release is essential to avoid ischaemic injury.

It is important to note a number of case reports which describe acute anterior compartment syndromes brought on by exercise rather than trauma.[68, 69] In many of these cases, the athlete continued to exercise through their initial pain, which was most likely an exertional compartment syndrome that would otherwise have gone away with rest. When pain does not subside within an appropriate time, conversion of an exertional compartment syndrome to an acute compartment syndrome should be considered.

Outcomes of exertional compartment syndrome surgery

As noted previously, the majority of patients undergoing surgery for CECS (80–90%) have a satisfactory result, with many being able to return to their previous level of sport.[70] However, some patients either fail to improve after surgery or, after a period of improvement, have a recurrence of symptoms. Micheli noted a slightly decreased rate of successful outcomes among female patients,[71] but others have not found any difference in outcome between sexes.[72] Some studies suggest that failure and recurrences are more common in the deep posterior compartment,[70, 73] possibly due to failure to release the tibialis posterior compartment.[70] Indeed, there are few studies looking at outcomes of isolated CECS of the deep posterior compartment.

Patient satisfaction rates for surgical fasciotomy of the deep compartment have been reported to be as low as 52%.[74-76] This has been attributed to surgical technique, anatomic variation, over-extensive release (e.g. all four compartments) and inaccurate diagnosis. Confounding factors which may lead to inaccurate diagnosis of posterior CECS include venous insufficiency, popliteal and peroneal entrapment, and tibial stress fracture/periostitis. Thus, accurate diagnosis and conservative management may play a key role in avoiding poor outcomes associated with fasciotomy of the deep posterior compartment.

Several other factors are also associated with surgical outcomes for isolated CECS of the deep compartment. Preoperative ICP measured at four different time intervals (pre, immediately, 1 minute post, 5 minutes post exercise) predict outcomes: a higher area under the 4-point curve is an indicator of likely surgical success.[72] In addition, a delayed diagnosis is associated with poorer outcomes.[72]

toxin resulted in significant reduction of ICP at 1 minute and 5 minutes post exercise in both the anterior and lateral compartments. Subjective exertional pain scores also decreased, with 15 out of 16 study participants reporting no exertional pain at nine-month follow-up. However, the level of evidence to support this treatment is currently low, with several questions remaining regarding the exact mechanism and long-term outcome.[66]

When conservative treatment fails, surgical release is required, especially when there are no obvious precipitating factors to correct. Fasiectomy is rarely necessary for the anterior or lateral compartments, as they release with minimal incision. Indeed, percutaneous and endoscopically assisted releases are approaching 90% success rates. Newer equipment including balloon catheters or endoscopic vein harvesting retractors have been used to make endoscopic-assisted techniques even safer.[67] Special care is essential to visualise the superficial peroneal nerve at the time of surgery to avoid iatrogenic injury.

In a study of 18 patients who underwent revision surgery, increased pressure was found only in a localised area at the site of the scar, whereas 40% had high pressures throughout the compartment.[75] The exuberant scar tissue was thicker, denser and more constricting than was the original fascia. Eight of the 18 patients had entrapment of the superficial peroneal nerve with numbness and paraesthesia over the dorsum of the foot with exertion, positive Tinel's sign, and localised tenderness over the nerve, exacerbated by active dorsiflexion and eversion, as well as passive inversion and plantar flexion. All those with peroneal nerve entrapment had a good result from the revision surgery, whereas only 50% of those without nerve entrapment had a satisfactory outcome.

Lessons from surgery with unsatisfactory outcomes

The foundation of a successful surgical result begins with a proper anatomic diagnosis. The diagnosis should be confirmed preoperatively with intracompartmental pressure measurement, and all associated or contributing factors should be addressed.

- Surgery should target the specific anatomic pathology and the release of all four compartments should be avoided to reduce the risk of surgical complications.
- Meticulous control of intraoperative bleeding will reduce the risk of postoperative haematoma and cellulitis.
- Perioperative antibiotics and postoperative cryotherapy can reduce the risk of postoperative cellulitis or infection. If identified in the postoperative period, the surgeon should have a relatively low threshold to return to the operating room and perform early irrigation.
- A common complication is postoperative stiffness, which can be avoided by early and aggressive postoperative mobilisation.
- The absolute indication for fasciectomy in contrast to fasciotomy is not clear, as the former may increase the risk of bleeding and postoperative stiffness.

Rehabilitation following compartment syndrome surgery

The following protocol is recommended:[4]

- perioperative antibiotics and cryotherapy to reduce complications of infection, haematoma and cellulitis
- range of motion exercises of the knee and ankle in the immediate postoperative period. Full plantar and dorsiflexion is encouraged
- three to five days of limited weight-bearing on crutches, then full weight-bearing as tolerated
- once wounds have healed, a strengthening program including cycling and swimming to commence
- gradual return to light jogging at about 4–6 weeks after surgery
- full sports participation anticipated at 6–8 weeks (if one compartment released) and 8–12 weeks (if both legs and multiple compartments released)
- athlete should be pain-free with 90% strength regained prior to full sports participation.

LESS COMMON CAUSES
Stress fracture of the fibula

Stress fractures of the fibula are not as common as stress fractures of the tibia. As the fibula plays a minimal role in weight-bearing, this stress fracture is usually due to muscle traction or torsional forces placed through the bone. In the athlete with excessive subtalar pronation, the peroneal muscles are forced to contract harder and longer during toe-off. Examination may reveal local tenderness and pain in springing the fibula proximal to the site of the stress fracture.

This injury is usually not as painful on weight-bearing as is a stress fracture of the tibia. It is treated symptomatically with rest from activity until bony tenderness settles. Due to poorer rotational control, knee-high pneumatic braces may not be as effective as on the tibia. There should then be a gradual increase in the amount of activity. Soft tissue symptoms should be treated. This injury is often associated with a biomechanical abnormality such as excessive pronation or excessive supination.

Referred pain

Referred pain is not a common cause of leg pain in athletes, but should be considered in cases with persistent and atypical pain. Pain may be referred from the lumbar spine, proximal nerve entrapment, the knee joint (Baker's cyst, meniscal cysts), the superior tibiofibular joint (instability or ganglion cyst), and, occasionally, the ankle joint (instability, Maisonneuve fracture).

Nerve entrapments

Within the leg itself, nerve entrapment of either the superficial peroneal nerve in the lateral compartment or the deep peroneal nerve in the anterior compartment can occur due to trauma or a tight brace or cast. Fascial entrapment at the level of the fibular head may also occasionally occur.

The tibial nerve in the deep posterior compartment is less commonly involved with entrapment, but can been injured with trauma. Pain and sensory changes may occur. This diagnosis may be suspected in the presence of motor or sensory changes, and it is confirmed with nerve conduction studies performed pre- and post-exercise. Surgery may be required to alleviate these conditions.

Vascular entrapments

Popliteal artery entrapment syndrome usually presents with calf pain and is therefore more fully described in Chapter 39, but may rarely present as pain in the anterior compartment.[77] It can be misdiagnosed as anterior compartment syndrome as they both present with claudication-type pain. However, the pain from popliteal artery entrapment disappears immediately on cessation of exercise, whereas compartment syndrome pain often persists for approximately 30 minutes as an aching sensation. While DVT is most commonly posterior, chronic venous stasis changes can occur anteriorly and may be evidence of systemic disease.

Developmental issues

Juvenile tibia vara (Blount disease) usually presents due to deformity rather than pain. Osgood–Schlatter disease is a traction apophysitis at the insertion of the patellar tendon onto the tibial tuberosity seen commonly among adolescent athletes. Patients usually present with pain and tenderness at the tibial tuberosity (Chapter 44). 'Growing pains' may affect the leg and are usually a diagnosis of exclusion. Intermittent achy pain exacerbated by periods of active growth with completely negative imaging and work-up are characteristic. The youngest reported patient treated with surgical release for pressure positive CECS was 12 years old and it is unclear whether this patient would have grown out of the problem at maturity.

Periosteal contusion

Periosteal contusion occurs as a result of a direct blow from a hard object such as a football boot. It can be extremely painful at the time of injury but the pain usually settles relatively quickly. Persistent pain may occur because of a haematoma having formed under the periosteum. There will be local tenderness and bony swelling. Treatment consists of rest and protection.

Fractured tibia and fibula

Combined fractures of the tibia and fibula are often due to indirect violence in landing from a jump on a twisted foot. The tibia or fibula may be injured individually by a direct blow. Weight-bearing will be impossible in cases of displaced fracture of the tibia. Fracture of the tibia is often compound and visible through damaged skin. An isolated fracture of the fibula may exhibit only local tenderness. An isolated fractured fibula (except where it involves the ankle joint) requires analgesia only. However, the ankle and knee joint must be carefully examined for associated injuries (see Maisonneuve fracture, Chapter 41). The management of a combined fracture is that for fracture of the tibia. Patients with compound (open) fractures should be admitted to hospital.

Many closed tibial fractures can be treated conservatively as long as angulation is minimal. This involves an above-knee plaster with the knee slightly flexed and the ankle in 90° of dorsiflexion. The limb is elevated for 3–7 days until swelling subsides. A check radiograph should be taken after casting. Patients should be reviewed at 6–8 weeks, at which time they may be able to be placed in a hinged knee cast.

Bony union requires 8–12 weeks; however, 16–20 weeks are required for consolidation. Physiotherapy after removal of the plaster is aimed at regaining full range of knee flexion and quadriceps muscle strength. Activities such as swimming can be resumed immediately after removal of the plaster but multidirectional running sports must wait until range of movement and muscle strength have returned to normal.

> **PRACTICE PEARL**
>
> There is a strong trend toward early surgical fixation of unstable tibial fractures with intramedullary nailing, which allows athletes earlier weight-bearing, conditioning activities and return to sport, and obviates the risk of potential mal-union.

REFERENCES

References for this chapter can be found at www.mhhe.com/au/CSM5e

Chapter 39

Calf pain

with TAMIM KHANBHAI, MATT HISLOP and JEFF BOYLE

Kompany remains sidelined with a calf injury, sustained after just seven minutes of City's goalless draw with Dynamo Kiev one month ago. Remarkably, it is the 14th time he has suffered a problem with his calf since joining the club in 2008–with five of them occurring this season–and his 32nd injury overall during the past eight years.

PhysioRoom, 12 April 2016

Calf pain is common and if not managed appropriately it can persist for months and cause frustration for both athlete and clinician. Both acute and chronic calf pain can stem from injury to the calf muscle.

ANATOMY

The anatomy of the posterior compartment of the leg (Fig. 39.1) will be covered here. The anterior and lateral aspects have been covered in Chapter 38.

The muscles in the posterior compartment of the leg comprise a superficial and deep group. The superficial group is composed of the triceps surae (gastrocnemius and soleus) and plantaris muscle. These form the bulk of the calf muscle. The deep group is composed of the tibialis posterior, flexor digitorum longus, flexor hallucis longus and popliteus muscles.

Gastrocnemius has two heads; the medial and larger head is attached to the posterior aspect of the medial epicondyle of the femur and the lateral head to the lateral femoral condyle (Fig. 39.1b) The muscle extends down to the mid-calf, following which it inserts into a broad aponeurosis which receives the tendon of the soleus to form the tendon of Achilles (TA). The two heads are overlaid by the tendon of biceps femoris and the common peroneal nerve laterally and the semimembranosus muscle medially. This latter area between the medial head and semimembranosus is the location of the 'Baker's cyst' (Chapter 37).

Soleus is a large flat broad muscle, deep to the gastrocnemius (Fig. 39.1c). It arises from a number of locations; the posterior aspect of the head and proximal shaft of the fibula, the soleal line (prominent ridge posterior tibia), medial aspect of the tibia and a fibrous band between the tibia and fibula. The muscle joins with the tendon of gastrocnemius and together they form the TA, inserting into the calcaneal tuberosity.

Both the gastrocnemius and soleus muscles in the calf have been noted to have intramuscular tendons. In the

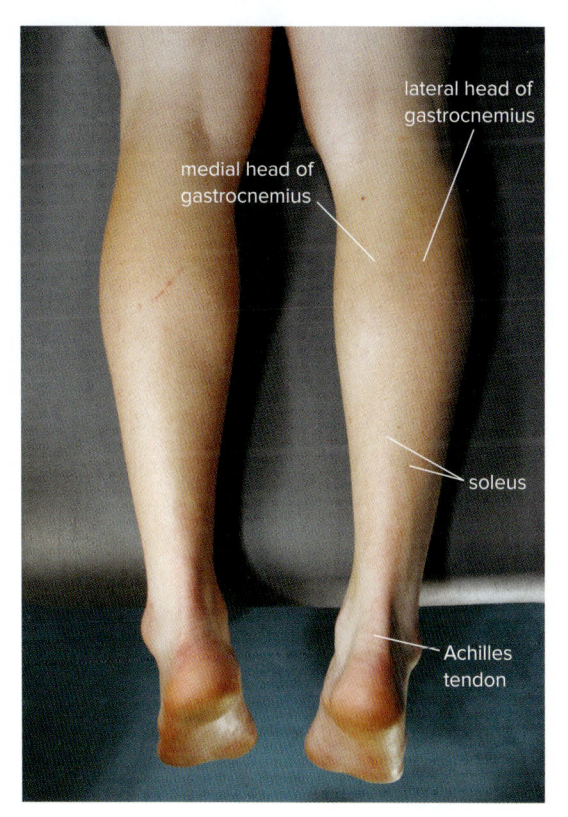

(a)

Figure 39.1 Anatomy of the calf (a) Surface anatomy

PART B Regional problems

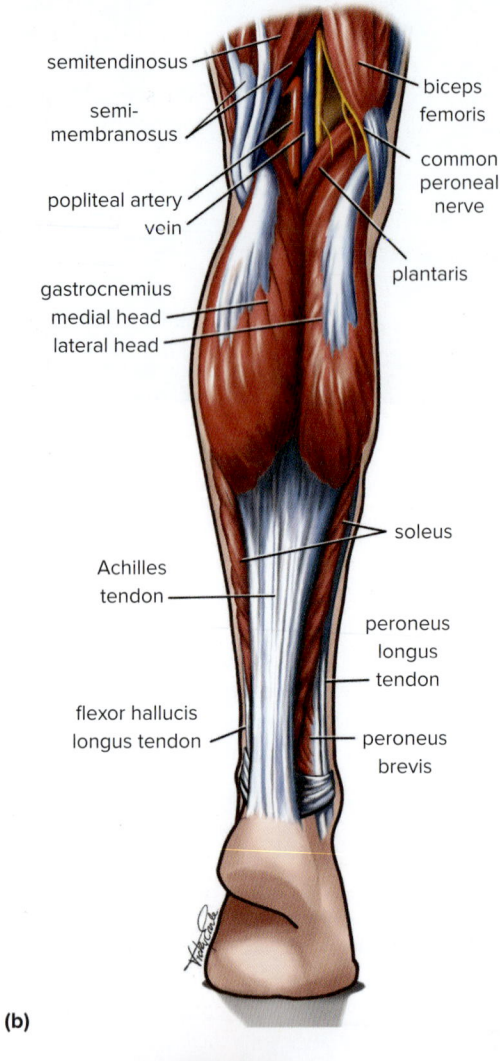

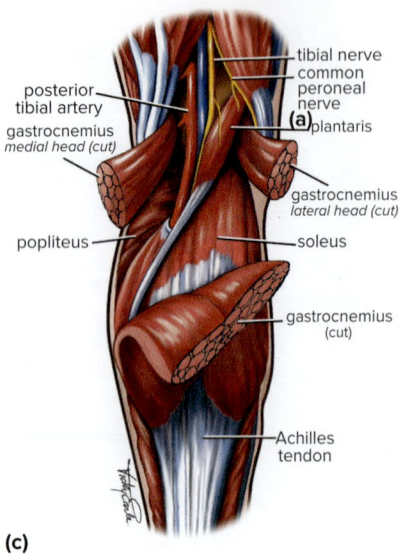

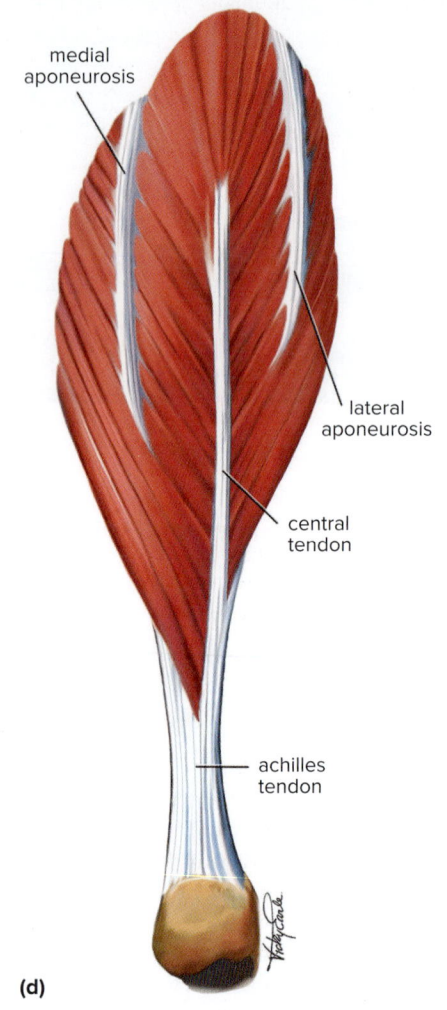

Figure 39.1 (cont.) (b) Superficial calf muscles (c) Removal of the gastrocnemius showing the underlying soleus and plantaris muscles (d) The intramuscular tendinous structures within the soleus muscle

gastrocnemius muscle, separate proximal medial and lateral tendons arise from the posterior aspects of the medial and lateral femoral condyles respectively.

There are three tendinous structures within the soleus muscle–medial and lateral 'aponeuroses' proximally, and a distal central tendon.[1] The medial and lateral aponeuroses (Fig. 39.1d) arise from the medial (tibial) and lateral (fibular) origins of the soleal epimysium and descend inferiorly, penetrating deep into the medial and lateral aspects of the soleal muscle belly, whilst simultaneously curving towards the midline of the muscle belly and distal central tendon. As they progress distally, the aponeuroses decrease in size until they can no longer be visualised. This most distal point is from where the lowest muscle fibres arise. As these aponeuroses are a continuation of the epimysium covering the soleus and act as rigid fibrous 'struts' from which the proximal soleus muscle fibres gain origin, they can indeed be considered as true intramuscular tendons from an anatomical, functional and pathologic perspective, albeit demonstrating a flattened and 'aponeurotic' morphology.

The central tendon (Fig. 39.1d) arises from the anterior aponeurosis and consequently represents the inferior muscular attachment; that is to say, the insertion of the soleal muscle fibres. This eventually forms the soleal contribution of the Achilles tendon, typically fusing along the most central aspect of the tendon, although it occasionally does so along the medial or lateral aspect.

CLINICAL APPROACH

Calf injuries are common, particularly in ball sports. For example, a large study of injuries in professional football found that 13% of all injuries were located in the calf.[2] Of these, 61% resulted in more than a week of time loss and 13% took more than 28 days to recover. The re-injury rate was also high at 13%.

The medial head of the gastrocnemius is the most common site of calf injury. In an MRI study of calf injuries by Koulouris and colleagues,[3] a total of 79 separate sites of strain injury were identified (39 solitary, 20 dual) in 59 patients. Of the 39 isolated strains, injury to the gastrocnemius was most common (49%), preferentially involving the medial head in 18 cases and the lateral head in one case. The soleus was also commonly involved (46%), with two cases (5%) of distal avulsions of the plantaris. Of the 20 dual injuries, a combination of gastrocnemius injury with soleus injury was the most frequent finding (60%). Dual injuries of both heads of the gastrocnemius muscles were demonstrated in four cases (20%), with the soleus and tibialis posterior injured in three cases (15%). A combination of soleus and flexor hallucis longus injury was seen in one case (5%).

Most calf muscle strains occur at the musculotendinous junction (MTJ)–either at the intramuscular tendon or the distal MTJ. Balius and colleagues found that musculotendinous junction strains involved all three of the soleus intramuscular tendons.[1] Of 31 strains considered musculotendinous, 14 (45%) were located at the medial aponeurosis, 10 (32%) at the central tendon and seven (23%) involved the lateral aponeurosis.

A sudden burst of acceleration, such as stretching to play a ball in squash or tennis, may precipitate injury. The classic mechanism is seen in middle-aged tennis players, normally over 40 years of age, with a sudden onset of acceleration, where the calf muscle is stretched eccentrically when the knee is extended and the foot in a dorsiflexed position, such as when overstretching for a ball. This results in immediate pain, tenderness (medial belly of gastrocnemius above the musculotendinous junction), a palpable defect and swelling. This is sometimes referred to as 'tennis leg'.

The calf region is also a common site of contusion caused through contact with playing equipment or another player. Muscle strains and contusions are acute injuries that present with typical histories that are usually easily distinguishable.

> **PRACTICE PEARL**
>
> The possibility of referred pain from the lumbar spine, neural or myofascial structures should always be considered. This is sometimes the underlying basis of calf strains, especially in the older athlete.[4]

The calf is the most common site in the body for muscle cramps (Chapter 3). Cramps may occur at rest, during or after exercise. Cramps are not specific to environmental conditions such as exercise in the cold or heat. They can occur in acclimatised and conditioned athletes. Cramps probably result from alterations in spinal neural reflex activity activated by fatigue in susceptible individuals.

The calf is also a common site of the phenomenon known as delayed onset muscle soreness (Chapter 4). This may occur after the first training session following a lay-off or a period of relative rest, or when excessive eccentric muscle contractions are performed, for example, during plyometric training. Lateral calf pain may be due to a direct blow, referred pain from the superior tibiofibular joint, peroneal muscle strain or fibular stress fracture. The causes of calf pain are listed in Table 39.1.

A variety of contributing factors can predispose an athlete to calf injury. These include:

- foot biomechanics (excessive pronation/supination)
- pelvic biomechanics (e.g. internal rotation femur)
- muscle imbalances (quadriceps, hamstrings, ankle everters and inverters)
- stiff ankle joint (decreased dorsiflexion)
- poor jumping and landing technique
- change in sporting environment (terrain, weather)
- poor nutrition and hydration
- change in sporting activity (cycling and swimming compared with running)
- change in footwear
- reduced muscle power, endurance and muscle fatigue
- lack of conditioning.

History

The most important aspect of the history is the description of the onset of pain. A sudden onset of a tearing or

PART B Regional problems

Table 39.1 **Causes of calf pain**

Common	Less common	Not to be missed
Muscle strains • Gastrocnemius • Soleus • Plantaris Muscle contusion • Gastrocnemius Muscle cramp Delayed onset muscle soreness	Superficial posterior compartment syndrome Deep posterior compartment syndrome (Chapter 38) Referred pain • Lumbar spine • Myofascial structures • Superior tibiofibular joint • Knee (Baker's cyst, posterior cruciate ligament, posterior capsular sprain) Vascular entrapment • Popliteal artery • Endofibrosis of external iliac artery Nerve entrapment • Tibial • Sural Stress fracture of the fibula Stress fracture of the posterior cortex of the tibia (Chapter 38) Varicose veins (e.g. superficial thrombosis)	Deep venous thrombosis

popping sensation in the calf is diagnostic of calf muscle strains. The patient is usually able to localise the site of the tear. The degree of disability, both immediately after the injury and subsequently, is a guide to the severity of the tear.

In athletes with chronic mild calf pain, a history of a previous acute injury may be significant and is a risk factor for calf injury in marathon runners and soccer referees.[5, 6] The practitioner should ask about the treatment and rehabilitation of the previous injury because inadequate rehabilitation will have an impact on recurrence rates.

Information about the training load, and especially running load, can be very helpful. Many runners now use GPS devices or mobile applications that provide extensive information about running distances, speed and total volume per week. This information can be very valuable.

A history of low back pain may be a clue to referred pain. The practitioner should also be alert to the possibility of referred pain if the calf pain is variable rather than constant. If there is no obvious precipitating cause of calf pain, the possibility of deep venous thrombosis after long car journeys, long flights or recent surgery needs to be explored.

Claudicant pain that comes on with exertion and then disappears may indicate proximal vascular occlusion by atheroma or entrapment (e.g. femoral or iliac artery stenosis) or exertional compartment syndrome. A ruptured Baker's cyst can also cause acute calf pain and swelling and should be considered as a differential diagnosis (refer to Chapter 37).

Physical examination

The aims of examination in the patient with acute calf strain are to determine the site and the severity of the injury as well as to detect any predisposing factors such as chronic calf tightness. Examination of a patient with chronic or intermittent calf pain requires not only palpation of muscles, but also assessment of possible neural contributors, ankle reflexes and examination of the lumbar spine. It is important to palpate the entire length and width of the muscle bellies and their associated aponeuroses for areas of muscle and fascial tightness and thickenings that may predispose to injury. Due to its deep position, the soleus can be difficult to palpate.

Clinical assessment should include both static and dynamic tests and should be performed in both knee flexion and extension. Comparing calf girth between left and right is also important. Foot alignment and biomechanics should also be considered.

1. Observation
    a. standing (foot posture, calf girth, swelling)
    b. walking (on toes, on heels)
    c. prone
2. Active ankle movements
    a. plantarflexion/dorsiflexion (standing) (Fig. 39.2a)
    b. plantarflexion/dorsiflexion (prone)
3. Passive ankle movements
    a. dorsiflexion (knee flexion) (Fig. 39.2b)
    b. dorsiflexion (knee extension) (Fig. 39.2c)

Calf pain   **CHAPTER 39**

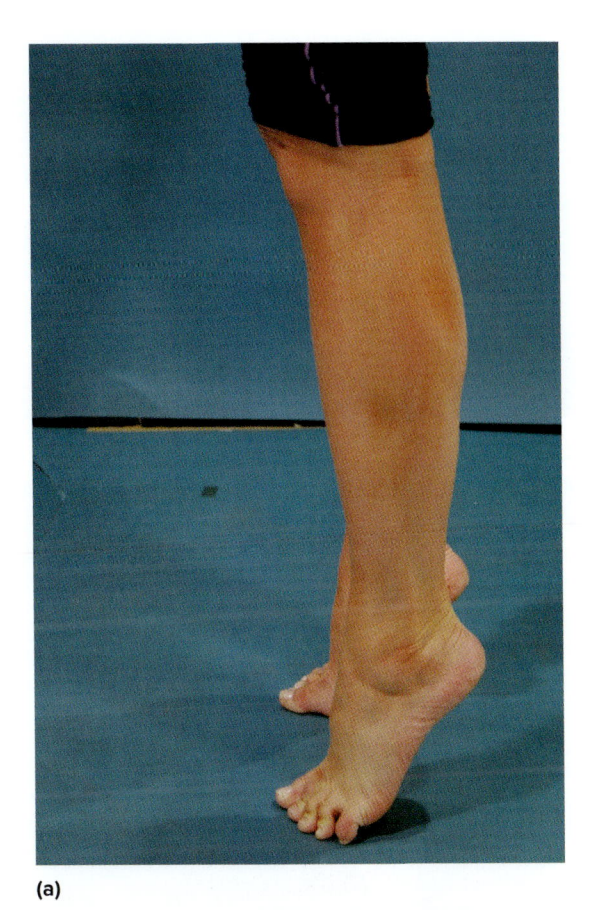

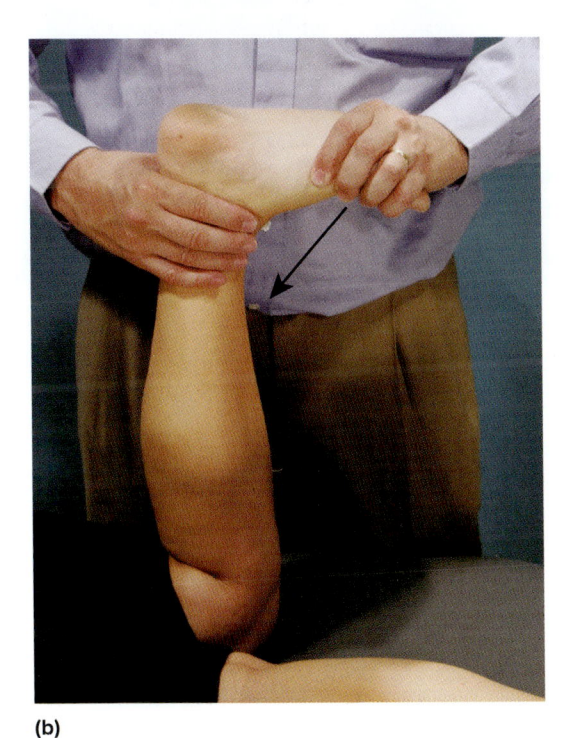

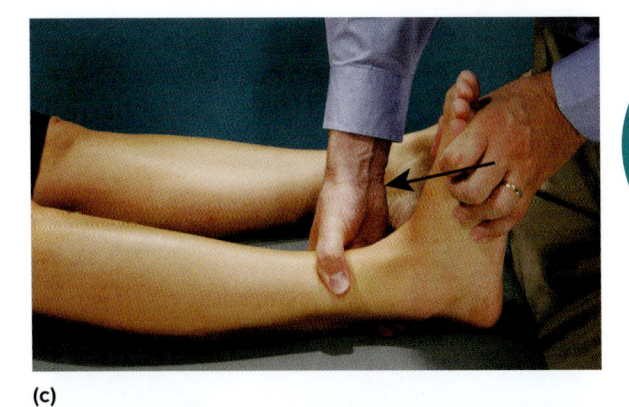

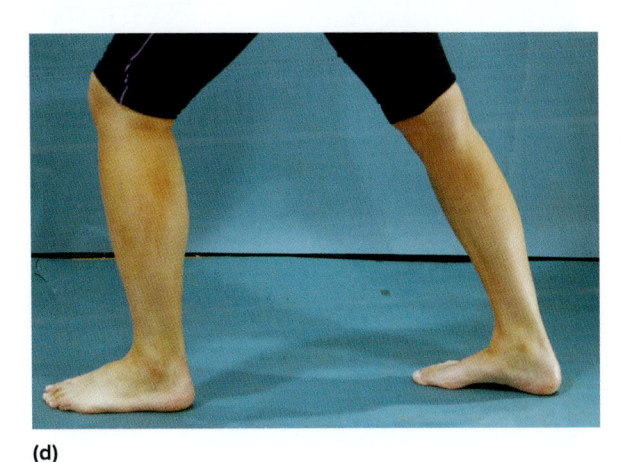

Figure 39.2 Examination of the patient with calf pain (a) Active movement—plantarflexion/dorsiflexion (standing). The functional competence can be assessed during a bilateral or unilateral heel raise-and-drop until pain is reproduced (b) Passive movement—ankle dorsiflexion (knee flexion). Examine with the knee flexed and add overpressure (c) Passive movement—ankle dorsiflexion (knee extension). Examine with the knee extended and add overpressure (Homan's sign) (d) Stretch—gastrocnemius (back leg). Examine with the knee in full extension and the heel on the ground

  c. muscle stretch
   i. gastrocnemius (Fig. 39.2d)
   ii. soleus (Fig. 39.2e)
4. Resisted movements
  a. dorsiflexion
5. Functional tests
  a. hop (hop for distance both straight leg and bent leg)
  b. jump (height, shock absorption)
  c. run
  d. calf raises to fatigue (both straight leg and bent leg)
6. Palpation
  a. gastrocnemius (Fig. 39.2f) (compare medial and lateral heads)

PART B Regional problems

(e)

(f)

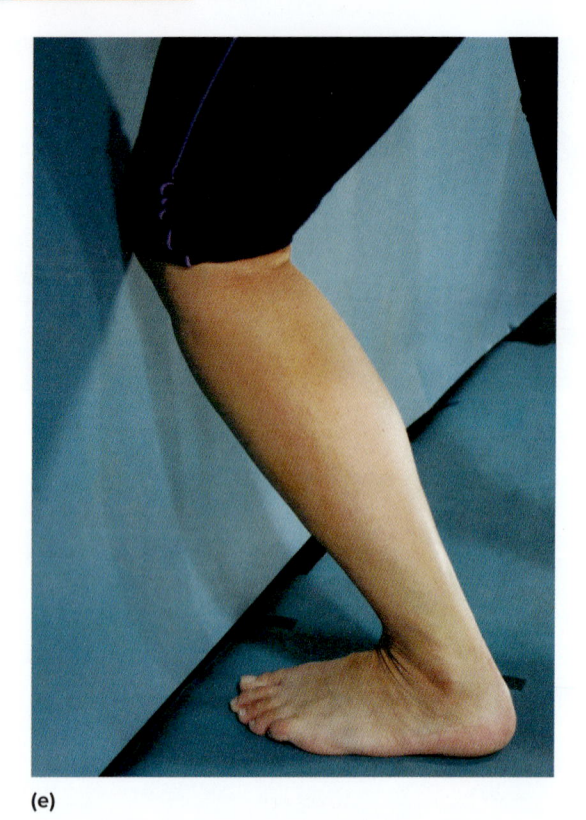

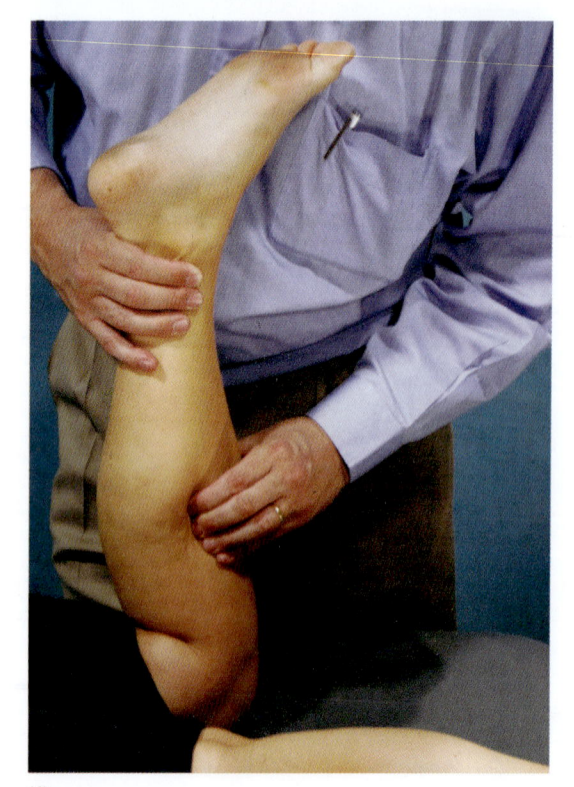

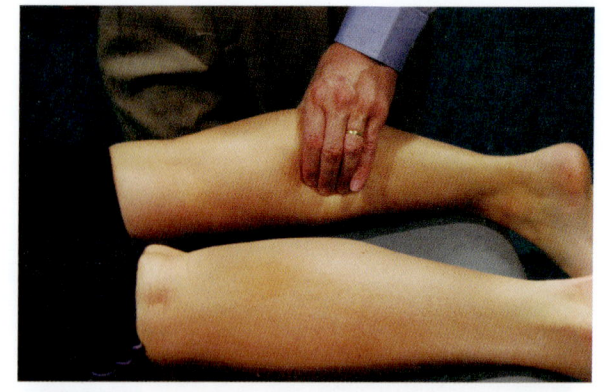

(g)

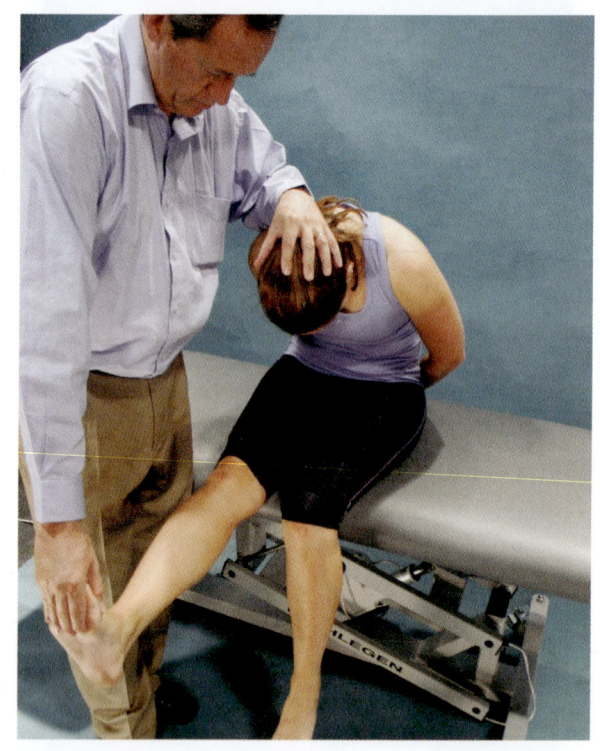

(h)

Figure 39.2 (cont.) (e) Stretch—soleus (lunge test). The patient should flex the knee so that it passes vertically over the third toe to prevent excessive pronation. Record the range of motion and compare both sides (f) Palpation. The patient should actively contract and relax the muscles and the ankle should be moved passively through dorsiflexion and plantarflexion during palpation. The gastrocnemius may be palpated in the relaxed position by placing the knee in flexion and the ankle in plantarflexion. Feel for swelling and defects in muscle or tendon tissue (g) Special test—calf squeeze test. The calf is squeezed. If no ankle plantarflexion occurs, there has been a complete tear of the Achilles tendon or musculotendinous junction (h) Special test—neurodynamic test (slump test)

Calf pain CHAPTER 39

   b. soleus
   c. posterior knee
   d. superior tibiofibular joint
   e. Achilles tendon
7. Special tests
   a. Calf squeeze test–for Achilles tendon rupture (Fig. 39.2g) (Chapter 40)
   b. Homan's sign–forced dorsiflexion in knee flexion may elicit pain in the presence of deep venous thrombosis (Fig. 39.2c). However, this is not a sensitive or specific test[7]
   c. neurodynamic test–slump test (Fig. 39.2h)
   d. gluteal trigger points
   e. lumbar spine (Chapter 29)
   f. biomechanical examination (Chapter 8)
   g. ankle jerk reflex
   h. popliteal artery auscultation after provocative manoeuvres.

Key outcome measures
There are no specific PROMs for calf strains. Generic measures such as a patient-specific functional scale or a numeric pain rating scale can be used to monitor progress (see Chapter 16).

Investigations
Ultrasound or MRI may be useful for evaluating a calf injury. These imaging modalities can localise pathology, identify presence of haematoma and scar tissue, and differentiate between a muscle strain and a contusion if not clinically evident. MRI is preferred because of its ability to identify intramuscular tendon injuries. If deep venous thrombosis is suspected, a Doppler scan may be required.

GASTROCNEMIUS MUSCLE STRAINS
Acute strain
Acute strain of the gastrocnemius muscle occurs typically when the athlete attempts to accelerate by extending the knee from a stationary position with the ankle in dorsiflexion, or when lunging forward, such as while playing tennis or squash. Sudden eccentric overstretch, such as when an athlete runs onto a kerb and the ankle drops suddenly into dorsiflexion, is another common mechanism.

The medial head of the gastrocnemius has a greater proximal attachment and a longer distal insertion into the Achilles tendon than the lateral head.[3] Therefore the medial head may have a greater capacity for force generation and may be more susceptible to injury compared to the lateral head.

History
The exact moment of injury was caught on video in the case of a famous Australian batsman whose gastrocnemius strain occurred when his entire body weight was over his foot on the injured side with the centre of mass well in front of the leg.[8] The gastrocnemius muscle tendon complex was at close to maximal length, and the muscle-tendon length was also constant at the time. Therefore, the injury probably occurred just as the muscle-tendon complex was moving from an eccentric to an isometric phase.

The athlete often complains of an acute, stabbing or tearing sensation, usually either in the medial belly of the gastrocnemius or at the musculotendinous junction.

Physical examination
Examination reveals tenderness at the site of a muscle strain and, in complete muscle tears, there may be a palpable defect. The athlete will walk with an antalgic gait. There may be skin changes such as bruising or discoloration and swelling. Assessing range of motion reveals pain on passive and active dorsiflexion (Fig. 39.2d), and on resisted plantarflexion with the knee extended. Assessment of the Achilles tendon and other structures in the calf and ankle are important.

If required, the functional competence of the injured muscle is assessed by asking the patient to perform a bilateral heel raise. If necessary, a unilateral heel raise, heel drop or hop may be used to reproduce the pain and to assess for weakness. Measuring the calf girth, comparing one side to the other in centimetres and a lunge test, when appropriate (not if examining the athlete acutely), can be useful objective markers during rehabilitation, and especially if there are baseline measurements for comparison.

Chronic gastrocnemius muscle strain may occur as an overuse injury or following inadequate rehabilitation of an acute injury. This results in disorganised, weak scar tissue that can predispose to further injury and compensatory movement patterns leading to muscle imbalances. Careful palpation of the muscle can reveal these tissue thickenings.

Treatment
Rehabilitation consists of a progressive program starting from the acute phase through to the athlete returning to sport. It is tailored to the individual, rather than a fixed time frame. Some athletes will recover faster than others, depending on the risk factors of the injury, presence of scar tissue, haematoma, previous injuries and the sport they need to return to. The aim is to return the athlete, at a minimum, to their pre-injury level, but ideally to use

853

this opportunity to correct other issues so they are in a better position than their pre-injury level. There are five stages to rehabilitation of gastrocnemius strains:

- Stage 1: Acute phase
- Stage 2: Improve ROM
- Stage 3: Power and endurance
- Stage 4: Coordination, agility, sport skills
- Stage 5: Return to sport.

Stage 1: Acute phase

Initial treatment of gastrocnemius strains aims to reduce pain, swelling and further injury. The initial approach is POLICE (protect, optimal loading, ice, compression, elevation)[9] and analgesics may be used if required, avoiding nonsteroidal anti-inflammatory drugs for the first 72 hours.[10, 11] Ice compression units may assist with this process, for 15–20 minutes every hour. Crutches may be necessary if the athlete is unable to bear weight, but should only be used for short periods as early mobilisation allows muscle fibres to regenerate and organise more effectively.[12]

A 6 mm heel raise may be used (on both the injured and uninjured side) to initially reduce calf length and off-load calf structures. There is no good quality evidence for electrotherapeutic modalities such as ultrasound therapy, but this can be used if the treating team is keen to incorporate this.

This stage can be achieved within a couple of days but can be longer depending on the severity of the injury. If the symptoms have failed to settle within 3–5 days, reassess and investigate further if required.

Stage 2: Improve ROM +/− flexibility

Once the pain and swelling has settled, ankle and knee active range of motion exercises should commence and exercises in a swimming pool can aid recovery.

Gentle stretching of the gastrocnemius to the level of a feeling of tightness (Fig. 39.3) can begin soon after the injury. Stretching is important to lengthen the muscle, which improves its elasticity and distends scar tissue appropriately.[12] Following this, unloaded isometric calf exercise should be incorporated.

Stage 3: Power and endurance

There are multiple facets to this stage. Within 10 days the scar tissue will have the same tensile strength as normal muscle and can be subjected to increased loading.[13] Progression from active ROM to strengthening of the plantarflexors can commence. This involves a progression of exercises starting with resistance band strengthening to concentric bilateral calf raises, unilateral calf raises and, finally, eccentric calf lowering. Weights can be

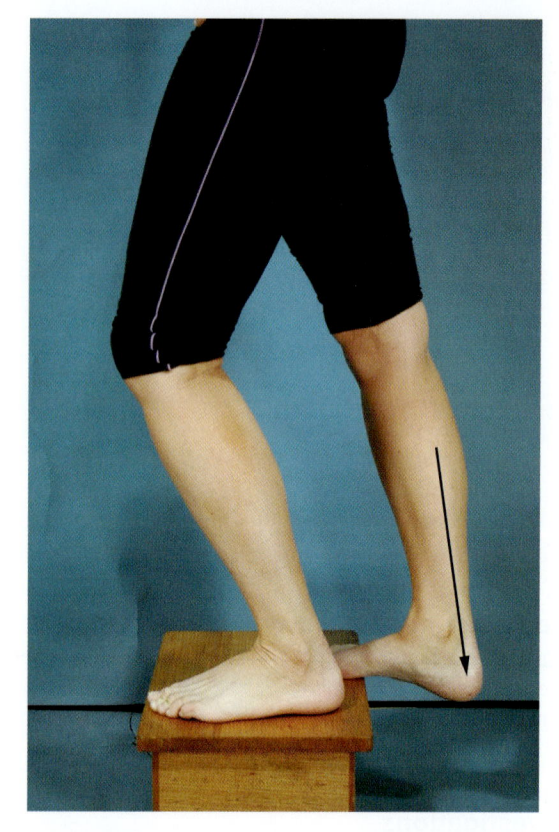

Figure 39.3 Stretching exercise for the right gastrocnemius muscle with the knee in full extension. This can be performed over a step or with the foot placed against a wall to increase the stretch

added gradually at each stage (Fig. 39.4). Strengthening routines should begin with open chain then closed chain exercises.

Prior to rehabilitation, ensure the muscle has been warmed up appropriately. Rehabilitation should concentrate on both gastrocnemius and soleus by varying knee extension and flexion. Stretching exercises will restore normal muscle length and should be held for at least 15 seconds. A systematic review of calf stretching on ankle dorsiflexion range of motion found an improvement of up to 2–3°,[14] but it is unknown whether this is clinically relevant. Measuring the lunge test is a useful indicator of posterior calf flexibility as a score <13 cm has been associated with lower limb injuries.[15]

Treatment may also include transverse friction and longitudinal gliding soft tissue therapy at the site of any excessive scar tissue and along the entire musculotendinous unit. When appropriate, sustained myofascial tension (Fig. 39.5) or digital ischaemic pressure can be applied to areas of increased tone.

Calf pain CHAPTER 39

(a)

(b)

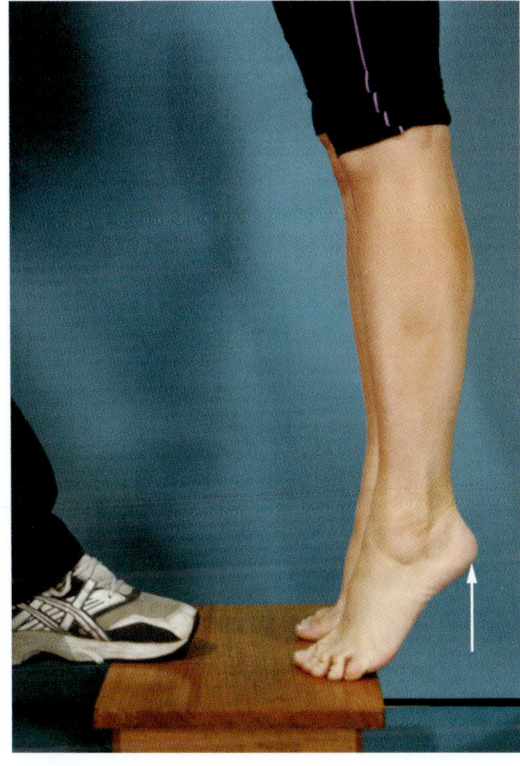

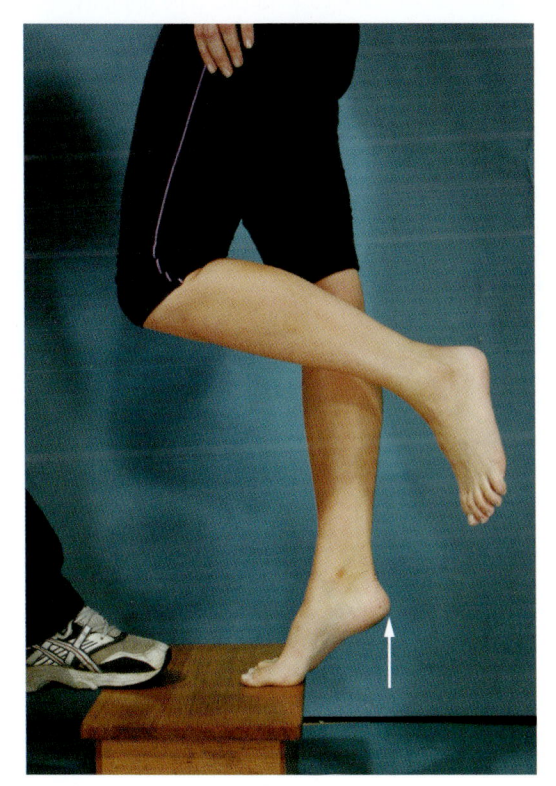

(c)

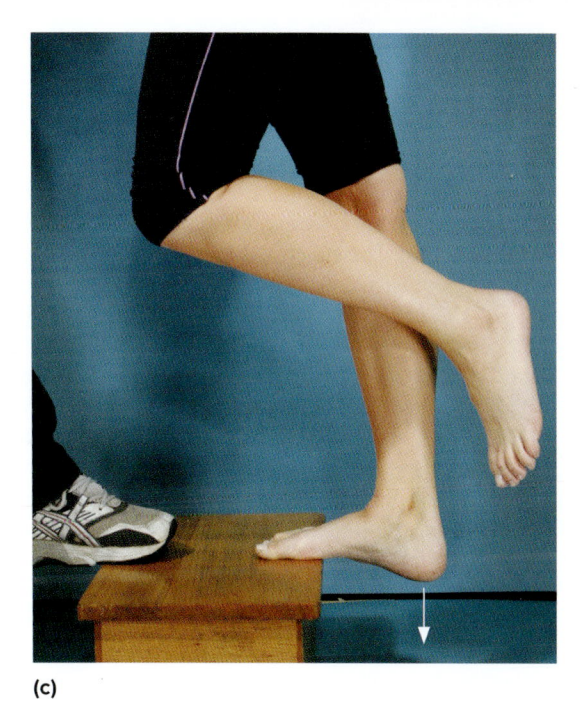

Figure 39.4 Strengthening exercises for the gastrocnemius muscle (a) Bilateral calf raise (b) Unilateral calf raise (c) Eccentric lowering

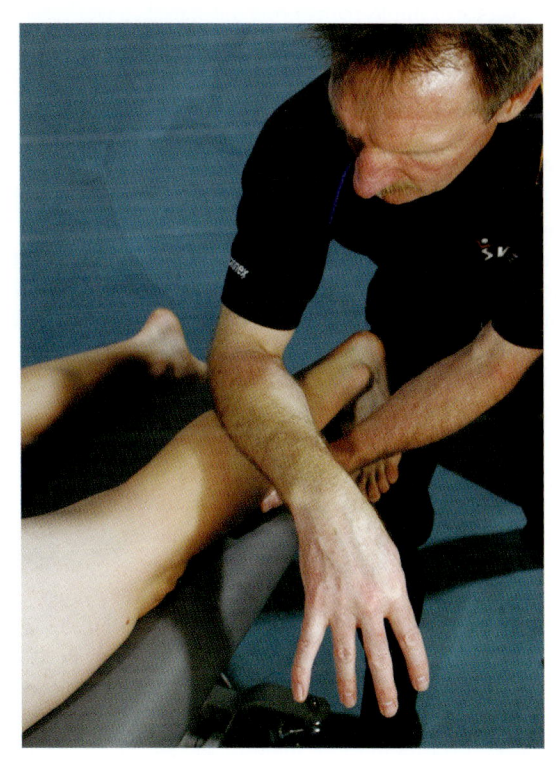

Figure 39.5 Soft tissue therapy—sustained myofascial tension to the muscle belly of the gastrocnemius

For favourable long-term results, treatment should address predisposing factors such as biomechanical factors, or risk factors that preceded the injury, such as calf muscle tightness, lumbopelvic dysfunction and knee or ankle-related abnormalities.

Normal, full weight-bearing gait should be achieved, following which proprioceptive exercises can be started. This begins with balancing on the injured leg, progressing through to a wobble board or BOSU® ball and incorporating functional movements like jumping onto or landing off the board once the strength in the calf is appropriate.

Increased amounts of cardiovascular exercise should be undertaken to maintain fitness levels. Low-impact cross training such as stationary cycling or swimming can be commenced as soon as pain allows. When active weight-bearing muscle contraction is pain-free, a cross trainer can also be used prior to running.

Stage 4: Coordination, agility, sport skills

By this stage, the strength on the injured side should be comparable to the non-injured leg. The aim now is to get the player ready for return to play. This involves continuing the gains made in the previous stage, such as strength work and proprioception. Now there needs to be a supervised, graduated running program, which should include sprint work, change of direction and change of pace. If the sport is football, for example, then during this stage ball work should be introduced, starting with short kicks and progressing to longer kicking drills. Athletes should undergo a supervised, graduated return-to-sport program.

Stage 5: Return to sport

This stage is often overlooked but is integral in a rehabilitation program (Chapter 19). Return to sport (RTP) needs a multidisciplinary approach, working with the coaching staff, informing and educating them about the injury. Often, coaches will feel that once a medical team hands a player back to them, they are ready to play. In fact, nothing in rehabilitation can replace or replicate the training and matches of team sport.

The aim should be to have a period of training with the team, the length of which is decided by the medical team and depends on factors such as the time out with that injury. Clearly if a player has been out for 1 week, they need less training time than if they are out for a period of 4-8 weeks. By this stage, strength, flexibility and proprioception should be equal to the uninjured site.

There is little evidence that a repeat MRI scan needs to be done to RTP as MRIs still show abnormalities 6 weeks after players had returned to play in Australian rules football.[16] The number of minutes the player participates in the sport should be lower than usual when the player first returns. This stage needs to be tailored to the individual, the injury and the sport. Re-injuries often occur because the importance of this stage is ignored.

> **PRACTICE PEARL**
>
> When a 'tennis leg' occurs in an older athlete it can take a few months before the individual is ready to return to sport. In such cases there is often fibrotic tissue between the gastrocnemius and soleus muscles, seen on follow-up ultrasound. This fibrotic tissue may increase the risk of recurrence. One of the aims with any treatment is to achieve optimal rehabilitation and to prevent the formation of fibrotic tissue or scarring.

Operative intervention

Surgery is rarely required for gastrocnemius tears. However, if there is a complete rupture of the medial gastrocnemius head or a large disruption of muscle or intramuscular tendon fibres then a surgical opinion should be sought. Likewise, a failure of conservative treatment or prolonged pain (4-6 months) with a contracture warrants a surgical opinion.[13] Surgical intervention is only indicated when the presentation is associated with acute compartment syndrome.[17] Reconstruction of the medial head of gastrocnemius has limited evidence, with few case reports, a small case series and no long-term follow up data.[18] It is thus reserved for the rarer cases of this type of injury.

SOLEUS MUSCLE STRAINS

The soleus muscle contains a high proportion of type I, slow-twitch muscle fibres, unlike the gastrocnemius, which contains a higher proportion of type II, fast-twitch muscle fibres. This allows the soleus muscle to have a significant role in posture control, especially in standing.

Soleus muscle strains occurring at the perimeter of the muscle, and not centred at the tendons, can be classified as myofascial (epimysial) strains. These may be at the myofascial junction of the soleus with the gastrocnemius (posterior myofascial), or at the junction between soleus with the deep posterior compartment of the leg (anterior myofascial). Musculotendinous junction strains can involve the distal intramuscular tendon, or the proximal medial and lateral aponeuroses (Fig. 39.1d).

Epidemiology

Strains of the soleus muscle were not thought to be common in the elite athlete,[17] but Koulouris who reviewed MRI findings rather than purely ultrasound found large numbers of soleus strains, and combination strains with gastrocnemius and other deep crural muscles to be common.[3] Of the 18 isolated soleus strains reported by Koulouris, 11 were described as myofascial, with the other seven as musculotendinous junction injuries, all medial.

Calf pain CHAPTER 39

Table 39.2 Distribution of soleus muscle strains

Myofascial vs musculotendinous strains		
	Myofascial	Musculotendinous
Koulouris et al[3]	11	7
Balius et al[1]	24	31
Distribution of musculotendinous strains		
	Medial	Lateral	Central
Koulouris et al[3]	7	0	0
Balius et al[1]	14	7	10

Balius reported a series of 55 cases of soleus muscle strains, of which 31 strains were considered musculotendinous and 24 were myofascial.[1] The distribution of the soleus strains in the two studies is shown in Table 39.2.

MRI demonstrates the differences between the myofascial (epimysial) strains (Fig. 39.6) and the more serious musculotendinous tear involving damage to the aponeurosis (Fig. 39.7).

Clinical assessment

Patients with acute soleus strains may present with sudden onset pain, or alternatively with a history of increasing calf tightness over a period of days or weeks. Often walking and jogging are more painful than sprinting. The medial third of the fibres of the soleus and its aponeurosis are prone to becoming hard and inflexible, particularly in athletes with excessive subtalar pronation. This focal tissue can be more susceptible to strain, especially at its junction with adjacent 'normal' tissue. Therefore, careful assessment by palpation as well as assessment of foot biomechanics is essential.

Examination often reveals tenderness deep to the gastrocnemius, usually in the medial aspect of the soleus muscle. Often, both the soleus stretch (Fig. 39.2e) and resisted soleus contraction reproduce the athlete's pain. This can be differentiated from the stretch and contraction that provoke pain in gastrocnemius strains (Fig. 39.2d).

Management

Treatment of soleus muscle strains is similar to gastrocnemius strains above and rehabilitation should target both muscles. It is important to note that activation of the soleus requires the knee to be partially flexed (lunge position). Soft tissue therapy is often directed at the site of the lesion as well as tissue proximally and distally (Fig. 39.8). Strengthening exercises are performed with the knee flexed, initially in a seated position (Fig. 39.9). If foot biomechanics are assessed to be a predisposing factor to injury, orthoses may be required.

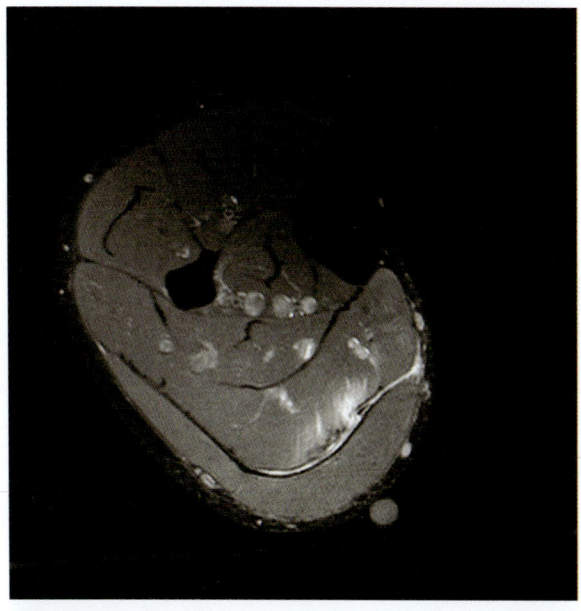

(a)

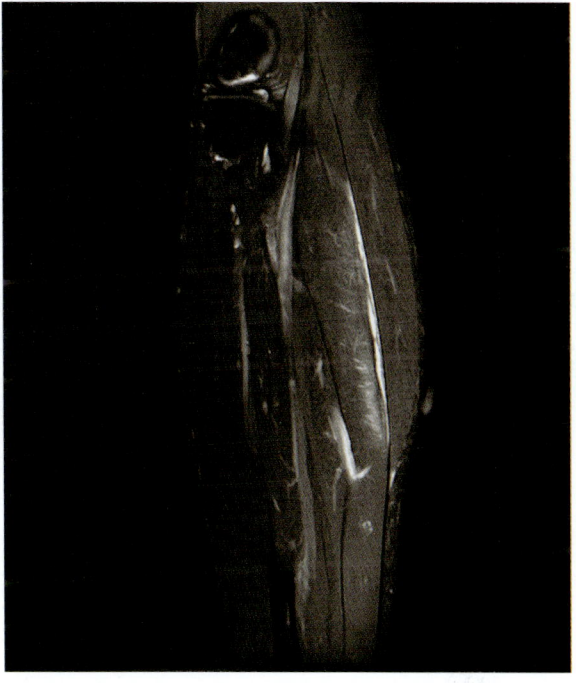

(b)

Figure 39.6 MRI of a 24-year-old running athlete presenting with sudden onset of calf symptoms (a) Axial fat-suppressed image shows epimysial tear of the superficial covering of medial soleus with tearing of the myofibrils from the connective tissue surface (arrow). The medial gastrocnemius epimysial surface is intact. Blood fluid products separate the two discrete layers (b) Sagittal fat-suppressed image

PART B Regional problems

(a)

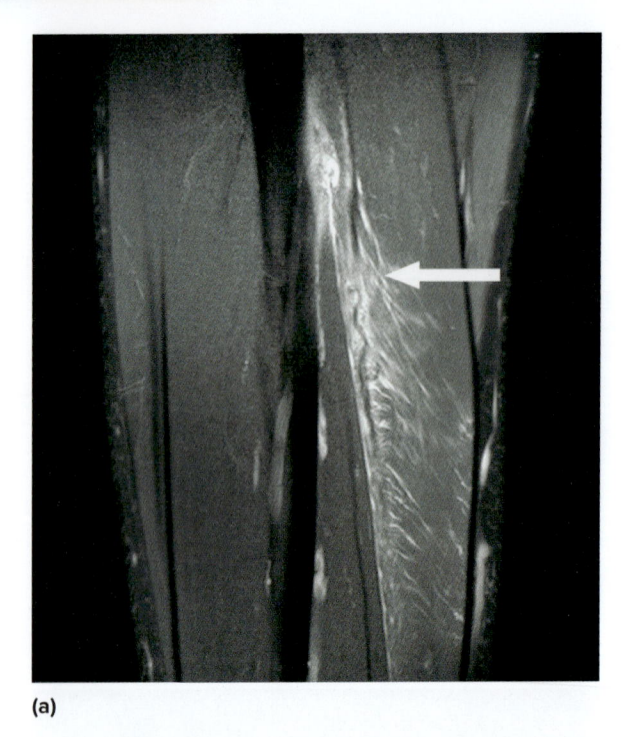

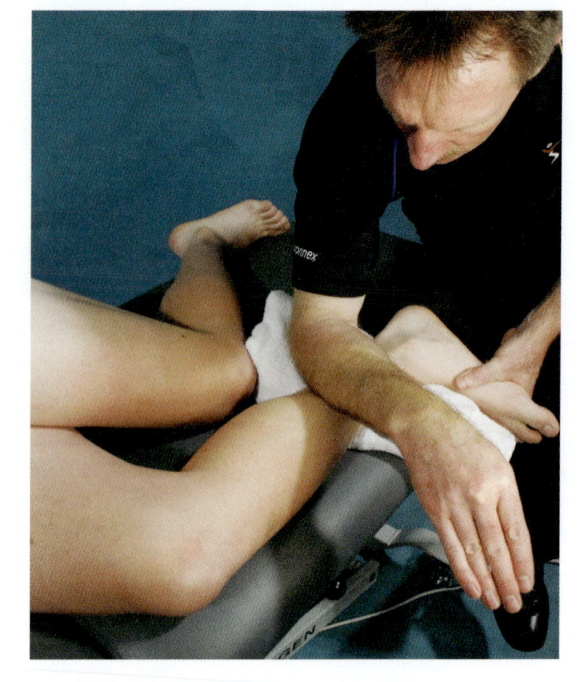

Figure 39.8 Soft tissue therapy—sustained myofascial tension to the soleus muscle

> **PRACTICE PEARL**
>
> When the soleus strain involves a lesion to the soleal aponeuroses (Fig. 39.7), rehabilitation time frames will be extended and management should be based on tendon treatment principles (see Chapter 4).

Accessory soleus

The soleus accessory muscle is a relatively rare anatomical variant (0.7–5.5%) and is bilateral in 10% of cases. It appears as a soft tissue mass bulging medially between the distal part of the tibia and the Achilles tendon, and may be mistaken for a tumour or an inflammatory lesion.[19] Athletes may have a fullness on inspection of their Achilles region from behind.

It may be asymptomatic (25%), or associated with chronic exertional compartment syndrome or posterior tibial nerve compression (tarsal tunnel syndrome). Athletes can present with ankle pain and soft tissue swelling.[20,21]

Presentation is usually in adolescence during periods of rapid muscle hypertrophy. Rapid muscle hypertrophy can lead to compartment-type syndrome, posterior tibial nerve compression, tendinopathy and/or partial accessory muscle strain.[20,21]

Plain radiography generally shows soft tissue swelling between the deep compartment and the Achilles tendon, which obscures or obliterates Kager's triangle on the

(b)

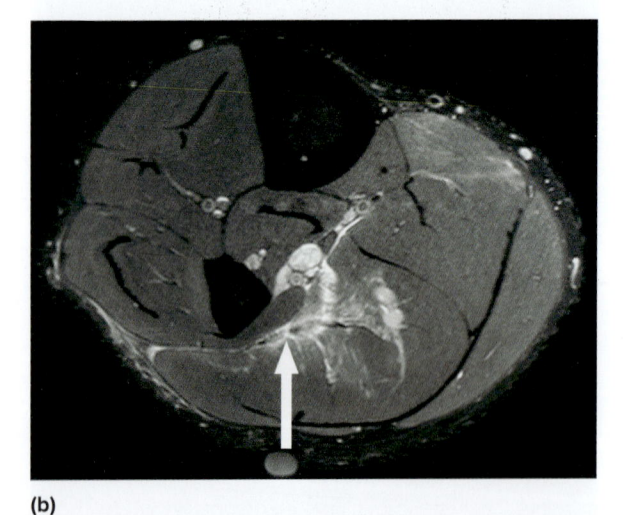

Figure 39.7 Musculotendinous strain involving the lateral aponeurosis with damage to the aponeurosis itself (a) Sagittal MR image shows disruption of the intramuscular aponeurosis (arrow) of the right lateral soleus muscle with retraction of the aponeurosis to create a wavy appearance. Oedema and blood fluid products track into the torn muscle fibres (b) Axial fat-suppressed image shows a discrete gap at the site where the aponeurosis has torn (arrow). The aponeurosis of the medial soleus muscle is intact

Calf pain CHAPTER 39

and improvement of ankle range when limited.[20] Surgery (involving either fasciotomy alone or with excision of the accessory muscle) is recommended when conservative measures fail.[19, 20]

CLAUDICANT-TYPE CALF PAIN

Another common presentation is the patient who complains of a claudicant-type calf pain with exercise. The differential diagnosis in this patient is a vascular cause (popliteal artery entrapment, atherosclerotic disease, endofibrosis), neuromyofascial causes (referred pain or nerve entrapment) or compartment syndrome (deep posterior or superficial).

Vascular causes

Vascular causes of exercise-induced lower limb pain were originally thought to be uncommon but the incidence may be greater than previously recognised, and it is possible that these conditions are under reported.[23]

The pain of vascular entrapment is brought on by exertion, like chronic exertional compartment syndrome, but has subtle differences in that it can be present at rest (positional), will typically develop more quickly and (usually) dissipate more quickly.[24]

Post-exercise examination of the peripheral pulses and arterial bruits is vital and the diagnosis can be confirmed by Doppler ultrasound, ankle–brachial ratios and angiography. It may also be important to perform compartment pressure tests and nerve conduction studies to rule out coexisting conditions.

Popliteal artery entrapment

Popliteal artery entrapment syndrome (PAES) is often not recognised, and misdiagnosed as a compartment syndrome.[25, 26] The syndrome was first described as a cause of exercise-induced leg pain in 1879. There are two types of popliteal artery entrapment syndrome: anatomical and functional (acquired).

The classically described anatomical (congenital) abnormality is a variation in the anatomical relationship between the popliteal artery as it exits the popliteal

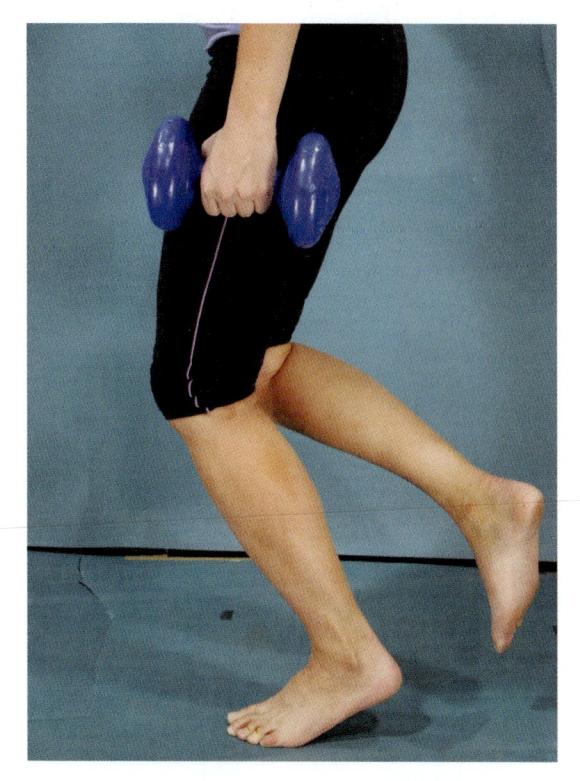

Figure 39.9 Strengthening exercises for the soleus muscle—calf raise with bent knee. This can be made more difficult by adding weights or having the patient drop down over the end of a step

lateral radiograph of the ankle. The appearance of normal muscle on MRI allows the clinician to distinguish it from both abnormal muscle and soft tissue tumours.[20, 22] Additionally, intrafascial fluid collection and perimuscular oedema have been associated with symptomatic accessory soleus muscle presentation on MRI.[21]

Asymptomatic cases require no treatment. If pain or discomfort is present, conservative treatment is trialled first. Conservative treatment can include soft tissue therapy, stretching and strengthening of the calf muscles

Table 39.3 Popliteal Vascular Entrapment Forum classification for popliteal entrapment syndrome (adapted from di Marzo and Cavallaro[29])

Type I	Popliteal artery running medial to the medial head of gastrocnemius
Type II	Medial head of gastrocnemius laterally attached
Type III	Accessory slip of gastrocnemius/fibrous bands arising from medial head of gastrocnemius
Type IV	Popliteal artery passing below popliteus muscle/fibrous bands arising from popliteus
Type V	Primarily venous entrapment
Type VI	Other variants
Type VII	Functional entrapment

PART B   Regional problems

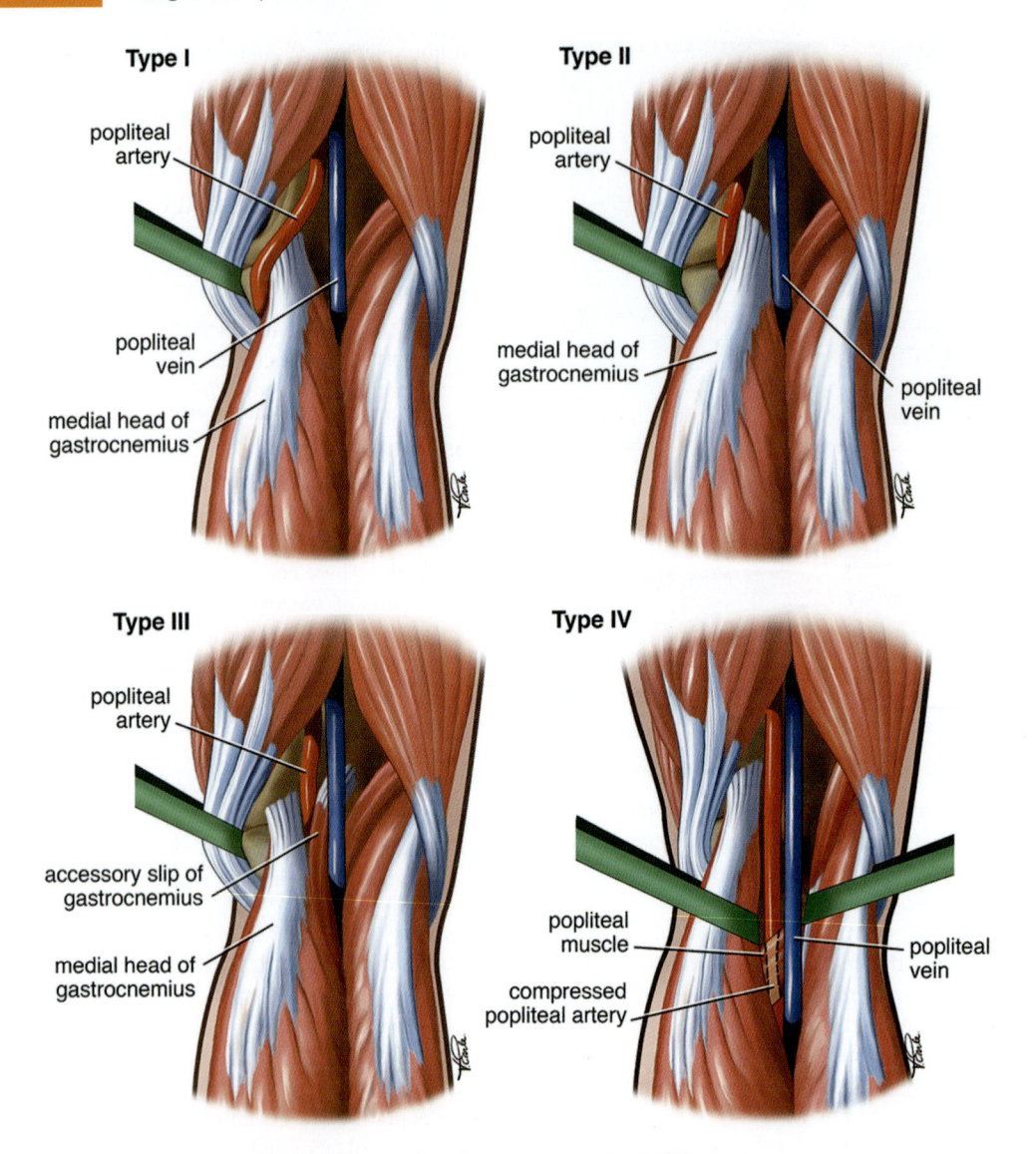

Figure 39.10 Popliteal Vascular Entrapment Forum classification system for PAES.
REDRAWN FROM PILLAI[30]

fossa and the medial head of the gastrocnemius muscle. It is quite rare, with an estimated prevalence of between 0.6% and 3.5%. Popliteal artery entrapment syndrome can be classified into seven categories according to the anatomical relationship between the popliteal artery and the adjacent muscular or fibrous bands in the popliteal fossa (Table 39.3 and Fig. 39.10).[26-28]

The most common abnormality describes an abnormal medial head of the gastrocnemius muscle, the accessory part of which passes behind the popliteal artery. Other observed abnormalities include a tendinous slip arising from the medial head of the muscle, an abnormal plantaris muscle and multiple muscle abnormalities involving the lateral and medial heads of the gastrocnemius and the plantaris. Rarer anatomical variations of popliteal artery entrapment syndrome include entrapment of the artery at the level of the adductor hiatus and an isolated entrapment of the anterior tibial artery as it passes through the interosseous membrane.

The term 'functional' or 'acquired' PAES was first described by Rignault et al. in 1985,[31] and describes a situation where no anatomical abnormality is visible at surgical exploration. Studies have shown that the medial head of gastrocnemius typically 'rests' in a lateral or intercondylar position, leading to crowding of the popliteal vessels and occlusion during muscle contraction (Fig. 39.11).[30] This syndrome is commonly seen in healthy young athletes and military recruits with hypertrophied gastrocnemius muscles.[25, 27]

Clinically, athletes present with claudication-type calf or anterior aspect of leg pain, which can be bilateral. The

Calf pain CHAPTER 39

Differentiating artery entrapment from chronic compartment syndrome

With artery entrapment, cessation of exercise brings about rapid relief from the pain. This compares with the classic pain pattern of compartment syndrome, which is related to the volume of exercise and tends to settle over a period of around half an hour after exercise. If exercise is attempted on consecutive days, the pain from compartment syndrome is often more severe on the second day. The pain from PAES is unaffected by exercise on the previous day. The pain can be paradoxically more severe on walking than on running. This is believed to be due to the more prolonged contraction of the gastrocnemius muscle while walking.

pain is brought on by exercise, and the severity of the symptoms is related to the intensity of exercise. Signs of ischaemia in the lower limb are uncommon.[32]

Examination of the distal pulses (dorsal pedis and posterior tibial) may be unremarkable at rest. Assessing the pulses while the athlete actively plantarflexes or passively dorsiflexes the ankle may reveal a popliteal artery bruit, but this may be unreliable.[27] Examining the athlete immediately post-exercise is important in making the diagnosis. Immediately post-exercise, a popliteal artery bruit may be heard and the peripheral pulses will be either weak, decreased or absent.

Ankle-brachial indices are useful for the more rare underlying vascular abnormalities, but not for functional PAES.[33] Doppler ultrasound is the initial investigation of choice, as it allows real-time assessment and can be performed during provocative manoeuvres. Angiography can rule out differential diagnoses such as aneurysms and emboli, and can be performed while the athlete actively plantarflexes, and actively and passively dorsiflexes the ankle.[27,28]

MRI and MR angiography may be more useful with multiplanar views, non-ionising radiation and high soft tissue contrast, and also allow much greater visualisation of the surrounding anatomy.[27]

There is some suggestion that the presence of chronic entrapment of the popliteal artery can lead to endothelial damage, which may lead to accelerated atherosclerotic disease in later life, especially in cases of anatomical PAES, where early surgical treatment is recommended.[34] In cases of functional PAES, the treatment is less clear. A pilot study on the use of ultrasound guided Botox® at the site of entrapment is showing promising initial results but requires further research.

Atherosclerotic vessel disease

Atherosclerotic vessel disease classically affects middle-aged sedentary patients. However, some athletes, particularly in the veteran or masters class, fall into the category of middle-aged or elderly and possess risk factors that predispose them to atherosclerosis.

Pain may be felt in the thigh or the calf and is typically claudicant. With progression of the disease, the intensity of exercise needed to produce symptoms decreases. At rest, the peripheral pulses may be difficult to palpate or

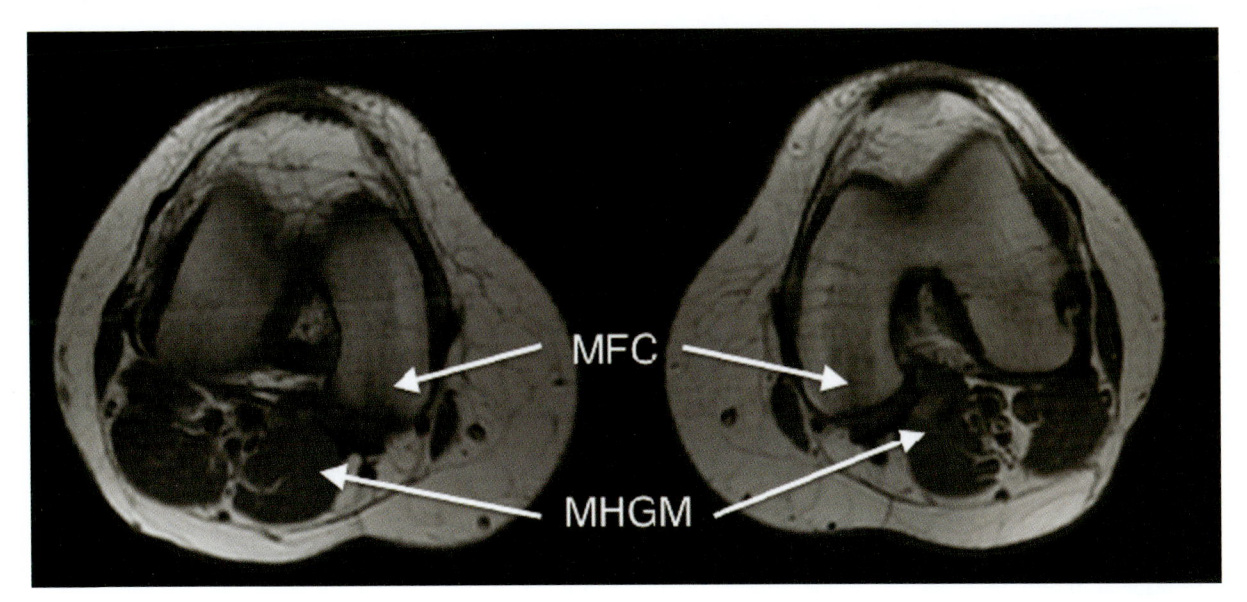

Figure 39.11 Axial MRI images of the popliteal region of both knees. The medial head of gastrocnemius muscle (MHGM) is seen to arise from a more lateral position off the posterior aspect of the medial femoral condyle (MFC) leading to 'crowding' of the popliteal vessels

absent. An arterial bruit may also be heard at rest. The presence of such bruits may be enhanced by examining the patient post-exercise.

The gold standard diagnostic test is Doppler ultrasound, although pre- and post-exercise ankle–brachial ratios can be used as a non-invasive screening test. Angiography can confirm the diagnosis.

Surgical treatments include angiographic balloon catheter dilatation or stenting, open endarterectomy or bypass surgery. Bypass surgery is the most commonly used surgical technique for atherosclerotic vessel disease and its success depends on the extent of the disease and on the viability of the smaller distal vessels.

Endofibrosis

Endofibrotic disease can cause exercise-related calf pain, although more commonly the pain is felt in the thigh. Typically the lesion occurs in the proximal external iliac artery, but may extend distally towards the origin of the femoral artery beneath the inguinal ligament. It is bilateral in 15% of cases.

External iliac artery endofibrosis has been described in endurance athletes and professional cyclists, and causes exercise-related thigh or calf pain that is related to the intensity of cycling.[35, 36] The pain is therefore most commonly felt while racing, climbing a hill or riding into a strong wind. The pain is typically relieved rapidly by a drop in the intensity of exercise.

In cyclists, it is postulated that the cycling position may cause repetitive stress and folding of the artery during high flow rates associated with extreme exercise. As a result, micro-traumatic lesions lead to thickening of arterial walls.[36] Psoas hypertrophy may also have a direct effect on the stresses around the external iliac artery.

Examination at rest may reveal a positional bruit heard over the femoral artery with the hip held in flexion. The diagnosis is made clinically by examining the patient immediately post-exercise, detecting a bruit over the femoral artery, and weak or absent distal pulses. Pre- and post-exercise ankle–brachial ratios screen for the diagnosis, which is anatomically confirmed with angiography. Arterial ultrasound or echography can also be useful in visualising the endofibrotic lesion.

Non-surgical techniques for the treatment of external iliac artery endofibrosis include angioplastic balloon catheter dilatation and stenting, which can be planned for and performed at the time of angiography. Surgical techniques include bypass surgery and open endarterectomy. In the short term, use of these techniques has made a return to top-level cycling and triathlon possible in patients.[37] However, long-term follow-up of such patients has not been carried out.

The natural history of this pathology is not certain. However, Abraham et al. suggest that it is non-progressive once high-level sport is ceased.[38] They advise that an athlete who is reducing his or her sporting level, and who is asymptomatic with activities of daily living and submaximal, be managed conservatively but followed up regularly.

LESS COMMON CAUSES
Neuromyofascial causes

The neural component of calf pain can be assessed with the use of the slump test (Fig. 39.2h). This may reproduce the patient's calf pain. If pain is relieved by cervical extension, neural structures may be contributing to the patient's pain.

The joints of the lumbar spine may occasionally refer pain to the calf. This should be suspected clinically if the pain is somewhat variable in location or if there is a history of recurrent 'calf strains'.

Another source of referred pain is myofascial trigger points in the gluteal muscles. Myofascial pain may present as an episode of sudden sharp pain and mimic a calf strain, as pain of more gradual onset accompanied by tightness, or as muscle cramps. Treatment consists of ischaemic pressure or dry needling to the trigger points followed by muscle and neural stretching.

The knee joint may also refer pain to the calf (Chapter 35). This may be due to a Baker's cyst, or a posterior cruciate ligament injury. Bleeding may track down into the calf from a strain of the posterior capsule of the knee joint or a popliteus muscle injury.

Nerve entrapments

Nerve entrapments around the calf include:

- tibial nerve entrapment secondary to a Baker's cyst (rare)
- popliteal artery aneurysm or ganglion resulting in ankle inverter and toe flexor weakness and paraesthesia to the sole of the foot
- sural nerve entrapment, which may result from compression (ski boots, casts), mass lesions, trauma or thrombophlebitis causing pain and paraesthesia in the lateral heel and foot.

The sural nerve may be compressed in a fibrous arch that thickens the superficial sural aponeurosis around the opening through which the nerve passes. Intense physical training may lead to an increase in the sural muscle mass, which in turn compromises the sural nerve in its trajectory through the unyielding and inextensible superficial sural aponeurosis. The nerve may also become trapped in scar tissue.[39]

Investigations can include nerve conduction studies +/− MRI to detect a space-occupying lesion. Management includes conservative measures such as neural stretches, fascial massage or corticosteroid injections, and failing this, consideration of surgical exploration and/or neurolysis.

Superficial compartment syndrome

Patients with superficial posterior compartment syndrome, the least common of the lower leg compartment syndromes, present with calf pain. The superficial compartment contains the gastrocnemius and soleus muscles, which are enclosed in a fascial sheath. Symptoms are similar to those of the other compartment syndromes with pain aggravated by activity and relieved by rest. An elevated compartment pressure confirms the diagnosis during and after exercise. Treatment consists of soft tissue therapy or, if this is unsuccessful, surgery.

Patients with either deep posterior compartment syndrome or stress fracture involving the posterior cortex of the tibia may present with calf pain instead of, or as well as, shin pain (Chapter 38).

CONDITIONS NOT TO BE MISSED

Deep venous thrombosis occurs occasionally in association with calf injuries. The post-injury combination of lack of movement, disuse of the muscle pump and the compressive effect of swelling may all lead to venous dilatation, pooling and a decrease in the velocity of blood flow. Certainly athletes who sustain a calf muscle injury should avoid travelling on long flights in the days after injury.

Deep venous thrombosis is a rare, but potentially fatal, risk after arthroscopy.[40] The diagnosis should be suspected when the patient has constant calf pain, tenderness, increased temperature and swelling. Homan's sign (passive dorsiflexion) (Fig. 39.2c) may be positive. Homan's test is taught to all medical students but has poor diagnostic utility. The best test for deep vein thrombosis is Wells' clinical prediction rule.[41] The presence of deep venous thrombosis may be confirmed by Doppler scan and venography.

REFERENCES

References for this chapter can be found at www.mhhe.com/au/CSM5e

Chapter 40

Pain in the Achilles region

with JILL COOK, KARIN SILBERNAGEL, STEFFAN GRIFFIN, HÅKAN ALFREDSON and JON KARLSSON

> *The anger is rage. Why the hell did this happen?!? ... Now I'm supposed to come back from this and be the same player or better ... How in the world am I supposed to do that?? ... Maybe this is how my book ends. Maybe Father Time has defeated me ... Then again maybe not!*
>
> Kobe Bryant, LA Lakers shooting guard and five-time NBA champion, after rupturing his Achilles tendon in a game against the Golden State Warriors in 2013. He returned to play until his retirement in 2016

The Achilles tendon is prone to injury when subjected to unaccustomed repetitive high loads.[1,2] Runners, for example, have a 15 times greater risk of Achilles tendon rupture and 30 times greater risk of tendinopathy as they age than do sedentary controls.[3] In this chapter, we review the approach to assessment (history, examination, investigation). We then outline the specific treatment approaches.

> **PRACTICE PEARL**
>
> Patients most commonly present with gradual (overuse) pain in the Achilles region due to pathology in the midportion of the Achilles tendon (Fig. 40.1a).

Other important conditions in order of prevalence at a sports clinic with a broad-based clientele are:

- pain at the insertion of the Achilles tendon and associated retrocalcaneal bursa ('enthesis organ')
- posterior impingement (an important differential diagnosis)
- Achilles pain related to the plantaris tendon
- pain related to friction between the Achilles tendon and surrounding tissues (peri-tendinopathy).

Achilles tendon pathology can also manifest in a very different, dramatic manner: via acute rupture of the Achilles tendon. This immediately disabling condition is captured in the chapter opening quote. The management of cases like that of Kobe Bryant is discussed in the last section of this chapter.

CLINICAL PERSPECTIVE

The key areas of pain in the Achilles region (posterior heel and proximal toward the calf) are illustrated in Figure 40.1.

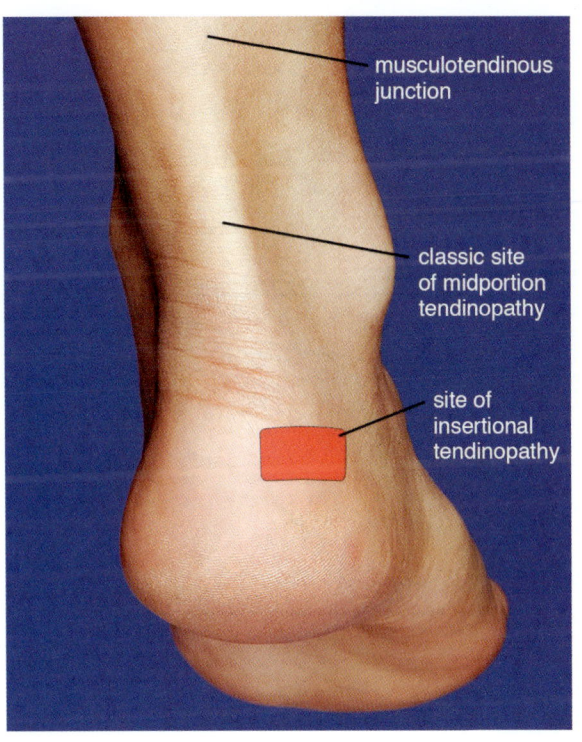

(a)

Figure 40.1 The Achilles region (a) The midportion of the tendon is clearly distinct from the insertion—an important clinical feature

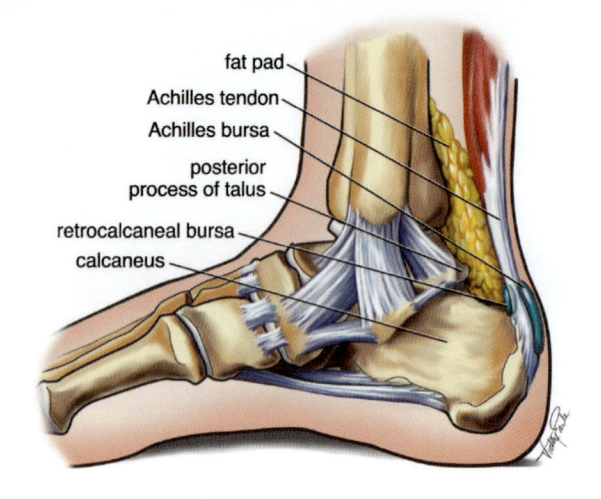

PART B   Regional problems

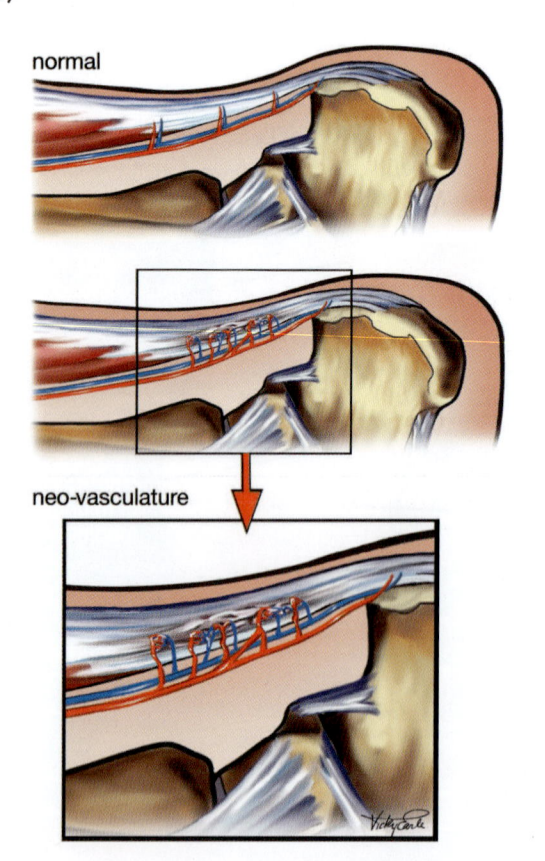

The Achilles tendon is the combined tendon of the gastrocnemius and soleus muscles, and is the thickest and strongest tendon in the human body.[4] Anteriorly, the deep surface of the tendon is supported by a fat pad (Fig 40.1b) through which most of the vessels and nerves enter the tendon (Fig. 40.1c). The tendon has no synovial sheath, but has a peritendon which is continuous with the perimysium of the muscle and the periosteum of the calcaneus, and which enfolds the anterior fat pad of the tendon. The tendon attaches to the inferior half of the calcaneus. The plantaris tendon is located medial to the Achilles and has variable anatomy, which is discussed later. The posterosuperior process of the calcaneus approximates the Achilles, usually with a bursa between.

The vast majority of patients who present with gradual onset of Achilles region pain can be treated successfully non-operatively. Experienced clinicians can quickly home in towards a diagnosis by following the clinical reasoning outlined in Figure 40.2. The first step is to rule out recent acute rupture by listening to the patient's history and performing one simple clinical test (see Physical examination, below). In many cases of acute Achilles tendon rupture, the patient or a friend has diagnosed the condition before reaching the clinician's office.

Among the conditions that manifest with more gradual onset of Achilles region pain, the most common is midportion tendinopathy. Have the patient point to the location of pain during the history–that part of the leg is easily accessible during the office consult with most types of clothing. If the history and location of pain do not fit the typical pattern for midportion tendinopathy, use the location of pain to consider other diagnoses. Broadly speaking, the second most prevalent condition is insertional tendinopathy and its associated bursitis, but in settings like a ballet school, posterior impingement will be more common than insertional tendinopathy (and more common than midportion tendinopathy too!).

History

The standard presentation is with the patient reporting a gradual onset of pain around the midportion of the Achilles, often first noticed on waking and generally associated with a recent increase in load volume or intensity.[1] Patients complain of pain at the start of activity and pain and stiffness the following morning.

> **PRACTICE PEARL**
>
> The combination of morning stiffness and pain confined to the tendon is a hallmark of Achilles tendinopathy. If these are not present, the clinician should consider alternative diagnoses.

Figure 40.1 (cont.) (b) The anatomy of the Achilles midportion, Achilles insertion and posterior process of talus (c) Stylised illustration to show the blood supply of the normal Achilles tendon (top) and in tendinopathy (middle and below)

Pain in the Achilles region CHAPTER 40

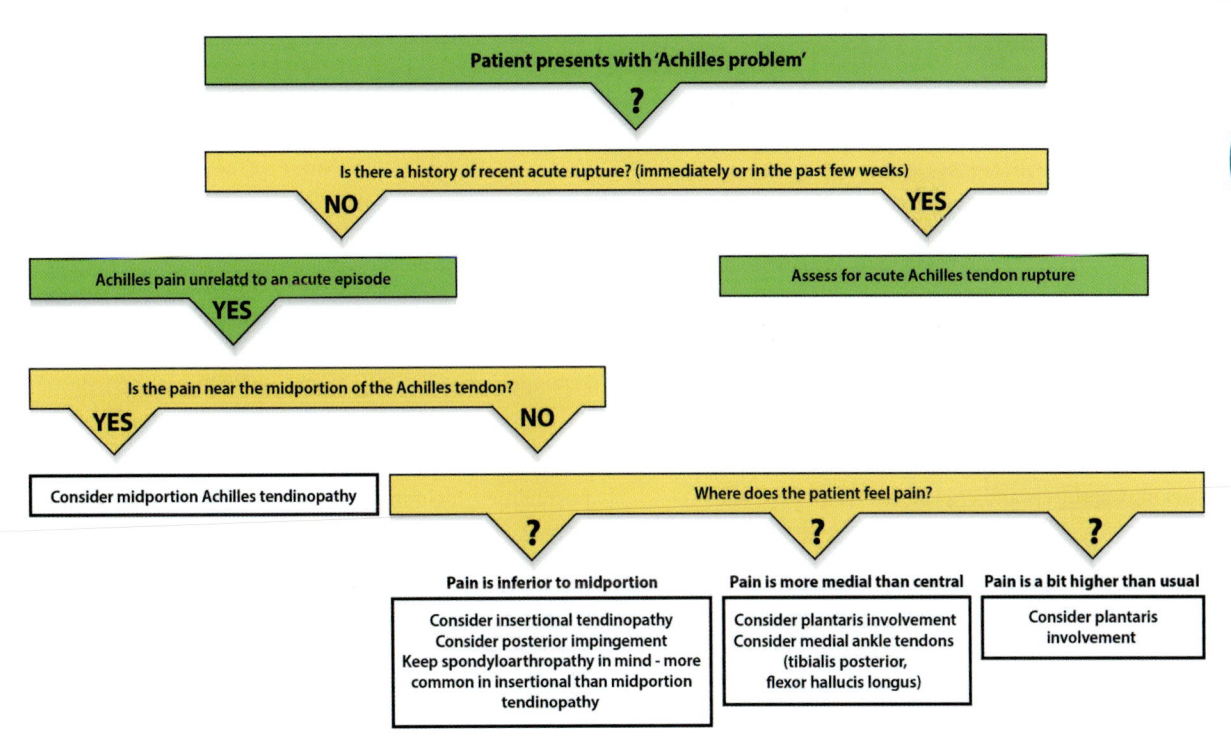

Figure 40.2 Flow diagram showing how to rapidly subgroup patients with various presentations of pain in the Achilles region

If the patient gives a history of typical midportion Achilles pain, the clinician can follow up with questions aiming to identify the cause. Was the main inciting factor a sudden increase in loading–for example, due to an increased volume, intensity or type of exercise, or a change in surface or footwear? Commonly, return to loading after a layoff for another injury is the catalyst; this also reflects a relative increase in load. Or is there a systemic condition underpinning tendinopathy (e.g. consider the possibility of Type 2 diabetes mellitus, especially in older and overweight people)?.

Careful history taking is important in case the gradual-onset Achilles region pain arises from neighbouring anatomy. For example, pain medial to the Achilles tendon or deep to the Achilles tendon with a pain pattern that is not typical of Achilles tendon suggests an alternative diagnosis.

As highlighted in Figure 40.2, the location of pain provides important diagnostic information. Pain closer to the musculotendinous junction than the standard midportion Achilles pain (Fig. 40.1a) can arise from the plantaris tendon being pathological itself or causing local Achilles tendon pathology.

Table 40.1 Causes of pain in the Achilles region

Common	Less common	Not to be missed
Midportion Achilles tendinopathy (including tendinosis—with or without partial tears—and peritendinopathy)	Plantaris tendon involvement	Achilles rupture—partial/total accessory soleus muscle
Insertional Achilles tendinopathy (at the superior lateral calcaneum, pathology includes retrocalcaneal bursitis)	Flexor hallucis longus and tibialis posterior tendinopathy (Chapter 42)	Referred pain • Peripheral neural structures • Lumbar spine
	Subcutaneous bursitis	Sever's disease (in adolescents)
	Posterior ankle joint impingement	Metabolic condition (potentially undiagnosed) • Hypercholesterolaemia • Type 2 diabetes mellitus
	Tightness of the posterior Achilles retinaculum, compressing the tendon (rare)	Spondyloarthropathy (Chapter 7)

PART B Regional problems

> **PRACTICE PEARL**
>
> If the patient offers a history of repeated soleus strains (low calf pain that comes and goes), has proximal, *medial* Achilles pain and is intolerant of dorsiflexion loading, be alert to the possibility of plantaris tendon involvement.

If the patient engages in activities that involve repeated end-range plantarflexion, posterior impingement is the key differential diagnosis for pain approximately at the midportion. The textbook activity with high prevalence of this condition is ballet (pointe/demi-pointe), but it is a common presentation to the clinic in football players (kicking), sprinters and cricket fast bowlers.

A key alternate diagnosis

Anatomically, the impingement (of the os trigonum or the posterior process of the talus, Fig 40.10 below) takes place anterior and inferior to the Achilles midportion. Some patients appreciate that the pain feels 'deeper' than at the Achilles tendon, but many do not offer that distinction, so the clinician must bracket the midportion Achilles diagnosis with the possibility of posterior impingement. It is not uncommon for a patient to have wasted time and 'failed' prolonged Achilles rehabilitation when the true diagnosis was posterior impingement. Having considered these two conditions together, the clinician can easily distinguish them during physical examination (see passive plantarflexion).

The patient may report pain medially at about the level of the Achilles tendon; this can be due to tibialis posterior peritendinopathy (proximal to the flexor retinaculum of course) or flexor hallucis tendinopathy (a common ballet pathology). These two conditions generally present more inferiorly and more medially than typical midportion Achilles tendinopathy. These two conditions are discussed in Chapter 42.

If the patient gives a history of relatively unloaded plantarflexion and dorsiflexion, such as an inexperienced cyclist spiking his or her load, consider peritendinopathy.

A sudden explosive event

A sudden, disabling sensation or pain and inability to function is often due to complete tendon rupture. The greatest prevalence is among men aged between 30 and 50.[5,6] It occurs in sports with explosive movements like basketball, tennis and Ultimate (Frisbee®), but it can arise in people with underlying degenerative (but asymptomatic) tendon pathology as simply as a result of stepping off a curb awkwardly. The patient often reports hearing a noise like a gunshot or feeling like he or she was kicked on the tendon.

> **PRACTICE PEARL**
>
> Many textbooks suggest that complete Achilles rupture prevents active plantarflexion. This is wrong! Patients can often plantarflex weakly in non weightbearing positions using intact accessory plantar flexors such as tibialis posterior, plantaris, flexor digitorum longus and flexor hallucis longus. It is a naive error to rule out Achilles tendon rupture from patient reports of plantarflexion. The key diagnostic test is the 'calf squeeze test' (also called Simmond's or Thompson's test)[7,8] (see Fig. 40.3h).

When the patient reports an acute episode, other possibilities include (i) partial rupture of the Achilles tendon and (ii) plantaris tendon rupture. The latter presents with acute onset of pain on the medial side of the upper Achilles midportion. In athletes, this typically occurs during sprinting. If the presentation to the clinic is not acute, the patient may report having had a short period (3–5 days) with disabling pain and then being able to run again.

Physical examination

If there is no suspicion of tendon rupture, the examination should begin with the patient standing. The clinician should first assess the muscles for signs of wasting, then examine how the patient copes with loading tasks likely to provoke pain. In most patients, simple double or single-leg heel raises will cause pain. In more active individuals whose tendon can tolerate higher loads, ask the patient to hop on the spot or hop forward to reproduce pain.

In some athletes, repeated loading tests (multiple hops, jumps) or examination after a training session will be valuable to fully evaluate the tendon. Record not only the function of the calf and Achilles tendon, but also note how the lower limb kinetic chain is performing. Longstanding symptoms can cause substantial unloading (favouring the unaffected side) and impair the function of the entire kinetic chain (see Chapter 8).

After assessing function, assess strength and strength endurance, and seek possible predisposing factors such as unilateral calf tightness, reduced dorsiflexion and abnormal lower limb biomechanics. This may require analysis of treadmill running or video analysis of jump and other sporting movements that are provocative (Chapter 8).

Finally, compare the resting muscle tone between sides and palpate around the tendon for specific areas of tenderness (e.g. ventral, superficial, medial tendon), crepitus (a 'crackling' feeling that arises because of the fibrinous exudate in the peritendon) and tendon thickening.

Pain in the Achilles region CHAPTER 40

> **PRACTICE PEARL**
>
> Palpation tenderness in the Achilles is not a diagnostic or prognostic sign. Achilles tendons are always sore to touch. (Tenderness—pain on palpation—has a very poor positive likelihood ratio (LR+). See Chapter 14.)

A focused examination relevant to the patient who presents with Achilles pain includes:

1. Observation
   a. standing and walking: Observe soleus and gastrocnemius muscle bulk on both sides. Look for wasting of quadriceps femoris and gluteal muscles
   b. ask the patient to identify the location of pain (midportion, distal, specific to Achilles tendon or more medial/lateral) (Fig. 40.1a). You may see thickening at site of pain or you may be able to feel crepitus
   c. if Achilles tendon rupture is a possibility, inspect for obvious swelling (Fig. 40.3a). If the patient is seen acutely, the tendon defect is evident beneath the skin at the site of rupture. This defect fills rapidly with blood but if the patient is lying supine, the unsupported foot rests in excessive dorsiflexion due to loss of resting calf muscle (plantarflexion) tone (see also special tests, below).
2. Functional tests
   a. plantarflexion–double- and single-leg calf raises for pain
   b. hopping/forward hopping (if clinically indicated–in higher-functioning patients while testing their capacity) (Fig. 40.3b)
   c. strength/endurance–examine the patient's capacity to repeat single-leg heel raises with full height. Record the number as a baseline
   d. biomechanics (see also Chapter 8 for general biomechanical assessment)
      i. Active dorsiflexion (lunge)
      ii. Gastrocnemius stretch (Fig. 40.3c)
      iii. Soleus stretch (Fig. 40.3d)
3. Supine/prone
   a. active movements (only useful if rupture suspected)
      i. plantarflexion and dorsiflexion
      ii. first-toe flexion and extension in full ankle plantarflexion for flexor hallucis longus tendinopathy (Fig. 40.3e)

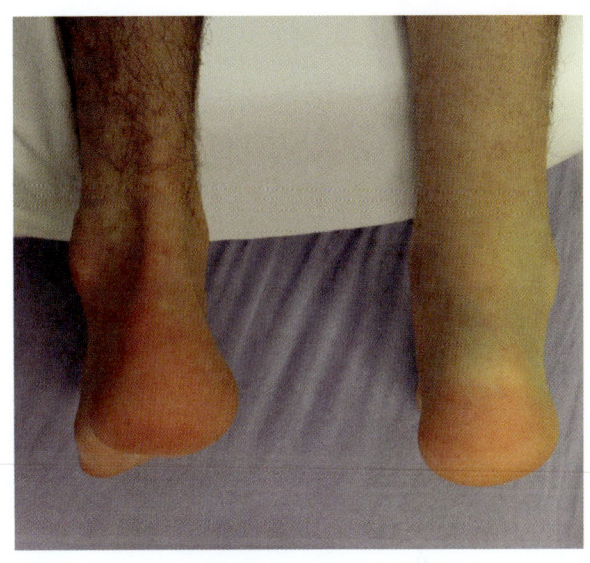

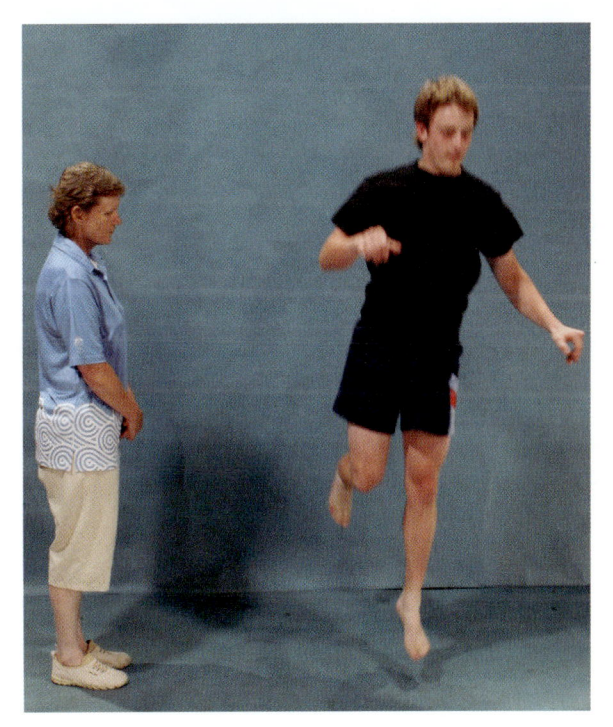

(a)

(b)

Figure 40.3 Examination of the patient with pain in the Achilles region (a) Inspect for Achilles tendon rupture if this is a possibility. In this case the right side has a ruptured Achilles tendon (b) Functional tests. These can be used to reproduce pain, if necessary, or to test strength. Tests include double-leg and single-leg calf raises, hops (illustrated), hops forward, eccentric drops and lunge

PART B   Regional problems

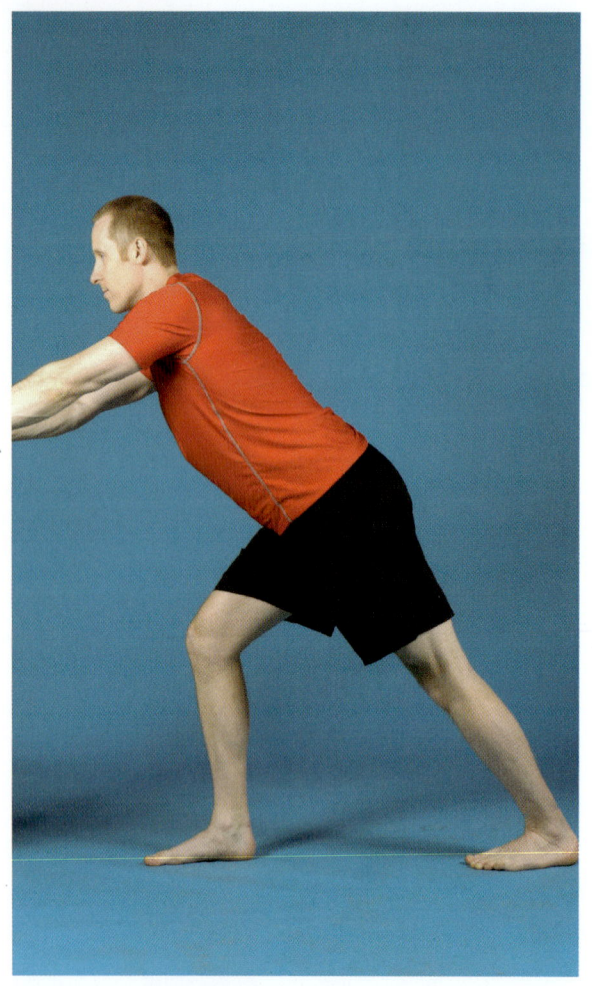

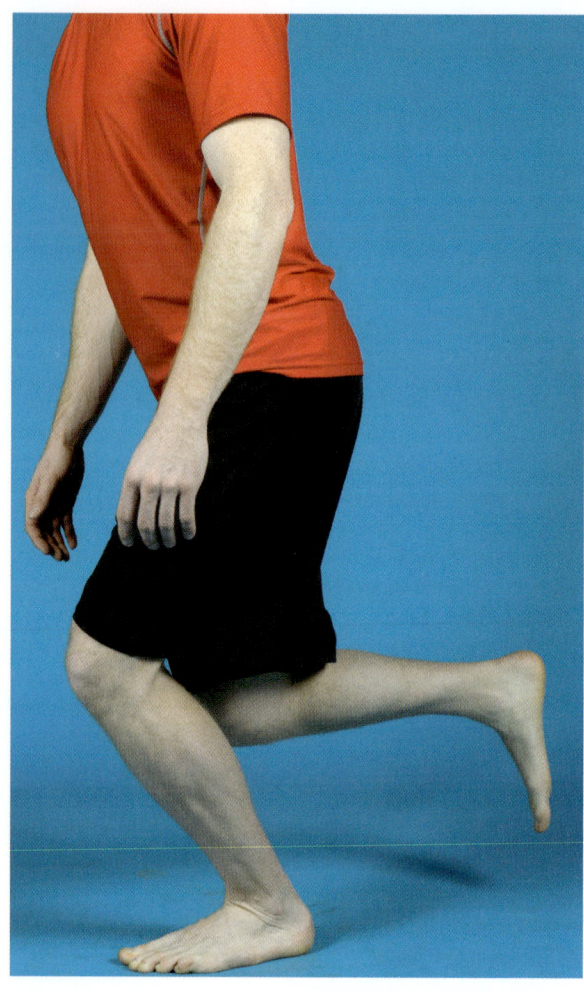

(c)   (d)

Figure 40.3 (cont.) (c) Passive movement—muscle stretch (gastrocnemius). The patient stands so that body weight causes overpressure. The knee must remain extended and the heel (back foot) keeps contact with the floor. The foot remains in neutral if the patient keeps the patella in line with the second metatarsal. Compare the stretch on both sides (d) Passive movement—muscle stretch (soleus). The patient stands upright and keeps the knee flexed. The foot should remain in a neutral position

b. Passive movements
   i. plantarflexion with and without overpressure (Fig. 40.3f) to assess posterior impingement)
   ii. inversion and eversion

c. Palpation
   i. firm palpation of the Achilles tendon is not recommended as normal tendons are tender–they are painful to touch
   ii. palpation may identify associated pathologies (such as the more proximal medial tenderness if the plantaris is a cause of pain/contributing to Achilles tendinopathy)
   iii. Posterior talus may be tender in posterior impingement but the key test is the passive plantarflexion text
   iv. Palpate more inferiorly and medial to the midportion Achilles tendon for flexor hallucis longus tendinopathy
   v. Palpate the tibialis posterior tendon before it passes under the flexor retinaculum to ensure it is not contributing to symptoms
   vi. Assess the flexor hallucis longus, which is a differential for posterior impingement

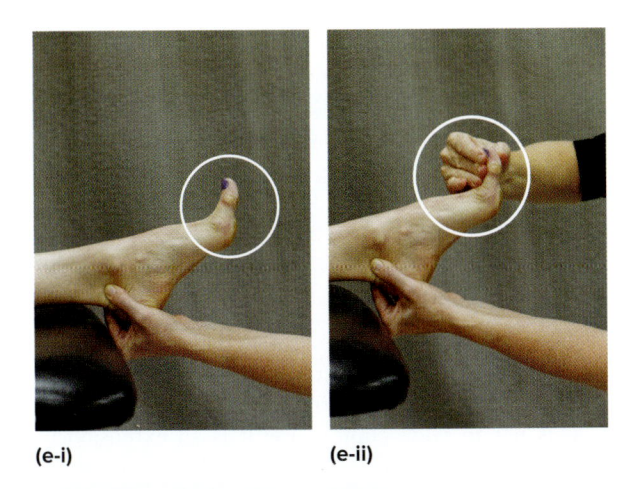

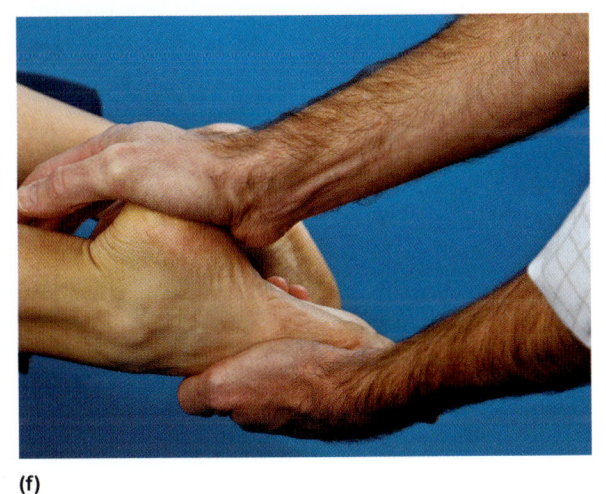

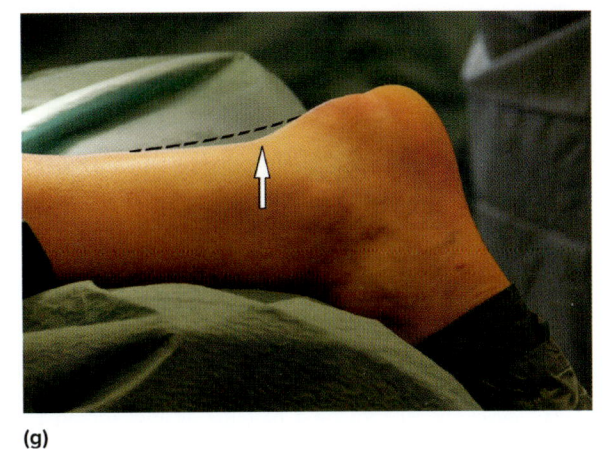

Pain in the Achilles region CHAPTER 40

(e-i) (e-ii) (g)

Figure 40.3 (cont.) (e) Active first-toe flexion and extension in full ankle plantarflexion for flexor hallucis longus tendinopathy (e-i) Active movement without resistance (e-ii) Movement against the examiner's resistance. Examiner is feeling for FHL swelling or crepitus with her left hand (f) Passive movement—plantarflexion. This will be painful if posterior impingement is present. Overpressure can be applied (g) Observation (prone)—for suspected Achilles tendon rupture. The Achilles tendon would normally bridge the space from the superior calcaneum through to the muscle tendon junction (normal anatomical skin/tendon position shown by dotted line). In cases of tendon rupture (arrow), the tendon is not connected to the calcaneum and rests on underlying soft tissue. (h) Special test—the calf squeeze test. (h-i) At rest. The ruptured Achilles (right leg, white arrow) hangs more vertically compared to the uninjured leg (red arrows). (h-ii) Squeeze. The ruptured Achilles (right leg) fails to plantar flex (red arrow), while the normal leg plantar flexes on squeeze (green arrow)

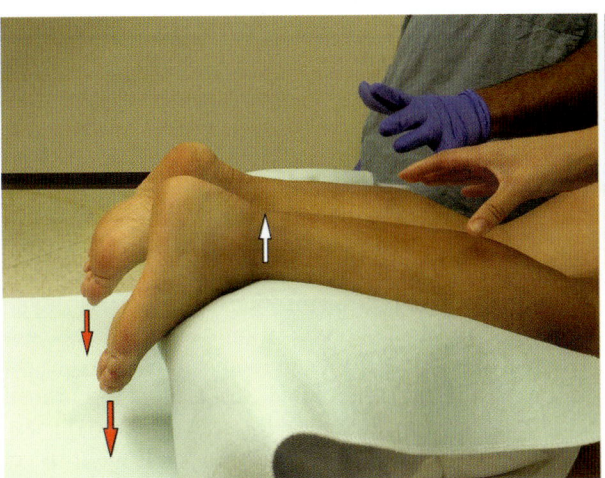

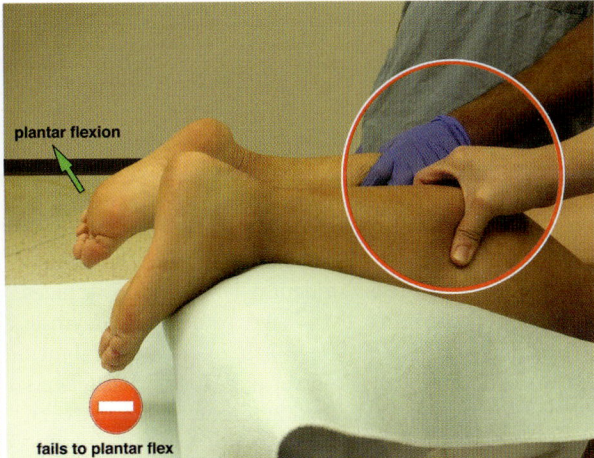

(f)

plantar flexion

fails to plantar flex

(h-i) (h-ii)

871

vii. Achilles tendon insertion and retrocalcaneal bursa (insertional tendinopathy)
viii. Tightness in the posterior retinaculum
ix. Crepitus associated with peritendinopathy

4. Special tests
   a. Inspect for tendon defect and loss of resting tone for tendon rupture (Fig. 40.3a, g)
   b. Simmond's/Thompson's calf squeeze test[7, 8] (Fig. 40.3h).

> **PRACTICE PEARL**
>
> Under careful diagnostic scrutiny, imaging such as colour and power Doppler examinations and MRI have been disappointing for clinicians who had hoped they could offer prognostic information or guide response to treatment[15, 23–25] (see also Table 40.4 and Chapter 15).

Key outcome measures (PROMs)

Functional tests mentioned and depicted above (number of calf raises, hops) provide a baseline against which to compare treatment response. In addition, the Victorian Institute of Sport Assessment–Achilles (VISA-A) has been widely used since 2001 to monitor the clinical progress of Achilles tendinopathy[17] (Table 40.2). It takes less than 5 minutes to complete and once patients are familiar with it they can complete it themselves. Scores range from 0–100, where 100 represents no pain, full function and no limitation of training or competition. Baseline values for Achilles tendinopathy patients can be expected to be between 24 and 60, and scores above 90 represent full recovery.[18] The minimum clinically important difference (MCID) of the VISA-A score is in the range of 12–20.[19-21] The VISA-A should be administered monthly rather than daily or weekly as 40% of the score comes from capacity to complete higher-load activities.

Investigations

Plain radiographs are of limited value–they do not improve the positive likelihood ratio (Chapter 14) of making the diagnosis of a form of Achilles tendinopathy (either midportion or insertional).[22] Tendon calcification is not a predictor of current symptoms of prognosis (Fig. 40.4a). The patient should be managed according to symptoms. A radiographic finding of a prominent superior projection of the calcaneus (Haglund's morphology) is normal. See discussion of this condition below. Anatomical changes responsible for posterior impingement may also be evident on plain radiographs (see posterior impingement section later in this chapter); such anatomy does not predict current symptoms or prognosis.

In patients with Achilles tendon pain, ultrasound examination can help distinguish whether the Achilles or the peritendon or both have pathology. Greyscale ultrasound examination (Fig. 40.4b, c) can be combined with colour and power Doppler (Fig. 40.4d) that reflects blood flow inside and outside the tendon. MRI can demonstrate abnormal tendon morphology (Fig. 40.4e) but it did not prove a good predictor of current or future symptoms.[15]

Ultrasound tissue characterisation (UTC) (Fig. 40.4f) is not grouped with ultrasound modalities above as it is not in wide clinical use. It is an extension of traditional ultrasound[19] (Chapter 15) that allows intra-tendinous structure to be quantified. As with other imaging modalities, an abnormal UTC appearance does not guarantee that the tendon is the source of pain; experienced clinicians believe that the appearance of abnormal collagen may increase the positive likelihood ratio (Table 40.3). UTC can demonstrate changes in Achilles tendon structure with loading rehabilitation (i.e. the effect of mechanotherapy, Chapter 17),[23] in cases of tendinopathy and also after tendon rupture. UTC is not yet useful to guide treatment; rehabilitation should be guided by clinical assessment and functional testing.

MIDPORTION ACHILLES TENDINOPATHY

This section outlines (i) pathology so that it can be explained to patients, (ii) relevant risk factors and (iii) treatment principles including a four-stage exercise program based on the concept of tendon capacity (Chapter 4, Fig. 4.14).

Pathology

The macroscopic changes seen at surgery for chronic midportion Achilles tendinopathy are characterised by a poorly demarcated dull-greyish discolouration of the intratendinous collagen with a focal loss of normal fibre structure.[26, 27] Partial ruptures may occur in regions of pre-existing pathology.[28] Peritendinous structures may be normal, oedematous or scarred. If scarred, the peritendon may adhere to the tendon.

Under the light microscope, pathological tendon reveals abnormal proliferation of tendon cells (fibroblasts), increases in ground substance, collagen fibre disarray and increased vascularity as outlined in Chapter 4 (see box and Figs. 4.10 and 4.11). These regions of tendon disarray correspond to areas of increased signal on MRI and hypoechoic regions on ultrasound[29] (Fig. 40.4c, d, e).

Pain in the Achilles region CHAPTER 40

Table 40.2 Victorian Institute of Sport Assessment—Achilles (VISA-A) questionnaire[17]

1. For how many minutes do you have stiffness in the Achilles region on first getting up? POINTS

   100 min | 0 | 1 | 2 | 3 | 4 | 5 | 6 | 7 | 8 | 9 | 10 | 0 min

2. Once you have warmed up for the day, do you have pain when stretching the Achilles tendon fully over the edge of a step? (keeping knee straight) POINTS

   Strong severe pain | 0 | 1 | 2 | 3 | 4 | 5 | 6 | 7 | 8 | 9 | 10 | No pain

3. After walking on flat ground for 30 minutes, do you have pain within the next 2 hours? (If unable to walk on flat ground for 30 minutes because of pain, score 0 for this question.) POINTS

   Strong severe pain | 0 | 1 | 2 | 3 | 4 | 5 | 6 | 7 | 8 | 9 | 10 | No pain

4. Do you have pain walking down stairs with normal gait cycle? POINTS

   Strong severe pain | 0 | 1 | 2 | 3 | 4 | 5 | 6 | 7 | 8 | 9 | 10 | No pain

5. Do you have pain during or immediately after doing 10 (single-leg) heel raises from a flat surface? POINTS

   Strong severe pain | 0 | 1 | 2 | 3 | 4 | 5 | 6 | 7 | 8 | 9 | 10 | No pain

6. How many single-leg hops can you do without pain? POINTS

   0 | 0 | 1 | 2 | 3 | 4 | 5 | 6 | 7 | 8 | 9 | 10 | 10

7. Are you currently undertaking sport or other physical activity? POINTS
   - 0 ☐ Not at all
   - 4 ☐ Modified training ± modified competition
   - 7 ☐ Full training ± competition but not at same level as when symptoms began
   - 10 ☐ Competing at the same or higher level as when symptoms began

8. Please complete *either* A, B or C in this question.
   - If you have no pain while undertaking Achilles tendon loading sports, please complete Q8A only.
   - If you have pain while undertaking Achilles tendon loading sports but it does not stop you from completing the activity, please complete Q8B only.
   - If you have pain that stops you from completing Achilles tendon loading sports, please complete Q8C only.

   A. If you have no pain while undertaking Achilles tendon loading sports, for how long can you train/practice? POINTS

Nil	1–10 min	11–20 min	21–30 min	>30 min
0	7	14	21	30

   B. If you have some pain while undertaking Achilles tendon loading sports but it does not stop you from completing your training/practice, for how long can you train/practice? POINTS

Nil	1–10 min	11–20 min	21–30 min	>30 min
0	4	10	14	20

   C. If you have pain that stops you from completing your training/practice in the Achilles tendon loading sports, for how long can you train/practice? POINTS

Nil	1–10 min	11–20 min	21–30 min	>30 min
0	2	5	7	10

   TOTAL SCORE ☐ /100

Reproduced with permission of British Journal of Sports Medicine

Table 40.3 Diagnostic accuracy of clinical tests in patients with tendinopathy and rupture

Assessment finding	What is a positive finding?	Sensitivity	Specificity	Likelihood ratio −	Likelihood ratio +
History					
Tendinopathy					
Pain[9]	Patient points to site	78	77	0.50	3.39
Morning stiffness[9]	Pain worse in morning	89	58	0.19	2.12
Physical examination					
Tendon rupture					
Palpation of gap in tendon[10]	Tendon gap	73	89	0.30	6.64
Tendinopathy					
Palpation (tenderness)[11]	Patient reports tenderness	64	81	0.48	3.15
Palpation of tendon thickening[9]	Subjective tendon thickening	59	90	0.46	5.9
Palpation of crepitus[9]	Subjective crepitation with passive ankle movement	3	100	0.97	>10*
Arc sign[11]	Swelling moves during ankle dorsi/plantarflexion	42	88	0.68	3.24
Special tests					
Tendon rupture					
Thompson's calf squeeze test[7]	Ankle remains still	40	–	–	–
Calf squeeze test[10]	Ankle remains still	96	93	0.04	13.71
Matles test[10]	Neutral or dorsiflexed ankle	88	85	0.14	6.29
Tendinopathy					
Royal London Hospital test[11]	Tenderness on palpation in end-range dorsiflexion	54	86	0.54	3.84
Imaging					
Tendon total rupture					
Ultrasound[12] Radiologist interpretation		100	83	0	5.88
MRI[13] Radiologist interpretation		91	–	–	0.91
Tendon partial rupture					
Ultrasound[14] Radiologist interpretation		50	81	0.62	2.63
Tendinopathy					
Ultrasound[15] Radiologist interpretation		80	49	0.39	1.57
MRI[15] Radiologist interpretation		95	50	0.1	1.9
Combination of findings	*Number of variables present*				
Tendinopathy[16]					
+ Palpation (tenderness)	3/3	59	83	0.49	3.47
+ Arc sign					
+ Royal London Hospital test					

Sn = Sensitivity; = Sp Specificity; LR − = Negative likelihood ratio; LR + = Positive likelihood ratio
Blue − Large change in likelihood (LR − <0.1, LR + >10)
Red − Rarely important change in likelihood (LR − >0.5, LR + <2.0)
* Positive likelihood ratio cannot be calculated when specificity equals 100

Pain in the Achilles region   CHAPTER 40

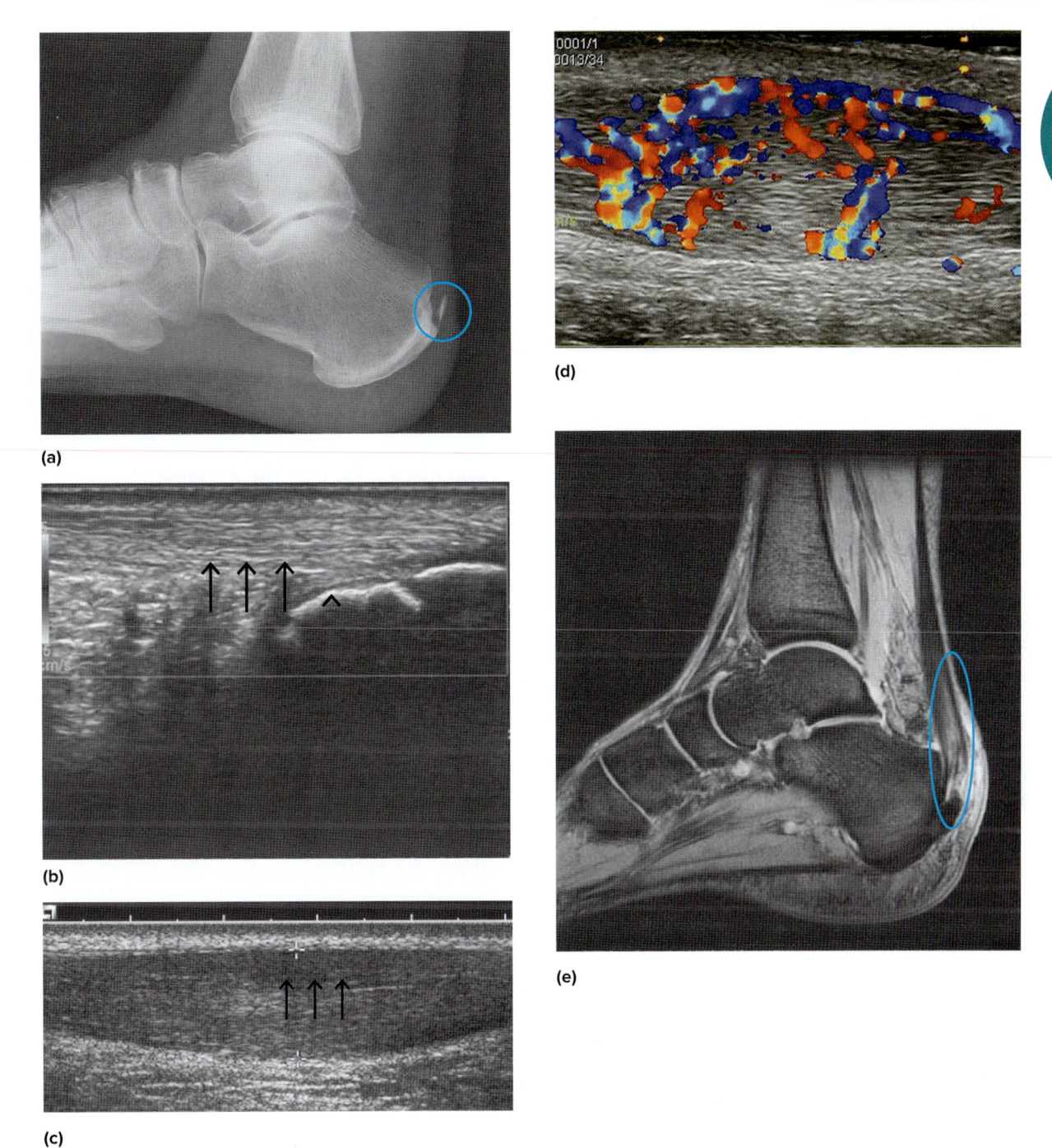

Figure 40.4 Imaging findings in the Achilles region (a) Calcification is a common finding in pathological tendons. It should not influence management and a bone spicule (circle) is very difficult to find in surgery. The take-home message is to manage according to symptoms and function; do not manage the radiograph (b) Greyscale ultrasound of a normal Achilles tendon (arrows). The superior calcaneum (arrowhead) prevents sound waves from penetrating, hence the acoustic 'shadow' deep to the calcaneal margins (c) Greyscale ultrasound of an Achilles tendon with mild morphological abnormality (arrows)—thickening of the tendon and less echodensity (because of increased matrix ground substance and associated fluid) (d) Colour Doppler ultrasound showing abnormal vessels in symptomatic tendinopathy. Appearances do not mirror symptoms enough to provide definitive clinical support (e) MRI appearance of increased signal in the distal Achilles tendon extending into the insertion (blue oval)

PART B   Regional problems

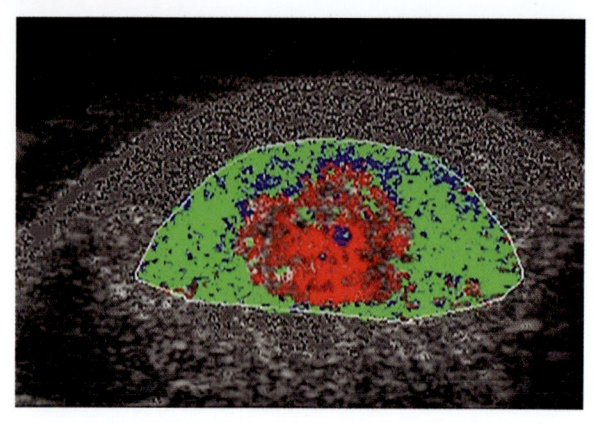

(f)

Figure 40.4 (cont.) (f) Ultrasound tissue characterisation (UTC). This ultrasound modality has been most used in Achilles tendinopathy as the subcutaneous tendon anatomy is well suited to the linear probe. Whether the instrument will have widespread clinical utility remains to be seen

Table 40.4   Imaging findings in overuse Achilles tendinopathy (i.e. not a complete rupture). Imaging appearances do not equate with symptoms nor do they predict time to return to sport (recovery). See also Figure 40.4

Imaging appearance	Variations seen in clinical practice
Normal appearance on ultrasound/MRI	It is possible, but unusual, to have a normal imaging with symptoms of Achilles tendinopathy. Carefully evaluate alternative structures as a potential source of pain
Ultrasound and MRI tendon swelling	Tendon thickening varies, but there is often a fusiform swelling. Evaluate contribution of peritendon to swelling
Ultrasound discontinuity of tendon fascicles	Hypoechoic regions are often seen inside the thickened tendon. This corresponds to a fluid-rich region with irregular collagen fascicle arrangement
Doppler ultrasound evidence of high blood flow	May be extensive or absent and may vary in amount when imaged after rest or activity, and on different days
Increased MRI signal	Abnormal high signal, best seen on T2-weighted sequences (see also Chapter 15 for more advice for clinicians on interpreting MRI)

Inflammatory cells are few in midportion Achilles tendinopathy.[26, 30] Intratendinous microdialysis[31, 32] and analysis of appropriately prepared biopsy tissue using cDNA-arrays and real-time quantitative polymerase chain reaction (PCR)[33] all failed to show prostaglandin-mediated inflammation.[34] The debate around whether Achilles tendinopathy has an inflammatory component or not[35] is complicated because of the various definitions of inflammation.[36]

Biopsy specimens from midportion Achilles tendinopathy show increases in some cytokines and neuropeptides, such as substance P and calcitonin gene-related peptide (CGRP). Activated tendon cells can produce substances that can cause pain that may be detected by nerves in the peritendon.[37] Tendon pain is complex and the source is often unknown.[38] (See Chapters 5 and 6 for more on pain biology.)

Predisposing factors for Achilles tendinopathy

Midportion Achilles tendinopathy is most common among active people, but it also occurs in inactive individuals. Irrespective of the baseline level of activity, relative tendon overload is the main trigger. This may occur in a single episode or, more often, over a period of time. Athletes, for example, may overload their tendon during an intensive period of competition or training, whereas for inactive people the commencement of a new exercise regimen may be sufficient. Although overload is considered to be the primary inciting event for tendinopathy, tendons' response to load is also influenced by a range of intrinsic and extrinsic risk factors.

Intrinsic risk factors
Modifiable intrinsic risk factors include central adiposity in men and peripheral adiposity in women,[39] increased BMI,[40, 41] hypercholesterolaemia and diabetes mellitus (type 1 and 2).[42, 43] Non-modifiable factors include previous injury/tendinopathy,[44, 45] genetic predisposition (certain genes coding for collagen),[46, 47] exposure to fluroquinolones[48] or steroids,[49] and (for insertional tendinopathy) inflammatory arthritis.[50] Older age may also be a risk factor; however, the current evidence is conflicting, suggesting that other specific factors such as cumulative load may influence this association.[51]

There are also a number of modifiable biomechanical factors associated with Achilles tendinopathy, shown in Table 40.5. These either increase strain on the tendon or reduce its ability to bear load. Contrary to popular belief, there is little evidence of an association between subtalar joint pronation and Achilles tendinopathy.[52] In fact, a *supinated and rigid foot* is associated with tendinopathy.[53-55]

Extrinsic risk factors

In active individuals, the main extrinsic risk factor for Achilles tendinopathy is a recent change in tendon loading, such as increasing distance, speed or frequency of training/competition with insufficient recovery between loading periods.[61-64] In particular, a sudden increase in activities involving high energy storage, such as jumping and landing, is thought to be important. In sedentary individuals this stimulus may be significantly less but the principles still apply. Other extrinsic risk factors such as changes in footwear or training surface may be important, especially in elite athletes, but are secondary to load.

Treatment of midportion Achilles tendinopathy

Experienced clinicians begin conservative treatment by identifying and correcting possible aetiologic factors. Most importantly, this involves management of the patient's tendon load (first decrease load to control symptoms and then increase load to improve tendon capacity). Biomechanical limitations such as restricted ankle dorsiflexion and hallux rigidus should also be addressed if possible. Below, we outline common treatments for Achilles tendinopathy including targeted exercises (mechanotherapy,[65] see Chapter 17), injections and surgery.

Focused rehabilitative exercise training: the hub of tendinopathy treatment

Exercise training is at the hub of effective treatment for midportion Achilles tendinopathy (Fig. 40.5). Such treatments became the preferred non-surgical management for Achilles tendinopathy after Alfredson published his eccentric loading program in 1998.[66] Repeated and, initially, pain-provoking exercise led to patients being pain-free in about 12 weeks. This program was a landmark in moving treatment away from rest and passive approaches. In addition to the good clinical results, ultrasound and MRI follow-up demonstrated that patients' tendons improved in appearance and decreased in thickness, although they did not return to a normal appearance.[67]

> **PRACTICE PEARL**
>
> Various types of exercise programs are effective for tendinopathy—there does not appear to be anything 'magical' about eccentric exercise in this setting.[68, 69] The combination of eccentric and concentric movements may be as beneficial as eccentric movements alone.[69-71]

Doing both concentric and eccentric exercises may also promote muscle strength and endurance adaptation.[69, 72] In addition, the inclusion of more dynamic exercise may not adversely affect the outcome.[73]

The take-home message in 2017 appears to be that progressively loading the muscle tendon unit (kinetic chain) to promote recovery of full-capacity tendon is likely the effective stimulus; this argues against 'recipe

Table 40.5 Biomechanical factors that are associated with Achilles tendinopathy and their possible mechanisms

Factor	Possible mechanisms	Assess by
Relative weakness in plantarflexion strength[53]	Increased load on tendon by failing to attenuate load	Single-leg heel raise, single-leg hop, dynamometer or strength/endurance tests (heel raise to fatigue)
Increased dorsiflexion range of motion[53]	Increased tendon load (via longer loading period) and longer levers Possible collagen abnormalities (e.g. benign hyperlaxity syndrome/Ehlers–Danlos syndrome)	Weight-bearing (knee to wall) and non weight-bearing assessment of dorsiflexion ROM
Reduced dorsiflexion range of motion with or without supinated foot type[54, 56]	Increased tendon load (due to faster loading time)	Weight-bearing (knee to wall) and non weight-bearing assessment of dorsiflexion ROM
Reduced knee flexor strength[57]	Increased tendon load by increasing demand on plantarflexors	Dynamometry or clinical strength/endurance tests (bridging)[58]
Poor quality tendon structure[59, 60]	Reduced capacity to tolerate load Less effective load-bearing tissue	Ultrasound, Ultrasound Tissue Characterisation (UTC), MRI

877

PART B Regional problems

physiotherapy' ('Do X of these exercises twice a day like a robot'). The 'capacity' concept[74] is illustrated and discussed in Chapter 4 (see Fig. 4.14). That key diagram can be photocopied and marked up to show patients their current capacity (triangle at bottom left of the figure) and their required capacity (triangle at top right of the figure). Different exercises are prescribed to improve the patient's capacity (Chapter 4, four-stage training program).

Four-stage, progressive Achilles exercise program adapted to the clinical assessment

In this chapter, the broad 'capacity' concept is customised for Achilles tendinopathy in Figure 40.6. The four stages of treatment include three relating to developing tendon capacity and one that provides analgesia (isometric exercises). The four stages are outlined in the box.

Prevention: Can exercises prevent tendinopathy?

Eccentric exercise appears to be ineffective as a prophylactic treatment to prevent Achilles tendinopathy. Soccer players who performed eccentric exercise and stretches during the playing season were no more likely to be free of Achilles tendon injury than those who did not.[59]

Beware: Is the plantaris tendon a culprit?

The plantaris tendon is usually a tiny benign tendon medial to and removed from the Achilles (Fig. 40.8a) In some people, it enlarges and compresses the Achilles tendon, in others it can be ensheathed in the Achilles peritendon (Fig. 40.8 b, c, d) In both cases the variable properties of the plantaris and Achilles cause compression of the Achilles tendon and may provoke tendinopathy.[77–79] The plantaris was first identified as a potential contributor to midportion Achilles region pain around 2011.[80] The clinical clues to this culprit are pain and tenderness that are more medial and more proximal to the 'classic' midportion Achilles tendinopathy symptoms and pain aggravated by loading in dorsiflexion.

If this diagnosis is suspected, imaging (ultrasound or MRI) is indicated.

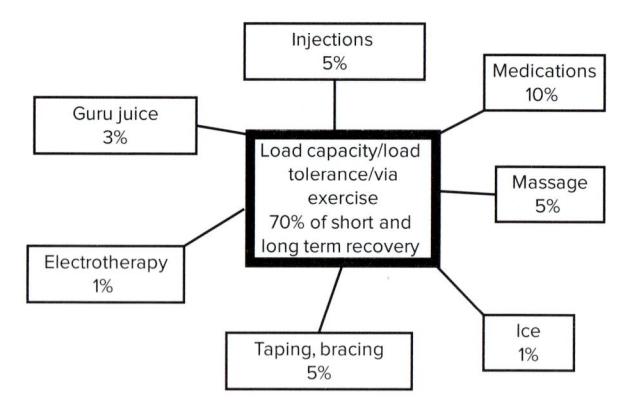

Figure 40.5 Treatment of midportion Achilles tendinopathy. Warning! Warning! The numbers in this conceptual figure are not to be taken literally. There are many possible treatment options for Achilles tendinopathy. Systematic reviews indicate that various forms of exercise prescription provide superior pain relief over control treatments (level 1 evidence). The relative effect sizes suggested in this figure should be considered estimates and will vary from patient to patient. The estimates of relative importance reflect the chapter authors' expert clinical experience (level 5 evidence). It highlights that not all treatments are created equal

Plantaris management

Conservative management of this condition follows the loading principles of the four-stage program (outlined in the box below, Figs. 40.6 and 40.7) while reducing compression of the plantaris against the Achilles tendon. This is achieved by ensuring the patient completes all exercises with a moderate degree of ankle plantarflexion, and avoids loads in dorsiflexion, especially in the early stages of rehabilitation. Using a high heel raise similar to those used for insertional Achilles tendinopathy (see below) will allow the patient to complete these exercises pain-free. At stages 3 and 4 of the rehabilitation program, it is appropriate to gradually reduce the heel height until the exercise can be completed through the full range.

The four-stage program for midportion Achilles tendinopathy

This four-stage rehabilitation program incorporates the exercises from various published programs and is clinically effective for Achilles tendinopathy. The key elements are its (i) stages, (ii) progressive nature, and (iii) flexibility (to adapt it to clinical re-assessment).

Stage 1—Pain relief. Isometric exercises
Patients focus on isometric calf raise exercises that relieve pain. These can be done with simple body-weight holds (single- or double-leg depending on strength and pain), but athletes require weights in a standing heel raise machine.

Pain in the Achilles region CHAPTER 40

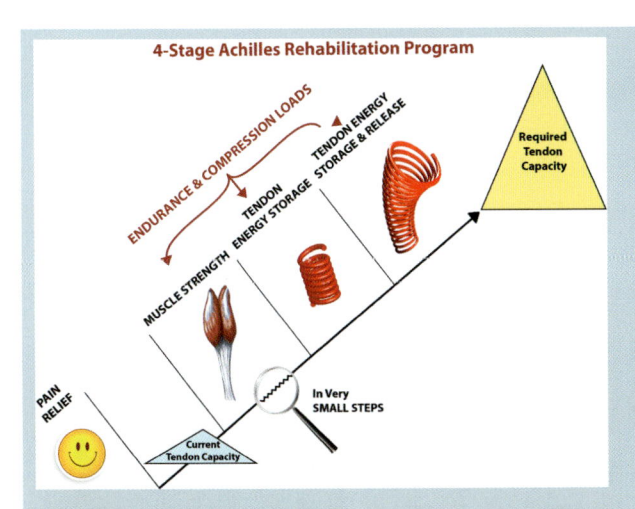

Figure 40.6 The four-stage program for midportion Achilles tendinopathy. Pain relief (with isometric exercise) allows the patient to undertake exercises to improve tendon capacity (see also Fig. 4.14)
REPRODUCED WITH PERMISSION OF BRITISH JOURNAL OF SPORTS MEDICINE

The isometric holds should be long (up to 45 seconds) with the load that can be held without perturbation in the muscle. Four to five repetitions interspersed with 2 minutes rest have proven effective in our clinical experience. This exercise can be repeated several times a day to provide the patient with pain relief as needed.

In those who have substantial pain and pathology, the seated heel raise exercise offers the opportunity to use loads that are below body weight; it is possible to find an isometric load that is suitable for even the most compromised tendon.

Stage 2—Isotonic strength endurance where appropriate

Progress the patient to this stage when Achilles tendon pain has settled and the patient is competent at isometrics and slowly building both (i) hold time (45 s, as above) and (ii) weights (adjusted based on what the patient can do and hold steady). Isotonic exercise (slow concentric and eccentric heel raises) with body weight or additional weights with a weight-based machine strengthens muscle and provides beneficial load to tendon. Aim to go from full plantar flexion to plantar grade (i.e. neutral). Only lower into dorsiflexion for athletes who need strength in this range.

> **PRACTICE PEARL**
>
> Remember: Isometrics can be done prior to isotonic loading as they may relieve cortical motor inhibition that will assist with strength gains.[75,76]

Ensure the patient reaches full range (maximal) plantar flexion without using trick movements such as supination. When is strength adequate for progress? High-functioning patients will be able to raise (using a single leg) up to 1.5 times their body weight as additional load; patients whose demand is lower can progress when they can raise (using a single leg) the equivalent of their own body weight as additional load. Be sure to train endurance with high-quality movement (no trick movements) before progressing to stage 3. There should be evidence of muscle bulk returning at this point. Stage 2 exercises must be maintained at least twice a week for the remainder of the person's active life.

If necessary, a strength endurance exercise can be added, where one set to fatigue of repeated heel raises is completed each night. A functional alternative is stair climbing with the foot maintained in sustained plantarflexion; that is, the heels do not touch the steps while climbing.

Stage 3—Energy storage exercises

Exercises in this stage place faster loads on the tendon and this causes the tendon to store energy and begin to act as a spring. In stages 3 and 4 (see below) the patient does not carry additional weight; body weight is sufficient and provides close to maximum load for the tendon. Any fast exercise, particularly if it includes eccentric loading, will induce energy storage, so exercises such as slow skipping-type activities and faster stair climbs are ideal. Stage 3 and 4 loads should be completed a maximum of three times a week. The remaining days can be used to continue strength work and cross-training.

Stage 4—Energy storage and release exercises

These exercises are a progression of stage 3, where the speed increases and the release of energy from the tendon occurs. Faster skipping, running drills and change of direction drills begin to prepare the athlete for return to training.

Return to training and competition—as after all injuries

This is an essential, and often neglected, element of successful tendon rehabilitation (see also Chapters 18 and 19). We distinguish this final element from the four-stage tendon rehabilitation so as not to dilute the tendon-specific elements of that program. Return-to-training or return-to-play exercises are constructed with the athlete's specific functional requirements in mind. Thus, there is no recipe because the demands of an elite track athlete and recreational runner are very different even within the one activity/sport (running). Transition to training is permitted when the person can complete stage 4 exercises repeatedly without an increase in symptoms the morning after the rehabilitation session.

PART B   Regional problems

How does exercise promote tissue repair in tendinopathy?

Exercise therapy can affect any tissue at the cellular level through the process of mechanotherapy,[65] and this is detailed in Chapter 17.

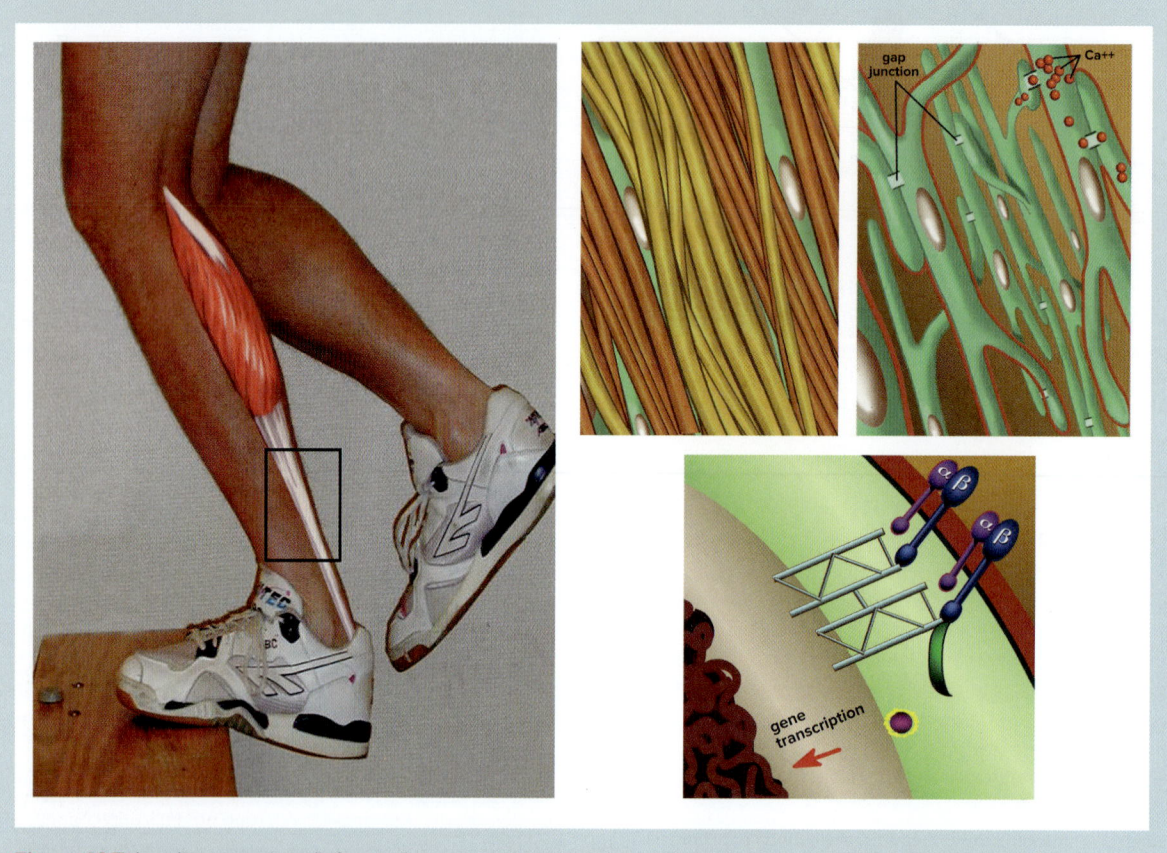

Figure 40.7 Loading exercises (left panel), cause sliding of collagen fibres (illustration of the microscopic view, top centre panel) leading to intercellular[65] communication via gap junctions (top right panel), and intracellular communication with the cell nucleus (lower right panel).
REPRODUCED WITH PERMISSION OF BRITISH JOURNAL OF SPORTS MEDICINE

Because the aberrant plantaris can be fixed to the Achilles tendon (Fig. 40.8), conservative management may not be successful. Sweden's Professor Håkan Alfredson was a pioneer in identifying this pathology in patients with painful Achilles tendons.[80] Surgery is performed under ultrasound and Doppler guidance. The symptomatic pathological region is approached using a medial incision and the adherent tendons are separated or the plantaris tendon is extirpated (divided and removed).[81]

Other interventions used in conjunction with staged progressive exercise therapy

We summarise interventions that have been used in conjunction with an exercise program (Table 40.6) and note two things. First, exercise is excellent for tendons and, second, added interventions add minimally to exercise therapy. It is important to apply the 'exercise is medicine' message from public health to tendons.

Pain in the Achilles region CHAPTER 40

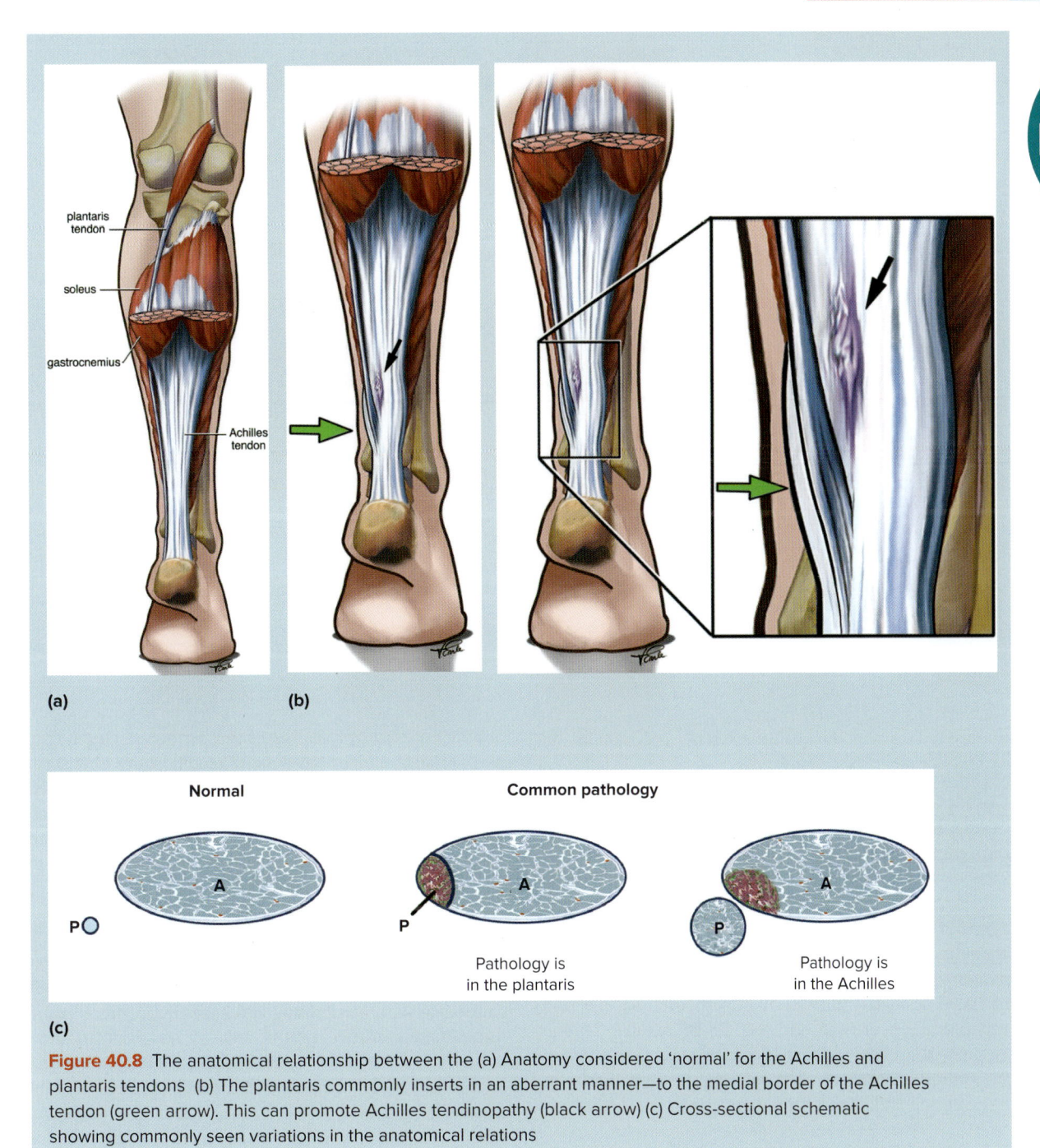

Figure 40.8 The anatomical relationship between the (a) Anatomy considered 'normal' for the Achilles and plantaris tendons (b) The plantaris commonly inserts in an aberrant manner—to the medial border of the Achilles tendon (green arrow). This can promote Achilles tendinopathy (black arrow) (c) Cross-sectional schematic showing commonly seen variations in the anatomical relations

It is unfortunate that among many patients and clinicians, exercise is incorrectly assumed to be less effective than traditional medical therapies such as medication or injection.

Injections

There are a range of substances that have been used both in and around the Achilles tendon. The basis for injection is variable, but should only be used when there is failure

881

PART B   Regional problems

(d)

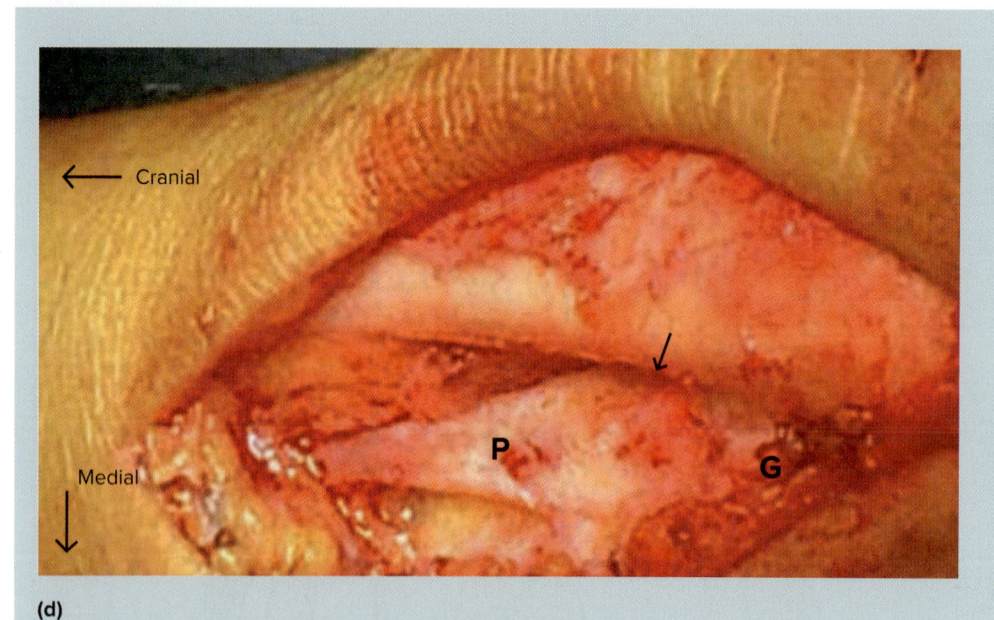

Figure 40.8 (cont.) (d) Plantaris tendon (P) adherent to the medial aspect of the Achilles tendon (arrow) with prominent richly vascularised fat tissue that (G) contains sympathetic and sensory nerves

to respond to a good quality exercise program for an extended time.

Corticosteroid injections
Corticosteroid injections are falling out of favour for long-term management of tendinopathy.[86] Corticosteroid has an immediate and short-term pain-relieving effect (for up to 8 weeks). The mechanism for cortisone potentially healing a tendon has not been clearly articulated and clinical trials of the medication consistently point to poorer long-term outcomes than 'wait and see' in various tendons. There has been no high-quality study of corticosteroid injection versus placebo or 'wait and see' at the Achilles tendon as there has been at the elbow. Longer-term outcomes at various anatomical sites are poorer than both no intervention and exercise interventions.[86]

Autologous blood and platelet-rich plasma (PRP)
With ROBERT-JAN DE VOS

Autologous blood and platelet-rich plasma (PRP) has become popular in recent years. They have been proposed to improve tendon healing because of the growth factors and cytokines present in blood.[97, 98] There are many protocols for the preparation and injection of the blood products and cells, making it harder to compare studies. A number of clinical trials have been performed on patients with chronic midportion Achilles tendinopathy. One small randomised study did not show benefit of PRP compared to eccentric exercise therapy.[99] One placebo-controlled randomised trial on the effectiveness of PRP combined with eccentric exercises did not show differences in clinical recovery or improvement of tendon structure.[19, 100]

Sclerosing
This treatment consists of injecting a vascular sclerosant (polidocanol, an aliphatic nonionised nitrogen-free substance with a sclerosing and anaesthetic effect) using ultrasound guidance in the area of neo-vascularisation anterior to the tendon. In a small double-blind, randomised controlled study comparing the effects of injections of a sclerosing and a non-sclerosing substance (lidocaine plus adrenaline), the sclerosing therapy had superior results to placebo.[83] In a 2-year clinical and ultrasound follow-up, good clinical results persisted and the tendon had decreased in thickness.[84] Whether the sclerosant decreases vascularity or pain is not known. Sympathetic and sensory nerves run alongside blood vessels.[101] Short-term follow-up of tendons that have had vessels sclerosed demonstrated an increase in both short- and medium-term vascularity.[102] This, in combination with

Pain in the Achilles region   CHAPTER 40

Table 40.6 Best available evidence for treatments of midportion Achilles tendinopathy

Intervention	Level of evidence	References
Mechanotherapy		
Eccentric exercise	1	66, 69, 82
Isotonic concentric/eccentric exercise	1	69, 73
Isometric exercise	5	76
Injections		
Sclerosing	2	83, 84
Platelet-rich plasma (PRP)	1	19
Corticosteroid	1	85, 86
High volume imaging guided (HVIG)	2	87
Cell injections	(Rabbit model)	88
Electrotherapy		
Shockwave therapy	1	89, 90
Laser	1	21, 91, 92
Surgery		
Ultrasound-guided scraping	2	93, 94
Open surgical revision	4	95

Blue = use supported by meta-analyses (systematic reviews) or randomised controlled trials
Orange = use supported by non-randomised studies and case series
Black = use supported by expert opinion or clinical guidelines
Red = current evidence does not support common clinical use

the anaesthetic properties of polidocanol, suggests that a change in vascularity is not necessary for a change in pain. Complications include a small risk of rupture and infection; they are very rare if small volumes of poliocanol are used.

High-volume imaging-guided (HVIG)
Despite the general lack of success of injection therapies for Achilles tendinopathy, optimists continue to trial various combinations of compounds in low-quality case series. One combination, called high-volume image-guided injection (HVIGI), includes normal saline, local anaesthetic and corticosteroid. Uncontrolled case series have reported decreases in patient pain over time and improvements in VISA-A scores.[87] A 2016 study acknowledged fatal (in the research sense of that word) confounding in study design; investigators were unable to draw conclusions from a retrospective series using high-volume injection.[103] As summarised in Table 40.6, current evidence does not support such treatments. One can always speculate as to possible mechanism of action for any physical agent (volume) or compound (pharmaceutical or naturopathic). See Chapter 2 for discussion of 'evidence' in contemporary medical practice.

Cell-based therapies
Therapies that inject cells (stem, fibroblasts) into the tendon are nascent but currently only supported in humans by case series.[104] It is critical to remember that tendon pathology is largely a pathology of hyper-cellularity, so the underlying premise for the use of additional cells is not obvious. Most biological processes need a careful interplay of elements (cells, hormones, cytokines). Because the ideal tendon milieu for healing has not been identified, it appears that a lot more research will be needed before clinicians can customise cell therapy (biologics) to match the healing stage of the underlying tendon. Inventors and investors stand to make large profits in the biotechnology arena. It is also important to be explicit that some healthcare systems provide financial incentives (fee for service) for clinicians to offer permitted, but unproven, treatments.

Medications

Nonsteroidal anti-inflammatory medications have failed to improve patient outcomes in tendinopathy. This is supported by individual randomised controlled trials (RCTs), one systematic review[105] and clinical impression. Leading SEM physicians do not prescribe NSAIDs for long-term treatment of tendinopathy in the routine clinical setting. They may consider these medication as an adjunct for short-term pain relief or if a player continues to compete with tendinopathy because of a short-term goal.

Professional sport is a different context and players often seek the analgesic effect of NSAIDs.[106] The ethical issues of using pain-relieving medication in sport are beyond the scope of this chapter.

Electrophysical agents

There is evidence that extracorporeal shock wave therapy (ESWT) is effective in treating lower limb tendinopathies including Achilles tendinopathy (AT).[89, 107–109] This mechanical treatment is described in Chapter 17. Studies have shown small benefits over and above eccentric exercise in treating midportion tendinopathy.[89] The mechanism of action of ESWT is unknown, but it may affect the nerves or provide a physical stimulus to tendon cells. The modality caused disorganisation of tendon collagen in Shetland ponies.[110] It damages renal tissue when used in humans for lithotripsy. Because it is a physical agent, collateral damage is inevitable. Whether this damage is clinically relevant in human tendons has not been studied.

One RCT found that laser therapy was an effective adjunct to eccentric exercise compared to a placebo.[91] Placing laser therapy in a clinical context is difficult as how it has an effect on tendon pathology and pain is unknown.

Surgical treatment

A systematic review of Achilles tendon surgery identified 23 studies with almost 1200 patients in total who underwent five different categories of types of surgery.[111] The main types of surgery, and those common in clinical practice, were open surgical debridement (11 studies) and minimally invasive procedures (7 studies). Patient satisfaction and complication rates were the main reported outcomes.

> **PRACTICE PEARL**
>
> It is difficult to draw conclusions about Achilles tendinopathy surgery because no study has yet (as of November 2016) compared surgical intervention with non-surgical or placebo intervention.

The minimally invasive procedures yielded lower complication rates with similar patient satisfaction in comparison with open procedures.[111] In clinical practice, it is clear that Achilles tendon surgery is not a quick fix for patients.

If a patient is not making progress with an exercise program, it would be reasonable to refer the patient to a fellow clinician who is expert in treating tendinopathy (e.g. specialist physiotherapist, sport and exercise physician, or other non-surgical specialist) rather than opting to refer to a surgeon who is not expert in treating tendinopathy. There are of course, expert sports surgeons who provide excellent advice (Chapter 1). The key is to find tendon-specific expertise from among the disciplines in our community.

INSERTIONAL ACHILLES TENDINOPATHY INCLUDING RETROCALCANEAL BURSITIS—THE 'ENTHESIS ORGAN'

There has been confusion regarding the terminology in this region (see box). To aid new clinicians, we first consider three separate diagnoses: (i) insertional Achilles tendinopathy, (ii) retrocalcaneal bursitis and (iii) Achilles (superficial calcaneal) bursitis. In clinical practice the first two commonly occur together because they have a shared aetiology–excessive tendon load in compression against the calcaneum.

The key concept is that at the Achilles insertion, the tendon, bursa and bone are intimately related so that in dorsiflexion (compression) they operate in partnership to *reduce* strain on the insertion itself[112]–the 'enthesis organ'[113] (Fig. 40.9). Excessive dorsiflexion, especially with high tensile loads, will predispose to mechanical irritation of the bursa and the tendon just proximal to the insertion.[114] In response to such irritation, the tendon adapts with increased fibrocartilage and, if the loads are excessive, tendon pathology. If the compression is sufficient and over an extended time period, the tendon may develop foci of ossification. This is how the body responds to high compressive loads.

Anatomy and the key role of compression

At the Achilles tendon insertion, the fibrocartilaginous walls of the retrocalcaneal bursa extend into the tendon (Fig. 40.9b) and the adjacent cartilage-covered calcaneum. Let us examine each element in turn. First, the calcaneum and the 'Haglund deformity'.

Historically, much has been made of the so-called Haglund deformity (see box below). However, this is normal anatomy, the way the greater trochanter serves as a cam for the gluteal tendons and the ischial tuberosity plays that role for hamstring tendons.[117, 118] Tendons insert at an angle into a hollow over a bony prominence to obtain mechanical advantage (i.e. a cam) and to protect the insertion from high loads. This is

Pain in the Achilles region   CHAPTER 40

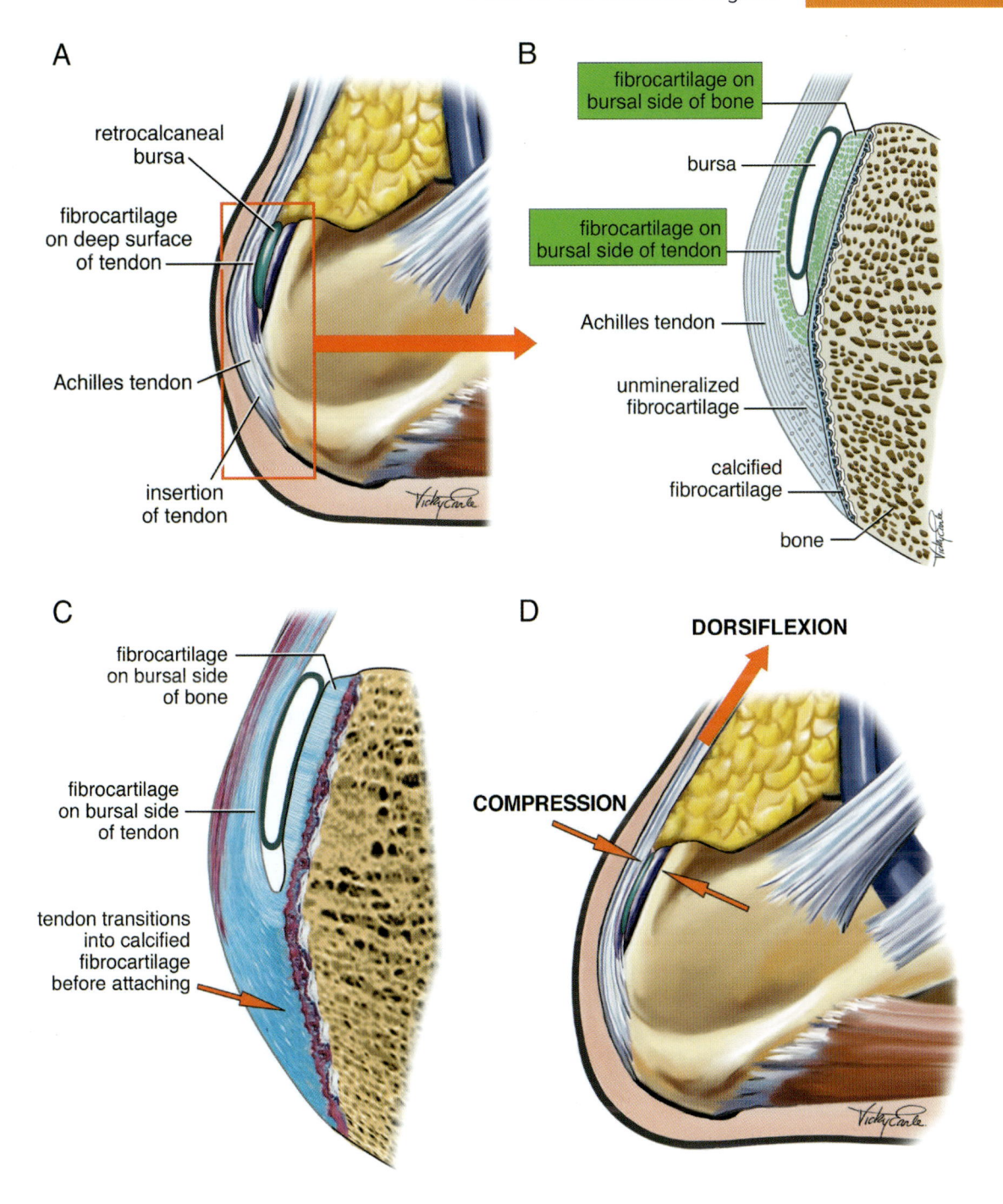

Figure 40.9 The critical role of compression in 'retrocalcaneal bursitis' (a) The anatomy represents an 'enthesis organ'. A prominent calcaneum greatly predisposes to mechanical irritation of the bursa and development of excess fibrocartilaginous tissue on both sides of the bursa (b). Note that fibrocartilage is normal at that site, but it can become thickened with excessive compression (c) Shows the microscopic appearance of the tendon insertion (red and blue, [from photomicrograph]) attaching to the artist's rendition of the calcaneum (d) This image highlights the effect of dorsiflexion—excessive compression. This underpins the treatment principle of limiting dorsiflexion (compression) with a substantial heel raise

885

PART B   Regional problems

> ### Haglund: time to take this eponym out of the books?
>
> There has always been considerable confusion about the terminology associated with pain in this region. Originally, Haglund described pain in the hindfoot caused by a prominent posterosuperior corner of the calcaneus in combination with wearing a rigid low-back shoe.[115] Since then, various terms have been used incorporating Haglund's name.
>
> 'Haglund-type calcaneus' or 'Haglund deformity' or 'Haglund's exostosis' is a descriptive label for a protuberance of the posterolateral calcaneum, where a calcaneal prominence can often be palpated. This is also known as 'pump bump', with alternative names such as calcaneus altus, high prow heels, knobbly heels, and cucumber heel. This deformity is frequently present in asymptomatic patients. There is a school of thought that considers it normal and thus better referred to as a Haglund *morphology*.
>
> Haglund's syndrome involves a painful swelling of an inflamed retrocalcaneal bursa, sometimes combined with insertional tendinopathy of the Achilles tendon. It must be distinguished from Haglund's disease, which is the term for osteochondrosis of the accessory navicular bone.
>
> It has been proposed[116] that terms such as Haglund's disease, Haglund's syndrome, Haglund's deformity, pump bump, calcaneus altus, high prow heels, knobbly heels and cucumber heel no longer be used.

the point where the tendon is compressed against the calcaneus in dorsiflexion; this load can induce pathology at this site.

Much of the pathology is seen at the upper calcaneal/bursa/tendon interface (the cam), where the compression of the tendon against the upper calcaneus occurs.

Clinical assessment

Good clinical practice includes evaluation of the tendon and tendon insertion by taking a careful history and performing functional tests in addition to inspecting and palpating the region for bony prominence and local swelling. Discriminating between pain with tensile, compressive and combined loads can help with diagnosis. For example, hopping on the toes (tensile loads) may give some pain, but a hop-lunge into dorsiflexion (compression and tensile loads) may be more painful at the insertion.

> **PRACTICE PEARL**
>
> A heel raise of 30–50 mm is a good practical way of reducing compressive loads.

Ultrasound and MRI can help to assess the extent of pathology in the tendon and the bursa. Ultrasound + Doppler (US + DP) examination can image the bursa and tendon insertion (thickening and localised high blood flow).

Symptoms of insertional Achilles tendinopathy, as with any enthesopathy, should raise suspicion about the possibility of rheumatoid arthritis or spondyloarthropathy, and this is particularly true if symptoms are bilateral.

Treatment

Treatment must consider the enthesis organ as a unit. Isolated treatment of a bursitis is generally unsuccessful. They key principle is to use a staged loading program with particular attention to avoiding dorsiflexion (to avoid compression of the tendon).[119]

Repeated stretching is not recommended as it provides compression load to the insertion.

Alternative treatments for chronic insertional tendinopathy include sclerosing of regions with high blood flow and nerves with polidocanol.[121]

Treatment of insertional tendinopathy with extracorporeal shock wave therapy (ESWT) showed more benefit than a low-quality exercise,[122] but the eccentric program used was designed for mid-Achilles tendinopathy, and better benefits from exercise are evident when using the specific insertional protocol.[119]

> **PRACTICE PEARL**
>
> Conservative management is usually successful, while surgery can require long-term rehabilitation. Our clinical experience includes elite middle-distance runners who were unable to return to their previous level of competition after surgery. Some case series report unflattering outcomes.[123]

Only a few case series have reported outcomes after surgery for insertional Achilles tendinopathy.[124-126]

Retrocalcaneal bursitis

The reader coming to this subheading 'cold' from the index will also need to read the section above. Retrocalcaneal bursitis is not generally an isolated condition in the sports medicine setting. Inflammation of the retrocalcaneal bursa (Fig. 40.9a) results in a painful soft tissue swelling, medial and lateral to the Achilles tendon at the level of the posterosuperior calcaneus.

> **PRACTICE PEARL**
>
> Histopathologically, the fibrocartilaginous bursal walls show degeneration and/or calcification, with hypertrophy of the synovial infoldings and accumulation of damaged fibrocartilaginous cells and fluid in the bursa itself.[127]

Rarely, but not to be missed, this condition may signal an underlying infectious bursitis due to an inflammatory arthropathy.[116]

To determine whether tendon or bursa is the primary pain generator, one of the clues suggesting retrocalcaneal bursitis is irritable pain and symptoms on low-load activities such as heel raises or end-range compression in dorsiflexion. A lot of fluid or thickening of the bursa on imaging (ultrasound or MRI) may be associated with the bursa being a pain generator. Conversely, a little fluid on imaging is normal in active populations.

For treatment of the combined 'enthesis organ'– the bursa and associated tendon–see the section above and note the need to avoid compression (see Fig. 40.9). Principles of quality tendon management apply (see the four-stage Achilles rehabilitation program above).

Injection of corticosteroid into the bursa, preferably under ultrasound guidance, can be effective in relieving symptoms[128] but is associated with an increased risk of Achilles tendon rupture.[129] This may be due to the presence of a connection between the retrocalcaneal bursa and the anterior fibres of the Achilles tendon.

If conservative treatment fails, then surgery to remove the bursa and any associated bony prominence is often advocated;[123, 130] Our reasons for making that an absolute last resort have been laid out.

Achilles (superficial calcaneal) bursitis

The Achilles or superficial calcaneal bursa (Fig. 40.1b) is located between a calcaneal prominence or the Achilles tendon and the skin, resulting in a visible, painful, solid swelling and discolouration of the skin. It is most often located at the posterolateral aspect of the calcaneus. Histopathologically, the subcutaneous bursa is an adventitious bursa, which is acquired after birth, and develops in response to friction. Unlike the retrocalcaneal bursa, which is lined by fibrocartilaginous cells, this bursa consists of hypertrophic synovial tissue and fluid. A superficial calcaneal bursitis can be further specified by its location; that is, posterior, posterolateral or posteromedial.

It is generally caused by excessive friction, such as by heel tabs, or wearing shoes that are too tight or too large. Various types of stiff boots (skating, cricket bowling, etc.) can cause such friction. Removing the source of the friction by using a punch to widen the heel of the boot, or providing 'donut' protection to the area of bursitis as it resolves is generally successful. As with many conditions, corticosteroid injection was considered a quick fix in the 1990s but is falling out of favour as a definitive treatment. The underlying cause of the pathology (the culprit) needs to be addressed.

POSTERIOR IMPINGEMENT SYNDROME

with SUSAN MAYES

Posterior impingement syndrome of the ankle refers to impingement of soft tissue or bony structures between the posterior aspect of the tibia and the superior aspect of the calcaneus in extremes of plantarflexion. Gradual onset of posterior pain may arise from impingement of an enlarged posterior tubercle of the talus (Fig. 40.10a) or an os trigonum (Fig. 40.10b), but is usually the result of impingement of the synovium or capsuloligamentous structures. This condition is common among ballet dancers, gymnasts, cricket bowlers and football players, all of whom maximally plantarflex their ankles in a loaded position. It is also seen secondary to ankle plantarflexion or inversion injuries. It can also arise from an acute presentation–when a forceful hyperplantarflexion fractures the posterior process of the talus (Chapter 41).

The diagnosis of posterior impingement syndrome is suggested by pain at the posterior aspect of the ankle and confirmed by a positive posterior impingement test– pain reproduced on passive plantarflexion of the ankle (Fig. 40.3f). Flexor hallucis longus (FHL) tenosynovitis commonly coexists with posterior impingement in dancers (Chapter 42). Pain with active first-toe flexion and extension in full ankle plantarflexion indicates FHL tenosynovitis (Fig. 40.3e). Another differential in ballet dancers is Achilles tendinopathy. The posterior impingement test is pain-free (negative) in that condition.

In ballet dancers, forcing turnout or 'fishing' the foot (Fig. 40.11) can predispose to this condition. Forced turnout occurs when the feet are planted in greater external rotation than is available at the hips–this places excessive rotary forces at the posterior ankle (and knee). 'Fishing' is a ballet term referring to foot deviation away from the ideal leg/foot alignment as shown in Figure 40.11.

Technique assessment, and strength and endurance training of the hip external rotators, calf complex and foot intrinsic muscles are an essential part of treatment. Treatment of posterior impingement syndrome includes modified workload, manual mobilisation of the subtalar, talocrural and midfoot joints as well as NSAIDs or paracetamol (acetaminophen) for symptomatic relief. Ballet dancers can cross-train via Pilates and gradually

PART B   Regional problems

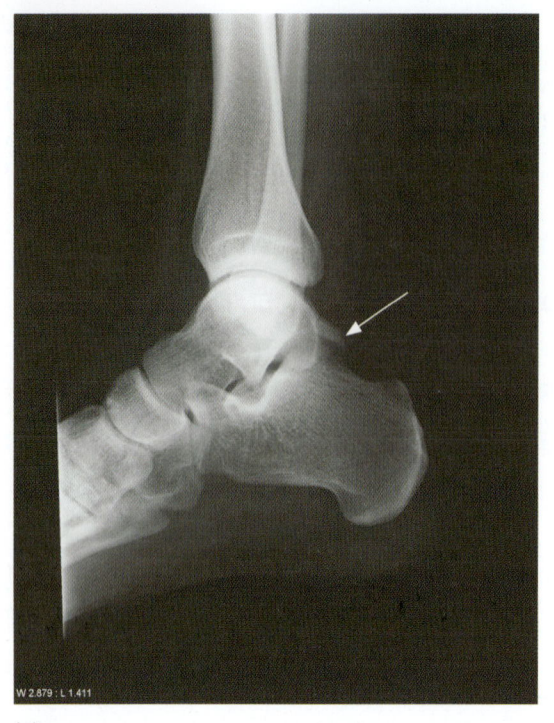

(a)

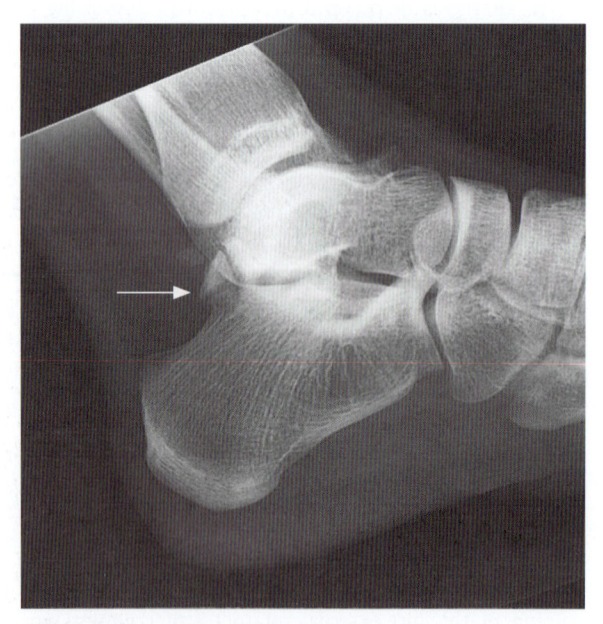

(b)

Figure 40.10 Anatomy that underpins posterior impingement when symptoms are present. These anatomical changes can be asymptomatic (a) A prominent posterior process of the talus (arrow) (b) The os trigonum (arrow)

progress their training from working flat (no raising) to *en pointe* during the treatment phase.

If the condition persists, a corticosteroid injection around the area of maximal tenderness may reduce pain. This is best done from the lateral side, as the medial aspect of the ankle contains the neurovascular bundle.

If posterior impingement does not respond to conservative management, then arthroscopic or open removal of the enlarged posterior process or the os trigonum is indicated. For dancers, the modal time it takes to return to full performance is around 4 months.

SEVER'S DISEASE

Sever's disease or calcaneal apophysitis is a common insertional enthesopathy among adolescents (Chapter 44). It can be considered the Achilles tendon equivalent of Osgood-Schlatter disease at the patellar tendon insertion. It should be treated by reducing load until pain is settled, (a heel raise is helpful) increasing strength and endurance, and then gradually reintroducing load.

OTHER CAUSES OF PAIN IN THE ACHILLES REGION (GRADUAL ONSET)
Accessory soleus

A rare cause of Achilles region pain in the sports medicine setting, an accessory soleus is present in about 5–10% of people.[131, 132] The condition is more common among men than women, and average age of presentation is 20 years. The true accessory soleus inserts into the calcaneum, but it may also insert into the distal part of the tendon. It generally occurs unilaterally, but it may occur bilaterally.[133]

The primary presenting patterns are pain in the Achilles region during exercise (a 'compartment' type pain) with swelling, or a painless swelling. There is an obvious muscle bulk very low, deep to the Achilles, on both the medial and lateral sides which is often tender on palpation. The main differential diagnosis is soft tissue tumour. Imaging findings are characteristic; plain radiographs have poor sensitivity for this condition but, when positive, show a soft tissue shadow posterior to the tibia obscuring the pre-Achilles fat pad. MRI is the investigation of choice[132] and confirms a mass with the same signal intensity as muscle; ultrasound can also confirm that there is a low-lying soleus (or accessory) soleus. In cases that are a symptomatic, observation is an appropriate treatment, but if symptoms warrant, surgical removal of the accessory soleus is probably the best treatment.[134] Botulinum toxin has been trialled in a case series.[123]

Referred pain

Referred pain to this region from the lumbar spine or associated neural structures is unusual, but always warrants consideration in challenging cases.

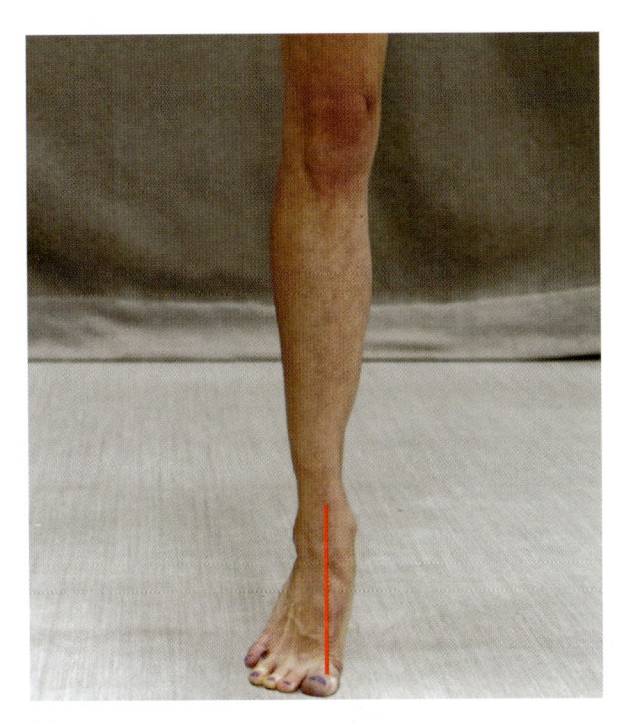

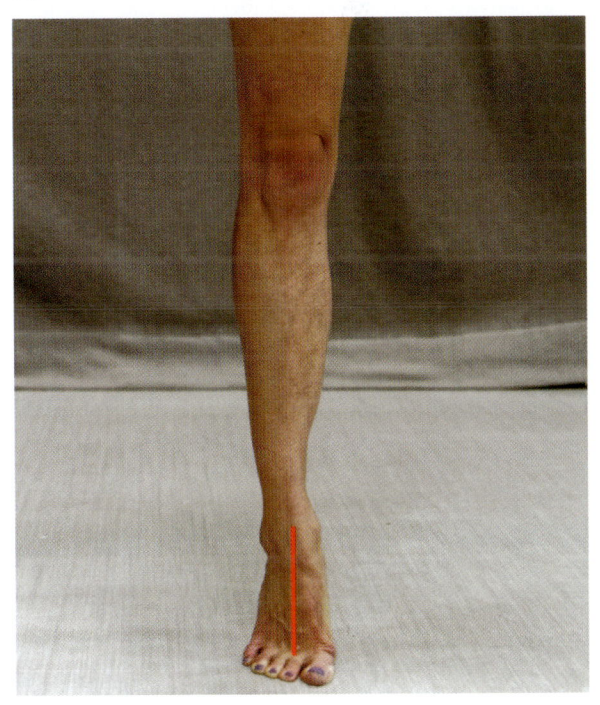

Pain in the Achilles region CHAPTER 40

ACUTE ACHILLES TENDON RUPTURE (COMPLETE)

Clinical approach
Complete rupture of the Achilles tendon (Fig. 40.12) classically occurs in athletes in their 30s or 40s, and the male:female ratio is 10:1. The typical patient is a 40-year-old sports-active male. The incidence is reported to be 5–36 in 100 000 and is increasing, especially over the last 10 years, with 60–90% of all Achilles tendon ruptures occurring during sports. The majority of the patients have not had any symptoms from the Achilles tendon region prior to injury. We address the debate around conservative versus surgical treatment of Achilles rupture below. Regardless of treatment, long-term deficits in strength and function are common and approximately only 30–40% of athletes return to their previous pre-injury level.[135]

History
Usually the rupture occurs when the person performs a quick change of direction and the ankle is forced into dorsiflexion while the calf muscle contracts. The patient describes feeling 'as if I was hit or kicked in the back of the leg'; pain might not always be the strongest sensation. This is immediately followed by grossly diminished function. A snap or tear may be audible and the patient has difficulty walking. However, the ability to resume walking with short steps returns quickly, but without power in the push-off phase.

The patient will usually have an obvious limp, but may have surprisingly good function through the use of compensatory muscles such as plantaris and the long toe flexors. That is, the patient may be able to walk, but not on

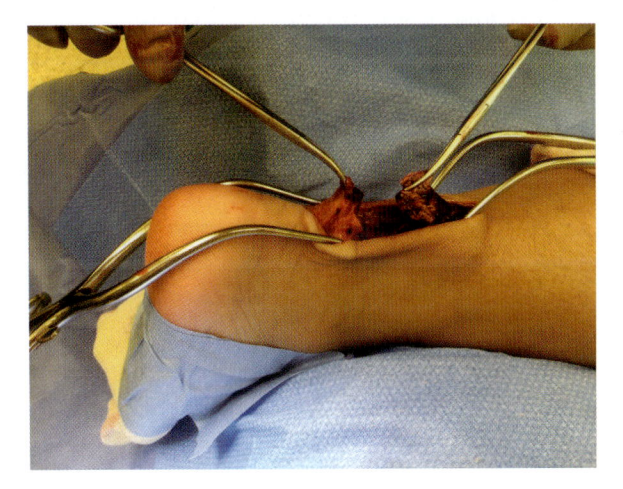

Figure 40.11 'Fishing' at the ankle can predispose to posterior impingement in a ballet dancer (a) 'Fished' position. The midline (second metatarsal) of the foot deviates laterally to the midline of the ankle (b) Correct demi-pointe position. The midline of the foot is aligned with the midline of the ankle

Figure 40.12 Achilles tendon rupture presents very differently from overuse Achilles tendinopathy. This intraoperative photograph highlights the severity of this injury. Not all cases need to be operated on (see below)

889

his or her toes. During the initial assessment, the clinician should take time to ask about risk factors for Achilles tendon rupture (including previous Achilles rupture, other major tendon rupture, recent local corticosteroid injection, or clues to other collagen diseases, diabetes mellitus type 2, etc.).[136]

Physical examination

Four clinical tests greatly simplify examination for complete Achilles tendon rupture (Fig. 40.3):

1. The calf squeeze test (also known as Simmond's or Thompson's test) (see Fig. 40.3h) has a sensitivity of 0.96, a specificity of 0.93, a positive likelihood ratio of 13.7 and a negative likelihood ratio of 0.04.[10]
2. Matle's test has a sensitivity of 0.88, a specificity of 0.85, a positive likelihood ratio of 6.3 and a negative likelihood ratio of 0.14.[10]
3. Copeland's test has a sensitivity of 0.78 (specificity and likelihood ratios are unreported).[10]
4. Palpation for a gap in the tendon has a sensitivity of 0.73, a specificity of 0.89, a positive likelihood ratio of 6.6 and a negative likelihood ratio of 0.3.[10] The gap in the tendons becomes increasingly difficult to palpate as time between rupture and clinical assessment increases.

Key outcome measures

The Achilles tendon total rupture score (ATRS) is a patient-reported outcome measure developed to evaluate outcome after an Achilles tendon rupture.[137, 138] ATRS evaluates aspects of symptoms and physical activity. The score consists of 10 questions, where the score for each item ranges from 0–10 on a Likert scale, with a maximum score of 100. It has been shown to have excellent reliability (ICC 0.98-0.99), an effect size of 0.87-2.21 and a minimal detectable change of 6.75 points. The score in patients varies from 17-100 depending on the stage of recovery (approximately a mean of 40/100 at 3 months, 70/100 at 6 months and 80-100/100 at 12 months).

A heel raise test to measure both calf-muscle endurance and the maximal heel raise height is commonly used to measure outcome in this population. For this test the person is asked to perform as many high single-leg heel raises at a standardised frequency (usually 30 reps/min) as possible to evaluate the endurance of the calf muscles. The maximal heel raise height is measured by evaluating how high the patient can lift the heel off the floor. This test has good reliability (ICC 0.78-0.84) and has been used to evaluate recovery over time in patients with Achilles tendon rupture.[137, 139-143] The side-to-side differences in maximal heel raise height, when comparing the injured and healthy sides in patients with an Achilles tendon rupture, correlated[141] with the occurrence of tendon elongation on the injured side.

Outcome measures that evaluate higher-level function, such as single-leg jump tests for distance or height, are used later in rehabilitation, and the performance on the injured side can be compared to the healthy side.

Investigations

Investigations such as ultrasonography and magnetic resonance imaging (MRI) are sometimes used as adjuncts to clinical investigation. However, such investigations are seldom necessary if the clinical history and clinical examination are thorough. Ultrasonography and MRI are needed only in doubtful cases, such as re-ruptures and when there is a long delay from the index injury. However, they are not needed in routine healthcare to establish the diagnosis of a torn Achilles tendon.

Rehabilitation of Achilles tendon ruptures

Historically, there was a fear of loading the Achilles tendon during the initial 6-8 weeks because of a putative risk of re-rupture and other complications. Systematic

---

Treatment of the acutely ruptured Achilles tendon: To operate or not to operate

Surgical management

With a 2–3% re-rupture rate, open surgical treatment of Achilles tendon rupture has approximately 10% lower risk of re-rupture compared with non-surgical treatment, which stands at just under 13%.[144] Promising new surgical techniques may further reduce the rate of postoperative re-rupture (see below). However, open operative treatment is associated with an increased risk of complications, including superficial wound infection, adhesions and disturbed skin sensitivity.[146] Another approach to reduce these surgical complications is to perform surgery percutaneously, but this does not entirely eliminate the risk of complications.

The postoperative treatment regimen has a significant effect on the outcome.[146] Comparisons of rigid cast immobilisation with a short period of rigid cast and then use of a functional brace after surgical intervention, indicates that early mobilisation decreases re-rupture rates without an increased risk of other complications. Furthermore, patient satisfaction is higher with the functional brace. Postoperative management is usually with an immobilising brace for the first 6–8 weeks; however, the period of postoperative immobilisation may very well be shortened and recent studies have used short or even no immobilisation after surgery. Because range of movement and strength can be difficult to regain after rupture repair, the earliest possible mobilisation and rehabilitation is recommended.

Surgery using stable core sutures and local augmentation has good results with no re-ruptures.[147] This technique is based on the principle of using the strongest possible suture material to make the surgical construct as strong as possible and enable the patient to start early range-of-motion training, even without any immobilisation at all. Early weight-bearing is encouraged as well.

Non-surgical management

Historically, non-surgical management of an Achilles tendon rupture has been recommended in older patients or patients with low levels of activity.[144] Early mobilisation for non-surgically treated patients also decreases the re-rupture rate compared with rigid cast immobilisation.[146] When both surgically and non-surgically treated patients received identical mobilisation protocols (cast for 2 weeks and then a functional brace), there was no difference in patient-reported outcome. Non-surgical treatment leads to a high success rate, provided no re-rupture occurs, and may therefore be considered a valid option for all patients (Fig. 40.13).

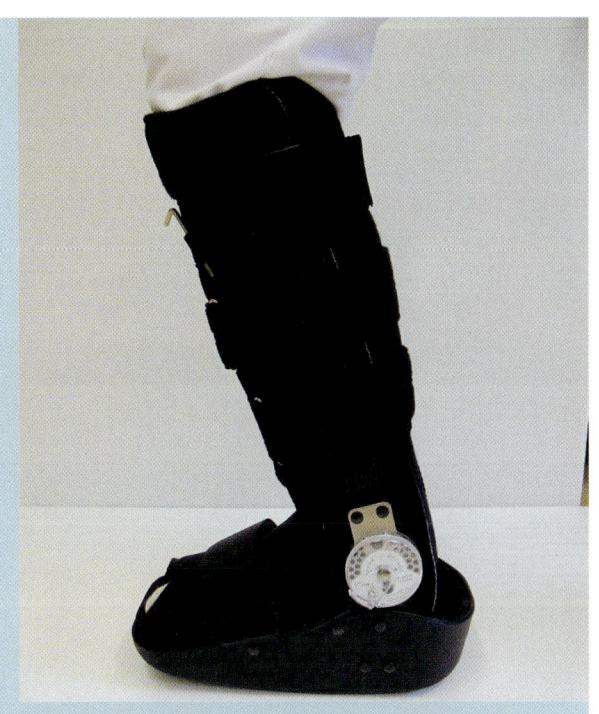

Figure 40.13 There is increasing evidence that non-surgical management with appropriate rehabilitation can be effective

reviews[146] report that simple and early mobilisation while in the functional brace improved outcomes. Thus, patients are often instructed to move the toes and perform light plantar flexion isometrics or active range of motion (if the brace allows for it). This advice applies whether the patient has undergone surgical repair of the tendon or is being managed non-surgically.

After the removal of the brace or cast, the goal for the patient is to regain calf-muscle strength and achieve normal gait while limiting the chance of re-rupture. It is usually at this stage that the formal rehabilitation starts. It is important to understand that the load on the Achilles tendon can be increased both by increasing the external load and by increasing the speed of movement. Therefore, during the initial 4 weeks of rehabilitation, slower and controlled movements are recommended. All the muscles around the ankle need to be strengthened and this can be progressed through the use of exercise tubing (Fig. 40.14a). Moreover, the calf muscle is strengthened by progressively increasing the load through sitting heel raises (Fig. 40.14b) and bilateral heel raises, and ultimately the patient should be able to perform a single-leg heel raise.

> **PRACTICE PEARL**
>
> Achieving full ankle range of motion (as compared with the healthy side) is important in all cases of Achilles rupture treatment. It should not be achieved by stretching the calf musculature in the first 3–4 weeks in the rehabilitation period. Such stretching can leave the Achilles tendon to heal in an elongated position.[147, 148] Instead, full ankle range of motion can be achieved through joint mobilisation and stretching into dorsiflexion with the knee in a flexed position.

Timing to return to jogging and sports

Whether or not treatment is surgical or non-surgical, the decision to return to jogging and sports is often time-based. Traditional recommendations are that jogging can be started after 12–16 weeks, return to non-contact sports after 16–20 weeks and contact sports after 20–24 weeks.

Time criteria may be inadequate, and it is essential that the key criteria for return to jogging and sports be functional, such as the recovery of the capacity of the tendon to store and release energy in sports-specific

PART B Regional problems

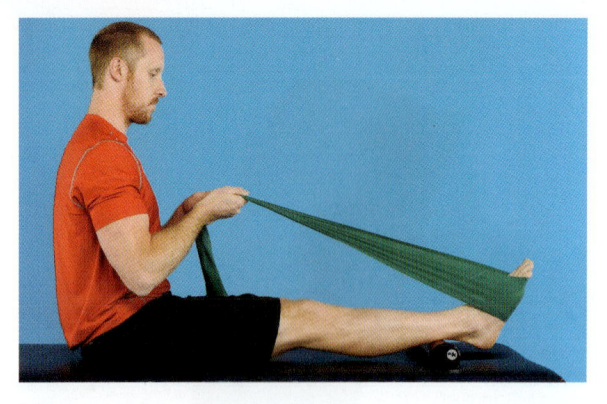

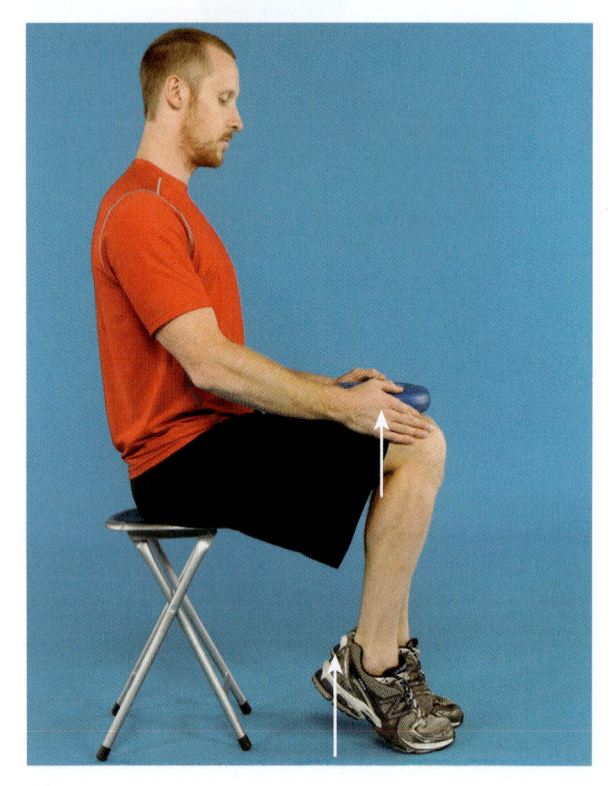

loading, as well as the patient having excellent calf-muscle strength and ankle range of motion. Muscle bulk may lag many months behind these functional criteria and should not be used to delay return to sport. The patient should be able to hop similarly to the unaffected side, and repeatedly store and release energy (repeated hopping) in the tendon adequately for their sport. Strength, measured with single-leg heel raises, should be at least 20, reps but can range from 6–70 reps in healthy individuals.[149]

Longer-term rehabilitation deficits

Regardless of whether initial treatment was surgical or non-surgical, complications such as calf-muscle weakness, tendon elongation and gait abnormalities can persist for at least a year after injury. Because of individual differences, rehabilitation should be tailored to each patient's deficits. Often the patient cannot raise the heel as high on the injured side as the uninjured side. The clinician should test whether this is due to tendon elongation, weakness or both. This does not appear to limit return to physical activity in the majority of patients, and whether it has any long-term implications is not known.

About 50% of patients can perform a single-leg heel raise 3 months after their injury. Between 3 and 6 months after injury, the majority of patients can achieve this milestone. However, it is common to have a strength deficit of 10–30% in the calf musculature on the injured side compared with the healthy side, and this commonly becomes permanent.

Thus, it is important to encourage the patient to persist with a comprehensive functional rehabilitation program and ideally return to full activity. The clinician needs to be alert to identifying any specific barriers to this successful return to activity. The early phase of rehabilitation in particular should be closely monitored. Studies have shown very limited improvement between 1 and 2-year follow-ups.

Additional studies are needed to garner better evidence about the appropriate and most beneficial type of exercises both in the initial immobilisation period (if any) and during rehabilitation. The issue of tendon lengthening after treatment, especially non-surgical treatment, leading to insufficient power in the calf muscles is still not well studied.

Figure 40.14 Calf muscle strengthening after Achilles tendon rupture (a) Early rehabilitation includes low-load ankle plantarflexion with knee extended (e.g. with Thera Band™) (b) Seated heel raise against resistance loads the soleus preferentially

REFERENCES

References for this chapter can be found at www.mhhe.com/au/CSM5e

Chapter 41

Acute ankle injuries

with PIETER D'HOOGHE, EVERT VERHAGEN and JON KARLSSON

Total rupture of left ATFL (ankle ligament) and associated joint capsule damage in a soccer kickabout with friends. Continuing to assess extent of injury and treatment plan day by day. Rehab already started.
World golf number 1 Rory McIlroy on Instagram, nine days before the British Open, 6 July 2015

Ankle injury is arguably the most common sporting injury. In 24 of the 70 sports for which there are quality data, ankle injury holds the number 1 spot.[1] In sports such as volleyball, ankle injuries account for nearly half of all injuries.[2]

Ankle injuries include, but are not limited to 'ankle sprains'. The first half of this chapter focuses on anatomy, clinical assessment and management of lateral ligament injuries after ankle sprain and their sequelae. We address less common immediate diagnoses for ankle sprains: medial ligament injury and significant ankle fractures.

Importantly for clinicians who work in sport, a 'sprained ankle' can mask damage to other structures, such as subtle fractures around the ankle joint, osteochondral fractures of the dome of the talus, and dislocation or longitudinal rupture of the peroneal tendons. Such injuries and their complaints persist longer than would be expected with a straightforward lateral ligament sprain. This is often referred to as 'the difficult ankle' and it is the focus of the second half of this chapter.

FUNCTIONAL ANATOMY

The ankle contains three joints (Fig. 41.1):

1. talocrural (ankle) joint
2. inferior tibiofibular joint (syndesmosis)
3. subtalar joint.

The talocrural or ankle joint (Fig. 41.1a) is a hinge joint formed between the inferior surface of the tibia and the superior surface of the talus.

The medial and lateral malleoli provide additional articulations and stability to the ankle joint. The ankle joint can plantarflex and dorsiflex. As the ankle is least stable in plantarflexion, where most stability is provided by the ligaments, injuries are more common when the foot is in this position.

The distal parts of the fibula and tibia articulate at the inferior tibiofibular joint where they are supported by the inferior tibiofibular ligaments or syndesmosis. The small amount of movement present at this joint is extremely important for normal walking and running. Injuries to this joint are more common than previously recognised.

The subtalar joint (Fig. 41.1b), between the talus and calcaneus, is divided into an anterior and posterior articulation separated by the sinus tarsi.

(a)

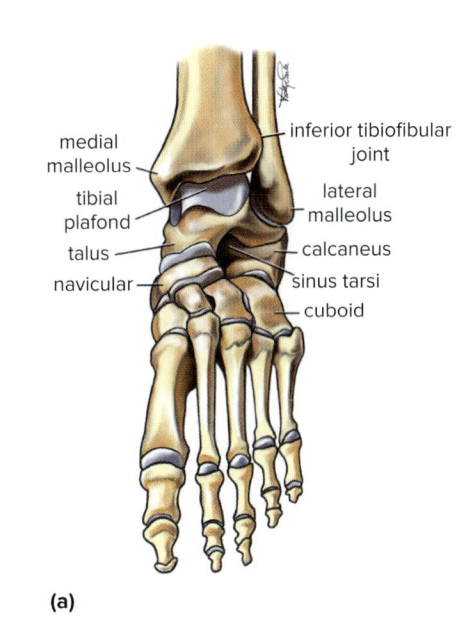

Figure 41.1 Anatomy of the ankle. (a) Talocrural (ankle) joint

PART B   Regional problems

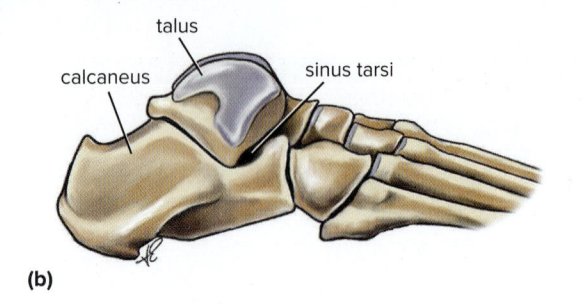

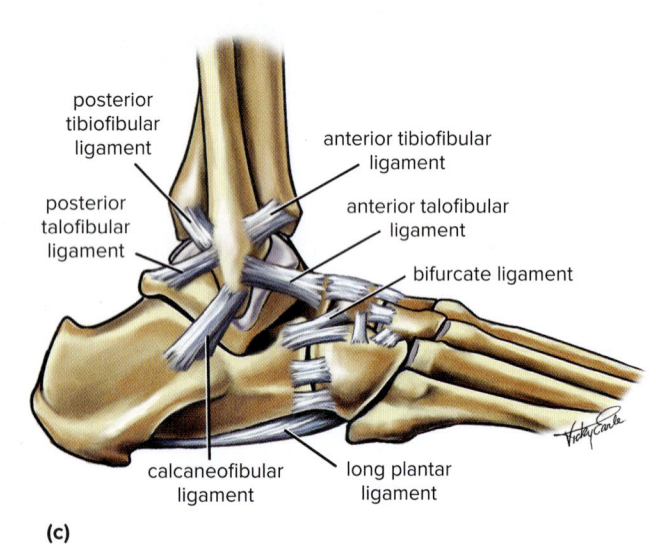

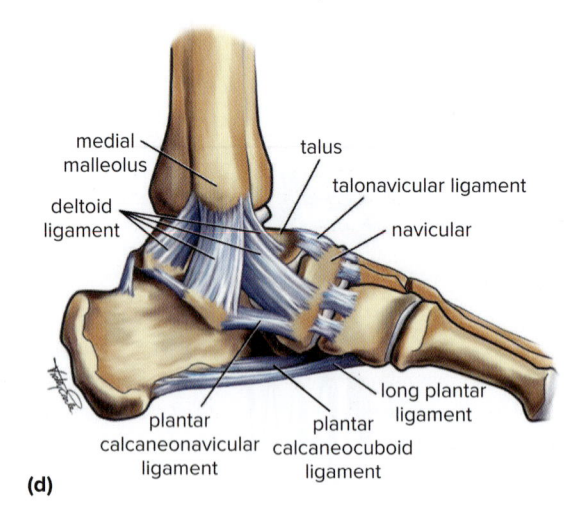

Figure 41.1 (cont.) (b) Subtalar joint (c) Ligaments of the ankle-lateral view (d) Ligaments of the ankle-medial view

Inversion and eversion occur at the subtalar joint. It provides shock absorption and permits the foot to adjust to uneven ground. The subtalar joint allows the foot to remain flat on the ground when the leg is at an angle to the surface.

The ligaments of the ankle joint are shown in Figures 41.1c and d.

The lateral ligament consists of three parts:

- anterior talofibular ligament (ATFL), which passes as a flat and rather thin band from the anterior aspect of the fibula anteriorly to the lateral talar neck
- calcaneofibular ligament (CFL), a cord-like structure directed inferiorly and posteriorly
- posterior talofibular ligament (PTFL), a short structure running posteriorly from the fibula to the talus.

The medial or deltoid ligament of the ankle is a fan-shaped ligament extending from the medial malleolus anteriorly to the navicular and talus, inferiorly to the calcaneus and posteriorly to the talus.

It can be differentiated into the anterior tibiotalar ligament (most commonly affected), tibiocalcaneal ligament, posterior tibiotalar ligament and the tibionavicular ligament. This strong ligament is composed of two layers, one deep and the other more superficial.

The syndesmosis consists of the anterior and posterior inferior tibiofibular ligament (AITFL/PITFL) and the interosseous tibiofibular ligament (IOTFL). In almost 75% of cases, there are contact facets with articular cartilage between the distal tibia and fibula, forming a true synovial joint. The PITFL provides approximately 40% of the resistance to lateral displacement, the AITFL 35% and the IOTFL 22%. The remaining stability is provided by the interosseous membrane.

Relevant nerves for the ankle originate from the lower lumbar and higher sacral spinal roots (L4–S2). Efferent fibres of the deep peroneal nerve innervate the anterior muscles of the leg, the superficial peroneal nerve innervates the peroneal muscles on the lateral side, and the tibial nerve innervates the muscles on the posterior side of the leg. The afferent path consists of all nerves that send proprioceptive information from mechanoreceptors around the ankle to the central nervous system.

CLINICAL PERSPECTIVE

It is estimated that 10 ankle sprains occur per 1000 exposures.[1] Inversion injuries are at least four times more common than eversion injuries due to the relative instability of the lateral joint and weakness of the lateral ligaments compared with the medial ligament.[3] Around 80% of ankle sprains are ligamentous caused by sudden inversion or supination.[1] The injury motion often happens at the subtalar joint and tears the ATFL which is the weakest of the lateral ankle ligaments.

Acute ankle injuries   CHAPTER 41

Table 41.1 Acute ankle injuries

Common	Less common	Not to be missed
Lateral ligament sprain • ATFL • CFL • PTFL	Osteochondral lesion of the talus Ligament sprain/rupture • Medial ligament injury • AITFL injury Fractures • Lateral/medial/posterior malleolus (Pott's—bimalleolar) • Tibial plafond • Base of the fifth metatarsal • Anterior process of the calcaneus • Lateral process of the talus • Posterior process of the talus • Os trigonum Dislocated ankle (fracture/dislocation) Tendon rupture/dislocation • Tibialis posterior tendon • Peroneal tendons (longitudinal rupture)	Complex regional pain syndrome type 1 (post-injury) Greenstick fractures (children) Syndesmosis injury Tarsal coalition (may come to light as a result of an ankle sprain)

ATFL = anterior talofibular ligament; AITFL = anteroinferior tibiofibular ligament; CFL = calcaneofibular ligament; PTFL = posterior tibiofibular ligament

As the stronger medial ligament requires a greater force to be injured, these sprains almost always take longer to rehabilitate. The differential diagnoses that must be considered after an ankle injury are listed in Table 41.1. The aim of the initial clinical assessment is to rule out ankle fractures (see Ottawa ankle rules, below), and if possible, to diagnose the site of abnormality as accurately as possible.

History

> **PRACTICE PEARL**
>
> The mechanism of the ankle sprain is an important clue to diagnosis. An inversion injury suggests lateral ligament and medial compression damage. Eversion injury suggests medial ligament damage. If the injury involved ankle compression, the clinician should consider osteochondral injury.

The onset of pain is very important. A history of initial ability to weight-bear after an injury followed by a subsequent increase in pain and swelling with continued activity suggests a ligament injury rather than a fracture. The location of pain and swelling generally indicates which ligaments were injured. The most common site is over the anterolateral aspect of the ankle involving the ATFL, in approximately two-thirds of all injuries.

In inversion injuries the ATFL is the first ligament to tear, and is torn in 97% of cases. The CFL can then subsequently tear after the ATFL. Isolated rupture of the CFL occurs in only 3% of inversion injuries. The last ligament to tear is the PTFL, which is usually uninjured unless there is a frank dislocation of the ankle. In severe injuries, both medial and lateral ligaments may be damaged; however, this is infrequent. The degree of swelling and bruising is usually, but not always, an indication of the severity of injury.

The degree of disability, both immediately following the injury and subsequently, indicates the severity of the injury (Fig. 41.2). The practitioner should ask about initial management, the use of the POLICE regimen (Chapter 17) and the duration of restricted weight-bearing after the injury, as a poorly managed injury will appear 'more significant' in terms of swelling and long-term disability than a similar injury that has been managed appropriately. An example of severe swelling and bruising in an ankle managed without POLICE is shown in Figure 41.2.

The practitioner should ask about a previous history of ankle injury and assess whether the post-injury rehabilitation was adequate. Did the athlete use protective tape or braces for the first 3–6 months after the previous injury, or until the end of the season?

Examination

The aims of ankle examination are to:

- assess the degree of instability present (grade the ligamentous injury)
- detect functional deficits (i.e. loss of range of motion, reduced strength and reduced proprioception)

895

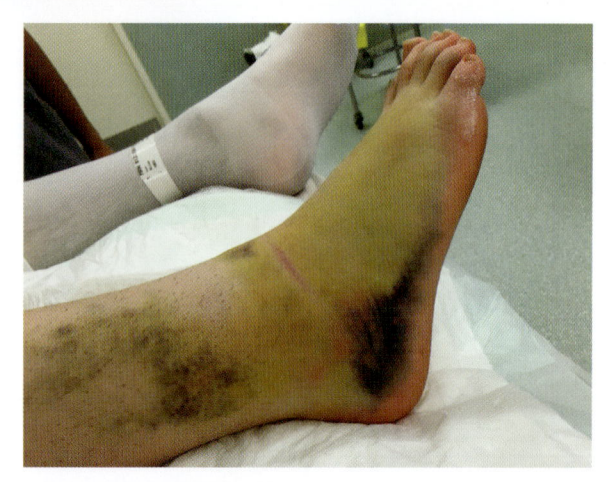

PART B   Regional problems

Figure 41.2 Severe swelling and bruising in an ankle

- detect any associated injuries (e.g. avulsion fracture of the base of the fifth metatarsal is commonly overlooked but is easily detected by palpation. Also, injury to the peroneal tendons may lead to longstanding disability and is easily missed during the acute phase.).

Examination involves:

1. Observation
    a. standing
    b. supine
2. Active movements
    a. plantarflexion/dorsiflexion (Fig. 41.3a)
    b. inversion/eversion
3. Passive movements
    a. plantarflexion/dorsiflexion
    b. inversion/eversion (Fig. 41.3b)
4. Resisted movements
    a. eversion (Fig. 41.3c)
5. Functional tests
    a. lunge test (Fig. 41.3d)
    b. hopping
6. Palpation
    a. distal–and proximal–fibula
    b. lateral malleolus
    c. lateral ligaments (Fig. 41.3e)

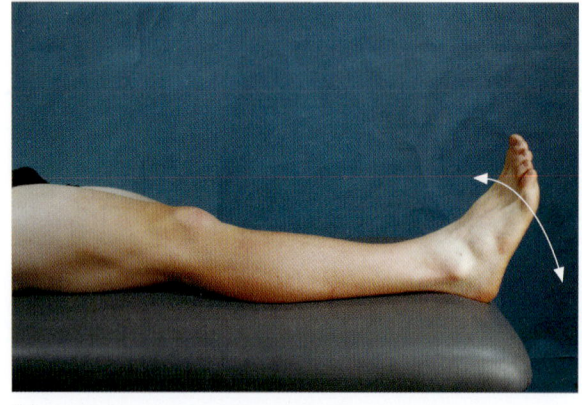

(a)

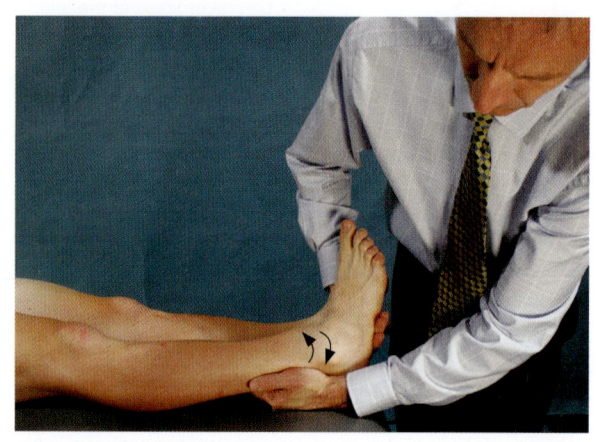

(b)

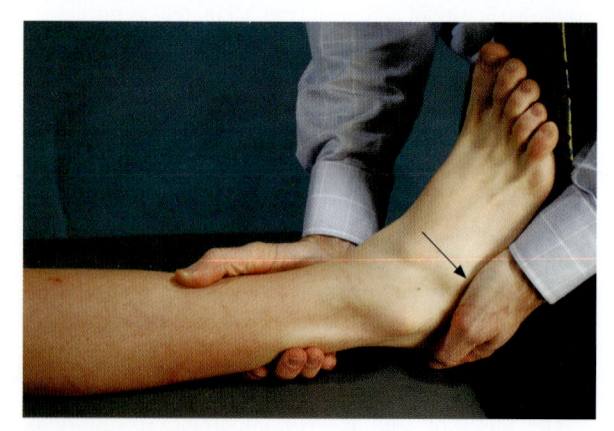

(c)

Figure 41.3 (a) Active movement—plantarflexion/dorsiflexion. Assessment of dorsiflexion is important as restriction results in a functional deficit. Range of motion can be compared with the uninjured side. Tight calf muscles may restrict dorsiflexion. This can be eliminated by placing the knee in 70–90° flexion

(b) Passive movement—inversion/eversion. Inversion is frequently painful and restricted in lateral ligament injury, while eversion is painful following injuries to the medial ligament. Increased pain on combined plantar flexion and inversion suggests ATFL injury (c) Resisted eversion—this can be difficult in the acute setting. In cases of persistent pain, weakness of the evertors (peroneal muscles) should be assessed

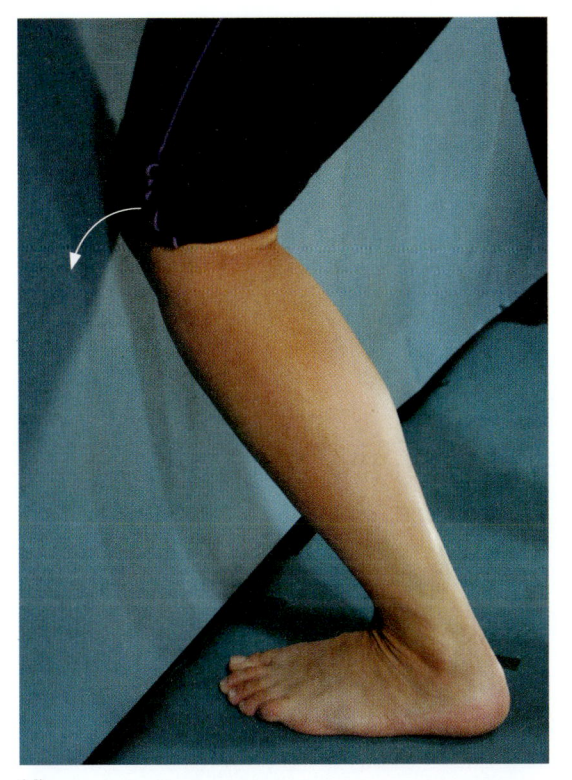

Acute ankle injuries CHAPTER 41

h. medial ligament
i. sustentaculum tali
j. sinus tarsi
k. anteroinferior tibiofibular ligament

7. Special tests (comparison with other side necessary; however, it should be borne in mind that there is no obvious correlation between increased anterior drawer and/or lateral talar tilt and symptoms of ankle insufficiency)
   a. anterior drawer (Fig. 41.3f)
   b. lateral talar tilt (increased inversion) (Fig.41.3g)
   c. proprioception (Fig. 41.3h).

Investigations

Should the clinician order a radiograph? Clinicians can use Ottawa ankle rules to assist them in making this decision (Fig. 41.4).[4,5]

Radiographs of the ankle joint should include the base of the fifth metatarsal to exclude avulsion fractures. If damage to the lower tibiofibular syndesmosis (AITFL) is suspected, special ankle mortise or syndesmosis views are required.

An osteochondral lesion of the talus–especially the medial side–may not be apparent on initial radiograph. If significant pain and disability persist despite appropriate

(d)

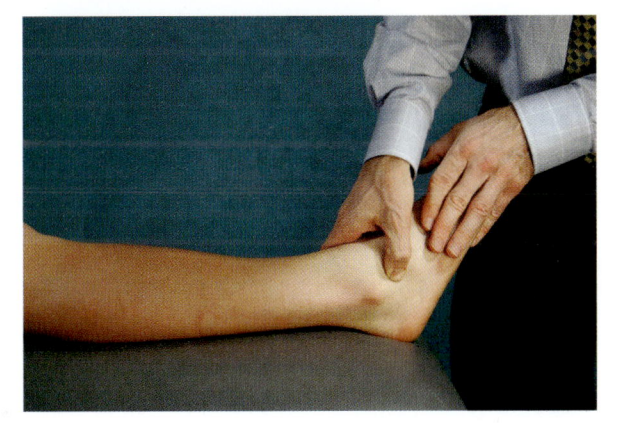

(e)

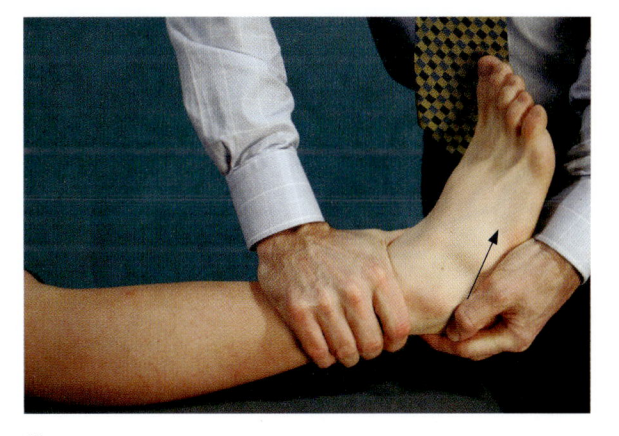

(f)

Figure 41.3 (cont.) (d) Functional test—lunge test. Assess ankle dorsiflexion compared with the uninjured side. Note any pain. Other functional tests may be performed to reproduce the patient's pain if appropriate (e.g. single-leg standing, hopping) (e) Palpation—lateral ligament

d. talus
e. peroneal tendon(s)
f. base of fifth metatarsal
g. anterior joint line

(f) Ligament testing—anterior drawer test. The ankle is placed in slight plantarflexion and grasped as shown. Pressure is exerted upwards and the degree of excursion (anterior drawer) is noted and compared with the uninjured side. This test assesses the integrity of the ATFL and CFL. Pain on testing should also be noted; if painful it may indeed mask injury to the ligament. Then the test should be repeated after five days. The optimal time to test the integrity of the lateral ligaments is on the fifth post-injury day

PART B   Regional problems

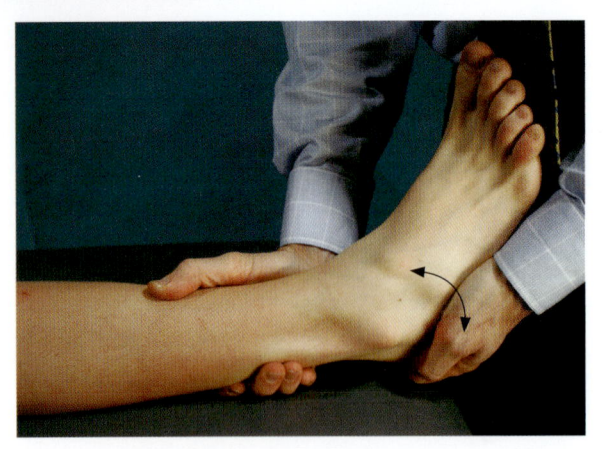

(g)

Figure 41.3 (cont.) (g) Ligament testing—talar tilt. This tests integrity of the anterior talofibular and calcaneofibular ligaments laterally and the deltoid ligament medially. The ankle is grasped as shown and the medial and lateral movement of the talus and calcaneus are assessed in relation to the tibia and fibula. Pain on this test must also be noted (h) Special test—proprioception. Single-leg standing with eyes closed may demonstrate impaired proprioception compared with the uninjured side

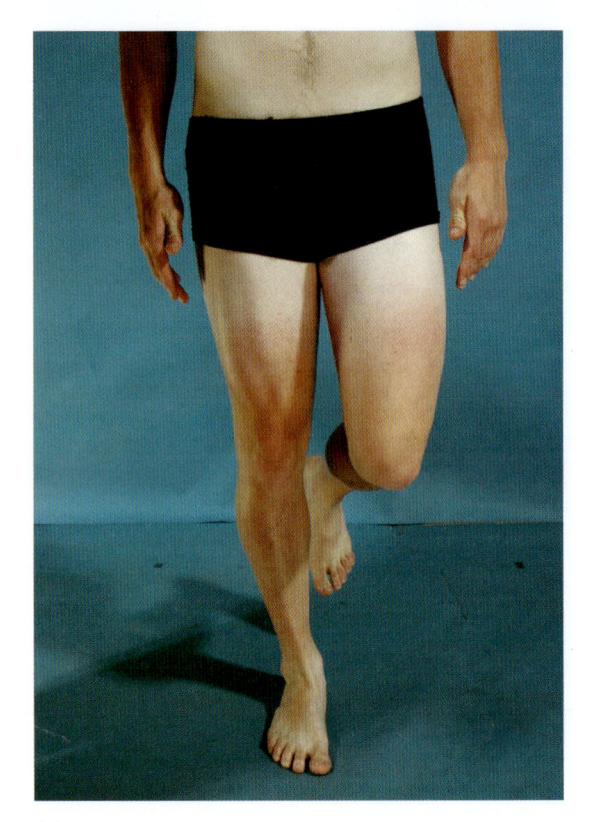

(h)

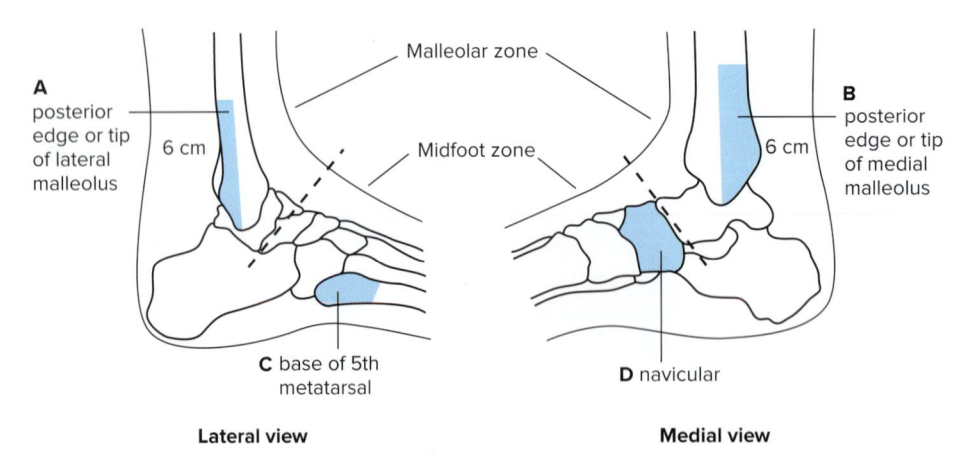

A posterior edge or tip of lateral malleolus   6 cm
Malleolar zone
Midfoot zone
B posterior edge or tip of medial malleolus   6 cm
C base of 5th metatarsal
D navicular

Lateral view   Medial view

Figure 41.4 Ottawa ankle rules X-ray recommendation[4]—Ankle X-rays are only required if there is any pain in the malleolar zone, and any one of these findings: bone tenderness at A; bone tenderness at B; inability to bear weight both immediately and at the clinical assessment (four steps). Foot X-ray recommendation—foot X-rays are only required if there is any pain in the midfoot zone, and any one of these findings: bone tenderness at C; bone tenderness at D; inability to bear weight both immediately and at the clinical assessment (four steps)

treatment 4–6 weeks after an apparent 'routine' ankle sprain, MRI is the investigation of choice to exclude an osteochondral lesion, especially when dealing with the 'difficult ankle', that is, longstanding pain/disability without obvious cause or pathology. If MRI is not available a radioisotopic bone scan or CT can be used.

898

Acute ankle injuries CHAPTER 41

LATERAL LIGAMENT INJURIES

Lateral ligament injuries often occur during activities requiring rapid changes in direction, especially if these take place on uneven surfaces (e.g. grass fields). They also occur when a player, having jumped, lands on another competitor's foot. They are very common in basketball, volleyball, netball and most football codes.

The usual mechanism of lateral ligament injury is inversion and plantarflexion, and this damages the ATFL before the CFL.[6] This occurs because the ATFL is taut in plantarflexion and the CFL is relatively loose (Fig. 41.5).

Also, the ATFL can only tolerate half the strain of the CFL before tearing. A complete tear of the ATFL, CFL and PTFL is rare and results in a dislocation of the ankle joint (Fig. 41.6). Isolated ligament ruptures of the CFL and especially the PTFL are also rare.

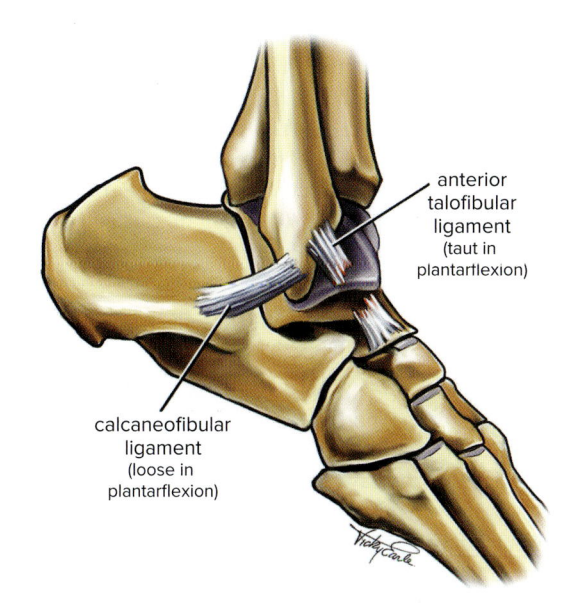

Figure 41.5 A plantarflexion injury generally leads to injury of the anterior talofibular ligament before the calcaneofibular ligament

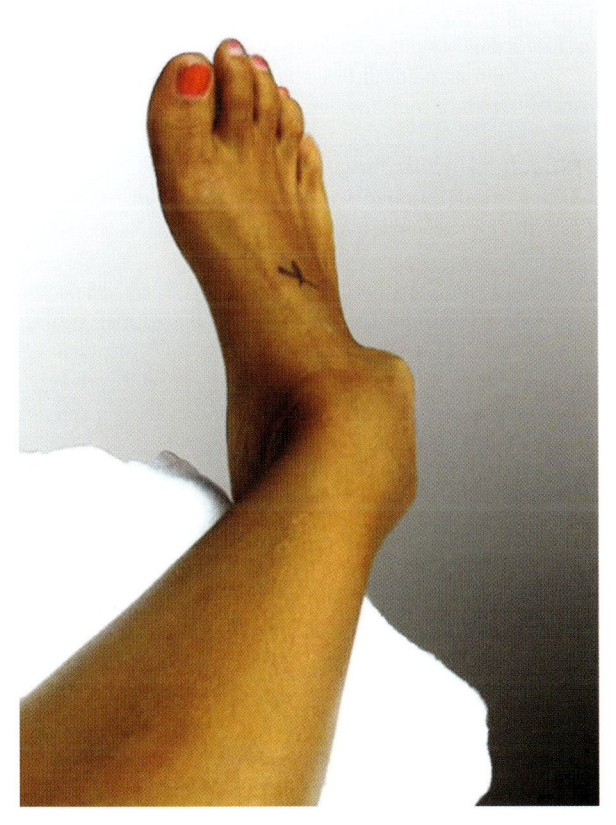

Figure 41.6 A posteromedial ankle dislocation

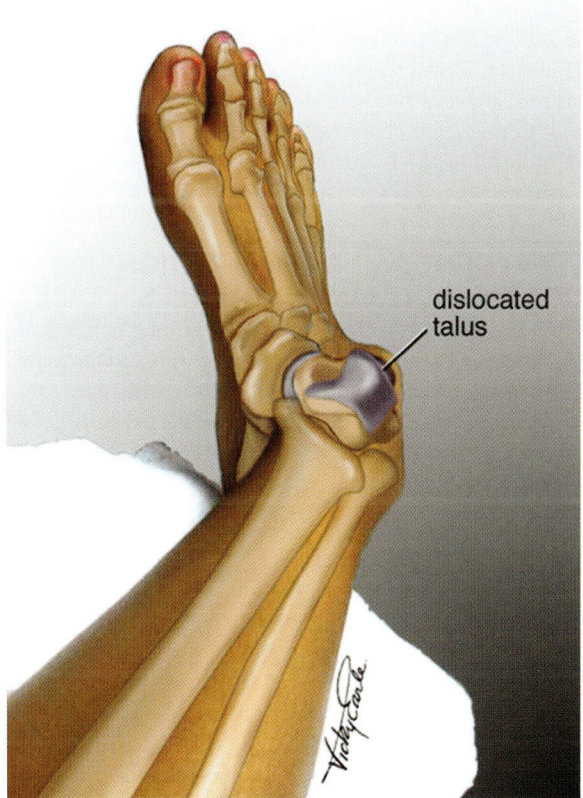

Ankle sprain may be accompanied by an audible snap, crack or tear, which, although often of great concern to the athlete and onlookers, has no particular diagnostic significance. This is unlike the case in knee ligament injuries where a 'pop' has profound implications (see Chapter 35). Depending on the severity of the injury, the athlete may continue to play or may have to stop immediately. Swelling usually appears rapidly, although occasionally it may be delayed some hours.

To assess lateral ligament injuries, examine all three components of the ligament and determine the degree of ankle laxity:

- A grade I tear has normal ligament laxity. It is important to compare both sides (assuming the other side has not been previously injured) as there is a large inter-individual variation in normal ankle laxity.
- A grade II tear reveals some degree of laxity but with a firm end point.
- A grade III tear shows gross laxity without a discernible end point.

All three grades are associated with pain and tenderness, although grade III tears may be least painful after the initial episode has settled. Grading of these injuries guides prognosis and helps determine the rate of rehabilitation. Grading also affects selection of the acute treatment. Note that in the acute phase, the reliability and validity of manual stress tests (e.g. anterior drawer or talar-tilt test) are very low. Manual stress tests are more reliable and valid when performed 5-7 days post injury. But keep in mind the limitations of 'special tests' in general (Chapter 14).[7]

TREATMENT AND REHABILITATION OF LATERAL LIGAMENT INJURIES

The management of lateral ligament injuries regardless of the grade follows the same principles. After minimising initial haemorrhage and reducing pain, the aims are to restore range of motion, muscle strength and proprioception, and then prescribe a progressive, sport-specific exercise program.

Initial management

Lateral ligament injuries require POLICE treatment where the letters ICE represent ice, compression and elevation (Chapter 17). This limits the haemorrhage and subsequent oedema that can cause an irritating synovial reaction and restrict joint range of motion for a long period of time. The injured athlete should avoid things that promote blood flow and swelling, such as hot showers, heat rubs or excessive weight-bearing. Gradually increased weight-bearing will, however, help reduce the swelling and increase the ankle motion, and enhances recovery.

Reduction of pain and swelling

Analgesics and/or NSAIDs may be required. After 48 hours, gentle soft tissue therapy and mobilisation may reduce pain. By reducing pain and swelling, muscle inhibition around the joint is minimised, permitting the patient to begin range of motion exercises.

The indications for the use of NSAIDs in ankle injuries are unclear. Many clinicians prescribe these drugs after lateral ligament sprains although their efficacy has not been proven (Chapter 17). The rationale for commencing NSAIDs 2-3 days after injury is to reduce the risk of joint synovitis with early return to weight-bearing.

Restoration of full range of motion

If necessary, the patient may be non weight-bearing on crutches for the first 24 hours, but then should commence partial weight-bearing in normal heel-toe gait. This can be achieved while still using crutches or, in less severe cases, by protecting the damaged joint with strapping or bracing.[8] Thus, partial and, ultimately, full weight-bearing can take place without aggravating the injury. Lunge stretches, and accessory and physiological mobilisation of the ankle (Fig. 41.7a), subtalar (Fig. 41.7b) and midtarsal joints should begin early in rehabilitation.

As soon as pain allows, the clinician should prescribe active range of motion exercises (e.g. stationary cycling).

Muscle conditioning

Active strengthening exercises, including plantarflexion, dorsiflexion, inversion and eversion (Fig. 41.8), should begin as soon as pain allows.

The exercises should be progressed by increasing resistance (a common method is to use rubber tubing). Strengthening eversion with the ankle fully plantarflexed is particularly important in the prevention of future lateral ligament injuries. Weight-bearing exercises (e.g. shuttle [Fig. 41.9] and wobble-board exercises [Fig. 41.10a]) are encouraged as soon as pain permits, preferably the first or second day after injury.

Proprioception

Proprioception is invariably impaired after ankle ligament injuries. The assessment of proprioception is shown in Figure 41.3h. The patient should begin proprioceptive retraining (Chapter 18) early in rehabilitation and these exercises should gradually progress in difficulty. An example of a common progression is balancing on one leg, then using the wobble board (Fig. 41.10a) or mini-trampoline, and ultimately performing functional activities while balancing (Fig. 41.10b).

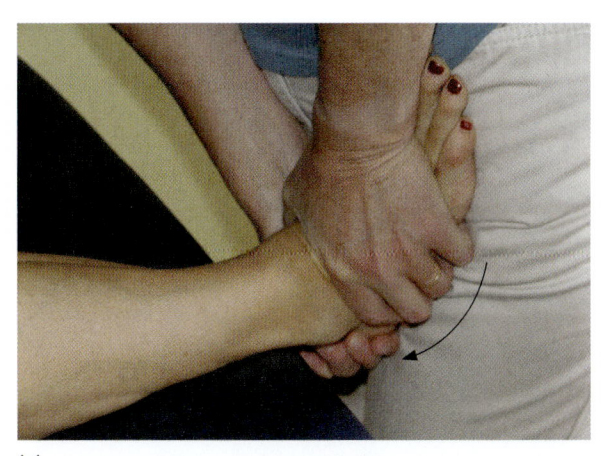

Acute ankle injuries CHAPTER 41

(a)

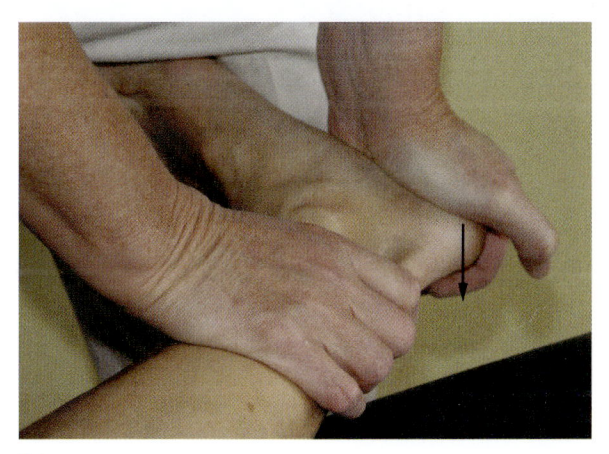

(b)

Figure 41.7 Mobilisation of the ankle joint (a) ankle dorsiflexion. The calcaneus and foot are grasped to passively dorsiflex the ankle (b) eversion mobilisation techniques to restore subtalar joint movement after ankle sprain

Functional exercises

Functional exercises (e.g. jumping, hopping, twisting, figure-of-eight running) can be commenced once an athlete is pain-free, has full range of motion, and adequate muscle strength and proprioception. Specific technical training can accelerate a player's return to sport and substantially reduce the risk of re-injury.[9, 10, 11] Remember that approximately 75% of those who sustain an ankle ligament injury have had a previous injury. In many cases this old injury was not fully rehabilitated.

> **PRACTICE PEARL**
>
> The high risk of recurrent injury means that all ankle ligament injuries should be fully rehabilitated.

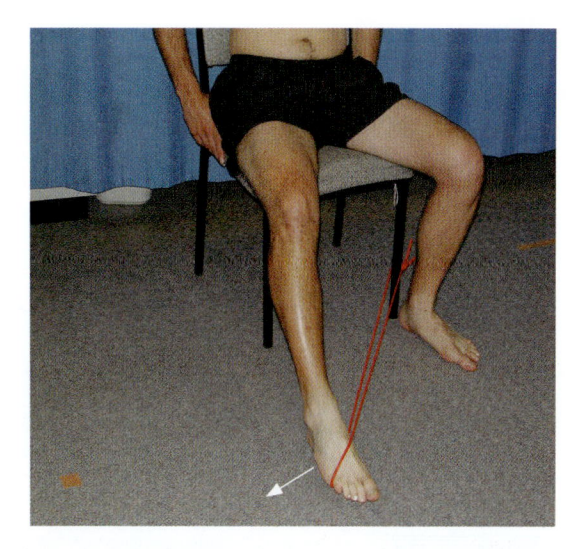

Figure 41.8 Strengthening exercises—eversion using a rubber tube as resistance

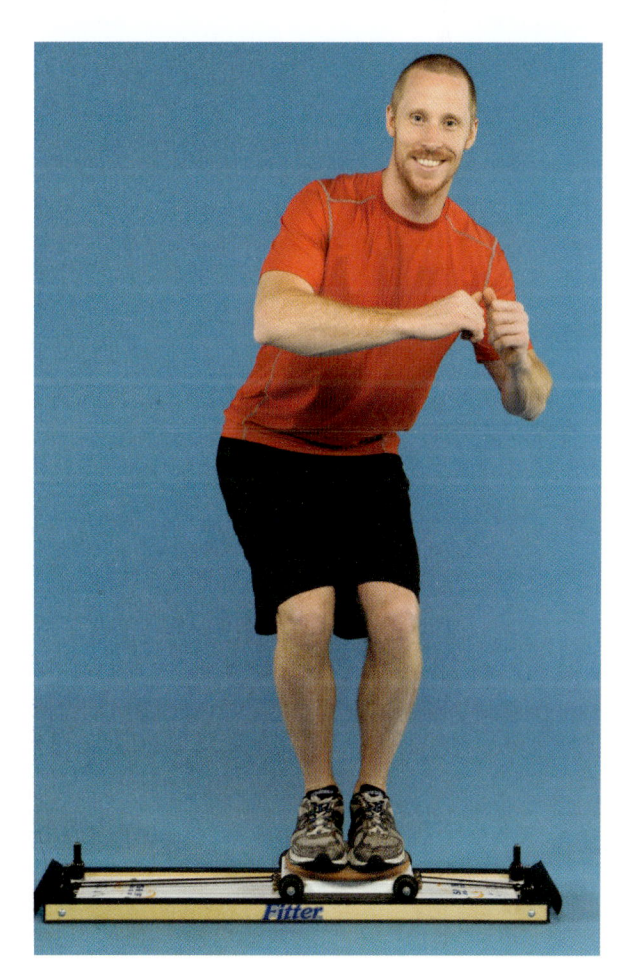

Figure 41.9 Strengthening exercises—weight-bearing shuttle exercises

901

PART B   Regional problems

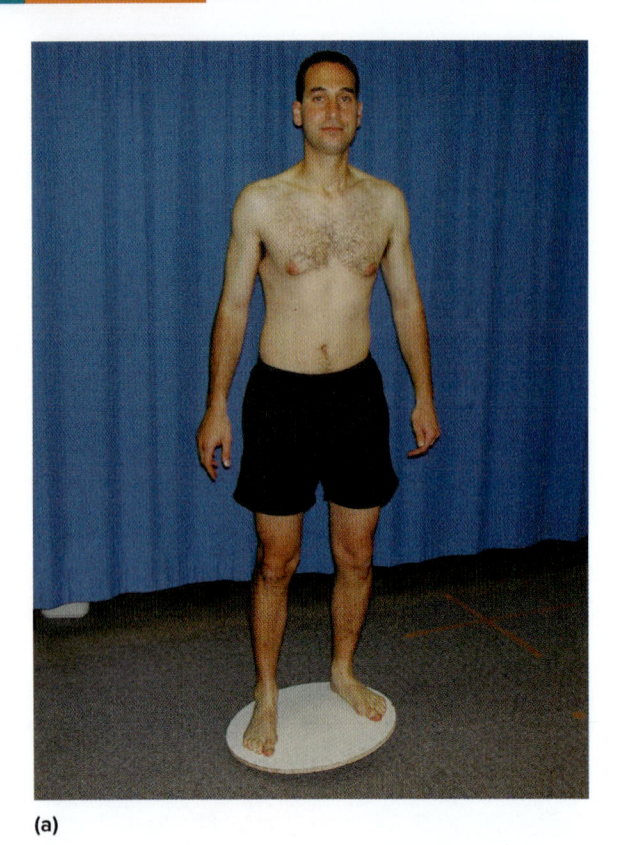

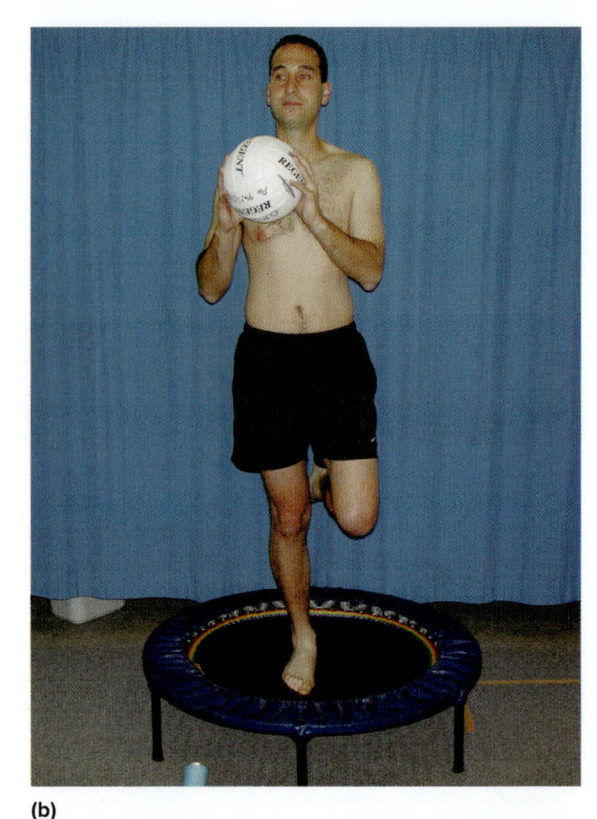

Figure 41.10 (a) Proprioceptive retraining following acute ankle injury using wobble board (b) Proprioceptive retraining following acute ankle injury using functional activity while balancing

Return to sport

Return to sport is advised when functional exercises can be performed without pain during or after activity. However, any athlete who has had a significant lateral ligament injury has an increased risk of injury recurrence post injury for a minimum of 6–12 months post-injury.[2, 12, 13] There are a number of methods to protect against these subsequent inversion injuries. Both external prophylactic measures (i.e. tape or brace), as well as neuromuscular training, seem equally effective in reducing the increased risk of ankle sprain recurrences after an index ankle sprain.[14, 15] They have seemingly different pathways through which they achieve this secondary preventive effect.

The relative advantages of taping and bracing have been discussed in Chapter 12. As both seem equally effective, the choice of taping or bracing depends on patient preference, cost, availability and expertise in applying tape.[16]

The three main methods of tape application are stirrups (Fig. 41.11a), heel lock (Fig. 41.11b) and the figure of six (Fig. 41.11c). Usually at least two of these methods are used together.

Braces have the advantage of ease of fitting and adjustment, lack of skin irritation and reduced cost compared with taping for a lengthy period. There are a number of different ankle braces available. Lace up and/or Velcro braces are the most common (Fig. 41.12).

External measures (e.g. braces/tape) act primarily by temporarily enhancing proprioception after an ankle sprain, rather than by restricting ankle range of motion.[17-20] This support is immediately available. Nonetheless, external measures only support the impaired ankle and do not rehabilitate the underlying impaired neuromuscular function. As such, their preventive effects are limited to the period when the athlete is wearing the external measure. This means that an athlete should brace or tape for the entire 6–12 month healing period during which risk is increased to fully benefit from any preventive effects.[21]

In contrast neuromuscular training targets the underlying impairment by re-establishing and strengthening the ligament, muscles and protective reflexes of the ankle.[22, 23] After completion of the training the athlete's increased recurrence risk is reduced and, in theory, no

Acute ankle injuries CHAPTER 41

(a)

(b)

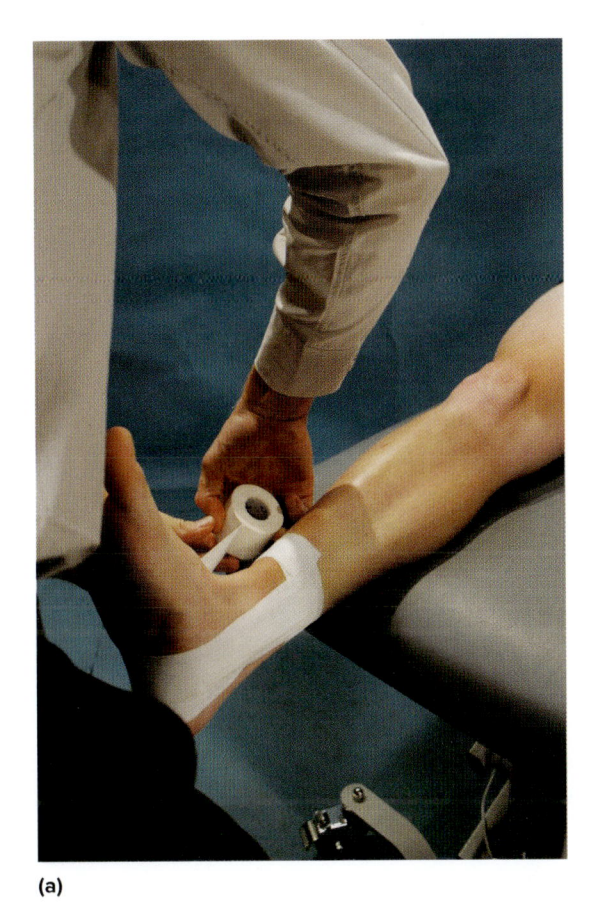

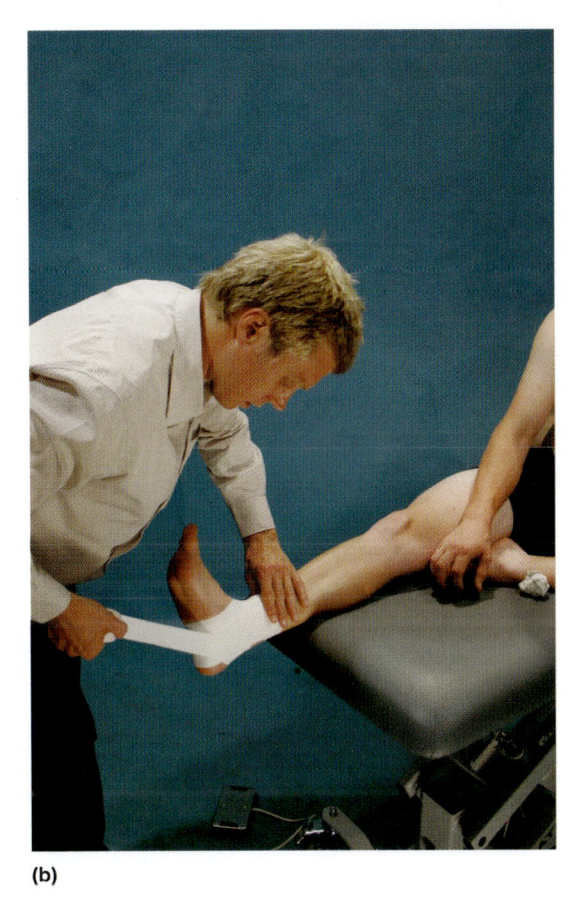

Figure 41.11 Application of ankle tape (a) stirrups. After preparation of the skin, anchors are applied circumferentially. The ankle should be in the neutral position. Stirrups are applied from medial to lateral, and repeated several times until functional stability is achieved (b) heel lock. To limit inversion, taping is commenced at the front of the ankle and then angled inferiorly across the medial longitudinal arch, then diagonally and posteriorly across the lateral aspect of the heel, and then continued medially over the back of the Achilles tendon to loop back anteriorly. Tape direction is thereafter reversed to restrict eversion

further preventive means are necessary. However, these exercises do not reduce injury risk immediately with the first training session.

> **PRACTICE PEARL**
>
> It takes 8–10 weeks for more intensive neuromuscular training programs to achieve an effect.[9, 24]

When external measures are employed during a period of intensive neuromuscular training after return to sport, the patient benefits from an immediate risk-reducing effect while targeting the underlying causes of an increased recurrence risk. This results in full reduction of the risk of a recurrent sprain within 10 weeks after return to sport.

Treatment of grade III injuries

Systematic reviews support non-surgical treatment of grade III ankle sprains.[25, 26] Functional recovery (as measured by return to work) was quicker in those treated with rehabilitation, subsequent rate of ankle sprains was no different between groups, and there was more ankle stiffness in those treated surgically.[26]

Finnish researchers compared surgical treatment (primary repair plus early controlled mobilisation) with early controlled mobilisation alone in a prospective study of 60 patients with grade III lateral ankle ligament injuries.[27] Of the patients treated with rehabilitation alone, 87% had excellent or good outcomes compared with 60% of patients treated surgically. Thus, early mobilisation alone provided a better outcome than surgery plus mobilisation in patients with complete tears of the lateral

PART B   Regional problems

(c)

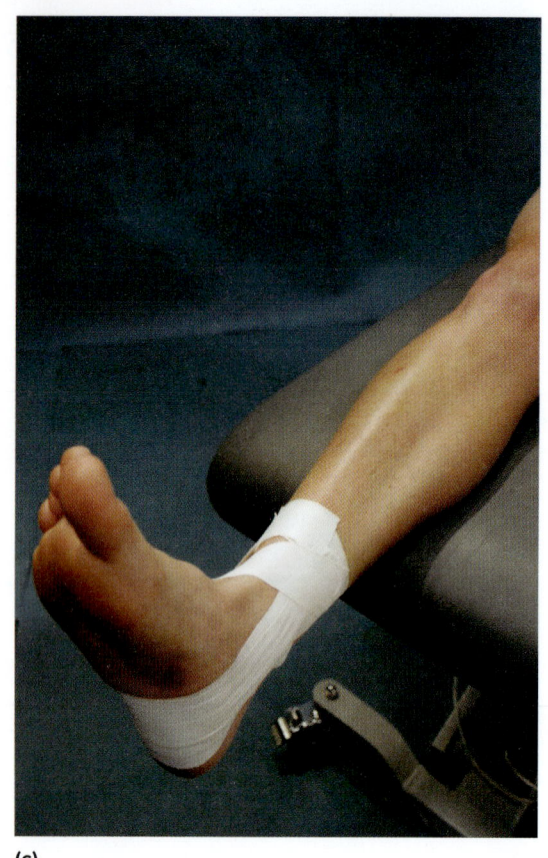

Figure 41.11 cont. Application of ankle tape (c) figure of six. This is applied over stirrups. Tape runs longitudinally along the medial ankle, under the heel and is pulled up to loop back around the medial ankle as shown

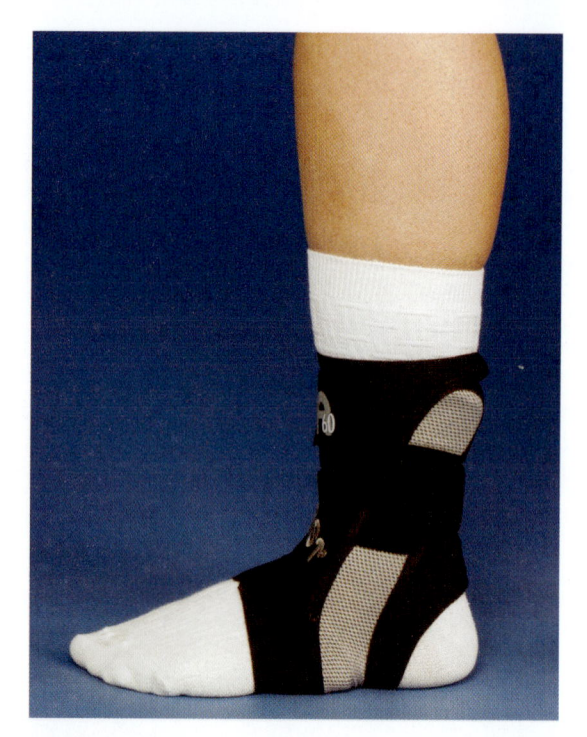

Figure 41.12 Ankle braces—a variety of braces are available

ankle ligaments. Dutch investigators have reported better long-term outcomes after surgery for lateral ligament rupture compared with rehabilitation, but this conclusion was controversial.[28] Differences in rehabilitation protocols may explain such contradictory study results.

> **PRACTICE PEARL**
>
> Thus, grade III ankle injuries warrant a trial of initial conservative management over at least a 6–12 week period, irrespective of the level of the athlete.

If, despite appropriate rehabilitation and protection, there is recurrent instability or persistent pain, then surgical reconstruction of the lateral ligament is indicated.

The preferred surgical method is anatomical reconstruction using the damaged ligaments; this method produces good functional results in several studies, with low risk of complications. The ligaments are shortened and reinserted to bone. If the ligament tissue is extremely damaged or even absent, other methods can be considered. Postoperatively, early range of motion training, such as using an air-cast stirrup, is recommended.

Following surgery, it is important for the patient to undertake a comprehensive rehabilitation program to restore full joint range of motion, strength and proprioception. The principles of rehabilitation outlined earlier are appropriate.

Anatomical reconstruction produces good clinical results in more than 90% of patients. There is, however, increased risk of inferior results in cases of very longstanding ligament insufficiency and generalised joint laxity.

LESS COMMON CAUSES

Medial (deltoid) ligament injuries

As the medial ligament is stronger than the lateral ligament, and probably because eversion is a less common mechanism of ankle sprain, medial ankle ligament injuries are less common than lateral ligament injuries.

The classical injury mechanism of a medial ligament lesion is forced eversion of the foot, such as a direct trauma to the lateral aspect of the foot and ankle. It is relatively uncommon that an inversion trauma causes combined lateral and deltoid ligament injuries.

Physical examination reveals swelling and pain on palpation of the medial ligament with signs of talar subluxation in complete lesions. Standard radiographs are frequently normal. The sensitivity of MRI to detect medial ligament lesions is high. However, there is a risk of over-diagnosing medial ligament lesions–which can be seen after a classical inversion trauma (with lateral ligaments injuries) in 60% of the cases, but this frequently does not match the clinical findings.

Medial ligament injuries may occur together with fractures (e.g. medial malleolus, talar dome, articular surfaces) and the treatment will depend on these associated injuries. Isolated medial ligament sprains should be treated in the same manner as lateral ligament sprains. In cases of gross laxity, elite athletes can be advised to consider a surgical option.

> **PRACTICE PEARL**
>
> After a medial ligament injury, return to activity takes about twice as long (or more) as would be predicted were the injury on the lateral side.

Significant ankle fractures

A fracture affecting one or more of the malleoli (lateral, medial, posterior) can be difficult to distinguish from a moderate-to-severe ligament sprain because both conditions result from similar mechanisms of injury and cause severe pain and inability to weight-bear. Careful and gentle palpation can generally localise the greatest site of tenderness to either the malleoli (fracture) or just distal to the ligament attachment (sprain). Radiographs should be ordered; the Ottawa ankle rules (Fig. 41.4) are useful to avoid missing fractures or performing unnecessary investigations in these cases.

Treatment of ankle fractures (sometimes called Pott's fractures) requires restoration of the anatomy of the superior surface of the talus and the ankle mortise (inferior margins of the tibia and fibula). If the anatomy has been disrupted with dislocation of the joint surface, internal fixation is almost always required. When using stable internal fixation, early range of motion training can be started early.

Isolated undisplaced spiral fractures of the lateral malleolus (without medial ligament instability) and posterior malleolar fractures involving less than 25% of the articular surface are usually stable. These fractures can be treated symptomatically with early mobilisation using crutches in the early stages for pain relief.

Lateral malleolar fractures associated with medial instability, undisplaced medial malleolar fractures or larger undisplaced posterior malleolar fractures are potentially unstable, but may be treated conservatively with six weeks of immobilisation using a walking boot (Fig. 41.13) that extends to include the metatarsal heads. In cases of undisplaced or minimally displaced fractures, the immobilisation time may be shortened considerably, using an ankle brace and early range of motion training.

Displaced medial malleolar, large posterior malleolar, bimalleolar or trimalleolar fractures, or any displaced fracture that involves the ankle mortise, require orthopaedic referral for open reduction and internal fixation. A comprehensive rehabilitation program should be undertaken following surgical fixation. The aims of the rehabilitation program are to restore full range of motion, strengthen the surrounding muscles and improve proprioception. Refer to guidelines provided earlier.

Lateral malleolar fracture with syndesmotic injury (Maisonneuve fracture)

This injury is more common in patients presenting to emergency departments than in the sports setting, but occasionally high-impact sports injuries can cause this variant of the syndesmosis sprain.

> **PRACTICE PEARL**
>
> The injury involves complete rupture of the medial ligament, the AITFL (see below) and interosseous membrane, along with a proximal fibular fracture.

Surprisingly, non weight-bearing X-rays may not demonstrate the fracture, and the unstable ankle can reduce spontaneously. Urgent referral to an orthopaedic surgeon is necessary.[29]

PERSISTENT PAIN AFTER ANKLE SPRAIN— 'THE DIFFICULT ANKLE'

Most cases of ankle ligament sprain resolve satisfactorily with treatment–pain and swelling settle and function improves. However, as ankle sprain is such a common condition, a substantial number of patients do not progress well and complain of pain, recurrent instability, swelling and impaired function 3-6 weeks after injury, or even longer. This is a common presentation in sports medicine practice and the key to successful management is accurate diagnosis. The ankle may continue to cause problems because of an undiagnosed fracture or other bony abnormality (Table 41.2). Alternatively, there may be ligament, tendon, synovial or neurological dysfunction (Table 41.3). Here we discuss a clinical approach to managing patients with the difficult ankle before detailing management of specific conditions.

PART B Regional problems

Table 41.2 Fractures and impingements that may cause the 'difficult ankle'—persistent ankle pain after ankle injury

Fractures	Bony impingements[a]
Anterior process calcaneus	Anterior impingement
Lateral process talus	Posterior impingement
Posterior process talus (also os trigonum fracture)	Anterolateral impingement
Osteochondral lesion	
Tibial plafond chondral lesion	
Fracture of base of fifth metatarsal	

(a) Although impingements are included here in the bony causes, pain commonly arises from soft tissue impingement between bony prominences.

Clinical approach to the difficult ankle

The clinician should take a detailed history: clarify whether pain or impairment started following an ankle sprain (the true 'difficult ankle') or if it is longstanding and arose without a history of injury (see Chapter 42). The patient who has had inadequate rehabilitation will usually complain of persistent pain, reduced range of motion and limitation of function with increasing activity. The clinician should determine whether the rehabilitation was adequate by asking the patient to demonstrate the exercises he or she performed in rehabilitation. Did therapy include range of motion exercises (particularly dorsiflexion), strengthening exercises (with the foot fully plantarflexed to engage the peroneal tendons/muscles) and proprioceptive retraining?[30]

Examination of the inadequately rehabilitated ankle reveals decreased range of motion in the ankle joint (especially dorsiflexion), weak peroneal muscles and impaired proprioception. These findings can be reversed with mobilisation of the ankle joint (Fig. 41.7a), muscle strengthening (Fig. 41.8) and training of proprioception (Fig. 41.10). Other abnormalities can also cause this constellation of examination findings—remember that the ankle may be inadequately rehabilitated because of the pain of an osteochondral lesion of the talus.

If rehabilitation has been appropriate and symptoms persist, it is necessary to consider the presence of other abnormalities. Was it a high-energy injury that may have caused a fracture? Symptoms of intra-articular abnormalities include clicking, locking and joint swelling. The clinician should palpate all the sites of potential fracture very carefully to exclude that condition. See also the section on Ottawa ankle rules (Fig. 41.4).

Soft tissue injuries that can cause persistent ankle pain after sprain include chronic ligament instability, complex regional pain syndrome type 1 and, rarely, tendon dislocation or subluxation, or even tendon rupture (partial or total). Inflammation of the sinus tarsi (sinus tarsi syndrome) can also cause persistent ankle pain, but this can also occur secondary to associated fractures. Thus, even if there are features of the sinus tarsi syndrome, the clinician should still seek other injuries too.

Appropriate investigation is a key part of management of patients with the difficult ankle. MRI is preferred to bone scan as it can detect bony and soft tissue abnormalities. Clinicians must remember that a subluxing tendon can appear normal on MRI.

> **PRACTICE PEARL**
>
> Isotope activity in the bone phase is normal in soft tissue problems and increased if bony damage is present.

Osteochondral lesions of the talar dome

An osteochondral lesion of the talus is an important cause of residual pain after an ankle sprain. It is defined as the separation of a fragment of articular cartilage, with or without subchondral bone. Its incidence after an ankle sprain has been reported to be around 6.5%, and is probably underestimated because these lesions often remain undetected. The grading of osteochondral fractures of the talar dome is shown in Figure 41.15.

History

Osteochondral fractures of the talar dome usually occur in association with ankle sprains when there is a compressive

Table 41.3 Ligamentous, tendon and neurological causes of the 'difficult ankle'—persistent ankle pain after ankle injury

Atypical sprains	Tendon injuries	Other soft tissue and neural abnormalities
Chronic ligamentous instability	Chronic peroneal tendon weakness	Inadequate rehabilitation
Medial ligament sprain	Peroneal tendon subluxation/rupture	Chronic synovitis
Syndesmosis sprain (AITFL sprain)	Tibialis posterior tendon subluxation/rupture	Sinus tarsi syndrome
Subtalar joint sprain		Complex regional pain syndrome type 1

Acute ankle injuries CHAPTER 41

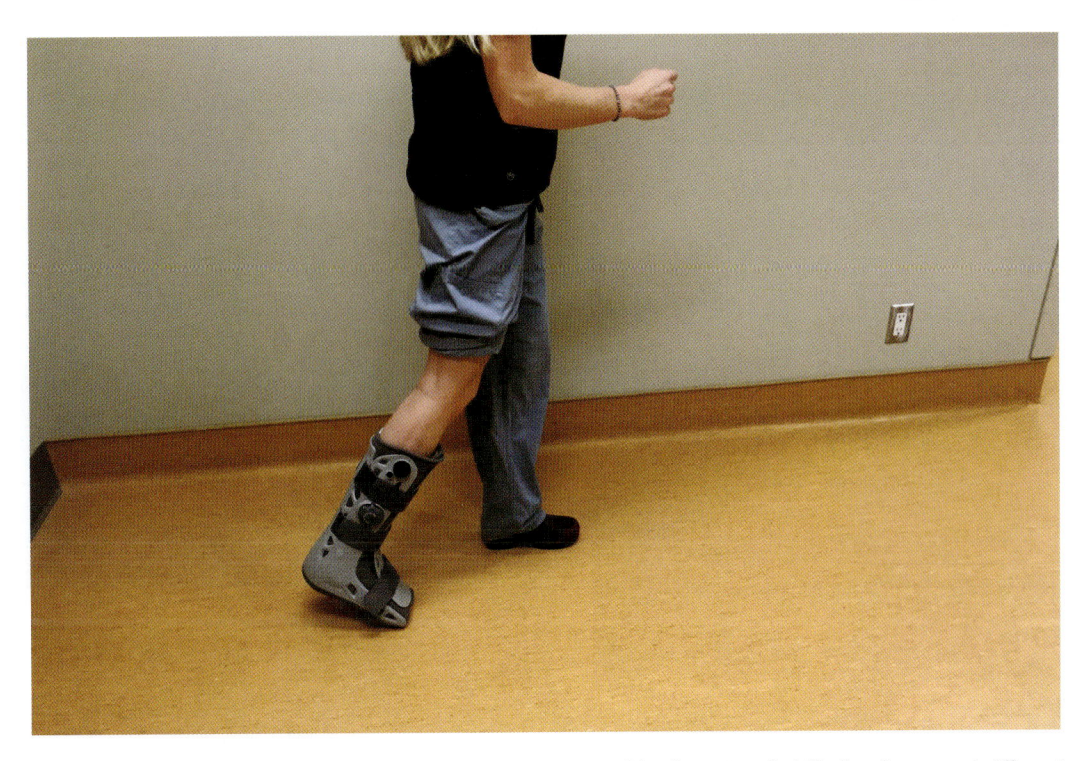

Figure 41.13 A CAM (Controlled Ankle Movement) walker boot is a useful adjunct to rehabilitation for several different ankle injuries

component to the inversion injury, such as when landing from a jump. The talar dome is compressed by the tibial plafond, causing damage to the osteochondral surface. The lesions are usually in the superomedial corner of the talar dome, and are less common superolaterally.

Large fractures may be recognised at the time of injury. The fracture site will be tender and may be evident on plain radiography (Fig. 41.14a).

Often an osteochondral lesion of the talus is not detected initially and the patient presents later with unremitting ankle aching and locking or catching, despite appropriate treatment for an ankle sprain. The patient often gives a history of initially progressing well following a sprain, but then developing symptoms of increasing pain and swelling, stiffness and perhaps catching or locking as activity is increased. Reduced range of motion is often a prominent symptom. The reason why an osteochondral lesion of the talus produces these symptoms is poorly understood. It has been hypothesised that a focal loss of structural support of the talar dome or cyclical change in intra-osseous pressure with gait, triggers pain receptors in the richly innervated subchondral bone.

Examination
Examination with the patient's foot plantarflexed at 35° to rotate the talus out of the ankle mortise may reveal tenderness of the dome of the talus. This may, however, be difficult due to pain. The diagnosis of osteochondral lesion of the talus requires a high index of suspicion. Focal chondral and osteochondral defects may eventually progress to ankle joint osteoarthritis.[31]

Investigations
Plain radiographs often appear normal or show only minor changes resulting in a delayed diagnosis. If osteochondral lesion of the talus is suspected, an MRI (Fig. 41.14b) should be requested.

A CT scan (Fig. 41.14c) can be used to determine the exact degree of skeletal injury.

MRI provides anatomical and pathological data, and is the investigation of choice. MRI has a benefit of being positive in grade I lesions. The grading of osteochondral fractures of the talar dome is shown in Figure 41.15.

Treatment
The treatment of an osteochondral lesion of the talus is complex and numerous non-surgical and surgical options including marrow stimulation techniques and tissue transplantation have been reported. All options have some limitations, mainly due to the poor regenerative capacity of the articular cartilage and the limited access to the ankle joint.

907

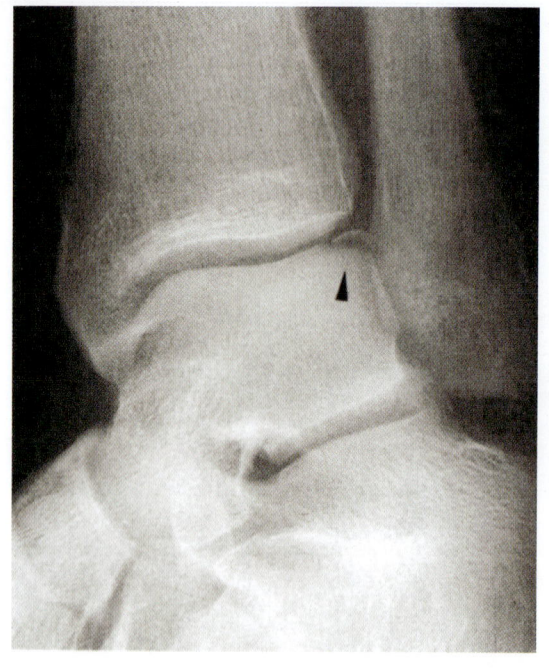

PART B Regional problems

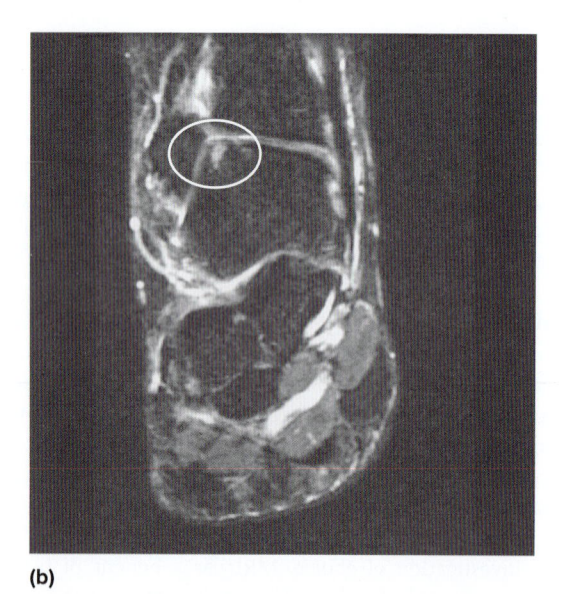

Figure 41.14 Osteochondral lesion of the talar dome (a) radiograph (arrow) (b) MRI (circle) (c) CT scan (grade IV)

Chronic grade I and II lesions should be treated conservatively. Patients should avoid activities that cause pain and ride an exercise bike with low resistance. Cast immobilisation has now been replaced with early joint motion without significant loading to promote articular cartilage. If there is pain, symptoms of clicking, locking or giving way persisting after 2–3 months of conservative management, ankle arthroscopy is indicated in order to remove or fix loose bodies. A grade IIa, III or IV lesion also requires arthroscopic removal of the separated fragment or cyst, and curetting and drilling of the fracture bed down to bleeding bone. After surgical treatment of osteochondral lesions, a comprehensive rehabilitation program is required. Tibial plafond chondral lesions (see below) are managed identically.

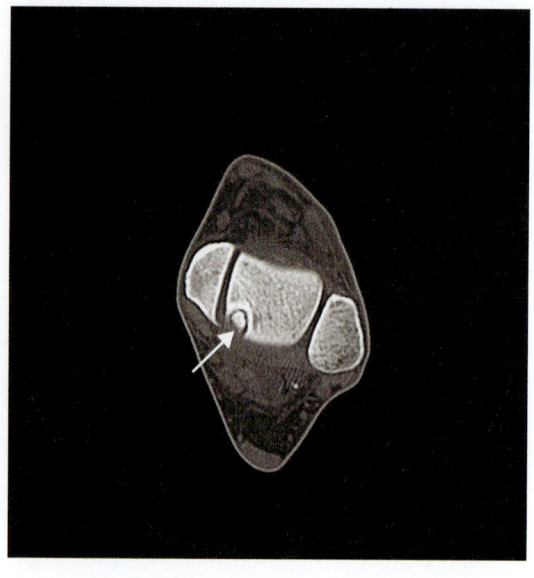

Clinical outcome studies have identified some prognostic parameters, such as the size of the lesion. However, there is only limited information available to predict the individual patient outcomes when treating osteochondral lesions of the talus.

Avulsion fracture of the base of the fifth metatarsal

Inversion injury may result in an avulsion fracture of the base of the fifth metatarsal. This benign fracture can occur in isolation or, more commonly, in association with a lateral ligament sprain. The fracture results from traction of the peroneus brevis tendon attachment at the base of the fifth metatarsal.

Plain radiographs should be examined closely. Avulsion fracture is characterised by its involvement of the joint surface of the base of the fifth metatarsal (Fig. 41.16).

A potentially confusing fracture is the fracture of the proximal diaphysis of the fifth metatarsal that does not involve any joint surfaces. This fracture is known as the Jones fracture and may require internal fixation (Chapter 43).

Acute ankle injuries CHAPTER 41

Grade I Subchondral fracture   Investigation: MRI

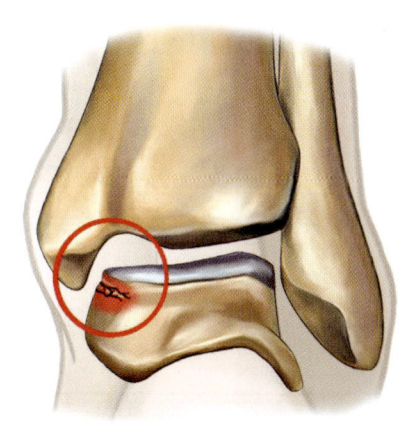

Grade II Chondral fracture   Investigation: CT/MRI

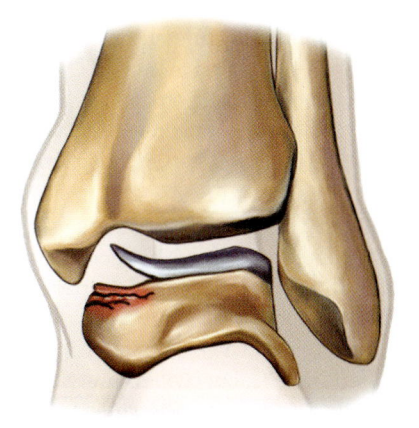

Grade IIa Subchondral cyst   Investigation: CT/MRI

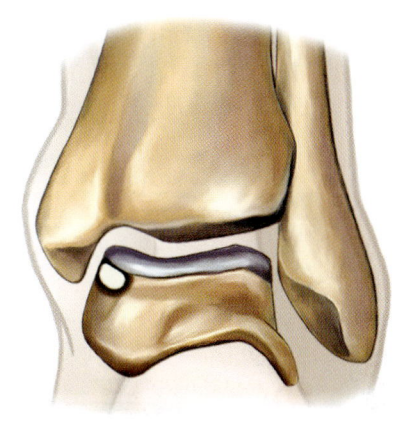

Grade III Chondral fracture with separated but not displaced fragments   Investigation: CT/MRI

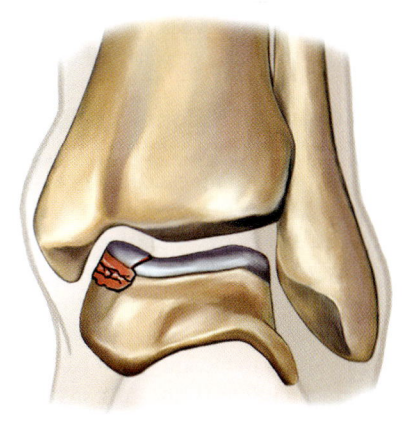

Grade IV Chondral fracture with separated and displaced fragment(s)   Investigation: X-ray/CT/MRI

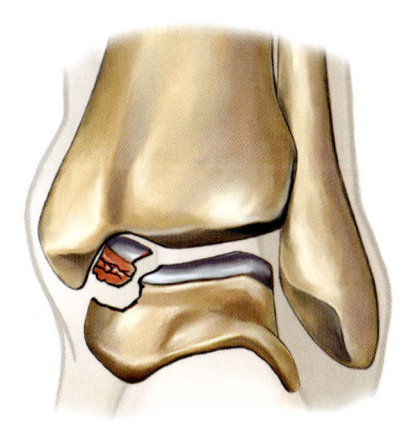

Figure 41.15 Grading of osteochondral fracture of the talar dome

909

PART B   Regional problems

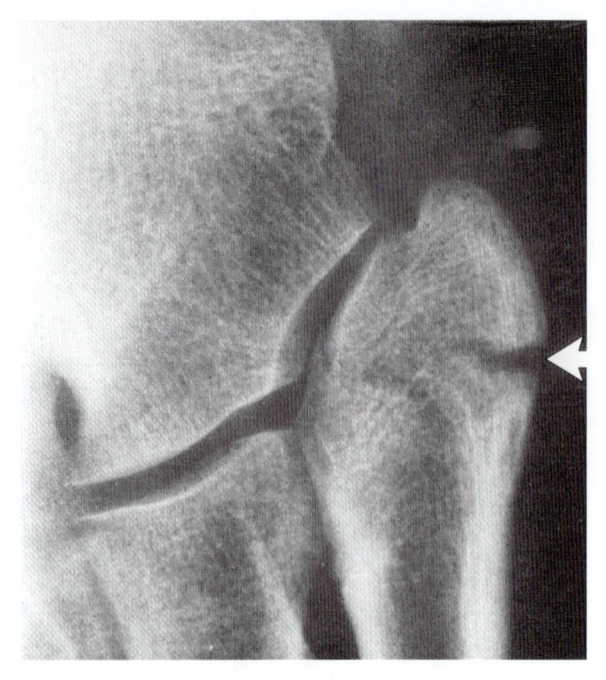

Figure 41.16 Avulsion fracture of the base of the fifth metatarsal

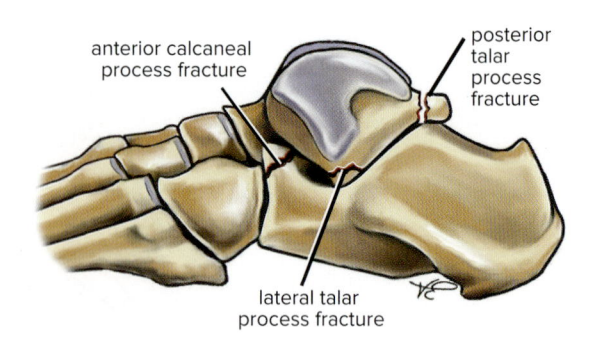

Figure 41.17 Fractures around the talus and calcaneus

> **PRACTICE PEARL**
>
> It is important to distinguish between the benign fracture of the base of the fifth metatarsal and a Jones fracture. Refer to Chapter 43 for more information.

Although the mechanism can appear to be one of 'acute' injury, in most cases the Jones fracture is a result of repetitive overuse (i.e. a stress fracture) of the proximal diaphysis of the fifth metatarsal.

Other fractures
A number of other fractures can occur as a result of acute ankle injuries (Fig. 41.17), alone or in association with ligamentous injury. They may be undetectable or subtle on plain radiograph.

Fractured lateral talar process
The lateral talar process is a prominence of the lateral talar body with an articular surface dorsolaterally for the fibula and inferomedially for the anterior portion of the posterior calcaneal facet (Fig. 41.17). Patients with a fracture of this process may present with ankle pain, swelling and inability to weight-bear for long periods. Examination reveals swelling and bruising over the lateral aspect of the ankle and tenderness over the lateral process, immediately anterior and inferior to the tip of the lateral malleolus. The fracture is best seen on the mortise view radiograph of the ankle. Undisplaced fractures may be treated in a short leg cast. Fractures displaced more than 2 mm require either primary excision or reduction and internal fixation. Comminuted fractures may require primary excision, which is a safe treatment, followed by short immobilisation only.

Fractured anterior calcaneal process
Fractures of the anterior calcaneal process may cause persistent pain after an ankle sprain. Palpation of the anterior calcaneal process, just anterior to the opening of the sinus tarsi (Fig. 41.17), is painless in patients with a tear of the ATFL, but will cause considerable pain in those with a fracture of the anterior process. If plain radiographs (including oblique foot views) fail to show a fracture that is suspected clinically, MRI or CT is indicated (Fig. 41.18).

If the fracture is small, symptomatic treatment may suffice. If large, it requires four weeks of non weight-bearing cast immobilisation or surgical excision of the fragment.

Tibial plafond chondral lesions
Tibial plafond (the inferior tibial articular surface) injuries may occur with vertical compression forces, such as a fall from a height. However, they can also result from straightforward ankle sprains. The patient complains of difficulty weight-bearing, and examination reveals swelling and restricted dorsiflexion. As with talar dome lesions, plain radiograph can be normal, so MRI or CT are necessary to demonstrate the lesion (Fig. 41.19).

If imaging and clinical features are consistent with bony damage, arthroscopic debridement, including microfracturing is indicated but ankle pain can persist for months to a year, even after treatment.

Acute ankle injuries CHAPTER 41

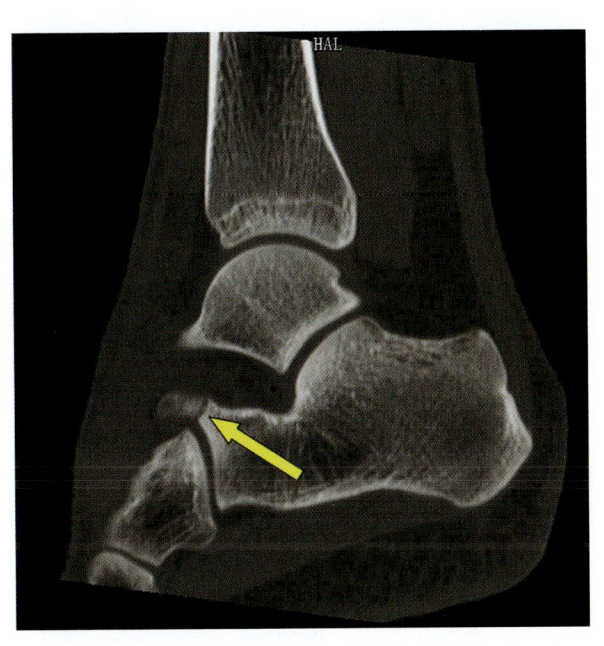

Figure 41.18 Sagittal CT image showing an anterior process calcaneal fracture

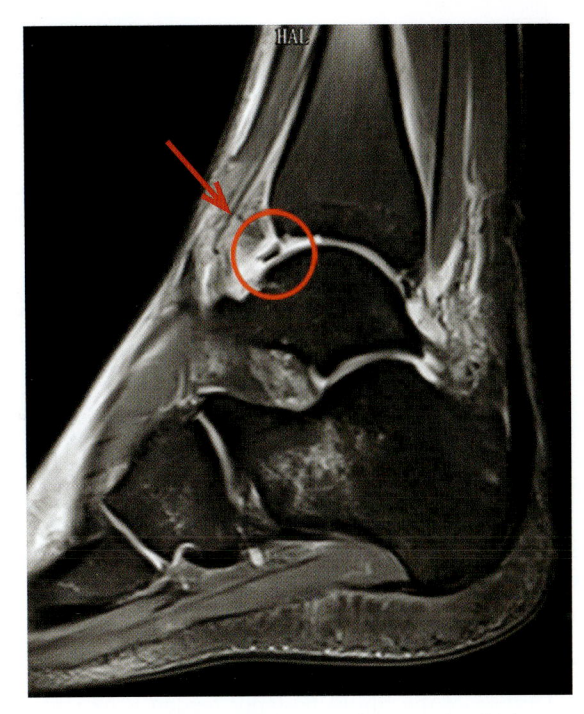

Figure 41.19 Sagittal T2 MRI image of an anterior tibial plafond cartilage lesion with a loose fragment of cartilage in the joint

Fractured posterior process of the talus
Posterior process fractures occur usually as a result of forced plantar flexion injuries and are even less common than lateral process fractures (Fig. 41.17). This mechanism is often seen during kicking and has been reported in fencing.

Routine AP and lateral radiographs may not show the acute fracture and can be wrongly interpreted. CT scanning remains the mainstay of diagnosis, but a high index of suspicion is required.

Most of these injuries will be treated initially with conservative treatment. Acute fractures of the posterior process of the talus may require surgical excision.

Medial tubercle fractures
Fractures of the medial tubercle of the posterior process talus are rare in sports. They can occur due to a dorsiflexion avulsion by the posterior talotibial ligament (posterior aspect of the deltoid ligament) and eversion (Cedell fracture), or by direct traumatic compression.

In contrast to lateral tubercle injuries, pain and swelling is usually present between the Achilles tendon and the medial malleolus, but there may be limited pain on walking or moving the ankle. It is difficult to visualise fractures of the medial tubercle on plain AP and lateral radiographs, and it has been suggested that the addition of two oblique views at 45° and 70° of external rotation may significantly aid detection prior to resorting to a CT or MR imaging. The fracture can be treated arthroscopically with a posterior approach.

Impingement syndromes
Ankle impingement syndromes are usually the result of overuse, but can occur following acute ankle injuries. For example, ballet dancers often suffer posterior impingement following lateral ankle sprain, due to the presence of an os trigonum, processus posterior of the talus and/or posterior osteophytes. In the acute ankle a blocked kicking action can cause posterior impingement. Posterior impingement syndrome is discussed in detail in Chapter 40. Anterior and anterolateral impingement syndromes and their treatment are discussed in Chapter 42.

Tendon dislocation or rupture
Dislocation or longitudinal rupture of the peroneal tendons (in most cases peroneus brevis tendon) can cause persistent lateral ankle symptoms. Tibialis posterior injury can cause similar symptoms on the medial side but is very uncommon in sport.

Dislocation of the peroneal tendons
The peroneal tendons are situated behind the lateral malleolus and held there by the superior peroneal

retinaculum. They are occasionally dislocated as a result of forceful passive dorsiflexion with rupture of the retinaculum from the posterior edge of the lateral malleolus. This may occur when a skier catches a tip and falls forward over the ski. Rupture of the peroneal retinaculum allows one or both of the tendons to move out of their groove. The dislocated tendon(s) may remain in a dislocated position or spontaneously relocate and subsequently become prone to recurrent subluxation. Examination reveals tender peroneal tendons that can be dislocated by the examiner, especially with ankle plantarflexion.

Treatment of dislocation of peroneal tendons is surgical replacement of the tendons in the peroneal groove and repair of the retinaculum, using bone anchors or drill holes. If the peroneal groove is shallow, then retinacular repair should be accompanied by deepening of the groove or rotation of the malleolus (not often recommended). Soft tissue repair, however, produces a good result in most cases.

Dislocation of the tibialis posterior tendon

Dislocation of the tibialis posterior tendon is extremely rare in sport. It occurs with ankle dorsiflexion and inversion, where forceful contraction of the tibialis posterior muscle pulls the tendon out of its retinaculum using the malleolus as a fulcrum. The patient may complain of moderate medial ankle pain and inability to weight-bear. Examination reveals swelling and bruising around the medial malleolus with tenderness along the course of the tibialis posterior tendon. The tendon can be subluxed anteriorly and subsequently relocated posteriorly with the foot in the fully plantarflexed position. The diagnosis is clinical, but ultrasonography or MRI (Fig. 41.20) may reveal fluid around the tendon.

Immediate surgical treatment is indicated to minimise the time that the tendon is dislocated while permitting primary repair of the flexor retinaculum and reattachment of the tibialis posterior sheath.[32] Postoperatively the ankle is immobilised in a CAM walker for a total of six weeks' non weight-bearing. Once the walking boot is no longer required an ankle brace can be used to support the ankle with active ankle motion permitted three times daily while taking care to avoid resisted inversion. Weight-bearing can recommence at six weeks under physiotherapy supervision followed by strengthening and functional rehabilitation.

Rupture of the tibialis posterior tendon

An athlete with a ruptured tibialis posterior tendon presents with pain in the region of the tubercle of the navicular extending to the posterosuperior border of the medial malleolus and along the posteromedial tibial border. Examination reveals thickening or absence (less

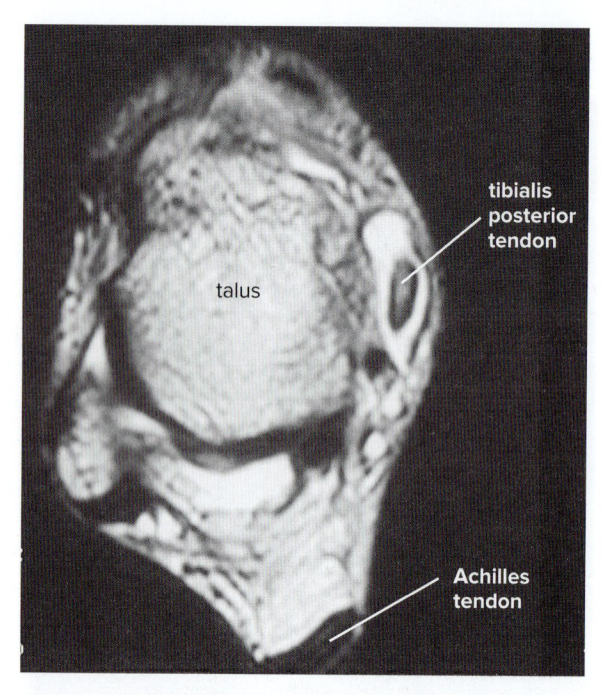

Figure 41.20 MRI appearance (T2-weighted) shortly after tibialis posterior tendon dislocation shows the tibialis posterior tendon (dark) in cross-section surrounded by abnormal fluid (high signal intensity). The tendon is in its normal position during this examination. If imaging had been delayed sufficiently, fluid would have been absent and the MRI appearance may have been normal

frequent) of the tibialis posterior tendon and inability to raise the heel. A flattened medial arch is a classic sign. MRI is the investigation of choice in this condition, although ultrasound may also be helpful. However, there is low correlation between MRI findings and symptoms. Surgical repair, often including major reconstruction of the midfoot anatomy is indicated as the tibialis posterior tendon is essential to maintain the normal medial arch of the foot.

Other causes of the difficult ankle
Anteroinferior tibiofibular ligament injury/syndesmotic injury

The distal tibiofibular joint is a fibrous syndesmotic articulation consisting of the concave surface of the distal tibia and convex shape of the distal fibula.[33] The syndesmosis is a complex ligamentous structure including three different portions. The anterior syndesmosis consists of the anterior inferior tibiofibular ligament (AITFL); the middle part consists of the interosseous ligament (IOL); and the posterior syndesmosis includes the posterior inferior tibiofibular and the transverse ligaments (PITFL and TL). Each structure plays a critical role to provide stability of the ankle mortise. The resistance to diastasis comes from the PITFL and TL for 40–45%, the AITFL for 35% and the IOL for 20–25%.[34]

Injuries to the distal tibiofibular syndesmosis (Fig. 41.21) account for 11–17% of the ankle sprains in athletic populations.[35] Acute syndesmotic injuries have been reported especially in football and skiing. They can range from stable minor sprains to significant fractures (e.g. Maisonneuve fracture) of the distal fibula with combined syndesmotic disruption. Syndesmotic injuries usually present with more pain and disability than a typical lateral ankle sprain.

The mechanism of syndesmotic injury can be an isolated hyperdorsiflexion force, but is most commonly due to an external rotation injury, in combination with axial loading of the ankle. In patients with a combined deltoid injury or medial malleolar fracture, an abduction force is the main cause of the associated syndesmotic lesion.

Syndesmotic injuries can be isolated or associated with bony or ligamentous ankle injuries. The term 'isolated' is commonly used for syndesmotic injuries without ankle fractures, although concomitant ligamentous or soft tissue injuries and tibiofibular avulsion fractures may be present.[36]

If there is pain on palpation over the anterior and posterior tibiofibular ligaments, the more proximal the pain, the greater the extent of the lesion. It is also important to check the entire fibula up to the knee if there is any suspicion of syndesmotic/Maisonneuve fracture. Swelling is less marked in syndesmotic injury compared with a normal ankle sprain and bruising is usually more proximal to the ankle joint.

> **PRACTICE PEARL**
>
> There is no pathognomonic clinical test to evaluate a syndesmotic injury but the external rotation test is the most helpful test. The test is performed by stabilising the leg with the knee flexed at 90° and then rotating the foot externally.

A positive test will elicit pain at the syndesmosis. During physical examination, it is important to palpate the medial ankle in addition to determine the integrity of the deltoid ligament, since it can highlight a more significant unstable syndesmotic injury.

Radiographic imaging must include an AP view and a mortise view of the syndesmosis to rule out the tibiofibular clear space, medial clear space overlap, tibial width and fibular width. In acute syndesmotic lesions, MRIs have a sensitivity and specificity that are about 100%.[37] Furthermore, injury to the distal tibiofibular syndesmosis has a significant association with a number of secondary findings on MRI, including bone bruises, osteochondral lesions, tibiofibular joint congruity and height of the tibiofibular recess.

Acute ankle injuries with an isolated lesion of the syndesmosis should be classified as stable or unstable.

- The stable ankle sprain is characterised by a lesion of the AITFL with or without interosseous ligament (IOL) with a continent deltoid ligament.
- The unstable ankle sprain should be classified as latent or frank diastasis. The latent diastasis is characterised by a rupture of the AITFL with or without IOL and deltoid ligament. It can be detected on MRI and/or arthroscopic assessment. The frank diastasis is characterised by a rupture of all the syndesmotic and deltoid ligaments, and it is visible on standard radiographs.[33]

Syndesmotic sprains without instability should be treated non-operatively with a CAM walker (Fig. 41.13) or brace. Syndesmosis injuries frequently require almost twice as much time rehabilitating compared with patients who have lateral ankle sprains. An acute syndesmotic ligament rupture with instability of the ankle should be managed operatively.[33]

Post-traumatic synovitis

Some degree of synovitis will occur with any ankle injury due to the presence of blood within the joint. This

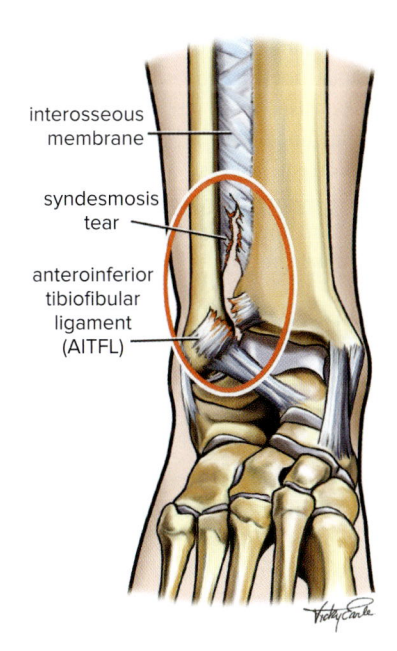

Figure 41.21 Anatomy of a syndesmosis sprain. This injury may be associated with medial malleolar fracture (not illustrated)

PART B Regional problems

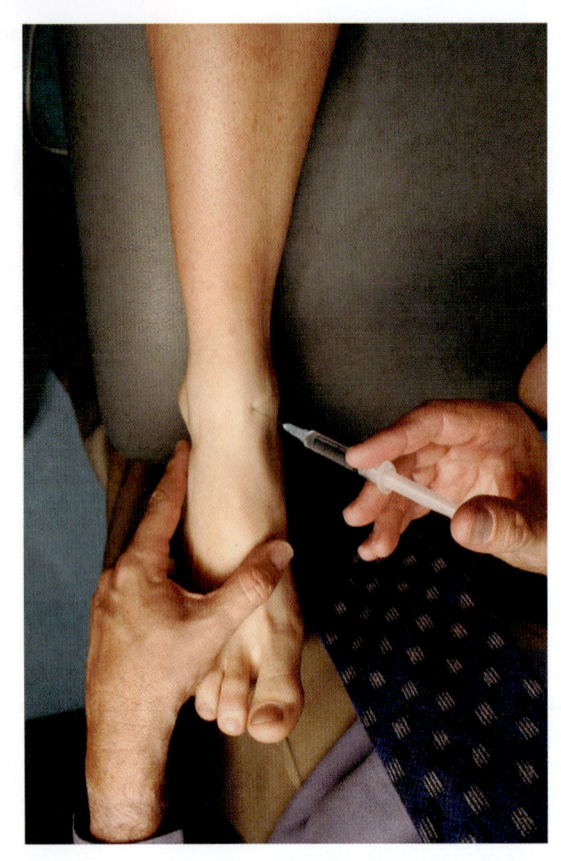

Figure 41.22 Corticosteroid injection into the ankle joint in the treatment of post-traumatic synovitis. The needle is inserted medial to the tibialis anterior tendon and directed posterolaterally

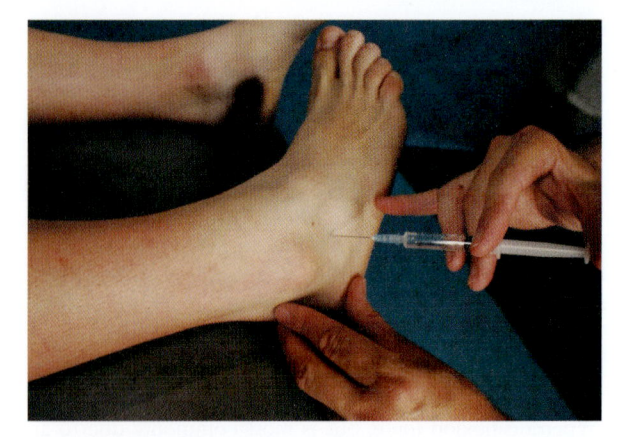

Figure 41.23 Injection into the sinus tarsi. The lateral opening of the sinus is maintained when the foot is inverted. The needle is directed towards the tip of the medial malleolus

usually resolves in a few days, but may persist if there is excessive early weight-bearing, typically in athletes eager to return to training soon after their ankle sprain, or due to insufficient rehabilitation. These athletes will often develop persistent ankle pain aggravated by activity and associated with swelling. Synovitis of the ankle joint is also seen in athletes who have chronic mild instability because of excessive accessory movement of the ankle joint during activity.

Treatment of synovitis includes NSAIDs, rest from aggravating activity and local electrotherapy. A corticosteroid injection into the ankle joint (Fig. 41.22) may be required. An injection should be followed by 48 hours of limited weight-bearing and gradual resumption of activity. Sometimes arthroscopy with synovectomy may be indicated.

When synovitis is associated with a degree of chronic instability, treatment involves taping or bracing. Such patients can have significant relief when wearing a brace for activities of daily living as well as sport. These patients may also benefit from ankle ligament reconstructive surgery.

Sinus tarsi syndrome

Sinus tarsi syndrome may occur as an overuse injury secondary to excessive subtalar pronation (Chapter 42) or following an ankle sprain. Pain occurs at the lateral opening of the sinus tarsi (Fig. 41.1b). The pain is often more severe in the morning and improves on warming up.

Forced passive inversion and eversion may both be painful. The most appropriate aid to diagnosis is to monitor the effect of injection of a local anaesthetic agent into the sinus tarsi under fluoroscopy (Fig. 41.23).

Treatment consists of relative rest, NSAIDs, electrotherapeutic modalities, subtalar joint mobilisation and taping to correct excessive pronation if present. If conservative management is unsuccessful, injection of corticosteroid and local anaesthetic agents may help resolve the inflammation.

Complex regional pain syndrome type 1

Complex regional pain syndrome (CRPS) type 1, formerly known as RSD (Chapters 5, 6 and 7), may occasionally complicate ankle injury. Initially, it appears that the patient with a 'sprained ankle' is improving but then symptoms begin to relapse. The patient complains of increased pain, swelling recurs and the skin may become hot or, more frequently, very cold. There may also be localised sweating, discoloration and hypersensitivity.

As early treatment substantially improves the prognosis in CRPS type 1, early diagnosis is imperative. Initial radiographs are normal. Later, patchy demineralisation occurs and this can be seen as regions of decreased opacity on plain radiograph and areas of increased uptake on bone scan or increased signal on MRI.[38] Tests of sympathetic function may confirm the diagnosis.[38]

It is most important that the specific nature of the condition be explained to the patient as it may be very painful, even at rest. It remains difficult to treat and there have been few controlled treatment trials for established CRPS type 1.[39] Physiotherapy may play a role[40] and ultrasound and hydrotherapy may facilitate range of movement exercises. Gabapentin, an anticonvulsant with a proven analgesic effect in various neuropathic pain syndromes, has shown mild efficacy as treatment for pain in patients with CRPS type 1.[41] As CRPS type 1 is associated with regional osteoclastic overactivity (excessive bone turnover, as shown by increased uptake on radionuclide bone scan), a bisphosphonate medication (alendronate) was trialled in 39 patients.[42] In contrast to placebo-treated patients, all of the alendronate-treated patients had substantially reduced pain and improved joint mobility as early as the fourth week of treatment.

If the pain does not settle, chemical or surgical blockade is indicated. However, a Cochrane systematic review failed to support this therapy for relieving pain.[43] CRPS type 1 remains a very difficult condition to treat.

REFERENCES

References for this chapter can be found at www.mhhe.com/au/CSM5e

Chapter 42

Ankle pain

with KAREN HOLZER and JON KARLSSON

Dance is the hidden language of the soul.
Martha Graham, dancer and choreographer, 1894–1991

Sportspeople, particularly ballet dancers, footballers, basketballers and high jumpers, may complain of ankle pain that is not related to an acute ankle injury (Chapter 41). Clinical management of such 'overuse' injuries is simplified if the presentations are further divided into:

- medial ankle pain
- lateral ankle pain
- anterior ankle pain
- posterior ankle pain: defined in this book as the 'Achilles region' (Chapter 40).

It is important to note that clinically, patients often present with combinations of pain, such as anterolateral ankle pain in soccer players. In those circumstances, the systematic clinical approach outlined in this chapter still aids in diagnosis and management.

MEDIAL ANKLE PAIN

Although there are numerous causes of medial ankle pain, the most common is tendinopathy, in particular of the tibialis posterior tendon, and to a lesser degree the flexor hallucis longus tendon. Another important cause of medial ankle pain is tarsal tunnel syndrome, where the posterior tibial nerve is compressed behind the medial malleolus. This may present as medial ankle pain with sensory symptoms distally. Posterior impingement syndrome of the ankle can also present as medial ankle pain (Chapter 40).

The causes of medial ankle pain are listed in Table 42.1. The anatomy of the region is illustrated in Figure 42.1.

History

In patients with medial ankle pain there is usually a history of overuse, especially running or excessive walking (tibialis posterior tendinopathy), toe flexion in ballet dancers and high jumpers (flexor hallucis longus tendinopathy) or plantarflexion in dancers and footballers (posterior impingement syndrome). In the case of tibialis posterior tendinopathy, pain may radiate along the line of the tendon to its insertion on the navicular tubercle, or in tarsal tunnel syndrome the arch of the foot. Associated sensory symptoms such as pins and needles or numbness

Table 42.1 Causes of medial ankle pain

Common	Less common	Not to be missed
Tibialis posterior tendinopathy	Medial calcaneal nerve entrapment	Navicular stress fracture (Chapter 43)
Flexor hallucis longus tendinopathy	Calcaneal stress fracture	Complications of acute ankle injuries (Chapter 41)
	Tarsal tunnel syndrome	Complex regional pain syndrome type 1 (following knee or ankle injury) (Chapter 5)
	Talar stress fracture	
	Medial malleolar stress fracture	
	Posterior impingement syndrome (Chapter 40)	
	Referred pain from lumbar spine	

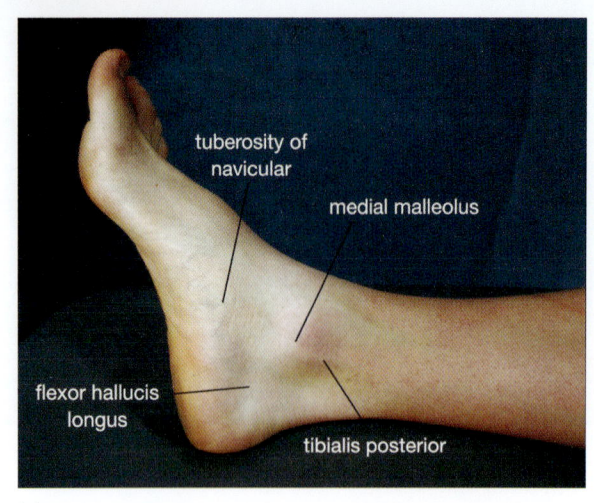

PART B Regional problems

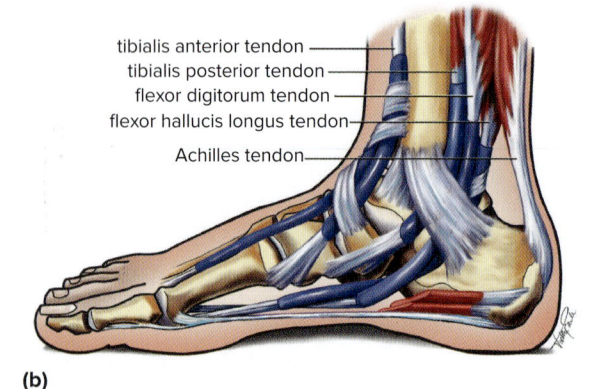

Figure 42.1 Medial aspect of the ankle (a) Surface anatomy (b) Anatomy of the medial ankle

may suggest tarsal tunnel syndrome. Crepitus is commonly associated with flexor hallucis longus and occasionally tibialis posterior tendinopathy.

Examination
Careful palpation and testing of resisted movements is the key to examination of this region.

1. Observation
    a. standing
    b. walking
    c. supine
2. Active movements
    a. ankle plantarflexion/dorsiflexion
    b. ankle inversion/eversion
    c. flexion of the first metatarsophalangeal joint
3. Passive movements
    a. as for active
    b. subtalar joint
    c. midtarsal joint
    d. muscle stretches
        i. gastrocnemius
        ii. soleus
4. Resisted movement
    a. inversion (Fig. 42.2a)
    b. first toe flexion; check for crepitation (Fig. 42.2b)
5. Functional tests
    a. hop
    b. jump
6. Palpation
    a. tibialis posterior tendon (Fig. 42.2c)
    b. flexor hallucis longus; behind the medial malleolus
    c. navicular tubercle
    d. ankle joint
    e. midtarsal joint
    f. Achilles tendon
7. Special tests
    a. Tinel's test (Fig. 42.2d)
    b. sensory examination; especially for nerve entrapment of the calcaneal branches (Baxter's nerve) (Fig. 42.2e)
8. biomechanical examination (Chapter 8)
9. lumbar spine examination (Chapter 29).

Key outcome measures
The key patient-reported outcome measures (PROMs) used in ankle pain are shown in Table 42.2.

Investigations
Plain radiograph is indicated when the following conditions are suspected:

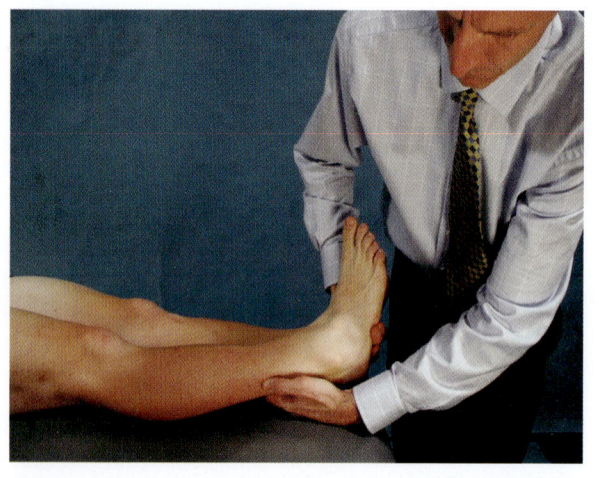

Figure 42.2 Examination of the patient with medial ankle pain (a) Resisted movement—inversion (tibialis posterior)

Ankle pain CHAPTER 42

(b)

(c)

(d)

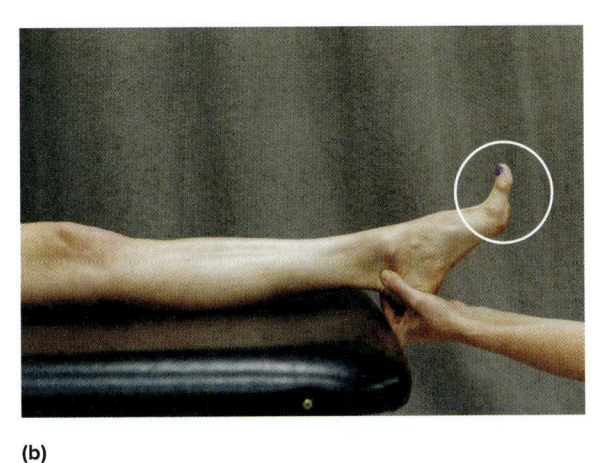

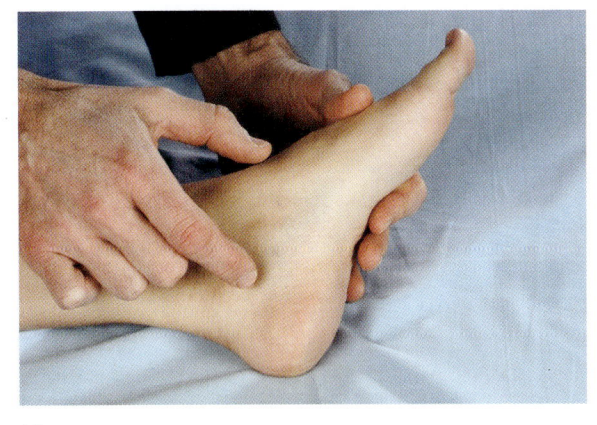

(e)

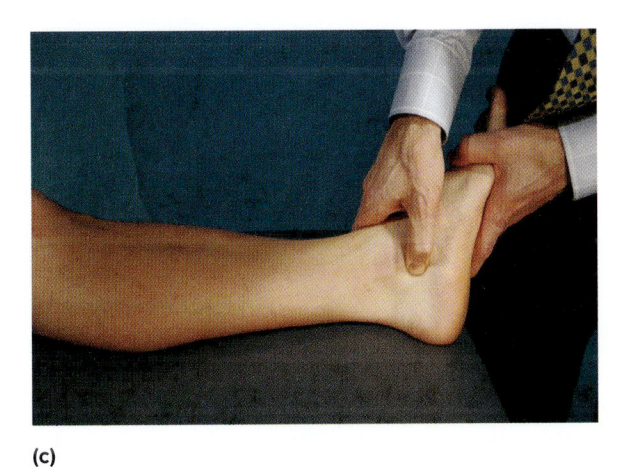

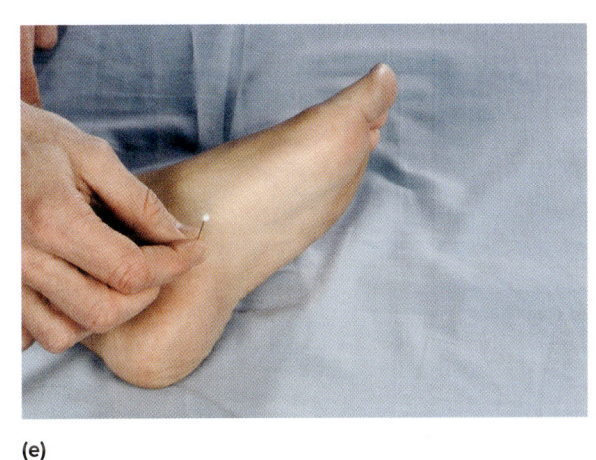

Figure 42.2 (cont.) (b) Resisted movement—toe flexion (flexor hallucis longus) (c) Palpation—tibialis posterior tendon. The tibialis posterior tendon is palpated from posteromedial to the medial malleolus to its insertion at the navicular tubercle (d) Special tests—Tinel's test. Tapping over the posterior tibial nerve in the tarsal tunnel may reproduce symptoms (e) Special tests—sensory examination especially for nerve entrapment of the calcaneal branches (Baxter's nerve). (See also Chapter 43, and refer to Figure 43.7.)

- Posterior impingement: to confirm the presence of either a large posterior process of the talus/fracture of the posterior process of the talus or an os trigonum. A lateral view with the foot in a maximally plantarflexed position (posterior impingement view) can be useful to determine if bony impingement is occurring.
- Anteromedial impingement: anteroposterior views may reveal osteophytes with joint narrowing between the medial talus and medial malleolus, or the anteromedial aspect of the medial tibial plafond.
- Stress fracture of the medial malleolus: often a delayed diagnosis, and as such sclerosis and/or a fracture line may be seen.

Ultrasound can assist in the diagnosis of tibialis posterior or flexor hallucis longus tenosynovitis or tendinopathy. MRI assists in the diagnosis of most medial ankle conditions including impingements, tenosynovitis and tendinopathies, and bony injuries.

Nerve conduction studies may be performed if tarsal tunnel syndrome is suspected. However nerve conduction studies are seldom diagnostic.

PART B Regional problems

Table 42.2 Patient-reported outcome measures for the ankle

Generic foot and ankle pain measures

Foot and Ankle Ability Measure (FAAM)[1]

- Self-administered questionnaire evaluating difficulty with activities of daily living (ADL) and sporting activities for patient with foot and ankle pain
- Two subscales: ADL and Sports subscales
- 29 items (21 on difficulty with ADL, 8 on difficulty with sporting activities)
- Score range: 0–100 for each subscale
- Test-retest reliability:
  - ADL subscale: 0.89
  - Sports subscale: 0.87
- Construct validity:
  - ADL subscale: SF-36′ PF subscale and PCS subscale: both 0.84[1]
  - Higher ADL subscale scores for healthy athletes (M=100, SD=0) compared to patients with chronic ankle instability (M=88, SD=7.7)
  - Sports subscale: SF-36′ PF subscale and PCS subscale: 0.78 and 0.80 respectively[1]
  - Higher Sports subscale scores for healthy athletes (M=99, SD=3.5) compared to patient with chronic ankle instability (M=76, SD=12.6)
- Minimal detectable change (MCD95%):
  - ADL subscale: 5.7
  - Sports subscale: 12.3
- Minimal clinically important difference (MCID):
  - ADL subscale: 8
  - Sports subscale: 9* (* as determined with optimal sensitivity/specificity in ROC curve)
- Developed and validated in American English, cross-culturally validated to Brazilian Portuguese,[3] Dutch,[4] German,[5] Italian,[6] Japanese,[7] Korean,[8] Persian,[9] Thai[10] and Turkish[11]

Oxford Ankle Foot Questionnaire[12,13]

- Self-administered questionnaire evaluating disability in children with foot and ankle problems (5–16 years of age)
- 15 items (6 on physical domain, 4 on school and play domain, 4 on emotional domain and 1 on footwear)
- Score range:
  - Physical domain: 0–24 (0–100 if transformed to)
  - School and Play domain: 0–16 (0–100 if transformed to %)
  - Emotional domain: 0–16 (0–100 if transformed to %)
- Test-retest reliability:
  - Physical domain: 0.62[12] and 0.85[13]
  - School and Play domain: 0.87 and 0.95
  - Emotional domain: 0.83 and 0.78
  - Footwear item: 0.76[13]
- Construct validity[12]
  - Physical domain: Kidscreen physical wellbeing: 0.60
  - School and Play domain: Kidscreen physical wellbeing and school: 0.54 and 0.31 respectively
  - Emotional domain: Kidscreen psychological wellbeing: 0.46
  - Footwear item: N/A
- MDC90%:
  - Physical domain: 7.1[13]
  - School and Play domain: 5.4[13]
  - Emotional domain: 8.0[13]

Generic foot and ankle pain measures (cont)

- MCID:
  - Physical domain: 10.0[13]
  - School and Play domain: 8.7[13]
  - Emotional domain: 8.3[13]
- Developed and validated in British English,[12–14] cross-culturally validated to Danish[15] and Italian[16]
- Available online at www.orthopaedicscore.com/scorepages/foot_and_ankle_disability_index_fadi.html

Foot and Ankle Disability Index (FADI) Score

- Self-administered questionnaire that evaluated ADL and sporting activities
- 34 items (26 on ADL and 8 on sports)
- Score range:
  - FADI ADL 0–104[17]
  - FADI Sport 0–32[17]
  - Score transformation to 0–100%; 100% means no dysfunction
- Test-retest reliability:
  - FADI ADL: 0.89 and 0.93[17]
  - FADI Sport: 0.84 and 0.92[17]
- Developed[18] and validated[17] in American English
- Available online at www.orthopaedicscore.com/scorepages/foot_and_ankle_disability_index_fadi.html

American Academy of Orthopaedic Surgeons (AAOS) Foot and Ankle Module

- Self-administered questionnaire evaluating symptoms and function of the foot and ankle
- 25 items (20 global foot ankle scale; 5 items shoe comfort scale)
- Scores are transformed to 0–100% for each scale; 100% means no dysfunction
- Test-retest reliability; global rating scale, r = 0.79; shoe comfort scale, r = 0.87[19]
- Construct validity:
  - Foot and Ankle Module (both subscales): FAAM 0.92,[20] AOFAS 0.81,[20] SF-12 Physical 0.69,[20] Foot function index -0.85[20]
  - Global Foot and Ankle Scale: physician-assessed function: 0.43;[19] physician-assessed pain: 0.49;[19] SF-36 Physical Health: 0.65[19]
- Developed and validated in American English,[19] cross-culturally validated to Spanish[21] and Korean[22]

American Orthopaedic Foot & Ankle Society (AOFAS) Clinical Rating System

- Clinician-administered, region-specific questionnaires evaluating pain, function and alignment in patients with foot and ankle pain
- Four separate scales:[23]
  - Ankle-Hindfoot Scale (9 items)
  - Midfoot Scale (7 items)
  - Hallux Metatarsophalangeal-Interphalangeal Scale (8 items)
  - Lesser Metatarsophalangeal-Interphalangeal Scale (8 items)
- 0–100 points; 100 = no dysfunction, for all scales
- Test-retest reliability:
  - Ankle-Hindfoot Scale: 0.71[24]
  - Midfoot Scale: N/A
  - Hallux Metatarsophalangeal-Interphalangeal Scale: 0.95[25] and 0.82[24]
  - Lesser Metatarsophalangeal-Interphalangeal Scale: 0.80[25]
- Construct validity:
  - Ankle-Hindfoot Scale:
    - SF-36: Physical component scale: 0.27;[26] Bodily pain: 0.53;[26] Physical functioning: 0.34;[26] Vitality 0.41[26]

continued

Table 42.2 Cont.

Generic foot and ankle pain measures (cont)

American Orthopaedic Foot & Ankle Society (AOFAS) Clinical Rating System

- Manchester-Oxford Foot Questionnaire: Walking/standing: −0.56;[27] Pain: −0.60[27]
- Generic Health quality-adjusted life-year (QUALY) Score: 0.24–0.47[28]
- Self-reported Foot and Ankle Score: 0.49[24]
– Midfoot Scale:
  - Generic Health QUALY Score: 0.23–0.37[28]
– Hallux Metatarsophalangeal-Interphalangeal Scale:
  - Foot Function Index: −0.81[25]
  - Generic Health QUALY Score: 0.35–0.58[28]
  - Self-reported Foot and Ankle Score: 0.67[24]
– Lesser Metatarsophalangeal-Interphalangeal Scale
  - Generic Health QUALY Score: 0.22–0.67[28]
- MDC 90%:
  – Ankle-Hindfoot Scale: 6.30[29]
  – Midfoot Scale: 6.74[29]
  – Hallux Metatarsophalangeal-Interphalangeal Scale: 7.10[29]
  – Lesser Metatarsophalangeal-Interphalangeal Scale: 7.12[29]
- MCID:
  – Ankle-Hindfoot Scale: 8.90[29]
  – Midfoot Scale: 12.40[29]
  – Hallux Metatarsophalangeal-Interphalangeal Scale: 24.75[29]
  – Lesser Metatarsophalangeal-Interphalangeal Scale: 11.33[29]
- Developed and validated in American English,[23–26, 28, 29] cross-culturally validated to Brazilian Portuguese,[30, 31] German[32] and Italian[33]

Foot and Ankle Outcome Score

- Self-administered questionnaire evaluating pain, symptoms, ADL, sport and recreation function, and foot and ankle-related quality of life (QOL)
- 42 items (9 on pain, 7 on symptoms, 17 on ADL, 5 on Sport and Recreation and 4 on foot and ankle QoL)
- Score range 0–100 (100 = no problem)
- Test-retest reliability:
  – Pain: 0.78[34]
  – Symptoms: 0.86[34]
  – ADL: 0.70[34]
  – Sport and recreation: 0.85[34]
  – Foot and Ankle QoL: 0.92[34]
- Construct validity: Karlsson Score 0.58–0.67[34]
- Developed and validated in Swedish, cross-culturally validated to Dutch,[35–37] German,[38] Korean,[39] Persian[40] and Turkish[41]
- Validated in American English, without cross-cultural translation process[21, 42–45]
- Non-validated versions available in Arabic, Brazilian Portuguese, Chinese, Danish, Norwegian, Polish and Portuguese
- Available online in multiple languages: www.koos.nu

Lower limb pain measures

Lower Extremity Functional Score (LEFS)

- Self-administered questionnaire: difficulty with various activities
- 20 items
- Score ranges from 0–80 (80 = no difficulty)[46]
- Test-retest reliability: intraclass correlation coefficient (ICC) = 0.87–0.96[46, 47]
- Construct validity: SF-36 physical function: $r = 0.80$; SF-36 physical component: $r = 0.80$;[46] Olerud Molander Ankle Score: $r = 0.80–0.87$,[48] LLFI: 0.88[49]

Lower limb pain measures (cont)

- MDC 90%: 9,[46] 9.4,[47] 13;[50] MDC 95%: 15[50]
- MCID: 9[46]
- Developed and validated in American English,[46] cross-culturally translated and validated in Arabic,[51] Brazilian Portuguese,[52] Dutch,[53] Finnish,[54] French,[55] Italian,[56] Persian,[57] Spanish,[58] Taiwanese[59] and Turkish[60]

Lower Limb Functional Index (LLFI)

- Self-administered questionnaire evaluating lower limb function
- 25 items
- Score ranges from 0–100 (100 = no difficulty)
- Test-retest reliability: ICC = 0.97[49]
- Construct validity: LEFS: 0.88[49]
- MDC 90%: 6.63[49]
- Developed and validated in a mixed Australian/American population,[49] cross-culturally translated and validated in Spanish[61] and Turkish[62]

Lower Limb Task Questionnaire

- Self-administered questionnaire evaluating ADL and recreational activities
- Two subscales, both scores range from 0–40 (40 = no difficulty)
- Test-retest reliability:
  – ADL, ICC = 0.96[63]
  – Recreational activities, ICC = 0.98[63]
- Construct validity:
  – ADL: Motor activity scale, r = 0.62[63]
  – Recreational activities: Motor activity scale, r = 0.72[63]
- MDC95%: N/A
- MCID:
  – ADL: 10.1[63]
  – Recreational activities: 7.7[63]
- Developed and validated in New Zealand[63]

Ankle Joint Functional Assessment Tool

- Self-administered questionnaire evaluating ankle function
- Score ranges from 0–48 (48 = full function)[64]
- Developed in American English; no validation studies were found

Tibialis posterior tendinopathy

The tibialis posterior tendon is the largest and most anterior structure that passes behind the medial malleolus (Fig. 42,1b). It then divides and sends attachments to the navicular tuberosity, the cuboid, cuneiforms, bases of the second to fourth metatarsals and the spring ligament.

The functions of the tibialis posterior include:

- inversion of the subtalar joint
- dynamic stabilisation of the hindfoot against valgus (eversion) forces
- support of the medial longitudinal arch
- locking the transverse tarsal joints, thus allowing the gastrocnemius to support heel raise, and assisting the Achilles tendon in plantarflexion of the ankle.

Causes

Acute injuries of the tibialis posterior tendon are rare. Thus, tibialis posterior tendinopathy is usually related to overuse and is most often seen in middle-aged women, and in ballet dancers. It comes on slowly, and is not self-limiting.

1. Overuse, often related to:
   a. excessive walking, running or jumping
   b. excessive subtalar pronation. This increases eccentric tendon loading during supination for toe-off
2. Acute:
   a. direct trauma–laceration
   b. indirect trauma–eversion ankle sprain, ankle fracture
   c. acute avulsion fracture

3. Inflammatory conditions:
   a. tenosynovitis secondary to rheumatoid arthritis and seronegative arthropathies.

Chronic tendinopathies are characterised by collagen disarray and interstitial tears, and may eventually lead to total tendon rupture.

Clinical features

The clinical features of tibialis posterior tendinopathy are as follows.

- Medial ankle pain often arising from behind the medial malleolus and extending towards the medial midfoot to the insertion of the tendon at the navicular bone.
- Swelling is very unusual in the early stages and if present may suggest a substantial tendon injury or an underlying seronegative arthropathy. In the later stages, however, swelling is more pronounced and is often diffuse around and below the medial malleolus.
- Tenderness along the tendon is usual, most prominent posterior and inferior to the medial malleolus or at the insertion onto the navicular bone.
- Crepitus is only occasionally present.
- Resisted inversion (Fig. 42.2a) will elicit pain and relative weakness compared with the contralateral side.
- A single heel raise test viewed from behind will reveal lack of inversion of the hindfoot, and if severe the patient may have difficulty performing a heel raise. In the normal ankle, the calcaneus moves into varus position during a single heel raise; in patients with tibialis posterior tendinopathy, this does not happen and the heel remains in the valgus position.

Investigations

MRI (Fig. 42.3) or ultrasound may confirm the diagnosis and reveal the extent of tendinosis, including the presence of tears. MRI is the imaging modality of choice for the evaluation of tibialis posterior tendinopathy dysfunction. MRI has a sensitivity of 95%, a specificity of 100% and an accuracy of 96% in identifying disorders of the tendon.[65] It also has the ability to recognise injuries associated with longer-term tibialis posterior dysfunction, such as spring ligament failure, sinus tarsi inflammation and midfoot degeneration.[66]

Treatment

In milder cases conservative treatment is recommended; however, in more severe cases surgery may be required. Frequently the patient presents with an acute painful tendon, termed a 'reactive tendinopathy' which should be treated with rest, ice and non-steroidal anti-inflammatory drugs (NSAIDs) in the initial phase. Once the pain and inflammation has settled, treatment includes the following.

- Deep soft tissue therapy to the tibialis posterior muscle.
- Footwear: a stability shoe is recommended and often the wearing of an orthoses to control excessive pronation.
- Progressive concentric and eccentric tendon loading exercise program once the inflammation has settled (Fig. 42.4).[67-69]

> **PRACTICE PEARL**
>
> Corticosteroid injections should never be used in the management of tibialis posterior tendinopathy due to poor long-term outcomes and an increased risk of total tendon rupture.

The use of platelet rich plasma (PRP) injections has no biological rationale and no trial evidence (see also Chapter 17).

Surgery is recommended if there is tendon rupture (Chapter 41) or if conservative management fails to settle the condition. In the case of tenosynovitis, a synovectomy may be performed, while in cases of severe tendinopathy or tendon rupture a reconstruction may be required. There is often need for large corrective surgical treatment. This treatment is directed towards correct alignment of the heel, and may include tendon transfer, calcaneus osteotomy, and/or midfoot corrective osteotomy/arthrodesis.

One major problem with the management of tibialis posterior tendinopathy is the long time from injury to final treatment which can result from delayed presentation or delay in diagnosis.

Flexor hallucis longus tendinopathy

The flexor hallucis longus (FHL) tendon flexes the big toe and assists in plantarflexion of the ankle. It passes posterior to the medial malleolus, and runs between the two sesamoid bones to insert into the base of the distal phalanx of the big toe.

Causes

FHL tendinopathy may occur secondary to overuse, a stenosing tenosynovitis, a pseudocyst or tendon tear. The tendon tear may be partial or total. A common cause is overuse in a ballet dancer, as dancers repetitively go from flat-foot stance to the *en pointe* position when extreme plantarflexion is required. Wearing shoes that are too big and require the athlete to 'toe-grip' may also result in flexor hallucis longus tendinopathy.

Ankle pain   CHAPTER 42

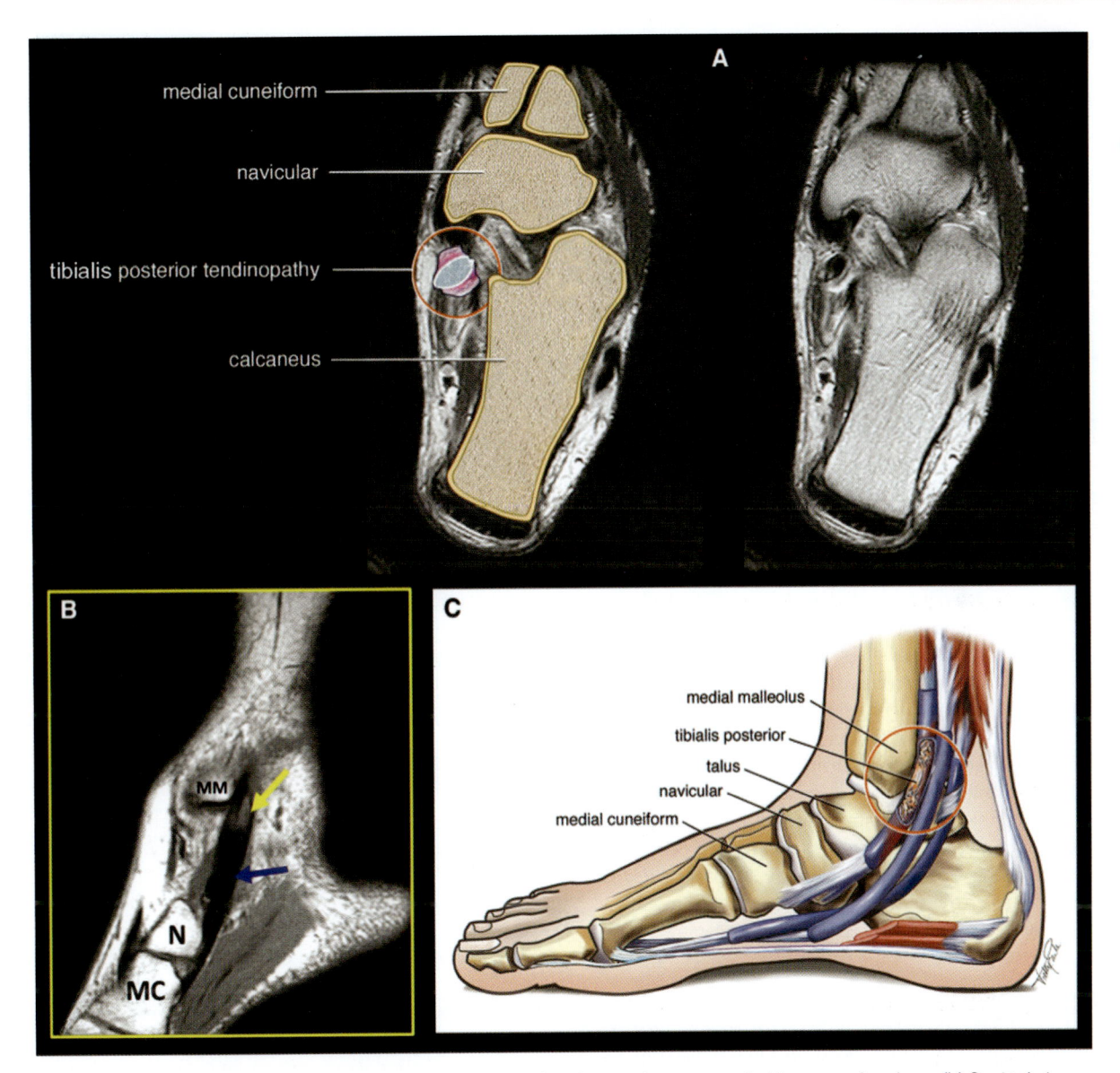

Figure 42.3 Tibialis posterior tendinopathy (a) Axial view showing tendon surrounded by area of oedema (b) Sagittal view showing abnormal (yellow arrow) and normal (blue arrow) tendon appearance (c) Anatomy

This condition is often associated with posterior impingement syndrome (Chapter 40) as the flexor hallucis tendon lies in a fibro-osseous tunnel between the lateral and medial tubercles of the posterior process of the talus. Enlargement or medial displacement of the posterior process of the talus or os trigonum compresses the flexor hallucis longus at the point where the tendon changes direction from a vertical course dorsal to the talus to a horizontal course beneath the talus (Fig. 42.5). This can cause tendon thickening and may result in 'triggering' of the tendon with loud and painful crepitation, as a consequence of partial tearing and subsequent healing of the tendon with excessive scar tissue production.

Clinical features

The clinical features of FHL tendinopathy are as follows.

- Pain is on toe-off or forefoot weight-bearing (e.g. rising in ballet), maximal over the posteromedial aspect of the medial malleolus and the calcaneus around the sustentaculum tali.
- Pain landing from jumps (key differentiator from posterior impingement syndrome)

PART B Regional problems

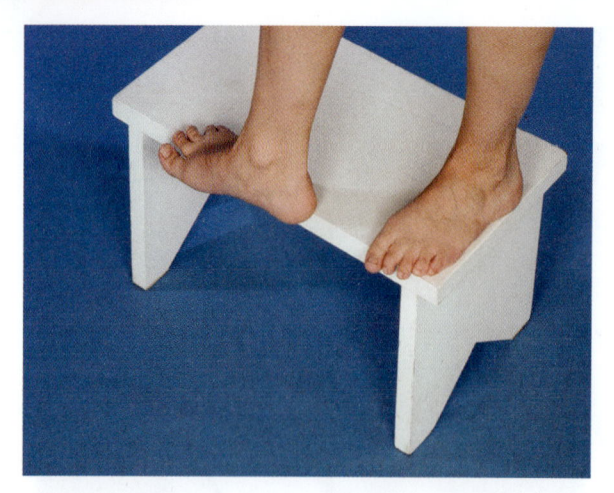

Figure 42.4 Eccentric exercises—tibialis posterior. Patient stands on the edge of a step and drops down into eversion, eccentrically contracting the tibialis posterior muscle

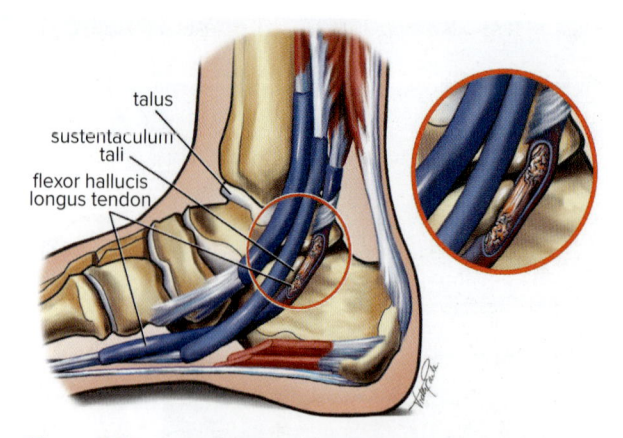

Figure 42.5 Flexor hallucis longus tendinopathy showing the tendon irritated near the medial malleolus

- Pain may be aggravated by resisted flexion (Fig 42.2b) or passive stretch into full dorsiflexion of the hallux.
- Prominent crepitus in the sheath of flexor hallucis longus
- In more severe cases, there may be 'triggering' of the first toe, both with rising onto the ball of the foot (e.g. in ballet) and in lowering from this position. Triggering occurs when the foot is placed in plantarflexion and the athlete, unable to flex the hallux, is able to extend the interphalangeal or metatarsophalangeal joints of the toe with forcible active contraction of the FHL. A snap or pop (crepitus) occurs in the posteromedial aspect of the ankle when this happens. Subsequent passive flexion or extension of the interphalangeal joint produces a painless snap posterior to the medial malleolus.

Investigations
MRI and ultrasound may both reveal pathology. However, the diagnosis is primarily based on clinical signs as the correlation between imaging findings and symptoms is often limited. The characteristic MRI sign (Fig. 42.6) in the case of tendon pathology, such as partial rupture, is abrupt fluid cut-off in the tendon sheath; excessive fluid is found located around a normal-appearing tendon proximal to the fibro-osseous canal.[70]

Treatment
In the acute phase, treatment may include:[65]

- ice
- avoidance of activities that stress the flexor hallucis longus tendon (e.g. dancer working at the barre but not rising *en pointe*)
- flexor hallucis longus strengthening and stretching exercises

- soft tissue therapy to the proximal muscle belly
- correction of subtalar joint and 1st MTP joint hypomobility with manual mobilisation and orthoses
- control of excessive pronation during toe-off with tape or orthoses–this may be helpful but is difficult to achieve in dancers.

> **PRACTICE PEARL**
>
> To prevent recurrences of FHL tendinopathy, the dancer should focus on slightly reducing the amount of hip turnout thus ensuring that the weight is directly over the hip, avoiding hard floors, and using firm, well-fitting pointe shoes, so that the foot is well supported and no additional strain is placed on the tendon. Technique correction is important in ballet dancers as the tendinopathy arises not only from excessive ankle eversion or inversion with pointe work, but also from proximal weakness, such as poor trunk control.[65]

If symptoms persist after consultation with an expert ballet clinician, surgical treatment should be considered when persistent synovitis or triggering prevents dancing. Arthroscopic surgery involves exploration of the tendon and release of the tendon sheath with a posterior approach. The fibrous band around the tendon is cleaned off and the tendon released. Progressive return to ballet after such surgery takes in the order of 2–3 months.

Tarsal tunnel syndrome
Tarsal tunnel syndrome occurs as a result of entrapment of the posterior tibial nerve in the tarsal tunnel where

Ankle pain CHAPTER 42

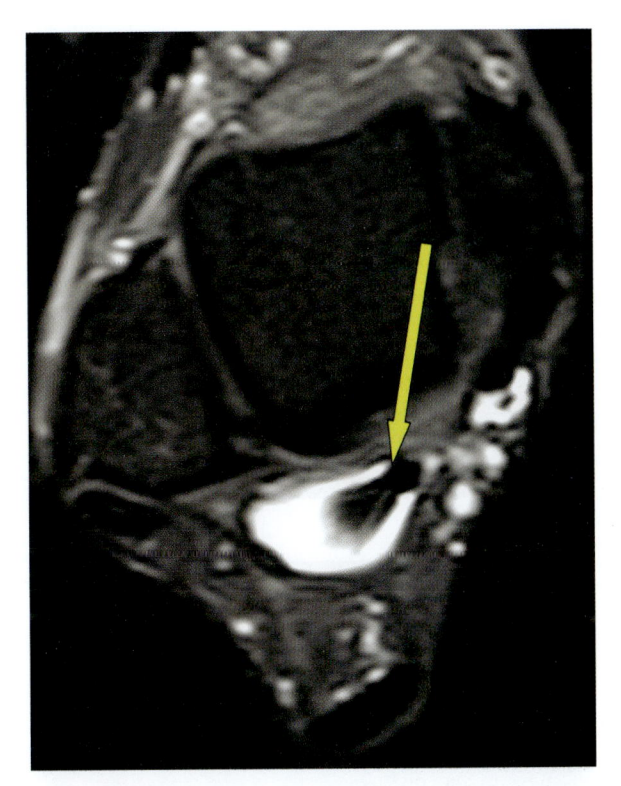

Figure 42.6 Flexor hallucis longus tendinopathy. Axial short tau inversion recovery (STIR) MRI demonstrates a large amount of fluid along the flexor hallucis longus at the level of the myotendinous junction (arrow)

the nerve winds around the medial malleolus.[72] It may also involve only one of its terminal branches distal to the tarsal tunnel. In such cases, the clinical presentation is pain in the medial part of the heel and sensory disturbance in the same region.

Causes

In approximately 50% of cases, the cause of tarsal tunnel syndrome is idiopathic. It may also occur as a result of trauma (e.g. inversion injury to the ankle, direct blow to the ankle with significant bleeding) or overuse associated with excessive pronation. Other less common causes include:

- ganglion
- talonavicular coalition
- varicose veins
- synovial cyst
- lipoma
- accessory muscle–flexor digitorum accessorius longus
- tenosynovitis; often associated with arthritis (sero-negative rheumatoid arthritis)
- fracture of the distal tibia or calcaneus.

Clinical features

The clinical features of tarsal tunnel syndrome are as follows.

- Poorly defined burning, tingling or numb sensation on the plantar aspect of the foot, often radiating into the toes.
- Pain is usually aggravated by activity and relieved by rest. The location of the pain can be diffuse and poorly defined.
- In some patients, the symptoms are worse in bed at night, and relieved by getting up and moving, or massaging the foot.
- Swellings, varicosities or thickenings may be found on examination around the medial ankle or heel.
- A ganglion or cyst may be palpable in the tendon sheaths around the medial ankle.
- Tenderness in the region of the tarsal tunnel is common.
- Tapping over the posterior tibial nerve (Tinel's sign) may elicit the patient's pain and very occasionally cause fasciculations; however, this 'classic' sign is not commonly seen.
- There may be altered sensation along the arch of the foot.
- The distribution of the sensory changes in the foot needs to be differentiated from the typical dermatomal distribution of S1 nerve root compression.

Investigations

Nerve conduction studies should be performed.[66, 67] These not only help to confirm the diagnosis but they can also guide the surgeon as to the location of the nerve compression. However, it must be borne in mind that tarsal tunnel syndrome is primarily a clinical diagnosis and nerve conduction studies are negative in approximately 50% of patients. Ultrasound or MRI may be required to assess for a space-occupying lesion as a cause of the syndrome. A plain radiograph and, if required, a computed tomography (CT) scan should be performed in the case of excessive pronation or if a tarsal coalition is suspected.

Differential diagnoses

Differential diagnoses include entrapment of the medial and/or lateral plantar nerves (or both), plantar fasciopathy, intervertebral disc degeneration and other causes of nerve inflammation or degeneration. The diagnosis of tarsal tunnel is often difficult and the symptoms and signs are often vague.[68] This is important to bear in mind, at least before deciding on surgical intervention.

Treatment

Non-surgical treatment should be attempted in those with either an idiopathic or biomechanical cause. If neurodynamic tests prove positive, then appropriate gliding treatments are indicated (Chapter 17). If excessive pronation is present, initially taping, and if successful an orthosis, may be required.

Surgical decompression of the posterior tibial nerve and its branches may be indicated in selected cases, but only after both the diagnosis and site of nerve entrapment have been confirmed.

> **PRACTICE PEARL**
>
> Surgery should be reserved as the last resort, if all other treatment fails, symptoms are severe and the clinician is confident of mechanical pressure on the nerve. Results of surgery have not been encouraging,[69] with a high perioperative complication rate.[70]

Medial malleolar stress fracture

Medial malleolar stress fractures are rare, but should be considered in runners or footballers presenting with persistent medial ankle pain aggravated by activity.[73] Although the fracture line is frequently vertical from the junction of the tibial plafond and the medial malleolus, it may arch obliquely from the junction to the distal tibial metaphysis.

Clinical features

Athletes with medial malleolus stress fractures typically present with anterior and medial ankle pain that progressively increases with running and jumping activities. The onset of pain may be acute or gradual. Examination reveals tenderness overlying the medial malleolus, frequently in conjunction with a mild ankle effusion.

Investigations

In the early stages, X-rays may be normal, but with time a linear area of hyperlucency may be apparent, progressing to a lytic area and fracture line (Fig. 42.7a). If the X-ray is normal, an MRI is recommended (Fig. 42.7b).

Treatment

For most fractures 4-6 weeks NWB in a CAM boot is required. Following fracture healing, the practitioner should assess biomechanics and footwear. A graduated return to activity follows and usually takes around 12 weeks.[74] In the case of complete fracture, surgical intervention with internal screw fixation (percutaneous screw fixation) followed by immobilisation in plaster for 3 weeks and air-cast for a further 3 weeks is advisable. A recent systematic review showed that non-operative and operative interventions have proven to be successful with regard to healing and return to play for medial malleolar stress fractures in the recreational and competitive athlete.[75] However, early operative intervention can possibly create a higher likelihood of early healing, decrease in symptoms, and return to play.

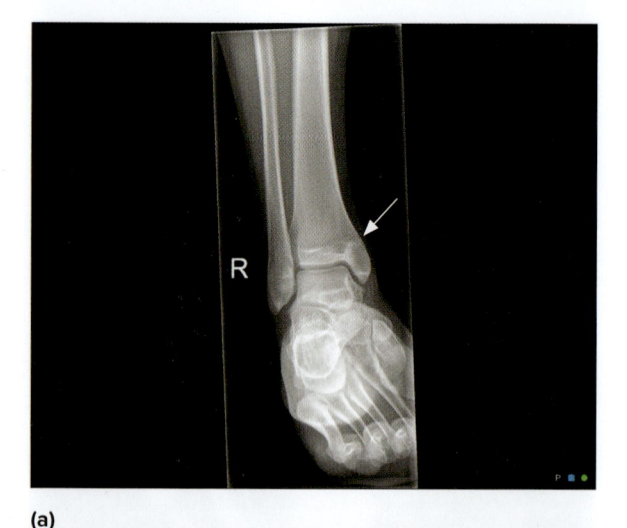

Figure 42.7 Medial malleolar stress fracture (a) X-ray showing sclerotic line (arrow) through medial malleolus indicating a stress fracture (b) MRI. Fat suppressed T2-weighted image showing bright T2 signal (arrow) at the site of the stress fracture

Medial calcaneal nerve entrapment

The medial calcaneal nerve is a branch of the posterior tibial nerve arising at the level of the medial malleolus or below, and passing superficially to innervate the skin of the heel. Occasionally it may arise from the lateral plantar nerve, a branch of the posterior tibial nerve. It has been theorised that a valgus hindfoot may predispose joggers to compression of this nerve branch. This nerve entrapment is often termed 'Baxter's nerve' (see Chapter 43).

Clinical features

Entrapment or irritation of the nerve causes burning pain over the infero-medial aspect of the calcaneus, which often radiates into the arch of the foot, and is aggravated by running. Examination reveals tenderness over the medial calcaneus and a positive Tinel's sign. There is frequently associated excessive pronation of the hindfoot.

Investigations

The diagnosis may be difficult to establish. Nerve conduction studies can be helpful, and injection of local anaesthetic at the point of maximal tenderness with a resultant disappearance of pain will help confirm the diagnosis.

Treatment

Treatment involves minimising the trauma to the nerve with a change of footwear or the use of a pad over the area to protect the nerve. If this is not successful, injection of corticosteroid and local anaesthetic into the area of point tenderness may be helpful. If this fails to settle, other treatment options include radiofrequency denervation (RFD) of the nerve and surgical decompression.[76]

Other causes of medial ankle pain

Two conditions that generally cause foot pain, but may present as medial ankle pain, are stress fractures of the calcaneus and the navicular bone (Chapter 43). Referred pain from neural structures may occasionally present as medial ankle pain. Entrapment of the medial plantar nerve (Chapter 43) generally causes midfoot pain, but may present as medial ankle pain.

LATERAL ANKLE PAIN

Non-traumatic lateral ankle pain is generally associated with a biomechanical abnormality. The two most common diagnoses are peroneal tendinopathy and sinus tarsi syndrome. The causes of lateral ankle pain are listed in Table 42.3. The anatomy of the region is illustrated in Figure 42.8.

Examination

Examination is as for the patient with acute ankle injury (Chapter 41) with particular attention to testing resisted eversion of the peroneal tendons (Fig. 42.9a) and careful palpation for tenderness, swelling and crepitus (Fig. 42.9b).

Peroneal tendinopathy

The most common overuse injury causing lateral ankle pain is peroneus brevis tendinopathy. The peroneus longus and peroneus brevis tendons cross the ankle joint within a fibro-osseous tunnel, posterior to the lateral malleolus (Fig 42.8a). The peroneus brevis tendon inserts into the tuberosity on the lateral aspect of the base of the fifth metatarsal. The peroneus longus tendon passes under the plantar surface of the foot to insert into the lateral side of the base of the first metatarsal and medial cuneiform. The peroneal tendons share a common tendon sheath proximal to the distal tip of the fibula, after which they have their own tendon sheaths. The peroneal muscles serve as ankle dorsiflexors in addition to being the primary evertors of the ankle.

Causes

Peroneal tendinopathy may occur either as a result of acute or recurrent ankle inversion injuries, or as an overuse injury. Soft footwear may predispose to the development of peroneal tendinopathy.

Common causes of an overuse injury to the peroneal tendons include:

- excessive eversion of the foot, such as occurs when running on a cambered surface[77]
- excessive pronation of the foot
- secondary to tight ankle plantarflexors (most commonly soleus) resulting in excessive load on the lateral muscles
- excessive loading of the peroneals (e.g. dancing, basketball, volleyball).

An inflammatory arthropathy may promote peroneal tenosynovitis and subsequent peroneal tendinopathy. Peroneal tendinopathy may also be due to the excessive pulley action and abrupt change in direction of the peroneal tendons at the lateral malleolus. In some cases, peroneal tendinopathy is correlated with peroneal tendon instability in the retromalleolar groove of the lateral malleolus.

There are three main sites of peroneal tendinopathy:

1. posterior to the lateral malleolus (most common)
2. at the peroneal trochlea
3. at the plantar surface of the cuboid.

Clinical features

The athlete commonly presents with:

- lateral ankle or heel pain which is aggravated by activity and relieved by rest
- local tenderness of the peroneal tendons, sometimes associated with swelling and crepitus (a true paratenonitis)

PART B Regional problems

Table 42.3 **Causes of lateral ankle pain**

Common	Less common	Not to be missed
Peroneal tendinopathy Sinus tarsi syndrome	Impingement syndrome • Anterolateral • Posterior Recurrent subluxation/dislocation of peroneal tendons Stress fracture of the talus Referred pain • Lumbar spine • Peroneal nerve • Superior tibiofibular joint	Stress fracture of the distal fibula Cuboid syndrome Complex regional pain syndrome type 1 (following knee or ankle trauma)

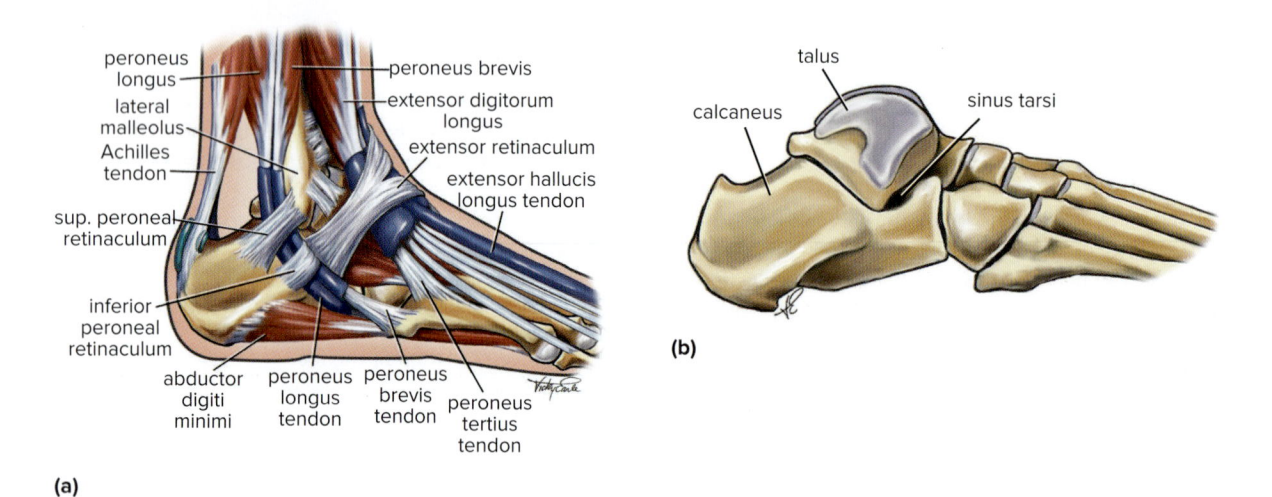

Figure 42.8 Lateral aspect of the ankle (a) Anatomy of the lateral ankle (b) Sinus tarsi

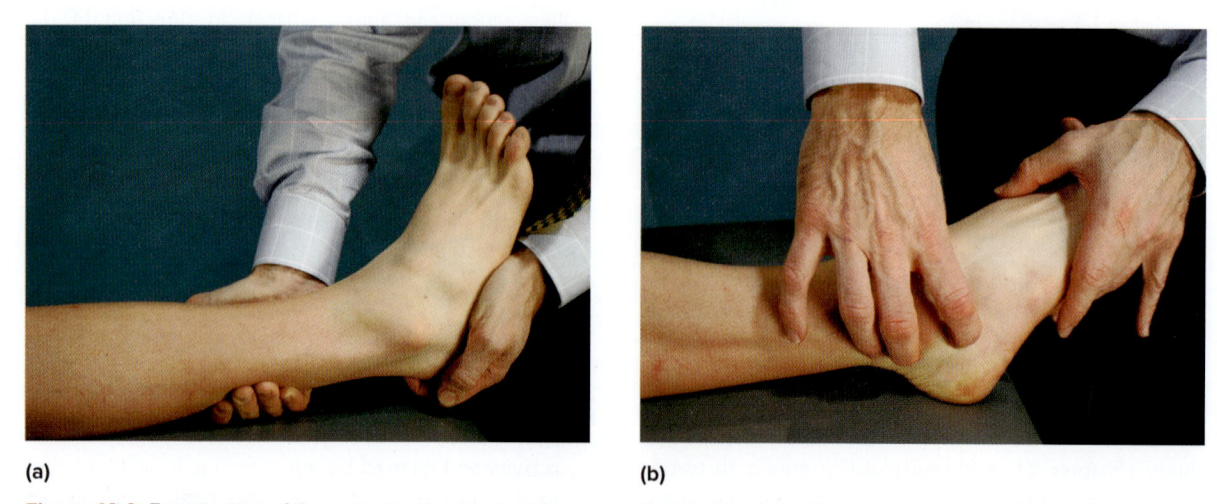

Figure 42.9 Examination of the patient with lateral ankle pain (a) Resisted movement—eversion (peroneal muscles) (b) Palpation—the peroneal tendons are palpated for tenderness and crepitus

Ankle pain CHAPTER 42

- painful passive inversion and resisted eversion, although in some cases eccentric contraction may be required to reproduce the pain
- calf muscle tightness
- excessive subtalar pronation or stiffness of the subtalar or midtarsal joints that is demonstrated on biomechanical examination.

Investigations

MRI is the recommended investigation and shows characteristic features of tendinopathy–increased signal and tendon thickening (Fig. 42.10)–and may show longitudinal tears.[78] If MRI is unavailable, ultrasound provides similarly good results. If an underlying inflammatory arthropathy is suspected, blood tests should be obtained to assess for rheumatological and inflammatory markers.

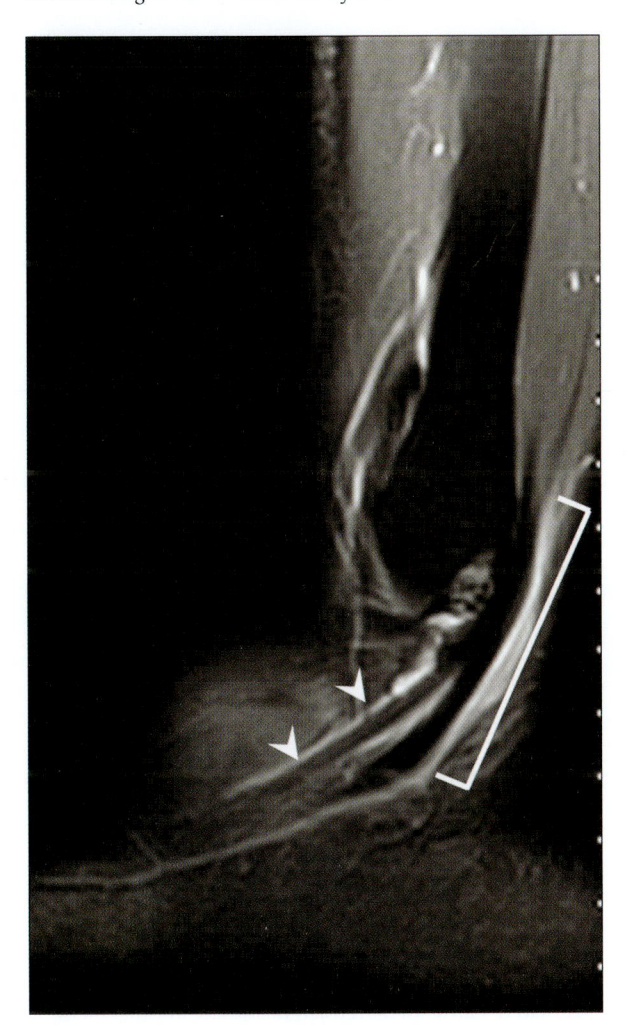

Figure 42.10 Peroneal tendinopathy. MRI showing oedema around the peroneus longus (bracket) and peroneus brevis (arrowheads)

Treatment

Treatment initially involves:

- rest from weight-bearing and loading activities; the use of a controlled ankle motion (CAM) boot may be required
- if a reactive tendinopathy is present, NSAIDs and regular icing
- soft tissue therapy to the peroneal muscles
- mobilisation of the ankle, subtalar and midtarsal joints
- footwear assessment: the use of lateral heel wedges or orthoses may also be required to correct biomechanical abnormalities
- strengthening exercises: should be introduced once the pain and inflammation has settled and should include resisted eversion (e.g. rubber tubing, rotagym), especially in plantarflexion as this position maximally engages the peroneal muscles.

PRP injections may be considered as an adjunct to a comprehensive rehabilitation program; however, there is currently little supporting evidence. In severe cases, or with failure of conservative management, surgery may be required, which may involve a synovectomy, tendon debridement, or repair of the tendon in case of longitudinal rupture.[79] If peroneal tendinopathy is associated with tendon instability, ligament reconstruction should address the instability of the tendon at the same time as the tendon is repaired.

Sinus tarsi syndrome

The sinus tarsi (Fig. 42.6b) is a small osseous canal running from an opening anterior and inferior to the lateral malleolus in a posteromedial direction to a point posterior to the medial malleolus. The interosseous ligament occupies the sinus tarsi and divides it into an anterior portion, which is part of the talocalcaneonavicular joint, and a posterior part, which represents the subtalar joint. It is lined by a synovial membrane and in addition to the ligament it contains small blood vessels, fat and connective tissue.

The sinus tarsi contains abundant synovial tissue that is prone to synovitis and inflammation when injured. An influx of inflammatory cells may result in the development of a low-grade and long-standing inflammatory synovitis. Although injury to the sinus tarsi may result from chronic overuse secondary to poor biomechanics (especially excessive pronation), approximately 70% of all patients with sinus tarsi syndrome have had a single or repeated inversion injury to the ankle. It may also occur after repeated forced eversion to the ankle, such as high jump take off. Other causes of sinus tarsi syndrome may include chronic inflammation in conditions such as gout, inflammatory arthropathies and osteoarthritis.

PART B Regional problems

Clinical features
The symptoms of sinus tarsi syndrome include:

- pain which may be poorly localised and vague but is most often centred just anterior to the lateral malleolus
- pain that is often more severe in the morning and may diminish with exercise
- pain that may be exacerbated by running on a curve in the direction of the affected ankle; the patient may also complain of ankle and foot stiffness, a feeling of instability of the hindfoot and occasionally of weakness
- difficulty–often marked–walking on uneven ground
- full range of pain-free ankle movement on examination but the subtalar joint may be stiff
- pain on forced passive eversion of the subtalar joint; forced passive inversion may also be painful due to damage to the subtalar ligaments
- tenderness of the lateral aspect of the ankle at the opening of the sinus tarsi and occasionally also over the anterior talofibular ligament; there may be minor localised swelling.

Investigations
MRI may show an increased signal and fluid in the sinus tarsi, but is not often helpful. The most appropriate diagnostic test is injection of 1 mL of a short-acting local anaesthetic agent (e.g. 1% lignocaine [lidocaine]) into the sinus tarsi; ideally this should be done using fluoroscopy to ensure correct location (Fig. 42.11). In sinus tarsi syndrome, this injection will relieve pain so that functional tests, such as hopping on the affected leg, can be performed comfortably (for diagnosis). An ankle radiograph may be performed to exclude degenerative changes of the subtalar joint.

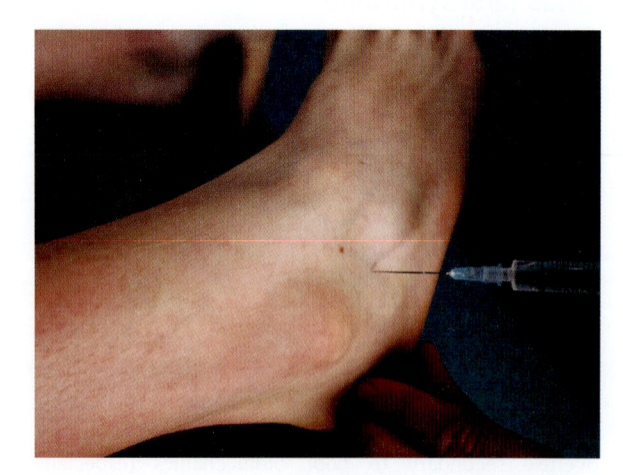

Figure 42.11 Diagnostic local anaesthetic injection under fluoroscopic guidance. The needle is introduced into the lateral opening of the sinus tarsi with the foot in passive inversion. The needle should be directed medially and slightly posteriorly. Corticosteroid can be added if treatment required

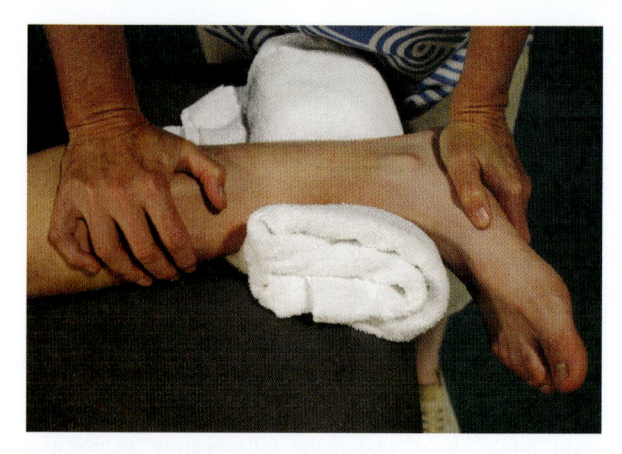

Figure 42.12 Mobilisation of the subtalar joint is performed by medial-to-lateral transverse glide of the calcaneus on the talus

Treatment
Surgery is rarely indicated. Non-surgical management includes:

- relative rest
- short-term use of NSAIDs and ice
- mobilisation of the subtalar joint; this is essential (Fig. 42.12)
- direct infiltration of the sinus tarsi with corticosteroid (Fig. 42.11)
- correction of footwear and biomechanics
- proprioception and strength training.

Anterolateral impingement
Repeated minor ankle sprains or a major sprain involving the anterolateral aspect of the ankle may cause anterolateral impingement. An inversion sprain to the anterior talofibular ligament may promote synovial thickening. Usually this is subsequently resorbed, but sometimes this is incomplete and the residual tissue becomes hyalinised and moulded by pressure from the articular surfaces of the lateral aspect of the talus and lateral malleolus, where it may be trapped during ankle movements. A meniscoid lesion thus develops in the anterolateral gutter. Another postulated cause of anterolateral ankle impingement is chondromalacia of the lateral wall of the talus with an associated synovial reaction.

Clinical features
The classic presentation is pain at the anterior aspect of the lateral malleolus and an intermittent catching sensation in the ankle in an athlete with a previous history of ankle inversion injuries.

Examination may reveal tenderness in the region of the anteroinferior border of the fibula and anterolateral surface of the talus. End range dorsiflexion, such as in a lunge position, is often reduced and painful. Proprioception may be poor.[80]

Investigations
Clinical assessment is more reliable than MRI to diagnose this lesion.[81] An arthroscopic examination confirms the diagnosis.

Treatment
In milder cases corticosteroid injection into the anterolateral gutter combined with physiotherapy and correction of biomechanics may be helpful. In more severe cases arthroscopic removal of the fibrotic, meniscoid lesion is required. Results after arthroscopic removal of the impinged tissue are encouraging and soccer players often return to sport after a short period (3-4 weeks) of rehabilitation. Surprisingly for a condition that limits dorsiflexion, it takes ballet dancers about 3 months to regain full pointe position (plantarflexion) after this operation.

Posterior impingement syndrome
Posterior impingement syndrome sometimes presents as lateral ankle pain, but more commonly as pain in the posterior ankle (Chapter 40).

Stress fracture of the talus
Stress fractures of the posterolateral aspect of the talus have been described in track and field athletes, triathletes, Australian rules footballers,[82] elite female gymnasts[83] and a soccer player.[84]

Causes
These stress fractures may develop secondary to excessive subtalar pronation and plantarflexion, resulting in impingement of the lateral process of the calcaneus on the posterolateral corner of the talus. In pole vaulters, this injury is usually acute and is attributed to 'planting' the pole too late.

Clinical features
The main symptom is that of lateral ankle pain of gradual onset, made worse by running and weight-bearing. Clinical examination reveals marked tenderness and occasionally swelling in the region of the sinus tarsi or posterior aspect of the ankle.

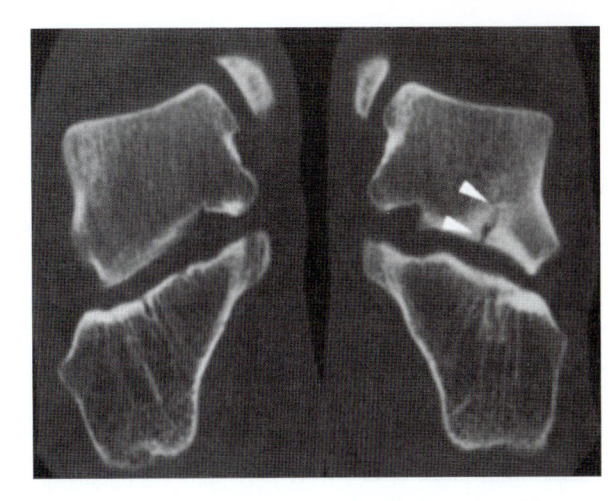

Figure 42.13 Stress fracture of the talus (arrowheads) demonstrated by coronal CT scan

Investigations
Typical CT scan appearance is shown in Figure 42.13. MRI will also reveal the fracture, with the STIR sequence being most helpful (see Chapter 15).

Treatment
Treatment requires 6-8 weeks non weight-bearing immobilisation and then a supervised graduated rehabilitation. In elite athletes, when a rapid recovery is required, or in the case of failure of non-surgical management, surgical removal of the lateral process has been performed.

> **PRACTICE PEARL**
>
> As talar stress fractures are frequently associated with excessive pronation, biomechanical correction with orthoses is required before activity is resumed.

Referred pain
A variation of the slump test (Chapter 15) with the ankle in plantarflexion and inversion can be performed to detect increased mechanosensitivity in the peroneal nerve. If the test is positive, this position can be used as a glide or stretch in addition to soft tissue therapy to possible areas of restriction (e.g. around the head of the fibula).

PART B Regional problems

ANTERIOR ANKLE PAIN

Pain over the anterior aspect of the ankle joint without a history of acute injury is usually due to either tibialis anterior tendinopathy or anterior impingement of the ankle. The surface anatomy of the anterior ankle is shown in Figure 42.14.

Anterior impingement of the ankle

Anterior impingement of the ankle joint (anterior tibiotalar impingement) is a condition in which additional soft or bony tissue is trapped between the tibia and talus during dorsiflexion. This may be the cause of chronic ankle pain or may result in pain and disability persisting after an ankle sprain. Although this syndrome has been called 'footballer's ankle', it is also seen commonly in basketballers and ballet dancers.

Anterior impingement occurs secondary to the development of exostoses (bone spurs) on the anterior rim of the tibia and on the upper anterior surface of the neck of talus (Fig. 42.15). The exostoses were initially described in ballet dancers and thought to be secondary to a traction injury of the joint capsule of the ankle that occurs whenever the foot was repeatedly forced into extreme plantarflexion. Subsequently, the development of the exostoses has been attributed to direct osseous impingement during extremes of dorsiflexion, as occurs with kicking in football and the *plié* (lunge) in ballet. As these exostoses become larger, they impinge on overlying soft tissue and cause pain.

Ligamentous injury and instability following ankle inversion injuries may also result in anterior ankle impingement; it has been shown that the distal fascicle of the anterior inferior tibiofibular ligament may impinge on the anterolateral aspect of the talus.[85]

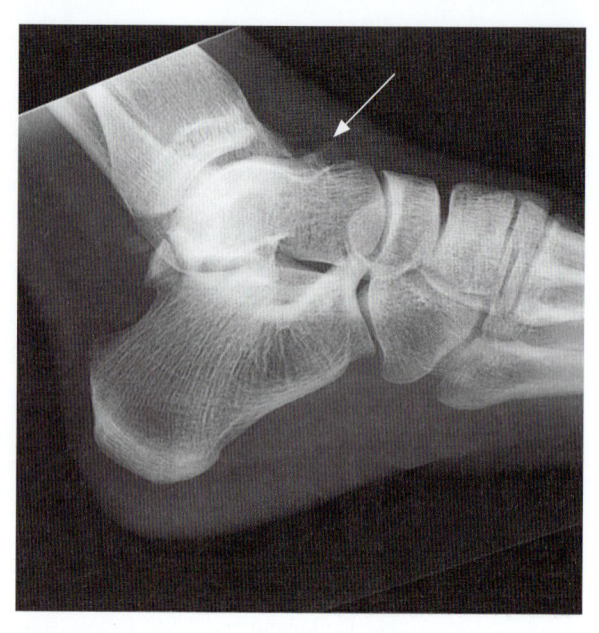

Figure 42.15 X-ray showing bony exostosis on the anterior talus

Clinical features

The patient complains of:

- anterior ankle pain, which initially starts as a vague discomfort
- pain ultimately becomes sharper and more localised to the anterior aspect of the ankle and foot, especially on dorsiflexion of the foot
- pain that is worse with activity, particularly with running, descending *plié* (lunge) in classical ballet, kicking in football or other activities involving dorsiflexion.

As the impingement develops, the patient complains of ankle stiffness, a limitation of *plié*, and in athletes a loss of take-off speed.

Examination reveals tenderness along the anterior margin of the talocrural joint. If the exostoses are

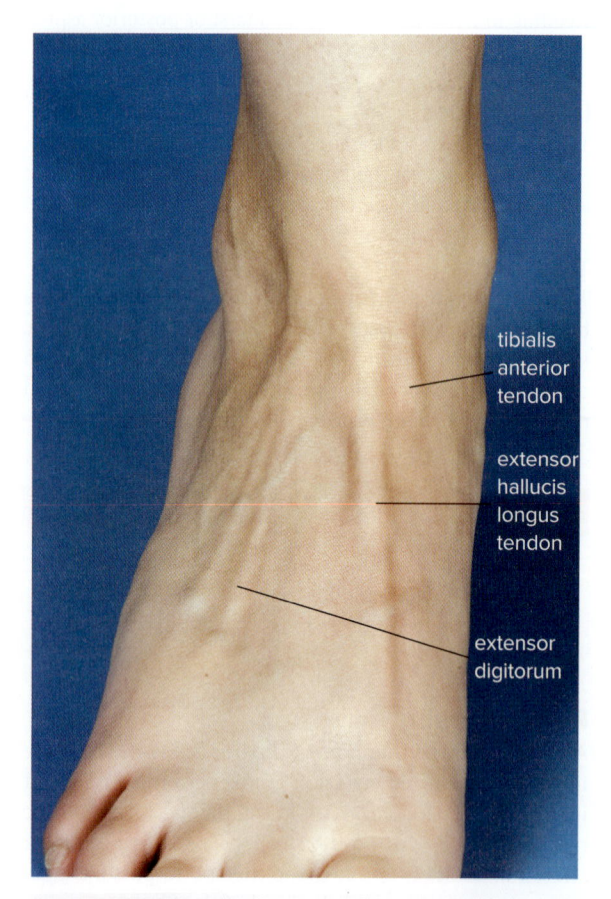

Figure 42.14 Surface anatomy of the anterior ankle showing tendons

(labels: tibialis anterior tendon, extensor hallucis longus tendon, extensor digitorum)

Ankle pain   CHAPTER 42

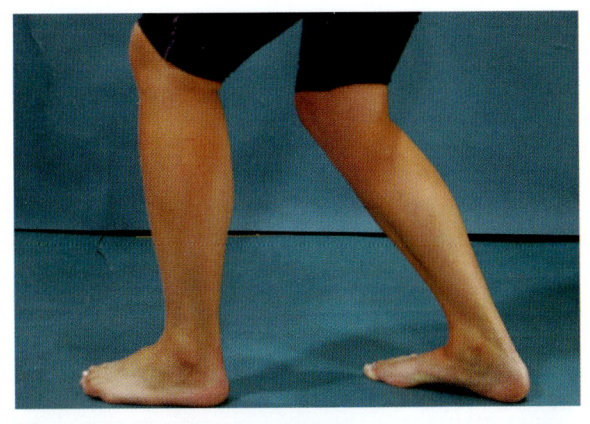

(a)

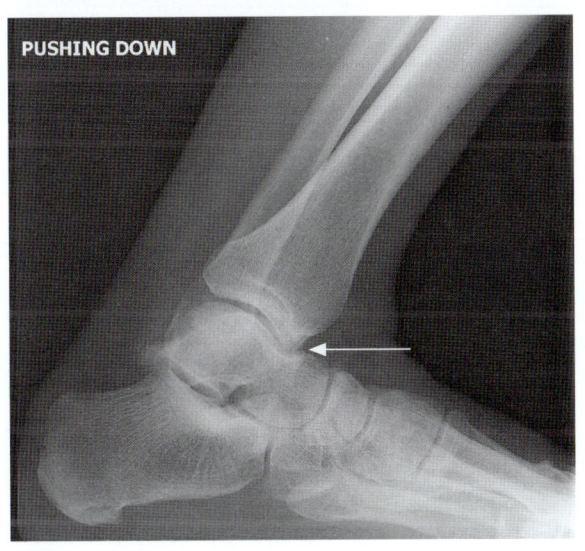

(b)

Figure 42.16 The anterior impingement test (a) The patient lunges forwards maximally and, if this reproduces the pain, the test is positive and suggests the diagnosis of anterior impingement (b) The same position is used to take a lateral X-ray. A positive test reveals bone-on-bone impingement (arrowed) when the patient adopts the lunge position that reproduces pain

large, they may occasionally be palpable. Dorsiflexion of the ankle is restricted and painful. The anterior impingement test (Fig. 42.16a), where the patient lunges forwards maximally with the heel remaining on the floor, reproduces the pain.

Investigations
Lateral X-rays in flexion and extension show both exostoses and abnormal tibiotalar contact. Ideally performed weight-bearing in the lunge position, bone-on-bone impingement confirms the diagnosis (Fig. 42.16b).

Treatment
In milder cases, non-surgical treatment consists of a heel lift, rest, modification of activities to limit dorsiflexion, NSAIDs and manual therapy, including accessory anteroposterior glides of the talocrural joint at the end of range of dorsiflexion. Taping or orthoses may help control the pain if they restrict ankle dorsiflexion or improve joint instability, which has been shown to contribute to the development of anterior impingement.[86]

More prominent exostoses may require arthroscopic removal. The clinical results after arthroscopic removal are encouraging, and the majority of patients become pain-free with increased range of ankle motion.[87-89]

Tibialis anterior tendinopathy
The tibialis anterior tendon is the primary dorsiflexor of the foot, in addition to adducting and supinating (inverting) the foot. It passes medially over the anterior ankle joint and runs to insert into the medial and plantar aspects of the medial cuneiform bone and the adjacent base of the first metatarsal.

Causes
Tendinopathy of the tibialis anterior may result from overuse of the ankle dorsiflexors secondary to restriction in joint range of motion, as may occur with a stiff ankle. It may also be due to downhill running, playing racquet sports involving constant change of direction, or with excessive tightness of strapping or shoelaces over the tibialis anterior tendon.

Clinical features
The main symptoms are pain, swelling and stiffness in the anterior ankle. These symptoms are aggravated by activity, especially running, and walking up hills or stairs. On examination, there is localised tenderness, swelling and occasionally crepitus along the tibialis anterior tendon, especially over the anterior joint line. There is pain on resisted dorsiflexion and eccentric inversion. Long-standing and non-treated tendinopathy may eventually lead to partial or even total rupture of the tendon (under the extensor retinaculum).

Investigations
Ultrasound or MRI may be used to confirm the diagnosis and assess the severity of the tenosynovitis/tendinopathy.

Treatment
Treatment involves:

- rest from weight-bearing and loading activities
- the use of a CAM boot, if required

935

PART B   Regional problems

- if reactive tendinopathy present, NSAIDs and regular icing in the short term
- soft tissue therapy focusing on the tibialis anterior muscle in conjunction with ankle and subtalar joint mobilisation
- reducing running stride length; taking shorter steps decreases the functional length of the tibialis anterior and subsequently reduces the pull of the muscle on the tibia
- correction of biomechanics with the use of footwear and orthoses, if required
- eccentric strengthening and proprioception, required once the pain has settled.

In case of partial or total rupture, surgical reconstruction may be required.

Anterior inferior tibiofibular ligament (AITFL) injury

This injury is discussed in Chapter 41 because it results from an acute ankle injury (and often a fracture). If missed, it will present as persistent pain and loss of function after an ankle sprain.

REFERENCES

References for this chapter can be found at www.mhhe.com/au/CSM5e

Chapter 43

Foot pain

with KARL LANDORF, STEPHEN SIMONS, CHRISTOPHER JORDAN and MICHAEL RATHLEFF

Plantar fasciitis sucks. It feels like you have needles underneath your feet while you're playing.
Joakim Noah, NBA Chicago Bulls, 2013

Injuries to the foot, both acute and chronic, can be extremely challenging for the clinician, largely due to the complex anatomy (Figs 43.1 and 43.2). If the foot is considered in its three distinct regions (Fig. 43.1)– the rearfoot (calcaneus and talus), the midfoot (the navicular proximally and medially, the cuboid laterally, and the cuneiforms distally and medially), and the forefoot (the metatarsals and phalanges)–the bony anatomy is greatly simplified. Soft tissue anatomy can then be superimposed on the regional division of the foot (Figs 43.2c-e).

In this chapter we will consider the three different clinical presentations:

- rearfoot pain (mainly the heel)
- midfoot pain
- forefoot pain.

REARFOOT PAIN

The most common cause of rearfoot (inferior heel) pain is plantar fasciopathy/fasciitis, often mistakenly referred to as 'heel spur'. This condition occurs mainly in runners and the older adults, and may be associated with a biomechanical abnormality, such as excessive pronation or supination.[1] Another common cause of heel pain is fat pad syndrome or fat pad contusion. This is also known as a 'bruised heel' or a 'stone bruise'.

Less common causes of heel pain are stress fracture of the calcaneus and conditions that refer pain to this area such as tarsal tunnel syndrome or medial calcaneal nerve entrapment (Chapter 42). Causes of rearfoot pain are listed in Table 43.1.

History

The pain of plantar fasciopathy is usually of insidious onset, whereas fat pad damage may occur either as a result of a single traumatic episode (e.g. jumping from a height onto the heel) or from repeated heel strike (e.g. on hard surfaces with inadequate heel support). Plantar fasciopathy pain is typically worse in the morning, improves with exercise at first and is aggravated by standing.

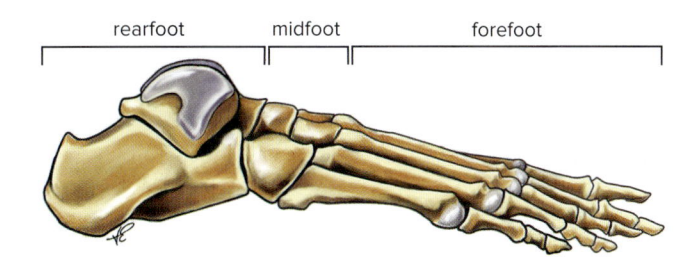

Figure 43.1 The regions of the foot: rearfoot, midfoot and forefoot

PART B Regional problems

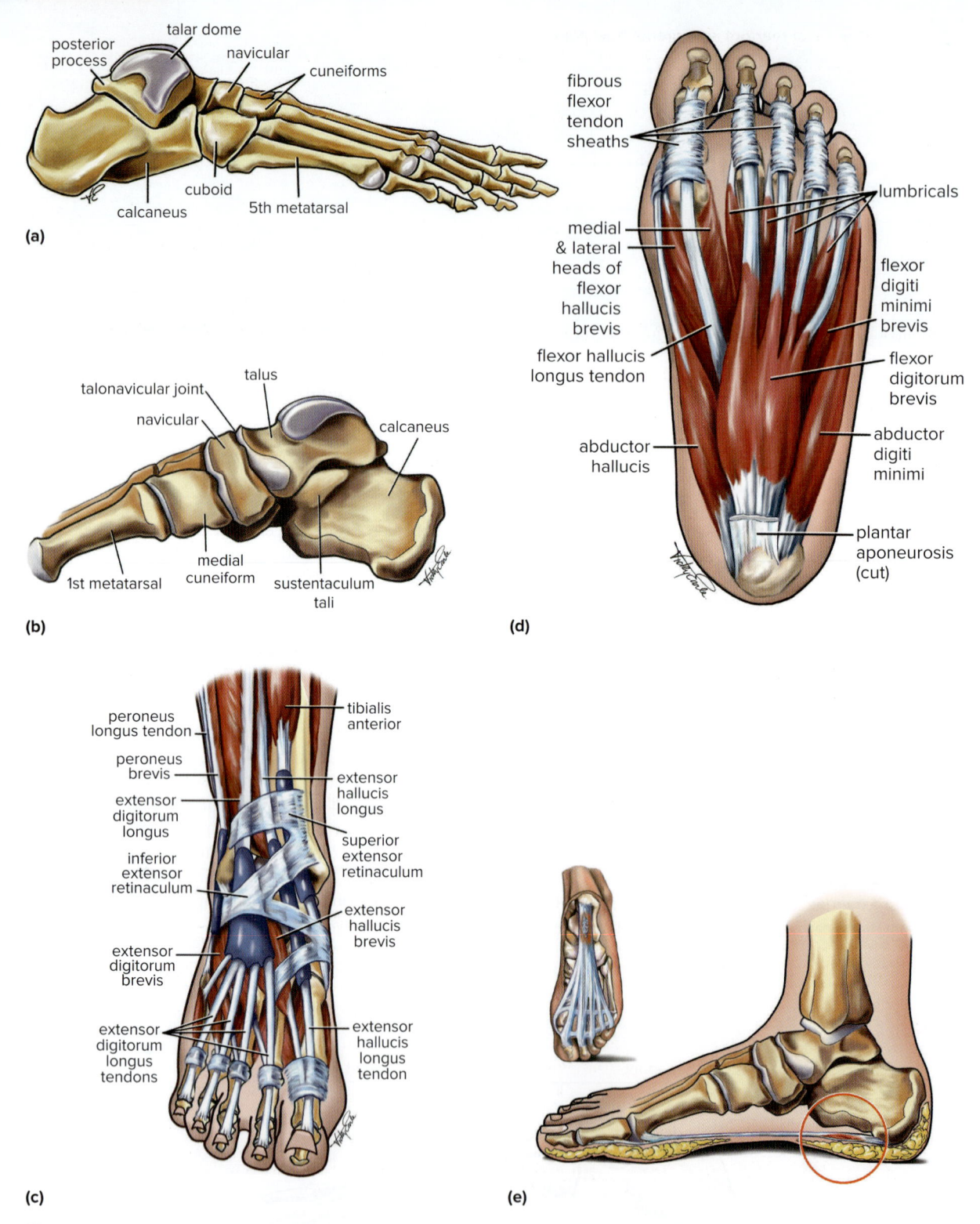

Figure 43.2 Anatomy of the foot (a) Lateral view of the bones of the foot (b) Medial view of the bones of the foot (c) Dorsal view of the soft tissues of the foot (d) Plantar view of the soft tissues of the foot: first layer (e) Plantar fascia

Foot pain   CHAPTER 43

Table 43.1 Causes of rearfoot and inferior heel pain

Common	Less common	Not to be missed
Plantar fasciopathy (fasciitis)	Calcaneal stress fracture	Spondyloarthropathies
Fat pad contusion	Medial calcaneal nerve entrapment (Chapter 42)	Osteoid osteoma
	Lateral plantar nerve (Baxter's nerve) entrapment	Complex regional pain syndrome type 1 (after knee or ankle injury)
	Tarsal tunnel syndrome (Chapter 42)	
	Talar stress fracture (Chapter 42)	
	Retrocalcaneal bursitis (Chapter 40)	

Examination

Examination of the rearfoot is shown in Figure 43.3. The windlass (or Jack's) test (passive dorsiflexion of the first metatarsophalangeal joint that provokes pain) is a quick and highly specific test for the plantar fascia (Fig. 43.3c).[2]

Biomechanical assessment is an important component of the examination and should include ankle, subtalar and midtarsal joint range of motion. Also assess function of the forefoot and first metatarsophalangeal (MTP) joint range of motion. Examine footwear, looking for asymmetrical wear of the sole which may indicate differences in function between left and right sides.

Investigations

Radiographs only contribute to the clinical work-up of rearfoot pain in a small proportion of cases. It may reveal a calcaneal spur which is associated with increased risk of heel pain. Plain radiograph is generally normal in stress

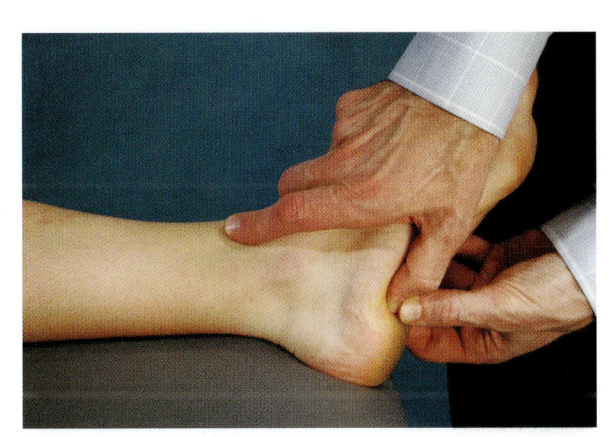

(a)

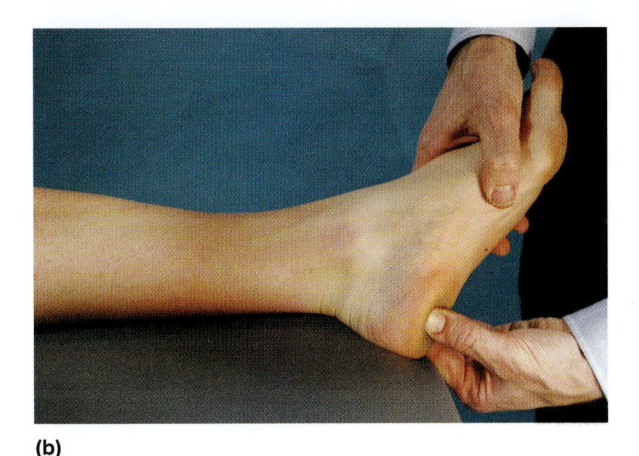

(b)

(c)

Figure 43.3 Examination of the rearfoot (a) Palpation—medial process of calcaneal tuberosity. Palpate plantar fascia attachment (b) Palpation—heel fat pad

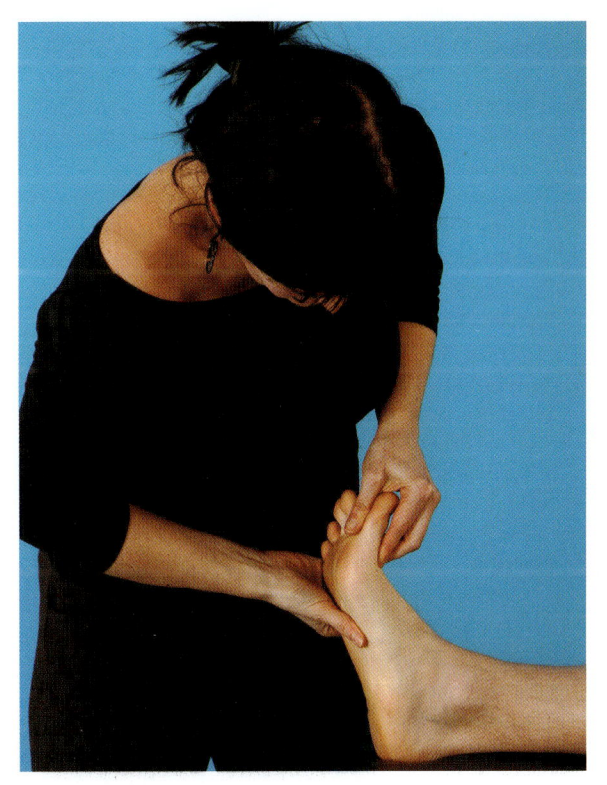

Figure 43.3 (cont.) (c) The windlass (or Jack's) test—passive dorsiflexion of the first metatarsophalangeal joint

fractures of the calcaneus, but if the injury has been present for many weeks, there may be a line of sclerosis (increased opacity).

Magnetic resonance imaging (MRI) is the investigation of choice for stress fracture. MRI and ultrasound can each confirm the presence of plantar fasciopathy. MRI reveals increased signal intensity and thickening at the attachment of the plantar fascia to the calcaneus at the medial calcaneal tuberosity, often with oedema in the adjacent bone. Ultrasound reveals a characteristic region of hypoechogenicity.

Patient-reported outcome measures

There are a number of patient-reported outcome measures (PROMs) which are relevant for patients with foot pain. Combined Foot and Ankle PROMs have been described in Chapter 42. The foot specific PROMs are shown in Table 43.2.

Table 43.2 Patient-reported outcome measures for the foot

Foot Function Index (FFI)

- Self-administered questionnaire evaluating pain, disability and activity restrictions
- 23 items (9 on pain, 9 on disability and 5 on activity limitation)
- Score range 0–100 for all subscales (100 = maximal impairment)[3]
- Test-retest reliability:
  - Total score, ICC = 0.87[3]
  - Pain subscale, ICC = 0.70[3]
  - Disability subscale, ICC = 0.84[3]
  - Activity limitation subscale, ICC = 0.81[3]
- Construct validity:
  - Pain subscale: SF-36: bodily pain subscale: –0.61; physical component summary scale: –0.45[4]
  - Disability subscale: SF-36: physical component summary scale: –0.67; physical functioning: –0.69; role-physical: –0.62; bodily pain: –0.64[4]
  - Activity limitation subscale: physical component summary scale: –0.53; physical functioning: –0.55; role-physical: –0.64; social functioning: –0.57[4]
  - Total score: SD-36; physical component summary scale: –0.64;[5] AOFAS, Hallux Metatarsophalangeal-Interphalangeal Scale: –0.81
- Developed and validated in American English[3] and there is a revised-FFI version available with 34 items[6]
- The original FFI was cross-culturally validated to Danish,[7] French,[8] German,[9] Italian,[10,11] Korean,[12] Spanish[13] and Taiwan Chinese[14]

Rowan Foot Pain Assessment Questionnaire

- Self-administered questionnaire evaluating pain in sensory, affective and cognitive dimensions
- 36 items (16 on the sensory, 10 on the affective and 10 on the cognitive dimension)
- Score ranges from 0–5 for each subscale
- Test-retest reliability:
  - Sensory subscale: Spearmans $\rho = 0.88$[15]
  - Affective subscale: Spearmans $\rho = 0.93$[15]
  - Cognitive subscale: Spearmans $\rho = 0.82$[15]
- Construct validity:
  - Sensory subscale: $FFI_{pain} = 0.88$[15]
  - Affective subscale: $FFI_{pain} = 0.69$[15]
  - Cognitive subscale: $FFI_{pain} = 0.70$[15]
- Developed and validated in English

Foot Health Status Questionnaire

- Self-administered questionnaire evaluating foot pain, foot function, footwear and general foot health
- 13 items (4 items on foot pain, 4 items on foot function, 3 items on footwear, 2 items on general foot health)
- Score range 0–100 (100 = no health problem)

- Test-retest reliability:
  - Foot pain: ICC = 0.86
  - Foot function: ICC = 0.92
  - Footwear: ICC = 0.74
  - General foot health: ICC = 0.78
- MCID:
  - Foot pain: 13[16]
  - Foot function: 7[16]
  - Footwear: 2[16]
  - General foot health: 0[16]
- Developed and validated[17] in Australian English; cross-culturally validated to Brazilian Portuguese[18] and Spanish[19]

Podiatric Health Questionnaire

- Self-administered questionnaire evaluating walking, hygiene, nail care, foot pain, worry/concern QoL and general foot status
- 6 items + 1 visual analogue scale (VAS) regarding foot status
- 6 items score range: VAS Score range 0–100 (100 = best possible foot health)
- Construct validity:
  - Walking: $EQ\text{-}5D_{mobility}$: 0.54; $EQ\text{-}5D_{usual\ activities}$: 0.45; $EQ\text{-}5D_{pain/discomfort}$: 0.49[20]
  - Hygiene: $EQ\text{-}5D_{self\text{-}care}$: 0.58[20]
  - Nail care: $EQ\text{-}5D_{self\text{-}care}$: 0.37[20]
  - Foot pain: $EQ\text{-}5D_{pain/discomfort}$: 0.40[20]
  - Worry/concern: $EQ\text{-}5D_{anxiety/depression}$: 0.21[20]
  - Quality of life: $EQ\text{-}5D_{mobility}$: 0.54, $EQ\text{-}5D_{usual\ activities}$: 0.34[20]
- Developed and validated in British English

Plantar fasciopathy (formerly called 'plantar fasciitis')

Plantar fasciopathy (also known as plantar heel pain or plantar fasciitis/fasciosis) is an overuse condition of the plantar fascia at its attachment to the calcaneus.

> **PRACTICE PEARL**
>
> The histology is of degenerative changes at the plantar fascia enthesis, including a deterioration of collagen fibres, increased secretion of ground substance proteins, focal areas of fibroblast proliferation and increased vascularity.[21–23]

The plantar fascia consists of type 1 collagen and has common tendinopathy traits, hence we recommend using the term 'fasciopathy' rather than the former 'plantar fasciitis'. Plantar fasciopathy is the most common cause of plantar heel pain, which has an estimated prevalence of 4–7%.[24, 25] It commonly affects very physically active people (e.g. runners) or people with high amounts of standing occupational work (who may also have a high BMI). Through this section we try to differentiate between the two groups and discuss how treatment strategies might be tailored to each overarching group.

Risk factors

Only one true prospective study has investigated risk factors for plantar fasciopathy. The study was conducted in a cohort of 166 runners followed over 5 years.[26, 27] The study found the overall incidence of plantar fasciopathy over the 5-year period to be 31%. Four risk factors that were significantly associated with an increased risk of plantar fasciopathy: varus knee alignment (OR 5.63); use of spiked athletic shoes (OR 5.49); cavus foot posture (OR 5.52); and greater number of days of practice per week (OR 2.59). High BMI was not a risk factor for developing plantar fasciopathy in this cohort of runners with low BMIs. This suggests that high training volumes that increase load or vertical force on the plantar fascia may increase a runner's risk of plantar fasciopathy which fits well with the belief that it is an overuse type injury.

Weight and BMI

One of the most common findings is that patients with plantar fasciopathy have a high BMI, although many of the studies that contribute to this evidence are cross-sectional.[27] Increased mechanical load due to higher BMI is a plausible source of increased plantar fascial stress. However, an important point is that high BMI was not a risk factor in the study in runners,[26] which may suggest that a high BMI increases risk in more sedentary people and in people with occupational work that requires many hours of standing, particularly on harder surfaces.

PART B Regional problems

Alignment of the foot
Cross-sectional studies that have investigated the association between foot type and plantar fasciopathy provide conflicting evidence.[27] One prospective study found that runners with a cavus foot have a higher risk of plantar fasciopathy, but cross-sectional research fails to identify a strong link between foot type and plantar fasciopathy.[26] It may be that in some patient types (e.g. those with standing work and high BMI), foot type is important. Nevertheless, a recent systematic review found that overall, the evidence supporting associations for foot and ankle range of motion and strength, kinematic and kinetic factors, and foot posture was either inconsistent or inconclusive.[27]

Training volume
Plantar fasciopathy in the younger, athletic population is associated with activities that cause a dose-dependent repetitive stress to the plantar fascia, such as running.[26, 28] Accordingly, one of the most important management strategies in these cases may be to adjust training volume and educate the patient with plantar fasciopathy to adjust training load for a period.

Standing work
People who spend the majority of their work day on hard surfaces and on their feet may be at higher risk for developing plantar fasciopathy.[27] This has only been shown in cross-sectional data, but it fits well with the proposition that high mechanical loads may increase an individual's risk of developing plantar fasciopathy. This may have implications for occupational interventions (more in the section on treatment).

Flexibility and strength
Plantar fasciopathy may be associated with decreased flexibility of the ankle joint and hamstrings, as well as decreased plantar flexion peak torque. Likewise, patients with plantar fasciopathy may have significantly lower toe flexor strength. It is unknown if this is a cause or an effect of longstanding plantar fasciopathy.[27] However, these findings may be important as treatment may need to address these strength and flexibility deficits.

Plantar fasciopathy may be associated with tightness in the proximal myofascial structures, especially the calf, hamstring and gluteal regions. Tightness in these muscle groups can alter foot biomechanics.[29]

Clinical features
The pain related to plantar fasciopathy is usually of gradual onset and felt classically on the inferior medial aspect of the heel. Initially, it is worse in the morning when getting out of bed (referred to as 'first-step pain') and decreases with activity, only to return with an ache post-activity. Periods of inactivity during the day are generally followed by an increase in pain as activity is recommenced. As the condition becomes more severe, the pain may be present when standing and worsen with activity. Some patients may also experience atypical pain when non weight-bearing, for example, when they go to bed at night.

Examination reveals pain or tenderness along the medial tuberosity of the calcaneus, and this may extend some centimetres along the medial and central components of the plantar fascia. Stretching the plantar fascia via dorsiflexion of the hallux, such as during the windlass test, may reproduce pain and may assist with palpation of the plantar fascia (Fig. 43.3c).

Investigations
If the patient has the classic history and examination findings, and there is no other suggestion of a 'red flag' (Chapter 7 and Table 43.1), then medical imaging or other investigations are not indicated. Further investigation is recommended however, if pain is particularly persistent without responding to treatment (e.g. >1 month, raising suspicion of other pathologies; Table 43.1) or if the nature of the pain is atypical for plantar fasciopathy (acute onset of pain, persistent pain even at rest, systemic symptoms, night pain). Blood tests may be warranted to rule out inflammatory arthritis, which can cause symptoms in the heels, although frequently symptoms will be more widespread. The primary imaging modalities that are useful include plain radiographs, ultrasound and MRI.

Plain radiographs, primarily the lateral view (Fig. 43.4a) are mainly used to investigate for the presence of a plantar calcaneal spur. The radiograph appearance of 'calcaneal spur' is eight times more likely in patients with plantar fasciopathy compared to those without plantar fasciopathy.[30] However, calcaneal spurs are also common in people without heel pain, and the presence of a spur does not indicate that this is the cause of pain. Plain radiographs of both feet are useful as they may show spurs bilaterally and allow comparison between feet in the situation of unilateral symptoms. Fractured spurs have also been reported, and although the findings may be subtle, plain radiographs can be used in the first instance to investigate whether a spur has, indeed, fractured.[31] Lastly, plain radiographs can be used to rule out other bone pathology (e.g. bone cysts).

Ultrasound is particularly useful for detecting pathological changes within the plantar fascia itself. Ultrasound may reveal thickening, hypoechogenicity and heterogeneity, delamination and tears (Fig. 43.4b). A systematic review and meta-analysis found that patients with plantar fasciopathy are 105 times more likely to have a fascia greater than 4.0 mm thick and 204 times

Foot pain CHAPTER 43

more likely to have hypoechogenicity compared to controls without fasciopathy.[30] Ultrasound can also be used to assess for other soft tissue pathologies associated with plantar fasciopathy, such as tissue change within the plantar fat pad, myopathies (e.g. of the deeper intrinsic musculature) and neuroma (e.g. of the medial calcaneal nerve).

MRI is the investigation of choice if there are atypical symptoms and if a wider selection of tissues (e.g. bone) are of interest. Similar to ultrasound, MRI will detect thickening of the plantar fascia, as well as heterogeneity, delamination and tears (Fig. 43.4c). MRI signs of plantar fasciopathy include hyperintensity within and around the plantar fascia, and delamination and tears within the plantar fascia. MRI is also useful for determining acute versus more chronic pathological change via the intensity of the signal on sagittal fat-suppressed short tau inversion recovery (STIR)/T2 images (lower signal signifying more chronic pathology). In addition, there is some evidence to suggest that a subsection of patients with plantar fasciopathy have bone marrow oedema on MRI, and this may be associated with atypical symptoms such as night pain.[32] MRI can also identify stress fractures of the calcaneus. Finally, MRI is particularly useful for detecting other soft tissue pathologies that may be associated with a painful heel, including soft tissue tumours, medial tendinopathy and plantar fat pad pathology.

Treatment

Treatment is often multi-faceted and generally starts with conservative interventions, progressing to more invasive interventions if conservative care fails to improve the condition. Treatment can be thought of in terms of three

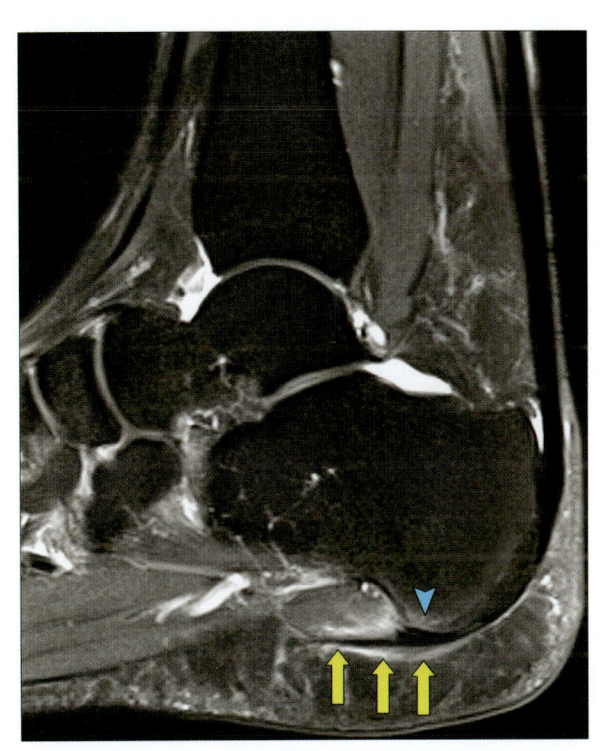

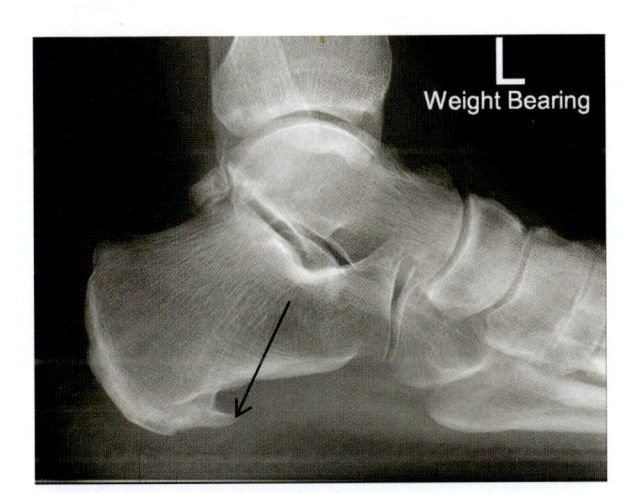

Figure 43.4 (a) Lateral plain radiograph highlighting a large plantar calcaneal spur (b) Ultrasound scan highlighting a thickened plantar fascia (0.902 cm), heterogeneity and hypoechogenicity within the plantar fascia (deep hypoechogenicity representative of a tear within the fascia) (c) MRI of plantar fasciopathy. Sagittal fat-suppressed T2-weighted MRI demonstrates thickening of the plantar fascia and hyperintense signal in the adjacent perifascial soft tissues (arrows). There is bone marrow oedema in the calcaneal attachment (arrowhead)[33]

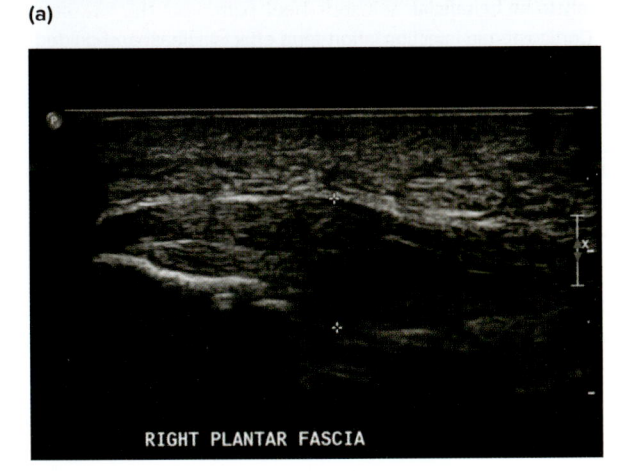

(c) IMAGING IN SPORTS-SPECIFIC MUSCULOSKELETAL INJURIES 2016, P. 528. ALI GUERMAZI, FRANK W ROEMER, MICHEL D CREMA. © SPRINGER INTERNATIONAL PUBLISHING SWITZERLAND 2016. WITH PERMISSION OF SPRINGER

tiers, which essentially equate to short-, medium- and long-term options.[34] The tiers also relate to the complexity, cost and invasiveness of the intervention. The following interventions are listed, taking into account evidence from two systematic reviews, unless otherwise indicated.[35, 36] The evidence is summarised in Table 43.3.

First tier/short term

Minimise the aggravating activity and educate the patient about the potential causes of their heel pain. If the patient is a runner, it is essential that you also discuss training loads, and regression and progression of their training volumes. The following is some of the generic advice that we give to patients.

- You should not begin to run before your heel has been pain-free for 4 weeks and you can walk 10 km without pain during the walk or the morning after.
- If you need to wear dress shoes, you might consider using soft silicone gel heel pads or contoured prefabricated foot orthoses in your shoes.
- It is important that you decrease or avoid activities that cause your heel pain to worsen.
- When you want to start activities again, you should be careful and progress slowly.

If your patient is a factory worker with many hours of standing work each day, it is important that you discuss potential options on how to decrease the number of hours of standing per day. The following points of advice are generic and should be individualised to the patient.

- Advise the patient to wear appropriate footwear (offering both cushioning for the heel and support for the rearfoot and midfoot). Although there is little evidence for footwear, it is a good starting point for long-term treatment.[36, 41]
- Two types of taping have been advocated. The first is low-Dye taping (Fig. 43.5a), which involves the application of rigid tape to the plantar aspect of the foot with the aim of supporting the plantar fascia.[37, 38] This is sometimes augmented with the second type, calcaneal taping (Fig. 43.5a).
- Recommend appropriately contoured prefabricated foot orthoses.[39, 40]
- Provide strengthening exercises for proximal muscle groups (e.g. tibialis posterior and hip abductors/external rotators).
- A silicone gel heel pad may be beneficial (Fig. 43.5b) although the evidence is unclear.
- Recommend stretching of the plantar fascia[42-44] (Fig. 43.5c), gastrocnemius and soleus.
- Suggest self-massage with a frozen bottle or golf ball (Fig. 43.5d). This is commonly used but there is no supporting evidence.
- Suggest soft tissue therapy (minimal evidence), both to the plantar fascia (Fig. 43.5e) and proximal myofascial regions including calf, hamstrings and gluteals.[45]

Table 43.3 Evidence table

Interventions	
Conservative	*Non-conservative*
Likely to be beneficial • Taping (e.g. low-Dye): limited evidence for up to 1 week • Customised and prefabricated foot orthoses (up to 12 months): note that there is no difference between customised and appropriately contoured prefabricated orthoses	**Likely to be beneficial** • Corticosteroid injection (short-term effects): ultrasound-guided injections have been found to be more effective than placebo
Unknown effectiveness • Heel pads • Night splints • Stretching exercises	**Unknown effectiveness** • Corticosteroid injection plus local anaesthetic (short term) • Extracorporeal shock wave therapy • Surgery
Likely to be ineffective or harmful	**Likely to be ineffective or harmful** • Corticosteroid injection (long-term effects) • Corticosteroid injection plus local anaesthetic injection (long-term effects)

Note: No evidence from high-quality systematic reviews is available for dry needling, strengthening exercises, weight loss and non-steroidal anti-inflammatory drugs (NSAIDs) so they have not been included in this table.
ADAPTED FROM LANDORF [35]

Foot pain   CHAPTER 43

(a) (i)

(a) (ii)

(b)

(c)

(d)

(e)

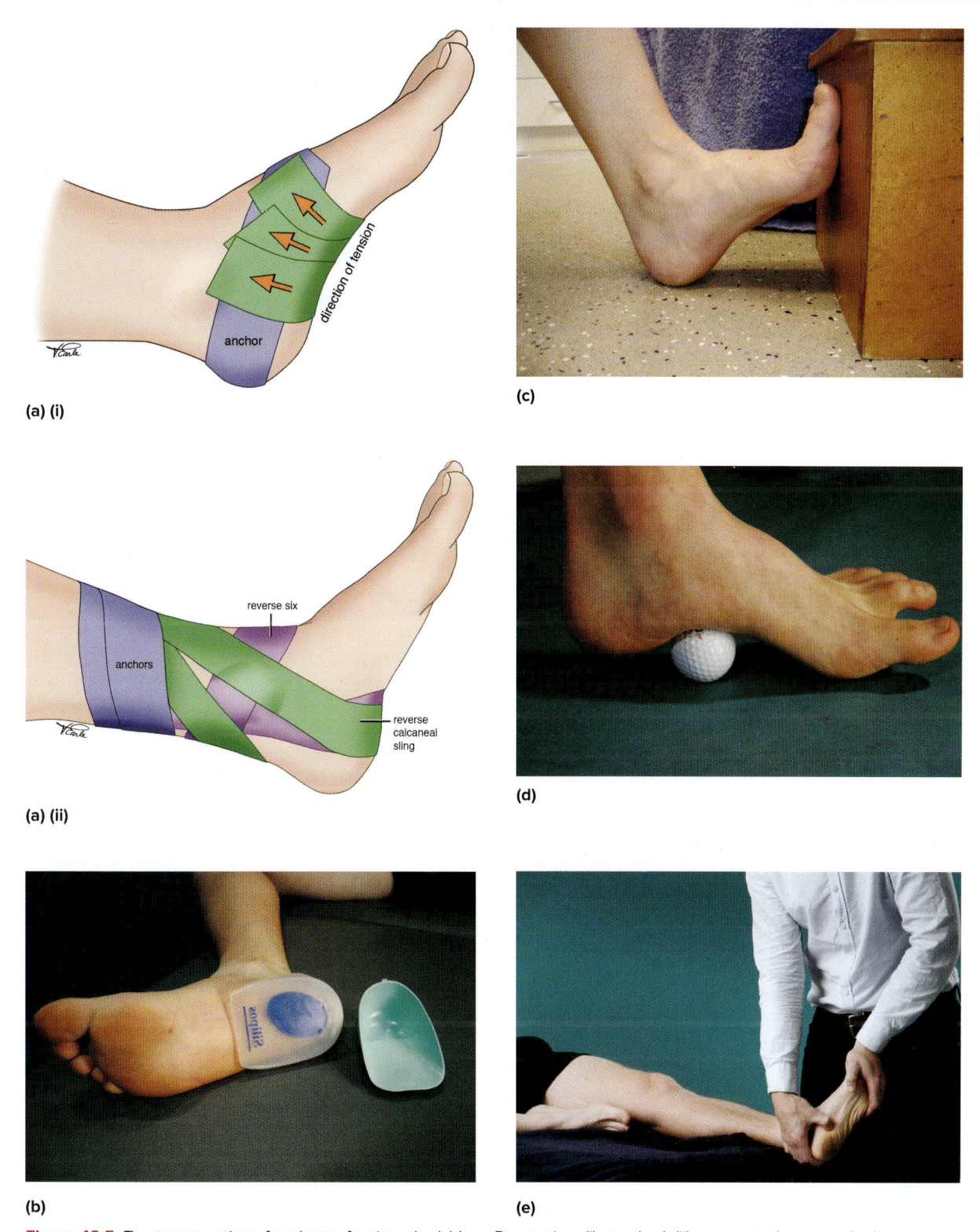

Figure 43.5 Treatment options for plantar fasciopathy (a) Low-Dye taping: (i) standard; (ii) augmented tape applied over standard low-Dye taping (b) Silicone gel heel pad and cup (c) Stretching of the plantar fascia (d) Self-massage with a golf ball (e) Soft tissue therapy to plantar fascia

PART B   Regional problems

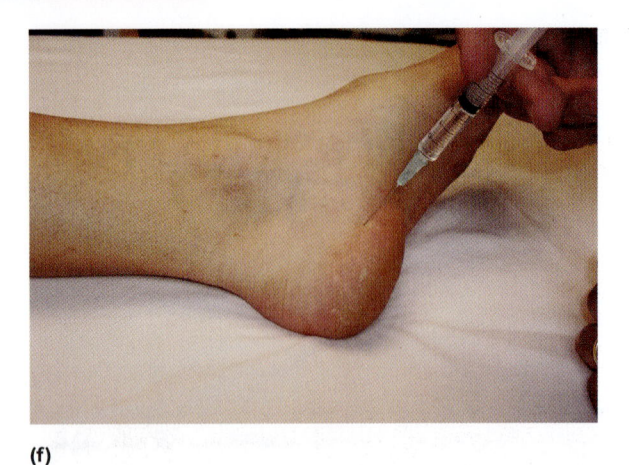

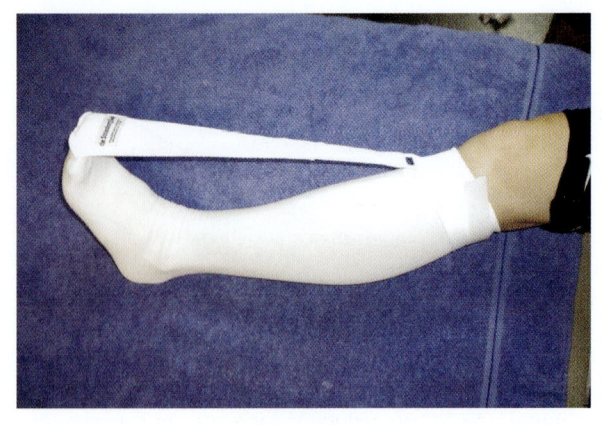

Figure 43.5 (cont.) (f) Corticosteroid injection (g) Strasbourg sock

- Recommend the use of non-steroidal anti-inflammatory drugs (NSAIDs)[46]
- Advise the patient to lose weight. Although there is no evidence for weight loss as being effective, it is biologically plausible that it may be effective given that plantar fasciopathy is highly associated with increased BMI.

Second tier/medium term
The following are recommended second-tier interventions.

- Dry needling of related lower limb muscles is effective.[47]
- Customised foot orthoses may be considered; although there is no evidence that customised foot orthoses are more beneficial than appropriately contoured prefabricated foot orthoses.
- Corticosteroid injection (Fig. 43.5f): evidence supports the use of corticosteroid injection for pain relief in the short term (4–6 weeks).[35, 48, 49] Ultrasound-guided injections were more effective than palpation-guided injections.[50] It should always be combined with other treatments such as stretching, foot orthoses or other evidence-based treatments to prevent recurrence. There is some concern that corticosteroid injections are associated with an increased risk of rupture and fat pad atrophy.[51, 52] However, this is likely related to the solubility and duration of the corticosteroid. Lateral plantar nerve injury is a potential adverse event.[53]
- High-load strength training consisting of unilateral heel-raises with a towel inserted under the toes to further activate the windlass mechanism may potentially be effective for longstanding cases of plantar fasciopathy. This has been evaluated in one RCT.[54]

Third tier/long term
The following are recommended third-tier interventions.

- Night splints[55-57] or a Strasbourg sock (Fig. 43.5g) should be considered for patients with pain of over 6 months in duration, although the evidence is unclear and some patients will not tolerate them. One RCT found this to be effective in reducing pain that had been present for more than 6 months.[1]
- Extracorporeal shockwave therapy (ESWT) may be of benefit for longstanding cases, although the evidence is still unclear and it may cause substantial pain for some patients while being applied.[35, 58]
- As the evidence for surgery is unclear and of low quality, it should only be considered in severe longstanding cases that do not respond to any of the evidence-based treatments available. Surgical options include plantar fasciotomy ± nerve release, plantar fasciectomy with neurolysis of the nerve to the abductor digiti quinti muscle,[59] and minimally invasive endoscopic plantar fascia release.[60, 61]

Fat pad contusion
The heel fat pad, elastic fibrous tissue septa separated by closely packed fat cells, absorbs the shock of heel strike. Contusion can occur acutely after a fall onto the heels from a height, but is more common chronically because of poor heel cushioning or repetitive stops, starts and changes in direction.

The patient often complains of marked heel pain, particularly during weight-bearing activities. The pain is felt laterally in the heel due to the pattern of heel strike, which may help differentiate this condition from plantar fasciopathy. Examination reveals tenderness in

Foot pain   CHAPTER 43

the posterolateral heel region. MRI often demonstrates oedematous changes in the fat pad, with ill-defined areas of decreased signal intensity on T1-weighted images that increase in signal intensity on T2-weighted images.

The patient should avoid aggravating activities. NSAIDs or paracetamol (acetaminophen) may provide short-term pain relief. Athletes can maintain cardiovascular fitness by cross-training with low-impact activities such as cycling and swimming. Training on soft surfaces can assist athletes with returning to sport.

As the pain settles, the use of a silicone gel heel pad (Fig. 43.5b) and good footwear are important as the athlete resumes activity. A well-fitting heel counter in athletic footwear can reduce shear stress and tension in the fat pad.[62] Heel-lock taping (see Fig 41.11b) will often provide symptomatic relief.

Calcaneal stress fracture

Calcaneal stress fracture is the second most common tarsal stress fracture. It occurs at either the upper posterior margin of the calcaneum or adjacent to the medial tuberosity, at the point where calcaneal spurs occur. First described among the military as a marching injury (Chapter 45), calcaneal stress fractures occur in runners, ballet dancers and jumping athletes.

Patients give a history of insidious onset of heel pain that is aggravated by weight-bearing activities, especially running. Examination should include viewing the patient perform the causative activity if feasible (i.e. gait analysis in a runner). Palpation reveals localised tenderness over the medial or lateral aspects of the posterior calcaneus and pain that is reproduced by squeezing the posterior aspect of the calcaneus from both sides simultaneously.

Investigations

Plain radiography is often normal, but may show a typical sclerotic appearance on the lateral radiograph, parallel to the posterior margin of the calcaneus (Fig. 43.6a). Stress injury was only visible in 15% of plain radiographs.[63] The majority of calcaneal stress fractures are posterior. MRI reveals an area of high signal on a T2-weighted image (Fig. 43.6b).

Use the level of pain to guide how much the patient must reduce activity. If pain is marked, a short period of non weight-bearing may be required. Soft heel pads can contribute to immediate pain relief. Weight-bearing can be reintroduced gradually once pain settles.

As with every training-related injury, assess sport technique to determine if abnormal biomechanics may have contributed to the injury. If indicated, prescribe rigid or soft orthoses. Expert foot clinicians consider that joint mobilisation and stretching of the calf muscles and plantar fascia contribute to recovery.

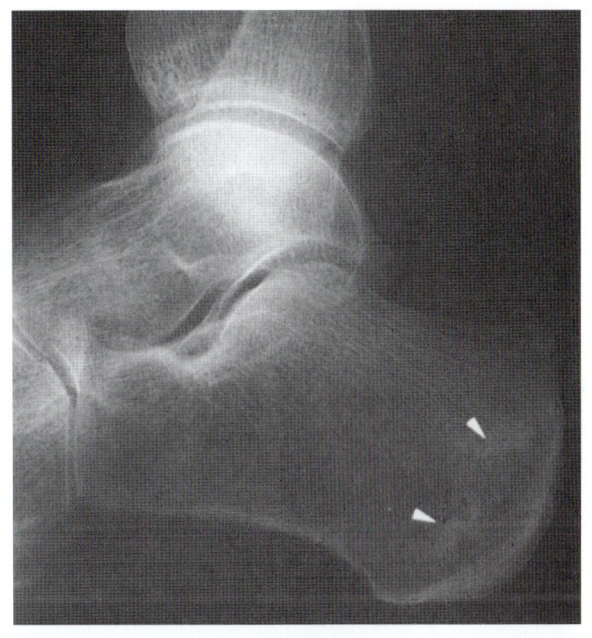

(a)

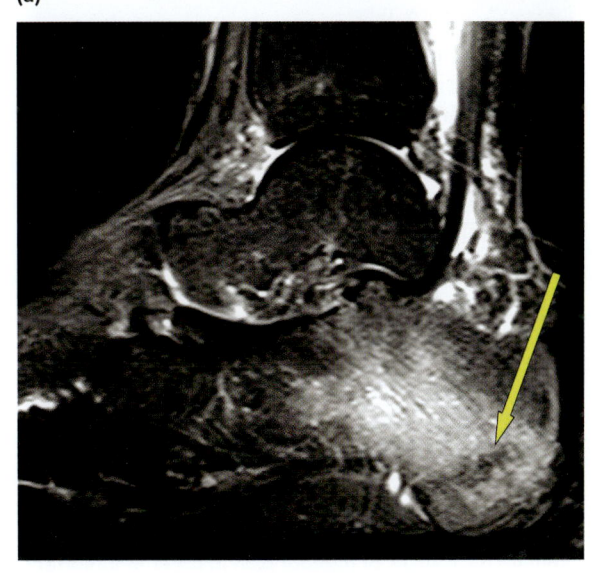

(b)

Figure 43.6 (a) Plain radiograph appearance of a calcaneal stress fracture. The white arrowheads indicate typical sclerotic appearance (b) T2-weighted MRI showing characteristic appearance[33] of a stress fracture
(b) IMAGING IN SPORTS-SPECIFIC MUSCULOSKELETAL INJURIES 2016, P. 655,: ALI GUERMAZI, FRANK W ROEMER, MICHEL D CREMA. © SPRINGER INTERNATIONAL PUBLISHING SWITZERLAND 2016. WITH PERMISSION OF SPRINGER

First branch of lateral plantar nerve (Baxter's nerve) entrapment

An overlooked cause of rearfoot pain is entrapment of the first branch of the lateral plantar nerve (Fig. 43.7). This

PART B Regional problems

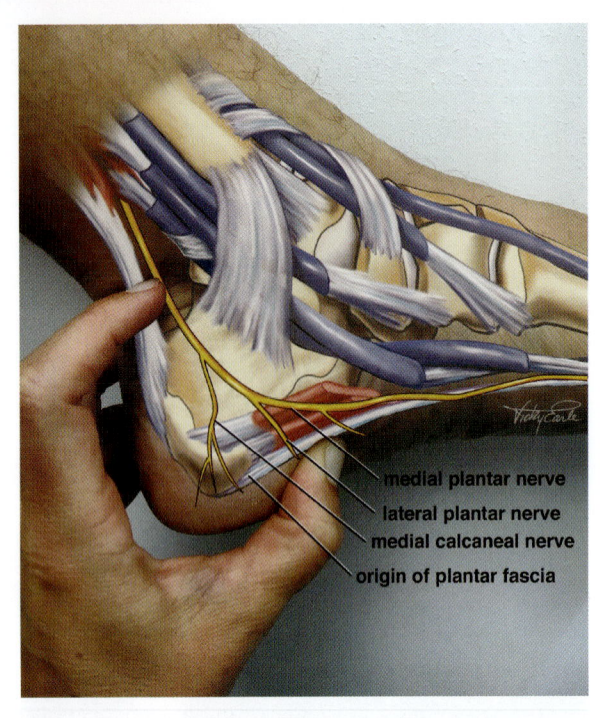

Figure 43.7 The lateral plantar nerve. The nerve is one of three terminal branches of the posterior tibial nerve arising distal to the tarsal tunnel

terminal branch of the posterior tibial nerve arises distal to the tarsal tunnel and it can become trapped between the deep fascia of the abductor hallucis longus and the medial caudal margin of the quadratus plantae muscle.[64]

Pain radiates to the medial inferior aspect of the heel and proximally into the medial ankle region. Patients do not normally complain of numbness in the heel or foot. Often confused with plantar fasciopathy, the two conditions were shown to coexist in 52% of patients with this nerve entrapment.[65]

Examination is nonspecific with maximal tenderness at the plantar medial heel just proximal to the plantar fascia. A Tinel's sign at this location may reproduce pain. Theoretically, the condition is associated with 'subtle weakness of fifth toe abduction'[66] and atrophy to the abductor digiti quinti muscle, although this is an example of a clinical test that would have very low sensitivity if tested formally (Chapter 14). Some authors claim that atrophy can be identified on MRI or ultrasound exam.[67, 68]

In the clinic, a diagnostic injection with local anaesthetic, ideally performed using ultrasound to identify the nerve, can increase the clinician's confidence in the diagnosis (increased positive likelihood ratio, Chapter 14).[69] Referral for nerve conduction tests may be helpful for diagnosis and to determine the location of compression in the lateral plantar tunnel, Baxter's nerve or more proximally in the tarsal tunnel.[67] This is particularly important if surgery is being considered.

Treatment consists of using soft-soled shoes, heel cups or arch support, tape or an orthosis for athletes with excessive pronation. A corticosteroid injection, best ultrasound-guided as described earlier, may be helpful. Radiofrequency denervation of the nerve may give short- to medium-term pain relief. Surgical release would be indicated if conservative measures have failed.[64]

MIDFOOT PAIN

The midfoot consists of the three cuneiform bones, the cuboid and the navicular bones as well as the surrounding soft tissues (Figs 43.1 and 43.2). The most common cause of midfoot pain is midtarsal joint sprain after ankle injury, but the most important cause of midfoot pain is stress fracture of the navicular bone. Tendinopathy of the extensor tendons is another common cause of midfoot pain. The causes of midfoot pain are listed in Table 43.4.

Table 43.4 Causes of midfoot pain in order of importance (clinical relevance)

Common	Less common	Not to be missed
Navicular stress fracture	Cuneiform stress fracture	Lisfranc's joint injury (fracture or dislocation)
Midtarsal joint sprain	Cuboid stress fracture	Osteoid osteoma
Lisfranc joint injury (sprain)	Stress fracture base second metatarsal	Complex regional pain syndrome type 1 (after knee or ankle injury)
Tibialis posterior tendinopathy	Extensor tendinopathy	Referred pain
Plantar fascia strain	Peroneal tendinopathy	
	Abductor hallucis strain	
	Cuboid syndrome	
	Tarsal coalition (in adolescents)	
	Köhler's disease (in young children)	
	Accessory navicular bone	

Foot pain CHAPTER 43

Clinical approach to midfoot pain

Acute midfoot pain results from a sprain of the midtarsal joint or plantar fascia. Gradual pain is a sign of overuse injury, such as extensor tendinopathy, tibialis posterior tendinopathy or navicular stress fracture. In most conditions, pain is well localised to the site of the injury, but in navicular stress fracture, pain is poorly localised.

Examination involves palpation of the area of tenderness and a biomechanical examination to detect factors that predispose to injury. Examination of the midfoot is shown in Figure 43.8.

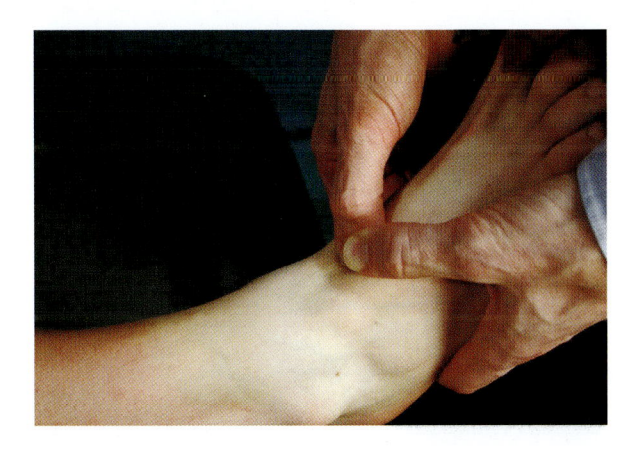

Investigations

If there is a clinical suspicion of a stress fracture of the navicular or a cuneiform, plain radiographs are indicated. This rarely reveals a fracture, even if one is present, but it is useful to rule out tarsal coalition, to show bony abnormalities such as talar beaking (osteophytes at the talonavicular joint) and accessory ossicles, and to exclude bony tumours. MRI should be performed if X-ray fails to reveal a stress fracture.

Navicular stress fracture

Stress fractures of the navicular are among the most common stress fractures seen in the athlete, especially in sports that involve sprinting, jumping or hurdling.[70] The stress fracture commonly occurs in the middle third of the navicular bone (Fig. 43.9). This site is a relatively avascular 'watershed area' of bone as the blood supply comes from the lateral and medial sides of the navicular. This is thought to contribute to poor healing of these stress fractures.

Spikes in training load are thought to be the most common cause of navicular stress fractures. It is likely that the navicular bone is jammed between the talus proximally and the cuneiforms distally. Many clinicians speculate that reduced ankle dorsiflexion may cause excessive midfoot dorsiflexion and thus increase the load at the talonavicular joint with subsequent failure of the slightly concave proximal lip of the navicular at that site.[71]

Clinical features

The onset of symptoms is usually insidious, consisting of a poorly localised midfoot ache associated with activity. The pain typically radiates along the medial aspect of the

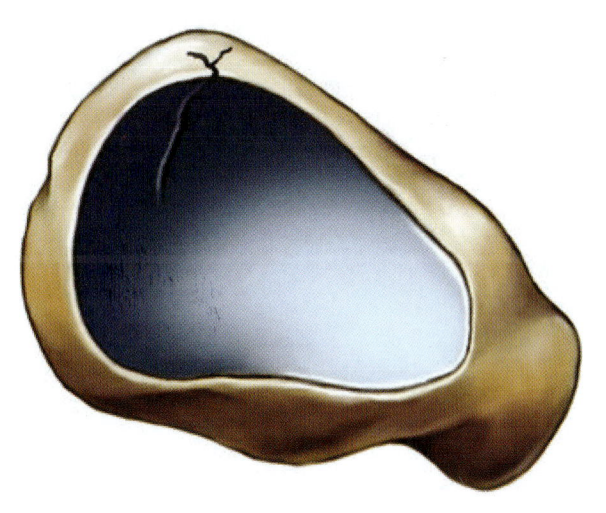

(a)

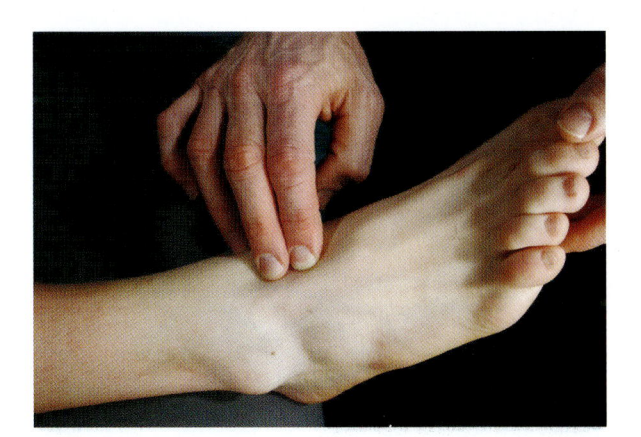

(b)

Figure 43.8 Examination of the midfoot (a) Palpation—N spot. The proximal dorsal surface of the navicular is tender when a stress fracture is present (b) Palpation—extensor tendons. These may be tender as they pass under the extensor retinaculum

Figure 43.9 Navicular stress fractures occur at a characteristic proximal site on the bone. This N-spot corresponds with the point of tenderness on palpation

949

PART B Regional problems

longitudinal arch or the dorsum of the foot. The symptoms abate rapidly with rest, unfortunately often contributing to diagnostic delays. Examination reveals localised tenderness at the N-spot: the proximal dorsal portion of the navicular.[72] If palpation confirms tenderness over the N-spot, particularly when compared to a symmetric location on the contralateral foot (Fig. 43.8a), the athlete should be considered to have a navicular stress fracture until proven otherwise.

> **PRACTICE PEARL**
>
> The pain of navicular stress fracture is often poorly localised.

The astute clinician assesses the patient for factors that predispose to the condition, such as tarsal coalition, excessive pronation and restricted ankle dorsiflexion. Any factors that need to be corrected should be attended to at the appropriate time in the management program (see below).

Investigations
Plain radiographs lack sensitivity to detect navicular stress fractures.[72] MRI (Fig. 43.10a) is the investigation of choice. Computed tomography (CT) scan can further clarify the morphology of this fracture (Fig. 43.10b and c). Poor positioning of the patient's foot and scanning with slice thickness >2 mm can lead to a navicular stress fracture being missed on CT scan.[73]

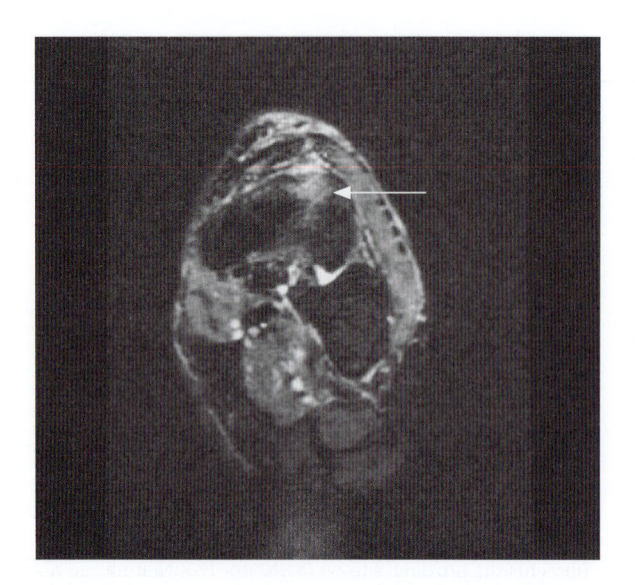

Management of navicular bone stress injuries
We consider treatment according to whether the diagnosis is: 1. stress reaction; 2. typical (uncomplicated) stress fracture; and 3. complicated stress fracture (e.g. delayed diagnosis, delayed union). (See also Chapter 4–Bone stress injuries.)

Stress reaction
If a patient has only had symptoms for a relatively short time (days, <2 weeks), he or she may not have a full

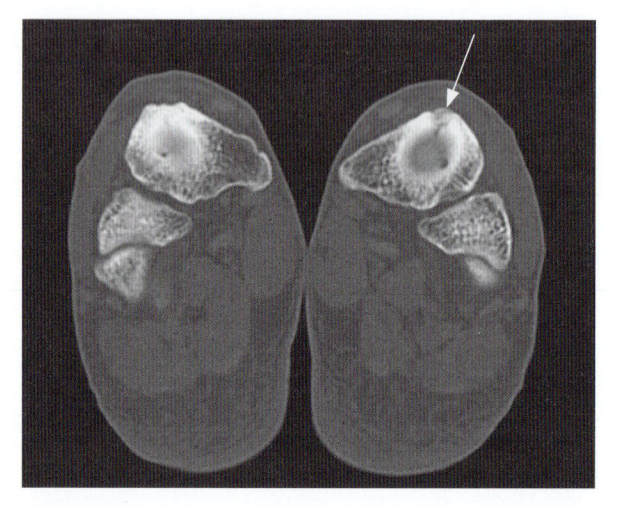

(a)

(b)

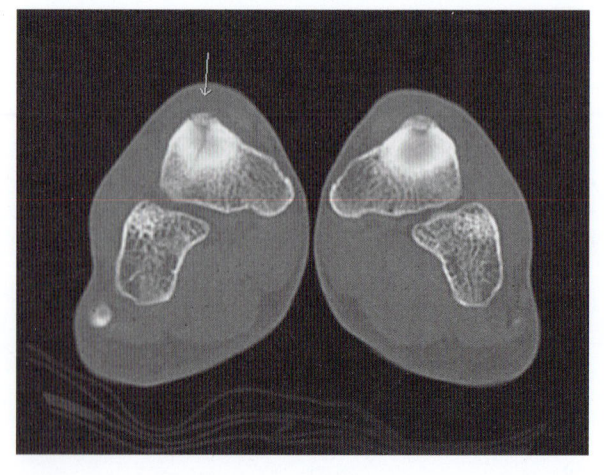

(c)

Figure 43.10 Navicular stress fracture (a) T2-weighted MRI showing bone marrow oedema (b) CT scan showing undisplaced fracture (arrow) (c) CT scan showing more extensive Y-shaped fracture

950

Foot pain   CHAPTER 43

stress fracture but only a stress reaction. A positive MRI combined with a normal CT scan (skilfully executed, as mentioned in the previous section) confirms the diagnosis of navicular stress *reaction* (no cortical breach). This can be treated with weight-bearing relative rest which means the patient can take weight through the part but cannot play sport. This is generally done by having the patient wear a CAM boot for 1–3 weeks until pain is absent and the N-spot is no longer tender. This is then followed by a graduated return to activity (aim for increases in the acute:chronic workload to be <1.1 or 10%) over 2–3 months (Chapter 12).

Typical stress fracture
In the majority of cases, patients who present with midfoot pain and navicular tenderness have a frank stress fracture visible on both MRI and CT scan. Remember that bone pathology (failure) begins before the patient feels pain, so day 1 of pain is not day 1 of relative excessive load and microfractures (which precede frank stress fracture).

> **PRACTICE PEARL**
>
> The typical non-displaced stress fracture should be treated with absolute non weight-bearing.

Non weight-bearing can be achieved with patient education and a rigid fibreglass boot.[72] This period of non weight-bearing is ideally carried through a *minimum* of 6 weeks but many clinicians recommend 8 weeks so as to lower the risk of recurrence.

At the end of the period of non weight-bearing immobilisation, the boot should be removed and the N-spot palpated for tenderness. Generally, the N-spot will be non-tender; however, if tenderness is present, the patient should have a further 2 weeks of non weight-bearing immobilisation. Management is primarily based on the clinical assessment, as there is poor CT and MRI correlation with clinical union of the stress fracture (Fig. 43.11).[70, 74]

Following removal of the boot, it is essential for a skilled clinician to mobilise the stiff ankle and the subtalar and midtarsal joints. The calf muscles require soft tissue therapy and a progressive strengthening program. This rehabilitation must precede return to running.

Activity must begin gradually, slowly building up to full training over a period of 6 weeks. Return to sport often takes 3 months in the ideal case where the athlete has maintained fitness with cross-training and meets all his or her rehabilitation landmarks smoothly. Taking 4 months to return to play is within normal limits for this injury.[75] Note that even if a player rested for 8 weeks

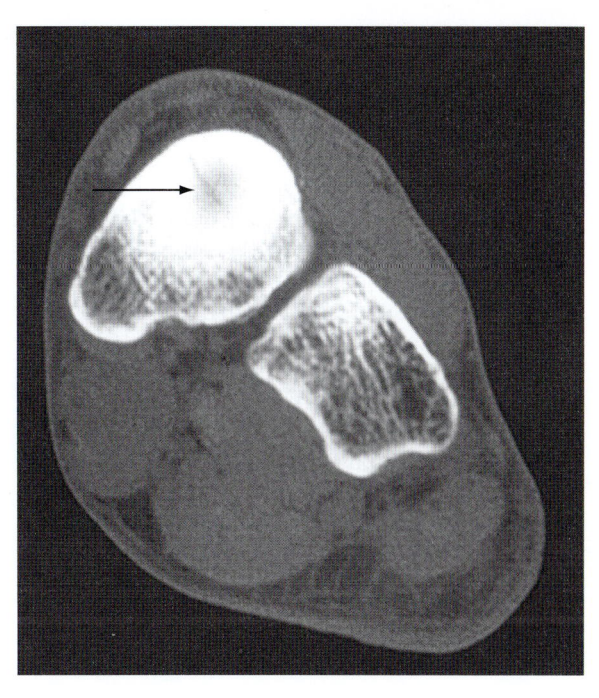

Figure 43.11 Imaging of navicular stress fracture does not necessarily mirror clinical recovery. This CT scan of a 26-year-old runner shows that the fracture line is still evident (arrow) but the patient had returned pain-free to all competition and had no further recurrences of stress fracture

(without any injury), it would take 3 months to return to a high level of training merely to avoid spiking training loads.[76]

> **PRACTICE PEARL**
>
> **WARNING:** A recipe for navicular disaster is for the patient to think that 'non weight-bearing' is merely an aspirational goal or a guideline. Countless athletes have had their careers ruined by navicular stress fracture recurrence. The fracture is notorious for non-union if the first treatment attempt is a failure.[72]

Complicated stress fracture
Often, patients with a stress fracture of the navicular present after a long period of pain or after a period of weight-bearing rest. There is no evidence to suggest these patient should have immediate surgical treatment. Patients who have been unsuccessfully treated with weight-bearing rest or short-term boot immobilisation should undergo non weight-bearing immobilisation for 8 weeks. This method of

treatment is associated with an 80% successful return-to-sport rate and may be successful even in cases where the patient has had longstanding (>6 months) pain.[70, 74]

Failure of rigorous conservative treatment is an indication for surgery. Which type of surgery is best has not been tested. Some surgeons favour internal fixation, others prefer to excise the facture and perform a bone graft. As the fracture involves a joint surface (proximal navicular, at the talonavicular joint; Fig. 43.10) surgery is not universally successful.

A 2010 systematic review and meta-analysis found no significant difference between non weight-bearing conservative treatment and surgical treatment in terms of pain reduction.[74, 77]

Midtarsal joint sprains

The midtarsal joint (Chopart's joint) consists of the talonavicular and calcaneocuboid joints. Other joints in the midtarsal area are the naviculocuneiform, cuboid cuneiform and intercuneiform joints. Injuries to the midtarsal joints are most commonly seen in gymnasts, jumpers and footballers.

Individual ligamentous sprains to the midtarsal joints are uncommon and if they occur usually affect the dorsal calcaneocuboid or bifurcate ligament, comprising the calcaneonavicular and calcaneocuboid ligament.

Dorsal calcaneocuboid ligament injury

Patient presents with pain in the lateral midfoot following an inversion injury. Examination reveals localised tenderness and swelling at the dorsolateral aspect of the calcaneocuboid joint. Stress inversion of the foot elicits pain.

Plain radiography is required to exclude fracture and MRI may confirm the diagnosis. Taping may provide additional support while orthoses may help to de-load the painful ligaments. A joint sprain can sometimes lead to secondary joint inflammation. This generally responds well to NSAIDs but if inflammation persists the patient may benefit from a corticosteroid injection into the painful midtarsal joints.

Bifurcate ligament injuries

Injuries to the bifurcate ligament may be associated with fractures to the anterior process of the calcaneus secondary to violent dorsiflexion, forceful plantarflexion and inversion injuries (Chapter 41). Patients present with lateral midfoot pain and swelling, usually following an ankle sprain or injury. Examination reveals local tenderness and occasionally swelling overlying the ligament, with pain elicited at the site with simultaneous forefoot supination and plantarflexion.

Plain radiograph may reveal a fracture of the anterior process of the calcaneus but it can miss one, so never rely on X-ray to rule out a fracture. An MRI scan can be used to confirm the joint/ligament sprain. If a fracture is present, a CT scan may be required for further assessment (see Fig. 41.17).

Treatment is similar to the dorsal calcaneocuboid sprain mentioned previously. If a non-displaced or mildly displaced fracture of the anterior process of the calcaneum is present, 4 weeks immobilisation is required. If the fracture is displaced, surgery is required.

Lisfranc joint injuries

The eponymous Lisfranc joint refers to the tarsometatarsal joints: the bases of the five metatarsals with their corresponding three cuneiforms and cuboid (Fig. 43.12). The spectrum of injuries of the Lisfranc joint complex ranges from partial sprains with no displacement, to complete tears with separation (diastasis) of the first and second metatarsal bones and, depending on the severity, different patterns of tarsal and metatarsal displacement (Fig. 43.13).

> **PRACTICE PEARL**
>
> Be alert! Although Lisfranc joint injuries ('midfoot sprains') are not common in the general population, they are the second most common foot injury in athletes. In sport, they generally occur via low-velocity indirect force.

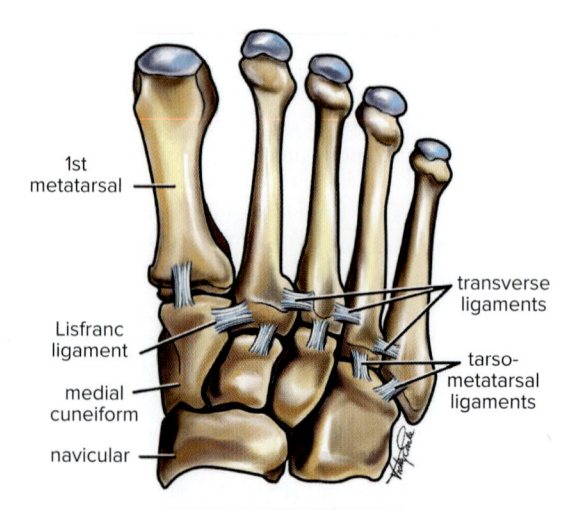

Figure 43.12 Ligamentous attachments of the Lisfranc joint articulation

Foot pain CHAPTER 43

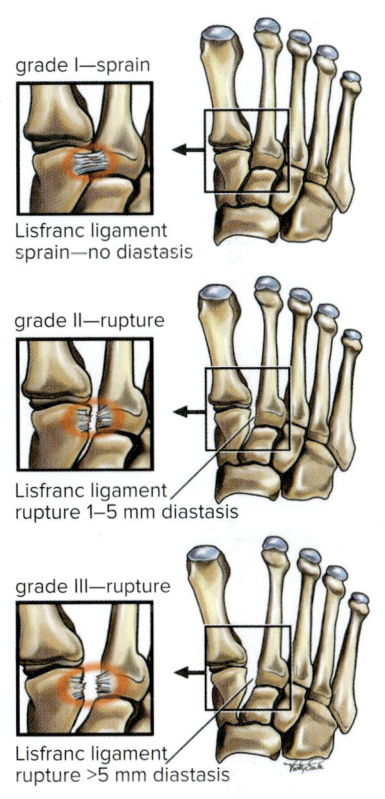

Figure 43.13 Lisfranc joint injury classification system

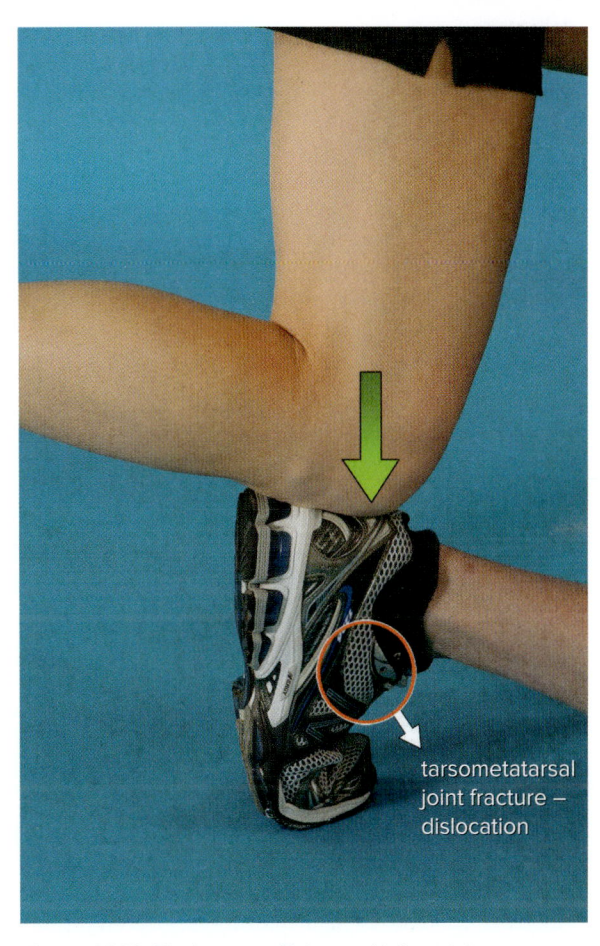

Figure 43.14 Mechanism of injury to Lisfranc joint—longitudinal compression

Lisfranc joint fracture–dislocation is rare in sport, but, because of its disastrous consequences if untreated, the diagnosis must be considered in all cases of 'midfoot sprain' in the athlete.

Causes
There are two main mechanisms of injury.

- *Direct*. This injury is relatively uncommon and occurs as a simple crush injury to the tarsometatarsal joint region. There is no specific pattern of damage or distinctive appearance with a direct injury.
- *Indirect*. This mechanism is more common and generally occurs secondary to a longitudinal force sustained while the foot is plantarflexed and slightly rotated. There are three common injury situations: longitudinal compression (Fig. 43.14); a backward fall with the foot entrapped; and a fall on the point of the toes.[78]

The extent of the damage depends on the severity of the injury. In milder injuries, the weak dorsal tarsometatarsal ligaments are ruptured; with more severe injuries, there may also be fractures of the plantar aspect of the metatarsal base, or the plantar capsule may rupture and the metatarsal may displace dorsally. Thus, a fracture at the plantar base of a metatarsal can be a clue to a subtle Lisfranc joint injury.

Clinical features
A patient with Lisfranc joint injury may complain of midfoot pain and difficulty weight-bearing, following an acute injury by the mechanisms described above. Pain is classically aggravated by forefoot weight-bearing–the patient is unable to run on the toes and feels pain on the push-off phase of running (and sometimes during walking) and on calf raises. Often the presentation may be delayed, and the patient presents with ongoing midfoot pain and swelling, aggravated by running.

> **PRACTICE PEARL**
>
> Midfoot pain that persists for more than 5 days post injury should raise suspicion of a Lisfranc joint injury.

953

Examination reveals:

- tenderness with or without swelling on the dorsal midfoot, often with associated bruising in this region
- pain with combined eversion and abduction of the forefoot while the calcaneus is held still
- plantar medial ecchymosis may be observed in a delayed diagnosis[79]
- neurovascular examination is mandatory as the dorsalis pedis artery can be compromised in the initial injury or by subsequent swelling of the foot.[78]

Investigations

Plain weight-bearing radiographs are recommended. Diastasis between the first and second metatarsal bases of greater than 2 mm. (Fig. 43.15a) suggests a Lisfranc joint injury, although in patients with a metatarsus adductus a 3 mm separation may be normal. In such cases, it is essential to take comparative weight-bearing X-rays of the non-injured side, as a difference in diastasis of greater than 1 mm between the two sides is considered diagnostic.

Other radiological signs that may indicate an injury to the Lisfranc joint include a 'fleck sign', which appears as a fleck fracture near the base of the second metatarsal or medial cuneiform or, in the lateral view, either dorsal displacement of the metatarsal bases relative to the tarsus or flattening of the medial longitudinal arch. However, a dislocation may reduce spontaneously, and the foot may appear normal on plain X-rays despite severe soft tissue disruption. There was a high correlation between rupture or grade II sprain of the plantar ligament between the first cuneiform and the bases of the second and third metatarsals, and true midfoot instability.

If injury is suspected, and X-ray is normal, both CT (Fig 43.15b) and MRI (Fig 43.15c) can help the clinician make the diagnosis. MRI is more sensitive and specific than CT to demonstrate all the components of the Lisfranc complex.[80, 81]

Static and dynamic ultrasound examination of the dorsal cuneiform metatarsal (C1–M2) ligament is a sensitive indicator of stable or unstable sprains. Thickening to this ligament without joint space widening is consistent with a grade 1 sprain. Absence of this ligament and joint space wider than 2.5 mm, plus increased spacing upon weight-bearing, suggests Lisfranc ligament tear.[82]

Treatment

The treatment of a Lisfranc joint injury depends on the degree of instability present.[83] In grade I injuries, where there is no instability (diastasis), conservative management is recommended with non weight-bearing in a CAM boot or Aircast® for 6 weeks. The goal of this treatment is to restore the integrity of the tarsometatarsal ligaments and hence the stability of the midfoot. Following removal of the cast, mobilisation of the ankle and a calf-strengthening program are required. Orthoses may be needed to correct the intrinsic alignment of the foot and to support the second metatarsal base. A graded return to activity is required. Recovery time from diagnosis to activity return is prolonged, often requiring 3–4 months of total treatment.[79]

Due to instability, injuries of grade II or greater severity require surgical reduction and fixation. This may be performed percutaneously or, in more difficult cases, an open operation may be needed. There has also been consideration for primary arthrodesis as opposed to open reduction internal fixation (ORIF); however, this is a less-preferred method.[84] In the situation of a delay in diagnosis, similar treatment protocols are required, however grade II or grade III Lisfranc injury is a significant injury that has a much better prognosis if managed correctly initially, rather than being salvaged once there is prolonged joint malalignment and non-union.

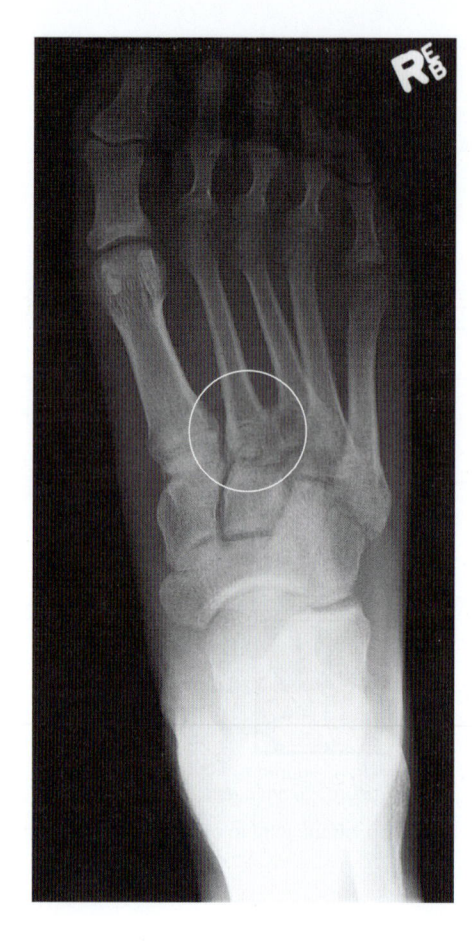

Figure 43.15 Lisfranc fracture–dislocation (a) Plain radiograph

Foot pain CHAPTER 43

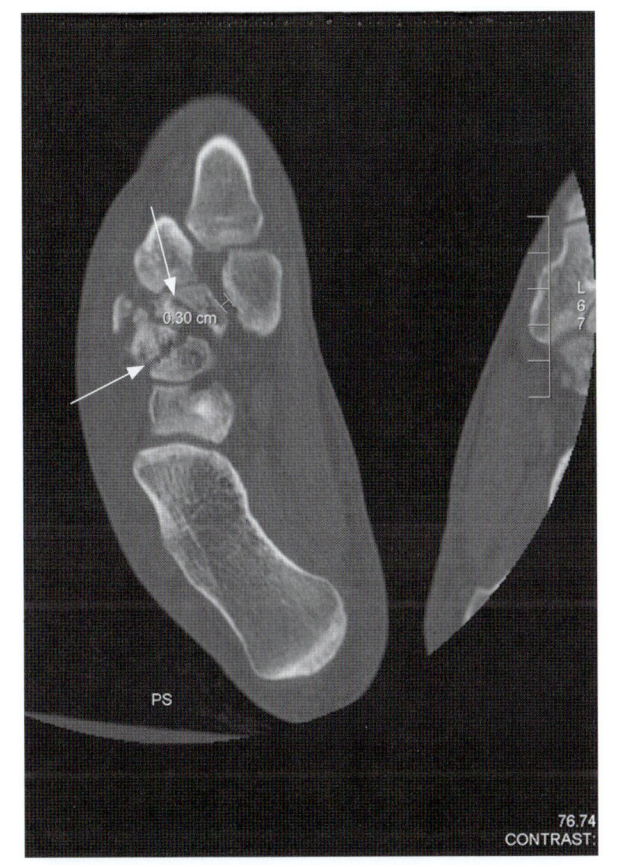

A delay in diagnosis has been associated with a poor outcome, a prolonged absence from sport, and chronic disability due to ligamentous instability of the tarsometatarsal joint.

Tibialis posterior tendinopathy (distal pain presentation)

Tibialis posterior tendinopathy is described in the previous chapter on ankle pain (Chapter 42), but tendinopathy at the distal insertion of the tendon into the navicular may present primarily as medial foot pain. In younger patients, the accessory ossicle, the os navicularis (Fig. 43.16), may be avulsed. This requires orthoses and gradual return to activity. Surgery is rarely indicated as the tibialis posterior has a complex insertion into all bones of the foot.

Less common causes of midfoot pain
First tarsometatarsal joint pain

A prominent first metatarsal–cuneiform joint may cause pain to the dorsomedial midfoot. Most often, constricting shoelaces or excessively tightly fitting shoes will compress a dorsally protuberant first tarsometatarsal joint. The prominent base of the first metatarsal may be anatomically determined or developed due to degenerative changes at the joint. Dorsal cutaneous nerve compression can also result from this prominent dorsal bump. Suggested treatments focus to reduce pressure at this site. Modified lacing patterns, shoes with soft leather through the midfoot,

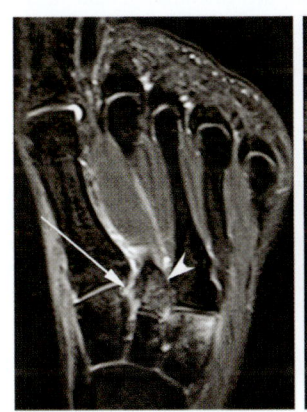

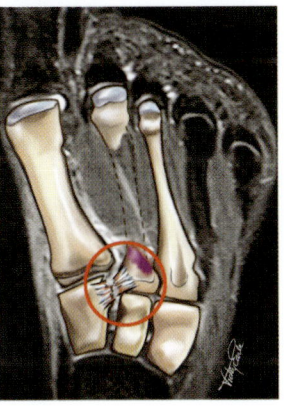

(b)

(c)

Figure 43.15 (cont.) (b) CT scan showing fractures of middle and lateral cuneiforms (arrows) with 0.30 cm of diastasis in the Lisfranc joint (c) Axial STIR MRI highlights torn Lisfranc ligament (arrow) and associated cuboid and metatarsal base contusion (arrowhead)[33]

(c) IMAGING IN SPORTS-SPECIFIC MUSCULOSKELETAL INJURIES, 2016, P. 660: ALI GUERMAZI, FRANK W ROEMER, MICHEL D CREMA. © SPRINGER INTERNATIONAL PUBLISHING SWITZERLAND 2016. WITH PERMISSION OF SPRINGER

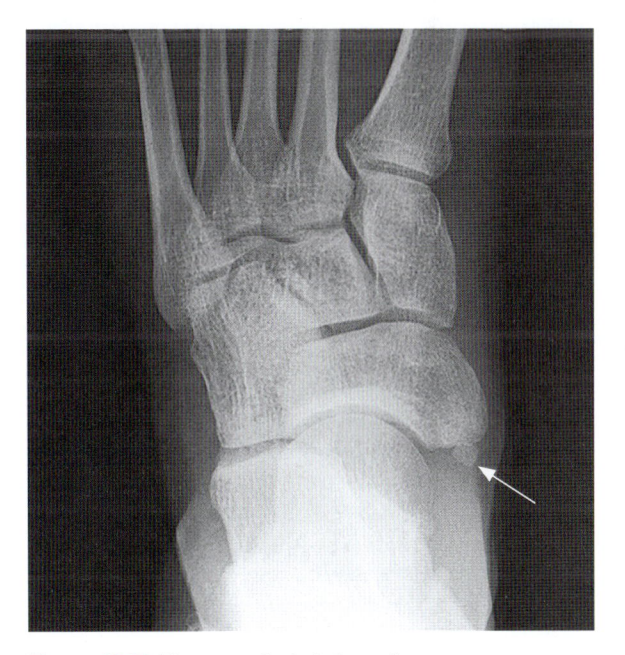

Figure 43.16 The os navicularis (arrow)

PART B Regional problems

and accommodative padding around the bump can all be attempted before more aggressive treatments. Surgery may be required to remove persistently painful bony exostoses.

Extensor tendinopathy

The extensor (dorsiflexor) muscles of the foot comprise the tibialis anterior, extensor hallucis longus and brevis, as well as extensor digitorum longus and brevis. Tibialis anterior tendinopathy is the most common tendinopathy occurring in the extensor muscles of the foot. Tendinopathies of the extensor hallucis longus and brevis and extensor digitorum longus and brevis muscles are rare.

The tibialis anterior muscle eccentrically controls plantarflexion and eversion of the foot at heel strike and its tendon is therefore susceptible to overuse injury. Tendinopathy generally occurs because of excessive training load in relation to background preparation. Experienced clinicians believe that stiffness of the first MTP joint and midfoot joints may contribute.

Generally, after a period of overuse, the patient with extensor tendinopathy complains of burning or aching medial midfoot pain. Examination may reveal tenderness, often with mild swelling, at the insertion of the tibialis anterior tendon at the base of the first metatarsal and the cuneiform. Pain may be elicited by passive plantar flexion combined with eversion, abduction and dorsiflexion. This is otherwise known as the tibialis anterior passive stretch (TAPS) test.[85] Resisted dorsiflexion and eccentric inversion may also exacerbate symptoms. Functional assessment may reveal excessive heel strike or over-striding during running. Both ultrasound and MRI may reveal swelling of these tendons and exclude the presence of a degenerative tear.

Popular clinical treatment includes relative rest and soft tissue therapy to the extensor muscles. Extensor muscle strengthening is advocated as is the case with other tendinopathies. The underlying precipitating cause needs to be addressed. If this is load, then training load needs to be considered. Local treatment may include mobilisation of the first ray, and tarsometatarsal and midtarsal joints, if the first MTP joint and midfoot is stiff. Modification of running technique may be required (reduce stride length) and footwear may need to be replaced.

Peroneal tendinopathy

Peroneal tendinopathy is an overuse injury of the peroneal tendons associated with running, dancing and in those with chronic lateral ankle instability. The management of this condition is described in Chapter 42.

Abductor hallucis strains

Abductor hallucis strains result in pain along the medial longitudinal arch and are often associated with excessive pronation. The abductor hallucis tendon is tender to palpate. Treatment consists of local electrotherapeutic modalities and taping.

Cuboid syndrome

The renowned physiotherapist from the American Ballet Theatre in the 1990s, Peter Marshall, brought this condition to the mind of clinicians who specialise in foot pain.[86, 87] Marshall argued that due to excessive traction of the peroneus longus, the cuboid becomes 'subluxated'. The term 'subluxated' is still challenging, 35 years after Marshall used it; certainly there have never been imaging changes captured to confirm subluxation or dislocation. Cuboid syndrome may also manifest following an acute plantarflexion and inversion ankle injury, and is common among professional ballet dancers. Pain is experienced with lateral weight-bearing. Most patients with this syndrome have excessively pronated feet but it is also seen in patients with lateral ankle instability.

The peroneus longus subluxates the cuboid bone so that the lateral aspect is rotated dorsally and medially. There may be a visible depression over the dorsal aspect of the cuboid. Treatment involves a single manipulation to reverse the subluxation.[88] The cuboid should be pushed upwards and laterally from the medial plantar aspect of the cuboid, as shown in Figure 43.17. In the largest case series, athletes returned to sport immediately following cuboid manipulation without any recurrences.[89]

Stress fracture of the cuboid

Stress fractures of the cuboid are uncommon and occur secondary to compression of the cuboid between the calcaneus and the fourth and fifth metatarsal bones when exaggerated plantarflexion is undertaken with or without inversion. Diagnosis is often delayed due to non-specific signs or symptoms clinically and typically normal plain radiography. MRI is the preferred choice of imaging (Fig. 43.18).[90, 91] Treatment of the uncomplicated stress fracture requires non-weight-bearing for 4–6 weeks, followed by a graduated return to activity.

Stress fracture of the cuneiforms

Stress fractures of the cuneiform bones are quite rare. We reported one in 1993 and have seen less than a handful between us since then.[92] Theoretical risk factors are large body habitus, plantar fascia injury,[93] overuse and altered gait pattern. Limited weight-bearing rest is treatment for medial cuneiform stress fractures; however, stress fractures of the intermediate cuneiform require surgical reduction and fixation for adequate healing.[94]

Köhler's disease

Köhler's disease, or osteochondritis of the navicular, is found in children aged 2–8 years (Chapter 44).

Foot pain CHAPTER 43

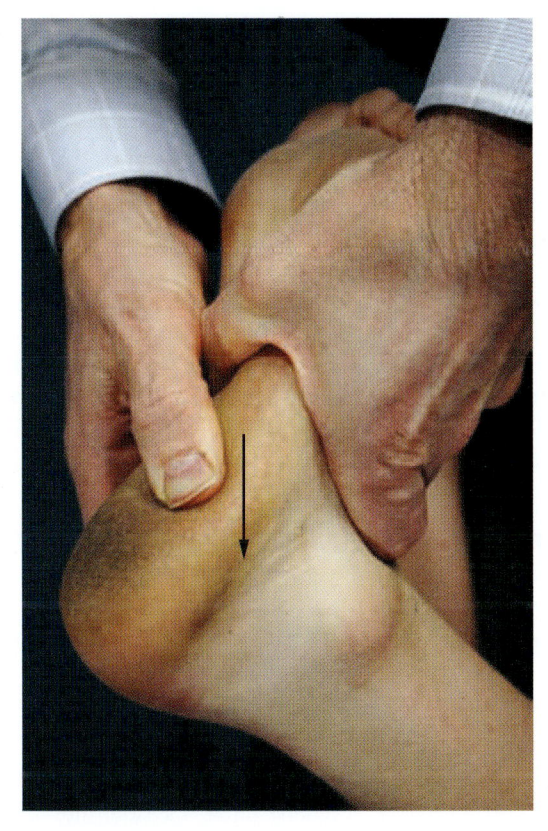

Figure 43.17 Manipulation of the cuboid in a superior and lateral direction in cuboid syndrome

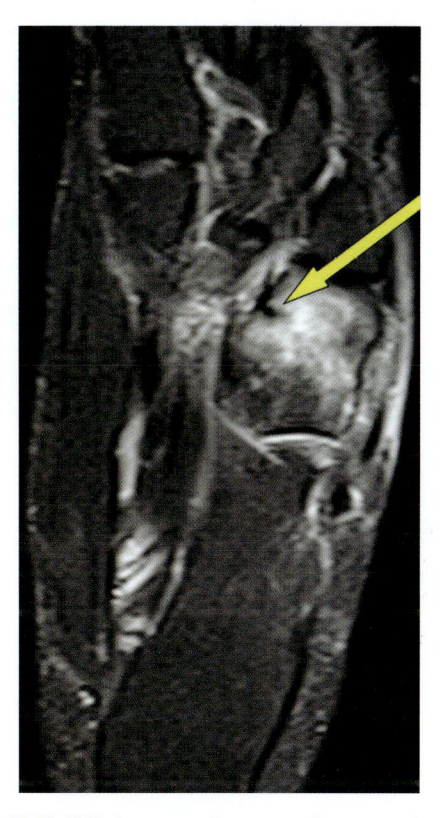

Figure 43.18 MRI demonstrating stress fracture cuboid (arrow)[33]
IMAGING IN SPORTS-SPECIFIC MUSCULOSKELETAL INJURIES, 2016, P. 659, ALI GUERMAZI, FRANK W ROEMER, MICHEL D CREMA.
© SPRINGER INTERNATIONAL PUBLISHING SWITZERLAND 2016. WITH PERMISSION OF SPRINGER

Tarsal coalition

Congenital fusions of the foot bones usually present as midfoot pain. Tarsal coalitions may be osseous, cartilaginous (synchondrosis), fibrous (syndesmosis) or a combination. The estimated prevalence is 1–2%, although a recent CT and cadaver dissection study found 12.7%.[95] A fibrous coalition is relatively mobile and therefore may not cause any pain on limited motion. As fibrous or cartilaginous coalitions ossify during adolescence, rearfoot or midfoot joint range of motion decreases, placing additional stress on the talocrural (ankle) joint. Accounting for 90% of coalitions, the two most common tarsal coalitions occur at the calcaneonavicular joint and the talocalcaneal joint; 50–60% occur bilaterally.

Clinical presentation usually occurs during the adolescent/young adult years coinciding with ossification of the cartilaginous coalitions and more vigorous sports and physical activity.[96] Patients can also present after minor trauma such as an ankle sprain that does not clinically improve (Chapter 41). Because tarsal coalition causes subtalar restriction, adjacent joints may function abnormally and thus the patient presents with joint spurs and symptoms remote from the coalition (Fig. 43.19).

Examination usually reveals limited range of subtalar and midtarsal joint movement that may be painful at end range. Plain radiographs remain the initial test of choice and are the most useful diagnostic tool for osseous coalitions. A Harris-Beath view may detect a talocalcaneal coalition. A complete C-sign seen on a lateral X-ray is highly correlated with bony talocalcaneal coalition (Fig. 43.19), although the absence of this sign does not rule out the possibility of this condition.[97] CT scan provides the most complete diagnostic imaging for bony tarsal coalition, while MRI can identify fibrous coalition.

Asymptomatic cases do not require treatment. For symptomatic cases, initial conservative management includes a period of relative rest to allow inflamed joints to settle. NSAIDs may provide a short-term palliative effect as can paracetamol (acetaminophen). Orthoses may alter biomechanics favourably but they can also eliminate

PART B Regional problems

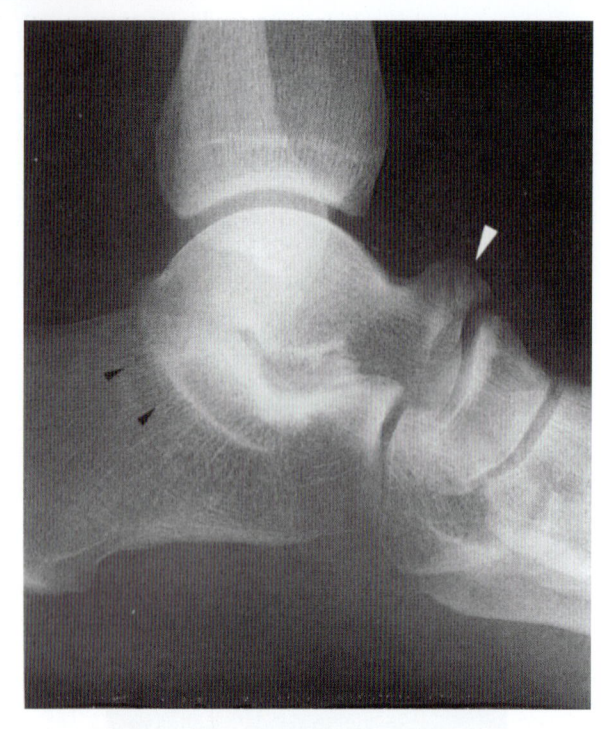

Figure 43.19 Radiograph showing talocalcaneal coalition (black arrows) with a continuous cortical line, the C-sign, joining the talus and sustentaculum tali, and talar beaking (white arrow) that results from abnormal subtalar movement

movement at joints that provide motion so they need to be considered carefully and their effects monitored. Corticosteroids are mentioned in sports medicine texts but we do not see a compelling case in tarsal coalition.[96]

Surgery may be required for recalcitrant or disabling pain. As always, an experienced subspecialist foot surgeon is likely to provide better advice and have superior clinical outcomes compared to a general orthopaedic surgeon who is essentially unfamiliar with the intricacies of the procedure or its postoperative rehabilitation.

FOREFOOT PAIN

Forefoot problems that can severely compromise dancers' and athletes' performance include stress fractures and soft tissue injuries such as the plantar plate tear. Common problems that are far more significant in a competitive athlete's life than in a 'weekend warrior' include corns, calluses and nail problems. Causes of forefoot pain are listed in Table 43.5 and that list guides the order in which we discuss the conditions in the chapter.

Clinical perspective

Accurate diagnosis in the forefoot often requires the clinician to combine the evidence from a careful history (mechanisms, time course), with careful palpation and understanding of the limitations of investigations (e.g. Morton's neuroma will likely come with a normal MRI).

History

Most causes of forefoot pain result from training errors and thus have an insidious onset. Occasionally, acute forefoot pain may result from a sprain of the first MTP joint ('turf toe'). Sensory symptoms may indicate that a neuroma is present.

Examination

The key to examination of the patient with forefoot pain is precise palpation to identify the site of maximal tenderness. Biomechanical examination is necessary.

Table 43.5 Causes of forefoot pain

Common	Less common	Not to be missed
Stress fracture of the neck of metatarsals I–IV	Stress fracture of the great toe	Referred pain
Stress fracture of the base of the second metatarsal	Joplin's neuritis	
Fractures of the fifth metatarsal	Freiberg's osteochondritis	
MTP joint synovitis	Toe clawing	
First MTP joint sprain ('turf toe')	Subungual haematoma	
Hallux limitus	Subungual exostosis	
Hallux valgus ('bunion')		
Sesamoid injuries including stress fracture		
Plantar plate tear		
Morton's neuroma		
Corns, calluses		
Plantar wart		
Onychocryptosis (ingrown toenail)		

1. Observation (Fig. 43.20a)
2. Palpation:
   (a) metatarsals (Fig. 43.20b)
   (b) first MTP joint (Fig. 43.20c)
   (c) sesamoid bone of the foot (Fig. 43.20d)
   (d) space between third and fourth metatarsal (Fig. 43.20e)

Investigations

Plain radiographs may show evidence of a healing stress fracture or acute fracture, the presence of hallux abducto-valgus, hallux limitus or a subungual exostosis. MRI may confirm the diagnosis of a stress fracture. Both MRI and ultrasound have limited utility to identify a neuroma[98] (see section on Morton's neuroma below).

Stress fractures of the neck of metatarsals I–IV

Stress fractures of the metatarsals are the second most common stress fractures of all.[99] Training errors (sudden increase in load, change in training conditions or footwear) or poor biomechanics can load the forefoot to failure.[100] Fatigue of the gastrocnemius muscle increases forefoot loading.[101, 102]

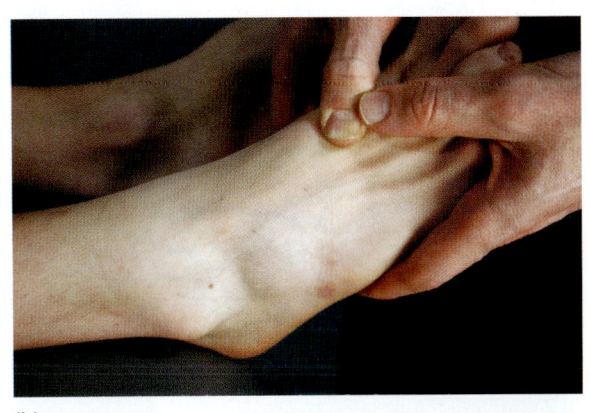

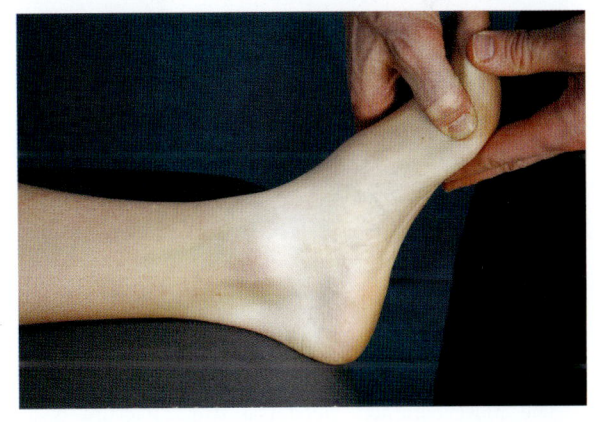

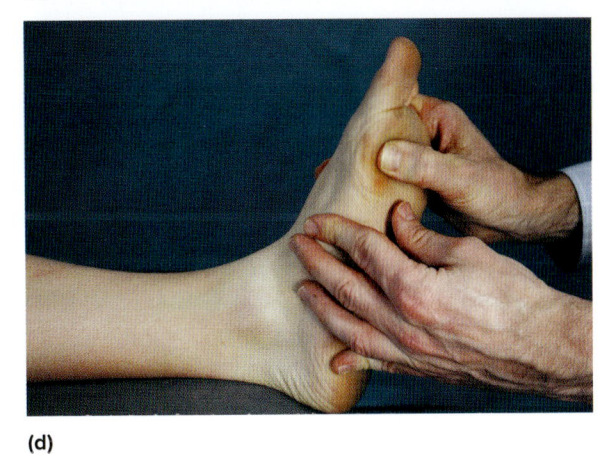

Figure 43.20 Examination of the patient with forefoot pain (a) Observation for the presence of obvious abnormalities (e.g. hallux abducto-valgus, claw toes, Morton's foot, plantar warts, onychocryptosis, corns, callus) (b) Palpation—metatarsals (c) Palpation—first MTP joint (d) Palpation—sesamoid

PART B   Regional problems

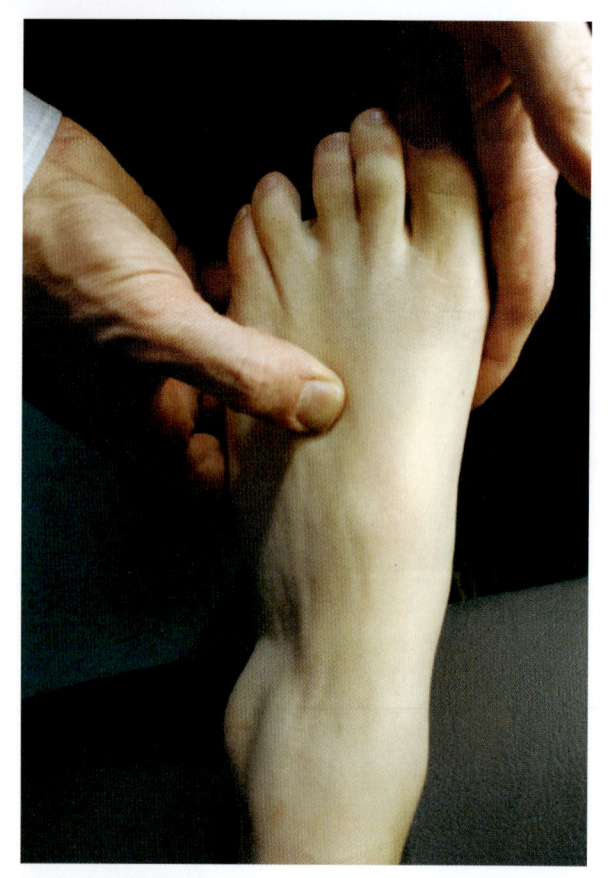

(e)

Figure 43.20 (cont.) (e) Palpation—space between third and fourth metatarsal

The most common metatarsal stress fracture is at the neck of the second metatarsal. This occurs in the pronating foot, when the first ray is dorsiflexed and the second metatarsal becomes subjected to greater load. The second metatarsal is also susceptible to stress fracture in the case of a Morton's foot, where the second ray is the longest ray (Fig. 43.21). The base of the second metatarsal is firmly fixed in position next to the cuneiform bones, further increasing the likelihood of fracture. Stress fracture of the second metatarsal is common in ballet dancers. Stress fractures of the other metatarsals also occur, particularly in the third metatarsal if it is longer than the second.

Plain radiograph is not sensitive to detect early stress fractures but may reveal a radiolucent line or periosteal thickening if the fracture has been present for a few weeks (Fig. 43.22). MRI is the investigation of choice.

The management of most stress fractures is straightforward, involving rest from weight-bearing aggravating activities for approximately 4 weeks, and addressing any underlying contributing factors. If the patient is required to be on his or her feet excessively, the use of a CAM boot may be required for 1–2 weeks until pain settles.

The athlete should be allowed to recommence activity when he or she does not experience pain when walking and there is no local tenderness at the fracture site. A graduated exercise program should be instituted to return the athlete to full training and competition. Orthoses may

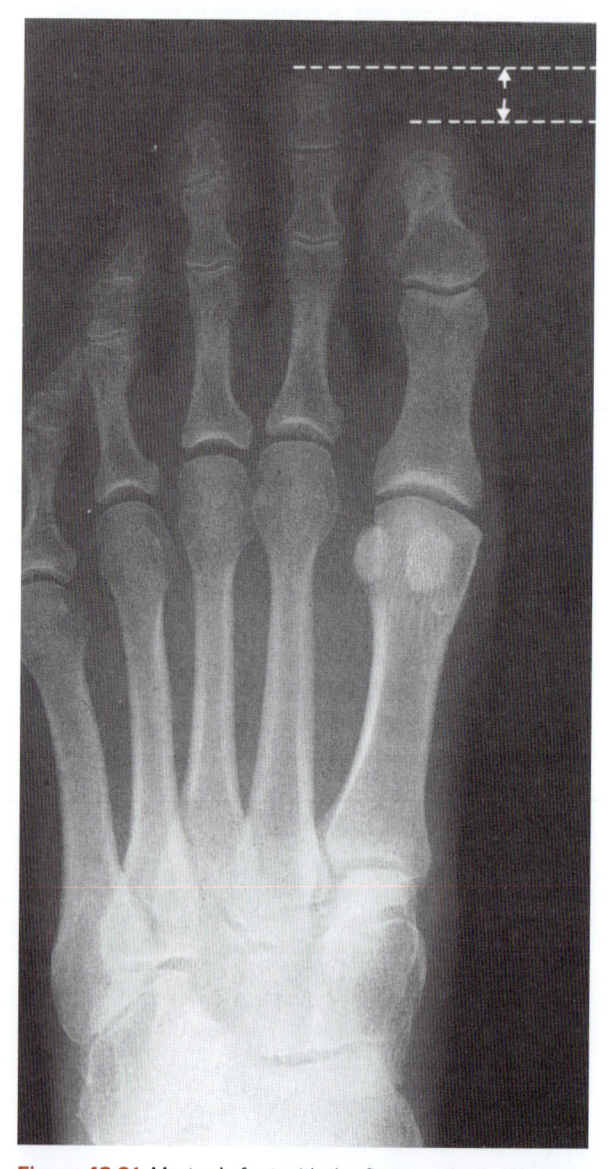

Figure 43.21 Morton's foot with the first ray shorter than the second. The patient with a metatarsal stress fracture complains of forefoot pain aggravated by activity such as running or dancing. The pain is not severe initially but gradually worsens with activity. Examination reveals the presence of focal tenderness overlying the metatarsal

Foot pain CHAPTER 43

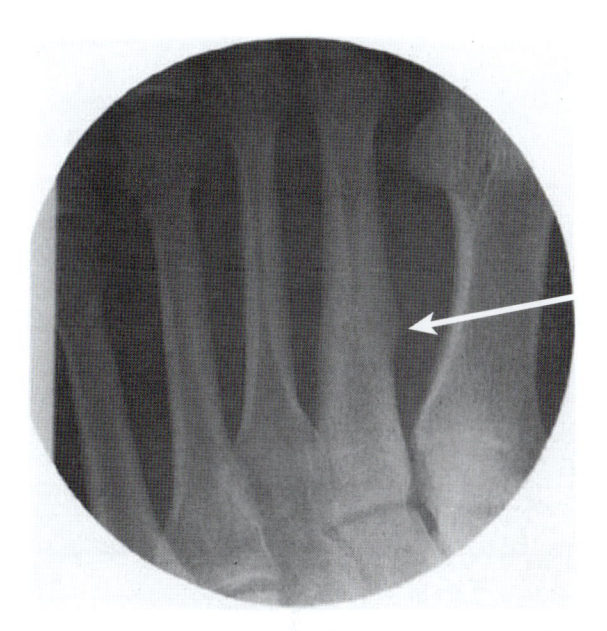

Figure 43.22 Stress fracture of the second metatarsal. X-ray appearance—arrow points to new bone formation at the site of the stress fracture. This ballet dancer's metatarsal displays generalised cortical hypertrophy

be required to control abnormal foot mechanics; however, it is still unclear from current research whether orthoses can prevent metatarsal stress fractures.[103] Any instability during forefoot weight-bearing may predispose to the development of a stress fracture. Intrinsic and extrinsic foot muscle strengthening exercises may help prevent recurrence.

> **PRACTICE PEARL**
>
> Two metatarsal stress fractures require special treatment: fractures of the base of the second metatarsal and the stress fracture in the Jones position of the fifth metatarsal.

Special metatarsal stress fracture: base of the second MT

An unusual fracture of the base of the second metatarsal (Fig. 43.23a) involving the joint occurs in ballet dancers.[99, 104-106] The fracture can sometimes be seen on plain X-ray (Fig. 43.23b), however MRI is the investigation of choice (Fig. 43.23c). This fracture should be treated by having the dancer remain non weight-bearing on crutches until tenderness settles, usually at least 4 weeks. The differential diagnosis of proximal second metatarsal stress fracture is chronic joint synovitis.

These stress fractures may be associated with Achilles tightness, low bone mass and high training loads.[107]

Clinicians expert in managing metatarsal fractures advocate soft tissue therapy to the calf muscles in addition to strengthening of all foot muscles including the peroneals.

Fractures of the fifth metatarsal

Ever since Sir Robert Jones described[108] in 1902 a fracture 2 cm from the base of the fifth metatarsal that he himself sustained (while maypole dancing!), there has been considerable confusion regarding the different types of fractures and their definitions. For many years, fractures at the base of the fifth metatarsal were simply divided into avulsion fractures of the tuberosity, and all others, which were collectively known as Jones fractures.

In 1993, Lawrence and Botte were the first to introduce a classification distinguishing three different fracture types based on mechanism of injury, fracture location, treatment options and outcome.[109] They described the 'Jones fracture' being located more proximally, and assigned it at the level of the entire fourth-fifth intermetatarsal articulation

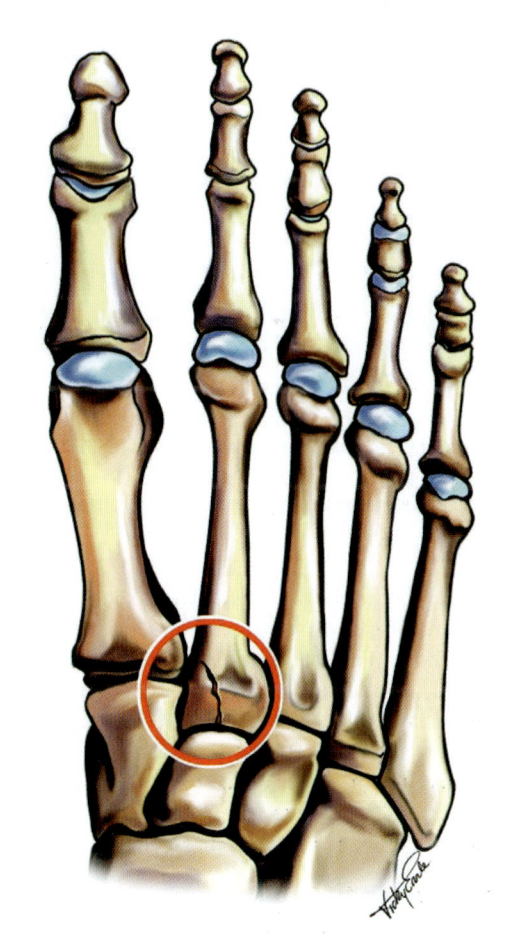

(a)

Figure 43.23 (a) Stress fracture of the base of the second metatarsal

961

PART B   Regional problems

(b)

(c)

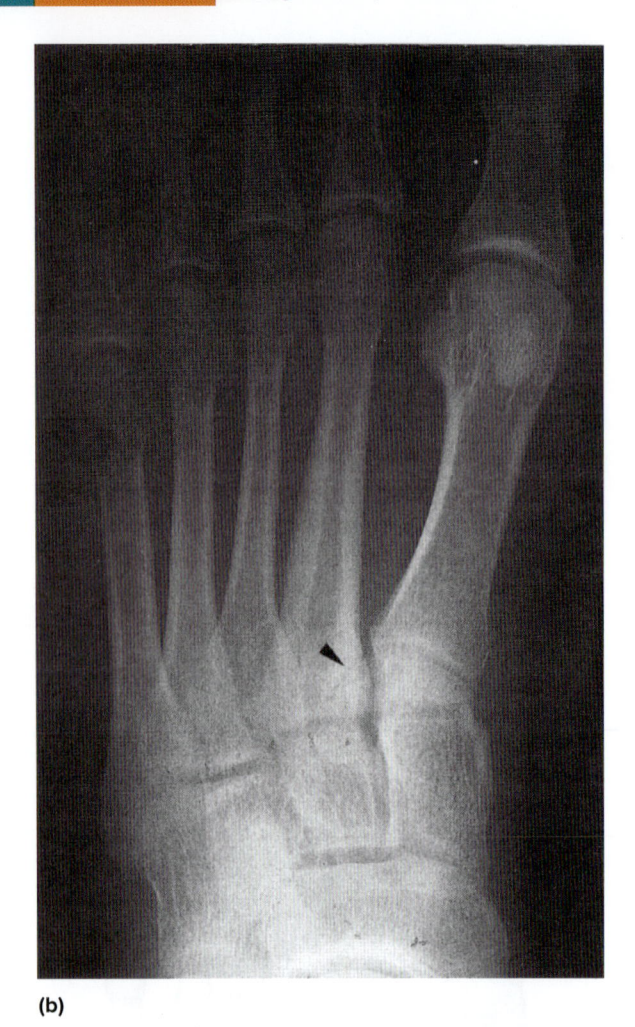

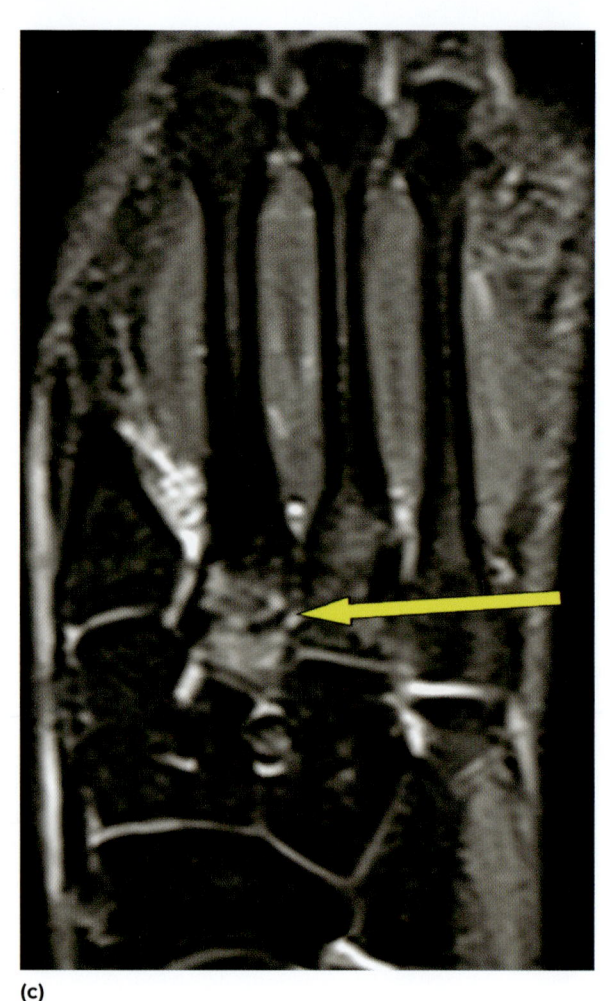

Figure 43.23 (cont.) (b) Stress fracture of the base of the second metatarsal involving the joint. The fracture line (arrowhead) extends to the second tarsometatarsal joint (c) MRI of stress fracture (arrow) at base of second metatarsal. This is a common site of stress fractures in ballet dancers[33]
(c) IMAGING IN SPORTS-SPECIFIC MUSCULOSKELETAL INJURIES 2016, P. 659, ALI GUERMAZI, FRANK W ROEMER, MICHEL D CREMA. © SPRINGER INTERNATIONAL PUBLISHING SWITZERLAND 2016. WITH PERMISSION OF SPRINGER

(Zone 2). The location formerly known as 'Jones fracture' at the proximal diaphysis was renamed as 'diaphyseal stress fracture' (Zone 3). Fractures to the most proximal part of the fifth metatarsal were named 'tuberosity avulsion fracture' (Zone 1).

Still today, the most common classification of fractures to the proximal fifth metatarsal bone is into 'tuberosity avulsion fractures' (Zone 1), 'Jones fractures' (Zone 2) and 'diaphyseal stress fractures' (Zone 3) as shown in Figure 43.24a.

Fracture of the tuberosity

The fracture of the tuberosity at the base of the fifth metatarsal (Fig. 43.24b) has been described in Chapter 41 and is usually an avulsion injury that results from an acute ankle sprain. This uncomplicated fracture does well treated with weight-bearing as tolerated with an elastic wrap circumferentially placed around the midfoot.[110]

Jones fracture

The fifth metatarsal fracture at the level of the articulation of the fourth and fifth metatarsals (Zone 2) is the Jones fracture (Fig. 43.24c). A Jones fracture may occur as the result of an acute plantarflexion/inversion mechanism or a medially directed force on a planted foot, and thus create an acute fracture. There may be a history of prodromal symptoms suggesting that the fracture may occur in an area already suffering bone stress. In Ekstrand's UEFA study of professional footballers with fifth metatarsal fractures, 45% reported pain on the lateral side of the foot prior to the acute fracture.[111]

Foot pain   CHAPTER 43

In 1984, Torg proposed managing these fractures on the basis of a radiographic (Fig. 43.24c) classification into three types.[112]

- Type 1: acute fractures characterised by a narrow fracture line and absence of intramedullary sclerosis.
- Type 2: those with delayed union, with widening of the fracture line and evidence of intramedullary sclerosis.
- Type 3: those with non-union and complete obliteration of the medullary canal by sclerotic bone.

Jones fractures can be treated operatively or non-operatively. In the 1990s, most Jones fractures were managed non-operatively with 6-8 weeks of non-weight-bearing.

However, there is now compelling evidence for screw fixation (Fig. 43.24d) of Jones fractures in sports medicine. Superior outcomes include both faster return to play (as early as 2-4 weeks) and fewer recurrences compared with cast treatment.[113-115] The average time to return to sport following primary screw fixation is 7.5 weeks.[116]

Non-union may occur with this type of fracture because of the location of the nutrient artery (Fig. 43.24e).[115]

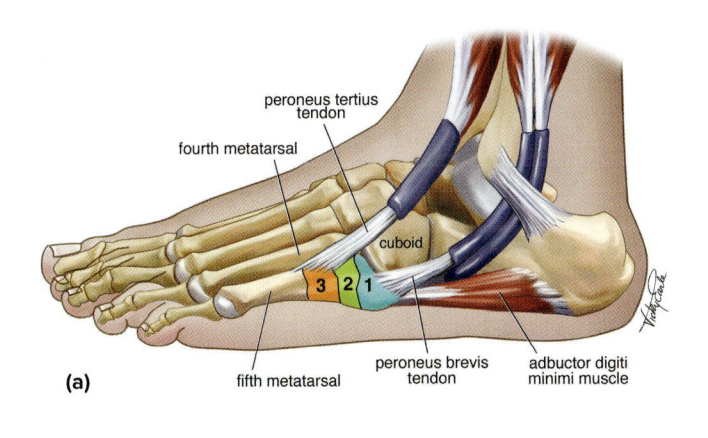

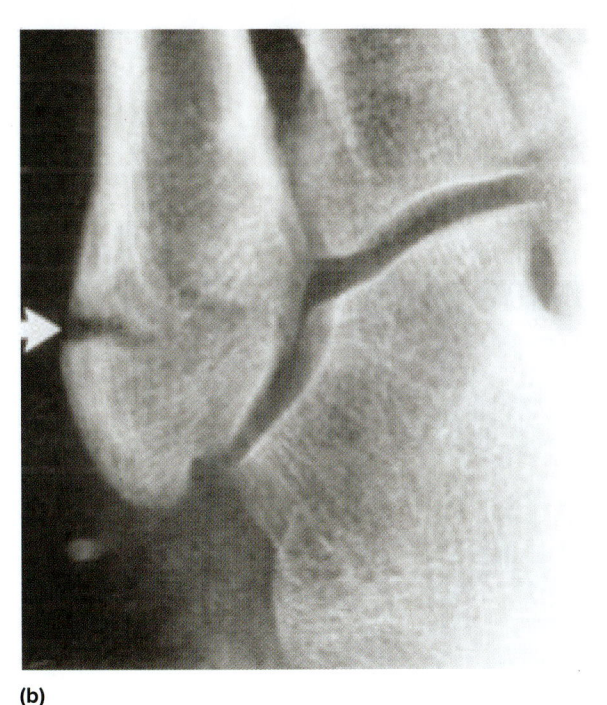

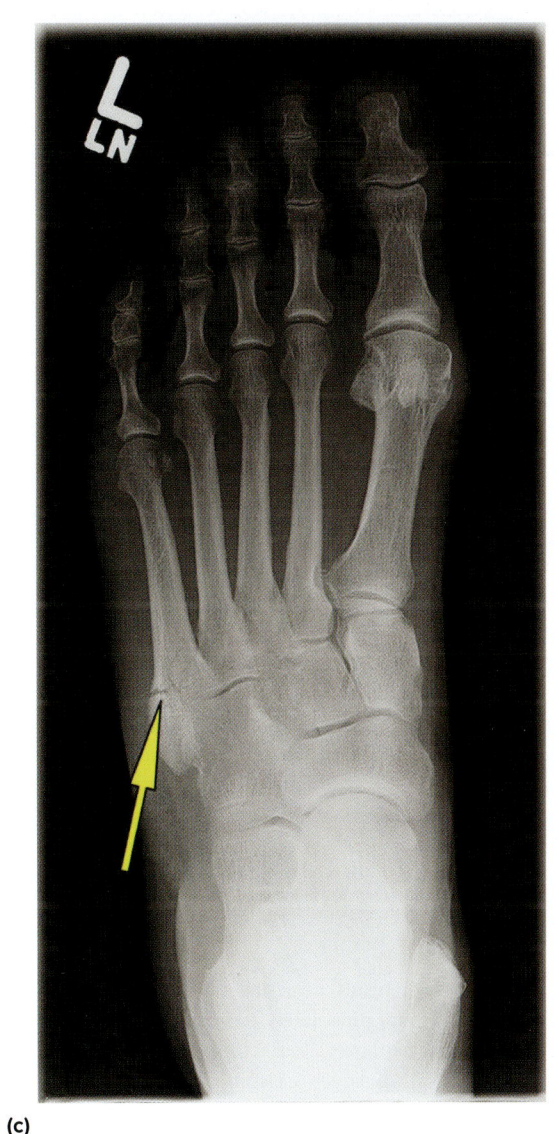

Figure 43.24 (a) Anatomical locations of the different types of proximal fifth metatarsal fractures. Zone 1 tuberosity avulsion fractures, Zone 2 Jones fractures and Zone 3 diaphyseal stress fractures (b) Fracture of the tuberosity of the fifth metatarsal (c) Jones fracture at the level of the fourth–fifth metatarsal articulation

963

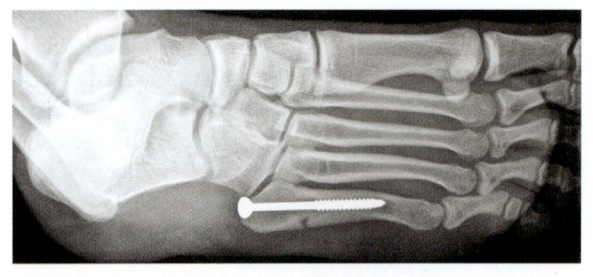

PART B Regional problems

(d)

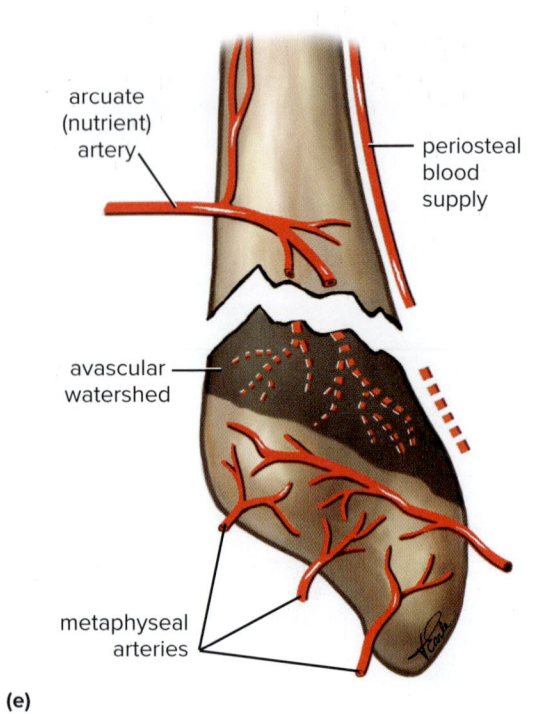

(e)

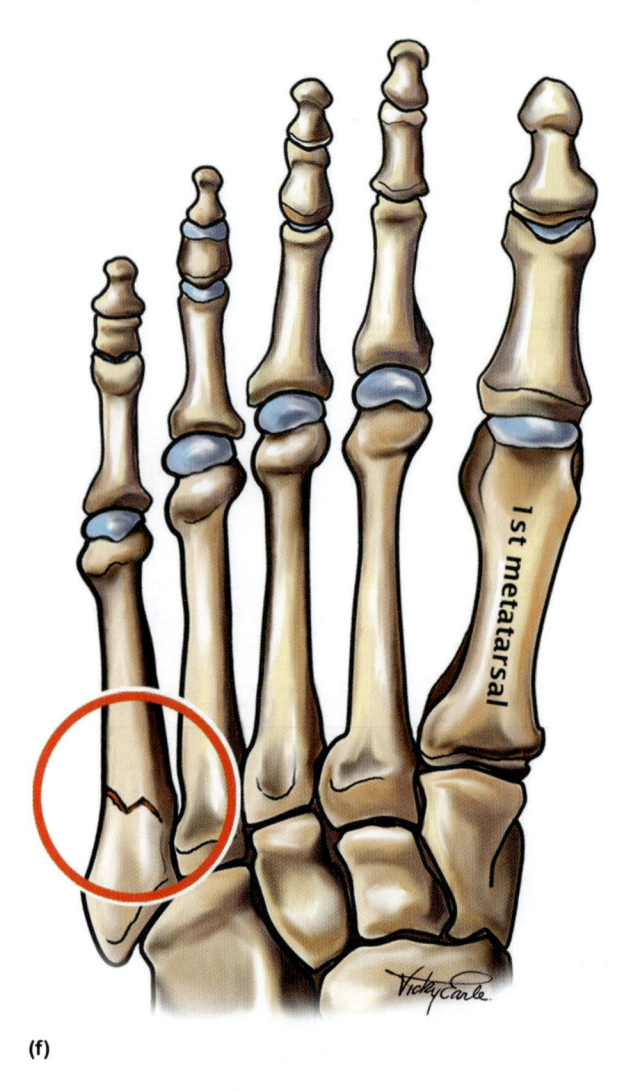

(f)

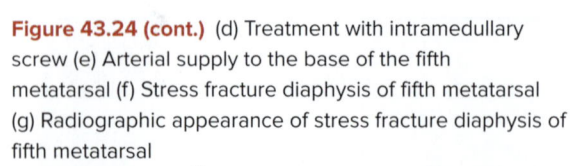

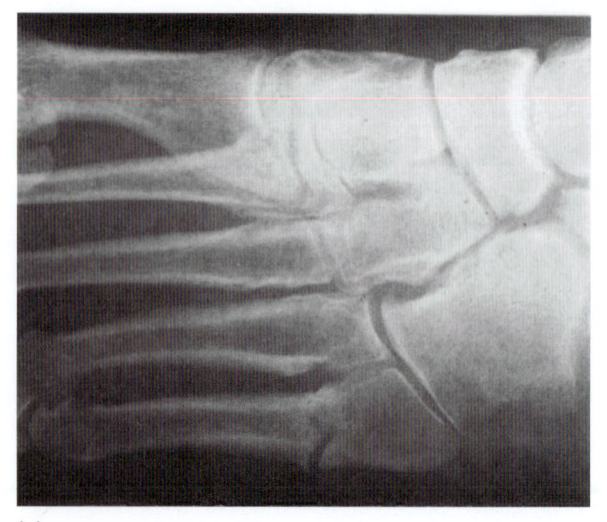

Figure 43.24 (cont.) (d) Treatment with intramedullary screw (e) Arterial supply to the base of the fifth metatarsal (f) Stress fracture diaphysis of fifth metatarsal (g) Radiographic appearance of stress fracture diaphysis of fifth metatarsal

(e) FROM DEN HARTOG.[161] ADAPTED FROM DAMERON TB JR. FRACTURE OF THE PROXIMAL FIFTH METATARSAL: SELECTING THE BEST TREATMENT OPTION. J AM ACAD ORTHOP SURG 1995;3:110–14

Re-fractures as a result of screw failure are fortunately uncommon, but are most likely to occur soon after return to full unrestricted sport. Re-fractures and non-unions are best treated with a large, 5.5 mm or larger, solid screw and bone grafting.[117] The average time to return to sport following revision is 12 weeks. Early return to sport may predispose the athlete to re-fracture[118] and it may be wise to wait for full radiographic healing before return to sport.[119]

(g)

Stress fracture of the diaphysis

Diaphyseal stress fractures occur distal to the intermetatarsal articulation (Zone 3) in the diaphysis of the bone (Fig. 43.24f and g). Similarly to Jones fractures, these fractures are prone to non-union and treatment with screw fixation (Fig. 43.24d) has been found to both reduce the incidence of non-union and result in improved return-to-sport times (6.9 weeks compared to 14.5 weeks in a non-operative group).[114]

Spiral fracture (distal third)

An acute spiral fracture of the distal third of the fifth metatarsal is seen, especially in dancers who suffer this fracture when they lose their balance while on demi pointe and roll over the outer border of the foot–the 'fouetté fracture' (Fig. 43.25). Non-displaced fractures may be treated with a plastic cast shoe, short leg walking boot or firm-soled shoe with weight-bearing as tolerated. Fractures that are displaced more than 3-4 mm or angulated more than 10° in the sagittal plane should be reduced.[110]

Approximately 25% of individuals who sustain a fifth metatarsal fracture–of any kind–continue to have some non-limiting pain up to one year later. Despite this low-level pain there were no functional impairments in a cohort of patients prospectively followed for one year.[120]

MTP joint synovitis

MTP joint synovitis (commonly referred to as 'metatarsalgia') is a common painful condition occurring most frequently in the second, third and/or fourth MTP joints, or isolated in the first MTP joints. Tenosynovitis of the flexor tendon sheath is a potential differential diagnosis.[121]

The synovium of the MTP joints becomes painful, usually due to excessive pressure over a prolonged period. It is often related to:

- pes cavus or high-arched foot
- excessive pronation of the foot
- clawing or hammer toes
- tight extensor tendons of the toes
- prominent metatarsal heads
- Morton's foot (Fig. 43.21): there is a shortened first metatarsal, which results in weight going through the second MTP joint.

The patient complains of pain aggravated by forefoot weight-bearing, particularly in the midstance and propulsion phases of walking. Pain onset is usually gradual.

Examination reveals local tenderness on palpation. Pain is aggravated by passive forced flexion of the toe. The V sign is sometimes seen in the early stages of metatarsal joint synovitis. A separation of the toes can create a V shape that may indicate underlying dysfunction.[122]

There may be an associated skin lesion (e.g. a callus) over the plantar surface of the affected joint due to the excessive load. This injury may be caused by uneven distribution of load, especially with excessive pronation.

Treatment involves addressing the most likely biomechanical contributing factors, as well as providing

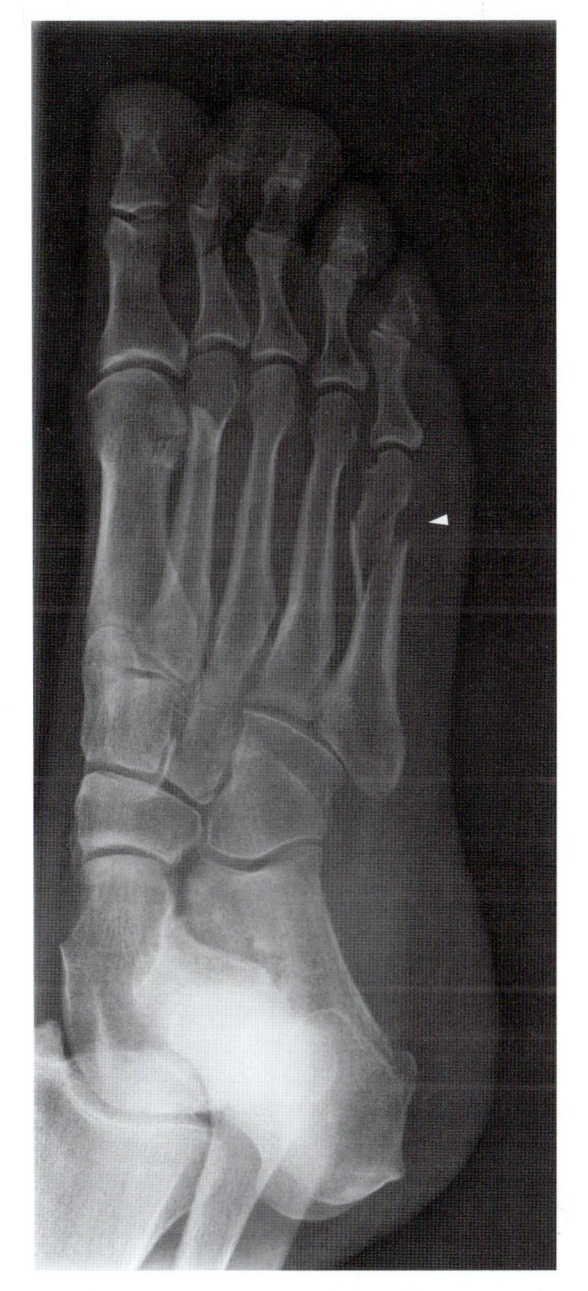

Figure 43.25 Spiral fracture of the distal fifth metatarsal

symptomatic relief. Padding to redistribute weight from the painful areas can provide short-term relief. Footwear that has adequate midsole cushioning is essential. NSAIDs may be helpful and corticosteroid injection is occasionally required. The joint is injected via the dorsal surface, while longitudinal traction is placed on the toe to open the joint space.

First MTP joint sprain ('turf toe')

A sprain to the first MTP, otherwise known as a 'turf toe', is a common injury occurring in athletes in which the plantar capsule and ligament of the first MTP joint is damaged. The classic mechanism of injury is usually that of a forced hyperextension to the first MTP joint, although occasionally a plantarflexion injury to the joint may result in this injury.

Turf toe injuries are classified on the basis of their severity into grade I (mild), grade II (partial plantar capsule and ligament disruption) and grade III (complete plantar capsule and ligament disruption) (Table 43.6). Grade III injuries are often associated with injury of other structures such as the plantar plate or the flexor hallucis longus/flexor hallucis brevis tendons.[123]

Predisposing risk factors include:

- competing or training on artificial turf
- pes planus or excessive pronation
- decreased pre-injury ankle range of motion
- decreased pre-injury MTP range of motion
- soft flexible footwear.

The athlete usually complains of localised pain, swelling and occasional redness at the first MTP joint following a 'bending' injury to the joint. The pain is classically aggravated by weight-bearing or movement of the big toe.

Examination reveals localised swelling and tenderness at the first MTP joint. In mild injuries plantar or plantar medial tenderness is present; in more severe injuries, dorsal tenderness occurs. Passive plantarflexion and dorsiflexion of the first MTP joint are generally painful and there may be a reduction in the range of movement in both directions. Passive gliding of the joint in a dorsal to plantar direction can be used to evaluate the plantar plate. Resisted plantarflexion and dorsiflexion can be used to evaluate the integrity of the flexor and extensor tendons.[123]

Plain radiographs are generally unremarkable, although occasionally small periarticular flecks of bone are noted, most likely indicating avulsion of the MTP capsule or ligamentous complex. If injury to the plantar plate is suspected, lateral views in forced dorsiflexion can be used. This view may demonstrate a lack of distal sesamoid excursion, which is indicative of complete disruption of the plantar ligament structures.[123] MRI may be appropriate for elite athletes with grade II and III injuries to outline the extent of ligamentous, osseous and cartilage damage.[124]

Treatment consists of ice, NSAIDs, electrotherapeutic modalities and decreased weight-bearing for at least 72 hours. Additional treatment may include taping (Fig. 43.26) and the use of stiff-soled shoes or a CAM walker boot to protect the first MTP joint from further injury. Treatment of the various grades of injury is summarised in Table 43.6. Recovery from grade I and II turf toe injury generally takes 3–4 weeks. Surgical indications for grade III injuries include:[123]

- large capsular avulsion and vertical instability
- retraction of sesamoids
- loose body
- chondral injury.

A possible long-term sequel to this injury is the development of hallux limitus, discussed in the next section.

Table 43.6 Turf toe grading and treatment

Grade	Description/Findings	Treatment	Return to play
I	Attenuation of plantar structures Localised swelling Minimal ecchymosis	Symptomatic	Return as tolerated
II	Partial tear of plantar structures Moderate swelling Restricted motion due to pain	Walking boot Crutches as needed	Up to 2 weeks May need taping on return to play
III	Complete disruption of plantar structures Significant swelling/ecchymosis Hallux flexion weakness Frank instability of hallux MTP	Long-term immobilisation in boot or cast OR Surgical reconstruction	6–10 weeks depending on sport and position Likely need taping on return to play

ADAPTED FROM MCCORMICK AND ANDERSON[169] REPRODUCED WITH PERMISSION OF JOURNAL OF CLINICAL SPORTS MEDICINE

Foot pain CHAPTER 43

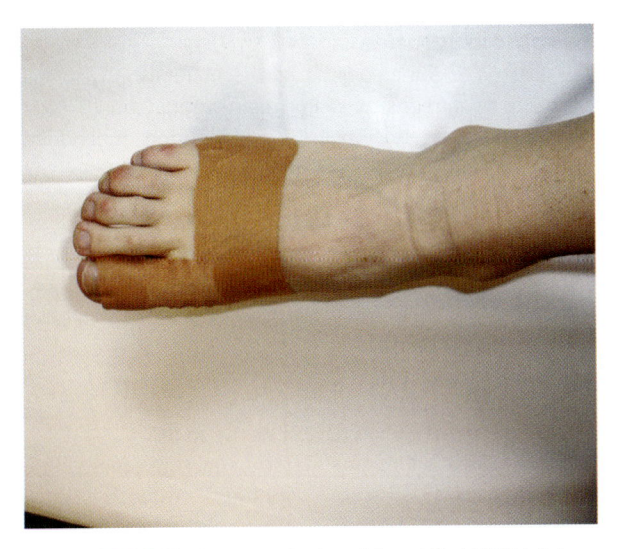

Figure 43.26 Taping to protect an injured first MTP joint

Hallux limitus

Hallux limitus refers to restriction in dorsiflexion of the hallux at the first MTP joint secondary to exostoses or osteoarthritis of the joint. Often the term 'hallux rigidus' is used to describe the final progression of hallux limitus as ankylosis of the joint occurs.

The primary role of the hallux is to enable dorsiflexion of the first metatarsal during the propulsive phase of gait. Approximately 60° of dorsiflexion is required for normal gait. Limitation of this range of motion results in problems with gait. Normal dorsiflexion is achieved via the action of peroneus longus, which helps to stabilise and maintain plantarflexion of the first ray.[125]

There is some evidence that the following may contribute to development of hallux limitus:

- trauma: secondary to chondral damage
- excessive load: via absolute loading or due to excessive pronation of the foot which increases the stresses on the joint and promotes development of exostoses
- repetitive weight-bearing dorsiflexion of the first MTP joint
- autoimmune arthropathy or metabolic conditions (e.g. rheumatoid arthritis, psoriatic arthritis, ankylosing spondylitis, gout)[125]
- hypermobile first ray (e.g. reduced plantarflexion of the first ray can increase compressive forces in the joint during propulsion).[125]

The main symptom is usually pain around the first MTP joint–often described as a deep aching sensation. Pain is aggravated by walking, especially in high heels, or activities involving forefoot weight-bearing. Dorsal joint hypertrophy can cause footwear to impinge on the joint and may lead to pain secondary to skin or soft tissue irritation. In patients with longstanding hallux limitus, a distinct shoe wear pattern is seen: the sole demonstrates wear beneath the second MTP joint and the first interphalangeal joint.

Examination reveals tenderness over the dorsal aspect of the first MTP joint, often with palpable dorsal exostoses. There is a painful limitation of joint motion. Some with this condition may develop chronic subungual haematoma due to repetitive compensatory dorsiflexion in the interphalangeal joint.[125]

Plain radiographs display the classic characteristics of degenerative osteoarthritis and the degree of degeneration. Features include joint space narrowing, sclerosis of the subchondral bone plate, osteophytic proliferation, flattening of the joint, sesamoid displacement and free bony fragments.

Conservative management consists of an initial reduction in activity, NSAIDs, a corticosteroid injection as adjuvant therapy, passive joint mobilisation before the joint fully fuses, correction of abnormal biomechanics with orthoses and/or footwear, and dynamic splinting.[126] Conservative treatment often fails when hallux dorsiflexion is less than 50°.

If conservative treatment fails, cheilectomy (resection of all bony prominences of the metatarsal head and base of the proximal phalanx) is required. Occasionally, arthroplasty of the first MTP joint is indicated.

Hallux valgus

Hallux valgus refers to static subluxation of the first MTP joint. It is characterised by valgus (lateral) deviation of the great toe and varus (medial) deviation of the first metatarsal (Fig. 43.27). Bony exostoses develop around the first MTP joint, often with an overlying bursitis. In severe cases, exostoses limit first MTP joint range of motion and cause pain with the pressure of footwear. Hallux valgus is common, affecting 23% of adults aged between 18 and 65 years.[127] It is more common in women. Although it is more common in older athletes, it can also develop in adolescence.[128]

The development of hallux valgus appears to occur secondary to a combination of intrinsic (genetic) and extrinsic causes. There is some evidence for an association of the condition with:

- constricting footwear (e.g. high heels)
- excessive pronation: increased pressure on the medial border of the hallux, resulting in deformation of the medial capsular structures
- increased length of the first metatarsal and hallux[129]
- trauma to the medial and plantar ligament complex and medial sesamoid bone[123]
- others including cystic degeneration of the medial capsule, Achilles tendon contracture, neuromuscular disorders and collagen-deficient diseases.

967

PART B   Regional problems

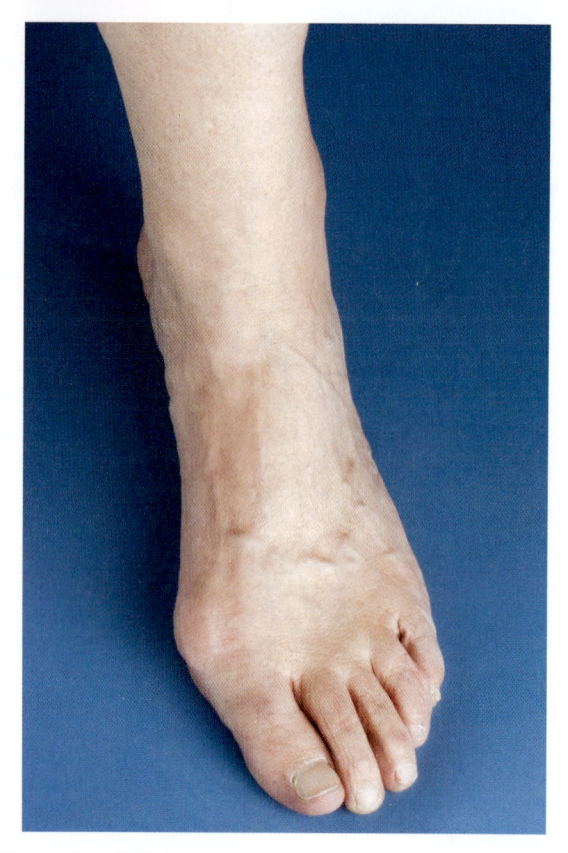

Figure 43.27 Hallux valgus

In the early phases, hallux valgus is often asymptomatic but as the deformity develops, pain arises at the medial eminence. The pain is typically relieved by removing shoes or by wearing soft, flexible, wide-toed shoes. Blistering of the skin or development of an inflamed bursa over the medial eminence may occur. In severe deformity, lateral metatarsalgia may occur due to the diminished weight-bearing capacity of the first ray.

Examination reveals the hallux valgus deformity often with a tender swelling overlying the medial eminence. Plain radiographs can image both the severity of the deformity and the degree of first MTP joint degeneration.

Initial treatment involves appropriate padding and footwear to reduce friction over the medial eminence. Correction of foot function with orthoses is essential. In more severe cases, surgery may be required to reconstruct the first MTP joint and remove the bony exostoses.

Minimally invasive surgical techniques for hallux valgus have been developed.[130] Orthoses are often required after surgery and gait re-education is needed to restore normal weight-bearing through the first ray.[131]

Sesamoid injuries

The first MTP joint consists of the metatarsophalangeal joint and two regularly occurring sesamoid bones, that play a significant role in great toe function. Embedded within the two tendons of the flexor hallucis brevis, the sesamoids:

- functionally lengthen the first metatarsal
- protect the tendon of flexor hallucis longus
- transfer weight-bearing from the lateral to the medial aspect of the forefoot.

Bipartite sesamoids occur in approximately 30% of individuals and are bilateral 25% of the time.

The sesamoid bones can suffer stress fracture, sesamoiditis ('chondromalacia'), acute fracture, osteochondritis, osteoarthritis and bursitis.[132] Sesamoid stress fractures may occur in many sporting activities, but particularly in basketball players, tennis players and dancers. Most sesamoid abnormalities involve inflammatory changes and osteonecrosis. The medial sesamoid is more frequently affected. Injury may be caused by landing after a jump, increased forefoot weight-bearing activities (e.g. sprinting and dancing) or after traumatic dorsiflexion of the hallux. Pronation and progressive hallux valgus positioning may cause lateral displacement or subluxation of the sesamoids within the plantar grooves of the first metatarsal. This subluxation of the sesamoids may lead to erosion of the plantar aspect of the first metatarsal, resulting in pain underneath the first metatarsal head and arthritic changes reminiscent of patellofemoral pathology.

The patient complains of pain with forefoot weight-bearing and may display a supinated antalgic gait to avoid painful toe-off. Examination reveals marked local tenderness and swelling overlying the medial or lateral sesamoid. Movement of the first MTP joint is usually painful and often restricted. Resisted plantar flexion of the great toe is weak and painful.

Plain radiographs for this bone require an anteroposterior (AP), lateral and axial sesamoid view but radiographs are often not diagnostic for stress injury. They may show an acute fracture or bony sclerosis of sesamoid necrosis. MRI is often required to detect early stress fractures or more specific pathologies as mentioned above.

Recent onset or mild cases of sesamoid pain are traditionally treated with load modification, ice and possibly NSAIDs. Appropriate accommodative padding can partially relieve direct pressure to the sesamoids (Fig. 43.28). Orthoses can include this accommodation within the cushioning layer of the device. A carefully placed corticosteroid injection may provide pain relief for those athletes who must delay a rest period but it is not recommended. Ideal initial treatment of sesamoid

Foot pain   CHAPTER 43

with the previously discussed orthosis which unloads the first MTP and places the foot into a laterally directed supinated position thereby reducing the toe-off force through the first MTP.

Non-operative management is preferable, but a few cases will fail this approach. Surgical fixation or sesamoidectomy is reserved for these recalcitrant few. Sesamoidectomy does risk developing hallux deformities. A recent surgical series estimated approximately 12 weeks to return to sport.[133]

Plantar plate tear

with KENT SWEETING

Tears of the plantar plate may be the most common cause of pain under the second MTP joint, though it can occur at any of the MTP joints. It is also referred to as pre-dislocation syndrome, crossover toe deformity and floating toe syndrome. A fibrocartilaginous thickening of the MTP joint (Fig. 43.29a), the plantar plate:

- stabilises the MTP joint
- assists in the windlass mechanism due to its attachment to the plantar fascia
- resists hyperextension of the MTP joint
- absorbs compressive loads.

The second MTP joint is most likely to be affected as it is the longest metatarsal and has unopposed lumbricals and no plantar interossei insertions. Plantar plate tears usually result from repetitive overload from abnormal forefoot loading patterns resulting from hallux valgus, excessive pronation, short first metatarsal or long second metatarsal. The tear usually arises from the base of the proximal phalanx.[134]

The athlete usually complains of localised pain under the MTP joint. Swelling may be present, extending to the dorsal aspect of the joint. Neuroma-like symptoms may be experienced by patients due to irritation of the plantar digital nerve from the localised oedema.

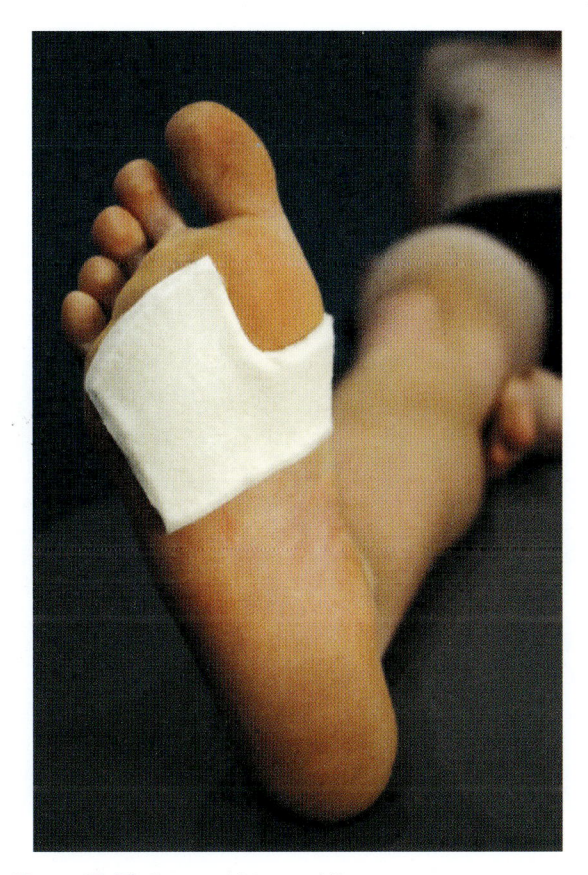

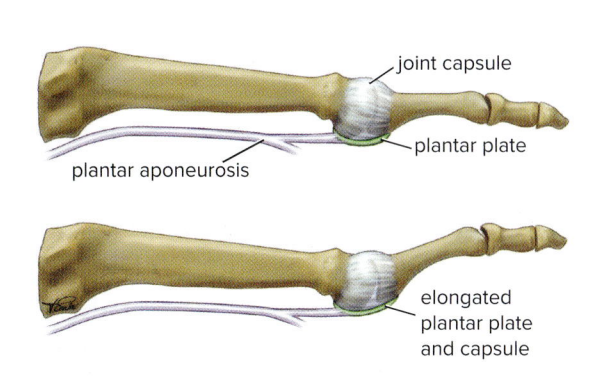

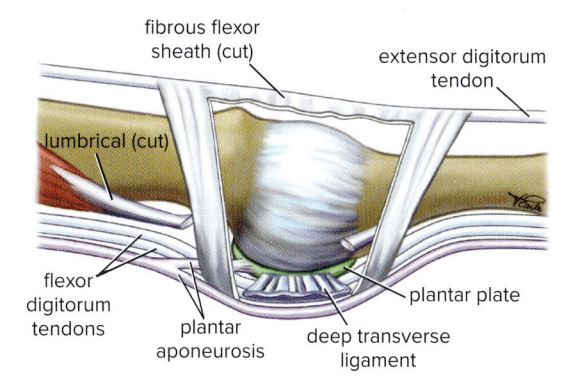

Figure 43.28 Sesamoiditis—padding

stress fractures includes a several-week period of non weight-bearing in a boot or short leg cast. The duration is determined by frequent examination awaiting resolution of tenderness by firm palpation.

Gradual return to full weight-bearing can be bridged by using a highly curved stiff shoe or rocker bottom shoe. Transition to athletic activities should also be assisted

Figure 43.29 (a) Anatomy of the MTP joint demonstrating the plantar plate

969

PART B Regional problems

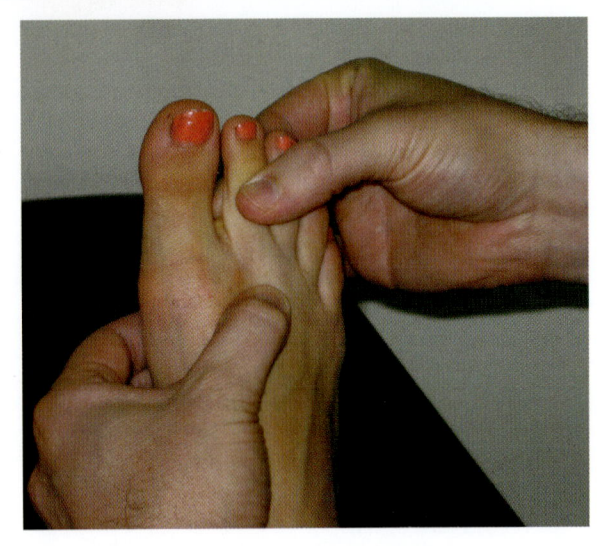

(b)

Figure 43.29 (cont.) (b) Modified Lachman's anterior-posterior drawer test. The metatarsal head is stabilised and the proximal phalanx is dorsally translocated. A 2 mm or 50% joint displacement is a positive sign of plantar plate laxity (c) Taping. Plantarflexion strapping of the digit

(c)

Examination reveals pain at the base of the proximal phalanx which may be aggravated by dorsiflexion of the joint. In relaxed stance, a dorsiflexion deformity of the toe may be noted. This is often accompanied by a crossover deformity. The modified Lachman's test (anterior-posterior drawer) can also be utilised. The metatarsal head is stabilised and the proximal phalanx is dorsally translocated (Fig 43.29b). A 2 mm or 50% joint displacement is a positive sign of plantar plate laxity.

Ultrasound may reveal a hypoechoic defect in the plantar plate, usually at the distal attachment. Historically arthrography was used to demonstrate synovial hypertrophy and extravasation of dye into the flexor tendon sheath. Today, MRI is helpful to demonstrate a tear of the plantar plate. There is increased signal intensity within the plate, along with a loss of continuity.[135]

Treatment initially consists of ice, NSAIDs, relative rest, plantarflexion strapping of the digit (Fig 43.29c) and accommodative padding to reduce loads under the affected MTP joint. Orthoses and a stiff-soled shoe or rocker bottom shoe are also required. Some clinicians consider an extra-articular corticosteroid injection may also be useful but there have been no quality trials of this treatment. Primary repair of the plantar plate with or without a flexor tendon transfer may be required in patients that fail to respond to conservative measures.

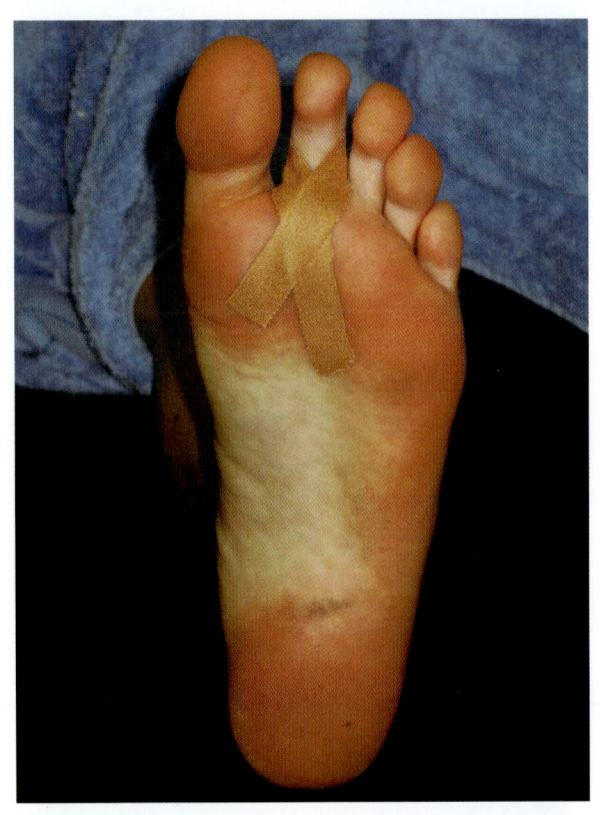

Corns and calluses

Excessive pressure on the skin may cause hypertrophy of the squamous cell layer of the epidermis, which manifests as corns and calluses. In the feet, corns and calluses result from uneven weight distribution and thus indicate abnormal foot biomechanics or poorly fitting footwear.

Treatment involves the removal of circumscribed corns and diffuse areas of callus with a scalpel, the wearing of well-fitting footwear and, if abnormal foot mechanics are present, orthoses. Petroleum jelly over the corn or callus and on the outside of the sock can also help.

Morton's interdigital neuroma

So-called Morton's neuroma is not a true neuroma, but a swelling of nerve and scar tissue arising from compression of the interdigital nerve, usually between the third and fourth metatarsals (Fig. 43.30a). Excessive pronation contributes to metatarsal hypermobility and impingement of the interdigital nerve.

The patient complains of pain radiating into the toes, often associated with pins and needles, and numbness. A clicking sensation may be noticed. Pain is increased by forefoot weight-bearing activities and with narrow-fitting footwear, and is often relieved by removing the shoes.

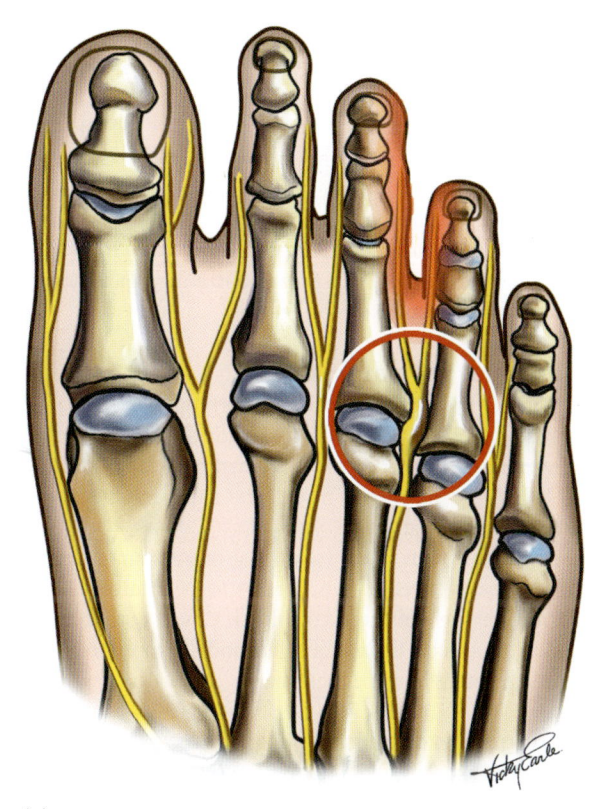

Foot pain CHAPTER 43

Examination reveals localised tenderness and, in cases of extensive chronic proliferation, there may be a palpable click on compression of the metatarsal heads. Web space tenderness and toe tip sensation deficit may be present.[136]

Diagnostic confirmation with imaging can be performed for chronic cases considering surgical management. MRI demonstrating a neuroma greater than 5 mm is generally significant. Ultrasound has emerged as a viable technique to diagnose and distinguish an interdigital nerve from an intermetatarsal bursa.[137, 138]

Treatment consists initially of ice to alleviate acute tenderness. Plantar metatarsal padding to subtly separate the metatarsals and shoes with a wide toe box are used to reduce the side-to-side compression of the metatarsals (Fig. 43.30b). However, in chronic cases, little improvement is seen with padding. Intrinsic and extrinsic foot muscle strengthening exercises are indicated to maintain or improve the transverse arch and control of foot pronation. The use of orthoses is essential if excessive pronation is present.

Various interventions have been proposed.[139] Injection of corticosteroid and local anaesthetic agents in conjunction with the padding may provide lasting relief. An ultrasound-guided corticosteroid injection via a distal interdigital approach provided at least 9 months significant relief of symptoms for the majority of patients.[140] Injection with alcohol is also an option.[141, 142]

If the patient obtains no relief, radiofrequency ablation of the nerve appears to be a promising new therapy.[143] Recently, sonographically guided cryoneurolysis improved four of five Morton's neuroma patients.[144]

Surgical management is quite successful for those cases not responding to conservative care. Pain relief remains the principal goal of treatment; however, a resected neuroma will result in permanent numbness and this needs to be discussed with the patient prior to surgery. Decompression by neurolysis has been described as a successful intraoperative decision to preserve the nerve in some cases.[145]

Plantar warts

The papovavirus causes plantar warts when it enters the skin. The warts can be particularly painful on weight-bearing. They should be differentiated from corns. Applying lateral pressure or pinching will be painful in warts, whereas corns are more painful with direct pressure. Gentle paring with a scalpel will also reveal the characteristic appearance of a plantar wart with fine black dots within a defined margin of white or brown tissue.

Plantar warts are best treated with chemical solutions containing salicylic acid. The overlying hyperkeratosis should be removed weekly to allow the chemicals to penetrate the wart. Blistering and abscess formation occur and require debridement with a scalpel and the application of a dressing.

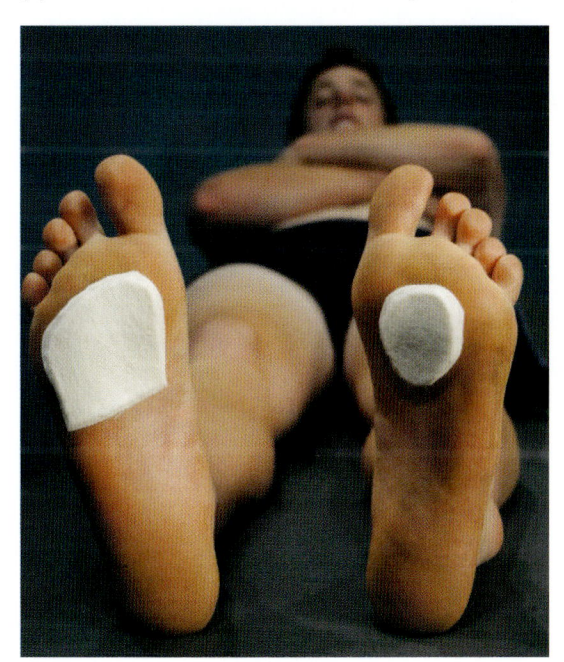

Figure 43.30 Morton's neuroma (a) Location of nerve entrapment in Morton's neuroma (b) Plantar metatarsal padding

Onychocryptosis

Onychocryptosis (ingrown toenail) arises from abnormal nail growth or poor nail cutting. Patients often present in acute pain with tenderness on gentle palpation. Nails are often infected. Treatment with local and oral antibiotic therapy is required. Conservative treatment involves elevating the offending corner of the nail plate from the soft tissue, cutting a small 'V' into the middle of the nail distally (to take pressure off the edges) and stretching the soft tissue away from the nail with a cotton bud.

Surgical management consists of resection of the outer aspect of the nail to prevent the nail border injuring the soft tissue. Resection involves anaesthetising the toe and removing the nail border with appropriate nail splitters and forceps. All abnormal tissue is removed and the nail matrix treated with phenol to prevent regrowth.

Less common causes of forefoot pain

Stress fracture of the great toe

Stress fractures of the proximal phalanx of the great toe have been reported in adolescent athletes.[99, 146] Stress fractures in the distal phalanx can occur in ballet dancers. There appears to be an association with hallux valgus. Treatment involves a period of non weight-bearing rest of 4–6 weeks followed by graduated return to activity.

Joplin's neuritis

Joplin's neuritis involves compression and irritation of the dorsal medial cutaneous nerve over the first metatarsal and first MTP joint. It usually occurs because of irritation from footwear and is common in patients with hallux abducto-valgus or exostoses around the first MTP joint.

The patient complains of pain radiating along the first ray into the hallux. Wearing appropriate footwear and using foam and felt to redistribute the load from the affected area generally provides relief. Orthoses may be required to prevent excessive pronation.

Freiberg's osteochondritis

Freiberg's disease or osteochondritis of the metatarsal head affects adolescents between the ages of 14 and 18 years (Chapter 44). The metatarsal head appears fragmented on radiograph. Offloading of the metatarsal heads using padding and orthoses is essential to prevent permanent metatarsal head flattening that may predispose to adult osteoarthritis.

Toe clawing

Toe clawing occurs secondary to short, tight long flexor tendons (Fig. 43.31). During the propulsive phase of gait, the long flexors contract to stabilise the toes. In the unstable foot, these long flexors contract excessively during the propulsive phase and the toes claw the surface in an attempt to maintain stability.

Clawing of toes does not result in pain itself but excessive pressure on the prominent joints and ends of toes often causes painful skin lesions.[88]

Subungual haematoma

Subungual haematoma occurs when direct trauma or repetitive pressure from footwear leads to bleeding under the toenails. Pain arises from increased pressure under the nail and the nails appear black. The nail may eventually loosen from the nail bed.

Treatment of an acute subungual haematoma involves using a heated needle or paperclip to perforate the nail and release the collection of blood. Cover with a small dressing. Correctly fitting footwear and appropriate lacing techniques may prevent recurrence.

Subungual exostosis

A subungual exostosis develops because of direct trauma. The patient presents with pain on direct pressure to the nail. The nail plate may be displaced from the nail bed due to elevation from the exostosis. Treatment requires the wearing of loose-fitting footwear, appropriate cutting of the nail and padding. Surgery may be required to remove the bony exostosis.

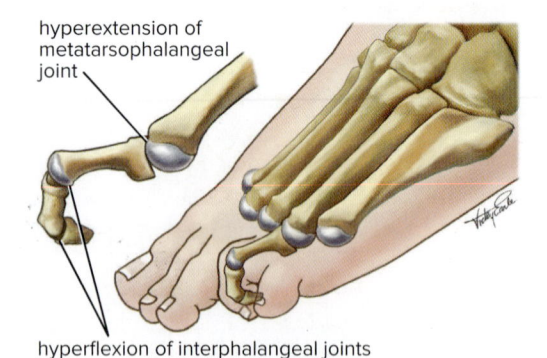

Figure 43.31 Toe clawing

REFERENCES

References for this chapter can be found at www.mhhe.com/au/CSM5e

PART C

Practical sports medicine

Chapter 44

The younger athlete

with NEBOJSA POPOVIC, BOJAN BUKVA, NICOLA MAFFULLI and DENNIS CAINE

Youth is full of sport, age's breath is short; Youth is nimble, age is lame; Youth is hot and bold, age is weak and cold; Youth is wild, and age is tame.
William Shakespeare (1564–1616) 'Crabbéd Age and Youth'

Participation in youth (i.e. child and adolescent) sports is popular and widespread. Many youngsters train year-round and specialise in their sports in childhood, and during adolescence some may reach peak performance and compete nationally or internationally. It is not uncommon for preteens to train 20 or more hours each week at regional training centres in tennis or gymnastics, to compete in triathlons, or for youngsters as young as 6–8 years of age to play organised hockey or soccer and travel with select teams to compete against other teams of similar calibre. Thus, knowledge about specific physiologic characteristics, management of orthopaedic conditions, injury prevention guidelines, and information regarding non-orthopaedic concerns is imperative to all individuals involved in the healthcare of young athletes.

THE YOUNG ATHLETE IS UNIQUE

Engaging in sports activities at a young age has numerous health benefits, but also involves risk of injury. Indeed, the young athlete may be particularly vulnerable to sport injury due to the physical and physiological processes of growth. Injury risk factors that are unique to the young athlete include specifics of the musculoskeletal system such as an immature skeleton, nonlinearity of growth, maturity-associated variation, the adolescent growth spurt and the response to skeletal injury.[1] Young athletes might also be at increased risk because of immature or underdeveloped coordination, skills and perception, in addition to psychological issues. Although problems do not ordinarily arise at normal levels of activity, the more frequent and intense training and competition of young athletes today may create conditions under which this susceptibility exerts itself.

Nonlinearity of growth

The normal growth pattern is nonlinear; that is, differential growth of the body segments (head, trunk and lower extremities) occurs throughout growth and influences body proportions accordingly.[2] At birth, the relative contribution of head and trunk to total stature is highest and declines through childhood into adolescence. Thus, the child is characterised by a proportionally larger head and trunk, and shorter legs compared to an adult. In some events, for example rodeo 'mutton busting', one can anticipate that a young 'top-heavy' child would be at increased risk of falling off a sheep compared to an older child with proportionally longer legs.

One of the features of the child's skeleton is the existence of the epiphyseal growth zones (physis). It has traditionally been divided into four zones: the resting or germinal zone, the proliferation zone, the zone of hypertrophy and the zone of enchondral ossification, which is continuous with the metaphysis (Fig. 44.1).

In each segment of the young skeleton, for example the femur or humerus, the contribution to growth of distal and proximal parts are not equal. This is the concept of the 'fertile physis'. The proximal part of the humerus and distal part of the femur contribute much more in skeletal growth, an important factor in the treatment approach after skeletal injuries.

It could also be argued that under a given physical load, for example over a distance run, a child's locomotor

The younger athlete CHAPTER 44

apparatus would be exposed to greater stress: hence to a higher risk of overuse injury than that of an adult. Yet, often child athletes progress rapidly to training regimens, skills and stunts that were originally introduced and intended for more mature individuals.

Maturity-associated variation

Maturity-associated variation depends on the sex of the young athlete. In general, girls are more mature than boys at a given age. Early-maturing boys have structural, functional and performance advantages in sports requiring size, strength and power over late maturers.

> **PRACTICE PEARL**
>
> Children of the same chronological age may vary considerably in biological maturity status, and individual differences in maturity status influence measures of growth and performance during childhood and adolescence.[2]

Chronological age (CA) may add yet another dimension of individual variation given that most youth sports are categorised by CA. Within a single age group (e.g. 12 years of age), the child who is 12.9 years of age is likely to be taller, heavier and stronger than the child who is 12.0 years of age, even though both are classified as 12 years of age. The fear is that an unbalanced competition between early and late-maturing and/or older and younger boys in contact sports such as martial arts and wrestling contributes to at least some of the serious injuries in these sports. A matching system based on physical attributes, although logistically difficult to implement, may be beneficial to equalising competition, to maintaining interest in participation, and to reducing potential for injury.[3]

Unique response to skeletal injury

Often, the mechanism of injury in young athletes and adult athletes is the same. However, there are some significant differences in the type of injuries sustained by children and adolescents because of the differences in the structure of growing bone compared with adult bone. The different components of growing bone are indicated in Figure 44.1b.

The differences between growing and adult bone (Fig. 44.2) are summarised below.

- The periosteum is thicker in children and has considerable healing potential.
- The articular cartilage of growing bone is a thicker layer than in adult bone and can remodel.

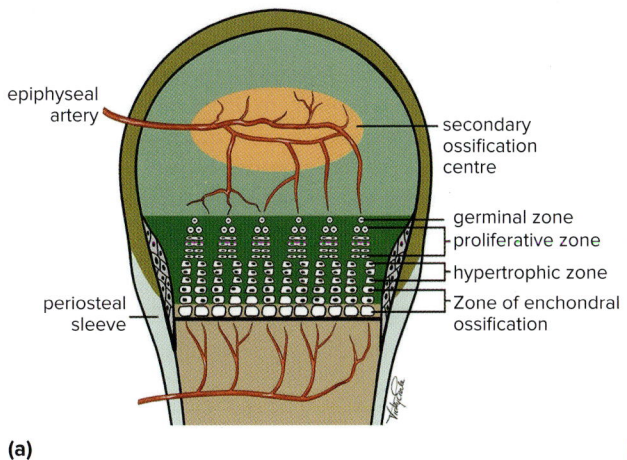

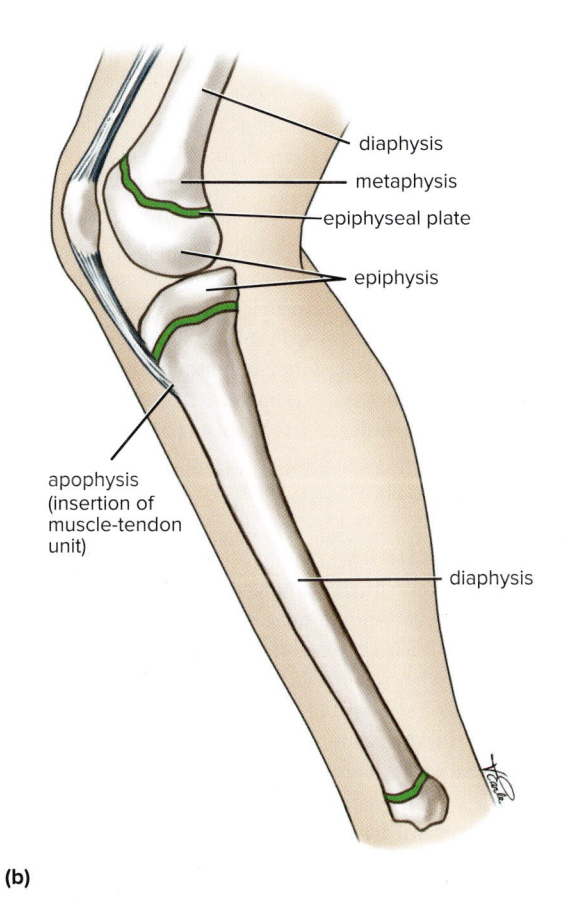

Figure 44.1 (a) Anatomy of the physis (b) Different parts of the growing bone—the metaphysis, epiphysis, diaphysis and epiphyseal plate

975

PART C Practical sports medicine

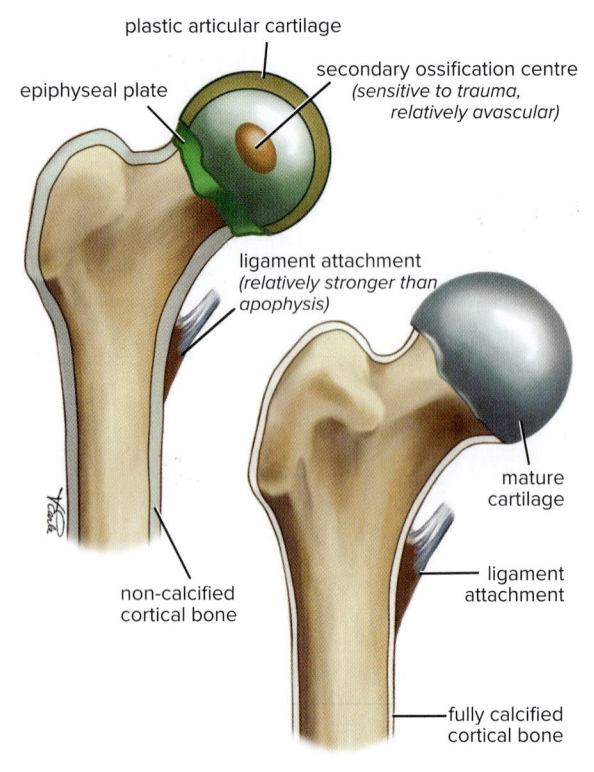

Figure 44.2 Contrasting features of growing bone (left) and adult bone (right)

- The junction between the epiphyseal plate and the metaphysis in children is vulnerable to disruption, especially from shearing forces.
- Tendon attachment sites–apophyses–are cartilaginous plates that, in children, provide a relatively weak cartilaginous attachment, predisposing to the development of avulsion injuries.
- The cortex of long bones in children is more resilient and elastic than adult bone, withstanding greater deflection without fracture. Thus, children tend to suffer incomplete fractures of the greenstick type, which do not occur in adults.
- During the adolescent growth spurt, structural changes in physeal cartilage occur that result in a thicker and more fragile epiphyseal plate.[4] Studies of the incidence of physeal fractures indicate an increased occurrence of fractures during pubescence.[5, 6]
- It has been proposed that the adolescent growth spurt may also increase susceptibility to physeal injury by causing an increase in muscle-tendon tightness about the joints and loss of flexibility.[7] However, this concept is controversial.[8]
- The vascular supply is different especially in very young athletes.

As a result of these differences, a particular mechanism of injury may result in different pathological conditions in the younger athlete compared with the mature adult. The younger athlete is more likely to injure cartilage and bone or completely avulse an apophysis than to have a significant ligament sprain or tendinopathy. Some examples of different injuries in children and adults that are the result of similar mechanisms are shown in Table 44.1.

> **PRACTICE PEARL**
>
> Younger athletes have a greater healing potential than adult athletes.

MANAGEMENT OF MUSCULOSKELETAL CONDITIONS

In children, traumatic injuries may result in fractures of the long bones or the growth plates, or soft tissue damage. Strong, incoordinate muscle contractions are more likely to lead to an avulsion fracture at the site of attachment of the muscle or tendon rather than to a tear of the muscle or tendon itself.

The osteochondroses are a group of conditions affecting secondary ossification centres of the growing bones. Although the aetiology of the osteochondroses is not well understood, non-articular osteochondroses may well be related to overuse (Table 44.2).

Each of the following common paediatric injury presentations are discussed in this chapter: acute fractures, shoulder pain, elbow pain, wrist pain, back pain or postural abnormality, hip pain, knee pain, painless abnormalities of gait and foot pain.

Acute fractures

Fractures occur in the young athlete due to the line of weakness between the epiphyseal plate and the formed bone, the relative weakness of apophyseal cartilage compared with the musculotendinous complex, and the direction and strength of the force. Four types of fractures are seen in the younger athlete: metaphyseal, physeal, diaphyseal and apophyseal avulsion fractures.

Metaphyseal fractures

Metaphyseal fractures occur especially in the forearm and lower leg. The most common type of fracture seen is a buckling of one side of the bone. The management of metaphyseal fractures in children depends on age, gender, the degree and plane of displacement, and the distance from the joint. The treatment usually simply consists of cast immobilisation and complications are very rare. Occasionally, angular or rotational deformity is present and requires open reduction and internal fixation.

The younger athlete

Table 44.1 Comparison of injuries that occur with similar mechanisms in children and adults

Site	Mechanism	Injury in adult	Injury in child
Thumb	Valgus force as in 'skier's thumb'	Sprain of ulnar collateral ligament	Fracture of proximal phalangeal physis (usually Salter–Harris type III)
Distal interphalangeal joint of finger	Hyperflexion injury	Mallet finger	Fracture of distal phalangeal epiphysis Salter–Harris (type II or III)
Hand	Punching injury as in boxing	Fracture of metacarpal head	Fracture of metacarpal epiphysis Salter–Harris (type II)
Shoulder	Fall on point of shoulder	Acromioclavicular joint sprain	Fracture of middle third of clavicle epiphysis
	Abduction and external rotation force	Dislocated shoulder	Fracture of proximal humeral epiphysis Salter–Harris (type I or II)
Thigh/hip	Acute flexor muscle strain or extensor strain	Quadriceps strain or hamstring strain	Apophyseal avulsion of anterior inferior iliac spine or ischial tuberosity
Knee	Overuse injury	Patellar tendinopathy	Osgood–Schlatter disease or Sinding–Larsen–Johansson disease
	Acute trauma (e.g. skiing) injury	Meniscal or ligament injury	Fractured distal femoral or proximal tibial epiphysis, avulsion of tibial spine
Ankle	Acute inversion	Lateral ligament sprain	Salter–Harris type I or II fracture of tibia or fibula
Heel	Overuse	Achilles tendinopathy	Sever's disease

Table 44.2 Types of osteochondroses

Type	Condition	Site
Articular	Perthes' disease	Femoral head
	Kienböck's disease	Lunate
	Köhler's disease	Navicular
	Freiberg's disease	Second metatarsal
	Osteochondritis dissecans	Medial femoral condyle, capitellum, talar dome
Non-articular	Osgood–Schlatter disease	Tibial tubercle
	Sinding-Larsen–Johansson disease	Inferior pole of patella
	Sever's disease	Calcaneus
Physeal	Scheuermann's disease	Thoracic spine
	Blount's disease	Proximal tibia

Physeal (growth plate) fractures

Approximately 15% of all fractures in children involve the physis[9] or growth plate, and more than a third of these occur in organised sport settings. Fractures of the growth plate are of particular concern because of the dangers of interruption to the growth process via injury to the cells in the zone of hypertrophy.

Although more elaborate systems for describing acute physeal injuries are available,[9] the system most widely used was developed by Salter and Harris[10] (Fig. 44.3). Salter-Harris types I and II fractures usually heal well. However, these injuries are not as innocuous as originally described and may occasionally be associated with local growth plate closure and osseous bridging.[9]

PART C Practical sports medicine

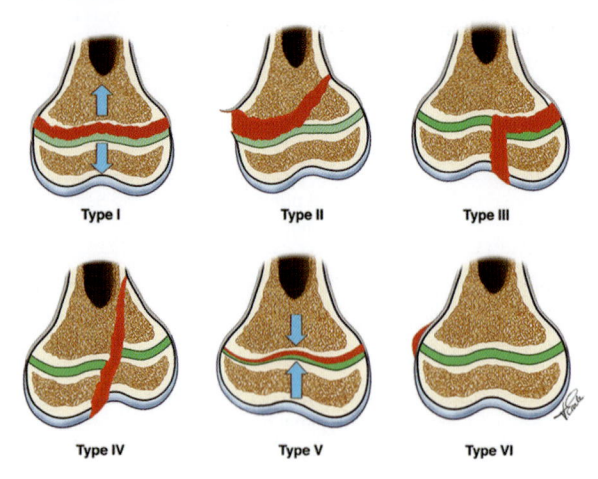

Figure 44.3 Salter–Harris classification of physeal (growth plate) fractures

Type III and IV fractures involve the joint surface as well as the growth plate and have a high complication rate. If these fractures are not recognised, they could produce permanent injury to the growth plate, resulting in growth disturbances. When recognised, accurate anatomical reduction must be performed to reduce the possibility of interference in growth and to minimise the possibility of long-term degenerative change. However, occasionally the initial insult can produce permanent growth arrest despite subsequent anatomical reduction.

Type V fractures are compressive force fractures of the physis and can lead to growth zone lesions. Type VI fractures are lesions of the periosteal attachment (Ranvier zone) and can also lead to growth zone disturbances.

Management of physeal fractures depends on the age and gender of the athlete, grade and plane of the displacement and the distance from the joint. In the paediatric population, they mostly require cast immobilisation only, or closed reduction and cast immobilisation (types I and II). Types III and IV may require percutaneous fixation using Kirschner wires.

> **PRACTICE PEARL**
>
> The common sites of physeal fractures in the younger athlete with recommended management and potential complications are shown in Table 44.3.

It is most important to recognise a physeal fracture. Radiographs should be obtained of both limbs (for comparison) if clinical features suggest growth plate injury. A normal radiograph does not exclude a growth plate fracture. A history of severe rotational or shear force with accompanying localised swelling, bony tenderness and loss of function should be regarded as a growth plate fracture until proven otherwise. If there is any doubt regarding the diagnosis or management of these injuries, specialist orthopaedic referral is mandatory.

Diaphyseal fractures

Most fractures of the shaft of long bones do not involve the growth plate and metaphysis of the bone, but only the diaphysis of the long bone (especially in the forearm and lower leg). In younger athletes, fractures are often incomplete due to the thicker periosteum. They are referred to as 'greenstick' fractures. The treatment of diaphyseal fractures is usually through cast immobilisation only. Indications for surgical treatment depend on the degree of displacement, age and gender of the athlete.

Apophyseal (avulsion) fractures

Avulsion fractures occur at the apophyseal attachments of large musculotendinous units, that is, large tendons to bones or, less frequently, at ligament insertions. The common sites are at the attachment of the:

- sartorius muscle to the anterior superior iliac spine
- rectus femoris muscle to the anterior inferior iliac spine
- hamstring muscles to the ischial tuberosity
- iliopsoas tendon to the lesser trochanter of the femur
- gluteus medius to the greater trochanter of the femur
- anterior cruciate ligament to the tibial plateau
- patellar tendon to the tibial tubercle
- peroneus brevis to the base of the 5th metatarsal bone
- triceps to the olecranon
- forearm flexors and pronator to the medial epicondyle humerus.

In the younger athlete, apophyseal fractures are the equivalent of acute muscle strains in the adult. Instead of a tear of the muscle fibres in the mid-substance of the muscle or at the musculotendinous junction, the tendon is pulled away with its apophyseal attachment. Many patients will describe a 'pop' with the onset of discomfort. This is confirmed on plain radiographs (e.g. Fig. 30.17). Even though injury involving the apophyseal growth plate does not normally result in length discrepancy, angular deformity or altered joint mechanics, it may adversely affect training and performance as well as the long-term health of young athletes. The most common site of an avulsion fracture is the tibial tubercle at the attachment of the patella tendon, especially in football and basketball players. Radiographs should be performed in all cases.

Management depends on the degree of the displacement of the avulsed fragment of bone. It involves cast immobilisation and, in more displaced fragments, surgical reattachment. In general, apophyseal fractures around

The younger athlete — CHAPTER 44

Table 44.3 Management and possible complications of physeal (growth plate) fractures in young athletes

Site	Management	Potential complications
Distal radius fracture	Cast immobilisation (3–4 weeks)	Not recognised, growth disturbance
Supracondylar fracture of the elbow (undisplaced)	Sling (3 weeks)	Vascular compromise of brachial artery, median nerve damage, malalignment
Distal fibular fracture	Cast, non weight-bearing (4–6 weeks)	Growth disturbance can occur up to 18 months later
Distal tibial fracture	Cast, non weight-bearing (4–6 weeks)	Premature closure of physis can lead to angulation and leg length discrepancy
Distal femur fracture	Anatomical reduction	Greater incidence of growth discrepancies than in other fractures, Salter–Harris types I and II fractures; must be observed closely

the pelvis do not need surgical treatment because the displacement is mostly not significant and the continuity of the periosteum is preserved.

One common site of an avulsion fracture at a ligamentous attachment is at the attachment of the anterior cruciate ligament to the tibia. An acute rotational injury to the knee may present with the symptoms and signs of an anterior cruciate ligament tear. Instead of the in-substance tear common in adults, the more common injury in children is avulsion of the tibial spine or distal femoral attachment. Radiographs should be performed in all cases of acute knee injuries accompanied by haemarthrosis. Management involves surgical reattachment of the avulsed fragment and ligament.

The most commonly reported acute apophyseal sport injuries in the upper extremity involve the olecranon and medial epicondyle of the humerus. The vertebral ring apophysis is the site most often involved in the spine.

Management of avulsion fractures is identical to that for grade III tears of the muscle. It involves initial reduction of the pain and swelling, restoration of full range of motion with passive stretching and active range of motion exercises as symptoms settle, as well as a graduated program of muscle strengthening. Any biomechanical abnormalities that may have predisposed the athlete to this injury should be corrected. Reattachment is occasionally required when there is a large displacement of the avulsed fragment.

Overuse injuries of the physis

Trends in children's and youth sports include increased numbers of participants, greater duration and intensity of training, and earlier specialisation and year-round training. Increased involvement and repetition of skills practiced at an early age and continued through the years of growth raises concern about risk of injury. In particular, there is concern that the tolerance limits of the physis (growth plate) may be exceeded by the repetitive physical loading required in many sports, particularly during the adolescent growth spurt. Physeal growth disturbance as a result of injury can result in length discrepancy, angular deformity, or altered joint mechanics, and may cause significant long-term disability.

Physeal stress injuries are thought to develop when repetitive loading of the extremity disrupts metaphyseal perfusion which may inhibit ossification of the chondrocytes in the zone of provisional calcification. The hypertrophic zone continues to widen as the chondrocytes transition from the germinal layer to the proliferative zone. Widening of the physis may be seen radiographically, whereas physeal cartilage extension into the metaphysis has been shown with magnetic resonance imaging (MRI).

Physeal stress injuries were first recognised in baseball pitchers and are also found in other young athletes involved in overhead sports, including cricket, gymnastics, badminton, swimming and volleyball.

Treatment for physeal stress injury is straightforward: rest from loading of the extremity. However, in cases involving growth disturbance, corrective surgery may be required. Clinicians need to educate parents and coaches as to the existence of overuse physeal injury and the need for rest to ensure proper recovery and return to sport participation.

Shoulder pain

Acute trauma to the shoulder in children may result in fracture of the proximal humerus, the clavicle or proximal humeral physis. Fractures of the acromion or the coracoid process are rare.

Dislocation of the glenohumeral joint is common in the adolescent but uncommon in the younger child. Dislocations in adolescents are associated with a high incidence of recurrence and development of post-traumatic instability. The management of acute dislocation of the shoulder is discussed in Chapter 24.

Stress fracture of the proximal humeral physis (growth plate) was first observed in young baseball pitchers, but has since been reported in young athletes representing a variety of sports including cricket, gymnastics, badminton, swimming and volleyball.[11] Radiographs may show widening of the proximal humeral physis. Metaphyseal sclerosis and demineralisation or fragmentation of the epiphysis may also be present.[12] MRI should be performed if the X-ray is negative and clinical suspicion high. In most cases, subjects improved with rest and were able to return to their sport.

Shoulder impingement is also seen in the younger athlete. In the young athlete involved in throwing sports, the impingement is usually secondary to atraumatic instability, which develops because of repetitive stress to the anterior capsule of the shoulder joint at the end range of movement (Chapter 24). Impingement and rotator cuff tendinopathy also occur in swimmers where excessive internal rotation causes a tendency to impinge. The aetiology of these problems in throwers and swimmers is discussed in Chapters 8 and 9.

Elbow pain

Delineating injury patterns to the elbow in children can be challenging, given the cartilaginous composition of the distal humerus and the multiple secondary ossification centres which appear and unite with the epiphysis at defined ages. The pitching motion in baseball, serving in tennis, spiking in volleyball, passing in American football, and launching in javelin throwing can all produce elbow pathology caused by forceful valgus stress, with medial stretching, lateral compression and posterior impingement.

The valgus forces generated during the acceleration phase of throwing (Chapter 8) result in traction on the medial elbow structures and compression to the lateral side of the joint. This may injure a number of structures on the medial aspect of the joint. Injuries include chronic apophysitis of the medial epicondyle, acute or chronic strain of the ulnar collateral ligament (also referred to as the medial collateral ligament) or avulsion fracture of the medial epicondylar apophysis. The ulnar nerve may also be damaged.

> **PRACTICE PEARL**
>
> Acute ulnar collateral ligament (UCL) injuries are increasing in young baseball pitchers at an alarming rate. Children who are still growing are more likely to injure the growth area of the elbow, but older adolescents are more likely to present with a frank UCL tear.

Some young athletes have avulsion injuries where the ligament stays intact but pulls off a piece of bone. If the UCL is torn, non-operative treatment is attempted but if the ligament fails to heal, the patient often undergoes reconstructive Tommy John surgery if he or she wishes to continue throwing at a high level (Chapter 25).[13]

The lateral compressive forces may damage the articular cartilage of the capitellum or radial head. The long-term sequelae of these repetitive valgus forces include bony thickening, loose body formation and contractures.

Flexion contractures can occur because of repeated hyperextension. The majority of these contractures are relatively minor (less than 15°). Significant contractures (greater than 30°) should be treated with active and active-assisted range of motion exercises accompanied by a lengthy period of rest (e.g. 3 months).

Osteochondritis dissecans of the capitellum is also seen in pitchers and, more commonly, in gymnasts. Osteochondritis dissecans is a localised area of avascular necrosis on the anterolateral aspect of the capitellum. Initially, the articular surface softens and this may be followed by subchondral collapse and formation of loose bodies in the elbow. X-rays will frequently demonstrate the lesion. In cases with suspicious radiographic changes, MRI is critical to confirm the diagnosis as well as to characterise the extent and stability of the osteochondral lesion. The early stages of osteochondritis dissecans may respond well to rest. Surgical procedures include removal of loose bodies, joint debridement and fixation of stable fragments. The results of surgical management of this condition are variable.[14]

The younger child (under 11 years) may develop Panner's disease. This self-limiting condition is characterised by fragmentation of the entire ossific centre of the capitellum. Loose bodies are not seen in Panner's disease and surgery is not required.

Wrist pain

Wrist pain in children may be acute or chronic. In acute conditions, it is mostly related to a distal radial fracture/epiphiseolysis or, rarely, scaphoid fracture.

Chronic dorsal wrist pain is commonly seen in gymnasts where pain is aggravated by weight-bearing with the wrist extended. The gymnast complains of tenderness over the dorsum of the hand and perhaps swelling. An often reported cause among gymnasts is a stress injury to the distal radial physis involving compromise of the metaphyseal and/or the epiphyseal blood supply.[11] Longstanding injuries are associated with typical radiographic changes, including widening, irregularity, haziness or cystic changes of the growth plate. Other causes of dorsal wrist pain include scaphoid impaction syndrome, dorsal impingement syndrome/capsulitis, tear of the triangular fibrocartilage complex and stress fractures.

Management of the younger gymnast with dorsal wrist pain includes relative rest, and splinting. Strengthening of the wrist flexors may also be useful in association with tape and pads to decrease hyperextension of the wrist. Most gymnasts with stress injuries involving the distal radial physis recover with rest; however, there are also reports of stress-related premature closure of the distal radial growth plate leading to positive ulnar variance.[15]

Kienböck's disease of the wrist (Chapter 26) is an osteochondrosis of the lunate bone. It occurs generally in older patients (20 years old) and rarely in adolescents.

Back pain and postural abnormalities

Younger athletes may present with pain or postural abnormalities, such as 'curvature' of the spine, or both.

Low back pain

Common causes of back pain in the younger athlete are similar to those in the mature adult. Minor soft tissue injuries to the intervertebral disc, the apophyseal joints and associated ligaments, and muscle strains in the paravertebral muscles usually respond well to reduction in activity. Manipulative treatment in the management of these conditions in the younger athlete is probably contraindicated.

Back pain is more common among young athletes participating in sports with high demands on the back, such as wrestling, gymnastics and American football, than other athletes or non-athletes.[16] Back pain in the young athlete may be associated with one or more of the following conditions: idiopathic scoliosis, spondylolysis, spondylolisthesis, disc degeneration, disc herniation, Schmorl's nodes, vertebral end-plate fracture and atypical Scheuermann's lesion (vertebral apophysitis). The spine, as with the rest of the skeleton, is at greater risk of injury during the adolescent growth spurt.[16]

Severe disc injuries and tumours are occasionally seen in the lumbar spine of the adolescent athlete. Biomechanical abnormalities such as leg length discrepancy, pelvic instability and excessive subtalar pronation may also indirectly lead to low back pain.

Idiopathic scoliosis

Idiopathic scoliosis accounts for 80% of structural scoliosis and is the most common cause of back discomfort in young athletes. Nearly 32% of adolescents with idiopathic scoliosis complain of back discomfort.[17] The pain is not related to the size or location of the curve and usually does not interfere with the patient's ability to perform daily activities.

Non-predictive but predisposing factors for the progression of the scoliosis before skeletal maturity include a family history of scoliosis, patient height-to-weight ratios, lumbosacral transitional anomalies, thoracic kyphosis, lumbar lordosis and spinal balance.

In general, the rate of progression of scoliosis in adulthood is much slower than that in adolescence and depends on the size of the curve once skeletal maturity has been reached.

The screening protocol for scoliosis in young athletes is the most important issue in the assessment of spine disorders. On physical examination the most common findings are: shoulder asymmetry, unequal scapular prominence, appearance of an elevated or prominent hip, greater space between the arm and body on one side (with the arms hanging loosely on the side), head not centred over the pelvis, and a positive forward-bending test (Adam's test). A plain radiograph in anteroposterior and lateral view plays an important part in assessment.

In selecting appropriate treatment, the clinician must take into consideration the adolescent's remaining growth potential, the severity of the curve, as well as the pattern and location of the scoliosis. The available treatment choices are observation, non-surgical intervention and surgical intervention. It is imperative that clinicians know which option is appropriate for each individual patient.

Actively growing adolescents (Risser grade 2 or lower) with curves between 30° and 45° should be started on brace therapy at the time of the initial visit. In very immature patients (Risser grade 0 and pre-menarcheal if female) with curves exceeding 25° degrees, bracing should be started immediately. In most cases, growing adolescents with curves exceeding 45-50° require operative treatment (stabilisation) because other forms of treatment are ineffective to control or correct the scoliosis. Skeletally mature individuals with curves exceeding 50-55° also are at risk for curve progression and should be considered for surgical treatment.

Spondylolysis

Spondylolysis has received particular attention due to its high prevalence among athletes (Chapter 29). This condition may also occur in the younger athlete, particularly because of repeated hyperextension of the lumbar spine. This injury is typically seen as a result of participation in ballet, gymnastics, diving, volleyball, fast bowling in cricket and serving in tennis. The management of this condition is discussed in Chapter 29. The amount of hyperextension activity must be reduced and this may involve some alteration in technique.

There is considerable debate whether these defects in the pars interarticularis are congenital or acquired. They are probably acquired, even though this may occur at an extremely young age. A fibrous union develops across the defect and this is susceptible to injury. The presence of a pars interarticularis defect does not automatically mean that this is the cause of the patient's pain. MRI may confirm that the pars interarticularis defect is the site of an acute fracture.

Spondylolisthesis

Spondylolisthesis is defined as the forward slippage of one vertebra on its adjacent caudal segment (Chapter 29). Spondylolisthesis is one of the most variable conditions affecting the paediatric spine. The severity of its clinical manifestation ranges from a coincidental radiographic finding in asymptomatic patients, to a disabling deformity that produces severe postural and gait disturbances, pain and neurologic impairment affecting the lower extremities, the bowel and the bladder. Just as the initial symptoms can vary, so does the radiographic severity of the slippage, which ranges from a few millimetres of anterior displacement to complete dislocation of L5 anteriorly over the sacrum (called *spondyloptosis*). Unabated controversy continues regarding optimal surgical treatment in severe cases.

Spondylolisthesis is divided into five types based on the radiographic findings and age at onset: the dysplastic, isthmic, degenerative, post-traumatic and pathologic types. The age of the patient and the degree of listhesis determine whether observation, non-operative management, or immediate surgical stabilisation is necessary. It has been commonly believed that the younger the patient, the greater the risk of progression of the deformity.

Low-grade spondylolisthesis (<50% slip) is treated conservatively, with surgical treatment reserved for patients with continued symptoms, disability, or in the case of juvenile onset, evidence of progressive listhesis. High-grade spondylolisthesis (>50% slip) generally requires surgical treatment. Objective opinions that reduction of the slip angle and L5 incidence correlate with better clinical outcome suggest that this is becoming the treatment of choice, although the degree of reduction is still being debated. Current expert opinion favours *partial* reduction–by postural means if possible–maintained by internal fixation as the appropriate middle ground to achieve neurologic safety, sagittal realignment and a high fusion rate.[17]

Postural abnormalities

The commonest postural abnormality of the spine in the younger athlete is excessive kyphosis of the spine due to an osteochondrosis (Scheuermann's disease). This condition occurs typically in the thoracic spine, but is also seen at the thoracolumbar junction. The thoracolumbar form of Scheuermann's disease, which encompasses both the thoracic and lumbar regions of the spine, is more common in athletes than non-athletes and also is considered to be associated more frequently with back pain.[16] Children can present with acute pain. It usually presents in later years as an excessive thoracic kyphosis in association with a compensatory excessive lumbar lordosis.

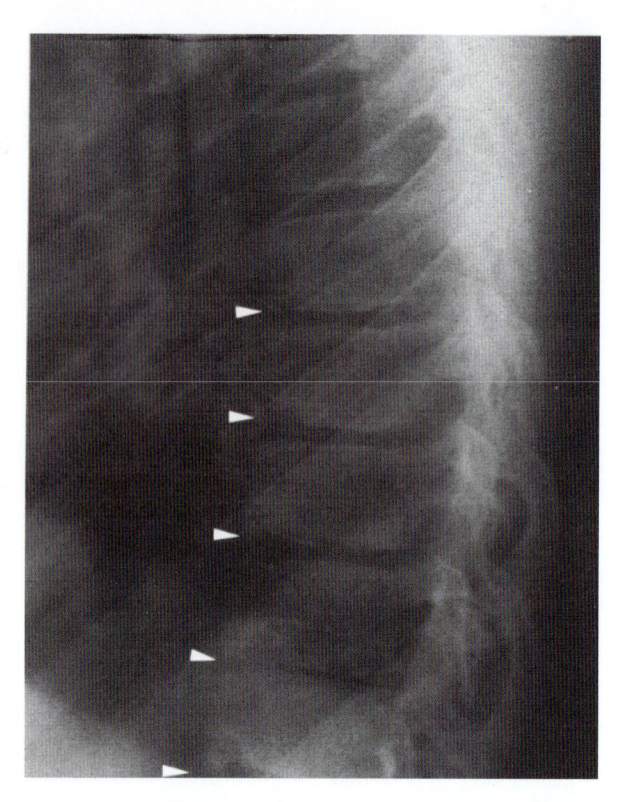

The typical radiographic appearance of Scheuermann's disease is shown in Figure 44.4. This demonstrates irregularity of the growth plates of the vertebrae. The radiological diagnosis of Scheuermann's disease is made on the presence of wedging of 5° or more at three adjacent vertebrae.

Management is aimed at preventing progression of the postural deformity and involves a combination of joint mobilisation, massage therapy to the thoracolumbar fascia, stretching of the hamstring muscles and abdominal muscle strengthening. A brace may be worn to decrease the thoracic kyphosis and lumbar lordosis. Surgery may be indicated if the kyphosis is greater than 50° or if signs of spinal cord irritation are present.

Figure 44.4 Radiographic appearance of Scheuermann's disease

Hip pain

Hip pain is a more common presenting symptom in the younger athlete than the mature adult. The causes of hip pain in the younger athlete are shown in Figure 44.5. There are a number of possible causes of persistent hip pain and decreased range of motion in the younger athlete, in addition to those seen in the older athlete such as FAI, labral tears, stress fractures and snapping hip (all discussed in Chapters 31 and 32). MRI plays an important role in the diagnosis of the young athlete with hip pain.

Apophysitis

A number of large musculotendinous units attach around the hip joint. Excessive activity can result in a traction apophysitis at one of these sites, usually the ischial tuberosity at the attachment of the hamstring muscles, the anterior inferior iliac spine at the attachment of the rectus femoris, the anterior superior iliac spine at the attachment of the sartorius, or the iliopsoas attachment

The younger athlete   CHAPTER 44

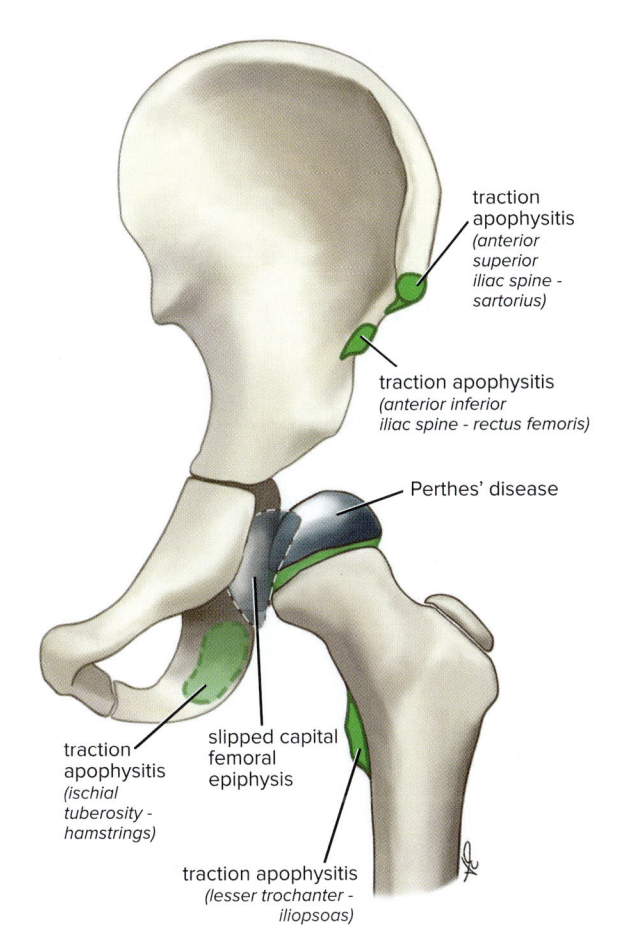

Figure 44.5 Causes of hip pain in children

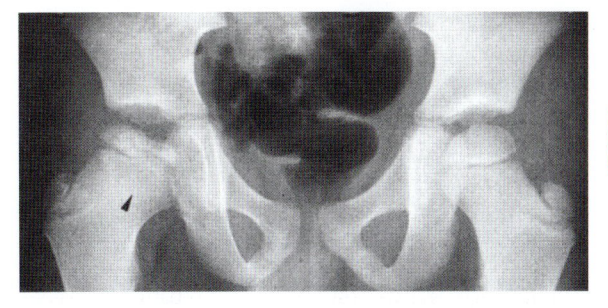

Figure 44.6 Radiographic appearance of Perthes' disease

to the lesser trochanter. Conservative therapy, including relative rest and modification of the athlete's activity level and strengthening, is usually effective.[18]

Perthes' disease

Perthes' disease is an osteochondritis affecting the femoral head. Perthes' disease is usually unilateral. It typically affects children between the ages of 4 and 10 years, is more common in males, and may be associated with delayed skeletal maturation. It presents as a limp or low-grade ache in the thigh, groin or knee.[19] On examination there may be limited abduction and internal rotation of the hip. Radiographs vary with the stage of the disease, but may show increased density and flattening of the femoral capital epiphysis (Fig. 44.6).

Management consists of rest from aggravating activity and range of motion exercises, particularly to maintain abduction and internal rotation. The age of the child and the severity of the condition according to radiographic findings (Herring or Catarell scale) will affect the intensity of the management. For initial stages in children under 6 years of age, pain killers, and avoiding jumping and running are sufficient to control the disease. In older children (over 6 years) with lateral pillar collapse of the femoral head over 50%, surgical treatment is indicated.

Various surgical techniques are used to cover the femoral head and protect it from further damage. Most frequently, femoral osteotomy or iliac augmentation techniques (or both) are used. In borderline cases, usage of orthoses is indicated. It is important for parents to prevent their children from engaging in sports that involve running and jumping, especially during the healing period of the femoral head (lasting approximately 2–3 years).

The condition usually resolves and return to sport is possible when the child is symptom-free and radiographs show some improvement. The main long-term concern is the development of osteoarthritis due to irregularity of the joint surface.

Slipped capital femoral epiphysis

A slipped capital femoral epiphysis (SCFE) may occur in older children, particularly between 12 and 15 years,[20] but can also be observed in younger children. Radiographs in SCFE have a similar appearance to a Salter-Harris type I fracture.

A slipped capital femoral epiphysis is associated with endocrinological disorders, biomechanical stress on the proximal femoral physis and high body mass index (BMI). It occurs typically in overweight boys who tend to be late-maturing, and thus is of increased concern given the trend towards adolescent obesity and selection for heavy boys in sports like American football and rugby. It has also been suggested that increased physical stress associated with intense sports participation may precipitate this condition.[21]

The slip itself may occur suddenly or, more commonly, as a gradual process. There is sometimes associated pain, frequently in the knee, but the most common presenting symptom is a limp. Examination reveals shortening and external rotation of the affected leg. Hip abduction and internal rotation are reduced. During flexion the hip moves into abduction and external rotation.

Bilateral involvement is common (approximately 20% of cases). Slips may compromise the vascular supply to the femoral head and lead to avascular necrosis.

983

PART C Practical sports medicine

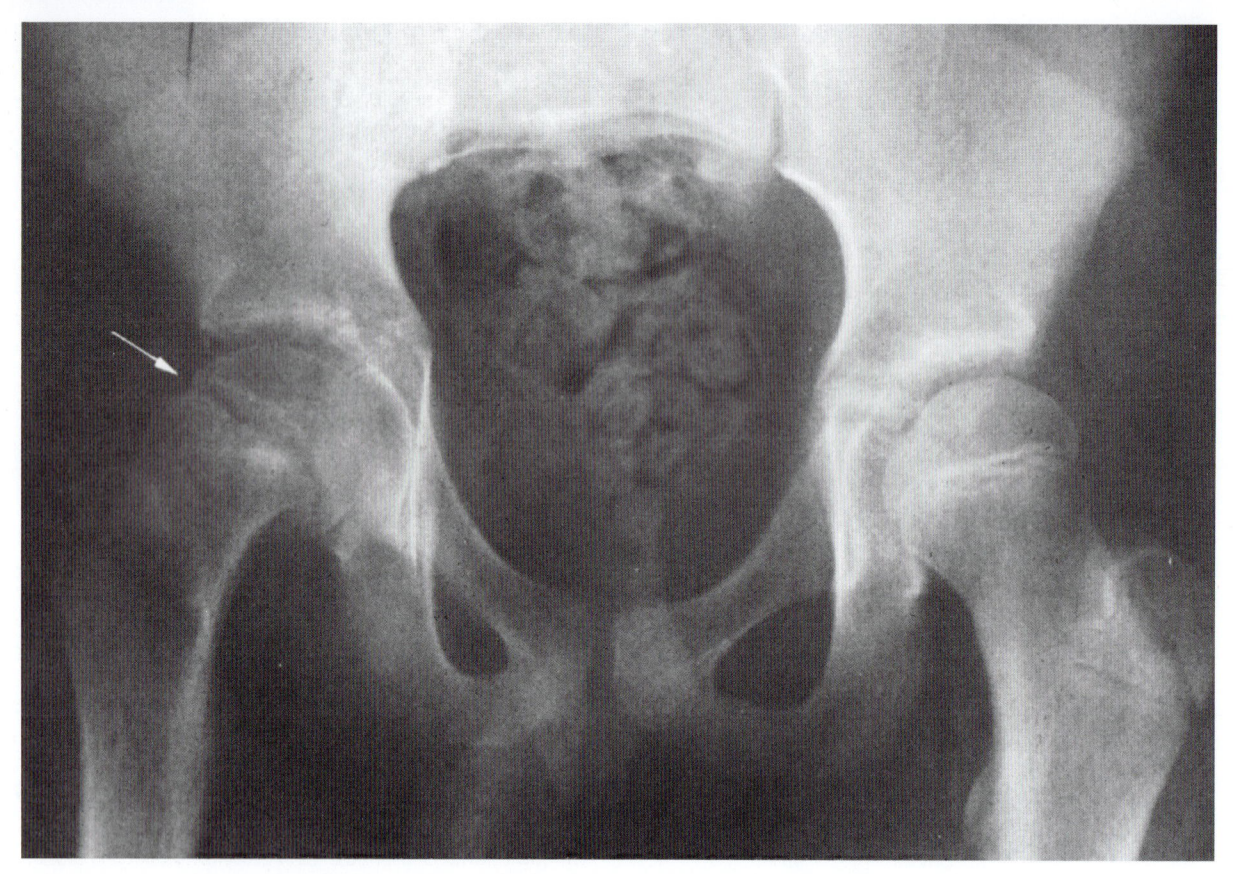

Figure 44.7 Radiographic appearance of slipped capital femoral epiphysis

> **PRACTICE PEARL**
>
> Radiographs show widening and irregularity of the growth plate, cystic changes in the proximal femoral metaphysis and a line continued from the superior surface of the neck of the femur does not intersect the growth plate (Fig. 44.7).

Avascular necrosis is the most common and severe complication of a slipped capital femoral epiphysis and requires orthopaedic assessment. A gradually progressing slip is an indication for surgery. The aim is to prevent further slipping of the epiphysis by transcervical fixation using one or more cannulated screws. An acute severe slip occurs occasionally. This is a surgical emergency.

Irritable hip

'Irritable hip' or transitory synovitis is common in children, but should be a diagnosis of exclusion. It is often related to a respiratory, often viral, infection. The child presents with a limp and pain that may not be well localised. Examination reveals painful restriction of motion of the hip joint, particularly in extension and/or abduction in flexion. Radiographs, and blood tests are usually normal. Ultrasound may demonstrate fluid in the joint capsule and MRI can help in challenging cases.

In the majority of cases, a specific cause is never identified and the pain settles after a period of bed rest and observation.[22]

Knee pain

Knee pain, especially anterior knee pain, is a common presentation in the younger athlete. Common causes of anterior knee pain include: Osgood-Schlatter disease, Sinding-Larsen-Johansson disease, patellofemoral joint pain (Chapter 36), patellar tendinopathy (Chapter 36), and referred pain from the hip.

Osgood–Schlatter disease

Osgood-Schlatter disease is an osteochondritis that occurs at the growth plate of the tibial tuberosity. Repeated

The younger athlete CHAPTER 44

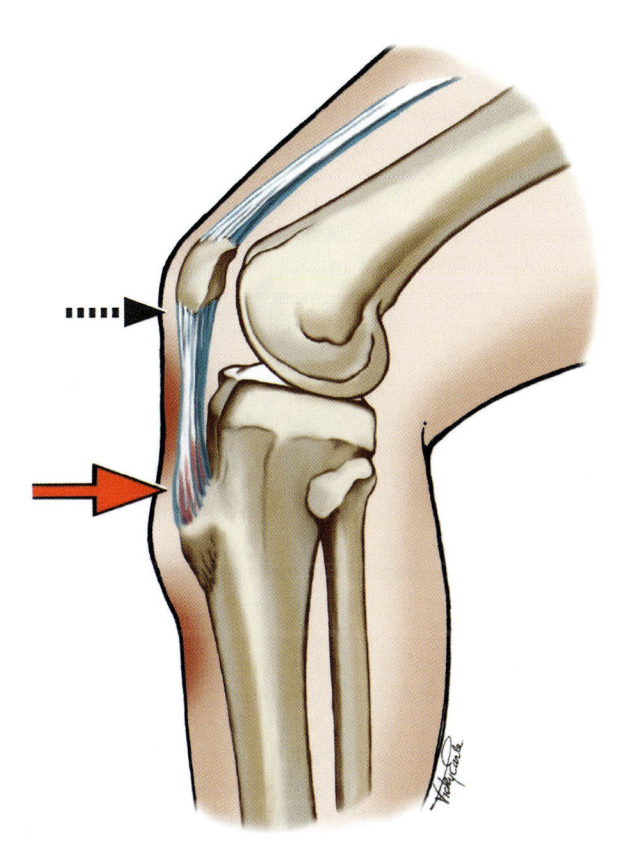

Figure 44.8 Sites of maximal tenderness in Sinding–Larsen–Johansson disease (black arrow) and Osgood–Schlatter disease (red arrow)

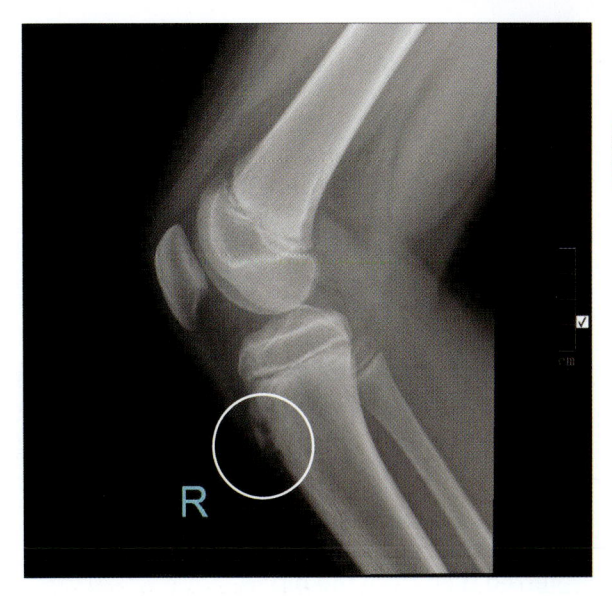

Figure 44.9 Radiographic appearance of Osgood–Schlatter disease

contraction of the quadriceps muscle mass may cause softening and partial avulsion of the developing secondary ossification centre.

This condition is extremely common in adolescents at the time of the growth spurt. It is usually associated with repeated forced knee extension, especially in sports involving running and jumping, such as basketball, football or gymnastics. Pain around the tibial tuberosity is aggravated by exercise.

Examination reveals tenderness over the tibial tuberosity (Fig. 44.8). There may be associated tightness of the surrounding muscles, especially the quadriceps. The presence of excessive subtalar pronation may predispose to the development of this condition.

The diagnosis of Osgood–Schlatter disease is clinical and radiographs are usually not required. In cases of severe anterior knee pain with more swelling than expected, a radiograph may be indicated to exclude bony tumour. Although all bone tumours are rare, the knee is a site of osteogenic sarcoma in the 10–30 year age group. The typical radiographic appearance of Osgood–Schlatter disease is shown in Figure 44.9.

Osgood–Schlatter disease is a self-limiting condition that settles at the time of bony fusion of the tibial tubercle. Its long-term sequel may be a thickening and prominence of the tubercle. Occasionally, a separate fragment develops at the site of the tibial tubercle. Athletes and parents need to understand the nature of the condition as symptoms may persist up to full maturity.

Management

Management of this condition requires activity modification. While there is no evidence that rest accelerates the healing process, a reduction in activity will reduce pain.

> **PRACTICE PEARL**
>
> As this condition occurs in young athletes with a high level of physical activity, it may be useful to suggest they eliminate one or two of the large number of sports they generally play. There is no need to rest completely. Pain should be the main guide as to the limitation of activity.

Symptomatic management via relative load reduction is key. The athlete may consider a stretching program and some massage therapy to the quadriceps muscle. Muscle strengthening can be introduced as pain allows.

Correction of any predisposing biomechanical abnormality, such as excessive subtalar pronation, is necessary. Neither injection of a corticosteroid agent nor surgery is required. Very occasionally, the skeletally mature person may continue to have symptoms (e.g. with work-related kneeling) due to non-union. The separate fragment should then be excised.

Sinding-Larsen–Johansson disease
This is a similar condition to Osgood-Schlatter disease. It affects the inferior pole of the patella at the superior attachment of the patellar tendon (Fig. 44.8). It is much less common than Osgood-Schlatter disease, but the same principles of management apply.

Patellar tendinopathy
Although symptomatic tendinopathy was thought to be rare in children, Professor Jill Cook showed that patellar tendinopathy is prevalent in junior basketball players.[23, 24] Management is as per the tendinopathy management principles in adults (Chapter 36).

Referred pain from the hip
Conditions affecting the hip, such as a slipped capital femoral epiphysis or Perthes' disease, commonly present as knee pain due to the innervation by the obturator nerve. Examination of the hip joint is mandatory in the assessment of any young athlete presenting with knee pain.

Popliteal cysts
Popliteal cysts (called 'Baker's cysts') are cystic formations filled with gelatinous mass developing in the popliteal fossa. The usual presenting complaint in children is the presence of a mass at the back of the knee. The most common site of origin is the bursa of the gastrocnemius and semimembranosus muscle. The cyst often appears gradually and may be fairly large when first noticed. Occasionally, it is found after an injury. Popliteal cysts in children are usually minimally symptomatic or asymptomatic, and not related to an intra-articular pathologic process.

Physical examination reveals a firm cystic mass in the popliteal fossa, often medially located and usually distal to the popliteal crease. It is most prominent when the knee is hyperextended with the patient in a prone position. Plain radiographs and ultrasound are the imaging techniques of choice. MRI should be obtained if an atypical history or abnormal physical findings are present.

In the vast majority of cases, popliteal cysts do not require treatment. The cyst usually resolves spontaneously over a period of months to a few years. Surgical excision of a popliteal cyst is indicated only when symptoms are severe and limit the range of motion of the knee, and have not resolved with at least several months of follow-up.

Less common causes of knee pain
Osteochondritis dissecans may affect the knee. This generally presents with intermittent pain and swelling of gradual onset. Occasionally, it may present as an acute painful locked knee. This acute presentation is associated with haemarthrosis and loose body formation. Radiographs may reveal evidence of a defect at the lateral aspect of the medial femoral condyle. Osteochondritis dissecans requires orthopaedic referral for possible fixation of the loosened fragment or removal of the detached fragment.

In juvenile rheumatoid arthritis (Still's disease) of the knee, there is a persistent intermittent effusion with increased temperature and restricted range of motion. There may be a family history of rheumatoid arthritis. Investigation requires serological examination, including measuring the level of rheumatoid factor and the erythrocyte sedimentation rate and, if indicated, serological examination of joint aspirate. The child's activity should be adapted to avoid using the painful joints while exercising other body parts and promoting cardiovascular fitness.

A differential diagnosis in paediatric arthritis that is relatively rare but is increasing in the developed world is acute rheumatic fever.[25] As there may be no history of sore throat and carditis may be silent, the diagnosis can only be made if the practitioner maintains an index of suspicion for this condition. Investigations should include markers of inflammation (erythrocyte sedimentation rate, C-reactive protein), serology for streptococci (anti-streptolysin-O titre, anti-DNaseB titres) and echocardiography. Penicillin and aspirin taken orally remain the mainstays of management.

A partial discoid meniscus may cause persistent knee pain and swelling in the adolescent athlete. A complete discoid meniscus is characterised by a history of clunking in the younger child (approximately 4 years). There is usually marked joint line tenderness, and a palpable snapping at the joint line with flexion/extension and/or rotation. MRI will demonstrate the lesion. Arthroscopy may be diagnostic and therapeutic.

Adolescent tibia vara (Blount's disease) is an uncommon osteochondritis that affects the proximal tibial growth plate. It usually affects tall, obese children around the age of 8-10 years. It is generally unilateral and radiographs show a reduced height of the medial aspect of the proximal tibial growth plate. Surgery may be required to correct any resultant mechanical abnormality.

Painless abnormalities of gait
It is not uncommon for a child to present with an abnormality of gait. The child is typically brought in by a parent who has noticed an unusual appearance of the lower limb or an abnormal gait while walking or running. The child may complain of foot pain (see below). However, in many instances, the abnormal gait is painless.

It is not sufficient to say that the child will 'grow out of it'. The child requires a thorough biomechanical

CHAPTER 44

The younger athlete

Anterior cruciate ligament (ACL) injuries in the skeletally immature athlete
with HÅVARD MOKSNES

Instability and functional impairments following ACL tears in skeletally immature children have been increasingly recognised.[26–32] Intrasubstance ACL ruptures are most worrisome due to the serious long-term health effects of potential early osteoarthritis.[33] Furthermore, the open growth plates on both sides of the knee joint warrant particular caution before surgical interventions with ACL reconstruction are performed.[34, 35]

Risk factors
It seems that boys may be more prone to rupturing their ACL before maturity, while girls have an increased risk through and after puberty,[36, 37] and most authors state that the incidence of these injuries is rising. However, no epidemiological studies are available with historical or new data to support this assumption. The perceived increased occurrence of ACL tears in children and adolescents may be due to higher participation and early specialisation in sports; however, it can also be caused by increased awareness and advances in diagnostic methods.

Treatment
Treatment algorithms for ACL ruptures in skeletally immature children vary around the world.[28-40]

> **PRACTICE PEARL**
>
> One of three different treatment algorithms is traditionally recommended to skeletally immature children after ACL injury:[38, 39, 41]
> - a transphyseal (adult) surgical reconstruction
> - non-operative treatment with active rehabilitation and an optional delayed ACL reconstruction if specific criteria are met
> - a physeal-sparing ACL reconstruction.

Unfortunately, the methodological quality in research on treatment of ACL injuries in younger populations has been poor.[42] Thus, there is a need for adequately sized prospective multicentre studies to heighten the scientific base for which treatments should be offered to children after suffering an ACL injury. Specific decision criteria with regard to which of these algorithms a child should be recommended have not been established, and treatment decisions are traditionally based on the experiences and practice of the individual orthopaedic surgeon or institution.

(i) Surgical reconstruction
Surgical reconstruction of the ACL in a skeletally immature patient is usually advocated to provide ligamentous knee joint stability, and to potentially protect the menisci from subsequent injury. However, surgical treatment may also damage the epiphyseal growth plates and result in various growth disturbances.[34, 35, 43] Furthermore, development of the graft during the remaining skeletal growth is unknown, and different authors have discussed the possibility of increased risk of re-injuries in adulthood due to impaired biomechanical properties.[31, 44, 45]

(ii) Primary active rehabilitation without surgical reconstruction
Conversely, primary active rehabilitation without surgical reconstruction has been documented to give favourable functional outcomes for a majority of children who have undergone supervised active rehabilitation programs.[30] Still, between one-third and half of these children report a change in their preferred sports activities from level 1 to level 2 activities (e.g. abandoning pivoting sports). Studies reporting comparable numbers following surgical treatment have not yet been reported. Either way, paediatric ACL injuries should be thoroughly assessed on an individual basis and treatment algorithms should be presented in a balanced fashion to the child and his or her parents.

(iii) Physeal-sparing ACL reconstruction
Intercondylar tibial eminence avulsion fractures involving the ACL are frequent and have long been assumed to be the most common injury involving the ACL in skeletally immature children.[46] Since a paper on surgical treatment of tibial spine avulsion injuries with involvement of the ACL from Roth in 1928,[47] consensus has developed that the majority of these injuries should be treated surgically with fixation to the bone without intervening with the epiphyseal growth plate.[48, 49]

Surgery or rehabilitation?
The clinical challenges with treatment for paediatric ACL injuries are related to the weighing of risks and benefits between primary surgical treatment and primary active rehabilitation without surgical intervention.[50] Regardless of whether the child is advised to undergo surgical treatment or not, there is substantial support in the literature that supervised rehabilitation should be performed exhaustively through all phases before the ultimate treatment decision is taken (Chapter 35).

Rehabilitation
Paediatric rehabilitation has to be performed in close collaboration with the parents. Exercises and goals have to be adjusted compared to traditional rehabilitation

continued

protocols because children are not small adults, and they cannot be expected to perform unsupervised training independently. Rehabilitation exercises are primarily focused on neuromuscular stimulation and control, with less focus on muscular strength and hypertrophy.[50, 51] Throughout the first two phases the child should be guarded from pivoting activities, and possibly should also wear a protective brace in school and training. Training sessions including exercises to facilitate proper alignment and adequate landing techniques have been successfully implemented in injury prevention programs,[52–54] and are also recommended through phases 2 and 3 of an ACL rehabilitation protocol.

Similarly, rehabilitation after surgical interventions has to be thorough and individualised with regard to the child's physiological and psychological maturity to achieve successful outcomes. Additionally, a longer time from surgery to return to sport should be advocated as emerging data from international registries suggest that young athletes have a high risk of suffering a second ACL injury following an ACL reconstruction.[55–59]

assessment, which may reveal a structural abnormality. The most common biomechanical problems in children are rotational abnormalities originating from the hip and the tibia causing either in-toed or out-toed gait.

If the child is asymptomatic and biomechanical abnormalities are not marked, no treatment is indicated. If abnormalities are marked or if the child is symptomatic, management may involve physiotherapy, as well as the use of braces or night splints when the child is very young and during periods of rapid growth. In the older child, orthoses can be used to compensate for the deformity.

Foot pain

Foot pain of gradual onset is a common presenting symptom in the younger athlete. The causes of foot pain are either acquired and congenital foot deformities such as flat feet, metatarsus adductus, clubfoot, vertical talus, pes calcaneovalgus or toe abnormalities, or osteochondroses of the foot such as Köhler's disease and Freiberg's disease. Examination of younger athletes with foot pain requires precise determination of the site of maximal tenderness.

Sever's disease

Heel pain is a common complaint in the skeletally immature athlete. Sever originally described[60] this condition as an inflammatory condition to the apophysis (Sever's apophysitis). It is a self-limited disease.

The patient complains of activity-related pain and examination reveals localised tenderness and swelling at the site of insertion of the Achilles tendon. There may be tightness of the gastrocnemius or soleus muscles, and dorsiflexion at the ankle is limited. Biomechanical examination is necessary. Radiographic examination is usually not required except in persistent cases.

Management consists of activity modification so that the child becomes pain-free. The patient should be advised that the condition will typically always settle, usually within 6-12 months, but occasionally symptoms will persist for as long as 2 years. A heel raise should be inserted in shoes. Stretching of the calf muscles is also advisable. Any biomechanical abnormalities should be corrected. Orthoses may be required. Strengthening exercises for the ankle plantarflexors should be commenced when pain-free and progressed as symptoms permit. Corticosteroid injections and surgery are contraindicated in this condition.

There is MRI evidence that this condition is not an inflammation within the apophysis, but rather is a chronic (repetitive) injury to the actively remodelling trabecular metaphyseal bone.[61,62] This condition should be treated as a stress fracture with a limited period of partial or non weight-bearing[61] and temporary discontinuation of the offending activity.

Tarsal coalitions

Congenital fusions of the bones of the foot may be undetected until the child begins participation in sports. The most common form is a bony or cartilaginous bar between the calcaneus and navicular bone. The second most common coalition is between the calcaneus and talus. Calcaneocuboid coalition is the least common form. There is often a family history. The adolescent may present with midfoot pain, after recurrent ankle sprains or after repetitive running and jumping. The pain may be associated with a limp.

Examination reveals restriction of subtalar joint motion. There may be a rigid flat-foot deformity. Radiographs taken at 45° oblique to the foot may confirm the diagnosis, but if these are normal and clinical suspicion persists, a CT scan or MRI should be obtained.

Management may require orthotic therapy. Surgical excision may be necessary in a young patient with severe symptoms or after failure of conservative therapy. The bony or cartilaginous bar may recur after surgery.

Köhler's disease

Köhler's disease is a form of osteochondrosis affecting the navicular bone seen in young children, especially between the ages of 2 and 8 years, and more frequently in boys. The exact cause of Köhler's disease is not known. It has been suggested in the literature that because of its late ossification relative to the other tarsal bones, the navicular is vulnerable to mechanical compression injury.

The child complains of pain over the medial aspect of the navicular bone and often develops a painful limp. Tenderness is localised to the medial aspect of the navicular bone. Radiographs reveal typical changes of increased density and narrowing of the navicular bone. Management in a walking cast for 6 weeks may accelerate relief of the symptoms. Orthoses should be used if biomechanical abnormalities are present. The natural history of the disease is spontaneous resolution of clinical symptoms and the radiographic abnormalities over time.

Apophysitis of the tarsal navicular bone

Pain on the medial aspect of the tarsal navicular in the older child may result from a traction apophysitis at the insertion of the tibialis posterior tendon to the navicular. This condition is often associated with the presence of an accessory navicular (Fig. 43.16) or a prominent navicular tuberosity. Management involves modification of activity, local electrotherapy and NSAIDs, with orthoses to control excessive pronation if this is present.

The accessory navicular which is found in 2.5% of children can cause pain by itself. Throughout early childhood, this condition is not noticed. However, in adolescence, when the accessory navicular begins to calcify, the bump on the inner aspect of the arch becomes noticed. For most, it is never symptomatic. However, for some, there is some type of injury, whether a twist, stumble or fall, that makes the accessory navicular symptomatic.

Apophysitis of the fifth metatarsal

A traction apophysitis at the insertion of the peroneus brevis tendon to the base of the fifth metatarsal is occasionally seen. Examination reveals local tenderness and pain on resisted eversion of the foot. Management consists of modification of activity, stretching and progressive strengthening of the peroneal muscles.

Freiberg's disease

Freiberg's disease (infarction) is an osteochondrosis causing collapse of the articular surface and adjacent bone of the metatarsal head. It is commonly thought to be due to avascular necrosis of the metatarsal head as demonstrated by destructive radiographic changes. The second metatarsal is most commonly involved (especially in ballet dancers), the third occasionally, and the fourth rarely. It occurs most frequently in adolescents over the age of 12 years.

Standing on the forefoot aggravates pain. The head of the second metatarsal is tender and there is swelling around the second metatarsal joint. Radiographs reveal a flattened head of the metatarsal with fragmentation of the growth plate. However, these changes may lag well behind the symptoms. Isotopic bone scan or MRI are more sensitive investigations.

If Freiberg's disease is diagnosed early, management with activity modification, padding under the second metatarsal and footwear modification to reduce the pressure over the metatarsal heads may prove successful. If the symptoms persist, surgical intervention may be necessary.

Flat foot

The exact incidence of flat foot in children is unknown. It is undoubtedly one of the most common 'deformities' evaluated by sports medicine clinicians. Most often, flat foot is a reflection of ligamentous laxity in the foot resulting in an abnormally low or absent arch.

In asymptomatic paediatric patients with a hypermobile flat foot, no treatment is indicated. Orthopaedic shoes, including various heel modifications, moulded heel cups, medial arch support and other orthoses, have traditionally been prescribed, even though there is no scientific evidence that such measures are efficacious.

In symptomatic patients, arch support and other orthoses may be of benefit. In some cases, where bony abnormalities caused by tarsal coalition (rigid type of flat foot) are present, surgical intervention is indicated if conservative treatment does not achieve satisfactory results.

REFERENCES

References for this chapter can be found at www.mhhe.com/au/CSM5e

Chapter 45

Military personnel

with STEPHAN RUDZKI, TONY DELANEY and ERIN MACRI

The limbs of soldiers are in as much danger from the ardor of young surgeons as from the missiles of the enemy.

Confederate surgeon Julian John Chisholm's observations on the limitations of medical care for military personnel in the American Civil War (1861–1865)

In the United States (US) Army, injuries and injury-related musculoskeletal conditions are responsible for more than 660 000 visits annually.[1] Injuries are the biggest cause of disability in the US Army.[1]

In this chapter, we discuss the principles of sport and exercise medicine that will help you provide services to a military population.

We introduce:

- the special culture of the military environment
- epidemiology of military injuries
- common military injuries with a sport and exercise medicine focus (i.e. not major trauma).

SPECIAL MILITARY CULTURE

Clinicians who provide medical and physiotherapy care in a military setting have a challenging task. An important difference between civilian and military practice is the compulsory nature of physical training. All military recruits undergo exercise regimes that are designed not only to improve their fitness, but also to prepare them physically and psychologically for extreme environments, discomfort and pain (Fig. 45.1). Military trainees have not always had a background of physical training. Increasingly, young adults come into the military with little experience of contact sports or regular physical activity. It is challenging to bring them to a required level of strength and aerobic fitness without causing injury.

The traditional military culture generally encouraged personnel to continue exercising despite early warning signs of pain that would cause civilian athletes to stop or slow down. Many recruits conceal injuries until graduation for fear of medical 'back squadding' (recruits held back in training) and derision from fellow recruits and their superiors. A soldier who finishes a forced march by walking on a broken ankle for 20 km with a fully weighted rucksack receives accolades and respect from peers and superiors.

Further to the drive towards pushing through pain, soldiers with a history of previous injury demonstrate an increased pain threshold–they feel less pain for a given stimulus compared to controls.[2,3] Pain thresholds may also be related to environmental and psychological factors

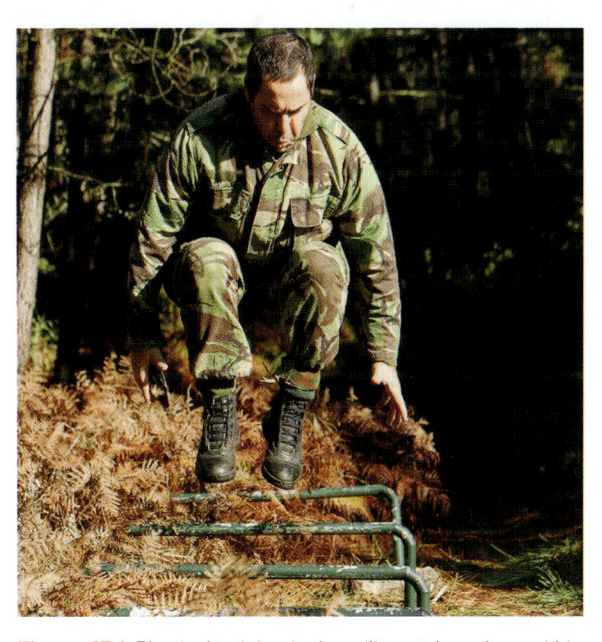

Figure 45.1 Physical training in the military takes place within a distinct culture and environment
ISTOCKPHOTO

(e.g. the common experience of World War II soldiers reporting no pain during the heat of battle despite severe injuries).[4]

As a consequence of these changes in experiencing or reporting of pain, military members often present to clinics with musculoskeletal injuries that are severe and debilitating, requiring longer periods of rehabilitation. Patients may present stoically, making it challenging to determine the true severity of pain or injury.

Because of the cultural overlay and late presentation in at least some military settings, it is common for patients to present with multiple concurrent pathologies. It is therefore very important to take a thorough history and physical examination (Chapter 14 and 15) on the initial presentation even if under time pressures. Concurrent pathology should always be considered in a patient whose progress is slow or who does not respond to treatment considered appropriate for the initial diagnosis.

EPIDEMIOLOGY OF MILITARY INJURIES

Recruit populations have an especially high incidence of injury and attrition. In New Zealand, the injury rate for recruits was more than five times that of trained personnel.[5] High attrition rates represent a significant cost. An injured soldier cannot perform his or her duties even if physically fit, and a moderate level of injury can impinge on the combat readiness of individual units.

US military studies have shown that training injury incidence rates range from 120 to 144 injuries/100 soldiers/year[6] in infantry, special forces and ranger units and 360/100/year for Naval Special Warfare training.[7]

These rates are far greater than the rates of injury in wars themselves. The Watson Institute monitors the cost of war: more than 970 000 Iraq and Afghanistan veteran disability claims were registered with the US Department of Veterans Affairs as of April 2016.[8] Rates of musculoskeletal injury in combat are estimated at around 3 per 1000 deployed soldiers per year. However, when a group of soldiers is monitored prospectively the rate is 10 times as high.

One of the larger reports of the type of musculoskeletal injuries highlights the proportion of fractures when soliders are in the combat setting (as distinct from the training setting when soft tissue injuries dominate) (Fig 45.2).[9] The most common sites of fracture are humerus, femur, tibia and fibula.

Injuries are not just a problem within a barracks setting. Non-battle injuries in US service personnel have been a major cause of medical evacuation from Iraq and Afghanistan. Referred to as DNBI (disease and non-battle injury), these conditions had an incidence rate of 130 per 1000 combat years and resulted in over 80% of the evacuations required from Afghanistan and Iraq in 2001-2012.[9,11] The importance of rehabilitation is underscored

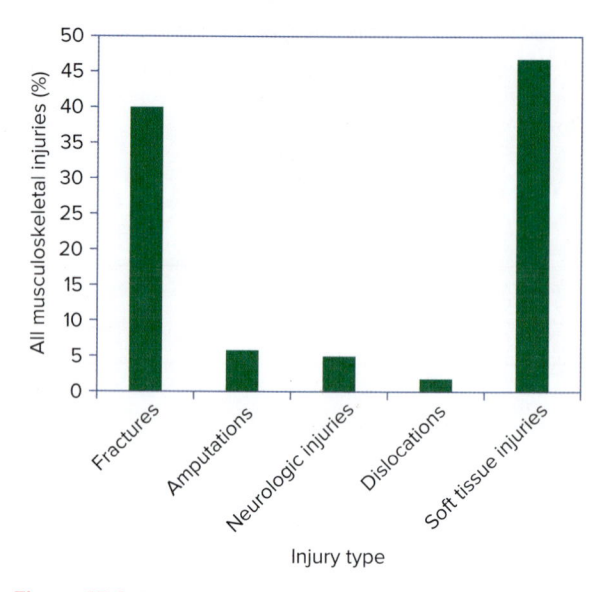

Figure 45.2 Fractures and soft tissue injuries provide the bulk of military injuries in the combat setting[10]
ADAPTED FROM BELMONT ET AL.[9]

by the fact that >90% of these injured military personnel returned to duty. Also relevant to the sports medicine community is that 50 000 anterior cruciate ligament (ACL) injuries were sustained among almost 2 million US troops during 10 years in Afghanistan and Iraq.[9]

Historically, the lower limb comprised the bulk of combat injuries (Table 45.1a), but recent wars have seen an increase in spinal/trunk injuries and spinal cord injury as a result of more powerful explosives.[9,17] The back, knee and wrist/hand are body regions commonly affected in those medically evacuated. This pattern of military injuries (i.e. being primarily lower limb in nature) presents in contrast to the Australian civilian workplace where back injury is the most common injury (25%) followed by the hand (14.3%) and finally lower limb injuries (10.8%).[18] Overuse is the most common cause of military training injuries.[6,7,14,15]

Wearing combat body armour is a risk factor in the development of low back pain during a military deployment.[19,20] In a prospective cohort study of US troops who deployed to Afghanistan for 12 months, moderate or worse low back pain occurred in 22% (175/805) and there was some back pain in 77% of the soldiers. Risk of back pain was sharply increased (relative risk >4.0) if the combatant wore body armour for greater than 6 hours a day or wore equipment weighing >32 kg. The incidence of low back pain in deployed US troops increased 20 times from 1.5/1000 in 2001 to 29.8/1000 in 2010. See Chapter 29 for discussion of the biopsychosocial factors that contribute to back pain.

Military personnel CHAPTER 45

Table 45.1 (a) Types and incidence of injuries by country

Body part	US infantry[12]	US military[13]	Australian recruits[14]	Australian Army[14]	South African recruits[15]	New Zealand recruits[4]
Ankle/foot	11.6%/20.8%	13%	18.3%/11.9%			35%
Knee/lower leg	17.6%/15.1%	22%	32.1%/7.3%			16%
Low back	10.2%	20%				
Spine				15.2%		
Lower limb				39.6%	80%	
Upper limb				19.4%		

(b) Cause of injuries by country

Cause	US infantry[12]	Afghanistan/Iraq medical evacuations[13]	Australian recruits[14]	Norwegian recruits[16]	New Zealand recruits[4]
Training-related	47%	19–21%	19.2%		
Falls/jumps		18%			
Motor vehicle-related		12–16%			
Running			36.6%		28%
Obstacle course			14.6%		
Basic training				20–25%	
Acute overexertion					37%
Team sports					25%

Injuries cause disproportionate morbidity in young military populations. In a US military population, injuries accounted for 56% of sick-call diagnoses, but caused nearly 10 times the number of limited-duty days as illness. Soldiers with lower extremity running injuries spent seven times more days on a restricted duty profile than those with non-running injuries.[21] In outpatient clinics, 80–90% of all limited-duty days accrued by US Army trainees and infantry soldiers were the result of training-related injuries (Table 44.1b).[6]

COMMON MILITARY INJURIES

The range of injury and illness facing clinicians who serve the military greatly exceeds that usually seen in civilian medicine. In the military, individuals are exposed to extremes in temperature, biological and chemical agents, and communicable diseases (e.g. sexually transmitted, tropical). Traumatic injuries can result in concussion or traumatic brain injury, spinal cord injury, limb amputation, and injuries that can affect multiple systems and often require urgent medical care. For example, significant risk for injury occurs in diving operations, including submariner evacuation and rescue. However, the majority of the injuries tend to be related to environmental exposure (e.g. barotrauma, decompression illness, cold exposure, marine life exposure) rather than to mechanical mechanisms of injury, and thus most diving injuries are of a non-musculoskeletal nature.[22, 23]

Psychosocial factors can influence the recovery trajectory of military sports injuries (see also Chapter 5). Experiencing deployment can affect emotional and psychological health, even in situations of peacekeeping missions, resulting in issues ranging from fatigue and exhaustion to depression, post-traumatic stress disorder and suicidal ideation. Mental health is a major issue in military medicine and suicide rates are higher among military populations than among civilians.[9]

The following discussion will address musculoskeletal and sports injuries. However, maintain a broad perspective when assessing sports injuries as often these other factors present at the same time. Many 'injury' chapters (Part B) in this volume are relevant to the military population. This chapter highlights common specific military issues and treatment that is particular to this population.

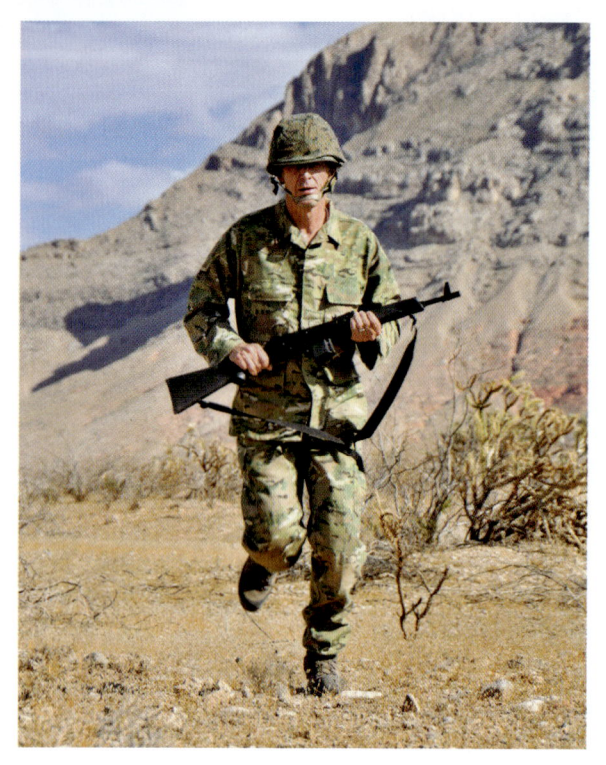

Figure 45.3 Running is a predominant source of exercise in many forces. Competition is high and environments are usually extreme compared with recreational running programs ISTOCKPHOTO

Overuse injuries of the lower limb

There are three peaks of overuse lower limb injuries in the military. The first and greatest is among recruits, the second in trained soldiers preparing for special forces selection (Fig 45.3) and the third is older soldiers training to pass annual fitness assessments.

The most common lower limb overuse injury is leg pain due to medial tibial stress syndrome (see Chapters 4 and 38). Early identification with correction of training errors and biomechanical factors often leads to rapid resolution. Recalcitrant medial tibial stress syndrome may require customised orthoses, gait retraining and more appropriate footwear where possible.

A significant proportion of recalcitrant medial tibial stress syndrome may be due to underlying exertional compartment syndrome (see Chapter 38). We have encountered resting compartment pressures >50 mmHg (normal resting <15 mmHg) in military trainees with largely medial tibial pain and tenderness. Changes in running technique (shortening stride length, landing more towards the forefoot) decreased leg pain and increased pain-free running distance in US Army recruits

at the United States Military Academy at West Point (see Chapter 38).[24–26]

The incidence of stress fracture in military recruits varies from 1–30%, with female rates generally higher than male rates.[15, 27-32] The most common sites of stress fracture are the tibia, metatarsals, pelvis and femur.[33] Previous stress fracture and lower baseline levels of weekly exercise are well-recognised risk factors.[32] There may be genotypic predisposition.[32]

To prevent stress fractures, as well as other injuries, aim to have recruits enter physical training with a reasonable level of fitness (as measured by the 20 m shuttle run). The issue of fitness at entry and injuries is discussed in more detail later in this chapter. Correction of biomechanical faults, and reduction of training to 60-70% of the injury-causing load, will contribute to rapid recovery and return to full training. Complete rest is contraindicated as this leads to loss of cardiorespiratory fitness and often depression. Training should change from large marching and running volumes to cycling, rowing and swimming pool work. For more on stress fracture aetiology see Chapter 4 and for treating specific stress fractures, please see the index. Medial tibial stress syndrome, exertional compartment syndromes and bone stress injuries can coexist. All personnel presenting with lower limb injuries should be evaluated for referred pain from the spine (Chapters 5, 6 and 29).

Blister injuries

Blister injury from endurance marching has been a major problem for infantry soldiers throughout history. Among Canadian military, there was a 43% incidence of blisters during a 56 km night march carrying an 11 kg load.[34, 35] High rates of blister injury occur in recruits in the US Marine Corps and US Navy.[36] The morbidity associated with blisters should not be underestimated.[37]

Blisters are caused by shear forces acting on the skin, mainly due to friction while braking. This causes a mechanical split in the skin layers, which subsequently fills with fluid. Moist (sweaty) skin is most prone to blister formation because of increased friction and softening of the hard outer layer of skin (stratum corneum).[38] Braking forces on the foot increase with increased rucksack load.[39]

Sock type reduces the incidence of blisters. During a 3-day road march in the United Kingdom (UK), soldiers wearing a nylon inner sock had fewer blisters per person than those with either a single or double woollen sock.[40] A study in runners suggests that an acrylic sock results in fewer and smaller blisters than a cotton sock.[38] A joint US military task force recommended the use of synthetic-blend socks to prevent blisters.[41]

In addition to type of sock, use of an inner sock can reduce the severity and associated morbidity of blister

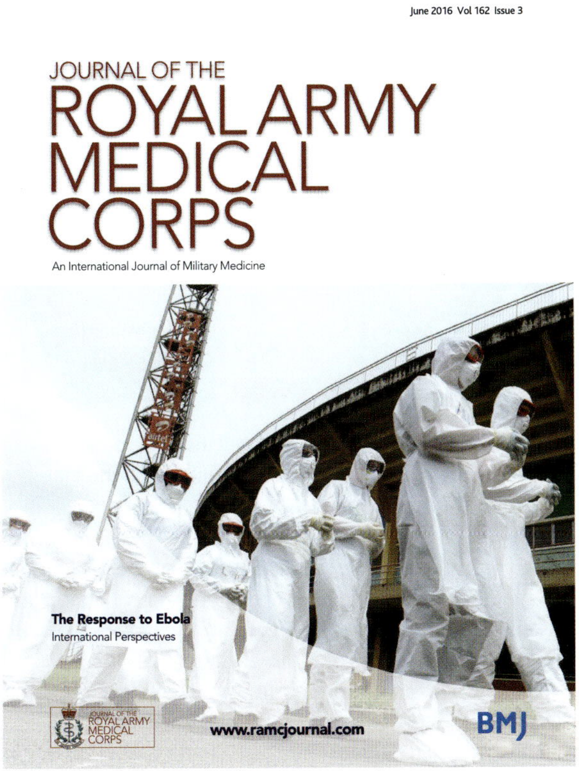

Military personnel   CHAPTER 45

Fig 45.4 The *Journal of the Royal Army Medical Corps* (cover shown) along with *Military Medicine* provide valuable research and education
A 2016 COVER IMAGE, COURTESY OF THE *JOURNAL OF THE ROYAL ARMY MEDICAL CORPS*

- use off-the-shelf heat-mouldable orthoses to reduce shearing loads to the sole of the foot
- reduce heel lift and blistering by tightening boot laces over the dorsum of the foot and tying a reef knot to lock the lace at the anterior ankle joint.

Parachuting injuries

Military parachuting has the potential to cause severe injuries.[46] Military parachutists use static line parachutes with limited manoeuvrability. In conditions where the prevailing winds exceed 5-8 knots, the parachutist has limited ability to reduce speed on landing. Dirt landing strips and airports are hazardous landing areas. Night descents are associated with a greater rate and severity of injury.[46] Paratrooper body weight influences risk of injury, particularly when the drop zone is on land.[47] There appears to be a relatively high rate of thoracic spine injuries in military parachutists jumping with operational loads.

Military round parachutes should not be used in wind conditions over 10 knots for trainees and 13 knots for trained static line paratroopers. If the wind on a drop zone is a steady 10 knots, there is a high probability of 15-18 knot gusts every 10-15 minutes. A 20 knot wind carries a parachutist into an obstacle at four times the force of a 10 knot wind (i.e. $F = 1/2mv^2$). There is often real or perceived pressure to complete training or military exercise jumps in marginal wind conditions. Most military mass parachuting injuries occur when a strong wind gust comes through after the jump has been initiated. Our experience is that the cost of aborting a jump due to wind is dwarfed by the financial and human cost of injuring highly trained paratroopers or special forces operators, many of whom will not return to pre-injury duties.

injuries compared to a single sock.[42] Foot powder does little to reduce blister incidence in recruits and may even increase the incidence of blister formation.[43]

Boots have traditionally been blamed for the problem of blisters, but changes in boot fit, style and composition have had little effect on blister incidence.[40, 44, 45] Nevertheless, the following strategies are recommended for boot fitting and blister prevention:[42]

- wear a sock, sock liner and insoles (if applicable)
- have a load on your back when fitting boots
- measure both feet; length and width
- fit length first
- push the foot forwards in unlaced boot; ensure 1.5 cm space behind the heel
- push the foot backwards; ensure 1.5 cm from the longest toe to the end of boot
- ensure the boot width over the arch is snug but not tight
- fit the boots at the end of a day's activity, when the foot has spread
- apply sports tape directly to the feet before a long march; this may prevent blisters

> **PRACTICE PEARL**
>
> Prophylactic ankle bracing significantly reduced ankle sprains and fractures in US Army paratroopers.[48]

Prophylactic ankle bracing significantly reduced ankle sprains and fractures in US Army paratroopers[48] and it also reduced the amount of time spent on medically restricted duties.[49] It has been estimated that for every dollar expended on a parachute ankle brace, a saving of between US$7-9 could be achieved in medical and personnel costs.[50]

The ageing defence forces

Retirement ages are extending to 60 for full-time defence personnel and up to 65 for some reservists. With ageing, incidence of injury may increase as may risk of

995

PART C Practical sports medicine

central obesity, insulin resistance, hyperlipidaemia, hypertension, cardiovascular disease and neoplasia. Attention to lifestyle, exercise and diet is equally as important as in the general population.

INJURY PREVENTION IN THE MILITARY

This chapter extends the principles of injury prevention outlined in Chapter 12 and in specific injury chapters (e.g. Chapter 35, prevention of ACL injuries) to focus on prevention in the military setting. Risk factors for injury can be divided into intrinsic (specific to an individual, e.g. age, height, foot shape, sex and body weight) or extrinsic (training errors, footwear or environmental considerations such as weather or running surface). This distinction is important in a military context because military forces must recruit from a civilian pool with a wide range of physical and athletic abilities, and seek to train these new members to achieve and maintain a standard of fitness relevant to the physical demands of the profession. There is little or no scope to select out applicants with intrinsic risk factors, as most military forces are required to take applicants from the broadest possible pool.

During recruit training, very high rates of injury lead to medical discharge and a loss of personnel. Australian recruits who developed an injury during recruit training were 10 times more likely to fail to complete training than those who were not injured.[51] US male recruits who were discharged during training sustained injuries three times more frequently than those not discharged; discharged females sustained injuries at twice the rate of non-discharged females.[52]

As it is costly to attract and process new recruits, minimising recruit attrition during basic training is an important objective for all military forces. Addressing modifiable extrinsic factors can provide the greatest yield in terms of decreasing injury levels and allowing the broadest range of entrants to successfully enter into a military career.

Injury surveillance

Injury surveillance is the necessary precursor to injury prevention; it allows for the identification of incidence, location, nature and cause of injury. Population-based data are necessary in order to target interventions appropriately.

Ideally, military services should adopt a public health approach to injury prevention as a framework.[53] The public health approach is characterised by four steps:

1. surveillance
2. risk factor identification
3. intervention implementation
4. evaluation (Fig. 45.5).[54]

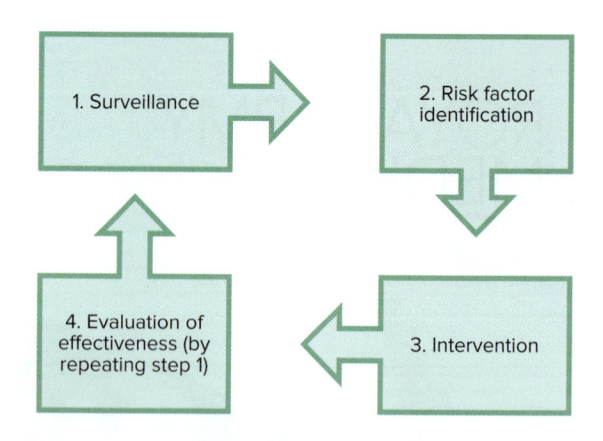

Figure 45.5 The public health model that is appropriate for the military setting. Note the similarities with the injury prevention model outlined in Chapter 12

Surveillance data are fundamental to priority setting, but are dependent on reliable and valid data collection and dissemination. Without such data, it is nearly impossible to measure the impact of interventions.[53]

The aim of any military injury surveillance system should be to provide commanders with accurate and reliable information on the type, nature and cause of injury, in conjunction with well thought out strategies for injury prevention. The army dictum 'do not come to me with problems, just solutions' is especially pertinent in military settings.

The public health approach to injury prevention was utilised to identify and eliminate ACL ligament ruptures at an Australian Army Recruit Training Centre as detailed below.[55, 56]

1. *Surveillance:* data identified a greater than expected number of ACL ruptures occurring in an obstacle course landing area.
2. *Risk factor analysis:* rubber matting installed to provide shock absorption was causing ACL injuries due to increased friction and 'stickiness' on landing.
3. *Intervention:* removal of the rubber matting and its replacement with river pebbles.
4. *Evaluation:* no further ACL ruptures at this particular location after removal of the rubber matting.

The success of this approach highlights the utility of following a public health approach. A similar approach has been adopted with other key risk factors including initial level of aerobic fitness and running distance (see relevant sections below).

Despite evidence to support strategies to prevent injuries in a military setting, effecting change is challenging as in all walks of life.[57] Officers and non-commissioned officers (NCOs) may seek to maintain and honour traditions, and may resist changes in training regimes or minimum fitness standards. For example, there are conflicting opinions within the military as to whether fitness standards should be different for men and women if they are working in the same trade. One argument is that a combat engineer needs to meet the standards for being a combat engineer regardless of gender.

To summarise, the implementation of changes must consider the cultural environment of the military and a strategic plan implemented in order to ensure a smooth and effective transition.[58] In recent times, Western militaries have moved towards gender-free assessments of physical capability that are valid predictors of work performance. Australia has removed all sex barriers to military employment in 2016. All jobs in the Australian Defence Force are open to women who are able to pass the relevant occupation-specific tests. The effects this change will have on injury type, frequency and severity will be the subject of prospective study and evaluation.

Sex as a risk factor for injury

In Australian, British and American troops, there are higher rates of injury and illness among female soldiers than their male counterparts.[59-62] Overall morbidity of injury in women is also greater.[63] Medical discharge rates are higher among women in both Australia and Britain.[60, 61]

An increased risk of injury was first identified in 1976 at the US Military Academy at West Point with the introduction of female cadets.[64] On average women had lower aerobic fitness than men (VO_2max, 46 mL/kg/min versus 59 mL/kg/min) and this variable was associated with injury incidence.[65]

When stratified by 1 mile run time, the risk of injury between men and women was comparable, with the highest risk of injury in the slowest group.[63] Of note was that 51% of the women were in the group with the longest run time compared to 1% of the men. Lower peak VO_2 is also an independent risk factor for time-loss injury.[66] For a standardised level of physical activity, UK male recruits worked at a lower cardiovascular strain than females (24% vs 33% of heart rate reserve), and this additional cardiovascular strain is believed to increase fatigue, thus predisposing to injury.[62] Sex is therefore not an independent risk factor for injury when controlled for aerobic fitness levels among recruits.[61]

Aerobic fitness

The initial level of aerobic fitness of a recruit has been shown to be a predictor of both injury and successful completion. In an Australian Army recruit cohort, aerobic fitness was measured using the 20 m shuttle run test (SRT).[67, 68] Lower scores on the 20 m SRT were related to increased risk of attrition (Fig. 45.6a) as well as increased risk of injury (Fig. 45.6b).[51] The least fit soldiers (20 m SRT score 3.5) were 20 times more likely to not complete training than the fittest recruits (score 13.5). If injured, fit subjects were 25 times more likely to recover from their injury than the least fit subjects with an injury. Similar relationships between fitness, injury rates and attrition have been seen in British Navy and Army recruits.[61, 69]

One and 2 mile run times (both proxies for aerobic fitness) are significant predictors of injury in US Army and infantry recruits, respectively.[12, 63, 71] As mentioned above, recruits of equivalent aerobic capacity have similar rates of injury. However, in a female cohort of US Marine Corps recruits, a slower 2 mile run time was associated with increased incidence of stress fractures. It was suggested that stress fractures may be reduced if women participated in pre-training activities designed to improve aerobic fitness.[33]

It should not be surprising that faster runners get fewer injuries. They are, almost by definition, good runners, and therefore less likely to sustain a running-related injury. Fitter individuals also do not experience

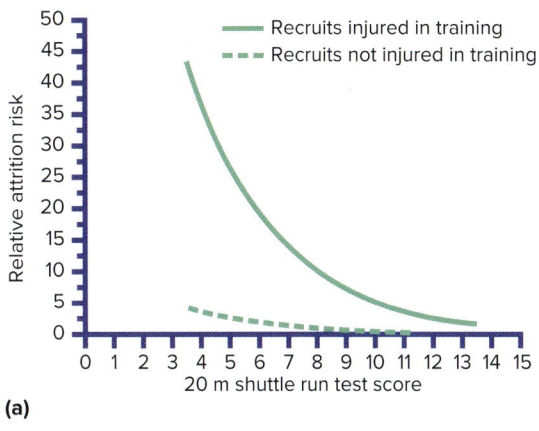

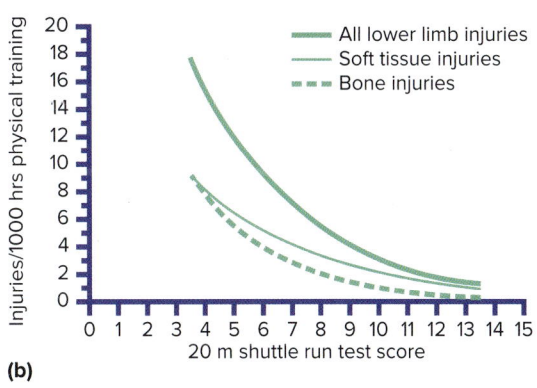

Figure 45.6 (a) The risk of recruit attrition based on 20 m SRT (b) The rate of recruit injury based on 20 m SRT
REPRODUCED FROM POPE[70] WITH PERMISSION

the same level of physiological strain during recruit training as those with lower levels of aerobic fitness. Less-fit individuals work closer to their maximum workload during recruit training and thus are at increased risk of injury.

The situation of a variable aerobic fitness start point and fixed endpoint could be viewed as a recipe for injury.[51,63] Ensuring that recruits arrive at training centres with a minimum level of aerobic fitness is a logical strategy to reduce the risk of injury and subsequent attrition. A screening 20 m SRT test was introduced at all Australian Army recruiting centres in 1997, and only recruits who scored higher than level 7.5 on the 20 m SRT were allowed to proceed to the recruit training battalion. The Royal Navy used a 2.4 km treadmill run to assess initial aerobic fitness.[72] Following introduction of the screening test, the pass rate in recruit training increased by 10%. and the number of recruits applying for voluntary release decreased from 15% to 6%. Overall, pre-enlistment aerobic testing positively impacted on recruit training pass rates.

The US Army tried a slightly different approach, in which they identified recruits with poor aerobic fitness at entry and then provided them with an in-service remedial physical fitness program before starting basic combat training (BCT). Women who undertook this remedial training then began BCT with similar mean 2 mile run times compared with non-remedial women, and had similar graduation success and time-loss injury rates.

Men with poor aerobic fitness (slower 2 mile run time) also undertook remedial training, but they did not improve their fitness to the level of normal entry male recruits. These men began BCT with considerably slower mean 2 mile run times than normal entry male recruits, and were ultimately less likely to graduate and more likely to suffer a time-loss injury.[52] Thus, the remedial program improved initial fitness levels in female, but not male, recruits within a predetermined time period.

These data suggest to us that encouraging potential recruits to achieve a minimum level of aerobic fitness before presenting to a recruit training centre may result in better outcomes than investing in remedial training once enlisted. Regardless of the method employed, overall evidence suggests that improving aerobic fitness levels prior to basic training could help to decrease the risk for injury and attrition.[33]

Body composition

If aerobic fitness level influences risk of injury and subsequent attrition rates in the military, would body composition also be a contributing factor? It has been noted that, in the US Army's view, 'obesity is associated with being unfit and unsoldierly'.[63] This is a view shared by many military forces, and most have programs in place to assist members to maintain their weight within prescribed ranges of body mass index (BMI) or percentage body fat.

The US Army weight control program has the stated aims of ensuring that soldiers are physically fit for their combat mission and that they present 'a trim military appearance'. US Army regulations consider body composition to be a subcomponent of fitness.[63] Using defined body fat standards, it has been estimated that 5% of eligible men and 30% of eligible women would be excluded from enlistment in the US military based on failing to meet these standards.

There is a clear relationship between body composition and performance on run tests: 1 and 2 mile run times increase with increasing percentage body fat.[63] For males, the highest percentage body fat group had more injuries; however, in females, the leanest had more injuries.[63]

Current cohorts of young adults are less fit than previous generations of young adults entering military service in the US, as mean times for 1 and 2-mile runs have increased since 1987.[73] US Army recruit height, weight and BMI values have progressively increased, with increases of both body fat and fat-free mass in male recruits. Body composition data on female recruits does not show a consistent trend.[73]

In Norwegian recruits, BMI was an independent risk factor for injury, while height and weight were not associated with injury.[16] In Australian recruits, none of these measures predicted injury.[51] Also, despite the US Army's views on obesity, there were no significant differences in attrition between Army recruits who met body weight standards and those who did not, regardless of sex, provided they met physical fitness standards on entry.[74]

> **PRACTICE PEARL**
>
> In considering the conflicting evidence available regarding BMI as an independent risk factor for injury, it is important to recognise that efforts might best be served focusing on overall fitness levels rather than body composition per se in assessing suitability for entry into the forces.

Previous injury

Many studies have linked history of injury and likelihood of a new injury. After adjusting for weekly distance, there was a 65% increased risk of injury in runners with a history of previous injury[75] and a doubling of the risk in those with previous injury.[76] After adjusting for age and sex, previous injury was a strong predictor of injury with an odds ratio of 1.5.[77] In one study of runners training for a marathon, half of the participants who reported an injury had sustained a previous injury and 42% had not completely rehabilitated before starting a training program.[78, 79] Controlled rehabilitation reduced the number of injuries in soccer.[80]

Previous injury and incomplete rehabilitation are therefore strong risk factors for recurrent injury. Rehabilitation is complete when an athlete is free from pain, muscle strength has returned to the pre-injury level and joint range of motion is restored.[80]

Clinicians responsible for the care of soldiers have a responsibility to ensure that complete recovery from injury has occurred before clearing them to return to full duties. Sports medicine clinicians appreciate that musculoskeletal injuries can only recover fully with adequate functional training.

> **PRACTICE PEARL**
>
> Consistent with the principle of specificity, a soldier will only recover sufficiently to return to full duties if given a functional training regime to prepare for full duties.[81]

Weekly running distance

Overtraining, and in particular, excessive running distance, is the most significant underlying cause of lower limb injuries in athletic populations.[82, 83] The only risk factor for injury consistently identified in running studies is weekly running distance. There is an almost linear relationship between increasing weekly distance and the incidence of injury in both men and women.[75, 76, 84-87] A sudden increase in weekly distance without a gradual build-up (or 'spike' of >10% per week) is considered a training error.[87, 88] Training errors such as running too frequently, too fast or for too long are major causes of injury in both beginner and experienced runners, accounting for up to 60% of injuries.[82, 87, 89, 90] We recommend Dr Tim Gabbett's review of sports injuries and training loads to all who work in the military setting (Chapter 12).[91]

Reducing weekly run distance

Most military forces use running tests ranging from 1.6 km (1 mile) to 5 km (3 miles) to assess physical fitness. The distance of the Australian Army physical training test has been reduced from 5 km to 2.4 km on the basis that reducing the test distance might reduce the training distances and result in a concomitant reduction in overtraining. However, attempts such as these have met with varying degrees of success worldwide.

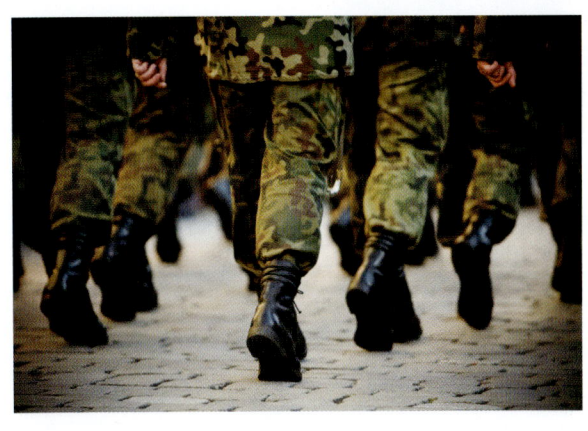

Figure 45.7 Marching has historically been a mainstay of military forces, both in training and in active deployments
ISTOCKPHOTO

In US studies spanning the Marine Corps, Army and Navy, recruits given lower mileage running programs sustained fewer injuries with no subsequent differences in performance on run tests or other physical fitness tests.[92-95] One study demonstrated a 54% reduction in stress fracture incidence compared to the high-mileage group.[92] The US Department of Defense estimated in 1995 that the reduction in running mileage had saved US$4.5 million in medical care costs and nearly 15 000 training days annually by preventing stress fractures alone.[96]

Cross-training and other program modifications

There are effective alternatives to running to condition recruits. Marching with rucksacks in place of running was investigated in Australia with subsequent reduction in injury rates and morbidity, while improvements in performance on run tests and VO$_2$max were as good as a group given a traditional running program (Fig. 45.7).[14, 97] Load bearing or pack marching is more occupation-specific to the military environment than distance running in a singlet, shorts and shoes. There is considerable gain in aerobic conditioning from shorter, high-intensity training. Given the variety of careers in the military, with varying physical and intellectual demands, imposing a single rigid training regime on all recruits, regardless of physique, sex, age and aspiration, is unrealistic.

Some level of running is essential in military training programs, but the design of running programs may reduce the risk of injury. Interval training and periodisation are other training modifications that have been successfully used to reduce injuries.[60, 94, 98]

In Australia, sport and exercise physician Dr Stephan Rudzki published the results of an intervention that consisted of:

- discontinuing road runs as formed groups
- introducing 400–800 m interval training
- reducing test run distance from 5 km to 2.4 km
- standardising route march speed, and
- introducing deep water running as an alternate aerobic activity.

The incidence of injuries decreased 46% among men but increased in women. Overall, there was a striking cost saving because of the much lower rates of medical discharge and medical investigation.[60]

In a US study, recruits were divided into ability groups based on initial 2 mile run times. Running speed was managed to keep effort at between 70–83% of VO_2max. This modified program was compared with a traditional training program. The proportion of recruits who failed the Army Physical Fitness Test (APFT) was lower in the modified program than the traditional training group (1.7% vs 3.3%). After adjustment for initial fitness levels, age and body mass index, the relative risk of an injury in the traditional training group was about 50% greater in both men and women.[99]

Training modifications nearly abolish the incidence of pelvic stress fractures in female recruits.[98] Interventions included a reduction in route march speed from 7.5 km/h to 5 km/h and placing shorter women at the head of the column to reduce stride length. Individual step length was promoted instead of marching in step, march and run formations were more widely spaced, and interval-running training replaced traditional middle-distance runs. The rate of pelvic stress fractures fell from 11% to 0.6%.[98]

Deep water running is an aerobic activity that can rest the lower limbs and periodise impact loading.[100] It is performed in the deep end of a swimming pool, normally with the aid of a flotation vest or belt. This form of training will maintain existing aerobic performance for up to 6 weeks.

To summarise, a comprehensive review of injuries in the US Armed Forces stated that:

> *Military and civilian research indicates that high running volume significantly increases the risk for lower extremity injury. During initial military training, about 25% of men and about 50% of women incur one or more training-related injuries. About 80% of these injuries are in the lower extremities and are of the overuse type—a condition brought about by training volume overload (generally excessive running relative to initial fitness level and running capability of the individual).*[41]

> **PRACTICE PEARL**
>
> Reducing running distances among recruits is a logical strategy to reduce injury rates while still attaining minimal physical fitness standards. Ideally, recruits come to training in good condition; this has been associated with fewer injuries.[101]

Running experience

The risk of running injuries declines with increased running experience.[75] This appears contradictory in the context of the clear association between running distance and injury, but may be related to experience (i.e. chronic adaptation of tissues to long-term running programs, improved running mechanics with experience) and/or the 'healthy runner' effect.[82, 90, 102] The 'healthy runner' describes the phenomenon that only those without injury can continue with a running program on a long-term basis. This suggests that 'healthy runners' have the intrinsic characteristics required to become long-term runners in the first place, while others will stop running due to an inability to tolerate the sport. Alternatively, if experience causes reduced injury rates over time, then this would suggest that the reason military recruits tend to have higher injury rates is because they are new to the intensity of the training regime. Either way, runners with less than 3 years of regular running experience have twice the risk of lower limb injury than those with more than 3 years running experience.[76]

Competitive behaviours

Injury incidence is associated with motivation score.[103] Higher scores correlate with higher incidence of medically treated injury. Runners who compete have higher injury rates than recreational runners, even when adjusting for mileage.[75, 77] More motivated runners may ignore the first signs of injury.

In military populations, every activity is highly competitive. The US Army places great emphasis on the APFT. Better scores influence prospects for promotion and most US soldiers strive to achieve the maximum score. The Australian Army now utilises a pass/fail result instead of a score, to reduce competitive behaviours and subsequent risk of injury.

Warm-up/stretching

The role of stretching as a component of a pre-activity warm-up, and in preventing injuries in the military, is unclear. As outlined in Chapter 12, in the general sporting population an acute bout of stretching prior to activity results in short-term loss of muscular strength, power and endurance[104, 105] and does not reduce overall injury risk[106]

Military personnel CHAPTER 45

> ### Military recommendations for injury prevention initiatives
>
> The evidence base for injury prevention recommendations has been reviewed by a joint US military task force.[41] Six interventions had strong enough evidence to be recommended for implementation in the military services and two interventions were not recommended due to evidence of ineffectiveness or harm.
>
> #### Recommended interventions (sufficient scientific evidence)
> 1. Prevent overtraining.
> 2. Perform multiaxial, neuromuscular, proprioceptive and agility training.
> 3. Wear mouth guards during high-risk activities.
> 4. Wear semi-rigid ankle braces for high-risk activities.
> 5. Consume nutrients to restore energy balance within 1 hour following high-intensity activity. (High carbohydrate/protein replacement within 15–30 minutes of finishing high-intensity exercise leads to more rapid muscle and liver glycogen restoration and preservation of muscle mass.)
> 6. Wear synthetic-blend socks to prevent blisters.
>
> #### Interventions not recommended (evidence of ineffectiveness or harm)
> 1. Wear back braces, harnesses or support belts.
> 2. Take anti-inflammatory medication prior to exercise.
>
> While physical training is necessary to condition soldiers for their occupational tasks, the authors noted that 'in classic military tradition, however, efforts to exceed the standards have contributed to the injury epidemic present today'.[41]

In a randomised controlled study in Australian military recruits there was no effect of pre-exercise static stretches on all-injury risk, soft tissue injury risk or bone injury risk.[107] Among Japanese recruits, the total injury rate was the same between those who conducted static stretches and those who did not. However, the incidences of muscle/tendon injury and low back pain were significantly lower in the stretching group.[108]

As it is clear that traditional static stretches do not reduce overall injury rate, warm-ups today should be incorporating light cardiovascular activities such as jogging and dynamic range of motion activities, and progress to sport-specific drills.[104, 109-111]

> **PRACTICE PEARL**
>
> The wise military physician should never assume that all apparent musculoskeletal pain in the young soldier is due to overuse injury.

Conclusion

Injury is a major problem for most Western military forces, and female recruits bear a disproportionate burden. Although the military population usually is fit and has access to high-quality healthcare, they can still have the systemic, metabolic, infective and neoplastic diseases found in the wider population.

Reducing running distance reduces both the incidence and severity of injury in military recruit populations, without affecting overall physical performance. The entry level of aerobic fitness is a key modifiable risk factor, and screening for physical fitness prior to clearing to participate in basic training programs has reduced both injury and attrition rates. Early identification of injuries and counselling trainees about achievable career paths is an important part of rehabilitation. Not all somatotypes or psyches are suited for infantry, marines or special forces, regardless of pre-recruitment dreams.

Injury prevention strategies should be based on robust surveillance systems using a public health approach to accurately identify risk factors, implement interventions and evaluate outcomes. While the nature of the profession comes with inherent risk, it is possible to reduce injury and improve retention.

REFERENCES

References for this chapter can be found at www.mhhe.com/au/CSM5e

Chapter 46

Periodic medical assessment of athletes

with STEPHEN TARGETT and BEN CLARSEN

To screen or not to screen, that is the question.
adapted from *Hamlet*, William Shakespeare (1564–1616)

Sports medicine clinicians commonly perform standardised health evaluations of athletes and many different organisations around the world require that athletes undergo a pre-participation evaluation to be allowed to participate in sport. However, organisations rarely provide guidance regarding the content of the required evaluation and the effectiveness of the approach in reducing the risk of injury, illness or sudden death in athletes remains controversial.

There are many different templates available, such as the Fédération Internationale de Football Association (FIFA) pre-competition medical assessment (PCMA),[1] the International Olympic Committee periodic health examination (PHE)[2] and the American Academy of Paediatrics pre-participation physical evaluation (PPE).[3] It should be emphasised, however, that these are designed for different target groups and there is no one universal template that suits all situations.

In order to avoid any confusion in terminology in this chapter, we use the term 'periodic medical assessment' (PMA) to refer to the standardised medical assessment of athletes, without being specific to any group's recommended template.

The development of a template for the PMA of an athlete, whether elite or recreational, requires careful planning, and gives an opportunity for all of the members of the sports medicine team and coaching staff to work in collaboration. Establishing the optimum template for each situation can be achieved by considering the following questions in turn.

- Why perform the medical assessment?
- Who is being assessed?
- When and where should the assessment be performed, and by whom?
- What should be included in the assessment?
- Are there any other issues to consider?

WHY PERFORM THE MEDICAL ASSESSMENT?

The first step in planning a PMA template is to determine why you are performing the medical assessment. The primary goal of the PMA is to make participation in sport safer, but there are a number of other valid reasons for wanting to perform a PMA such as assessing the status of known injuries and illnesses, screening for risk factors, reviewing medications and supplements, baseline testing, athlete education and establishing rapport with athletes.

Identification of medical conditions that contraindicate participation in sport

There are some medical conditions that may contraindicate participation in certain sports or recreational activities; for example, uncontrolled epilepsy in motor racing, cycling or swimming; or human immunodeficiency virus (HIV) infection in an amateur boxer. In many cases, such as asthma in a scuba diver, the medical condition is not an absolute contraindication and athletic participation should be decided on a case-by-case basis. It is therefore important that the medical professional performing the PMA understands the physical and mental demands of the sport in question, as well as its regulations. Table 46.1 shows examples of medical conditions that warrant special attention or contraindicate participation in certain sports.

It is important to identify medical conditions that may be made worse by intense exercise; for example, uncontrolled type 1 diabetes, poorly controlled asthma or uncontrolled hypertension. Although such conditions are usually not absolute contraindications to sports participation, optimal control should be established prior to commencing intense training and competition.

PART C Practical sports medicine

Table 46.1 Medical conditions affecting sports participation (adapted from Bernhardt et al.[4])

Medical condition	Sport/activity participation recommendations
Atlantoaxial instability	Medical evaluation necessary
Bleeding disorder, blood thinning medications	Medical evaluation necessary. Contact sport usually discouraged
Cardiovascular disease*	
Myocarditis/cardiomyopathy	All exercise contraindicated
Hypertension	Those with severe hypertension (>99th percentile for age plus 5 mmHg) should avoid heavy weight and power lifting, bodybuilding, strength training and sports with a high static component. Those with sustained hypertension (>95th percentile for age) need medical evaluation
Congenital heart disease	Medical evaluation necessary
Dysrhythmia	Medical evaluation necessary
Heart murmur	Medical evaluation necessary
Structural/acquired heart disease	
Hypertrophic cardiomyopathy	All exercise normally contraindicated
Coronary artery anomalies	All exercise normally contraindicated
Arrhythmogenic right ventricular cardiomyopathy	All exercise normally contraindicated
Acute rheumatic fever with carditis	All exercise normally contraindicated
Ehlers-Danlos syndrome, vascular form	All exercise normally contraindicated
Marfan syndrome	Medical evaluation necessary
Mitral valve prolapse	Medical evaluation necessary
Anthracycline use	Medical evaluation necessary
Vasculitis/vascular disease	Medical evaluation necessary
Cerebral palsy	Medical evaluation necessary
Diabetes mellitus	Participation normally allowed with proper attention to diet, blood glucose concentration, hydration and insulin therapy
Infectious diarrhoea	All sports normally contraindicated, unless symptoms are mild and the athlete is fully hydrated
Eating disorders	Medical and psychological evaluation necessary. Sports participation contraindicated when athlete is not compliant with therapy and follow-up, or where there is evidence of diminished performance or potential injury because of eating disorder
Eye conditions	
Functionally one-eyed athlete	Medical evaluation necessary. Protective eyewear may be appropriate, although in some sports (e.g. boxing, martial arts) it is not permitted
Loss of an eye	
Detached retina or family history of retinal detachment at a young age	
High myopia	
Connective tissue disorder, such as Marfan or Stickler's syndromes	
Previous intraocular eye surgery or serious eye injury	
Infectious conjunctivitis	Swimming contraindicated

Periodic medical assessment of athletes CHAPTER 46

Table 46.1 Cont.

Medical condition	Sport/activity participation recommendations
Fever	All exercise contraindicated
Gastrointestinal conditions	
Malabsorption syndromes (coeliac disease, cystic fibrosis)	Medical evaluation necessary
Short bowel syndrome or other disorders requiring specialised nutritional support including parenteral or enteral nutrition	Medical evaluation necessary
Hepatitis, infectious	Participation normally allowed in all sports where the athlete's state of health permits. Athletes should receive hepatitis B immunisation and universal precautions should be used when handling blood or body fluids with visible blood
Human immunodeficiency virus (HIV) infection	Participation normally allowed in all sports where the athlete's state of health permits. Universal precautions should be used when handling blood or body fluids with visible blood. Sports with a high risk of viral transmission (e.g. boxing and wrestling) should be avoided
Infectious mononucleosis—acute or with splenic enlargement	Moderate/intense exercise and participation in collision and contact sports contraindicated
Absence of one kidney	Medical evaluation necessary for collision, contact and limited-contact sports. Protective equipment may be available to protect the remaining kidney.
Acute liver enlargement	All exercise normally contraindicated
Chronic liver enlargement	Medical evaluation necessary, particularly for collision, contact and limited-contact sports
Malignant neoplasm	Medical evaluation necessary
Neurological disorders	
History of serious head or spine trauma or abnormality, including craniotomy, epidural bleeding, subdural haematoma, intracerebral haemorrhage, second-impact syndrome, vascular malformation and neck fracture	Medical evaluation necessary
History of simple concussion (mild traumatic brain injury), multiple simple concussions and/or complex concussion	Medical evaluation necessary. Research supports a conservative approach to concussion management, including no athletic participation while symptomatic or when deficits in judgment or cognition are detected, followed by a graduated, sequential return to full activity (see Chapter 20)
Myopathies	Medical evaluation necessary
Recurrent plexopathy (burner or stinger) and cervical cord neuropraxia with persistent defects	Medical evaluation necessary for collision, contact or limited-contact sports; regaining normal strength is an important benchmark for return to play
Seizure disorder with risk of seizure during participation	Athlete needs individual assessment for collision, contact or limited-contact sports. The following non-contact sports should be avoided: archery, shooting, swimming, weight or power lifting, strength training, or sports involving heights or high velocities (e.g. cycling, motor racing). In these sports, occurrence of a seizure during the activity may pose a risk to self or others
Organ transplant recipient (and those taking immunosuppressive medications)	Medical evaluation necessary, particularly for collision, contact and limited-contact sports

Continued

1005

PART C Practical sports medicine

Table 46.1 Cont.

Medical condition	Sport/activity participation recommendations
Pregnancy	Medical evaluation necessary. As pregnancy progresses, modifications to usual exercise routines will be necessary. Activities with a high risk of falling or abdominal trauma, scuba diving and activities posing a risk of altitude sickness should be avoided. Postpartum, physiologic and morphologic changes of pregnancy take 4–6 weeks to return to baseline
Respiratory conditions Pulmonary compromise, including cystic fibrosis	Medical assessment necessary, participation normally allowed. Athletes with cystic fibrosis have an increased risk of heat illness
Asthma	Medical assessment necessary prior to scuba diving
Acute upper-respiratory infection	Upper-respiratory obstruction may affect pulmonary function. Athlete needs individual assessment for all but mild disease. If fever is present, all exercise is contraindicated
Rheumatologic diseases Juvenile rheumatoid arthritis, juvenile dermatomyositis, idiopathic myositis or systemic lupus erythematosus	Medical assessment necessary
Raynaud's phenomenon	Care should be taken when exposing hands and feet to cold
Sickle cell disease	Medical assessment necessary. In general, if status of the illness permits, all sports may be played; however, any sport or activity that entails overexertion, overheating, dehydration and chilling should be avoided. Participation at high altitude, especially when not acclimatised, also poses risk of sickle cell crisis.
Skin infections—including herpes simplex, molluscum contagiosum, verrucae (warts), staphylococcal and streptococcal infection (furuncle/boils, carbuncle, impetigo, methicillin-resistant *Staphylococcus aureus*/cellulitis/abscess/necrotising fasciitis), scabies, tinea	During contagious period, participation in gymnastics with mats, martial arts, wrestling or other collision, contact or limited-contact sports is contraindicated
Enlarged spleen	If the spleen is acutely enlarged, participation should be avoided because of risk of rupture. If the spleen is chronically enlarged, individual assessment is needed before collision, contact or limited-contact sports are played

*All suspected cases should be evaluated by a cardiologist. The 36th Bethesda Conference,[5] the European Society of Cardiology consensus statements[6] and the recommendations from the American Heart Association and American College of Cardiology[40] provide detailed recommendations for sports participation for cardiovascular conditions

Assessment of known injuries and illnesses

Athletes often have persisting or recurrent injury problems and the PMA is a good opportunity to check that they are receiving optimal treatment. Recent studies of American college athletes and professional footballers in Qatar found that 11% and 17% of athletes had a current injury at the time of the PMA, respectively.[7, 8]

All medical personnel involved in the care of each existing injury should be listed. The current level of symptoms should be ascertained, as well as athlete's compliance to ongoing rehabilitation or prevention exercises. It is also important to check that exercises are being performed correctly.

It is equally important to address chronic or recurrent illnesses. This involves checking for optimum treatment (e.g. measurement of blood pressure for those with hypertension, asking about breakthrough symptoms in asthma or epilepsy, checking blood glucose control for diabetics), monitoring compliance with treatment (e.g. taking of medication, inhaler technique and attending follow-up appointments) and checking whether the athlete has any questions and/or adequately understands their condition.

Review of current medications and supplements

This involves checking prescribed medications as well as 'over-the-counter' medications or supplements that an athlete is currently taking, takes occasionally or is considering taking. Athletes sometimes neglect to inform their team medical staff about any changes and these should be checked to ensure compliance with the current World Anti-Doping Agency (WADA) regulations and be updated in their medical records.

While discussing medication, it may also be a good opportunity to remind athletes of their responsibilities under the WADA code (www.wada-ama.org). In particular, it should be emphasised that they are ultimately responsible for all substances they ingest and may be required to report their whereabouts to anti-doping authorities. They should also be reminded about the potential hazards associated with taking supplements, minerals and non-prescription medications without first checking with medical staff.

Education

In addition to providing education about anti-doping, medication use and supplements, other issues may be worth discussing with athletes depending on the local circumstances. Although cardiac screening is a hot topic at present, the leading cause of death in teenagers and young adults is accidents, in particular road traffic accidents, meaning that education on drink driving, wearing seatbelts and safe driving practices should be considered.[9] Other lifestyle practices that may have a negative effect on health and/or performance include abuse of alcohol, the use of recreational drugs or 'legal highs', smoking (tobacco or shisha) and unsafe sexual practices.

Careful consideration should be given to the best mode of delivery of these messages; for example, whether done on a one-to-one basis during the PMA or at a later date as a group lecture or interactive workshop. This will vary from situation to situation.

Other general health topics that may affect performance include basic nutrition advice and the importance of sleep and recovery, and should be discussed.

Baseline testing

The PMA can be used to perform baseline tests for a range of purposes if appropriate. Examples include:

- neuropsychological testing for athletes involved in contact sports to be used as a baseline following head injury (see Chapter 20)
- tests used in the monitoring of fatigue and recovery in athletes throughout a season, such as blood and/or saliva biochemical, hormonal or haematologic tests, aerobic or anaerobic fitness tests, psychological tests such as profile of mood states (POMS) or tools to assess sleep and recovery (see Chapter 13)
- physical measures to be used as post-injury reference values (these can be important when making return-to-play decisions; see Chapter 19), such as:
  - muscle strength (Fig. 46.1)
  - single-leg hop tests (see Chapter 35)

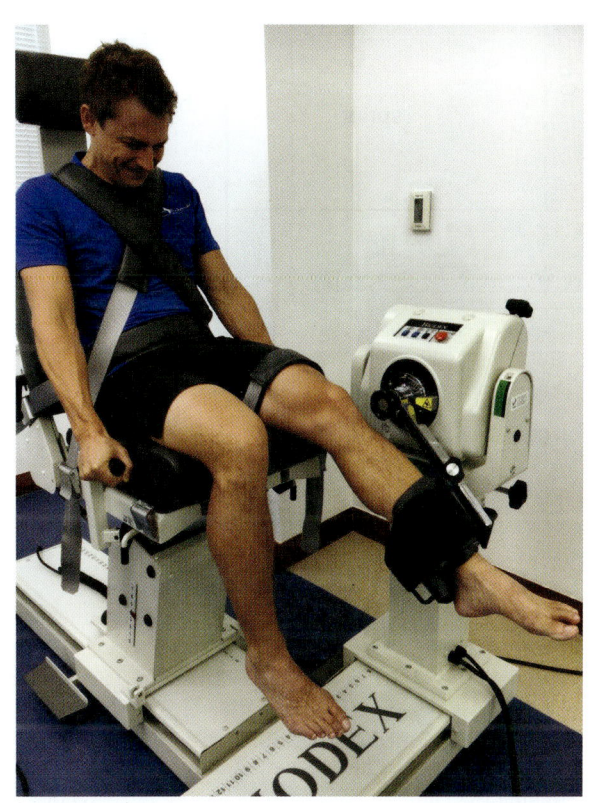

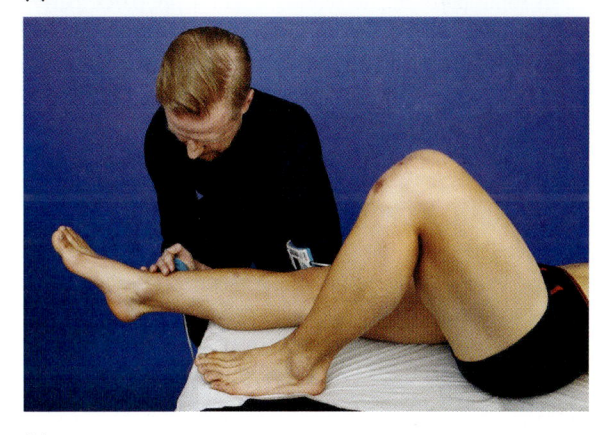

Figure 46.1 Strength testing (a) Quadriceps strength testing using an isokinetic dynamometer (b) Testing hip abductor strength with a hand-held dynamometer

PART C   Practical sports medicine

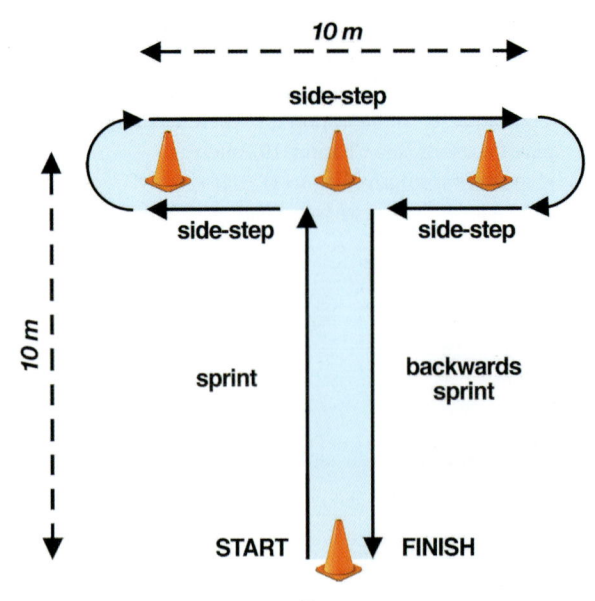

Figure 46.2 The agility T-test[10]

- vertical jump (counter movement jump)
- agility T-test (Fig. 46.2)[10]
- 30 m sprint time
- glenohumeral joint range of motion (Chapter 24).

Development of athlete rapport
The PMA is often the only time that team medical personnel have an opportunity to have a one-on-one consultation with athletes and to be proactive rather than reactive. It is an opportunity for athletes to ask questions or discuss any matters that they have been hitherto unwilling to discuss and helps in improving rapport and building the clinician-patient relationship.

In some parts of the world, where a pre-participation evaluation is required for recreational athletes, the PPE is the only contact that some athletes will have with the healthcare system and is an opportunity to establish a 'medical home' and discuss general health issues, especially if performed by a family physician.

Screening
Screening is traditionally defined as the identification of disease among apparently well persons. In 1968, Wilson and Jungner described 10 principles of early disease detection that are still relevant today when considering a screening program for athletes (see box).[11]

Although these principles are universal, two of them are worth considering more closely in the context of sport, as they may be interpreted differently in athletes than in the general population.

Ten principles of early disease detection

1. The condition should be an important health problem.
2. There should be an accepted treatment for patients with recognised disease.
3. Facilities for diagnosis and treatment should be available.
4. There should be a recognisable latent or early symptomatic stage.
5. There should be a suitable test or examination.
6. The test should be acceptable to the population.
7. The natural history of the conditions, including development from latent to declared disease, should be adequately understood.
8. There should be an agreed policy on whom to treat as patients.
9. The cost of case-finding (including diagnosis and treatment of patients diagnosed) should be economically balanced in relation to possible expenditure on medical care as a whole.
10. Case-finding should be a continuing process and not a 'once and for all' project.

Wilson and Jungner state that the ability to be able to treat the condition adequately when discovered is perhaps the most important. For those conditions where there is no treatment or intervention that will offer a better prognosis, alerting a person to such a condition may cause actual harm. In order to know whether a treatment offers benefit, the natural history of a condition needs to be known.[11]

First, the condition being screened for should be deemed 'important'. For athletes, particularly elite competitors, anything that negatively affects performance or leads to lost training time may be seen as very important, particularly during crucial periods of the season. In the general population, however, a 2% reduction in 5 km time or a 10% loss of strength may be insignificant.

Second, the screening program must be cost-effective. In professional sport, where athletes are often paid many thousands of dollars per week, even short periods of time loss or small performance reductions can be very costly. Prevention of minor injuries and illnesses among professional athletes may therefore be highly cost-effective.

Screening is therefore commonly considered to be a valuable process for athletes and is standard practice in many elite sports. However, the actual preventive value of mass screening programs for athletes has been questioned.[12–15] We will examine this in greater detail in the following section where we review the most common types of athlete screening: cardiac screening, screening for unknown injuries and illnesses, and screening for risk factors for future injury.

Cardiac screening

Several high-profile cases of sudden cardiac death in athletes over recent years, such as that of Norwegian swimmer Alexander Dale Oen, as well as the case of English professional footballer Fabrice Muamba, who survived a sudden cardiac arrest after prolonged resuscitation, have stimulated a healthy debate in both the medical community and the popular press about the pros and cons of cardiac screening.

Despite all this debate, there is no universal consensus on whether or how cardiac screening should be performed. The lack of agreement is because the context in which the PMA is being performed will affect the decision on whether or not to offer cardiac screening and thus this decision will likely remain an individual one for each organisation or country.

Some of the many factors that have to be considered when deciding whether or not to offer cardiac screening and/or how to screen are the population being studied (numbers, age group, gender, prevalence of conditions predisposing to sudden cardiac death), the screening tests being used (sensitivity and specificity) and the resources available (money, equipment and access to cardiologists with expertise in conditions that predispose to sudden cardiac death).

When considering mass screening funded by the public purse, the cost-benefit of screening for conditions predisposing to sudden cardiac death versus other demands for the health dollar also needs to be considered. Many countries simply do not have the resources to be able to offer a large-scale screening program particularly if it might place barriers to people partaking in exercise, which will actually reduce public health costs.

Cardiac screening usually consists of the following elements:

- targeted history for symptoms suggestive of cardiac disease, and for personal or family history of cardiac disease
- physical examination of the cardiovascular system
- special tests such as electrocardiograph (ECG), echocardiograph or stress test.

As mentioned, there is no international consensus on which special tests should routinely be used. Most of the debate, however, centres on the routine use of an ECG as part of cardiac screening. Those against the routine use of ECG in cardiac screening point out that there is a high false positive rate, there may be undue stress associated with further investigations of 'abnormal' results, expertise is required to interpret the ECG and the costs are high. Those in favour of the routine use of ECG argue that:

- ECG is more sensitive and specific than history and examination alone; a study of college athletes showed that 30% responded positive to at least one of the American Heart Association cardiac questions, which reflects the high rate of false positives[8]
- the use of standardised ECG criteria to interpret ECGs can improve the accuracy of ECG interpretation[16]
- athletes feel reassured by ECG screening, not unduly stressed.[17,18]

Echocardiograph and stress tests are usually only routinely used as part of cardiac screening by professional sporting teams with sufficiently large budgets and access to expertise, or when further investigation is indicated by an initial screening assessment.

> **PRACTICE PEARL**
>
> An important part of the topic that often gets overlooked when considering cardiac screening is being adequately prepared for a sudden cardiac arrest should one occur. Even a comprehensive cardiac screening program will not identify all persons with conditions predisposing to sudden cardiac death.

High school studies in the United States clearly show the benefit of having an automated external defibrillator (AED) on site (Fig. 46.3) and that sudden cardiac arrest (SCA) is survivable with an AED program. A study published in 2013 looking prospectively at 2149 US high schools, 87% of which had an AED program, reported that 89% of the athletes (including students and older athletes) survived to hospital discharge because of prompt CPR and early defibrillation.[19] Being prepared for SCA involves more than just having an AED on site.

Screening for unknown illnesses

In some situations, screening for the presence of unknown or subclinical medical conditions may be worthwhile. For example, these include any medical conditions that:

- have a negative effect on performance, such as iron deficiency anaemia or exercise-induced asthma
- predispose athletes to injury; for example, there is an association between vitamin D deficiency and stress fractures in military populations[20]
- might be hazardous to other athletes or medical staff, such as hepatitis B.

Screening for risk factors for future injury

A comprehensive musculoskeletal examination is among the most common elements of a PMA. Typically,

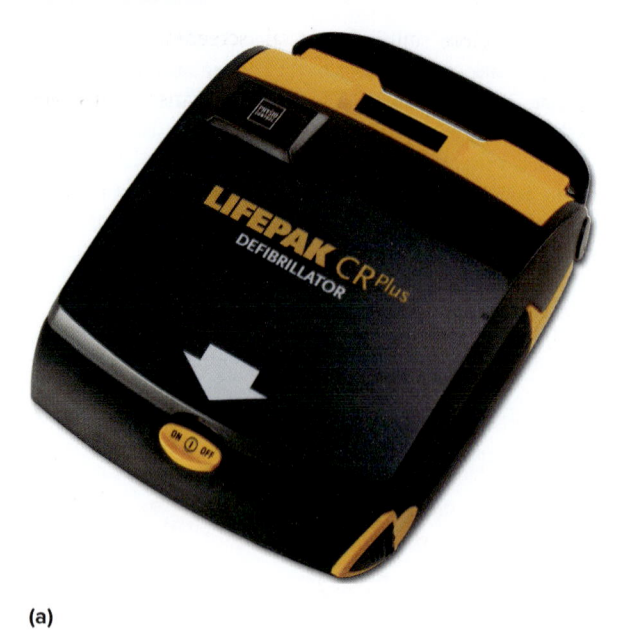

PART C Practical sports medicine

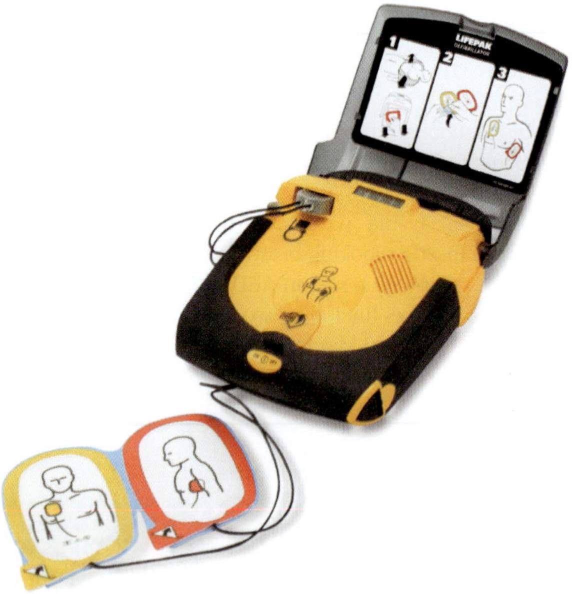

athletes' strength and flexibility are measured and compared to normative values or pre-determined cut-off values to determine whether the athlete is at risk of future injury. Specific orthopaedic tests may also be performed in order to identify unknown existing injuries. In recent years, however, there has been a trend away from static clinical measurements towards dynamic screening of the athletes' ability to perform a range of functional tasks. A number of similar systems are currently popular, all of which aim to identify 'weak links' in strength, flexibility or motor control, which can be targeted by individualised injury prevention programs. These include the Functional Movement Screen (FMS),[21–23] the United States Tennis Association High-Performance Profile[24] and the 9+ test battery developed by physiotherapists at the Swedish Sports Confederation (Fig. 46.4).[25]

Irrespective of whether traditional clinical measurements or a qualitative approach are used, the goals of musculoskeletal screening remain the same–to identify athletes at risk of specific injuries and guide the development of individualised injury prevention training programs. Although this is a theoretically appealing approach, there are several reasons why it may not deliver the desired results in practice.

First, for most injuries very few intrinsic modifiable risk factors have been identified and screening cut-off values are often based on expert opinion or assumed associations with injury risk. For example, athletes with poor hamstring flexibility are commonly advised to stretch in order to avoid hamstring strains. However, research into the link between hamstring flexibility and injury is inconclusive, and there is no cut-off value for hamstring flexibility that can identify players at risk for future injury.[26, 27] This is the case for the majority of physical measures currently used to screen athletes.

Second, even in cases where significant associations between risk factors and injury have been established, such as eccentric knee flexor weakness for hamstring strains[28] or glenohumeral joint stiffness for shoulder injuries in throwing athletes,[29–32] intrinsic risk factors are poor predictors of future injury. This is because they typically only explain a small part of an athlete's overall injury risk and because cut-off values are likely to have low sensitivity (many false negatives) and/or low specificity (many false positives), depending on which value is used.[15]

Clearly, more high-quality research into injury risk factors is required, in particular into the combination of test findings in order to maximise their predictive value. It is likely that dynamic predictive models are necessary before athletes at risk of future injury can be successfully identified.[33]

Figure 46.3 A functioning automated external defibrillator (AED) is essential equipment at venues that host sporting events. (a) AED closed, showing on/off switch (b) AED open, showing simple instructions on the flap and electrodes ready to be placed on the patient's chest

COURTESY OF PROFESSOR JONATHAN DREZNER, UNIVERSITY OF WASHINGTON CENTER FOR SPORTS CARDIOLOGY, WITH PERMISSION FROM PHYSIO-CONTROL, INC.

Periodic medical assessment of athletes **CHAPTER 46**

Nevertheless, musculoskeletal screening remains a popular and potentially valuable tool, particularly in helping sports medicine personnel familiarise themselves with each athlete's physical attributes and limitations. Care should be taken, however, in telling athletes that they are not at risk of injury or that they don't need to perform injury prevention training, because they passed a particular screening test.

WHO IS BEING ASSESSED?

There are numerous factors to consider about the population being assessed that can affect the content of the PMA.

Sport and position

The incidence and type of injuries or medical issues varies widely between sports. For example, in soccer the major injuries are knee injuries (ligament and meniscal tears), ankle ligament sprains, thigh muscle strains (hamstrings and quadriceps) and groin injuries; this is different to many other sports.[34] In some sports such as rugby, the incidence of injuries differs between positions. A study of professional rugby union players in the United Kingdom showed that anterior cruciate ligament (ACL) injuries caused the most time loss for forwards and hamstring injuries for backs.[35]

It is important to know about the injury and illness epidemiology for the particular athlete's sport and position as the PMA should specifically look for any risk factors associated with the important injuries or medical issues associated with each athlete's sport, and seek to address any of those that are modifiable. Some sporting bodies require athletes taking part in international competitions to undergo a medical assessment prior to competing, such as the FIFA football World Cup, the World Rugby (IRB) World Cup and the Olympics. A set template will usually be provided and should be followed.

Geographical location

In some countries, legislation dictates that some athletes require a medical assessment prior to playing sport. The Italian Government has required the screening and medical clearance of athletes since 1971 with an annual physical examination, personal and family history, and 12-lead ECG for all athletes aged 12–35 years participating in competitive sport.

Local patterns of disease, both infective and genetic, vary around the world and should be taken into account when designing a PMA. For example, in certain parts of the world there is a high prevalence of hepatitis B. The most recent guidelines from the US Preventive Task Force recommend mass population screening for hepatitis B in areas with a prevalence of over 2% in the

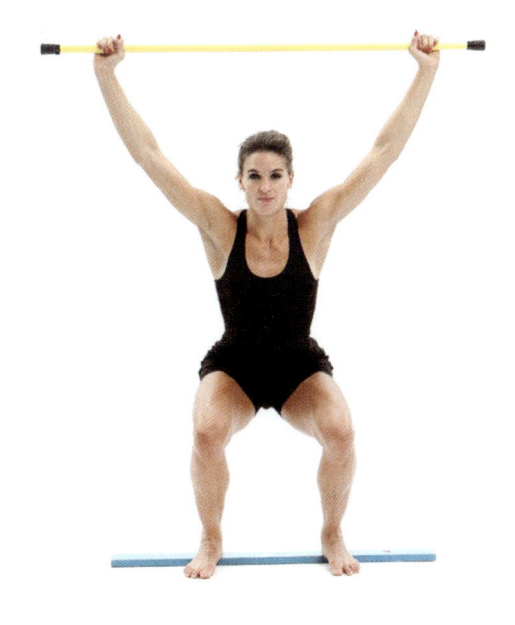

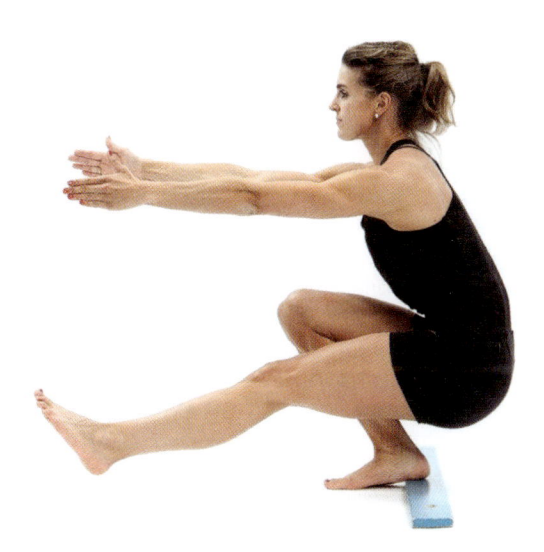

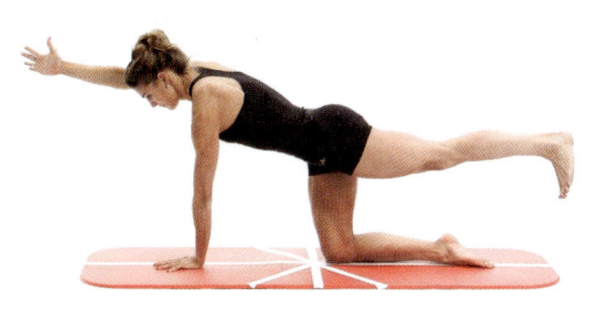

Figure 46.4 Examples of tests within the 9+ test battery. A full description of the tests and scoring criteria can be found in Frohm et al.[25]
COURTESY OF A FROHM, SWEDISH SPORTS CONFEDERATION

general population.[36] However, screening for hepatitis B immunity in order to be able to offer immunisation to those who are non-immune may be appropriate, even in countries with a lower prevalence rate for athletes involved in contact sports.

Extreme environmental conditions such as heat, cold and altitude can be experienced by some athletes as part of their sport when played in some geographical locations. Any previous history of complications associated with such conditions should be explored in the history when athletes are likely to encounter such environmental stresses.

Age

There is no consensus on what age to start performing PMAs. The American Academy of Paediatrics recommends annual routine health screening for all healthy children and adolescents from age 6, but there is no evidence to support starting PMAs in sporting groups at any particular age. As mentioned previously, in Italy an annual cardiac screening is mandatory for all competitive athletes from age 12. The European Society of Cardiology recommends pre-participation cardiac screening from ages 12 to 14, and Cardiac Risk in the Young (CRY) in the UK recommends screening from age 14.

Some sports have an increased risk of overuse injuries to certain growth plates (epiphysitis or apophysitis); for example, the proximal humeral epiphysis or medial humeral epicondyle epiphysis in pitchers and the distal radial epiphysis or calcaneal apophysis in gymnasts (Chapter 44). Symptoms of growth plate injuries associated with the particular sport being played should be enquired about during the PMA in young athletes who are between the ages at which these different conditions occur and a change in technique or training load may be required. Although the majority of these heal with adequate rest, there have been case reports of growth arrest of epiphyses when not treated properly.

If at all practicable, a parent or legal guardian should accompany a child to the PMA. Studies of high school students undergoing a PPE have shown that only 19-33% of athletes' responses were the same as those given by their parents or legal guardians when completing the same form.[37, 38] If a parent is unable to attend, then the previous medical history and family history sections of the questionnaire should be completed by them prior to the consultation.

Sex

Female athletes will generally have the same basic PMA template as males playing the same sport; however, the range of conditions associated with relative energy deficiency needs to be considered in female athletes, particularly in those who are involved with high-risk sports (those with weight categories to meet or where the aesthetic can be judged, such as gymnastics or ballet).[39] Several screening tools have been proposed to identify the athlete with relative energy deficiency. However, none have been validated and a high index of suspicion is required. It should be noted that, although much less common, relative energy deficiency may also occur in male athletes.

It is known that female athletes have a 2-3-fold higher incidence of ACL injury than their male counterparts and that male athletes have a higher incidence of hamstring injuries. Such differences in injury rates, when present, should be reflected in the medical assessment.

Available resources

At the end of the day, the available budget will usually dictate the content of the PMA, irrespective of the desired components. A major hurdle for organisations considering developing a publicly funded PMA cardiac screening program for large numbers of athletes is the availability of cardiologists with expertise in sports cardiology who will be needed to follow up those with cardiovascular symptoms, abnormal physical examination findings or abnormal ECGs.

In elite or professional sport, where money may be less of an issue and there are often full-time medical staff available to perform medical assessments, access to equipment (e.g. for isokinetic or VO_2max testing) or expertise (cardiologists with expertise in sports cardiology) may instead limit the content of the PMA.

WHEN TO PERFORM A PMA

The PMA is typically performed in the pre-season period. This is often the first time that the medical staff get to meet any new members of the squad who have joined in the off-season and is a good opportunity to develop a working relationship with new players.

It is a good idea for medical staff to engage coaching staff and management in the development and planning of the PMA so that they understand the goals (and limitations) and are encouraged to think about injury prevention. This makes them more likely to allow adequate time for medical staff to perform the medicals and be supportive of the delivery of any recommendations that might come out of the PMA, such as individual or team-wide injury prevention programs.

The value of engaging coaching staff has been clearly shown with the ACL injury prevention program in elite female handball players in Norway.[40] Despite an intervention study showing that a series of rehabilitation exercises done routinely as a part of team training significantly reduced the incidence of ACL injury, most teams stopped performing the exercises once the study was completed and the study personnel driving the injury prevention exercises were removed from the clubs; ACL rates consequently rose in subsequent seasons. A reduction of injury rate was seen after the introduction of education sessions for coaches and a sport-specific website on injury prevention.[40]

Ideally, a shorter modified PMA is also performed at the end of the season to review any injuries that might have occurred during the season (including ones that may not have been reported to medical staff), to possibly repeat some of the baseline musculoskeletal and/or laboratory measurements that were performed earlier in the season and to formulate a treatment or rehabilitation program over the off-season.

No research has conclusively shown that more frequent PMAs reduce the incidence of death or injury and recommendations on frequency vary. The most common recommendation is that a comprehensive assessment be performed every 2-3 years with a shorter, annual questionnaire and targeted examination in between. However, practice varies depending on the context and available resources.

WHAT TO INCLUDE IN THE TEMPLATE

The basic structure of the medical template will consist of history, examination and investigations. A detailed history is an important part of the assessment because the most consistent risk factor for injury across injury types is a previous history of injury. Defining the goals of the PMA (which, as referred to earlier, can vary depending on the stage of the season) and taking into account the unique factors associated with the population in question (including the available resources) will allow you to select the appropriate tools for the task.

The PPE monograph from the American Academy of Paediatrics is an excellent resource for anyone designing a PMA. It contains sections on the history and a systems-based examination, and has an example of a PMA form.[3]

The temptation when designing a PMA template is to include too much, particularly in the musculoskeletal examination. For example, taking reliable measurements of strength or joint range of movement is time consuming and may be a waste of time if no action is going to be taken for 'abnormal' results (what is 'abnormal' is often not even considered), if the data are not going to be used as a baseline post injury or if the data are not being used as part of a research project.

OTHER ISSUES TO CONSIDER

Consent

The PMA form should contain a consent section that the athlete should sign covering the following points, if appropriate:

- the athlete consents to undergo a medical assessment to assess their fitness to safely participate in sport
- the athlete understands that clearance may not be given if any significant medical issues or injuries are discovered
- the athlete certifies that their answers to all PMA questions are true to the best of their knowledge
- the athlete agrees to inform the medical professional if their medical situation changes significantly after the completion of the PMA
- the athlete consents to the use of data collected as part of the PMA for research purposes as long as the results do not in any way identify the athlete
- a parent or legal guardian should sign the consent form for athletes under the age of consent (18 in most countries).

Clearance or restriction from play

A very small percentage of athletes undergoing a PMA will be diagnosed with a medical condition that is associated with an increased risk of sudden cardiac death. In such cases, a cardiologist with the appropriate experience should review the athlete. The assessment of risk, however, is not a precise science and may differ between physicians. In order to make the decisions more consistent, guidelines have been produced for participation in sport with different cardiovascular conditions; however, the guidelines do differ in places and the decision on whether to allow the athlete to participate should be individualised once all the relevant information is available.[6, 41]

If clearance to participate is not given, the athlete may ask to sign a 'risk release' acknowledging that they have been fully informed of the risks and assume the risk of participating against medical advice; however, this may not be appropriate in all cases. It is important that documentation of any risk release is completed correctly and some experts recommend that the athlete and/or parents write in their own words their understanding of the risks of continued participation to prove that they have been fully informed of the risks. A decision to withhold clearance from participation may be subject to legal challenge. The success of a challenge will depend on the circumstances of the individual case and the local legislation, which varies widely from country to country.

Who should perform the PMA?

Although some parts of the PMA are often performed by other health professionals (e.g. nurses may take history and vital signs, physiotherapists may perform musculoskeletal assessments), the overall responsibility to review all the PMA components and make recommendations on clearance and follow-up should lie with a medical doctor who has the clinical training to deal with the wide variety of issues that might arise as part of the assessment.

Pre-employment medical assessment

Many professional athletes will be required to undergo a medical before their employment contract becomes valid. The principles for creating a template for the medical assessment are the same as for any PMA; however, there are some differences that are worth considering.

The biggest difference is the doctor-patient relationship. The person performing the medical assessment is often the athlete's team physician, with whom they have a normal doctor-patient relationship. When completing a new contract medical assessment, the doctor is acting on behalf of a third party (the club/employer). The fact that the athlete understands this difference and that that athlete agrees to the doctor providing a report on the athlete's ability to play sport to the employer using medical information from the assessment needs to be reflected in the consent form.

Even though the consent form requires athletes to promise to provide honest answers, there is a temptation for athletes to be economical with the truth (or even to lie) during a new contract medical, especially if the contract is worth large amounts of money. The physician performing the assessment should bear this in mind and if possible attempt to see the previous medical records. For some sports, injury information as well as matches and minutes played is freely available on the internet and is a valuable source of information and should be obtained if possible.

For high-value contracts, some clubs routinely ask for multiple magnetic resonance imaging (MRI) scans as part of the new contract medical (e.g. both knees, ankles, groin and lumbar spine in soccer players). The value of this approach is unknown as an MRI scan often picks up asymptomatic findings, such as a chondral defect in a knee that may have little or no practical prognostic value when taken in the context of a 1-year contract, but can be useful as a baseline when repeating imaging at a later date. Clubs can also use this information to negotiate a clause in the contract to protect themselves against prolonged future time loss from identified abnormalities.

In addition to the usual goals of a standard PMA, the role of the medical team performing a new contract medical is to provide the potential employer with an estimated level of risk that any identified medical and/or injury issues might preclude the athlete from being able to perform at their best for the duration of their contract. Some studies show a link between previous injury and future playing ability or length of career, such as the reduced performance of running backs in National Football League (NFL) after ACL reconstruction,[42] or the effects of previous injury history noted at the NFL Combine medical assessment on future career length.[43] The Combine study also showed, however, that athlete talent was a big factor that also had to be taken into account.

The prediction of future injury risk is complex and likely depends on a number of different factors in addition to injury history. This was highlighted by a recent pilot study at the Aspetar Orthopedic and Sports Medicine Hospital in Qatar (as yet unpublished), where a group of experienced sports physicians were asked to predict the risk of future injury for a series of case scenarios. The responses showed markedly different estimations of risk (from high to low) for almost all cases.

Once the risk has been conveyed to the potential employer, which is best done verbally so that any questions can be answered, it is up to the employer to decide whether they offer the athlete a contract. This can be quite a complex decision and involves many different factors such as depth of squad in the athlete's chosen position, the experience and talent of the athlete, the contract cost and duration, and the sport or position played.

Insurance medical assessment

Many athletes take out income protection insurance and will require a medical certificate to be completed by a doctor. In the majority of occasions, the insurance company will provide a form with the required template. If the athlete does not provide a form, they should be instructed to contact their insurance company to provide one as the requirements can vary between different companies.

It is important that the form is completed accurately as any incorrect answers can render the insurance void and may place the doctor at risk of legal action if there is any suggestion that there was any attempt to be economical with the truth. If the athlete is putting undue pressure on the team doctor to withhold certain information, the medical might be better performed by an independent doctor.

Action points from the PMA

Any action points identified as a result of the PMA should be discussed with the athlete and written on a discharge summary, which is then given to the athlete. This should also clearly indicate who is responsible for initiating the various action points and when follow-up is required (if possible, a follow-up appointment should be given at the same time). If appropriate, the discharge summary could also be sent to any relevant stakeholders, such as team medical staff or the athlete's personal physician. However, it is important to get the athlete's consent prior to sharing any health information.

For some athletes who spend a lot of time travelling and/or are members of several teams, there can be some challenges around distribution of the results of the PMA to the various medical teams looking after them to avoid any unnecessary duplication of tests or to refer to when required. There is no one solution that will suit all athletes and this should be dealt with on a case-by-case basis.

SUMMARY

The PMA can have many uses that have been outlined in this chapter. There is no one PMA that suits all situations. Care should be taken when designing a PMA to ensure that it meets the required goals for your particular situation and also avoids performing unnecessary (and possibly time consuming and expensive) examinations or tests. Communication of the results to the athlete and an action plan to address any identified issues are important to maximise the benefits of the assessment.

REFERENCES

References for this chapter can be found at www.mhhe.com/au/CSM5e

Chapter 47

Working and travelling with teams

with LIAM WEST

Talent wins games, but teamwork and intelligence win championships.
Michael Jordan

Within sports medicine, involvement in team care is a very rewarding yet challenging experience. Working alongside other clinicians and disciplines enables individuals to build upon their own skills and translate this into their everyday practice. Working with athletes on a regular basis helps the clinician to understand the psychological pressures placed upon them and appreciate the physical demands of the particular sport.

Clinicians working in a team environment must adapt and fit into the 'team chemistry'. This involves adhering to team rules and customs while appreciating that the clinician is a small cog in a very large wheel, where the players and the coach are the key people.[1] To be accepted by the coaches, athletes and other members of the medical team, the clinician needs to be in regular attendance during training sessions and competition. This in return offers the relatively unique opportunity to closely observe and understand mechanisms of injury before monitoring the progress of these injuries during rehabilitation.

Travelling with a team presents the sports medicine clinician with a considerable challenge.[2] In order to provide quality medical support on the road, clinicians must be flexible, innovative and fulfil a number of roles, as not all members of the medical team will be able to travel and less equipment will be available. Travelling with a team often involves working long hours in less than ideal conditions with sportspeople and coaches who are under great stress due to the demands of competition and travel.[3] Nonetheless, travelling with a team is fun, a great opportunity to learn, and offers the chance to broaden your horizons by seeing the world.

THE MEDICAL SUPPORT TEAM

The size and make-up of the medical support team often depends on the size of the sporting team, the competition standard and financial considerations. Frequently, the support team will consist of just one individual, who may be a physiotherapist, physician, massage therapist or trainer. Specialists from various branches of medicine can contribute to the sports and exercise medicine (SEM) team.[4-6] It is imperative that a solo clinician develops a network of colleagues who can assist where additional specialised management is indicated. Not all members of the medical support team will be remunerated and the ethical issues facing professional teams' clinicians are slightly different from those of volunteer clinicians'.[7-10]

KEY ATTRIBUTES OF A SUCCESSFUL MEDICAL TEAM

In order to add value to athletes, the medical team often consists of representatives from different health disciplines. In an ideal scenario, the professional sporting team should have access to the services of an SEM physician, physiotherapist, massage therapist, podiatrist, dietitian, psychologist, orthopaedic surgeon, cardiologist and sports trainer as well as the coaching, sports science and fitness staff. Whoever is responsible for assembling such a support team must ensure that all individuals have high professional standards and work well collectively.[11] This leader does not necessarily need to be the team physician; often the physiotherapist or sports scientist is better placed to lead the medical team as they work full time with the sporting team. The appointed medical team lead should take ultimate responsibility for difficult management decisions and the smooth running of the group.

The best medical teams have clearly defined roles and duties that help to avoid conflict. The clinician has a primary responsibility to the athlete, but must determine and define his or her responsibilities to the coach, the team management and the fellow support staff before taking up the position. Medical teams should actively encourage the 'cross pollination' of ideas from different medical disciplines. Effective communication with each other, the athletes and the coaching staff is the cornerstone of success for a medical team.

MEDICAL INDEMNITY AND TRAUMA TRAINING

We live in a world of litigation, and the sports medicine arena is not exempt. It is imperative that sports clinicians arrange medical indemnity to cover their entire scope of practice. Without this cover, the financial and reputational risks can be devastating. It is the responsibility of the team clinician to ensure that his or her medical indemnity is not only current, but also indemnifies them in any state, county or country to which team competition may take them. In addition to indemnity, it is important that medical team members (not just the physician) undertake an appropriate advanced resuscitation and emergency aid course for their sport so that they can competently care for a seriously injured or ill athlete. Without adequate training, indemnity may be null and void.

WHERE DOES THE MEDICAL TEAM WORK?

The medical team is required to operate in various settings including at the training ground, at competition venues, and during travel. At each location the team must ensure that it has adequate equipment for each member to perform his or her role–see below for information on the pitchside medical bag. The club medical room should ideally be a clean room that has a door that can be locked to enable privacy and confidentiality. It should have at least one examination couch, facilities to enable the clinician to clean his or her hands at a sink or with alcohol hand gel, and all the medical equipment required for the particular sport.

The team clinician must ensure that medications and other medical equipment, such as oxygen, are stored safely and securely. If the clinician is expected to perform procedures such as suturing, he or she should aim to have an area to do so under sterile conditions while being able to safely dispose of sharps and blood-contaminated products. Clinicians should consider decorating the medical room with anatomy posters to help explain injuries, and evidence-based infographics to educate athletes about various topics within sports medicine such as the importance of sleep or adequate hydration.

MEDICAL EQUIPMENT

The contents of the medical bag will vary depending on the type of sport, access to other facilities, and the clinician's own preferences. It is often impossible to carry all required items in one bag and therefore equipment should be organised into storage within the medical room, a pitchside suitcase, a medical bag and a hip bag that contains the essentials to provide athletes with symptom relief or immediate care until a more comprehensive kit can be accessed.[12] An exhaustive list of contents of medical equipment for a contact sports team without immediate access to more sophisticated facilities can be found in the box below. When travelling with a team, the contents of the medical kit will vary depending on the make-up of the medical support team, the size of the overall team and the local facilities available.

TEAM CARE THROUGHOUT THE SEASON

The team clinician must tailor athlete care according to the stage of competition – pre-competition, during competition and post-competition. In the pre-competition phase there should be a full assessment of all team members based around a comprehensive history and examination (Chapter 46). This screening should evaluate for medical illness and musculoskeletal conditions that may need further follow-up. This screening will often be carried out in conjunction with a fitness assessment. A similar assessment should be performed on new team recruits and also on the entire team at the end of a season to plan appropriate individual off-season treatment and rehabilitation programs. Arrangements for how this will be monitored by the sports clinician should also be made. During the season, post-game/competition injury clinics help to diagnose and plan treatment of acute injuries and illnesses. Where possible, these clinics should be attended by both a team physician and physiotherapy staff.

Core principles providing care for a team

The medical team should look to develop various core 'team principles' that underpin good sports medicine care. An athlete's right to confidentiality must be strictly adhered to by ensuring that their medical problems are not discussed with other team members, officials or the media without the player's permission.[13] Good record keeping is important for patient care and medico-legal purposes. There are many excellent software programs that allow practitioners to maintain records on a laptop computer, which is particularly useful when travelling with a team. The sports clinician should consider keeping two sets of password-encrypted notes: one for musculoskeletal injuries that can be seen by other members of the treating medical team, and the other for medical and mental health issues to which only

Working and travelling with teams — CHAPTER 47

Contents of the medical bag

Diagnostic instruments
Oral/rectal thermometer
Stethoscope
Blood pressure cuff
Ophthalmoscope
Otoscope (auroscope) & ear pieces
Pencil torch
Tongue depressors
Oxygen saturation (SATS) probe
Tendon hammer
Portable ultrasonography device
Snellen eye chart & Ishihara plates
SCAT3™ forms

Medications
Oral analgesics (e.g. paracetamol [acetaminophen], aspirin, codeine, tramadol)
Intravenous analgesics (morphine, tramadol)
Adrenaline (epinephrine) for anaphylaxis (& hydrocortisone)
NSAIDs (nonsteroidal anti-inflammatory drugs)
Antibiotics (e.g. amoxycillin, erythromycin, flucloxacillin, doxycycline, metronidazole)
Antacid tablets
Anti-nausea tablets (e.g. prochlorperazine [oral/IM], metoclopramide)
Antidiarrhoeal agent (e.g. loperamide)
Faecal softeners
Antihistamines
Bronchodilators (e.g. salbutamol inhaler, beclomethasone inhaler)
50% glucose solution
Sedatives and hypnotics
Nasal spray decongestants
Eye and ear antibiotic solutions
Ear wax softener
Throat lozenges
Cough mixture
Creams/ointments: antifungal, antibiotic, corticosteroid, anti-inflammatory
Tetanus toxoid
GTN sublingual spray
Corticosteroid injections

Sutures/dressings
Needle holders
Forceps
Scissors: nail clippers, small sharp scissors, tape scissors
Syringes (various sizes)
Needles (various sizes)
Sutures (various sizes), absorbable & non-absorbable
Suture cutters
Scalpels
Local anaesthetics: lignocaine (lidocaine) with and without adrenaline (epinephrine)
"Steri-strips"™ (various sizes)
Alcohol swabs
Gauze swabs
Dressings packs
Antiseptic solution
Tincture of benzoin
Dressing pads (various sizes)
Low-adherent dressing (e.g. Jelonet™)
Band-Aid® plastic strips
Crepe bandages
Tube gauze (Tubigrip™)
Sterile gloves, goggles & mask

Resuscitation and emergency equipment
Defibrillator
Resuscitation medications (e.g. adrenaline, amiodarone)
Oropharyngeal & nasopharyngeal airways (various sizes)
Bag valve mask (BVM)
Oxygen with suitable delivery masks
Emergency cricothyroid set
Portable suction device
Cannulation equipment
Intravenous (IV) sodium chloride
Intravenous (IV) giving set
Rectal diazepam (for seizures)
EpiPen®

Blood management
Gauze swabs
Klatostat® for lacerations
Klatostat strings & Rapid Rhino™ for epistaxis
Blood tape (Coban™)
Co-phenylamine/tranexamic acid nasal spray
Betadine® spray
Vaseline®

Other equipment
Bolt cutters/screwdriver
Air/box splints
Triangular bandages (sling)
Cotton-tipped applicators
Rigid sports tape (various sizes)
Elastic adhesive tape (various sizes)
Compression bandage (various sizes)
Adhesive foam pad
SAM splint
Blister pads
Coolant spray
Crutches
Deep Heat® muscle warming spray
Finger splints
Adjustable cervical collar (soft & hard)
Spinal board with straps
Eye kit: irrigation solution, fluorescein, eye patches, local anaesthetic/dilating eye drops, contact lens container
Sunscreen
Bonjela mouth ulcer cream
Massage oil/heat rubs
Electrotherapy (e.g. TENS, portable laser)
Portable couch
Alarm clock
Plaster of Paris/thermoplastic casting equipment

Miscellaneous equipment
Pen and paper
Urine reagent strips and urine sample pots
Safety pins
Tampons
Condoms
Contaminated needle container
Acupuncture needles
Foam rollers & rehabilitation equipment
Spare shoelaces
Spare mouth guard
Flexible orthoses
Batteries
Safety razor
Plastic bags & cling film for ice
Transformer & dual voltage connector (if appropriate)
Glucose sweets (for hypoglycaemia)
Alcohol hand gel
Heel-raise foam pads
List of WADA banned substances

the clinician has access. A simple overview of player availability using a traffic-light coloured coding system (green = available, orange = available with conditions, red = unavailable) can help communication with coaching staff while maintaining confidentiality.

Working with a team provides an ideal opportunity to educate sportspeople and coaches. The medical team should look to create 'teaching moments' throughout the season during opportunities such as the pre-season health assessment, treatment sessions or team presentations. Experienced team clinicians have found that relevant topics of education include the following.

- Sexual activity: Team members should be warned of the dangers of acquiring sexually transmitted infections such as chlamydia, gonorrhoea, hepatitis B and HIV. Abstinence guarantees prevention, but condoms should be made available.
- Hygiene: Players should be encouraged to wash their hands regularly with alcohol hand gel and to avoid contact with any ill team members or loved ones. Travelling to foreign countries or participating in large sporting events places both athletes and support staff at risk of endemic disease and outbreaks of infectious diseases.[14]
- Vaccinations: Team members should be educated about the need for vaccinations depending on the countries they will compete in. Immunisations for the athlete are listed in Table 47.1. Team clinicians should use websites to gain up-to-date information on vaccination and illness prevention, especially in destinations where disease pattern is rapidly evolving.[15]
- Anti-doping: Team members must ensure they have a sound appreciation of those medications that are currently banned by the World Anti-Doping Agency (WADA). Up-to-date information can be obtained from national sporting organisations and Olympic federations—some useful contacts are listed in Table 47.2. Medical team members need to educate players so they understand that many over-the-counter medications used in the treatment of coughs and colds are banned, and they should not take any medications or supplements without consulting their medical team.[16]

EMERGENCY ACTION PLANS

Emergency action plans (EAPs) are extremely useful documents that can help the sports clinician prepare for difficult scenarios that can arise within sports medicine. EAPs containing, but not limited to, the below information should be created for home training and competition venues in addition to all the locations you may travel to with your team:

- Contact details of the entire medical and coaching staff
- Address and contact details of all sporting and accommodation venues
- Distances from these locations to various specialist medical services and their contact details:
    - emergency department
    - trauma unit
    - orthopaedic surgery
    - plastic surgery
    - cardiac services
    - neurosurgery
    - burns unit
- National consulates and embassies are useful for foreign travel to source information on the quality of local medical personnel and facilities
- For each venue, entry points for emergency services (i.e. ambulances) should be determined so that clear instructions can be given to locate the team

Table 47.1 Immunisations suitable for the athlete according to the World Health Organization in May 2016

Routine vaccination	Selective use for travellers	Mandatory vaccination in particular countries
• Diphtheria, tetanus, pertussis	• Cholera	• Yellow fever (depending on the country)
• Hepatitis B	• Hepatitis A	• Meningococcal disease and polio (required by Saudi Arabia for pilgrims; updates are available on www.who.int/wer)
• Haemophilus influenzae type b	• Japanese encephalitis	
• Influenza (seasonal)	• Meningococcal disease	
• Measles, mumps, rubella	• Rabies	
• Pneumococcal disease	• Tick-borne encephalitis	
• Human papillomavirus (females)	• Typhoid	
• BCG	• Dengue (CYD–TDV)	

Working and travelling with teams
CHAPTER 47

Table 47.2 Contact details for obtaining drug information in various countries

Country	Drug information website address
World Anti-Doping Agency (WADA)	www.wada-ama.org www.wada-ama.org/en/Anti-Doping-Community/NADOs/List-of-NADOs/ lists all of the antidoping organisations in alphabetical order by country
Australia	Australian Sports Anti-Doping Authority, www.asada.gov.au
Brazil	Brazilian Agency for Doping Control, www.cob.org.br
Canada	Canadian Centre for Ethics in Sport, www.cces.ca
France	Agence française de lutte contre le dopage, www.afld.fr
India	National Anti-Doping Agency, India, www.nada.nic.in
Japan	Japan Anti-Doping Agency, www.anti-doping.or.jp
New Zealand	Drug Free Sport NZ, www.drugfreesport.org.nz
South Africa	SA Institute for Drug-Free Sport, www.drugfreesport.org.za
Spain	Agencia Estatal Antidopaje, www.aea.gob.es
United Kingdom	UK Sport, www.uksport.gov.uk
United States	US Anti-Doping Agency (USADA), www.usada.org

- All medical team staff should have completed an emergency life support training course that involves education regarding cervical spine immobilisation and transferring the athlete from the pitchside to hospital safely. The team should then make, and frequently practise, plans for caring for a medically unstable athlete in various situations
- A pitchside extrication plan should be created and practised regularly throughout the year. This plan should be exhaustive and address questions such as:
  - Who will perform what duties during pitchside extrication (such as cervical spine immobilisation, positions within a log roll, and positioning the spinal board)?
  - What will the instructions be during a log roll?
  - Does the defibrillator have scissors attached to it to facilitate quick removal of a jersey so pads can be applied to the chest?
  - Where are the defibrillator and other emergency equipment located is this equipment locked and if so who has the key?
  - Who will call for an ambulance?
  - How do you carry the athlete off the pitch?
  - Where will the athlete be taken to once on the spinal board?
  - Is this designated place warm or do blankets need to be stored there?
- Consider which member of the medical team will stay with an athlete during drug testing procedures or in the event that he or she is unable to travel back from a destination due to injury or illness.

PREPARING TO TRAVEL

When travelling to any venue away from home, the usual medical support structure is lost and the nature of existing medical support services in different countries varies substantially.[17] In order to become self-sufficient, a detailed plan must be constructed before travelling with sports teams.[18] Team clinicians may find it useful to split preparation into the following four stages;

1. Before travel

- *Travel destination.* The team clinician needs to have a good understanding of the climate, altitude, level of pollution, water supplies, security, recent health epidemics and natural disasters at the destination.[19-21]
- *Accommodation.* In hot climates, air conditioning may be advantageous for comfort although it may delay heat acclimatisation. It may also cause respiratory issues if used excessively as it can dry out the upper respiratory tract mucosa. Particularly tall athletes will require extra-long beds. Try to have a dedicated medical room when travelling with a large team to allow for privacy and confidentiality.
- *Vaccinations.* As discussed earlier (Table 47.1), vaccinations and malaria prophylaxis must be considered before embarking upon travel.[15]
- *Equipment and travel logistics.* It is important that the weight allowance for travel is considered when packing medical equipment so that everything can be transported to the destination. The local destination

medical services should be researched to decide whether medical equipment and medications can be sourced locally or need to be transported. It is important to note that medications may have different compositions in different countries. An advance visit to the competition location is extremely advantageous, if feasible, for the team physician to inspect local medical facilities, hotel kitchens and the like.[22] Formulas exist within the literature to assist in estimating the pharmacological needs for a trip,[23] and it is important that all the medications be accompanied by a prescription or doctor's letter as well as being kept in the original containers.[24]

- *EAPs*. As discussed above, creating EAPs to prepare for travelling with a team is invaluable.
- *Fitness to travel assessments*. Contact all team members, including coaches and officials, to ask about present and past injuries or illnesses. Often officials are older than the athletes and can cause anxiety for a travelling clinician because of medical conditions such as coronary artery disease. These individuals must be reminded to bring their own medications. Attempts must be made to treat injuries or illnesses prior to departure.
- *Nutrition*. It is challenging for athletes to maintain good dietary habits when travelling and they should be counselled on wise food choices before travel.[25] At large competitions, athletes often eat in village communal restaurants where buffet-style dining practices may lead to overeating. In addition to food intake, adequate hydration–especially when travelling to warm climates–is important.[21] To minimise the risk of traveller's diarrhoea, athletes should eat only food that has been cooked, and avoid shellfish, salads, unpasteurised milk products and unpeeled fruit.
- *Jet lag*. This is discussed in the following section.
- *Insurance and indemnity*. As described earlier, your policies must cover you to practice at your destination. If any minors are in attendance, it is important to travel with the appropriate permission documents to treat them, as well as their guardian's contact information.[26]
- *SAMPLE forms*. It is useful to create a history and treatment sheet for each athlete prior to travel in case she or he should need to be transfer to hospital during the trip. This sheet can be pre-filled with certain details such as their past medical history, regular medications, allergies, personal details and next of kin details. The SAMPLE format is a useful format for this sheet: **S**igns and symptoms, **A**llergies, regular **M**edications, **P**ast medical history, **L**ast meal/drink and **E**vents (including examination and treatment/intervention).

- *Injury prevention*. It is important to ensure that despite travelling, the team conduct proper warm-ups, stretching/yoga and strength maintenance, and receive regular soft tissue therapy.

2. During travel

Sports physicians should create a medical travel bag that contains medications to deal with travel sickness and simple analgesic medications. They must ensure that the athletes have sufficient water and food for the duration of their trip, especially if they are to compete soon after reaching their destination. If travelling long distances via road or aeroplane, the use of thromboembolism-deterrent (TED) stockings, electronic calf stimulators, earplugs, eye masks and facemask air humidifiers can help athletes to sleep in comfort and reduce the risk of venous thrombosis.

3. On arrival

A medical room should be established soon after arrival. Ideally, this should be a large room separate from any bedrooms. Treatment hours should be specified using an appointment sheet so that the practitioner has adequate time for meal and exercise breaks. This must be strictly enforced as athletes have a tendency to extend these hours. The clinician should ensure that athletes know the room number of the medical staff in case of emergencies. It is important that the team manager know how to contact the medical staff if the room is unattended. It also helps to obtain an athlete room list from the team manager.

For trips involving a single venue, a portable examination couch (treatment table) is invaluable for the comfort of both the athlete and the treating clinician. A low, soft bed may not be an appropriate site for massage or spinal mobilisation. On trips involving multiple venues, the advantage of having a treatment couch must be weighed up against the inconvenience of transporting it.

Traveller's diarrhoea is very common when travelling for sports,[27] and while the infection is usually self-limiting, team physicians should institute oral fluid replacement as the mainstay of treatment

4. Journey home

Preparation for the return journey is important as some injuries or illnesses incurred while away may need specialist arrangements for travel or referral for specialist follow up.[28] Thought must be given to the thromboembolic risk of various injuries, such as fractures, and whether anticoagulation should be used prior to return travel. Once back in the home country, the medical staff should have a debriefing session to review any issues during the trip to enable changes to be implemented for future medical care.[18]

JET LAG

Jet lag presents a major challenge for clinicians travelling long distances with teams.

Air travel and jet lag

Air travel is an important part of professional and international sports. Short-distance air travel (up to 3 hours) does not appear to present any problems for the athlete.[29] However, extended air travel, often required for major events such as Olympic Games or World Championships, can provide significant problems.[30] Thus travelling athletes, team officials and team physicians will benefit from education on how to decrease the harmful effects of long-distance travel, such as jet lag, on performance (Table 47.3).

Jet lag is when the body is unable to adapt rapidly to a time zone shift and normal body rhythms lose synchrony with the environment. In general, it is a benign and self-limited condition. The major complaints of the condition are poor sleep, daytime fatigue and poor performance.[31] The sleep deprivation secondary to the flight can be mostly made up in a day, whereas jet lag lasts much longer.[32] A number of factors influence the severity of jet lag symptoms.[33-34] These include: individual differences, number and direction of time zones crossed, temporal and seasonal timing of flight, age, impaired health, lack of previous travel experience, sleep deprivation, dehydration, stress, alcohol and excessive food intake.[35]

Pathophysiology

The suprachiasmatic nuclei (SNC), located in the hypothalamus, produce a timing signal that modulates circadian rhythms of sleep and alertness, core body temperature and certain hormonal secretions such as melatonin and cortisol. The SNC, via the eyes, senses darkness and sends a timing signal to the pineal gland. This maintains the nocturnal secretion of melatonin for 10-12 hours. Beta blockers can inhibit melatonin secretion. Although the SNC signal is important, melatonin secretion requires darkness. Light intensity of >50 lux can cause some melatonin inhibition and light of >2000 lux completely suppresses it. Therefore, summer's long days and short nights will suppress melatonin secretion despite the 12-hour SNC 'on' signal.

The 12-hour SNC 'on' signal, despite melatonin inhibition by light, is considered an operational definition for biological night. Therefore, the nocturnal SNC signal synchronised to home night time (biological night) may result in melatonin secretion if the unadapted, jet-lagged traveller is placed in a dimly lit room. Melatonin can be measured in saliva, plasma and urine.[31]

The circadian rhythm is regularly synchronised to the 24-hour day by environmental time cues, termed 'zeitgebers', such as alternation of light and darkness, ingestion of melatonin, sleep/awake schedules, physical activity and meal timing.[31, 35]

Travelling across multiple time zones (>3 time zones) causes a temporary misalignment between the circadian clock (lag) and the sleep/wake schedule at the destination time zone, that is slow to reset. The symptoms of jet lag dissipate as the circadian clock gradually resets (adjusts) to the time cues at the new destination time zone.[31, 32, 35, 36] Although there is considerable individual variability, it is estimated that it takes about 1 day per time zone for the biological clock to resynchronise with the sleep/wake schedule.[25, 31]

Prevention of jet lag

The faster the biological clock adapts to the new time zone, the shorter the symptomatic period. Thus, speeding up the adaptation is the primary goal.[35] When travelling in more than three time zones for a stay longer than five days, circadian adaptation is desirable (Table 47.3).[35, 37] Pre-flight adjustment to travel may speed up adaption and is discussed below.[38] Experienced practitioners and many successful athletes also suggest that low-intensity physical activity early after arrival helps promote adjustment to the new time zone. Seasoned air travellers have developed a series of guidelines to minimise the adverse effects of long-distance travel (Tables 47.3 and 47.4).

Timed light exposure and avoidance

Light intensity and timing are the two most important factors that influence phase shift. Exposure to bright light (sunlight at approximately 3000-100 000 lux, light box at 1500-3500 lux or room light at 100-550 lux) can help phase shifting. The magnitude of shift is greater as we get closer to the Tmin (the body's minimum core temperature, which is estimated to occur at 3-5 am in most individuals). Light has more shifting effect at night when bright light is absent.

> **PRACTICE PEARL**
>
> Light exposure late in the sleep episode or in the early morning (i.e. after the Tmin phase advances) will promote phase shifting. The same light stimulus, when applied early in the sleep episode (i.e. before the Tmin) will delay phase shifting.[31, 32, 35, 39]

Table 47.3 General guidelines for adaptation strategies based on the length of stay at destination and numbers of zones crossed[35]

Length of stay at destination	Recommended strategy
Long (>5 days)	• Pre-travel adaptation of sleep schedule to that of the destination • Timed light exposure and avoidance • Timed melatonin intake
Intermediate (3–4 days) OR Short (1–2 days) OR Game aligned with circadian time of peak performance	• Work around sleep and alertness times • Schedule critical activity to daytime in the departure zone • Airplane light exposure/avoidance strategy • Short-term measure to maintain alertness (caffeine) and sleep (naps and short-acting hypnotics)

Table 47.4 General principles to help clinicians customise jet travel schedules for athletes travelling in any direction across multiple time zones

Goal: Get Tmin within sleeping episodes and avoid being awake at the sleepiest time (Tmin)

Eastward jet lag	Westward jet lag
Differences	
• Requires advancing the circadian clock • Harder and slower to adjust (1 h/day) • Abrupt 12-h time zone shift, takes 8–9 days to adjust • Destination Tmin=origin Tmin+number of time zones crossed	• Requires delaying the circadian clock • Easier and quicker to adjust (1.5–2 h/day) • Abrupt 12 h time zone shift, takes 4–5 days to adjust • Destination Tmin = origin Tmin − number of time zones crossed
Similarities	
• Maximum or largest shift is 12 h time zones • Traveller feels sleepy in hours surrounding Tmin and difficulty sleeping at hours far from the Tmin • Traveller will experience impaired daytime activity near Tmin • Phase shifting needs to be applied daily for several days to produce results	

Tmin origin = minimum core temperature, estimated to occur at 3–5 am (hours before wake-up time) for most individuals, 2–4 am for larks (morning type, M-type), and 5–7 am for owls (evening type, E-type) based on the sleep pattern for the last week. Tmin coincides roughly with the maximum nocturnal melatonin level in the circulation

Timed light avoidance is equally important. Light avoidance can be achieved by staying in a dim light room (<10 lux) or wearing dark sunglasses.[39] Light exposure should be augmented with light avoidance during flight or on arrival to a new destination as it ensures a unidirectional phase shifting. For instance, an eastward-travelling athlete needs to maximise light exposure after Tmin and avoid or minimise light before Tmin to ensure phase advancement of the circadian clock, and vice versa for the westward travelling athlete.[38] On the other hand, exposure to light before and after Tmin would result in no phase shifting.

Timed melatonin pills
Despite being marketed as an over-the-counter sleep aid, melatonin is not associated with sleep or increased sleepiness. Instead, melatonin is considered a darkness signal. The timing of melatonin pills is more important than dose. It has more of a phase-shifting effect when there is less endogenous melatonin in the circulation. Therefore, a timed melatonin pill (3 mg) can help produce the greatest phase advance of the circadian clock when taken in the afternoon (approximately 5 hours before dim light melatonin onset [DLMO] or 12 hours before Tmin) while phase delays occur when taken in the morning.[32, 35]

Pre-travel sleeping schedule

Adjusting sleep schedule in 1–2 days (depending on the number of time zones to be crossed) prior to travel to gradually match the destination schedule may help with phase shifting. Sleep on flights should be avoided unless it is night at destination.[40]

Synergistic approach

When combined with a pre-travel sleep schedule for the destination, timed light exposure/avoidance and melatonin pills can have a synergistic phase-shifting effect.

Symptomatic treatment for jet lag

If the travelling athlete still suffers jet lag symptoms despite the gradual shifting, stimulants such as slow-release oral caffeine (300 mg) could be helpful to induce daytime alertness, and hypnotics such as oral zolpidem (10 mg) could be used to counteract night insomnia.

REFERENCES

References for this chapter can be found at www.mhhe.com/au/CSM5e

Chapter 48

Career development

by MICHAEL DAVISON

If you don't build your dream, someone else will hire you to help them build theirs!
Dhirubhai Ambani

The first thing to realise is that, irrespective of the industry in which you work, the fundamental responsibility for your career lies with you. You are in charge. Of course you can let fate play its part, and without certain qualifications and experience you may find obstacles in your path. All of this considered though, it will be your determination and persistence that creates your career opportunities. It is important to think big about where you would like to be and to have the dream, but within this dream you need both a plan (which can change over time) and the stepping stones to achieve it.

In this chapter we explore the context in which careers in sport and exercise medicine (SEM), sports therapy and physiotherapy operate. This landscape has changed greatly in the past decade and is set to evolve even further in the next. The main driver has been the globalisation of medicine to support sport which has mirrored the globalisation of sport.

Furthermore we want to focus readers' attention, in particular that of future sports clinicians, on the key behaviours that are important to both potential employers and other people who will help with career progression.

We then reflect on some career advice provided by five members of the SEM community: two international sports physiotherapists; a young SEM doctor; one of the most controversial characters in SEM; and finally, a leading figure in injury prevention. All of their stories and advice provide invaluable real life guidance and inspiration.

DEVELOPMENT OF SPORT AND EXERCISE MEDICINE

Sport and exercise medicine has become an all-encompassing term for many subdisciplines and types of practitioners. Sports medicine is a multidisciplinary way of thinking based around three core themes or approaches:

1. Work as a team.
2. Communicate internationally.
3. Reach the top with your patients or athletes, where you seek to achieve the maximum functional recovery possible.

Across the world, SEM has developed at different rates and with different styles of leadership and personality. Now, however, the effect of globalisation is felt more strongly through the diaspora of the playing talent in sport and increased global travel to compete in both professional and amateur events, such as marathons and triathlons. Following this pattern, clinicians have begun to move internationally to practise and so cross-pollination is taking place. There has never been a better time for an international career in SEM.

The internationalisation of the discipline is not constrained to the travels of individual athletes. In fact, in the past decade international governing bodies such as FIFA (Fédération Internationale de Football Association) and the IOC (International Olympic Committee) have created international networks of clinics and scientific research centres or hubs (48 in the case of FIFA and nine in the case of the IOC), with the key driver of promoting international collaboration. Both groups also support large conferences, such as the annual Football Medicine Strategies Conference organised by Isokinetic Medical Group and the IOC World Conference on Prevention of Injury and Illness (held every three years). More than 1000 sports medicine practitioners from more than 70 countries come together at these conferences to share their experiences, network and seek collaboration for future multicentre studies.

This explosion in interest in the discipline has led to the need to establish a common method of communication, and sports medicine has adopted English as its base language. To support and stimulate further cross-border sharing of information and experience, the *British Journal of Sports Medicine* (BJSM) has been proactive in co-opting well over 20 professional member bodies from countries as diverse as The Netherlands, South Africa, Australia and Switzerland, and has extended its editorial board to embrace 35 nations (at the time of publication).

Against this backdrop of movement of people and information, two other macro trends are positively impacting upon the cultural development of the discipline and the number of career opportunities. These are an increase in televised sport and its associated investment, and a growing understanding of the dangers of physical inactivity, which has led to the view that 'exercise is medicine'.

The adoption of exercise medicine in the sports medicine movement

In many countries, sports medicine has become known as 'sport and exercise medicine'. This term provides an apt description of the discipline, blending management of sports injuries and medicine in the sporting population with promotion of the beneficial effects of exercise and its positive contribution to world health.

Treatment of the effects of physical inactivity is outside the scope of this volume (see Volume 2: *Exercise Medicine*), but it is widely recognised that insufficient physical activity is a key risk factor for non-communicable diseases (NCDs) such as cardiovascular disease, cancer and diabetes.[1] There is mounting scientific evidence that physical activity may be a most important public health intervention to prevent NCDs. Evolving national health systems and structures, and public health policies, will increasingly shape the way in which investment is targeted to deal with the mounting burden of NCDs. This will lead to wider and more specialised career opportunities. The private sector will support this, especially where there are sporting injury comorbidities or a patient wishes to regain functional capacity. Additionally, as the population ages and the importance of sporting activities and participation among the older generation increases, the demand for specialised, private sports medicine services will increase.

Increased resources in sport

Television companies are now able to access global markets through digital and internet-based channels, resulting in a huge inflow of money into sport. This has triggered an increase in investment in both SEM and research. Not only are there now more resources available to club management to spend on player support and welfare, the economic rationale and business case for the role of SEM is better understood. Now, in a premier league football clinical team you would expect to see at least:

- a full-time SEM doctor
- two or three part-time doctors across all teams
- a ratio of one physiotherapist to five first team players
- osteopaths and chiropractors
- a sessional sports psychologist, a dietitian/nutritionist and a podiatrist
- sports therapists and other soft tissue specialists
- a medical administrator.

These roles, although they may be well paid, are also very demanding, often requiring availability across the full week. (See also Chapter 1.)

Proficiency in a second or third language

Another trend, in European football clubs in particular, is that language skills within the SEM team are increasingly required and valued. Considering that the playing group of most UEFA Champions League football teams is drawn from more than a dozen countries and mother tongues, it is difficult for SEM practitioners to communicate and build a bond of trust if they do not fully understand the cultural heritage of the players and their medical history. Added to this is the requirement to communicate effectively with the national team SEM staff for acute injury management, workload modifications and return-to-play (RTP) considerations. This additional workload on top of normal day-to-day club commitments is becoming more common in football as there are more international 'friendlies' and larger national team squads. Within football, Spanish and French are probably the most valuable second languages to learn. This allows for better communication with players from North and West Africa, and Central and South America.

Widening the scope of practice—dual qualifications and subspecialist courses

In addition to the increased demands that are placed upon SEM teams in professional sport, employers expect practitioners to have a wider vision than would be provided by a single educational experience. For example, within a rehabilitation-focused setting, classical physiotherapy training is not considered sufficient to help a patient to reach the maximum functional recovery possible.

If a practitioner has a secondary qualification, the scope of practice widens and there is a greater benefit for both the patient and the team. Among the staff at the Isokinetic Clinic in London practitioners hold the following dual qualifications: sports therapy BSc and fast-track physiotherapy BSc; physiotherapy BSc and sport and exercise medicine MSc; engineering science BSc and physiotherapy BSc; human movement science BSc and sports physiotherapy MSc. After the base university

Career development CHAPTER 48

education, the next development steps are in specialist courses and certification. For example, a SEM physician, doctor, or physiotherapist may be able to add value by doing an MSc in ultrasound or injections. This is a way of adding value to patients' treatment and at the same time becoming more employable. Another example might be a physiotherapist undertaking a course in the management of non-specific low back pain, if this is what is being seen in their clinical practice.

Sports therapy, sports and exercise science, and sports rehabilitation

There is a well-identified need for a blended skill-set and perspective, whether as an individual practitioner or among the wider SEM team. After graduating from undergraduate physiotherapy or physical therapies degree courses, the clinician has not yet received sufficient training to be effective in SEM settings. To meet this need, many clinicians undertake sports physiotherapy masters degrees.

There has also been an explosion in the number of new courses designed specifically to train students in the management and treatment of sports injuries. In the United Kingdom, sports therapy, sports and exercise science and sports rehabilitation courses have been among the fastest growing university courses over the past five years.

Overall, however, systems in public and private medicine and in team sports have not kept pace with this change, especially in the areas of state registration, professional indemnity insurance and identifying where they fit in the clinical governance model. In the United Kingdom, for example, because of a lack of state registration by the Health and Care Professions Council, (HCPC) sport and exercise clinicians are unable to be registered with private medical insurers (PMI) for work in the private sector and cannot always assume highly responsible roles in team settings. Fortunately it does seem that change is just around the corner and future accreditation processes will open up new avenues of career opportunities.

Men and women have a place in sport and exercise medicine

One final but important dimension to the development of SEM over the past decade has been the increasing participation of female doctors, physiotherapists, osteopaths and other clinicians in the discipline. Sport has historically been male-dominated and resistant to change. Women were (and many still are) disadvantaged in many settings. This is beginning to change, not simply in an age of equal opportunities, but as sporting teams recognise that medical teams need to be selected on merit and not prejudice.

KEY BEHAVIOURS FOR A SUCCESSFUL AND INTERESTING CAREER

My personal career path in sports medicine has been far from traditional. Three key points that contributed to my being in the position of responsibility I have are: (i) gaining skills that would *add value* to a sports medicine setting (business management in my case), (ii) adopting a *flexible attitude*–embracing change, and (iii) working to develop a network of top experts who support me and to whom I contribute. Turning the mirror to face the reader, I suggest the following five key behaviours are critical to developing a successful career:

- willingness to make yourself available to patients and colleagues
- open, honest and timely communication
- problem solving
- determination to reach the optimal result
- attention to detail.

Surrounding this is the development of self-awareness, which is built through an evolutionary process of maturation. These phases do not have to be sequential and they often run in parallel. There may be times when you reflect and revisit an earlier phase, especially as your self-awareness grows. Don't be afraid to go back to run forward.

In the first phase of your career you should seek to develop your technical skills and knowledge. This knowledge increases over time, but mainly as a result of practice. 'Miles on the clock' are important (Fig. 48.1).

Being an 'expert' is a dangerous time for a clinician. It may be a time of making clinical errors in advance of developing greater insight into one's limitations (Fig. 48.2).

A positive next step and second phase of your career is to develop your 'softer' skills, such as effective communication, negotiation, conflict resolution and problem solving (both through specific courses and also by talking with those close to you). To really develop in this area you

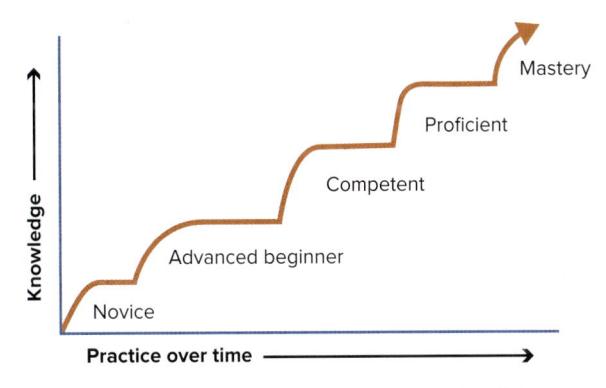

Figure 48.1 A schematic of how we can describe different levels of development as a health professional

PART C   Practical sports medicine

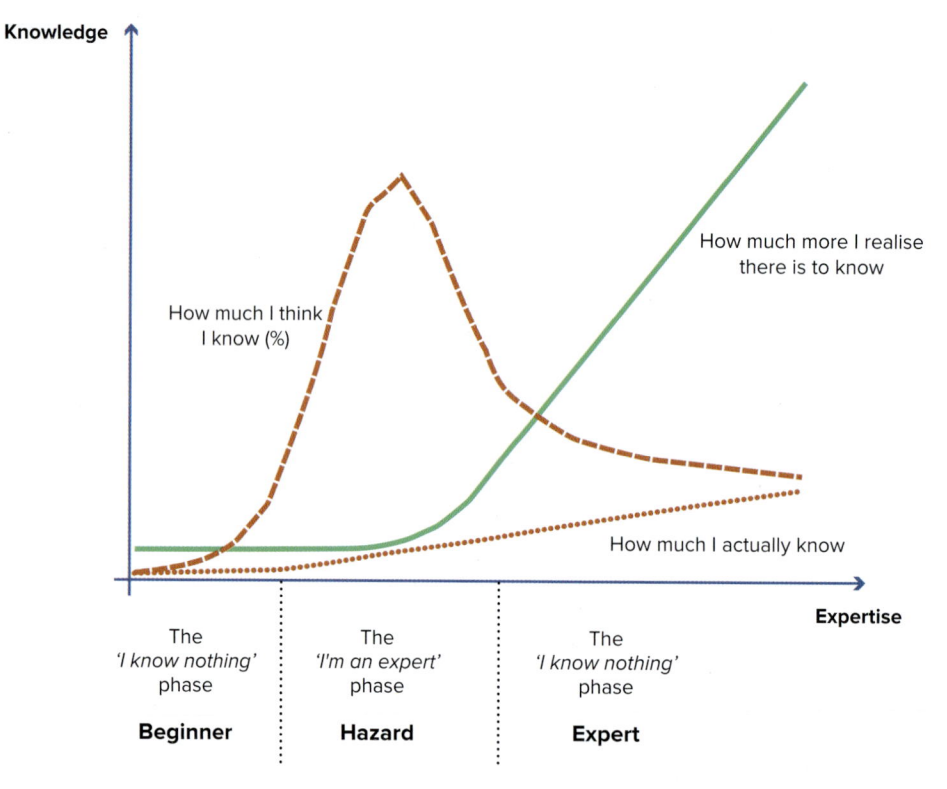

Figure 48.2 Depicts a common feeling where a learner's feeling of knowing nothing changes into feeling that he or she knows everything, before soon realising that even the most expert really knows very little

need not to be afraid of making mistakes and you need to seek out constructive criticism.

This then leads you into a critical SEM phase—that of understanding what it really means to work in a team. It means *collective action over self-interest*. Much easier said than done. There are countless examples of dysfunctional medical teams due to the inability of team members to find a simple working consensus.

At all times in your life and particularly as you start making your own decisions, you need to recognise the role of others close to you in your career development. This can be your parents, but is more likely to be your partner or spouse. Including that individual(s) in any decision making and being very clear about the likely impact on your time together (especially as sports medicine often involves travel with a team or long or anti-social hours in the working environment), will provide stability for you to grow. It is not a normal career that you are looking to develop, so you will need extraordinary support, understanding and encouragement around you.

Last, and while this sounds the easiest, the greatest challenge you will have is working on yourself. This is not in relation to developing knowledge or skills, nor is it the teamwork that is required inside and outside work. It is about making sure you have a good relationship with yourself. One where you actively critique and score yourself, and drive yourself to live in the present, understanding the importance of the past and how it seeds the future. You need to have a relationship with yourself where you reflect on your actions honestly and with humility.

Complementing my perspective, here is an American perspective on how you could break into the world of sports medicine, especially team medicine, and succeed:[2]

- Pay your dues. Start working with local sports teams to gain experience.
- Create visibility. Make yourself known to team decision makers.
- Communicate clearly. Professional communication training is a plus.
- Build relationships. Sport is like life: it's all about relationships.
- Create protocols. A disorganised doctor is an ineffective doctor.
- Establish a chain of command. Let others know who to talk to and when.

Career development CHAPTER 48

- Direct the flow of information. A team needs to speak with one voice.
- Clarify expectations. Determine the needs and wants of each stakeholder.
- Let the coaches coach. Don't stick your nose where it doesn't belong.
- View each player as an individual. That goes for visiting players, too.
- Be wary of the media. If you must talk to them, stick to the facts.

LESSONS FROM AROUND THE WORLD

Below, five members of the international sport and exercise medicine community offer their advice to others about developing a career in sports medicine.

Ummukulthoum Bakare—football medicine enthusiast and sports injury prevention strategist West Africa

Ummukulthoum Bakare is based in Lagos, Nigeria. She is a member of the Medical and Scientific Commission of the Nigerian Olympic Committee. Alongside this role she is a senior physiotherapist at Lagos Teaching Hospital and one of the few accredited FIFA 11 For Health and FIFA 11+ (injury prevention program) instructors in Africa.

Like many successful SEM professionals before her, she understands that it is important to engage in continuous self-improvement and professional development.

Her advice to aspiring SEM clinicians is:

- Be willing to shadow, undertake work experience, learn and do a large amount of volunteer work to get the necessary hands-on exposure and experience. Practice makes perfect.
- Never be tired of being a part of the knowledge continuum and always share information. It does not make you any less intelligent!
- Don't think you know everything and want to be in the spotlight. Even professors are still learning–so should you.
- The light will shine on you when the time is right.
- Procrastination is the thief of time. Poor time management is the bane of any professional.

Dr Liam West—the rookie doctor Northern Europe and Australia

Liam is based in Melbourne, Australia, but completed his junior medical jobs in Oxford, England, and his undergraduate medical training in Cardiff, Wales. At the time of publication he was planning to start his specialist training in SEM medicine. He has a passion

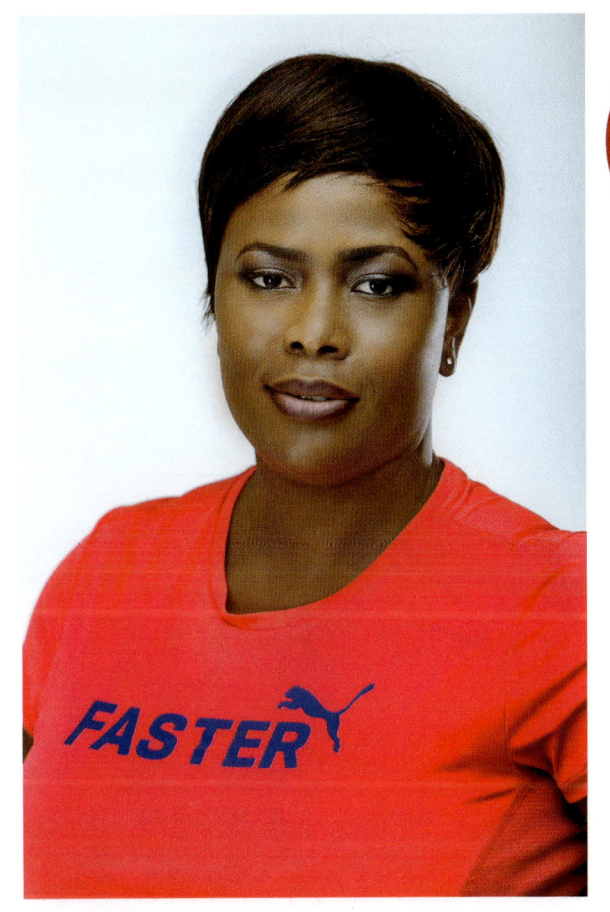

Ummukulthoum Bakare
COURTESY OF OBE TOLULOPE O. CROSSHAIRS PHOTOGRAPHY

Once you identify what goal you want to achieve as an upcoming sports physiotherapist, you have to seek out and surround yourself with senior colleagues who can help you on your path—mentors in the profession or a related field. An orthopaedic surgeon acted in this role early in my career (undergraduate university) and helped me identify my interest of specialisation in sport and exercise medicine. Let passion be your driving momentum and all the glitz and glamour may follow, but it is not guaranteed unless you make it count!   Ummukulthoum Bakare

for increasing the opportunities and education in SEM for undergraduates and junior doctors. To help achieve this he founded societies: at local level while at Cardiff Medical School; at national level in the UK with USEMS (Undergraduate Sport & Exercise Medicine Society)–and at European level, with ECOSEP (European College of Sports

1031

PART C   Practical sports medicine

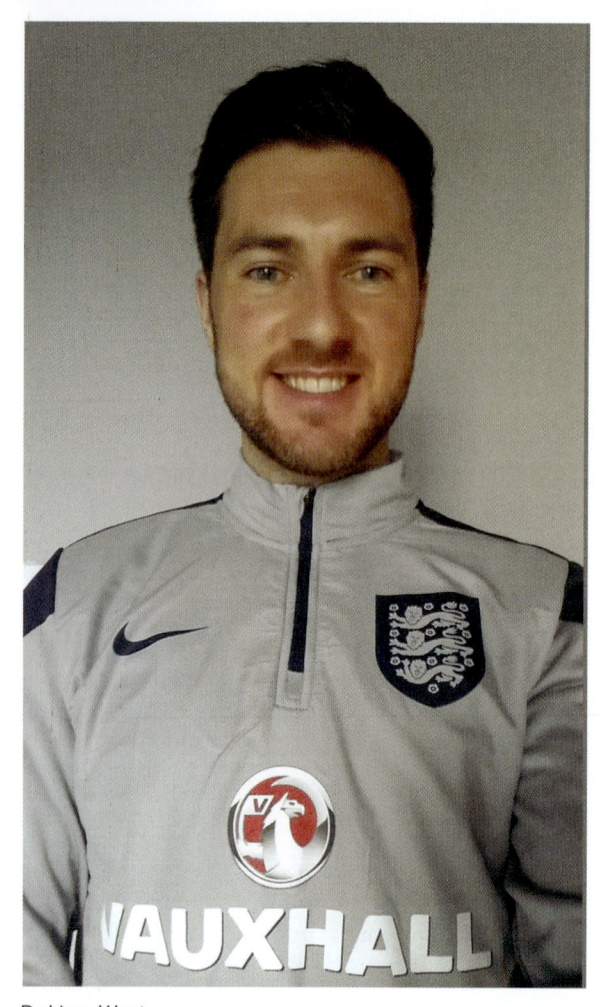

Dr Liam West

& Exercise Physicians). He is a Senior Associate Editor for the BJSM, produces insightful podcasts for the journal, and coordinated the BJSM 'Undergraduate Perspective on Sport and Exercise Medicine' blog series.

Liam recognises the value of developing an international network. During his undergraduate elective, he gained experience at the Olympic Park Sports Medicine Centre, Melbourne and the Stadium Orthopaedic and Sports Medicine Centre, Sydney, followed by time at the Aspetar Orthopaedic and Sports Medicine Hospital, Qatar.

Liam's suggestions for juniors wanting to develop a career in SEM include the following.[3]

- You need energy and motivation, especially to seize opportunities.
- How do you get these opportunities? By approaching medical or physiotherapy schools in the first instance to see what they can offer. Ask if they have lectures on SEM and if they have faculty working there who are involved in sport.
- When you are there, find out if there is a local student society. If there is, then get involved. If not, make one. Aim to get on the committee to learn valuable skills while meeting key individuals in SEM.
- Networking is key. You can network in a general way (i.e. online) but the most effective way is at conferences—choose five names on the program and don't leave until you have their email addresses. Email them that night explaining it was nice to meet them and include something interesting about either what you said or did while with them. Then in the no-so-distant future, when you're looking for SEM experience, reply to that initial email and they will remember who you are from your story. This will help your request stand out from the weekly emails for shadowing opportunities the clinician receives. Wait until your chosen contacts are with at least two of their colleagues—you will meet more people this way for less effort. Networking should be fun!
- Offer to work at conferences for free admission—pack bags, etc. This gets you networking opportunities and plenary education for free!
- Remember to network within your peer group, not just the big guns. In 15 years time, hopefully you and your colleagues will be the leaders of the clinical and research arms of SEM so forge lasting relationships early.
- Once networked, get your hands dirty and try to get as much experience as possible in sport. You need to start viewing long weekends in the rain as good things. When shadowing, be polite, gently inquisitive, energetic and offer to help at every opportunity—do NOT be a burden and, importantly, do NOT be a fan. Doctors are employed to provide clinical care for athletes, not to scream abuse at a referee or celebrate a goal.
- People don't owe you this experience—you don't get it handed to you like cardiology or respiratory medicine during your undergraduate studies—you need to offer value to those giving the experience. Sitting in on a clinic may be achieved by doing an audit for the company, etc. Create your self-directed study modules or elective placements in SEM. Travelling for these experiences should not put you off.
- Adding value can also be in the form of targeted learning—if you are interested in a certain sport, learn about the common injuries—spines and fingers in cricket, groins and ankles in football, anterior cruciate ligament injuries in netball, etc.

Career development CHAPTER 48

Hans-Wilhelm Müller-Wohlfahrt—the team and celebrity doctor Bavaria, Central Europe

The oldest of our interviewees, Müller-Wohlfahrt (or MW as he is often referred to) is one of the most renowned sports doctors in the world. Aged in his 70s, he has been challenging the status quo and the orthopaedic medicine paradigm over the past 40 years. Often talked about with an air of controversy (due to his use of homoeopathic medicine to treat players), there is no doubt that he has pushed forward SEM's understanding of muscle injuries in particular. Along with his roles with Bayern Munich and the German national team, he has been a magnet for many celebrities from the world of sport and beyond. This includes Usain Bolt, Paula Radcliffe, Ronaldo, Steven Gerrard, Michael Owen and many more. Orthopaedically trained with a specialisation in sports medicine, his approach is one of conservative management and the avoidance of surgery until there is no other option.

For him, the advice for career development is simple and summed up in three principles shown in Figure 48.3. He believes that your career is defined by your ability to manage and win with patients.

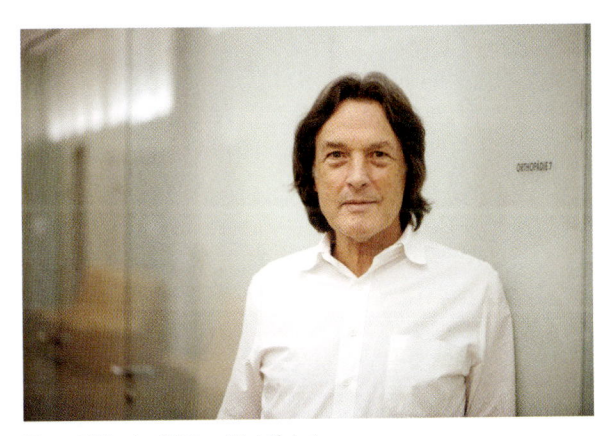

Hans-Wilhelm Müller-Wohlfahrt

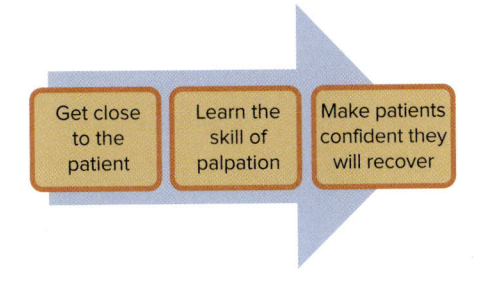

Get close to the patient → Learn the skill of palpation → Make patients confident they will recover

Figure 48.3 Dr Müller-Wohlfahrt's keys to career development

Rod Whiteley—sports physiotherapist who has moved across continents for his career Middle East via Australasia and Major League Baseball

Rod Whiteley is a sports physiotherapist working at Aspetar Orthopaedic and Sports Medicine Hospital in Qatar as a research and education physiotherapist. His primary clinical interest is in upper limb injuries, stemming in large part from having played baseball for over 30 years, from which point his PhD in throwing-related injury seemed almost inevitable. He was physiotherapist to the Australian Baseball Federation for 20 years prior to joining Aspetar and recently was the first non-American to be an invited keynote speaker at Major League Baseball's Winter Medical Meeting.

For him, the overall perspective to share is that 'there is no formula'. Reflecting on his career, he says the underlying theme 'is that you will need to very early suck up the idea that you are not going to be driving a Porsche, so if that's your motivation, get out while you can. If, on the other hand, your motivation is curiosity, an open ended career where things are constantly evolving, and the opportunity to be around other people who are also striving to get as far as they can largely through hard work, then come in, the water's fine'.

He also has some cautionary tales regarding fan syndrome, and losing sight of clinical and professional objectivity. He believes in the importance of honest and frequent self-appraisal and addressing one's own deficits. He is not sure if you could work properly in sport medicine if you are not athlete-centred rather than it all being about how wonderful you are as a clinician.

Finally he also recognises the phenomenon of 'How much I actually know'. He reflects: 'I keep reminding myself of whatever I was doing five years ago and how embarrassed I am about this now, which of course makes me realise that in five years from now I will think exactly the same about what I am now doing'.

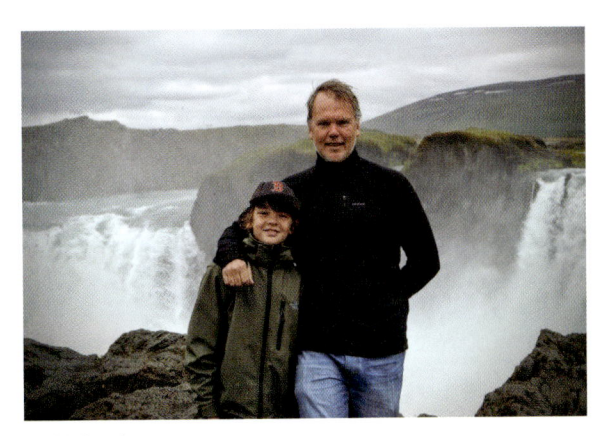

Rod Whiteley

PART C   Practical sports medicine

Roald Bahr—Professor of Sports Medicine
The Nordic countries

Last but far from least, is one of the editors of this book, Roald Bahr, Professor of Sports Medicine in the Department of Sports Medicine at the Norwegian School of Sport Sciences and the Chair of the Oslo Sports Trauma Research Center. He is also the Chief Medical Officer for Olympiatoppen and Chair of the Medical Department at the National Olympic Training Center. Additionally he is the Head of the Aspetar Sports Injury and Illness Prevention Programme.

Roald is more than these titles though. Professionally he is a world leader in sports injury prevention research having published more than 300 original research articles, review papers and book chapters, in addition to several books. More importantly though he is one of the most warm and generous human beings you could meet.

As is so often the case with those who have been very successful in their careers, the simple advice is built on a deep understanding of those things that really work. For him, the advice he would wish to share is shown in Figure 48.4.

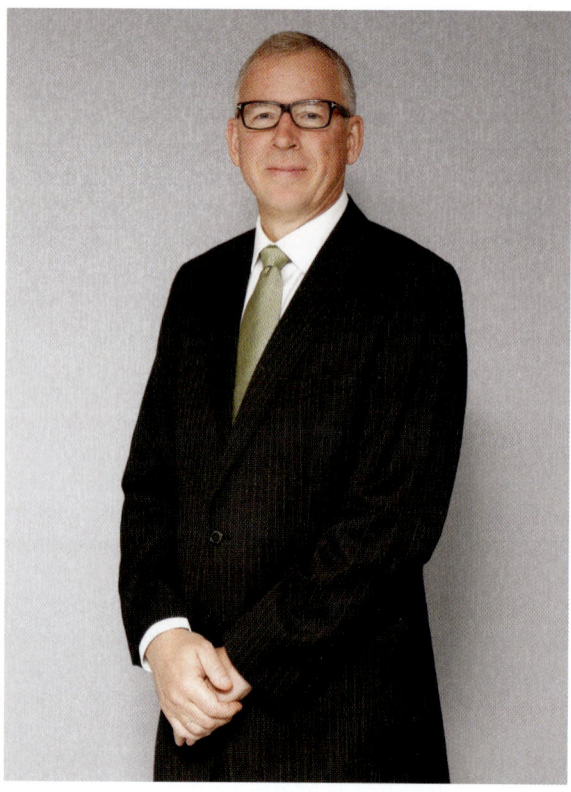

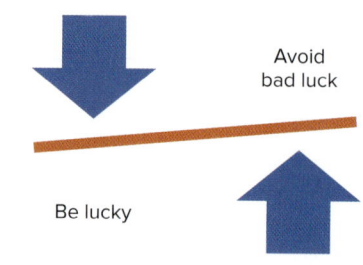

Roald Bahr

Figure 48.4 Professor Roald Bahr's keys to success

Avoid bad luck

Be lucky

But chance favours the prepared mind . . .

REFERENCES

References for this chapter can be found at www.mhhe.com/au/CSM5e

Quotation sources

Chapter 1
You may have the greatest bunch of individual stars in the world, but if they don't play together, the club won't be worth a dime.

Babe Ruth (1895-1948)

Chapter 2
Incredibly, some scientifically educated medical school graduates still see evidence as inferior to intuition and experience: those are the ones who give me chills.

Dr Harriet Hall, www.sciencebasedmedicine.org, 29 May 2012

Chapter 3
After feeling discomfort in my hamstring after the first round last night and then again in the semi-final tonight, I was examined by the Chief Doctor of the National Championships and diagnosed with a grade 1 tear.

Usain Bolt, posted on Twitter 6 weeks before the Rio 2016 Olympic Games

Chapter 4
During training, I suffered a stress fracture. It was madness that I carried on and ran the 800 metres and 1500 metres, but because it's the Olympics, you run through the pain. You never know if you'll have another chance at the Olympics, so unless you can't actually walk you carry on, because you don't want to be asking yourself, 'What if?'

Dame Kelly Holmes, MBE, DBE, 800 and 1500 m gold medallist, Athens 2004 Olympic Games

Chapter 5
... then, [Mr Hammerhead Shark] his shirt covered in blood, spun around and hit his knee on the table, at which point he swore and yelled 'My knee! My knee!', the whole time unfussed about the hammer stuck in his neck.

G Lorimer Moseley, *Painful Yarns. Metaphors and stories to help understand the biology of pain*, Dancing Giraffe Press 2007

Chapter 6
Understanding pain biology changes the way people think about pain, reduces its threat value and improves their management of it.

David Butler & Lorimer Moseley, *Explain Pain*, 2nd ed, Noigroup Publications 2013

Chapter 7
Belgian decathlete Thomas Van der Plaetsen had testicular cancer diagnosed because abnormal levels of the HCG hormone were detected on a routine doping test in 2014. After treatment, 2016 saw him win the European Championships and compete at the Rio 2016 Olympic Games.

Authors

Chapter 8
Mo Farah has nine key elements to his running technique that have allowed him to become Britain's greatest ever runner.

R Gray, 'The secrets of Mo Farah's success', www.telegraph.co.uk, 16 September 2013

Chapter 9
Nothing compares to the simple pleasure of riding a bike.

John F Kennedy (1917-1963)

Chapter 10
In football as in watchmaking, talent and elegance mean nothing without rigour and precision.

Lionel Messi, www.thewatchquote.com, 7 September 2012

Chapter 11
Core strength and stability is very important to me. Tennis is all about rotation of the body and my ability to create power. I incorporate a lot of abdominal, back and glute exercises into my gym sessions.

Samantha Stosur.
A Proszenko, 'New attitude, new Sam', www.smh.com.au, 6 June 2010

Chapter 12
An ounce of prevention is worth a pound of cure.

Benjamin Franklin (1706-1790)

Chapter 13
Paul Quantrill will never forget the feeling of pure exhaustion at the most important moment of his career. It was the fourth game of the 2004 American League Championship Series, at Fenway Park, with the Yankees trying to finish a sweep of the Boston Red Sox. The teams were tied, 4-4, heading into the bottom of the 12th. It was Quantrill's 100th relief inning of the season. 'We were done',' Quantrill said. 'We were wrecked. We battled, but we just weren't where we needed to be.'

T Kepner, 'The Endangered Species of Baseball' *New York Times*, 31 March 2016

Chapter 14
Listen: the patient is telling you the diagnosis.

Sir William Osler, Canadian physician (1849-1919)

Quotation sources

Chapter 15
Wherever the art of medicine is loved, there is also a love of humanity.

Hippocrates (c.460-370 BCE)

Chapter 16
The operation was entirely successful, but the patient succumbed.

Manual of Operative Surgery, published 1887

Chapter 17
Healing is a matter of time, but is sometimes also a matter of opportunity.

Hippocrates (c.460-370 BCE)

Chapter 18
The pearl of long-term rehabilitation is to build a small team of core people who collaborate with other professions. Never walk alone!

Kjetil Jansrud, alpine skiing gold medallist at the 2014 Sochi Winter Olympic Games, 13 months after rupturing his anterior cruciate ligament

Chapter 19
Perhaps the most common question for every active but injured patient is 'When can I return to play?'

Authors

Chapter 20
I've been knocked out a few times in there, but I have no idea how many concussions I've ever had.

Hulk Hogan, Ewrestling News, 2 January 2015

Chapter 21
In the beginner's mind there are many possibilities, in the expert's mind there are few.

Shunryu Suzuki, Zen Mind, Beginner's Mind, T Dixon and R Baker (eds), Weatherhill NY, 1970

Chapter 22
Having looked at it on YouTube, I don't like to look at it too much because it freaks me out a bit. The bail hit me in the eye and went two centimetres back.

South African cricket player Mark Boucher on his career-ending eye injury
F Moonda, 'Boucher finally says goodbye', www.espncricinfo.com, 16 February 2013

Chapter 23
It makes your arm very hot, heavy and difficult to move. Stingers don't tend to last too long: you get pins and needles down your arm as the heaviness goes away. Sometimes it's 10 seconds, sometimes maybe a minute.

England Rugby star Jonny Wilkinson, who required neck surgery after recurrent injuries
P Rees, The Guardian, 7 February 2004

Chapter 24
When I dislocated my shoulder back in 2005 and (went through) rehab throughout 2006, I was told by Dr Andrews 'you're always going to have to stay on top of that shoulder. You're always going to have to do a little bit extra to keep it at the level you want to keep it at'. In a lot of ways it was the best thing that ever happened to me because I started doing things that I'd never done before. So I learned so much about my shoulder and how to manage my shoulder.

Drew Brees, NFL quarterback
J Bennett, 'Drew Brees updates shoulder injury', www.raycomgroup.worldnow.com, 24 September 2015

Chapter 25
Throwing warmup pitches to start the bottom of the second inning, Hudson felt some tightness around his elbow. On the second pitch that inning, he felt that something was seriously wrong. His fastball dipped to about 85 mph, and he became hittable. He stayed in the game and completed the inning ... but that ... would be Hudson's last pitch for another year.

Report on major league baseball pitcher Daniel Hudson's return from two ulnar collateral ligament surgeries
M Hendley, 'After Two Tommy John Operations, Daniel Hudson Hopes to Rejoin the D-backs' Starting Rotation', www.phoenixnewtimes.com, 1 April 2015

Chapter 26
Laura Robson admits she will have to start her career all over again after she recovers from major wrist surgery. Robson said she 'felt like a child again' in the aftermath of her operation, struggling to dress herself and cut her own food. Itching to return to action, Robson said she has been reduced to tears, at times frustrated with rehabilitation while her peers train and compete.

Sky Sports, 20 June 2014

Chapter 27
Star midfielder Daniel Kerr says he's willing to risk permanent damage to his injured finger if it means helping the Eagles reach and win another Grand Final. West Coast's bid for a third straight grand final, and back-to-back premierships, was dealt a shattering blow last week when Kerr had to undergo surgery on a ruptured tendon in the ring finger of his left hand.

T Clarke, 'Daniel Kerr willing to risk permanent damage to finger', Superfooty AFL, www.Perthnow.com, 29 August 2007

Chapter 28
I want to apologise to my fans. I broke my rib and again I am out of the fight. I really wanted to come back, I'm not sure if I will ever come back.

Khabib Nurmagomedov, UFC, October 2015

Chapter 29
My MRI shows I have a damaged disc at L5/S1. I am disappointed that I can never play basketball, golf and go for a

run ever again. A neurosurgeon says he can perform a fusion. Is there anything else I can do?

24-year-old athlete with disabling low back pain

Chapter 30

Running has substantially shaped human evolution, it is one of the most transforming events in human history. We have literally evolved to run and our big incredible butts are evidence of this.

Professor Dan Lieberman, evolutionary biologist, Harvard University, *Nature*, November 2004, p.345

Chapter 31

... Lionel Messi returned to Barcelona early from international break due to an inflammation in his hip, pain that has also plagued other players such as Raul, Xabi Alonso, Aduriz, Busquets and a host of Athletic Club's current squad. There are different options in terms of treatment, and each player has undergone their own decision towards recovery to get back onto the pitch as quickly as possible.

J Rincón, 'Messi not the only one to suffer from hip pain', www.Marca.com, 4 September 2016

Chapter 32

Soccer was my first love, and I enjoyed playing on the left wing until a groin injury forced me out of the game in 2008.

Chad le Clos, South African swimming gold medallist 'Chad's in le Clos of his own', *City Press*, www.News24.com, 19 November 2011

Chapter 33

It was the quad in my right leg, the tendon just kept tearing. I couldn't get back to the point of playing and obviously after having a really good start last season, and not playing again, it was frustrating.

Joel Paris, promising Australian cricket fast bowler L Jolly, 'Paris primed for Warriors' campaign', www.cricket.com.au, 1 October 2015

Chapter 34

You know, this is a different hamstring—I did my left hamstring, I've done the right side of my back, I've just done my right hammy... obviously I've got injury concerns at the moment, now I have to go back and do what the experts tell me to give myself the best chance of being fully fit.

Michael Clarke, Australian cricket captain A Burnett, 'Clarke openly ponders playing future', www.cricket.com, 13 December 2014

Chapter 35

The thing is I have no ACL. So unless I get surgery, there's nothing really magical that I can do that's going to make it better. I just can get my leg stronger, my muscle stronger and try and support it a little more. But that has a small impact.

My knee is loose and it's not stable and that's the way it's going to be from here on out.

Lindsey Vonn, Olympic gold medal skier 'Vonn: Knee fine after skiing off in downhill', www.abclocal.go.com, 21 December 2013

Chapter 36

The New York Knicks announced today that Carmelo Anthony will have season-ending left knee surgery. The procedure, which will be performed by Team Orthopedist Dr. Answorth Allen, includes a left knee patella tendon debridement and repair.

www.NBA.com, 18 February 2015

Chapter 37

When I listened to other people–who seemed to have trouble even though their [knee replacements] went well–[I learned that] they didn't make the commitment to rehab ... I can walk forever now–pain-free ... I can hit a tennis ball again.

Billie Jean King, 6 years after her 2010 knee replacements M Cartel, 'Billie Jean King: Life after knee replacements', www.lifescript.com, 23 January 2016

Chapter 38

I saw it once like two years ago ... And that was it, I didn't need to see any more after that.

Kevin Ware, commenting on his gruesome complete tibial fracture that occurred while contesting a loose ball in NCAA in 2013
R Barrigon, 'Kevin Ware: "I saw the injury once two years ago, I didn't need to see any more after that"', www.Hoopshype.com, 27 March 2016

Chapter 39

Kompany remains sidelined with a calf injury, sustained after just seven minutes of City's goalless draw with Dynamo Kiev one month ago. Remarkably, it is the 14th time he has suffered a problem with his calf since joining the club in 2008 - with five of them occurring this season - and his 32nd injury overall during the past eight years.

PhysioRoom, 12 April 2016

Chapter 40

The anger is rage. Why the hell did this happen?!? ... Now I'm supposed to come back from this and be the same player or better ... How in the world am I supposed to do that?? ... Maybe this is how my book ends. Maybe Father Time has defeated me ... Then again maybe not!

Kobe Bryant, LA Lakers shooting guard and five-time NBA champion, after rupturing his Achilles tendon in a game against the Golden State Warriors in 2013. He returned to play until his retirement in 2016 www.kobebryant.com

Quotation sources

Chapter 41
Total rupture of left ATFL (ankle ligament) and associated joint capsule damage in a soccer kickabout with friends. Continuing to assess extent of injury and treatment plan day by day. Rehab already started.

World golf number 1 Rory McIlroy on Instagram, nine days before the British Open, 6 July 2015
www.instagram.com

Chapter 42
Dance is the hidden language of the soul.

Martha Graham, dancer and choreographer (1894-1991)

Chapter 43
Plantar fasciitis sucks. It feels like you have needles underneath your feet while you're playing.

Joakim Noah of the Chicago Bulls (NBA)
D.L. Moore, 'Plantar fasciitis knocking top athletes off their feet', www.usatoday.com, 21 August 2013

Chapter 44
Youth is full of sport,
Age's breath is short;
Youth is nimble,
Age is lame;
Youth is hot and bold,
Age is weak and cold;
Youth is wild, and age is tame.

From William Shakespeare, 'Crabbèd Age and Youth'

Chapter 45
The limbs of soldiers are in as much danger from the ardor of young surgeons as from the missiles of the enemy.

Confederate surgeon Julian John Chisholm's observations on the limitations of medical care for military personnel in the American Civil War (1861-1865)

Chapter 46
To screen or not to screen, that is the question.

Authors (adapted from *Hamlet*, William Shakespeare)

Chapter 47
Talent wins games, but teamwork and intelligence win championships.

Michael Jordan

Chapter 48
If you don't build your dream, someone else will hire you to help them build theirs!

Dhirubhai Ambani

A G KRISHNAMURTHY, 'Against all Odds: A story of courage perseverance and hope', McGraw-Hill Education Leadership Essentials Series, 2008

Index

A

abductor hallucis strains, 956
accelerating tissue healing, 40
acceleration/deceleration injury (whiplash), 375
accessory soleus, 888
acetabular labrum, 594-5
Achilles pain, 865-92
   accessory soleus, 888
   acute Achilles tendon rupture (complete), 889-92
   autologous blood and platelet rich plasma (PRP), 882
   causes, 867
   cell-based therapies, 883
   clinical assessment, 878-9, 886
   clinical perspective, 865-72
   compression, 884-6
   corticosteroid injections, 882
   electrophysical agents, 884
   gradual onset, 888
   history, 866-8
   insertional Achilles tendinopathy, 884-7
   investigations, 872
   medications, 884
   midportion Achilles tendinopathy, 872-84
   pathology, 872-6
   physical examination, 868-72
   posterior impingement syndrome, 887-8
   PROMs, 872
   referred pain, 888
   rehabilitation exercise training, 888
   rehabilitation of Achilles tendon ruptures, 890-1
   retrocalcaneal bursitis (enthesis organ), 884-5, 886-7
   return to sport, 891-2
   sclerosing, 882-3
   Sever's disease, 888
   surgical treatment, 884
   tendinopathy, 872-84
   treatment, 886
Achilles (superficial calcaneal) bursitis, 887
acquired sport-specific instability (AIOS), 407, 408, 411, 412, 418
acromioclavicular joint injuries, 426-8
active movement tests (neck pain), 355-7
active recovery, 189-91, 200

high-duration short-duration exercise, 190
long-duration exercise, 190-1
psychological effects, 191
active spondylolytic bone stress injury, 541-2
activity history and injury, 213
actovegin, 269
acupuncture, 256-8
   lateral elbow tendinopathy, 447
acute Achilles tendon rupture (complete), 889-92
acute acromioclavicular joint injuries, 426
acute ankle injuries, 893-915
   anteroinferior tibiofibular ligament injury/syndesmotic injury, 912-13
   anterior calcaneal process fracture, 910
   avulsion fracture of the base of the fifth metatarsal, 908-10
   causes, 906, 908, 912-14
   clinical approach, 906
   clinical perspective, 894-8
   common/less common, 895
   complex regional pain syndrome type 1, 914-15
   examination, 895-7
   fractures, 910-11
   functional anatomy, 893-4
   grade III injuries (treatment), 903-4
   history, 895
   impingement syndromes, 911
   investigations, 897-8
   lateral ligament injuries, 899-900
   lateral talar process fracture, 910
   maisonneuve fracture, 905
   medial (deltoid) ligament injuries, 904-5
   medial tubercle fractures, 911
   osteochondral lesions of the talar dome, 906-8
   Ottawa ankle rules, 895, 897, 898, 905
   peroneal tendons dislocation, 911-12
   persistent pain after ankle sprain, 905-15
   posterior process of the talus fracture, 911
   post-traumatic synovitis, 913-14
   Pott's fracture, 905
   rehabilitation, 900-4

sinus tarsi syndrome, 914
tendon dislocation/rupture, 911-12
tibial plafond lesions, 910
tibialis posterior tendon dislocation, 912
tibialis posterior tendon rupture, 912
treatment, 900-4, 907-908
see also ankle pain; ankle sprain
acute compartment syndrome, 24-5, 844
acute elbow injuries, 456-60
   fractures, 456-7
   hyperextension injuries, 460
   rupture of MLC, 459
   posterior dislocation, 457-9
   tendon ruptures, 459-60
acute groin injuries, 633, 642-3
   diagnosis, 642-3
acute hamstring muscle strains, 685-705
   criterion-related rehabilitation, 693
   epidemiology, 686
   manual therapy, 694-5
   medical therapies, 692-3
   muscle activation, 692
   prognosis, 689-703
   RICE, 692
   risk factors, 703-5
   stretching, 694
   type I and type II, 686-8
   type I: sprinting related, 688
   type II: stretch-related (dancer's), 689
acute knee injuries, 713-67
   acute patellar trauma, 762-5
   anterior cruciate ligament tears, 737-55
   articular cartilage damage, 760-2
   bursal haematoma, 767
   causes, 714
   clinical approach, 714-23
   fat pad impingement, 767
   fracture of the tibial plateau, 767
   functional anatomy, 713-14
   investigations, 722-3
   lateral collateral ligament tears, 759-60
   medial collateral ligament injury, 729-36
   meniscal injuries, 723-8
   patellar tendon rupture, 765, 767
   physical examination, 716-22
   posterior cruciate ligament (PLC) tears, 755-9

1039

Index

prevention, 177-81
rehabilitation, 727-88, 745-50
ruptured hamstring tendon, 767
superior tibiofibular joint injury, 767
surgical treatment, 742-4
time relationship of swelling to diagnosis, 715
treatment, 726-7, 729-36, 757-9, 765
acute patellar tendon pain, 801
acute patellar trauma, 762-5
acute radiculopathy +/-nerve root compression, 545-7
acute sports injuries *see* sports injuries, acute
acute wry neck, 374
adductor magnus strains, 711
adductor-related groin pain, 643-50
   acute/subacute phase, 647
   compression shorts, 650
   conditioning phase, 647-8
   diagnostic criteria, 643-50
   manual therapy, 650
   rehabilitation, 649
   return-to-sport phase, 649
   sports-specific phase, 648-9
   treatment, 644-5
adhesive capsulitis 'frozen shoulder', 429
Advanced Trauma Life Support (ATLS) 299
age and ACL injuries, 755
agility training, 144
amnesia and injury severity, 305-6
analgesics, 264
anatomical considerations (neck pain), 347-9
anatomical planes of the body, 86
ankle dorsiflexion, 98-9
ankle injuries *see* acute ankle injuries
ankle joint, 85-8
ankle pain, 917-36
   anterior, 934-6
   lateral, 929-33
   medial, 917-29
   posterior, 917
   see also Achilles pain; acute ankle injuries
ankle sprain, persistent pain after 'the difficult ankle', 905-15
   avulsion fracture of the base of the fifth metatarsal, 908-10
   causes, 912-14
   clinical approach, 906
   complex regional pain syndrome type 1, 914-15
   fractures, 910-11
   impingement syndromes, 911
   osteochondral lesions of the talar dome, 906-8
   post-traumatic synovitis, 913-14
   sinus tarsi syndrome, 914
   tendon dislocation or rupture, 911-12
ankle sprain prevention, 174-7
   injury mechanisms, 175
   programs, 175-7
   risk factors, 175
anterior ankle pain, 934-6
   anterior impingement of the ankle, 934-5
   anterior inferior tibiofibular ligament (AITFL) injury, 936
   tibialis anterior tendinopathy, 935-6
anterior calcaneal process fracture, 910
anterior cruciate ligament (ACL) injuries, 166, 714, 715
   age, 755
   anatomy, 737
   clinical features, 738-40
   gender difference, 754-5
   mechanism of injury, 737-8
   muscle weakness, 749-50
   osteoarthritis, 753-4
   partial tear, 755
   prevention, 755
   re-injury rate, 752-3
   return to sport, 751-2
   revision surgery, 753
   self-reported knee function, 750-1
   surgery, 748-50
   tears, 737-55
   treatment, 740-4
   treatment, outcomes after, 750-5
anterior cruciate ligament rehabilitation, 745-5
   instability, 748
   low back pain, 748
   low limb stiffness, 749
   muscle weakness, 749-50
   patellar region pain, 748-9
   postural control, 750
   psychological problems, 750
   soft tissue laxity, 749
   soft tissue stiffness, 749
   symptomatic meniscus tears, 748
anterior exertional compartment syndrome, 843-4
anterior impingement of the ankle, 934-5
anterior inferior tibiofibular ligament (AITFL) injury/syndesmotic injury, 912-13, 936
anterior knee pain, 769-803
   bursitis, 802-3
   causes, 770
   clinical approach, 770-5
   fat pad irritation/impingement, 801-802
   Osgood-Schlatter lesion, 802
   patellofemoral instability, 792-3
   patellofemoral pain, 775-91
   patient reported outcome measures, 774-5
   physical examination, 771-4
   quadriceps tendinopathy, 802
   Sinding-Larsen-Johansson lesion, 802
   synovial plica, 803
anterior thigh pain, 659-77
   biomechanics, 660-1
   causes, 660
   clinical approach, 661-4
   epidemiology, 660
   femoral nerve injury, 676-7
   functional anatomy, 660-1
   investigations, 664
   key outcome measures, 664
   lateral femoral cutaneous nerve injury ('meralgia paresthetica'), 676
   physical examination, 661-4
   quadriceps contusion, 664-71
   quadriceps strain, 671-4
   referred apin, 677
   stress fracture of the femur, 674-6
anterolateral impingement, 932-3
antibiotics, quinolone, 272
anti-doping, 1020
antidepressants, 267
anti-gravity treadmill training, 41
apophysitis, 982-3
   of the fifth metatarsal, 989
   of the tarsal navicular bone, 989
arm pain, 439-62
   forearm, 460-1
   upper, 461-2
arthroscopic surgery, 274-5
arthroscopy
   diagnosis (knee), 723
   diagnosis (shoulder), 402
   hip injury, 621-2
artificial turf *vs.* natural grass, 187-8
articular cartilage
   damage, 760-2
   and mechanotherapy, 245
atherosclerotic vessel disease, 861-2
athlete
   coach and the clinician (relationship), 5-6
   and importance of sport (injuries), 213
   overhead athletes and shoulder injuries, 433-8
   return to play, 285-93
   and return-to-play decisions, 292
athletes, periodic medical assessment (PMA), 1003-15
   action points, 1014-15
   age, 1012
   assessment of known injuries and illnesses, 1006

Index

available resources, 1012
baseline testing, 1007-8
cardiac screening, 1009
clearance or restriction from play, 1013
conditions affecting sports participation, 1003-6
consent, 1013
education, 1007
geographical location, 1011-12
identification of medical conditions, 1003-6
insurance medical assessment, 1014
pre-employment medical assessment, 1014
rapport development, 1008
review of current medications and supplements, 1007
risk factors for future injury, 1009-11
screening, 1008-11
sex, 1012
sport and position, 1011
when to perform a PMA?, 1012-13
who is being assessed, 1011-12
athletes and core stability, 164
atraumatic multidirectional instability (AMBRI), 411
auricular haematoma, 335
autologous blood and platelet rich plasma (PRP), 882
autologous blood injections, 273, 450
axillary nerve injury, 430-1
axillary vein thrombosis ('effort' thrombosis), 432
axio-scapular muscles (neck pain), 361-2, 372

B

back pain, 981-2
back pain, low, 521-65
   acute radiculopathy +/-nerve root compression, 545-7
   acute severe, 549-51
   clinical approach, 528-35, 563-5
   contributing factors, 526-8
   epidemiology, 521-3
   high-complexity profile, 562-3
   investigations, 534-5
   management of non-specific disorders, 548-63
   management of specific disorders, 535-48
   medium-complexity profile, 561-2
   multidimensional nature, 523
   passive treatments, 551-4
   patient-reported outcome measures (PROMs), 529-30
   physical examination, 530-4
   recurrent/persistent, 555-61
   rehabilitation, 563, 748
   spondylolisthesis, 543-4
   stress fracture of the pars interarticularis, 535-43
   subacute, 551
   triage, 523-6
   vertebral endplate oedema, 547-8
   young athlete, 981-2
Bahr, Roald, 1034
Baker's cyst, 822-3
Bankart lesion, 401, 407, 408, 409-10, 415
Bankart repair, 408
Baxter's nerve entrapment, 947-8
biceps femoris tendinopathy, 815, 823
biceps rupture, 429
bifurcate ligament injuries, 952
biomechanical aspects of injury in specific sports, 121-38, 166
   cricket fast bowling, 125-7
   cycling, 121-4
   golf, 128-30
   rowing, 130-3
   swimming, 133-6
   tennis, 136-8
biomechanical examination, 214, 221
biomechanics
   altering, 245-6
   bone stress injuries, 32
   and leg pain, 826
biomechanics, clinical, 85-120
   footwear assessment, 105-6
   lower limb, 85-90
   lower limb abnormalities, 108-14
   lower limb assessment, 95-105
   with movement, 90-5
   upper limb, 114-20
BioMed Central (BMC), 11
bisphosphonates, 272
blisters, 52
blood flow and massage, 191
bone injuries, 14, 15-17
   fracture, 14, 15-17
   and mechanotherapy, 245
   and NSAID, 266
bone scan, 35, 642
bone stress injury, 29-43
   apophysitis, 43
   articular cartilage, 43
   classification, 37-8
   diagnosis, 34-7
   epidemiology, 31
   examination, 35
   healing of, 42
   imaging, 35-7, 38
   osteitis and periostitis, 42-3
   pathophysiology, 30-1
bone stress injuries (management), 38-42
   accelerating tissue healing, 40
   healing, 42
   initial, 39-40
   and return to running, 40-2
bone stress injuries (risk factors), 31-4
   biomechanical factors, 32
   calcium and vitamin D status, 34
   energy availability, 34
   load applied to bone, 32-3
   muscle factors, 33
   physical activity history, 34
   playing surfaces, 33
   resist load without damage accumulation, 33-4
   shoes and inserts, 33
   specific treatment, 38
   training factors, 32-3
bone tumours, 78-80
botulinum toxin (botox) injection, 450
Boutonnière deformity, 503-4
brachial plexus injuries (stingers/burners), 375
bracing
   lateral elbow tendinopathy, 447-8
   patellofemoral pain, 788-9
'stinger' phenomenon (neck pain), 375
brain
   and pain, 59-61
   and persistent pain, 60-1
   and spinal cord, 60
bruise/contusion, fat pad, 26-7
'burners' phenomenon (neck pain), 375
bursa, 14, 26, 51-2
bursal hematoma, 767
bursitis, 802-3, 819
buttock pain, 567-91
   avulsion fracture of ischial tuberosity, 589
   causes, 567
   clinical approach, 567-74
   history, 568-9
   investigations, 573-4
   ischiofemoral impingement, 587
   myofascial, 574-6
   physical examination, 569-73
   piriformis syndrome, 585-7
   posterior thigh compartment syndrome, 587-8
   proximal hamstring tendinopathy, 577-81
   proximal hamstring tendon rupture, 588-9
   referred pain from lumbar spine, 576
   sacral and pubic ramus stress fractures, 590
   sacroiliac joint dysfunction, 581-5
   specificity and sensitivity of tests, 574
   spondyloarthropathies, 589-90

Index

C

calcaneal stress fracture, 947
calcium, bone stress injuries, 34
calf pain, 847-63
    anatomy, 847-9
    causes, 850, 862-3
    clinical approach, 849-53
    deep venous thrombosis, 863
    gastrocnemius muscle strains, 853-6
    investigations, 853
    nerve entrapments, 862-3
    neuromyofascial causes, 862
    physical examination, 850-3
    soleus muscle strains, 856-9
    superficial compartment syndrome, 863
career development, 1027-34
    key behaviours for a successful and interesting career, 1029-31
    lessons from around the world, 1031-4
    sport and exercise medicine, 1027-9
carpal bones, dislocation, 479
carpal tunnel syndrome, 471, 485-6
carpometacarpal joint dislocations, 498-9
case manager approach and SEM, 6-8
cell therapy, 274
Central Government Model (CGM) for the limits of performance 140-2
central nervous system (CNS), 70
central sensitization, 69-71
centrally dominated pain, 69-72
cervical arterial dysfunction, 364
cervical extensors, assessment of, 360-1
cervical flexors, assessment of, 358-60
cervical nerve injury, 374-5
cervical radiculopathy, 374-5
cervical sensorimotor function, tests for, 362-4
cervicogenic headache, 322-8
    classification, 323
    clinical features, 323-8
    examination, 324-5
    mechanism, 322-3
    and neck pain, 374
    treatment, 326-8
chest pain, 514-20
    cardiac origin, 515
    causes, 515
    clinical assessment, 516
    costochondritis, 518
    stress fracture to ribs, 518-19
    rib trauma, 516-17
    side strain, 519-20
    sternoclavicular joint problems, 517-18
    thoracic spine, 517

chest wall pain, 132
children and concussion in sport, 311-16
chondral injuries, 17-18, 818-19
chondral surfaces, 596
chondroitin, 272-3
chronic acromioclavicular joint pain, 426-8
chronic compartment syndrome (CCS), 45, 861
chronic exertional compartment syndrome (CECS), 834-6, 841-5
chronic temporomandibular injuries, 345-6
chronic traumatic encephalopathy (CTE), 310
claudicant-type calf pain, 859-62
    atherosclerotic vessel disease, 861-2
    endofibrosis, 862
    popliteal artery entrapment, 859-61
    vascular causes, 859-62
clavicle fractures, 424-6
clinical approach
    acute Achilles tendon rupture, 889
    acute knee injury 714-23
    anterior knee pain, 770-4
    anterior thigh pain, 661-4
    difficult ankle, 906
    headache, 318-20
    hip-related pain, 598-604
    lateral knee pain, 806-9
    leg pain, 823-24
    lower back pain, 528-35
    posterior thigh pain, 681-5
    wrist pain, 463-70
clinical assessment, 201-7
    Achilles tendon 886
    calculating an accurate diagnosis, 202-5
    chest pain, 516
    and concussion, 311
    differential diagnosis, 201-2
    differential diagnosis: three step process, 201-2
    facial injuries, 331-2
    formal diagnosis assessment, 206
    neurological, 357
    positive and negative predictive values, 202-3
    posterior knee pain, 820-2
    reliability, 202
clinical examination
    diagnosis, 4-5
    groin pain, 635-9
clinical features
    lateral elbow tendinopathy, 444-5
    lisfranc joint injuries, 955
    navicular stress fracture, 953-4
    plantar fasciopathy, 942-3

clinical measurement of headache, 319-20
clinical neurological examination, 357
clinical perspective
    Achilles pain, 865-72
    acute ankle injuries, 894-898
    forefoot pain, 958-9
    neck pain, 349-65
clinical utility, 203-4
clinical relevant pathology (lateral elbow tendinopathy), 443-4
clinicians
    coach, and the athlete (relationship), 5-6
    and recovery, 198-9
    and return-to-play decisions, 290-1
closed chain exercises, 146-8
coach
    athlete and the clinician (relationship), 5-6
    and return-to-play decisions, 292
Cochrane Library, 10, 12
codeine, 264
cognitive function and concussion, 308
cognitive therapy and pain, 75
cold water immersion (CWI), 195-6, 200
Colour Doppler ultrasound, 228
compartment syndrome
    acute, 24-5, 844
    chronic, 45, 861
    chronic exertional compartment syndrome (CECS), 834-6, 841-6
    of the posterior thigh, 711
    of the thigh, 670
    superficial compartment syndrome, 863
complex regional pain syndrome type 1, 914-15
compression
    acute injury management, 248-50, 692
    retrocalcaneal bursitis, 884-6
compression and recovery, 196, 200
compression shorts, 650
computed tomography (CT), 35, 37, 129, 221, 223, 229, 468-9, 642
concussion, 296-316
    acute, 306
    amnesia and injury severity, 305-6
    Child-SCAT3™, 312-15
    and children, 311-16
    chronic traumatic encephalopathy (CTE), 310
    clinical assessment, 311
    definition, 296-7
    diagnosis conformation, 300-6
    initial impact, 298
    investigations, 311
    management of the athlete, 298-310

Index

mental health issues, 310
on-field management, 298-300
prevention, 297-8
prolongation of symptoms, 310
return to play, 306-10
SCAT3™, 301-4, 311
second impact syndrome (SIS), 310
symptoms and signs, 300, 308
treatment, 311
concussive convulsions, 310
conditioning training, 142-50
agility, 144
endurance, 142-3
flexibility, 149-50
resistance, 144-9
speed, 143-4
contrast water therapy (CWT), 195-6, 200
contusion, muscle, 23-4
core stability, 153-64
in athletes, 164
introduction, 153-4
motor control training, 154-64
prevention of pain and injury, 164
corneal injuries, 338
corns and calluses, 970
coronoid fractures, 457
corticosteroid injection
lateral elbow tendinopathy, 448-9
midportion Achilles tendinopathy, 882
corticosteroid, 270-1
costochondritis, 518
costovertebral and costotransverse joint disorders, 511-12
counter irritants, 267-8
cramps, muscle, 25, 849
cranio-cervical flexion test (CCFT), 358-9
cricket fast bowling (biomechanical aspects of injuries), 125-7
cross-training, 143
cryotherapy modalities used to treat sports injuries, 249, 799
cuboid, stress fracture of the, 956
cuboid syndrome, 956
cuneiforms, stress fracture of the, 956
cupping, vacuum, 255
cycling (biomechanical aspects of injuries), 121-4
bike fitting, 124
knee pain, 121-3
low back pain, 123
risk factors and loading, 121

D

de Quervain's tenosynovitis 476-7
deep posterior compartment syndrome, 842-3

deep venous thrombosis, 824, 863
delayed onset muscle soreness (DOMS), 46, 146, 189, 191-2
dermatitis, 52
diagnosis, 209-29
accurate, 210-11
clinical questions, 12
description of symptoms, 211-12
examination, 4-5, 213-21
history, 211-13
radiological investigation, 223-9
sport and exercise medicine (SEM), 4-5
diagnostic assessment
clinical, 4-5, 201-7
formal, 206
diagnostic imaging, 221-3
diagnostic metrics, 206
differential diagnosis, 201-2
three step process, 201-2
digital ischaemic pressure, 253-4
dislocation/subluxation 14, 18-19, 457-9
distal quadriceps muscle strain, 671-2
distal radioulnar joint instability, 484
distal radius fracture, 470-2
dorsal calcaneocuboid ligament injury, 952
DRABC (danger, response, airway, breathing, circulation) 299
dry needling, 256-8
Dynamic Gait Index 364
dynamic movement assessment, 104-5
dynamic stretching, 150

E

ear injuries, 335-6
elbow pain, 980
elbow injuries, 439
acute, 456-60
elbow anatomy, 439-40
elbow pain, 439-62
lateral, 136-7, 440-51
medial, 451-4
posterior, 454-6
electromagnetic therapies, 16, 263
electrophysical agents, 261-4, 884
electrotherapeutic modalities (lateral elbow tendinopathy), 446
elevation (acute injury management), 247, 250, 692
emergency action plans and teams, 1020-1
Emergency Management of Severe Trauma (EMST) 299
endocrine disorders, 81-2
endofibrosis, 862
endurance, skill training as, 143

endurance training, 142-3
methods, 142-3
enthesopathy, 51
epidemiology
anterior thigh pain, 660
bone stress injuries, 31
groin pain, 631-2
low back pain, 521-3
equipment
and injury, 213, 221
injury prevention and protective, 187
evidence-based medicine (EBM), 9
evidence-based practice (EBP), 9-12
challenges to, 10
concept of, 10
definition, 9
implementing, 10-12
examination and injury, 213-21
biomechanical, 214, 221
examination routine, 214-21
functional testing, 214
groin pain, 635-9
lateral hip pain, 623-5
ligament testing, 215
palpation, 215
range of motion, 214-15
spinal, 214, 219-21
strength testing, 215-19
excessive lateral pressure syndrome, 814-15
exercise
hight-intensity short-duration, 190
long-duration, 190-1
exercise associated muscle cramps (EAMC), 25
exercise-induced anaphylaxis (EIA), 213
exercise-induced hypoalgesia, 246
exercise-induced muscle soreness, 45-6
exercise medicine, 1029
exercises see resistance exercises
exertional compartment syndrome surgery
outcomes, 844-5
rehabilitation, 845
extensor carpi ulnaris tendon injuries, 484-5
extensor tendinopathy, 956
external compression headache, 328
extracorporeal shockwave therapy (ECSWT), 263-4
eye injuries, 336-40
assessment, 336-8
corneal injuries, 338
hyphema, 339
lens dislocation, 339
prevention, 340
retinal detachment, 340

1043

Index

retinal haemorrhage, 339
subconjunctival haemorrhage, 338-9
vitreous haemorrhage, 339
eyelid injuries, 339

F

faceguards, 341
facial bones, fractures of, 343-6
   maxillary fractures, 344
   mandibular fractures, 344-5
   orbital fracture, 343-4
   temporomandibular injuries, 345-6
   zygomaticomaxillary complex, 344
facial injuries, 331-46
   clinical assessment, 331-2
   ear, 335-6
   eye, 336-40
   functional anatomy, 331
   lacerations and contusions, 332-3
   nose, 333-5
   prevention, 346
   in sport, 333
   teeth, 340-3
Fagan's nomogram, 203-4, 226
fascia
   tear/rupture, 14, 26
Fartlek training, 142-3
fat pad, 26-7
   contusion (rear foot pain), 946-7
   impingement, 767
   irritation/impingement, 801-802
fatigue and running biomechanics, 95
femoral nerve injury, 676-7
femoroacetabular impingement (FAI), 607-10
fibrocartilage injuries, 14, 18
fibula fracture, 845
finger injuries, 489-505
   Boutonnière deformity, 503-4
   carpometacarpal joint dislocations, 498-9
   chronic swan neck deformity, 503
   clinical approach, 489-92
   dislocation, 499
   fractures of phalanges, 497-8
   'jersey finger', 504
   ligament and tendon injuries, 499-504
   mallet finger, 501-3
   metacarpal fractures, 494-7
   overuse conditions, 504-5
   patient-reported outcome measures (PROMs), 493
first branch of lateral plantar nerve (Baxter's nerve) entrapment, 947-8
first tarsometatarsal joint pain, 955-6
flat foot, 989

flexibility in the rehabilitation process, 150
flexibility training, 149-50
flexion-pattern motor control dysfunction, 123
flexor hallucis longus tendinopathy, 924-6
fluid replacement and recovery, 197
foot
   biomechanical assessment, 96-8
   bones, 938
   first metatarsophalangeal joint (MTPJ) range, 98
   flat, 989
foot orthoses, 109-12
   comfort, 112
   custom-fabricated, 109-10
   effectiveness, 110-11
   fitting (contemporary approaches), 111-12
   mechanism of action, 110
   and over-use injuries, 183
   subtalar joint neutral, 111-12
   treatment direction test, 112
   types of, 109-10
foot pain, 937-72
   forefoot, 958-72
   midfoot, 948-58
   rear, 937-48
foot posture index, 96-8
footwear as therapy, 112-14
footwear assessment tool, 105-6
forearm compartment pressure syndrome, 461
forearm injuries and rowing, 132-3
forearm pain, 460-1
forefoot pain, 958-72
   causes, 958, 972
   clinical perspective, 958-9
   corns and calluses, 970
   first MTP joint sprain ("turf toe"), 966-7
   fractures of the fifth metatarsal, 961-5
   Frieberg's osterochondritis, 972
   hallux limitus, 967
   hallux valgus, 967-8
   Joplin's neuritis, 972
   Morton's interdigital neuroma, 970-1
   MTP joint synovitis, 965-6
   onychocryptosis 972
   plantar plate tear, 969-70
   plantar warts, 971
   sesamoid injuries, 968-9
   special metatarsal stress fracture: base of the second MT, 961
   stress fractures of the great toe, 972

   stress fractures of the neck of metatarsals I-IV, 959-61
   subungual exostosis, 972
   subungual haematoma, 972
   toe clawing, 972
fractures, 14, 15-16, 34
   acute, 976-9
   acute ankle injuries, 905, 907, 910-11
   acute elbow injuries, 456-7
   anterior calcaneal process, 910
   apopyseal (avulsion), 978-9
   avulsion fracture of the base of the fifth metatarsal, 908-10
   avulsion fracture of ischial tuberosity, 589
   clavicle, 424-6
   coronoid, 457
   diaphyseal, 978
   distal radius, 470-2
   facial bones, 343-6
   fibula, 845
   hook of hamate, 481-2
   lateral talar process, 910
   maisonneuve, 905
   medial tubercle, 911
   metacarpal, 494-7
   metaphyseal, 976-7
   nasal, 334
   olecranon, 456-7
   patella, 762
   phalanges, 497-8
   physeal (growth plate), 977-8
   posterior process of the talus, 911
   Pott's, 905
   radial head, 457
   radius and ulna, 460
   scaphoid, 472-5
   shoulder, 425, 432
   supracondylar, 456
   talus, 933
   tibia, 846
   tibial plateau, 767
   trapezium, 475-6
   triquetral, 482
   ulnar styloid, 481
   see also stress fractures
Freiberg's infarction, 989
Freiberg's osteochondritis, 972
'frozen shoulder', 429
fuel replacement and recovery, 197-8
function and injury, 212, 214
functional anatomy
   acute ankle injuries, 893-4
   anterior thigh pain, 660-1
   bones of the face, 331
   hip-related pain, 593-8
   posterior thigh pain, 679-81

Index

G

gabapentin, 267
gait, painless abnormalities of, 986-8
gait velocity and running, 94
ganglions, 478-9
gastrocnemius muscle strains, 853-6
    acute strain, 853-6
    operative intervention, 856
    physical examination, 853
    treatment, 853-6
gastrocnemius tendinopathy, 824
gender
    and ACL injuries, 755
    sport and exercise medicine, 1029
    and sports injuries, 166
general health and injury, 212
genetic disorders, 82
glenohumeral internal rotation deficit (GIRD), 382
    clinical evaluation, 394-5
    pathological, 417-19
    pathomechanics, 417
    treatment, 417-19
glenohumeral joint, posterior dislocation, 408
glucosamine, 272-3
glyceryl trinitrate (GTN) patches, 272
golf (biomechanical aspects of injuries), 128-30
    hip pain, 130
    low back pain, 130
    shoulder pain, 129
    wrist pain, 128-9
graded motor imagery and pain, 75
granulomatous diseases, 83
greater trochanteric pain, 622-3
green tea, 273
groin pain, 629-57
    acute groin injuries, 633, 642-3
    adductor-related, 643-50
    anatomy, 629-31
    assessment of severity, 635-9
    causes in athletes, 634
    classification, 633-4
    clinical examination, 635-9
    clinical overview, 634-42
    complete adductor avulsions, 654
    epidemiology, 631-2
    examination, 635-9
    hip adductors, 630
    hip flexors, 630
    iliopsoas-related, 650-1
    imaging, 639-42
    inguinal region, 631
    inguinal-related, 652-4
    injury prevention, 657
    longstanding groin pain, 633-4, 643-54
    nerve entrapments, 655
    obturator neuropathy, 654-5
    PROM, 639
    pubic symphysis, 629-30
    pubic-related, 654
    referred pain to the groin, 656-7
    risk factors, 632
    stress fractures of the inferior pubic ramus, 656
    stress fractures of the neck of the femur, 655-6
    terminology and definitions, 632-4
gymnast's wrist, 476

H

hallux limitus, 967
hallux valgus, 967-8
hamstring
    muscles, strengthening, 695-8
    proximal hamstring tendinopathy, 577-81
    proximal hamstring tendon rupture, 588-9
    tendon ruptures, 767
    upper hamstring tendinopathy, 710-11
    see also acute hamstring muscle strains
hamstring injuries
    acute management phase, 692-3
    intramuscular tendon injuries, 690
    management, 690-703
    nerve entrapments, 711
    rehabilitation, 693
    subacute/conditioning phase, 694-701
hamstring strains, prevention, 173-4, 705-7
    balance exercises/proprioception training, 705-6
    eccentric strength training, 705
    high-risk athlete, 706-7
    injury mechanisms, 173
    programs, 173-4
    risk factors, 173
    sport-specific training, 706
hamstring synergists, strengthening for, 698-9
hand injuries, 489-505
    Boutonnière deformity, 503-4
    carpometacarpal joint dislocations, 498-9
    chronic swan neck deformity, 503
    clinical approach, 489-92
    dislocation, 499
    exercises, 494
    finger joint dislocations, 499
    investigations, 492
    lacerations and infections, 504
    ligament and tendon injuries, 499-504
    mallet finger, 501-3
    metacarpal fractures, 494-7
    oedema control, 493-4
    overuse conditions, 504-5
    patient-reported outcome measures (PROMs), 493
    phalanges fractures, 497-8
    physical examination, 489-92
    sport-specific conditions, 490
    surgical referrals, 505
    taping and splinting, 494
    treatment principles, 492-4
hand pain, 485-6
HARM (heat, alcohol, running, massage), 250
headache, 317-29
    cervicogenic, 322-8, 374
    classification, 317
    clinical approach, 318-20
    clinical measurement, 319-20
    external compression, 328
    high-altitude, 328
    hypercapnia, 329
    measurement, 319-20
    migraine, 320-2
    post-traumatic, 328
    primary, 320-2
    primary exercise, 322
    secondary, 322-9
    in sport, 317-18
heel raise, single-leg, 102
herniation of nucleus pulposus from intervertebral disc, 18
high-altitude headache, 328
hight-intensity short-duration exercise, 190
hip adductors, 630
hip flexors, 630
Hip and Groin Outcome Score (HAGOS), 232, 233
hip
    control in functional task performance, 618-19
    instability, 614
    irritable, 984
    joint, 85
    lateral pain, 622-8
    ligaments, 596
hip-related pain, 593-628
    acetabular labrum, 594-5
    adverse loading, 620-1
    arthroscopy, 621-2
    balance and proprioception, 618
    biomechanics, 593-8
    causes, 599
    chondral surfaces, 596
    chondropathy, 613-14
    clinical approach, 598-604
    diagnostic imaging tests, 605
    distal factors, 607

Index

femoroacetabular impingement (FAI), 607-10
functional anatomy, 593-8
functional task performance, 620
gait biodynamics, 620
greater trochanteric pain, 622-3
iliac crest pain, 623
investigations, 603-4
labral tears, 610-12
ligamentum teres tears, 612
morphology, 594
muscle function, 596-8
muscle strength, 616-18
osteoarthritis, 610
physical examination, 601-3
predisposing factors, 604-7
PROMs, 603-4
proximal factors, 606
rehabilitation, 614-15, 621-2
remote factors, 606-7
restoring ROM, 615
surgical management, 621-2
synovitis, 612-13
systemic factors, 607
treatment, 614-22, 625-8
trunk muscle strength, 619-20
homunculi, motor and sensory, 66
hook of hamate fracture, 481-2
hyaline cartilage, 14, 17-18
hyaluronic acid, 269-70
hypercapnia headache, 329
hyperextension injuries (elbow), 460
hypertrophy training, 149
hyphema, 339

I

ice (acute injury management), 248, 692
idiopathic scoliosis, 981
iliac crest pain, 623
iliopsoas-related groin pain, 650-1
iliotibial band friction syndrome (IBTFS), 809-13
imaging
  bone stress injuries, 35-7
  groin pain, 639-42
  neck pain, 353
impingement syndromes, 481, 911
inciting event (injury causation), 166
individual needs
  sport and exercise medicine (SEM), 5
individualisation (training), 140
infections, 83
inferential stimulation, 262
inguinal hernia, 654
inguinal region, 631

inguinal-related groin pain, 652-4
  diagnostic criteria, 652
  treatment, 652-4
injection therapy, 268
injections
  autologous blood, 273
  corticosteroid injection (lateral elbow tendinopathy), 448-9
  high-volume, 269
  local anaesthetic, 268-9
  mechanical, 269
injured athlete
  from injury to return to play, 7
injuries see sports injuries
injury management, acute, 247-50
  compression, 248-50
  elevation, 250
  ice, 248
  initial management, 13-15
  optimal loading, 247-8
  pathophysiology, 13-15
  protection, 247
injury prevention, 165-88
  ankle sprains, 174-7
  conceptual approach, 165-6
  hamstring strains, 173-4
  knee, 177-81
  and managing load, 183-6
  overuse injuries, 181-3
  playing surfaces, 187-8
  protective equipment, 187
  risk management, 166-73
  targeted program, 172-3
input-dominated pain, 65-9
  from musculoskeletal tissues, 66
  neuropathic, 68-9
  referred pain, 66-8
instability and injury, 212
insurance medical assessment, 1014
integrated performance health management and coaching model, 4
intersection syndrome, 477-8
interval training, 142
intramuscular tendon injuries, 690
iontophoresis, 448
irritable hip, 984
ischial bursitis, 711
ischial tuberosity avulsion fracture, 589
ischiofemoral impingement, 587
isokinetic exercises
  for resistance, 146
isometric exercises
  for resistance, 144-5
  tendinopathy rehabilitation, 50-1
isotonic exercises
  for resistance, 145-6
  tendinopathy rehabilitation, 51

J

Jack's test for first metatarsophalangeal joint (MTPJ) range 97, 98, 101, 939
'jersey finger', 504
jet lag, 1023-5
  and air travel, 1023
  prevention, 1023-5
  symptomatic treatment for, 1025
joint motion, lower limb, 85-8
joints
  dislocation/subluxation, 14, 18-19
  overuse sports injuries, 43
Jones fracture, 962-4
Joplin's neuritis, 972

K

Kienböck's disease, 479-81
kinetic chain integration, 433-5
knee
  assessment, 102-3
  tibiofemoral alignment at the, 99
  see also anterior knee pain
knee injuries, acute
  injury mechanisms, 177
  prevention, 177-81
  prevention programs, 177-81
  risk factors, 177
knee joint, 85
knee pain
  and cycling, 121-4
  and rowing, 133
  and swimming, 136
  see anterior knee pain; lateral knee pain; medial knee pain; posterior knee pain
Köhler's disease, 956, 988-9

L

labral tears, 610-12
lacerations and contusions (facial injuries), 332-3
  immediate management, 332
  management of larger, 332-3
language and pain, 75
laser therapy, 262-3
lateral ankle pain, 929-33
  anterolateral impingement, 932-3
  causes, 929
  examination, 929
  peroneal tendinopathy, 929-31
  posterior impingement syndrome, 933
  referred pain, 933
  sinus tarsi syndrome, 931-2
  stress fractures of the talus, 933
lateral collateral ligament complex (LCLC), 440

1046

Index

lateral collateral ligament tears, 759-60
    posterolateral corner (PLC) injuries, 759-60
lateral elbow pain, 136-7, 440-51
    causes, 441, 451
    examination, 441-2
    history, 440-1
    investigations, 442-3
lateral elbow tendinopathy, 443-51
    acupuncture, 447
    autologous blood, 450
    botulinum toxin, 450
    bracing and taping, 447-8
    clinical features, 444-5
    clinical relevant pathology, 443-4
    correct predisposing factors, 450
    corticosteroid injection, 448-9
    electrotherapeutic modalities, 446
    exercises for strengthening and coordination, 445-6
    Iontophoresis, 448
    nitric oxide donor therapy, 449-50
    return to activity, 450-1
    soft tissue therapy, 446-7
    surgery, 450
    treatment, 445
    trigger points, 447
lateral exertional compartment syndrome, 843-4
lateral femoral cutaneous nerve injury ('meralgia paresthetica'), 676
lateral hip pain, 622-8
lateral knee pain, 805-16
    causes, 806, 814-16
    clinical approach, 806-9
    iliotibial band friction syndrome, 809-13
    investigations, 809
    lateral meniscus abnormality, 813-14
lateral ligament injuries, 899-900
    treatment and rehabilitation, 900-4
lateral meniscus abnormality, 813-14
lateral plantar nerve, 947-8
leg length assessment, 99-100
leg pain, 825-46
    biomechanics, 826
    causes, 827, 829
    chronic exertional compartment syndrome, 834-6, 841-45
    clinical approach, 825-36
    diagnostic questions, 830
    fractured tibia and fibula, 846
    investigations, 832-6
    medial tibial stress syndrome, 839-41
    nerve entrapment, 845-6
    outcome measures, 832
    patient-reported outcome measures, 833
    periosteal contusion, 846
    physical examination, 828-32
    referred pain, 845
    stress fracture of the anterior cortex of the tibia, 838
    stress fracture of the fibula, 845
    stress fracture of the tibia, 836-8
    vascular entrapments, 846
leisure activities and injury, 212
lens dislocation (eye injury), 339
ligament injuries
    bifurcate, 952
    classification of, 20
    dorsal calcaneocuboid, 952
    examination, 215
    hand and finger, 499-504
    hips, 596
    medial (deltoid), 904-5
    and NSAIDs, 266
    overuse sports injuries, 43
    sprain/tear, 14, 19-21
    see also lateral ligament injuries
ligamentum teres tears, 612
lisfranc joint injuries, 952-5
    causes, 953
    clinical features, 953-4
    investigations, 954
    treatment, 954-5
load management
    for performance enhancement, 150-1
    and prevention of injury, 183-6
load ratio, monitoring acute:chronic, 184-6
local anaesthetic injections, 268-9
local anaesthetic patches, 267
long-duration exercise, 190-1
long thoracic nerve injury, 430
low back pain
    and cycling, 123
    and rowing, 130-2
lower limb biomechanical abnormalities
    biofeedback, 108-9
    foot orthosis, 109-12
    management of, 108-14
    movement pattern retraining, 108-9
    taping, 112-14
lower limb biomechanics, 85-90
    common observations, 101
    conditions related to suboptimal, 106-8
    ideal neutral stance position, 88-90
    joint motion, 85-8
lower limb biomechanics assessment, 95-105
    dynamic movement, 104-5
    functional tests, 100-4
    structural ('static') assessment, 96-100
    summary, 105
lower limb joint motion, 85-8
    ranges of motion, 86
lower limb overuse injuries, 107-8
lower limb stiffness, 749
lower limb tests, functional, 100-4
    landing-specific considerations, 103-4
    single-leg heel raise, 102
    single-leg squat, 102-3
    single-leg stance with progressions, 100
low-level laser therapy (LLLT), 262-3
lubricants (soft tissue therapy), 255
lumbar spine, referred pain from, 576, 707-9
lumbopelvic control, 155-6
lumbopelvic dysfunction, 154-5
lumbopelvic pain, 162
lunotriquetral dissociation, 482-3

M

magnetic resonance imaging (MRI), 12, 35-7, 129, 221-3, 224-7, 306, 353, 469
    acute knee injuries, 722-3
    groin pain, 641-2
    shoulder investigations, 401
maisonneuve fracture, 905
mallet finger, 502
management
    bone stress injuries, 38-42
    of concussion, 298-310
    of mechanical neck pain, 365-74
    and return-to-play decisions, 292
    sport and exercise medicine (SEM), 4-5
    sports injuries, 13-15
mandibular fractures, 344-5
manual treatments (musculoskeletal conditions), 250-9
    joint techniques, 251-2
    neurodynamic techniques, 258-9
    soft tissue therapy, 252-8
manipulation (musculoskeletal conditions), 251-2
Marfan syndrome, 79, 82, 340
massage and recovery, 191-2, 200
maxillary fractures, 344
Maximal Aerobic Speed (MAS) training, 143
mechanotherapy, 241-5
medial ankle pain, 917-29
    causes, 917, 927
    examination, 918
    flexor hallucis longus tendinopathy, 924-6
    history, 917-18
    investigations, 918-19

1047

Index

medial calcaneal nerve entrapment, 928-9
medial malleolar stress fracture, 928
PROMs, 918, 920-23
tarsal tunnel syndrome, 926-8
tibialis posterior tendinopathy, 923-4, 955
medial calcaneal nerve entrapment, 928-9
medial collateral ligament (MCL) injury, 729-36, 816-17
  chronic, 819-20
  rehabilitation, 730-1
  treatment, 729-36
medial (deltoid) ligament injuries, 904-5
medial knee pain, 136, 816-20
  causes, 817, 819-20
  chronic, 819-20
  medial meniscus abnormality, 817-18
  patellofemoral syndrome, 817
  Pellegrini-Stieda syndrome, 819-20
  pes anserinus tendinopathy/bursitis, 819
medial malleolar stress fracture, 928
medial meniscus abnormality, 817-18
medial tibial stress syndrome, 839-1
medial tubercle fractures, 911
median nerve entrapment, 461
medical assessment, periodic (sports injuries), 171-2
medical equipment, 1018
medicine team
  attributes, 1017-18
  equipment, 1018
  indemnity and trauma training, 1018
  support team, 1017
  sport and exercise, 2-3
meniscal injuries, 723-8
  clinical features, 724-6
  non-surgical management, 727
  rehabilitation, 727-8
  surgical management, 727
  symptomatic meniscus tears, 748
  treatment, 726-7
meniscal lesions, degenerative, 724-5
mental health issues and concussion, 310
metacarpal fractures, 494-7
metatarsal, avulsion fracture of the base of the fifth, 908-10
midfoot pain, 948-58
  abductor hallucis strains, 956
  causes, 948, 955-8
  cuboid syndrome, 956
  extensor tendinopathy, 956
  first tarsometatarsal joint pain, 955-6
  investigations, 949

Köhler's disease, 956
lisfranc joint injuries, 952-5
midtarsal joint sprains, 952
navicular stress fracture, 949-52
peroneal tendinopathy, 956
stress fracture of the cuboid, 956
stress fracture of the cuneiforms, 956
tarsal coalition, 957-8
tibialis posterior tendinopathy (distal pain presentation), 955
midportion Achilles tendinopathy, 872-84
  biomechanical factors, 877
  cell-based therapies, 883
  four-stage program, 878
  pathology, 872-6
  predisposition factors, 876-7
  sclerosing, 882-3
  treatment, 877-84
midtarsal joint sprains, 952
migraine, 320-2
  post-traumatic, 328
military personnel, 991-1001
  aerobic fitness, 997-8
  blister injuries, 994-5
  body composition, 998
  common injuries, 991-6
  epidemiology of military injuries, 992-3
  gender, 997-8
  injury prevention, 996-1001
  injury surveillance, 996-7
  overuse of lower limb, 994
  parachute injuries, 995
  previous injuries, 998-9
  special culture, 991-2
  warm-up/stretching, 1000-1001
  weekly running distance, 999-1000
mobilisation (musculoskeletal conditions), 251-2
Morton's interdigital neuroma, 970-1
motion
  lower limb joint, 85-8
motor adaption to pain, 72-5
  education, 74
  exercise/progressive loading, 74-5
  graded motor imagery, 75
  manual therapy, 74
  medications, 74
  treatment options for patients, 72-3
motor control
  balance between movement and stiffness, 155
  and biology of pain, 158-9
  clinical principles, 160-4
  common misconceptions, 155
  and core stability, 154-64
  and the individual, 159
  lumbopelvic control, 155-6

lumbopelvic dysfunction, 154-5
lumbopelvic pain, 162
and motor learning, 157-8
and neck pain, 370-2
and treatments for musculoskeletal conditions, 245-6
and pain prevention, 164
and rehabilitation, 156-7
motor function (neck pain), 370-73
motor learning, 163
mouth guards, 341-3
movement assessment, dynamic, 104-5
movement biomechanics (running), 90-5
movement pattern retraining (lower limb biomechanics), 108-9
MRI *see* magnetic resonance imaging (MRI)
MTP joint synovitis, 965-6
Müller-Wohlfahrt, Hans-Wilhelm, 1033
multiskilling, 3
muscle cramps, 25, 849
muscle disorders, 81
muscular endurance, 149
muscle factors
  bone stress injuries, 33
muscle function in hips, 596-8
muscle function tests (neck pain), 358-62
muscle injuries
  acute, classification, 22
  acute compartment syndrome, 24-5
  chronic compartment syndrome (CCS), 45
  contusion, 23-4
  cramp, 25
  exercise-induced muscle soreness, 45-6
  gastrocnemius muscle strains, 853-6
  and mechanotherapy, 245
  myofascial pain, 43-5
  myositis ossificans, 24
  and NSAID, 266
  overuse sports injuries, 43-6
  shoulder, 429
  soleus muscle strains, 856-9
  strain/tear 14, 21-3
muscle soreness and NMES, 193
muscle weakness following ACL reconstruction, 749-50
musculoskeletal conditions, management of, 976-91
  acute fractures, 976-9
  overuse injuries of the physis, 979
musculoskeletal conditions, treatments for, 239-75
  actovegin, 269
  acute injury management, 247-50
  analgesics, 264

autologous blood, 273
bisphosphonates, 272
cell therapy, 274
chondroitin, 272-2
corticosteroid, 270-1
dry needling, 256-8
electromagnetic therapy, 263
electrophysical agents, 261-4
exercise-induced hypoalgesia, 246
extracorporeal shockwave therapy, 263-4
glucosamine, 272-3
green tea/polyphenols, 273
GTN patches, 272
hyaluronic acid, 269-70
interferential stimulation, 262
laser, 262-3
local anaesthetic injections, 268-9
manual treatments, 250-9
mechanical and high-volume injections, 269
mechanotherapy, 241-5
motor-control training, 245-6
neurodynamic techniques, 258-9
neuromuscular stimulators, 262
neuropathic pain, 267-8
neutraceuticals in injury management, 272-3
NSAIDs, 264-7
omega-s fatty acids, 272-3
platelet-rich plasma, 273
prolotherapy, 269
quinolone antibiotics, 272
sclerosant, 269
sleep medication, 271
soft-tissue therapy, 252-6
surgery, 274-5
taping, 259-61
TENS, 262
therapeutic exercise, 241-6
therapeutic medication, 264-72
therapeutic ultrasound, 261
traumeel, 269
vitamin D, 273
musculoskeletal symptoms and diagnosis, 212
musculoskeletal tissues and input-dominated pain, 66
myofascial, 574-6
myofascial pain syndrome, 43-5, 68
myofascial tension, sustained, 254
myositis ossificans, 24, 670-1

N

nasal fractures, 334
natural grass *vs.* artificial turf, 187-8
navicular stress fracture, 949-52
  clinical features, 949-50
  investigations, 950
  management, 950-52
neck extensors, 372
neck flexors, 370-1
neck pain, 347-75
  acceleration/deceleration injury (whiplash), 375
  active movement tests, 355-7
  acute wry neck, 374
  anatomical considerations, 347-9
  axio-scapular muscles, 361-2, 372
  biopsychosocial model for, 350
  brachial plexus injuries (stingers/burners), 375
  cervical arterial dysfunction, 364
  cervical extensors, assessment of, 360-1
  cervical flexors, assessment of, 358-60
  cervical nerve injury, 374-5
  cervical radiculopathy, 374-5
  cervical sensorimotor function, tests for, 362-4
  cervicogenic headache, 374
  clinical neurological examination, 357
  clinical perspective, 349-65
  conditions, 374-5
  education, 366-7
  imaging, 353
  maintenance program, 374
  manual therapy, 367-9
  mechanical, management of, 365-74
  motor control, 370-2
  muscle function, tests of, 358-62
  nervous system, tests of the, 357-8
  neural tissue mobilisation, 369-70
  pain management, 367
  passive tests, 357
  patient reported outcome measures (PROMs), 352
  performance-based outcome measures, 364-5
  physical examination, 353-64
  postural analysis, 354-5
  posture, 371-2
  presentations (red flags), 351
  psychological features, 352
  quantitative sensory testing, 357
  resistance training, 372-3
  social/sport factors, 352
  sport and functional modifications, 365-6
  symptoms and behaviours, 351
  training motor function, 370-73
  training sensorimotor control, 373-4
nerve entrapments
  calf pain, 862-3
  compartment syndrome, 844
  hamstring, 711
  groin pain, 655
  medial calcaneal, 928-9
nerve injuries, 26, 52
  cervical, 374-5
nerve tissue pain (neuropathetic pain), 68-9, 268
nervous system tests (neck pain), 357-8
neural mechanosensitivity, 214
neural tissue mobilisation, 369-70
neurodynamic techniques (musculoskeletal conditions), 258-9
neuromechanical sensitivity and injuries, 215-19
neuromuscular control exercises, 699-701
neuromuscular electrical stimulation (NMES), 193, 199, 262
neuromyofascial causes of calf pain, 862
neuropathic pain, 68-9
neuropraxia, 26
neuropsychological tests (cognitive function and concussion), 308-9
neurovascular injuries, 429-32
neutral stance position, 88-90
nociception, 56-9, 67
non-steroidal anti-inflammatory drugs (NSAIDs), 264-7
  adverse effects, 266-7
  hamstring injuries, 692-3
  use in sport, 265-6
  and musculoskeletal injury, 266
  and wrist injuries, 486
Nordic hamstring, 699
nose injuries, 333-5
  fractures, 334
  septal haematoma, 334-5
nosebleed, 333-4
nutraceuticals in injury management, 272-3
nutrition and recovery, 196-9, 200
nutritional factors and injury, 213
nutritional strategies
  and prevention of stress fractures, 182

O

obturator neuropathy, 654-5
olecranon fractures, 456-7
omega-3 fatty acids, 272-3
on-field management of concussion, 298-300
on-field rehabilitation, 8
onychocryptosis 972
open chain exercises, 146-8

1049

Index

open wounds, treatment of, 27
optimal loading (acute injury management), 247-8
orbital fracture, 343-4
orthoses, 109-12, 183, 788
Osgood-Schlatter disease, 802, 888, 984-6
osteoarthritis, 610, 762-3, 814
osteochondral injuries, 17-18
osteochondral lesions of the talar dome, 906-8
otitis externa, 336
Ottawa ankle rules, 897, 898, 905
overload (training), 140
overtraining and injury, 213
overuse injuries *see* sports injuries, overuse

P

pain, 55-62
  and the brain, 59-61
  biology of, 158-9
  centrally dominated, 69-75
  definition, 55-6
  and diagnosis, 211-12
  and language, 75
  persistent, 60-1, 154
  prevention, 164
  and PROMs, 231-7
  radicular, 67-8
  referred, 66-8, 576, 656-7, 677, 707-9, 816, 845, 888, 933
  syndromes, 83-4
  treating, 61-3
  treatment options, 72-5
  from trigger points, 44, 83
  see also individual locations and types of pain
pain, clinical aspects, 65-76
  centrally dominated, 69-72
  input-dominated, 65-9
palpation and injuries, 215
paratenonitis, 49-50
passive movement tests, 357
patellar
  acute patellar trauma, 762-5
  dislocation, 762-5
  fracture, 762
  pain, 748-9
  tendinopathy, 769-1, 791-9, 986
  tendon rupture, 765-7
  treatment, 765
patellofemoral instability, 792-3
patellofemoral pain, 769, 770, 771, 774-92
patellofemoral pain, treatment, 782-90
  braces, 789
  exercise, 783-90
  extrinsic contributing factors, 790

in-shoe foot orthoses, 788
manual therapies, 788
physical intervention, 789-90
surgery, 790
patellofemoral syndrome, 817
pathophysiology, 30-31
  and concussion, 298
patient-reported outcome measures (PROMs), 210, 231-8
  Achilles pain, 872
  anterior knee pain, 774-5
  considerations for 'good' use, 232-5
  definition, 231
  easiness to use, 232-3
  evaluation dimensions, 233
  groin pain, 639
  hand and finger injuries, 493
  hip-related pain, 603-4
  leg pain, 833
  low back pain, 529-30
  medial ankle pain, 918, 920-3
  and neck pain, 352
  patellofemoral pain, 775
  and patient changes, 233-5
  plantar fasciopathy, 941-6
  use in sports medicine, 231-2
  wrist pain, 471
pectoralis major tears, 429
Pellegrini-Stieda syndrome, 819-20
pelvis/hip function assessment, 102
perforated eardrum, 335-6
performance enhancement, training load management for, 150-1
periodic medical assessment (PMA), 171-2
periodisation (training), 139-40
periosteal contusion, 16-17
peroneal tendinopathy, 929-33, 956
persistent pain, 60-1
  contribution of body and mind, 154
Perthes' disease, 983
pes anserinus tendinopathy/bursitis, 819-20
phalanges fractures, 497-8
pharmacotherapy, 799
physical activity and clinician, 6
physical activity history
  bone stress injuries, 34
physical conditioning
  bone stress injury management, 40
physical examination
  Achilles pain, 868-72
  acute Achilles tendon rupture, 890
  acute knee injuries, 716-17
  anterior knee pain, 771-4
  anterior thigh pain, 661-4
  bone stress injuries, 35
  gastrocnemius muscle strains, 853
  hip-related pain, 601-3
  and injury, 213-21

and leg pain, 828-32
posterior thigh pain, 682-4
shoulder pain, 383-8
and wrist pain, 466
physical examination and neck pain, 353-65
  active movement tests, 355-7
  anterior knee pain, 771-4
  axio-scapular muscles, 361-2
  cervical arterial dysfunction, 364
  cervical extensors assessment, 360-1
  cervical flexors assessment, 358-60
  cervical sensorimotor function, 362-4
  clinical neurological examination, 357
  manual examination of segmental dysfunction, 357
  muscles function, 358-62
  nervous system, 357-8
  passive tests, 357
  patellofemoral pain, 775
  postural analysis, 354-5
  quantitative sensory testing, 357
Physiotherapy Evidence Database (PEDro), 10, 11-12
piriformis syndrome, 585-7
plantar fasciopathy, 941-6
  alignment of the foot, 942
  clinical features, 942-3
  flexibility and strength, 942
  investigations, 942-3
  PROMs, 940
  risk factors, 941-3
  standing work, 942
  training volume, 942
  treatment, 943-6
  weight and BMI, 941
plantar nerve, first branch of lateral (Baxter's nerve) entrapment, 947-8
plantar plate tear, 972-3
plantar warts, 971
platelet-rich plasma (PRP), 273
play, return to (RTP), 285-93
  StARRT, 285-93
playing surface
  bone stress injuries, 33
POLICE (protection, optimal loading, ice, compression, elevation), 247, 280
polyphenols, 273
popliteal artery entrapment syndrome (PAES), 859-61
popliteal cysts, 986
popliteus tendinopathy, 823
posterior cruciate ligament (PCL) tears, 755-9
  clinical features, 756-7
  treatment, 757-9

posterior dislocation (acute elbow injuries), 457-9
posterior knee pain, 820-24
    Baker's cyst, 822-3
    biceps femoris tendinopathy, 823
    causes, 821, 824
    claudication, 824
    clinical evaluation, 820-22
    deep venous thrombosis, 824
    examination, 821-2
    gastrocnemius tendinopathy, 824
    investigations, 822
    popliteus tendinopathy, 823
posterior impingement syndrome, 887-8, 933
posterior thigh compartment syndrome, 587-8
posterior thigh pain, 679-712
    acute hamstring muscle strain, 685-705
    adductor magnus strains, 711
    avulsion of the hamstring from the ischial tuberosity, 709-10
    causes, 682
    clinical approach, 681-5
    compartment syndrome, 711
    functional anatomy, 679-81
    hamstring strains prevention, 705-7
    investigations, 684-5
    ischial bursitis, 711
    lumbar spine, 708-9
    nerve entrapments, 711
    physical examination, 682-5
    referred pain, 707-9
    sacroiliac complex, 709
    trigger points, 707
    upper hamstring tendinopathy, 710-11
    vascular, 712
posterolateral corner (PLC) injuries, 759-60
post-traumatic headache, 328
post-traumatic migraine, 328
post-traumatic synovitis, 913-14
postural abnormalities and young athlete, 982
postural imbalance, 514
posture, 371-2
Pott's fracture, 905
power training, 148-9
pregabalin, 267
Pre-Hospital Emergency Care Course (PHECC), 299
Pre-Hospital Trauma Life Support (PHTLS), 299
PRICE (protection, rest, ice, compression and elevation), 247, 280
primary headache, 320-2
primary exercise headache, 322

Profile of Mood State (POMS) scores, 191
prolotherapy, 269
Proprioceptive Neuromuscular Facilitation (PNF) stretching, 150
protective equipment and injury prevention, 187
protection (acute injury management), 247
proximal hamstring tendinopathy, 577-81
proximal hamstring tendon rupture, 588-9
psychological effects
    of active recovery, 191
    of massage, 192
psychological factors and injury, 213
pubic ramus stress fractures, 590
pubic related groin pain, 654
pubic symphysis, 629-30
published appraisals and (EBP), 10-11
PubMed, 10, 11
pulsed electromagnetic field therapy (PEMF), 263

Q

quadriceps contusion, 664-71
    compartment syndrome, 670
    complications, 670-1
    distinguishing features, 665
    grading, 665
    myositis ossificans, 670-1
    treatment, 666-770
quadriceps strain, 671-4
    avulsion injury, 673-4
    complete rectus femoris tear, 673
    distal quadriceps muscle strain, 671-3
    prevention, 674
    proximal rectus femoris strain, 672-3
    treatment, 672
quadriceps tendinopathy, 802
Quality Assessment of Diagnostic Accuracy Studies (QUADAS), 206
quantitative sensory testing (neck pain), 357
quinolone antibiotics, 272

R

radial column presentations, 470-8
radial epiphyseal injury (gymnast's wrist), 476
radial head fracture, 456
radial sensory nerve compression, 478
radial tunnel syndrome, 460-1
radicular pain, 67-8
radiological investigation, 466-70

range of motion exercises and neck pain management, 368-9
range of motion testing
    active, 214
    passive, 215
randomised control trials (RCTs), 10, 11
rearfoot pain, 937-51
    calcaneal stress fractures, 947
    causes, 939
    clinical features, 942-3
    examination, 939
    fat pad contusion, 946-7
    first branch of lateral plantar nerve (Baxter's nerve) entrapment, 948-9
    history, 937
    inferior foot pain, 939
    investigations, 939-40
    plantar fasciopathy, 941-6
    PROMs, 940
    treatment, 943-6
recovery, 189-200
    active, 189-91, 200
    assessment, 189
    compression, 195, 200
    massage, 191-2, 200
    modalities, 200
    neuromuscular electrical stimulation (NMES), 193, 200
    nutrition, 196-9, 200
    practical considerations, 199-200
    sleep, 194-5
    stretching, 193-4, 200
    water immersion, 195-6, 200
rehabilitation, 239
    Achilles tendon ruptures, 890-2
    ACL injury, 745-50
    acute ankle injuries, 900-4, 908
    closed chain exercises, 147-8
    effective planning, 278
    and the flexibility process, 150
    goal setting, 279-80
    groin pain, 649
    hamstring muscle strains, 693
    hip-related pain, 614-15, 621-2
    isometric exercises, 50-1
    isotonic exercises, 51
    lateral ligament injuries, 900-4
    low back pain, 563, 748
    lower limb (tendinopathy) 50-1
    medial collateral ligament injury, 730-1
    meniscal injuries, 727-8
    open chain exercises, 147-8
    phases, 280-3
    principles of sports injury, 277-83
    and return to play (RTP), 285-93
    scapular dyskinesis, 420-4
    shoulder injuries, 402-7, 412-14
    and sleep, 271

Index

sports, 1029
targeted interventions, 279-80
tendon injuries, 145
when it doesn't go to plan, 283
wrist, 475, 487
rehabilitation gym, 8
research and (EBP), 10-12
resistance exercises
  classification, 146-8
  closed chain exercises, 146-8
  isokinetic exercises, 146
  isometric exercises 144-5
  isotonic exercises, 145-6
  open chain exercises, 146-8
  types of, 144-6
resistance training, 144-9
  hypertrophy training, 149
  loading patterns, 148
  muscular endurance, 149
  and neck pain, 372-3
  power, 148-9
  qualities of, 148-9
  strength, 148
rest (acute injury management), 692
retinal detachment, 340
retinal haemorrhage, 339
retrieving articles and EDP, 11
retrocalcaneal bursitis (enthesis organ), 884-7
return to play (RTP), 285-93
  ACL injury, 751-2
  acute Achilles tendon rupture, 889-2
  acute ankle injuries, 902-3
  additional perspectives, 289
  beyond risk for injury, 287
  and concussion, 306-10
  decision making, 290-3
  gastrocnemius muscle strains, 856
  lateral elbow tendinopathy, 451
  outcomes and probabilities, 288-9
  and PMA, 1014
  risk tolerance modifiers, 287
  and shoulder injuries, 437-8
  StARRT, 285-93
  tissue health, 286-7
  tissue stress, 287
return-to-sport phase
  groin pain, 649
  posterior thigh pain, 701-3
reverse Nordics, 669
rheumatological conditions, 80-1
RICE (rest, ice, compression, elevation) 692
rib stress fractures (RFS), 132, 515
rib trauma, 516-7
risk factors
  acute hamstring pain, 703-5
  bone stress injuries, 31-4

groin injuries, 632
plantar fasciopathy, 941-3
risk management and injury prevention, 166-73
Roland Morris Disability Questionnaire, 529-30
rotator cuff
  injuries, 402-7
  tears, 406-7
  tests, 390
rotator cuff tendinopathy, 402-6
rowing (biomechanical aspects of injuries), 130-3
  chest wall pain, 132
  knee pain, 133
  low back pain, 130-2
  wrist and forearm injuries, 132-3
running
  barefoot/minimalist, 183
running (bone stress injury management), 40-2
  anti-gravity treadmill training, 41
  gait retraining, 41-2
  program design, 42
  returning to, 40-2
running (movement biomechanics), 90-5
  angle and base of gait, 93
  comparing heel and forefoot strike patterns, 94-5
  influence of fatigue, 95
  influence of gait velocity, 94
  initial swing, 92-3
  landing point relative to centre of mass, 94
  loading (heel strike to foot flat), 90-1
  midstance (foot flat to heel off), 91-2
  propulsion (heel off to toe off), 92
  terminal swing, 93

S

scaphoid fracture, 472-5
scapholunate dissociation, 479
scapular
  involvement tests, 390
  in normal shoulder function, 379-80
  snapping scapular syndrome, 432-3
scapular biomechanics
  abnormal, 118
  normal biomechanics of the scapular, 117-18
  in shoulder injuries, 118-19
scapular dyskinesis, 419-24
  rehabilitation, 421-4
  and shoulder pain, 419-20
sacral and pubic ramus stress fractures, 590

sacroiliac complex, 709
sacroiliac joint dysfunction, 581-5
SCAT3™, 301-4, 312-15
Scheuermann's disease, 512
sclerosant, 269
sclerosing, 882-883
second impact syndrome (SIS), 310
secondary headache, 322-9
self-treatment of soft tissues, 256
sensation of primary nociceptors ('peripheral sensitisation'), 57-8
sensation of spinal nociceptors ('central sensitisation'), 58-9
sensorimotor control (neck pain), 373-4
sensory discrimination training and pain, 75
septal haematoma, 334
serotonin reuptake inhibitors, 267
sesamoid injuries, 968-9
Sever's disease, 888, 988
sex and periodic medical assessment, 1012
sexual activity and teams, 1020
shin pain, common causes, 827
'shin splints' 4
shoes and inserts
  bone stress injuries, 33
  patellofemoral pain, 788
  and preventing overuse injuries, 182-3
shoulder injuries
  anterior dislocation, 408
  Bankart repair, 408
  fractures, 425, 432
  neurovascular injuries, 429-32
  and overhead athletes, 433-8
  posterior dislocation of the glenohumeral joint, 408
  rehabilitation guidelines, 402, 412-14
  and return to play, 437-8
  rotator cuff injuries, 402-7
  scapular biomechanics in, 118-19
  and tennis, 137-8
  treatment, 402-7
shoulder instability, 407-14
  acquired sport-specific instability (AIOS), 408-12, 418
  atraumatic multidirectional instability (AMBRI), 411
  rehabilitation, 402, 412-14
  traumatic shoulder instability (TUBS), 407-8
shoulder pain, 377-438
  acromioclavicular joint injuries, 426-8
  acute vs. overuse, 380
  adhesive capsulitis 'frozen shoulder' 429

anatomy, 377-80
biceps-related pathology, 414-16
biomechanics, 377-80
causes, 380-2, 428-323
clavicle fractures, 424-6
dynamic stabilisers, 379
and golf, 129-30
impingement, 380-2, 388-9
muscle tears, 429
neurovascular injuries, 429-32
objective measurements, 397-9
patient-reported outcome measures, 400-1
pathological glenohumeral internal rotation deficit, 417-19
scapular dyskinesis, 419-24
scapular in normal shoulder function, 379-80
SLAP lesions, 394, 414-17
special considerations for the overhead athlete, 433-8
static stabilisers, 377-9
and swimming, 133-6
and tennis, 137-8
young athletes, 979-80
shoulder pain, clinical approach, 382-402
additional tests, 396
arthrography, 401
biceps pathology, 394
clinical evaluation of GIRD, 394-5
diagnostic testing, 388-96
diagnosis arthroscopy, 402
history, 383
impingement tests, 388-90
instability tests, 390
investigations, 397-402
MRI, 401
physical examination, 383-8
rotator cuff tests, 390
scapular involvement tests, 390
screening of the kinetic chain, 396
shoulder symptom modification procedure, 395-6
SLAP lesion tests, 394
ultrasound, 401
X-ray, 397-401
shoulder symptom modification procedure (SSMP), 395
side strain, 519-20
side-lying slump test, 664
Sinding-Larsen-Johansson disease, 986
Sinding-Larsen-Johansson lesion, 802
single-leg heel raise (functional lower limb test), 102
single-leg squat (functional lower limb test), 102-3
single-leg stance with progressions (functional lower limb test), 100
sinus tarsi syndrome, 914, 931-2

skill training
 as agility, 144
 as speed, 143-4
skin cancers, 52-3
skin infections, 52-3
skin injuries, 14, 27
 overuse sports injuries, 52-3
SLAP lesions, 380, 382, 394, 402, 411, 414-17
 treatment, 416-17
sleep and recovery, 194-5, 200
sleep hygiene strategies, 195
sleep medication, 271
slipped capital femoral epiphysis, 983-4
snapping scapular syndrome, 432
soccer and groin pain, 631
social/sport factors (neck pain), 352
soft tissue
 injuries, 16
 laxity, 749
 stiffness, 749
 tumours, 78-80
soft tissue therapy, 252-6
 combination treatments, 255
 depth of treatment, 255
 digital ischaemic pressure, 253-4
 friction, 254-5
 lubricants, 255
 self-treatment, 256
 sustained myofascial tension, 254
 treatment position, 252-6
 vacuum cupping, 255
soleus muscle strains, 856-9
somatic pain, 68
specificity (training), 140
speed intervals, 143
speed training, 143-4
 skill training as speed, 144
 technique training, 143
spinal cord and pain, 60
spinal examination, 214, 219-21
spiral fracture (distal third), 965
spondyloarthropathies, 589-91
spondylolisthesis, 543-5, 981-2
spondylolysis, 981
spondylolytic bone stress injury, 541-2
Sport Concussion Assessment Tool (SCAT3)™
 Child-SCAT3™, 312-15
 SCAT3™, 301-4, 311
sport and exercise medicine (SEM), 2-8
 case manager approach, 6-8
 challenges of management, 4-5
 clinician, 5-6
 coach, the athlete and the clinician, 5-6
 from injury to return to play, 7

model, 3-4
 team, 2-4
sports equipment
 and preventing overuse injuries, 183
sports injuries
 circumstances, 211
 classification, 14
 conditions that masquerade as, 77-84
 cryotherapy modalities used to treat, 249
 ear, 335-6
 and equipment, 213, 221
 examination, 213-21
 eye, 336-40
 facial, 333, 343-5
 and gender, 166
 HARM, 250
 headache, 317-18
 history, 211-13
 ligament testing, 215
 medical assessment, periodic, 171-2
 medical therapies, 692-3
 muscle activation, 692
 nose, 333-5
 and pain, 211-12
 palpation, 215
 POLICE, 247
 prevention models, 166-73
 prevention of re-injury, 282-3
 PRICE, 247
 range of motion testing, 214-15
 RICE, 692
 season analysis, 170-1
 soft tissue, 16
 spinal examination, 219-21
 and strength testing, 215
 and surgery, 274-5
 surveillance program, 168
 swelling, 212
 and technique, 221
 teeth, 340-3
 see also injury management, acute; injury prevention; rehabilitation
sports injuries, biomechanical aspects in specific sports, 121-38, 166
 cricket fast bowling, 125-7
 cycling, 121-4
 golf, 128-30
 rowing, 130-3
 swimming, 133-6
 tennis, 136-8
sports injuries, overuse, 29-53
 barefoot/minimalist running, 183
 biomechanical abnormalities, 214
 bone stress injury, 29-43
 bursa, 51-2
 hand and finger, 505
 joint, 43
 ligament, 43

1053

Index

lower limb, 107-8, 183
muscle, 43-6
nerve, 52
nutritional strategies to prevent stress fractures, 182
orthoses, 183
overuse injuries of the physis, 979
predisposing factors, 29
prevention, 181-3
shoe selection, 182-3
skin, 52-3
sports equipment, 183
stretching, 181-2
structured training programs, 182
technique modification, 182
tendon (tendinopathy), 46-51
sports medicine and PROMs, 210, 231-8
sports surfaces and injury prevention, 187-8
sport-specific assessment, 105
sport-specific biomechanical issues, 105
sport-specific hand conditions, 490
sport-specific rehabilitation programs, 6
sports-specific phase (adductor-related groin pain), 648-9
sprain
  ligament, 14, 19-21
  midtarsal joint sprains, 952
  muscle, 14, 21-3
Strategic Assessment of Risk and Risk Tolerance (StARRT), 285-93
  additional perspectives, 289
  beyond risk for injury, 287
  decision making, 290-3
  outcomes and probabilities, 288-9
  risk tolerance modifiers, 287
  tissue health, 286-7
  tissue stress, 287
static stretching, 149
sternoclavicular joint problems, 517-18
strength testing and injuries, 215
strength training, 148
strengthening exercises (lateral elbow tendinopathy), 445-6
stress fractures, 34, 38, 460
  anterior cortex of the tibia, 838
  calcaneal, 947-8
  cuboid, 956
  cuneiforms, 956
  diaphysis, 965
  femur, 674-6
  fibula, 845
  great toe, 972
  inferior pubic ramus, 656
  medial malleolar, 928
  navicular, 949-52
  neck of metatarsals I.IV, 959-61

neck of the femur, 655-7
pars interarticularis, 535-43
and preventing overuse injuries, 182
rib stress fractures (RFS), 132, 515
special metatarsal stress fracture: base of the second MT, 961
specific treatment of, 38
talus, 933
tibia, 836-8
stretching, 150
and preventing overuse injuries, 181-2
and recovery, 193-4, 200
structural ('static') biomechanical assessment, 96-100
  ankle dorsiflexion, 98-9
  foot, 96-8
  leg length, 99-100
  summary, 100
  tibiofemoral alignment at the knee, 99
subacromial impingement, 381
subconjunctival haemorrhage, 338-9
subluxation, 14, 18-19
suboptimal lower limb biomechanics, conditions related to, 106-8
subscapularis muscle tears, 429
subtler joint, 85-8
subungual exostosis, 972
subungual haematoma, 972
superficial compartment syndrome, 863
superior tibiofibular joint injury, 767, 815-16
supracondylar fractures, 456
suprascapular nerve entrapment, 429-30
surfaces, injury prevention and sports, 187-8
surgery
  Achilles tendon 884
  arthroscopic 274-5, 621-2
  hand injuries, 505
  hip injury, 621-2
  lateral elbow tendinopathy, 451
  meniscal injuries, 727
  open, 275
  and patellofemoral pain, 789-90
  and sports injuries, 274-5
  wrist, 486
sustained myofascial tension, 254
swelling and injury, 212
'swimmer's shoulder' see rotator cuff tendinopathy
swimming (biomechanical aspects of injuries), 133-6
  biomechanics 133
  freestyle techniques, 133
  medial knee pain, 136
  shoulder pain, 133-6

swimming biomechanics, 133
synovial plica, 803
synovitis 612-13
  post-traumatic 913-14

T

T_4 syndrome, 514
talar dome, osteochondral lesions of the, 906-8
talus, stress fracture, 933
taping
  finger injuries, 494
  lateral elbow tendinopathy, 447-8
  lower limb biomechanical issues, 112-14
  musculoskeletal conditions, 259-61
tarsal coalition, 957-8, 988
tarsal navicular bone, apophysitis, 989
tarsal tunnel syndrome, 926-8
team care throughout the season, 1018-20
  anti-doping, 1020
  core principles, 1018-20
teams, working and travelling with, 1017-25
  emergency action plans, 1020-21
  hygiene, 1020
  immunisation and WHO, 1020
  jet lag, symptomatic treatment for, 1025
  jet lag and air travel, 1023
  jet lag prevention, 1023
  medical equipment, 1018
  medical indemnity and trauma training, 1018
  medical support team, 1017
  medical team attributes, 1017-18
  sexual activity, 1020
  travel preparation, 1021-2
  vaccinations, 1024
tear
  fascia, 14, 26
  ligament, 14, 19-21
  muscle, 14, 21-5
  tendon, 14, 25-6, 50
technique training, 143
teeth injuries, 340-3
  dental management, 341
  emergency management, 340-1
  emergency treatment, 342
  prevention, 341-3
temporomandibular injuries, 345-6
tendinopathy, 46-51
  biceps femoris, 815, 823
  degenerative, 49
  extensor, 956
  flexor hallucis longus, 924-6
  gastrocnemius, 824
  lower limb rehabilitation, 50-1

1054

Index

midportion Achilles, 872-84
patellar, 771, 793-801, 986
peroneal, 929-31, 956
pes anserinus, 819
popliteus, 821
proximal hamstring, 577-81
quadriceps, 802
tibialis anterior, 935-6
tibialis posterior, 923-4, 955
upper hamstring, 710-11
tendinosis, 47
tendon
    dislocation/rupture (acute ankle injury), 911-12
    dysrepair, 49
    enthesopathy, 51
    extensor carpi ulnaris tendon injuries, 484-5
    hamstring ruptures, 767
    hand and finger injuries, 499-504
    and hyaluronic acid, 270
    intramuscular tendon injuries, 690
    and mechanotherapy, 245
    and NSAID, 266
    overuse injury (tendinopathy), 46-50, 143
    partial tears, 50
    peroneal dislocation, 911-12
    rupture (patellar), 765
    ruptures (acute elbow injuries), 459-60
    tear/rupture, 14, 25-6, 50
    tibialis posterior rupture, 912
    tibialis posterior tendon dislocation, 912
tennis (biomechanical aspects of injuries), 136-8
    lateral elbow pain, 136-7
    shoulder injuries, 137-8
tennis elbow, 136-7, 440
tenosynovitis
    de Quervain's, 476-7
thigh pain *see* anterior thigh pain; posterior thigh pain
therapeutic exercise, 241-6
therapeutic medication in musculoskeletal injury, 264-72
    actovegin, 269
    analgesics, 264
    bisphosphonates, 272
    central sensitisation, 267-8
    corticosteroid, 270-71
    GTN patches, 272
    hyaluronic acid, 269-70
    mechanical and high-volume injections, 269
    neuropathic pain, 267-8
    non-steroidal anti-inflammatory drugs (NSAIDs), 264-7
    prolotherapy, 269
    quinolone antibiotics, 272
    sclerosant, 269
    sleep medications, 271
    traumeel, 269
thoracic outlet syndrome (TOS), 430-1
thoracic pain, 507-20
    assessment, 508-11
    causes, 507
    costovertebral joint disorders, 511
    intervertebral disc prolapse, 512-14
    intervertebral joint disorders, 511
    postural imbalance, 514
    Scheuermann's disease, 512
    T_4 syndrome, 514
throwing
    abnormal biomechanics, 118
    acceleration, 115
    biomechanics, 114-17
    cocking, 114-15
    deceleration/follow-through, 116
    normal biomechanics of the scapular, 117-18
    scapular biomechanics in shoulder injuries, 118-19
    and shoulder injuries, 435-7
    wind-up, 114
tibia, stress fracture, 836-8, 846
    anterior cortex, 838
    assessment, 836-7
    medial tibial stress syndrome, 839-41
    prevention of recurrence, 837-8
    treatment, 838
tibial plafond lesions, 910
tibialis anterior tendinopathy, 935-6
tibialis posterior tendinopathy, 923-4, 955
tibialis posterior tendon dislocation, 911-12
tibialis posterior tendon rupture, 911-12
tibiofemoral alignment at the knee, 99
tibiofibular ligament injury/syndesmotic injury, anteroinferior, 912-13
tissue healing
    bone stress injury management, 42
tissue status (damage), 56-7, 66
toe clawing, 972
training
    agility, 144
    and bone stress injuries, 32-3
    Central Government Model (CGM) for the limits of performance, 140-2
    cross-training, 143
    endurance, 142-3
    Fartlek, 142-3
    flexibility, 149-50
    hypertrophy, 149
    individualisation, 140
    interval, 142
    load management for performance enhancement, 150-1
    Maximal Aerobic Speed (MAS), 143
    overload, 140
    periodisation, 139-40
    power, 148-9
    principles of, 139-42
    programming and prescription, 139-51
    resistance, 144-9
    specificity, 140
    speed, 143-4
    speed intervals, 143
    strength, 148
    technique, 143
    see also conditioning training; skill training
training history and injury, 213
training programs and preventing overuse injuries, 181-3
transient receptor potential (TRP), 267-8
transcutaneous electrical nerve stimulation (TENS), 262
trapezium fracture, 475-6
traumatic bursitis, 26
traumatic shoulder instability (TUBS), 407-11
traumeel, 269
treatment
    Achilles tendinopathy, 887
    acute Achilles tendon rupture, 889-92
    acute ankle injuries, 900-4, 907-8
    adductor-related groin pain, 644-7
    anterior impingement of the ankle, 935
    anterolateral impingement, 932
    chronic exertional compartment syndrome (CECS), 841-5
    and concussion, 311
    distal quadriceps muscle strain, 671-2
    flexor hallucis longus tendinopathy, 926
    gastrocnemius muscle strains, 853-6
    hip-related pain, 614-22, 625-8
    iliotibial band friction syndrome (IBTFS), 811-12
    iliopsoas-related groin pain, 650-1
    inguinal-related groin pain, 652-4
    lateral elbow tendinopathy, 445
    lateral ligament injuries, 899-900
    lisfranc joint injuries, 954-5
    medial calcaneal nerve entrapment, 929
    medial collateral ligament injury, 729-36

medial malleolar stress fracture, 928
medial tibial stress syndrome, 837
meniscal injuries, 726-7
midportion Achilles tendinopathy, 877-84
options for pain, 72-4
patellar dislocation, 765
patellofemoral pain, 782-92
peroneal tendinopathy, 931
plantar fasciopathy, 943-6
primary patellofemoral instability, 792-3
pubic-related groin pain, 654
quadriceps contusion, 666-770
sacroiliac joint dysfunction, 585
sinus tarsi syndrome, 932
sport and exercise medicine (SEM), 5
stress fracture of the tibia, 837-41
tarsal tunnel syndrome, 927-8
tibialis anterior tendinopathy, 935-6
tibialis posterior tendinopathy, 924
triangular fibrocartilage complex tear (TFCC), 483-4
tricyclic antidepressants, 267
trigger points
  lateral elbow tendinopathy, 447
  myofascial, 43-5, 68
  pain from, 44, 83
  posterior thigh, 707
  treatment, 44-5
triquetral fracture, 482
trunk function assessment, 102-5
tumours
  bone, 78-80
  soft tissue, 78-80
turf toe, 966

U

ulnar column presentations, 481-5
ulnar nerve compression, 486
ulnar styloid fracture, 481
ultrasound, 37, 40
  acute knee injuries, 723
  for diagnosis, 228-30
  groin pain, 642
  and injection therapy, 268
  shoulder investigations, 401
  therapeutic, 261
Ummukulthoum Bakare, 1031
upper arm pain, 461-2
upper limb 114-20
  abnormalities specific to throwing, 120
  changes in throwing arm with repeated throwing, 119-20
  biomechanics of the scapular in throwing, 117-18
  kinetic change, 116-17

neurodynamics test 215, 220, 258, 354, 396
  shoulder injuries, 118-19
  throwing, 114-17

V

vacuum cupping, 255
vascular disorders, 82
vascular entrapment, 846
vertebral endplate oedema, 547-8
vitamin D
  bone stress injuries, 34
  musculoskeletal injuries, 273
vitreous haemorrhage, 339

W

warm-up program, 178-81
water immersion and recovery, 195-6
West, Dr Liam, 1031-2
whiplash associated disorders (WAD), 357, 375
Whiteley, Rod, 1033
work activities and injury, 212
World Anti-Doping Agency (WADA), 1007
wounds, treatment of open, 27
wrist injuries and rowing, 132-3
wrist pain, 463-87
  carpal bone dislocation, 479
  carpal tunnel syndrome, 471, 485-6
  central column problems, 478-81
  clinical approach, 463-70
  de Quervain's tenosynovitis, 476-7
  distal radius fracture, 470-2
  ganglions, 478-9
  impingement syndromes, 481
  intersection syndrome, 477-8
  investigations, 466-70
  Keinböck's disease, 479-81
  numbness, 485-6
  outcome measures, 466
  patient-reported outcome measures, 471
  physical examination, 466
  plain radiography, 466-8
  radial column problems, 470-8
  radial epiphyseal injury (gymnast's wrist), 476
  radial sensory nerve compression, 478
  regions, 464
  rehabilitation, 475, 487
  scapholunate dissociation, 479
  scaphoid fracture, 472-5
  special imaging studies, 468-70
  surgery, 486
  trapezium fracture, 475
  triangular fibrocartilage complex tear (TFCC), 483

ulnar column problems, 481-6
ulnar nerve compression, 486
young athletes, 980
wrist pain and golf, 128-9
  leading wrist, 128-9
  trailing wrist, 129
wrist splinting, 487
wry neck, 374

X

X-ray, 401

Y

younger athlete, 974-89
  acute fractures, 976-9
  apophysitis, 982-3
  apophysitis of the fifth metatarsal, 989
  apophysitis of the tarsal navicular bone, 989
  back pain, 981-2
  elbow pain, 980
  flat foot, 989
  foot pain, 988-9
  Freiberg's infarction, 989
  hip pain, 982-4
  idiopathic scoliosis, 981
  irritable hip, 984
  knee pain, 984-6
  Köhler's disease, 988-9
  maturity-associated variations, 975
  musculoskeletal conditions, management of, 976-89
  nonlinearity of growth, 974-5
  Osgood-Schlatter disease, 984-6
  overuse injuries of the physis, 979
  painless abnormalities of gait, 986-8
  patellar tendinopathy, 986
  Perthes' disease, 983
  popliteal cysts, 986
  postural abnormalities, 981-2
  referred pain from the hip, 986
  Sever's disease, 988
  shoulder pain, 979-80
  Sinding-Larsen-Johansson disease, 986
  slipped capital femoral epiphysis, 983-4
  spondylolisthesis, 981-2
  spondylolysis, 981
  tarsal conditions, 988
  unique response of skeletal injury, 975-76
  uniqueness, 974-6
  wrist pain, 980-81

Z

zygomaticomaxillary complex, 344